NEONATAL-PERINATAL MEDICINE

NEONATAL-PERINATAL MEDICINE

Diseases of the Fetus and Infant

Edited by

AVROY A. FANAROFF, M.B., F.R.C.P. (Edinburgh), D.C.H.

Professor and Vice Chairman, Department of Pediatrics, Case Western Reserve University School of Medicine; Director of Neonatology, Rainbow Babies and Childrens Hospital, Cleveland, Ohio

RICHARD J. MARTIN, M.B., F.R.A.C.P., F.R.C.P. (Canada)

Associate Professor of Pediatrics, Case Western Reserve University School of Medicine; Co-Director of Neonatology, Rainbow Babies and Childrens Hospital, Cleveland, Ohio

FOURTH EDITION

with 572 illustrations

The C. V. Mosby Company

ST. LOUIS • WASHINGTON, D.C. • TORONTO 1987

MOSBY

A TRADITION OF PUBLISHING EXCELLENCE

Editor: Stephanie Bircher
Developmental Editor: Kathryn H. Falk
Assistant Editor: Ellen Baker Geisel
Project Editor: Sylvia B. Kluth
Manuscript editors: John Rogers, Sheila Walker, Joan Warrington
Book design: Gail Morey Hudson
Production: Florence Achenbach

FOURTH EDITION

Printed in the United States of America

The C.V. Mosby Company
11830 Westline Industrial Drive, St. Louis, Missouri 63146

Libary of Congress Cataloging-in-Publication Data

Neonatal-perinatal medicine.

Rev. ed. of: Behrman's neonatal-perinatal medicine. 3rd ed. 1983.
Includes bibliographies and index.
1. Infants-(Newborn)—Diseases. 2. Fetus—Diseases. I. Fanaroff, Avroy A. II. Martin, Richard J. III. Behrman's neonatal-perinatal medicine [DNLM: 1. Fetal Diseases. 2. Infant, Newborn, Diseases. WS 420 N438]
RJ254.N456 1987 618.92′01 87-7947
ISBN 0-8016-1583-6

GW/MV/MV 9 8 7 6 5 4 3 2 01/C/009

Contributors

STUART L. ABRAMSON, M.D., Ph.D.

Medical Staff Fellow, National Institute of Allergy and Infectious Disease, National Institutes of Health, Bethesda, Maryland

JACOB V. ARANDA, M.D., Ph.D., F.R.C.P. (C)

Professor of Pediatric and Pharmacology and Therapeutics, McGill University Faculty of Medicine; Director, Developmental Pharmacology and Perinatal Research Unit, Director, Apnea Treatment and Research Center, Attending Neonatologist, The Montreal Children's Hospital, Montreal, Quebec, Canada

JILL E. BALEY, M.D.

Assistant Professor of Pediatrics and Reproductive Biology, Rainbow Babies and Childrens Hospital, Case Western Reserve University; Director of Nurseries, MacDonald Hospital for Women, Cleveland, Ohio

WILLIAM F. BALISTRERI, M.D.

Dorothy M.M. Kersten Professor of Pediatrics, Director, Division of Pediatric Gastroenterology and Nutrition, Children's Hospital Research Foundation, Cincinnati, Ohio

RICHARD E. BEHRMAN, M.D.

Professor, Department of Pediatrics, and Dean, Case Western Reserve University School of Medicine, Rainbow Babies and Childrens Hospital, Cleveland, Ohio

KURT BENIRSCHKE, M.D.

Professor, Department of Pathology and Reproductive Medicine, University of California at San Diego; Chief, Autopsy Service, Department of Pathology, University Hospital, San Diego, California

JAY BERNSTEIN, M.D.

Director, Department of Anatomic Pathology, William Beaumont Hospital, Royal Oak, Michigan

THOMAS A. BLUMENFELD, M.D.

Associate Professor of Clinical Pathology, Columbia University College of Physicians and Surgeons; Vice-President, Medical Affairs, The Presbyterian Hospital, Columbia-Presbyterian Medical Center, New York, New York

JEFFREY L. BLUMER, Ph.D., M.D.

Associate Professor of Pediatrics and Pharmacology, Case Western Reserve University; Chief, Division of Pediatric Pharmacology & Critical Care, Rainbow Babies and Childrens Hospital, Cleveland, Ohio

HAYIM BOICHIS, M.D.

Professor of Pediatrics, Dean, Sackler Faculty of Medicine, Tel Aviv University; Director, Department of Pediatrics, The Pediatric Renal Unit, Chaim Sheba Medical Center, Tel Hashomer, Israel

ROBERT O. BOLLINGER, Ph.D.

Assistant Professor of Pediatrics, Wayne State University School of Medicine, Detroit, Michigan

ALFRED W. BRANN, Jr., M.D.

Professor, Pediatrics and Obstetrics & Gynecology, Emory University, Atlanta, Georgia

PATRICK J. BRYAN, M.D.

Associate Professor of Radiology, Case Western University; Director, Division of Ultrasound, University Hospitals of Cleveland, Cleveland, Ohio

JOHN C. BUCUVALAS, M.D.

Assistant Professor of Pediatrics, Division of Pediatric Gastroenterology and Nutrition, Children's Hospital Medical Center, Cincinnati, Ohio

LUIS A. CABAL, M.D.

Associate Professor of Pediatrics, University of Southern California; Director, Respiratory Therapy, Department of Newborn Pediatrics, Women's Hospital, Los Angeles County, Los Angeles, California

WALDEMAR A. CARLO, M.D.

Assistant Professor of Pediatrics and Reproductive Biology, Case Western Reserve University; Associate Director, Newborn Intensive Care Nursery, Rainbow Babies and Childrens Hospital, Cleveland, Ohio

LAWRENCE CHIK, Ph.D.

Director, Medical Database Informatics, Ob/Gyn, Wayne State University, Hutzel Hospital, Detroit, Michigan

MITCHELL B. COHEN, M.D.

Research Scholar, Division of Pediatric Gastroenterology and Nutrition, Children's Hospital Medical Center, Cincinnati, Ohio

KAREN D. CRISSINGER, M.D.

Fellow, Division of Pediatric Gastroenterology & Nutrition, Children's Hospital Medical Center, Cincinnati, Ohio

ROBERT K. DANISH, M.D.

Assistant Professor of Pediatrics, Case Western Reserve University School of Medicine; Pediatric Endocrinologist, Cleveland Metropolitan General Hospital, Cleveland, Ohio

HAROLD M. DICK, M.D.

Clinical Professor of Orthopaedic Surgery, Department of Orthopaedics, Columbia University College of Physicians and Surgeons; Chief of Pediatric Orthopaedic Surgery, Babies Hospital, Columbia-Presbyterian Medical Center, New York, New York

JOHN M. DRISCOLL, Jr., M.D.

Professor of Clinical Pediatrics, Columbia University College of Physicians and Surgeons; Director, Newborn I.C.U. and Nurseries, Department of Pediatrics, Babies Hospital, Columbia Presbyterian Medical Center, New York, New York

METHOD A. DUCHON, M.D.

Assistant Clinical Professor, Department of Reproductive Biology, Case Western Reserve University; Director, Division of Maternal-Fetal Medicine, Department of Obstetrics and Gynecology, Saint Luke's Hospital, Cleveland, Ohio

CHESTER M. EDELMANN, Jr., M.D.

Professor of Pediatrics and Associate Dean, Albert Einstein College of Medicine, Yeshiva University, Bronx, New York

MORVEN S. EDWARDS, M.D.

Associate Professor of Pediatrics, Department of Pediatrics, Infectious Diseases Section, Baylor College of Medicine; Active Staff Pediatrician, Texas Children's Hospital and Harris County Hospital District, Houston, Texas

NANCY BURTON ESTERLY, M.D.

Professor of Pediatrics and Dermatology, Northwestern University Medical School; Head, Division of Dermatology, Department of Pediatrics, Children's Memorial Hospital, Chicago, Illinois

PHILIP M. FARRELL, M.D., Ph.D.

Professor and Chairman, Department of Pediatrics, University of Wisconsin School of Medicine, Madison, Wisconsin

RALPH D. FEIGIN, M.D.

J.S. Abercrombie Professor and Chairman, Department of Pediatrics, Baylor College of Medicine; Physician-in-Chief, Texas Children's Hospital, Houston, Texas

BARRY D. FLETCHER, M.D.

Professor of Radiology, Case Western Reserve University; Director, Division of Pediatric Radiology, Rainbow Babies and Childrens Hospital, Cleveland, Ohio

WILLIAM W. FOX, M.D.

Professor of Pediatrics, University of Pennsylvania School of Medicine; Medical Director, Infant Intensive Care Unit, Staff Neonatologist, The Children's Hospital of Philadelphia, Philadelphia, Pennsylvania

ROGER K. FREEMAN, M.D.

Professor, Department of Obstetrics and Gynecology, University of California School of Medicine, Irvine; Medical Director, Women's Hospital, Memorial Medical Center of Long Beach, Long Beach, California

LAWRENCE M. GARTNER, M.D.

Professor and Chairman, Department of Pediatrics, The University of Chicago; Director, Wyler Children's Hospital, Chicago, Illinois

JUDITH GIBBS, M.D.

Former Director of Neonatology, Allentown Hospital, Allentown, Pennsylvania

STANLEY N. GRAVEN, M.D.

Professor and Chairman, Department of Community and Family Health, College of Public Health, University of South Florida, Tampa, Florida

GEORGE A. GREGORY, M.D.

Professor of Anesthesia and Pediatrics, University of California, San Francisco, San Francisco, California

MICHAEL T. GYVES, M.D.

Associate Professor of Obstetrics & Gynecology, Department of Reproductive Biology, Case Western Reserve University; Director, Department of Ob/Gyn, St. Luke's Hospital, Cleveland, Ohio

MAUREEN HACK, M.D.

Associate Professor of Pediatrics and Reproductive Biology, Case Western Reserve University; Director, High Risk Follow-Up Program, Rainbow Babies and Childrens Hospital, Cleveland, Ohio

BARBARA F. HALES

Associate Professor, Department of Pharmacology and Therapeutics, Centre for the Study of Reproduction, McGill University, Montreal, Quebec, Canada

NANCY ANDERSON HAMMING, M.D., M.S.

Assistant Professor, Department of Ophthalmology, Rush-Presbyterian-St. Luke's Medical Center, Chicago, Illinois

TIBOR HEIM, M.D., Ph.D.

Professor of Pediatrics and Nutrition, University of Toronto; Staff Physician, Director, Nutrition Research, Departments of Pediatrics and Surgery, Division of Clinical Nutrition and Research Institute, The Hospital for Sick Children, Toronto, Ontario, Canada

JOAN E. HODGMAN, M.D.

Professor of Pediatrics, University of Southern California, School of Medicine, Faculty, Newborn Division, Los Angeles County, University of Southern California Medical Center, Los Angeles, California

JOHN F. HUDDLESTON, M.D.

Clinical Professor, Department of Obstetrics and Gynecology, University of Florida College of Medicine, Gainesville; Director of Women's Services, Pavilion Women's Center at Baptist Medical Center, Jacksonville, Florida

SONIA E. HULMAN, M.D.

Assistant Professor of Pediatrics, Hahnemann University, Philadelphia, Pennsylvania

L. STANLEY JAMES, M.D.

Professor of Pediatrics and Obstetrics & Gynecology, Director, Division of Perinatal Medicine, Columbia University College of Physicians and Surgeons; Attending Physician, Department of Pediatrics, Presbyterian Hospital in the City of New York, Babies Hospital, New York, New York

MAJIDA N. JASSANI, M.D.

Associate Professor of Obstetrics and Gynecology and Radiology, Case Western Reserve University, Cleveland, Ohio

JOHN KATTWINKEL, M.D.

Professor of Pediatrics, University of Virginia Medical Center; Director, Newborn Services, University Hospital, Charlottesville, Virginia

JOHN H. KENNELL, M.D.

Professor of Pediatrics, Case Western Reserve University, Rainbow Babies and Childrens Hospital, Cleveland, Ohio

DOUGLAS H. KING, M.D.

Clinical Instructor of Pediatrics, Oregon Health Sciences University; Pediatric Cardiologist, Department of Pediatrics, Emanuel Hospital, Portland, Oregon

MARSHALL H. KLAUS, M.D.

Director of Academic Affairs, Children's Hospital of Oakland, Oakland, California

ROBERT M. KLIEGMAN, M.D.

Associate Professor of Pediatrics and Vice Chairman of Pediatrics for Education, Case Western Reserve University, Rainbow Babies and Childrens Hospital, Cleveland, Ohio

NEIL K. KOCHENOUR, M.D.

Director, Maternal-Fetal Medicine, Department of Obstetrics & Gynecology, University of Utah School of Medicine, Salt Lake City, Utah

THADDEUS W. KURCZYNSKI, M.D., Ph.D.

Associate Professor of Pediatrics and Neurology; Acting Chairman, Department of Pediatrics; Director, Genetics Center, Medical College of Ohio, Toledo, Ohio

KWANG-SUN LEE, M.D.

Professor of Pediatrics and Obstetrics and Gynecology, University of Chicago; Department of Pediatrics, Wyler Children's Hospital, Chicago, Illinois

MARTIN H. LEES, M.D., F.R.C.P. (London)

Professor of Pediatrics and Perinatology, Oregon Health Sciences University; Pediatric Cardiology, Department of Pediatrics, Emanuel Hospital, Portland, Oregon

LAWRENCE D. LILIEN, M.D.

Director of Neonatalogy, Department of Pediatrics, Fairview General Hospital, Cleveland, Ohio

HENRY H. MANGURTEN, M.D.

Associate Professor of Clinical Pediatrics, Abraham Lincoln School of Medicine, University of Illinois College of Medicine, Chicago, Illinois;
Director, Section of Neonatology, Department of Pediatrics, Lutheran General Hospital, Park Ridge, Illinois

UWE MANTHEI, M.D.

Assistant Professor of Pediatrics, Washington University School of Medicine; Assistant Pediatrician, Division of Allergy/Immunology, Children's Hospital, St. Louis, Missouri

JOHN S. McDONALD, M.D.

Professor and Chairman, Department of Anesthesiology, Professor of Obstetrics and Gynecology, Ohio State University, College of Medicine, Columbus, Ohio

MICHAEL T. MENNUTI, M.D.

Professor, Obstetrics and Gynecology, Pediatrics, and Human Genetics, University of Pennsylvania; Senior Physician, Department of Obstetrics/Gynecology, Hospital of the University of Pennsylvania, Philadelphia, Pennsylvania

IRWIN R. MERKATZ, M.D.

Professor and Chairman, Department of Obstetrics and Gynecology, Albert Einstein College of Medicine, Bronx, New York

MARILYN T. MILLER, M.D.

Associate Professor, Department of Ophthalmology, University of Illinois at Chicago; Associate Professor of Ophthalmology, University of Illinois Hospitals and Clinics, Chicago, Illinois

MARTHA J. MILLER, M.D., Ph.D.

Assistant Professor of Pediatrics, Case Western Reserve University; Neonatologist, Department of Pediatrics, Rainbow Babies and Childrens Hospital, Cleveland, Ohio

FRANCIS MIMOUNI, M.D.

Senior Fellow, Department of Pediatrics, University of Cincinnati College of Medicine, Children's Hospital Medical Center, Cincinnati, Ohio

RACHEL MORECKI, M.D.

Professor of Pathology and Pediatrics, Albert Einstein Research Center and the Marian Bassine Liver Research Center; Attending Physician, Department of Pathology, The Hospital of Albert Einstein College of Medicine, Bronx, New York

AKIRA MORISHIMA, M.D., Ph.D.

Associate Professor of Pediatrics, Director, Division of Pediatric Endocrinology, Columbia University College of Physicians and Surgeons; Associate Attending Pediatrician, Babies Hospital, New York, New York

JEFFREY P. MORRAY, M.D.

Associate Professor of Anesthesiology and Pediatrics, University of Washington School of Medicine; Medical Director, Pediatric Intensive Care Unit, Children's Hospital and Medical Center, Seattle, Washington

STUART C. MORRISON, M.B., Ch.B., M.R.C.P.

Assistant Professor of Radiology, Case Western Reserve University; Assistant Professor of Radiology, Division of Pediatric Radiology, University Hospitals of Cleveland, Cleveland, Ohio

MARTIN A. NASH, M.D.

Associate Professor of Clinical Pediatrics, College of Physicians & Surgeons, Columbia University; Associate Attending Pediatrician, Babies Hospital, Columbia-Presbyterian Medical Center, New York, New York

MICHAEL R. NEUMAN, M.D., Ph.D.

Associate Professor of Biomedical Engineering in Reproductive Biology, Department of Reproductive Biology and Department of Obstetrics and Gynecology, Cleveland Metropolitan General Hospital, Case Western Reserve University, Cleveland, Ohio

JOHN F. NICHOLSON, M.D.

Associate Professor of Pediatrics and Pathology, Columbia University College of Physicians and Surgeons; Associate Attending Physician, Department of Pediatrics, Presbyterian Hospital, New York, New York

JOHN P. O'GRADY, M.D.

Associate Professor of Reproductive Biology, Case Western Reserve University; Chief, Division of Maternal-Fetal Medicine, Department of Obstetrics and Gynecology, MacDonald Hospital for Women, Cleveland, Ohio

LU-ANN PAPILE, M.D.

Associate Professor of Pediatrics, and Obstetrics and Gynecology, University of New Mexico School of Medicine, Albuquerque, New Mexico

ROBERT H. PERELMAN, M.D.

Associate Professor of Pediatrics, University of Wisconsin School of Medicine, Madison, Wisconsin

PAUL H. PERLSTEIN, M.D.

Professor of Pediatrics and Obstetrics & Gynecology, Division of Neonatalogy, University of Cincinnati College of Medicine; Attending Neonatologist, University Hospital, Cincinnati Children's Hospital, Cincinnati, Ohio

DALE L. PHELPS, M.D.

Associate Professor, Department of Pediatrics and Ophthalmology, University of Rochester, Division of Neonatology, Department of Pediatrics, Strong Memorial Hospital, Rochester, New York

ROSITA S. PILDES, M.D.

Chairman, Division of Neonatalogy, Cook County Children's Hospital, Professor of Pediatrics, University of Illinois, Chicago, Illinois

RONALD L. POLAND, M.D.

Associate Professor of Pediatrics, Wayne State University School of Medicine; Director of Neonatal-Perinatal Medicine, Department of Pediatrics, Children's Hospital of Michigan, Detroit, Michigan

RICHARD A. POLIN, M.D.

Professor of Pediatrics, University of Pennsylvania School of Medicine; Neonatologist, Senior Physician, Department of Pediatrics, The Children's Hospital of Philadelphia, Philadelphia, Pennsylvania

STEPHEN H. POLMAR, Ph.D., M.D.

Professor of Pediatrics, Washington University School of Medicine; Director, Division of Allergy and Immunology, Children's Hospital, St. Louis, Missouri

JOHN T. QUEENAN, M.D.

Professor and Chairman, Department of Obstetrics and Gynecology, Georgetown University School of Medicine; Obstetrician and Gynecologist in Chief, Georgetown University Hospital, Washington, D.C.

JOHN E. READ, M.D., F.A.C.S.

Associate Clinical Professor, Department of Ophthalmology, Abraham Lincoln School of Medicine, University of Illinois, Eye & Ear Infirmary, Chicago, Illinois; Medical Staff, Porter Memorial Hospital, Valparaiso, Indiana

TOVE S. ROSEN, M.D.

Associate Professor of Clinical Pediatrics, Columbia University College of Physicians and Surgeons; New York, New York

FREDERICK C. RYCKMAN, M.D.

Assistant Professor of Surgery, Division of Pediatric Surgery, Children's Hospital Medical Center, Cincinnati, Ohio

JAMES F. SCHWARTZ, M.D.

Professor of Pediatrics and Neurology, Department of Pediatrics, Emory University School of Medicine; Chief, Pediatric Neurology Division, Henrietta Egleston Hospital for Children, Grady Memorial Hospital, Atlanta, Georgia

THOMAS H. SHAFFER, Ph.D.

Associate Professor of Physiology, Temple University, School of Medicine, Philadelphia, Pennsylvania

SUSAN B. SHURIN, M.D.

Associate Professor of Pediatrics, Case Western Reserve University, School of Medicine; Director, Division of Hematology, Rainbow Babies and Childrens Hospital, Cleveland, Ohio

BIJAN SIASSI, M.D.

Associate Professor of Pediatrics and Radiology, Department of Pediatrics, University of Southern California, Los Angeles, California

ROBERT J. SOKOL, M.D.

Professor and Chairman, Department of Obstetrics and Gynecology, Wayne State University School of Medicine; Chief, Department of Obstetrics and Gynecology, Hutzel Hospital, Detroit, Michigan

LAWRENCE M. SOLOMON, M.D.

Professor and Head, Department of Dermatology, University of Illinois, Chicago, Illinois

SHARON SPEAKS, R.N.

Assistant Director, Special Care Nurseries, Department of Maternal Child Health, Parkland Memorial Hospital, Dallas, Texas

ADRIAN SPITZER, M.D.

Professor of Pediatrics and Director, Division of Nephrology, Albert Einstein College of Medicine; Attending Pediatrician, Bronx Municipal Hospital Center, The Jack D. Wyler Hospital of the Albert Einstein College of Medicine/ Montefiore Hospital, Bronx, New York

EILEEN KANE STORK, M.D.

Assistant Professor of Pediatrics, Case Western Reserve University; Neonatologist, Department of Pediatrics, Rainbow Babies and Childrens Hospital, Cleveland, Ohio

JOHN E. STORK, M.D.

Assistant Professor of Pediatrics, Case Western Reserve University; Chief, Pediatric Nephrology, Rainbow Babies and Childrens Hospital, Cleveland, Ohio

PAUL R. SWYER, M.A., M.D. (Cantab), F.R.C.P. (C), F.R.C.P. (L)

Professor of Pediatrics, University of Toronto; Director, Division of Neonatology, Department of Pediatrics, The Research Institute, The Hospital for Sick Children, Toronto, Ontario, Canada

REGINALD C. TSANG, M.B.B.S.

Professor of Pediatrics, Obstetrics, and Gynecology, David G. and Priscilla R. Gamble Professor of Neonatology; Director, Perinatal Research Institute, Children's Hospital Medical Center, University of Cincinnati, Cincinnati, Ohio

JON E. TYSON, M.D.

Associate Professor of Pediatrics and Obstetrics & Gynecology, University of Texas Health Science Center, Dallas, Texas

JEAN-CLAUDE VEILLE, M.D.

Assistant Professor of Obstetrics & Gynecology and Reproductive Biology, Case Western Reserve University; Attending Physician, MacDonald Hospital for Women, Cleveland, Ohio

MICHELE C. WALSH, M.D.

Senior Fellow in Neonatology, Department of Pediatrics, Rainbow Babies and Childrens Hospital, Cleveland, Ohio

PHYLLIS I. WARKENTIN, M.D.

Assistant Professor of Pathology and Pediatrics, Case Western Reserve University; Physician, Pediatric Hematology/Oncology, Rainbow Babies and Childrens Hospital; Associate Medical Director, Northern Ohio Red Cross Blood Services, Cleveland, Ohio

BARRY S. YULISH, M.D.

Assistant Professor of Radiology, Case Western Reserve University; Radiologist, Division of Pediatric Radiology, University Hospitals of Cleveland, Cleveland, Ohio

FREDERICK P. ZUSPAN, M.D.

Richard L. Meiling Professor and Chairman, Department of Obstetrics and Gynecology, The Ohio State University; Obstetrician-Gynecologist-in-Chief, University Hospitals, Columbus, Ohio

To

Roslyn and **Patricia**

Preface

We would like to take this opportunity to thank Dr. Richard E. Behrman, a pioneer in perinatology, who offered us the privilege of editing this book. He continues to serve as a pathfinder in the field and has provided inspirational leadership for established as well as aspiring perinatologists. In keeping with the original intent, the goal of this fourth edition of *Neonatal-Perinatal Medicine* is to provide the reader with a current view of the philosophy and the technology relating to disorders of the fetus and newly born infant. All the contributors, including a significant number of new authors, have been instructed to balance their presentations, equally emphasizing advances in the basic and the clinical sciences. The result is a text that continues to focus on the pathophysiology, the clinical and laboratory presentations, and the prevention and treatment of disorders that have their onset in utero or during the neonatal period. New sections have been added to address the role of computers in perinatal care and the expanded role of ethical issues both before and after delivery. Each section and chapter has undergone significant revision and reflects the prevailing approaches to perinatal problems. We gratefully acknowledge the professionalism and dedicated hard work of our many contributors, as well as that of Bonnie Siner and Linda Ko who have served as in-house editors. Our task has been pleasurable as a result of the highly efficient and skilled publishing staff at Mosby, including Ellen Baker Geisel, Kathy Falk, Stephanie Bircher, Sylvia Kluth, Sheila Walker, and Florence Achenbach.

Avroy A. Fanaroff
Richard J. Martin

Contents

NEONATAL-PERINATAL MEDICINE

CHAPTER 1

The field of neonatal-perinatal medicine and neonatal risk

OVERVIEW

The term *perinatal* designates the period from the twelfth week of gestation through the twenty-eighth day after birth. The *neonatal period* is defined as the first 4 weeks of life and is the period of the greatest mortality in childhood, with the highest risk occurring during the first 24 hours of life. The continuing high mortality and morbidity during this period are closely related to the fact that it is part of a continuum of fetal growth and development. Factors acting during gestation and delivery, as well as during the postnatal period, have a major impact on the health of both the fetus and neonate. Social, economic, and cultural influences are superimposed on genetic, metabolic, and physiologic intrauterine and extrauterine environmental effects.

The high incidence of disease during the perinatal period and the excessive neonatal and perinatal death rates make it important to identify as early as possible those fetuses and infants who are at greatest risk. Of equal importance is the need to lower the morbidity, especially for handicapping conditions such as mental retardation, resulting from untoward prenatal and neonatal factors. Our development as a species ultimately depends on the quality of the babies who are produced and their potential talents. There is increasing evidence that early recognition of the high-risk pregnancy and high-risk infant and appropriate antenatal and intrapartum management along with special neonatal intensive care will reduce the incidence of handicapping conditions and will reduce both the perinatal and neonatal death rates.

Those who die are a source of anguish and grief to their parents and relatives for a varying but relatively brief period, whereas those who survive with disabilities and disease may be a continuing source of pain, anguish, and loss of resources for their parents and society, in addition to the personal suffering they may endure. They may also impose a very real biologic burden on future generations. In addition to the human tragedy, the fiscal impact of this problem on our society is estimated to be in the billions of dollars each year. The major problems of cerebral palsy, mental retardation, sensory and cognitive disabilities, and a diminished ability to successfully adapt socially, psychologically, and physically to an increasingly complex environment are some of the results observed in children and adults who were *low birth weight* (LBW) infants.

Infants who are born before attaining normal intrauterine growth and development are at greatest risk of dying during infancy and at significant risk of morbidity during childhood. LBW infants, weighing up to 2,500 gm, born prematurely or retarded in intrauterine growth are 40 times more likely to die than infants of normal birth weight; the relative risk of neonatal death is almost 200 times greater for *very low birth weight* (VLBW) infants, who weigh up to 1,500 gm. LBW survivors have an increased incidence of disability from a broad range of conditions, including neurodevelopmental handicaps, congenital anomalies, respiratory illnesses, and complications acquired during neonatal intensive care.

In the United States, LBW infants account for a relatively greater proportion of infant deaths (deaths within the first year of life) than in the past. Early in the twentieth century, two thirds of infant deaths occurred in the postneonatal period, primarily from infectious diseases. However, by 1950 7.5% of live-born infants weighed less than 2,500 gm, and two thirds of all infant deaths occurred in the neonatal period, secondary mostly to antenatal and intrapartum events such as birth injury, asphyxia, congenital malformation, and "immaturity." Awareness of the increased morbidity in surviving LBW infants, coupled with a greater understanding of fetal and

Table 1-1. Decline in low birth weight rates per 1000 deliveries

	Weight	1971	1976	1981
United States	VLBW*	11	12	12
	MLBW†	65	61	56
California	VLBW	9	9	10
	MLBW	57	52	49
Massachusetts	VLBW	10	9	9
	MLBW	61	57	50
Michigan	VLBW	12	13	13
	MLBW	64	62	57
North Carolina	VLBW	14	14	15
	MLBW	74	69	65
Oregon	VLBW	8	8	9
	MLBW	49	46	41

From Behrman, R.E.: J. Pediatr. **107:**842, 1985.
*Very low birth weight, ≤1500 gm.
†Moderately low birth weight, 1,501 to 2,500 gm.

infant nutrition, pharmacology, and pathophysiology, advanced the development of perinatal care in the 1950s and 1960s. The infant mortality rate decreased 47% from 1965 to 1980, primarily because of a decrease in neonatal mortality, a major factor of which was the increased survival of LBW high-risk infants. Providing perinatal intensive care units for geographically defined areas has contributed significantly to the increase in the proportion of LBW and VLBW infants cared for in tertiary centers and the consequent decrease in neonatal mortality.

However, at the start of the 1980s, despite their increased survival rates, LBW infants still accounted for two thirds of the neonatal deaths with the VLBW infants accounting for half. Surviving LBW infants also remained three times as likely as infants of normal birth weight to have untoward neurologic sequelae, the risk of which increases with decreasing birth weight. There is also increased risk of congenital anomalies, especially for those infants who are small for gestational age. Lower respiratory tract problems, particularly infections, are more common, as are complications of neonatal care. LBW infants are five times more likely to die in the first

Risk factors associated with low birth weight

I. Demographic risks
   A. Age (younger than 18, older than 35 years)
   B. Race (black)
   C. Low socioeconomic status
   D. Unmarried
   E. Low level of education

II. Medical risks predating pregnancy
   A. Parity (0 or more than 4)
   B. Low weight for height
   C. Genitourinary anomalies/surgery
   D. Selected diseases such as diabetes, chronic hypertension
   E. Nonimmune status for selected infections such as rubella
   F. Poor obstetric history including previous LBW infant, multiple spontaneous abortions
   G. Maternal genetic factors

III. Behavioral and environmental risks
   A. Smoking
   B. Poor nutritional status
   C. Alcohol and other substance abuse
   D. Diethylstilbestrol and other toxic exposures, including occupational hazards
   E. High altitude

IV. Health care risks
   A. Absent or inadequate prenatal care
   B. Iatrogenic prematurity

V. Medical risks in current pregnancy
   A. Multiple pregnancy
   B. Poor weight gain
   C. Short interpregnancy interval
   D. Hypotension
   E. Hypertension/preeclampsia/toxemia
   F. Selected infections such as symptomatic bacteriuria, rubella, cytomegalovirus
   G. First- or second-trimester bleeding
   H. Placental problems such as placenta previa, abruptio placentae
   I. Hyperemesis
   J. Oligohydramnios/polyhydramnios
   K. Anemia/abnormal hemoglobin
   L. Isoimmunization
   M. Fetal anomalies
   N. Incompetent cervix
   O. Spontaneous premature rupture of membranes

VI. Evolving concepts of risk
   A. Stress (physical and psychosocial)
   B. Uterine irritability
   C. Events triggering uterine contractions
   D. Cervical changes detected before onset of labor
   E. Selected infections such as mycoplasma and *Chlamydia trachomatis*
   F. Inadequate plasma volume expansion
   G. Progesterone deficiency

From Behrman, R.E.: J. Pediatr. **107:**842, 1985.

year of life, and their deaths account for about 20% of all postnatal deaths. The relationship of LBW to post-neonatal death is modified by socioeconomic factors. Unfortunately, the neonatal and infant mortality rates in the black population have remained almost twice as high as that of the white population throughout the 1980s.

In contrast to the dramatic decrease in neonatal mortality, the incidence of LBW births has declined a more modest 11%, from 1971 to 1981, to about 6.8%. This decline in LBW rates generally has been confined to the moderately LBW group (1,501 to 2,500 gm) with no significant decline in the VLBW rate or among preterm infants (Table 1-1). A difference of over 200% persists between the white and black races in the United States. The relative risk of a LBW birth is increased for blacks, teenage mothers, and unmarried persons; it is also increased for those who have less than 12 years of education, have late initiation of prenatal care, have a shortened interval between pregnancies, and those who have had a prior birth of an LBW infant (see box on p. 2).

In addition to these population and societal dimensions of the field of neonatal-perinatal medicine, it is becoming increasingly evident that important antecedents of many adult diseases, such as coronary artery disease, chronic renal and liver disease, obesity, and other human maladies, may be present in early development, at which stage there is real opportunity for prevention. Further improvement in longevity and decreased morbidity are likely to result from increased understanding of the origins of adult diseases in fetal life and infancy and the prevention and early management of these diseases.

HIGH-RISK INFANTS

Infants particularly at risk during the neonatal period should be identified as early as possible in order to decrease neonatal morbidity and mortality. These infants should be under close observation by experienced physicians and nurses. Although usually needed for only a few days, such observations may range from a few hours to several weeks or more. Some institutions find it advantageous to provide a special or transitional care nursery for high-risk infants, often within the labor and delivery suite. This facility should be equipped and staffed similarly to a neonatal intensive care area in order that well but high-risk infants can be observed and cared for immediately after birth without being separated from their mothers (Chapter 2, part one; Chapter 24, part four).

Infants in the high-risk category are listed in the box on the right; many of the factors contributing to their risks are also related to the risk of LBW (see box on p. 2). Examination of a fresh placenta, cord, and membranes may alert the physician to a newborn infant at high risk. However, many high-risk infants are born prematurely, have low birth weight for gestational age, have significant perinatal asphyxia, or are born with life-threatening congenital anomalies without exhibiting previously identified risk factors.

Generally, for any given duration of gestation, the lower the birth weight the higher the neonatal mortality, and for any given weight, the shorter the gestational duration the higher the neonatal mortality (Fig. 1-1). The lowest risk of neonatal mortality occurs among infants with birth weights of 3,000 to 4,000 gm and whose gestational age is 38 to 42 weeks. Nevertheless, approximately 40% of all *perinatal deaths* occur after 37 weeks' gestation in infants weighing 2,500 gm or more; many of these deaths occur in the period immediately before birth and are more readily preventable than those of smaller and more immature infants. In addition, neonatal mortality rates rise sharply for infants weighing over 4,000 gm and for those whose gestational period is 42 weeks or longer. Fig. 1-1 helps to quickly identify the mortality risk *at birth;* the prognosis improves rapidly with increasing postnatal duration of survival.

Infants categorized as high risk

1. Birth before 37 weeks' or after 42 weeks' gestation
2. Birth weight <2,500 or >4,000 gm
3. Deviations in expected size for stage of development
4. History of fetal or neonatal sibling deaths or serious illness
5. Poor condition at delivery (Apgar 0-4 at 1 min) or resuscitation required at delivery or subsequently
6. History of maternal infection or other illness during pregnancy, premature rupture of membranes, severe social problems (e.g., teenage pregnancy, drug addiction), absent or late prenatal care, abnormal gestational weight gain, prolonged infertility, four or more previous pregnancies, 35 years or more maternal age (especially if primiparous), or ingestion of drugs
7. Multiple pregnancy or gestation commencing within 6 months of a previous pregnancy
8. Delivery by cesarean section or any unusual obstetric complication, including hydramnios, abruptio placentae, placenta previa, or abnormal presentation
9. Significant malformation or suspicion of malformation
10. Anemia or blood group incompatibility
11. Severe maternal emotional problems such as hyperemesis gravidarum
12. Serious accidents or general anesthesia during pregnancy

From Kliegman, R., and Behrman, R.E.: The fetus and neonatal infant. In Nelson's textbook of pediatrics, ed. 13, Philadelphia, 1987, W.B. Saunders Co.

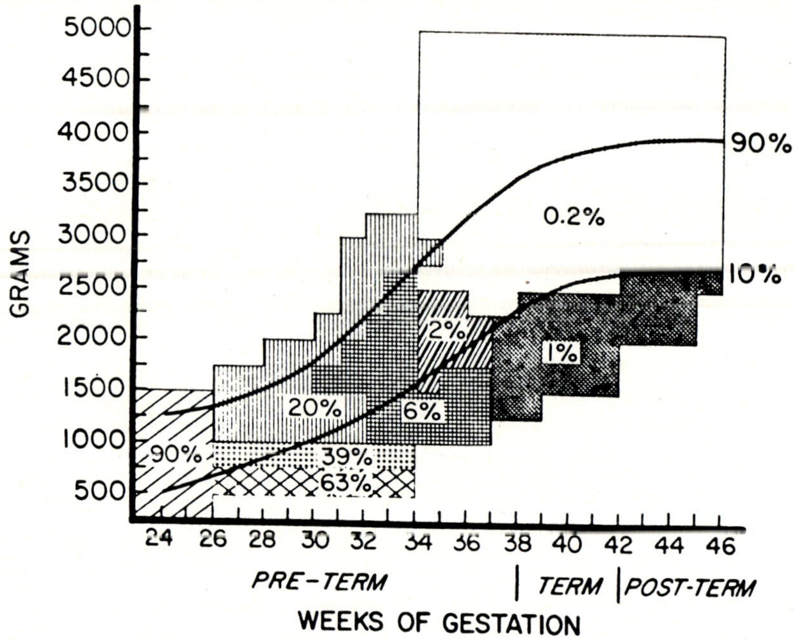

Fig. 1-1. Mortality risk according to birth weight–gestational age relationship. (From Sweet, A.Y.: Classification of the low birth weight infant. In Klaus, M.H., and Fanaroff, A.A., editors: Care of the high-risk neonate, ed. 3, Philadelphia, 1986, W.B. Saunders Co.)

Prematurity and intrauterine growth retardation

Definitions. Liveborn infants delivered before 37 weeks from the first day of the last menstrual period are termed *premature* by the World Health Organization. Premature is also often used to denote immaturity, and infants of extremely low birth weight, that is, less than 750 gm, have been referred to as immature neonates. Historically, prematurity was defined by a birth weight of 2,500 gm or less, but today these LBW infants are considered to be *premature* with an appropriately low weight for shortened gestational period or to be *intrauterine growth retarded* (IUGR) in fetal weight gain for their gestational age, or *both*. Prematurity and IUGR are associated with increased morbidity and mortality. LBW infants are also further subclassified as very low birth weight (VLBW: less than 1,500 gm) and moderately low birth weight (MLBW: 1,501 to 2,500 gm). The risk associated with the degree of LBW varies with different genetically and environmentally defined populations.

Incidence and mortality rates. Of the 6.8% of infants born weighing 2,500 gm or less in the United States (1981), the rate for whites was 5.7% and the rate for blacks was 12.5% (see Table 1-1). About one third of the LBW infants had a gestational age of 37 weeks or more. In general, at LBW rates above 10%, the majority of infants are IUGR and are commonly referred to as small for gestational age (SGA); at LBW rates of 5% to 7%, the majority are appropriate for gestational age (AGA). Except for term LBW infants, SGA infants generally have lower neonatal and postneonatal mortality than AGA infants of the same weight.

VLBW infants constitute about 1.2% of all births, and their survival is directly related to birth weight; about 2% survive at 501 to 600 gm, and 85% to 95% survive at 1,250 to 1,500 gm. Perinatal care and improved survival rate of these VLBW infants have assumed great importance because their survival rate has a significant impact on overall premature mortality rates. Furthermore, there is a great commitment of resources required to achieve lower mortality in the VLBW infant. Their decrease in mortality has not been associated with increased morbidity, but this possibility continues to be investigated. However, compared to larger infants, VLBW infants have a higher incidence of rehospitalization during the first year of life for causes such as inguinal hernias, infections, treatment of chronic sequelae of prematurity, and caretaking disorders.

Factors related to premature birth and LBW. It is difficult to completely separate factors associated with prematurity from those associated with IUGR (see box on p. 2). A strong positive correlation exists between both premature birth and IUGR and low socioeconomic status (SES). In families of low SES there are relatively high incidences of maternal undernutrition, anemia, and illness; inadequate prenatal care; drug addiction; obstetric complications; and maternal histories of reproductive inefficiency (relative infertility, abortions, stillbirths, premature or LBW infants). Other less clearly SES associated factors such as illegitimacy, teenage pregnancies, close spacing of pregnancies, and mothers who have borne more than four previous children also are encountered more frequently. Although systematic differences in fetal growth have been described in association with maternal size, birth order, sibling weight, social class, maternal smoking habit, and other factors, the degree to which the variance in birth weight between various subgroups is due to environmental (extrafetal) rather than to genetic differences in growth potential is unknown. The *premature birth* of infants whose LBW is appropriate for their preterm gestational age is generally associated with medical conditions in which there is inability of the uterus to retain the fetus, interference with the course of pregnancy, premature separation of the placenta, or a stimulus to effective uterine contractions before term. IUGR is associated with medical conditions that interfere with the circulation and efficiency of the placenta, with development or growth of the fetus, or with the general health and nutrition of the mother (Table 1-2).

Disease in LBW infants. Immaturity tends to increase the severity but reduce the distinctiveness of the clinical manifestations of most disease in LBW infants. The principal causes of death are respiratory distress syndrome (hyaline membrane disease), intraventricular hemorrhage, septicemia, asphyxia, birth injuries, and malformations.

Although substantial overlap exists, the incidence of certain neonatal risks varies with birth weight, gestational age, and birth weight for gestational age. Problems of major clinical significance associated with premature birth include respiratory distress (hyaline membrane disease, pulmonary hemorrhage, transient tachypnea, congenital pneumonia, pneumothorax, bronchopulmonary dysplasia), recurrent apnea, hypoglycemia, hypocalcemia, hyperbilirubinemia, anemia, edema, cerebral anoxia, circulatory instability, hypothermia, bacterial sepsis, and disseminated intravascular coagulopathies. In addition, preterm infants frequently have weak or uncoordinated ability to feed and prolonged failure to gain weight.

Infants with IUGR (SGA) are a heterogeneous population, even when those with congenital anomalies and infections are excluded. They tend to have problems related more to their gestational age than to their birth weight. Preterm IUGR infants have a lower incidence of hyaline membrane disease than expected for their birth weight. Problems encountered in IUGR infants include perinatal asphyxia, hypoglycemia, hypothermia, meconium aspiration, necrotizing enterocolitis, polycythemia, and illnesses related to congenital anomalies, syndromes, or infections. The prognosis depends, in part, on the etiology of their growth retardation (see Chapter 7). Head circumference less than the tenth percentile at birth and abnormal newborn neurologic examination are associated with poor growth, later microcephaly, and neurologic deficits.

Table 1-2. Maternal noninfectious disease affecting the fetus

Maternal disorder	Fetal or neonatal effects
Cholestasis	Preterm delivery
Cyanotic congenital heart disease	Intrauterine growth retardation
Diabetes mellitus	Large for gestational age infants, hypoglycemia, hypocalcemia, immaturity
Endemic goiter	Neonatal hypothyroidism
Graves disease	Transient neonatal thyrotoxicosis
Hyperparathyroidism	Hypocalcemia
Hypertension	Intrauterine growth retardation, stillbirth
Hypoparathyroidism	Hypercalcemia
Idiopathic thrombocytopenia	Thrombocytopenia, bleeding
Immune neutropenia	Fetal neutropenia
Malignant melanoma	Placental metastasis
Myasthenia gravis	Transient neonatal myasthenia
Myotonic dystrophy	Neonatal myotonic dystrophy
Obesity	Large for gestational age infant, hypoglycemia
Preeclampsia-eclampsia (toxemia)	Intrauterine growth retardation, stillbirth, asphyxia
Phenylketonuria	Microcephaly, mental retardation
Renal disease	Intrauterine growth retardation, abortion
Rhesus immunization	Fetal anemia, hydrops
Rickets	Hypocalcemia, rickets
Sickle cell anemia	Intrauterine growth retardation
Systemic lupus erythematosus	Congenital heart block, transient rash, anemia, leukopenia, thrombocytopenia, pericardial effusion

Modified from Kliegman, R., and Behrman, R.E.: The fetus and neonatal infant. In Nelson's textbook of pediatrics, ed. 13, Philadelphia, 1987, W.B. Saunders Co.

Hemorrhage is frequent and often severe in LBW infants. Subcutaneous ecchymosis and subependymal and intraventricular hemorrhage are frequent. Increased capillary fragility (including arterial and venous networks in friable periventricular germinal tissue), hypernatremia, and increased vascular pressure may be contributing causes. Sudden shock during the first few days of life is often due to massive intraventricular hemorrhage, which occurs predominantly in very small premature infants. Less severe degrees of hemorrhage may be associated with lethargy, seizures, apnea, and an acute fall in hematocrit. Pulmonary hemorrhage has a similar pattern of increased incidence and high mortality in preterm infants (Chapter 32, part one).

Hyaline membrane disease (respiratory distress syndrome) occurs most frequently, and mortality is highest, in infants of shortest gestation, and the incidence and mortality fall progressively with increasing gestational age (Chapter 28, part three).

There is a higher *congenital malformation rate* both in preterm LBW infants and in full-term SGA infants than in term-normal birth weight infants. Those with the slowest intrauterine growth rates have the highest incidence of malformations. The incidence of patent ductus arteriosus is much higher in LBW infants and in those whose gestational age is less than 34 weeks than among larger or older infants (Chapter 17).

Hypoglycemia may occur in 15% of premature infants and up to 65% of IUGR infants. *Hyperglycemia* is common in extremely small infants receiving large concentrations of glucose (Chapter 37, part one).

Recurrent apnea, necrotizing enterocolitis, and *retinopathy of prematurity* occur most commonly in VLBW infants and in those with shorter gestations.

Kernicterus is found at autopsy in 2% to 20% of premature infants. VLBW infants are at increased risk, particularly if they have infection.

Prevention of LBW. Preventing pediatric mortality and morbidity associated with LBW infants requires a broad range of activities involving patients, parents, health care professionals, and community groups. These include identifying prepregnancy risks; counseling for risk reduction; implementing school health and related education programs; increasing accessibility of early, high quality prenatal care services; and expanding the content of such care to meet the variable needs of individual women and selected high-risk groups; and in developing, implementing, and supporting a long-term public information program with a few, well-chosen messages targeted at LBW risks (i.e., stop smoking).

FUTURE PROGRESS

Most progress is likely to result from the continuing expansion of our understanding of and ability to measure embryonic and fetal physiologic and biochemical homeostasis. As our appreciation of the mechanisms controlling labor and the protective circulatory adjustments of the fetus to hypoxia continues to increase, along with our understanding of pharmacology, we are likely to develop new means not only to detect but also to medically treat the fetus before and during labor and to prevent premature labor. In 1960 our ability to detect *fetal asphyxia* consisted of clinical auscultation of the fetal heart rate during labor and observation of the amniotic fluid for meconium staining when the membranes ruptured. We now know the sequence of events in the fetus that occurs in response to maternal hypotension, or hypoxia. The heart rate and blood pressure initially increase; then with the rapid onset of fetal bradycardia and hypotension the fetus develops a mixed metabolic and "placental" respiratory acidosis. The cardiac output and umbilical blood flow decrease sharply. A greater portion of the oxygenated umbilical vein blood is shunted past the liver into the inferior vena cava and returned to the heart. The cardiac output to the brain, heart, and adrenals is preferentially maintained so that tissue perfusion of these organs does not decrease significantly. In contrast, the fetal lungs and cortex of the kidneys have a decreased perfusion. The oxygen consumption of the fetus decreases by over 50%. When this sequence of events becomes far enough advanced in the rhesus monkey, baboon, and probably in the human, the problem is detectable by continuous monitoring of the fetal heart rate and uterine pressure curves; characteristic high-risk patterns such as those for cord occlusion or placental insufficiency can be identified (see Chapter 8). Nevertheless, the treatments for fetal asphyxia currently available are limited to surgical intervention, oxygen, or position changes. Improved understanding of the hormonal and neural regulation of labor and the patterns of fetal pathophysiologic response may broaden our pharmacologic approach to treatment before birth. Our ability to diagnose and/or treat some diseases before birth, such as erythroblastosis, respiratory distress syndrome (hyaline membrane disease), and a large number of genetic defects, has changed dramatically in recent years.

Investigation of the cellular level of development and pharmacology of the uterus, placenta, and fetus may be critical to understanding the control of labor and thus, eventually, to our ability to decrease the incidence of LBW or premature infants. Prenatal diagnosis and biochemical and ultrasonic fetal monitoring may be the first steps to future treatments that may include hybridization of cells in the early blastocyst or embryo to correct inborn errors of metabolism, the stimulation of embryogenesis of organs, and the acceleration of organ maturation.

Finally, advances in the field of neonatal-perinatal medicine have focused attention on a number of ethical and legal issues. There is continuing concern about life and death decision making in neonatal intensive care units. New and complex physician-patient-family–nursing staff–societal relationships exist in these units, and this development has had an enormous impact on the process of making medical decisions. Regionalization has brought these issues into a sharper and more demanding focus. Criteria have to be formulated for making certain decisions that previously were made on a chance basis of access to the health system, which was strongly influenced by the economic position of a family. For example, should a 750 gm infant with a poor prognosis for intact survival be accepted in a regional neonatal intensive care unit when it means one cannot accept a 2,000 gm infant who is at high risk but has a good prognosis if he or she survives, just because the referring physician in the case of the 750 gm infant calls first or because the infant is born in the same hospital where the intensive care unit is located? The nature of the evolving customs or prelegal restraints differs in some important respects from those impinging on the traditional physician-patient relationship outside neonatal intensive care centers. Participation in discussions antecedent to decision making involves a diversity of people, the discussions are more explicitly informative, and the demands on the physician's ability to perceive what is meant from what is said are more exacting. Ironically, but not surprisingly, as the technology of care increases in these units, the difficult choices for the physician are not the technical medical decisions, but matters of judgment that require evaluating, analyzing, and interpreting the complex human interests and concerns of the relatives, their friends and advisors, and the staff, and the various consequences for the people involved. These have always been the most challenging and demanding decisions for physicians that cannot be delegated to others. The new elements are the frequency and complexity of these judgments in regional neonatal intensive care centers (Chapter 18).

Whatever decision-making process is used to improve the quality of care provided to the individual patient, certain principles are important, but often not easy to apply. The fundamental responsibility of all who are concerned is to do no harm or, at least, no harm without a reasonable expectation of a compensating benefit for the patient. A corollary principle is that there must be continuous objective, critical scientific evaluation of the care being currently provided and of proposed innovations. Activities should not be initiated or continued that on balance do harm to the well-being of a newborn infant. The definition of "well-being" is the major problem, since the varying ethical values, religious commitments, and life experiences of all those who care for and about the infant, as well as legal restraints, must be taken into consideration. In general, the elements of well-being include at the least a life prolonged beyond infancy, without excruciating pain, and with the potential of participating in human experience to a minimal degree.

Awareness of the above diverse considerations has contributed to the impetus for further clinical specialization within pediatrics, and obstetrics and gynecology, resulting in the formation of a field of clinical medicine for the fetus and neonatal infant: neonatal-perinatal medicine. This field has already expanded to encompass the developing embryo before, as well as after, organ formation and older infants whose immaturity or disease process makes them best cared for in neonatal intensive care centers.

Richard E. Behrman

BIBLIOGRAPHY

Behrman, R.E.: Preventing low birthweight: a pediatric perspective, J. Pediatr. **107**:842, 1985.

Behrman, R.E., and others: Distribution of the circulation in the normal asphyxiated fetal neonate, Am. J. Obstet. Gynec. **108**:956, 1970.

Janis, A.R., and others: Critical issues in newborn intensive care: a conference report and policy proposal, Pediatrics **555**:756, 1975.

Kliegman, R., and Behrman, R.E.: The fetus and the neonatal infant. In Behrman, R.E., and Vaughan, V.C., editors: Nelson's textbook of pediatrics, ed. 13, Philadelphia, 1987, W.B. Saunders Co.

Report and recommendation for research on the fetus, Pub. No. (05)76-127, Washington, D.C., 1975, The National Commission for the Protection of Human Subjects of Biomedical and Behavioral Research, Department of Health, Education and Welfare.

The prevention of low birthweight, Report of the Committee to Study the Prevention of Low Birthweight, Division of Health Promotion and Disease Prevention, Institute of Medicine, National Academy of Sciences, Washington, D.C., 1985, National Academy Press.

CHAPTER 2

Perinatal services and resources

PART ONE

The organization of perinatal health services

The successful delivery of high-quality care to perinatal patients requires not only excellence from physicians, nurses, and other health professionals as individuals, but also community involvement and a mechanism or system of organization that permits them to function as cohesive and well-coordinated teams.

> Regionalization implies the development, within a geographic area, of a coordinated cooperative system of maternal and perinatal health care in which, by mutual agreements between hospitals and physicians and based upon population needs, the degree of complexity of maternal and perinatal care each hospital is capable of providing is identified so as to accomplish the following objectives: quality care to all pregnant women and newborns, maximal utilization of highly trained perinatal personnel and intensive care facilities, and assurance of reasonable cost effectiveness.*

BACKGROUND AND HISTORICAL PERSPECTIVE

Before 1940 perinatal care services were delivered in the United States, Canada, and Europe without any particular organization or structure. Most of the care was provided by an individual physician or midwife. In many areas the majority of the deliveries occurred in the home. A number of maternity hospitals developed in the larger urban areas, usually serving as teaching hospitals. These maternity hospitals often had home delivery services and neighborhood clinics serving a geographic area.

During the 1940s and early 1950s a number of cities developed centers for the care of premature infants. Most of these centers were located in urban areas. In Illinois, premature centers were located to serve the rural areas as well. In the late 1940s and 1950s many of the European countries, particularly in Scandinavia and the Netherlands, developed systems of care for the perinatal patient based on the development of primary prenatal care clinics staffed largely by midwives with district and regional hospitals for the care of mothers with complications. During the 1950s a number of states developed maternal mortality committees. These committees developed data that were used as a basis for activities directed at preventing maternal mortality.

From 1964 to 1968 studies were undertaken in Massachusetts, Wisconsin, and Arizona to analyze causes of neonatal mortality and morbidity. In Massachusetts the studies led to the development of standards and regulations for maternity units. Their implementation resulted in a decrease in the number of maternity units in Massachusetts from 102 in 1967 to 65 in 1975. In Wisconsin the studies led to the development of a statewide education-consultation program and regional newborn intensive care centers. These units subsequently evolved into regional perinatal centers. In 1967, as a result of a study of premature mortality, Arizona developed a statewide transport program for premature and other high-risk neonates. Three additional factors that promoted the movement toward the development of regional care plans were the study and report of the Joint Committee of the Society of Obstetricians and Gynaecologists of Canada and the Canadian Paediatric Society, entitled "Regional Services in Reproductive Medicine"; the adoption of a statement on regionalization of perinatal care by the American Medical Association; and the report of the joint Committee on Perinatal Health of the American Medical Association, the American College of Obstetricians and Gynecologists, the American Academy of Family Physicians, and the American Academy of Pediatrics, entitled "Toward Improving the Outcome of Pregnancy." These reports, along with the data from Wisconsin, Massachusetts, and Arizona, have stimulated activities in most states toward development of regional organizations for perinatal care services. Additional impetus has been

*From Ryan, G.M.: Toward improving the outcome of pregnancy, Report of the Committee on Perinatal Health (AAFP, AAP, ACOG, AMA), 1976, Obstet Gynecol. **46**:375, 1975. Reprinted with permission from The American College of Obstetricians and Gynecologists.

derived from the establishment of regional perinatal centers in the United States by the Robert Wood Johnson Foundation.

NEED FOR AN ORGANIZED PERINATAL CARE SYSTEM

There are marked disparities in the perinatal mortality for various nations. These disparities are particularly striking among various European nations, the United States, and Canada. There are also marked differences between states or districts within a country and between areas within the same district or state. Marked differences in perinatal mortality exist between census tracts within the same urban area. Those nations with well-organized systems for perinatal care have better perinatal mortality and morbidity statistics.

Often high fetal and neonatal mortality is attributed to socioeconomic conditions, educational deficiencies, and related social factors. In some areas, however, high perinatal mortality may exist simultaneously with very low mortality for older age groups, suggesting that the lack of adequate health care services for the pregnant woman and neonate is a major factor responsible for the high perinatal mortality.

In the studies from Massachusetts and Wisconsin 30% to 65% of the fetal and neonatal mortalities were judged preventable. Of the preventable deaths, approximately half were judged preventable within the resources of the community hospital and its staff; the other half required the resources of a specialized regional center with team-derived resources. Studies of infants following neonatal intensive care have shown a marked reduction in the frequency of permanent neurologic sequelae. Thus the development of neonatal intensive care results not only in reduction in mortality but also in a reduction in serious morbidity. Maternal intensive care units and high-risk obstetric programs decrease fetal mortality and also reduce the frequency of neonatal problems requiring intensive care. The decrease in the number of deaths and improvement in the outcome for the survivors of both maternal and neonatal intensive care have justified the cost investment in these programs.

PRINCIPLES OF ORGANIZATION

There are general principles that form the basis for the development of regional health care services for perinatal patients. These principles derive from an understanding of the care needs of the mother, fetus, and family during pregnancy, and of the mother, newborn, and family following birth.

Accountability for population

Regionalization denotes a geographic area or population with definable care needs. The regional center and the network of related institutions are accountable for the overall perinatal health care for the region. The data on mortality and morbidity, frequency of problems, and quality of care are assessed for the entire population in the area. The availability and quality of care in any given institution become the responsibility of all the institutions, including the perinatal center.

One standard of quality

Regionalization is based on the premise that there should be a single standard of quality perinatal care. Any mother or infant should have equal access to all the components of a functioning perinatal system (Table 2-1).

Differing care capabilities of institutions

Institutions operating within a region will differ in their capability for providing perinatal care. These differences reflect number of patients, educational background and experience of medical and nursing staff, and availability of equipment and facilities. Each institution is expected to deliver high-quality care up to the level of its capability. When care requirements exceed its capability, the patient is referred to the closest facility that has the capability.

The majority (60% to 80%) of problems associated with increased risk for the mother, fetus, or newborn are detectable sufficiently in advance of the crises to permit either the appropriate care resources to be made available locally or transfer of the patient to where appropriate resources are available. Even under ideal circumstances certain patients will have to move from one facility to another during the course of care. Thus institutions within a region must be effectively linked to permit ease of patient movement.

Minimal patient movement

The organization of the regional care network should be designed to make it possible for patients to receive care appropriate to their needs as close to their homes as possible. Only those patients with care needs exceeding that of their community facility should need to be referred to another institution. Through outreach education (see Chapter 2, part two) and consultation programs, efforts should be made to continually develop and expand the care capabilities of each institution to minimize the number of patients who must be dislocated while receiving care.

Optimal use of facilities and personnel

The concept of regionalization is designed to permit optimal use of both facilities and personnel. With the use of a regional perinatal center it is possible to have sufficient numbers of high-risk mothers and neonates concentrated in a single location to economically justify

Table 2-1. Services provided by perinatal facilities

Services	Level I	Level II	Level III
Complete prenatal care for maternity patient with no complications or with minor complications	X	X	X
Complete prenatal care for maternity patients with most complications		X	X
A special diagnostic and management clinic for high-risk prenatal patients			X
Risk identification scoring system	X	X	X
Management of uncomplicated labor and delivery of normal term fetus	X	X	X
Prompt management of unexpected complications occurring during labor and delivery, including anesthesia, cesarean section, and blood administration	X	X	X
Management of complicated labor and delivery		X	X
Intrapartum intensive care			X
In-house anesthesia service		X	X
Electronic fetal monitoring	±	X	X
Physically separated facilities for obstetrics	X	X	X
Capability for resuscitation of depressed neonate at every delivery	X	X	X
Care for the healthy newborn	X	X	X
Stabilization and risk assessment of all neonates	X	X	X
Intravenous fluid administration to neonates	X	X	X
Management of most neonates who have complications up to short-term assisted ventilation		X	X
Continuous neonatal monitoring capability		X	X
Blood gases available on 24-hour basis		X	X
Neonatal intensive care including assisted ventilation and hyperalimentation			X
Neonatal surgical capability			X
Availability of pediatric subspecialists in cardiology, genetics, and hematology			X
Care of mothers with no postpartum complications	X	X	X
Management of unexpected postpartum complications including hemorrhage and sepsis	X	X	X
Management of most postpartum complications		X	X
Data collection on performance and outcome	X	X	X
Laboratory services for electrolytes, bilirubin, blood glucose, calcium on 24-hour basis	X	X	X
X-ray services with portable film capability on 24-hour basis	X	X	X
Laboratory services to assess fetal well-being and maturity		X	X
Diagnostic x-ray and ultrasound facilities		X	X
Nutritional consultation		X	X
Social service		X	X
Respiratory therapy consultation		X	X
Sterilization and family planning services	X	X	X
Follow-up developmental assessment clinic			X

the staffing and equipment necessary to meet their care needs. In addition, personnel who have frequent opportunities to use their skills are able to maintain and enhance these skills. Institutions with small patient loads can avoid the expense of developing staff and equipment for services that are infrequently used.

Differing care needs for different groups

Groups within a population have differing care needs by virtue of socioeconomic conditions, education, ethnic background, personal health care practices, age, and other factors. The organization of facilities and personnel involved in perinatal care must reflect these varying needs.

Perinatal care: a team service

The health care needs of the perinatal patient require a close working relationship between the various disciplines involved to prevent fragmentation and gaps in care.

ORGANIZATION

Those countries with better perinatal mortality and morbidity statistics have carefully organized and universally made available primary care for a mother during pregnancy and an established mechanism for referral of mothers and infants from primary care institutions to district or center hospitals when the needs of the patient indicate. They have placed less emphasis on tertiary care or intensive care because of the relatively low demand for such services. By contrast, the perinatal health services of the United States and Canada place great emphasis on the specialized hospital services for the perinatal patient, but the primary care services available to the mother during her pregnancy are disorganized and inconsistent. The number of perinatal patients requiring intensive in-hospital care is inversely related to the quality and availability of primary services, as well as to the general health status of the mothers before pregnancy.

An organized system for providing care to the maternity patient and her neonate consists of six types of units or facilities: physicians' offices and clinics, level I or community hospital facilities, level II hospital facilities, level III hospital facilities, regional perinatal centers, and specialized units such as children's hospitals and cardiac centers.

Physicians' offices and clinics

The basic or primary care units for care during pregnancy as well as for care of the mother and infant following delivery are physicians' offices and general clinics. These units need to have the capability for obtaining a complete health history, careful physical assessment of the mother or infant, systematic risk assessment (using one of the available risk scoring systems), and laboratory resources for determination of hematocrit or hemoglobin concentration and urinalysis.

Level I facilities

Level I (community hospital) facilities are those designed primarily for the care of the maternal and neonatal patients who have no complications. These units exist primarily because of geographic or cultural situations that limit access to units with greater care capabilities. Since even uncomplicated maternal and neonatal patients have a potential for unexpected complications, level I units must have the resources to provide competent emergency services when the need arises. The necessary services for a level I facility are shown in Table 2-1 and include a normal newborn nursery (see Chapter 24, part four).

Level II facilities

Level II facilities are those hospitals that have larger maternity and newborn services. These hospitals will be located in urban and suburban areas serving larger communities. In addition to providing a full range of maternal and newborn services for perinatal patients who have no complications, they will provide services for some of the obstetric and neonatal patients who have complications. The range of obstetric and neonatal complications that fall within the capabilities of a given institution will depend on the resources available. The services available in level II units are presented in Table 2-1 and include both a normal newborn nursery and a transitional care nursery (Chapter 21, part four).

Level III facilities

In addition to the resources and capabilities of a level II unit, level III facilities are able to provide for a full range of maternal complications and newborn intensive care. The neonatal intensive care unit needs to have a full range of services for the neonate, with the possible exception of an occasional infant with congenital heart disease or other complex congenital anomaly who requires a specialized unit. The services offered by level III facilities are listed in Table 2-1 and include a neonatal intensive care nursery (Chapter 8).

Regional perinatal center

A regional perinatal center is a level III facility that also has responsibility for coordination and management of special services, including transportation, that are needed for the region. In areas where there is only one level III facility, it is expected to function as the regional perinatal center. In areas where there is more than one unit with level III capabilities, one of the units would serve as the regional perinatal center. The regional perinatal center must offer outpatient and inpatient consultation and diagnostic services for level I and level II facilities within the region, including ultrasonography, laboratory analysis of amniotic fluid, gestational assessment, genetic studies, and other studies of fetal health. It also should provide specialized nursing services and consultation in nutrition, social services, respiratory therapy, and laboratory and radiology services. The center is responsible for carrying on an active outreach education program for the institutions, health professionals, and public within the region (see Chapter 2, part two).

A regional perinatal center has unique personnel needs. It should be directed by a full-time physician with extensive training and experience in perinatal medicine as well as in administration. There also should be a director of obstetric services and a director of neonatal services. The director of obstetric services should be a full-time physician with training and experience in fetal-maternal medicine, including maternal intensive care. The director of neonatal services should be a full-time neonatologist with training and experience in neonatal care, including newborn intensive care. The perinatal nursing services should be directed by a clinical nurse specialist with advanced experience in maternal and neonatal nursing and experience in administration. The center also may require a full-time director of the outreach education program to coordinate the active participation from physicians in obstetrics and newborn care, nurses in obstetrics and newborn care, nutritionists, social workers, and other specialized personnel. The obstetric and newborn care units, including the newborn intensive care unit, should have clinical nurse specialists in obstetrics and neonatal care, respectively, responsible for organizing the nursing programs and coordinating the patient care needs.

Frequency of risk problems

It is important to estimate the number of pregnant women who may need specialized obstetric and neonatal services within the area of a given regional perinatal center. The percentage of pregnancies at increased risk may vary from 10% for general populations, such as an entire state or country, to over 90% in some urban hospitals. In an Ontario perinatal study 32% of pregnancies had some increased risk factor that resulted in 60% of the neonatal problems. In the Nova Scotia Fetal Risk Project 11% of 9,483 patients accounted for 50% of the stillbirths and 75% of the neonatal deaths.

The number of neonatal care beds and neonatal intensive care days needed for a given population is most influenced by the frequency of premature birth and low birth weight. There are great differences in these frequencies between countries and between populations within a country. Low birth weight infants comprise less than 5% of the births in the Scandinavian countries and 6% to 9% of infants in some states in the United States; in some institutions the frequency may run as high as 15% to 20%. (See Chapter 1.)

Swyer calculated a need for neonatal intensive care beds at 0.7 beds per 1,000 live births on the basis of a 7% low birth weight rate. Transitional or intermediate bed and convalescent bed needs were approximately 4 per 1,000 live births. The Wisconsin Perinatal Care Program predicted a need for 12 intensive care beds for 6,000 live births (7% low birth weight rate). Data from Utah indicate a need for two beds per 1,000 annual live births in special care facilities. The estimated breakdown was 0.5 level I beds, 0.5 level II beds, and one bed per 1,000 annual live births at level III.

Other services in a regional care system

An effective public health nursing system and availability of public health services are essential ingredients for effective perinatal care. Home visits during pregnancy and after birth provide a dimension of care not met by physician's offices or community hospitals. Finally, a perinatal center and hospital network must develop close working relationships with regional blood banks and with state or regional laboratories that provide special services to meet the unique needs of the perinatal patient.

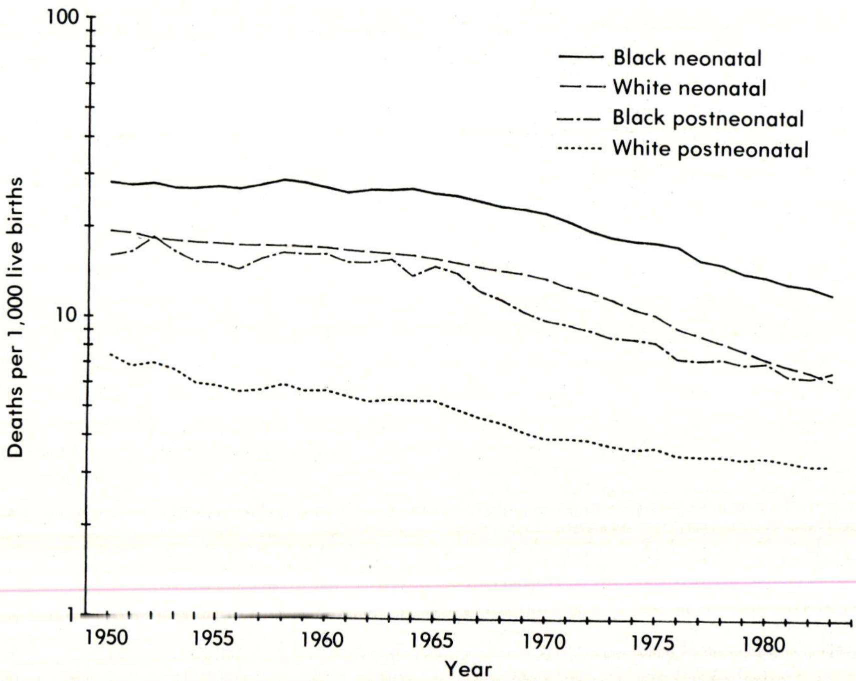

Fig. 2-1. Neonatal and postneonatal mortality rates, black and white, United States, 1950 to 1983. (From Wegman, M.E.: Pediatrics **76:**861, 1985. Reproduced by permission of Pediatrics.)

EFFECTS OF REGIONAL ORGANIZATION OF PERINATAL SERVICES

The development of newborn intensive care units and transport systems has been associated with marked reduction in neonatal mortality (Fig. 2-1), as well as reduction in the frequency of neurologic sequelae. In Quebec the perinatal mortality survey demonstrated reduced mortality in hospitals using referral to a neonatal intensive care unit. In Toronto the neonatal mortality was reduced nearly 50% over a 10-year period with the development of a neonatal intensive care unit. Similar reductions in mortality have been demonstrated in Halifax, Nova Scotia, and Madison, Wisconsin. The development of statewide regional perinatal programs in Wisconsin, Massachusetts, and Arizona has likewise produced marked statewide reductions in perinatal mortality attributed to the statewide teaching programs, as well as to the development of regional centers. Following the development of a statewide infant transport program for regional neonatal intensive care units in Arizona there was a decrease in the state neonatal mortality from 17.3 to 11.5 deaths per thousand live births over a 5-year period. Infant mortality decreased and care practices improved within 2 years of the development of a statewide perinatal care program in Iowa.

PROBLEMS OF REGIONALIZATION

One of the most common disorders of regionalization is centralization in place of regionalization. This is the end product of a regional center that operates with no outreach education program or other mechanisms for continuing the development and improvement of services in the other hospitals of the region. With such a system the central hospital continues to receive the referrals of high-risk mothers or high-risk noenates but makes no effort to help the referring hospital develop programs for preventing the problems. This may be particularly true in university medical centers where outreach education and service are not considered a regular academic or hospital activity. Recently this problem appears to have diminished, particularly with "reverse transports," in which neonates no longer requiring tertiary level care are transported back to their community hospitals.

A second common disorder of regionalization is unnecessary duplication of units. This includes the unnecessary duplication of both level I and level II units within rural or urban areas and competing level III units, particularly in the smaller urban areas. The duplication results in difficulties in recruiting and maintaining the necessary personnel for such care units as well as in increased cost per patient for such care. Such duplication invariably is a result of competing institutions and competing medical staffs who view maternal intensive care and neonatal intensive care units as important to their business, income, or institutional image.

Many regional centers are staffed with inadequate or inappropriately trained personnel. One of the most common problems is the staffing of maternal and infant intensive care nurseries with inexperienced house staff as the primary responsible physicians, particularly during night hours and weekends. Such units often have only a single neonatologist or fetal-maternal obstetrician available, thus placing a great reliance on house staff. In such circumstances house staff also may become involved in answering requests for consultations from outlying hospitals and in other activities for which they are inadequately prepared. An equally serious problem of medical supervision is seen in those intensive care units which operate with no full-time staff. The coverage and time commitment available from busy general pediatric practitioners does not permit the attention necessary for intensive care or the development of expertise. Inadequate or inappropriate staffing is also often manifested in the use of licensed practical nurses by hospitals in place of experienced professional nurses in the care of high-risk mothers and high-risk neonates. This is usually done as a cost-saving measure with inadequate understanding of the value of experienced professional nurses in the delivery of high-risk perinatal care. There is likewise a reluctance to use clinical nurse specialists and nurse clinicians because of the cost and lack of understanding of their role in patient care.

A number of regional networks have no integrated system for transportation. This results in many patients, particularly high-risk infants, being transported in poorly equipped vehicles with poorly trained or inexperienced staff. Such regions have consistently increased mortality and morbidity as a direct result of problems associated with transport.

Finally, in most regions there are some institutions and physicians that consistently fail to appropriately use the resources of a regional center when the care of the patient clearly indicates such a need. The hospitals that make least use of the center may be located closest to the center. Fear of loss of patients, physician ego, and failure to recognize problems promptly are the major inhibitors to appropriate use of perinatal center resources.

MEASUREMENTS OF EFFECTIVENESS OF CARE ORGANIZATION

When the effectiveness of any care system as well as of its individual components is measured, it is essential to analyze data for the entire region. There are many examples of dramatic changes in mortality or morbidity statistics for a given hospital in the course of a single year, not as a result of improvement of care, but as a result of movement of patients with particular problems to another institution. If the geographic boundaries of a region are well designed, there will be limited patient movement from region to region. This permits consistent year-to-year evaluation of the care within the region.

Maternal mortality has declined to the point that it is no longer a satisfactory index of quality care. Fetal and neonatal mortality is still a reasonable indicator of perinatal care. In their evaluation within a region, the data must link the hospital in which the death is recorded with the institution and community in which the birth occurred or the care was initiated. Fetal and neonatal mortalities should also be divided by weight groups. The weight groups should be in 500 gm increments or less, beginning with 500 gm. If possible, the gestational age distribution and cause of death for the fetal or neonatal deaths should be established. Such practices make it possible to identify those areas or institutions within a region in which there are major problems with care. Infant mortality (those deaths occurring between 28 days and 1 year after birth) is an indicator of socioeconomic conditions and living standards, as well as the availability and quality of health care.

When maternal, fetal, or neonatal mortality or morbidity rates are used, certain other information is necessary to permit useful interpretation. For maternal mortalities it is essential to separate those maternal deaths during or as a result of pregnancy associated with other maternal disease, such as severe cardiac disease or malignancy, from those deaths associated primarily with the pregnancy. This requires individual analysis of each death and assignment to preventable or nonpreventable categories. For evaluation of neonatal programs and regionalization, the frequency of 1-minute Apgar scores of 3 or under and 5-minute Apgar scores of 5 and under should be recorded. Also helpful in assessing effectiveness of care are the frequency of sepsis, traumatic delivery, respiratory distress syndrome, and neurologic problems, the number of intensive care days, and the number of patient transfers from community institutions to institutions of greater care capability.

All high-risk mothers and neonates should have systematic follow-up. Those infants at high risk for developmental, neurologic, or learning problems should be followed into school age with careful neurologic and educational testing. The incidence of child abuse and failure to thrive may also reflect parenting disorders having antecedents in the perinatal period.

EVALUATION OF TRANSPORT SERVICES

Despite the proliferation of neonatal coverage for level II nurseries, efficient maternal-fetal and neonatal transport services form a key component of regional perinatal care. Ideally, the delivery of an infant of less than 32 weeks' gestation or weighing less than 1.5 kg should occur at a perinatal center. Although comparisons of mortality statistics following maternal versus neonatal transfer suffer from many confounding variables, several studies have demonstrated a lower morbidity and shorter neonatal hospitalization following maternal-fetal transport.

It is estimated that antenatal maternal transfer is not possible in up to 50% of high-risk pregnancies. In these situations neonatal transport must be performed by specially trained teams skilled in adequate stabilization before and effective management during transport. Hood has documented a 60% greater mortality rate when neonates were transferred by an untrained vs. trained neonatal transport team. Hypothermia and acidosis in particular were more common after transfer by an untrained team. The transport team from the referral hospital also serves an important educational function and can both influence and improve methods of stabilization at the referring center, which in turn may influence mortality statistics (see Chapter 2, part two).

In many areas limited regional perinatal resources have hampered referrals and required the referring physician to make multiple calls until an available bed can be located. Central telephone operator systems have partially alleviated this problem. A computer-based coordination of telecommunications has been developed in North Carolina, which is linked to the state's nine tertiary centers and provides two hourly updates on neonatal and maternal bed availability, it appears cost-effective.

An effective means of managing overcrowding at the perinatal referral center is to encourage reverse transport of previously ill neonates to levels II and I nurseries for intermediate care. This can include not only babies with resolved acute medical problems but also those with continuing chronic problems such as bronchopulmonary dysplasia. The tertiary center must, however, be familiar with the capabilities, facilities, and resources of the hospitals to which reverse transport is occurring so that quality of care can be ensured. This evaluation can be combined with an outreach education program. Apart from the obvious cost effectiveness of reverse transport it can encourage family bonding and greater involvement of the pediatrician who will be offering continuing care to the infant.

FINANCIAL CONSIDERATIONS

The facilities within a regional network, including a regional perinatal center, are financially dependent on patient revenue or public support or both for the care of neonatal patients. With carefully coordinated use of resources and facilities the cost of care delivery can be contained. It is essential that the health insurance programs provide adequate coverage for obstetric and neonatal conditions and that charges reflect the cost of delivering the services. Medical assistance and other forms of payment, as well as direct support of state and county hospitals, must be adequate for the care needs. There must be adequate nursing staff, physician coverage, equipment, and supplies to achieve an acceptable quality of care. The reimbursement schemes should provide for patient transfer between institutions without multiplication of deductibles or major financial hardship to the patient. The cost of emergency transport of high-risk maternal and newborn patients should be covered. The financial incentives should promote the use of the resources appropriate to the patient care needs.

Diagnostic related grouping has been implemented as the method of federal reimbursement, and other third party payers will follow shortly. The limited initial data base to determine the reimbursement level did not take into account many variables that influence length of stay, particularly at a tertiary center. If the guidelines are not modified, major tertiary centers will be at a distinct financial disadvantage, particularly when providing care for extremely complicated and LBW infants. The system may also discourage transport of infants from both level I and II units if the referring hospitals perceive financial gain, hence quality of care may be compromised.

IMPLICATIONS FOR EDUCATION

In the organization of most perinatal regions the educational needs of health care professionals must be carefully integrated with the needs of the patient and family. It is essential that the patient's needs for privacy, care, professional attention, and time for personal interactions among infant, family, and other important caretakers be recognized by those participating in patient care: for example, nurses, medical students, and house staff. However, quality care is in large part dependent on undergraduate and graduate education programs that are an integral part of the responsibilities of a regional perinatal center. Senior staff physicians and nurses must accept direct responsibility for patient care and major management decisions while fulfilling their educational responsibilities toward those in training or in practice in the community.

FUTURE CONSIDERATIONS

Centers for newborn care have expanded at the level II institutions with large delivery services so that many have developed capabilities similar to those at university centers. In many areas competition exists between the tertiary and level II units, in others the two centers are working hand in hand. In all communities it is essential for mutually productive relationships to be reestablished between the academic and community hospitals. A majority of board-certified neonatologists in the United States now practice outside the traditional academic settings. These personnel needs are being met by the university-based training programs, however, with fewer training programs accredited and more trainees completing a third fellowship year it is conceivable that in the near future there will not be an adequate number of trained neonatologists to staff the ever expanding level II units. Today the major strategies relate to provision of cost-effective medical care, to compliance with regulations that dictate standards required for reimbursement, and above all to a strategy for the prevention of low birth weight and prematurity.

Avroy A. Fanaroff
Stanley N. Graven

BIBLIOGRAPHY

American Medical Association, House of Delegates: Report J, Atlantic City, N.J., 1971, The Association.

Aubry, R.H., and Nesbitt, R.E.L., Jr.: High risk obstetrics. 1. Perinatal outcome in relation to a broadened approach to obstetrical care for patients at special risk, Am. J. Obstet. Gynecol. **105**:241, 1969.

Bacola, E., and others: Perinatal and environmental factors in late neurogenic sequelae. 1. Infants having birth weights under 1500 grams, Am. J. Dis. Child. **112**:359, 1966.

Bostick, J.S., Hsiao, H.S., and Lawson, E.E.: A minicomputer-based perinatal/neonatal telecommunications network, Pediatrics **71**:272, 1983.

Callon, H.F.: Regionalizing perinatal care in Wisconsin, Nurs. Clin. North Am. **10**:263, 1975.

Committee on Perinatal Welfare: Report on perinatal and infant mortality in Massachusetts, 1967 and 1968, Boston, 1971, Massachusetts Medical Society.

Crenshaw, C., and others: Prematurity and the obstetrician, Am. J. Obstet. Gynecol. **147**:125, 1983.

Drillien, C.M.: Growth and development in a group of children of very low birth weight, Arch. Dis. Child. **33**:10, 1958.

Drillien, C.M.: The long term prospects for babies of low birth weight, Hosp. Med. **1**:937, 1967.

Erickson, S.: Infant I.C.U.'s save lives but too many units may add cost and hamper growth, Mod. Hosp. **15**:80, 1970.

Goodwin, J.W., Dunne, J.T., and Thomas, B.W.: Antepartum identification of the fetus at risk, Can. Med. Assoc. J. **101**:458, 1969.

Grassy, R.G., and Zachman, R.D.: The growth and development of low birth weight infants receiving neonatal intensive care, Clin. Pediatr. **15**:549, 1976.

Graven, S.N., and Callon, H.F.: Perinatal care in Wisconsin, 1964-1974 (unpublished report), 1976.

Graven, S.N., Howe, G., and Callon, H.F.: Perinatal health care studies and program results in Wisconsin, 1964-1970. In Stetson, J.B., and Swyer, P.R., editors: Neonatal intensive care, St. Louis, 1975, Warren H. Green, Inc.

Hackel, A.: Interregional transport of high risk infants, Columbus, Ohio, 1974, Sixty-sixth Ross Conference on Pediatric Research.

Hobel, C.J., and others: Prenatal and intrapartum high risk screening, Am. J. Obstet. Gynecol. **117**:1, 1973.

Hood, J.L., and others: Effectiveness of the neonatal transport team, Crit. Care Med. **11**:419, 1983.

Indyk, L.: Evaluation of equipment in transport systems, Columbus, Ohio, 1974, Sixty-sixth Ross Conference on Pediatric Research.

Jung, A.L., and Bose, C.L.: Back transport of neonates: improved efficiency of tertiary nursery bed utilization, Pediatrics **71**:918, 1983.

Jung, A.L., and Streeter, N.S.: Total population estimate of newborn special-care bed needs, Pediatrics **75**:993, 1985.

Knobloch, H., and others: Neuropsychiatric sequelae of prematurity: a longitudinal study, JAMA **161**:581, 1956.

Lagoe, R.J., Milliren, J.W., and Baader, M.J.: Impact of selected diagnosis-related groups on regional neonatal care, Pediatrics **77**:627, 1986.

Leonard, T.: History of the Wisconsin maternal mortality study and survey committee, Wis. Med. J. **69**:75, 1970.

Lubchenco, L.O., and others: Evaluation of premature infants of low birth weights at ten years of age, Am. J. Dis. Child. **106**:101, 1963.

Merkatz, I.R., and Fanaroff, A.A.: The regional perinatal network. In Caplan, R.M., and Sweeney, W.J., editors: Advances in obstetrics and gynecology, Baltimore, 1978, The Williams & Wilkins Co.

Meyer, H.B.P.: Regional perinatal care in Arizona, Columbus, Ohio, 1974, Sixty-sixth Ross Conference on Pediatric Research.

Ontario Perinatal Mortality Study Committee: Second report of the perinatal mortality study in ten university teaching hospitals in Ontario, Canada, 1967, Ontario Department of Health.

Pettigrew, A.H.: The role of the state department of health in regionalized perinatal care, Columbus, Ohio, 1974, Sixty-sixth Ross Conference on Pediatric Research.

Poland, R.L., and others: Analysis of the effects of applying federal diagnosis-related grouping (DRG) guidelines to a population of high-risk newborn infants, Pediatrics **76**:104, 1985.

Pomerance, J.J., and others: Cost of living for infants weighing 1,000 grams or less at birth, Pediatrics **61**:908, 1978.

Rawlings, G., and others: Changing prognosis for infants of very low birth weight, Lancet **1**:516, 1971.

Robertson, A.M., and Crichton, J.U.: Neurological sequelae in children with neonatal respiratory distress: infants with low birth weights, Am. J. Dis. Child. **117**:271, 1969.

Ryan, G.M.: Toward improving the outcome of pregnancy: recommendations for the regional development of perinatal health services, Obstet. Gynecol. **46**:375, 1975.

Ryan, G.M., and Fogerty, S.: Regionalization of perinatal health services (unpublished report), 1976.

Sandhu, B., and others: Cost of neonatal intensive care for very-low-birthweight infants, Lancet **1**:600, 1986.

Schneider, J.H., and Graven, S.N.: Regionalized obstetric/gynecology care in Wisconsin perinatal centers, Contemp. Ob/Gyn **3**:35, 1974.

Scott, K.E.: Report of the Committee on Maternal and Perinatal Health of the Province of Nova Scotia, Nova Scotia Med. Bull. **49**:81, 1970.

Segal, E.S., editor: Transport of high risk newborn infants, Toronto, 1972, The Foetus and Newborn Committee of the Canadian Paediatric Society.

Silverman, W.A.: Dunham's premature infants, New York, 1961, Harper & Row, Publishers.

Stewart, A.L., Reynolds, E.O.R., and Lipscomb, A.P.: Outcome for infants of a very low birthweight: survey of world literature, Lancet **1**:1038, 1981.

Swyer, P.R.: The regional organization of special care of the neonate, Pediatr. Clin. North Am. **17**:761, 1970.

Swyer, P.R., and Goodwin, J.W., editors: Regional services in reproductive medicine, Toronto, 1973, The Joint Committee of the Society of Obstetricians and Gynaecologists of Canada and the Canadian Paediatric Society.

Toward improving the outcome of pregnancy (report of Committee on Perinatal Health of the American Medical Association, American College of Obstetrics and Gynecologists, American Academy of Pediatrics, and American Academy of Family Physicians), New York, 1975, National Foundation–March of Dimes.

Vapaavuori, E.K., and Raiha, N.C.R.: Intensive care of small premature infants: indications and results of treatment, Acta Paediatr. Scand. **59**:353, 1970.

World Health Organization Technical Report, Series No. 457, p. 7, as reported by Swyer, P.R.: Pediatr. Clin. North Am. **17**:761, 1970.

PART TWO

Perinatal outreach education

RATIONALE

The basic tenet of regionalized perinatal care is that all fetuses and newborn infants should receive optimum care consistent with their degree of illness or risk and regardless of their place of residence. Since over 80% of pregnancies are managed outside of regional perinatal centers, the main responsibility for early identification of the high risk patient resides with community-based practitioners. These individuals must assume responsibility for providing optimum resuscitation and stabilization for the 20% to 40% of high-risk newborns not identified before delivery. In rural areas the number of babies requiring such stabilizing care is even higher because of the inadvisability of transporting a woman in advanced labor over long distances. Thus, if perinatal statistics are to improve, the community-based perinatal professionals should be the main target population for teaching optimum perinatal principles and techniques. It is with sound basis, therefore, that the regional perinatal concept assigns outreach education as one of the major responsibilities of each regional perinatal center.

CLASSIC APPROACHES

Most of the traditional programs of continuing education have been based on the regional center's perception of the community hospital's needs. The most familiar of these is the 1- to 3-day lecture series organized for referring physicians and held at the regional center. Content often covers those subject areas that are appealing to the program director or that are particularly current in the medical literature. Usually the mistaken assumption is that the audience has a significant and uniform background fund of knowledge on which the speakers can build fairly complex concepts. There is frequently little attempt made to evaluate the practitioners' needs and then to design a program around those needs.

A fairly recent form of continuing education has been the "mini-residency," in which practicing physicians and/or community hospital nurses visit the regional center for several days or even weeks to function as short-term staff members. Although this format gives the practitioner more "hands-on" experience than does the lecture approach, generally the patients cared for have more complex problems and the equipment used is more sophisticated than will be dealt with or needed in the participant's local environment.

Most regional centers have developed a traveling outreach program in which a neonatologist, perinatologist, and perinatal nurse spend several hours in each of their referring hospitals giving lectures, critiquing the hospital's perinatal facilities, and reviewing the course of patients recently referred to the regional center. This format is often more successful than the others because it makes a significant attempt to tailor the educational experience to the unique needs of the community hospital. Disadvantages are that it is a relatively brief educational experience, it tends to attract the least busy individuals who often need the teaching the least, it is viewed with skepticism by many busy practitioners, and it is relatively time consuming for regional center personnel.

In general, each of these classic approaches is structured after the traditional teaching model of medical education (e.g., classroom lectures, apprentice training, education of each professional group separately). However, modern perinatal medicine does not function in a classic format of a single physician treating a single patient. The obstetrician relies on consultation from the pediatrician, the practicing physician cannot prescribe rational therapy for the infant without the expertise of the nurse at the bedside, and the perinatal patient with complex problems requires an intricate interdigitation of respiratory therapist, laboratory technician, social worker, nutritionist, and perinatal nurses and physicians to receive quality care. Community hospital perinatal medicine may rely on a smaller team size, but the same interdigitation of medical, nursing, and support disciplines is essential. Thus, although many of the classic teaching methods may be quite useful, they are not likely to have a significant effect on altering care practices unless they are incorporated as part of a comprehensive program that is team oriented and uses local resources.

PRINCIPLES OF OUTREACH EDUCATION

Community base

It is important that program participants be able to relate what they learn to their available resources for new knowledge to be translated into altered care practices. Also, because of the nature of community hospital staffing patterns and private practice demands, it is virtually impossible for more than several individuals to leave their jobs at one time. Therefore, for a program to be effective in changing patient care and to reach the most individuals, it should require a minimum of off-the-job travel time. The community hospital/office-based program is ideal for this purpose.

Multidisciplinary orientation

The most successful perinatal educational program will be aimed at the same multidisciplinary team that is involved with taking care of the patient in the clinical setting. Thus pediatricians, obstetricians, perinatal nurses, and supporting professionals such as respiratory therapists must be exposed to the same concepts simultaneously. A program aimed at only nurses or only physicians will generally not be reflected in clinical practice without the endorsement of the other team members. Likewise, for maximum acceptability and practicality of subject matter, it is just as important that the program be developed and introduced to the community by the same type of multidisciplinary group. The minimum components of a regional center outreach education team include a perinatal physician and nurse. Optimally, all the disciplines just mentioned should be represented on this team.

Local participation in teaching process

It is extremely beneficial to have some of the program's activities coordinated by local personnel. This is particularly valuable if the program is anticipated to last several weeks or months or, preferably, to be a continuous experience. In most regional systems, geography and staffing limitations prohibit frequent interaction between center and community personnel. Also, in general, new concepts and skills will be more readily accepted and adapted to local care practices if first introduced by local community professionals. Therefore the most efficient and useful program will use selected local physicians and/or nurses as teachers and coordinators.

Content matched to patient care goals

Program content should be selected to match the complexity of care anticipated. If, for example, it is hospital practice and consistent with the state's regional plan for babies requiring respirator therapy or exchange transfusion to be referred to another center, then these subjects should be deleted from the program for that specific hospital. There are certain basic topics, such as resuscitation of the newborn, that are appropriate for all perinatal professionals; however, the overall content should be flexible to meet specific community patient care goals. In some regions these goals will have already been determined through the regionalization planning process. In others a process of identification of goals and resources must precede the educational program. An outline of the content for perinatal outreach education follows.

A. Fetal evaluation
   1. High-risk pregnancies
   2. Fetal maturity and well-being
      a. Skill: amniocentesis*
      b. Skill: ultrasonography*
   3. Fetal monitoring
      a. Skill: fetal monitoring techniques
B. Immediate newborn assessment
   1. Resuscitation
      a. Skill: Apgar scoring

*Optional unit or skill. Included only for those community hospitals with the appropriate facilities and patient care goals.

   b. Skill: bag and mask ventilation
   c. Skill: endotracheal intubation
   d. Skill: cardiac massage
   e. Skill: medication administration
2. Gestational age and size assessment
   a. Skill: physical/neurologic examination

C. Newborn care concepts and procedures
1. Temperature control
   a. Skill: operation of radiant warmers
   b. Skill: operation of incubators
2. Oxygen therapy
   a. Skill: measurement of oxygen concentration
   b. Skill: mixing, heating, and humidifying oxygen and compressed air
3. Respiratory distress and apnea
   a. Skill: arterial sampling/transcutaneous monitoring
   b. Skill: chest tube insertion
   c. Skill: continuous positive airway pressure*
   d. Skill: mechanical ventilation*
4. Umbilical catheters
   a. Skill: umbilical catheterization
5. Blood pressure
   a. Skill: blood pressure measurement
6. Hypoglycemia
   a. Skill: blood glucose screening
7. IV therapy
   a. Skill: starting peripheral IVs
8. Feeding
   a. Skill: tube feedings*
9. Hyperbilirubinemia
   a. Skill: exchange transfusion*
10. Infections
11. Preparation for transport
12. Continuing care for infants at risk

COMPONENTS OF A COMPREHENSIVE PROGRAM

The following items should be included in any comprehensive outreach education program. Each step builds on the accomplishments of the preceding one and anticipates the existence of the subsequent step. Therefore a regional center should have organized an entire plan (including provisions for funding, personnel, and software) before the potential participants are approached.

Initial contact

Unless a close rapport has already been developed between the community hospital and regional center, the proposed program often will be viewed with skepticism at this stage. Physicians will be concerned about regulation of care practices, nurses will anticipate unrealistic demands on staff time, and administrators will predict that the program will impose an unneeded expense on the hospital budget. Therefore community leaders from all three groups (medicine, nursing, and hospital administration) should be contacted simultaneously to prevent misconceptions from developing.

Commitment

Some general commitment to participate should be secured from the hospital and signed by the individuals just noted. At this time the commitment should be no more than an agreement between the community hospital and regional center to devote the staff time and funds (if any) to the program. Issues such as referral contracts or patient care agreements should be avoided or at least postponed until after the educational program. By that time a much closer working relationship will have developed, and all parties will be aware of the resources required for delivery of various intensities of care.

Inventory process

Before any education is provided, it is important to define goals and identify resources. It is pointless to teach procedures or concepts that will never be used, either because the appropriate type of patient will not be managed locally or because the necessary equipment will not be available in the local hospital. Therefore local practitioners should be encouraged to define their patient care goals and hospital personnel should be asked to define the facilities, staffing, and equipment available for patient care before any educational intervention. There should then be an attempt to compare the goals and resources so that the facilities can be expanded to accommodate the stated goals. In some cases the practitioners may elect to change their goals rather than acquire the recommended resources. As much as possible this process of goal setting and resource identification should take place at the local level with regional center personnel acting as advisors rather than prescribers.

Regional center workshop

At this point it is beneficial to have selected nurses and physicians visit the regional center to learn the new concepts and skills that will be introduced to the entire local staff during the upcoming program. This type of workshop differs from the classic mini-residency in that the participants should learn through structured sessions oriented toward community hospital medicine rather than through focus on care practices appropriate for a tertiary care center.

Cognitive program

Educational content areas for the program will vary depending on the patient care goals of each community

*Optional unit or skill. Included only for those community hospitals with the appropriate facilities and patient care goals.

hospital (see preceding outline). However, several areas (e.g., resuscitation of the newborn) are basic for any hospital with a delivery service. Several different formats have been developed (e.g., self-instructional books, mediated programs, programed texts, organized lecture series), and many are available commercially. Comparative studies indicating preference for one type of program over another have not been performed.

Skills acquisition

Many of the new concepts introduced in the cognitive program require the performance of newly acquired skills before they can be translated into altered care practices. Teaching of new skills often requires hands-on practice sessions in addition to a written or mediated lesson. Models such as manikins, sections of human umbilical cords, anesthetized cats, or preserved animal specimens can provide subjects for the practice of certain complex skills, such as umbilical catheterization, endotracheal intubation, or chest tube insertion.

Continuation (review/update)

All hospitals should have a comprehensive basic educational program available for orientation of new staff. The local professionals who have visited the regional center should be responsible for maintaining this availability. The regional center should periodically update the basic program, as well as provide a mechanism for teaching new concepts and skills to the individuals who have previously completed the basic program. One format that has been suggested for a periodic update is the transport-referral conference, in which physicians and nurses from the regional center and community hospitals meet to discuss the management of previously referred antenatal and neonatal patients. These conferences are particularly valuable after the community participants have been exposed to the basic program but may prove overly controversial and threatening if sufficient background knowledge has not been acquired.

EVALUATION

The type of evaluation process used should depend on three factors: the purpose of the evaluation, the size of the population being evaluated, and the extent of evaluation resources. Measures can be made of ultimate outcomes (such as changes in perinatal mortality and morbidity) or of intermediate outcomes (such as changes in patient care practices or referral patterns). Ultimate outcomes require longer analysis periods and larger populations and are therefore affected by more variables than are intermediate outcomes. On the other hand, if immediate outcomes are used as a measure of effectiveness, one must make the assumption that a change in intermediate outcome will lead to a corresponding change in ultimate outcome. (For example, one must assume that, if arterial oxygen tensions are measured more frequently, there will be a reduced incidence of retrolental fibroplasia.) In general, ultimate outcomes are of particular value for analyzing the effects of multifactorial programs on large populations (such as the statewide effects of a perinatal regionalization program), whereas intermediate outcomes are more valuable for measuring specific changes in a small population (such as the effects of an educational program on the perinatal care delivered by a specific hospital).

Baseline preprogram measurements

There are two purposes in obtaining baseline measurements. First, it is helpful to determine which communities are in greatest need of an educational program. Second, to measure the effects of a program, preintervention data must be collected for comparison with data obtained after program activities.

The perinatal mortality data are probably the simplest and most accessible data for determining which communities are in greatest need of an educational program. However, as just mentioned, mortality data are not reliable for small populations, and therefore one should be extremely cautious about interpreting mortality data collected from individual hospitals, particularly if the birth rate is low. Therefore, for the purposes of determining educational need, only perinatal mortality trends occurring over several years should be examined. Estimates of educational need may also be derived from an analysis of patient status at the time of referral or by preprogram administration of one of the instruments listed in Table 2-2.

Measures of program effectiveness

For an educational program to be truly effective, it must be used by the community professionals and result in improved knowledge; the hospital facilities required for delivery of optimum care must improve; the care delivered to patients must change; and, ultimately, the number of babies dying or damaged must decrease (Table

Table 2-2. Measure of program effectiveness

Evaluation measure	Instrument
Program use	Completion rate Evaluation forms
Changes in cognitive knowledge	Preprogram vs. postprogram test scores
Changes in facilities	Preprogram vs. postprogram inventory survey
Changes in care practices	Chart review Patient status at transport Referral patterns
Changes in patient outcome	Mortality Morbidity

2-2). Only two of these measures (changes in cognitive knowledge and facilities) require that prospective, preprogram measurements be made. The others (e.g., changes in patient records or referral patterns) are best analyzed retrospectively to avoid having the evaluation process directly affect the outcome.

Program use is easily assessed by comparing the number of program participants to the total number of available personnel in each professional group. Most programs also include an evaluation form asking for the participants' assessment of the programs' format and appropriateness.

Cognitive knowledge change is classically measured by a written test administered before and after the program. However, good test questions are difficult to prepare and require extensive validity analysis before one can be confident of the results. Tests can also be threatening to the community hospital participants, particularly if administered on a pass/fail basis. If possible, answers should be returned to the participants so that the test becomes part of the learning process. A particularly valuable form of testing is the patient management problem of the branching tree or algorithm format. However, again, it is difficult to prepare such problems without ambiguity, and considerable validation testing of large populations is advisable.

Changes in hospital facilities can be measured by a simple postprogram repetition of the self-inventory process suggested for analysis of the hospital's baseline resources.

Changes in care practices are the most important of the intermediate outcomes to measure. Unfortunately, they also require the most time-consuming and expensive evaluation techniques. Also, they generally will be among the slowest to show change as the result of an education effort. It is not unusual for perinatal professionals to know intellectually the appropriate clinical action but then not practice it in the field. For example, although a physician may answer a test question correctly regarding the increased incidence of hypoglycemia in infants large for gestational age, considerable time may pass before a change in hospital policy will result in all babies large for gestational age receiving a blood glucose screen. A hospital chart review or analysis of patient status at the time of transport can be used to document various care practices. Translation of learned knowledge into altered care practices can be facilitated by returning the analysis results to the participants (see section on continuation [review/update]).

Change in patient outcome cannot be measured reliably on a short-term basis and therefore is of limited value for assessing the results of a specific educational intervention. A reflection in mortality statistics will require many thousands of births to occur, and true morbidity cannot be tested reliably in neonates. However, with appropriate resources, large populations, and sufficient follow-up time these ultimate outcomes provide the most convincing evidence of true change.

John Kattwinkel

BIBLIOGRAPHY

American Academy of Pediatrics and American College of Obstetricians and Gynecologists: guidelines for perinatal care, Evanston, Ill., American Academy of Pediatrics and American College of Obstetricians and Gynecologists, Washington, D.C., 1983.

Clarke, T.A., Levy, L., and Mannino, F.: Use of the placenta as a teaching model, Pediatrics **62**:234, 1978.

Harlan, R.H., and others: Impact of an education program on perinatal care practices, Pediatrics **66**:893, 1980.

Hein, H.A.: Regionalization of perinatal care in rural areas based on the Iowa experience, Semin. Perinat. **1**:241, 1977.

Jennings, P.B., Alden, E.R., and Brenz, R.W.: A teaching model for pediatric intubation utilizing ketamine sedated kittens, Pediatrics **53**:283, 1974.

Kattwinkel, J., and others: Improved perinatal knowledge and care in the community hospital through a program of self-instruction, Pediatrics **64**:451, 1979.

Kattwinkel, J., and others: Perinatal outreach education: a continuation strategy for a basic program, Am. J. Perinat. **1**:335, 1984.

March of Dimes Proceedings of the Conference on Outreach Programs: Their integral parts and processes, White Plains, N.Y., 1978 and 1980, The March of Dimes Birth Defects Foundation.

Oh, W., and others: Role of an educational program in the regionalization of perinatal health care, Semin. Perinatol. **1**:279, 1977.

Ryan, G.M.: Toward improving the outcome of pregnancy. Recommendations for the regional development of perinatal health services, Obstet. Gynecol. **46**:375, 1975.

Task Force on Pediatric Education: The future of pediatric education, Evanston, Ill., 1978, American Academy of Pediatrics.

Wirtschafter, D.D., and others: Continuing medical education: an assessment of impact upon neonatal care in community hospitals, Annu. Conf. Res. Med. Educ. **18**:252, 1979.

PART THREE

Stress and the performance of neonatal intensive care unit staff

The ability of nurses and physicians to function effectively has a major bearing on the outcome of high-risk newborns. Near optimum performance is required of nursery staff to prevent death or handicap among the sickest infants. The awareness of this fact is but one stress experienced by nursery personnel. This section considers the sources of stress in the neonatal intensive care unit (ICU), the reaction of the staff to stress, the effect of stress on personnel performance, and the management of stress in the ICU.

SOURCES OF STRESS IN THE NEONATAL ICU

Neonatal ICU staff, like the staff in other intensive care units, are confronted with a variety of stresses, including patient suffering and death, excessive duty hours, complex and demanding responsibilities, interpersonal conflict, and ethical and legal uncertainties. In addition, neonatal staff face a number of stresses peculiar to neonatal units—congenital anomalies incompatible with extrauterine life, iatrogenic disorders specific to neonates (e.g., birth trauma, kernicterus, and retrolental fibroplasia), and disabling life-long effects of serious errors in care. Few work environments entail stress factors of this magnitude.

In most level III nurseries, 10% to 25% of infants requiring intensive care die, with as many as 20% of deaths occurring after more than 28 days of care. The strong feelings about suffering and death common to health care workers in general may be even more intense among those who work in neonatal units. Todres and associates reported that pediatricians expressed more distress associated with patient death than did anesthesiologists.

The severe fatigue experienced by many house staff in neonatal units is the predictable result of working in a highly stressful environment for 80 hours a week or more, with 24 to 32 hours of uninterrupted call every third to fourth night. The 96 neonatologists polled by Clarke and colleagues worked a mean of 72 hours per week. The chronic fatigue common among neonatal ICU nurses results from the combined effects of an excessive workload, extra duty, and frequent shift changes. Laube and Stehle surveyed 359 nurses in 30 randomly selected units and reported an occupancy rate exceeding 100% in 26% of the units. In 48% of units nurses worked 6 to 8 consecutive days, whereas in 70% of units nurses worked double shifts.

Despite their fatigue neonatal staff are expected to provide expert care for infants with complex medical problems or life-threatening emergencies. Any inadequacies in training or performance are stressful and often a source of conflict between house officers and nurses. Conflict between nurses and physicians (particularly house officers), role confusion, and changes in the traditional physician-nurse hierarchy have been a by-product of the increasing role of nurses in neonatal units. In a survey of randomly selected units Harper and colleagues noted that the responsibilities of staff or charge nurses extend to needle aspiration for pneumothorax in 26% of units, initiating ventilator changes in 19%, insertion of umbilical artery catheters in 17%, and insertion of endotracheal tubes in 7%. These tasks are regularly performed by neonatal nurse clinicians in those units that they staff.

Ethical problems remain an unavoidable source of major stress in the ICU (see Chapter 18). The attitudes of physicians toward ethical problems differ according to age, religious background, marital status, and specialty. Youngner and co-workers found that nurses in medical intensive care units were more often dissatisfied than physicians with the method of reaching ethical decisions and the communication between staff and family members. Lippincott has emphasized that discordant values within groups are particularly stressful to intensive care unit personnel. Increases in malpractice litigation and public scrutiny of ethical decision making in neonatal units have aggravated the staff distress associated with ethical problems.

To define interventions most likely to reduce staff stress, it is important to identify the most important sources of stress for physicians and for nurses. The neonatologists surveyed by Clarke and colleagues were asked to list their two most important sources of stress. Of those responding, 36% listed an excessive workload, 36% listed difficult aspects of patient care (e.g., death, chronic illness, and difficult clinical decisions), and 32% listed staff conflict. Of the nurses surveyed by Laube and Stehle, 29% noted neonatal death as their most stressful problem; 17%, a heavy workload; and 12%, conflict with other personnel. The nurses surveyed by Jacobson noted feelings of incompetence as a major cause of stress, even among experienced nurses. Lancaster and Korones found that admission of infants born outside the hospital at a time of high census was a frequent and severe source of stress. Moderately severe sources of stress included a generally heavy workload, ethical problems, a maldistribution of nurses among shifts, inadequate time for parental support, and conflict with house officers.

To compare physicians and nurses from the same unit, we have surveyed house officers and nursing staff of the Special Care Nursery at Parkland Memorial Hospital. This is a recently constructed unit that includes 15 intensive care beds and 35 intermediate care beds for a large delivery population (13,018 deliveries in 1985). A total of 70 nurses, 6 house officers, and 2 attending neonatologists staffed this unit at the time that our survey was conducted.

A questionnaire was completed by 61 of 66 house officers who had rotated through this unit and 28 of 33 nurses who regularly worked in the intensive care area. Eleven sources of stress were each rated from 0 (absolutely nonstressful) to 10 (unbearably stressful) based on the frequency and the intensity of stress produced.

The mean ratings for nurses and for house officers for each stress source are compared in Table 2-3 with the sources ranked in order of decreasing average score for nurses and house officers. The three factors rated as most stressful were (1) concern that an unreasonable work load would compromise patient care, (2) fatigue, and (3) feelings associated with brain-damaged survivors. Concern that one's level of expertise (relative to that expected for someone of the same experience) would compromise patient care was rated least stressful. We suspect that the

Table 2-3. Mean stress ratings for staff of the Parkland Memorial Hospital Neonatal ICU*

	Nurses n = 28	House officers n = 61
Concern that an unreasonable workload would compromise patient care	7.6	6.4†
Fatigue	6.0	7.1‡
Feelings associated with brain-damaged survivors	5.9	5.9
Feelings associated with death	5.6	5.6
Feelings associated with prolonged care of infants likely to die	5.8	5.3
Support service inadequacies	6.0	5.0
Ethical qualms about intensive care for very immature, chronically ill, or brain-damaged babies	5.2	5.4
Conflict between nurses, house officers, and/or attending physicians	5.5	4.0
Parental anger, guilt, grief, etc.	5.0	4.4
Physical environment (crowding, heat, noise, odors)	5.0	3.9
Concern that your level of expertise relative to that expected for your experience would compromise patient care	2.8	4.5†

*Source of stress listed in descending order of average intensity. (The standard deviations ranged from 1.9 to 2.8 for all ratings.)
†$p < 0.05$.
‡$p < 0.01$.

low scores on this item reflect the use of denial as a defense mechanisms by ICU staff.

Nurses and house officers generally gave similar ratings ($r = 0.69$ for stress rankings by physicians and by nurses; $p < 0.03$). However, nurses gave a higher stress rating than house officers for concern that an unreasonable workload would compromise patient care, a lower rating for concern that one's level of expertise would compromise patient care, and a marginally lower rating for fatigue. (Given multiple comparisons of interrelated items, a $p < 0.01$ was considered significant.) Nurse and house officer ratings were not influenced by sex, marital status, or whether they had children.

We also compared our findings with those in a survey reported in the previous edition of this text. Compared to our present unit, the unit at that time had one instead of two attending neonatologists assigned to the unit and approximately one half the number of beds, space per bed, and nursing staff and 33% fewer house officers for the number of deliveries. As might be expected, the neonatal mortality rate was higher than at the time of the present survey, (12 deaths versus 7 deaths per 1,000 live births). House officers recorded significantly lower mean stress scores (reductions of 1.3 to 2.2 points) in the recent survey than in the previous survey with respect to parental reactions, physical environment, staff conflict, and support service deficiencies. With the increasing nursing efforts for the care of infants who previously died and the increasing expectations for survival of very small or severely ill infants, none of the stress ratings recorded by the nurses diminished significantly. In fact, concern that an unreasonable work load would compromise patient care received a higher mean rating (7.6 versus 5.9; $p < 0.05$).

Although our results may not be relevant to all neonatal units, our findings that the greatest sources of stress are an excessive workload and staff fatigue are comparable to those in studies discussed earlier. Ostensibly, these problems would be managed simply by increasing the number of staff. However, our findings indicate that high stress levels may persist despite substantially increased staff number and reduced neonatal mortality.

REACTION OF INTENSIVE CARE UNIT STAFF TO STRESS

The reaction of physicians to stress in neonatal units has received little study. Todres and co-workers interviewed house officers in Boston about their experience in a pediatric intensive care unit. During the last week of their rotation, 41% reported discontent concerning staff relationships; 36%, excessive fatigue; 36%, depression related to death of patients; and 25%, feelings of incompetence. Frader reported similar feelings among pediatric residents in Philadelphia. Of the neonatologists surveyed by Clarke and colleagues, 34% reported moderately severe stress while 16% noted severe stress; 20% reported significant stress-related illnesses in the previous 5 years. Changing to another subspecialty had been considered by 58% (18% seriously); 49% planned to stay active in neonatology for 10 years or less. Laube and Stehle reported that 35% of neonatal intensive care nurses reported stress-related illnesses including headaches, gastrointestinal disturbances, and hypertension.

In our survey we explored the perceived effect of stress on the well-being and social relationships of house officers and nurses. Among 61 house officers, 5 (8%) reported stress in our ICU as having no effect on their well-being, 25 (41%) reported minor effects (mild stress-related ailments such as headaches or depression on fewer than 10% of days); 26 (43%) reported moderate effects (mild stress-related ailments on 10 to 50% of days); and 4 (8%) reported major effects (minor ailments on more than 50% of days or any serious ailment). Of the

28 nurses surveyed, 4 (14%) reported no effect on well-being, 16 (57%), mild effects, 7 (25%), moderate effects, and 1 (4%), major effects.

No effect of stress on relationships with friends and family was reported by 5 (8%) of our house staff. Twenty (33%) reported a mild effect (minor difficulties on a few days), 26 (43%) reported moderate stress (minor effects on multiple days), and 10 (16%) reported major effects (major difficulties among family members or persons most important to the house officer). The corresponding numbers for the 27 nurses who answered this question were 8 (30%) for no effect, 16 (60%) for mild effects, 2 (7%) for moderate effects, and 1 (4%) for major effects. By chi square analyses, moderate or major effects on interpersonal relationships were reported by a significantly greater percentage of house officers than nurses ($p < 0.01$). We interpret this finding as the result of a variety of factors, including the fact that nurses who experience the most adverse effects are unlikely to remain in our ICU. Indeed, the attrition rate among our nursing staff has been greater than 20% per year.

Other workers have attempted more objective evaluations of the psychologic effects of working in an ICU by comparing ICU nurses to nurses in other areas of the same hospital. These studies vary in their findings, and their interpretation is obscured by the multiple confounding variables that influence job selection and assignment among nurses. For physicians, as well as nurses, the extent to which stress is accompanied by objective evidence of stress-related disorders remains to be determined. Exposure to high stress and a high incidence of such disorders as hypertension, diabetes, and ulcer disease has been noted in nonmedical occupations (e.g., air traffic controllers). Nevertheless, whether stressful work, regardless of the personality and life-style of persons who choose such work, increases the likelihood of serious disorders is unclear. Caplan contends that exposure to high stress by persons who receive adequate support does not increase their risk of physical and mental illness.

Undoubtedly, appropriate coping mechanisms are important to minimize adverse effects of stress. According to Lippincott, physicians are notable for their poor stress management and their use of denial. Denial, rationalization, and preoccupation with technology and pathophysiology are often used by physicians to shield themselves from the awareness of stress. Oskins has studied the coping methods and defense mechanisms of 79 nurses working in various ICUs in five hospitals. In dealing with stressful situations, these nurses noted a variety of coping behaviors. The three most common behaviors involved direct efforts to eliminate the source of stress. For the most stressful situations they also reported palliative and sometimes detrimental responses that most commonly included anxiety, anger, and the use of humor. Laube and Stehle in their study of neonatal nurses noted that the two most common coping responses involved "talking it out" and direct efforts to reduce the stress. About one half of the nurses' responses involved such indirect methods of coping as exercise, hobbies, eating, and smoking. Gribbins and Marshall have emphasized the changing nature of stress and coping strategies used by nurses according to their length of ICU experience.

EFFECT OF STRESS ON PERSONNEL PERFORMANCE

Although an optimal level of stress may improve performance, stress of the kind and degree present in neonatal units may be expected to impair performance. Psychologists have shown deleterious effects of crowding, noise, and role conflict in nonmedical settings. Adverse effects of work load, work schedule, fatigue, and sleep loss have been extensively investigated in military, aerospace, and industrial personnel. Performance deteriorates at night among those who regularly work the night shift, as well as among those who rotate shifts. Optimal adaptation to night work cannot be expected with shift changes occurring every few weeks. The decline in mental and motor abilities at night is aggravated by extended periods of duty and sleep loss.

Little research has been performed to evaluate the effect of stress on the performance of medical and nursing personnel. The research that has been performed has focused on the effects of fatigue and sleep loss. A survey in England, Wales, and Scotland indicated that 49% of obstetric house staff and 40% of pediatric house staff believed that their work was always or often impaired by their long periods of duty. Friedman and co-workers reported that house staff errors in the interpretation of electrocardiograms increase following nights on call. Stanley and Alberman noted an increased neonatal mortality at night in London hospitals in association with diminished staffing during the same hours.

We have compared the quality and outcome of newborn intensive care during the day with that at night in a 22-bed neonatal unit at McMaster University, Hamilton, Ontario. At the time the study was conducted, nursing staff routinely worked 12-hour shifts in teams of 8 to 11 nurses. Often one less nurse worked at night than during the day. Nurses changed shifts every 2 weeks and worked 7 days and 7 nights during each 4-week period. Three residents and two to four fellows worked in the unit each weekday. At night and on weekends one resident and one fellow remained in the hospital on duty for a continuous period of 28 to 32 hours. Thus, as in other neonatal units, the number and supervision of staff declined at night as levels of fatigue increased.

As shown in Table 2-4, we found that during the night

(2101 to 0900 hours) intravenous infusions infiltrated more often, and the tidal volume of ventilators was regulated less often than during the day (0901 to 2100 hours). Blood pH values less than 7.20 (excluding values within 12 hours of admission) were recorded more often and in more patients at night. In addition, significantly more deaths occurred at night (even though deaths within 12 hours of admission were excluded). When weekdays were compared to weekends, pH values less than 7.20 tended to occur more often on weekends. However, neither acidosis nor death occurred significantly more often on weekends. The fewest deaths occurred in the middle of the week in the periods beginning at 0901 on Tuesday, Wednesday, and Thursday. A progressive increase in deaths occurred on Friday, Saturday, Sunday, and Monday.

The increased frequency of acidosis and death among newborns at night may result from endogenous diurnal rhythms unrelated to care and environment. However, such rhythms have not been identified in the first weeks after birth. A change in the quality of care seems the more likely explanation for the deterioration of infants at night during times of reduced staffing.

Table 2-4. Measures of patient care and outcome during the day (0901-2100) hours and night (2101-0900 hours) in the McMaster University Neonatal ICU

	Day	Night
IV infiltrations/patient/12h	0.38	0.60*
Calculations of tidal volume/patient/12h	2.13	1.19*
Patients with pH <7.20/12h	0.39	0.53†
Deaths during study period	23	40†

*$p < 0.01$.
†$p < 0.05$.

This explanation is supported by a study we performed using time-lapse photography to assess the effect of time-related and clinical variables on bedside care in the McMaster neonatal unit. The activities of physicians and random samples of nurses assigned to the four-bed study area were photographed. To allow staff to adjust to the presence of the camera, photographs taken during the first weeks were discarded. As shown for the residents in Fig. 2-2, physicians were observed providing bedside care significantly less often at night than during the day. Total resident and fellow time devoted to bedside care was also significantly less on weekends. Much of this difference was due to a reduced number of house officers on duty at night and on weekends. Physician time devoted to bedside care increased abruptly for patients with the greatest care needs as measured by our infant care score, which was calculated each day for each infant. This score was determined independently by a senior nurse and based on a detailed list of observations and treatment methods used in our unit.

In contrast to that observed for physicians, bedside nursing time was unaffected by time-related variables (day versus night, weekday versus weekend, consecutive days or nights of work, or various nursing rotations). Regression analysis showed a linear increase in bedside nursing with increasing infant care score.

The importance of individual differences among nursery personnel is suggested by multivariate analysis, which indicated that differences between individual nurses accounted for as much of the total variation of bedside care (30%) as did differences between infants in their care needs. The differences between nurses were not explained by traditional biographic information—age, marital status, rank in nursing school, nursing degree, and duration of ICU nursing experience.

The influence of the infant on his or her care is sug-

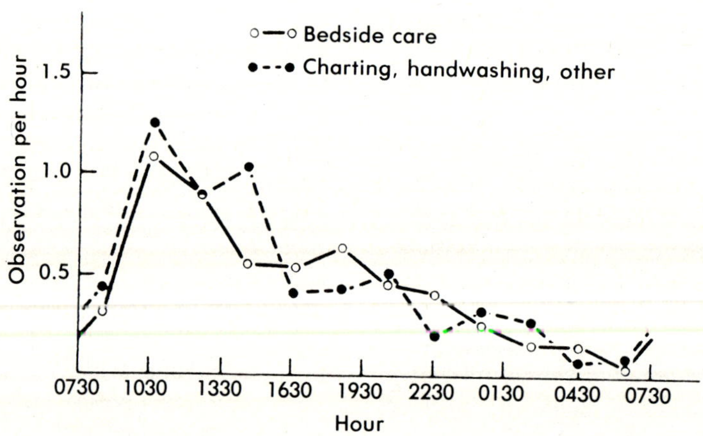

Fig. 2-2. Activities of neonatal residents during average 24-hour period at McMaster University Medical Centre.

gested by the observation that 7% of the total variation in bedside care resulted from differences among infants unrelated to care scores. Several infants acknowledged as nursing favorites consistently received more bedside care than expected from their infant care scores; one ventilator-dependent infant with end-stage bronchopulmonary dysplasia consistently received less than expected. This study suggests that the deterioration of infants at night is likely to relate to a marked reduction in physician time devoted to bedside care during hours of diminished mental and motor skills as a result of fatigue. Our observations also suggest that many as yet undefined factors affect the individual or group performance of nursery personnel.

METHODS TO MANAGE STRESS IN THE ICU

The deleterious effects of stress on the morale and performance of staff can be minimized by attention to the following areas.

Physical environment, staff number, and staff schedules

When asked to suggest one improvement for their ICU, 43% of nurses surveyed by Laube and Stehle indicated the need for either more space or more staff. The degree of responsibility and stress associated with intensive care would seem to justify fewer hours and greater pay. The cost of changes that increase retention of experienced nurses may be partly offset by a reduction in the cost of iatrogenic disease and, as shown by Consolvo, the cost of training new staff.

Physician staffing practices should be reconsidered. The education of house officers and the welfare of high-risk infants may be best served by fewer duties for house officers in neonatal units, more equitable staffing at night, and increased responsibilities for properly trained nurses.

Our stress surveys indicate that high stress levels may persist despite improvements in the physicial environment and staffing of neonatal units and a substantial reduction in neonatal mortality. Therefore other strategies of stress management should also be used.

Staff interaction

As emphasized by Marshall and Kasman, any effective program to manage stress in the ICU will include continuous attention to staff interaction. Increased interpersonal conflict is often the first symptom of the unusual stresses experienced by ICU staff members. Such conflict should be appreciated before an increase in staff illness, resignations, errors in patient care, or other obvious stress-related problems occur.

Some sources of staff conflict can be managed by measures that are not only inexpensive but cost saving. These measures include well-defined nursery policies, clear communication of treatment plans, adequate training and supervision of nursery staff, and recognition of skilled performance. Conflict between house officers and nurses should be minimized by emphasis on the team approach to patient care. Ethical dilemmas are more tolerable if the issues are clearly identified and discussed with a well-defined method of obtaining all appropriate consultations and designation of those responsible for reaching a decision.

Regularly scheduled meetings are widely recommended as a forum to improve communication and interaction among neonatal staff. Such meetings can be used to identify problems in the operation of the unit, to resolve unnecessary misunderstanding or misinterpretation, to increase the appreciation of individual staff members for the opinions and concerns of others, and to communicate that anxiety, guilt, and uncertainty are common and acceptable feelings among neonatal staff. However, attempts to establish regular group discussions between physicians and neonatal nurses have not been universally successful. Attendance often is limited by clinical demands and scheduling problems, especially if the meetings are not perceived as particularly helpful. Both Frader and Rosini found that a significant proportion of house officers were unenthusiastic about these meetings. The effectiveness of these discussions depends, in part, on whether there is sufficient leadership to maintain a healthy interaction between staff members and to improve problem areas once they are clearly identified. Even with expert leadership, difficult transition periods can be expected during the course of these meetings.

We have conducted a study to determine whether conventional nursing support groups improved the quality of care in neonatal units by reducing the adverse effects of stress on personnel performance. Two units were studied that had high, but differing, sources of stress. The unit at St. Paul Medical Center was newly opened, and the primary sources of stress were limitations in staff experience and education. Stress in the unit at Parkland Memorial Hospital was due primarily to limitations in staff number and resources. In neither unit were interactional problems within or between nursing and physician staff considered to be important problems. The support groups met once weekly or biweekly and were led by psychiatrists who had been successful in conducting similar groups in a large pediatric ICU in our center.

Contrary to our expectations, the support groups lasted only 6 to 7 months, were considered to have limited benefit by our staff, and had no discernible effect on detailed measures of quality of care in a comparison of intervention months and carefully selected control months. Although the failure of the support groups may be due to a number of factors, we suspect that the primary reason is that support groups may not be a successful method to deal with inadequacies in staffing or resources or in limitations in training or experience.

Support groups in neonatal units have been recommended without careful study of their limitations or proper purpose and conduct. In some circumstances reliance may be placed on support groups when more direct measures to reduce stress (e.g., improved staff training) are needed. Nevertheless, support groups may perform a useful function in dealing with some stress-related problems in neonatal units, although support groups or open staff meetings should not supersede private discussions that may be needed to promptly resolve strong personnel conflicts. Very stressful events (e.g., iatrogenic disease, ethical dilemmas, and neonatal deaths) often require immediate discussion between senior staff members and those experiencing the most distress. In some instances a series of discussions is helpful, especially for those coping with death or ethical dilemmas for the first time. After the death of infants, meetings between the parents and close staff members are often therapeutic for all involved. The strong relationships developed with families of seriously ill infants can be enriching and fulfilling to nursery staff and make the frequent occurrence of death in neonatal units more tolerable.

Professional stature and satisfaction of neonatal staff

The most important method to reduce staff stress in neonatal units may be the provision of sufficient training to facilitate highly expert care and ensure the confidence of the staff in their competence to deal with even the most difficult problems. Such training not only improves the quality of care but also reduces the levels of staff discomfort and guilt associated with the inevitable occurrence of handicap and death in ICUs. We have found it useful to develop an extensive ICU certification program, to conduct periodic resuscitation drills with house officers and nurses, to develop an active charge nurse system, and to carefully scrutinize the care given during emergencies.

A challenge in all neonatal units is to retain and enhance the skills of the most experienced nurses. Much of intensive care nursing involves highly repetitive activities, and an active ongoing in-service education program is essential to maintain the interest and increase the sophistication of nursing staff. Rotations to less stressful areas of the perinatal services are enjoyed by some, but not all, nurses. Nurses should be encouraged to attend conferences and workshops in other centers. Experienced nurses should be given new responsibilities to enhance their development and the development of the ICU (e.g., participation in the transport program, the follow-up clinic, or the in-service, outreach, or parent education programs). Lateral promotions should be feasible for experienced nurses who prefer bedside care to administration.

In university hospitals the house staff teaching program should be carefully designed to meet specified educational goals at each level of training. House staff enthusiasm and effectiveness are likely to be increased by the feeling that education is an important goal of those who direct the unit. If time permits, house officers should be encouraged to participate in teaching conferences and in the review of literature related to the management of difficult problems.

Although formal conferences may be quite educational, the greatest opportunity for professional growth for both house officers and nurses occurs at the bedside. Close supervision, encouragement, and evaluation from the attending physician are crucial to the continuing improvement of staff performance and professional satisfaction.

Investigation

Considerable research is needed to answer a variety of questions vital to the effective function of nursery personnel. What stresses most disrupt staff performance? What are practical ways to minimize serious stress and facilitate effective coping strategies? How can stress tolerance be predicted before selecting personnel to staff neonatal units? How can individual staff members having the most difficulty be identified and helped? What is the relationship of staff number to quality of care? What work schedule is most effective for neonatal personnel? What factors contribute most to personnel satisfaction, and how can they be used to maximize retention of experienced staff?

SUMMARY

Multiple sources of stress in neonatal units affect nursery personnel and compromise the outcome of seriously ill infants. With effective stress management the operation of neonatal units can be modified to support the best possible performance of nursery staff and an optimum outcome for high-risk infants.

Jon E. Tyson
Sharon Speaks

BIBLIOGRAPHY

General

Marshall, R., and Kasman, C.: Burnout in the neonatal intensive care unit, Pediatrics **65**:1161, 1980.

Marshall, R., Kasman, C., and Cape, L.: Coping with caring for sick newborns, Philadelphia, 1982, W.B. Saunders Co.

Walker, C.: Neonatal intensive care and stress, Arch. Dis. Child. **57**:85, 1982.

Sources of stress in the intensive care unit

Clarke, T., and others: Job satisfaction and stress among neonatologists, Pediatrics **74**:52, 1984.

Harper, R., Little, G., and Sia, C.: The scope of nursing practice in level III neonatal intensive care units, Pediatrics **70**:875, 1982.

Jacobson, S.P.: Stressful situations for neonatal intensive care nurses, Am. J. Matern. Child Nursing, **3**:144, 1978.

Laube, J., and Stehle, J.: Neonatal intensive care unit nurses: who are they? What are their stresses? How do they cope? Paper presented at the Mead Johnson Nursing Symposium in Perinatal and Developmental Medicine, Vail, Colo., June 1979.

McCue, J.: The distress of internship, N. Engl. J. Med. **312**:449, 1985.

Todres, I.D., and others: Pediatrician attitudes affecting decision making in defective newborns, Pediatrics **60**:197, 1977.;

Turner, A., King, C., and Craddock, J.: Measuring and reducing noise, Hospitals **49**:85, 1975.

White, L.P.: The self-image of physicians and the care of dying patients, Ann. N.Y. Acad. Sci. **164**:822, 1969.

Youngner, S., Jackson, D.L., and Allen, M.: Staff attitudes towards the care of the critically ill in the medical intensive care units, Crit. Care Med. **7**:35, 1979.

Reactions of intensive care unit staff to stress

Caplan, G.: Mastery of stress: psychosocial aspects, Am. J. Psychiatry **138**:413, 1981.

Frader, J.: Difficulties in providing intensive care, Pediatrics **64**:10, 1979.

Gentry, W., and Parker, K.: Psychologic stress in intensive care unit and nonintensive care unit nursing: a review of the past decade, Heart Lung **11**:43, 1982.

Gribbins, R., and Marshall, R.: Stress and coping in the NICU staff nurse: practical implications for change, Crit. Care Med. **10**:865, 1982.

Lancaster, J., and Korones, S.: Stress factors for nurses in iatrogenic problems in neonatal intensive care, Paper presented to the Sixty-ninth Ross Conference on Pediatric Research, 1975.

Lippincott, R.C.: Psychological stress factors in decision making, Heart Lung **8**:1095, 1979.

Maloney, J.: Job stress and its consequences on a group of intensive care and nonintensive care nurses, Adv. Nurs. Sci., p. 31, Jan. 1982.

Maloney, J., and Bartz, C.: Stress tolerant people: intensive care nurses compared with non-intensive care nurses, Heart Lung **12**:389, 1983.

Oskins, S.L.: Identification of situational stresses and coping methods by intensive care nurses, Heart Lung **8**:933, 1979.

Rahe, R.: Life change measurement as a predictor of illness, Proc. Roy. Soc. Med. **61**:1124, 1968.

Rose, R., Jenkins, C.D., and Hurst, M.W.: Health change in air traffic controllers: a prospective study. I. Background and description, Psychosomatics **40**:142, 1978.

Todres, I.D., Howell, M.C., and Shannon, D.C.: Physicians' reactions to training in a pediatric intensive care unit, Pediatrics **53**:375, 1974.

Effect of stress on personnel performance

Alluisi, E.: Sustained performance, work rest scheduling, and diurnal rhythms in man, Acta Psychol. **27**:436, 1967.

Asken, M., and Raham, D.: Resident performance and sleep deprivation: a review, J. Med. Ed. **58**:382, 1983.

Ax, A., and others: Quantitative effects of sleep deprivation, J. Exp. Psychol. **66**:439, 1963.

Conroy, R.T.W.L., and Mills, J.N.: Human circadian rhythms, London, 1975, J. and A. Churchill, Ltd.

Friedman, R.C., Bigger, J.T., and Kornfield, D.S.: The intern and sleep loss, N. Engl. J. Med. **285**:201, 1971.

Stanley, F.J., and Alberman, E.D.: Infants of very low birthweight. I. Perinatal factors affecting survival, Dev. Med. Child. Neurol. **20**:300, 1978.

Tyson, J., and others: Diurnal variation in the quality and outcome of newborn intensive care, J. Pediatr. **95**:277, 1979.

Tyson, J., and others: Analysis of newborn intensive care by time-lapse photography, Crit. Care Med. **9**:780, 1981.

Wilkinson, R.T.: After effect of sleep deprivation, J. Exp. Psychol. **66**:439, 1963.

Wilkinson, R.T., Tyler, P.D., and Varey, C.A.: Duty hours of young hospital doctors: effects on the quality of work, J. Occup. Psychol. **48**:219, 1975.

Williams, W.L., Lubin, A., and Goodnow, J.: Impaired performance with acute sleep loss, Psychol. Monogr. **73**:1, 1959.

Methods to manage stress in the intensive care unit

Consolvo, C.: Nurse turnover in the newborn intensive care unit, J. Obstet. Gynecol. Neonatol. Nurs. **8**:201, 1979.

Drotar, D.: Consultation in the intensive care nursery, Int. J. Psychiatr. Med. **7**:69, 1976.

Dubovsky, S., and others: Impact on nursing care and mortality: psychiatrists on the coronary care unit, Psychosomatics **18**:18, 1977.

Duxbury, M., and others: Head nurse leadership style with staff nurse burnout and job satisfaction in neonatal intensive care units, Nurs. Res. **33**:97, 1984.

Hay, D., and Oken, D.: The psychological stresses of intensive care nursing, Psychosom. Med. **34**:109, 1972.

Koran, L., and others: Changing hospital work environments: an example of a burn unit, Gen. Hosp. Psychiat. **5**:7, 1983.

Rosini, L.A., and others: Group meetings in a pediatric intensive care unit, Pediatrics **53**:371, 1974.

Tyson, J., and others: Effect of nursing-staff support groups on the quality of newborn intensive care, Crit. Care Med. **12**:901, 1984.

Weiner, M., and Caldwell, T.: Stress and coping in ICU nursing, II. Nurse support groups on intensive care units, Gen. Hosp. Psychiat. **3**:129, 1981.

PART FOUR

Computer applications in perinatal medicine

In preparing an appropriate overview of perinatal computing that encompasses computer applications both in obstetric perinatology and in neonatology, it is tempting to entitle it "In search of . . . ." If one does a formal literature search in this area, the results are disappointing. It is true that some collections of conference papers have been published; however, the literature is generally sparse. A more successful approach involves exploring perinatal units; then a very different picture emerges. The number and range of computer applications in place, particularly in tertiary centers, are considerable. Much of the work is developmental, in the engineering sense, rather than experimental, and much of it is being done by relatively junior individuals. It is perhaps these facts that account for the relative paucity of published results.

This chapter provides an overview of computer technology in the service of direct patient care, research, education, and administration in the perinatal setting. The goal is not to provide an exhaustive listing of specific applications, but rather to provide examples of what has been done and is being done as a basis for identifying promising areas for future applications in specific health care settings.

In the following sections sample applications, including some developed by the authors, will be presented. The first discusses clinical data manipulation and online data acquisition and analysis. Attention then will be turned to clinical information systems at the level of the hospital, the department, and "perinatal region." Applications involving medical knowledge retrieval, artificial intelligence, computer-assisted diagnosis, and computer-assisted education are followed by some brief comments concerning computerized billing systems and management information systems.

REPETITIVE AND COMPLEX PROCESSES
Clinical data manipulation

There are many tasks in the care of the pregnant woman and neonate that are repetitive, time consuming, and require accurate and sometimes complex calculations. Among them are:

1. Calculating drug doses, infusion rates, dilutions of drugs
2. Maintaining a detailed record of intake, output, and weight changes
3. Calculating fluid and dietary requirements and intakes
4. Computing various indices of fetal size, age, and well-being from ultrasonographic data
5. Keeping a record of complex clinical events for future retrieval and analysis

A number of clinical units in the United States now have terminals or microcomputers with programs that allow the user to enter the patient's weight and the name of a drug (often from a menu of drug names). The program then provides appropriate dosage regimens for the indicated drug(s), customized for the individual patient. The program may also accept data that may alter the recommended dosage, such as renal functional impairment or the presence of other factors, such as drugs or pregnancy that alter the metabolism of the drug in question. In addition, once circulating concentrations of a drug, such as gentamicin, are measured over a period after administration, computer programs can calculate factors, such as half-life and volume of distribution, that the clinician or the computer can use to prescribe an ideal dose and dosing interval.

One such program is called Mycin (devised by Shortliffe). Mycin acts as a consultant for antimicrobial management. It asks for information about the site and severity of the infection, prior drug reactions, and the laboratory data obtained thus far, including the renal function of the patient. It then recommends the type of antibiotic(s) for initial treatment and the dosage regimen (including loading and maintenance doses) that should be ideal for that patient. The user can choose the dosing interval, or the program will specify it. This program also generates a graph of expected serum drug concentrations over time, indicating the toxic concentration, as well as the minimal inhibitory concentration of the drug against the assumed organism(s). The user can request and receive a narrative explanation of the program's rationale for the selection of antibiotics and calculation of dosages.

Another innovation in the care of seriously ill patients has been the bedside computer, which is used to store and display many aspects of the patient's progress. Several of these systems are currently being marketed as stand-alone bedside tools, whereas others have been developed (e.g., at New York University and the University of Pennsylvania) as mainframe (central computer) systems with terminals at or near the bedside. Nursing and medical personnel can record observations, such as intake, output, and vital signs, directly into the computer as they are obtained. Summaries of these measurements are then available to the clinicians in easily digested forms (tables and graphs), facilitating the clinical decision-making process.

One of the most common applications of computer technology in the care of high-risk newborns is dietary calculations. The weight of a growing infant must be followed in relation to the number of calories consumed. The distribution of calories offered as fat, carbohydrate, and protein is also of interest to the clinician. In the usual microcomputer nutrition program a menu of possible sources of nutrition is provided (e.g., infant formulas, intravenous glucose, and intravenous alimentation solutions), the nutrient contents of which are contained in a data set within the program. The patient's weight is entered into the program along with the volume per day of each possible source of nutrient. The program then provides the user with a summary of intake by constituent, including volume, calories, and various caloric sources. In addition, some of these programs provide an analysis of other dietary or intravenous intake, such as electrolytes, trace minerals, and vitamins. Using these programs, the clinician can plot weight change versus caloric intake and know whether the minimal requirements for these nutrients are being provided.

Yet another area in which the computer has added speed and accuracy to clinical calculations is the use of measurements obtained by clinical ultrasonography. The data are entered either from a keyboard or automatically as the operator marks the two ends of a line to be measured on a display of the sonogram. Such systems are built into almost all state-of-the-art commercial ultrasound scanners. Formulas have been derived that relate the linear measurements one can obtain by using ultrasound technology to the size and (perhaps) maturity of the fetus.

On-line data acquisition

Data need not be entered into a bedside computer system (be it stand-alone or mainframe) by a human observer. The professional observer (physician, nurse, technician) supports the process of data entry by screening out data that make no clinical sense (e.g., a persistent heart rate of zero along with a normal temperature and respiratory rate). Electronic monitors with microprocessors also can screen out some uninterpretable data using algorithms that separate artifacts from true signals, but these devices cannot be programmed to screen out all possible nonsense, therefore they sometimes record unbelievable data. Nonetheless, most of today's electronic monitors have devices within them designed to communicate data to a computer. Thus continuous records of neonatal heart rate, respiratory rate, blood pressures, transcutaneous blood gas tensions, hemoglobin saturation, and many other clinical measurements can be stored for later analysis. Tabular or graphic summaries of such data can be displayed to help the clinician recognize trends and events that might better describe the patient's course in the hospital. In some instances the rate of change of a clinical variable is more important to the care of the patient than the absolute and static value of the variable. These same data also can be the basis of hypothesis formulation and testing (i.e., clinical research).

Gorski and colleagues reported the use of such a system that includes the continuous collection of physiologic data from electronic monitoring devices (including heart rate, respiratory rate, blood pressure, and transcutaneous oxygen tensions), as well as data (e.g., observational, laboratory, fluid balance) that could be entered by the observer via a keyboard. Some data were further summarized or transformed before storage. For example, heart rates were sampled once per second, and summaries of 30-second intervals were stored by the computer in the form of mean, maximum, and minimum heart rate for each interval. For other kinds of data (e.g., respiration) all of the data points were stored. This allowed the authors to analyze the physiologic and behavioral responses of small premature infants to external stimuli (e.g., auditory, tactile).

Since the 1970s on-line electronic fetal monitoring data acquisition and analysis have been the focus of perinatologists. It was believed that the use of computer assistance in electronic monitoring of the fetal heart rate and maternal uterine contractions, with automated pattern recognition, could lead to the early diagnosis of fetal distress. Our own preliminary work suggested that computer aided–risk assessment with fetal monitoring data could significantly improve neonatal outcome, although the effect might not have been as great as expected or desired.

Despite promising beginnings very little current investigation exists in this area, let alone clinical applications. There are probably several contributing factors. The first involves inherent statistical and biologic variance, leading to false-positive and false-negative diagnoses of fetal distress. A second and perhaps more important reason for failure to proceed with the design and application of "intelligent fetal monitors" is product and professional liability. Although at least two manufacturers of fetal monitoring equipment have performed developmental work in this area, it has been suggested that marketing efforts have been scrapped because of fear of liability. Therefore intelligent monitors may remain in the realm of academic investigation for the foreseeable future.

However, liability concerns may produce a less ambitious but very important computer application in obstetric perinatology, that of electronic data storage. The capture, storage, and retrieval of electronic fetal monitoring tracings is both a major concern and an important component of all obstetric perinatal programs; the inability to recover a specific, complete fetal monitoring tracing in the face of a lawsuit that is based on patient management of many years before can make such a suit nearly impossible to defend. The cost of mass storage of fetal monitoring data has decreased to the point that this application is clinically feasible. Potential media include cassette tape and "laser disk"; such systems may be available soon. If brought to market, many institutions probably would purchase such devices as a risk-management tool. In addition, electronically stored fetal monitoring data also would have considerable research potential.

CLINICAL INFORMATION SYSTEMS

Hospital information systems

The common hospital system of a decade ago provided only for logging the admission, discharge, or transfer of a patient, the collection of demographic and insurance information, and the generation of a hospital bill from manually entered charges when the patient was discharged. Now the computer is involved in the operation of virtually every hospital department, acting as a financial and clinical tool and as a means of interdepartmental communication.

The functions of these generalized hospital systems are not specific to perinatal medicine, but both neonatal and obstetric perinatologists have particular needs for the orderly management of clinical care information (prenatal, intrapartum, and postpartum) for the mother, fetus, and newborn. Several computerized systems have been designed to meet these special needs and to provide more extensive and defined data specific to perinatology. These systems provide for the recording, summarization, and analysis of risk factors that are significant to the care of mother, fetus, and infant. The storage requirements for perinatal data systems are enormous because of the complexity of the record and the length of time over which data must be collected. The Problem Oriented Perinatal Risk Assessment System (POPRAS) record, for example, has about 2,000 data elements. Nonetheless, computerized systems like POPRAS not only provide an easily accessible medical record, but they also automate the preparation of discharge summaries, letters to referring physicians and other clinical reports, and statistical summaries.

An example of a perinatal database

A third-generation perinatal data system has been placed in operation at Hutzel Hospital at Wayne State University. It is based on the POPRAS record developed by Hobel at the University of California at Los Angeles. This system was chosen in part because it was possible to validate it independently as a risk assessment methodology.

Because perinatal data for each pregnancy span approximately 9 to 10 months, covering multiple antenatal visits, as well as labor and delivery and the neonatal period, with a variety of data subsets that are often not relevant for many patients, a relational database management system is the system of choice for efficient surveys and clinical studies. Using a relational database management system, antenatal, intrapartum, postpartum, and neonatal data are stored separately in individual relations, or tables. A unique number to "join" all relevant data for a given pregnancy is needed; we have found that a unique joining key, produced by the date and the daily patient encounter sequence, is very useful for this purpose.

Clearly, obstetric and neonatal perinatal data for a single pregnancy may span a large number of domains. These are summarized as they are represented in our perinatal records system, based in turn on the contents of the POPRAS record (see box). In addition to the domains detailed, additional data are acquired in the system for all genetic consultations and ultrasound examinations performed.

There are several applications for a perinatal database, such as those described here. The first is for direct patient care. A sample antepartum summary is shown in Fig. 2-3. This summary is placed on the front of each gravida's antepartum record and serves as a quick overview of the problems the patient has during antenatal

Domains of perinatal data in a relational perinatal database*

ANTENATAL

Patient identification
Encounter identification
Care provider identification
Obstetric index
Past pregnancies
Health status indicators
Historical problem list
Physical examination
Medications
Laboratory database
Developing problem list
Prenatal flow chart
Treatment plans
Routine plans
Comments

INTRAPARTUM

Admission notes
Routine admission orders
Obstetric index (repeated)
Physical examination and laboratory data
Early labor problems

INTRAPARTUM cont.

Interim labor problems
Intrapartum flow chart including:
- Dilation, station, and labor graph
- Pelvic examination
- Medications, oxytocin
- Electronic fetal monitoring
- Fetal scalp microblood examination

Late labor problems
Delivery data
Recovery room
Postpartum data and plan
Postpartum problems
Operative procedures
Laboratory data
Diagnostic summary
Discharge plan

NEONATAL

Newborn delivery data
Newborn problem list
Newborn special treatment and procedures
Newborn physical/discharge

*Implemented at Hutzel Hospital, Wayne State University, Detroit, Mich.

HUTZEL HOSPITAL
OB/GYN COMPUTER LAB

MR#
DOB 10/26/48
University Health Center
Dr. O'Halloran

ANTENATAL RISK SUMMARY
Generated on: Sep 15 1986

____________ is a 37 year old divorced black female, obstetric index term 3, premature 3, aborta 2, living 5, with an EDC of 9/18/86. She was first examined on 07/03/86 by Dr. O'Halloran at University Health Center.

Of possible early dating parameters, the IMP was uncertain, there is no record of a positive pregnancy test, there is no record of the uterine size at the time of first examination on 07/03/86, and there is no record of the date of quickening.

There is a history of allergy to penicillin.

PROBLEM NUMBER	RISK SCORE	PROBLEM — Details
1	5	AGE >35
2	5	MULTIPARTY
5	10	HISTORY OF PREMATURE DELIVERY
8	10	HISTORY OF PERINATAL DEATH — Neonatal death.
10	10	HISTORY OF NEONATAL JAUNDICE — See chart for other cause of jaundice.
17	10	HISTORY OF CHRONIC HYPERTENSION — On drug therapy.
18	10	HISTORY OF HEART DISEASE — Arteriosclerotic.
19	5	HISTORY OF PULMONARY DISEASE — Asthma.
20	5	HISTORY OF GENITOURINARY INFECTIONS — Pyelonephritis. — Cystitis.
26	5	HISTORY OF PSYCHIATRIC PROBLEMS — Hospitalized. — On drug therapy.
27	5	HISTORY OF PREVIOUS OPERATIONS — See chart on other operations.
28	10	HISTORY OF SUBSTANCE ABUSE — Tobacco. — Narcotics.
29	5	POSITIVE MATERNAL FAMILY HISTORY — Hypertension. — Multiple births.
53	5	PSYCHO-SOCIAL PROBLEMS — See chart for other psycho-social problem.
58	10	SUPERIMPOSED PREECLAMPSIA — Mild (Persistent edema).

Fig. 2-3. Example of a computer-generated antepartum summary. Data are captured at the first antenatal visit and again at the beginning of the third trimester of pregnancy. A summary such as this one is placed on the front of each prenatal record to highlight important health problems for physicians and nurses in a very busy clinic.

Name:
Referring physician: Roberts
Birth date: 09/10/68
Examination date: 09/10/86
LMP: 04/01/86
Indication(s): Hypertension
Uncertain dates

Placenta: Anterior, not previa, grade 1, normal in appearance
AF volume: Normal, Maximum vertical pocket = 60 mm
Presentation: Transverse, variable

The fetus appears to have*:

Cerebral ventricles	n
Heart—four chambers	n
Cardiac rhythm	n
Stomach	n
Left kidney	n
Right kidney	n
Intestine	n
Bladder	n
Diaphragm	n
Spinal column	n
Extremities	n
Umbilical cord—three vessels	n

*n, normal, abn, abnormal.

Measurements (mm): BPD = 53; abdomen = 52; femur = 40

Dates (by weeks):	LMP	EDC	BPD	ABD	Femur	Mean US
	23	—	23	23	23	23

Conclusion(s) and recommendation(s):
Live intrauterine fetus corresponding in size to 23 ±2 weeks; no visible fetal anomalies; size of the fetus is within the range with LMP; follow-up examination in 4 weeks.

Fig. 2-4. Example of a typical report of an antenatal ultrasound examination as used at Hutzel Hospital, Wayne State University, Detroit, Mich.

care. These data may also be accessed online in the labor and delivery suite when the patient comes to the hospital for admission and labor. Fig. 2-4 shows a typical ultrasound report generated on our service. This form, signed by the examiner, serves as the official ultrasound report. The data forming the basis for this report are also available online in the labor and delivery suite. Similar reports are available covering the labor and delivery and the infant's course in the nursery. These forms are made available on both the maternal and infant chart, facilitating exchange of information between obstetricians and pediatricians.

A second application of this perinatal database involves the generation of service statistics on a monthly basis. A standard reporting format is used, the first page of which is shown in Fig. 2-5. Such reports can be cumulated for any given period. In addition, it is possible to generate such reports for patient population samples of interest (e.g., private patients, staff patients, or patients of a specific health maintenance organization). These statistical surveys form an extremely useful component of the quality assurance program operational in our institution.

A final and very important application of a perinatal database in the academic setting is the use of the database for research; however, the use of such a database is directly dependent on the quality of the data entered into the system. This, in turn, is largely dependent on the usefulness of the clinical reports to the physicians and nurses responsible for recording the data in the first place.

Regional information systems

In many areas of the country perinatal care is organized into working regions with primary, secondary, and tertiary care institutions that combine to offer a population of women and their offspring a wide range of services. Regional planning for perinatal care and risk assessment is facilitated by regional collection and analysis of data. In some areas hospitals have agreed to use a standardized system of data collection and analysis for mutual benefit.

	BIRTHS N	BIRTHS %
Total		
Deliveries	553	
Singleton	543	98.2
Multiple	10	1.8
Births	562	
Live births	559	
Birth weight		
<2,500 gm	90	16.0
2,501-4,000 gm	433	77.0
>4,000 gm	39	6.9
Not recorded	0	0.0
Gestational age (Ballard)		
<38 weeks	127	22.6
38-41 weeks	389	69.2
≥42 weeks	46	8.2
Not recorded	0	0.0
Growth		
SGA	43	7.7
AGA	458	81.5
LGA	58	10.3
Not recorded	3	0.5

	BIRTHS N	BIRTHS %
Prenatal care		
Private	332	59.1
Staff	178	31.7
None	51	9.1
Not recorded	1	0.2
Method of delivery		
Vaginal	420	74.7
Cesarean	138	24.6
Primary	87	15.5
Repeat	51	9.1
Not recorded	0	0.0
Not recorded	4	0.7
Neonatal care		
Private	192	34.2
Staff	276	49.1
Not recorded	94	16.7
Neonatal morbidity		
APGAR <7 at 1 minute	58	10.4
APGAR <7 at 5 minutes	14	2.5
NICU admission	24	4.3

Mortality	N	Rate
Perinatal deaths	6	10.7/1,000 births
Fetal deaths	3	5.3/1,000 births
Antepartum stillbirths	3	5.3/1,000 births
Intrapartum stillbirths	0	0.0/1,000 births
Neonatal deaths	3	5.4/1,000 live births
Still hospitalized/missing neonatal charts	90	16.1% live births

Fig. 2-5. First page summary of a preliminary perinatal monthly report of service statistics. By following these reports serially, emerging problems on the service can be detected readily.

This allows the pooling and sharing of data for regional studies related to quality control. Another approach to regional data collection has been the development of summary records that abstract prenatal, intrapartum, and postnatal events for high-risk births. Summary records, although not useful for day-to-day patient management, are less costly to maintain and store than complete medical records. They, too, are useful tools for research and regional planning.

MEDICAL KNOWLEDGE RETRIEVAL SYSTEMS

The MEDLARS system for cataloging the medical literature was one of the earliest effective applications of computers to medical problems. This system indexes citations to articles contained in the several hundred journals covered by *Index Medicus*. Several other indexing systems have since appeared, providing useful alternatives to MEDLARS. Some of these provide abstracts of articles in addition to citations (e.g., Biosciences Information Services, [BIOSIS]; Excerpta Medica [EMBASE]; and PSYCHINFO, the American Psychological Association database). Most of these services were originally designed to be used by librarians trained in the use of a cryptic command language for search logic and criteria. Today, a "user friendly" version of MEDLARS is available to help the novice through the appropriate steps of a computer literature search. Thanks to the ever-diminishing costs of electronic data storage, entire texts of published papers are now available on-line, rather than just citations or abstracts. This capability brings an entire medical library, cataloged and instantly available, into every physician's office via telephone lines.

ARTIFICIAL INTELLIGENCE AND COMPUTER-ASSISTED DIAGNOSIS

The application of computers to diagnosis and treatment begins with history-taking; several programs have been devised to guide the clinician in taking a history. The advantage of these programs is the discipline they impress on the process of history taking. Through the use of branching logic, answers to preliminary questions determine the depth and direction of the interview in some areas, while just screening in other areas. Questions inappropriate to the age, sex, or clinical condition are avoided, but relevant points are always covered. Although this kind of task is not difficult to program and implement, the need for widespread access to microcomputers and/or terminals and for patient acceptance has limited the proliferation of this type of system in the medical practice environment.

A second level of complexity in computer-assisted diagnosis is in algorithmic-diagnostic and clinical-decision support. It would appear that obstetric and neonatal-perinatal medicine would be an ideal area for such applications, because the number of diagnostic situations with which perinatal clinicians are faced is relatively limited compared, for example, with the general internist or general surgeon. From this perspective the number of such applications reported in the literature appears surprisingly limited. One such application in obstetric perinatology involves computer diagnosis of labor progression. Labor progress can be quantitated, in terms of time of onset, cervical dilation, station of the fetal presenting part, and change in the latter two parameters over time. Dysfunctional labor patterns, such as secondary arrest of dilation and arrest of the descent, have well-defined quantitative criteria for diagnosis. Furthermore, although it is surely true that appropriate management of labor progress remains an art, there is reasonable agreement concerning an appropriate approach to management of certain labor abnormalities. All of these considerations make management of labor progress a nearly ideal area for application of algorithmic support for clinical decision making. Components of such a system were first designed and applied in 1973. The program was first written in BASIC and required less than 8 kilobytes of storage—very compact, considering that microprocessors now typically have 256 to 512 kilobytes of online memory. The program was later converted to FORTRAN. In the early 1970s, online application, although tested, was impractical on the computers available at that time. However, offline application was possible, and over 30,000 consecutive labors have been analyzed using this program, making it possible to use the algorithm in support of a large number of specific research projects. Furthermore, the algorithm has been updated recently and demonstrated in the online setting. The impact on clinical decision making of this online application will require further study.

In the neonatal area an excellent example of a clinical test of algorithmic management has been published recently (Chapter 28, part four). The effectiveness of a computer program embodying an algorithm for mechanical ventilation of infants with respiratory distress syndrome was evaluated by examination of correction of deranged arterial blood gases in neonates. Arterial blood gas values improved more frequently in neonates managed with computer consultation than in two control groups. The investigators concluded that in teaching institutions more effective care of neonates with respiratory failure may be facilitated by computer-assisted management of mechanical ventilators. Another program facilitates sophisticated pulmonary function studies during mechanical ventilation of neonates.

The next level of complexity in the area of diagnostic and clinical decision support is the expert system. One successful example of this kind of facility is the Birth Defects Information System (BDIS) sponsored by the March of Dimes. It was developed in the 1970s to assist physicians with the diagnosis of known patterns of human malformation. This program provides a list of codes for specific physical findings and historical information arranged by system. Upon entering the appropriate codes for the patient's characteristics, the clinician is asked for additional information as may be available from historical or clinical sources. Then the computer lists the 10 most likely diagnoses (syndromes) for the given information using a complex system of Bayesian probability, based on the literature prevalence of signs and symptoms, along with a set of rules of diagnosis (e.g., Turner's syndrome is not possible in males who have XY chromosomes) that eliminate obvious errors. Individual cases can be updated as new information becomes available, and revised lists of likely diagnoses are then generated. This system also provides summary descriptions of each possible diagnosis.

Expert systems have not been applied widely to other areas of perinatal medicine to date, but another well-known example of an expert system is one developed by Jack Myers at the University of Pittsburgh called INTERNIST-I. This experimental computer program is capable of making multiple and complex diagnoses in internal medicine. In 1982 this program was tested in 19 clinicopathologic exercises from the case records of the Massachussetts General Hospital. It was found that the acumen of the program was similar to that of the physicians who originally cared for the cases, but inferior to the discussants selected for the exercises published in the *New England Journal of Medicine*. One of the deficiencies of the program was that it failed to take change over time into account in its decision making, and it did less well when there were multiple diagnoses.

Artificial intelligence (AI) is an area of computer research that may have widespread applications in medicine. Although definitions of AI vary widely, it is generally accepted to be the use of a computer to perform tasks that are considered to require intelligence when performed by humans. Part of the expectation for AI is that the program will "learn" from past errors and correct its own logic as information about its performance is received. Programs such as MYCIN and INTERNIST-I are steps toward a true artificial intelligence system for clinical use.

COMPUTER-ASSISTED EDUCATION

Programmed instruction did not originate with the use of computers. Many texts have been written in which the reader is presented with a set of facts that build on each other, and his or her knowledge of the facts presented so far is verified by testing devices within the text. Often, the device used was a piece of cardboard covering a column on the right side of the printed page that contained answers to questions posed on the remainder of the page.

The computer lends itself readily to this form of programmed instruction. Holley and Heller compared a pair of computer-assisted educational programs in acid-base balance with presentations of the same material by lectures with slides to two randomly selected groups of medical students. They found that both groups improved their knowledge of the subject to about the same extent (17% more correct answers on the posttest as compared to the pretest). The disadvantage of computer assisted instruction (CAI) was that students spent up to twice the time of the lectures learning the same amount of material. The advantages of the CAI method included time savings for faculty and convenience for the students, who were able to work with the program on their own schedules and at their own speed.

Programming languages such as PILOT are available to instructors to facilitate the construction of teaching modules. These modules generally present information to the student and allow the student to interact by selecting what he or she needs to review. The student then answers questions that verify mastery of the subject. The program itself can then redirect the student to areas of weakness and confirm for the student what has been accomplished in using the module. The languages currently available for programmning such instruction allow for the presentation of text and graphic displays of information, the asking and answering of factual questions, and the redirection of the student to various parts of the module according to the student's performance. The modules do not tire of repetitive tasks or appear annoyed at students who are slow or inattentive; they give a fair and factual estimate of performance to the student as he or she is learning the subject.

One of the most sophisticated of these languages is called PROF (for professor). With this language the author need not be particularly adept at computer programming. The author designs a patient-management problem on paper with diagnostic and therapeutic choices, as well as common mistakes and pitfalls in a branching-decision tree. The PROF language system leads the author through the process of entering the data for the patient simulation and requires little or no computer experience. The program starts by inviting the participant to ask questions after a brief case presentation. The participant starts by gathering information (as if questioning the patient). The student may ask and respond in conversational English. The program recognizes the content of the questions and answers through sets of key words (mostly noun-verb combinations), synonyms and word roots. In this system visual clues are presented on a television screen by the computer, which selects images from a compact laser disk.

Another even more sophisticated form of programmed instruction is that of the clinical simulation. This form of clinical exercise, too, existed before it was adapted to the computer. In the 1960s clinical simulations represented an innovative approach to the problem of testing a large number of students uniformly and simultaneously, not just for a measure of the facts that they might be able to repeat, but also for their ability to organize information and apply it to a clinical problem in a logical step-by-step fashion. The original version of this sort of exercise allowed for choices to be made at various stages of a clinical presentation. The candidates would indicate their preferred course of action by rubbing out an area of camouflage covering the text. The newly exposed text would provide data (e.g., if the action chosen was to obtain a particular test), or it might give a clue to the consequences of the last choice made by the candidate (e.g., "your patient responded to vigorous stimulation by going into shock"). As embodied in a computer-based system, the path the student takes to get to the end of the clinical problem is recorded. A review is presented to the student or to the instructor at the end of the process. This report notes the student's performance and indicates the "ideal solution" to the problem. The method requires careful and thoughtful programming, but once it is completed any number of students can benefit from the exercise and experience it at an individualized pace that cannot be matched by many other forms of instruction.

The computer can function as a great convenience for harried clinical instructors in the area of testing and evaluation. In addition, it can act as a storehouse for a large number of clinical test questions that can be accumulated over a period of years. A program can be used to allow the student to take a formal test based on a portion of questions stored. The question-and-answer process can be managed on-line with instant feedback to the student about right and wrong answers while the computer keeps a record of performance. If the store of questions is sufficiently large, so that only a small percentage of them is randomly selected for each student's examination, the instructor need not worry about the lateral spread of information about the test among the students. Records can also be kept about the effectiveness of individual questions in discriminating good students from poor students (reliability), allowing the test to be refined with each use. In addition, records of student performance can be stored on computer as scores and comments to assist with overall evaluation (averaging and summarizing) of a student's progress in the curriculum.

The computer offers the opportunity to present patient simulations to the examinee. An excellent example of this sort of test is the computer-based examination (CBX), which is under development by the National Board of Medical Examiners and the American Board of Internal Medicine. This simulation model works by having the examinee interact with the computer through a keyboard and a cathode-ray tube (CRT). A patient is presented whose clinical condition, laboratory values, and consultation results vary with time and treatment. The examinee is presented with a narrative description and then is allowed to obtain more information by requesting additional history and physical findings. Visual information is presented to the examinee via 35 mm slides projected on a screen beside the CRT. The examinee makes decisions about the timing and content of tests and therapies and is given the results of these over time. Tests can be ordered routinely or immediately, at the request of the examinee. The patient's status (deterioration, improvement, no change) then is reflected in the values of laboratory tests and symptoms. The exercise is scored on the basis of the efficiency of the diagnosis and treatment process. This includes endpoints, decision points, and process scores. Endpoints include factors such as the identification of the disease process and whether the patient benefited from the therapies recommended. Decision points represent those key decisions (e.g., gathering appropriate information, making appropriate judgments and instituting therapy) that an expert would deem necessary to achieve a satisfactory outcome. These decision points represent intermediate goals in the patient-management problem. Finally, a score is calculated for process that takes into account the expense to the patient in risk, dollars, and discomfort versus the benefit achieved. This score examines the efficiency, completeness, and appropriateness of the process used by the examinee. These simulations therefore attempt to test the thought processes needed for good patient care, an area not adequately tested by multiple-choice examinations. The use of these simulations has undergone extensive evaluation, and they offer a more representative picture of the clinician's behavior and effectiveness in the field than multiple choice examinations that test the ability of the examinee to recall facts.

OTHER PERINATAL COMPUTER APPLICATIONS

Practice management

Practice management may be regarded as medical accounting on a departmental scale or within a medical professional corporation. The key components of a practice management system are:

1. Appointment scheduling
2. Medical records
3. Financial accounting

Many commercial practice-management systems are available. Based on our experience, expertise in areas previously covered in this chapter does not guarantee wise decision-making in choosing such systems for application, particularly in the academic practice setting. Nonetheless, based on our experience, the most important features of a practice-management package to consider are the following.

Statement of accounts. This must conform to what is needed in a particular practice setting. If possible, it is important to avoid custom designs, since it invariably takes longer than expected to get custom programs running and working effectively.

Posting. The detailed steps in posting patient data in the system must be evaluated. In particular, how long does it take? Some systems appear to be considerably more effective than others, depending on methods in use in a given setting. We have found that a system suitable for one office manager may be totally unacceptable to another.

Insurance claim–form preparation. In addition to standard American Medical Association forms, which are accepted by many insurance carriers, different states have varying requirements for Medicare and Medicaid claim forms. Specific insurance carriers or health maintenance organizations also may require different formats for insurance claims. It is crucial to be sure you are getting what you need. Claim-form preparation can be further complicated by physicians not adhering to systematic procedures (e.g., acceptance of assignment, write-offs).

Medical records. In our experience, most practice-management packages have very limited capability for medical records beyond the simplest level. Medical record applications are better handled by an independent system.

User applications. If a practice-management system is not database oriented, experience indicates that it is unlikely that it will be able to support specific local applications.

Converting from one practice-management system to

another is a major problem. Therefore it is important to do it right the first time. We find it easy to write such a statement, but we haven't managed to accomplish it.

Management information systems

In our experience, those systems that are typically termed hospital management–information systems seldom generate information of use either in day-to-day management of the service, in terms of staffing, costs, financial performance, or other measures of activity. For example, perhaps a director of obstetric perinatology wishes to follow the activity of an antenatal diagnostic unit (e.g., the number of ultrasound examinations, nonstress tests, and contraction stress tests), or contributions to a dean's practice plan need to be documented to ensure continued academic support. Experience indicates that there are no systems specifically designed for managing such common problems on perinatal services. However, there are very powerful and useful systems readily available for use on microprocessors. We have found standard spread-sheet, graphic, and word processing programs extraordinarily useful in the perinatal environment. From the practical perspective, we have found a reasonable approach to be the initial development of a single useful output with progressive modification on a month-by-month basis, as the strengths and shortcomings of that particular application become obvious. One such minimal application tends to spawn several others, and over the period of a few years a custom-tailored system can be developed relatively easily and at minimal cost.

SUMMARY

Computers and software programs are emerging to facilitate patient care (decision-making), perinatal data management (particularly monthly statistical reports, morbidity and mortality data), education, and practice management. Caution must be exercised in selecting a system. The tendency is to want to collect too much information. Special attention must be directed to ensure that there is strict quality control of the data entered.

Ronald L. Poland
Robert J. Sokol
Robert O. Bollinger
Lawrence Chik

BIBLIOGRAPHY

General

Chik, L., and others: Development of a practical departmental computer system for ob/gyn, (scientific exhibit), Presented at the annual meeting of the Association of Professors of Gynecology and Obstetrics, New Orleans, La., March 1986.

Frayer, W.: First of four issues with articles from the International Symposium, 1984, Am. J. Perinatol. **2:** 1985.

Lindberg, D.A.B.: The growth of medical information systems in the United States, Lexington, Ky., 1979, Lexington Press.

Repetitive and complex processes

Clinical data manipulation

Shortliffe, E.H.: Computer based medical consultations: mycin, New York, 1976, Elsevier Science Publishing Co.

Wilson, F.E., and others: Computerized nutritional data management in neonatal intensive care, Arch. Dis. Child. **58:**732, 1983.

On-line data requisition

Chik, L., and Sokol, R.J.: Risk-intervention-outcome: a model for the evaluation of an on-line computer generated running risk score for intrapartum fetal monitoring, Acta Obstet. Gynecol. Scand. Suppl. **109:**94, 1982.

Chik, L., and others: Programmed identification of fetal heart rate deceleration patterns, Am. J. Obstet. Gynecol. **119:**816, 1974.

Chik, L., and others: Computer interpreted fetal monitoring data: discriminant function analysis of perinatal data for the classification of one year neurological outcome, J. Pediatr. **90:**985, 1977.

Gorski, P.A., and others: Direct computer recording of premature infants and nursery care: distress following two interventions, Pediatrics **72:**198, 1983.

Clinical information systems

Hospital information systems

Bahr, J.P., and Grausz, J.P.: An on-line perinatal data system. In Harris, T.R., and Bahr, J.P., editors: The use of computers in perinatal medicine, New York, 1982, Praeger Publishers.

Bollinger, R.O., Poland, R.L., and Cummings, G.D.: The design and implementation of a statewide perinatal automated medical network for Michigan (PAM/NET). In Ackerman, M.J., editor: Proceedings of the ninth annual symposium on computer applications in medical care, 1985, IEEE Computer Society.

Chik, L., and others: A perinatal database management system, Methods Inf. Med. **20:**133, 1981.

Hammond, W.E., and others: Functional characteristics of a clinical information system, Methods Inf. Med. **19:**38, 1980.

Hobel, C.J.: Have data systems: What for? Acta Obstet. Gynecol. Scand. Suppl. **109:**53, 1982.

Janik, D.S., and others: Computerized newborn intensive care data recording, reporting, and research. III. A practical microcomputer system, J. Pediatr. **97:**497, 1980.

Lindstrom, D.P., and Cotton, R.B.: Computer assisted neonatal data base designed primarily for clinical research. In Harris, T.R., and Bahr, J.P., editors: The use of computers in perinatal medicine, New York, 1982, Praeger Publishers.

Rosen, M., Sokol, R.J., and Chik, L.: The use of computers in the labor and delivery suite: An overview, Am. J. Obstet. Gynecol. **132:**589, 1978.

Stephan, P.D., and Merkatz, I.R.: A functional regional perinatal information system: The Cleveland experience. In Harris, T.R., and Bahr, J.P., editors: The use of computers in perinatal medicine, New York, 1982, Praeger Publishers.

Yamamoto, K., and others: Progress report on nationwide networking system of perinatal summary records, Asia Oceania J. Obstet. Gynecol. **11:**99, 1985.

Perinatal databases

Hobel, C.J.: Development of POPRAS: problem oriented perinatal risk assessment system. In Harris, T.R., and Bahr, J.P., editors: The use of computers in perinatal medicine, New York, 1982, Praeger Publishers.

Sokol, R.J., and others: Clinical application of high risk scoring on an obstetric service, Am. J. Obstet. Gynecol. **128:**652, 1977.

Regional information systems

Jennett, R.J., and others: A computerized perinatal data system for a region, Am. J. Obstet. Gynecol. **131**:157, 1978.

Sokol, R.J., and Chik, L.: Perinatal computing: an overview, Acta Obstet. Gynecol. Scand. Suppl. **109**:7, 1982.

Stephan, P.D., and Merkatz, I.R.: A functional regional perinatal informational system: the Cleveland experience. In Harris, T.R., and Bahr, J.P., editors: The use of computers in perinatal medicine, New York, 1982, Praeger Publishers.

Whiting-O'Keefe, Q.E., and others: A computerized summary medical record system can provide more information than the standard medical record, JAMA **245**:1185, 1985.

Medical knowledge retrieval systems

Collen, M.F., and Flagle, C.D.: Full-text medical literature retrieval by computer, JAMA **254**:2768, 1985.

Johnson, D.E.: Information containment: online searching for health care information. I. Getting started, Software in Health Care, **2**:628, 1984-1985.

Johnson, D.E.: Information containment: online searching for health care information. II. Doing an online search, Software in Health Care, **3**:40, 1985.

MEDLARS and health information policy: A technical memorandum, Office of Technology Assessment, United States Congress, Sept. 1985.

Artificial intelligence and computer-assisted programs

Carlo, W.A., and others: Efficacy of computer-assisted management of respiratory failure in neonates, Pediatrics **78**:139, 1986.

Chik, L., and others: Computers in obstetrics and gynecology. In Benson, R.C., and others: Current obstetrics and gynecologic diagnosis and treatment, ed. 6, Los Altos, Calif., 1987, Lange Medical Publications.

Kulikowski, C.A.: Artificial intelligence methods for expert medical consultant systems, Mt. Sinai J. Med. **52**:87, 1985.

Miller, R.A., Pople, H.E., and Myers, J.D.: INTERNIST-I: an experimental computer based diagnostic consultant for general internal medicine, N. Engl. J. Med. **307**:468, 1982.

Minsky, M.: Semantic information processing, Cambridge, Mass., 1968, M.I.T. Press.

Sokol, R.J., Miller, S., and Reed, G.: Alcohol abuse during pregnancy: an epidemiologic study, Alcoholism **4**:135, 1980.

Sokol, R.J., and others: Computer diagnosis of labor progression. I. Development of an on-line interactive digital computer program for the diagnosis of normal and abnormal cervical dilatation patterns, J. Reprod. Med. **11**:149, 1973.

Sokol, R.J., and others: Computer diagnosis of labor progression. IV. An on-line interactive digital computer subroutine for evaluating descent of the fetal presenting part during labor, J. Reprod. Med. **13**:177, 1974.

Sokol, R.J., and others: Risks preceding increased primary cesarean birth rates, Obstet. Gynecol. **59**:340, 1982.

Computer-assisted education

Abdulla, A.M., Watkins, L.O., and Henke, J.S.: The use of natural language entry and laser videodisk technology in CAI, J. Med. Educ. **59**:739, 1984.

Friedman, R.B.: Some results from the computer-based examination project. In Lloyd, J.S., editor: Computer applications in the evaluation of physician competence, Chicago, 1984, American Board of Medical Specialties.

Holley, H.S., and Heller, F.N.: Microcomputers for computer-assisted instruction in anesthesiology, J. Med. Educ. **59**:521, 1984.

CHAPTER 3

Diabetes in pregnancy

The challenges offered to the obstetric-neonatal team by the occurrence of diabetes in pregnancy have served to stimulate many of the recent advances in perinatal medicine. Maternal metabolic disturbances and those affecting both fetus and neonate fully test the integrated medical, nursing, nutritional, and supportive skills of a perinatal unit undertaking care of high-risk patients. Despite acknowledged challenges to both maternal and infant well-being, with no other condition has it been more readily demonstrated that comprehensive perinatal care can be effective in normalizing pregnancy outcome. Although many problems remain unsolved, the elucidation of the basic pathophysiology affecting the maternal-fetal relationship has led to better clinical results for both the diabetic woman and her offspring.

The scope of the problem of diabetes in pregnancy can be appreciated by a 1973 Health Interview Survey, which reported 443,000 women of childbearing age with diabetes mellitus in the United States. The prevalence of overt diabetes complicating pregnancy has been estimated to approximate 0.5% of all gestations in the United States; an additional 3% of women demonstrate transient biochemical abnormalities that are unmasked only during their pregnancies. Without appropriate care those women who are diabetic prior to pregnancy evidence a perinatal mortality 10 times that of a normal population, whereas those with diabetes only during gestation still have a twofold to threefold increase in rate of loss. The latter group requires special identification so that appropriate preventive efforts be initiated to ensure careful supervision of the developing fetus.

The overt or juvenile-onset diabetic woman presents more of a management than a diagnostic challenge. Under ideal circumstances, in her early reproductive years she will have been referred to an experienced center for contraceptive services, prepregnancy counseling, and advice with respect to later pregnancy supervision. However, a woman with a more subtle form of carbohydrate intolerance presents an additional problem of detection. Too often her diagnosis may be unsuspected or missed, and an unanticipated fetal death ensues. Unfortunately, there are as of yet no universally accepted criteria for a diagnosis of gestational diabetes. The Second International Workshop on Gestational Diabetes decided to maintain the term *gestational diabetes* to refer to a condition of "glucose intolerance with its recognition of onset during pregnancy."

In the past, much of the pregnancy-focused diabetic testing was inappropriately performed in the early puerperium, at a point when it is now understood that insulin antagonism is no longer operative. Furthermore, traditional glucose testing during pregnancy had usually been confined only to selected high-risk categories. Women with histories of stillbirth, macrosomic infants, or first-degree family members affected with diabetes were the ones most commonly suspected of having latent diabetes mellitus. Studies have now shown that such clinical risk factors are by themselves insensitive indicators for patients with gestational diabetes. Therefore routine diabetic screening is currently advocated for all pregnant women. Although not yet universally practiced, this approach appears to offer particular benefit in identifying those women at increased risk for carbohydrate-related perinatal loss, macrosomia, and birth injury.

The screening test involves a 50 gm oral glucose load and a venous plasma glucose determination 1 hour later (Table 3-1). This 1-hour screening test has the advantage of being applicable any time of day, irrespective of the fed or fasted state, and it is well tolerated by patients. A venous plasma glucose value of 140 mg/dl (7.8 mmol/

Table 3-1. Screening for diabetes in pregnancy: 1-hour-test*

Time	24-28 weeks gestation
Load	50 gm carbohydrate
Result	140 mg/dl (venous plasma)

*May be done any time of day. Patient need not be fasting.

Table 3-2. O'Sullivan-Mahan criteria for diabetes in pregnancy*

Fasting blood sugar	105 mg/dl
1 hour	190 mg/dl
2 hour	165 mg/dl
3 hour	145 mg/dl

*Based on overnight fast with 100 gm oral glucose load. Values are for plasma glucose with two abnormal values needed for diagnosis.

L) indicates a need for confirmatory testing. Confirmatory testing should conform to the 100 gm oral test employing the original published cirteria of O'Sullivan and Mahan (Table 3-2). Although it may eventually be proved that these values do not pertain to pregnant women at all ages, weights, and stages of gestation, they remain the most extensively studied.

The White classification groups pregnant diabetic women according to age of onset and duration of their disease and according to the presence or absence of vascular complications. Although generally helpful as a prognostic guide to care, the system has its greatest potential value in comparing outcome results of clinical series reported by various institutions. The classification should not be used by itself to set guidelines for the timing of a particular patient's delivery, since irrespective of the White class that decision is now more appropriately based on a concept of individualized patient management. Following is a breakdown of the White classification of diabetes.

Class A: Gestational diabetes
Class B: Age of onset over 20 or duration of disease under 10 years with no vascular disease
Class C: Age of onset between 10 and 20 or duration of disease between 10 and 20 years with no vascular disease
Class D: Age of onset under 10, disease longer than 20 years, or retinopathy
Class E: Calcification of pelvic vessels
Class F: Nephropathy
Class R: Proliferative retinopathy

Pedersen and Pedersen originally identified co-risk factors known as "prognostically bad signs during pregnancy" that could be shown to adversely affect the outcome of the diabetic pregnancy. They demonstrated in all White categories that a fetus remains at increased risk if the mother experiences pyelonephritis, ketoacidosis, toxemia, or neglect of care. The obstetrician must be vigilant in identifying such factors promptly and in taking aggressive therapeutic steps to ameliorate or prevent their deleterious effects.

Changes in carbohydrate metabolism are characteristic of the normal pregnant state. Early in gestation, improved glucose utilization is typical for all, so for the diabetic woman an episode of hypoglycemia may sometimes provide the first clue that conception has occurred. This physiologic alteration usually begins in the first trimester and lasts for about 8 to 12 weeks. In the second half of pregnancy there occurs a decrease in the ability of endogenous insulin to translocate glucose into cells. The diabetic woman evidences a progressive increase in her insulin requirement. Rising levels of maternal progesterone, estrogen, and human chorionic somatomammotropin (HCS) all appear to play a role in this "insulin resistance" of pregnancy, but HCS has been primarily implicated. After delivery of the placenta the typical insulin refractoriness is abruptly lost, and the diabetic patient then becomes exquisitely sensitive to exogenous therapy. Thus normal and diabetic women alike are subjected to a series of metabolic alterations throughout both gestation and the puerperium.

INTRAPARTUM COMPLICATIONS
Unstable metabolic condition

Recent physiologic studies conducted in the controlled environment of the metabolic unit have provided 24-hour profiles of blood insulin levels, glucose concentrations, amino acids, and other metabolic parameters throughout normal and diabetic pregnancies. In particular, the fasting blood glucose level has been clearly shown to be lower during pregnancy than in the nonpregnant state. Furthermore, there is a marked constancy of blood glucose levels throughout the day, with plasma levels rarely exceeding 100 mg/dl except during the first hour following meals. In diabetic pregnancies, on the other hand, there appears a much greater flux in the concentrations of all fuels between fed and fasted states. With respect to glucose there is a tendency toward hyperglycemia after breakfast and nocturnal hypoglycemia. Thus the extremely stable metabolic milieu for the fetus that appears to characterize normal pregnancy is lost in the pregnancy complicated by diabetes. These observations now provide the clinician with a rational basis of blood glucose regulation during both the gestational and overt diabetic pregnancy.

It is prudent in both of these pathologic situations that the maternal metabolic condition be stabilized by all available means to reapproximate the normal physiology of pregnancy. For the insulin-dependent patient dietary management, insulin therapy, and maternal activity are integrated to maintain euglycemia throughout the day. For most gestational diabetic patients dietary therapy alone suffices in achieving this objective. Although achieving normal blood glucose levels is important, the purpose of the diet is first to ensure an adequate maternal weight gain during pregnancy. Caloric intake is not restricted, since every attempt is made to meet both the calorie and protein requirements of normal gestation.

Most patients consume a 2,200- to 2,400-calorie diet to satisfy both their own and the fetal energy demands. With obesity or adolescence, more rather than fewer calories are often needed to prevent the potentially deleterious effects of ketonemia. A nutritionist experienced with pregnant diabetic patients thus becomes an essential member of the health care team. Diets are constructed and modified in accordance with individual needs and preferences. Attention is focused on the total caloric intake as well as its individual components at various times during the day. To avoid marked fluctuations in the blood glucose level, an even distribution of calories and carbohydrates is suggested among meals and snacks. At least 20% of the diet should comprise protein totaling up to 115 gm. Carbohydrates usually provide 45% or more of the total calories, but monosaccharides are to be avoided, except for those available in natural sources.

If, after the establishment of an appropriate diet, blood glucose levels are not normalized throughout the day, insulin therapy is instituted. The data currently indicate that about 15% of gestational diabetic women need insulin treatment comparable to that for the overt diabetic. Combinations of intermediate- and short-acting insulins divided between morning and evening doses appear to be most effective; approximately two thirds of the insulin is administered before breakfast and the remainder prior to the evening meal. Especially for patients unaccustomed to such insulin regimens, a period of adjustment and training in the hospital is often useful at midpregnancy. Corresponding to the times of peak insulin effect, four blood glucose determinations are obtained daily. Adjustments in one or more of the four insulin components can then be made in order to approximate the desired constant euglycemia.

It is, of course, difficult to simulate normal activity under such hospital conditions, so insulin requirements may be overestimated. Therefore, once a general strategy of dietary and insulin therapies has been established, continued ambulatory management is preferred. More exquisite metabolic control can be obtained when activity or frank exercise is used as a third therapeutic modality. As shown by Jovanovic and others, this ambulatory management has now become markedly facilitated through the availability of home glucose-monitoring techniques. The pregnant diabetic woman is currently able to closely supervise her own glucose profiles and to periodically adjust her diet, insulin, or activity accordingly. As pregnancy advances and the phenomenon of insulin antagonism becomes more influential, periodic modifications in the regimen are mandated. Blood glucose values in the range of 60 to 80 mg/dl fasting and less than 120 mg/dl postprandial reflect optimum maternal-fetal homeostasis. It should be underscored that oral hypoglycemic agents are not to be employed during pregnancy because of their potentially teratogenic effects in the first trimester and because of their capacity to induce profound and prolonged hypoglycemia in the neonate.

Fetal hyperinsulinism

Insulin has been implicated as the primary growth hormone for intrauterine development. For example, when fetal insulin is absent, marked intrauterine growth retardation occurs. On the other hand, when fetal hyperinsulinism is present as the result of maternal and fetal hyperglycemia, marked anabolic actions of insulin become manifest. There ensues an accelerated protein synthesis together with a deposition of excessive glycogen and fat stores. The typical macrosomic, plethoric infant of the diabetic mother results. This is the infant most at risk for the neonatal complications of hypoglycemia, hypocalcemia, hyperviscosity, and hyperbilirubinemia (Chapter 37, part one). Evidence from in vitro studies and from clinical observations among gestational diabetic women has recently been used to modify the original Pedersen hypothesis so that it now recognizes elevated maternal levels of amino acids and free fatty acids along with hyperglycemia as factors in promoting the development of fetal macrosomia. A surfeit of all metabolic fuels presented to the fetus in the presence of fetal hyperinsulinism is now understood to represent the basic pathologic mechanism in the diabetic pregnancy. Nevertheless, clinical efforts can as yet only be focused primarily on the control of maternal plasma glucose concentrations.

Maternal ketoacidosis

An episode of *maternal ketoacidosis* with its accompanying metabolic derangements represents the greatest threat to the life and well-being of the pregnant diabetic woman and her fetus. The mortality for the unborn baby resulting from such an episode may be as high as 50% or greater. With such a high degree of risk it must be concluded that only by early and aggressive management or, better still, through prevention will the contribution of diabetic ketoacidosis to overall perinatal mortality be significantly reduced. Each diabetic patient must be instructed to report early signs of infection and any suggestion of loss of metabolic control. A healthy dialogue must be established between physician and patient to ensure adherence to therapeutic regimens, and the entire obstetric team must be receptive to the patient's own concerns and observations. Maternal fasting and dehydration act in concert to augment the production of ketone bodies and to decrease their rate of eventual excretion. Superimposed on the normal accelerated physiologic ketosis of pregnancy, disturbances in oral intake coupled with nausea and vomiting serve to set the stage for a ketoacidotic episode. This risk is heightened particularly during protracted nausea and vomiting in late gestation. Patients may unwisely choose to eliminate an insulin dose. If there is a delay in diagnosis or continued disturbances in oral intake, serious decompensation of the diabetes may result. Therefore, when any potentially dangerous signs or evidence of serious alterations in metabolic regulation appear, the patient should be hospitalized and appropriately evaluated.

With overt ketoacidosis the maternal status, the insulin therapy, and fluid and electrolyte balance are best followed with a flow sheet. The fetal condition is appraised with external cardiotachometry. Maternal acidosis is often reflected in uterine hyperactivity together with a loss of fetal heart rate variability and/or the appearance of late decelerations. These changes usually resolve when maternal and fetal homeostasis has been restored. Intravenous insulin by bolus or continuous infusion is a primary component of therapy. The other principal need is for adequate replacement of body fluids, particularly to restore the depleted intravascular compartment. Therapy proceeds along physiologic lines to achieve metabolic stability. An initial use of isotonic (0.9%) saline solution is favored with a subsequent employment of more dilute fluids. Serum electrolytes, pH, and bicarbonate levels are followed closely. There is a reluctance to employ bicarbonate therapy in correcting maternal acidosis because of experimental data suggesting that it may paradoxically accentuate acidosis in the fetus. As metabolic equilibrium is restored, the diet and usual insulin regimen are resumed while antibiotics and other specific therapies are instituted to correct any underlying pathologic condition.

Stillbirth

Whether or not ketoacidosis, toxemia, polyhydramnios, or other serious complications develop during the course of a diabetic pregnancy, the risk of a sudden stillbirth at or near term cannot be totally discounted. For this reason, as the pregnancy advances, careful confirmation of fetal well-being is mandatory. The insulin-dependent patient may still have to be admitted to the hospital for a period of fetal surveillance prior to delivery. With more severe diabetes or with documentation of inadequate metabolic control, admission as early as 34 weeks' gestation may be prudent. When the maternal condition has been stable and there are no ominous signs, early admission may be delayed until much closer to term or omitted entirely. The gestational diabetic patient whose blood glucose profile remains normal with dietary regulation alone and who develops no other complication is typically followed on an ambulatory basis until labor begins spontaneously or until the duration of pregnancy becomes prolonged. If the pregnancy is to be carried much beyond 40 weeks, hospitalization should then be considered and the same intensive fetal surveillance provided as that for the insulin-dependent woman. Daily maternal plasma or 24-hour urinary estriol determinations are no longer widely used to assess these pregnancies. Stress or nonstress cardiotachometry (Chapter 8) provides the primary evidence of placental respiratory reserve and the status of fetal autonomic function. It has been sufficiently substantiated that this conservative approach is preferable to one that formerly recommended routine preterm delivery for all diabetic women.

Premature births

In the past, programmatic attempts to prevent intrauterine deaths resulted instead in many iatrogenic premature births with an attendant high rate of neonatal loss and long-term serious hazard. Contemporary control of maternal diabetes and the available tools permitting adequate fetal supervision now facilitate the prevention of such prematurity. In particular, through amniocentesis and the analysis of amniotic fluid, the degree to which fetal pulmonary development has progressed may be ascertained prior to birth (Chapter 9). An induction of labor or scheduled cesarean section is postponed unless indices of surfactant synthesis are available and indicative of functional pulmonary maturity. When blood biochemical control has been present during late gestation, the usual lecithin/sphingomyelin ratio appears dependable for the diabetic pregnancy. However, occasional respiratory distress in the newborn is encountered despite a lecithin/sphingomyelin ratio consistent with pulmonary maturity. Because of these false positive test results, the additional determination of amniotic fluid phosphatidylglycerol is now recommended prior to scheduled delivery.

Induction of labor is best initiated early in the morning when the entire perinatal team can be alerted and adequately prepared for delivery. From most reports it appears that, with modern management, as many as half of pregnant diabetics can now have safe vaginal deliveries.

Congenital anomalies

By correcting the metabolic abnormalities of diabetes in pregnancy and by individualizing the timing of delivery, we can minimize the incidence of stillbirths and neonatal deaths. Congenital anomalies, however, continue to be a significant problem for the offspring of diabetic woman. Infants with major anomalies are born to diabetic women two to three times more often than they are to women in the general obstetric population. These anomalies most commonly arise during the first 7 weeks of embryonic life, which is before most women come under the care of their obstetricians and also before metabolic control is normalized. Thus there remains an irreducible minimum of perinatal mortality and morbidity that is secondary to fetal anomalies. Poor control in early pregnancy as evidenced by elevated maternal hemoglobin A_{1c} is associated with an increased risk of major structural malformations. There is a growing body of evidence that the establishment of euglycemia prior to conception and through the first trimester will reduce the incidence of congenital anomalies to approximately that of the general obstetric population. Further reductions in perinatal mortality and morbidity beyond the "irreducible minimum" may in time be feasible but only when providers emphasize the need for prepregnancy planning and diabetes control.

POSTPARTUM CARE

After delivery, the diabetic woman must continue under close supervision. Because of her potential sensitivity to exogenous therapy, long-acting insulins are usually withheld for the first 24 hours or more, and usually as little as half the prepregnancy dosage is the starting point for resumption of therapy. A prompt return to oral feedings following cesarean delivery aids in the restoration of normal control.

Lactation

It has been observed for years that lactation may be poor with maternal diabetes, and the problem remains unsolved today. Considerable support by the nursing staff and encouragement by all professionals are essential in aiding the well-motivated woman to establish adequate milk production. Good nutrition and continued attention to metabolic control help to overcome initial obstacles to successful breast-feeding.

Family planning

Finally, comprehensive perinatal care for the diabetic patient must also provide appropriate family planning advice and services. The postpartum period is a time when patients are eager for contraceptive counseling and most receptive to educational efforts. In general, barrier methods entail the least medical risk along with satisfactory levels of effectiveness for the motivated diabetic woman. Studies have also shown that the IUD may be employed without undue risk of infection. Oral contraceptive treatment entails potential problems with diabetic regulation and long-term cardiovascular complications. Nevertheless, with careful supervision this contraceptive modality may also be considered.

Method A. Duchon
Michael T. Gyves
Irwin R. Merkatz

BIBLIOGRAPHY

Freinkel, N., editor: Second International Workshop-Conference on Gestational Diabetes, Diabetes **34:**(2), Entire issue, 1985.

Fuhrman, K., and others: Prevention of congenital malformations in infants and insulin-dependent diabetic mothers, Diabetes Care **6:**219, 1983.

Goodlin, R.C.: Maternal-fetal acidosis. In Care of the fetus, New York, 1979, Masson Publishing USA, Inc.

Gyves, M.T., and others: A modern approach to management of pregnant diabetics: a two year analysis of outcomes, Am. J. Obstet. Gynecol. **128:**606, 1977.

Hill, E.: Effect of insulin on fetal growth. In Merkatz, I.R., and Adam, P.A.J., editors: The diabetic pregnancy: a perinatal perspective, New York, 1979, Grune & Stratton, Inc.

Jovanovic, J., and others: Feasibility of maintaining normal glucose profiles in insulin-dependent pregnant diabetic women, Am. J. Med. **68:**105, 1980.

Linzey, E.M.: Controlling diabetes with continuous insulin infusion, Contemp. Ob/Gyn. **12:**43, 1978.

Merkatz, I.R., and others: A pilot community based screening program for gestational diabetes, Diabetes Care **3:**453, 1980.

Merkatz, R.B., Budd, K., and Merkatz, I.R.: Psychological and social implications of scientific care for pregnant diabetic women. In Merkatz, I.R., and Adam, P.A.J., editors: Diabetes in pregnancy, Semin. Perinatol. (2):373, 1978.

Miller, E., and others: Elevated maternal hemoglobin A_{1c} in early pregnancy and major congenital anomalies in infants of diabetic mothers, N. Engl. J. Med. **304:**1331, 1981.

O'Sullivan, J.B., and Mahan, C.M.: Criteria for the oral glucose tolerance test in pregnancy, Diabetes **13:**278, 1964.

Pedersen, J., Molsted-Pedersen, L., and Anderson, B.: Assessors of fetal perinatal mortality in diabetic pregnancy, Diabetes **23:**302, 1974.

Chapter 4

Preeclampsia-eclampsia

Preeclampsia-eclampsia (also referred to as *toxemia, pregnancy-induced hypertension*, or *acute hypertension*) is peculiar to pregnancy and is found only in humans. It occurs clinically after the twentieth week of pregnancy and is characterized by the sequential appearance of edema, hypertension, and proteinuria. Its onset is often subtle, and its etiology remains obscure. The pathophysiology of toxemia is well documented; toxemia affects both mother and fetus with the major component being vasospasm. It is the most significant medical problem the mother and fetus encounter during pregnancy, and it may cause death or serious morbidity.

DIAGNOSIS

Preeclampsia may resemble any of the following specific categorical diagnoses if the patient is seen for the first time in the third trimester of pregnancy:

1. True preeclampsia (glomeruloendotheliosis)
2. Chronic hypertension
3. Renal disease
4. Transient hypertension

The differentiation of these diagnoses is often difficult and can be accomplished by a retrospective evaluation of each case or a renal biopsy during the first 5 postpartum days. Renal biopsy is seldom done anymore but in the past has provided answers to many questions about which disease is present. We know that the renal lesion of glomeruloendotheliosis is reversible and subsides after pregnancy.

Mild preeclampsia is defined as the sequential development of more than one of the following conditions after the twentieth week of pregnancy:

1. Edema of the face or hands (a soft sign and not now used for diagnosis)
2. A systolic blood pressure of at least 140 mm Hg or a rise of 30 mm or more above the usual level
3. A diastolic pressure of 90 mm Hg or more or a rise of 15 mm above the usual level
4. Proteinuria of greater than 300 mg/L

The blood pressure during pregnancy should always be taken in the lateral recumbent position on each prenatal visit so that comparisons can be accurately made from various weeks of gestation without uterine pressure interference. Any rise in blood pressure is significant if the increase in systolic pressure exceeds 30 or the increase in diastolic pressure exceeds 15 mm Hg.

The proposed new classification of hypertensive and proteinuric disorders in pregnancy sponsored by WHO and The International Society for the Study of Hypertension in Pregnancy is as follows:

1. Gestational hypertension—hypertension without significant proteinuria (less than 0.3 gm/L) developing
   a. After 30 weeks of gestation
   b. In labor or within 48 hours of delivery
2. Unclassified hypertension in pregnancy—hypertension found when blood pressure is recorded for the first time
   a. After 20 weeks of gestation
   b. In labor or within 48 hours of delivery

   Unclassified hypertension should be reclassified as gestational hypertension if blood pressure returns to normal in the postnatal period, although some of these cases may have underlying hypertension or renal diseases
3. Gestational proteinuria—significant proteinuria (greater than 0.3 gm/L)
   a. After 20 weeks of gestation
   b. In labor or within 48 hours of delivery
4. Preeclampsia—gestational hypertension and significant proteinuria
   a. After 20 weeks of gestation
   b. In labor or within 48 hours of delivery
5. Eclampsia
   a. Antepartum
   b. Intrapartum
   c. Postpartum
6. Underlying hypertension or renal disease; for example, women may have hypertension only during preg-

nancies and be normotensive between pregnancies, but later in life develop sustained hypertension
   a. Underlying hypertension
   b. Underlying renal disease
   c. Other known causes of hypertension (such as pheochromocytoma)
7. Preexisting hypertension or renal hypertension and/or proteinuria in pregnancy; for example, in women known to have disease prior to pregnancy
   a. Preexisting hypertension
   b. Preexisting renal disease
   c. Preexisting proteinuria
   d. Preexisting other known causes of hypertension
8. Superimposed preeclampsia-eclampsia
   a. Preexisting hypertension with superimposed preeclampsia (an increase in hypertension of at least 15 mm Hg diastolic blood pressure above nonpregnancy values plus the development or worsening of proteinuria)
   b. Preexisting hypertension with superimposed eclampsia
   c. Underlying hypertensive disease
   d. Underlying renal disease
   e. Other known causes of hypertension

The term *superimposed preeclampsia* should only be used in cases in which hypertension has been known to be present before pregnancy or is discovered early in pregnancy and proteinuria develops in late pregnancy.

In general, the following chronologic sequence occurs in preeclampsia: edema, an increase in blood pressure, and the appearance of proteinuria. Edema is almost always present but is a soft sign and difficult to evaluate. (The WHO study group agreed not to use it because of this.) Variations in the blood pressure obtained by the same observer may be caused by the vasospasm present in the disease, different environment, position of the pregnant patient, anxiety, activity, and time of day. It is essential that the blood pressure be taken in the lateral recumbent position on each prenatal visit. If a significant increase in systolic pressure (i.e., greater than 30 mm Hg) or a significant increase in diastolic pressure (i.e., greater than 15 mm Hg) is observed, consideration should be given for the development of impending or overt preeclampsia. When the blood pressure is taken in the lateral recumbent position, the effect of the enlarging uterus on large vessels is eliminated, making comparisons in different weeks of gestation more equal. Proteinuria should be present in a clean-catch urine specimen. If proteinuria is present in a significant amount (2+), this most likely indicates the renal lesion of glomeruloendotheliosis and denotes seriousness of the problem.

The normal decrease in peripheral resistance and blood pressure in the middle trimester of pregnancy must be considered. We believe the dip in the midtrimester blood pressure is an artifact resulting from position and changes in cardiac output and blood pressure caused by the enlarging of the uterus. We have shown that if the blood pressure is always taken in the lateral recumbent position, no fall in blood pressure occurs; hence, a rise should be significant. The absolute values in blood pressure may not be as important as a change from baseline pressures. A recently observed phenomenon (roll test) is the increase in blood pressure when the position of a patient is changed. An increase of 20 mm Hg or more diastolic blood pressure from when the patient is on her side after stabilization to when she is rolled on her back (positive) correlates with an increased risk of subsequently developing preeclampsia. The test should be done on *all* primigravida patients on each visit (preferably no longer than 2 weeks apart) starting at 24 weeks of gestation and continuing to term. If the roll test remains negative, it is unusual for the patient to develop preeclampsia. If it is positive, the certainty of the problem is still obscure, but altered vascular reactivity may be present.

Severe preeclampsia is diagnosed if one of the following signs or symptoms is present.

1. Diastolic blood pressure greater than 100 mm Hg
2. Increase in liver enzymes or jaundice
3. Platelets less than 100,000
4. Oliguria less than 400 ml/24 hours
5. Proteinuria greater than 5 gm/L or + + on random sample
6. Epigastric pain
7. Scotomata, visual disturbances, or severe frontal headache
8. Pulmonary edema

The connotations for both mother and fetus are significant in severe preeclampsia.

Chronic hypertension is diagnosed by comparison of blood pressure values in a woman during pregnancy and in a nonpregnant state. In addition, pregnancy may unmask latent hypertension; a diastolic blood pressure of greater than 80 in the first or second trimester bears suspicion. A strong family history of hypertension is also helpful information. The long-term follow-up of patients who manifest hypertension during pregnancy is a means of retrospectively diagnosing whether the patient had preeclampsia or whether she had chronic vascular or renal disease with or without preeclampsia. Long-term studies have shown that preeclampsia does not cause hypertension in subsequent pregnancies or later in life.

ETIOLOGY AND ASSOCIATED FACTORS

The cause or causes of preeclampsia are still unknown. However, certain factors or associations must be included in any etiologic theory of preeclampsia. Preeclampsia is

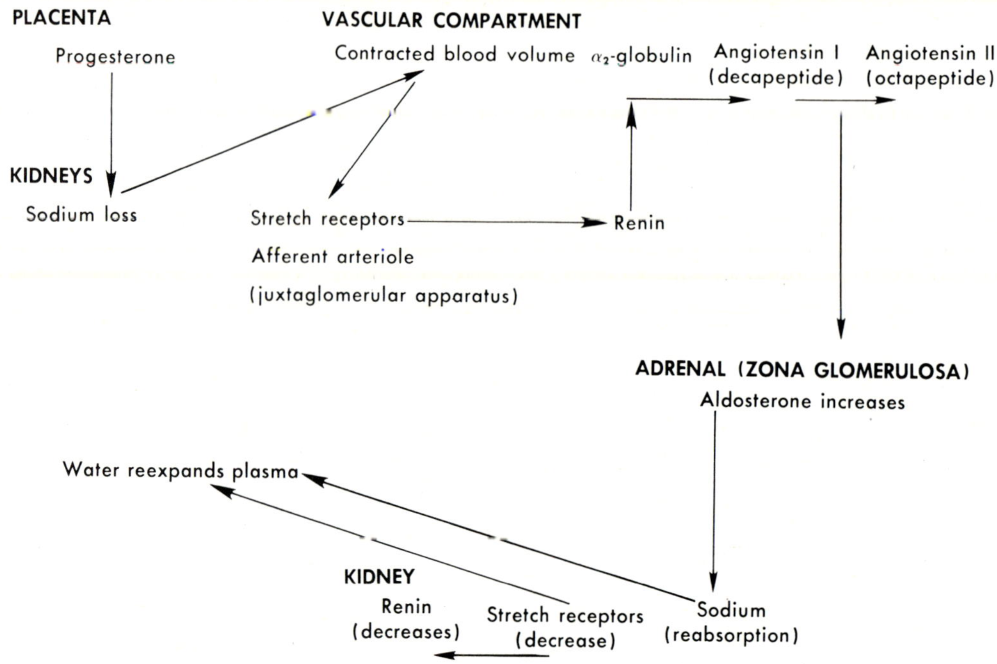

Fig. 4-1. Homeostatic relationships in normal pregnancy.

primarily a disease of the primigravida. Predisposing factors include a first pregnancy carried to term, hyperplacentosis that occurs in diabetes and multiple gestation, uterine anomalies, chronic hypertension and renal disease, and, in a small percentage of patients with recurrent hypertension, a genetic component.

Preeclampsia is seen more often in certain regions of the world, particularly in the southern regions of the United States. The condition occurs more frequently among indigent than private patients, and it is more prevalent as term approaches. It disappears once the uterus is empty. A renal lesion (glomeruloendotheliosis) and a uteroplacental lesion of less dilated spiral arteries are usually present and disappear after pregnancy. Some disruption of pregnancy homeostasis triggers events that eventually lead to preeclampsia (Fig. 4-1).

EPIDEMIOLOGY

The incidence of preeclampsia throughout the United States is estimated to be 5% to 7% of all pregnancies. Reliable statistics on the incidence for large segments of the United States are not available for the hypertensive diseases of pregnancy. The problem is compounded further by erroneous diagnoses often made in this disease syndrome, and the recording of statistics is customarily an inpatient hospital procedure rather than an outpatient responsibility. In their international survey of eclampsia, Doll and Hanington cite the incidence in different countries as varying between 1.2 and 2.6 per 1,000 deliveries. Most studies have only dealt with severe disease and not just preeclampsia. Fortunately, eclampsia in the United States is uncommon and occurs in less than 1 in 1,000 deliveries.

PATHOGENESIS

The normal homeostatic relationship during pregnancy (Fig. 4-1) becomes disrupted in preeclampsia. During uncomplicated pregnancies, the placenta produces an increased amount of progesterone, which contributes to a minor sodium loss because progesterone is a mild diuretic. This sodium loss results in contraction of the blood volume in the vascular compartment, which in turn activates the stretch receptor afferent arteriole and the juxtaglomerular apparatus to produce renin. Renin activates α_2-globulin in the blood, which is converted to angiotensin I and, by another enzyme, to angiotensin II. The angiotensin, in turn, acts on the zona glomerulosa of the adrenal gland to produce an increased amount of aldosterone as a compensatory mechanism. This increases the reabsorption of sodium from the renal tubule and subsequently reexpands the water in the vascular compartment, thus decreasing the stimulus on the stretch receptors, which then decreases renin production.

This homeostatic mechanism is altered by the pathophysiology seen in preeclampsia, including (1) a disease of arterioles, (2) a compromised metabolic function, (3) an increased central nervous system (CNS) irritability, (4) a decrease in renal function, (5) an increased catabolism, and (6) a decreased vascular volume. The scheme

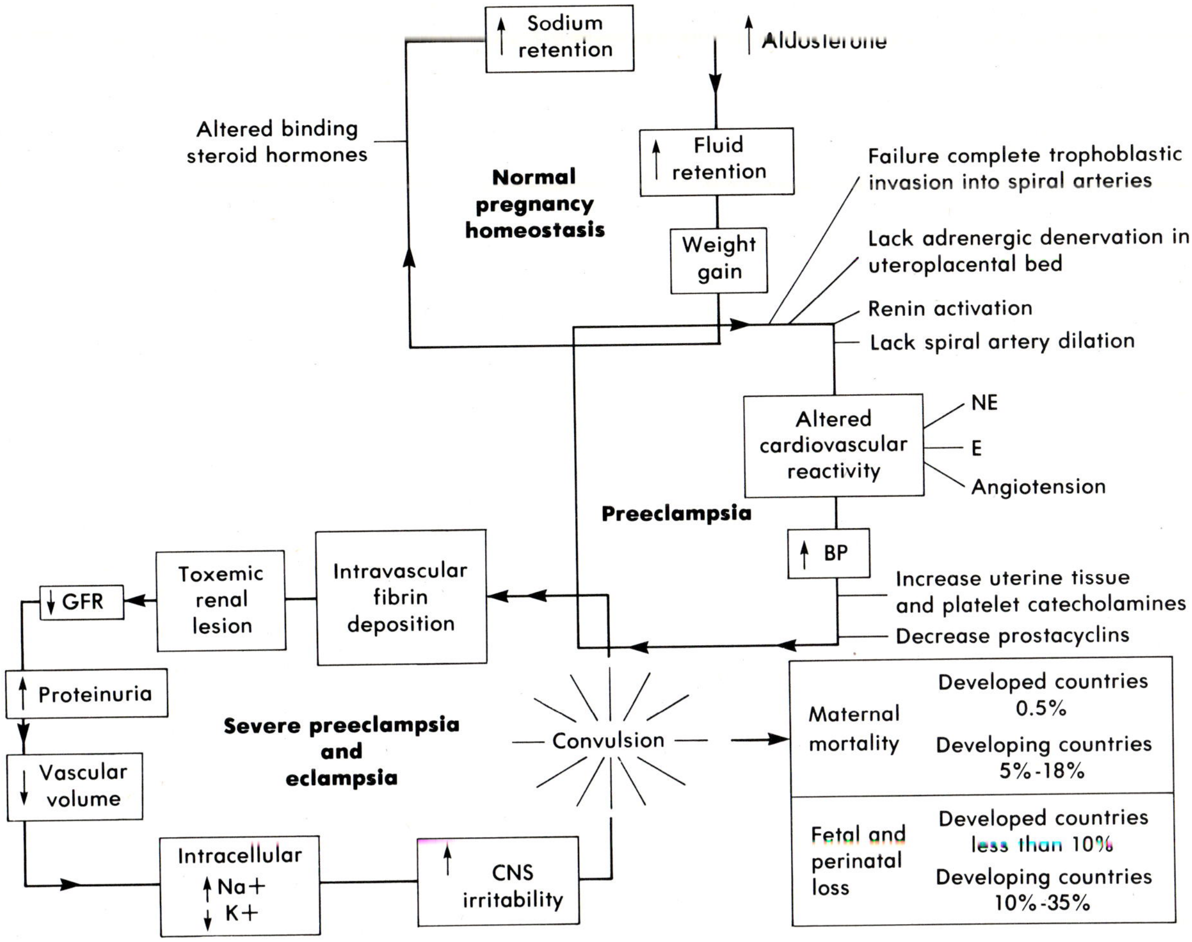

Fig. 4-2. Pathophysiology of preeclampsia-eclampsia.

in Fig. 4-2 represents the development of altered homeostasis in preeclampsia. The increased steroids and binding hormones contribute to the sodium retention and weight gain seen in normal pregnancy. There is also an increased aldosterone secretion rate in normal pregnancy, which is associated with an increased retention of fluid. The unaffected pregnant patient can easily handle this excess salt load until a renal lesion develops. The beginning of preeclampsia may be associated with an incomplete invasion of trophoblastic cells into the spiral arteries of the uterus with associated increase in tissue norepinephrine and decreased production of prostacyclin. Renin activation triggers events that, along with sodium retention in vessel walls, contribute to the altered cardiovascular reactivity. The preeclamptic patient hyperresponds to pressor infusions such as epinephrine, norepinephrine, and angiotensin. A lesion most likely exists in the uteroplacental bed involving the spiral arteries of the mother. The trophoblastic invasion of the spiral arteries is incomplete in patients who develop preeclampsia. This incomplete invasion of trophoblastic tissue, which replaces the musculoelastic tissue of the spiral artery, results in an inability of the spiral artery to dilate as much as seen in the physiologic dilation of the spiral artery. This, coupled with the relative lack of adrenergic denervation at the base of the spiral artery, further contributes to the vasospasm and constriction of the spiral artery, which ultimately results in a relative decrease in nutrients and gases to the fetus. Biopsies of the uteroplacental bed at the time of cesarean section in severe preeclamptic patients indicate elevated tissue levels of norepinephrine. This is probably part of the generalized vasospasm seen in preeclampsia. There is intravascular fibrin deposition, which may contribute to the development of the "toxemic lesion" (glomeruloendotheliosis); this may decrease the glomerular filtration rate and result in increased proteinuria. Glomeruloendotheliosis consists of a reversible swelling of the endothelial cytoplasm without involving other structures. The severe preeclamptic patient may also become oliguric.

Vasospasm and altered cardiovascular reactivity are hallmarks of preeclampsia. Endogenous pressor substances may contribute to this hyperreactivity. The vasospasm of the arterioles is associated with a decrease in dilating prostacyclins and an increase in constricting norepinephrine in uterine tissues and platelets. This decreases blood flow to vital organs, especially the uterus, compromising placental function and placing the fetus in a precarious position for survival. Intrauterine growth retardation indicates prolonged vasoconstriction and poor placental nutrition. In all probability this altered uterine blood flow and decreased placental nutrition contribute to the stillbirths that occur in the severe forms of preeclampsia-eclampsia.

Sodium is retained in patients with preeclampsia. There is an increase in the sodium space and in the total exchangeable sodium. Severe disease is associated with an increase in intracellular sodium concentration and a decrease in intracellular potassium concentration. These changes in sodium balance may explain both the increased cardiovascular reactivity in vessel walls and the increase in CNS irritability. The latter is easily demonstrated by testing for hyperactive reflexes. As preeclampsia worsens, the CNS irritability increases. Signs of CNS irritability, such as apprehension and anxiety, often precede a convulsion and are difficult to evaluate.

Hemoconcentration also occurs as the preeclamptic condition worsens. Fluid and electrolytes may shift to the third space and decrease the blood volume, but the serum electrolytes are normal. The blood volume of the relatively severe preeclamptic patient may approach that of a nonpregnant patient; a deficit of 1,000 ml or more is not unusual. The hematocrit value is high from hemoconcentration when the ill preeclamptic-eclamptic patient is initially seen. Subsequently, therapy and mobilization of fluid from the extracellular compartment, as diuresis occurs, lead to a decreased hematocrit value and can be viewed as a positive response to therapy. A positive nitrogen balance is usually seen in the unaffected pregnant patient; however, in the severe preeclamptic-eclamptic patient there is a negative antepartum nitrogen balance and a positive postpartum nitrogen balance.

CLINICAL MANIFESTATIONS

It is often difficult to distinguish between abnormal fluid retention in the pregnant patient and early signs of preeclampsia. Intrauterine growth retardation is not present in most cases of preeclampsia but has been observed in cases of severe preeclampsia and eclampsia in which the disease was present for some time; in these cases intrauterine growth retardation indicates prolonged vasoconstriction.

Laboratory studies in all but the severe cases are usually within normal limits except that the hematocrit reading may show hemoconcentration. As the disease progresses, more abnormal findings may appear, as indicated in Table 4-1.

The most severe maternal and fetal complications obviously result in death. Perinatal mortality is in the vicinity of 10% in developed countries. During the past four decades, maternal mortality associated with preeclampsia-eclampsia has gradually decreased to less than 1% in developed countries. The incidence of maternal and fetal mortality is in direct proportion to the severity of the toxemia, as well as whether it occurs in a developed or developing country. There is an increased frequency of prematurity and neonatal death in pregnancies complicated by severe toxemia. The overall perinatal mortality per 1,000 total births is increased two to three times over the expected perinatal mortality in unaffected patients. Perinatal mortality is partially dependent on the stage of gestation in which severe preeclampsia occurs and should be less than 10% in developed countries.

Abruptio placentae occurs more frequently in patients who have acute hypertension (preeclampsia) during pregnancy and is more common in patients who have chronic hypertension. A review of 39 cases of *hypofibrinogenemia* revealed that 54% were associated with abruptio placentae and 23% were associated with preeclampsia-eclampsia. Hypofibrinogenemia is not clinically diagnosed until the fibrinogen level is 100 mg or less. The patient with severe toxemia of pregnancy

Table 4-1. Positive laboratory findings with level of hypertension

Condition	Hematocrit	Electrolytes	Serum creatinine (mg/dl)	Liver enzymes	Fibrinogen and split enzymes	Proteinuria	Antithrombin III
Normal	↓	Normal	0.4-0.6	Normal	Normal	0	>80%
Mild preeclampsia	↓	Normal	0.4-0.6	Normal	Normal	1+	<80%
Severe preeclampsia	↑	Normal	0.6-0.8	Normal	Normal	2+	<70%
Eclampsia	↑↑	Normal	Above 0.8	Elevated	Occasional ↓ fibrinogen and ↑ split products	4+	<70%

should be followed with serial fibrinogen and other coagulation determinations, most importantly platelet determinations.

The severe preeclamptic patient occasionally may exhibit clinical signs of hemolysis as manifested by jaundice and dark-colored urine, which should be considered a bad omen. It is not known whether this represents hepatocellular damage or red blood cell destruction from other causes. These patients may have abnormal liver enzyme function and a decrease in fibrinogen. Periportal necrosis of the liver is a common autopsy finding in eclampsia and partial or complete rupture of the liver may be seen.

Cerebral hemorrhage and cerebral edema are the most common causes of death in preeclampsia-eclampsia. Convulsions may occur secondary to cerebral hemorrhage, cerebral edema, or electrolyte imbalance and create added risks of aspiration, pneumonia, and trauma. Temporary loss of vision lasting for as long as 7 days has been observed. Hemorrhage occasionally occurs in the eyegrounds of a patient and should warn the clinician of an impending vascular accident. These patients require vigorous antihypertensive therapy with parenteral hydralazine to control symptoms and blood pressure, maintaining a diastolic pressure under 100 and over 80 mm Hg.

Intrauterine growth retardation may be associated with preeclampsia-eclampsia if the disease is present for a protracted time period (see Chapter 7).

PREVENTION

To prevent toxemia of pregnancy, one would have to eliminate many of the ills of society, including poor nutrition with low protein intake, overcrowding, limited antenatal care, poor education concerning reproduction, and lack of bed rest. Therefore, the health care team's main effort in prevention must be in the identification and optimum management of those patients in whom the risk of preeclampsia is known to be greatest. All primigravidas should be considered at high risk. Prevention should include (1) a nutritious diet high in protein (1 gm protein/kg/day), (2) bed rest at noon for 45 minutes, then 1 additional hour prior to dinner, (3) recognition of patient responsibility for pregnancy, and (4) frequent prenatal visits to the physician (every 2 weeks after 28 weeks).

The characteristics of patients at risk are:

1. Primigravida
2. Poverty
3. Lower level of education
4. Poor protein intake
5. Teenage primigravida
6. Diabetes, renal disease, chronic hypertension
7. Uterine anomalies
8. Hyperplacentosis as seen in multiple gestation and diabetes
9. Hydramnios

Patients with the above profile should be seen more frequently (every 2 to 3 weeks) since intensive prenatal care is essential to prevent development of preeclampsia or to recognize its onset. The roll test should be used regularly after week 24 of pregnancy, and if it remains negative, it gives reassurance that impending preeclampsia is *not* present. When patients with risk factors are identified early in pregnancy and seen at frequent intervals, these patients can be managed with a regimen that will prevent severe forms of preeclampsia. Hospitalization should be considered once a patient progresses beyond the clinical stage of abnormal fluid retention and has proteinuric hypertension (preeclampsia). The incidence of severe preeclampsia-eclampsia can be significantly decreased by early recognition of preeclampsia and by its aggressive hospital management. *Outpatient diuretic and antihypertensive therapies have no place in the management of preeclampsia.*

TREATMENT

All therapy for preeclampsia-eclampsia is empiric because the basic etiologic mechanism is unknown. Early hospitalization and proper care will almost completely eliminate the severe manifestations of preeclampsia and decrease maternal and fetal mortality and morbidity. Long-term prophylactic use of diuretics in pregnancy does not alter the incidence of preeclampsia, hypertension, prematurity, congenital anomalies, or perinatal mortality and should not be used.

Once a patient is hospitalized and receiving therapy, convulsions should rarely occur. If reflexes are hyperactive, an intravenous infusion of magnesium sulfate is given. The concern in the preeclamptic patient is primarily for the fetus because maternal mortality is rare. The timing of delivery can be aided by evaluation of amniotic fluid for maturity as well as other clinical factors of the disease (see Chapters 9 and 28).

The *mild preeclamptic patient* should be placed in the hospital at complete bed rest but given bathroom privileges; she should be positioned on her side and weighed daily. She should be restricted to a sodium intake of less than 4 gm per day, given a protein intake of 70 gm or more per day, and given mild sedatives, such as phenobarbital (30 mg four times a day). Diuresis should begin by 36 hours with this regimen. If there is a mild blood pressure rise, it usually returns to normal. The disease usually improves symptomatically, and often in 3 to 5 days the patient may be discharged from the hospital *under careful outpatient care*. However, if the gestation period is 37 weeks or more, the patient should be considered for induction of labor following control of the preeclampsia.

The patient with *severe preeclampsia* should be hospitalized and placed on her side at bed rest with bathroom privileges. She is weighed daily; intake and output are recorded; baseline laboratory studies are done, including liver enzymes, hematologic studies, and renal function studies, which include a 24-hour urine specimen collected for protein. An amniocentesis should be performed to evaluate fetal maturity. A 4 gm sodium diet containing 70 gm of protein is given, and the patient is given mild sedatives, such as phenobarbital (30 mg four times a day). The blood pressure is observed every 4 hours. Diuresis can be expected to occur within 24 to 48 hours, and the patient's condition should improve. If the patient has preeclampsia, her weight loss while she is on this regimen should exceed 2 kg in 3 days.

Unfortunately, some patients do not improve, and their condition deteriorates in spite of hospital management. Delivery must be considered in these patients. If the mother's condition and therapeutic control permit, induction of labor should be delayed until fetal pulmonary maturity is documented in the amniotic fluid. We have used betamethasone (12 mg IM 12 hours apart for 2 doses) to mature the lungs if the patient is less than 34 weeks' gestation. No worsening of the hypertension occurred. If the patient is beyond 34 weeks' gestation or the pulmonary maturity is adequate, the fetus should be delivered. The fetus of a severely preeclamptic-eclamptic patient usually has few problems with respiratory distress syndrome. The toxemic patient may have a vaginal delivery by oxytocin induction regardless of the condition of the cervix; delivery should occur in less than 18 hours or a cesarean section is done. Abdominal delivery may be indicated for maternal reasons or for fetal distress or because of insufficient progress of labor with oxytocin induction.

The reflexes may be hyperactive in the severe preeclamptic patient, and this is an indication for magnesium sulfate therapy, which should be administered even if the diagnosis is not certain. The magnesium sulfate is administered by infusion pump or by an intravenous infusion: 10 to 20 gm of magnesium sulfate is added to 1,000 ml of 5% dextrose and water. The rate of administration is approximately 1 to 2 gm per hour after a slowly administered loading dose of 4 to 6 gm. If magnesium sulfate is administered, the reflexes are monitored at frequent intervals (hourly); urinary output should be in excess of 100 ml every 4 hours and respirations should be more than 12 per minute. Diuretics or hypotensive agents should not be used routinely in severe preeclampsia or eclampsia. Antihypertensive therapy should be given to prevent a cerebrovascular accident or if CNS symptoms persist. A diastolic pressure above 100 mm Hg should be an indication for hypotensive therapy. If a hypotensive agent is used, however, the diastolic pressure should not be reduced below 80 mm Hg. Hydralazine hydrochloride (Apresoline) by bolus injection (5 mg), later followed by infusion pump administration (100 mg in 200 ml saline) has been used successfully in controlling hypertension. Methyldopa (Aldomet) may also be given; this medication takes longer to act, however. Diazoxide is not indicated in these acute problems in pregnancy because hypotension often develops after therapy, which is especially hazardous to the fetus.

The uterus should be emptied within a short period of time when the patient is ill. When labor is induced, the severely preeclamptic patient delivers the fetus readily because of the characteristically increased uterine activity in the toxemic patient. Oxytocin is given by infusion pump in small doses starting at 0.5 mU, and increased to achieve the desired uterine activity. Uterine pressures and fetal heart rate should be monitored electronically during labor. Cesarean section is reserved for obstetric indications, not for preeclampsia-eclampsia itself, unless the fetus is less than 1,500 gm and the cervix unfavorable, then cesarean section might be considered (Fig. 4-3).

Once a patient with preeclampsia develops a convulsion and eclampsia is diagnosed, the survival statistics for both mother and fetus decrease dramatically. The following treatment regimen has resulted in near zero maternal mortality and less than 10% fetal mortality if the fetus was alive when the eclamptic patient was seen. The basic therapy is with magnesium sulfate. No diuretics are used, and antihypertensive therapy (hydralazine) is used if the diastolic blood pressure exceeds 100 mm Hg or if CNS symptoms persist.

Self-injury to the oral passages can be prevented during a convulsion by use of padded tongue blades. They should be available at the bedside in labor and delivery rooms. A plastic airway is inserted following the convulsion, and oxygen is administered. Adequate suctioning of the oral passages and the Trendelenburg position are necessary to prevent aspiration. The stomach contents should be aspirated by a nasogastric tube, preferably after adequate control with magnesium sulfate has been achieved. If this is done, an antacid should be instilled before removal of the tube. The antacid will increase the pH of the gastric contents and help prevent aspiration complications. Magnesium sulfate, 4 to 6 gm, is given *slowly* and intravenously over a period of 5 minutes to control the convulsion. A Foley catheter is inserted, and urinary output is recorded hourly; the specific gravity and albumin of the urine are determined every 6 to 8 hours and in pooled 24-hour specimens. If the patient is not convulsing, the initial loading dose of magnesium sulfate is 4 to 6 gm given intravenously, fol-

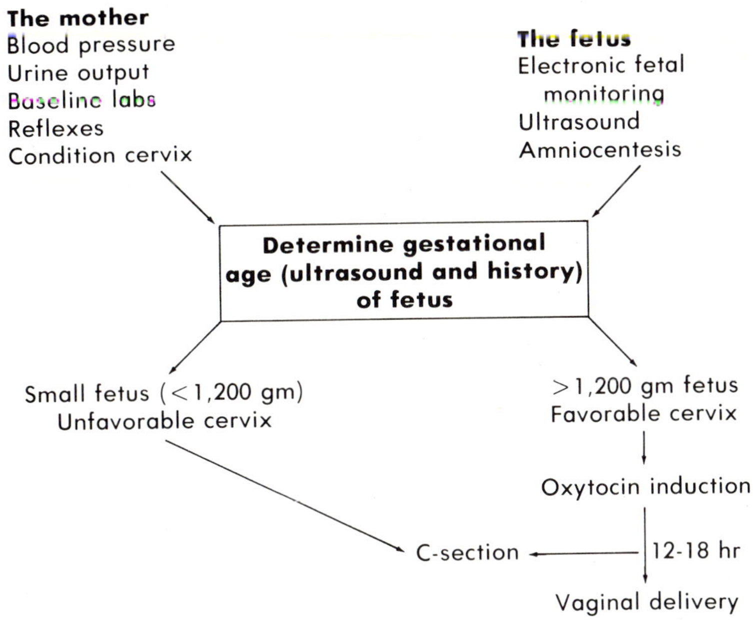

Fig. 4-3. Perinatal management of severe preeclampsia-eclampsia.

lowed by 1 to 2 gm per hour. Infusion pump administration is preferable. If additional magnesium sulfate is needed because of hyperactive patellar reflexes, it can be injected into the intravenous tubing. Therapeutic amounts of magnesium also act as a mild sedative. Calcium gluconate should be kept at the bedside and 1 gm administered intravenously for magnesium overdosage (rare). Patellar reflexes should always be present, but they should be hypoactive when optimum magnesium sulfate therapy has been achieved. The urinary output should exceed 25 to 30 ml per hour if magnesium sulfate is being administered. If urinary excretion decreases below this level, the magnesium sulfate dosage should be decreased or stopped; if diuresis occurs, the dosage should be increased since its excretion is predominantly by the kidney.

Because magnesium sulfate is a potentially dangerous drug, maternal reflexes, respiratory rate, blood pressure, heart rate, and urinary output must be monitored during its administration. The clinical manifestations of increasing levels of magnesium sulfate are a disappearance of knee jerks, a decrease in respiration, and cardiac arrest. Furthermore, it is synergistic when used with curare-like drugs. Although it is not a hypotensive drug, an initial transient decline in blood pressure may be observed, and it may decrease variability on a fetal heart pattern tracing. When administered for appropriate indications, in the optimum dose with adequate monitoring, the benefits of magnesium sulfate for the toxemic mother and her fetus outweigh the fetal and neonatal risks. The magnesium level in the newborn is the same as in the mother; thus, if a cord blood magnesium level is not measured, a maternal value is equally good. Most of the magnesium is excreted by the newborn in the first 12 hours of life, and it is completely excreted by 36 hours. Intensive observation of the newborn is indicated for signs of neuromuscular depression. (See Chapter 37, part two.)

The mild forms of preeclampsia are not associated with an increased fetal or maternal loss; however, the severe forms of preeclampsia-eclampsia are associated with an increase in fetal loss and in maternal mortality. If the cause of hypertension during pregnancy is not diagnosed, a renal biopsy may be indicated during the postpartum period. The long-term prognosis of both mother and fetus needs critical evaluation. Adequate studies on infants born of toxemic mothers have not been done. Follow-up studies on the long-term prognosis for the mother have shown that eclampsia does not contribute to residual cardiovascular disease.

Frederick P. Zuspan

BIBLIOGRAPHY

Brewer, T.H.: Role of malnutrition, hepatic dysfunction, and gastrointestinal bacteria in the pathogenesis of acute toxemia of pregnancy, Am. J. Obstet. Gynecol. **84**:1253, 1962.

Bryans, C.I., Jr., Southerland, W.L., and Zuspan, F.P.: Eclampsia; a longterm follow-up study, Obstet. Gynecol. **21**:701, 1963.

Chesley, L.C.: Toxemia of pregnancy in relation to chronic hypertension, West. J. Surg. **64**:284, 1956.

Cobo, E.: Uterine hypercontractility in toxemia of pregnancy, Am. J. Obstet. Gynecol. **90**:505, 1964.

Doll, R., and Hanington, E.: International survey of eclampsia and preeclampsia, 1958-1959: epidemiologic aspects, Pathol. Microbiol. (Basel) **24**:531, 1961.

Gant, N.F., and others: A clinical test useful for predicting the development of acute hypertension in pregnancy, Am. J. Obstet. Gynecol. **120**:1, 1974.

Iams, J.D., and others: Blood pressure response in hypertensive pregnancies treated with cortisol, Clin. Exp. Hyperten. Preg. **2**:923, 1980.

Madry, J.T.: Blood coagulation defects during pregnancy, Obstet. Gynecol. **20**:235, 1962.

O'Shaughnessy, R., and others: Plasma and platelet catecholamines in normal and preeclamptic pregnancy, Clin. Exp. Hyperten. Preg. **3B**:224, 1984.

Pritchard, J.A.: Changes in the blood volume during pregnancy and delivery, Anesthesiology **26**:393, 1965.

Pritchard, J.A., and Stone, S.R.: Clinical and laboratory observations on eclampsia, Am. J. Obstet. Gynecol. **99**:754, 1967.

Spargo, B., McCartney, C.P., and Winemiller, R.: Glomerular capillary endotheliosis in toxemia of pregnancy, Arch. Pathol. **68**:593, 1959.

Talledo, O.E., Chesley, L.C., and Zuspan, F.P.: Renin-angiotensin system in normal and toxemic pregnancies. III. Differential sensitivity to angiotensin II and norepinephrine in toxemia of pregnancy, Am. J. Obstet. Gynecol. **100**:218, 1968.

Talledo, O.E., and Zuspan, F.P.: Spontaneous uterine contractility in eclampsia, Clin. Obstet. Gynecol. **9**:910, 1966.

Weenink, G.H., and others: Plasma antithrombin III levels in preeclampsia, Clin. Exp. Hyperten. Preg. **2B**:145, 1983.

Weiner, C.P., and Brandt, J.: Plasma antithrombin III activity in normal pregnancy, Obstet. Gynecol. **56**:601, 1980.

Zuspan, F.P.: Treatment of severe preeclampsia and eclampsia, Clin. Obstet. Gynecol. **9**:954, 1966.

Zuspan, F.P.: Problems encountered in the treatment of pregnancy-induced hypertension, Am. J. Obstet. Gynecol. **131**:591, 1978.

Zuspan, F.P., and Bell, J.D.: Variable salt-loading during pregnancy with preeclampsia, Obstet. Gynecol. **18**:530, 1961.

Zuspan, F.P., Nelson, G.H., and Ahlquist, R.P.: Epinephrine infusions in normal and toxemic pregnancy. I. Nonesterified fatty acids and cardiovascular alterations, Am. J. Obstet. Gynecol. **90**:88, 1964.

Zuspan, F.P., and Talledo, O.E.: Factors affecting delivery in eclampsia: condition of the cervix and uterine activity, Am. J. Obstet. Gynecol. **100**:672, 1968.

Zuspan, F.P., and Ward, M.C.: Improved fetal salvage in eclampsia, Obstet. Gynecol. **26**:893, 1965.

CHAPTER 5

Erythroblastosis fetalis

Erythroblastosis fetalis is a condition of the fetus and newborn caused by the transplacental passage of maternal IgG antibodies, which react with antigens on the fetal red blood cells (RBCs). In most instances the mother becomes immunized by the antigen on the fetal erythrocytes from a previous pregnancy, abortion, or blood transfusion. During a subsequent pregnancy the destruction of the fetal RBCs by maternal antibodies causes a severe hemolytic anemia that may result in congestive heart failure and fetal death. Severely affected neonates show the characteristic stigmata of hydrops fetalis: edema, hepatosplenomegaly, cardiomegaly, and extramedullary erythropoiesis. Rh immunization generally progresses in severity with successive pregnancies. See Chapter 32 for a further discussion of this disorder and Chapter 6 for hydrops fetalis.

HISTORY

Accounts of erythroblastosis fetalis date as far back as 400 BC, when Hippocrates described a syndrome similar to hydrops fetalis. Although many descriptive reports appeared subsequently, the etiology of the condition was not discovered until 1939, when Levine and Stetson described an atypical agglutinin in the blood of a woman who had a transfusion reaction when transfused with apparently compatible blood following the birth of a stillborn, macerated fetus. They postulated that the maternal immunization was the result of a fetal antigen inherited from the father and lacking in the mother.

EPIDEMIOLOGY

Before the advent of passive immunization with Rh immune globulin, erythroblastosis fetalis occurred in approximately 1% of pregnancies. Increasing use of Rh immune globulin, beginning in 1968, has markedly decreased the frequency of this condition. However, there are many individuals still in their childbearing years who are already immunized. In addition, a significant number of newly immunized pregnancies occur each year due to three causes: immunizations occurring during pregnancy, failure to administer the Rh immune globulin after delivery, and failure to administer a dose of Rh immune globulin sufficient to cover a large antigenic stimulus. Before effective treatment of this condition, 20% of the affected infants were stillborn and another 50% died in the neonatal period or suffered permanent brain damage. Today the practices of early identification of the patient at risk, serial antibody titers, amniotic fluid analysis for bilirubin, fetal maturity studies, preterm delivery, neonatal exchange transfusions, and occasionally intrauterine transfusions have contributed to a lowered perinatal mortality of 8% to 9% of Rh-immunized patients.

DIAGNOSIS

Erythroblastosis fetalis encompasses a broad clinical spectrum. It can vary from mild disease that the newborn can overcome without therapy, to moderate disease requiring postnatal exchange transfusions, to severe fetal disease necessitating intrauterine transfusions. A careful history should include data on previous pregnancies and possible blood transfusions. ABO and Rh blood types should be determined in all patients, and antibody screening should be done on the initial antepartum visit regardless of the blood type of the individual. Today, the indirect Coombs' test is done at 28 weeks' gestation. If it is negative, the mother is given $Rh_o(D)$ immune globulin (RhIG). If the indirect Coombs' test is positive, the pregnancy is evaluated for the severity of the erythroblastosis fetalis. Although erythroblastosis fetalis is usually more severe in pregnancies following the initial immunization, as many as 20% of fetuses in the first Rh-immunized pregnancy are severely affected, and the perinatal mortality in this group is significant. The incidence of immunization in the first full-term pregnancy in the absence of a history of exposure to Rh-positive blood is 1% to 2% at the time of delivery if RhIG was not administered.

IgM (saline-reacting) antibodies may be detected in

early immunizations. These are generally transient. IgG (albumin-reacting) antibodies are detected when the IgM antibodies appear or shortly thereafter. Although the IgM antibodies disappear, the IgG antibodies do not. When a patient is immunized to the Rh antigen, she is immunized for life. The titer may decrease to a level where it is barely detectable, but further exposure to the Rh antigen generally invokes an anamnestic response with a substantial rise in the antibody titer.

In the *first immunized pregnancy* serial antibody determinations showing a rise in antibody titer indicate that the fetus is Rh positive. Serial antibody titers in this instance will usually reflect the condition of the fetus. Each laboratory should establish the "critical level" below which intrauterine death resulting from erythroblastosis fetalis has not occurred. For the optimum management of the Rh-negative patient, it is necessary to know when the anti-Rh_0(D) antibody first appeared. Once antibodies have been detected, titers should be repeated frequently until the "critical titer" is reached. At this point amniotic fluid analysis is required to assess the severity of the condition.

In *subsequent immunized pregnancies* the antibody titer may be of value only for indicating when other diagnostic procedures should be employed. If the antibody titer is low, a significant rise may indicate an Rh-positive fetus. If the antibody titer is high initially, the titer may rise, fall, or remain unchanged irrespective of the antigenic properties of the fetal RBCs. Therefore, in patients who have been previously immunized, serial antibody titers are not a reliable method of evaluating the status of the fetus. In these instances the amniotic fluid must be evaluated to assess the fetal condition. The time of the initial amniocentesis depends primarily on the patient's obstetric history and antibody titer. In general, the first amniocentesis should be performed at about 28 weeks' gestation unless a poor obstetric history or an antibody titer indicates that it should be performed earlier. Rarely is amniocentesis required before 22 weeks' gestation, since experience has shown that fetuses requiring an intrauterine transfusion earlier than 22 weeks' gestation are rarely saved. Once amniocentesis is initiated, it should be repeated at regular intervals until delivery.

CLINICAL MANIFESTATIONS

In 1956 Bevis reported a correlation between increased amniotic fluid blood pigments and the severity of erythroblastosis fetalis. There are several methods of analyzing amniotic fluid, all of which are based on the amount of indirect bilirubin pigment present; they provide an excellent index of the fetal condition. The various methods of analyzing the amniotic fluid have the same objectives: (1) to prevent intrauterine death of the affected fetus and (2) to prevent premature delivery of the unaffected or the mildly affected fetus. Most methods use a spectrophotometric scan of amniotic fluid to quantitate the amount of bilirubin pigments present. The pattern of these pigments is compared with the normal amniotic fluid pattern one would expect in an unaffected fetus at that stage of gestation. Based on the bilirubin values, the trend of these values, and studies of fetal maturity, a decision as to the appropriate time for delivery or the need for an intrauterine transfusion can be made. In general, rising bilirubin levels indicate a poor prognosis, whereas decreasing bilirubin levels indicate a good prognosis.

Most affected infants should be delivered before term. Mildly affected fetuses should be allowed to remain in utero until 38 weeks. More severely affected infants should be delivered as soon as fetal maturity is established or at that point at which the risk of infant death from prematurity is less than the expected mortality (5% per procedure by an experienced team) from intrauterine transfusions. In the very severely affected fetus requiring intrauterine transfusions, amniotic fluid frequently is not a reliable means of assessing the condition of the fetus after the first transfusion. The amniotic fluid may be contaminated with blood or meconium. In these instances, once an intrauterine transfusion has been performed, it is continued at regular intervals of 10 to 20 days until delivery. In addition to the analysis of amniotic fluid, some indication of fetal well-being can be obtained by observing fetal heart size, progressive absorption of blood, and absence of fetal ascites with ultrasound scanning. The oxytocin challenge tests (OCTs) may be helpful, but maternal estriol values (Chapter 8) are not. Although high maternal estriol levels indicate the adequacy of metabolic pathways, dependent on a well-functioning fetoplacental unit, the values themselves are not good indices of the severity of erythroblastosis fetalis.

MANAGEMENT

See Table 5-1.

Amniocentesis should always be preceded by placental localization with ultrasound to decrease the chance of placental injury. Fig. 5-1 is a transverse ultrasound section of a patient with a large anterior placenta. The transabdominal approach is always used. Fig. 5-2 shows how ultrasound scanning can be used to find a placenta-free window for amniocentesis. The needle is usually directed toward the area of the fetal small parts (Fig. 5-3). With careful ultrasound scanning, a placenta-free window can be found in most patients. Rarely, an amniocentesis may be done by displacing the fetal head upward, holding the head with one hand, and inserting the needle with the other. Objections to this technique are that it is cumbersome and manipulative and that the amniocentesis is done in the area of the maternal bladder. The needle puncture site is also closer to the cervix, and

Table 5-1. Management of erythroblastosis fetalis

Status	Management
No antibodies	No disease Repeat antibody determinations at 28 weeks, and if negative, give RhIG
First immunized pregnancy	Antibodies less than critical value indicate a good prognosis Follow every 2 to 3 weeks with Rh titer to detect significant rise and avoid amniocentesis Antibodies at critical level or greater Amniocentesis after 25 to 26 weeks' gestation; low values indicate repeat amniocenteses every 3 to 4 weeks; high values indicate repeat amniocenteses every 1 to 2 weeks to establish trend
Subsequent immunized pregnancy	Amniocentesis indicated after 21 weeks' gestation: low values indicate repeat amniocenteses every 2 to 3 weeks; high values indicate repeat amniocenteses every 1 to 2 weeks to establish trend and to determine if intrauterine transfusion is indicated

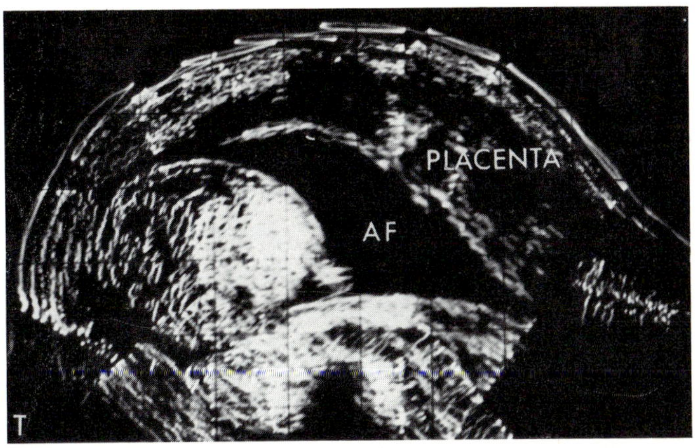

Fig. 5-1. Transverse ultrasound section of a patient with a large anterior placenta. Note the pocket of amniotic fluid *(AF)* and the fetal thorax on the patient's right side.

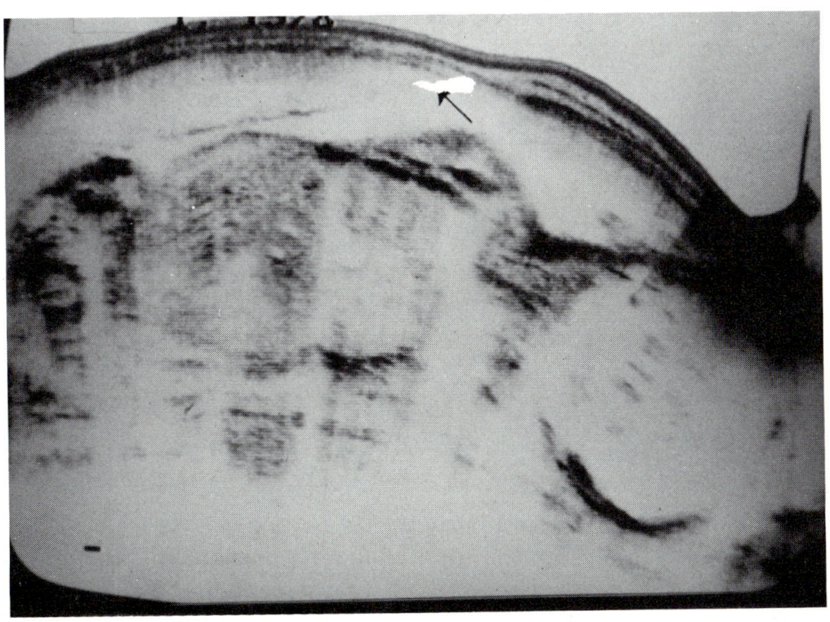

Fig. 5-2. Longitudinal ultrasound scan of patient with an anterior placenta. The arrow points to the lower edge of the placenta.

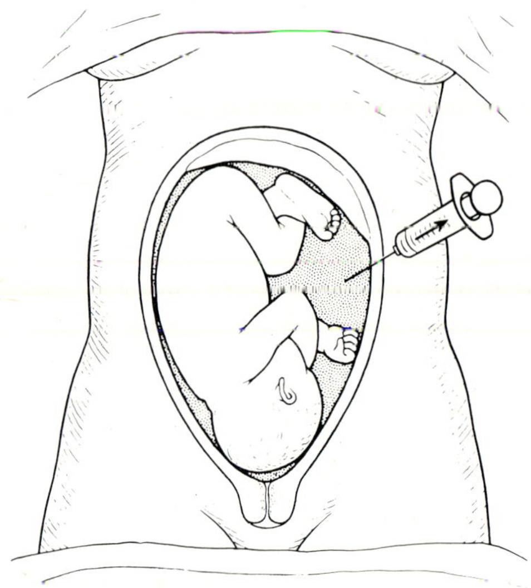

Fig. 5-3. Amniocentesis in the area of the fetal small parts. (From Queenan, J.T.: Clin. Obstet. Gynecol. **9:**491, 1966.)

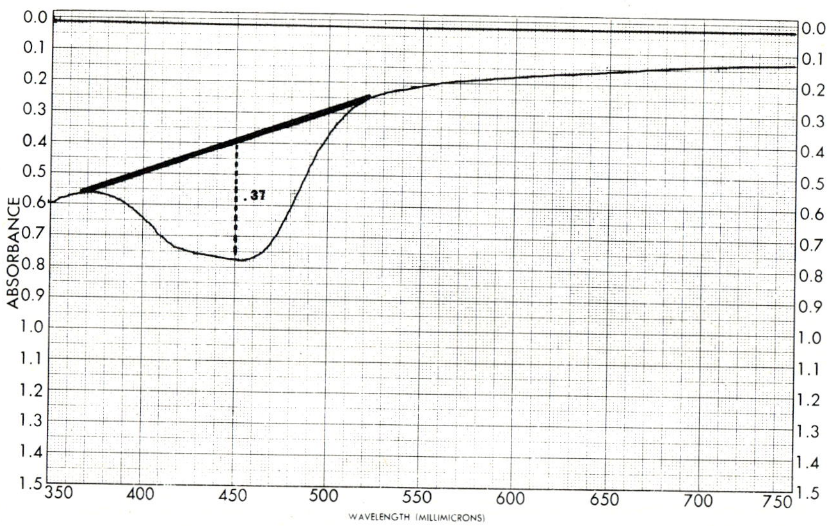

Fig. 5-4. Spectrophotometric scan demonstrating a typical "bilirubin hump" in a patient with severe erythroblastosis fetalis. The deviation in optical density at 450 nm is 0.37. (From Queenan, J.T.: Clin. Obstet. Gynecol. **9:**491, 1966.)

leakage of amniotic fluid may be more likely.

If a bloody specimen of amniotic fluid is obtained, a Betke-Kleihauer test smear should be done to determine if the blood is fetal. In 90% of instances the blood is maternal. There have been no reported cases of severe maternal hemorrhage caused by amniocentesis. If fetal blood is obtained and the fetus is viable, then the fetal heart rate (FHR) should be monitored for several hours to detect potential serious fetal hemorrhage.

A *spectrophotometric scan* is made of the amniotic fluid from 350 to 750 nm. The optical density (OD) or absorbance is plotted against the wavelength. To determine the magnitude of the deviation from normal, a line is projected from 375 to 525 nm delineating the approximate absorbance of amniotic fluid in the absence of bilirubin pigment. The deviation from normal is determined by calculating the increased absorbance caused by indirect bilirubin pigments at 450 nm. Fig. 5-4 is a spectrophotometric scan of a patient with severe erythroblastosis fetalis. The deviation in optical density (ΔOD) at 450 nm is 0.37. This value is used to evaluate the condition of the fetus.

Liley constructed a graph that he divided into three prognostic zones (Fig. 5-5). Zone 1, the low zone, indicates a nonaffected or mildly affected fetus. The upper zone, zone 3, indicates a severely affected fetus. In the middle zone, serial bilirubin values are used to assess the condition of the fetus. Those showing a decreasing

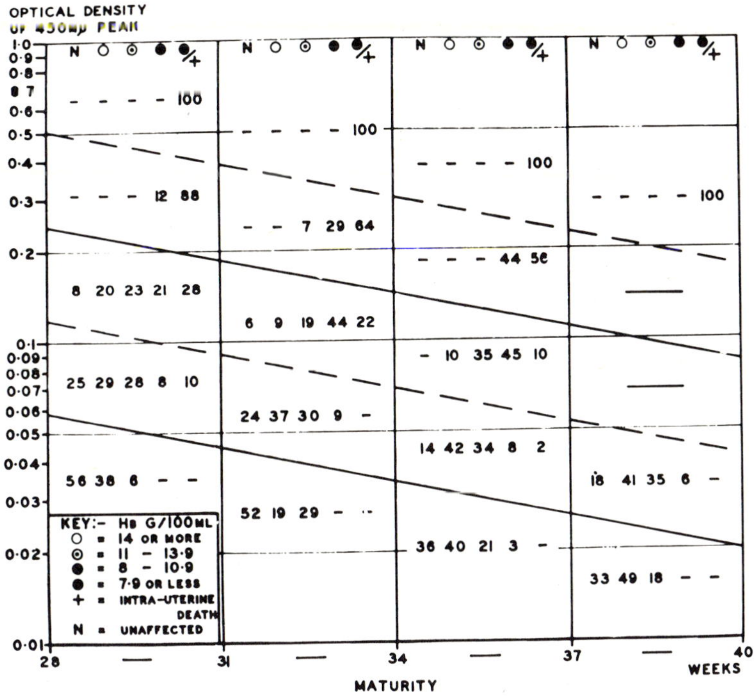

Fig. 5-5. Liley's graph with middle and upper zones (*solid lines*) divided into subzones (*hatched lines*). The percentage probability of various grades of affliction for the single amniotic fluid specimen is presented. (From Liley, A.W.: Am. J. Obstet. Gynecol. **82:**1359, 1961.)

trend of amniotic fluid bilirubin value usually have mild erythroblastosis fetalis. Those with increasing values have more severe disease.

Queenan and Goestchel noted, on serial determinations, a decreasing value of ΔOD at 450 nm with moderately affected, mildly affected, and unaffected fetuses. An increasing or horizontal trend occurred when the pregnancy terminated in intrauterine or neonatal death. A graph of their data is shown in Fig. 5-6. If the initial amniotic fluid bilirubin value is below the area of overlap, the fetus will almost certainly survive, but serial amniocenteses are still necessary to find the rare case in which the trend begins to rise later in gestation. Generally, two to four amniotic fluid samples are needed in these patients. If the initial value is above the area of overlap, the fetus is in danger of intrauterine or neonatal death. A repeat value in 1 week is indicated to verify the value and to determine the trend. If the value is constant or rising, the risk of an intrauterine transfusion must be weighed against the risk of the loss of the fetus resulting from complications of prematurity if delivered. If the risk to the fetus of delivery is greater than that of an intrauterine transfusion, then a transfusion is indicated unless the fetus is severely hydropic, as determined by ultrasonography. Generally, the earliest an intrauterine transfusion is performed is 22 weeks' gestation. If the fetus

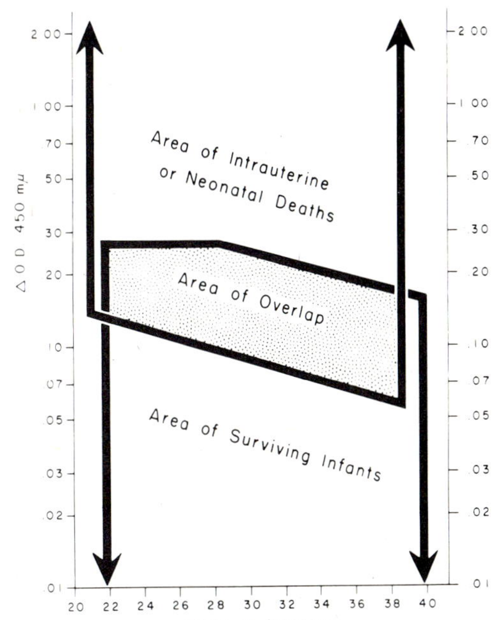

Fig. 5-6. Graphic representation of the distribution of amniotic fluid values from surviving infants and those with intrauterine and neonatal death. *ΔOD,* Change in optical density (absorbance). (Reprinted with permission from Queenan, J.T.: Modern management of the Rh problem, ed. 2, New York, 1977, Harper & Row, Publishers, Inc.)

is truly at risk of dying earlier in pregnancy, intraperitoneal intrauterine transfusions will not save the fetus. The latest that an intrauterine transfusion is initiated is 31 weeks' gestation. To be successful, the fetus must be sufficiently well to survive long enough to absorb the intraperitoneal blood.

Further study of amniotic fluid in Rh-immunized pregnancies has paid particular attention to the trend of amniotic fluid ΔOD at 450 nm values. Fig. 5-7 shows the trend of amniotic fluid bilirubin values in patients delivering Rh-negative (unaffected) babies. The trend is distinctly downward. When patients delivering mildly affected babies (cord blood hemoglobin 14 gm/dl or greater) were studied, the amniotic fluid bilirubin trends were almost identical. When patients delivering moderately affected babies (cord blood hemoglobin 10 to 14 gm/dl) were studied, the values were similar and the trend was almost always downward. When patients whose fetuses died in utero were studied, the trend was almost always horizontal or rising, as shown in Fig. 5-8. These findings led to the establishment of the method of determining fetal condition by the amniotic fluid bilirubin trend.

If the initial amniotic fluid bilirubin value is in the area of overlap, a single value is of little prognostic help, and repeat studies are necessary to establish a trend. Repeat amniocenteses indicating a decreasing trend denote a favorable prognosis. An exception to this generalization is seen in the case of polyhydramnios, which can dilute the bilirubin value and give a falsely low result. If the trend is horizontal or rising, the fetus is in jeopardy. Again, if the risk of intrauterine transfusion is less than the risk of perinatal death resulting from complications of prematurity, then an intrauterine transfusion should be performed.

Fetal exchange transfusion via the intravascular route, using the umbilical vein for venous access and sampling, allows direct access to the fetal circulation and circumvents the problem of unpredictable absorption of RBCs from the peritoneal cavity. This new approach holds considerable promise but requires extensive experience with ultrasound needle placement. The need for a fetal trans-

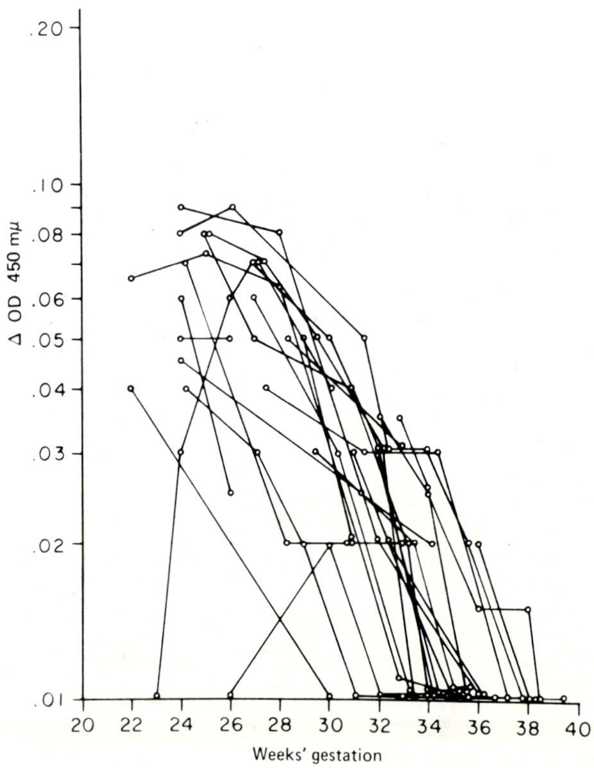

Fig. 5-7. Amniotic fluid bilirubin values from Rh-negative, immunized patients delivering Rh-negative (unaffected) infants. Values are recorded as change in absorbance at 450 nm *(mμ)* (ΔOD). Serial values are connected by lines; note downward trend. (Reprinted with permission from Queenan, J.T., editor: Modern management of the Rh problem, ed. 2, New York, 1977, Harper & Row, Publishers, Inc.)

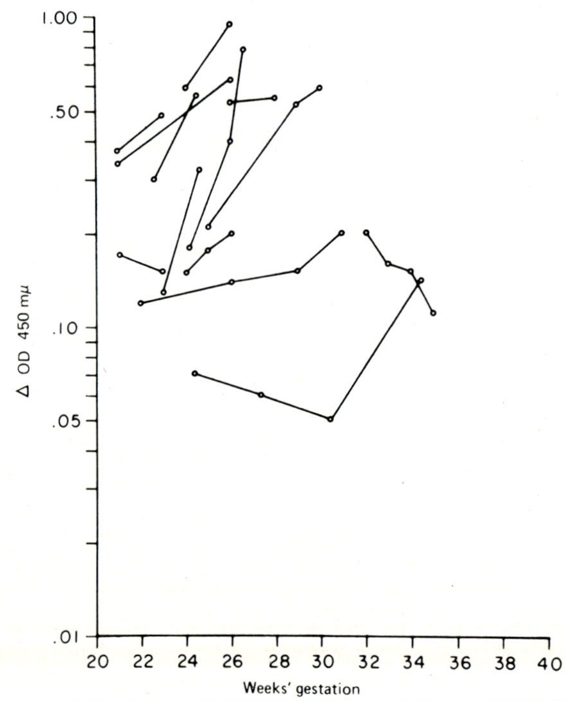

Fig. 5-8. Amniotic fluid bilirubin values from Rh-negative immunized patients whose fetuses died in utero. Serial values are connected by lines; note upward trend. (Reprinted with permission from Queenan, J.T., editor: Modern management of the Rh problem, ed. 2, New York, 1977, Harper & Row, Publishers, Inc.)

fusion is determined by sonographically directed percutaneous umbilical cord vessel aspiration to determine fetal hemoglobin.

CLINICAL APPLICATION

This method is based on the principle that the amniotic fluid bilirubin trend is extremely reliable in predicting the outcome of pregnancy in the Rh-immunized patient. The following protocol is suggested.*

1. Do an indirect Coombs' test every 2 to 3 weeks.
2. If the titer remains below critical level, perform delivery at 38 weeks' gestation with a neonatal team present and blood available for an exchange transfusion.
3. If the antibody level reaches or surpasses critical level, use amniotic fluid analyses to determine fetal condition.
4. Do initial amniocentesis at 28 to 29 weeks unless patient's obstetric history or antibody titer indicates it should be done earlier.
5. Repeat amniocentesis at 1- to 3-week intervals, depending on the ΔOD at 450 nm (Fig. 5-4).
6. Study serial ΔOD values to determine the trend (Fig. 5-9). If trend is falling, the fetus is safe until scheduled delivery at 38 weeks' gestation. If trend is rising between 23 and 31 weeks, do an intrauterine transfusion. If the trend is rising or horizontal after 31 weeks, perform preterm delivery.
7. Do amniotic fluid maturity studies in conjunction with ΔOD measurements to determine the optimum delivery time.
8. Coordinate delivery with the blood bank and neonatologist.

When amniotic fluid bilirubin levels indicate that the fetus is affected with erythroblastosis fetalis, the clinician should evaluate the fetal condition. The major fetal surveillance in erythroblastosis fetalis is done by ultrasound scanning. The heart size may be noted to increase when the fetus is developing congestive heart failure (Fig. 5-10). Additionally, fetal ascites suggests that the fetus may die in utero. Fig. 5-11 shows an ultrasound scan in cross section of a fetus without ascites. Fig. 5-12 shows an ultrasound scan of another fetus at the level of the umbilical vein with ascites present. Whereas amniotic fluid analysis will identify the fetus who is affected and will potentially die in utero, further information may be gained by ultrasound scanning.

Fetal activity, both perceived and observed, is very important in determining when a fetus may die in utero. In the setting of a severely compromised fetus, a marked

*From Queenan, J.T. In Queenan, J.T., and Hobbins, J.C., editors: Protocols for high-risk pregnancies, ed. 2, Oradell, N.J., 1987, Medical Economics Books.

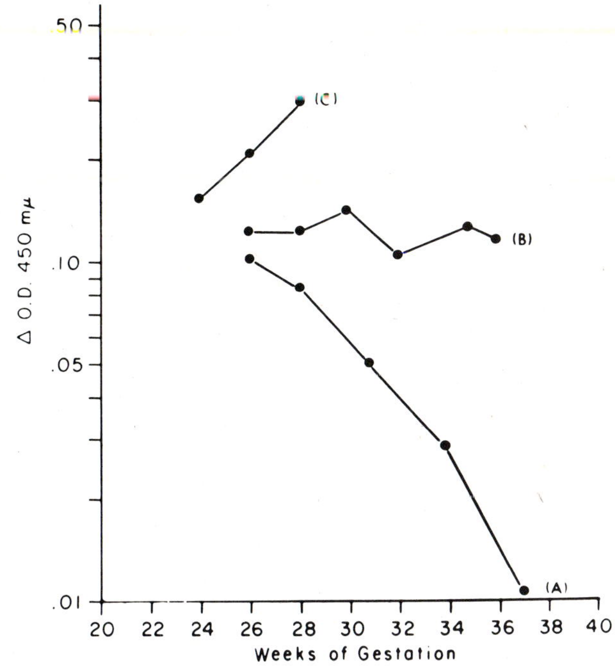

Fig. 5-9. Examples of various amniotic fluid bilirubin trend patterns. *A*, Decreasing trend, favorable outcome; *B*, horizontal or rising trend after 32 weeks indicates delivery; *C*, rising trend before 32 weeks may indicate intrauterine transfusion.

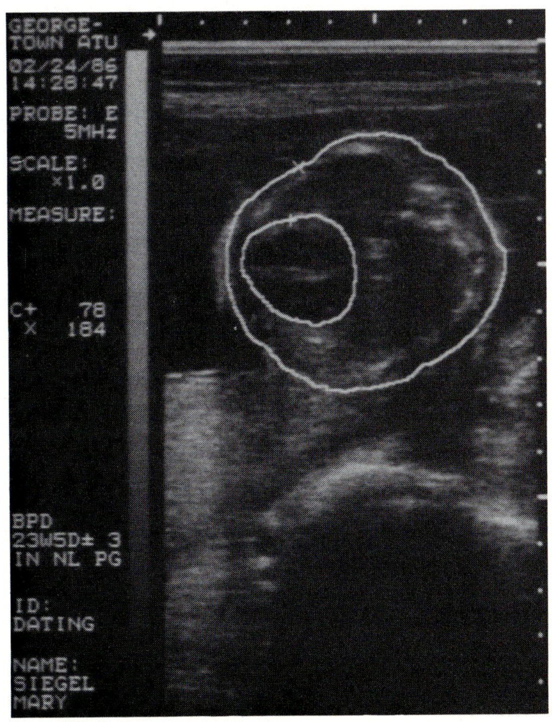

Fig. 5-10. Sonogram with heart and chest circumferences determined with onscreen electronic tracers.

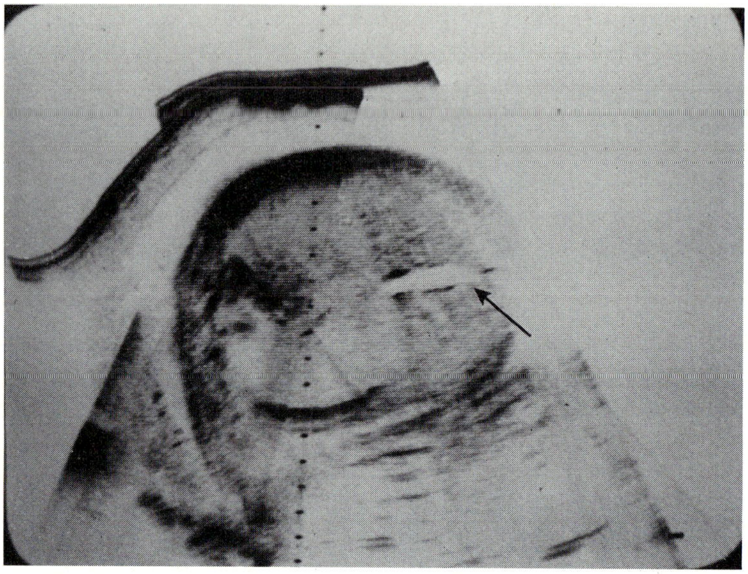

Fig. 5-11. Ultrasound cross section of the fetal abdomen in a normal pregnancy. The arrow points to the umbilical vein.

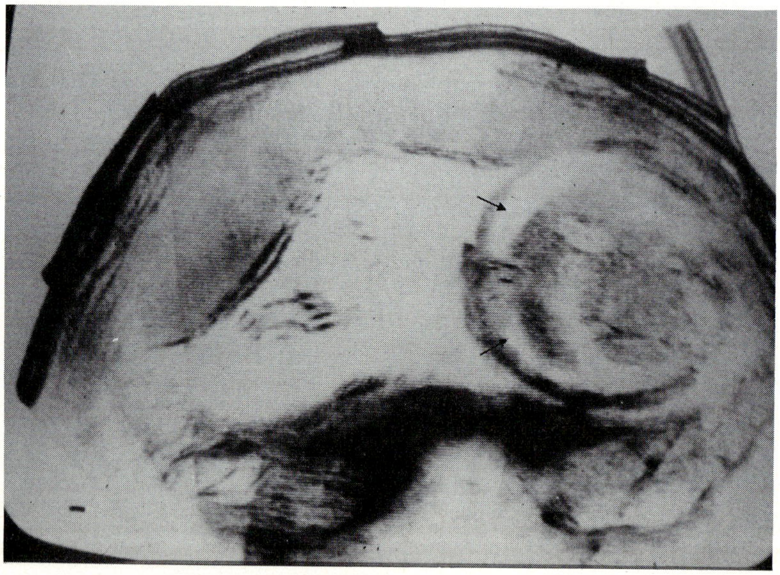

Fig. 5-12. Ultrasound scan of a fetus with moderate ascites *(arrows)*. Note that the placenta has a homogenous edematous appearance.

decrease in perceived fetal activity should warn the clinician that a fetal death could occur. Additionally, the decreased activity of a mildly hydropic fetus appears to be a bad prognostic sign.

When the decision to deliver the fetus has been made, the method of delivery must be chosen. If the fetal presentation and the condition of the cervix are favorable and continuous FHR monitoring is available throughout labor, an induction of labor is indicated. With an unfavorable fetal presentation, long uneffaced cervix, or a premature infant, cesarean section is indicated to prevent exposing the already compromised fetus to the risk of labor.

ABO INCOMPATIBILITY

Halbrecht was the first to describe ABO erythroblastosis in 1954. These infants may develop early severe jaundice but rarely show signs of fetal hemolysis. The mother's and infant's major blood groups are incompatible; the mother's is usually group O and the infant's group A or B. Coombs' test may be negative in ABO hemolytic disease. When a positive Coombs' test does occur, it is different from that seen in Rh hemolytic disease; a small weak agglutination appears after 3 to 8 minutes, rather than the complete agglutination that comes in less than 1 minute with Rh erythroblastosis fetalis. The antenatal prediction of ABO erythroblastosis is not possible with any degree of certainty. Since anti-A and anti-B occur naturally, they may be present in maternal serum without clinical disease in the infant. ABO erythroblastosis fetalis is about three times as common as Rh erythroblastosis fetalis. Since there is no risk of intrauterine death with ABO incompatibility, amniocentesis is not indicated and intrauterine transfusion is never required. There are no indications for preterm delivery of these infants. A history of previous ABO incompatibility can alert the obstetrician and pediatrician of an impending problem. Routine unbilical cord blood Coombs' tests at delivery and careful observation of the neonate are generally adequate to detect ABO disease. Because of the recent trend toward early discharge, the physician should be particularly careful to rule out the possibility of ABO incompatibility. Treatment of the newborn with this condition is the same in other types of erythroblastosis fetalis (Chapter 32).

OTHER ANTIBODIES

Theoretically, any blood group antigen present on the fetal RBCs and not present on maternal erythrocytes could cause erythroblastosis fetalis. The incidence of antibodies to other blood group antigens in an obstetric population is in the range of 1% to 2%. Some Rh(D)-negative women will be immunized to other antigens, and it is therefore important to identify the antibody present rather than to assume that an Rh-negative woman is immunized to $Rh_0(D)$. More than half the obstetric patients with other antibodies will be Rh positive; therefore it is important to screen Rh-positive and Rh-negative patients to detect the possibility of erythroblastosis fetalis. Anti-(C), anti-(E), anti-Fy^a, and anti-Kell have been shown to cause erythroblastosis severe enough to require exchange transfusion. Rh-positive women can be immunized to "c" to "e" if they have received a transfusion of O Rh-negative *(cde)* blood.

PREVENTION

The long-term solution is passive immunization through the administration of adequate amounts of antepartum and postpartum (RhIG). Maternal immunization usually occurs at delivery, and the administration to the patient of RhIG binds Rh-positive antigenic sites on transfused fetal RBCs. Spontaneous abortions carry a 3% to 4% risk of immunization, whereas induced abortions have a slightly higher risk. The first full-term pregnancy has approximately a 1% to 2% risk of immunization up to the time of delivery. Subsequent term pregnancies carry a 10% risk of immunization. Ectopic pregnancies can also result in immunization.

An antibody excess is required to protect the patient from Rh immunization. In general, a dose of 300 μgm of RhIG is in excess of the dose necessary for the prevention of maternal immunization. However, more than this dose of immunoglobulin should be given for suspected large transplacental hemorrhage. It is mandatory that all unimmunized, Rh-negative women delivering Rh-positive infants receive RhIG. Unimmunized, Rh-negative patients with either spontaneous or induced abortions as well as ectopic pregnancies should also receive prophylaxis.

In 1982 antepartum administration of RhIG was recommended to prevent immunization during the third trimester. When an Rh-negative patient undergoes genetic amniocentesis, she runs the risk of Rh immunization if the needle interrupts the integrity of the fetoplacental circulation. The phenomenon of immunization as a consequence of amniocentesis has been definitely demonstrated by numerous investigators. If RhIG is administered for a genetic amniocentesis from 15 to 17 weeks' gestation, the administration of RhIG should be repeated again at 28 weeks, thus maintaining an effective antibody level to prevent enhancement.

The standard of care today for unsensitized Rh-negative women is to administer RhIG at 28 weeks' gestation and after delivery if the baby is Rh positive. If the mother undergoes genetic amniocentesis at 15 to 17 weeks, 300 μgm of RhIG should be administered. Alternatively, if the mother has chorionic villus sampling at 8 to 10 weeks' gestation, 50 μgm of RhIG should be administered. If such a prophylaxis program is followed, the risk of immunization is negligible.

John T. Queenan

BIBLIOGRAPHY

Bevis, D.C.A.: Blood pigments in haemolytic disease of the newborn, J. Obstet. Gynaecol. Br. Emp. **63**:68, 1956.

Freda, V.J.: The Rh problem in obstetrics and a new concept of its management using amniocentesis and spectrophotometric scanning of amniotic fluid, Am. J. Obstet. Gynecol. **92**:341, 1965.

Goplerud, C.P., and others: The first Rh-isoimmunized pregnancy, Am. J. Obstet. Gynecol. **115**:632, 1973.

Grannum, P.A., and others: In utero exchange transfusion by direct intravascular injection in severe erythroblastosis fetalis, N. Engl. J. Med. **314**:1431, 1986.

Halbrecht, I.: Role of hemagglutinins anti-A and anti-B in pathogenesis of jaundice of the newborn (icterus praecox neonatorum), Am. J. Dis. Child. **68**:248, 1954.

Levine, P., and Stetson, R.E.: Unusual causes of intragroup agglutination, JAMA **113**:126, 1939.

Liley, A.W.: Liquor amnii analysis in management of pregnancy complicated by rhesus sensitization, Am. J. Obstet. Gynecol. **82**:1359, 1961.

Queenan, J.T.: Amniocentesis and transamniotic fetal transfusion for Rh disease, Clin. Obstet. Gynecol. **9**:491, 1966.

Queenan, J.T.: Role of spontaneous abortion in Rh immunization, Am. J. Obstet. Gynecol. **110**:128, 1971.

Queenan, J.T.: Modern management of the Rh problem, ed. 2, New York, 1977, Harper & Row, Publishers, Inc.

Queenan, J.T.: Management of high-risk pregnancy, ed. 2, Oradell, N.J., 1985, Medical Economics Co.

Queenan, J.T., and Goetschel, E.: Amniotic fluid analysis for erythroblastosis fetalis, Obstet. Gynecol. **32**:120, 1968.

Queenan, J.T., and others: Irregular antibodies in the obstetric patient, Obstet. Gynecol. **34**:767, 1969.

Queenan, J.T., and others: Role of induced abortion in Rh immunization, Lancet **1**:815, 1971.

CHAPTER 6

Polyhydramnios, oligohydramnios, and hydrops fetalis

POLYHYDRAMNIOS

Polyhydramnios (hydramnios) is a pathologic accumulation of excess amniotic fluid; an amniotic fluid volume exceeding 2,000 ml in the third trimester constitutes polyhydramnios. The amniotic fluid volume increases gradually during normal pregnancy, although the turnover of amniotic fluid is rapid. Fetal urine and tracheobronchial tree secretions contribute to the net increase in the amniotic fluid volume; fetal swallowing tends to reduce volume. In addition, water and solute are exchanged between the mother and the amniotic fluid across the placental membranes. In a normal patient this volume increases less than 10 ml/day until the thirty-fourth week of gestation, after which it slowly diminishes (Fig. 6-1). The volumes vary widely in normal pregnancies, a volume of 500 to 2,000 ml at term is normal. Various maternal and fetal conditions may disturb the dynamic equilibrium of the amniotic fluid volume. Esophageal atresia, which prevents normal swallowing, is usually associated with polyhydramnios, whereas fetal renal agenesis may be associated with oligohydramnios. Occasionally the volume increases without a recognizable maternal or fetal cause.

Clinical manifestations

The diagnosis of polyhydramnios is often first suggested by the patient's symptoms. She may complain of pressure, rapidly increasing size of the abdomen, or of a protuberant abdomen. Later she may complain of pain, contractions, dyspnea, or orthopnea. Physical signs include a rapidly enlarging uterus reflected in a disproportionate increase in fundal height, abdominal girth, weight gain, and abdominal striae. The fetal head can usually be ballotted, but the fetal extremities are difficult to outline. The fetal heart is difficult to hear; it is usually detectable with the Doppler ultrasound sensor, but the signal may be lost intermittently because of the mobility of the fetus in the abnormally large volume of amniotic fluid. The presentation may vary from examination to examination, and there is an increased frequency of breech and oblique lie with a single fetus.

The acute form of polyhydramnios is rare, occurring in 1 out of every 50 instances of polyhydramnios. The fluid accumulates rapidly, and the uterus is tense and tender. It is usually diagnosed by 23 to 25 weeks' gestation.

Chronic polyhydramnios, the most common form, is a problem of the third trimester. Occasionally the diagnosis is not made until the patient has a dysfunctional labor or until an abnormally large amount of amniotic fluid is noted during delivery. Most often the diagnosis is made by abdominal examination during the third trimester or by ultrasound scan. Prolonged pregnancy is rare except in association with anencephaly. The reported incidence of chronic polyhydramnios varies from 1 in 150 deliveries to 1 in 400 deliveries.

Ultrasound evaluation

Ultrasound is very useful in confirming the diagnosis of polyhydramnios. The increased amniotic fluid is evident as a large sonolucent echo-free area on the ultrasound scan (Fig. 6-2). Associated conditions, such as multiple gestations and congenital malformations, also may be appreciated.

Early in pregnancy, the amniotic fluid volume represents approximately 50% of the total intrauterine contents. The percentage decreases throughout pregnancy; at 40 weeks' gestation the amniotic fluid volume comprises only about 17%. Table 6-1 presents approximate fetal and placental weights and amniotic fluid volumes at several stages of pregnancy. The amniotic fluid percentages give an estimate of what portion the amniotic

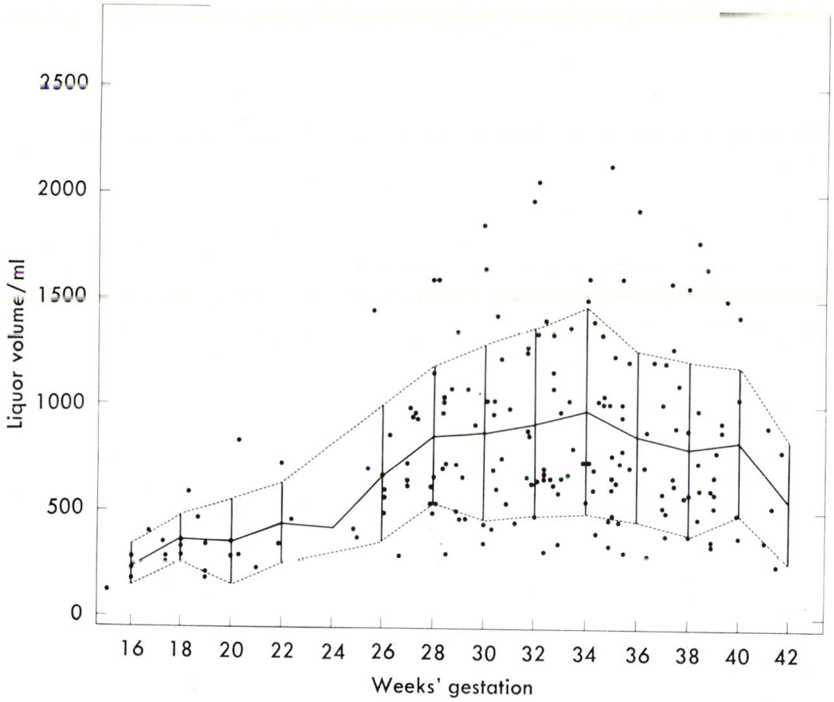

Fig. 6-1. Normal amniotic fluid volumes from 16 to 42 weeks' gestation determined by a dye dilution technique. (From Queenan, J.T., and others: Am. J. Obstet. Gynecol. **114:**34, 1972.)

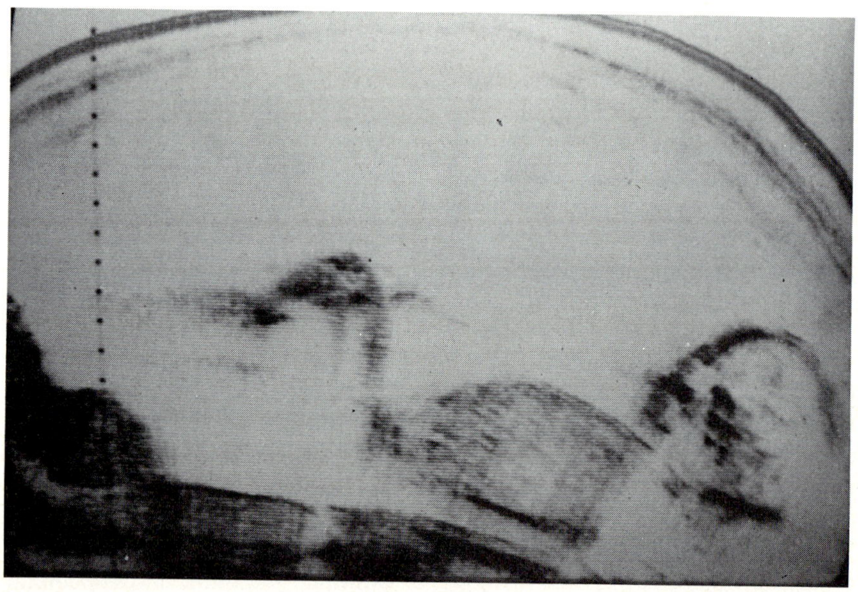

Fig. 6-2. Ultrasound scan showing severe polyhydramnios. Note the large sonolucent area.

Table 6-1. Fetal and placental weights and amniotic fluid volumes

Weeks	Fetus (gm)	Placenta (gm)	Amniotic fluid (ml)	Total	Amniotic fluid (%)
16	100	100	200	400	50
28	1,000	200	1,000	2,200	45
36	2,500	400	900	3,800	24
40	3,300	500	800	4,600	17

From Queenan, J.T. In Queenan, J.T., and Hobbin, J.C., editors: Protocols for high-risk pregnancies, ed. 2, Oradell, N.J., 1987, Medical Economics Books.

fluid volume should represent on a scan. The amniotic fluid volume would have to be pathologically increased to be diagnostic of polyhydramnios.

Associated conditions

In a study reported in 1970, 358 instances of polyhydramnios were found in 86,000 deliveries, a frequency of 0.41%. The associated conditions were diabetes mellitus (25%), congenital malformations (20%), erythroblastosis fetalis (11%), and multiple gestations (8%). Thirty-four percent had no apparent prenatal or postnatal cause. Acute polyhydramnios occurred in 2%. Polyhydramnios appeared to be more prevalent with severe diabetes than with mild disease.

When polyhydramnios is associated with erythroblastosis fetalis, there is usually hydrops fetalis. Multiple gestations, especially monochorionic twins, are more common than expected in pregnancies associated with polyhydramnios. There is also an increased incidence of postpartum hemorrhage resulting from overdistension of the uterus. The most frequently reported congenital anomaly is anencephaly; approximately 50% of pregnancies associated with anencephaly are found to have polyhydramnios. Hydrocephalus and both duodenal and esophageal atresia are also frequently associated with this condition. Ultrasound examination frequently can localize the site of gastrointestinal obstruction in the fetus. Neuromuscular disorders associated with impaired swallowing and reduced fetal activity frequently are complicated by polyhydramnios. Fig. 6-3 shows the interval between diagnosis and delivery according to diagnosis. The average birth weights are displayed on the vertical axis (see Chapter 16).

Treatment

If diabetes or erythroblastosis fetalis is the cause of polyhydramnios, appropriate therapy for these disorders should be undertaken. If twins are diagnosed, limitation of activity is indicated. Some major gastrointestinal anomalies can be corrected with prompt surgery during the neonatal period. However, if gross multiple anomalies are found, interruption of the pregnancy may be indicated.

Chronic polyhydramnios without underlying disease should be managed with bed rest, restricted activity, and a high-protein diet. An abdominal binder can sometimes relieve symptoms. Diuretics are not indicated. Rarely, amniocentesis is required to relieve maternal symptoms; fluid should be removed slowly to avoid causing premature labor or premature separation of the placenta. In contrast, acute recurrent polyhydramnios may require multiple amniocenteses. In one patient approximately 20,000 ml of amniotic fluid was removed during the third trimester, and the fetus developed to viability.

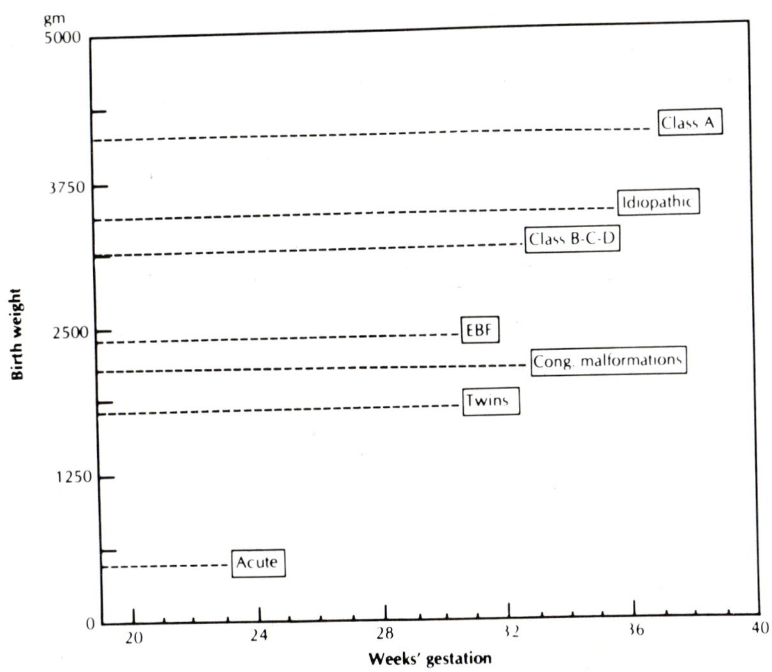

Fig. 6-3. Interval between diagnosis and delivery according to causes of polyhydramnios. EBF, Erythroblastosis fetalis. (From Queenan, J.T., and Gadow, E.C.: Am. J. Obstet. Gynecol. **108:**349, 1970.)

Prognosis

The overall prognosis for the fetus of a pregnancy complicated by polyhydramnios is poor. The incidence of stillborn infants is 10% to 20%. The perinatal mortality is 35% to 40%. The perinatal mortality is significantly higher with acute polyhydramnios. The prognosis for the infant depends on the associated conditions that are present. In 1970 Queenan reported a perinatal mortality in class A diabetic patients of 8%, whereas when class B, C, and D diabetes were associated with polyhydramnios, the perinatal mortality was 17.5%. The perinatal mortality in twin gestations associated with polyhydramnios was 45% in this study. Polyhydramnios associated with erythroblastosis fetalis portends a poor outcome for two reasons. Polyhydramnios is often associated with the development of hydrops fetalis, and second, the excess fluid can dilute the amniotic fluid bilirubin values and mask the severity of the disease. The perinatal mortality of patients with erythroblastosis fetalis and polyhydramnios in Queenan's series was 73%. In patients with polyhydramnios and congenital abnormalities the perinatal mortality reached 87%.

OLIGOHYDRAMNIOS

Oligohydramnios refers to diminished amounts of amniotic fluid. The occurrence of a very small amniotic fluid volume, a few ounces or less, is recorded less frequently than polyhydramnios. This can be attributed to the fact that generally the associated condition has caused no maternal distress and, if after rupture of the membranes during labor there is little fluid, it is often erroneously assumed that the rupture had occurred earlier and the fluid escaped. During the later stages of pregnancy the fetal urine is a major source of amniotic fluid, which is maintained in continuous equilibrium by being swallowed and reabsorbed by the fetus. A marked deficit of fetal urine production or excretion can lead to oligohydramnios. The clinical importance of significant decreases in amniotic fluid volume lies mainly in the increased incidence of fetal abnormality. Severe oligohydramnios is most often associated with major renal malformations, including renal aplasia with dysplastic kidneys and obstructive lesions of the lower urinary tract.

There has also been an association of small amniotic fluid volumes with fetal growth retardation attributed in initial reports to excessive fetal swallowing caused by fetal hunger. Liley, however, demonstrated that fetuses small for gestational age actually swallow at a low rate. Wallenberg documented ultrasonographically a decreased urine production and concluded that, in fetuses small for gestational age, the kidneys play a more important role in the regulation of amniotic fluid volume than in normally nourished fetuses. The underlying mechanism of the oligohydramnios in growth-retarded infants thus is not known.

The diagnosis of oligohydramnios is usually subjective, since precise values of amniotic fluid determinations are rarely available. Furthermore, because conditions associated with oligohydramnios other than premature rupture of membranes and prolonged leakage of amniotic fluid cause little or no distress to the mother, antenatal recognition may be difficult. More precise quantitation of amniotic fluid volume may be accomplished ultrasonographically, or the pathologist may confirm the diagnosis by documenting the presence of amnion nodosum (Chapter 11). These gray-yellow amniotic nodules consist histologically of clumps of vernix, desquamated fetal epidermal cells, and appendages of the skin on the amnion. The amniotic epithelium under the nodules may be completely intact. Amnion nodosum is thought to arise as a result of close contact between fetal skin and amnion resulting from oligohydramnios. Whereas amnion nodosum may imply oligohydramnios, oligohydramnios, especially when secondary to amniorrhea, does not necessarily imply amnion nodosum. Furthermore, although the oligohydramnios syndrome frequently accompanies renal agenesis, the features of the oligohydramnios syndrome may be absent if a defect in fetal swallowing coexists. The defects in fetal swallowing could compensate for fetal anuria, preventing oligohydramnios and its effects. The oligohydramnios tetrad of anomalies consists of facial anomalies, limb positioning defects, pulmonary hypoplasia, and fetal growth deficiency (Chapter 28, part five); when accompanied by bilateral renal agenesis, it is typically referred to as Potter's disease (facies) (Chapter 35). The characteristic facial appearance includes a flattened nose, recession of the chin, and a prominent fold that runs downward and outward from the inner canthus of the eye. The ears are often low set, aberrantly folded, and usually flattened to the side of the head. There are limb defects such as spadelike hands and talipes equinovarus. Additionally, these infants are usually growth deficient if delivered after 34 weeks, the lungs are hypoplastic, and there is most often a urinary tract defect such that urine production or flow is grossly deficient or absent. It has been assumed that the oligohydramnios that accompanies most cases of renal agenesis is the cause of the major nonrenal malformations, including pulmonary hypoplasia and the facial features (Fig. 6-4).

That oligohydramnios may cause fetal compression and so explain the facial appearance and limb defects is supported by the production of similar anomalies in rat fetuses subjected to amniocentesis. Fetuses unable to excrete urine into the amniotic space, but for unusual reasons having adequate amniotic fluid present, have none of these secondary features of Potter's disease. Furthermore, all the nonrenal features of Potter's disease can be present as a consequence of oligohydramnios secondary to chronic leakage of amniotic fluid in fetuses who have no problems of urine production. For any infant

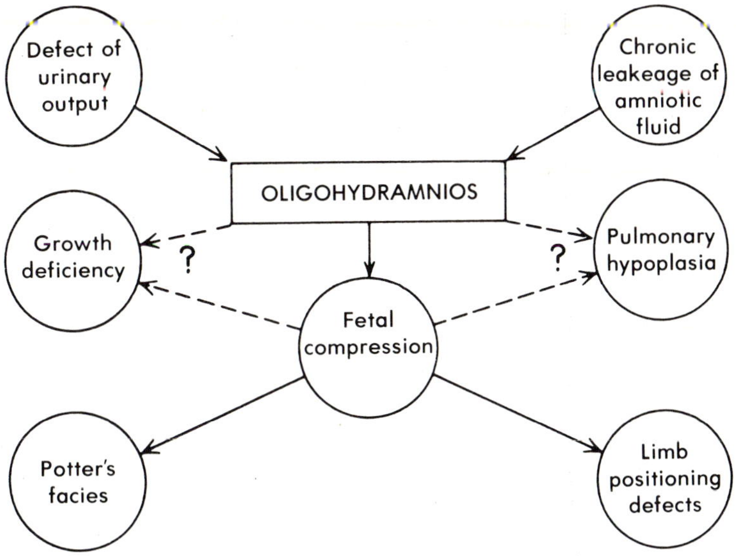

Fig. 6-4. Major nonrenal malformations caused by oligohydramnios. (From Thomas, I.T., and Smith, D.W.: J. Pediatr. **84:**811, 1974.)

who has a low Apgar score or severe respiratory distress together with features of the oligohydramnios tetrad, a detailed evaluation of the genitourinary tract should be undertaken.

HYDROPS FETALIS

Hydrops fetalis is characterized by generalized edema, frequently accompanied by cavity effusions. The severity of hydrops varies widely. With the advent of prophylaxis for Rh isoimmunization, there has been a steady decrease in the ratio of immunologic to nonimmunologic cases of hydrops fetalis. Although numerous maternal, fetal, and placental factors are now recognized to cause nonimmune hydrops, a substantial number remain idiopathic in etiology. The boxed material summarizes major causes of nonimmune hydrops fetalis.

Prognosis is compounded by the degree of immaturity, the presence of major congenital abnormalities, and the underlying etiology, if this is identifiable. Early recognition by ultrasound examination and aggressive perinatal management offer the best hope for an improved outcome, although the prognosis at present is not good. The suspicion of polyhydramnios warrants urgent ultrasound to exclude accompanying hydrops and evidence of malformations. In cases of Rh isoimmunization, hydrops is considered a poor prognostic sign. Although the timing of delivery may be influenced by fetal pulmonary maturity and maternal well-being, delivery of potentially viable neonates is usually via cesarean section. Vaginal delivery is complicated by the large size of both the fetus and the placenta, resulting in asphyxia and postpartum hemorrhage.

Major causes of nonimmune hydrops fetalis

HEMATOLOGIC
Fetal hemolytic anemia
α-Thalassemia
Fetomaternal or twin-to-twin transfusions

CARDIOVASCULAR
Structural congenital heart disease
Myocardial dysfunction
Supraventricular tachyarrhythmia or heart block

CONGENITAL INFECTION
Syphilis
Toxoplasmosis
Cytomegalovirus

PULMONARY MALFORMATIONS
Chylothorax
Lymphangiectasia
Hypoplasia
Cystic adenomatoid malformation

OTHER
Genitourinary obstruction
Chromosomal disorders
Congenital malformations and tumors
Placental anomalies

None of the suggested mechanisms for pathogenesis of hydrops fetalis has been universally accepted, although fetal hypoproteinemia and resultant decreased osmotic pressure appear to play a major role. Alternatively, increased capillary permeability, anemia, and congestive cardiac failure may be major contributing factors. The diagnosis of hydrops should be considered whenever ultrasound examination demonstrates tissue edema, pleural effusion, or ascites. The boxed material lists prenatal and postnatal laboratory tests that should be considered in the evaluation of hydrops fetalis. Echocardiography has been useful in making a prenatal diagnosis of heart failure or an arrhythmia, especially supraventricular tachycardia. Diagnosis of arrhythmia may require transplacental administration of digitalis or propranolol before birth. Holzgreve and associates were able to demonstrate an associated maternal, fetal, or placental problem in 84% of cases of nonimmune hydrops after extensive prenatal and postnatal study. Only 16% of cases were thus labeled as idiopathic. The authors recommended a vigorous approach to prenatal diagnostic evaluation, including ultrasound, echocardiography, and exclusion of isoimmunization. Serologic testing for congenital intrauterine infection and chromosomal evaluation should also be performed. Hematologic studies should comprise a complete blood count, red blood cell indices to search for evidence of α-thalassemia, and signs of fetomaternal hemorrhage. Nonetheless, for nonimmune hydrops, specific prenatal treatment is currently limited to cardiac tachyarrhythmias and possible selected cases of urinary tract obstruction.

The importance of vigorous cardiorespiratory stabilization for these infants at birth is emphasized in Chapter 22. This may include paracentesis, thoracentesis, and control of pulmonary edema by assisted ventilation and extremely cautious diuretic administration. With aggressive antenatal and postnatal management, an estimated 35% of infants with nonimmune hydrops fetalis beyond 28 weeks could survive without permanent disability.

Laboratory tests in evaluation of hydrops fetalis

- Complete ultrasound evaluation
- Blood cell count, platelet count
- Betke-Kleihauer test on maternal blood
- Electrolytes, renal and liver function tests
- Blood type, Coombs' (direct and indirect)
- Hemoglobin electrophoresis
- Imaging of chest, abdomen, long bones, and skull
- Echocardiography, electrocardiography
- Bacterial, viral cultures
- Serology for congenital infections (mother, infant)
- Diagnostic thoracentesis and paracentesis
- Placental anatomy and histology
- Chromosomal karyotype

Modified from Etches, P.C., and Lemons, J.A.: Pediatrics **64**:326, 1979. Reproduced by permission of Pediatrics.

John T. Queenan

BIBLIOGRAPHY

Polyhydramnios

Jacoby, H.E., and Charles, D.: Clinical conditions associated with hydramnios, Am. J. Obstet. Gynecol. **94**:910, 1966.

Kramer, E.E.: Hydramnios, oligohydramnios and fetal malformations, Clin. Obstet. Gynecol. **9**:508, 1966.

Kucera, M.: Rate and type of congenital anomalies among offspring of diabetic women, J. Reprod. Med. **7**:61, 1971.

Pitkin, R.M.: Acute polyhydramnios recurrent in successive pregnancies, Obstet. Gynecol. **48**:425, 1976.

Prindle, R.A., and others: Maternal hydramnios and congenital anomalies of the central nervous system, N. Engl. J. Med. **252**:555, 1955.

Queenan, J.T.: Recurrent acute polyhydramnios, Am. J. Obstet. Gynecol. **106**:625, 1970.

Queenan, J.T.: Polyhydramnios. In Queenan, J.T., and Hobbin, J.C., editors: Protocols for high-risk pregnancies, ed. 2, Oradell, N.J., 1987, Medical Economics Books.

Queenan, J.T., and Gadow, E.C.: Polyhydramnios chronic vs. acute, Am. J. Obstet. Gynecol. **108**:349, 1970.

Queenan, J.T., and Watkins, S.K.: Polyhydramnios. In Management of high-risk pregnancy, ed. 2, Oradell, N.J., 1985, Medical Economics Books.

Queenan, J.T., and others: Amniotic fluid volume in normal pregnancies, Am. J. Obstet. Gynecol. **114**:34, 1972.

Oligohydramnios

Brown, D.R., Doshi, N., and Taylor, P.M.: Oligohydramnios and fatal pulmonary hypoplasia without amnion nodosum, J. Reprod. Med. **20**:293, 1978.

Liley, A.W.: Disorders of amniotic fluid. In Assali, N.S., editor: Pathophysiology of gestation, New York, 1972, Academic Press, Inc.

Queenan, J.T.: Oligohydramnios. In Queenan, J.T., and Hobbin, J.C., editors: Protocols for high-risk pregnancies, Oradell, N.J., 1982, Medical Economics Books.

Thomas, I.T., and Smith, D.W.: Oligohydramnios, cause of the nonrenal features of Potter's syndrome, including pulmonary hypoplasia, J. Pediatr. **84**:811, 1974.

Wallenberg, H.C.S., and Wladimiroff, J.W.: The amniotic fluid. II. Polyhydramnios and oligohydramnios, J. Perinatol. Med. **6**:233, 1977.

Hydrops fetalis

Etches, P.C., and Lemons, J.A.: Nonimmune hydrops fetalis: report of 22 cases including three siblings, Pediatrics **64**:326, 1979.

Holzgreve, W., and others: Investigation of nonimmune hydrops fetalis, Am. J. Obstet. Gynecol. **150**:805, 1984.

Hutchison, A.A., and others: Nonimmunologic hydrops fetalis: a review of 61 cases, Obstet. Gynecol. **59**:347, 1982.

Kleinman, C.S., and others: Fetal echocardiography for evaluation of in utero congestive heart failure: a technique for study of nonimmune fetal hydrops, N. Engl. J. Med. **306**:568, 1982.

Quinlan, R.W., Cruz, A.C., and Martin, M.: Hydramnios: ultrasound diagnosis and its impact on perinatal management and pregnancy outcome, Am. J. Obstet. Gynecol. **145**:306, 1983.

Watson, J., and Campbell, S.: Antenatal evaluation and management in nonimmune hydrops fetalis, Obstet. Gynecol. **67**:589, 1986.

CHAPTER 7

Intrauterine growth retardation: determinants of aberrant fetal growth

Fetal development is characterized by sequential patterns of tissue and organ growth and maturation that are determined by the maternal environment, uteroplacental function, and the inherent genetic growth potential of the fetus. When circumstances are optimal, none of these factors has a rate-limiting effect on fetal growth and development. Thus the healthy fetus should achieve complete functional maturity and somatic growth, with the anticipation of an uncomplicated intrapartum course, and thus a smooth neonatal cardiopulmonary and metabolic adaptation to extrauterine life.

However, fetal growth and development do not always occur under optimum intrauterine conditions. Those neonates subjected to aberrant maternal, placental, or fetal circumstances that restrain growth are a high-risk group and are categorized as small for gestational age (SGA). The cumulative effects of both adverse environmental conditions and aberrant fetal growth (intrauterine growth retardation, IUGR) threaten continued intrauterine survival, and labor, delivery, and neonatal adaptation become increasingly hazardous. Similarly, postneonatal growth and development may be impaired as a result of IUGR and the subsequent problems encountered during the neonatal period. This chapter discusses normal and aberrant fetal growth and its sequelae.

Following is a list of synonyms for SGA*:

1. Small for dates
2. Small for gestational age
3. Light for dates
4. Chronic fetal distress
5. Hypotrophic fetus
6. Intrauterine growth retardation
7. Intrauterine malnutrition
8. Dysmature
9. Clifford syndrome
10. Postdates
11. Postmaturity
12. Failure to thrive in utero
13. Fetal deprivation syndrome
14. Pseudoprematurity

*From Brandt, I.: Growth dynamics of low birth weight infants with emphasis on the perinatal period. In Falkner, F., and Tanner, J.M., editors: Human growth, vol. 2: Postnatal growth, New York, 1978, Plenum Press.

FETAL GROWTH AND BODY COMPOSITION

Through anthropomorphic measurements that include fetal weight, length (crown-heel), and head circumference, fetal growth standards have been determined for different reference populations from various locations. Although the range of birth weight at each gestational age in these populations may vary (Table 7-1), the overall pattern of fetal growth (Fig. 7-1) is representative for each of these groups. Both early and late fetal growth appear to be linear beginning at approximately 20 weeks' gestation and lasting until 38 weeks; thereafter the rate of weight gain begins to decline. Reasonably equivalent data have been recorded when fetal dimensions are examined by ultrasound. Included in Fig. 7-1 are growth curves corrected for parity, race, and fetal sex, factors to be discussed in later sections. Fig. 7-2 demonstrates a similar linear relationship between fetal weight and gestational age. Near-term fetal weight gain appears to decelerate; following birth it again assumes the intrauterine rate. Fetal weight gain (grams per day) is constant during the second trimester, then accelerates during most of the third trimester, but declines near term. During the neonatal period the rate of gain accelerates again. This relative slowing of growth as the normal fetus approaches term is thought to be caused by some restraint of fetal growth. These restraining factors may be related to uterine size or placental function. Some fetuses, however, continue to grow in utero after week 40. During the

Table 7-1. Birth weights from six sources

Nearest week of gestation	Mean birth weight (gm) ± 1 standard deviation					
	Denver	Baltimore	Montreal	Portland	Chapel Hill	12 U.S. cities (cluster method)
28	1,150 ± 259	1,050 ± 310	1,113 ± 150	1,172 ± 344	1,150 ± 272	1,165 ± 109
29	1,270 ± 294	1,200 ± 350	1,228 ± 165	1,322 ± 339	1,310 ± 299	1,295 ± 94
30	1,395 ± 341	1,380 ± 370	1,373 ± 175	1,529 ± 474	1,460 ± 340	1,440 ± 115
31	1,540 ± 375	1,560 ± 400	1,640 ± 200	1,757 ± 495	1,630 ± 340	1,601 ± 117
32	1,715 ± 416	1,750 ± 410	1,727 ± 225	1,881 ± 437	1,810 ± 381	1,760 ± 128
33	1,920 ± 505	1,950 ± 420	1,900 ± 250	2,158 ± 511	2,010 ± 367	1,955 ± 138
34	2,200 ± 539	2,170 ± 430	2,113 ± 280	2,340 ± 552	2,220 ± 395	2,160 ± 202
35	2,485 ± 526	2,390 ± 440	2,347 ± 315	2,518 ± 468	2,430 ± 408	2,387 ± 208
36	2,710 ± 519	2,610 ± 440	2,589 ± 350	2,749 ± 490	2,650 ± 408	2,621 ± 274
37	2,900 ± 451	2,830 ± 440	2,868 ± 385	2,989 ± 466	2,870 ± 395	2,878 ± 288
38	3,030 ± 451	3,050 ± 450	3,133 ± 400	3,185 ± 450	3,030 ± 395	3,119 ± 302
39	3,140 ± 403	3,210 ± 450	3,360 ± 430	3,333 ± 444	3,170 ± 408	3,210 ± 434
40	3,230 ± 396	3,280 ± 450	3,480 ± 460	3,462 ± 456	3,280 ± 422	3,351 ± 448
41	3,290 ± 396	3,350 ± 450	3,507 ± 475	3,569 ± 468	3,360 ± 435	3,444 ± 456
42	3,300 ± 423	3,400 ± 460	3,513 ± 480	3,637 ± 482	3,410 ± 449	3,486 ± 463
43		3,410 ± 490	3,416 ± 465	3,660 ± 502	3,420 ± 463	3,473 ± 502

From Naeye, R., and Dixon, J.: Pediatr. Res. **12:**987, 1978. With permission.

neonatal period growth resumes and approaches the in utero rate once this restraint has been eliminated.

Although weight gain per day is maximum before term, when growth is expressed as percent increment per day, it is greatest during embryonic and early fetal development (Fig. 7-2). Interestingly, in the last half of pregnancy the fetus gains 85% of its birth weight. However, the nature of fetal growth is different during early and later fetal life. During the embryonic and early fetal growth period, tissues and organs increase in cell number rather than cell size (the hyperplastic phase of cell growth, when total deoxyribonucleic acid [DNA] content increases in new tissues). Later phases of growth include a period when cell size also increases (protein and ribonucleic acid [RNA] content), along with continued enhancement of cell number (mixed hyperplastic and hypertrophic phase). In muscle and brain (especially the cerebellum), this phase of growth may continue through adolescence and the second year of life, respectively. The final stage of growth is a purely hypertrophic phase, when only cell size increases.

The contribution of each tissue to body weight changes during fetal and postnatal development is depicted in Table 7-2. Muscle represents only 25% of fetal and neonatal body weight; once full adult maturity has been achieved, it accounts for 40% of the body's mass. Fetal muscle growth, as well as all protein synthesis in the fetus, depends on active transport of amino acids across the placenta. Once provided with these precursors, fetal protein synthesis is autonomous and results in the net synthesis of proteins that have amino acid patterns equivalent to those in the adult. Although the building blocks may be the same, developmentally the fetal muscle has a lower fibrillar protein content, whereas the sarcoplasmic protein concentration remains unchanged as maturation proceeds. Besides those immunoglobulins that cross the placenta, all protein present in the fetus has been synthesized de novo within fetal tissue.

Paralleling the patterns of fetal growth, the macromolecular composition of the body also undergoes sequential patterns of change. One general trend includes a decrease of total body and extracellular water content as the fetus and infant mature (Fig. 7-3; Table 7-3). Simultaneously, there is an increment of body protein and fat content (Fig. 7-4). Whereas the increase of tissue protein is gradual during development, the increment of fetal body fat is delayed until the third trimester. Once initiated, the deposition of subcutaneous and deep body adipose tissue accelerates more rapidly than the rate of protein accumulation.

Coinciding with the changes of the extracellular fluid space, the sodium and chloride concentration in the fetus declines, whereas the expansion of the intracellular fluid space results in an increase of potassium concentration. The decline of the total body sodium is less than that for chloride, since sodium is also a component of fetal bone. Calcium, phosphorus, and magnesium are nevertheless the major minerals in bone. By term the total body calcium/phosphorus ratio is 1.7:1.8 with 98% of calcium, 80% of phosphorus, and 60% of magnesium deposited within the bone.

To summarize, the composition and rate of new tissue deposited during each period of gestation varies (Fig. 7-4). As development proceeds toward term gestation, wa-

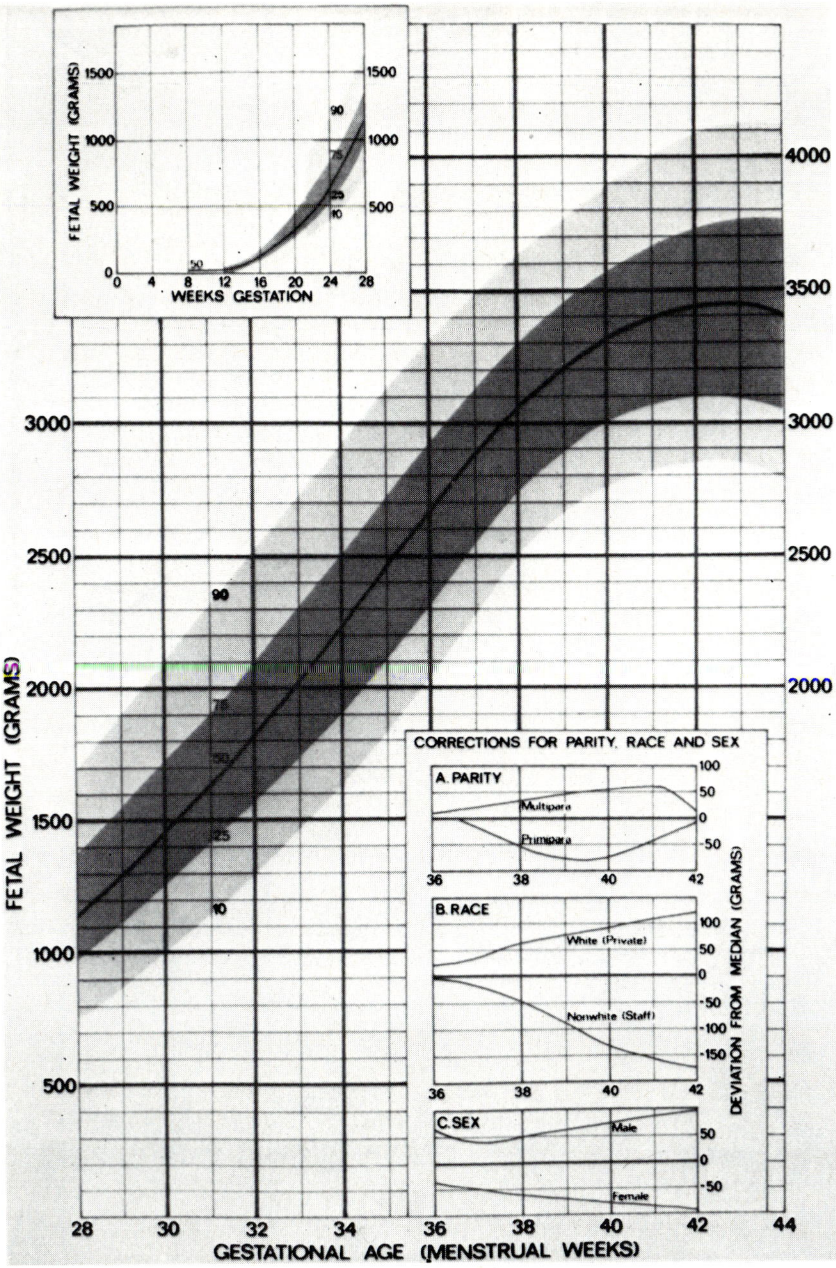

Fig. 7-1. Fetal weight with correction for parity, race (socioeconomic), and sex derived from 31,202 prostaglandin abortions and "spontaneous" deliveries. (From Brenner, W., and others: Am. J. Obstet. Gynecol. **126:**555, 1976.)

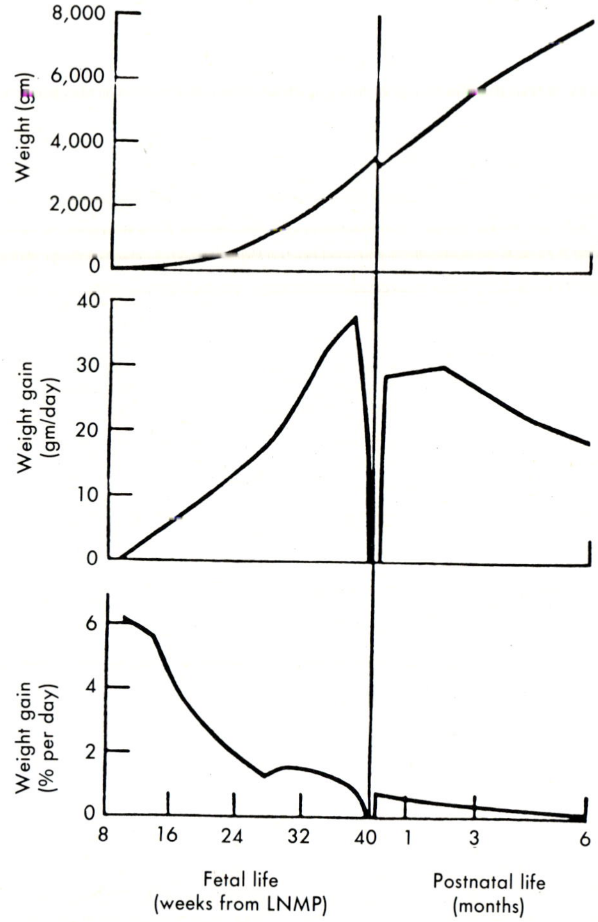

Fig. 7-2. Smoothed curves for fetal and postnatal growth in grams and grams gained per day and expressed as percent increment of body weight. (From Usher, R., and McLean, F. In Davis, J., and Dobbing, J., editors: Scientific foundations of pediatrics, Philadelphia, 1974, W.B. Saunders Co.)

Table 7-2. Contribution of organs to body mass during development

Tissue	Fetus 20-24 weeks (%)	Full-term baby (%)	Adult (%)
Skeletal muscle	25	25	43
Skin	13	15	7
Skeleton	22	18	18
Heart	0.6	0.5	0.4
Liver	4	5	2
Kidneys	0.7	1	0.5
Brain	13	13	2

From Widdowson, E. In Assali, N., editor: Biology of gestation, vol. 2, New York, 1968, Academic Press, Inc. With permission.

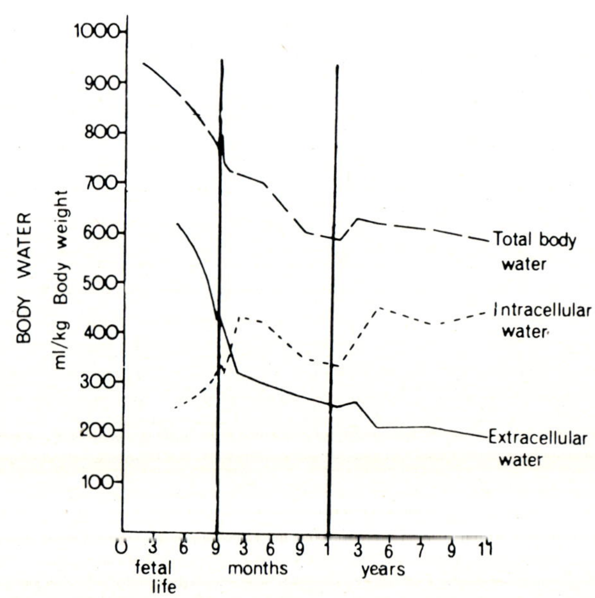

Fig. 7-3. Developmental alterations of fluid space distribution. (From Uttley, W., and Habel, A.: Clin. Endocrinol. Metabol. **5**:3, 1976.)

Table 7-3. Body composition of the reference fetus

		Per 100 gm body weight				Per 100 gm fat-free weight							
Gestational age (weeks)	**Body weight (gm)**	**Water (gm)**	**Protein (gm)**	**Lipid (gm)**	**Other (gm)**	**Water (gm)**	**Protein (gm)**	**Ca (mg)**	**P (mg)**	**Mg (mg)**	**Na (mEq)**	**K (mEq)**	**Cl (mEq)**
24	690	88.6	8.8	0.1	2.5	88.6	8.8	621	387	17.8	9.9	4.0	7.0
25	770	87.8	9.0	0.7	2.5	88.4	9.1	615	385	17.6	9.8	4.0	7.0
26	880	86.8	9.2	1.5	2.5	88.1	9.4	611	384	17.5	9.7	4.1	7.0
27	1010	85.7	9.4	2.4	2.5	87.8	9.7	609	383	17.4	9.5	4.1	6.9
28	1160	84.6	9.6	3.3	2.4	87.5	10.0	610	385	17.4	9.4	4.2	6.9
29	1318	83.6	9.9	4.1	2.4	87.2	10.3	613	387	17.4	9.3	4.2	6.8
30	1480	82.6	10.1	4.9	2.4	86.8	10.6	619	392	17.4	9.2	4.3	6.8
31	1650	81.7	10.3	5.6	2.4	86.5	10.9	628	398	17.6	9.1	4.3	6.7
32	1830	80.7	10.6	6.3	2.4	86.1	11.3	640	406	17.8	9.1	4.3	6.6
33	2020	79.8	10.8	6.9	2.5	85.8	11.6	656	416	18.0	9.0	4.4	6.5
34	2230	79.0	11.0	7.5	2.5	85.4	11.9	675	428	18.3	8.9	4.4	6.4
35	2450	78.1	11.2	8.1	2.6	85.0	12.2	699	443	18.6	8.9	4.5	6.3
36	2690	77.3	11.4	8.7	2.6	84.6	12.5	726	460	19.0	8.8	4.5	6.1
37	2940	76.4	11.6	9.3	2.7	84.3	12.8	758	479	19.5	8.8	4.5	6.0
38	3160	75.6	11.8	9.9	2.7	83.9	13.1	795	501	20.0	8.8	4.5	5.9
39	3330	74.8	11.9	10.5	2.8	83.6	13.3	836	525	20.5	8.7	4.6	5.8
40	3450	74.0	12.0	11.2	2.8	83.3	13.5	882	551	21.1	8.7	4.6	5.7

From Ziegler, E., and others: Growth **40:**329, 1976. With permission.

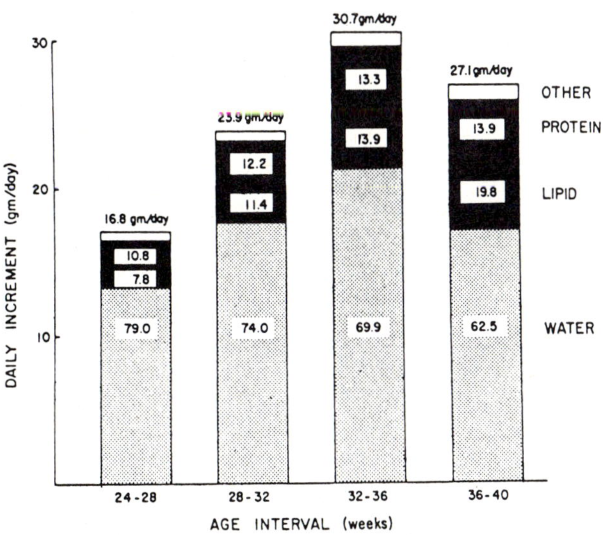

Fig. 7-4. Composition of fetal weight gain. (From Ziegler, E., and others: Growth **40:**329, 1976.)

ter represents a smaller component of each gram of fetal weight, whereas lipid and protein contribute a greater percentage to the mean increment of daily weight gain.

FETAL METABOLISM

Although the fetus is described as the perfect parasite, maternal and fetal nutritional deprivations can adversely affect fetal growth. The fetus depends on maternal nutrient intake and maternal endogenous substrate stores as precursors for fetal tissue synthesis and fuel for fetal oxidative metabolism. The oxygen consumed by the fetus in turn provides energy to support essential fetal "work," such as maintenance of transmembrane potentials and replacement of tissue components that are continuously being renewed. In addition, fetal oxygen consumption is required for net synthesis of complex macromolecules such as DNA, RNA, protein, and lipid. Each gram of protein synthesized requires the expenditure of 7.5 Cal, whereas a gram of triglycerides requires 11.6 Cal. Since 4.85 Cal use 1 L of oxygen, net tissue synthesis represents a substantial proportion of fetal oxygen consumption, which is approximately 4 to 6 ml/kg/minute. The energy cost of neonatal growth among premature infants constitutes the energy stored in tissue plus that expended for the synthesis of that tissue. Total energy cost per gram of new tissue is approximately 5.7 Cal, whereas that remaining in structural or depot macromolecules represents 4.0 Cal. Therefore 1.7 Cal are expended to produce 1 gm of new tissue. A similar relationship should occur in the third-trimester fetus, since energy requirements for growth should not change following birth.

Maternal metabolic adjustments during pregnancy are characterized by fuel and hormonal alterations that attempt to secure a continuous provision of substrates for use by the fetus. During periods of alimentation, sufficient substrates are presented to the uteroplacental circulation while maternal fuel stores are simultaneously enriched. During the third trimester maternal insulin resistance may partition ingested fuels toward the fetus. When fasting occurs during pregnancy, fuel mobilization is accelerated, as is evident by the rapid rise of maternal free fatty acids and ketone bodies. This accelerated mobilization of maternal adipose tissue stores is facilitated by a rapid decline of insulin levels and an enhanced secretion of human placental somatomammotropin. This latter placental hormone has lipolytic activity and may also diminish maternal glucose oxidation directly. In addition, maternal glucose utilization is attenuated because free fatty acids and ketones replace glucose as a fuel in maternal tissues, whereas hypoinsulinemia reduces glucose uptake in the insulin-dependent tissue of the mother. Thus fetal glucose provision may be continued. In addition, alternate substrates mobilized during maternal fasting, such as ketones, cross the placenta and may attempt to maintain fetal growth and development. Ketones may be oxidized or serve as precursors for fetal lipid or protein synthesis. This accelerated mobilization of fuels can ensure fetal growth during short periods of maternal fasting; however, prolonged periods of starvation will adversely affect fetal outcome.

The substrates used to maintain fetal oxygen consumption have been most accurately determined in the ovine fetus (Table 7-4). Glucose accounts for approximately 50% of fetal energy production in sheep when the mother is maintained in a high nutritional plane. Amino acids, in addition to functioning as precursors for fetal protein synthesis, serve as an oxidizable fuel; they may contribute to 25% of ovine fetal oxygen uptake. Taken together, lactate and acetate may supply an additional 25%. Data from human pregnancies suggest that glucose oxidation may contribute a greater proportion of fetal energy production than that in the ovine fetus.

Similarly, fetal respiratory quotient has been estimated to be close to 1.0 in other mammalian species, which suggests that carbohydrate oxidation is the predominant source for fetal oxidative metabolism. As discussed previously, fasting during human pregnancy may result in an alteration of substrates presented to the fetus when the level of maternal and subsequently fetal ketone

Table 7-4. Oxidizable substrates in the ovine fetus*

Substrate	Total oxygen consumption accounted for (%)
Glucose	50
Amino acids	25
Lactate	20
Acetate	5 to 10
Free fatty acids	Not significant
Fructose	Not significant
Glycerol	Not significant
Keto acids	Not significant

From Milley, J., and Simmons, M.: Clin. Perinatol. **6**:365, 1979. With permission.

*Sheep placenta is impermeable to free fatty acids and ketones, in contrast to that of other mammals, which may be permeable to these substrates.

bodies increase. Ketones may then serve as fuels for energy production and also as precursors for amino acids, proteins, and lipids. Although free fatty acids, especially the essential fatty acids, must cross the placenta, their role in fetal energy production is limited, since they probably are deposited in structural or depot tissues (Fig. 7-5).

In addition to the provision of substrates for fetal oxygen consumption and growth, tissue growth also depends on an appropriate fetal endocrine milieu (Table 7-5). Among the hormones, insulin has been implicated as the "growth hormone" of the fetus. Since insulin does not cross the placenta, this growth-enhancing hormone must be of fetal origin. Insulin promotes fetal deposition of adipose and glycogen stores while potentially stimulating amino acid uptake and protein synthesis in muscle. In the absence of fetal insulin production, as in conditions such as pancreatic aplasia, transient neonatal diabetes mellitus, or congenital absence of the islets of Langerhans, fetal growth is impaired. Also, when the peripheral action of insulin is attenuated by diminished receptor or postreceptor events, as in leprechaunism, fetal growth may be impaired. On the other hand, those neonates experiencing prolonged periods of hyperinsulinism in utero, such as infants of diabetic mothers or infants with Beckwith-Wiedemann syndrome or nesidioblastosis, demonstrate enhanced adipose and muscle tissue mass resulting in excessive birth weight (Chapter 37, part one). Amniotic fluid levels of C-peptide, a cleavage protein of proinsulin, vary directly with fetal growth status: C-peptide is reduced with intrauterine growth retardation and increased with fetal macrosomia.

Growth hormone probably does not influence fetal growth. The birth weight of a panhypopituitary fetus is not different from that of a normal fetus. However, the final common pathway of growth hormone action is mediated by the generation of insulin-like growth regulatory factors, the somatomedins (Table 7-5). The concentration

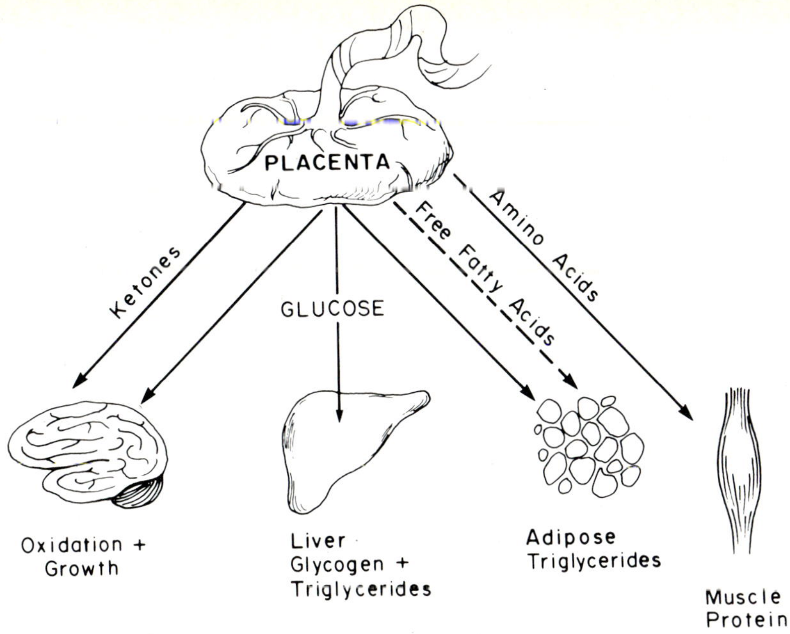

Fig. 7-5. Placental nutrient support and disposition of substrates. (Modified from Adam, P.A.J.: Metabolism in pregnant woman and fetus. In Falkner, F., and Tanner, J.: Human growth, vol. 1, New York, 1978, Plenum Press.)

Table 7-5. Hormonal effect on fetal growth

Hormone	Concentration*	Growth effect	Comment
Growth hormone	High	None	Absent tissue receptor
Thyroid	Low	None on growth ↑ Epiphyseal maturation	Fetus inactivates thyroxine (T_4) to reverse triiodothyronine (T_3) Postreceptor defect Stimulates epidermal growth factor
Androgens	High	Minimal	Specific receptors on gonadal tissue
Insulin	Normal	Major	Action by: ↑ Nutrient uptake ↑ Binding to type I insulin-like growth factor (IGF) receptor ↑ Release of IGF I
Vitamin D			
24,25-D_3	High	Anabolic for bone	Receptors on cartilage
1,25-D_3	Low		
Somatomedins (A, B, C)	High ↑ Levels with ↑ birth weight	Anabolic	Receptors present May ↑ growth independent of growth hormone ↑ In Beckwith-Wiedemann syndrome ↓ In IUGR
Insulin-like growth†:			
Factor I (IGFI)	Low	Unknown	Levels ↑ with gestational age
Factor II (IGFII)	Low	Purported growth factor	Levels ↑ before term but low at term
Epidermal growth factor (EGF) (urogastrone)	Unknown	Mitogen for epidermal cells and fibroblasts	Effects eye opening and tooth eruption in mice
Multiplication growth factor	High	Similar to IGF II	May be specific "fetal" somatomedin
Nerve growth factor	High	Mitosis of ganglion and glial cells	Maturation of adrenergic neurons and sympathetic nervous system
Platelet-derived growth factor	Unknown	Mitogenic for connective tissue	Related to tumor growth factors

*Compared with postnatal values.
†IGF II is identical to somatomedin C. IGF I and IGF II bind to specific receptors, stimulate mitosis, and are the mediators of growth hormone's effect on postnatal growth. These growth factors may function at the site of origin (paracrine) or through an endocrine mechanism by circulating on specific binding proteins. Type I IGF receptors are structurally similar to the insulin receptor and have high affinity for IGF I and IGF II and low affinity for insulin. Type II IGF receptors have less affinity for insulin. In utero growth hormone exerts little or no regulation of somatomedins or IGF, whereas other hormones (fetal insulin or placental lactogen) or substrates (glucose) may regulate somatomedin or IGF II secretion. Placental lactogen stimulates IGF II but not IGF I production by fetal fibroblasts. Furthermore, IGF II production predominates the fetal state, whereas IGF I is postnatal. Pygmy dwarfism is caused by an isolated IGF II deficiency; Laron type dwarfism is caused by low somatomedin levels. IGF II and insulin levels are reduced in IUGR with transient neonatal diabetes. Following postnatal malnutrition, low levels of IGF I increase with nutritional rehabilitation. Also, growth retardation in fetal alcohol syndrome may result from reduced receptor binding of somatomedins. Somatomedin and IGF levels have also correlated with a reduction in IUGR and an increase in large for gestational age (LGA) status. These hormones do not cross the placenta and are released by fibroblasts or hepatocytes.

of these substances in cord blood correlates with fetal weight. SGA infants may have diminished somatomedin values. Additional growth hormone–dependent "growth factors" include multiplication stimulating action factor and insulin growth factors I and II. Other growth hormone–independent factors, such as fibroblast growth factor, nerve growth factor, and epidermal growth factor, may have more specific effects on growth or differentiation.

The role of other hormones, notably corticosteroids and thyroid hormone, has not been well defined for fetal growth. With thyroid hormone deficiency, in the human athyrotic cretin, birth weight is not altered. These hormones, however, probably have a more significant role as regulatory signals for the initiation of maturation and differentiation in fetal tissues.

EPIDEMIOLOGY OF LOW BIRTH WEIGHT

See also Chapter 1.

The term *low birth weight* refers to infants born weighing less than 2,500 gm. Neonatal mortality is directly related to the low birth weight rate in a given population. These high-risk infants are a heterogenous group consisting of infants born preterm (less than 37 weeks) and those born at term but of reduced weight.

IUGR is the predominant etiology of low birth weight among developing areas and nations with low birth weight rates above 10%. Socioeconomic improvement decreases the proportion of IUGR. Between 20% to 30% of preterm infants also have decreased growth for gestational age. Although there appear to be differences in the relative incidence of IUGR and premature birth between countries, risk factors associated with birth of a low birth weight infant are similar (boxed material).

The rate of reduced weight at term gestation is probably twice as great among black infants as white. This may be independent of socioeconomic variables (which are of paramount importance), since black infants often have lower birth weight than infants of Hispanic or Oriental parents of similar socioeconomic status. Interestingly, the risk for low birth weight is related not only to the occupation of the future child's parents, but also to that of the grandparents. Provision of adequate nutrition and other environmental factors to the future mother may alter her growth and future reproductive capability. This intergenerational effect explains in part the observation that mothers of low birth weight infants were themselves low birth weight neonates. Although medical complications of pregnancy occur equally in all socioeconomic groups, many adverse behavioral attitudes or practices contribute to the greater low birth weight rate among women of low socioeconomic status.

Overview of risk factors* for low birth weight

DEMOGRAPHIC
- Race (black)
- Present low socioeconomic status
- Socioeconomic status of infant's grandparents

PREGNANCY
- Multiple gestation
- Birth order
- Anemia
- Elevated hemoglobin concentration (inadequate plasma volume expansion?)
- Fetal disease
- Preeclampsia and hypertension
- Infections
- Placental problems
- Premature rupture of membranes

PREPREGNANCY
- Low weight for height
- Short stature
- Chronic medical illness
- Poor nutrition
- Low maternal weight at mother's birth
- Previous low birth weight infant
- Uterine or cervical anomalies
- Parity (none or more than five)

BEHAVIORAL (maternal choices)
- Low educational status
- Smoking
- No care or inadequate prenatal care
- Poor weight gain during pregnancy
- Alcohol abuse
- Illicit and prescription drugs
- Short interpregnancy interval (less than 6 months)
- Age (less than 16 or over 35)
- Unmarried
- Stress (physical and psychologic)

Modified from Committee To Study the Prevention of Low Birthweight: Prevention of low birthweight, Washington, D.C., 1985, Institute of Medicine, National Academy Press.

*Many of these variables are risk factors for *both* IUGR and prematurity. These variables are not necessarily univariant risk factors, but rather interact in a complex relationship. Only a few factors exert an independent effect. The relationship between black race and low birth weight remains a significant factor, with a twofold increase in the incidence of prematurity and IUGR when controlled for other risks.

MATERNAL CONTRIBUTIONS TO ABERRANT FETAL GROWTH

Physical environment

Certain otherwise normal mothers are prone to repeated delivery of SGA infants; the recurrence rate may be 25% to 50%. Many of these women themselves were born SGA, raising the possibility of nongenetic intergenerational transmission of a physical regulator of fetal growth. A proportion of these women also remain small throughout life and are identifiable by low prepregnancy weight and stature. These women may exert a restraint on fetal growth by some unknown regulator, possibly related to their own stature, previous nutritional status, or uterine capacity. This may be analogous to the breeding experiments between Shetland ponies and Shire horses. The offspring resulting from breeding a male Shire to a female Shetland is similar in birth weight to a Shetland pony, whereas that born to a cross between a male Shetland and a female Shire approaches the birth weight of a Shire. The smaller Shetland female apparently exerts a growth restraint on the genetic potential derived from the larger Shire male.

Maternal genetic factors have a major direct effect on fetal growth. This influence depends on a transfer of maternal genes, but also on other unexplained maternal genetic factors related in part to uteroplacental function. The observations that sisters of sisters with SGA infants are at higher risk for having SGA infants than their sisters-in-law give further evidence of maternal genetic influences on fetal growth.

Paternal factors have less effect on fetal growth. Paternal genes affect fetal growth directly by transfer of genetic material, which may be modified (accelerated or inhibited) by maternal factors. Paternal genotypic potential is best expressed as a function of postnatal growth.

Other constraints on fetal growth may be exerted during multiple gestations, since fetal growth declines when the number of fetuses increases. The onset of growth retardation in multiple gestations is also related to the number of fetuses, since growth restraint begins sooner with triplets than twins (Fig. 7-6). In multiple gestations the uterine constraint appears to occur when combined fetal size approaches 3 kg. Placental implantation site, uterine anomalies, vascular anastomoses, and nutritional factors may also interfere with growth in these pregnancies. The uterine capacity itself may also place a constraint on optimum fetal growth.

Maternal nutrition

Prepregnancy weight and pregnancy weight gain are two important independent variables that affect fetal growth. Underweight mothers and those affected with malnutrition deliver infants with diminished birth weight. Weight gain during pregnancy in nonobese patients correlates significantly with fetal birth weight. The effect of prepregnancy weight in obese women is inde-

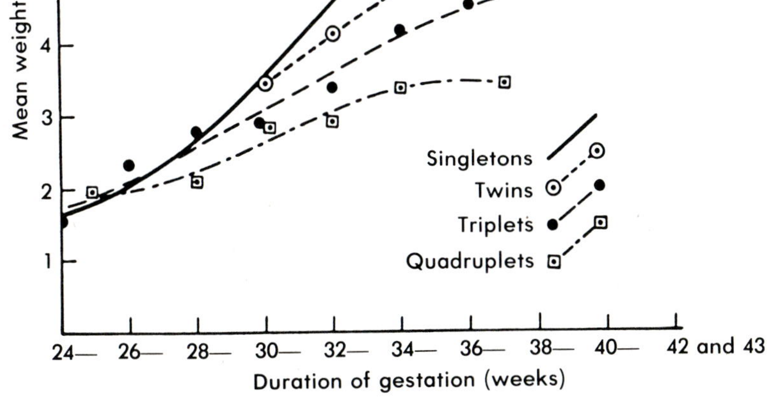

Fig. 7-6. Birth weight–gestational age relationships in multiple gestation denoting origin of aberrant fetal growth. (From McKeown, T., and Record, R.: J. Endocrinol. **8:**386, 1952.)

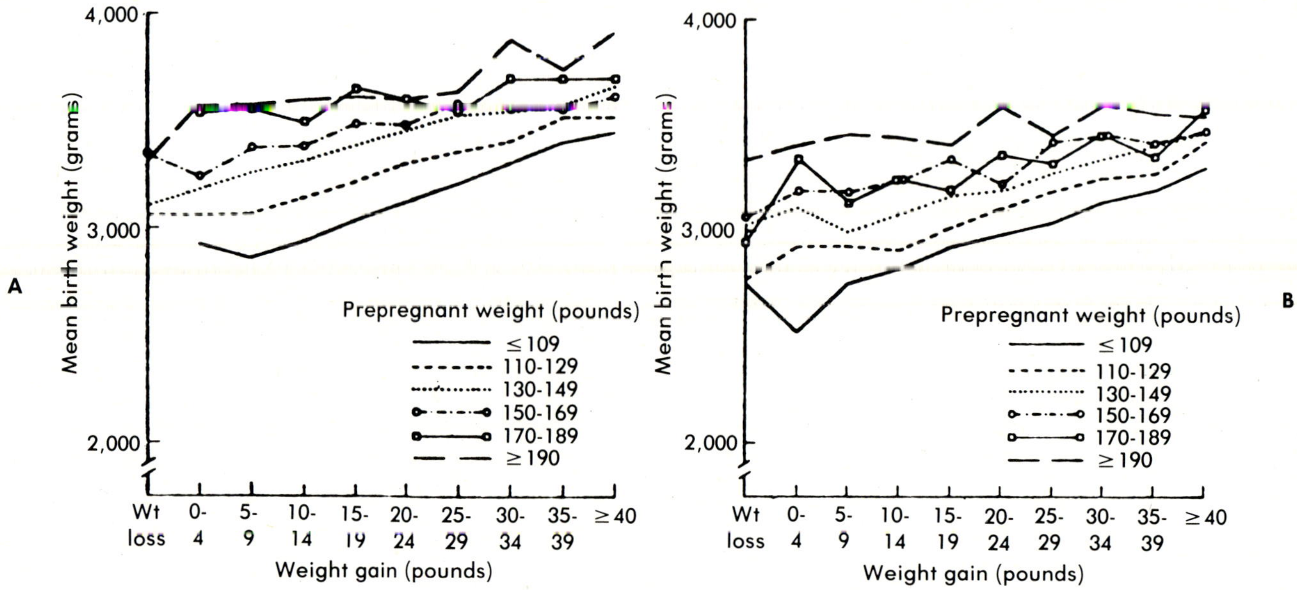

Fig. 7-7. Effect of prepregnancy weight and weight gain during pregnancy among white women (**A**) and black women (**B**). Note the reduced birth weight at term at all levels of maternal weight variables among black women. Also note that weight gain during pregnancy has its most positive effect on birth weight among lean women. Nonetheless, prepregnancy weight among obese, usually nondiabetic women has the greatest effect on birth weight. (From Niswander, K., and others: Obstet. Gynecol. **33:**482, 1969. Reprinted with permission from The American College of Obstetricians and Gynecologists.)

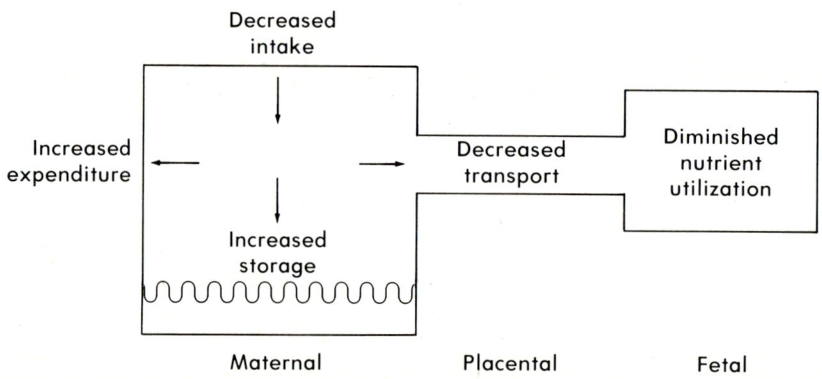

Fig. 7-8. Interrelationship of caloric intake and expenditure and fetal nutrient availability.

pendent of pregnancy weight gain and offsets the frequently observed poor weight gain of these overweight women (Fig. 7-7). SGA infants are unusual for obese women, whereas macrosomia is common. This may be related to large maternal nutrient stores.

The effects of maternal nutritional status on fetal growth are minimal during the first trimester of pregnancy. This is related to the large surfeit of nutrients presented to the relatively small, undemanding embryo and early fetus. As fetal growth accelerates, the requirements for fetal growth increase and may not be sufficiently provided by an inadequate maternal diet. Earlier attempts to limit weight gain in pregnancy with a 1,200 kcal diet to prevent preeclampsia resulted in a ten fold increase in growth retardation. In an otherwise healthy population of Dutch women experiencing a short period of famine during the Hunger Winter of 1944-1945, fetal growth was most severely affected when deprivation occurred in the third trimester. Substrate deficiency during this period resulted in an overall reduction of birth weight of 300 gm. Maternal weight gain and placental weight were even more drastically reduced, demonstrating preferential use of nutrients for the fetus. Poor nutrition may also reduce uterine blood flow, placental transport, and villous surface area (Fig. 7-8). Observations similar to the Dutch experience occurred during a more severe and prolonged famine in Leningrad, where birth weight was reduced by 500 gm at term.

As illustrated in Fig. 7-8, decreased caloric uptake below critical caloric needs may result in diminished fetal growth. Increased caloric expenditure may occur by two pathways: excessive physical activity and greater waste of calories. The nutritional aspects of cigarette smoking may be an example of the second path. Furthermore, the diminished heat expenditure that occurs among obese women may result in caloric storage and explain in part their excessively large babies. Increased maternal storage of calories may be exemplified by "selfish mother" hypothesis. These women may not develop usual insulin resistance during pregnancy and may direct ingested calories toward own tissue stores. These women have fasting hypoglycemia and/or accelerated disappearance of glucose following intravenous glucose tolerance test. Opposite of this occurs among women of low socioeconomic status who receive food supplementation; their skinfold thickness decreases as fetal weight increases. Decreased transport may reflect placental defects in function, nutrient supply, or blood flow. Decreased blood flow may be caused by peripheral vascular disease or failure to expand blood volume and cardiac output, as occurs in normal pregnancy. Fetuses with decreased numbers of cells may not be able to grow despite adequate nutrient supply. Examples include rubella embryopathy, autosomal trisomies, and other genetic causes of IUGR.

Attempts at improving the low birth weight outcome in high-risk populations (characterized by having poor nutritional histories) have demonstrated a positive effect of nutritional supplementation. Additional calories, rather than protein supplementation, correlate best with enhanced fetal weight. Caloric supplements greater than 20,000 calories per pregnancy reduced the number of low birth weight infants; each 10,000 calories supplemented above the standard diet improved fetal weight by an average of 29 gm. In Gambia, supplementation during seasonal periods of food shortage resulted in a net positive caloric intake of more than 400 kcal/day. This increased fetal weight 224 gm and reduced the low birth weight rate from 28% to under 5%. A threshold of 1,500 kcal/day was observed, which augmented fetal weight when the mother was in positive caloric balance.

Protein supplementation may even have adverse neurodevelopmental effects on the fetus. Aside from periods of famine and geographic areas where malnutrition is endemic, other conditions associated with poor maternal nutrition and suboptimum fetal growth are included in the following list.* Adolescent women, in particular, are at risk because of their own growth requirements in addition to those of the fetus.

1. Adolescents, especially those who are not married
2. Women with low prepregnancy weights
3. Women with inadequate weight gain during pregnancy
4. Women who have low income or problems purchasing food
5. Women with a history of frequent conceptions
6. Women with a history of infants having low birth weight
7. Women with diseases that influence nutritional status: diabetes, tuberculosis, anemia, drug addiction, alcoholism, or mental depression
8. Women known to be dietary faddists or with frank pica
9. Women who do heavy physical work during pregnancy

Certain maternal metabolic aberrations are associated with suboptimum fetal growth. Mothers who demonstrate excessively low fasting blood glucose values and those who fail to elevate their blood glucose sufficiently following an oral glucose tolerance test are at risk to deliver an SGA infant. A "selfish mother" hypothesis has been proposed to explain the poor growth of these infants. Additional nutrition variables affecting fetal weight are noted in Fig. 7-8.

*From Christaksis, G.: Am. J. Public Health **63**(suppl.):57, 1973.

Chronic disease

Of all disease mechanisms that interfere with fetal growth, those resulting in uterine ischemia and/or hypoxia have the most extreme effect. Chronic maternal hypertension caused by either primary renal parenchymal disease, such as nephritis, or those conditions extrinsic to parenchymal disorders, such as essential hypertension, significantly alters fetal growth and well-being. This effect is related to the duration of hypertension and to the absolute elevation of the diastolic pressure and is most severe in the presence of end-organ disorders, such as retinopathy. Well-controlled hypertension without the development of preeclampsia may not affect fetal growth.

Pregnancy-induced hypertension is of paramount importance to perinatologists in relation to its effect on fetal growth and well-being (Chapter 4). This disease, which may affect uteroplacental perfusion and fetal growth long before clinical signs of edema, proteinuria, and hypertension develop, reduces uterine blood flow, as determined by ^{24}Na and dehydroisonandrosterone clearance studies. Preeclampsia is characterized by an unusual sensitivity of maternal blood vessels to vasoactive compounds, resulting in enhanced and pathologic vasoconstriction. Low-dose aspirin, by reducing thromboxane production, may prevent platelet aggregation and arterial vasoconstriction and may improve fetal growth. In preg-

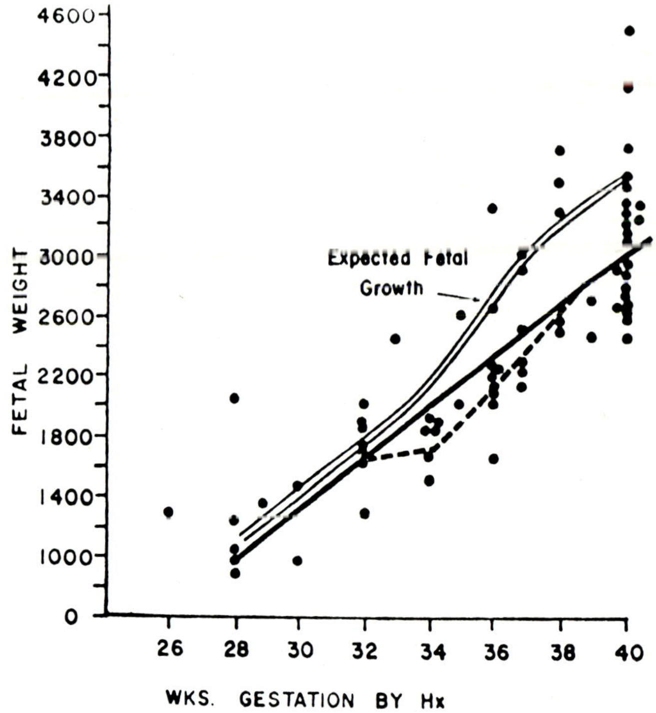

Fig. 7-9. Fetal weight following eclampsia. Broken line demonstrates mean weight alteration. (From Zuspan, F.: Clin. Obstet. Gynecol. **9**:954, 1966.)

nancies complicated by eclampsia, fetal growth deviates from the expected norm from 32 weeks onward (Fig. 7-9). Vascular insufficiency resulting from advanced maternal diabetes mellitus, especially in the presence of end-organ disease in the kidney or retina, also produces IUGR despite the presence of maternal hyperglycemia (Chapter 3). Women with serious autoimmune disease associated with the lupus anticoagulant are also a high-risk population for preeclampsia and IUGR.

Another major category associated with diminished fetal weight gain is that resulting from maternal hypoxemia. Severe cyanotic congenital heart disease, such as tetralogy of Fallot or Eisenmenger's complex, is the best example of this mechanism, whereas sickle cell anemia is representative of diseases that can produce local uterine hypoxia and ischemia. Nutritional anemias are not usually associated with aberrant fetal growth. In sickle cell anemia the abnormal cells may interfere with local uterine perfusion during episodes of sickling, and growth retardation is observed.

A common and nonpathologic factor related to maternal hypoxia is the diminished environmental oxygen saturation that is present at high altitudes. Infants born in the mountains of Peru demonstrate lower birth weights than do Peruvian infants born at sea level. Placental mass has hypertrophied in these newborns in an attempt to compensate for the lower circulating maternal oxygen concentration. Interestingly, these neonates are not born with polycythemia as a response to fetal hypoxia, as proposed in other SGA infants.

Drugs

The effects of maternal drug administration on the fetus are usually considered primarily in terms of teratogenicity. However, a continuum of fetal compromise may be present, since many malformation syndromes are associated with diminished birth weight, whereas other agents may interfere only with fetal growth. Drugs associated with intrauterine growth retardation are included in the following list:

1. Amphetamines
2. Antimetabolites (aminopterin, busulfan, methotrexate, etc.)
3. Bromides
4. Cigarettes (carbon monoxide, thiocyanate, nicotine)
5. Cocaine(?)
6. Ethanol (acetaldehyde)
7. Heroin
8. Hydantoin
9. Methadone
10. Phencyclidine
11. Polychlorinated biphenyls (PCBs)
12. Propranolol
13. Steroids (prednisone)
14. Toluene
15. Trimethadione (Tridione)
16. Warfarin

Many of the typically abused drugs have been implicated as agents producing fetal growth retardation by reducing maternal appetite and by being associated with lower socioeconomic groups. However, at least for heroin, methadone, and ethanol, a cellular toxic effect acting directly on cell replication and growth appears to be involved. This is most evident in the fetal alcohol syndrome, since the prenatal onset of growth retardation persists during postnatal periods despite adequate food intake. A placental transfer block for specific amino acids has been observed, resulting in the fetal alcohol syndrome.

Cigarette smoking during pregnancy reduces eventual fetal birth weight and is related directly to the amount of cigarettes consumed. Birth weight at term is reduced an average of 170 gm if more than 10 cigarettes are consumed per day; consumption of more than 15 per day may reduce weight by 300 gm. The mechanism of fetal growth retardation is uncertain, but nicotine and subsequent catecholamine release may produce uterine vasoconstriction and fetal hypoxia, whereas carbon monoxide and cyanide may cause a more direct effect. Following binding to hemoglobin, carbon monoxide and cyanide may diminish oxygen unloading from the mother to the fetus and from the fetus to its tissues. Nutritional supplementation does not completely eliminate the reduced fetal weight. Also, the effects of cigarettes may be greatest at advanced maternal age.

Drugs such as propranolol and corticosteroids probably have a direct effect on the fetus, although the confounding influences of the chronic maternal illness for which these agents are prescribed may also contribute to IUGR.

Socioeconomic status

Poor environmental conditions related to lower socioeconomic status have been associated with infant malnutrition of both prenatal and postnatal onset. With improvement of these conditions, birth weight is enhanced. This was extensively studied following the improvements in living conditions that occurred in postwar Japan. The improvement of birth weight during this era occurred only in infants born during the latter part of the third trimester, since nutritional or environmental effects seem greatest during this period of fetal growth.

Many of the maternal factors, such as drug abuse, poor nutritional habits, and cigarette smoking, are interrelated and are covariables associated with poor socioeconomic status. Factors such as adverse environmental living conditions and low levels of education are more prevalent among reproductive-age women of lower socioeconomic status. Adolescent and single-parent families and those who seek little prenatal advice are also more common variables among women in this bracket. Many investigations have demonstrated that these groups of women are at risk for IUGR. Evidence has been proposed suggesting that if chronic maternal illness and certain behavioral characteristics are eliminated, the remaining women of lower socioeconomic status do not have a higher incidence of SGA infants. The specific behavioral characteristics more common among poor women are noted in the previous boxed material.

These behavioral variables may be related to an attitude difference among these women, who choose a different life-style and constitute a subgroup, and may not specifically represent the entire population. Thus these behaviors may be based on choice and not necessarily environment.

PLACENTAL DETERMINANTS

Optimum fetal growth depends on efficient placental function as both nutrient supply line and organ of gaseous exchange. Placental functional integrity requires additional energy production, since placental oxidative metabolism may equal that of the fetus. This large energy requirement is essential to maintain fetal growth-promoting roles, which include the active transport of amino acids, synthesis of protein and steroid hormones, and support of placental maturation and growth. Placental growth parallels that of the fetus; however, toward term there is a greater decline in the rate of placental weight gain than that in the fetus. During this decline of placental weight, the fetus also exhibits a decrement in rate of weight change, suggesting that placental function, as well as weight, has declined and led to reduced fetal growth, as previously noted. However, despite the change in placental weight, the placenta continues to mature. Placental villous surface area continues to increase with advancing gestational age (Fig. 7-10); simultaneously, the syncytial trophoblast layer continues to thin out and vascularization of the terminal villi continues to improve. Functionally, urea clearance is enhanced toward term in the ovine placenta (Fig. 7-11), suggesting that permeability and diffusing distance improve as the placenta approaches term. Birth weight has been correlated to placental weight (Fig. 7-12) and villous surface area (Fig. 7-10), suggesting that macroscopic and microscopic events are related to optimum placental function. Uterine blood flow, and thus placental oxygen or nutrient transfer, may be reduced if maternal blood volume is contracted. Failure to expand plasma volume, which normally occurs in the last half of gestation, has been associated with IUGR. These high-risk women may be identified through an elevated hemoglobin level.

When placental insufficiency occurs, there may be a functional failure of the placenta as a respiratory or nutritive organ or both. Placental insufficiency associated with maternal nutritional deficiency has more than one effect on fetal growth. In addition to diminished fetal substrate provision, placental metabolism will be altered directly, as proposed in Fig. 7-8. Diminished placental

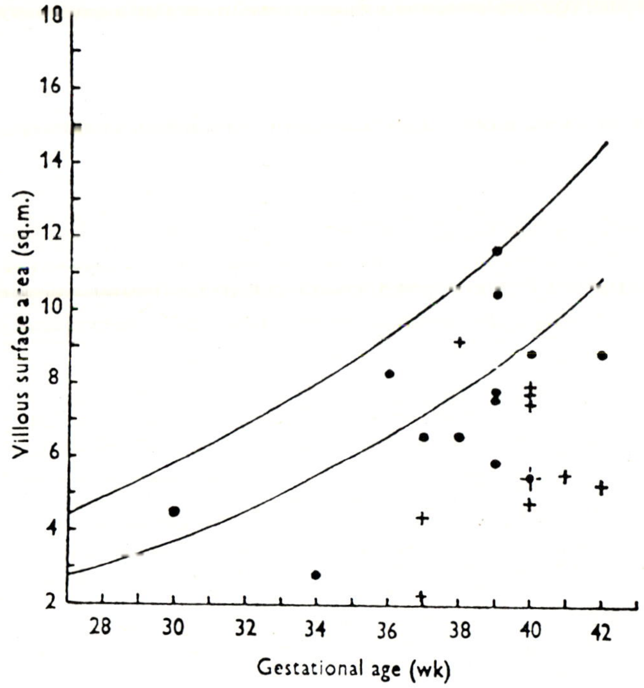

Fig. 7-10. Area of chorionic surface area in normal and abnormal pregnancies. ●, Maternal hypertension; +, normotensive, IUGR. (From Aherne, W., and Dunnill, M.: J. Pathol. Bacteriol. **91:**132, 1966.)

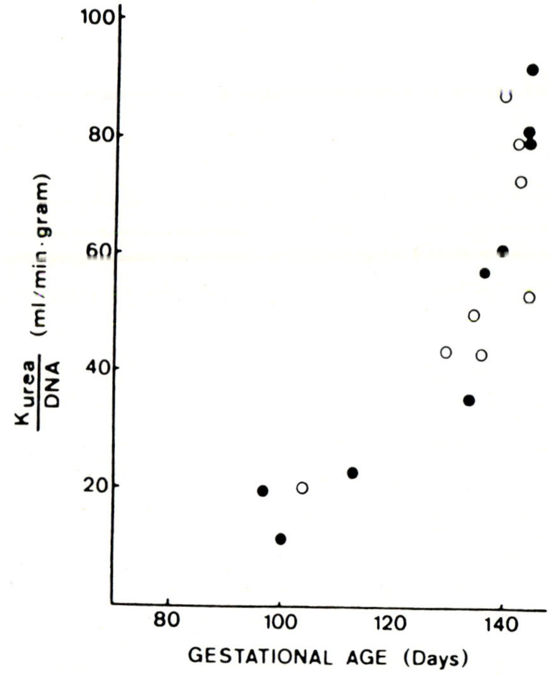

Fig. 7-11. Urea permeability per gram of the ovine placenta. ●, Singletons; ○, twins. (From Kulhanek, J., and others: Am. J. Physiol. **226:**1257, 1974.)

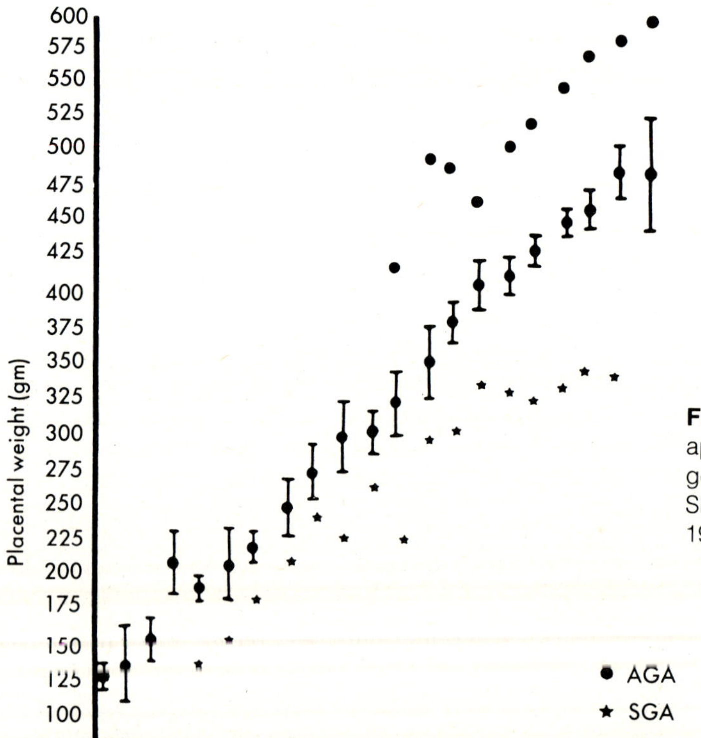

Fig. 7-12. Placental weight–gestational age relationship in appropriate for gestational age *(AGA)*, *SGA*, and large for gestational age *(LGA)* neonates. Mean placental weight ± SEM. (From Molteni, R., and others: J. Reprod. Med. **21:**327, 1978.)

growth will adversely affect total nutrient transfer, whereas reduced placental production of chorionic somatomammotropin will attenuate maternal mobilization of fuels to her fetus. Reduced placental energy production and protein synthesis will limit active transport of amino acids and facilitative transport of glucose.

When placental insufficiency complicates maternal vascular disease such as preeclampsia, placental weight and volume also diminish. In addition, a decline in villous surface area (Fig. 7-10) and a relative increase of nonexchanging tissue occur. At the same time, these placentas demonstrate thickening of the capillary basement membrane.

Following is a list of common findings in placental disorders associated with diminished birth weight:

1. Twins (implantation site)
2. Twins (vascular anastomoses)
3. Chorioangioma
4. Villitis (TORCH)
5. Villitis (unknown etiology)
6. Avascular villi
7. Ischemic villous necrosis
8. Multiple infarcts
9. Syncytial knots
10. Chronic separation (abruptio placentae)
11. Diffuse fibrinosis
12. Hydatidiform change
13. Abnormal insertion
14. Single umbilical artery
15. Fetal vessel thrombosis
16. Circumvallate placenta

Multiple gestations may produce significant placental disorders, both in suboptimum sites of implantation or, more often, related to abnormal vascular anastomoses in diamnionic monochorionic twinning (Fig. 7-13). As a result of arteriovenous interconnections, one twin serves as the donor and develops intrauterine growth retardation, losing nutrient supplies, whereas the other is the recipient and has satisfactory growth. These anastomoses may be detectable on careful gross examination of the placenta. Other detectable potential causes related to aberrant fetal growth include chorioangiomas, large retroplacental infarcts and hemorrhages, abnormal cord insertion patterns, and (questionably) single umbilical ar-

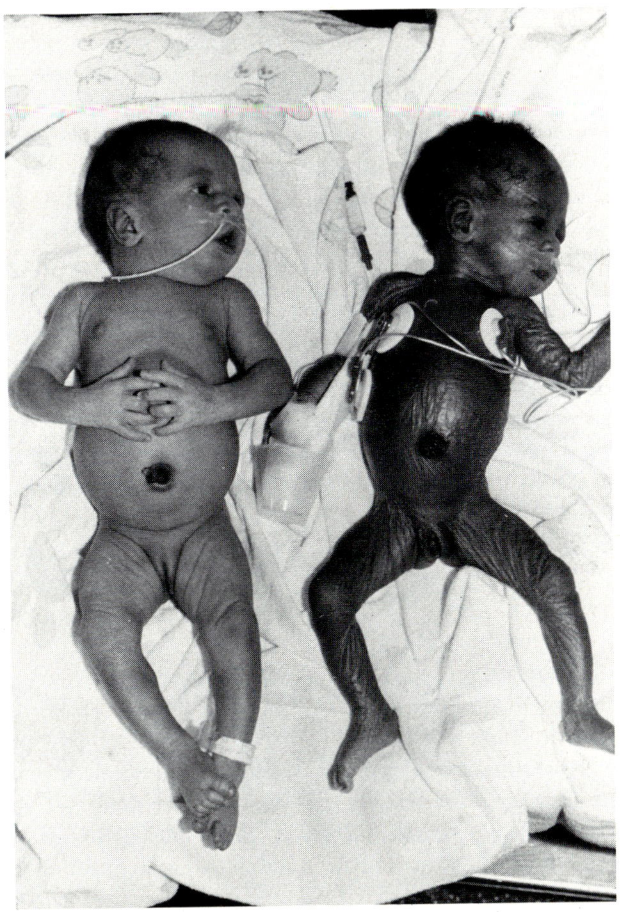

Fig. 7-13. Diamnionic monochorionic twins, 36 weeks' gestational age, with birth weights of 1.3 and 2.0 kg.

Table 7-6. Abnormalities of uteroplacental and fetal blood flow in IUGR pregnancies

Observation	Comment
50% ↓ uteroplacental flow	^{113}InCl to mother
↓ Uterine flow in malnutrition	Failure to increase cardiac output with pregnancy
↓ Placental nutrient transfer	
↑ Uterine artery systolic/diastolic waveform ratio	Suggests increased uterine artery resistance
↑ Umbilical artery velocity waveform	
↑ Fetal descending aortic pulsatile index*	Suggests increased peripheral vascular resistance
↓ Fetal descending aortic end-diastolic velocity	
↑ Fetal descending aortic resistance index	
↓ Fetal descending aortic peak velocity	Suggests decreased cardiac output, shunting away from descending aorta to brain, and fetal distress
↓ Umbilical venous flow	Associated with impending fetal distress
↓ Placental prostacyclin production	May promote platelet aggregation or diminish uterine vessel dilation

*Pulsatile index (PI) = $\frac{\text{Peak velocity} - \text{End-diastolic velocity}}{\text{Mean blood flow velocity}}$

tery. Combined reductions of uterine and umbilical blood flow have also been detected in IUGR. Furthermore, increased vascular resistance has been demonstrated in these circulations (Table 7-6). In addition, reduced placental prostacyclin (a potent vasodilator) production may be present in IUGR.

FETAL DETERMINANTS

Optimum fetal growth depends on adequate provision of substrates, their effective placental transfer, and the inherited regulatory factors within the fetal genotype. In addition to substrates, oxygen must be transferred and an appropriate hormonal milieu must be present. There must also be sufficient room within the uterus. In the absence of adverse environmental effects, the inherent growth potential of the fetus may be achieved.

Genetic determinants of fetal growth are inherited from both parents, and population norms must be established to detect aberrant fetal growth. For example, the average birth weight of Cheyenne Indians is 3,800 gm at term, whereas that for the New Guinea Luni tribe is 2,400 gm. Such genetic potentials are the major determinants of early fetal growth, since nutritional and environmental problems should not affect the fetus until the requirements for tissue growth increase during the third trimester.

Approximately 20% of birth weight variability in a given population is determined by the fetal genotype; maternal hereditary and environmental factors contribute an additional 65%; the remaining contributing factors are unknown. Birth order affects fetal size: Infants born to primiparous women weigh less than subsequent siblings (Fig. 7-1). The second and each additional child weigh an average of 180 gm more than the firstborn. This relationship is not true for multiparous adolescent pregnancies, in which subsequent births during adolescence produce neonates with lower term weights than the firstborn. Male sex of the fetus is associated with enhanced birth weight, beginning to become predominant after 28 weeks' gestation (Fig. 7-1). At term males weigh approximately 150 gm more than female infants. A male twin, in addition to affecting its own somatic growth, can also enhance the growth of its female co-twin. Androgenic hormonal stimulation of fetal growth may contribute to these observed differences. A theory also states that maternal-fetal antigenic (HL-A, ABO) differences are responsible for this effect. These antigenic differences result in enhanced placental trophoblastic invasion of the decidua, improving placental and subsequent fetal growth. As a corollary, interference with maternal immunologic function may inhibit this antigenic growth advantage and explain in part the diminished birth weights following maternal immunosuppressive therapy.

Alternately, chromosomes may carry growth-determining genes, since genetic material on the Y chromosome may enhance the growth of the male fetus. Similarly, chromosomal deletions or imbalances result in diminished fetal growth. For example, Turner's syndrome (XO) is associated with diminished birth weight. The converse is not true, since additional X chromosomes beyond the norm are associated with reduced fetal growth. For each additional X chromosome (in excess of XX), birth weight may be reduced 300 gm. Similarly, autosomal trisomies such as Down's syndrome are also associated with abnormal fetal growth. Chromosomal aberrations often result in diminished fetal growth by interfering with cell division. An intrinsic defect in cultured fibroblasts from trisomy 21 patients has been observed in tissue culture. In addition, placental function may be altered. Single-gene defects may also reduce fetal growth. The inborn errors most notably associated with diminished fetal weight are included in the following outline. Many syndromes with either autosomal recessive, dominant, polygenetic, or unknown inheritance are also associated with poor fetal growth and occasionally may produce marked intrauterine growth retardation.

Infectious agents are typically sought as being responsible for early onset of IUGR. Of these, cytomegalovirus and rubella virus are the most important identifiable agents associated with marked fetal growth retardation. Following maternal viremia, both agents invade the placenta, producing varying degrees of villitis, and then subsequently gain access to fetal tissues. The effects of placentitis itself on fetal growth are unknown, but once congenital fetal infection has occurred, these viral agents have direct adverse effects on fetal development. Intracellular rubella virus inhibits cellular mitotic activity in addition to producing chromosomal breaks and subsequently cytolysis. In addition, this virus produces an obliterative angiopathy that further compromises cell viability. Cytomegalovirus also causes cytolysis, resulting in areas of focal tissue necrosis. These viral agents therefore reduce cell number and subsequent birth weight by simultaneously inhibiting cell division and producing cell death.

Following are examples of factors affecting fetal growth:

A. Chromosome disorders associated with IUGR
   1. Trisomies 8, 13, 18, 21
   2. Short-arm deletion 4
   3. Long-arm deletion 13
   4. Long-arm deletion 21
   5. Triploidy
   6. XO
   7. XXY, XXXY, XXXXY
   8. XXXXX

B. Metabolic disorders associated with diminished birth weight
   1. Agenesis of pancreas
   2. Congenital absence of islets of Langerhans
   3. Congenital lipodystrophy
   4. Galactosemia (?)
   5. Generalized gangliosidosis type I
   6. Hypophosphatasia
   7. I cell disease
   8. Leprechaunism
   9. Maternal phenylketonuria
   10. Maternal renal insufficiency
   11. Maternal Gaucher's disease
   12. Menkes' syndrome
   13. Transient neonatal diabetes mellitus

C. Syndromes associated with diminished birth weight
   1. Aarskog-Scott syndrome
   2. Anencephaly
   3. Bloom's syndrome
   4. Cornelia de Lange syndrome
   5. Dubowitz syndrome
   6. Dwarfism (achondrogenesis, achondroplasia, etc.)
   7. Ellis-van Creveld syndrome
   8. Familial dysautonomia
   9. Fanconi's pancytopenia
   10. Meckel-Gruber syndrome
   11. Microcephaly
   12. Möbius' syndrome
   13. Osteogenesis imperfecta
   14. Potter's disease
   15. Prader-Willi syndrome
   16. Progeria
   17. Prune belly syndrome
   18. Radial aplasia; thrombocytopenia
   19. Robert's syndrome
   20. Silver syndrome
   21. Seckel's syndrome
   22. Smith-Lemli-Opitz syndrome
   23. VATER and VACTERL syndromes
   24. Williams syndrome

D. Congenital infections associated with IUGR.
   1. Rubella
   2. Cytomegalovirus
   3. Toxoplasmosis
   4. Malaria
   5. Syphilis
   6. Varicella
   7. Chagas' disease

THE SGA INFANT

Definition

Since the introduction of gestational age assessment and further subdivision of each neonatal age period into large, appropriate, and small for gestational age categories, it has become increasing apparent that the low birth weight infant (<2,500 gm) is not always premature (<37 weeks). On a worldwide basis, more than 20 million infants are born less than 2,500 gm. Between 30% and 40% of these infants are born at term gestation and are therefore undergrown, or SGA. As discussed previously, population norms need to be determined for each specific genetic group, especially those characterized by unusual inherited patterns of fetal growth. In general, these population norms established in various North American and European cities describe the usual fetal growth pattern for industrial societies and may be used as the reference norms for similar ethnic groups (Fig. 7-1; Table 7-1). Each curve defines either standard deviations or percentile units that include the normal variability or distribution of birth weights at each gestational age. By definition, infants less than two standard deviations or those less than the third percentile (tenth for Denver curves because of the lower birth weight at higher altitudes) will be classified as SGA. Therefore, between 2.5% and 10% of each population are SGA. The use of population means, however, is at times misleading. Within a sibship, fetal birth weight is less variable and more consistent than that for an entire population. Compared with family members, 80% of infants with congenital rubella infection were classified as SGA, whereas only 40% were SGA using population standards. Fetal growth assessment must therefore be considered in the context of both prior reproductive history and clinical examination of the newborn.

Aberrant fetal growth patterns

Fetal growth retardation may have its origins early or late during fetal development. Infants who demonstrate reduced fetal growth early in gestation constitute approximately 30% of all SGA infants. They are symmetrically growth retarded, since head circumference, weight, and length are proportionately affected to equivalent degrees. These fetuses and infants continue to grow, albeit with reduced net effect (Fig. 7-14, *A*). Besides inherent genetic growth constraint, other factors may produce diminished growth potential in these neonates. Congenital viral infections usually have their worst effect if infection occurs during the first trimester, when they have a significant effect on cell replication and subsequently birth weight. Similarly, abnormal genetic factors such as single gene deletions and chromosomal disorders also reduce the intrauterine growth rate at an early stage of development. Very early onset of growth delay has been reported in anomalous infants of diabetic mothers. The boxed material lists characteristics and examples of IUGR.

Growth retardation of a later onset is usually associated with impaired uteroplacental function or nutritional deficiency during the third trimester (Fig. 7-14, *B*). Nutrient supplies and uteroplacental perfusion are in excess of their requirements during early fetal development and should not interfere with fetal growth until the growth rate exceeds the provision of substrates and/or oxygen. During the last trimester the fetal growth rate and net tissue accretion increase markedly; if the uteroplacental supply line is compromised, IUGR will develop. The anthropomorphic findings among these infants demonstrate a relative sparing of head growth, whereas body

Characteristics and examples of IUGR

CHARACTERISTICS	
Early onset	Late onset
Symmetric	Asymmetric
Constitutional	Environmental
Low-profile biparietal diameter	Late flattening biparietal diameter
↓ Growth potential	Growth arrest
EXAMPLES	
Genetic	Preeclampsia
TORCH	Chronic hypertension
Chromosomal	Diabetes classes D to F
Syndromes	Nutrition

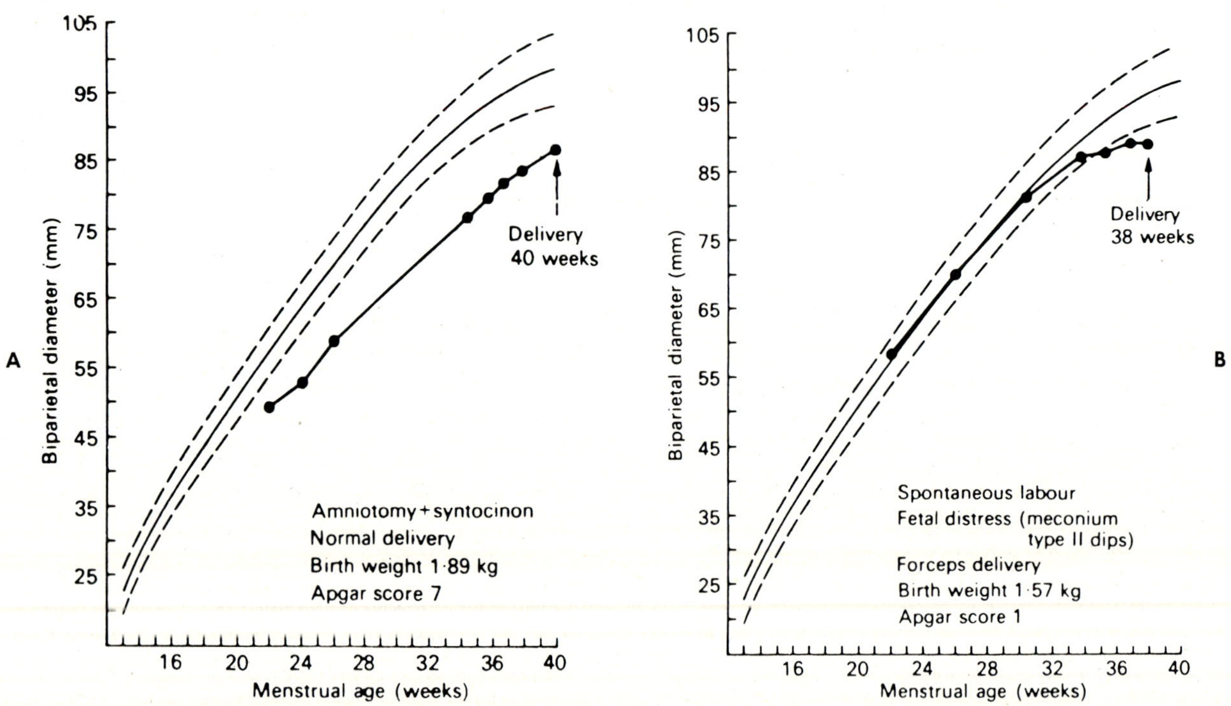

Fig. 7-14. Low profile **(A)** and late flattening **(B)** patterns of IUGR. (From Campbell, S. In Beard, R., and Nathanielsz, P., editors: Fetal physiology and medicine, Philadelphia, 1976, W.B. Saunders Co.)

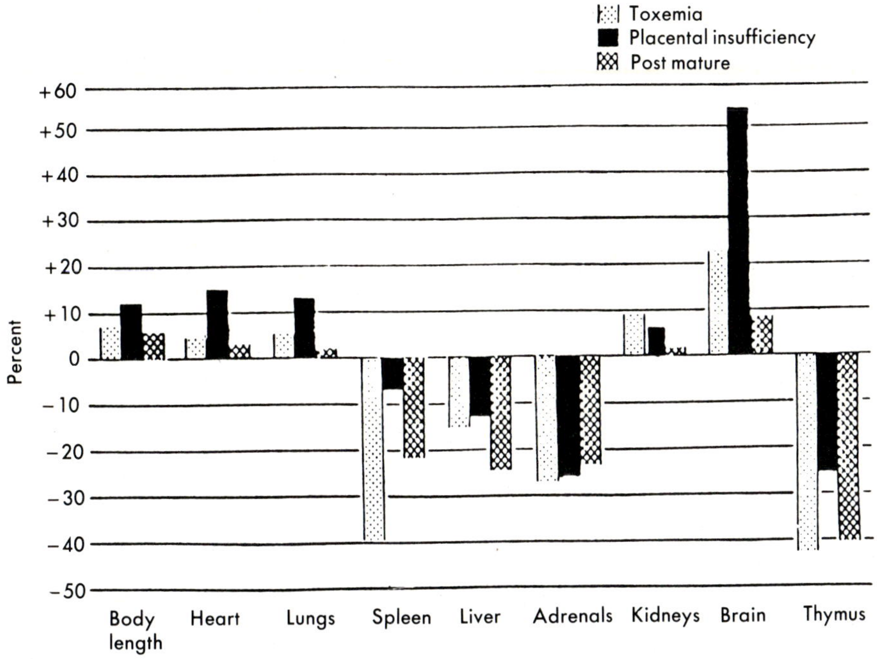

Fig. 7-15. Deviation of organ weights following IUGR. (From Naeye, R., and Kelly, J.: Pediatr. Clin. North Am. **13:**849, 1966.)

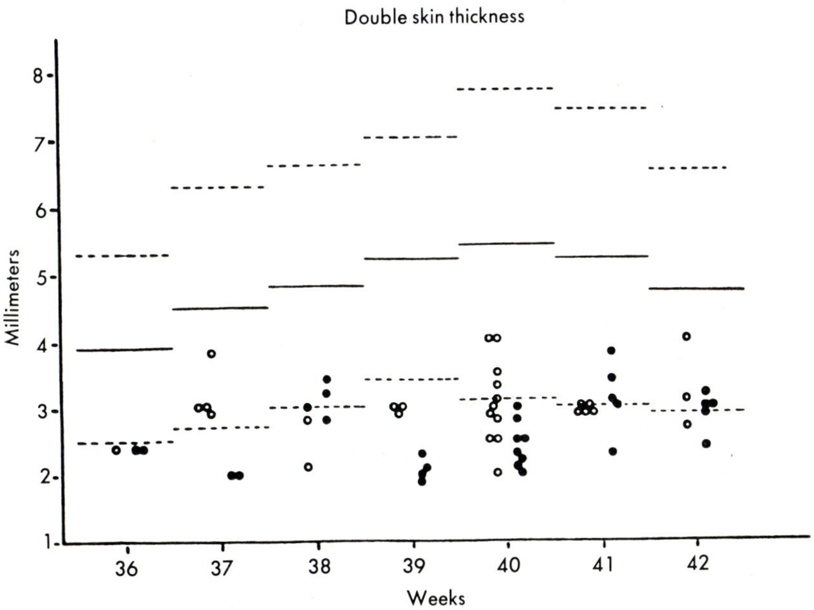

Fig. 7-16. Skinfold thickness is a major determinant of neonatal subcutaneous fat deposits. Fetal malnutrition with (●) and without (○) severe clinical signs of wasting. (From Usher, R.: Pediatr. Clin. North Am. **17:**169, 1970.)

weight and somatic organ growth are more seriously altered. Spleen, liver, adrenal, thymus, and adipose tissue growth is affected to the greatest extent in these late-onset SGA newborns (Figs. 7-15 and 7-16). The relative sparing of fetal head (brain) growth may be caused by preferential perfusion of the brain with well-oxygenated blood containing adequate substrates following redistribution of the cardiac output during periods of fetal distress. Infants with IUGR resulting from unknown or nutrition causes may have successfully adapted to a "hostile" in utero environment with reduced growth. After birth, in a more favorable environment, catch-up growth ensues.

ANTENATAL CARE

Diagnosis

Antenatal diagnosis of IUGR has proved an extremely difficult task. Usually these infants deliver at or beyond term without prior antenatal detection. At the very best, when looked for with careful maternal physical examination, accurate dating, and risk assessment analysis, only 50% of these infants may be detected before birth. Antenatal detection is an essential component of care for these infants, since they require intensive obstetric and neonatal management to reduce their excessive perinatal morbidity and mortality. This poor outcome is associated with unexplained antepartum fetal demise, intrapartum fetal death, neonatal asphyxia, and other major neonatal adaptive problems. Antenatal detection and intensive perinatal care of mother, fetus, and, later, the neonate are imperative components that result in improved outcome for these infants.

Currently, careful measurement and recording of the fundal height at each antenatal visit is the best clinical screening aid for the diagnosis of IUGR. When dates are confirmed by onset of quickening, audible heart tones, and accurate menstrual history, size-date discrepancy (i.e., fundal height smaller than or lagging behind gestational age) is suggestive of IUGR. Historic findings that may be components of a risk assessment score for IUGR include a past history of an SGA infant, vaginal bleeding, multiple gestation, low prepregnancy weight, and poor pregnancy weight gain, as noted earlier. Chronic maternal illness and preeclampsia are also high-risk situations indicating possible IUGR.

Laboratory tests potentially helpful in detecting IUGR include analysis of serum human placental lactogen concentration and serum or urinary estriol (E_3) determinations. Both are placental hormones secreted into the maternal circulation and in part related to placental mass, gestational age, and birth weight. However, these are not consistently helpful. Other determinants of fetal well-being and growth include maternal plasma assays of Schwangerschaft's protein, a pregnancy-specific glycoprotein; pregnancy-associated plasma protein A, which is increased with preeclampsia; and placental protein 5, which is similar to antithrombin III and increases with placental damage. These newer tests need further clin-

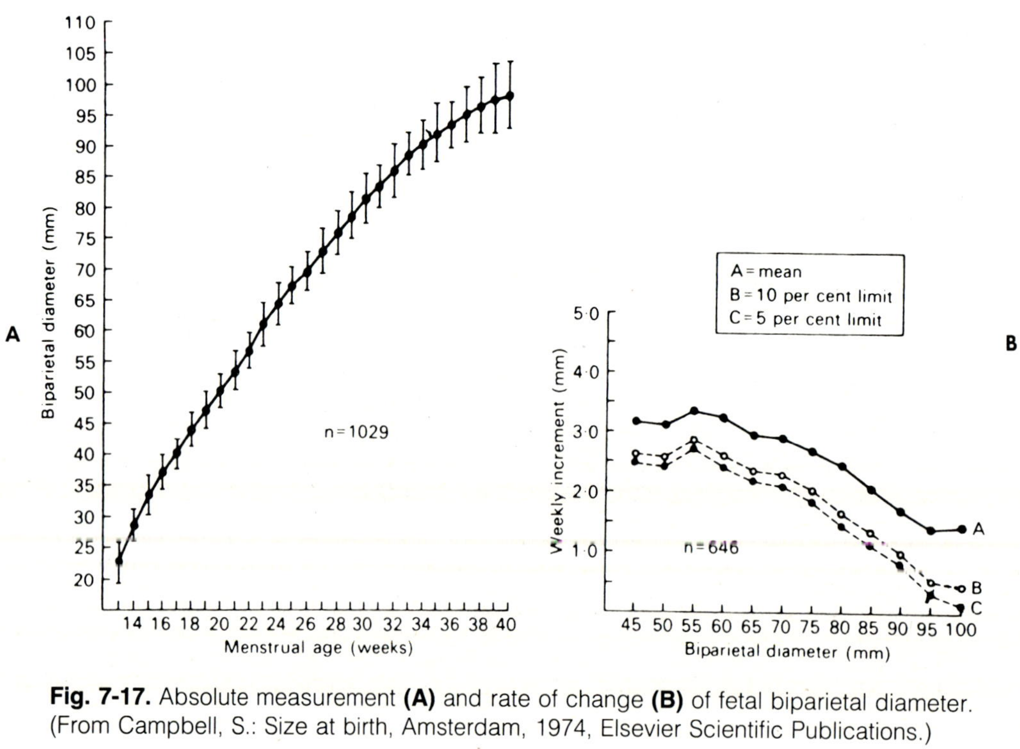

Fig. 7-17. Absolute measurement **(A)** and rate of change **(B)** of fetal biparietal diameter. (From Campbell, S.: Size at birth, Amsterdam, 1974, Elsevier Scientific Publications.)

ical evaluation. Since amniotic fluid C-peptide is low and the 3 methylhistidine/creatinine ratio is increased with IUGR, both these tests are also useful. In addition, the presence of phosphatidylglycerol helps separate IUGR from appropriately grown but preterm infants.

On the basis of maternal risk assessment and size-date discrepancy, fetal body measurement by ultrasonography is the best available method for the estimation of fetal weight and the diagnosis of IUGR retardation (Chapter 12). In addition to small size, the SGA fetus may have a smaller placenta; reduced fetal urine production may also result in less amniotic fluid. These individual components result in a diminished total uterine volume. The determination of this volume is tedious but useful in diagnosing IUGR. Demonstration of oligohydramnios with less than 1 cm pockets of fluid correlates highly with IUGR.

Classically, serial biparietal diameters (BPD) before 32 weeks' gestation, analyzed according to their absolute numeric values and to rate of change, have been established as a reliable means to determine fetal weight, maturity, and aberrant growth patterns (Figs. 7-14, 7-17, and 7-18). However, in asymmetric growth retardation, fetal head growth is spared relative to the degree of wasting of extracerebral tissues. Serial BPD determinations may not detect such affected infants. Truncometry may be employed by measuring the abdominal circumference at the level of the umbilical vein (Fig. 7-19). This permits more accurate determination of the asymmetrically growth-retarded fetus. Combining these data and investigating the ratio between fetal head and abdominal circumference has added even greater accuracy to the determination of IUGR (Fig. 7-20).

Fetal weight can be determined accurately with various equations that consider abdominal circumference, femur length, head circumference, and the BPD. This is less cumbersome and probably more accurate than determining the total intrauterine volume. These data can also be helpful in determining the fetal ponderal index (FPI):

$$\text{FPI} = \frac{\text{Weight}}{\text{Length}} \times 100$$

In addition, combing Doppler and real-time ultrasound can evaluate fetal vascular resistance, which is elevated in IUGR (Table 7-6).

Antenatal management

Once the diagnosis of IUGR is suspected and strengthened by ultrasonography, it is essential to institute appropriate maternal-fetal care and closely monitor the well-being of the fetus. With severe IUGR, maternal activity should be limited and bed rest initiated with the mother assuming a left lateral recumbent position to ensure optimum uterine blood flow. Chronic illness should be strictly managed to prevent further deterioration of the fetal environment; nutritional intake should be optimal. Serial ultrasonography will help define the pattern of growth retardation and the degree of growth arrest. An integral part of ultrasonography is to search carefully

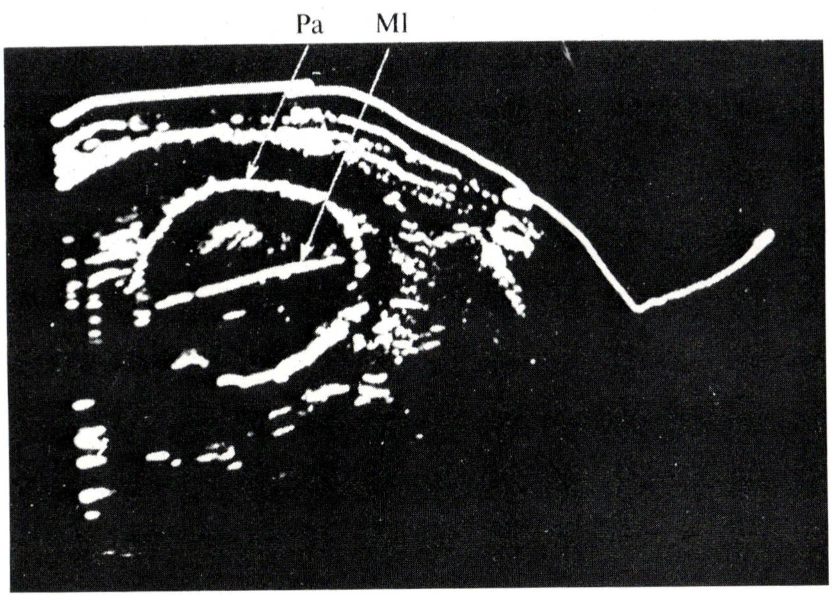

Fig. 7-18. Sonogram demonstrating determination of the biparietal diameter. *Pa,* Parietal bone; *Ml,* midline echo. (From Campbell, S. In Beard, R., and Nathanielsz, P., editors: Fetal physiology and medicine, Philadelphia, 1976, W.B. Saunders Co.)

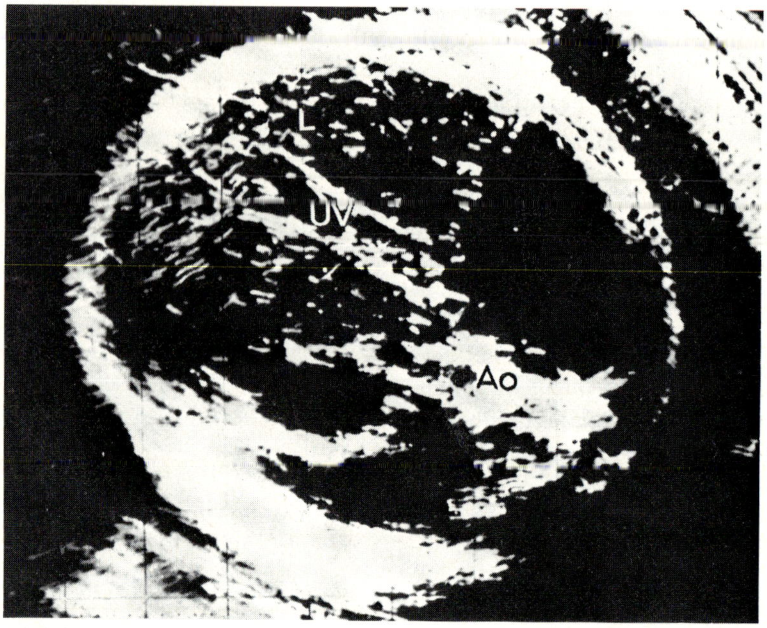

Fig. 7-19. Truncometry at the level of fetal liver *(L),* umbilical vein, *(UV),* and aorta *(Ao).* (From Campbell, S.: Size at birth, Amsterdam, 1974, Elsevier Scientific Publications.)

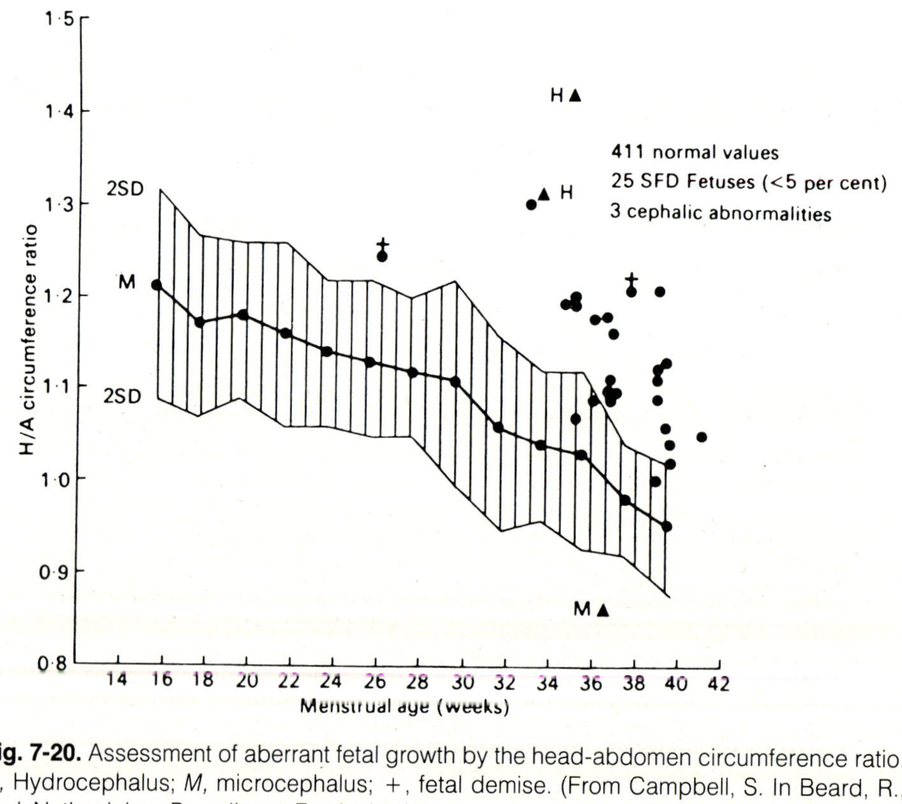

Fig. 7-20. Assessment of aberrant fetal growth by the head-abdomen circumference ratio. *H,* Hydrocephalus; *M,* microcephalus; +, fetal demise. (From Campbell, S. In Beard, R., and Nathanielsz, P., editors: Fetal physiology and medicine, Philadelphia, 1976, W.B. Saunders Co.)

for evidence of congenital malformations, since these anomalies are common among the early onset, low-profile group of SGA infants.

Assessment of fetal well-being should be instituted once the diagnosis is suspected and the fetus has approached a gestational age compatible with extrauterine survival. An inexpensive screening procedure is for the mother to record a log of fetal activity, since this is a reasonable sign of well-being. A specific period should be monitored, such as after a meal, and fetal activity recorded each day. In addition to this maternal record, a systematic approach to fetal evaluation should be performed routinely and frequently. Classically, the oxytocin challenge test (OCT) has been used to predicit the potential for fetal demise or an acute intrapartum death in a marginally oxygenated, compromised fetus. This test requires the intravenous administration of oxytocin, which must result in three uterine contractions within 10 minutes (Chapter 8). Late decelerations denote relative uteroplacental insufficiency and suggest that the oxygenation of the fetus may be impaired. A positive OCT (three late decelerations with three contractions) also suggests that the fetus may not tolerate the contractions that occur during labor. This is not a universal observation, since 50% of these infants may be able to withstand spontaneous or oxytocin-induced labor, without the development of fetal acidosis. Any decelerations less than that of a positive OCT should be considered suspicious and be repeated (along with technically unsatisfactory tracings) within the next 24 to 48 hours.

Because technical and time difficulties are related to the OCT and because contraindications exist for its use, such as a previous classic cesarean section, placenta previa, and concern about inducing premature labor, nonstress testing (NST) has been employed. This test examines fetal well-being by determining the acceleration of the fetal heart rate following spontaneous fetal movement. A healthy fetus (nonhypoxic) will respond to its own body movements with a mean acceleration of 15 beats/minute above baseline heart rate. In addition, the frequency of fetal movements should be ascertained; at the same time, examination of beat-to-beat and long-term variability can offer additional useful information. The NST can also supplement the OCT, since fetuses with a positive OCT but a reactive NST and normal beat-to-beat variability are more likely to tolerate labor without untoward problems. Under stable maternal conditions and signs of fetal well-being (negative OCT and/or reactive NST) these test may be repeated weekly.

The false-positive rate for OCT (25%) and NST (20%) is high compared with the false-negative rate for OCT (0.4 in 1,000) and NST (6.8 in 1,000). Intrauterine fetal demise is high following a positive OCT (32%) but lower with the NST (12%). Therefore, the contraction stress test is more predictive of fetal demise and has fewer false negatives. However, more false positives occur than with the NST.

Adjunct use of biochemical determination of plasma estriols has not added to the management of IUGR pregnancies. Nonetheless, biophysical determinants have been employed to assess fetal well-being successfully. The combined analyses of fetal breathing movements, gross body movements, fetal tone, fetal heart reactivity to movement, and qualitative amniotic fluid volume have improved the antenatal management of IUGR (Table 7-7). This biophysical profile (BPP) provides a nonweighted score that can identify the fetus at risk. A BPP score of 8 to 10 carries a 0.8% chance of fetal demise, whereas a score of 0 predicts a fetal mortality of 40%. This analysis takes approximately 30 minutes and should be repeated weekly with scores of 8 to 10. If the score is less than 8, the BPP should be repeated that afternoon. If again less

Table 7-7. Biophysical profile scoring: technique and interpretation*

Biophysical variable	Normal (score = 2)	Abnormal (score = 0)
Fetal breathing movements	≥1 episode of ≥30 seconds in 30 minutes	Absent or no episode of ≥30 seconds in 30 minutes
Gross body movements	≥3 discrete body or limb movements in 30 minutes (episodes of active continuous movement considered as single movement)	≤2 episodes of body or limb movements in 30 minutes
Fetal tone	≥1 episode of active extension with return to flexion of fetal limb(s) or trunk (opening and closing of hand considered normal tone)	Either slow extension with return to partial flexion or movement of limb in full extension or absent fetal movement
Reactive fetal heart rate	≥2 episodes of acceleration of ≥15 beats/min and of ≥15 seconds associated with fetal movement in 20 minutes	<2 episodes of acceleration of fetal heart rate or acceleration of <15 beats/min in 20 minutes
Qualitative amniotic fluid volume	≥1 pocket of fluid measuring ≥1 cm in two perpendicular planes	Either no pockets or a pocket <1 cm in two perpendicular planes

Modified from Manning, F.A., and others: Am. J. Obstet. Gynecol. **151:**343, 1985.
*See Manning, F.A., and others: Am. J. Obstet. Gynecol. **136:**787, 1980.

than 8, a OCT should be performed and a decision made to deliver the infant, regardless of gestational age, unless severe anomalies are determined. Assessment of fetal aortic flow with the pulsatile index (Table 7-6) may also help determine optional timing for delivery. If fetal lung maturity is present and aortic blood flow is reduced with other evidence of fetal distress, the fetus may need to be delivered before term.

With continued careful fetal surveillance and a stable maternal-fetal environment, a course of nonintervention is indicated.

The mode of delivery is not necessarily dictated by the abnormalities recorded by biophysical or electrophysiologic surveillance of the fetus. Many patients can tolerate labor following a positive OCT, with oxygen administration and a left lateral recumbent position. However, it would be judicious to avoid labor in those situations complicated by a nonreactive NST, a flat baseline, and a positive OCT. Similarly, SGA premature infants, in particular those with a breech presentation, and those whose mothers have a completely unfavorable cervix should be delivered by the abdominal route. Particular attention should be given to the asymmetrically (late flattening) growth-retarded fetus, who tolerates labor poorly and readily develops signs of fetal distress, compared with both the symmetrically undergrown and the normal fetus. Whether labor is induced or spontaneous, continuous intrapartum fetal heart rate monitoring combined with appropriate use of fetal scalp pH determinations must be employed (Chapter 8). If late decelerations become evident, scalp blood pH must be evaluated and, if fetal acidosis has developed, delivery should be expedited.

During labor, uterine contractions may further compromise marginal placental perfusion and fetal gas exchange. The myocardium of these fetuses may have diminished glycogen stores, a key energy source partially responsible for the fetal ability to withstand asphyxia. Because there is a high incidence of intrapartum birth asphyxia, it is essential that the delivery be coordinated with the neonatal team, who should be prepared to resuscitate a depressed or asphyxiated newborn. In addition, combined obstetric-pediatric management is indicated if meconium is present in the amniotic fluid. This event often follows periods of fetal hypoxia and stress, occurring with greatest frequency in the SGA term or postterm neonate. Obstetric management should include oropharyngeal suctioning immediately following delivery of the head. Immediately after the birth, the neonatal team should further clear the oropharynx and then the trachea of additional meconium (Chapter 37, part five).

One problem in managing these pregnancies is what to do when the fetus stops growing. Unfortunately, under stable maternal conditions and if the fetus demonstrates no other detectable signs of compromise, the best alternative is to leave the fetus in utero, ensure bed rest (preferably in-hospital), provide good nutrition, and continue fetal surveillance. The question of whether to deliver these fetuses should be tempered by the accuracy of the diagnosis and the ability to manage all potential neonatal problems efficiently, including appropriate alimentation. Although lung maturity may be present, many other problems are associated with prematurity that should temper a decision for delivery before 30 weeks. These additional risks of prematurity must be balanced against the risk of fetal demise in an adverse environment.

APPROACH TO THE SGA INFANT

Following birth, the SGA infant may develop significant neonatal problems (Table 7-8). In the delivery room it is essential to ensure optimum neonatal cardiopulmonary physiologic adaptation while ensuring minimum heat loss in a warm environment. Once stabilization has been established, a careful physical examination should be performed.

Table 7-8. Perinatal adaptive problems

Problem	Pathogenesis	Prevention
Perinatal asphyxia	↓ Placental reserve (insufficiency) ↓ Cardiac glycogen stores	Antepartum, intrapartum FHR monitoring
Meconium aspiration	Hypoxic/stress phenomenon	Oral-pharyngeal-tracheal suction
Fasting hypoglycemia	↓ Hepatic glycogen ↓ Gluconeogenesis	Early alimentation
Alimented hyperglycemia	"Starvation diabetes"	Avoid excessive carbohydrate loads
Polycythemia-hyperviscosity	Fetal hypoxia, ↑ erythropoietin Placental transfusion	Neonatal partial exchange transfusion
Temperature instability	↓ Adipose tissue ↑ Heat loss	Ensure neutral thermal environment
Pulmonary hemorrhage (rare)	Hypothermia, ↓ O_2/DIC	Avoid cold stress, hypoxia
Immunodeficiency	"Malnutrition" effect	Unknown

When infants with obvious anomalies and syndromes and those born to mothers with severe illness or malnutrition are excluded, there still remains a heterogeneous population of SGA infants. These infants have a characteristic physical appearance; the heads look relatively large for their undergrown trunks and extremities, which seem wasted. The abdomen is scaphoid, misleading one to suspect a diaphragmatic hernia. The extremities have a paucity of subcutaneous tissue and fat, best exemplified by a reduced skinfold thickness (Fig. 7-16). In addition, the skin appears to hang; is rough, dry, and parchmentlike; and desquamates quite easily. Fingernails may be long, and the hands and feet of these infants tend to look too large for the rest of the body. The facial appearance suggests the look of a "wise old person," especially in reference to that of premature infants (Fig. 7-21). Cranial sutures may be widened or overriding; the anterior fontanel is larger than expected, representing diminished membranous bone formation. Similarly, epiphyseal ossification at the knee (chondral bone) is also retarded. When meconium is passed in utero, there is often yellow-green staining of the nails, skin, and umbilical cord, which may also appear thinner than usual.

Gestational age assessment of the SGA infant may result in misleading data when based on physical criteria alone. Vernix caseosa is frequently reduced or absent, resulting from diminished skin perfusion during periods of fetal distress or from depressed synthesis of estriol, which enhances vernix production. In the absence of this protective covering, the skin is continuously exposed to amniotic fluid and will begin to desquamate following birth. Sole creases are determined in part by exposure to amniotic fluid and therefore will appear more mature. Breast tissue formation also depends on peripheral blood flow and estriol levels and will become markedly reduced in SGA infants. In addition, the female external genitalia will appear less mature because of the absence of the perineal adipose tissue covering the labia. Ear cartilage, as noted in bone ossification, may also be diminished.

Neurologic examination for gestational age assessment may be affected less by IUGR than the physical criteria. IUGR infants functionally achieve appropriate neurologic maturity. Peripheral nerve conduction velocity and visual- or auditory-evoked responses correlate well with gestational age in normal neonates and are not impaired following IUGR. These aspects of neurologic maturity are not sensitive to deprivation, and occasionally maturity may even become accelerated. Determinants of active or passive tone and posture may be reliable in SGA infants, assuming that those infants with significant central nervous system and metabolic disorders are excluded.

Specific organ maturity occurs despite diminished somatic growth. Cerebral cortical convolutions, renal glomeruli, and alveolar maturation all relate to gestational age and are not retarded with IUGR. As a result of stress in utero, these infants may occasionally accelerate the maturity of specific organ systems, such as the lung, thus explaining the paucity of respiratory distress syndrome in SGA preterm neonates.

When examined in closer detail, SGA infants do demonstrate specific behavioral characteristics that suggest, despite the presence of electric neurologic maturity, that functional central nervous system maturity may be impaired. In the absence of significant central nervous system disease these neonates demonstrate abnormal sleep cycles and diminished muscle tone, reflexes, activity, and excitability. This hypoexcitability suggests an adverse effect on polysynaptic reflex propagation and implies that central nervous system functional maturity does not necessarily proceed independently on the intrauterine events that result in IUGR.

Once stabilized and assigned a gestational age, the SGA neonate should be examined in more detail to direct the diagnostic work in a rational manner, as detailed in the following outline.

A. History and physical examination
B. Accurate growth parameters
C. Findings
   1. Dysmorphic features suggest:
      a. Chromosomes
      b. Syndrome
      c. Drugs
   2. Blueberry-muffin rash, petechiae, hepatosplenomegaly, and ocular pathology suggest:
      a. Rubella
      b. Cytomegalovirus (CMV)
      c. Other
   3. Neither 1 nor 2 suggests:
      a. Constitutional
      b. Genetic
      c. Nutritional
      d. Toxins
      e. Placenta twins
      f. Unknown

Dysmorphic features; "funny looking faces"; abnormal hands, feet, and palmar creases, in addition to gross anomalies, suggest congenital malformation syndromes, chromosomal defects, or teratogens. Ocular disorders such as chorioretinitis, cataracts, glaucoma, cloudy cornea, in addition to hepatosplenomegaly, jaundice, and a blueberry-muffin rash, should suggest a congenital infection (Chapter 31). The remaining infants constitute a heterogenous group that represents most SGA neonates. Multiple gestations are the most recognizable etiology in this category. TORCH infections resulting in SGA infants are unusual in the absence of other clinical signs of congenital infection; however, a screening determi-

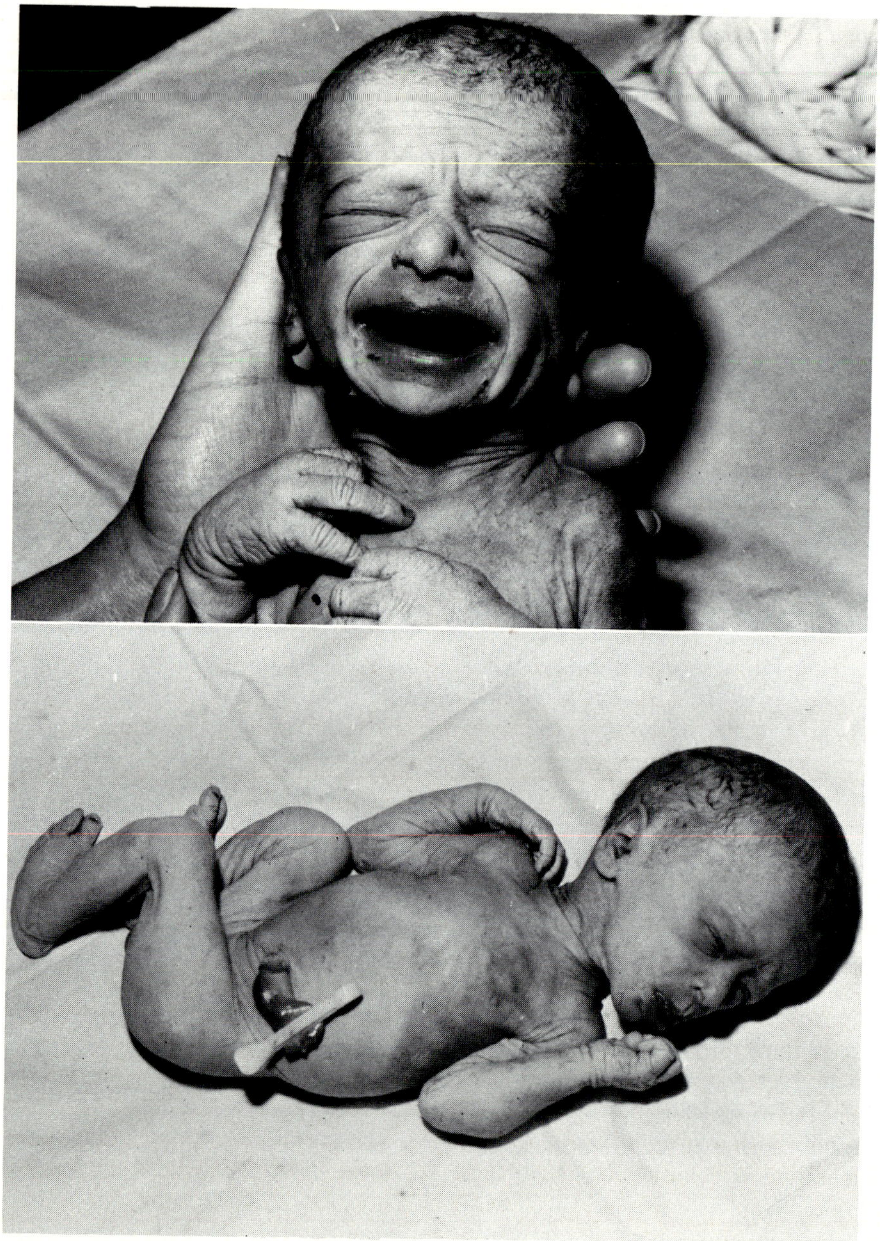

Fig. 7-21. Term SGA infant, demonstrating wizened facies and dry, desquamating, hanging skin. Birth weight: 1,500 gm.

nation on cord blood for IgM values and urine culture for CMV may be indicated. Radiographic examination of long bones and skull (or ultrasonography of the head) may be diagnostically useful. Careful data related to the present and past reproductive history of the mother, in addition to ongoing neonatal management and close observation, are indicated in the remaining large number of SGA neonates whose underlying diagnoses may never be determined.

NEONATAL PROBLEMS (Table 7-8)

Asphyxia

Perinatal asphyxia and its sequelae constitute the most significant immediate problem of SGA infants. As discussed, uterine contractions may add an additional hypoxic stress on the marginally functioning placenta. The ensuing fetal hypoxia, acidosis, and cerebral depression may result in fetal demise or neonatal asphyxia. IUGR represents a large proportion of stillborn infants experiencing hypoxia in utero. Myocardial infarction, amniotic fluid aspiration, and signs of cerebral hypoxia are noted in the IUGR stillborn infants. With repeated episodes of fetal asphyxia or persistent hypoxemia, myocardial glycogen reserves are depleted, further limiting the fetal cardiopulmonary adaptation to hypoxia. If inadequate resuscitation occurs at birth and Apgar scores are low, both intrapartum and neonatal asphyxia place the infant in double jeopardy for a continuum of central nervous system insult. The sequelae of perinatal asphyxia include multiple organ system dysfunction potentially characterized by ischemic-hypoxic encephalopathy, ischemic congestive heart failure, meconium aspiration pneumonia, persistent fetal circulation, gastrointestinal perforation, and acute tubular necrosis. Concomitant with these sequelae there may be metabolic derangements such as hypoglycemia. Hypocalcemia is partly caused by excessive phosphate release from damaged cells, acidosis, and its correction with sodium bicarbonate and diminished calcium intake. Hypocalcemia does not occur more often with IUGR unless these problems are present. Meconium aspiration syndrome, if managed inappropriately in the delivery room, may complicate the clinical picture and further embarrass respiratory function and oxygenation with the development of pneumonitis and pneumothorax.

Neonatal metabolism

Fasting hypoglycemia develops in SGA infants more than any other neonatal subgroup or category. The propensity for hypoglycemia is greatest during the first 3 days of life; however, some of these infants develop ketotic hypoglycemia months later. Key to the occurrence of hypoglycemia is the diminished hepatic glycogen stores (Fig. 7-22). Glycogenolysis constitutes the predominant source of glucose for the neonate during the immediate hours after birth. Later in the day, when

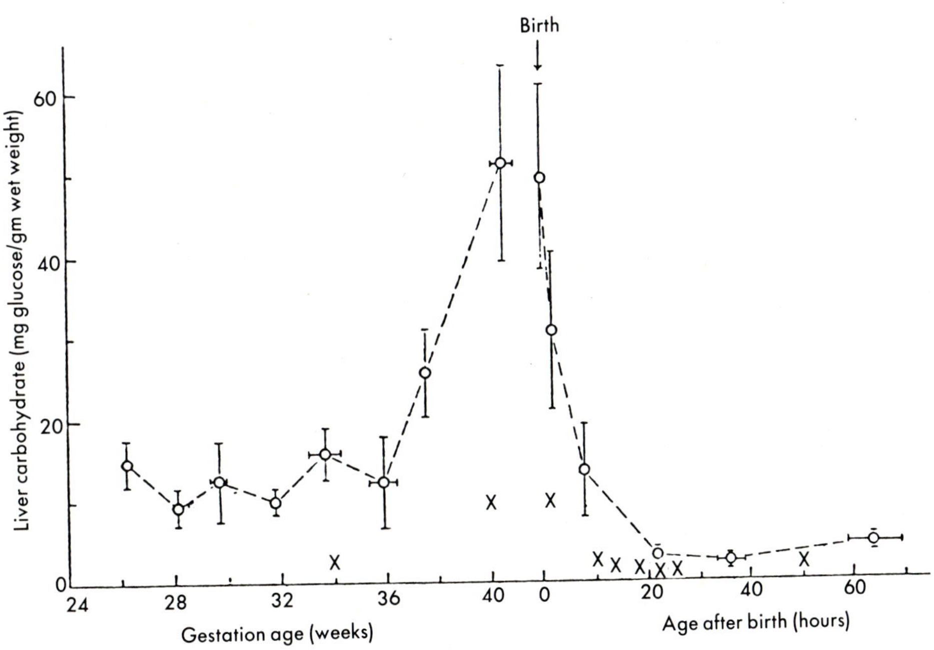

Fig. 7-22. Fetal and neonatal hepatic glycogen content *(X)* in IUGR patients. (From Shelly, H., and Neligan, G.: Br. Med. Bull. **22:**34, 1966.)

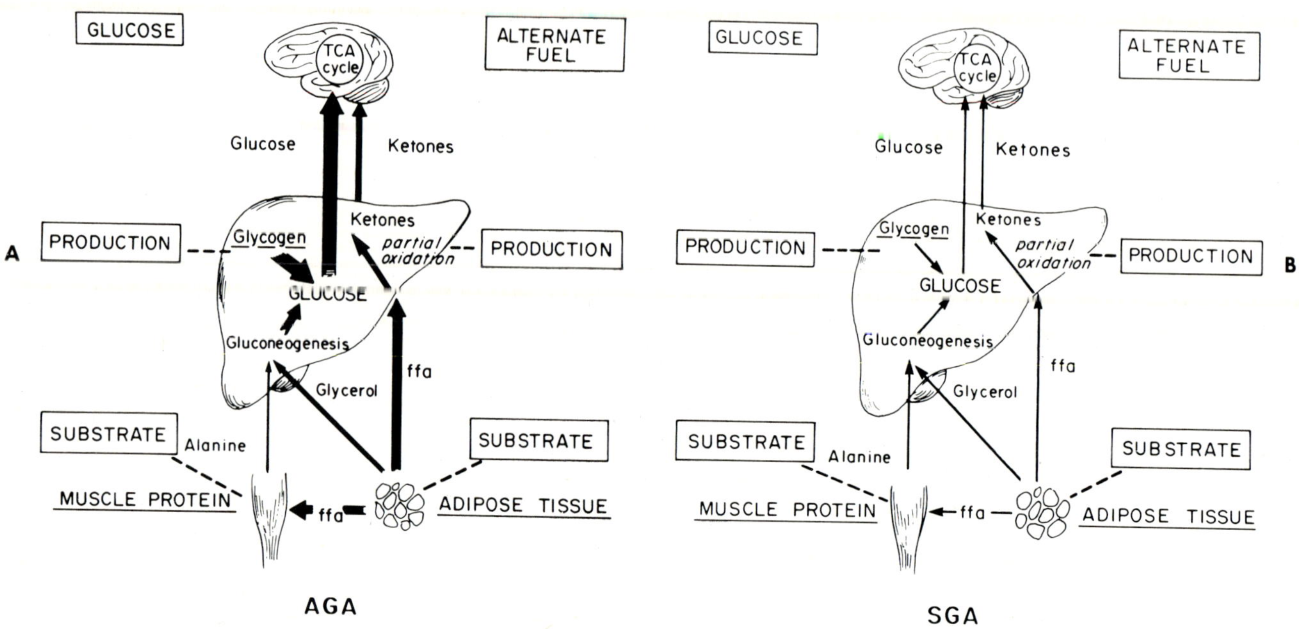

Fig. 7-23. Postnatal glucose and fatty acid metabolic relationships in AGA **(A)** and SGA **(B)** neonates. Arrows depict magnitude of flux. SGA infants demonstrate both diminished glycogen stores and gluconeogenesis. In addition, they may have attenuated fatty acid oxidation. (Modified from Adam, P.A.J.: Metabolism in pregnant woman and fetus. In Falkner, F., and Tanner, J.: Human growth, vol. 1, New York, 1978, Plenum Press.)

glycogen stores become depleted, fasting glucose production results from the incorporation of lactate and gluconeogenic amino acid precursors into glucose. SGA infants demonstrate an inability to increase blood glucose concentration following oral or intravenous administration of the key gluconeogenic amino acid, alanine. Hypoglycemic SGA infants have elevated alanine and lactate levels, suggesting that substrate availability is not rate limiting for gluconeogenesis and that the enzymes or cofactors are not active. Nonhypoglycemic SGA infants do demonstrate equivalent rates of gluconeogenesis from alanine compared with nonhypoglycemic AGA neonates.

Immediately following birth, fasting SGA infants may develop lower plasma free fatty acid levels than normally growing infants. Fasting blood glucose levels in SGA infants directly correlate with plasma free fatty acid levels. In addition, once fed, SGA infants have a deficient utilization of intravenous triglycerides. Following the intravenous administration of triglyceride emulsion, SGA infants develop high free fatty acid and triglyceride levels, but ketone body formation is attenuated. This suggests that the utilization and oxidation of free fatty acids and triglycerides are diminished in SGA neonates. Free fatty acid oxidation is important because it spares peripheral tissue use of glucose, whereas the hepatic oxidation of free fatty acids may contribute the reducing equivalents and energy required for hepatic gluconeogenesis. Deficient provision and/or oxidation of fatty acids may partly be responsible for the development of fasting hypoglycemia in these infants (Fig. 7-23).

Endocrine alterations have also been implicated in the pathogenesis of hypoglycemia in SGA infants. Hyperinsulinemia or excessive sensitivity to insulin may be one factor. Catecholamine release is deficient in these neonates during periods of hypoglycemia. Although basal glucagon levels may be elevated, exogenous administration of glucagon fails to enhance glycemia. These data suggest an abnormality of counterregulatory hormonal mechanisms during periods of neonatal hypoglycemia in SGA infants.

With improved standards of care and attempts at early feeding or intravenous alimentation, fasting hypoglycemia in the SGA neonate is a rare event. Before the onset of alimentation, careful monitoring with Dextrostix for determination of blood glucose values will detect infants with asymptomatic hypoglycemia. If whole blood glucose concentrations decline to less than 30 mg/dl during the first 3 days in term infants or 20 mg/dl in preterm infants and no untoward symptoms have occurred, glucose infusion initially at 4 to 8 mg/kg/minute should be commenced. Following this initial rate, the infusion should be titrated until blood glucose values achieve normal levels. If the hypoglycemia is symptomatic, particularly when seizure activity intervenes, an intravenous minibolus of D10W at 200 mg/kg should be given, followed by an infusion as just described. Infants at greatest risk

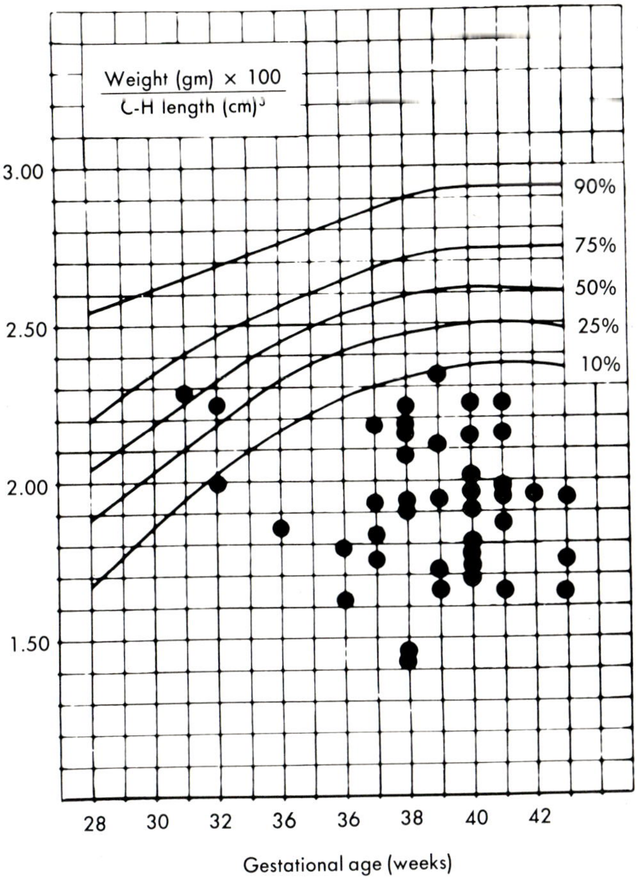

Fig. 7-24. Relationship between ponderal index and neonatal hypoglycemia in IUGR. ●, Hypoglycemic infants. (From Jarai, I., and others: Early Hum. Dev. **1**:25, 1977.)

for the development of hypoglycemia are those who have been asphyxiated and those who appear most undergrown according to the ponderal index (Fig. 7-24). Similarly, breast-fed twins who are not supplemented with a carbohydrate source are at risk, particularly the smaller co-twin, and should be monitored carefully.

Temperature regulation

See also Chapter 24, part two.

Following the birth of an infant complicated by utero-placental insufficiency, the neonate's initial body temperature may actually be elevated. When placental function fails, the neonate's heat-eliminating capacity also becomes deficient, resulting in fetal hyperthermia. On exposure to the cold environment of the delivery room, SGA infants can increase their heat production (oxygen consumption) appropriately, since brown adipose tissue stores are not necessarily depleted during IUGR. However, their core temperature drops if the cold stress continues, implying that heat loss has exceeded heat production. Heat loss in these infants is partly caused by the large body surface area exposed to cold and the deficiency of an insulating layer of subcutaneous adipose tissue stores. The SGA infant therefore has a narrower neutral thermal environment than full term infants but a broader one than that in premature neonates. In SGA infants hypoglycemia and/or hypoxia interferes with heat production and may contribute to their thermal instability. In all infants, particularly the SGA infant, a neutral thermal environment should be sought to prevent excessive heat loss and to promote appropriate postnatal weight gain.

When nursed in a neutral thermal environment, SGA infants demonstrate the usual decline of the respiratory quotient following birth, representing a shift toward free fatty acid oxidation. During the first 12 hours after birth, basal oxygen consumption may be diminished in SGA neonates. Similar observations have been recorded in utero among spontaneously SGA fetal lambs, suggesting in both situations that there is a deficiency of potentially oxidizable substrates. Supporting this hypothesis is the marked increment of oxygen consumption that occurs in well-alimented SGA infants. This latter observation is also analogous to the rise of energy production following the nutritional rehabilitation of infants with marasmus-kwashiorkor. The increment of oxygen consumption following fetal or infantile malnutrition represents the energy cost of growth. SGA infants have a significantly smaller postnatal weight loss because they are maturationally capable of achieving an adequate caloric intake earlier than premature neonates. Because of this enhanced caloric intake, SGA infants have a higher oxygen consumption than less mature neonates. Nutritional balance studies of premature SGA infants demonstrated an increase of fecal fat and protein loss despite faster rates of growth compared with premature AGA infants. Energy storage was lower with IUGR, suggesting less fat deposition.

A group of SGA neonates do not demonstrate an elevation of oxygen consumption following appropriate caloric intake. These infants have had low-profile intrauterine growth and may be considered examples of "primordial fetal growth retardation." Their growth is set and fixed at a slower rate, and their eventual growth potential is reduced. The diminished body cell number in congenitally infected infants and those with chromosomal disorders exemplifies these primordial growth-retarded neonates.

Hyperviscosity-polycythemia syndrome

The plasma volume of SGA infants immediately following birth averages 52 ml/kg, as opposed to 43 ml/kg in AGA infants. Once equilibrated at 12 hours of life, the plasma volume becomes equivalent in the two groups. In addition to an enhanced plasma space, the circulating red blood cell mass is expanded. Fetal hypoxia and subsequent erythropoietin synthesis may induce excessive red blood cell production. Alternately, a placental-fetal transfusion during labor or periods of fetal asphyxia may result in a shift of placental blood to the fetus. Nonetheless, the elevation of the hematocrit potentially increases blood viscosity, which interferes with vital tissue perfusion. The altered viscosity adversely affects neonatal hemodynamics and results in an abnormal cardiopulmonary and metabolic postnatal adaptation, producing hypoxia and hypoglycemia. These infants are at increased risk for necrotizing enterocolitis. In the event polycythemia is present (central hematocrit >65%) with such symptoms, appropriate therapy should be directed at correcting hypoxia and hypoglycemia, and a partial exchange transfusion to reduce blood viscosity and improve tissue perfusion should be considered (Chapter 32).

Other problems

Recent evidence has demonstrated that the immunologic function of SGA infants may be depressed, as it is in older infants with the postnatal onset of malnutrition. Neonates with congenital rubella syndrome have functional deficiencies of both T and B lymphocytes. This may, however, be related to continued intracellular viral infection. Other SGA infants may also manifest varying degrees of immunologic dysfunction that persists into childhood. Deficiencies have been demonstrated in lymphocyte number and function, which include decreased spontaneous mitogenesis and reduced response to phytohemagglutinin. Similarly, these infants tend to develop lower immunoglobulin levels during infancy and demonstrate an attenuated antibody response to oral polio vaccine. At birth, cord prealbumin and bone mineral content are low in term SGA infants. Thrombocytopenia, prolonged thrombin and partial thromboplastin times, and elevated fibrin degradation products are also problems among SGA infants. Sudden infant death syndrome (SIDS) may be more common following IUGR. Inguinal hernias also typically follow preterm IUGR. Additional problems and their management are noted in Table 7-8.

FOLLOW-UP

Excluding the severely affected SGA infants with serious congenital malformations and viral infections, the remaining neonates should benefit from optimum antenatal detection, exquisite management of pregnancy, and avoidance of hypoxic fetal distress. In addition, with ideal neonatal intensive care the morbidity and mortality of SGA infants should be reduced to a minimum, and postnatal developmental handicaps should be diminished. Unfortunately, in the best medical centers only 50% of these infants are recognized before delivery. These infants will continue to contribute to the excessive fetal and neonatal morbidity and mortality associated with IUGR. Neonatal mortality is greater than that of full-term but less than that in premature neonates, whereas the incidence of fetal demise remains higher than in both other groups. Besides the etiologic events that lead to the development of IUGR, these infants have additional multisystem problems that further compromise survival and future growth or development. Among these fetuses the perinatal mortality is 10 times that of appropriately grown infants. Intrauterine fetal demise is greatest among the most severely undergrown infants. Both antepartum and intrapartum events contribute to fetal mortality. Lethal congenital malformations and birth asphyxia are the two leading causes of death among SGA neonates.

Developmental outcome

When infants with congenital infections and severe malformations are excluded, there remains a heterogenous group of undergrown neonates. Intellectual and neurologic function in these remaining infants depends heavily on the presence or absence of adverse perinatal events, in addition to the specific etiology resulting in IUGR. Cerebral morbidity will be adversely affected by the hypoxic-ischemic encephalopathy subsequent to birth asphyxia and the postnatal problems of hypoxia and hypoglycemia. Therefore the prognosis must consider all the adverse perinatal circumstances in addition to IUGR. When these perinatal problems are minimal or are avoided, the SGA neonate may still demonstrate cerebral developmental handicaps, especially in the presence of relative head growth retardation (microcephaly). If term AGA neonates are used as a standard, term SGA infants demonstrate developmental problems when they are examined at follow-up at 2 years, 5 years, and older. Even when compared with premature neonates, term SGA infants continue to have developmental disadvantages. Follow-up of these term SGA infants reveals little differences in intelligence quotient or neurologic sequelae; however, their school performance is poor, partly because of behavioral and learning disorders. Preterm SGA infants may have an even greater percentage of abnormal neurodevelopmental outcomes than term SGA neonates. Those early-onset SGA infants demonstrating decreased BPD growth before 26 weeks' gestation and those with symmetric growth retardation have diminished developmental quotients in infancy. However, some follow-up observations on both term and preterm SGA neonates are very favorable, since these neonates compared well to their AGA counterparts. SGA infants are a heterogenous group, and the different populations investigated may vary in the severity of neurodevelopmental handicap; similarly, antenatal detection and perinatal management vary among high-risk centers. It would therefore appear that these latter favorable reports may

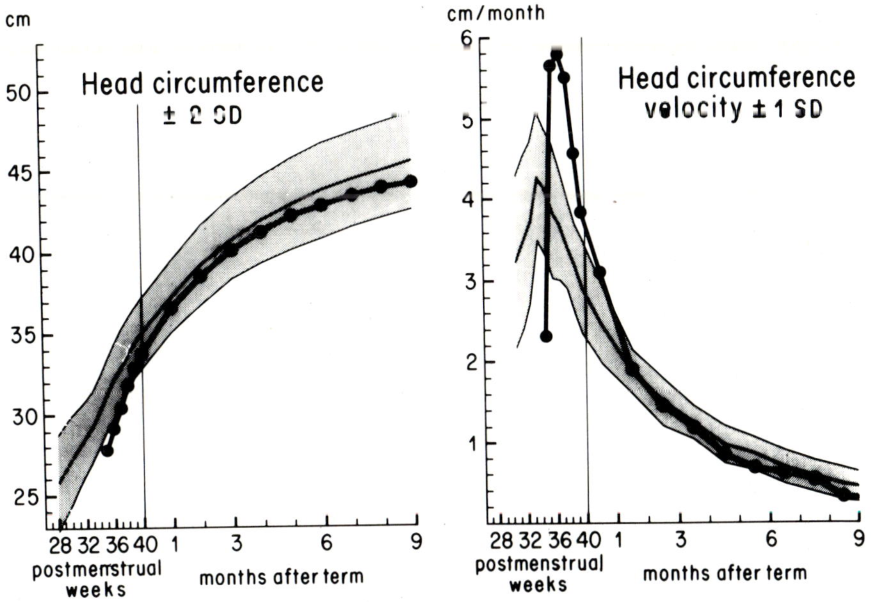

Fig. 7-25. Postnatal catch-up growth following IUGR. (From Brandt, I.: Growth dynamics of low birth weight infants with emphasis on the perinatal period. In Falkner, F., and Tanner, J., editors: Human growth, vol. 2, Postnatal growth, New York, 1978, Plenum Press.)

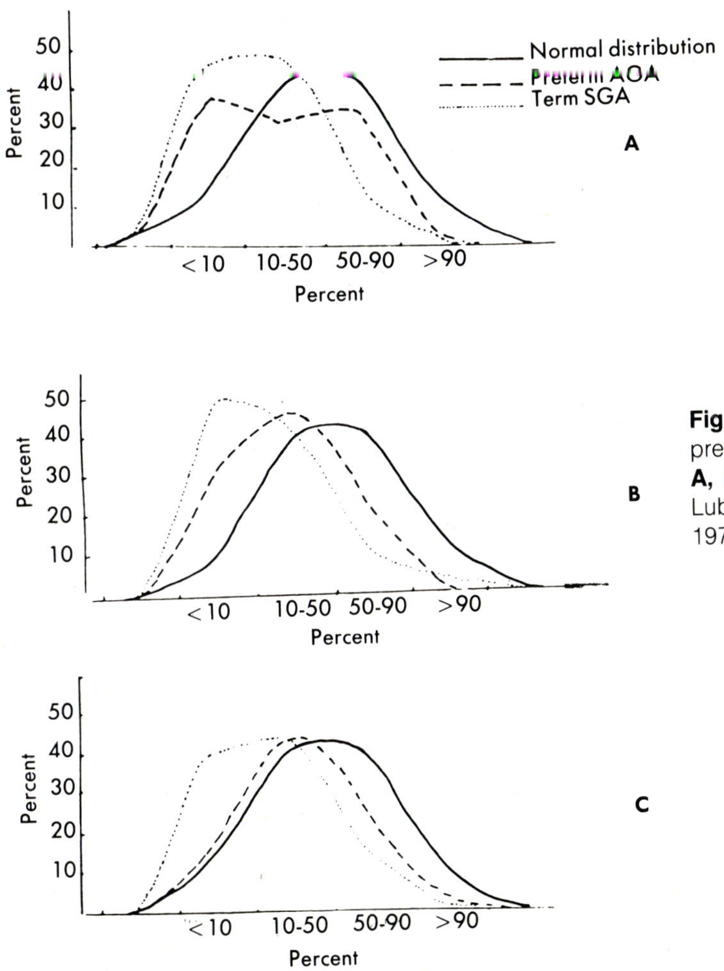

Fig. 7-26. Eventual physical growth of SGA term, AGA premature, and AGA term neonates at 4 years of age. **A,** Height; **B,** weight; **C,** head circumference. (From Lubchenco, L.: The high-risk infant, Philadelphia, 1976, W.B. Saunders Co.)

represent the outcome following optimum obstetric management and neonatal care.

Another major determining influence on neonatal neurodevelopmental outcome in SGA infants is the family's socioeconomic status. Parent educational background, place of rearing, and environmental conditions all have a strong effect on outcome. SGA infants born to families of higher socioeconomic status demonstrated little developmental differences on follow-up, whereas those born to poorer families have significant developmental handicaps.

Growth

Postnatal growth following IUGR depends in part on the cause of the growth retardation, the postnatal nutritional intake, and the social environment. Although birth weight correlates best to maternal weight, postnatal growth is related to both maternal and paternal growth characteristics. SGA neonates who have primordial growth retardation related to congenital viral, chromosomal, or constitutional syndromes will remain small throughout life. Those infants whose intrauterine growth was inhibited late in gestation because of uterine constraint, placental insufficiency, or nutritional deficits will have catch-up growth after birth and approach their inherited growth potential when provided with an optimum environment. These infants with low ponderal, indexor asymmetric growth retardation have an accelerated growth phase once adequate postnatal caloric intake has been established, suggesting release of an in utero constraining factor following birth (Fig. 7-25). This postpartum acceleration of growth occurs within the first 6 months of life, placing the infant on a new percentile growth tract (Fig. 7-25). Despite the catch-up period, some of these infants remain smaller than appropriately grown neonates (Fig. 7-26), especially those who had the onset of growth retardation before 26 weeks.

The goal of future management plans for the improvement of the growth and developmental outcome of SGA neonates must have its origins close to the onset of IUGR. Once growth retardation has developed, early identification and careful avoidance of undue hypoxic stress and nutritional deficits should enhance the survival and quality of these high-risk neonates.

Robert M. Kliegman
Sonia E. Hulman

BIBLIOGRAPHY

General

Cheek, D.: Fetal and postnatal cellular growth, New York, 1975, John Wiley & Sons, Inc.

Ciba Foundation Symposium 27: Size at birth, Amsterdam, 1974, Elsevier.

Committee To Study the Prevention of Low Birthweight: Preventing low birthweight, Washington, D.C., 1985, Institute of Medicine, National Academic Press.

Creasy, R., and Resnick, R.: Intrauterine fetal growth retardation. In Milunsky, A., Friedman, E., and Gluck, L., editors: Advances in perinatal medicine, vol. 1, New York, 1981, Plenum Press.

Falkner, F., and Tanner, J.: Human growth, vols. 1 and 2, New York, 1978, Plenum Press.

Goldenberg, R., and others: Low birth weight, intrauterine growth retardation and preterm delivery, Am. J. Obstet. Gynecol. **152**:980, 1985.

Lin, C., and Evans, M.: Intrauterine growth retardation, New York, 1984, McGraw-Hill Book Co.

Miller, H., and Merritt, T.: Fetal growth in humans, Chicago, 1979, Year Book Medical Publishers, Inc.

Usher, R., and McLean, F.: Normal fetal growth and the significance of fetal growth retardation. In Davis, J., and Dobbin, J., editors: Scientific foundations of pediatrics, Philadelphia, 1974, W.B. Saunders Co.

Villar, J., and Belizan, J.: The relative contribution of prematurity and fetal growth retardation to low birth weight in developing and developed societies, Am. J. Obstet. Gynecol. **143**:793, 1982.

Warshaw, J.: Intrauterine growth retardation: adaptation or pathology? Pediatrics **76**:998, 1985.

Fetal growth

Brenner, W., Edelman, D., and Hendricks, C.: A standard of fetal growth for the United States of America, Am. J. Obstet. Gynecol. **126**:555, 1976.

Lubchenco, L., and others: Intrauterine growth as estimated from liveborn birth weight data at 24 to 42 weeks of gestation, Pediatrics **32**:793, 1963.

Naeye, R., and Dixon, J.: Distortions in fetal growth standards, Pediatr. Res. **12**:987, 1978.

Robinson, J.: Growth of the fetus, Br. Med. Bull. **35**:137, 1979.

Seeds, J.: Impaired fetal growth: definition and clinical diagnosis, Obstet. Gynecol. **64**:303, 1984.

Vorherr, H.: Factors influencing fetal growth, Am. J. Obstet. Gynecol. **142**:577, 1982.

Ziegler, E., and others: Body composition of the reference fetus, Growth **40**:329, 1976.

Fetal metabolism

Adam, P.A.J., and Felig, P.: Carbohydrate, fat, and amino acid metabolism in the pregnant woman and fetus. In Falkner, F., and Tanner, J., editors: Human growth, vol. 1, New York, 1978, Plenum Press.

Battaglia, F., and Meschia, G.: Principal substrates of fetal metabolism, Physiol. Rev. **58**:499, 1978.

Brooke, O., Alvear, J., and Arnold, M.: Energy retention, energy expenditure, and growth in healthy immature infants, Pediatr. Res. **13**:215, 1979.

Kliegman, R., and Fanaroff, A.: Developmental metabolism and nutrition. In Gregory, G., editor: Pediatric anesthesia, New York, 1983, Churchill Livingstone, Inc.

Milley, J., and Simmons, M.: Metabolic requirements for fetal growth. Clin. Perinatol. **6**:365, 1979.

Simmons, M.: Intrauterine growth retardation, Semin. Perinatol. **4**, 1984.

Fetal endocrinology

Brinsmead, M., and Liggins, G.: Somatomedins and other growth factors in fetal growth. In Scarpelli, E., and Cosmi, E., editors: Reviews in perinatal medicine, vol. 3, New York, 1979, Raven Press.

Fisher, D.: Intrauterine growth retardation: endocrine and receptor aspects, Semin. Perinatol. **8**:37, 1984.

Gluckman, P., and Liggins, G.: Regulation of fetal growth. In Beard, R., and Nathanielsz, P., editors: Fetal physiology and medicine, New York, 1984, Marcel Dekker, Inc.

Hill, D.: Insulin and fetal growth. In Diabetes and other endocrine disorders during pregnancy and in the newborn, New York, 1976, Alan R. Liss, Inc.

Liggins, G.: Regulation of fetal growth. In Beard, R., and Nathanielsz, P., editors: Fetal physiology and medicine, New York, 1984, Marcel Dekker, Inc.

Maternal factors

Andrews, M., and Jones, H.: Impaired reproductive performance of the unicornuate uterus: intrauterine growth retardation, infertility and recurrent abortion in five cases, Am. J. Obstet. Gynecol. **144**:173, 1982.

Bakketerg, L., Hoffman, H., and Harley, E.: The tendency to repeat gestational age and birth weight in successive births, Am. J. Obstet. Gynecol. **135**:1086, 1979.

Branch, D., and others: Obstetric complications associated with the lupus anticoagulant, N. Engl. J. Med. **313**:1322, 1985.

Johnstone, F., and Inglis, L.: Familial trends in low birth weight, Br. Med. J. **3**:659, 1974.

Ounsted, M., and Ounsted, C.: Maternal regulation of intra-uterine growth, Nature **220**:995, 1966.

Visser, G., and others: Early fetal growth retardation: obstetric background and recurrence rate, Obstet. Gynecol. **67**:40, 1986.

Nutrition

Campbell, D., and Gillmer, S.: Nutrition in pregnancy, New York, 1983, Perinatal Press.

Campbell, D., and MacGillivray, I.: The effect of low calorie diet or a thiazide diuretic on the incidence of preeclampsia and on birth weight, Br. J. Obstet. Gynecol. **82**:572, 1975.

Hytten, F.: Nutrition in pregnancy, Postgrad. Med. J. **55**:295, 1979.

Metcoff, J.: Association of fetal growth with maternal nutrition. In Falkner, F., and Tanner, J., editors: Human growth, vol. 1, New York, 1978, Plenum Press.

Miller, H., and Hassanein, K.: Fetal malnutrition in white newborn infants: maternal factors, Pediatrics **52**:504, 1973.

Naeye, R., Blanc, W., and Paul, C.: Effects of maternal nutrition on the human fetus, Pediatrics **52**:494, 1973.

Niswander, K., and others: Weight gain during pregnancy and prepregnancy weight, Obstet. Gynecol. **33**:482, 1969.

Prentice, A., and others: Prenatal dietary supplementation of African women and birthweight, Lancet **i**:489, 1983.

Stein, Z., Susser, M., and Rush, D.: Prenatal nutrition and birth weight: experiments and quasi-experiments in the past decade, J. Reprod. Med. **21**:287, 1978.

Tafari, N., and others: Effects of maternal undernutrition and heavy physical work during pregnancy on birth weight, Br. J. Obstet. Gynecol. **87**:222, 1980.

Maternal disease and socioeconomic status

Clarren, S., and Smith, D.: The fetal alcohol syndrome, N. Engl. J. Med. **298**:1063, 1978.

Cnattingius, S., and others: Smoking, maternal age and fetal growth, Obstet. Gynecol. **66**:449, 1985.

Editorial: Diabetes and malformation, Lancet **ii**:587, 1982.

Gruenwald, P., and others: Influence of environmental factors on fetal growth in man, Lancet **1**:1026, 1967.

Kuzma, J., and Sokol, R.: Maternal drinking behavior and decreased intrauterine growth, Alcoholism: Clin. Exp. Res. **6**:396, 1982.

Sibai, B., and Anderson, G.: Pregnancy outcome of intensive therapy in severe hypertension in first trimester, Obstet. Gynecol. **67**:517, 1986.

Turner, G.: Recognition of intrauterine growth retardation by considering comparative birth weights, Lancet **2**:1123, 1971.

Usher, R.: Clinical and therapeutic aspects of fetal malnutrition, Pediatr. Clin. North Am. **17**:169, 1970.

Placental factors

Fleischer, A., and others: Uterine artery doppler velocimetry in pregnant women with hypertension, Am. J. Obstet. Gynecol. **154**:806, 1986.

Jogee, M., and others: Decreased prostacyclin production by placental cells in culture from pregnancies complicated by fetal growth retardation, Br. J. Obstet. Gynecol. **90**:247, 1983.

Lee, M., and Yeh, M.: Fetal microcirculation of abnormal human placenta: scanning electron microscopy of placental vascular casts from small for gestational age fetus, Am. J. Obstet. Gynecol. **154**:1133, 1986.

Tonge, H., and others: Blood flow velocity waveforms in the descending fetal aorta: comparison between normal and growth retarded pregnancies, Obstet. Gynecol. **67**:851, 1986.

Fetal factors

Hersh, J., and others: Toluene embryopathy, J. Pediatr. **106**:922, 1985.

Hoff, C., and Bixler, C.: Maternal-fetal ABO/Rh antigenic relationships and human fetal development, Am. J. Obstet. Gynecol. **154**:126, 1986.

Merimee, T., and others: Dwarfism in the pygmy: an isolated deficiency of insulin-like growth factor I, N. Engl. J. Med. **305**:965, 1981.

Antenatal diagnosis

Bastide, A., and others: Ultrasound evaluation of amniotic fluid: outcome of pregnancies with severe oligohydramnios, Am. J. Obstet. Gynecol. **154**:895, 1986.

Gross, T., and others: Using ultrasound and amniotic fluid determinations to diagnose intrauterine growth retardation before birth: a clinical model, Am. J. Obstet. Gynecol. **143**:265, 1982.

Hadlock, F., and others: Estimation of fetal weight with the use of head, body, and femur measurements—a prospective study, Am. J. Obstet. Gynecol. **151**:333, 1985.

Parker, A., and others: The ultrasound estimation of sex related variations of intrauterine growth, Am. J. Obstet. Gynecol. **149**:665, 1984.

Vintzileus, A., and others: Value of fetal ponderal index in predicting growth retardation, Obstet. Gynecol. **67**:584, 1986.

Warsof, S., and others: Routine ultrasound screening for antenatal detection of intrauterine growth retardation, Obstet. Gynecol. **67**:33, 1986.

Antenatal management

Lagrew, D., and Freeman, R.: Management of postdate pregnancy, Am. J. Obstet. Gynecol. **154**:8, 1986.

Manning, F.: Assessment of fetal condition and risk: analysis of single and combined biophysical variable monitoring, Semin. Perinatol. **9**:168, 1985.

Manning, F., and others: Fetal assessment based on fetal biophysical profile scoring: experience in 12,620 referred high risk pregnancies. I. Perinatal mortality by frequency and etiology, Am. J. Obstet. Gynecol. **151**:343, 1985.

Platt, L., and others: A prospective trial of the fetal biophysical profile versus the nonstress test in the management of high risk pregnancies, Am. J. Obstet. Gynecol. **153**:624, 1985.

SGA infant

Morrison, I., and Olsen, J.: Weight specific stillbirths and associated causes of death: an analysis of 765 stillbirths, Am. J. Obstet. Gynecol. **152**:975, 1985.

Oh, W., and Coustan, D.: Intrauterine fetal growth retardation: perinatal diagnosis and management, Ann. Nestle **40**:17, 1982.

Paul, R., and others: Fetal injury prior to labor: does it happen? Am. J. Obstet. Gynecol. **154**:1187, 1986.

Neonatal metabolism

Andrew, G., Chan, G., and Schiff, D.: Lipid metabolism in the neonate, J. Pediatr. **92**:995, 1978.

Chessex, P., and others: Metabolic consequences of intrauterine growth retardation in very low birthweight infants, Pediatr. Res. **18**:709, 1984.

Collins, J., and Leonard, J.: Hyperinsulinism in asphyxiated and small for dates infants with hypoglycemia, Lancet **ii**:311, 1984.

Frazer, T., and others: Direct measurement of gluconeogenesis from [2, $3^{13}C_2$] alanine in the human neonate, Am. J. Physiol. **615**, 1981.

Harris, R.: Plasma nonesterified fatty acid and blood glucose levels in healthy and hypoxemic infants, J. Pediatr. **84**:578, 1974.

Haymond, M., Karl, I., and Pagliara, A.: Increased gluconeogenic substrates in the small for gestational age infant, N. Engl. J. Med. **291**:322, 1974.

Jarai, I., and others: Body size and neonatal hypoglycemia in intrauterine growth retardation, Early Hum. Dev. **1**:25, 1977.

LeDune, M.: Response to glucagon in small for dates hypoglycemic and nonhypoglycemic newborn infants, Arch. Dis. Child. **47**:754, 1972.

Sabel, K., and others: Interrelation between fatty acid oxidation and control of gluconeogenic substrates in small for gestational age (SGA) infants with hypoglycemia and with normoglycemia, Acta Paediatr. Scand. **71**:53, 1982.

Shelly, H., and Neligan, G.: Neonatal hypoglycemia, Br. Med. Bull. **22**:34, 1966.

Stern, L., Sourkes, T., and Raiha, N.: The role of the adrenal medulla in the hypoglycemia of fetal malnutrition, Biol. Neonatal. **11**:129, 1967.

Williams, P., and others: Effect of oral alanine on blood glucose, plasma glucagon, and insulin concentration in small for gestational age infants, N. Engl. J. Med. **292**:612, 1975.

Other neonatal problems

Bard, H.: Neonatal problems of infants with intrauterine growth retardation, J. Reprod. Med. **21**:359, 1978.

Bhakoo, O., and Scopes, J.: Minimal rates of oxygen consumption in small for dates babies during the first week of life, Arch. Dis. Child **49**:583, 1974.

Chandra, R.: Fetal malnutrition and postnatal immunocompetence, Am. J. Dis. Child. **128**:456, 1975.

Chandra, R.: Serum thymic hormone activity and cell-mediated immunity in healthy neonates, preterm infants, and small-for-gestational-age infants, Pediatrics **67**:407, 1981.

Ferguson, S.: Prolonged impairment of cellular immunity in children with intrauterine growth retardation, J. Pediatr. **93**:52, 1978.

Mehta, P., and others: Thrombocytopenia in the high risk infant, J. Pediatr. **97**:791, 1980.

Minton, S., and others: Decreased bone mineral content in small for gestational age infants compared with appropriate for gestational age infants: normal serum 25-hydroxyvitamin D and decreasing parathyroid hormone, Pediatrics **71**:383, 1983.

Perlman, M., and Dvilansky, A.: Blood coagulation status of small for dates and postmature infants, Arch. Dis. Child. **50**:424, 1975.

Sinclair, J.: Heat production and thermoregulation in the small for date infant, Pediatr. Clin. North Am. **17**:147, 1970.

Spiers, P.: Does growth retardation predispose the fetus to congenital malformation? Lancet **1**:312, 1982.

Tsang, R., and others: Studies in calcium metabolism in infants with intrauterine growth retardation, J. Pediatr. **86**:936, 1975.

Follow-up

Brandt, I.: Growth dynamics of low birth weight infants with emphasis on the perinatal period. In Falkner, F., and Tanner, J., editors: Human growth, New York, 1978, Plenum Press.

Chamberlain, R., and Simpson, R.: Cross sectional studies of physical growth in twins, postmature, and small for dates children, Acta Pediatr. Scand. **66**:457, 1977.

Fancourt, R., and others: Follow-up study of small for dates babies, Br. Med. J. **1**:1435, 1976.

Fitzhardinge, P., and Steven, E.: The small-for-date infant. I. Later growth patterns, Pediatrics **49**:671, 1972.

Fitzhardinge, P., and Steven, E.: The small-for-date infant. II. Neurological and intellectual sequelae, Pediatrics **50**:50, 1972.

Francis-Williams, J., and Davies, P.: Very low birthweight and later intelligence, Dev. Med. Child. Neurol. **16**:709, 1974.

Harvey, D., and others: Abilities of children who were small for gestational age babies, Pediatrics **69**:296, 1982.

Hill, R., and others: The effect of intrauterine malnutrition on the term infant: a 14 year progressive study, Acta Paediatr. Scand. **73**:482, 1984.

Keet, M., and others: Follow-up study of physical growth of monozygous twins with discordant within pair birth weights, Pediatrics **77**:336, 1986.

Lipper, E., and others: Determinants of neurobehavioral outcome in low birth weight infants, Pediatrics **67**:502, 1981.

Low, J., and others: Intrauterine growth retardation: a preliminary report of long-term morbidity, Am. J. Obstet. Gynecol. **130**:534, 1978.

Low, J., and others: Intrauterine growth retardation: a study of long-term morbidity, Am. J. Obstet. Gynecol. **142**:620, 1982.

Lubchenco, L.: The high-risk infant, Philadelphia, 1976, W.B. Saunders Co.

Neligan, G., and others: Born too soon or born too small, London 1976, Spastics International Medical Publications.

Sable, K., Olegard, R., and Victorin, L.: Remaining sequelae with modern perinatal care, Pediatrics **57**:652, 1976.

Villar, J., and others: Heterogeneous growth and mental development of intrauterine growth retarded infants during the first 3 years of life, Pediatrics **74**:783, 1984.

Vohr, B., and others: The preterm small for gestational age infant: a two-year follow-up study, Am. J. Obstet. Gynecol. **133**:426, 1979.

CHAPTER 8

Estimation of fetal well-being

From the time pregnancy is confirmed, all couples typically anticipate a baby that is structurally and functionally intact. Some will be disappointed, however; abortion, stillbirth, malformation, or a genetic defect may interdict. In addition, the neonatal consequences of preterm delivery may result in damage to the initially intact but immature baby. From the moment of conception, the fetus is clearly vulnerable to a variety of stresses that occasionally may have permanent, adverse effects. Today's obstetrician has technologic refinements available that usually can permit the identification of deteriorating fetal state, presumably at a time when appropriate intervention can prevent damage. This chapter addresses fetal evaluation, initially from the more established intrapartum perspective, and then extends the lessons learned from intrapartum assessment into third-trimester surveillance of fetuses designated at risk for uteroplacental insufficiency.

PART ONE

Evaluation of the intrapartum fetus

Sudden, unanticipated, and sometimes unrelenting fetal distress can occur at any time during labor. Therefore, to prevent perinatal morbidity or mortality, every obstetrician must be familiar with the diagnosis and proper management of this condition. This implies a knowledge of relevant physiology and pathophysiology, an ability to accurately interpret data from fetal monitoring devices, a familiarity with the treatment of fetal distress, and the avoidance of circumstances that may worsen or even cause such distress.

IMPORTANCE OF RECOGNIZING INTRAPARTUM DISTRESS

The labor and delivery process resulting in vaginal birth is one of the most physiologically stressful events a human being faces. Although most fetuses seem to tolerate this stress without detectable, adverse consequences, some are not so fortunate. A few may sustain damage from hypoxic insults inherent in uterine contractions; extreme forms of this damage may result in perinatal death. Much less frequently, survivable damage may be associated with various degrees of organ insult, the most clinically obvious being to the central nervous system. The spectrum of such damage may range from severe (resulting in cerebral palsy with mental retardation), to mild (leading to such clinical problems as learning disabilities), to forms undetectable by available clinical assessments. The response of an individual fetus to intrapartum *stress* and the eventual outcome relative to any resultant *distress* depends on several factors; the most notable include preexisting fetal status, the intensity and duration of the stress, and the ability of the labor room team to assess fetal condition accurately and to react appropriately. All professionals concerned with intrapartum care would welcome the ability to identify precisely the distressed but as yet uncompromised fetus in imminent danger of suffering irreversible damage. Although our abilities in such identification remain imprecise, they are improving.

The importance of identifying the fetus in such a premorbid state is embodied in the following definition of distress: a precarious fetal condition that, if allowed to persist, *may* lead to permanent damage or perinatal death. This definition suggests that if the distress is recognized promptly and treated appropriately within a reasonable time, damage may be averted. Thus it would seem unreasonable and even counterproductive to insist on diagnostic criteria so strict as to encourage postponing appropriate intervention until the actual or probable occurrence of damage.

Before the development of modern methods of intrapartum fetal assessment, fetal distress usually was diagnosed through criteria now considered faulty or erroneous. For example, simple *baseline* (e.g., between

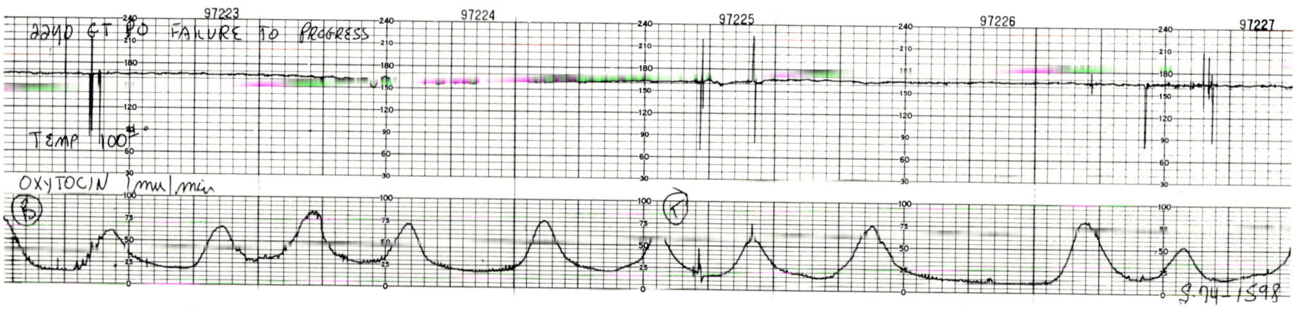

Fig. 8-1. Fetal tachycardia; heart rate is 165 beats per minute. This tachycardia is associated with maternal fever (note temperature). Also note the associated loss of variability. The absence of associated decelerations and presence of an explanation (fever) makes hypoxia an unlikely cause. (From Freeman, R., and Garite, T.: Fetal heart rate monitoring, Baltimore. Copyright 1981, The Williams & Wilkins Company. Reproduced by permission.)

contractions) tachycardia or bradycardia of the fetal heart rate (FHR) may occur with circumstances (e.g., maternal fever or β-sympathomimetic drugs) in which the fetus is not in jeopardy at all (Fig. 8-1). Meconium-stained amniotic fluid, in the absence of accepted FHR criteria for distress, is recognized now as an indicator for aggressive airway management at delivery, but not alone as diagnostic or distress (Chapter 28, part five).

Although not infallible, widely available methods can now identify fetal distress reasonably accurately. These methods employ electronic FHR monitoring and, when appropriate, the measurement of fetal scalp pH. Such identification then justifies an orderly sequence of maneuvers designed to relieve the distress; if these methods are unsuccessful, prompt delivery is justified. From the perinatal perspective the most important intrapartum goal is the atraumatic delivery of the fetus before any intrauterine compromise. The constant availability of oxygen in preventing such compromise is critical.

UTEROPLACENTAL EXCHANGE AND FETAL OXYGENATION

The placental interface may be considered a semipermeable membrane that separates the circulations of mother and fetus. Across this membrane all substances essential for fetal survival and growth must cross. Because of the storage capacities for such nutrients, a fetus might be able to tolerate brief interruptions in the provision of glucose, the primary energy source, or amino acids, the primary anabolic sources. However, oxygen must be provided without significant interruption, since the fetus has no capacity to store this element. A rather continuous supply of oxygen is necessary for the efficient catabolism of glucose and the maintenance of an appropriate intracellular pH.

When adequate amounts of oxygen are available, the reduced flavin and adenine nucleotides produced by glycolysis and by the Krebs cycle can be oxidized within the mitochondria to produce abundant chemical energy in the form of adenosine triphosphate (ATP). If cellular oxygenation is inadequate, glycolytic metabolism is diverted at the pyruvic acid step toward the production of lactic acid. This diversion results in the production of only one-nineteenth as much ATP from each mole of glucose. Moreover, an accumulation of lactic acid and a consumption of bicarbonate follow. Unlike carbon dioxide, which rapidly traverses the normally functioning placenta, lactic acid is nonvolatile and crosses only slowly. The consequent fall in pH may hinder function of, or even render inoperative, many enzymes necessary for the maintenance of vital cellular functions. The consequences of such cellular dysfunction might include cell death, fetal damage, especially neurologic damage, and even fetal death. Therefore a basic understanding of fetal oxygenation is fundamental to the diagnosis and treatment of fetal distress.

ELECTRONIC MONITORING OF THE FETAL HEART RATE

Electronic FHR monitoring during labor has been common practice in the United States for almost 15 years. The principle involves continuous, instantaneous beat-to-beat FHR recording on one channel of a two-channel recorder with simultaneous recording of uterine activity on the other channel. The original and still most effective method involves a direct fetal scalp electrode application after membranes have ruptured to provide a fetal ECG complex for counting the heart rate. The uterine activity is measured directly by a transvaginal uterine catheter connected to a strain gauge. External techniques for heart rate monitoring are less accurate but allow recording when membranes are intact or the fetal presenting part is not accessible. The methods include phonocardiography, Doppler ultrasound technique, and abdom-

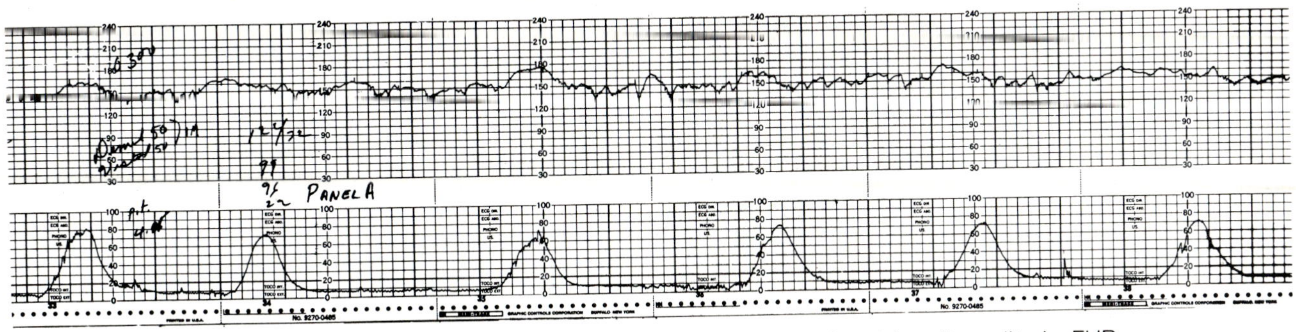

Fig. 8-2. Normal, reassuring FHA pattern. Note pertubations of FHR (small amplitude, FHR variability; larger amplitude, FHR reactivity). If seen during antepartum testing, this tracing would be interpreted as a reactive, negative contraction stress test. (From Freeman, R., and Garite, T.: Fetal heart rate monitoring, Baltimore. Copyright 1981, The Williams & Wilkins Company. Reproduced by permission.)

inal fetal electrocardiography. The Doppler technique is the only indirect external method that currently works adequately for labor monitoring. Uterine activity is measured by a tocodynamometer from the mother's abdominal wall when external uterine activity recording is desired. This gives only qualitative information about the frequency and duration of contractions and does not provide quantitative data on the amplitude of contractions.

Baseline fetal heart rate

The average FHR between periodic changes is referred to as the baseline FHR. Generally one needs to observe a tracing for 20 minutes or more to establish the true baseline FHR, especially if frequent periodic changes are occurring. The normal baseline range is usually considered to be between 120 and 160 beats per minute (Fig. 8-2). However, when the baseline heart rate is outside this so-called range, one must consider the possibilities for the causes of this deviation, since often it does not represent any intrinsic fetal problem. When the baseline FHR rises, it is referred to as tachycardia, either relative or absolute. When the baseline FHR is low, it is referred to as bradycardia, either absolute or relative. Later periodic changes refer to accelerations and decelerations. It is important to use this terminology. (See Chapter 21.)

Fetal tachycardia is most often caused by maternal fever and is a normal fetal response to hyperthermia (Fig. 8-1). Sometimes fetal tachycardia will be seen even before the mother becomes febrile, as in chorioamnionitis. Certain drugs will also cause the FHR to rise. These include parasympatholytic agents such as atropine, sympathomimetic agents such as ritodrine, and other drugs that may cause uterine blood flow to decrease, producing fetal hypoxia and secondary tachycardia. Rarely, a patient who is pregnant has hyperthyroidism; in a small percentage of these patients there will be fetal tachycardia, perhaps due to the presence of long-acting thyroid stimulator, which crosses the placenta, whereas T_4 and T_3 do not cross sufficiently to produce fetal tachycardia.

The most significant cause of fetal tachycardia is fetal hypoxia. The mechanism probably represents β-adrenergic activity stimulated by the hypoxemia itself. It is usually seen following a hypoxic episode and often is part of the recovery process. Sometimes, however, tachycardia will be seen during a more gradual onset of fetal hypoxemia and, if the uterus is not contracting, may even precede the development of late decelerations. For the clinician, a rising baseline FHR may signify developing or recovering hypoxemia in the fetus as well as maternal fever, drug effects, or hyperthyroidism in the mother. It is therefore a nonspecific change that should be interpreted along with other clinical information available, as well as other aspects of the FHR tracing.

Very rarely a fetus may have an FHR in the range of 220 to 300 beats per minute. This usually represents supraventricular tachycardia, which may be either paroxysmal or constant. Such fetuses are at great risk for death in utero. Maternal digitalization may be helpful for the fetus. Death appears to be caused by fetal heart failure, since the fetuses typically are hydropic. It is therefore recommended to deliver such fetuses if evidence of lung maturity exists; if not, they may be followed with serial sonograms, looking for fetal ascites, placental thickening, and fetal edema. If the fetus begins to become hydropic, it would seem best to deliver, even in the absence of confirmed fetal lung maturity. (See Chapter 6.)

Fetal bradycardia was originally thought to be a sign of fetal hypoxemia. However, except in preterminal situations where the FHR has previously been higher and there is no FHR variability, fetal bradycardia with good FHR variability is not a sign of fetal hypoxemia. Many times a baseline FHR of 90 to 120 beats per minute may be just the normal heart rate (Fig. 8-3).

Another feature of the baseline FHR is its variability. FHR variability (FHRV) has two characteristics. The short-term FHRV represents the actual beat-to-beat interval differences. Long-term variability is defined as FHR change that has a cycle of 3 to 6 per minute. Thus FHRV includes a series of FHR changes in a positive or negative direction.

Derivation of the heartbeat

Contractions of the fetal heart, as in the adult heart, derive from an autonomous atrial pacemaker. This intrinsic FHR is monotonous but is usually slightly increased or decreased on a beat-to-beat basis by normal sympathetic and parasympathetic influences, respectively. These autonomically generated FHR pertubations, or FHRV, presumably are responses to instantaneous changes in needs for cardiac output. As such, the FHRV is considered indicative of a functionally intact and metabolically normal central nervous system (Fig. 8-2). Even with a finding such as baseline fetal bradycardia, normal FHRV can be reassuring).

Problems with assessing fetal heart rate variability

Depressed FHRV does not automatically imply that the fetus is ill (Fig. 8-4). During sleep the fetus typically has reduced FHRV. In addition, most analgesic or sedative drugs administered to the mother will cross the placenta and to a greater or lesser extent will depress the fetal central nervous system and consequently the FHRV. Thus the intrapartum use of narcotics, barbiturates, benzodiazepines, and phenothiazines, as well as parasympatholytic drugs such as atropine and scopolamine, seriously diminishes the potential value of FHRV assessment. However, the FHRV depression related to these drugs generally should begin to resolve within 20 to 30 minutes after an intravenous dose. The same or similar drugs obtained illicitly also may produce the same effects on FHRV, and a gravida taking these drugs may not admit to having used them.

Also important is the very limited extent to which most external (ultrasonic) FHR monitors allow for an assessment of FHRV. The ultrasonic (Doppler) signal is derived from numerous mechanical cardiac events. Compared with the precise FHR determinations obtained from the fetal ECG signal by a scalp electrode, such determinations from the ultrasonic signal typically are highly irregular and may result in the deceptive introduction of apparently normal FHRV. On the other hand, if the FHRV appears depressed with external FHR assessment, it would prove to be at least as depressed on a simultaneously measured determination from a scalp electrode. However, FHR reactivity (FHR accelerations with fetal movement) determined externally, as is typically used for fetal assessment during a nonstress test, is another reflection of fetal autonomic function generally considered as reassuring as true FHRV. The latest generation of fetal monitors employs techniques that electronically compare the externally derived FHR signals from successive beats, and the FHRV displayed may prove to be more representative of true FHRV than that obtained with earlier machines.

Decelerations of the fetal heart rate

Late decelerations

Of the possible negative influences on fetal oxygenation, the most common and physiologic is that associated with normal uterine contractions. Even though fetal oxygen pressure (PO_2) is usually only 25 to 30 mm Hg, sufficient oxygen delivery is maintained because of the high fetal hematocrit and cardiac output and because of the favorable dissociation curve of fetal hemoglobin. It is well known from both human and animal studies that uterine blood flow, specifically that portion perfusing the intervillous space, essentially *ceases* during contractions of normal intensity. As a result, fetal oxygenation begins to fall as the contraction intensity increases. Oxygenation begins to return to its basal level only after the contraction is resolving and flow through the intervillous space is reestablished. The clinician should appreciate that the fetal PO_2 curve is thus temporally displaced from the associated contraction. For the fetus with normal basal oxygenation, or a normal resting PO_2 level before the stress of a contraction, the FHR is generally unaffected by contractions and maintains its normal, autonomically modulated rate, or FHRV (Fig. 8-2).

On the other hand, for the fetus with a reduction in basal oxygenation, the PO_2 during a contraction may be driven below a certain critical level and consequently the FHR slows. This slowing and subsequent return of the FHR follows the PO_2 curve, since it is delayed relative to the contraction. This is the FHR pattern of *late deceleration*, which has been demonstrated both in human and the rhesus monkey studies to reflect basal fetal hypoxemia reliably. Myers and associates noted that even the fetus remaining acidotic after restoration of PO_2 levels does not continue to demonstrate the late deceleration pattern. FHRV in such reoxygenated fetuses might be expected to remain depressed until normal acid-base status is reestablished. Martin and co-workers have found that the late deceleration pattern is vagally mediated initially but is caused by direct depression of myocardial rhythmicity when hypoxia is sufficiently prolonged for metabolic acidosis to supervene (Fig. 8-5).

Early decelerations

The uncommon *early deceleration* pattern resembles the late, except that the decelerations are concurrent

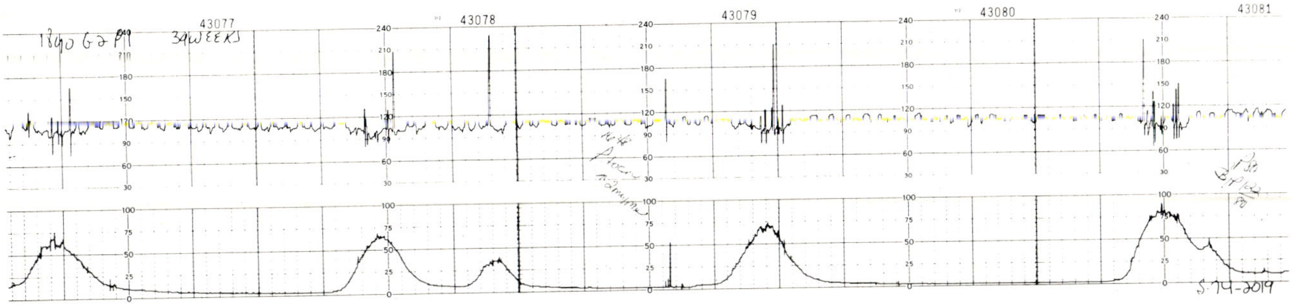

Fig. 8-3. Fetal bradycardia; heart rate is 110 beats per minute. Normal variability is present by direct (internal scalp electrode) monitoring. Four hours later, the patient delivered a 3,025 gm baby with Apgar scores of 9 at 1 minute and 10 at 5 minutes. Mother and baby did well. (From Freeman, R., and Garite, T.: Fetal heart rate monitoring, Baltimore. Copyright 1981, The Williams & Wilkins Company. Reproduced by permission.)

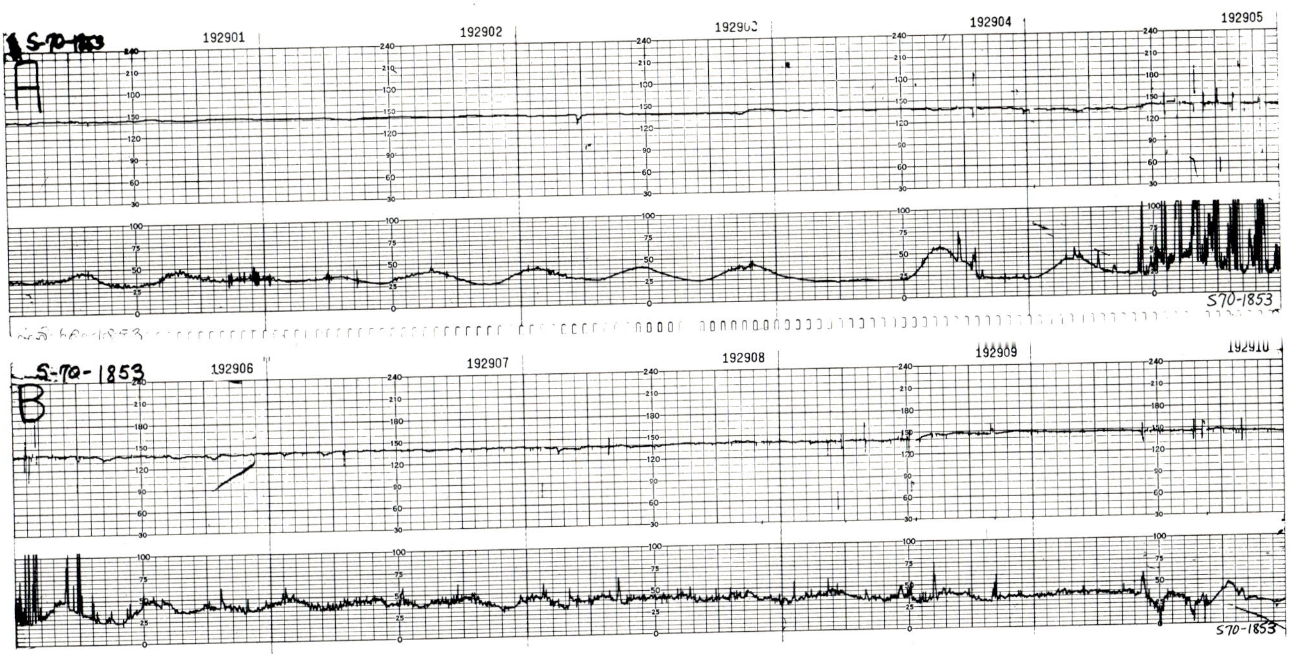

Fig. 8-4. Complete absence of FHR variability, without decelerations. The absence of late decelerations suggests that fetal hypoxemia does not currently exist. (From Freeman, R., and Garite, T.: Fetal heart rate monitoring, Baltimore. Copyright 1981, The Williams & Wilkins Company. Reproduced by permission.)

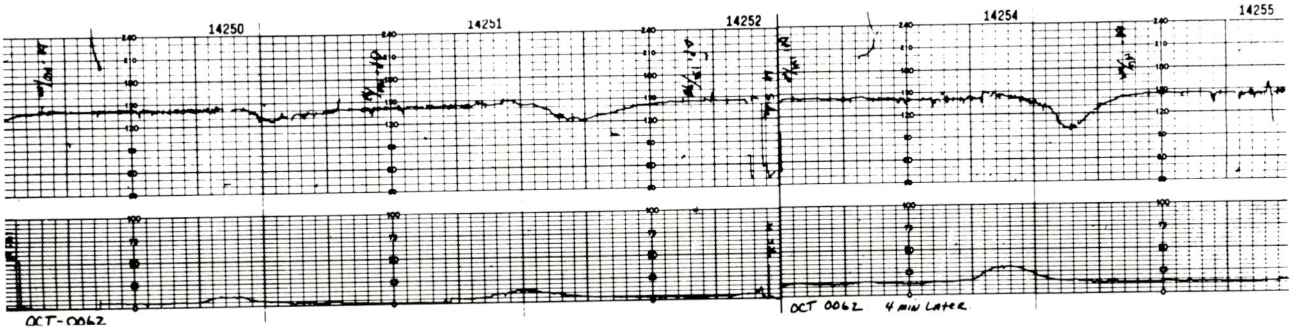

Fig. 8-5. Late decelerations with absent variability. (From Freeman, R., and Garite, T.: Fetal heart rate monitoring, Baltimore. Copyright 1981, The Williams & Wilkins Company. Reproduced by permission.)

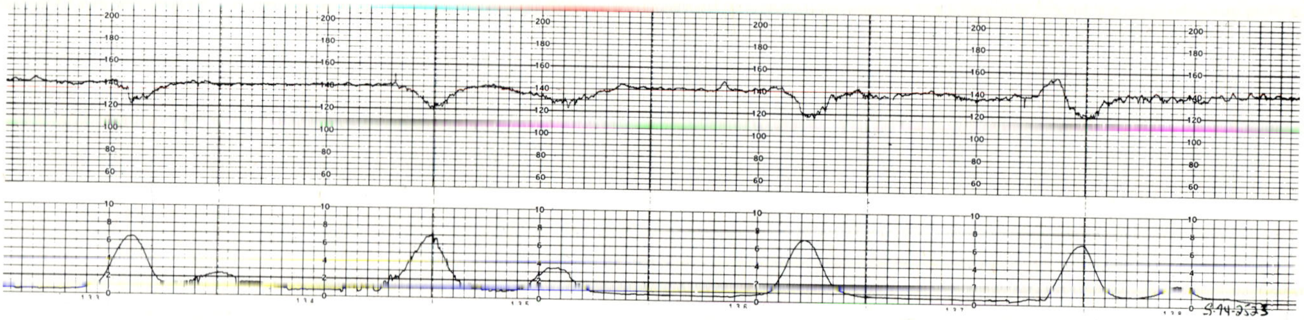

Fig. 8-6. Early decelerations are seen with each contraction on this panel. They are uniform, mirror the contractions, and decelerate only 10 to 20 beats per minute. (From Freeman, R., and Garite, T.: Fetal heart rate monitoring, Baltimore. Copyright 1981, The Williams & Wilkins Company. Reproduced by permission.)

with contractions (Fig. 8-6). The chief importance of recognizing the early pattern is that it is benign, whereas the similar late pattern is not. Early deceleration is characterized as a uniform pattern with gradual onset and gradual offset, resembling a mirror image of the uterine contraction. It tends to be uniform in shape from one contraction to the next and tends to parallel the amplitude of the contraction, with higher-amplitude contractions eliciting deeper decelerations and lower-amplitude contractions eliciting more shallow decelerations. The deceleration begins early in the contraction, has its nadir simultaneously with the peak of the contraction, and returns to baseline during the decline of the contraction so that the FHR is back to baseline by the time the contraction is over. The baseline FHR is usually in the normal range, and the FHR variability is most often normal. The FHR deceleration is quite shallow, and the nadir seldom drops below 120 beats per minute.

Clinically, early deceleration is usually seen between about 4 and 7 cm dilation. This corresponds to the time that the edge of the cervix is crossing the anterior fontanel. This pattern has been reproduced in neonates by exerting pressure with doughnut pessaries sized 4 to 7 cm over the fetal vertex. Since the anterior fontanel is the area most vulnerable to external pressure that may affect cerebrovascular hemodynamics, this clinical observation fits well with physiologic studies showing that the mechanism for early deceleration appears to be central vagal stimulation caused by altered cerebral blood flow. In direct proportion to the pressure being exerted on the fontanel, the vagal impulses then cause FHR slowing, which results in the uniform pattern previously described. Both animal and human studies have shown that this pattern is blocked or greatly altered by the administration of atropine; such data confirm the vagal reflex nature of the early deceleration pattern.

The clinical importance of this pattern relates to its similarity in appearance to late deceleration. Early deceleration is associated with normal fetal pH, normal Apgar scores, and no other evidence of fetal compromise. To the clinician it is a reassuring FHR pattern and should not indicate any form of intervention.

Variable decelerations

The variable FHR deceleration pattern is a normal response to umbilical cord compression. This pattern is characterized by an abrupt fall followed by an abrupt rise in the FHR and, most frequently, by its temporal concordance with a contraction (Fig. 8-7). Variable decelerations are seen at least occasionally in about one half of monitored labors. This FHR pattern usually is not viewed with great concern.

The pattern of variable deceleration also is characterized by a rapid and profound descent of the FHR to levels that are usually well below 120, often below 60, beats per minute. The duration, shape, and timing of the pattern are not uniform. It is often associated with acceleration preceding the development of this pattern, and after the variable deceleration again another acceleration, referred to by some as "shoulders."

The acceleration portion represents umbilical venous occlusion and a sympathetic response to the consequently decreased right atrial return. The variable deceleration is caused by compression of the umbilical arteries as the contraction intensity peaks. Physiologically, it is believed that, when the umbilical arteries are occluded, sudden and rapid fetal hypertension results from the cutoff of the low-resistance placental circuit. This brings forth a baroreceptor response, resulting in a vagal FHR deceleration. It has been shown that atropine will alter this response.

During variable deceleration there may be a rapid decline in the fetal PO_2, a rapid rise in the fetal carbon dioxide pressure (PCO_2), and a concomitant fall in the fetal pH. This transient fetal hypoxemia and respiratory acidosis are reversed as soon as the umbilical artery is

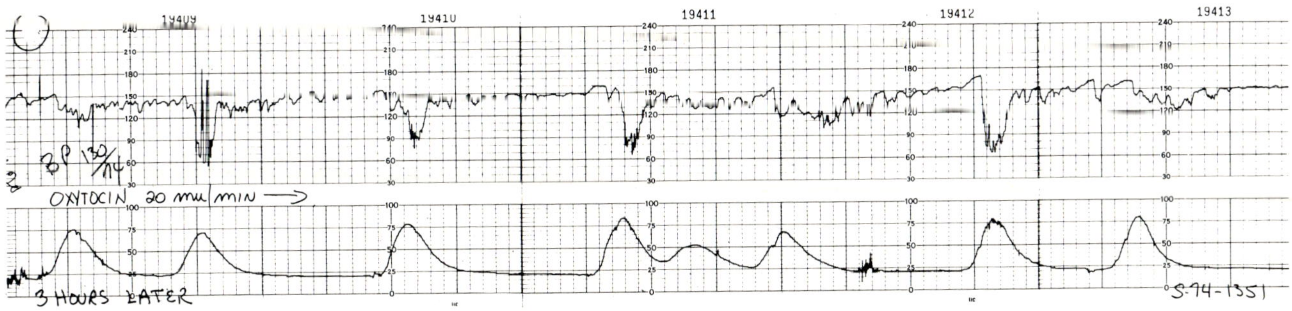

Fig. 8-7. Mild variable decelerations are seen in this panel. Baseline heart rate and variability are normal. (From Freeman, R., and Garite, T.: Fetal heart rate monitoring, Baltimore. Copyright 1981, The Williams & Wilkins Company. Reproduced by permission.)

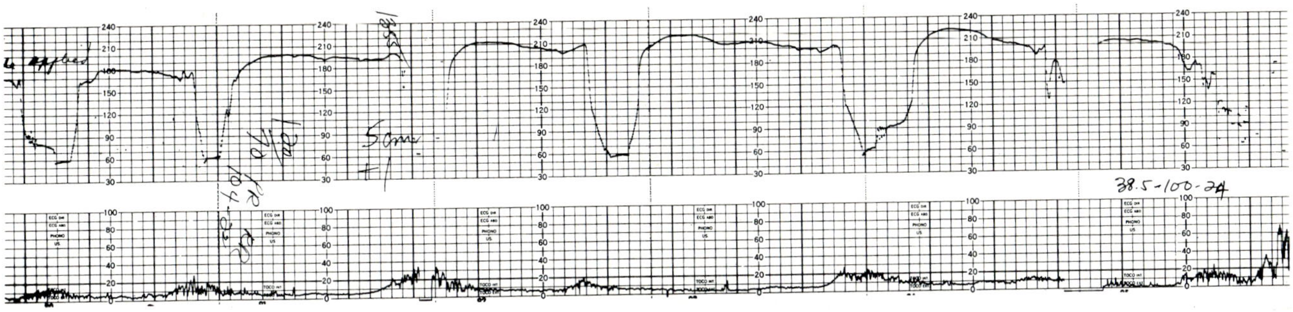

Fig. 8-8. Severe, ominous variable decelerations are seen with rising baseline heart rate to 210 beats per minute and virtually absent variability. A premature baby was delivered by cesarean section with Apgar scores of 1 at 1 minute and 2 at 5 minutes. (From Freeman, R., and Garite, T.: Fetal heart rate monitoring, Baltimore. Copyright 1981, The Williams & Wilkins Company. Reproduced by permission.)

released and circulation is restored to the intact placenta, where gas exchange and equilibration are rapid.

If cord compression is persistent or if it occurs together with suboptimal basal oxygenation, the FHR may take on characteristics that justify the label of *severe* variable deceleration, the most widely accepted of which is a slow return of the FHR to baseline. This feature of the severe variable pattern may be considered a combination of the variable and late deceleration patterns and should be viewed with the same concern as late deceleration. Depressed FHRV and/or baseline tachycardia may follow either of these patterns and should heighten concern. Another ominous pattern of variable deceleration involves an "overshoot," a smooth acceleration lasting 1 minute or more following the deceleration (Fig. 8-8).

AVOIDING CIRCUMSTANCES STRESSFUL TO THE FETUS

Although most antepartum and intrapartum fetal distress is associated with high-risk pregnancies, it is important to realize that it can occur in low-risk pregnancies as well. Such distress especially may occur in otherwise normal pregnancies unless particular attention is paid to those controllable circumstances that can cause reduced fetal oxygenation.

Maternal positioning

It has been demonstrated radiologically that at term nearly all women who lie supine have total occlusion of the vena cava because of pressure from the enlarged uterus. Whether a woman manifests the well-known supine hypotensive syndrome depends on the ability of her collateral venous system to permit sufficient cardiac return to maintain adequate cardiac output. Despite some of these women therefore having no symptoms, the abdominal aorta may be similarly compressed by the gravid uterus with resultant uterine arterial hypotension. Consequent reduction in intervillous space perfusion may then embarrass fetal oxygenation, despite normal readings of concurrently measured brachial arterial pressure. Thus no woman in late gestation should be asked to lie strictly supine for more than brief periods. The lateral position, especially the left, and possibly the semi-Fowler's position will avoid such posture-related fetal compromises. Even external fetal monitoring techniques will function well with the woman in other than a supine position. Typically one hip is elevated with a rolled sheet or a specially designed foam cushion wedge during antepartum testing or labor. These techniques, or delivery tables that will tilt laterally, are also important in the intrapartum period, especially if signs of fetal distress have been detected before delivery.

Effects of conduction anesthetics

Although spinal and epidural techniques are widely and safely used in obstetrics, some degree of sympathetic blockade regularly occurs with all these methods. Unless appropriate attention is directed to expanding the intravascular volume, such blockade can result in severe hypotension, depressed intervillous space perfusion, and fetal hypoxemia (Chapter 14). These effects will be exaggerated if the patient is lying supine. Thus, unless the patient has disease, such as mitral stenosis, placing her at risk for pulmonary edema, 500 to 800 ml of an appropriate intravenous solution (e.g., Ringer's lactate) should be administered immediately preceding the conduction anesthetic techniques. These techniques must be used with extreme care in the presence of the pathologic volume deficiency often seen with severe pregnancy-induced hypertension.

Undesirable actions of oxytocin

As previously noted, even normal uterine contractions cause recurrent hypoxic stresses to the fetus. Even in small doses exogenous oxytocin can sometimes prolong contractions as well as increase their frequency. Both effects can decrease the intervals during which the uterus is relaxed and normal intervillous space perfusion occurs. Late (Fig. 8-9) or prolonged (Fig. 8-10) decelerations can occur, the latter particularly with sustained hypercontractility. Another more subtle effect of oxytocin is its propensity to increase the resting uterine tonus insidiously above the normal 10 to 15 mm Hg. Blood flow to the intervillous space can be reduced seriously whenever resting intrauterine pressure exceeds normal. Moreover, subtle elevations of the baseline uterine tone cannot be ascertained by external contraction monitoring and frequently may escape detection by palpation, par-

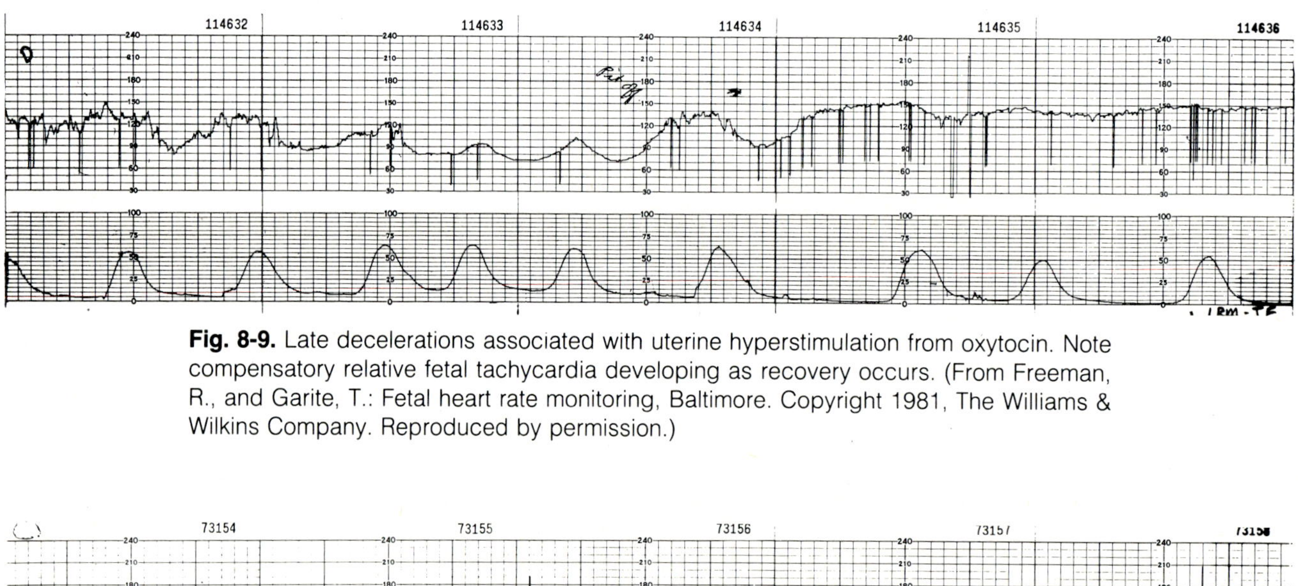

Fig. 8-9. Late decelerations associated with uterine hyperstimulation from oxytocin. Note compensatory relative fetal tachycardia developing as recovery occurs. (From Freeman, R., and Garite, T.: Fetal heart rate monitoring, Baltimore. Copyright 1981, The Williams & Wilkins Company. Reproduced by permission.)

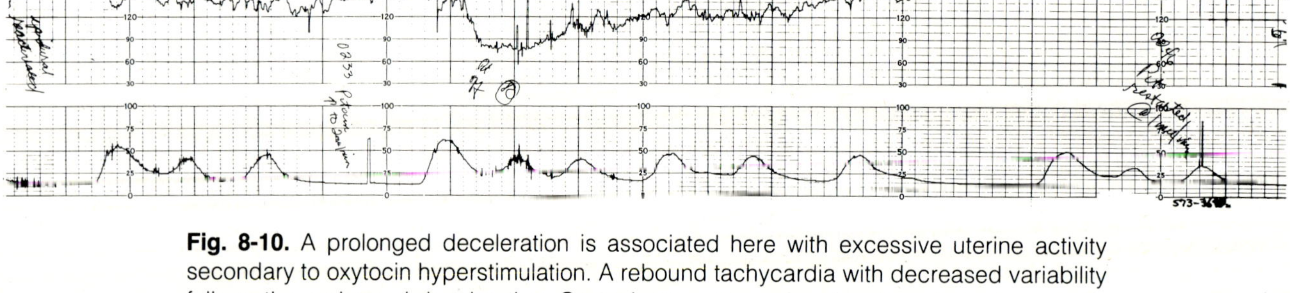

Fig. 8-10. A prolonged deceleration is associated here with excessive uterine activity secondary to oxytocin hyperstimulation. A rebound tachycardia with decreased variability follows the prolonged deceleration. Oxytocin was stopped and restarted at a lower rate, and the heart rate subsequently returned to normal. (From Freeman, R., and Garite, T.: Fetal heart rate monitoring, Baltimore. Copyright 1981, The Williams & Wilkins Company. Reproduced by permission.)

ticularly in obese women. It follows that intrauterine pressure catheters are advisable whenever labor is induced and the fetal membranes can safely be ruptured. These catheters are especially advisable to document uterine activity before any decision to augment spontaneous labor. Oxytocin should only be given intravenously and should be controlled accurately with precision, flow-regulating devices. Because uterine response to this drug may be highly variable, the initial infusion rate should be only 0.5 to 1.0 mU/minute and increments of 1.0 mU/minute made no more than every 20 to 30 minutes. Once achieved, the desired level of uterine activity typically can be maintained by decreasing the infusion rate, thereby reducing the likelihood of hypertonus.

Improper coaching

Although various breathing techniques may assist the pregnant woman in coping with the discomforts of labor, such teaching must avoid hyperventilatory breathing during contractions. Hyperventilation will result in hypoventilation between contractions, and the attendant fall in Po_2 could be detrimental to the fetus. The lowered Pco_2 produced has been shown in some studies to increase fetal blood lactate levels, although other studies did not find a clearly detrimental effect from maternal hyperventilation. During maternal bearing-down efforts in second-stage labor, the mother is apneic and her Po_2 falls. Caldeyro-Barcia has shown that encouraging such pushing efforts for longer than the mother spontaneously would choose results in deranged umbilical arterial blood gases. Thus one must weigh the relative merits of a delivery occurring a few minutes earlier against the possible adverse effects of being overzealous in one's coaching efforts.

INTRAUTERINE RESUSCITATION

Whenever the FHR decreases for more than a few seconds, the potential for developing or worsening fetal distress increases, since the umbilical blood flow and uteroplacental exchange depend directly on the FHR for perfusing the fetal side of the placenta. Fetal distress thus may become increasingly severe unless prompt measures are taken to reverse the process.

Once recognized, fetal distress should be treated aggressively to decrease the chances of fetal damage. The treatment of fetal distress, or intrauterine resuscitation, is directed primarily toward improving uterine and thus intervillous space blood flow and secondarily toward increasing the maternal-fetal oxygen gradient.

Avoiding the supine position

As explained earlier, the supine position should be avoided during labor. The lateral decubitus positions, especially the left, minimize compressive effects on the great vessels and therefore should be maintained if any fetal distress is evident. Mild-to-moderate variable decelerations may be resolved by having the gravida assume other positions. Because umbilical cord compression is the mechanism, variable decelerations can often be eliminated by maneuvers designed to alter the spatial relationships between the uterine wall, fetus, and umbilical cord. Right or left lateral decubitus, Trendelenburg's, and knee-chest positions may all be attempted, particularly if the variable deceleration pattern is either persistent or severe. Oxygen is generally administered by mask, although relief of cord compression is much more important. Overt cord prolapse should be excluded by prompt vaginal examination (Fig. 8-11). Occult cord prolapse should be suspected if the variable pattern resolves temporarily with elevation of the presenting part during vaginal examination.

Decreasing uterine activity

If oxytocin is being administered, it should be discontinued at once; it is inappropriate simply to decrease the rate of infusion. Because the half-life of oxytocin in serum is only a few minutes, its uterotonic effects should abate quickly.

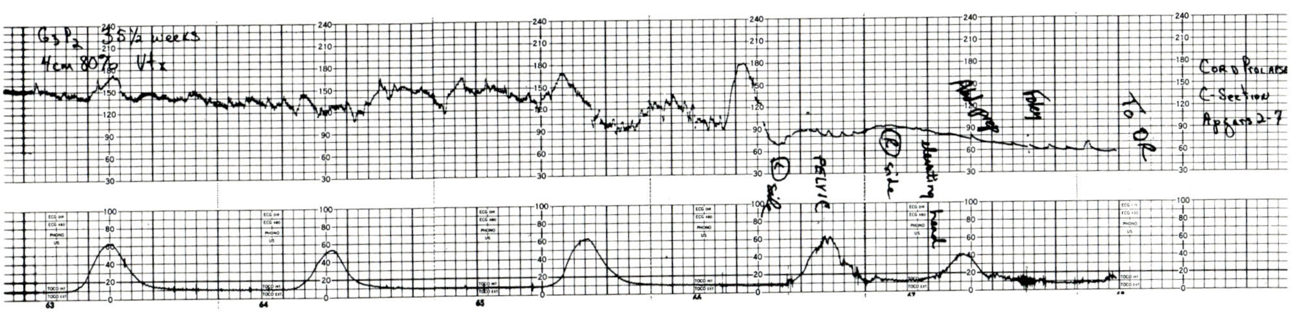

Fig. 8-11. A sudden, prolonged deceleration is seen in this patient in the early active phase of labor. Immediate pelvic examination revealed cord prolapse, and cesarean delivery was performed. (From Freeman, R., and Garite, T.: Fetal heart rate monitoring, Baltimore. Copyright 1981, The Williams & Wilkins Company. Reproduced by permission.)

β-Sympathomimetic drugs have been reported to inhibit uterine contractions during intrauterine resuscitation, although the technique currently should be considered experimental. Another potentially tocolytic drug used widely in the management of pregnancy-induced hypertension is magnesium sulfate. When a 4 gm dose is given intravenously over about 10 minutes, this drug may impressively decrease uterine activity without the risk of hypotension sometimes seen with rapid infusion of a β-sympathomimetic agent. (See Chapter 9.)

Correcting hypotension

Hypotension may result from acute hemorrhage, the supine position, or the sympatholytic effects of conduction anesthesia. Severe acute hemorrhage is managed most appropriately by the rapid infusion of blood. Hypotension, even in the presence of hemorrhage, may initially be treated by elevation of the woman's legs. Blood pooled in the legs, especially with sympathetic blockade, will then drain quickly into the central venous circulation and augment the effective intravascular volume. The intravenous fluid rate should be increased acutely and another intravenous line established, if necessary. If oxytocin has been inappropriately infusing directly through the primary intravenous line, instead of as a "piggyback" connection near the indwelling needle, increasing the fluid rate initially may cause a profound, counterproductive increase in uterine activity. Such a possibility underscores the importance that any oxytocin be infused piggyback and that the primary infusion not contain this drug.

Administering oxygen

The administration of oxygen is considered last because the maternal-fetal gradient usually is favorable. Also, the maneuvers designed to improve intervillous space flow are more urgent. When fetal distress is initially diagnosed, it is inappropriate to reach for an oxygen mask as the first step. This comment is not to disparage the value of augmenting maternal oxygenation. Although the Po_2 of fetal blood cannot be increased strikingly by this maneuver, the oxygen content can be impressively changed. This apparent contradiction occurs because fetal hemoglobin has a greater affinity than maternal hemoglobin for oxygen at low Po_2 levels.

CLINICAL DIAGNOSIS OF FETAL DISTRESS

As the earlier definition of fetal distress suggested, this diagnosis should be based on criteria that encourage interventions before possible fetal damage. A diagnosis of fetal distress is not justified simply on the basis of an occasional late deceleration, an infrequent severe variable deceleration, or even a transient loss of FHRV. The generally accepted FHR criteria for fetal distress are (1) persistent late decelerations, regardless of the deceleration depth; (2) persistent severe variable decelerations, especially with a slow return to the FHR baseline; or (3) prolonged decelerations, generally considered a variant of severe variable decelerations (Fig. 8-11).

If hypoxemia is severe and protracted, fetal acidosis may result and FHRV usually becomes depressed. For this reason depressed FHRV together with any of the three distress criteria listed may represent a more serious situation than if FHRV is normal. As indicated, external FHR monitoring may result in false reassurance because of apparently normal FHRV. Thus one should strongly consider applying an internal fetal electrode whenever better assessment seems necessary.

How is fetal scalp pH assessment appropriately used in fetal monitoring? In most obstetric units scalp pH assessment is used rarely or may not be available at all. Under most circumstances careful FHR and contraction monitoring are satisfactory to assess fetal status. One may be confident that a fetus is well oxygenated if the FHR tracing is normal; that is, none of the distress criteria is present and FHRV or reactivity is normal. On the other hand, if the FHR pattern is confusing, pH assessment may clear the confusion. A scalp pH value less than 7.25 generally is considered abnormal and, particularly if confirmed on repeat sampling, should suggest the need for immediate delivery. Also, when initial monitoring demonstrates loss of FHRV without late decelerations, the fetus may at that time be normally oxygenated but recovering from a previous severe hypoxic insult. Alternatively, such a fetus may be sleeping or the mother may have taken sedative or narcotic drugs, including those obtained illicitly. Again, pH assessment may be useful in making the distinction. As a general rule, however, the clinician can be reassured by a tracing that initially is normal by all criteria and that remains normal except for the development of depressed FHRV, provided there has not been an intervening segment with late or severe variable decelerations. Such FHRV depression will almost always be temporary and related to fetal sleep state.

Fetal scalp blood sampling is technically exacting and generally cannot be performed until the cervix is dilated 3 or 4 centimeters. The clinician also must be aware that a scalp pH measurement is a static point that must be reevaluated frequently, probably about every 15 minutes, as long as the abnormality prompting the initial measurement persists and delivery is not imminent.

Clark and associates reported that scalp stimulation during vaginal examination may evoke acceleration of the FHR in the fetus with otherwise poor FHRV and reactivity. This response was found to correlate well with normal scalp pH and is now frequently used as an alternative to the more invasive scalp blood sampling.

RESULTS OF INTRAUTERINE RESUSCITATION

Most often the resuscitative efforts described result in rapid resolution of the FHR abnormalities. The fetal distress in such cases may be considered *transient*. Labor usually can be allowed to proceed safely, sometimes even if oxytocin stimulation is needed. In the absence of correctable factors, such as hypotension related to epidural anesthesia, a fetus demonstrating transient distress should be considered at risk for redeveloping distress; if such adversity is not observed, however, a favorable outcome almost certainly can be expected. To discourage recurrence of distress, the intrauterine resuscitative measures instituted should be maintained until delivery.

If these resuscitative efforts initially are unsuccessful or if distress patterns subsequently recur despite these efforts, the potential for fetal damage must be realized and prompt delivery considered. Such fetuses are then considered to have *persistent* distress, which then justifies intervention.

Persistent distress

The urgency for delivering a fetus manifesting persistent distress may depend on several factors. Traumatic vaginal delivery must be avoided, although rapid atraumatic vaginal delivery is appropriate whenever feasible. Frequently, cervical dilation and descent of the presenting part may be incomplete and a decision must be made either to effect abdominal delivery promptly or to await conditions more favorable for vaginal delivery. Normal FHRV is most reassuring under such circumstances and may at times justify such a delay. If reduced FHRV is associated with FHR patterns showing persistent distress and no obvious pharmacologic explanation exists for such depression, delivery probably should occur, unless frequent scalp pH assessments or FHR acceleratory responses to scalp stimulation remain reassuring. If the distress pattern resolves at any point, FHR vigilance is continued and a normal outcome is expected. The availability of anesthetic methods appropriate to the specific problems must be considered in all these decisions (Chapter 14).

MOBILIZATION FOR CESAREAN DELIVERY

As the previous discussion and clinical experience have shown, the management of a woman whose fetus is in distress may involve minute-by-minute decisions regarding fetal status and the possible necessity for expedient delivery. At times a decision to proceed with abdominal delivery may be abrupt. Unless adequate preparations have been made prophylactically, time precious to the distressed fetus may be lost. Such preparations include obtaining permission for the procedure, placing an indwelling Foley catheter, and preparing the lower abdomen. The personnel necessary for cesarean delivery should be alerted and mobilized whenever a definitive diagnosis of fetal distress is made and while attempts at intrauterine resuscitation are being instituted. This usually includes personnel from anesthesia, nursing, and pediatrics. Although such mobilization may sometimes seem in vain because the distress FHR patterns frequently resolve with intrauterine resuscitation, it may be life saving for those few fetuses when resuscitation fails and expedient cesarean delivery is clearly indicated. For those hospitals with large- or moderate-sized obstetric services, in-house availability of such personnel should be encouraged and should largely alleviate potential delays. For hospitals with smaller delivery services and without such in-house availability, education of support persons and hospital administrators about the necessity for ready availability should decrease the potential for ill will resulting from the mobilization calls not resulting in abdominal delivery. The ability to perform cesarean delivery rapidly for fetal distress ranks among the most important surgical emergencies.

Nothing in this section is intended to suggest that any damage seen in any child *must* have had its antecedent in the intrapartum period. Genetic defects, maternal illness or exposure to toxic agents, episodes of cord occlusion, fetal hypoxia from maternal tobacco abuse or supine positioning, and other factors could have occurred and resulted in fetal injury before the application of a fetal monitor in early labor. Moreover, particularly in the very premature infant, neonatal morbidity, such as hyaline membrane disease with neonatal asphyxia, can occur in a child delivered atraumatically and with initially normal acid-base status. The need for documenting such normal fetal acid-base status by obtaining cord blood samples and measuring pH and blood gas values is evident. This can be accomplished easily at the time of either vaginal or abdominal delivery. Two pairs of umbilical cord or Kelly clamps are applied quickly to the cord before the onset of neonatal breathing. The pair closer to the placenta should be placed first to allow the fetal arterial pressure to keep the umbilical arteries distended while the second pair is being applied. After cutting between each pair, a 7 to 8 cm cord segment is handed to the nurse, who then draws 0.5 to 0.8 ml of blood anaerobically into a previously heparinized 1 ml tuberculin syringe. The syringe is then capped, placed on ice, and transported at once to the laboratory. The cord arterial gas values are frequently normal even when the Apgar scores are low, indicating that a low Apgar score is not synonymous with perinatal asphyxia.

John F. Huddleston
Roger K. Freeman

BIBLIOGRAPHY

Borell, U., and others: Effect of uterine contractions on the human uteroplacental blood circulation, Am. J. Obstet. Gynecol. **89**:881, 1964.

Caldeyro-Barcia, R.: The influence of maternal bearing-down efforts during second stage on fetal well-being, Birth Fam. J. **6**:17, 1979.

Carson, B.S., and others: Combined obstetric and pediatric approach to prevent meconium aspiration syndrome, Am. J. Obstet. Gynecol. **126**:712, 1976.

Clark, S.L., Gimovsky, M.L., and Miller, F.C.: The scalp stimulation test: a clinical alternative to fetal scalp blood sampling, Am. J. Obstet. Gynecol. **148**:274, 1984.

Cohen, W.R., Schifrin, B.S., and Doctor, G.: Elevation of the fetal presenting part: a method of intrauterine resuscitation, Am. J. Obstet. Gynecol. **123**:646, 1975.

Fabian, M., Forsling, M.L., and Jones, J.J.: The clearance and antidiuretic potency of neurohypophyseal hormones in man, and their plasma binding and stability, J. Physiol. **204**:653, 1969.

Fields, L.M., Entman, S.S., and Boehm, F.H.: Correlation of the one-minute Apgar score and the pH value of umbilical arterial blood, South. Med. J. **76**:1477, 1983.

Goldenberg, R.L., Huddleston, J.F., and Nelson, K.G.: Apgar scores and umbilical arterial pH in preterm newborns, Am. J. Obstet. Gynecol. **149**:651, 1984.

Hon, E.H., Bradfield, A.H., and Hess, O.W.: The electronic evaluation of the fetal heart rate. V. The vagal factor in fetal bradycardia, Am. J. Obstet. Gynecol. **82**:291, 1961.

Hon, E.H., and Quilligan, E.J.: Classification of fetal heart rate. II. A revised working classification, Conn. Med. **31**:779, 1967.

Huddleston, J.F.: Intrapartum fetal distress. In Fadel, H.E., editor: Diagnosis and management of obstetric emergencies, Menlo Park, Calif., 1982, Addison-Wesley Publishing Co.

Huddleston, J.F.: Intrapartum fetal distress. In Quilligan E.J., editor: Current therapy in obstetrics and gynecology, vol. 2, Philadelphia, 1983, W.B. Saunders Co.

Huddleston, J.F., Perlis, H.W., and Harris, B.A., Jr.: The case for electronic fetal monitoring, J. Reprod. Med. **25**:47, 1980.

Knox, G.E., Huddleston, J.F., and Flowers, C.E., Jr.: Management of prolonged pregnancy: results of a prospective randomized trial, Am. J. Obstet. Gynecol. **134**:376, 1979.

Lipshitz, J.: The use of a β_2-sympathomimetic drug as a temporizing measure in the treatment of acute fetal distress, Am. J. Obstet. Gynecol. **129**:31, 1977.

Low, J.A., Boston, R.W., and Cervenko, F.W.: Effect of low maternal carbon dioxide tension on placenta gas exchange, Am. J. Obstet. Gynecol. **160**:1032, 1970.

Martin, C.G., deHann, J., and van der Wildt, B.: Mechanisms of late decelerations in the fetal heart rate: a study with autonomic blocking agents in fetal lambs, Eur. J. Obstet. Gynecol. Reprod. Biol. **9**:361, 1979.

Meschia, G.: How oxygen is transferred across the placenta, Contemp. Ob/Gyn **14**(4):151, 1979.

Miller, F.C., Sachs, D.A., and Yeh, S.Y.: Significance of meconium during labor, Am. J. Obstet. Gynecol. **122**:578, 1975.

Miller, F.C., and others: Hyperventilation during labor, Am. J. Obstet. Gynecol. **120**:489, 1974.

Myers, R.E., Mueller-Heubach, E., and Adamsons, K.: Predictability of the state of fetal oxygenation from the quantitative analysis of the components of late deceleration, Am. J. Obstet. Gynecol. **115**:1083, 1973.

Parer, J.T.: Normal and impaired placental exchange, Contemp. Ob/Gyn **7**(2):117, 1976.

Paul, R.H., and others: Clinical fetal monitoring. VII. The evaluation and significance of intrapartum FHR variability, Am. J. Obstet. Gynecol. **123**:206, 1975.

Paul, W.M., Quilligan, E.J., and MacLachlan, T.: Cardiovascular phenomena associated with fetal head compression, Am. J. Obstet. Gynecol. **90**:824, 1964.

Pose, S.V., Escarcena, L., and Althabe, O.: The influence of uterine contractions on the partial pressure of oxygen of the human fetus, In Effects of labour on the foetus and newborn, Oxford, 1967, Pergamon Press, Inc.

Pose, S.V., and others: Test of fetal tolerance of induced uterine contractions for the diagnosis of chronic fetal distress. In Perinatal factors affecting human development, Washington, D.C., 1969, Pan American Health Organization.

Ramsey, E.M.: Uteroplacental circulation during labor, Clin. Obstet. Gynecol. **11**:78, 1968.

Rudolph, A.M.: How the fetal circulation responds to stress, Contemp. Ob/Gyn **21**(6):145, 1983.

Scott, D.B., and Kerr, M.G.: Inferior vena caval pressure in late pregnancy, J. Obstet. Gynaecol. Br. Commonw. **70**:1044, 1963.

Selzer, M.E., Myers, R.E., and Holstein, S.B.: Prolonged partial asphyxia: effects on fetal brain water and electrolytes, Neurology **22**:732, 1972.

PART TWO

Antepartum fetal surveillance

Even though steady and respectable improvement has occurred in perinatal outcome during recent years, a small percentage of pregnancies continues to terminate in either fetal mortality or serious morbidity. Many of these pregnancies end in antepartum stillbirth or are associated with severe distress, as evidenced by initial monitoring in early labor. Although not all potentially disastrous outcomes can be predicted, most pregnancies with such potential can be identified through screening methods, such as the history, the physical examination, and laboratory tests, and thus can be labeled as high risk.

THE CONCEPT OF HIGH-RISK PREGNANCY

See also Chapter 1.

Identification of pregnancies at risk

Over the past two decades several surveillance methods, generally based on techniques of intrapartum surveillance discussed in part one of this chapter, have been developed and used in managing high-risk pregnancies. Because of factors justifying the high-risk label, such pregnancies would be expected, without effective antepartum surveillance methods and selective intervention, to produce most cases of perinatal morbidity and mortality.

A pregnancy can be designated as high risk because of various undesirable outcomes. For instance, the woman who has lost several babies because of recurrent preterm labor in the midtrimester presents a management problem different from the diabetic woman who has had several stillbirths near term. Another pregnancy in the woman with diabetes would be at risk for the inadequate provision of nutrients and of oxygen, that is, uteroplacental insufficiency.

Significance of uteroplacental insufficiency

Pregnancies considered at risk for uteroplacental insufficiency carry a serious threat for fetal growth retardation, intrauterine fetal demise, intrapartum fetal distress, and various types of neonatal morbidity. Conditions such as insulin-dependent diabetes and hypertensive disorders can interfere with uterine blood flow, intervillous space perfusion, and placental exchange, thereby possibly interfering with fetal nutrition and oxygenation. The potential for perinatal morbidity or mortality thus increases. Of the general types of surveillance methods that have been introduced, those using electronic monitoring of the fetal heart rate (FHR) have become the most widely used and accepted for fetal assessment in the management of such pregnancies. Through assessment of the fetus at risk through antepartum FHR and at times biochemical and sonographic monitoring, those pregnancies with normal uteroplacental exchange, as evidenced by repetitively reassuring tests, can confidently be managed with a "hands-off" policy while awaiting fetal maturity and perhaps cervical changes that allow easy induction of labor. Of this large majority with normal tests, most may be carefully followed to term and undergo spontaneous labor and delivery. For those few fetuses with abnormal tests suggesting deteriorating uteroplacental function, corrective efforts can be instituted either to improve uterine blood flow or to remove these infants from their unfavorable environments.

INDICATIONS FOR TESTING

As the boxed material shows, maternal conditions placing a pregnancy at risk for uteroplacental insufficiency include chronic and pregnancy-induced hypertension, chronic renal disease, insulin-dependent diabetes mellitus, cyanotic congenital heart disease, isoimmunization, sickle cell diseases, maternal cigarette abuse, and history of a previous pregnancy terminating in unexplained stillbirth. Evolving obstetric problems that place a pregnancy at such risk include fetal growth retardation, postdatism (42 or more gestational weeks), hydramnios, and oligohydramnios. Fetal surveillance should also be considered when there are maternal sensations of decreased fetal movement and in cases of multiple gestation near term.

Primary emphasis in this section is given to electronic testing because it is used more extensively today. For the sake of completeness, biochemical testing methods still being used are also outlined.

Suggested indications for antepartum fetal assessment

- Chronic hypertension
- Pregnancy-induced hypertension
- Chronic renal disease
- Insulin-dependent diabetes mellitus
- Cyanotic congenital heart disease
- Rh or other isoimmunization
- Homozygous hemoglobinopathies
- Maternal abuse of cigarettes, alcohol, or drugs
- Previous unexplained stillbirth
- Fetal growth retardation
- Postdatism
- Hydramnios, oligohydramnios
- Decreased fetal movement
- Multiple gestation
- Premature rupture of membranes
- Third-trimester bleeding
- Sickle cell anemia
- Maternal collagen vascular diseases

PHYSIOLOGIC PRINCIPLES FOR ELECTRONIC TESTING METHODS

Any fetus considered to be at risk for uteroplacental insufficiency is a candidate, as early as 26 to 28 weeks' gestation, for electronic fetal evaluation. The time chosen to begin testing depends on both the circumstances surrounding each pregnancy and the neonatal survival data for tiny babies at a particular hospital or referral center. Typically, for at-risk pregnancies that are progressing well by clinical criteria, testing is begun at about 32 to 34 weeks. The lower gestational age limit to begin testing can be considered as that age when, after careful consultation with the patient and her husband, a cesarean delivery would be considered for fetal indications. In most tertiary referral centers, this lower limit currently is about 26 weeks.

Two types of electronic FHR evaluations have achieved widespread acceptance for antepartum surveillance. The first one introduced was the contraction stress test (CST), which relies on the FHR response to uterine contractions for its interpretation. Since even normal uterine contractions will exert some hypoxic stresses to the fetus through impairment of uterine blood flow, uteroplacental function can be assessed through performance of the CST. If such function and thus fetal oxygenation become depressed, these temporary interruptions of uterine blood flow will disturb fetal oxygenation sufficiently to cause repetitive late decelerations. A negative CST (*no* late decelerations with a contraction frequency of three in 10 minutes) has been found highly predictive of intrauterine survival for 7 subsequent days

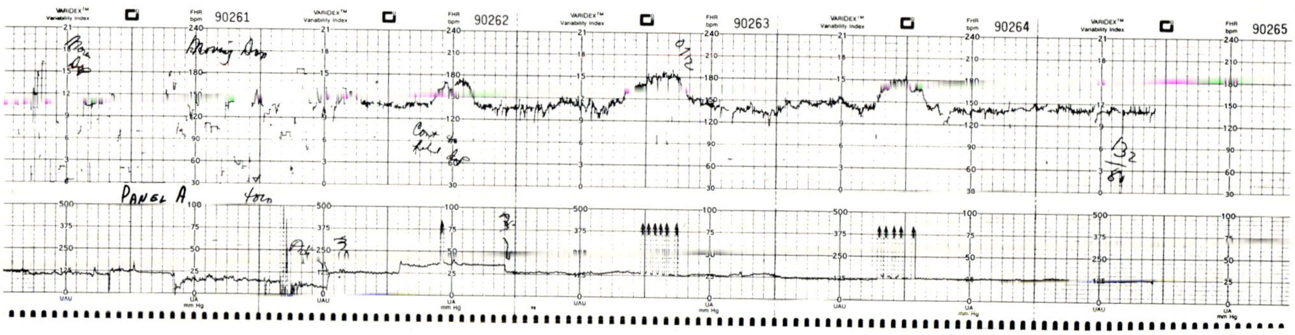

Fig. 8-12. Accelerations occurring with fetal movement, which is noted by arrows on contraction channel. (From Freeman, R., and Garite, T.: Fetal heart rate monitoring, Baltimore. Copyright 1981, The Williams & Wilkins Company. Reproduced by permission.)

(see Fig. 8-2). Gabbe and associates found CST results to be reliable even in the early third trimester.

The second of these electronic tests of FHR is the nonstress test (NST), which relies for its interpretation on FHR reactivity, or accelerations of the heart rate found in response to fetal movements (Fig. 8-12). As with the negative CST, a reactive NST is also highly predictive of intrauterine survival for 7 days subsequent to the test. However, finding a nonreactive pattern may imply that the fetus is already or is becoming acidotic, a result of prolonged suboptimal oxygenation. In the evolution of FHR changes caused by hypoxia, Murata and co-workers demonstrated in the rhesus monkey fetus that the appearance of late decelerations in response to contractions (positive CST) precedes loss of heart rate reactivity (nonreactive NST). However, since a nonreactive pattern frequently exists for other usually benign reasons, a follow-up CST is usually performed to explain a nonreactive pattern. A positive CST suggests that the nonreactive pattern results from protracted fetal hypoxia; a negative CST suggests that the nonreactivity is explained by some other factor, such as fetal sleep or maternal ingestion of narcotic or sedative drugs.

Of these electronic tests used for fetal surveillance, the NST has become the primary test in many institutions because it is simpler, requires less time, and is less costly than the CST. In our opinion, however, definite indications for the CST remain. Not only is this test used to define fetal status when a nonreactive NST is found, but some institutions rely on the CST for primary testing of either all high-risk pregnancies or those at highest risk, such as those complicated by severe chronic hypertension, insulin dependent diabetes, fetal growth retardation substantiated by ultrasound, and oligohydramnios. In addition, data now available from the CST/NST Collaborative Study suggest that the CST may be a better predictor of fetal reserve, since its use for primary fetal surveillance seems to be associated with slightly but statistically significantly fewer stillbirths when compared with primary use of the NST. Also, recent methods employing maternal nipple stimulation to produce uterine contractions may encourage more widespread use of the CST, since this test now compares favorably with the NST with regard to simplicity, time, cost, and acceptability among patients.

CONTRACTION STRESS TEST

Basic principles

For the CST the woman is placed comfortably in the left lateral or semi-Fowler's position in an attempt to prevent aortic and vena caval compression. Such compression can reduce uterine blood flow and result in temporary fetal hypoxemia and an abnormal test, independent of the reason for which the pregnancy is being tested. External fetal monitoring devices are then applied. Blood pressure is measured initially and at 10- to 15-minute intervals for the duration of the test. Any maternal hypotension is noted and corrected by positional change. Baseline FHR and spontaneous uterine contractions are assessed for 15 to 20 minutes after application of the external FHR transducer and the tocotransducer. Care must be taken in positioning and tightly securing the tocotransducer to ensure that uterine activity and fetal movements will be reliably recorded. After the baseline recording has been obtained, uterine activity (if any) is assessed as to adequacy. If spontaneous activity is inadequate, arbitrarily defined as less than three palpable 40- to 60-second contractions in 10 minutes, either oxytocin delivery is begun with an intravenous infusion pump or contractions are initiated by intermittent nipple stimulation.

A few relative contraindications should be considered before administering the CST. These contraindications include placenta previa, previous transmyometrial myomectomy, previous *vertical* cesarean delivery, history of preterm labor, incompetent cervix, multiple gestation, hydramnios, and premature rupture of the membranes.

Oxytocin administration by intravenous infusion pump

If spontaneous uterine activity is deemed inadequate during the 15- to 20-minute baseline period, a small intravenous infusion is begun, generally with either normal saline or Ringer's lactate solution. A controlled-rate infusion pump is then used to regulate the oxytocin infusion, which is administered "piggyback" into the intravenous line. Oxytocin, diluted in normal saline, is begun initially at a rate of 0.5 to 1.0 mU/minute and then increased by 1.0 mU/minute approximately every 20 to 30 minutes until an adequate contraction frequency is achieved. The typical rate of oxytocin delivery required to elicit adequate uterine activity is 2 to 4 mU/minute; rarely will a woman require more than 8 mU/minute. The average duration of a CST employing this method of oxytocin delivery has been reported to be 80 to 90 minutes.

Contractions evoked by intermittent nipple stimulation

As a result of impulses transmitted via thoracic sensory nerve roots, nipple stimulation in the lactating woman causes the posterior pituitary to release oxytocin. Nipple stimulation in the pregnant woman is an alternative to intravenous oxytocin delivery for achieving uterine contractions for the CST. However, the mechanism by which nipple stimulation causes contractions is uncertain and may not be a result of oxytocin release. Women wearing light clothing are instructed to rub gently *one* nipple through their clothes and with the palmar surfaces of their fingertips for 2 minutes, then to cease stimulation for 5 minutes. If a woman is wearing several layers of clothing, she is instructed to stimulate one nipple through her brassiere. Stimulation is stopped immediately whenever a contraction commences during the 2 minutes of stimulation, since uterine hyperstimulation may occasionally occur with prolonged stimulation. A gravida may alternate nipples during stimulation to decrease the chance of causing nipple tenderness. A 7-minute cycle is composed of the 2 minutes of nipple stimulation plus 5 minutes to rest. On the average only one or two nipple stimulation cycles are required to elicit adequate uterine activity; the average length of a CST using this technique is about 40 minutes, including the initial 15 to 20 minutes of observation. Techniques of continuous nipple stimulation have been reported as well.

Interpretation

Negative

CST results are interpreted in the classic manner. The test is negative only when there are *no* late decelerations present on the tracing *and* uterine contractions have been adequate to stress the fetus sufficiently: three 40- to 60-second palpable contractions in 10 minutes *or* a prolonged contraction lasting more than 90 seconds. Usually but not invariably, FHR reactivity is found (see Fig. 8-2). With a negative CST, testing is repeated every 7 days until delivery, unless severe clinical decompensation occurs (e.g., diabetic ketoacidosis or exacerbation of hypertensive disease). However, some authorities are advocating testing patients with insulin-dependent diabetes, gestational diabetes with a previous stillborn, postdate pregnancy, or intrauterine growth retardation (IUGR) twice a week. With this strict interpretation for the negative test, some authorities have noted a false-negative CST (fetal death occurring within 7 days of a negative test) rate of only 1 to 2 in 1,000 cases. Thus it is not considered necessary to shorten the interval between tests. About 80% to 90% of tests will be negative.

Positive

In the absence of uterine hyperstimulation, the presence of late decelerations with 50% or more of the contractions during a period of adequate uterine activity constitutes a positive CST. However, it is unnecessary and even undesirable to continue efforts to achieve three contractions in 10 minutes if recurrent late decelerations are evident with contractions occurring less frequently. Reactivity may or may not be concurrently present (Fig. 8-13).

From 2% to 5% of CSTs have been classified as positive. The fetus with a positive test is probably suboptimally oxygenated, at least at the time of testing. Thus management of the positive-CST fetus generally will include prompt intervention. The fetus at term or postterm is most frequently delivered. The route of delivery will depend on the presence of reactivity and other obstetric factors, such as the condition of the cervix and fetal lie. If such conditions are favorable and the fetus is treated prophylactically for fetal distress (i.e., mother placed in the left lateral position, hydrated intravenously, and given oxygen by mask), about half of these fetuses can safely tolerate the induction of labor without developing fetal distress. However, if the positive CST is also nonreactive, the fetal condition is generally such that labor will not be tolerated; cesarean delivery is generally but not always employed in a preemptive manner for these few patients. If fetal maturity is in doubt and if FHR reactivity, defined as two accelerations in 20 minutes increasing 15 beats above the baseline and lasting 15 seconds, is present on the positive CST tracing, an amniocentesis may be done for studies of pulmonary maturity. If such studies suggest that the fetus is quite immature and if the frequently assessed FHR reactivity remains reassuring, such a woman temporarily may be managed by bed rest in the left lateral position. Under such conditions some physicians consider the use of glucocorticoids in an attempt to hasten fetal pulmonary maturity. The management of such an immature fetus in-

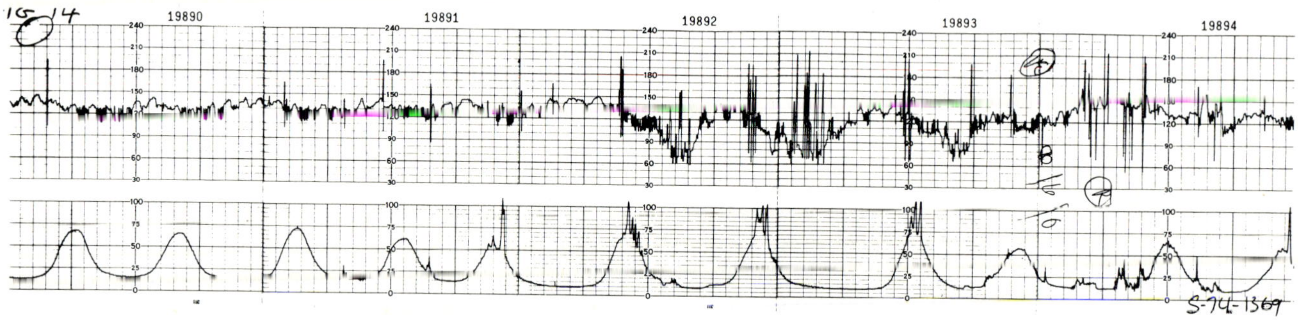

Fig. 8-13. Late decelerations with good variability. (From Freeman, R., and Garite, T.: Fetal heart rate monitoring, Baltimore. Copyright 1981, The Williams & Wilkins Company. Reproduced by permission.)

cludes daily assessments for FHR reactivity and/or daily biophysical profile assessments (see following discussion). If these tests become nonreassuring, however, the preterm fetus generally is transferred from its hostile intrauterine environment to a neonatal intensive care unit.

Equivocal

About 15% to 20% of CSTs will be neither negative nor positive. These tests are designated as equivocal and impart little useful information concerning well-being of the fetus. They should be repeated within 24 hours in an attempt to achieve a definitive test result. Equivocal tests may be further categorized as either suspicious, hyperstimulatory, or unsatisfactory.

A CST is designated as *suspicious* when late decelerations only intermittently are present with an adequate but not excessive contraction frequency (e.g., present with fewer than half of the contractions). Usually FHR reactivity is present. Since only about one fifth of these suspicious tests will become positive on repeat testing, and since a delay of 24 hours to repeat a suspicious test almost never will result in fetal loss, such repeat testing is generally employed. Decisions to intervene are typically not made on the basis of equivocal tests alone.

In the presence of excessive uterine activity (contractions occurring more often than every 2 minutes or lasting more than 90 seconds) with associated late deceleration(s), a CST is interpreted as *hyperstimulatory*. As uterine sensitivity to oxytocin varies, extreme care must be taken when introducing intravenous oxytocin or when beginning the intermittent nipple stimulation. However, excessive uterine activity may occur even in the gravida who is contracting spontaneously.

Rarely the quality of a tracing will be such that an interpretation of the CST cannot be made confidently; such tests are termed *unsatisfactory*. Factors that may increase the chance for an unsatisfactory CST result include extreme obesity, hydramnios, and a very active fetus. The effect of these factors can be reduced if the nurse doing the testing remains with the patient and monitors the tracing. At times actually holding the FHR transducer in a certain position may be necessary. Very rarely an adequate contraction frequency may not be obtainable, and such a CST is also classified as unsatisfactory. This latter type seems limited to those tests using exogenous oxytocin; our experience to date with the CST by intermittent nipple stimulation is that adequate uterine activity can be achieved in virtually all cases. Most of these gravidas will readily achieve an adequate frequency of contractions on follow-up testing within 24 hours.

NONSTRESS TEST
Basic principles

The NST is conducted in much the same manner as the CST, except that there is no need for a means to elicit uterine contractions. The woman is placed in the left lateral or semi-Fowler's position, and the external fetal monitoring transducers are applied. Blood pressure is recorded initially and at 10- to 15-minute intervals during testing, and any maternal hypotension is noted and corrected, generally by maternal positional change. Observations are made of the baseline FHR, of any spontaneous contractions, and of any decelerations (most often the variable type) evident on the monitor strip. At times the woman undergoing an NST will be spontaneously contracting at a frequency sufficient to give a "bonus": the added reassurance of a negative CST. Fetal movements are noted on the monitor strip. Fetal movements usually are appreciated as a spike on the uterine activity channel and are generally audible over the monitor's speaker. Since some gravidas, even in late pregnancy, are unaware of any but the strongest fetal movements, it is important that both patient and nurse seek to determine fetal activity.

Sleeping fetus

Since sleep/rest cycles probably occur at about 30- to 40-minute intervals, the sleeping fetus may be encoun-

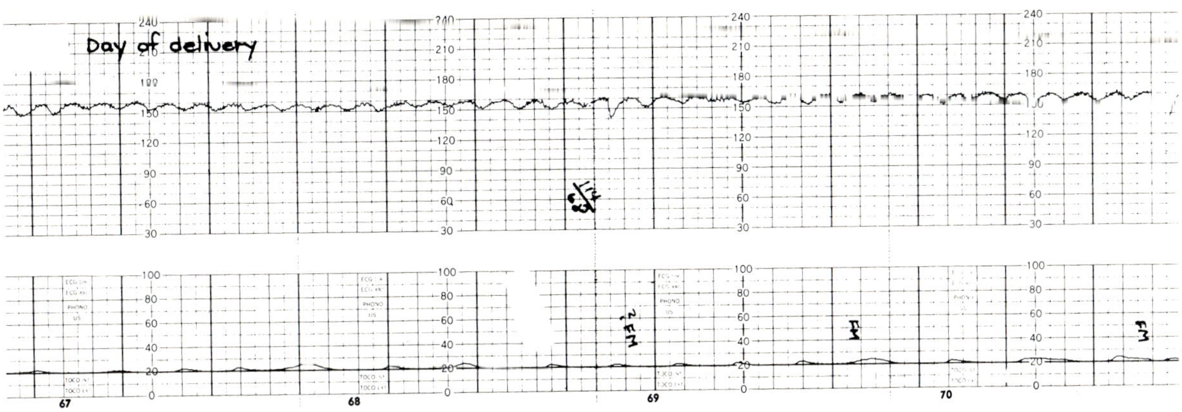

Fig. 8-14. Sinusoidal FHR pattern in patient with fetal hydrops from Rh sensitization. (From Freeman, R., and Garite, T.: Fetal heart rate monitoring, Baltimore. Copyright 1981, The Williams & Wilkins Company. Reproduced by permission.)

tered during an NST. Usually, gentle manipulation by the mother or the nurse or an external stimulus such as loud noise will awaken the healthy but sleeping fetus and elicit fetal movements with FHR reactivity. Such fetal stimulation will generally suffice to differentiate a sleeping fetus from a fetus that is hypoactive because of deterioration due to reduced uteroplacental exchange.

Interpretation

General considerations

The pattern of autonomic influences on the FHR, and thus by deduction fetal metabolic health, can be evaluated through FHR patterns of beat-to-beat variability and accelerations associated with fetal movements (reactivity). With chronic suboptimal oxygenation, both a reduction of FHR reactivity *and* a flattening of normal beat-to-beat variability will be exhibited. The latter assessment is generally achievable only during the intrapartum period, when the FHR is derived from a scalp electrode. Interpretation of the antepartum NST is based on the grosser changes of FHR reactivity, which are of sufficient magnitude and duration so as not to be confused with the smaller FHR changes of variability. FHR reactivity implies that, at the time of testing, the fetus is metabolically normal from an acid-base perspective.

Reactive

With the reactive NST there are accelerations of the FHR, in response to fetal movements, of at least 15 beats per minute and lasting at least 15 seconds (Fig. 8-12). Numerous criteria have been published concerning the number of FHR accelerations within a certain time required to justify a designation of reactive. We consider that two accelerations, meeting the criteria just listed, within 20 minutes qualify a test as reactive. Less stringent criteria for amplitude and duration may suffice for the very preterm fetus (i.e., less than 30 weeks). A reactive NST, without variable decelerations, using whatever criteria one elects, is a good predictor of fetal well-being for 1 week, unless severe clinical decompensation occurs. As with the CST, some workers are advocating testing twice a week for pregnancies involving insulin-dependent diabetes, gestational diabetes, a previous stillborn, postdatism, or IUGR. However, if variable decelerations are present (see Fig. 8-7), one should suspect oligohydramnios, and further evaluation, generally ultrasound and a CST, should be strongly considered.

Nonreactive

If the criteria for reactivity are not present, the NST is termed nonreactive. It must be ascertained, however, whether fetal sleep or a sedative drug, including ones that may have been obtained illicitly, may be responsible for the nonreactivity. In such cases prolonging the NST for an additional 20 minutes may reveal a reactive test. Since a nonreactive NST alone provides little or no useful information as to fetal well-being, a CST should then be performed. At the time of the CST, produced either by intravenous oxytocin or through intermittent nipple stimulation, the fetus may begin to stir and the test may become reactive. In these cases it is not necessary to continue with the CST unless there is some other clinical indication for this test.

Keegan and co-workers found that if the nonreactive NST is repeated later in the same day, 78% of those tests become reactive. Therefore some hospitals are now repeating the NST a few hours after an initial nonreactive test and before proceeding to the CST.

Sinusoidal

Sinusoidal patterns (Fig. 8-14) are seen as baseline oscillations at a frequency of two to five per minute, varying from 5 to 15 beats per minute, with an *absence* of FHR reactivity. Thus the sinusoidal pattern is a variant of the nonreactive test, and the presence of good reactivity either before or after the sinusoidal-like pattern (pseudosinusoidal) should preclude serious consideration of its being truly sinusoidal. The truly sinusoidal pattern is found usually with Rh-sensitized fetuses or with fetuses compromised by severe fetomaternal bleeding. This pattern is rare and ominous. The pseudosinusoidal pattern has been reported to follow maternal opiate administration.

PATIENT CONSIDERATIONS FOR NONSTRESS AND CONTRACTION STRESS TESTS

Before initiating NST/CST testing, the procedure is fully explained to the patient by a member of the obstetric team. In some hospitals a consent form, which covers either a single test or the series of tests, is obtained before testing. A thorough explanation of the reasons for and the methods of testing will help prevent most anxieties typical in these patients. Testing on a weekly basis, or more often if required, will be necessary for most women for the duration of the pregnancy. These rare exceptions for which testing is not repeated include gravidas who no longer have an indication for testing, such as those who were complaining on initial testing of now-resolved decreased fetal movement or those who were considered to have fetal growth retardation but for whom sonographic assessment has shown no evidence of this problem. Patients are encouraged to eat before testing, because this may promote greater fetal activity. The anticipated time requirement for testing should be explained, and for the patient's convenience testing should be scheduled on the same day as her medical appointment whenever possible. Patients may resume their previous level of activity immediately following testing.

Testing of multiple gestations can be accomplished by sequentially testing each fetus; one must be certain that different FHR baselines are distinguishable. Alternatively, two recordings can be performed at the same time, although with some instrumentation the two ultrasound signals may interfere with each other.

BIOPHYSICAL PROFILE

Methods

The biophysical profile (BPP) was developed by Manning and associates as another test to help discriminate between fetuses that are well and those whose physiologic status is deteriorating.

The BPP is derived from five observations. The first assessment is the NST. The other four are determined by ultrasonography: (1) the presence of fetal body movements (three movements within 30 minutes); (2) the presence of fetal chest wall (breathing) movements (30 seconds of continual breathing within 30 minutes); (3) the observation of good fetal tone (one extension/flexion cycle of a fetal limb with rapid return to the flexed posture within 30 minutes); and (4) the presence of a normal amount of amniotic fluid (a "pocket" of fluid greater than 1 cm in two perpendicular planes).

Interpretation

Each observation receives 2 points if present and 0 points if absent (or nonreactive); the highest score is 10, the worst 0. Scores of 8 to 10 are considered reassuring, and testing can be repeated in a week unless fetal or maternal circumstances suggest earlier retesting. A score of 4 to 6 is considered equivocal and requires that testing be repeated within 24 hours. Scores of 0 to 2 are abnormal and indicate immediate evaluation or delivery. Recently Manning and others, after reviewing a large series of BPPs, suggested that the NST be omitted and that the ultrasound observations, with a highest score of 8, be used. The ultrasound component of the BPP should be accomplishable within 30 minutes.

A theoretic concern with the BPP is that it measures only steady-state conditions and therefore might not be as predictive of uteroplacental reserve as a test requiring a fetal stress, such as the CST. A study comparing the relative efficacies of the BPP and the CST has not been reported.

The BPP may also be useful in following the very preterm fetus with a positive CST. In this case frequent, probably daily, reassuring BPPs might justify procrastination. The BPP also might lead to the discovery of unsuspected anomalies.

BIOCHEMICAL FETAL EVALUATION

General considerations

Numerous biochemical assays have been proposed for assessing fetoplacental function. Some obstetricians still use two: estriol and human placental lactogen (HPL), renamed human chorionic somatomammotropin. Currently the most common situation for use of these tests is when the fetal monitoring test results are nonreassuring and the pregnancy is preterm. Even for those physicians regularly ordering estriol or HPL assays, electronic fetal monitoring tests are generally performed as well. The serum or plasma concentrations of both hormones increase as pregnancy advances, and sharp or progressive decreases in concentration may indicate fetal jeopardy. Serial sampling is therefore essential for determining sequential changes and detecting fetal deterioration. Estriol values correlate with fetal weight in late pregnancy, and increasing HPL values parallel increasing placental mass.

Estriol

Production of the C_{18} steroid estriol by the placenta depends on proper functioning of the fetal adrenal gland

and liver, and the amount produced is influenced by many factors. Length of gestation, multiple gestation, fetal and placental size, certain drugs (particularly glucocorticoids), maternal activity, maternal renal function, and glycosuria may affect urinary or serum estriol levels and must be considered when interpreting values. In addition, some maternal diseases may affect test results. Low values from assays in a diabetic gravida may be more serious than low values in a hypertensive patient. A single assay is essentially valueless in assessing fetal condition unless the value is so low that imminent fetal demise is suspected. Either 24-hour urinary or plasma radioimmunoassays should be done two or three times weekly—daily in diabetic patients—so that any impending fetal disaster may be predicted and delivery performed if indicated. Any sharp (50% to 60% less than preceding measurements) or progressive decrease in serial values suggests fetal jeopardy. The normal range of daily 24-hour urinary estriol excretion at term is from 10 to 30 mg, and the normal range for plasma estriol concentration is 9 to 22 μgm/dl. Results of 24-hour urinary estriol excretion are generally available in about 12 hours, but measurement of plasma estriol levels may be accomplished within 1 to 2 hours.

Human placental lactogen

HPL is a single-chain peptide hormone released by the cytotrophoblast into the maternal circulation, where it can be detected as early as 20 days after implantation. Production of this peptide slowly increases until about 37 weeks' gestation, after which it remains the same or decreases slightly. By 42 weeks' gestation an impressive decrease is normally seen. As a result of associated increases in placental mass, higher HPL values are seen in multiple gestation, erythroblastosis, and poorly controlled diabetes. With these conditions prediction of fetal well-being by HPL seems to be especially inaccurate. Conversely, lower values have been reported in pregnancies complicated both by IUGR and maternal hypertension. Radioimmunoassays for HPL generally are performed weekly, and the normal range in maternal serum near term is 5.4 to 7.0 μgm/ml. Values lower than 4.0 μgm/ml may represent an increased risk for fetal compromise after 30 weeks' gestation, and consistently low values may be as serious as decreasing values. It has been suggested that serial HPL radioimmunoassays be done on specific high-risk pregnancies as an adjunct to other fetal surveillance methods.

Indications for estriol and HPL radioimmunoassays

Some fetuses at risk for uteroplacental insufficiency may be considered candidates for these estriol or HPL radioimmunoassays. Both assays have been claimed to help identify possible postmaturity in postdate pregnancies and to have some benefit in the management of hypertensive disorders of pregnancy. However, many doubt the value of HPL in predicting postmaturity. Estriol assays may be of value for fetal surveillance when maternal diabetes is present; HPL assays, however, have been reported to be of limited value in the management of this disorder. The diagnosis of IUGR may be suspected from HPL determinations, but probably not as readily from plasma assays for estriol. In addition, neither assay is considered to be of value in the management of Rh isoimmunization. Although these biochemical surveillance methods are still used in some obstetric centers, there has been a progressive decrease in their clinical use over the last several years.

SUMMARY

Approximately 15% of pregnancies seen in a high-risk obstetric service will have indications placing them at risk for uteroplacental insufficiency, and antepartum fetal surveillance methods play an important role in the obstetric management of these women. Although electronic evaluations of the FHR are more often used, some clinicians still rely on estriol and HPL radioimmunoassays in managing these pregnancies. Use of the BPP also is gaining acceptance.

The CST and NST have achieved widespread acceptance for antepartum fetal surveillance. These tests of the FHR can identify with reasonable accuracy in these high-risk pregnancies those fetuses (with negative CSTs and/or reactive NSTs) tolerating their intrauterine environments acceptably. These normal tests usually need be repeated only weekly. Such reassuring tests are comforting to both patient and clinician, and test results are available immediately. Those few fetuses whose test results are abnormal and who are in possible jeopardy can be identified immediately so that corrective measures can be undertaken. Moreover, a policy of nonintervention can be followed safely in approximately 95% of these high-risk pregnancies undergoing FHR testing, since only a small percentage—those with positive CSTs—will be at serious risk for impending disaster.

John F. Huddleston
Roger K. Freeman

BIBLIOGRAPHY

Aubry, R.A., and Pennington, J.C.: Identification and evaluation of high-risk pregnancy: the perinatal concept, Clin. Obstet. Gynecol. **16**:3, 1973.

Berkowitz, R.L., and Hobbins, J.C.: A reevaluation of the value of hCS determination in the management of prolonged pregnancy, Obstet. Gynecol. **49**:156, 1977.

Bishop, E.H.: Pelvic scoring for elective induction, Obstet. Gynecol. **24**:266, 1964.

Braly, P.S., and Freeman, R.K.: The significance of fetal heart rate reactivity with a positive oxytocin challenge test, Obstet. Gynecol. **50**:689, 1977.

Braly, P.S., and others: Incidence of premature delivery following the oxytocin challenge test, Am. J. Obstet. Gynecol. **141**:5, 1981.

Bruce, S.L., Petrie, R.H., and Yeh, S.Y.: The suspicious contraction stress test, Obstet. Gynecol. **51**:415, 1978.

Cobo, E.: Neuroendocrine control of milk injection in women. In Josimovich, J.F., Reynolds, M., and Cobo, E., editors: Lactogenic hormones, fetal nutrition, and lactation, New York, 1974, John Wiley & Sons, Inc.

Evertson, L.R., and others: Antepartum fetal heart rate testing. I. Evolution of the nonstress test, Am. J. Obstet. Gynecol. **133**:29, 1979.

Freeman, R.K.: The use of oxytocin challenge test for antepartum clinical evaluation of uteroplacental respiratory function, Am. J. Obstet. Gynecol. **121**:481, 1975.

Freeman, R.K.: Contraction stress testing for primary fetal surveillance in patients at high risk for uteroplacental insufficiency, Clin. Perinatol. **9**:265, 1982.

Freeman, R.K., Anderson, G., and Dorchester, W.: A prospective multi-institutional study of antepartum fetal heart rate monitoring. I. Risk of perinatal mortality and morbidity according to antepartum fetal heart rate test results, Am. J. Obstet. Gynecol. **143**:771, 1982.

Freeman, R.K., Anderson, G., and Dorchester, W.: A prospective multi-institutional study of antepartum fetal heart rate monitoring. II. Contraction stress test versus nonstress test for primary surveillance, Am. J. Obstet. Gynecol. **143**:778, 1982.

Freeman, R.K., and others: An evaluation of the significance of a positive oxytocin challenge test, Obstet. Gynecol. **47**:8, 1976.

Freeman, R.K., and others: Ensuring optimum outcome for postdate pregnancy, Contemp. Ob/Gyn **22**(6):187, 1983.

Gabbe, S.G., Freeman, R.K., and Goebelsmann, U.: Evaluation of the contraction stress test before 33 weeks' gestation, Obstet. Gynecol. **52**:649, 1978.

Goebelsmann, U., and others: Estriol in pregnancy. II. Daily urinary estriol assays in the management of the pregnant diabetic woman, Am. J. Obstet. Gynecol. **115**:795, 1973.

Goodwin, J.W., Dunne, J.T., and Thomas, B.W.: Antepartum identification of the fetus at risk, Can. Med. Assoc. J. **101**:458, 1969.

Green, J.W., Jr., and Touchstone, J.C.: Urinary estriol as an index of placental function, Am. J. Obstet. Gynecol. **85**:1, 1963.

Hoebel, C.H., and others: Prenatal and intrapartum high-risk screening. I. Prediction of the high-risk neonate, Am. J. Obstet. Gynecol. **117**:1, 1973.

Huddleston, J.F., and Freeman, R.K.: Assessment of fetal well-being by antepartum fetal heart rate testing. In Bolognese, R.J., Schwarz, R.H., and Schneider, J., editors: Perinatal medicine: management of the high-risk fetus and neonate, ed. 2, Baltimore, 1982, Williams & Wilkins.

Huddleston, J.F., Sutliff, G., and Robinson, D.: Contraction stress test by intermittent nipple stimulation, Obstet. Gynecol. **63**:669, 1984.

Huddleston, J.F., and others: Oxytocin challenge test for antepartum fetal assessment: report of a clinical experience, Am. J. Obstet. Gynecol. **135**:609, 1979.

Keegan, K.A., and others: Antepartum fetal heart rate testing. V. The nonstress test—an outpatient approach, Am. J. Obstet. Gynecol. **136**:81, 1980.

Kochenour, N.K.: Estrogen assay during pregnancy, Clin. Obstet. Gynecol. **24**:659, 1982.

Liggins, G.C., and Howie, R.N.: A controlled trial of antepartum glucocorticoid treatment for prevention of the respiratory distress syndrome in premature infants, Pediatrics **50**:515, 1972.

Manning, F.A., Platt, L.D., and Sipos, L.: Antepartum fetal evaluation: development of a fetal biophysical profile, Am. J. Obstet. Gynecol. **136**:787, 1980.

Manning, F.A., and others: Fetal assessment based on biophysical profile scoring: experience in 12,620 referred high-risk pregnancies, Am. J. Obstet. Gynecol. **151**:343, 1985.

Martin, C.B., Jr.: Regulation of the fetal heart rate and genesis of FHR patterns, Semin. Perinatol. **2**:131, 1978.

Martin, C.B., Jr., and Schifrin, B.S.: Prenatal monitoring. In Aladjem, S., and Brown, A.K., editors: Perinatal intensive care, St. Louis, 1977, The C.V. Mosby Co.

Mendenhall, H.W., O'Leary, J.A., and Phillips, K.O.: The nonstress test: the value of a single acceleration in evaluating the fetus at risk, Am. J. Obstet. Gynecol. **136**:87, 1980.

Miller, F.C., Skiba, H., and Klapholz, H.: The effect of maternal blood sugar levels on fetal activity, Obstet. Gynecol. **52**:662, 1978.

Modanlou, H.D., and others: Sinusoidal FHR pattern and severe anemia, Obstet. Gynecol. **49**:537, 1977.

Murata, Y., and others: Fetal heart rate accelerations and late decelerations during the course of intrauterine death in chronically catheterized rhesus monkeys, Am. J. Obstet. Gynecol. **144**:218, 1982.

Myers, R.E., Mueller-Heubach, E., and Adamsons, K.: Predictability of the state of fetal oxygenation from the quantitative analysis of the components of late deceleration, Am. J. Obstet. Gynecol. **115**:1083, 1973.

Parer, J.T.: Normal and impaired placental exchange, Contemp. Ob/Gyn **7**(2):117, 1976.

Platt, L.D., and others: Further experience with the fetal biophysical profile, Obstet. Gynecol. **61**:480, 1983.

Pose, S.V., and others: Test of fetal tolerance to induced uterine contractions for the diagnosis of chronic distress. In Perinatal factors affecting human development, Washington, D.C., 1969, Pan American Health Organization.

Poseiro, J.J., and others: Effect of uterine contractions on maternal blood flow through the placenta. In perinatal factors affecting human development, Washington, D.C., 1969, Pan American Health Organization.

Ray, M., and others: Clinical experience with the oxytocin challenge test, Am. J. Obstet. Gynecol. **114**:1, 1972.

Read, J.A., and Miller, F.C.: Fetal heart rate acceleration in response to acoustic stimulation as a measure of fetal well-being, Am. J. Obstet. Gynecol. **129**:512, 1977.

Resnik, R., and others: NST or CST? What's best for spotting the high-risk fetus? Contemp. Ob/Gyn **19**(4):92, 1982.

Rochard, F., and others: Nonstressed fetal heart rate monitoring in the antepartum period, Am. J. Obstet. Gynecol. **126**:699, 1976.

Schifrin, B.S.: Antepartum fetal heart rate monitoring. In Gluck, L., editor: Intrauterine asphyxia and the developing fetal brain, Chicago, 1977, Year Book Medical Publishers, Inc.

Scott, D.B., and Kerr, M.G.: Inferior vena caval pressure in late pregnancy, J. Obstet. Gynaecol. Br. Commonw. **70**:1044, 1963.

Spellacy, W.N.: Human placental lactogen in high-risk pregnancy, Clin. Obstet. Gynecol. **16**:298, 1973.

Thacker, S.B., and Berkelman, R.L.: Assessing the diagnostic accuracy and efficacy of selected antepartum fetal surveillance techniques, Obstet. Gynecol. Surv. **4**:121, 1986.

Varner, M.W., and Hauser, K.S.: Human placental lactogen and other placental hormones as indicators of fetal well-being, Clin. Obstet. Gynecol. **25**:673, 1982.

Zlatnik, F.J., Varner, M.W., and Hauser, K.S.: HPL: physiologic and pathophysiologic observations, Obstet. Gynecol. **54**:314, 1979.

CHAPTER 9

Obstetric management of prematurity

The pregnant woman is like a ship upon a stormy sea; full of white caps, and the good pilot who is in charge must guide her with prudence if he is to avoid shipwreck.

Francois Mauriceau

Traité des maladies des femmes grosses, 1668

PATHOGENESIS OF PRETERM LABOR

Despite the development and widespread use of effective tocolytic drugs since the early 1980s, a significant reduction in the incidence of preterm delivery, at least as judged by perinatal statistics, has not occurred. Preterm delivery remains the major uncontrolled element in perinatal mortality and morbidity. Drug therapies alone are not a complete answer. As Boylan and Papiernik have shown, it is possible to markedly improve perinatal statistics through long-term changes in obstetric management without primary resort to tocolytics. Preterm neonates represent only 8% of births nationally, yet they account for as much as 75% of neonatal losses other than those caused by congenital anomalies. In the last 10 years, preterm delivery has shown the lowest proportional decline of all the major causes of perinatal mortality. New and more effective management schemes are required if the high financial and social costs of preterm delivery are to be minimized.

A discussion of preterm delivery must distinguish between the truly preterm infant, that is, the newborn delivered at a gestational age of less than 37 completed weeks (less than 259 days) regardless of weight, and neonates who are actually growth-retarded but who are delivered at more than 37 weeks of gestational age (260 days or more) and weigh 2,500 gm or less at birth. This latter group comprises approximately one third of all infants with birth weights of less than 2,500 gm. The growth-retarded group is best excluded from discussions of preterm delivery because abnormalities in growth may well have different antecedents than those associated with prematurity (see Chapter 7). New technical improvements create clinical dilemmas beyond those of defining disordered fetal growth. The lower limit of gestational age and fetal weight compatible with potential survival has been pushed progressively to earlier weeks of pregnancy. Currently at MacDonald Hospital for Women in Cleveland, Ohio, pregnancies beyond 25 weeks with a fetal weight estimated at 600 gm or more are considered potentially viable. How much further these numbers will continue to decline is unknown. For purposes of this discussion, the period from 141 to 259 days of gestation (or 20 to 37 completed weeks) is considered to encompass preterm gestation.

The mechanism that triggers normal labor at term is under intensive study. Uterine activity during pregnancy is known to be influenced by myometrial stretch, the ratio of progesterone to estrogen, prostaglandin synthesis, changes in uterine blood flow, oxytocin release, and other factors. However, the actual trigger for the onset of human labor has not been identified. There is increasing evidence that endocrine changes initiated by the fetus influence the onset of parturition. It is also clear that a number of other factors (e.g., antepartum hemorrhage, genital tract infection, and membrane rupture) may intervene at an inappropriate time to initiate premature uterine activity. However, of those pregnancies that terminate in spontaneous preterm labor, only 25% have a clearly identified obstetric contributory factor (see boxed material on p. 124). Most have no abnormality that can be currently identified. Therefore, in the majority of instances, preterm labor occurs under circumstances when accurate identification of at-risk pregnancies is at best difficult and when the physiology is not completely known.

This chapter reviews the problems in the diagnosis, evaluation, and treatment of preterm birth. Limitations of current treatment and management plans for reducing the incidence of premature delivery are critically summarized. An understanding of the physiology of the onset of labor is an important initial step to an understanding of how this system functions.

Risk factors for preterm delivery

HISTORICAL (PREPREGNANCY)	DEVELOPING DURING PREGNANCY
Obstetric	**Medical-surgical**
Müllorian anomaly	Nephritis
Incompetent cervix	Pyelonephritis
Prior preterm delivery (two or more)	Liver disease
Prior fetal or neonatal death	Appendicitis
Prior antepartum hemorrhage	
Isoimmunization	**Obstetric**
Prior labor <3 hours	Anemia (Hb ≤8 gm)
Previous abortion or dilation and curettage	Pregnancy-associated hypertension
	Placental abnormalities (abruptio placentae, placenta previa)
Social	Multiple pregnancy
Single or divorced	Hydramnios
Low socioeconomic class	Poor weight gain (<10 lb) or weight loss
Poor nutrition and hygiene	Early dilation of cervix
Employed or long commute	Thinning of lower uterine segment
	Uterine irritability
Physical	Early descent of presenting part
Age: ≤17 or ≥40 years	
Weight: <45 kg	
Height: <160 cm	

Based on data from Hobel, 1984; Kaltreider, 1980; Johnson, 1980; and Berkowitz, 1981.

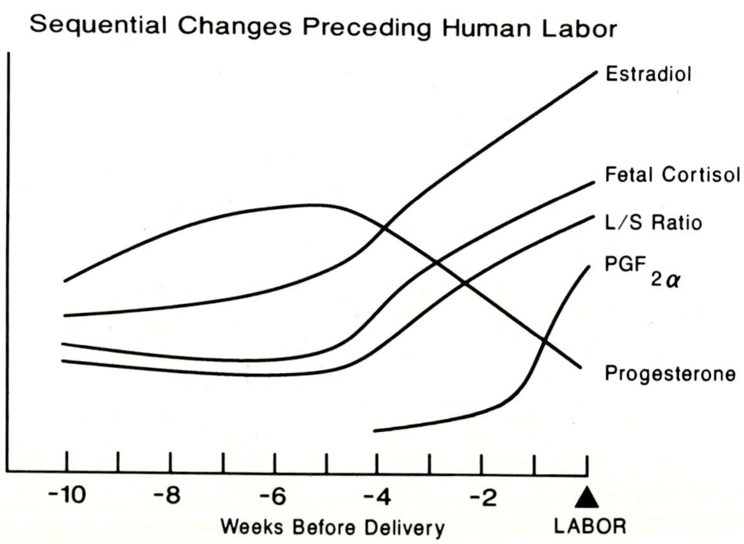

Fig. 9-1. Endocrine events preceding human parturition. Progesterone declines and estradiol rises, beginning several weeks before the onset of labor. (From Speroff, L.: Personal communication, 1985, with permission.)

Physiology of parturition

The principal model for the onset of parturition has been developed in sheep. In the ovine model, fetal cortisol production provides the trigger for the onset of labor, initiating a series of rapid endocrine events. Evidence supporting a similar mechanism in women is poor. In both humans and monkeys, exogenous administration of corticosteroids fails to induce labor except in postmature pregnancies. Although fetal cortisol may not trigger parturition in humans, evidence exists that fetal glucocorticoids do stimulate enzymatic development (such as the lung and liver) that is important in extrauterine life. The rapid endocrine events noted in sheep do not occur in humans; however, progressive increases in estradiol concentrations in the maternal plasma can be measured during the final 5 to 6 weeks of term gestation in normal human pregnancies (Fig. 9-1). A more rapid increase in estradiol concentration in amniotic fluid is observed during the last 3 weeks before the onset of labor. This rise in concentration of estradiol is similar in amniotic fluid samples from both preterm and term labor patients. The major role for estrogen in the onset of labor appears to be the increase of prostaglandin production. There is strong evidence that the ubiquitous prostaglandins, especially E_2 and $F_{2\alpha}$, are the final arbitrators of labor.

Prostaglandin production in humans occurs primarily within the decidua and the chorioamniotic membranes with the major rate-limiting step being the availability of the lysosomal enzyme phospholipase A_2. Therefore substances such as steroids might regulate phospholipid activity through their effects on the stability of lysozymes. Contractions of the uterus both at term and preterm can be induced by administration of prostaglandins intraamniotically, intravenously, and intracervically. Preterm and term labor also can be suppressed by inhibitors of prostaglandin synthesis such as indomethacin. Increases in production rate for prostaglandins are observed with the onset of spontaneous labor. For example, the metabolites of prostaglandin $F_{2\alpha}$ rise progressively in urine throughout late pregnancy and in the peripheral blood at the onset of labor. Finally, during active labor, both prostaglandin E_2 and $F_{2\alpha}$ increase in amniotic fluid, correlating with progressive cervical dilation. These complex relationships are best reviewed in graphic form (Fig. 9-2).

Endocrine changes and prostaglandin production would not result in effective parturition without accompanying physiologic changes in the myometrium. Incoordinate uterine activity (Braxton Hicks contractions), characteristic of the nonlaboring uterus, becomes rhythmic and coordinated as labor approaches through

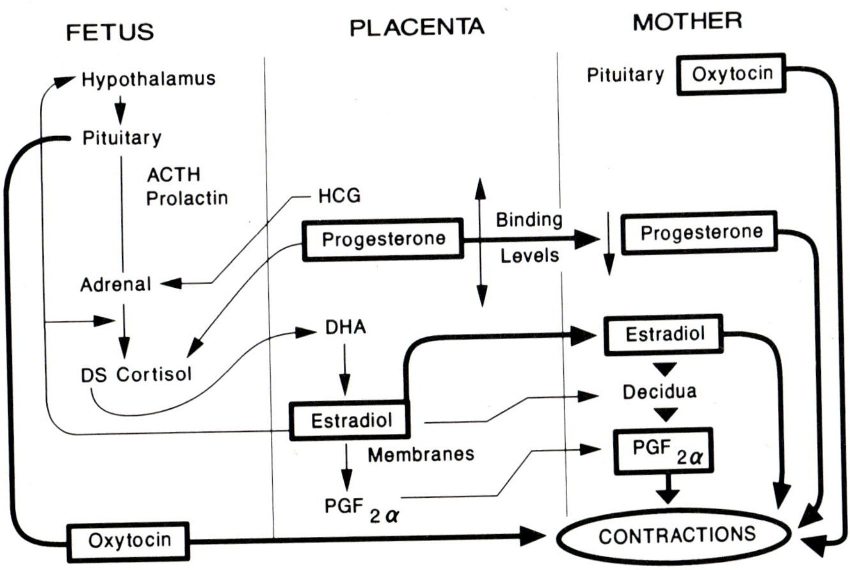

Fig. 9-2. Hormonal events in human parturition divided by compartments: fetal, placental, and maternal. Oxytocin is permissive in the onset of labor with fetal oxytocin probably more important than maternal. Oxytocin is active only in the second stage of labor, aiding expulsion of the infant. The role of fetal cortisol is unestablished. Fetal dehydroepiandrosterone sulfate (DS) increases placental estradiol production. Before the onset of labor, progesterone availability declines perhaps by alteration in receptor binding. Increases in placental and maternal estradiol lead to prostaglandin production by membranes and decidua. (From Speroff, L.: Personal communication, 1985, with permission.)

changes in the physiology of the uterus, including formation of myometrial gap junctions. These junctions are specific intracellular connections that can be identified by electron microscopy. They act to enhance electrical conductivity through the myometrium and are presumably critical for the development of effective uterine contractions. The area of gap junction contact between myometrial cells is small before the onset of contractions, but it increases during labor and declines only after parturition. In vitro studies indicate that increasing the estrogen/progesterone ratio favors the formation of gap junctions. Additional experiments suggest that it is the number of estrogen and progesterone membrane receptors, rather than the actual level of the circulating steroids, that is most important in governing gap junction formation. Furthermore, the prostaglandins E_2 and $F_{2\alpha}$ stimulate junction production, whereas prostaglandin inhibitors such as indomethacin inhibit this activity. Although junction formation progressively promotes coordinate uterine activity, actual contractions ultimately depend on actin/myosin interaction and calcium/cyclic AMP availability.

Myometrial smooth muscle is composed of two contractile proteins, actin and myosin, embedded in a connective tissue. Myosin, the most important protein, is composed of two heavy chains (200,000 daltons) and two light chains (20,000 daltons). Contraction occurs as the chemical energy of adenosene triphosphate is converted into mechanical energy at the junction between actin and myosin. This process requires the action of an enzyme, myosin light-chain kinase, activated by both calcium ion and calmodulin, a calcium regulatory protein. Dephosphorylation of the light chains by a specific phosphatase terminates the contraction. Control of the enzyme activity of the myosin light-chain kinase is the principal regulatory step in smooth muscle contraction (Fig. 9-3).

The availability of myosin light-chain kinase is itself dependent on the concentrations of both calcium and cyclic AMP that are under complex control. Cyclic AMP apparently dephosphorylates and thus inactivates myosin light-chain kinase through a cyclic AMP-dependent protein kinase enzyme. Either activation or inactivation of the enzymes of adenylate cyclase and phosphodiesterase determines the availability of cyclic AMP and, indirectly, the activity of myosin light-chain kinase. Increased cyclic AMP concentration and thus smooth muscle relaxation result from either stimulation of adenylate cyclase by β-mimetic agonists or by inhibition of phosphodiesterase by drugs such as theophylline. There is also a role for

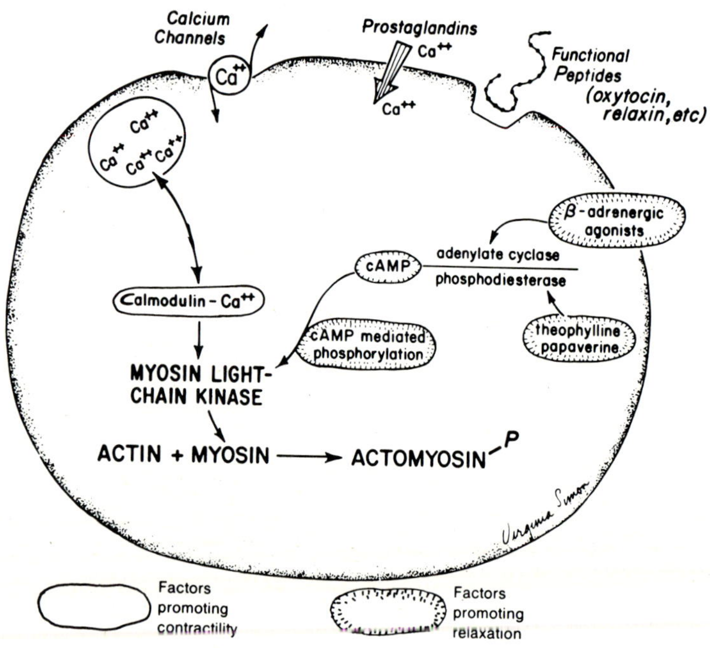

Fig. 9-3. The physiology of uterine smooth muscle contraction mechanism. Myosin light-chain kinase is the rate-controlling enzyme. Calcium availability and cyclic AMP govern kinase availability. Magnesium, prostaglandin and functional peptides act predominately at membrane sites. (From Huszar, G., In Preterm Birth: Causes, Prevention, and Management, edited by Fritz Fuchs and Phillip Stubblefield. Copyright © 1984 by Macmillan Publishing Company. Reproduced by permission of the publisher.)

the insulin-like peptide hormone, relaxin, which acts to increase cellular cyclic AMP levels, thus promoting myometrial relaxation.

Calcium ion, the critical cofactor in contractility, is derived from both intracellular and extracellular sources. Intracellular calcium is located in storage vesicles, including the endoplasmic reticulum and mitochondria. Postaglandin $F_{2\alpha}$ and oxytocin increase intracellular calcium, and both progesterone and cyclic AMP reduce its availability. Transmembrane calcium flux is also important in the availability of this ion and is probably antagonized by calcium channel blockers and magnesium sulfate. As yet, these mechanisms are not well understood.

It is becoming increasingly clear that the ultrastructural and biochemical alterations occurring in the myometrium are coordinated with progressive changes in the cervix. Successful parturition depends on both organized activity in the upper contractile portion of the uterus and changes in distensibility in the lower uterine segment. In concert, these changes facilitate eventual expulsion of the products of conception (Fig. 9-4).

The human cervix is composed of collagen, connective tissue, and varying amounts of smooth muscle. Factors influencing alterations in the cervix include the estrogen/progesterone ratio and local release of prostaglandins. The possible role of relaxin in human cervical maturation is not established. In vitro the combination of progesterone and relaxin decreases myometrial tone, suggesting that the role of relaxin is to maintain pregnancy. However, local administration of relaxin to the cervix promotes cervical dilation. Thus there is at least indirect evidence that relaxin is active in myometrial and cervical changes before the onset of parturition, although its complete role is uncertain.

Within the cervix as ripening progresses, the collagen framework and cervical matrix are disrupted by alterations in their chemical structure. There is an observable increase in hyaluronic acid and a decline in dermatan sulfate and chondroitin sulfate concentrations, accompanied by an increase in the solubility of collagen. The cervix becomes progressively swollen and soft as a result of an increase in hyaluronic acid and accompanying water content. Cervical softening and progressive loss of rigidity develop that, accompanied by the loss of collagen and dermatan sulfates, increase distensibility.

Thus, at least under normal circumstances, myometrial contractility and cervical ripening are under coordinate endocrine regulation by the ratio of estrogen to progesterone, and the various prostaglandins and relaxin are identified as important additions. The implication for the clinician is that attention to cervical changes will prove a reliable indicator of the progressive hormonal and biochemical alterations heralding the onset of either preterm or term labor.

Precipitants of preterm labor

Uterine activity

Spontaneous uterine activity occurs with increasing frequency in normal pregnancy as term approaches. There is evidence that both spontaneous uterine activity and the sensitivity of the uterus to various agents are inappropriately increased in patients who eventually develop preterm labor. Takahashi reported that patients who developed preterm labor were significantly more sensitive to oxytocin than patients who delivered either at term or postterm, implying that an acceleration of sensitivity to oxytocin-like substances occurs in patients with early labor. Clinically, inappropriate early uterine

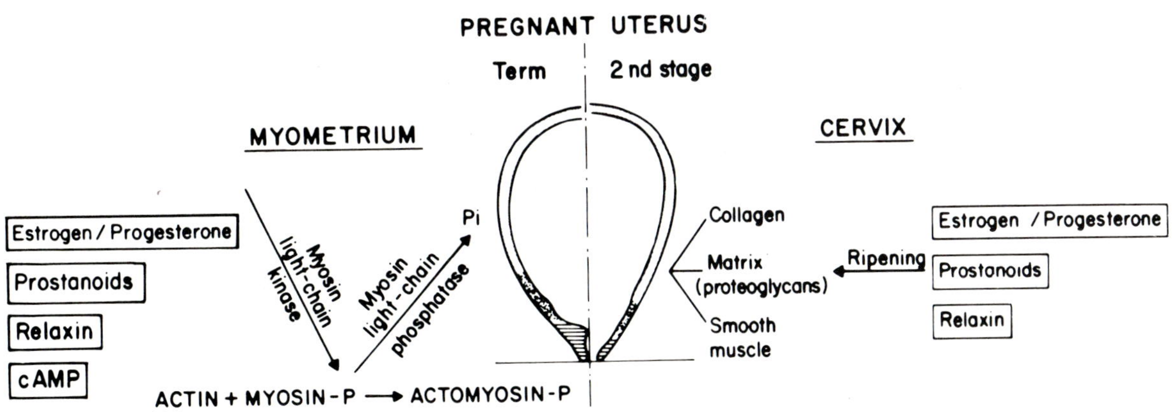

Fig. 9-4. Interaction between myometrial and cervical events in the onset of labor. Myosin light-chain kinase is the rate-controlling enzyme for uterine contractions. Enzyme availability is controlled by calcium/calmodulin and cyclic AMP concentration. (From Huszar, G., and Naftolin, F.: N. Engl. J. Med. **311:**571, 1984. Reprinted by permission of New England Journal of Medicine.)

activity, uterine irritability, and accompanying early cervical changes are associated with the development of preterm labor. Recent work by Katz, in a program in which patients at high risk for preterm labor wore external tocodynamometers that recorded uterine activity, suggests that such devices may be useful in the identification of those at high risk for preterm labor. However, the numbers in this original study were limited, and an appropriate control group was not clearly delineated.

Early anatomic change in the cervix is also observed with more frequency in patients with preterm labor than those delivering at term. For example, early cervical dilation and effacement assessed by clinical examination are associated with an increased risk of preterm delivery. The relationship of inappropriate cervical changes to preterm labor has been evaluated by ultrasound. In sonograms focusing on the degree of cervical shortening, dilation of the cervical canal, funneling of the lower uterine segment, and thinning of the anterior uterine wall, Bartolucci has shown that the risk of preterm labor is markedly increased when these signs are present. Thus both uterine irritability and early, inappropriate cervical change evaluated by ultrasound and clinical examination are associated with an increased risk of preterm delivery. However, these observations document the results, not causes, of inappropriate and premature preparation for labor. The factors initiating these physiologic events have not yet been clearly identified, although both genital tract infection and stress have been implicated as important triggers to preterm parturition.

Cervical insufficiency

Passive dilation of the cervix at midgestation is associated with premature membrane rupture and preterm delivery. Classically, painless cervical dilation resulting in pregnancy loss is termed cervical incompetence or insufficiency. The contributing factors are many and, for purposes of discussion, are easily grouped into congenital and acquired causes. Isolated congenital cervical incompetence is at best a rare condition. However, there is an association between müllerian duct abnormalities and cervical incompetence. For example, women exposed in utero to diethylstilbestrol (DES) frequently combine uterine anomalies (T-shaped uterus) with abnormalities in cervical structure, resulting in rates of preterm delivery and perinatal mortality higher than those seen in women of similar age who were not exposed to DES. Acquired cervical insufficiency is largely the result of surgical trauma, cervical conization, cauterization, and excessive cervical dilation at the time of curettage. Occasionally, obstetric trauma associated with difficult instrumental delivery or with delivery of a macrosomic infant can damage the cervix as well. There is controversy about the role of induced abortion in cervical insufficiency. If laminaria or prostaglandins are not used to soften the cervix before dilation, especially in more advanced gestations, damage to cervical tissue leading to an increase in incompetence may occur. However, termination of first-trimester pregnancy by suction technique, preceded by laminaria, results in minimal cervical damage or risk.

Diagnosis is the most important initial step. A history of painless midtrimester losses with minimal bleeding, with or without uterine contractions, is suggestive of cervical insufficiency. Careful pelvic examination with close attention to the endocervical canal can note unusual dilation even in the nonpregnant state. Early in pregnancy ultrasonic examinations at 6 to 8 weeks and again at 12 to 16 weeks may document early subclinical cervical changes compatible with thinning and weakening of the internal os. Frequently, serial pelvic examinations from 8 to 16 weeks of gestation are performed in the attempt to clinically identify the same phenomenon. Classically, the optimal time for surgical intervention of cervical incompetence is 12 to 14 weeks of gestation. However, this standard dates from the pre-ultrasound era. Spontaneous miscarriage is uncommon after 12 weeks of gestational age, and clinically observable cervical changes often do not occur until after this period. In selected patients with a strong or documented history, ultrasonic evaluation and placement of a cerclage before 12 weeks are indicated. If the gestational sac appears normal and if a crown rump length consistent with dates is measured and fetal cardiac activity observed, the spontaneous miscarriage rate after 8 to 9 weeks of gestational age does not exceed 4%.

Different surgical approaches have been attempted to reinforce the cervix. In all of these surgical techniques, patient choice, accuracy and rapidity of surgery, and minimization of trauma and blood loss are more important than the type of procedure or the choice of suture material. The simplest technique is described by McDonald. A purse-string suture, generally of a large nonabsorbable material, is placed as high as possible in the cervix without advancing the bladder. This is a simple procedure and requires only 10 to 15 minutes to complete. Historically, heavy silk had been the primary material used for this procedure. However, Dacron tape and other nonabsorbable suture materials have become increasingly popular. Shirodkar was the first to attempt to correct cervical insufficiency, and modifications of his original procedure are common. In this technique, anterior and posterior incisions are made at the cervical-vaginal junction and a 5 mm mersilene band is placed around the cervix. The bladder flap is mobilized and advanced to be certain that the stitch is placed as high as possible. The principal disadvantages of the Shirodkar technique are that more dissection is required and blood loss is greater than with the McDonald procedure. Further, there is a risk of inadvertent entry into the bladder or membranes. Finally, a second anesthetic is usually necessary to remove the Shirodkar cerclage. Other techniques have been described but are rarely used. Lash and Lash performed excision and plastic repair of the cervix in a nonpregnant state, and Wurm described a cerclage in which mattress sutures were placed at right angles to each other to essentially occlude the cervical os. These techniques, however, are of more historic than practical interest. There also has been interest in the use of vaginal pessaries for the treatment of cervical insufficiency, but this therapy has failed to achieve substantial popularity.

In certain circumstances, if the cervix is congenitally short or if little cervical tissue remains as a result of late diagnosis or prior conization, a transabdominal procedure may be required. Novy has described this technique in detail. A 5 mm mersilene band is placed around the cervix at the anatomic internal os at laparotomy. An avascular space is developed between the uterine artery and the wall of the uterus. The suture band is passed around the cervix and, once correctly in place, is firmly tied. This procedure is clearly more invasive than the others described. If early delivery or abortion occurs, repeat laparotomy is often necessary to sever the cerclage, unless the stitch can be reached from below.

The results of cervical cerclage operations are difficult to evaluate. With both the McDonald and Shirodkar techniques, 85% to 90% success rates are reported. Physicians often apply stitches to patients with histories of recurrent midtrimester loss where the etiology is obscure. The indications for cerclage are many. Clinical studies are contaminated by large numbers of patients who receive stitches unnecessarily. There are no good prospective, randomized studies with firm entry criteria to prove the efficacy of cerclage, although there is abundant clinical evidence to attest to the importance of sutures in maintaining pregnancies in individual cases. Thus there is little evidence that one suture technique is clearly superior to another. The majority of clinicians now favor the simplest possible technique, the McDonald procedure. Despite limitations in supporting data, surgical procedures for insufficiency are useful in prolonging carefully selected pregnancies.

Genital tract infection

The complex bacterial field of the genital tract is important in influencing inappropriate or early labor. Large numbers of predominantly commensal bacteria and yeast are normally present in the genital tract and produce no symptoms. However, when these lower genital tract organisms are introduced into the upper genital tract or amniotic fluid, severe infection may ensue. Although normal vaginal flora can be associated with clinical infection, their role in preterm labor is not established. Other clearly pathologic species observed in the vaginal flora (e.g., gonorrhea) are capable of initating infection and labor by disruption of membrane integrity or by direct contamination.

Genital tract infection may predispose to preterm labor by directly damaging fetal or maternal membranes, or by release of oxytocics by the inflammatory process itself. Both events can initiate prostaglandin production by phospholipase A_2. The type of bacteria involved also may be important, since there are substantial differences in the ability of different varieties of microorganisms to synthesize phospholipase A_2. Particular activity is noted among specific anaerobic species (e.g., *Bacteroides fragilis*, *Peptostreptococcus* organisms, and *Streptococcus viridans*). Thus it is possible that women who harbor high concentrations of certain anerobic bacteria within the vagina or genital tract are at increased risk for preterm labor. There is direct objective evidence for a link between infection (histologic chorioamnionitis) and preterm labor. For example, histologic evidence of inflammation is present in 60% to 90% of midtrimester deliveries but in only 5% of placentas from term gestations.

Microorganisms can be recovered from the amniotic fluid in 20% to 50% of women in preterm labor with intact membranes. In a study of 54 preterm labors with singleton gestation and intact membranes, bacteria and yeast (*Candida albicans*) were recovered at amniocentesis in 6 patients (11%) and genital *Mycoplasma* in 7 (13%). Prolongation of pregnancy by at least 7 days occurred in 80% or more of patients with sterile amniotic fluid and in five of the six patients whose amniotic fluid contained genital *Mycoplasma* only. However, tocolysis failed in all patients whose amniotic fluid was infected with either bacteria or yeast. Thus it seems possible that unrecognized and subclinical amniotic fluid infection predisposes to preterm labor or that, alternatively with the onset of premature labor, colonization promptly occurs.

Several well known genital pathogens also are implicated in preterm labor. *Neisseria gonorrhea* is associated with an increased incidence of both preterm rupture of membranes and puerperal infection. It is unclear whether the gonococcus actually invades the amniotic membranes primarily or if it interacts with other bacteria. As occurs with pelvic inflammatory disease, the gonococcus may only initiate the process of clinical infection by genital tract invasion. Thereafter, normal vaginal flora can enter the upper genital tract to establish an opportunistic infection.

Another organism, *Chlamydia trachomatis*, can frequently be isolated when the gonococcus is present. At MacDonald Hospital for Women, 18% (240 of 1,327 women) surveyed in outpatient clinics have a positive culture for *Chlamydia*. However, no association has been noted between antenatal infection and either prematurity or perinatal death. This differs from the tenfold increase in these antenatal complicatons reported by some investigators.

Another organism associated with prematurity is group B β-*Streptococcus*. Maternal carriage in the vaginal flora ranges from 8% to 31% in varying studies depending on population screened and methods of culture used. Transmission to the neonate at delivery is low with an attack ratio of 1.9:1,000 live births or less. However, in preterm delivery, the attack rate is as high as 45:1,000. This fact has led to programs for antenatal β-*Streptococcus* screening and selective intrapartum antibiotic therapy. Unfortunately, there is still no diagnostic test to identify which pregnancies colonized with group B β-*Streptococcus* will go into premature labor or produce maternal or neonatal septicemia. The validity of the use of prophylactic antibiotics in pregnancies with asymptomatic, culture-documented, β-*Streptococcus* is unsettled and controversial (Chapter 31).

Whether normal bacteria of the lower genital tract can precipitate preterm labor is not established. So-called nonspecific vaginitis has been associated with both premature rupture of the membranes and preterm uterine activity. Gravett reported clinical vaginitis in 49% of women who delivered infants under 37 completed weeks of gestational age or with a birth weight of less than 2,500 gm but in only 24% of consecutively selected comparison women delivering at term. In addition, Gravett's study found that clinical amniotic fluid infection and premature rupture of the membranes were more frequent in patients with vaginitis than in patients who did not have this infection.

Unfortunately, vaginitis is a poorly defined clinical entity. This disorder was initially believed to be caused by an infection from *Gardnerella vaginalis*. However, *G. vaginalis* is now thought to be an indicator organism, and new data imply that vaginitis is more likely caused by mixed anaerobic organisms and newly-described organisms such as *Mobiluncus* species. It is also possible, but less likely, that genital tract infection can ascend through intact fetal membranes, infect the amniotic fluid, and predispose to premature labor.

The relationship of sexual activity to premature labor is similarly controversial. Coitus could be associated with amniotic fluid infection by the sexual transmission of

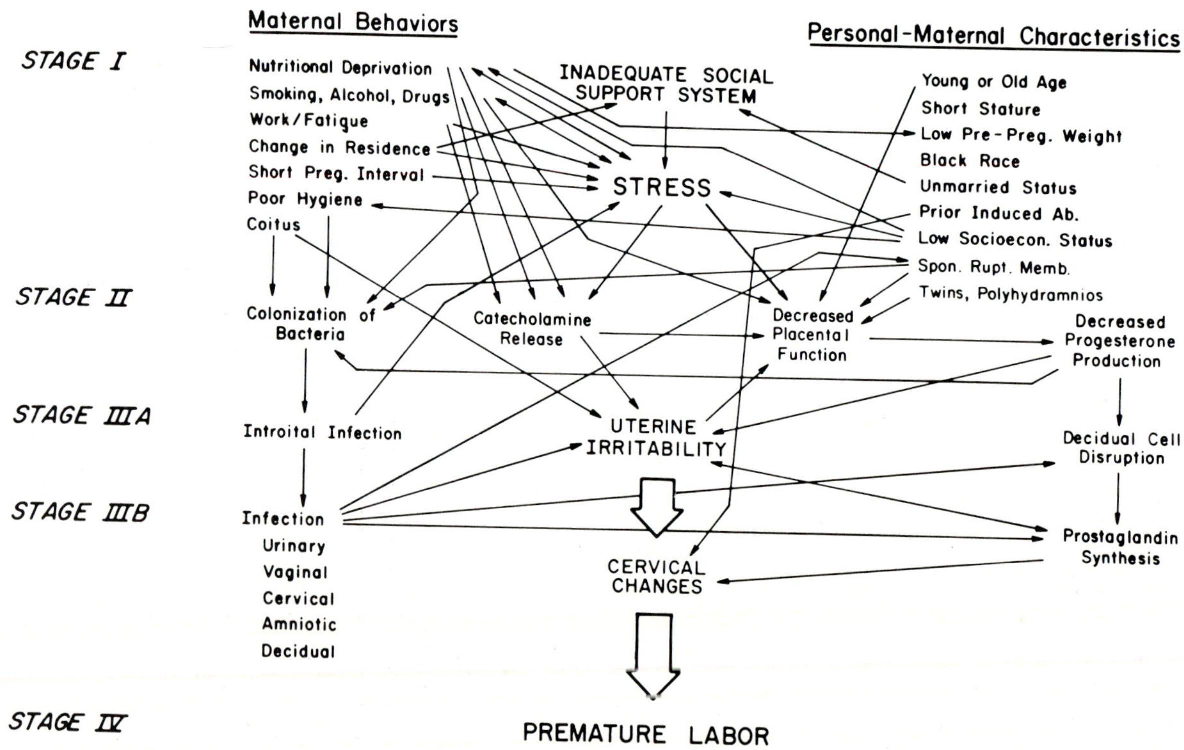

Fig. 9-5. A model for the interaction of behavior and personal-maternal characteristics predisposing to uterine irritability and preterm labor. (From Hobel, C.J., Beard, R.W., and Nathanielex, P.W., editors: Fetal physiology and medicine, New York, 1984, Marcel Dekker, Inc. Reprinted courtesy Marcel Dekker, Inc.)

specific pathogens. Alternatively, sexual activity might traumatize the cervix and membranes, rendering them susceptible to invasion by endogenous vaginal microorganisms. Also orgasm, by producing active uterine contractions, possibly augmented by seminal prostaglandins, could predispose to membrane rupture in patients with anatomically weak membranes or with cervical dilation. Although there are abundant theoretic reasons why sexual activity may initate labor, firm clinical data are scanty. Most clinicians advise patients at high risk for prematurity to avoid coitus or any sexual activity that leads to orgasm. The validity of such prohibition is controversial, but reasonable, in light of current knowledge.

In summary, maternal genital tract infection is an important cause of prematurity and may be responsible for up to 25% of preterm deliveries. The inability to successfully inhibit labor or delay delivery among patients whose amniotic fluid is infected with bacteria or yeast suggests that such organisms have an important role in preterm labor. Since maternal and genital tract infections can be readily diagnosed and treated, they represent a major cause of potentially preventable preterm labor.

Stress

Psychosocial variables of stress have been increasingly implicated in triggering preterm labor. The mechanisms by which life stresses predispose to uterine activity are poorly understood. It is apparent that many individuals show a significant adrenal cortical activation with increases in catecholamine production when they are exposed to major changes in their environment. If accompanied by declines in progesterone concentration, these changes could predispose to myometrial activation. This is clinically observed as uterine irritability and cervical change presumably mediated by prostaglandin synthesis.

Hobel has constructed a model or hypothesis for the onset of preterm labor that is useful in formulating programs and in testing ideas about the causes of preterm labor (Fig. 9-5). His scheme involves three stages: stages one and two are termed the silent stages of preterm labor in which a number of social and demographic features interact to produce biochemical changes predisposing to uterine contractions. In stage three, these factors produce uterine irritability and cervical change leading eventually to active labor.

An important factor in Hobel's scheme is the adverse effect of stress on conception, pregnancy, labor, and delivery. The core of his argument is that interaction exists between stress and maternal behavior, promoting catecholamine release, uterine irritability, and decreased uterine blood flow.

Stress also leads indirectly to preterm labor by contributing to inappropriate maternal behavior such as poor diet and hygiene, smoking, and alcohol or drug abuse, which, in and of themselves, have a demonstrable relationship to early labor.

Prevention of preterm labor

Despite our increased knowledge about the physiology of uterine activity and the development of potent tocolytic agents, little impact has been made on the overall incidence of preterm birth. This is the result of two factors. First, tocolytics are useful only in a small percentage of patients in preterm labor (see discussion later in chapter). Substantial numbers of those women with premature uterine activity have obstetric conditions, including antepartum hemorrhage or infection, which make tocolysis inappropriate. Second, tocolytics are not successful in all cases, and they carry significant side effects for a small but substantial number of recipients. These facts have led to analysis of the causes for preterm delivery in an attempt to determine if antepartum intervention in either patient education or specific therapy can reduce the incidence of prematurity.

The most impressive work has been done by Papiernik and co-workers. Over a 12-year period from 1971 to 1982 in Hagunenau, France, they achieved a 31% reduction (from 5.4% to 3.7%) in preterm births. These reductions were divided disproportionately among preterm infants. The major reduction was in infants with very low birth weight (less than 1,500 gm) and in very premature infants (less than 32 weeks of gestational age). It is interesting in reviewing Papiernik's work to speculate what may or may not be possible with an aggressive prevention program. It is apparent that there is a basal level of prematurity below which the rate probably cannot be depressed (about 3%). Patients contributing to this population include those with antepartum hemorrhage, hypertension, and probably those with a history of prior preterm birth. Papiernik has observed that the major improvement in preterm delivery occurred among women who did *not* have histories that included obstetric complications or prior premature deliveries. This implies that a risk system identifying patients largely on their obstetric history is not likely to impact greatly on the incidence of preterm delivery. Papiernik's method is to identify factors believed to promote uterine activity that could be modified during the course of pregnancy, including physical activity, life-style and habits, and stresses. The thrust of the work of Papiernik and others is that premature labor cannot be divorced from the larger social context. Poor life-styles and habits, smoking, absence of prenatal care, poor diet, and inappropriate living conditions contribute to and are probably additive in promoting early uterine activity.

The medical and social situation in France is different from that of the United States. In the French system, prenatal care and hospitalization are available at government expense. A national health authority disseminates information about premature birth and its prevention. Moreover, work laws permit leaves, restriction of work, or modification of work load or schedule without loss of economic benefit. The March of Dimes has been a leader in attempts to introduce Papiernik's techniques into the United States. Despite early reported success in trials in San Francisco and Ohio, recent studies in Philadelphia suggest that current methods are not invariably successful in reduction of preterm delivery. The ability of the caregivers, the type of social support systems that are available, and the socioeconomic status of the patients at risk all influence the likelihood of success for a given program.

A great deal more work needs to be done in studying the prevention of preterm delivery. There have been only a limited number of prospective studies dealing with psychosocial variables and stress. Much of the work has been retrospective or has involved only white patients or patients late in pregnancy. Moreover, most studies include retrospective data with study designs that fail to evaluate the problem adequately. Schemes like Hobel's (Fig. 9-5) are dependent partially on conflicting data in the interpretation of catecholamine levels and in the clinical importance, if any, of circulating progesterone levels during pregnancy. Finally, the studies of prevention by both Papiernik and Creasy, by their design, lack parallel controls to gauge effectiveness.

INITIAL EVALUATION FOR PRETERM LABOR

Parturition is a natural process characterized by uterine contractions that may or may not be perceived as uncomfortable. It is accompanied by progressive cervical dilation and effacement with eventual expulsion of the products of conception. The onset of labor may be insidious. Once labor is advanced, especially in the face of membrane rupture, it is difficult, if not impossible, to inhibit. Thus it is imperative to identify early signs of labor and to treat premature contractions promptly. A study of the natural history of parturition is complicated by the fact that many patients admitted with a presumptive diagnosis of preterm labor are not in true labor at all but have uterine irritability only and respond to bed rest with or without sedation. The problem in distinguishing true from false labor is common and confuses the interpretation of many clinical studies.

Appropriate management is difficult in patients remote from term who have regular uterine contractions. Even without cervical change, if the contractions are perceived as uncomfortable but observed to be regular, the clinician is pressed to consider tocolytics. To wait for definitive clinical evidence of dilation and effacement is correct given the high percentage of placebo responders. Although waiting risks cervical progression and may compromise membrane integrity, treating without necessity results in inappropriate anxiety, expense, and inflated statistical success.

Clinical evaluation of preterm labor

HISTORY

Cardiovascular disease, hypertension, membrane integrity, hemorrhage

EXAMINATION

General: physical examination
Pelvic: dilation/effacement, membrane integrity, evidence of bleeding
Real-time ultrasound: position and anatomy of placenta and fetus; estimate of gestational age and fetal weight

LABORATORY

CBC with differential count, glucose, electrolytes
Urinalysis, cervical culture

OBSERVATION

Progressive cervical change, increasing discomfort
Recurrent uterine contractions
Bleeding

When a woman with suspected preterm labor is admitted, physical examination with maternal vital signs, urinalysis, pelvic examination with cervical culture, and a complete blood count are indicated (see boxed material). Continuous external electronic fetal monitoring or fetal heart tone auscultation and careful abdominal palpation should be initiated by a trained observer. If uterine activity is persistent and is unresponsive to intravenous hydration, or if cervical dilation or effacement occurs, more extensive evaluation is necessary. Blood should be drawn for measuring baseline levels of electrolytes, hematocrit, hemoglobin, and white cell count including differential and serum glucose. Fetal and placental position, measurements for the estimation of fetal weight, and review of fetal anatomy by real-time ultrasound are indicated. Finally, amniocentesis should be considered if infection is suspected or if fetal pulmonic maturity is questioned.

The aggressive use of parenteral tocolytic drugs in patients beyond 34 weeks of gestational age or with documented pulmonic maturity is rarely indicated because the risks of such therapy outweigh the potential benefits. Further, the presence of such factors as insulin-requiring diabetes, severe hypertension, and fetal abnormalities will clearly influence the use of tocolytics. Before any agent is administered, a period of observation is appropriate. From 20% to 50% of women with preterm uterine activity will respond to bed rest or infusion of intravenous fluid. These responses may be the result of beneficial effects of lateral recumbency on uterine blood flow, cervical tension, or prostaglandin release. Whether patients responding to hydration and lateral recumbency would have ceased their uterine activity spontaneously is problematic. Valenzuela studied the use of bed rest, intravenous hydration (500 ml of 5% dextrose to 0.45% sodium chloride solution), and parenteral morphine sulfate (8 mg intramuscularly) in 184 consecutive singleton pregnancies admitted for suspected premature labor. Fifty-five percent of the patients with cervical dilation less than 4 cm, intact membranes, and no chorioamnionitis stopped contracting. However, when these women were followed to parturition, they had a 2.6 times increased likelihood of preterm delivery and/or tocolytic drug use than the general obstetric population. Thus uterine activity marked enough to cause patients to seek hospital evaluation is not necessarily normal.

Bed rest and fluid infusion may not be a placebo. Lateral recumbency increases uterine blood flow and, when accompanied by hydration, inhibits uterine activity. Women whose false labor responds to such measures do need continued close clinical observation and should not be assumed to be normal.

Techniques for the pharmacologic inhibition of preterm labor vary substantially from institution to institution. At MacDonald Hospital for Women, three parenteral agents are used as tocolytics: ritodrine hydrochloride, terbutaline sulfate, and magnesium sulfate. Oral terbutaline and ritodrine also are employed (see discussion later in chapter). Diazoxide, prostaglandin inhibitors, calcium blocking agents, or progestational compounds are not used as tocolytics in MacDonald Hospital except under rare circumstances.

Establishment of gestational age

Uncertainty as to the actual length of pregnancy is a common problem in evaluation of suspected preterm gestation. Classically, the period of gestation is calculated from the last normal menstrual period (LMP). The estimation of the date of confinement (delivery) is calculated by adding 7 days to the date of the first day of the LMP and then counting back 3 months (Naegle's rule). Thus menstrual dating assumes ovulation on day 14 of the cycle, with fertilization and implantation following. By these calculations the period estimated for length of gestation is 2 weeks longer than the actual elapsed period since ovulation. Since the time of ovulation or fertilization is unknown but the menstrual cycle is easily and often correctly recalled, menstrual dating of pregnancy is universal. The span of normal gestation is 280 days divided into 10 lunar months of 4 weeks each. The 40 weeks of pregnancy are divided into three parts or trimesters, each slightly more than 13 weeks or 3 calendar months each. Classically, the division into trimesters is for clinical convenience, since obstetric complications divide themselves into several groups when this convention is followed.

Given current pregnancy tests and ultrasound, the problem facing the obstetrician is no longer to determine if a given patient is pregnant but to calculate how far in gestation her pregnancy has advanced. Estimation of the true period of gestation is dependent on menstrual dating as just described, clinical parameters of quickening (the subjective report when the woman first feels fetal motion), palpation of uterine size, and ultrasound measurements. Menstrual irregularity, usually as the result of irregular ovulation, is common. Patients may become pregnant immediately following a delivery and before the resumption of regular menses, after a prolonged period of amenorrhea from other reasons, or immediately following discontinuation of oral contraceptives without an intervening cycle. Also, it is possible that threatened miscarriage may have occurred early in pregnancy and may have been mistaken for a menstrual cycle; thus menstrual dating can be unreliable.

A pelvic examination in the first trimester of pregnancy to palpate the uterus for size is helpful in the correct assessment of gestational age. However, early examination is not infallible and is subject to many variables, including the skill of the examiner, patient obesity, and uterine pathology (e.g., leiomyoma). Auscultation of the fetal heart is frequently suggested as a reasonable indication of gestational age (17 to 20 weeks). However, many clinicians now use Doppler devices to detect fetal heart activity. When such an instrument is used, it is not uncommon to detect the fetal heart at 12 weeks or occasionally, even earlier, depending on the skill of the observer and patient obesity.

The most reliable estimate of gestational age is provided by ultrasound (see Chapter 12). This is particularly true for patients who may have had little or late prenatal care. There is no modern indication for radiographic studies in establishing the period of gestation. Regardless of the presumed reliability of menstrual dating, ultrasound studies are important in patient evaluation if preterm labor is suspected. First, ultrasonic scans are unrivaled in the ability to localize the placenta and determine fetal position. Antenatal hemorrhage is frequently accompanied by premature uterine irritability or frank labor, and the early diagnosis of placenta previa or abruptio placentae has clear impact on the management choices made in individual cases. Ultrasound is also extremely useful in the evaluation of amniotic fluid volume in cases in which there are questions of membrane integrity. Normally, rupture of the fetal membranes is determined by a history of leaking or gushing of fluid combined with pelvic examination (presence of a pool, ferning, and positive nitrazine paper test). However, if the membranes have been ruptured for a prolonged period of time, or if the patient is a nulliparous woman whose history is uncertain, both sterile speculum examination and a dye study can be required. Between 2 and 3 ml of indigo carmine dye are injected at amniocentesis. A sterile tampon is placed in the vagina. Presence or absence of tampon staining over the subsequent 1 to 2 hours establishes the diagnosis of membrane rupture. Anatomic evaluation of the fetus is also important. Fetal abnormalities incompatible with life are a contraindication to attempts at tocolysis. Also, previously unrecognized multiple gestation would complicate clinical management.

Ultrasound is useful predominantly in estimation of fetal gestational age and weight. The important measurements are the biparietal diameter and the cranial circumference, the abdominal diameter and circumference, and the length of long bones (femur and tibia). With a combination of these measurements, the fetal weight can be calculated with good accuracy, and a reasonable estimate of fetal gestational age can be established. If rupture of the membranes is suspected, or if it is elected to perform an amniocentesis to rule out occult amnionitis or to determine fetal pulmonic maturity, ultrasound is extremely useful in safely directing the procedure. Although ultrasonic evaluation can give a good estimate of the period of gestation, only direct studies of the amniotic fluid can provide consistently reliable predictions about the status of fetal pulmonary function.

Assessment of lung maturity

See also Chapter 28.

Type II alveolar pneumocytes synthesize surfactant, a phospholipid substance that decreases the surface tension at the air/fluid interface in the alveoli of the neonatal lung. Surfactant lowers surface tension, preventing collapse of the small alveolar spaces during expiration and permitting the lung to retain residual air. If surfactant is not present during attempts at respiration, alveolar spaces collapse and acidosis, hypoxia, and progressive lung damage ensue (hyaline membrane disease). Thus a lack or deficiency of surfactant is the principal abnormality in the infant respiratory distress syndrome (RDS). Investigative work has identified a series of surface active substances from alveolar washings. Human surfactant contains a combination of lipid proteins and carbohydrates, the most important surface active component of which is lecithin. The accompanying phospholipids, phosphatidylglycerol (PG) and phosphatidylinositol (PI), act as surfactant-stabilizing substances, helping to prevent alveolar collapse. Lecithin is biosynthesized in the type II pneumocyte through the choline incorporation pathway. The enzymes responsible for the production of surfactant are glucocorticoid induced, providing a mechanism for induction of lecithin biosynthesis. The development of surfactant is closely tied to the early development of the fetal lung, and surfactant production may begin by weeks 24 to 25 of gestation.

The most common studies for the determination of fetal pulmonic maturity are tests for surfactant. Gluck originally described techniques by which lecithin levels in amniotic fluid could be measured and correlated with functional lung maturity. It soon became apparent that the determination of the amniotic fluid concentration of lecithin with sphingomyelin, a phospholipid that lacks surface activity and that does not vary substantially in concentration during gestation, permitted expression of increases in lecithin as a convenient ratio. Before week 30 of gestational age, the sphingomyelin concentration exceeds that of lecithin in amniotic fluid. After weeks 34 to 35, lecithin rises sharply and the ratio of lecithin to sphingomyelin (L/S ratio) reaches or exceeds 2:1. Depending on the laboratory, an L/S ratio of 2:1 or greater is consistent with maturity.

There are innumerable variations of the original method, and there is considerable confusion in the literature over the interpretation of the L/S ratio and functional pulmonic maturity. However, when the L/S ratio is 2 or greater in normal cases, as reported by the method of Gluck, the risk for respiratory distress is low. If the L/S ratio is between 1.5 to 2, RDS occurs in approximately 40% of neonates. When the L/S ratio is less than 1.5, approximately 75% of infants develop RDS, and the condition may be serious or fatal in 10% to 15% of those affected infants.

The L/S ratio is not without problems both in interpretation and performance. A number of maternal conditions have been identified that accelerate fetal pulmonic maturation (see boxed material). These include conditions associated predominantly with intrauterine hypoxia. In addition, to perform the L/S ratio requires a quality control laboratory, trained technicians, and 2 to 4 hours of laboratory time. Because of these limitations, the L/S ratio may not be available 24 hours a day, and the process is relatively expensive. The ratio may be unreliable in certain complicated pregnancies, including diabetes mellitus (classes A, B, and C) and Rh sensitization. The prediction of fetal pulmonic maturity in patients with insulin-requiring diabetes is controversial. In diabetes (classes A, B, and C), where vascular disease is not present, the consensus is that L/S ratio is not a highly reliable predictor of stable pulmonic maturity unless PG is also present in the test specimen (Chapter 3).

Hallman emphasizes the clinical importance of PG,

Factors accelerating pulmonic maturity
MATERNAL DISEASES
Hypertensive disease
Sickle cell anemia
Narcotic addiction
Diabetes mellitus (classes D, F, R)
PLACENTAL CONDITIONS
Circumvallate placenta
Chronic retroplacental bleeding (abruptio)
Placenta insufficiency (IUGR)
Premature rupture of membranes (≥24 hours)

Note: In certain other settings the appearance of a mature L/S ratio may be delayed, including diabetes mellitus (classes A, B, C) and hydrops fetalis/isoimmunization.

the surface-acting stabilizing factor. The presence of PG in amniotic fluid specimens, when the L/S ratio exceeds 2 is a strong predictor that RDS will not occur. For example, in the study of Whittle, respiratory distress did not develop if PG was present, even when the L/S ratio was less than 2. A further advantage for PG is that specimens contaminated by meconium, blood, or vaginal secretions are still suitable for analysis. Unfortunately, PG does not normally develop until late in gestation, generally after week 35, but, in stressed pregnancies, PG occasionally may be detected even before week 30. Its presence is reassuring in documenting pulmonic maturity; however, because of its appearance late in the third trimester, PG is frequently absent in pregnancies sampled before week 35. In summary, the absence of PG indicates gestational immaturity and some possibility of neonatal respiratory distress if delivery occurs. Recently, a slide agglutination test (Amniostat FLM) has been developed for PG. Preliminary experience with this rapid and nonquantitative test is favorable and false positives are rare. However, more information is necessary to ensure the reliability of this method in general clinical use.

Other surfactant studies include variants of the foam stability or shake test originally described by Clements. Such tests combine amniotic fluid and absolute ethanol to determine the ability of the preparation to form stable bubbles. When agitated in appropriate concentrations and with a surfactant present, a stable foam will form at the air/liquid interface. In the original description of the test, presence of a completely circular ring of bubbles for 15 minutes was found to be indicative of fetal pulmonic maturity. The shake test was initially described as a bedside test for maturity. However, many falsely negative tests occur, resulting largely from inconsistencies in technique. To overcome the limitations of the original shake test, a prepackaged test, the Foam Stability Index (FSI), has been developed. The test uses a plastic cartridge provided with a series of prefilled wells containing a known quantity of absolute alcohol. When a study is to be performed, amniotic fluid is added to each well to a premarked level. The cassette is then agitated vigorously. The top of each well is inspected for a complete ring of bubbles. Lung maturity is established when the bubble ring is stable in tube dilutions of 0.48 or greater. The FSI is reliable if it predicts fetal lung maturity. However, immature values are not as reliable because of the large number of false negative results.

Fluorescent polarimetry, measuring the microviscosity of the amniotic fluid, also can be used to estimate pulmonary maturity. The lower the value, the more likely that pulmonic maturity is present. This is a rapid and reliable test when it indicates maturity. The major drawback is the expense of the reading device.

It is possible also to measure the optical density of amniotic fluid at 650 nm using a standard spectrophotometer. After centrifugation, the phospholipids of the amniotic fluid give an optical density peak at 650 nm. This test has the advantage of speed and availability. However, reliability is questionable and contamination is a major problem. Other studies of amniotic fluid used in previous years for estimation of gestational age, including Nile blue staining of cells, determination of creatinine concentration, optical density at 450 nm, and osmolality are less reliable than surfactant tests and are not performed routinely.

The principal screen for lung maturity in perinatal laboratories remains a variant of the L/S ratio, with accompanying determination of PG. PG is important in diabetic pregnancies and in pregnancies complicated by isoimmunization or hydrops fetalis to adequately document stable pulmonic maturity. It is also useful in contaminated fluid and has value in amniotic fluid obtained from the vaginal pool and in fluid stained by meconium.

Use of corticosteroids

The most controversial treatment in cases of threatened preterm delivery is the use of corticosteroids for enhancement of fetal pulmonic maturity. Exogenous corticosteroids are known to enhance maturity in animal models including the rabbit, lamb, monkey, baboon, and rat. Mechanisms whereby endogenous corticosteroids influence fetal lung maturity are slowly becoming understood. Chronic in utero stress may accelerate fetal lung maturity, and a parallel rise in corticosteroids and catecholamines is observed in normal pregnancy. In cultures of fetal lung cells, addition of corticosteroids results in increased lecithin production. Corticosteroid receptors are present in the type II alveolar pneumocyte that is responsible for the production of lamellar bodies containing surfactant. Corticosteroids also inhibit phosphodiesterase activity in the fetal lung. This leads to increased cyclic AMP, which stimulates phosphatidylcholine production by the choline incorporation pathway. Corticosteroids also increase choline phosphotransferase activity in the fetal lung, and they may cause structural alterations in lung collagen and directly increase activity of other enzymes, leading to enhanced biosynthesis of PG.

Reasonable evidence indicates that administration of corticosteroids affects the L/S ratio. Morrison removed amniotic fluid before initiating hydrocortisone therapy in 70 patients; 7 hours to 9 days later, a marked increase in the L/S ratio was observed following the administration of hydrocortisone but none with placebo. In fetal monkeys, Socol noted a peak effect in L/S ratio some 2 to 3 days after the administration of dexamethasone. This pharmacologic effect disappeared by day 5 following dosing.

A number of different steroid compounds have been administered to enhance maturity. Most popular have been betamethasone, dexamethasone, and hydrocortisone. Betamethasone therapy has commonly consisted of 12 mg given intramuscularly in two doses 24 hours apart. Dexamethasone doses have varied from 4 to 12 mg intramuscularly given twice to three times a day for 2 to 7 days. Hydrocortisone treatments have ranged from 500 to 1,000 mg once or twice a day for 1 to 2 days. There are limited comparative studies contrasting these various dosage schedules. In studies in which a positive response was observed, the maximum benefit occurs in fetuses between 28 to 32 weeks of gestational age. In general, limited advantage has been seen for steroid use in pregnancies between 32 to 34 weeks but none in gestations beyond 34 weeks. It is also difficult to demonstrate clearly the benefit in fetuses less than 28 weeks of gestational age largely because of the small numbers reported. Usually no advantage is seen for steroid administration, if the drug has been given for less than 24 hours. Maximum benefits occur when at least 48 hours have elapsed from initiation of therapy. Variable benefit is noted between 24 to 48 hours and may be lost after 7 days. Factors other than gestational age may influence the response to steroids. The Collaborative Study claimed benefit for corticosteroid administration for nonwhites and for females only. A sex-specific effect favoring females also has been described by Papageorgiou. A critical review of the literature indicates that most other studies are reported in a manner that does not allow an analysis of steroid efficacy based on either race or sex.

In studies involving over 1,500 patients, reductions in the incidence off RDS are observed, but marked variation in the benefits occurs (Table 9-1). Part of the difficulty is that the various reports differ in the gestational ages chosen for treatment, the criteria for diagnosis of RDS, the steroids, and the dosage schedule chosen.

Clinicians have used corticosteroids less frequently in recent years. This is partially the result of evidence that steroids are unnecessary if membrane rupture has occurred and also the expression of concerns about potential adverse fetal side effects. Results of a 6-year follow-up in children treated by the original Liggins protocol reported no difference in physical examination, illness, speech, fine motor development, neurologic development, intelligence, or any other parameters studied. In the studies of both Garite and Taeusch there was an indication of increased maternal infection and a trend toward increased neonatal infection, but such deleterious effects of steroids have not been recorded by most observers. In Liggin's original series, it was suggested that steroid use was associated with a higher fetal death rate in patients who were chronically hypertensive. This association has not been confirmed in cases in which modern fetal surveillance was performed.

The possible adverse effects of corticosteroids have been extrapolated from animal models in which growth retardation, decreased growth of thymus, liver, lung, and brain, and decreased brain incorporation of DNA and RNA have been observed. In neonatal animals born after exposure to corticosteroids, decreased antibody responses, decreased brain growth, decreased brain and organ DNA, thymic evolution and pulmonary susceptibility to oxygen damage have also been noted. However, careful studies in humans have failed to document such effects. Further, administration of corticosteroids to nonhuman primates in schedules similar to those used for human RDS prophylaxis has not indicated adverse effects on fetal brain development.

A number of studies suggest that premature rupture of the fetal membranes alone results in a reduction in the expected incidence of RDS. In this setting, administration of corticosteroids is of little or no benefit. Although reports in the literature are variable, Iams (5.7% versus 23.7%), Garite (11% versus 29%), and Tauesch (12% versus 27%) reported an increased incidence of postpartum infection in women receiving corticosteroids in comparison to matched controls. Thus the fetal benefit from maternal administration of corticosteroids in the face of membrane rupture is at best limited, and some maternal risk does exist. Most clinicians have elected expectant management without use of steroids in this situation.

In summary, there is currently less clinical enthusiasm for the administration of corticosteroids than in the last several years. Most clinicians now restrict antenatal steroid use to pregnancies between 28 to 32 weeks of ges-

Table 9-1. Selected studies of corticosteroids in RDS prevention*

Author	Steroid†	Gestational ages or weights	Percent of RDS	
			Control	Steroid
Liggins/Howie (1972)	Beta	≤24-36	18/75 (24.0%)	4/93‡ (4.3%)
Liggins (1976)	Beta	≤30-32	29/51 (56.9%)	12/59‡ (20.4%)
Block (1976)	Beta	≤32	12/44 (27.3%)	5/49‡ (10.2%)
Morrison (1978)	Hydrocortisone	26-35	14/59 (24.0%)	6/67‡ (9.0%)
Taeusch (1979)	Dex	26-36	14/65 (22.0%)	7/50 (NS) (14.0%)
Papageorgiou (1979)	Beta	24-34	19/32 (59.4%)	6/29‡ (20.7%)
Doran (1980)	Beta	24-34	10/60 (17.0%)	4/80 (NS) (5.0%)
Collaborative Group (1981)	Dex	26-37	59/328 (18%)	42/335‡ (12.6%)

Modified from Garite, 1984, and Doran, 1980.
*Data based on randomized, prospective trials.
†Beta; betamethasone; dex, dexamethasone.
‡$p \le 0.05$.

Table 9-2. Administration of tocolytic drugs: primary agents

β-Mimetic drugs	Dosage/timing	Comments
Ritodrine (Yutopar)	Oral: 10 to 20 mg orally every 2 to 4 hours Parenteral: 0.150 to 0.350 mg/min by IV infusion pump	Dose titrated against effect on contractions and maternal pulse; careful control of total intravenous intake and restriction to brief courses are important in avoidance of complications.
Terbutaline sulfate (Brethine, Bricanyl)	Oral: 2.5 to 10 mg orally every 2 to 4 hours Parenteral: 0.250 mg subcutaneously every 1 to 4 hours	Subcutaneous doses are appropriate for obstetrical manipulations, treatment of hyperstimulation, and to slow labor to permit initial evaluation; oral doses may substitute for ritodrine
Magnesium sulfate ($MgSO_4$)	Loading dose: 4 to 6 gm/20 minutes Maintenance: 1 to 3.5 gm/hour	Infusion titrated to maintain a level of 4.5 to 6.5 mg/dl; careful attention to output and vital signs is essential.

Modified from O'Grady, J.P. In Rathi, M.V., editor: Clinical aspects of perinatal medicine, New York, 1985, Macmillan Publishing Co., Inc.

tational age, with intact membranes, when it is anticipated that delivery will not occur within 24 hours.

USE OF TOCOLYTICS IN PRETERM LABOR

After a woman is admitted for suspected preterm labor, clinical evaluation involves several steps. Patients admitted to the hospital at less than 34 weeks gestational age, with or without intact membranes and in apparent active labor, are given 0.250 mg of terbutaline subcutaneously to arrest labor initially and to permit evaluation (Table 9-2). Fetal distress, active maternal bleeding, hypertension, arrhythmia, or history of cardiac disease preclude the immediate use of this or any other β-mimetic drugs (see boxed material). Ultrasound, amniocentesis, and appropriate clinical and laboratory studies then can

Tocolysis: contraindications

RELATIVE	ABSOLUTE
Hypertension Twin or multiple gestation Insulin-dependent diabetes mellitus Antenatal hemorrhage Membrane rupture	Nonviable fetus Eclampsia or severe preeclampsia Septicemia/amnionitis Hyperthyroidism Abruptio placentae Cardiac arrhythmia or myocardial dysfunction

Modifed from O'Grady, J.P. In Rathi, M.V., editor: Clinical aspects of perinatal medicine, New York, 1985, Macmillan Publishing Co., Inc.

proceed as indicated. The terbutaline dose may be repeated at 1 to 4 hour intervals if contractions persist. Similar dosing for transfer patients is preferred when maintenance of an infusion pump and intravenous line during ambulance or air transport is difficult. Both intramuscular (5 to 10 mg) and small intravenous doses of ritodrine (4 to 6 mg) have the same effect and are equally safe.

If long-term tocolysis is chosen following initial evaluation, intravenous ritodrine is administered by infusion pump. The dose is increased in stepwise fashion until either intolerance or control of uterine activity occurs. Procedures are followed that are similar to those outlined by Lipshitz, where the maternal pulse (maximum acceptable 120 beats per minute) is used as a clinical marker of drug effect. Occasionally, doses in excess of 0.300 mg per minute of ritodrine will be administered, if the maternal pulse rate is less than 120 beats per minute and if the parturient is otherwise tolerating the infusion well. After a uterine-controlling dose has been established, the rate of administration is usually maintained for 6 hours and then progressive tapering to a lower dose is attempted. Every effort is made to avoid parenteral drug administration for longer than 12 hours. If a controlling dosage of the β-mimetic drug is accompanied by persisting maternal tachycardia or other unacceptable symptoms, the drug is stopped. In selected cases, ritodrine and magnesium sulfate can be administered concurrently. Some patients are candidates for tocolysis but have relative or absolute contraindications to the use of β-mimetics. In patients who are hypertensive or who have insulin-requiring diabetes, magnesium sulfate is administered as the drug of choice. If control is adequate, patients are reassessed at 12 to 24 hours (depending on the agent used) for conversion to an oral drug.

The β-mimetics in common use are ritodrine and terbutaline. Other agents including isoxsuprine, albuterol (salbutamol), nylidrin, fenoterol, hexoprenaline, and metaproterenol have been studied for tocolytic effect. Hexaprenaline *may* prove to have fewer cardiovascular side effects than other agents and will soon be approved for clinical use. However, a healthy skepticism is appropriate, since similar claims were made initially for each of the agents currently available.

The efficacy of ritodrine in inhibiting preterm labor is supported by controlled, double-blind studies conducted in both Europe and the United States. The American study, although flawed in experimental design, involved 313 singleton pregnancies. There were statistically significant reductions in neonatal death and RDS in the group treated with ritodrine in comparison to the controls. Treated patients were more likely to reach 36 weeks of gestational age and to deliver neonates exceeding 2,500 gm. Finally, ritodrine treatment prolonged gestation by a mean of 32.6 days in treated pregnant women versus 21.3 days for gravidas in the control group ($p < 0.001$). Terbutaline has also proved effective and safe in halting preterm labor in placebo-controlled, double-blind studies. Additional control studies and comparison studies matching terbutaline against other agents have also proved its clinical efficacy.

Metabolic and cardiovascular abnormalities have been observed in neonates exposed in utero to β-mimetics. Fetal tachycardia occurs occasionally. Increases in concentrations of umbilical cord insulin have been observed in response to maternal hyperglycemia followed by subsequent neonatal hypoglycemia. Side effects of major consequence, including marked hypotension and hypocalcemia, have been associated almost exclusively with isoxuprine and not the newer agents. In general, neonates appear to tolerate in utero exposure to β-mimetics with minimum complications. Follow-up studies of 1 to 9 years among individuals who had been exposed in utero to ritodrine reveal no differences in growth, structural anomalies, incidence of disease, or psychomotor development when compared with matched controls.

Ritodrine is the only pharmacologic agent approved for tocolytic use in the United States; however, it is not appropriate in all clinical settings. For example, patients intolerant of the side effects of ritodrine may tolerate effective doses of terbutaline. In patients with hypertension or insulin-requiring diabetes, when the β-sympathomimetics are relatively contraindicated, another agent such as magnesium sulfate is a better choice. When such drugs are used as tocolytics, there is a common misconception among physicians, pharmacists, or nurses that these agents are "unapproved" and therefore inappropriate for clinical use.

Regardless of indications in the package insert, a physician's best professional judgment is required in the decision to use a drug in a particular clinical setting. The use of an approved drug for an unapproved indication is the clinical practice of medicine. In the setting of preterm labor, choice of a tocolytic agent is governed by considerations of greatest efficacy and lowest possible fetal and maternal risk with clear goals in mind, regardless of the agent used.

Magnesium sulfate

Magnesium sulfate, administered principally as an anticonvulsant to patients with preeclampsia, has a long history in American obstetrics. Interest in magnesium as a tocolytic grew from clinical observations. Uterine hypertonicity was observed to respond to rapid infusions of magnesium, and patients treated with magnesium for preeclampsia often slowed labor and frequently required augmentation with oxytocin to achieve delivery. This anticonvulsant affects the myometrium by blocking calcium availability to myosin light-chain kinase, probably at the level of the cell membrane (Fig. 9-4). Of interest, maternal serum levels of magnesium have been reported to be low normal in patients with preterm labor. The implication of this observation on the mechanism of uterine activity remains unclear at best. In high doses, magnesium progressively blocks neuromuscular transmission at motor endplates. Thus overdosage results in progressive muscular paralysis, which is reversible by calcium administration. For use as a tocolytic agent, magnesium is given intravenously in a manner similar to that used for seizure prophylaxis (Table 9-4). An intravenous dose of 4 gm is administered over 20 minutes, and a maintenance infusion of 2 gm per hour is begun thereafter. Hourly checks of urinary output and maternal deep tendon reflexes follow. Levels of 4.5 to 6.5 mg/dl are maintained by adjustment of the infusion rate or by administration of further 1 to 2 gm boluses. Since magnesium is a peripheral vasodilator, patients often experience transient flushing and warmth during infusion. With rapid injection, palpitations, headache, or nausea also may occur briefly. Once labor has been halted for 12 to 24 hours, magnesium therapy is discontinued and administration of an oral β-mimetic is considered. Since magnesium salts are absorbed poorly or incompletely from the gastrointestinal tract (leading to their principal oral use as cathartics), it is unlikely that oral magnesium therapy will prove either successful or well tolerated.

Maternal complications from treatment are rare but potentially serious. Magnesium is renally excreted, and overdose can occur as a result of inadequate magnesium excretion in patients with reduced kidney function. In Elliott's review, the incidence of side effects to magnesium was 7%. However, in only 2% of 355 patients did side effects necessitate discontinuation of the drug. Pulmonary edema has been reported as complication of the use of magnesium sulfate as a tocolytic, but the incidence is extraordinarily low. Clinical studies by Elliott, Steer, Petrie, and Spisso provide data indicating that as a tocolytic, magnesium sulfate is successful in delaying delivery by 24 hours or more in 60% to 85% of patients treated. Miller and co-workers compared magnesium with terbutaline in a randomized study of 29 patients. Although the numbers were small, the drugs equally delayed delivery, but significant side effects were more prevalent in terbutaline-treated patients. Magnesium has definite advantages as a tocolytic agent. Physicians and nurses are accustomed to its administration and to treatment of its complications. Also, magnesium is suitable for patients with diabetes and hypertension. Finally, there is reasonable evidence of efficacy, and maternal side effects severe enough to curtail therapy are uncommon. However, there are also some distinct disadvantages; for example, there is no acceptable oral form. Further, magnesium crosses the placenta and may affect the fetus-depressing neuromuscular function and the neonate's Apgar scores. The clinical importance of transplacental transfer is debatable, and it is not usually a factor in neonatal depression. Adverse effects of magnesium in premature neonates are more common if mothers have received prolonged, continuous infusion (more than 24 hours). Clearance of magnesium is prolonged in neonates with a biologic half-life of more than 40 hours (see Chapter 33).

In summary, magnesium sulfate is the tocolytic agent of choice in limited circumstances. In consideration of extensive clinical experience with this agent and because of its limited potential for maternal and fetal complications, magnesium is probably the safest effective tocolytic drug available.

β-Sympathomimetics

β-Sympathomimetics inhibit preterm labor by reducing the availability of intracellular calcium and inhibit the phosphorylation of myosin light-chain kinase. The β-sympathomimetics were synthesized to avoid B_1 stimulation (predominantly cardiovascular) while acting more or less selectively on B_2 receptors (uterus, vascular smooth muscle, and bronchioles). However, available drugs lose beta specificity progressively when administered in high doses, tending to offset the advantages of selectivity. These drugs have major metabolic effects that limit their use. β-Sympathomimetics stimulate adrenocorticosteroid release, initiating gluconeogenesis. Lipolysis in adipose tissue also occurs, increasing serum free fatty acids and glycerol. Insulin also rises by direct action on β-mimetic receptors in the pancreas. The net result is a prompt rise in serum glucose accompanied by increased output of lactate, pyruvate, and ketone bodies. Both hyperglycemia in otherwise normal patients and rapid development of ketoacidosis in insulin-requiring diabetics have been observed with the administration of β-sympathomimetics. When these drugs are administered intravenously the serum potassium level drops rapidly. Total body potassium does not decline; instead, potassium simply shifts into other body compartments. This is partially the result of cell membrane hyperpolarization as intracellular sodium is exchanged for extracellular potassium. With no specific therapy the serum potassium levels return to normal after several hours. The measured hemoglobin/hematocrit also declines during β-sympathomimetic treatment. This is due to hydration, intravascular recruitment of extravascular fluid, and inhibition of renal sodium excretion. Common side effects include nausea and vomiting, headache, tremor, nervousness, and palpitations, but these are usually mild. β-Sympathomimetic drugs have been associated with serious complications including cardiac arrhythmia, ketoacidosis, cerebral vasospasm (in patients with a migraine history), hypotension (especially in the face of maternal hemorrhage), angina, and, rarely, maternal death.

The complication that has received the most attention, yet remains most elusive in etiology, is pulmonary edema. This potentially serious side effect has been reported for all the major β-sympathomimetics including fenoterol, ritodrine, and terbutaline. The causes of pulmonary edema have not been established; however, some clinical associations have been identified. Pulmonary edema is unusual with periods of drug use under 12 hours. Further, patients with pulmonary edema are frequently found to be overhydrated, experience prolonged tachycardia, and may have complications of amnionitis. Large doses of epinephrine are known to produce pulmonary edema in both human and animal models. In dogs, this effect is apparently the result of ventricular failure, although evidence for this in humans is lacking. In studies involving direct intravascular pressure measurements with flow-directed, balloon-tipped catheters, normal pulmonary capillary wedge and pulmonary artery pressures have been recorded in patients with β-mimetic associated pulmonary congestion. These data with concomitant evidence of increased cardiac output and *enhanced* ventricular performance do not indicate cardiac failure. In patients with both ritodrine and terbutaline-induced pulmonary edema, normal pulmonary capillary artery wedge pressures, evidence of increased cardiac output, and enhanced ventricular performance without evidence of ventricular failure have been observed. Further, the onset and rapid recovery of patients with β-mimetic-related pulmonary edema is not consistent with membrane injury (e.g., adult respiratory distress syndrome) as seen in clinical settings. The best evidence implies that progressive transudation of fluid across pulmonary capillaries, aided by vascular overexpansion and declining colloid osmotic pressure, is the major factor in promoting pulmonary congestion. All clinical evidence points toward a relatively slow process that close observation can frequently detect and prevent.

Treatment of β-mimetic pulmonary edema should not be directed to enhancing myocardial contractility but, instead, to reducing heart rate and cardiac output demands by judicious use of diuretics and termination of β-mimetic therapy. The principal treatment for pulmonary edema is avoidance. Most often edema occurs in a subclass of patients who have had prolonged drug administration accompanied by moderate to generous fluid infusion, with a corresponding decline in central hematocrit and, not infrequently, drug-induced hypokalemia. Therefore parenteral β-mimetic administration beyond 12 hours must be closely monitored with careful attention given to the patient's symptoms. Persisting, symptomatic tachycardia, restlessness, complaints of dyspnea, and clinical findings of bronchial breath sounds are all signs of a patient who is being pressed too vigorously, and infusion should be stopped or tapered. If pulmonary edema develops, the correct treatment is symptomatic. The infusion should be stopped, oxygen administered, and the parturient sat upright. Although small doses of furosemide (10 to 20 mg) may be administered, they are not often required. Digitalis, corticosteroids, dopamine, and a number of other potentially dangerous agents have been administered to these women. However, such polypharmacy is usually unnecessary and may be dangerous. The practice at MacDonald Hospital is to restrict intravenous fluids to 2 L per 24 hours in patients treated with β-mimetics and to restrain from treating women parenterally for more than 12 hours. These changes alone and an increased attention to patient symptoms have resulted in virtual disappearance of pulmonary edema as a complication of tocolysis.

The reported association between pulmonary edema and corticosteroid administration is accidental. Most patients who developed pulmonary edema were treated aggressively to prevent delivery for short time spans, thus permitting an enhancement of fetal pulmonic maturity. Therefore clinicians may have preselected patients for tocolysis with a particular goal in mind. In this setting, practitioners have been more willing to continue aggressive tocolysis in the face of increasing maternal symptoms than they would have been in the absence of corticosteroid treatment.

The serious and sometimes fatal cardiovascular complications associated with β-mimetics are due to their use in patients with unrecognized cardiovascular disease or to heroic attempts to control premature uterine activity. As mentioned previously, both terbutaline and ritodrine lose beta selectivity at higher dose ranges, and they may exhibit potent inotropic and chonotropic effects as the infusion rate increases. Since rate and contractility

Clinical management of patients undergoing β-mimetic tocolysis

- Frequent vital signs (every 30 min to 1 hour)
- Close observation of intake and output (total intake of <2,000 ml/24 hours)
- Continuous monitoring of uterine activity and fetal heart rate
- Careful notation of maternal signs and symptoms (shortness of breath, chest pain, tachycardia)
- Initial serum electrolytes and blood glucose (repeat at 1 to 3 hours)

are important determinants of myocardial oxygen demand, β-mimetics should be used sparingly, if at all, in patients with arrhythmias or structural and ischemic heart disease. Serious problems with hyperglycemia also can complicate β-mimetic therapy. These drugs should rarely be administered to insulin-requiring diabetics. Occasionally the administration of these agents may also unmask class A diabetes. Thus care also should be exercised in apparently normal patients, since vigorous β-mimetic therapy may evoke rapid onset of hyperglycemia in women who have no documented prior history of glucose intolerance. Coadministration of corticosteroids will enhance this effect. All patients receiving these drugs need a baseline blood glucose determination before initiating infusion, one or more repeated determinations after several hours of therapy, and especially close monitoring (see boxed material).

Prostaglandin synthetase inhibitors

As a result of the major importance of prostaglandins in the initiation of parturition, it is not surprising that various prostaglandin synthetase inhibitors have been investigated as potential tocolytics. Clinical evidence for the effects of synthetase inhibitors on labor was first observed in patients undergoing high-dose acetylsalicylic acid therapy during pregnancy. Both the average length of gestation and the mean duration of spontaneous labor were significantly lengthened in the aspirin-taking women. A number of additional studies have indicated clinical efficacy as tocolytic agents for several newer, more potent synthetase inhibitors, including naproxen, indomethacin, and flufenamic acid.

Clinical interest in the use of prostaglandin inhibitors has been slowed by concern over potential neonatal complications, particularly premature closure of the ductus arteriosus. Other concerns have centered on maternal side effects. Because of their important effects on platelet adhesiveness, these drugs are contraindicated in women with known bleeding disorders, aspirin allergy, and chronic renal or gastrointestinal disease (e.g., peptic ulcer). Prostaglandin inhibitors also have a potent antipyretic effect that might mask infection.

The drug most studied has been indomethacin (Table 9-3). Oral or rectal administration produces effective pharmacologic levels with peak plasma concentrations occurring 1 to 2 hours after administration. The potential complications of prostaglandin inhibitors restrain most clinicians from their use. Yet brief courses with the protocols described by Neibyl and Dudley have proved effective and have not produced significant maternal or neonatal complications. As long as the drug administration is relatively brief, mild maternal gastrointestinal side effects are those most frequently observed. The advantages of oral administration for a potent tocolytic are substantial, since potential problems with excessive intravenous hydration and the expense and problems associated with maintenance of intravenous lines can thus be avoided.

The principal neonatal problems associated with the administration of prostaglandin inhibitors have been persistent fetal circulation, premature closure of the ductus arteriosus, and neonatal platelet dysfunction. Persistent fetal circulation is a syndrome with a number of recognized causes including perinatal asphyxia, sepsis, and pulmonary hypoplasia—all of which may occur independent of drug therapy (see Chapter 29). There is evidence that administration of prostaglandin synthetase inhibitors to pregnant animals is followed by in utero ductal closure. In rats differences are observed in drug sensitivity, indicating less marked effects in premature versus mature animals. This may be due to maturational differences in the ability of indomethacin to cross the placenta. Thus placental transport of drugs, rather than changing sensitivity of the ductus arteriosus, may be the telling factor.

Both prostaglandins E_1 and $F_{2\alpha}$ promote dilation of the ductus arteriosus in newborns. In normal fetal physiology, as gestation proceeds, the ductus becomes progressively sensitive to oxygen. The effects of oxygen exposure are mediated apparently by prostaglan-

Table 9-3. Administration of tocolytics: second line drugs

	Dosage/timing	Comments
Indomethacin (Indocin and Indo-Lemmon)	100 mg by suppository, repeat every 1 to 2 hours; thereafter 25 mg orally every 6 to 8 doses 50 mg orally at once, then 25 mg every 4 hours for 6 doses	Best treatment schedule is not established; at present only brief courses are suggested
Diazoxide (Hyperstat)	5 mg/kg dose administered at 0.5 mg/kg per minute; repeat in 2 to 4 hours as required	Close cardiovascular monitoring is required Preadministration hydration with 500 ml of an isotonic solution is appropriate
Ethanol	Initial: 7.5 ml/kg body weight/2 hours Maintenance: 1.5 ml/kg body weight/hour for 10 hours	Desired blood concentration is 0.12% to 0.18% by breathalyzer, or 155 mg/dl by blood determination

dins. When the neonate breaths, oxygen tension rises, prostaglandin levels decline, and ductal closure occurs. Since this response to rising oxygen tension is less well developed in the premature infant, the higher incidence of incomplete ductal closure is expected (Chapter 29).

There is also concern about the effects of prostaglandin synthetase inhibitors on renal function. In nonpregnant women, indomethacin decreases the glomerular filtration rate and lowers plasma renin activity. In a study of the long-term administration of indomethacin to rhesus monkeys, Novy noted adverse effects on renal development. Although chronic drug administration was associated with a 50% fetal mortality, oligohydramnios, meconium staining, and maternal anemia, such effects have not been reported in humans.

Theoretically, prostaglandin inhibitors might promote increases in maternal blood loss with parturition as a result of the inhibition of platelet adhesiveness and uterine contractility. Aspirin has been implicated as a risk in hemorrhage because of its irreversible inactivation of cyclooxygenase in the prostaglandin biosynthesis pathway. Other nonsteroidal antiinflammatory agents such as indomethacin act reversibly, and presumably their use results in less severe effects on maternal and fetal platelet function. Most of these concerns are theoretic and have no real clinical consequence.

There are recent clinical data to place these concerns in context. In Dudley's study involving 167 patients, no evidence was noted of neonatal platelet dysfunction, persistent fetal circulation, or premature closure of the ductus. Only three patients (1.7%) were observed with postpartum hemorrhage. Further, these women delivered more than 4 weeks after receiving the drug. Thus indomethacin was highly unlikely to be the cause of their bleeding disorder.

The proper role for indomethacin and other prostaglandin inhibitors in the inhibition of preterm labor is unsettled. Although the total number of cases treated approaches 700, several different agents, including naproxen, indomethacin, flufenamic acid, and aspirin, have been administered by varying dosage schedules and usually in an uncontrolled manner. Maternal side effects have been minimal, usually restricted to gastrointestinal upset. The studies vary so greatly in dosage schedule and route of administration, choice of patients, and gestational ages that it is difficult to draw firm conclusions to facilitate comparison of this agent with other available substances. Dudley and Neibyl present persuasive evidence that brief periods of indomethacin administration in pregnancies before 33 to 34 weeks of gestational age are effective and do not result in significant maternal or fetal side effects. Indomethacin deserves consideration as a second-line tocolytic agent. Other synthetase inhibitors need to be investigated for tocolytic effect before a totally acceptable prostaglandin inhibitor is identified for widespread clinical use.

Other agents

A number of compounds including ethanol, isoxsuprine, calcium channel blockers, and diazoxide are in limited clinical use as tocolytics (Table 9-3). Extensive literature attests to the efficacy of ethanol in inhibiting uterine activity, but this compound is not used commonly. Alcohol infusion results in maternal intoxication and is associated with lower Apgar scores and a higher incidence of neonatal RDS, if delivery occurs before the ethanol load can be metabolized. Isoxsuprine was the first β-mimetic to be widely used as a tocolytic. It has been almost entirely superseded in the United States by the newer β-mimetics, principally as a result of its occasionally adverse neonatal (RDS, hypocalcemia, and hypotension) and maternal side effects (hypotension). This combination of side effects for both ethanol and isoxsuprine is unacceptable when compared with results with newer drugs. There is little current justification for their use as primary agents.

Investigation of diazoxide and newer calcium channel blockers is promising and may identify drugs useful as future tocolytics. Diazoxide is a compound of high plasma protein affinity, chemically derived from thiazide diuretics. Presently it is the only antihypertensive agent known to have tocolytic effects. It is believed that diazoxide activates adenylcyclase, reducing the activity of myosin light-chain kinase and leading to myometrial relaxation. The drug is nonselective and inhibits contraction of all smooth muscle. Metabolically, this compound inhibits insulin secretion, reduces cellular glucose uptake, and enhances sodium reabsorption. With the exception of transient hyperglycemia with episodic use, these effects are not clinically significant. Diazoxide differs from other tocolytic agents in that, when it is given in intermittent infusions, the tocolytic effect extends beyond the biologic half-life of the agent.

Diazoxide is administered by intravenous infusion at a dose of 5 mg/kg at a rate of 0.5 mg/kg per minute. Before infusion the patient's intravascular volume is expanded with 500 ml of isotonic saline. Close cardiovascular monitoring is required. If labor recurs in less than 2 hours after the initial infusion, no further tocolytic therapy is administered. However, if labor recurs after 2 to 4 hours, the diazoxide infusion is repeated. Diazoxide has been associated with development of pulmonary edema. As with the β-mimetics, the incidence of pulmonary complication is low and appears to be related to the total volume of fluid infused.

Adamsons and Wallach report insignificant side effects from the infusion of diazoxide, noting a mean fall in maternal diastolic pressure of 23% and systolic pressure of 13%, accompanied by mild increases in heart rate.

During the monitoring of more than 300 cases of diazoxide administration, no abnormal fetal heart rate patterns were identified. Minimum adverse neonatal effects were observed with the exception of one case of transient neonatal hyperglycemia. Diazoxide has interesting possibilities as an alternative tocolytic agent, but its potential cardiovascular side effects demand careful maternal observation during administration.

Calcium channel blockers or antagonists are a group of compounds of varying chemical structure that interfere with calcium passage through cell membranes. The various calcium channel antagonists differ substantially in their molecular structure. Their varying effect is believed to be the result of differences in calcium channel receptors. These drugs are effective as tocolytics due to a partially selective effect on smooth muscle. Striated muscle is much more resistant to calcium antagonism than smooth muscle, presumably because of its larger stores of calcium. Clinical study of calcium channel blockers as tocolytics has just begun, and initial investigations show substantial promise. The drug most commonly used is nifedipine. It is administered by giving 30 mg at once, with subsequent doses of 20 mg at intervals of 8 hours or more. Minimum maternal side effects are reported (transient headache, rapid pulse, and flushing) and neonatal complications have not been observed with this regimen, although the number of pregnancies treated is small.

Safety of the calcium channel blockers remains unsettled. In experiments conducted by Ducsay and Novy in which a nifedipine preparation was infused in an awake rhesus monkey, progressive fetal hypoxemia and acidosis developed despite close physiologic monitoring. The exact mechanism responsible is uncertain. The effects of calcium channel blockers on uterine blood flow and circulation of the placenta need to be carefully reviewed before these drugs are promoted for widespread human use. The selectivity of these agents may be manipulated to develop compounds that are more uterine selective and less permeable into the placenta than currently available drugs. The theoretic potential for calcium channel blockers is great; however, at present, their use in humans should be restricted to short courses of oral administration under experimental protocol until the neonatal effects of parenteral administration are further examined.

Progestational agents

Progesterone is important both in development of myometrial gap junctions and in initiation of anatomic changes in the cervix. Limited evidence indicates reduced progesterone levels in pregnancies complicated by preterm delivery. Thus various progestational agents have been studied as prophylactic agents to block preterm labor. Johnson and co-workers administered 17α-hydroxyprogesterone capronate weekly to 43 patients at high-risk for preterm delivery in a randomized, placebo-controlled study. The study population included women who had prior spontaneous abortions or preterm deliveries. The authors reported that preterm delivery was prevented in 86% of 21 gravidas receiving the drug in contrast to 59% of the 22 women receiving placebo. Perinatal mortality was 27% for the placebo group versus zero in the drug group. No complications were attributed to the use of progesterone. In a subsequent study, the same authors reported on 70 patients. Both prematurity and perinatal mortality were again significantly lower in the treated versus the placebo group. Kauppila studied 24 women in preterm labor, administering intravenous cortisol for 10 days, followed by weekly injections of 17α-hydroxyprogesterone capronate. The steroid treated women were compared with 24 women who received intramuscular and intravenous ritodrine. Although ritodrine was more rapid in terminating preterm labor, delivery was postponed at least 1 week in equal proportions of patients in both groups. Again, no adverse fetal effects were reported for the steroid administration. A similar study of twin pregnancies by Hartikainin-Srri failed to note any benefit from chronic prophylactic administration of 17α-hydroxyprogesterone capronate.

Yemini and co-workers reported on a prospective randomized study of 80 women whose previous obstetric history included two preterm deliveries, two spontaneous miscarriages, or a combination of both. Patients were randomly divided into groups. One group was given weekly injections of 250 mg 17α-hydroxyprogesterone capronate, the second received a placebo injection. The physicians and nurses were blinded to the agent given. Interestingly, a cervical cerclage was performed in all women as soon as the fetal heart tones were audible by Doppler fetascope. The incidence of miscarriage and premature rupture of membranes was not statistically significant between groups, but what the authors described as "imminent premature delivery" (evidence of preterm labor) occurred in a significantly smaller number of patients in the treated group (29%) than in the control group (59%). Also, the rate of actual premature delivery was significantly lower in the treatment group (16.1%) than in the control group (37.8%). There were no perinatal deaths or fetal malformations in either group.

The role for progestational agents in preterm labor management is unclear. Prophylatic therapy suggested by Johnson and co-workers has not achieved popularity, as a result of concerns over the use of progestational agents in early pregnancy. However, treatment with progestational compounds after the first trimester deserves some consideration in patients with histories of preterm delivery, documented fetal normality, and the absence of uterine anomalies. Further, recent study indicates such treatment is safe for fetal development. Whether combinations of parenteral progestational agents will prove useful to control active labor remains unsettled.

CONCLUSIONS

As Hobel points out, the incidence of low birth weight in the United States has remained essentially stable since the 1970s. It is clear that perinatal mortality has declined in the United States, largely as a result of better survival statistics for preterm infants. Neonatal care has improved rapidly, albeit at great expense, ensuring better care for cases where tocolysis fails or is inappropriate. Thus many very premature infants (1,000 gm or less) who would have been lost or severely damaged in years past are now saved.

The problem in our attempts to control preterm labor is that many of the causes of prematurity are embedded in social and economic factors that are difficult for clinicians to influence effectively. We have reached the point in which there is widespread availability of potent tocolytic agents. However, only a small percentage of the total number of patients in preterm labor are candidates for tocolysis, and further, contractions cannot be inhibited in all patients regardless of the agents used. The challenge now for health workers is to investigate the factors promoting preterm delivery and develop management schemes helpful in prevention. Continued efforts to improve diagnosis and therapy of preterm labor are appropriate but necessarily limited.

The work of Papiernik is useful in directing future efforts. He points out that the significant reductions in preterm delivery observed in his study populations in France occurred in that portion of the population that did not have antecedent histories of hemorrhage, preterm delivery, or hypertension. In patients with these obstetric complications, he was unsuccessful in reducing prematurity. The implication for planning is that preterm delivery prevention must be aimed at a wide population, not simply at the clearly high-risk patient. Programs for prevention of prematurity are not likely to prove successful, unless they are integrated into routine obstetric care.

John P. O'Grady
Jean-Claude Veille

BIBLIOGRAPHY

General

Berkowitz, G.S.: An epidemiologic study of preterm delivery, Am. J. Epidemiol. **113**:81, 1981.

Boylan, P., and O'Driscoll, K.: Improvement in perinatal mortality rate attributed to spontaneous preterm labor without use of tocolytic agents, Am. J. Obstet. Gynecol. **145**:781, 1983.

Creasy, R.K.: Prevention of preterm birth, Birth Defects **19**:97, 1983.

Creasy, R.K.: Gummer, B.A., and Liggins, G.C.: System for predicting spontaneous preterm birth, Obstet. Gynecol. **55**:692, 1980.

Goujon, H., Papiernik, E., and Maine, D.: The prevention of preterm delivery through prenatal care: an intervention study in Martinique, Int. J. Gynaecol. Obstet. **22**:339, 1984.

Goujon, H., and others: Prevention of preterm birth: a perinatal study in Haguenau, France, Pediatrics **76**:154, 1985.

Hemminki, E., and Starfield, B.: Prevention and treatment of preterm labor by drugs: review of controlled clinical trials, Br. J. Obstet. Gynaecol. **85**:411, 1978.

Herron, M.A., Katz, M., and Creasy, R.K.: Evaluation of a preterm birth prevention program: preliminary report, Obstet. Gynecol. **59**:452, 1982.

Hobel, C.J.: Prevention of preterm delivery. In Beard, R.W., and Nathanielex, P.W., editors: Fetal physiology and medicine, New York, 1984, Marcel Dekker, Inc.

Iams, J.D., Johnson, F., and Creasy, R.: Preliminary report of prospective random trial of a preterm birth prevention program, Abstract no. 81, p. 97, Society of Perinatal Obstetricians annual meeting, Las Vegas, Nev., Feb. 1985.

Johnson, J.W.C., and Dubin, N.H.: Prevention of preterm labor, Clin. Obstet. Gynecol. **23**:51, 1980.

Kaltreider, D.F., and Kohl, S.: Epidemiology of preterm delivery, Clin. Obstet. Gynecol. **23**:17, 1980.

Katz, M., Newman, R.B., and Gill, P.J.: Assessment of uterine activity in ambulatory patients at high risk of preterm labor and delivery, Abstract no. 13, p. 29, Society of Perinatal Obstetricians annual meeting, Las Vegas, Nev., 1985.

Maine, D.M., and others: Can preterm deliveries be prevented? Am. J. Obstet. Gynecol. **151**:892, 1985.

Papiernik, E., and Berkhauer, E.: Coefficient de risque d'accouchement premature (C.R.A.P.), Presse. Med. **77**:793, 1969.

Papiernik, E., and Kaminski, M.: Multifactorial study of the risk of prematurity at 32 weeks of gestation. I. A study of the frequency of 30 predictive characteristics, J. Perinat. Med. **2**:30, 1974.

Papiernik, E.: Proposals for a programmed prevention policy of preterm birth, Clin. Obstet. Gynecol. **27**:614, 1984.

Tejani, N.A., and Verma, U.L.: Effect of tocolysis on incidence of low birth weight, Obstet. Gynecol. **61**:556, 1983.

Zlatnik, F.: The applicability of labor inhibition to the problem of prematurity, Am. J. Obstet. Gynecol. **113**:704, 1972.

Labor: physiology

Challis, J.R.G., and Mitchell, B.F.: Hormonal control of preterm and term parturition, Semin. Perinat. **5**:192, 1981.

Cousins, L.M., and others: Serum progesterone and estradiol-17α levels in premature and term labor, Am. J. Obstet. Gynecol. **127**:612, 1977.

Csapo, A.I.: The "seesaw" theory of parturition, Ciba Found. Symp. **47**:159, 1977.

Drover, J.W., and Casper, R.F.: Initiation of parturition in humans, Can. Med. Assoc. J. **128**:387, 1983.

Huszar, G.: Biology and biochemistry of myometrial contractility and cervical maturation, Semin. Perinatol. **5**:216, 1981.

Huszar, G.: Physiology of myometrial contractility and cervical dilatation. In Fuchs, F., and Stubblefield, P.G., editors: Preterm birth: causes, prevention and management, New York, 1984, Macmillan Publishing Co., Inc.

Huszar, G., and Naftolin, F.: The myometrium and uterine cervix in normal and preterm labor, N. Engl. J. Med. **311**:571, 1984.

Liggins, G.C.: Premature delivery of foetal lambs infused with glucocorticoids, J. Endocrinol. **45**:515, 1969.

Liggins, G.C.: Adreno cortical-related maturational events in the fetus, Am. J. Obstet. Gynecol. **126**:931, 1976.

Thornburn, G.D.: Past and present concepts on the initiation of parturition. In MacDonald, P.C., and Porter, J., editors: Initiation of parturition: prevention of prematurity, Report of the fourth Ross Conference on Obstetric Research, Columbus, Ohio, Ross Laboratories, 1983.

Verhoeff, A., and others: Electrical and mechanical uterine activity and gap junctions in peripartal sheep, Am. J. Obstet. Gynecol. **153**:447, 1985.

Preterm labor: etiology

Anderson, A.B.M., and Turnbull, A.C.: Relationship between the length of gestation and cervical dilatation, uterine contractility, and other factors during pregnancy, Am. J. Obstet. Gynecol. **105**:1207, 1969.

Anderson, L.F., and Fuchs, F.: Sexual activity and preterm birth. In Fuchs, F., and Stubblefield, P.G., editors: Preterm birth: causes, prevention, and management, New York, 1984, Macmillan Publishing Co., Inc.

Baker, C.J., Barrett, F.F., and Yow, M.D.: The influence of advancing gestation on group B streptococcal colonization in pregnant women, Am. J. Obstet. Gynecol. **120**:820, 1975.

Bartolucci, L., and others: Ultrasonography in preterm labor, Am. J. Obstet. Gynecol. **149**:52, 1984.

Bejar, R., and others: Premature labor: bacterial sources of phospholipase, Obstet. Gynecol. **57**:479, 1981.

Bell, N.: Prediction of preterm labor by recording spontaneous antenatal uterine activity, Br. J. Obstet. Gynaecol. **90**:884, 1983.

Bobitt, J.R., Hayslip, C.C., and Damateo, J.D.: Amniotic fluid infection as determined by transabdominal amniocentesis in patients with intact membranes in premature labor, Am. J. Obstet. Gynecol. **140**:947, 1971.

Bobitt, J.R., and Ledger, W.J.: Unrecognized amnionitis in prematurity: preliminary report, J. Reprod. Med. **19**:8, 1977.

Boyer, K., and others: Selective intrapartum chemoprophylaxis of neonatal group B streptococcal early-onset disease. I. Epidemiologic rationale, J. Inf. Dis. **148**:795, 1983.

Chin, K., and others: A mean content of vaginal fluid from untreated and treated patients with nonspecific vaginitis, J. Clin. Invest. **68**:828, 1979.

Goodlin, R.C., Schmidt, W., and Creevy, D.L.: Uterine tension and fetal heart rate during maternal orgasm, Obstet. Gynecol. **39**:125, 1972.

Goodrich, J.T.: Pelvic inflammatory disease: consequence related to therapy, Rev. Inf. Dis. (suppl. 788):788, 1982.

Gravett, M.G.: Causes of preterm delivery, Semin. Perinatol. **8**:246, 1984.

Gravett, M.G., and others: Abnormal amniotic fluid in vaginal flora associated with preterm labor, Abstract no. 15, Society of Perinatal Obstetricians, San Antonio, Tex., 1983.

Gravett, M.G., and others: Preterm labor with subclinical amniotic fluid infection and with bacterial vaginosis, Obstet. Gynecol. **67(2)**:229, 1986.

Guzick, D.S., and Winn, K.: The association of chorioamnionitis with preterm delivery, Obstet. Gynecol. **65**:11, 1985.

Hammill, H., Sutter, V., and Citron, D.: Quantitative vaginal cultures in patients with recurrent nonspecific vaginitis and *in-vitro* susceptability (abstract), twenty-third Interscience Conference on Antimicrobial Agents and Chemotherapy, Las Vegas, 1983.

Hawkinson, J.A., and Schulman, H.: Prematurity associated with cervicitis and vaginitis during pregnancy, Am. J. Obstet. Gynecol. **98**:898, 1966.

Heggie, A., and others: *Chlamydia trachomatis* infections in mothers and infants: a prospective study, Am. J. Dis. Child **135**:507, 1981.

Lamont, R.F., Rose, M., and Elder, M.G.: Effect of bacterial products on prostaglandin E production by amnion cells, Lancet **2**:1331, 1985.

Lash, A.F., and Lash, S.R.: Habitual abortion: the incompetent internal os of the cervix, Am. J. Obstet. Gynecol. **59**:68, 1950.

Malmstrom, H., and Axelsson, O.: Results of cervical cerclage operations in pregnant women during a five-year period, Ann. Chir. Gynaecol. **70**:75, 1981.

Martin, D., and others: Prematurity and perinatal mortality in pregnancies complicated by maternal *Chlamydia trachomatis*, JAMA **247**:1585, 1982.

McDonald, I.A.: Suture of the cervix for inevitable abortion, J Obstet. Gynaecol. Br. Emp. **64**:346, 1957.

Naeye, R.L., and Ross, S.: Coitus and chorioamnionitis: a prospective study, Early Hum. Dev. **6**:91, 1982.

Novy, M.J.: Transabdominal cervicoisthmic cerclage for the management of repetitive abortion and premature delivery, Am. J. Obstet. Gynecol. **143**:44, 1982.

Ornoy, A., and others: Placental findings in spontaneous abortions and stillbirths, Semin. Perinatol. **24**:243, 1981.

Papiernik, E., and others: Precocious cervical ripening and preterm labor, Obstet. Gynecol. **67**:238, 1986.

Quinlan, R.W., and Cruz, A.C.: Reproductive failure and cervical incompetence in women exposed to diethylstilbestrol, South Med. J. **73**:89, 1980.

Russell, P.: Inflammatory lesions of the human placenta. I. Clinical significance of acute chorioamnionitis, Am. J. Diag. Gynecol. Obstet. **1**:127, 1979.

Sarrell, P., and Pruett, K.: Symptomatic gonorrhea during pregnancy, Obstet. Gynecol. **32**:670, 1968.

Shirodkar, V.N.: A method of operative treatment for habitual abortions in the second trimester of pregnancy, Antiseptic **52**:299, 1955.

Spiegel, C., and others: Curved anaerobic bacteria in bacterial (nonspecific) vaginosis and the response to antimicrobial therapy, J. Infect. Dis. **148**:817, 1983.

Spielberger, C.D., and Jacobs, G.A.: Stress and anxiety during pregnancy and labor. In Carenza, L., Panchei, P., and Zurchella, L., editors: Clinical psychoneuroendocrinology in reproduction, New York, 1978, Academic Press, Inc.

Stray-Pedersen, B., and Stray-Pedersen, S.: Etiologic factors and subsequent reproductive performance in 195 couples with prior history of habitual abortion, Am. J. Obstet. Gynecol. **148**:140, 1984.

Takahashi, K., and others: Uterine contractility and oxytocin sensitivity in preterm, term, and post-term pregnancy, Am. J. Obstet. Gynecol. **136**:774, 1980.

Wood, K., and others: The prediction of premature labor by observation of the cervix and external tocography, Am. J. Obstet. Gynecol. **91**:396, 1965.

Preterm labor: maturity and corticosteroids

Ballard, P.L., and Ballard, R.A.: Glucocorticoids in prevention of respiratory distress syndrome, Hosp. Pract. **81**:87, 1980.

Berkowitz, R.L., and others: Results of a management protocol for premature rupture of the membranes, Obstet. Gynecol. **60**:271, 1982.

Clements, J.A., and others: Assessment of the risk of the RDS by a rapid test for surfactant in the amniotic fluid (shake test), N. Engl. J. Med. **286**:1077, 1972.

Collaborative Group on Antenatal Steroid Therapy: Effective antenatal dexamethasone administration on the prevention of respiratory distress syndrome, Am. J. Obstet. Gynecol. **141**:276, 1981.

Doran, T.A., and others: Results of double blind control study on the use of betamethasone in the prevention of respiratory distress syndrome, Am. J. Obstet. Gynecol. **136**:313, 1980.

Epstein, M.E., and Farrell, P.M.: The choline incorporation pathway: primary mechanism for *de novo* synthesis in fetal primate lung, Pediatr. Res. **9**:658, 1975.

Fuller, W.E.: Management of premature labor, Clin. Obstet. Gynecol. **21**:533, 1978.

Garite, T.J.: Obstetrical prematurity, World Symposium of Perinatal Medicine, Washington, D.C., Sept. 8-12, 1984.

Gluck, L., and Kulovich, M.V.: Lecithin/sphingomyelin ratios in amniotic fluid in normal and abnormal pregnancy, Am. J. Obstet. Gynecol. **115**:539, 1973.

Gluck, L., and others: Diagnosis of the respiratory distress syndrome by amniocentesis, Am. J. Obstet. Gynecol. **109**:440, 1971.

Hallman, M., Feldman, B., and Gluck, L.: RDS: the absence of phosphatidylglycerol in surfactant, Pediatr. Res. **9**:936, 1975.

Iams, J.D., and Barrows, H.: Management of preterm, prematurely ruptured membranes: a retrospective comparison of observation versus use of steroids in timed delivery, Am. J. Obstet. Gynecol. **150**:977, 1984.

Iams, J.D., and others: Management of preterm prematurely ruptured membranes: a prospective randomized comparison of observation versus use of steroids and timed delivery, Am. J. Obstet. Gynecol. **151**:32, 1985.

Jeanty, P., and Romero, R. Obstetrical ultrasound, New York, 1984, McGraw-Hill, Inc.

Johnson, J.W.C.: Betamethasone: do side effects outweigh benefits? Contrib. Gynecol. Obstet. **15**:195, 1980.

Johnson, J.W.C., Mitzner, W., and Beck, J.C.: Long-term effects of betamethasone on fetal development, Am. J. Obstet. Gynecol. **141**:1053, 1981.

Johnson, J.W.C., and others: Betamethasone and the rhesus fetus: multisystemic effects, Am. J. Obstet. Gynecol. **133**:677, 1979.

Johnson, J.W.C., and others: High risk prematurity: progestin treatment and steroid studies, Obstet. Gynecol. **54**:412, 1979.

Kessler, D.L., and others: Experimental hyaline membrane disease in the premature monkey, Am. Rev. Respir. Dis. **126**:62, 1982.

Liggins, G.C., and Howie, R.N.: A controlled trial of antepartum glucocorticoid treatment for prevention of the respiratory distress syndrome in premature infants, Pediatrics **50**:515, 1972.

Lipshitz, J., Whybrew, W.D., and Anderson, G.D.: Comparison of Lumadex-Foam stability index test, lecithin:sphingomyelin ratio, and simple shake test for fetal lung maturity, Obstet. Gynecol. **63**:349, 1984.

Morrison, J.C., and others: Injection of corticosteroids into mother to prevent neonatal respiratory distress syndrome, Am. J. Obstet. Gynecol. **131**:358, 1978.

O'Grady, J.P.: Control of uterine activity: a clinical approach. In Rathi, M.V., editor: Clinical aspects of perinatal medicine, New York, 1985, Macmillan Publishing Co., Inc.

Papageorgiou, A.N., and others: The antenatal use of betamethasone in the prevention of respiratory distress syndrome: a controlled, double blind study, Pediatrics **63**:73, 1979.

Papageorgiou, A.N., and others: Incidence of respiratory distress syndrome following antenatal betamethasone: role of sex, type of delivery, and prolonged rupture of membranes, Pediatrics **67**:614, 1981.

Plauche, W.C., Faro, S., and Letellier, R.: Phosphatidylglycerol and fetal lung maturity, Am. J. Obstet. Gynecol. **144**:167, 1982.

Resnik, R.: Phospholipid analysis of amniotic fluid in maternal-fetal medicine. In Creasey, R.K., and Resnik, R., editors: Principles and practice, Philadelphia, 1984, W.B. Saunders, Co.

Sbarra, A.J., and others: Relation between optical density at 650 nm and L/S ratio, Obstet. Gynecol. **50**:723, 1977.

Sher, G., and Statland, B.E.: Assessment of fetal pulmonary maturity by the lumadex-foam stability index test, Obstet. Gynecol. **61**:444, 1983.

Shields, J.R., and Resnik, R.: Fetal lung maturation and the antenatal use of glucocorticoids to prevent the respiratory distress syndrome, Obstet. Gynecol. Surv. **34**:343, 1969.

Simon, N.V., and others: Prediction of fetal lung maturity by amniotic fluid fluorescence polarization, L/S ratio, and phosphatidylglycerol, Obstet. Gynecol. **57**:295, 1981.

Singh, E.J., Nejia, A., and Zuspan, F.P.: Studies of human amniotic fluid phospholipids in normal, diabetic and drug abuse pregnancies, Am. J. Obstet. Gynecol. **119**:623, 1974.

Socol, M.L., and others: Effect of corticosteroids on the lecithin/sphingomyelin ratio in the rhesus monkey, Am. J. Obstet. Gynecol. **140**:709, 1981.

Sumi, S.M., Truog, W.E., and Kessler, D.M.: Maternal corticosteroid therapy and the fetal brain in experimental hyaline membrane disease, Pediatr. Res. **18**:440, 1984.

Tauesch, H.W.: Glucocorticoid prophylaxis for respiratory distress syndrome: a review of potential toxicity, J. Pediatr. **87**:617, 1975.

Tauesch, H.W., and others: Risk of respiratory distress syndrome after prenatal dexamethasone treatment, Pediatrics **63**:64, 1979.

Tropper, P.J., and Petrie, R.A.: Corticosteroids to prevent RDS? Contrib. Gynecol. Obstet. **19**:177, 1982.

Valenzuela, G., Cline, S., and Hayaski, R.H.: Follow-up of hydration and sedation in the pretherapy of premature labor, Am. J. Obstet. Gynecol. **147**:396, 1983.

Weichsel, M.R.: Therapeutic use of glucocorticoid hormones in the prenatal period: potential neurological hazards, Ann. Neurol. **2**:364, 1977.

Whitt, G.G., and others: A comparison of two glucocorticoid regimens for acceleration of fetal lung maturation in premature labor, Am. J. Obstet. Gynecol. **124**:479, 1976.

Whittle, M.J., and others: Amniotic fluid phosphatidylglycerol and the lecithin/sphingomyelin ratio in the assessment of fetal lung maturity, Br. J. Obstet. Gynaecol. **89**:727, 1982.

Preterm labor: treatment

Abramovich, H., and others: Maternal pulmonary edema occurring after therapy with ritodrine for premature uterine contractions, Acta Obstet. Gynecol. Scand. **59**:555, 1980.

Adamsons, K., and Wallach, R.C.: Diazoxide and calcium antagonists in preterm labor. In Fuchs, F., and Stubblefield, P.G., editors: Preterm birth: causes, prevention, and management, New York, 1984, Macmillan Publishing Co., Inc.

Andersson, K.E., and others: Inhibition of prostaglandin-induced uterine activity by nifedipine, Br. J. Obstet. Gynaecol. **86**:175, 1979.

Barden, T.P., Peter, J.B., and Merkatz, I.R.: Ritodrine hydrochloride: a beta mimetic agent for use in preterm labor. I. Pharmacology, clinical history, administration, side effects, and safety, Obstet. Gynecol. **56**:1, 1980.

Benedetti, T.J.: Maternal complications of parenteral β-sympathomimetic therapy for premature labor, Am. J. Obstet. Gynecol. **145**:1, 1983.

Brezy, J.E., Little, V., and Grimm, J.: Isoxuprine in the perinatal period. II. Relationships between neonatal symptoms, drug exposure, and drug concentration at the time of birth, Pediatrics **98**:146, 1981.

Brezy, J.E., and others: Risk/benefit considerations for the use of isoxuprine in the treatment of premature labor, Obstet. Gynecol. **58**:207, 1981.

Brodey, P.A., Fisch, A.E., and Huffaker, J.: Acute pulmonary edema resulting from treatment for premature labor, Radiology **140**:631, 1981.

Brown, E.R., Torday, J.S., and Tauesch, H.W.: Pharmacologic control of fetal lung development, Clin. Perinatol. **5**:243, 1978.

Caspi, E., and Schreyer, P.: Prevention of respiratory distress syndrome by antepartum dexamethasone, Lancet **1**:973, 1976.

Creasy, R.K., and Katz, M.: Basic research in clinical experience with beta-adrenergic tocolytics in the United States. In Fuchs, F., and Stubblefield, P.G., editors: Preterm birth: causes, prevention, and management, New York, 1984, Macmillan Publishing Co., Inc.

Csapo, A.I., and Herczog, J.: Arrest of premature labor by isoxuprine, Am. J. Obstet. Gynecol. **129:**482, 1977.

Csapo, A.I., and others: Deactivation of the uterus during normal and premature labor by the calcium antagonist nicardipine, Am. J. Obstet. Gynecol. **142:**483, 1982.

Dangman, B.C., and Rosen, D.S.: Magnesium levels in infants or mothers treated with $MgSO_4$, Pediatr. Res. **11:**415, 1977.

Desir, D., and others: Ritodrine-induced acidosis in pregnancy, Br. Med. J. **2:**1194, 1978.

Domenichini, Y., and Thoulon, J.M.: The cardiovascular complications of the use of beta mimetic drugs in obstetrics, J. Gynecol. Obstet. Biol. Reprod. **11:**861, 1982.

Ducsay, C.A., and others: Nifedipine tocolysis in pregnant rhesus monkeys: maternal and fetal cardiorespiratory effects, Abstract no. 79, Society of Perinatal Obstetricians annual meeting, Las Vegas, Nev., Feb., 1985.

Dudley, D.K.L., and Hardie, M.J.: Fetal and neonatal effects of indomethacin used as a tocolytic agent, Am. J. Obstet. Gynecol. **151:**181, 1985.

Elliott, H.R., and Abdulla, U.: Pulmonary edema associated with ritodrine infusion and betamethasone administration in premature labor, Br. Med. J. **2:**799, 1978.

Elliott, J.P.: Magnesium sulfate as a tocolytic agent, Am. J. Obstet. Gynecol. **147:**277, 1983.

Ersoz, N., and Finestone, S.C.: Adrenaline-induced pulmonary edema and its treatment: a report of two cases, Br. J. Anaesth. **43:**709, 1971.

Finley, J., and others: Cardiovascular consequences of beta-agonist tocolysis: an echocardiographic study, Obstet. Gynecol. **64:**787, 1984.

Forman, A., Andersson, K.E., and Ulmsten, U.: Inhibition of myometrial activity by calcium antagonists, Semin. Perinatol. **5:**288, 1981.

Freyze, H., and others: A long term evaluation of infants who received a beta mimetic drug while *in utero*, J. Perinat. Med. **5:**94, 1977.

Fuchs, F., and Fuchs, A.R.: Ethanol for the prevention of preterm birth. In Fuchs, F., and Stubblefield, P.G., editors: Preterm birth: causes, prevention, and management, New York, 1984, Macmillan Publishing Co., Inc.

Garite, T.J., and others: Prospective randomized study of corticosteroids in the management of premature rupture of the membranes and premature gestation, Am. J. Obstet. Gynecol. **141:**508, 1981.

Garite, T.J., and others: A new rapid slide agglutination test for amniotic fluid PG: laboratory and clinical correlation, Am. J. Obstet. Gynecol. **147:**681, 1983.

Gross, T.L.: How tocolytics affect mother, fetus, and neonate, Contemp. Obstet. Gynecol. **19:**1, 1982.

Guernsey, B.G., and others: Pulmonary edema associated with the use of beta mimetic agents in preterm labor, Am. J. Hosp. Pharm. **38:**1942, 1981.

Hartikainin-Srri, A.L., Kauppila, A., and Tuimala, R.: Inefficacy of 17α-hydroxyprogesterone capronate in the prevention of prematurity in twin pregnancy, Obstet. Gynecol. **56:**692, 1980.

Hatjis, C.G., and others: Addition of magnesium sulfate improves effectiveness of ritodrine in preventing premature delivery, Am. J. Obstet. Gynecol. **150:**142, 1984.

Hawker, F.: Five cases of pulmonary oedema associated with B_2 sympathomimetic treatment of premature labor, Anaesth. Intensive Care **12:**159, 1984.

Hosenpud, J.D., Morton, M.J., and O'Grady, J.P.: Cardiac stimulation during ritodrine hydrochloride tocolytic therapy, Obstet. Gynecol. **62:**52, 1983.

Huisjes, H.J., and Touwen, B.C.L.: Neonatal outcome after treatment with ritodrine: a controlled study, Am. J. Obstet. Gynecol. **147:**250, 1983.

Ingemarsson, I.: Effect of terbutaline on premature labor, Am. J. Obstet. Gynecol. **125:**520, 1976.

Ingemarrson, I.: Use of β-receptor agonists in obstetrics, Acta Obstet. Gynecol. Scand. (suppl.) **108:**29, 1982.

Ingemarrson, I., and Bengtsson, B.: A five year experience with terbutaline for preterm labor: low rate of severe side effects, Obstet. Gynecol. **66:**176, 1985.

Johnson, J.W.C., Austin, K.L., and Jones, G.S.: Efficacy of 17α-hydroxyprogesterone capronate in the prevention of premature labor, N. Engl. J. Med. **293:**675, 1975.

Karlsson, K.: β-receptor agonists in pregnancy: long term effects in preterm children, Acta Obstet. Gynecol. Scand. (suppl.) **108:**71, 1982.

Katz, M., Robertson, P.A., and Creasy, R.K.: Cardiovascular complications associated with terbutaline treatment for premature labor, Am. J. Obstet. Gynecol. **139:**605, 1981.

Katz, Z., and others: Teratogenicity of progestogens given during the first trimester of pregnancy, Obstet. Gynecol. **65:**775, 1985.

Kaul, A.F., and others: The management of preterm labor with a calcium channel blocking agent nifedipine combined with a beta mimetic terbutaline, Drug Intell. Clin. Pharm. **19:**369, 1985.

Kauppila, A., and others: Suppression of threatened premature labor by administration of cortisol and 17α-hydroxyprogesterone capronate: comparison with ritodrine, Am. J. Obstet. Gynecol. **138:**404, 1980.

Kirkpatrick, C., Quenon, M., and Desir, D.: Blood anions and electrolytes during ritodrine infusion in preterm labor, Am. J. Obstet. Gynecol. **138:**523, 1980.

Korenbrot, C.C., Aalto, L.H., and Laros, R.K.: The cost-effectiveness of stopping preterm labor with beta-adrenergic treatment, N. Engl. Med. **310:**691, 1984.

Landesman, R., and others: The inhibitory effect of diazoxide in normal term labor, Am. J. Obstet. Gynecol. **103:**430, 1969.

Lewis, R.B., and Schulman, J.D.: Influence of acetylsalicylic acid, an inhibitor of prostaglandin synthesis, on the duration of human gestation and labor, Lancet **2:**1159, 1973.

Lipshitz, J.: Beta-adrenergic agonists, Semin. Perinatol. **5:**252, 1981.

Lipsitz, P.J.: The clinical and biochemical effects of excess magnesium in the newborn, Pediatrics **57:**501, 1971.

Maclennan, F.M., and others: Fatal pulmonary oedema associated with the use of ritodrine in pregnancy. Case Report, Br. J. Obstet. Gynaecol. **92:**703, 1985.

McAllister, R.G.: Clinical pharmacokinetics of calcium channel antagonists, J. Cardiovasc. Pharmacol. (suppl.) **4:**340, 1982.

Merkatz, I.R., Peter, J.B., and Barden, T.P.: Ritodrine hydrochloride: a beta mimetic agent for use in preterm labor. II. Evidence of efficacy, Obstet. Gynecol. **56:**7, 1980.

Miller, J.M., Jr., Keane, M.W.D., and Horger, E.O.: A comparison of magnesium sulfate and terbutaline for the arrest of premature labor: a preliminary report, J. Reprod. Med. **27:**348, 1982.

Milliez, J., and Sureau, C.: A case report of maternal death associated with beta mimetics and betamethasone administration in premature labour, Eur. J. Obstet. Gynaecol. Reprod. Biol. **11:**95, 1980.

Neibyl, J.R.: Drugs for inhibition of premature labor, Clin. Pharmacol. **6:**53, 1979.

Neibyl, J.R.: Prostaglandin synthetase inhibitors, Semin. Perinatol. **5:**274, 1981.

Neibyl, J.R., and Johnson, J.W.C.: Inhibition of preterm labor, Clin. Obstet. Gynecol. **23:**115, 1980.

Neibyl, J.R., and others: The inhibition of premature labor with indomethacin, Am. J. Obstet. Gynecol. **136:**1014, 1980.

Novy, M.J., and Liggins, G.C.: Role of prostaglandins, prostacyclin and thromboxanes in the physiologic control of the uterus and in parturition, Semin. Perinatol. **4**:45, 1980.

Petrie, R.H.: Stopping premature labor with magnesium sulfate, Contemp. Obstet. Gynecol. **11**:187, 1978.

Petrie, R.H.: Tocolysis using magnesium sulfate, Semin. Perinatol. **5**:266, 1981.

Philipsen, T., Eriksen, P.S., and Lynggard, F.: Pulmonary edema following ritodrine-saline infusion in premature labor, Obstet. Gynecol. **58**:304, 1981.

Polowczyk, D., and others: Evaluation of seven to nine year-old children exposed to ritodrine *in utero*, Obstet. Gynecol. **64**:485, 1984.

Schenken, R.S., and others: Treatment of premature labor with beta sympathomimetics: results with isoxuprine, Am. J. Obstet. Gynecol. **137**:773, 1980.

Schilthnis, M.S., and Aarnoudse, J.G.: Fetal death associated with severe ritodrine induced ketoacidosis, Lancet **1**:1145, 1980.

Shinitzky, M., and others: A new method for assessment of fetal lung maturity, Br. J. Obstet. Gynaecol. **83**:838, 1976.

Souney, P.F., Kaul, A.F., and Osathanondh, R.: Pharmacotherapy of preterm labor, Clin. Pharm. **2**:29, 1983.

Spellacy, W.N., and others: The acute effects of ritodrine infusion on maternal metabolism measurements of levels of glucose, insulin, glucagon, triglycerides, cholesterol, placental lactogen, and chorionic gonadotropin, Am. J. Obstet. Gynecol. **131**:637, 1978.

Spellacy, W.N., and others: Treatment of premature labor with ritodrine: a randomized controlled study, Obstet. Gynecol. **54**:220, 1979.

Spisso, K.R., Harbert, G.M., and Thiagarajah, S.: The use of magnesium sulfate as the primary tocolytic agent to prevent premature delivery, Am. J. Obstet. Gynecol. **142**:840, 1982.

Steer, C.M., and Petrie, R.H.: A comparison of magnesium sulfate and alcohol for the prevention of premature labor, Am. J. Obstet. Gynecol. **128**:1, 1977.

Stone, S.R., and Pritchard, J.A.: Effects of maternally administered magnesium sulfate on the neonate, Obstet. Gynecol. **35**:574, 1970.

Stubblefield, P.G.: Neonatal effects of tocolytic therapy. In Fuchs, F., and Stubblefield, P.G., editors: Preterm birth: causes, prevention, and management, New York, 1984, Macmillan Publishing Co., Inc.

Stubblefield, P.G., and Heyl, P.S.: Treatment of premature labor with subcutaneous terbutaline, Obstet. Gynecol. **59**:457, 1982.

Tinga, D.J., and Aarnoudse, J.G.: Post-partum pulmonary edema associated with preventative therapy for premature labor (letter), Lancet **1**:1026, 1070.

Tye, K.H., Desser, K.B., and Benchimol, A.: Angina pectoris associated with use of terbutaline for premature labor, JAMA **224**:692, 1980.

Ulmsten, U.: Treatment of normotensive and hypertensive patients with preterm labor using oral nifedipine, a calcium antagonist, Arch. Gynecol. **236**:69, 1984.

Ulmsten, U., Andersson, K.E., and Wingerup, L.: Treatment of premature labor with the calcium antagonist nifedipine, Arch. Gynecol. **229**:1, 1980.

Van Lierde, M., and others: Administration intraveineuse de ritodrine chez la diabetique insulino-dependante enceinte. J. Gynecol. Obstet. Biol. Reprod. **2**:869, 1982.

Veille, J.C., and others: The effect of a calcium channel blocker (nifedipine) on uterine blood flow in the pregnant goat, Am. J. Obstet. Gynecol. **154**:1160, 1986.

Wesselius-de Casparis, A., and others: Results of double-blind multicentre study with ritodrine in premature labour, Br. Med. J. **3**:144, 1971.

Wilson, K.H., and others: Effects of diazoxide and beta adrenergic drugs in spontaneous and induced uterine activity in the pregnant baboon, Am. J. Obstet. Gynecol. **118**:499, 1974.

Yemini, M., and others: Prevention of premature labor by 17α-hydroxyprogesterone capronate, Am. J. Obstet. Gynecol. **151**:574, 1985.

CHAPTER 10

Obstetric management of multiple pregnancy and postmaturity

MANAGEMENT OF MULTIPLE PREGNANCY

For centuries multiple births have been regarded with mysticism, awe, and apprehension. This concern is well placed. Multiple births account for disproportionately high perinatal morbidity and mortality, caused primarily by the increased likelihood of low birth weight infants as a result of prematurity, intrauterine growth retardation, or both. Congenital malformations, abnormal presentation, and prolapsed umbilical cord also contribute to the excessive risk. In addition, maternal risk is also increased by polyhydramnios, preeclampsia, placenta previa, postpartum hemorrhage, and anemia, which are all more common in multiple than singleton pregnancies.

Twinning normally occurs in approximately 1 of 80 pregnancies; triplets in 1 of 8,000 pregnancies; and the frequency of multiple births of a higher number can be estimated by applying Hellin's hypothesis that the frequency of births of n infants can be expressed by the equation $f = 80^{(n-1)}$. For example, the frequency of quadruplets ($n = 4$) is equal to 80^3 or 1 in 512,000. The frequency of monozygous (MZ) twinning appears to be constant throughout the world (3.5 per 1,000), whereas the frequency of dizygous (DZ) twinning is influenced by a number of factors. Dizygous twinning increases with advancing maternal age and parity and varies with race. (See Chapter 11.)

Because of the widespread use of ovulation-inducing medications, the incidence of multiple gestations in the United States has increased. The use of clomiphene increases the rate of twinning to between 6% and 8% of pregnancies. Gonadotrophin therapy increases the frequency of multiple pregnancy even more.

The perinatal death rate for twin gestations is approximately four times that for singleton pregnancies and increases correspondingly for gestations of higher number. The perinatal death rate for MZ twins is approximately 2.5 times that for DZ twins, and the death rate for monoamniotic twins has been estimated to be as high as 50%. Low birth weight is the major cause of perinatal mortality and morbidity in multiple gestations. McKeown and Record found that the mean birth weight of singletons with a mean gestational age of 280 days is about 3,400 gm, and the mean birth weight of twins with a mean gestational age of 262 days is about 2,400 gm. Triplets have a mean birth weight of 1,800 gm and an average gestation of 247 days. Caspi and associates ascertained precisely the time of ovulation for 111 pregnancies in women whose ovulation was induced. They found the average length of gestation in twin pregnancies was 35 completed weeks and with triplets, 33 completed weeks.

The possible long-term disadvantages that result from multiple pregnancy remain somewhat controversial. In Norway, Nilsen and associates evaluated the physical and intellectual development of male twins at 18 years of age. Compared to singletons, twice as many were found to be physically unfit for military service. They attributed this finding to preterm delivery rather than twinning per se. In the Nilsen study, general intelligence did not appear to be affected. In studying monozygous twins who were dissimilar in size at birth, Babson and Phillips found that the undersized twin continued to be inferior in both growth and intelligence into adult life.

Several significant maternal complications occur more frequently in multiple gestations because the normal maternal physiologic adaptations to pregnancy are greater in multiple gestations. In some cases, such as maternal heart disease, these adaptations may pose a clinically significant increase in risk. For instance, the average increase in maternal blood volume in singleton pregnancies is 40% to 50% in late pregnancy, but the mean increase in twin gestations is 50% to 60%. The incidence of anemia is also increased, in part because of the exaggerated physiologic anemia that results from the greater increase in plasma volume relative to red cell mass. The incidence of pregnancy-induced hypertension rises in multiple gestations, occurring in as many as one third of twin pregnancies. Polyhydramnios accompanies approximately 12% of multiple gestations and is associated with an increased rate of premature labor and congenital anomalies. Premature rupture of the membranes also occurs more frequently in multiple gestations, often leading to premature labor.

Diagnosis

Historically, a large number of twin gestations were not recognized until the time of labor (up to 40% to 50% in some studies). This failure undoubtedly contributed to the increased morbidity and mortality. With the availability of diagnostic ultrasound, the diagnosis is now being made earlier and more frequently. The use of ovulation-inducing drugs or implantation of multiple ova that have undergone in vitro fertilization, should always raise the question of a multiple pregnancy; however, other factors should alert the physician to this possibility. A significant discrepancy between the menstrual age and the size of the uterus requires further evaluation (more than 75% of the women who subsequently deliver twins will have a uterine measurement of 4 cm, or more, greater than the weeks of gestation indicate).

Auscultation of two or more heartbeats that differ by more than 10 beats per minute suggests a multiple pregnancy. Severe nausea and vomiting and a uterus larger than expected early in pregnancy should cause some suspicion of a multiple gestation or hydatid mole. An elevated maternal serum α-fetoprotein level early in the second trimester may be the result of a multiple gestation; the early diagnosis of multiple gestations is one of the advantages of routine maternal serum α-fetoprotein screening. Late in pregnancy, anemia that is unresponsive to customary iron and multiple-vitamin therapy or mild preeclampsia in a multiparous patient should raise the possibility of a multiple pregnancy.

Whenever multiple gestation is suspected, ultrasound examination should be used to establish the diagnosis. An ultrasound examination carefully performed should detect almost all sets of twins and can often determine whether there is one amniotic sac or two. As the number of fetuses increases, the accuracy of diagnosis about the number and the morphologic measurements decreases.

Antepartum evaluation and management

To reduce the perinatal morbidity and mortality associated with multiple gestations, steps should be taken to:

1. Provide an optimum uterine environment to assure fetal growth potential
2. Decrease the number of very premature infants
3. Identify the fetuses who are not thriving in their uterine environment so as to deliver them prior to permanent impairment
4. Avoid fetal trauma during labor and delivery
5. Provide experienced neonatal care at delivery

As soon as a multiple pregnancy is recognized, the patient should be told about her high-risk status and about the efforts that are necessary to increase the chance of a good pregnancy outcome. The dietary requirements for calories, proteins, minerals, vitamins, and essential fatty acids are increased. Dietary supplementation and counseling should be provided to ensure these needs are being met. Iron supplementation should be given to all patients, and although an adequate diet will probably supply the required folate, most authorities recommend folic acid supplementation for women with a multiple gestation.

Numerous methods have been tried in an attempt to decrease the incidence of prematurity. Several retrospective studies have suggested that bed rest may be of value in the management of twin pregnancies. Some have suggested that delivery is delayed as a consequence of bed rest; others have failed to confirm this finding but suggest that birth weight is increased by bed rest even if the duration of the pregnancy is not prolonged. Several recent prospective, randomized trials have failed to confirm the benefit of hospitalization early in the third trimester in twin gestations. Criticisms of the hospitalization trials include the following: (1) patients were hospitalized at 32 weeks' gestation (although retrospective studies suggest that to be of value bed rest should begin during the second trimester of pregnancy) and (2) the stress of hospitalization in itself may counteract any beneficial effects of bed rest. Whether bed rest is effective and, if so, how strictly and at what stage of gestation it should be instituted are still not clear. For gestations of more than two, the conventional wisdom is that bed rest should be liberally used and most physicians recommend hospitalization early in the third trimester.

The role that periodic cervical examinations should play in the management of multiple gestations is not well defined. Recent studies in the management of singleton pregnancies at high risk for premature labor have suggested that frequent cervical examinations do not predispose to premature rupture of the membranes or to infection and do aid by identifying patients with premature effacement or dilation of the cervix. Early identification of these women allows a more agressive approach to limiting activity, planning for early hospitalization, or tocolysis.

Although the prophylactic use of β-sympathomimetic drugs to decrease the incidence of preterm labor has been recommended in multiple pregnancies, prospective randomized trials using relatively low doses of these medications have failed to establish any benefit for their use. Serial injections of 17-hydroxyprogesterone caproate and the prophylactic placement of a cervical cerclage have been advocated to prevent prematurity; however, again there is no evidence that either of these is effective (see Chapter 9).

Surfactant production, as measured by lecithin sphingomyelin (L/S) ratio and phosphatidylglycerol (PG) in the amniotic fluid, is usually similar in both twins when their growth is similar. In multiple pregnancies when there is discordant growth, however, pulmonary maturation may differ markedly among fetuses.

The availability of ultrasound, with its capability of measuring multiple morphologic parameters, has made it possible to evaluate fetal growth throughout gestation. During the first two trimesters, fetal growth is similar in singleton and multiple gestations. During the third trimester, the growth of multiple fetuses, as determined by either ultrasound parameters or birth weight, is less than the growth of comparable singleton fetuses. In general, the greater the number of fetuses, the greater the growth retardation. In addition to the general decreased fetal growth seen in multiple gestations, occasionally one or more of multiple fetuses will show more severe growth retardation. Several studies have demonstrated that twins of dissimilar size are at increased risk prenatally, intrapartum, and in the neonatal period. Once the diagnosis of multiple pregnancy has been made, serial ultrasound examinations should be performed to assess fetal growth.

In addition to monitoring fetal growth during gestation, it also is important that fetal well-being be regularly assessed. Such biochemical measures of fetal well-being as urinary and serum estriol and human placental lactogen (HPL) have not been effective in evaluating multiple gestations and have been almost universally replaced by such biophysical methods as the nonstress test (NST) and the biophysical profile. Ultrasound and NSTs have greatly improved our ability to identify the fetus in jeopardy. Some recent evidence suggests that twin fetuses do not thrive in utero beyond 40 weeks; however, the data available do not permit an accurate assessment of the risks inherent in the twin gestation continuing beyond 40 weeks. (See Chapter 8.)

The antepartum death of one twin is an uncommon occurrence. When it does occur, it is most commonly associated with MZ twinning. Maternal disseminated intravascular coagulation has been described following prolonged death of one twin in utero. A syndrome in which the surviving fetus develops multicystic encephalomalacia has been the subject of a number of reports. The frequency of either of these severe complications is unknown, but the possibility of their occurrence underscores the importance of continued careful evaluation when one fetus of a multiple gestation dies in utero.

Intrapartum evaluation and management

The intrapartum management of multiple pregnancies begins as soon as the diagnosis has been made. Plans should include delivery at an institution having the facilities and personnel to provide adequately for the number of infants anticipated. The mother should be informed of the signs and symptoms of preterm labor and encouraged to report their occurrence immediately. Medical personnel responsible for her care should be appraised of her high-risk status.

If the patient begins premature labor, the decision must be made whether to attempt to inhibit labor. Such a decision should be based on the gestational age of the fetuses, any associated pregnancy complications, the degree of cervical dilation, the state of the membranes, and the well-being of the fetuses as assessed by fetal monitoring and the potential complications of the tocolytic agent. Because of the maternal cardiovascular adaptations in multiple pregnancies, maternal complications of β-sympathomimetic agents are increased. When delivery is anticipated, the presentations of the fetuses must be determined. Real-time ultrasound is preferred for making this determination. If there is any confusion about the presentations, a single x-ray film may be helpful. With twins, all possible combinations of fetal positions occur.

The optimum route of delivery for twins has not been clearly established. When both fetuses are in the cephalic presentation, an attempt at vaginal delivery is universally favored. When the presenting fetus is breech, cesarean delivery is recommended because of (1) the risks of a prolapsed cord with positions other than frank breech, (2) the risks of a trapped head with small infants, and (3) the possibility that a large fetus will exceed the capacity of the birth canal. There is no consensus about the optimum route when the first twin is cephalic and the second a noncephalic presentation. This difference of opinion results from a large body of literature demonstrating a poorer outcome for the second twin. Much of the data were collected when internal version and extraction was a common procedure, and before fetuses were routinely monitored during labor. More recent data confirm that the outcome of the second twin is not as good as that of the first twin, but this does not appear to be as dependent on presentation or route of delivery as previously thought. If vaginal delivery is to be attempted, both fetuses should be continuously monitored during labor, preparations should be made for immediate cesarean delivery if it becomes necessary, and the second fetus should be continuously monitored after the delivery of the first twin. Whichever route of delivery is selected, it is essential that appropriate medical personnel be present to provide immediate care to the infants. Careful examination of the placenta is important at delivery, especially if evidence for twin-to-twin transfusion is sought (see Chapters 11 and 32). The preferred route of delivery for three or more fetuses is by cesarean section.

In summary, the patient with a multiple pregnancy is at risk for increased perinatal morbidity and mortality and for a number of maternal complications. Pregnancy management should be directed toward optimizing the intrauterine fetal environment, decreasing the incidence of prematurity, evaluating fetal growth and well-being, avoiding traumatic delivery, and providing skilled neonatal care.

MANAGEMENT OF THE POSTTERM PREGNANCY

The postterm pregnancy dramatically illustrates the importance of precisely determining the gestational age in managing pregnancy. The postterm pregnancy persists for more than 280 days after ovulation; in women with 28-day cycles who normally ovulate about day 14, the pregnancy persists more than 42 weeks beyond the onset of the last menstrual period. Although this definition would include approximately 10% of all pregnancies, some are not actually postterm but rather are the result of ovulation after the fourteenth day or an error in the estimation of gestational age.

The fetus of the postterm pregnancy may continue to grow in utero and thus be unusually large at birth. At the other extreme, the uterine environment may be unfavorable for fetal growth with the result that the infant at birth appears to have lost considerable weight, especially from loss of subcutaneous fat and muscle mass (Chapter 7). Although the large infant is at greater risk for birth trauma, it is the small, dysmature infant who is at greatest risk for fetal death, distress in labor, and neonatal morbidity. These pregnancies are frequently accompanied by oligohydramnios and thick meconium, leading to an increased risk of meconium aspiration.

Although the dysmature infants resulting from postterm pregnancies were recognized early in this century, it was not until 1945 that the clinical findings characteristic of these infants (wasting and staining of the skin, nails, and umbilical cord) were organized into a syndrome by Clifford. Browne emphasized the significance of this condition in 1963 when he reported that by 43 weeks' gestation the perinatal mortality rate doubled and by 44 weeks trebled when compared to the perinatal mortality rate between 39 and 41 weeks.

The pregnancy that persists beyond 42 weeks has been termed *postdate* or *postterm*, whereas the infant who is born with this syndrome has been labeled *postmature* or *dysmature*. Use of the term *dysmature* emphasizes the fact that the fetus need not be postterm to develop the characteristic features of this condition, which is thought by most obstetricians to be the result of placental insufficiency.

The causes of the postterm pregnancy are unknown. Several uncommon conditions, such as anencephaly and placental sulfatase deficiency, are associated with prolonged gestation. Nevertheless, in most postterm pregnancies the cause is not apparent. Until the mechanism governing the onset of normal spontaneous labor is determined (Chapter 9), the causes of prolonged gestation will probably continue to elude us. Evidence that the fetus itself plays an important role in the onset of labor is accumulating, and it may well be that the postterm pregnancy is of fetal origin.

Management of the postterm pregnancy has been the subject of considerable investigation and debate. Unfortunately, most reports have described the results of specific management protocols or the inability of a given antepartum fetal surveillance test to identify the fetus at risk. Prospective, randomized trials comparing management schemes and surveillance methods are rare. No consensus has emerged on the ideal management of this condition; nevertheless, numerous protocols have been devised. All address the issues, presented in the following list, that make the management of this condition difficult.

1. Although an important principle of prenatal care is the accurate determination of gestational age, this is not always possible and a pregnancy may not be as advanced as thought.
2. Most fetuses, even after 280 days of gestation, are not in jeopardy.
3. Current methods for fetal surveillance are not totally reliable in identifying the fetus at risk for fetal death or serious morbidity.
4. No safe, consistently effective method of cervical ripening is currently available.
5. Induction of labor is not always successful, and induced labors are usually longer than spontaneous labors.
6. Cesarean delivery increases maternal risk.

In the patient with well-established dates, concern about the postterm pregnancy begins at about 42 weeks' gestation. If at this time the cervix is favorable for induction, many obstetricians recommend induction of labor. When induction of labor is attempted in patients with a favorable cervix, induction will be successful over 95% of the time. Labor can be induced with intravenous oxytocin, or by rupturing the membranes and using oxytocin only if spontaneous labor does not begin.

What should be done for the patient with well-established dates but an unfavorable cervix is more controversial. Although some researchers recommend induction of labor at 42 weeks regardless of the state of the cervix, published studies do not support this approach. Most recommend that induction of labor not be attempted but rather that fetal surveillance be undertaken. Options for fetal evaluation include a nonstress test two to three times a week, a contraction test weekly, a biophysical profile weekly, or a combination of these tests. Because of the increasing perinatal morbidity and mortality with advancing gestational age and because some patients never develop a favorable cervix, most protocols call for delivery at a specified gestational age (43 or 44 weeks) regardless of the state of the cervix. Investigations into the efficacy and safety of prostaglandin gel for cervical ripening are in progress. If these studies lead to the availability of this substance, management of the patient with a postterm pregnancy and an unfavorable cervix may well become more aggressive.

When patients have uncertain dates but are suspected of being postterm, the management tends to be more conservative than when the dates are well established. In the absence of any identified complication of pregnancy, if the amount of amniotic fluid volume is adequate and if fetal well-being has been demonstrated, the risk of intervention is probably greater than the risk posed by possible postterm gestation.

Fetal surveillance

Antepartum fetal surveillance has proved to be essential in the postterm pregnancy. The complex array of biochemical and biophysical parameters enables us to identify the fetus at risk (Chapter 8). No single test is optimum for all high-risk situations, and no single test has been shown to be completely reliable in identifying the compromised fetus in the postterm pregnancy.

Biochemical methods

Historically, the most commonly used biochemical test of fetal well-being has been the measurement of serum or urinary estriol. Although these tests have been almost universally replaced by biophysical measurements, the postterm pregnancy was the high-risk situation in which estriol measurement was most reliable in identifying the fetus at risk. The incidence of dysmaturity in pregnancies beyond 42 weeks' gestation is approximately 50% in women with low estriol levels. Conversely, the chance of delivering a dysmature infant in patients whose estriol levels are in the normal range is very small.

Biophysical methods

Fetal movement is one of the oldest variables used in evaluating the condition of the fetus. Maternal assessment of fetal movement is simple, universally available, convenient, inexpensive, and a reasonably accurate predictor of fetal well-being. Fetal movement, as perceived by the mother, is frequently used with other measures of fetal well-being in high-risk patients.

Numerous studies have confirmed that fetal heart-rate acceleration associated with fetal movement is a good predictor of fetal well-being. This observation forms the basis of the nonstress test (NST). This test is performed at weekly intervals in most high-risk situations; however, the evidence indicates that a 1-week interval between NSTs is too long to permit detection of all fetuses at risk in postterm pregnancies. Miyazaki reported an 8% incidence of falsely reactive NSTs in a group of 125 postterm patients. The presence of spontaneous decelerations, even with a reactive NST, is ominous in patients with a postterm pregnancy. (See Chapter 8.)

Analysis of the patterns of fetal heart-rate deceleration during labor led to the identification of late decelerations as a presumptive sign of uteroplacental insufficiency. Subsequent research demonstrated that late decelerations resulted from an impaired oxygen transfer across the placenta. With each uterine contraction, a decrease or cessation of blood flow in the intervillous space occurs, resulting in a diminished respiratory gas exchange between mother and fetus. This observation led to the development of the contraction stress test (CST). In the CST, during a period when contractions are induced by the intravenous administration of oxytocin or, more recently, by nipple stimulation, the fetal heart rate is monitored externally. Theoretically, the occurrence of repetitive, late decelerations during the CST (positive CST) depicts a fetus at risk. Conversely, the absence of repetitive late decelerations (negative CST) is indicative of fetal well-being. Experience has demonstrated that fetal death resulting from placental insufficiency within 1 week is extremely rare. The incidence of false-negative CSTs is very low; however, about 25% of fetuses with a positive CST whose mothers are allowed to labor show no evidence of late decelerations during the intrapartum period. Freeman and others recommend the CST as the primary method of fetal surveillance in pregnancies that go beyond 280 days. In a series of 679 postterm pregnancies, there were no perinatal deaths and perinatal morbidity was no greater than in a control population. Seventy-five percent of the postterm patients went into spontaneous labor.

The evaluation of several biophysical variables may better predict fetal health. The biophysical profile measures five variables: the nonstress test, fetal breathing movements, fetal tone, fetal movements, and quantitative evaluation of amniotic fluid. An advantage of the biophysical profile in the management of postterm pregnancies is that it evaluates the amount of amniotic fluid. The presence of oligohydramnios has been shown to be a good predictor of fetal compromise in these women. After studying 727 women with postterm pregnancies,

Leveno and others concluded that the cause of fetal distress in postterm pregnancies is typically oligohydramnios leading to cord compression rather than the prevailing theory of uteroplacental insufficiency. The presence of oligohydramnios is thought by many obstetricians to be an indication for delivery in the postterm patient (Chapter 6).

Intrapartum management

The fetus of the postterm pregnancy is more susceptible to distress during labor than the fetus in a normal term pregnancy. These women should be cautioned to come to the hospital as soon as labor begins. Continuous electronic fetal monitoring should be used throughout labor. If real-time ultrasound is available, the amount of amniotic fluid should be evaluated. The question of whether to rupture the membranes is controversial. Reducing the amount of amniotic fluid by amniotomy can certainly increase the possibility of cord compression. However, amniotomy usually will permit the identification of thick meconium if present. Knowledge of the presence of thick meconium is important for several reasons: (1) it is evidence of fairly recent fetal distress; (2) if aspirated by the fetus, it can lead to a syndrome with a high neonatal mortality; and (3) suspicious fetal heart-rate tracings have an even more ominous significance in the presence of thick meconium. Also, rupture of the membranes allows placement of an internal fetal electrode, which provides more accurate information than the external system. Biochemical monitoring with fetal blood scalp sampling can be helpful in the intrapartum evaluation of these fetuses.

The postterm fetus is particularly vulnerable at the time of delivery. Aspiration of meconium can be minimized by suctioning of the pharynx as soon as the head is delivered but prior to the delivery of the thorax (Chapter 28, part five). In the face of hypoxia and dysmaturity, the postterm infant may be at considerable risk for the adverse effects of asphyxia, as discussed in Chapter 22. Finally, hypoglycemia may be a manifestation of depleted nutrient stores secondary to postmaturity (Chapter 7).

In summary, the postterm pregnancy is associated with increased perinatal morbidity and mortality. Management begins with the accurate determination of gestational age. At 42 weeks' gestation, induction of labor should be considered in women with a favorable cervix, and intensive fetal surveillance should begin if the cervix is unfavorable for induction. A marked decrease in the amount of amniotic fluid is an especially ominous sign in these pregnancies. The postterm fetus is susceptible to hypoxic damage before and during labor, and to meconium aspiration during labor and at the time of delivery. Although the optimum management for this condition has not been determined, a number of clinical protocols have been shown to reduce considerably the perinatal morbidity and mortality of the postterm pregnancy.

Neil K. Kochenour

BIBLIOGRAPHY

Multiple pregnancy

Babson, S.G., and Phillips, D.S.: Growth and development of twins dissimilar in size at birth, N. Engl. J. Med. **289**:937, 1973.

Barrett, J.M., and others: The effect of type of delivery upon neonatal outcome in premature twins, Am. J. Obstet. Gynecol. **143**:360, 1982.

Benirschke, K., and Kim, C.K.: Multiple pregnancy, N. Engl. J. Med. **288**:1276, 1329, 1973.

Caspi, E., and others: The outcome of pregnancy after gonadotropin therapy, Br. J. Obstet. Gynaecol. **83**:967, 1976.

Chervenak, F.A., and others: Is routine cesarean section necessary for vertex-breech and vertex-transverse twin gestations? Am. J. Obstet. Gynecol. **148**:1, 1984.

Crane, J.P., Tomich, P.G., and Kopta, M.: Ultrasonic growth patterns in normal and discordant twins, Obstet. Gynecol. **55**(6):678, 1980.

Divers, W.A., and Hemsell, D.L.: The use of ultrasound in multiple gestations, Obstet. Gynecol. **53**(4):500, 1979.

Enbom, J.A.: Twin pregnancy with intrauterine death of one twin, Am. J. Obstet. Gynecol. **152**:424, 1985.

Haney, A.F., Crenshaw, M.C., Jr., and Dempsey, P.J.: Significance of biparietal diameter differences between twins, Obstet. Gynecol. **51**(5):609, 1978.

Hartikainen-Sorri, A.L., Kauppila, A., and Risto, T.: Inefficacy of 17-hydroxyprogesterone caproate in the prevention of prematurity in twin pregnancy, Obstet. Gynecol. **56**:692, 1980.

Houlton, M.C.C.: Divergent biparietal diameter growth rates in twin pregnancies, Obstet. Gynecol. **49**(5):542, 1977.

Houlton, M.C.C., Marivate, M., and Philpott, R.H.: Factors associated with preterm labour and changes in the cervix before labour in twin pregnancy, Br. J. Obstet. Gynaecol. **89**:190, 1982.

Iffy, L., and others: The rate of early intrauterine growth in twin gestation, Am. J. Obstet. Gynecol. **146**:970, 1983.

Jeffrey, R.L., Bowes, W.A., Jr., and Delaney, J.J.: Role of bed rest in twin gestation, Obstet. Gynecol. **43**:822, 1974.

Komaromy, B., and Lampe, L.: The value of bed rest in twin pregnancies, Int. J. Gynaecol. Obstet. **15**:262, 1977.

Leveno, K.J., and others: Sonar cephalometry in twins: a table of biparietal diameters for normal twin fetuses and a comparison with singletons, Am. J. Obstet. Gynecol. **135**:727, 1979.

Marivate, M., De Villiers, K.Q., and Fairbrother, P.: Effect of prophylactic outpatient administration of fenoterol on the time of onset of spontaneous labor and fetal growth rate in twin pregnancy, Am. J. Obstet. Gynecol. **128**:707, 1977.

McKeown, T., and Record, R.G.: Observations on foetal growth in multiple pregnancy in man, J. Endocrinol. **5**:387, 1952.

Medearis, A.L., and others: Perinatal deaths in twin pregnancy, Am. J. Obstet. Gynecol. **134**:413, 1979.

Misenhimer, H.R., and Kaltreider, D.F.: Effects of decreased prenatal activity in patients with twin pregnancy, Obstet. Gynecol. **51**:692, 1978.

Naeye, R.L., and others: Twins: causes of perinatal death in 12 United States cities and one African city, Am. J. Obstet. Gynecol. **131**:267, 1978.

Nilsen, S.T., Bergsjo, P., and Nome, S.: Male twins at birth and 18 years later, Br. J. Obstet. Gynaecol. **91**:122, 1984.

O'Connor, M.C., Murphy, H., and Dalrymple, I.J.: Double blind trial of ritodrine and placebo in twin pregnancy, Br. J. Obstet. Gynaecol. **86**:706, 1979.

Powers, W.F., and Miller, T.C.: Bed rest in twin pregnancy: identification of a critical period and its cost implications, Am. J. Obstet. Gynecol. **134**:23, 1979.

Romero, R., and others: Prolongation of a preterm pregnancy complicated by death of a single twin in utero and disseminated intravascular coagulation, N. Engl. J. Med. **310**(12):772, 1984.

Rovinsky, J.J., and Jaffin, H.: Cardiovascular hemodynamics in pregnancy. III. Cardiac rate, stroke volume, total peripheral resistance, and central blood volume in multiple pregnancy: synthesis of results, Am. J. Obstet. Gynecol. **95**:787, 1966.

Saunders, M.C., and others: The effects of hospital admission for bed rest on the duration of twin pregnancy: a randomised trial, Lancet **2**:793, 1985.

Skjaerris, J., and Abert, A.: Prevention of prematurity in twin pregnancy by orally administered terbutaline, Acta Obstet. Gynecol. Scand. (Suppl.) **108**:39, 1982.

Spellacy, W.N., and others: Amniotic fluid L/S ratio in twin gestation, Obstet. Gynecol. **50**:66, 1977.

Veille, J.C., Morton, M.J., and Burry, K.J.: Maternal cardiovascular adaptations to twin pregnancy, Am. J. Obstet. Gynecol. **153**:261, 1985.

Weekes, A.R.L., Menzies, D.N., and De Boer, C.H.: The relative efficacy of bed rest, cervical suture, and no treatment in the management of twin pregnancy, Br. J. Obstet. Gynaecol. **84**:161, 1977.

Yoshioka, H., and others: Multicystic encephalomalacia in a liveborn twin with a stillborn macerated co-twin, J. Pediatr. **95**:798, 1979.

Young, B.K., and others: Differences in twins: the importance of birth order, Am. J. Obstet. Gynecol. **151**:915, 1985.

Postterm pregnancy

Browne, J.C.M.: Post maturity, Am. J. Obstet. Gynecol. **85**:573, 1963.

Cario, G.M.: Conservative management of prolonged pregnancy using fetal heart rate monitoring only: a prospective study, Br. J. Obstet. Gynaecol. **91**:23, 1984.

Clifford, S.H.: Clinical significance of yellow staining of the vernix caseosa, skin, nails, and umbilical cord, Am. J. Dis. Child. **69**:327, 1945.

Clifford, S.H.: Post maturity—with placental dysfunction, J. Pediatr. **44**:1, 1954.

Devoe, L.D., and Sholl, J.S.: Postdates pregnancy — assessment of fetal risk and obstetric management, J. Reprod. Med. **28**:576, 1983.

Eden, R.D., and others: Comparison of antepartum testing schemes for the management of the postdate pregnancy, Am. J. Obstet. Gynecol. **144**:683, 1982.

Elliott, J.P., and Flaherty, J.F.: The use of breast stimulation to prevent postdate pregnancy, Am. J. Obstet. Gynecol. **149**:628, 1984.

Fleischer, A., and others: Antepartum nonstress test and the postmature pregnancy, Obstet. Gynecol. **66**:80, 1985.

Granados, J.L.: Survey of the management of postterm pregnancy, Obstet. Gynecol. **63**:651, 1984.

Goldkrand, J.W., and Benjamin, D.S.: Antepartum fetal heart testing: a clinical appraisal, Obstet. Gynecol. **63**:48, 1984.

Harris, B.A., and others: The unfavorable cervix in prolonged pregnancy, Obstet. Gynecol. **62**:171, 1983.

Knox, G.E., and others: Management of prolonged pregnancy: results of a prospective randomized trial, Am. J. Obstet. Gynecol. **134**:376, 1979.

Kochenour, N.K.: Estrogen assay during pregnancy, Clin. Obstet. Gynecol. **25**(4):659, 1982.

Kohouzami, V.A., and others: Comparison of urinary estrogens, contraction stress tests and nonstress tests in the management of postterm pregnancy, J. Reprod. Med. **28**:189, 1983.

Manning, F.A., and others: Fetal biophysical profile scoring: a prospective study in 1,184 high-risk patients, Am. J. Obstet. Gynecol. **140**:289, 1981.

Miller, F.C., and Read, J.A.: Intrapartum assessment of the postdate fetus, Am. J. Obstet. Gynecol. **141**:516, 1981.

Miyazaki, F.S., and Miyazaki, B.A.: False reactive nonstress tests in postterm pregnancies, Am. J. Obstet. Gynecol. **140**:269, 1981.

Moya, F., and others: Ultrasound assessment of the postmature pregnancy, Obstet. Gynecol. **65**:319, 1985.

Nwosu, U.C., and others: Possible adrenocortical insufficiency in postmature neonates, Am. J. Obstet. Gynecol. **122**:969, 1975.

Nwosu, U.C., and others: Adrenocortical response to ACTH stimulation in postmature newborns, Obstet. Gynecol. **52**(2):213, 1978.

Phelan, J.P., and others: Continuing role of the nonstress test in the management of postdate pregnancy, Obstet. Gynecol. **64**:624, 1984.

Rayburn, W.F., and others: Antepartum prediction of the postmature infant, Obstet. Gynecol. **60**:148, 1982.

Spellacy, W.N., and others: Macrosomia—maternal characteristics and infant complications, Obstet. Gynecol. **66**:158, 1985.

Stubblefield, P.G., and Berek, J.S.: Perinatal mortality in term and postterm births, Obstet. Gynecol. **56**:676, 1980.

Yeh, S., and Read, J.A.: Plasma unconjugated estriol as an indicator of fetal dysmaturity in postterm pregnancy, Obstet. Gynecol. **62**:22, 1983.

Yeh, S., Huang, X., and Phelan, J.P.: Postterm pregnancy after previous cesarean section, J. Reprod. Med. **29**:41, 1984.

CHAPTER 11

Placental pathology

Neonatal diagnosis and therapy are greatly enhanced by the availability of the placenta. This organ may reflect many of the intrauterine events that affect the infant's health, and a quick but knowledgeable examination of this organ before it is discarded can save valuable hours of differential diagnosis and laboratory work. The neonatologist should know what the normal placenta looks like so that the pathologic specimen can be recognized immediately.

EXAMINATION

The placenta is examined in the fresh state, before fixation or freezing. Its cord and membranes are positioned to assume approximately the shape they occupied in utero before a systemic examination is begun. The external surface of the membranes, the chorion laeve, is examined for presence of old or fresh blood; the point of rupture of the membranes is noted; and the membranes are trimmed off the edge of the placenta proper. Next, the cord is studied. Its normal position is near the center of the organ; less commonly it inserts at the margin or even on the membranes. If the latter occurred, then the blood vessels that ramify from this velamentous cord must be examined for tears, thrombi, or calcification. The cord is cut and the number of vessels counted on a fresh-cut surface. Next, the fetal surface of the placenta is inspected carefully. Is it shiny, opacified, or discolored? Are there possible needle punctures from amniocentesis, and can nodules of amnion nodosum be identified? Similarly, the surface of the umbilical cord should be inspected for the presence of nodules that may signify *Candida* infection, and its color is noted. Thereafter the placenta should be weighed and the maternal surface inspected after removing the loosely attached jellylike clots that form after delivery. In my experience, a majority of *retroplacental hematomas* are overlooked clinically, and this is the time when they may be recognized. The old retroplacental blood appears brown and has a dry, granular appearance. Often a hue of yellow or green from blood breakdown pigments is present, and the villous tissue beneath may be firmer and infarcted. Calcification is noted as fine yellow stippling and has no known pathologic significance, even when excessive; it connotes maturity of the organ. Finally, the placenta is sectioned into strips with a long, sharp knife. The color is noted and abnormalities such as infarcts, thrombi, and chorangiomas are both palpated and visualized. Unusual congestion suggests the possibility of maternal glucose intolerance; unusual pallor connotes fetal anemia. At this point sections are taken for fixation and future histologic analysis because some lesions, such as inflammatory ones, often cannot be suspected by macroscopic examination.

MEMBRANES

The inner surface is composed of the amnion. It can easily be stripped off the chorion; such disruption occurs often at the time of delivery, so inspection of the sac may be confusing. The amnion contains no blood vessels, and its integrity depends on nutrition from the underlying chorion and its adjacent tissue. Between amnion and chorion lies the yolk sac, whose minute (0.3 cm) yellow remnants must not be considered a pathologic lesion. The chorionic sac is covered on the outside by remains of villi, trophoblast enmeshed in fibrin, and decidua capsularis. The latter often shows extensive degeneration and is yellow and friable. The membranes may tear with greater or lesser ease at examination, but this feature has not been correlated with any specific pathologic lesion and is not indicative of inflammation or time of rupture of membranes in the course of delivery.

The point of rupture of the membranes identifies approximately the position of the placenta within the uterus. Thus, when a margin of membranes exists all around a vaginally delivered placenta, the examination rules out placenta previa. On rare occasion one can determine from the shape of the membranous sac, particularly when it is distended under water as Torpin ad-

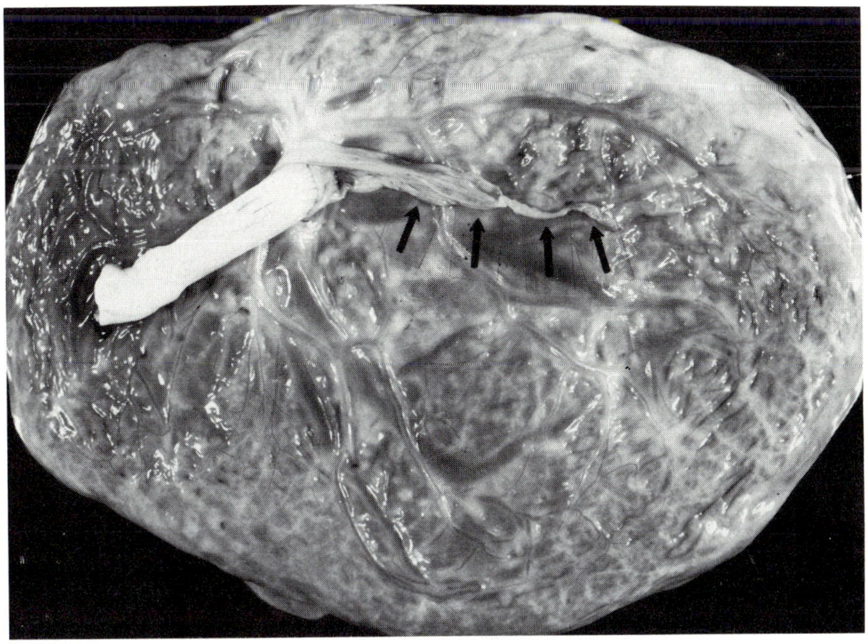

Fig. 11-1. Placenta from a term infant with amputation of terminal phalanx, several toes, and deep constriction of muscles in the calf. There were clubbed feet and only 60 ml of dark amniotic fluid. Remains of amnion are extending into thin band at arrows.

vocates, that a uterine anomaly, such as a bicornuate uterus, was present. The presence of succenturiate lobes on the membrane also may indicate an anomaly of implantation, but for the neonatologist it is more important to ascertain whether the fetal vessels that supply this extra lobe have become disrupted by the tear in the membranes, leading to fetal anemia.

A final but significant deduction that may be made from observations of the rupture of the membranes is the rare event of extramembranous gestation. In such patients the hole within the membranes is too small for the passage of the fetus; only the cord emanates through the opening. The fetus had its growth within the endometrial cavity, having escaped earlier through a tear in the membranes, which then collapsed. Fetal growth retardation, pulmonary hypoplasia, misshapen extremities, circumvallate placentation, and amniorrhea are all sequelae of this abnormal event.

The amnion alone may tear before delivery during the first 3 months of development. Remnants of amnion are frequently found, particularly around the cord (Fig. 11-1), as bands or sheets with stringlike extensions. *Amniotic bands* may strangulate the cord, leading to abortion; they may entangle the extremities, leading to amputations, severe constrictions, or other deformities (Chapter 40); they may adhere to the skull of anencephalics; and their presence may be correlated with other anomalies. Since the fetus resides within the chorionic sac, outside the (destroyed) amnion, the chorionic surface and its vessels are opacified and thickened. The etiology of amnion ruptures is obscure.

Oligohydramnios secondary to deficient fetal urine production or prolonged amniorrhea is associated with *amnion nodosum*. Pulmonary hypoplasia is the common cause of neonatal respiratory distress of infants with this placental abnormality (Chapter 6). Amnion nodosum represents the deposition of impacted granules of vernix on the degenerating amnion. Usually the amnion epithelium undergoes necrosis first, and then the vernix is deposited. It is most readily recognized on the placental surface but also can be seen on the free membranes. The surface sheen of the amnion is usually lost, the membranes are slightly opacified, and yellow-brown granules of irregular size are found. They must be differentiated from the normal nodules of squamous metaplasia (Fig. 11-2). The latter are present in most mature placentas and are distributed primarily around the insertion of the cord. They are rarely found in the periphery of the placenta and never on the membranes.

Discoloration of the fetal surface occurs frequently. Fresh meconium may be wiped off. After a short time the pigmented material is taken in by a large number of resident macrophages within the amnion, and then after some 3 hours or more it is passed into the chorionic macrophages. Thus a very rough guide exists from examining the placenta as to how long meconium was present in the sac. Bilirubin stains the cord and membranes green-yellow, whereas yellow-brown colors are imparted by hemosiderin and hematoidin from marginal or retromembranous hemorrhages as well as from fetal hemorrhages into the amniotic sac.

Inflammation is the only other important process to be observed in the membranes. Polymorphonuclear leukocytes migrate into the amniotic cavity exclusively in response to infection of the amniotic fluid. The older concept that chorioamnionitis also represents a response to hypoxia or changes in pH can no longer be accepted. Polymorphonuclear leukocytes come from the decidual (maternal) vessels in the free membranes, from the intervillous space (maternal) on the placental surface, and

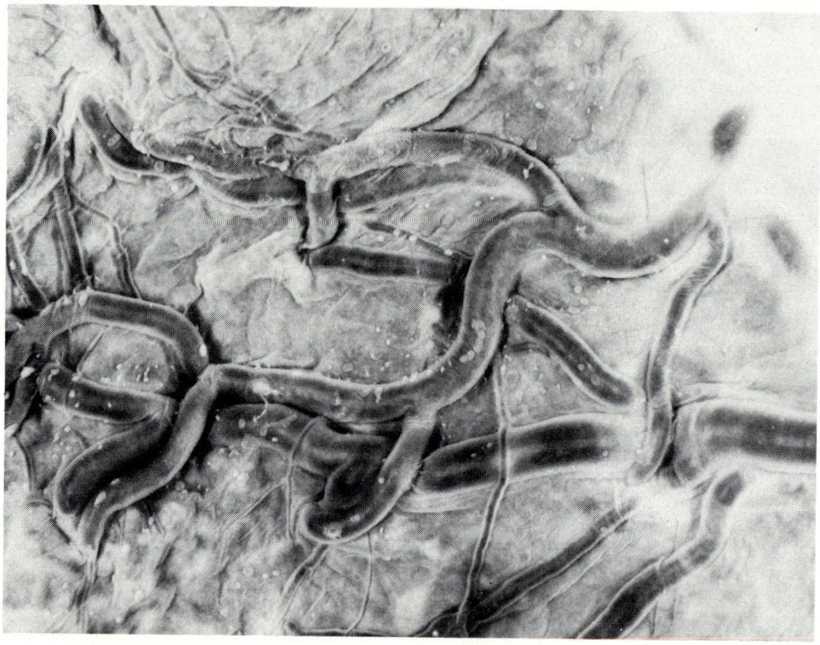

Fig. 11-2. Plaques of squamous metaplasia on the amnion of a normal placenta are prominent over fetal vessels near the insertion of umbilical cord. This must not be confused with amnion nodosum secondary to oligohydramnios (see text).

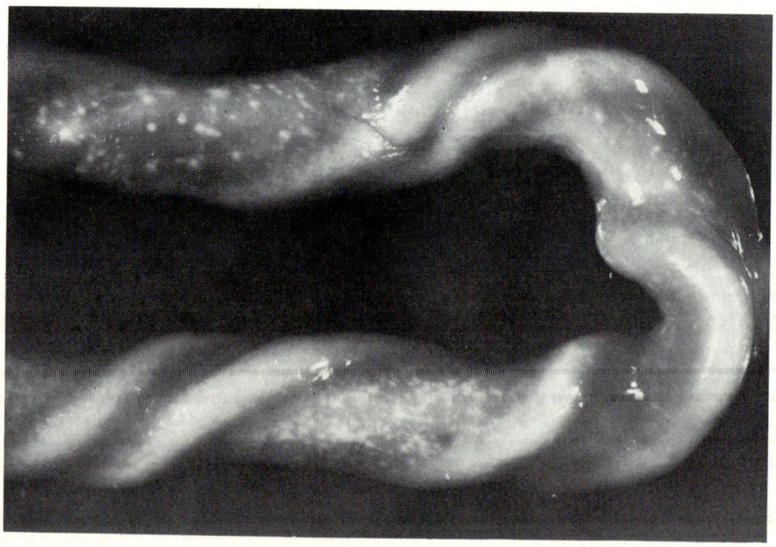

Fig. 11-3. Typical small granules of candidiasis on surface of a discolored umbilical cord.

from the cord and its vascular ramifications (fetal). In general, the most severe infiltration usually exists around the point of rupture of the membranes; it is inferred from this and other correlations that it is usually related to an ascending, transcervical infection. Organisms may be found in large numbers at times, while at other times they cannot be identified at all. A significant degree of inflammation can be identified grossly because it renders the surface of the placenta opaque. In particular, the normally blue fetal vessels appear whitish, and the luster of the surface is gone. At times the surface is malodorous. To assess the nature and degree of this inflammation more accurately, one must prepare histologic sections. Touch preparations and smears prepared from a clean placental surface or after removal of the amnion may also identify the polymorphonuclear leukocytes. A late sequel of severe inflammation is mural thrombosis of surface vessels, which then appear to have yellow-white streaks. Lymphocytic infiltration of the membranes is most uncommon, but a plasmacellular response is, on occasion, seen with virus infections or with syphilis.

Infection with *Candida albicans* is a special form of amniotic sac infection that is readily recognized by placental examination. It is more common than hitherto recognized and may be accompanied by a diffuse or pustular rash in the neonate. Aside from the chorioamnionitis, the surface of the cord has a characteristic appearance (Fig. 11-3). Small whitish nodules appear distributed irregularly on a brownish discolored Wharton's jelly. These nodules are composed of inflammatory exudate and fungi. While the hyphae of *C. albicans* are nearly always present, infections with *C. parapsilosis* (lacking hyphae), a fungus with wide distribution, are now recognized.

UMBILICAL CORD

Normally the cord measures between 50 and 60 cm, but extremes occur in association with abnormal fetal development. Thus unusually *short cords* exist in some chromosomal anomalies and with omphalocele; they occasionally tear on delivery, with fetal blood loss. Excessively *long cords* are prone to knot or entangle around fetal parts; thrombosis and fetal death may be sequelae. Nothing is known of the factors that regulate the length of the cord except that, in rats, removal of amniotic fluid leads to short cords and various fetal positional anomalies.

Angiomas occur on occasion within the cord, usually at its placental insertion, and present a grave prognosis (Fig. 11-4). They may partially calcify or thrombose and probably represent a variation of the more common *chorangioma* of the placental tissue.

The most common anomaly of the cord is a *single umbilical artery* (Fig. 11-5). In the collaborative Perinatal Study, single umbilical artery occurred in 0.9% of deliveries; it is slightly more frequent in white than in black infants and in multiple pregnancies (my own observations indicate a frequency of 3.5%; Soma and associates found 6.2%). Single umbilical artery is an indicator of possible hidden anomalies. The Collaborative Perinatal Study indicated that 14% of infants with this anomaly die perinatally and that 53% of these infants

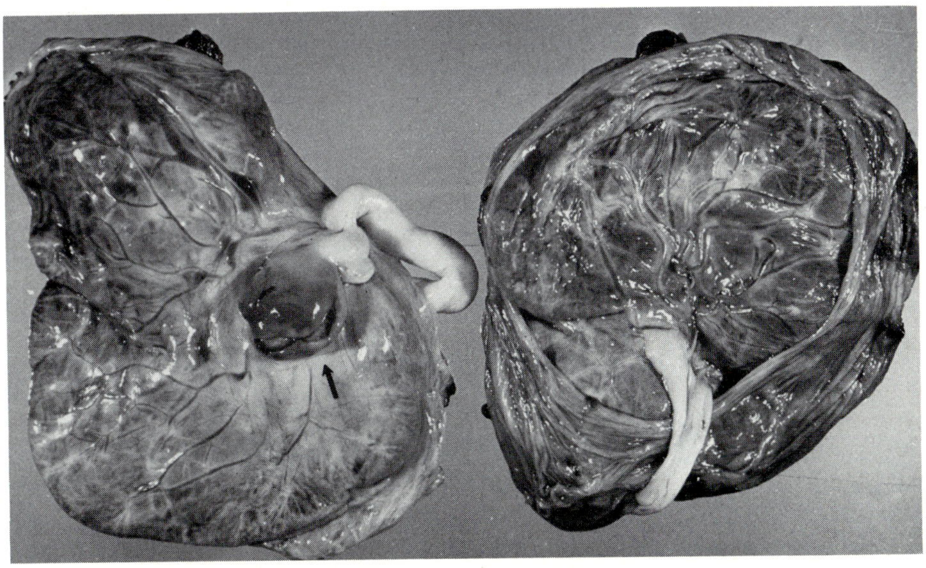

Fig. 11-4. Placentas of premature dizygotic twins. The arrow at left points to an angioma at the insertion of the umbilical cord. This infant had no congenital anomalies but died in the neonatal period.

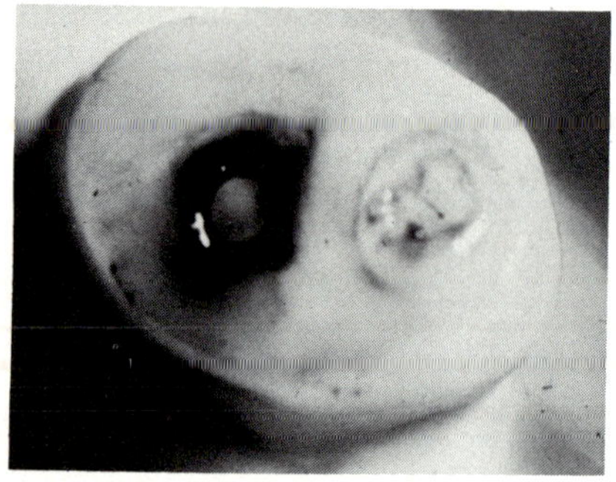

Fig. 11-5. Single umbilical artery of newborn with renal agenesis and velamentous insertion of cord.

A

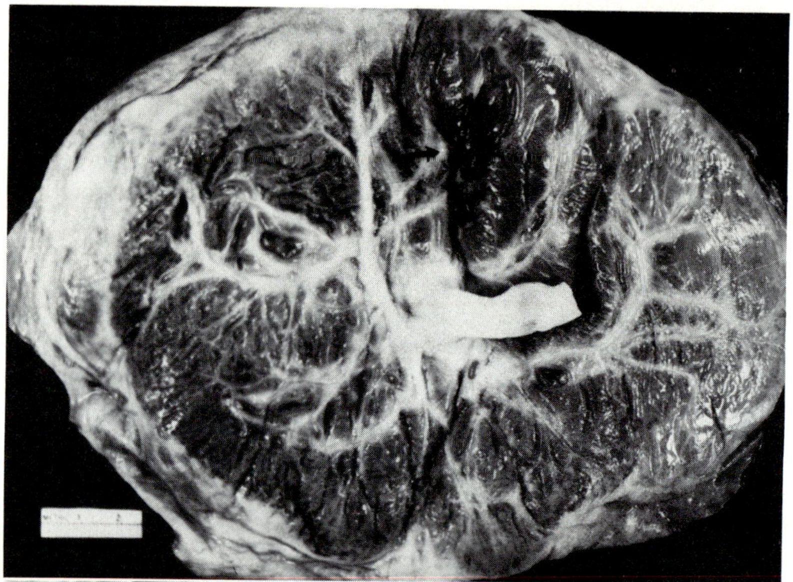

B

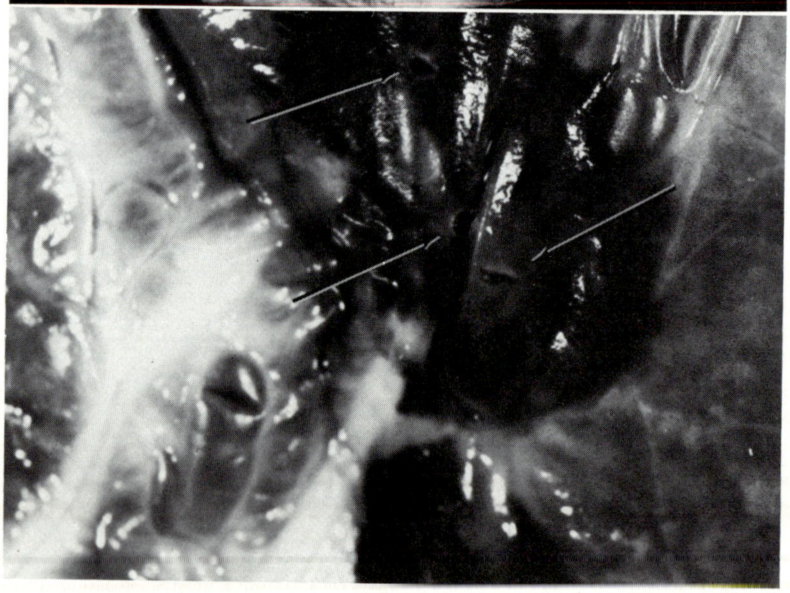

Fig. 11-6. A, Placenta of 38 weeks' gestation following cesarean section performed to ascertain the lecithin/sphingomyelin ratio in a patient with class B diabetes; the fourth amniocentesis led to recognition of fetal bleeding. Infant survived following neonatal transfusion. A small area of subamnionic hemorrhage is seen at arrow. **B,** Higher magnification of hemorrhagic area from **A**. At arrows are three distinct puncture sites of fetal vessels from which fetal bleeding occurred.

have congenital abnormalities; among the survivors, anomalies are identified in only 4%, and when followed to age 4 years there is a significant increase of inguinal hernias. When single umbilical artery is diagnosed, the pediatrician should be notified so that there may be a detailed search for congenital anomalies. Urogenital anomalies are not more common than other types of maldevelopment. Sections of the cord frequently reveal remnants of an atrophying second artery; the frequency of anomalies is the same as with complete single umbilical artery.

Single umbilical artery often occurs with *velamentous cords*. Normally the cord comes from near the center of the placenta, but in about 7% of placentas it inserts marginally—the battledore placenta. In velamentous cords (1.6% of singletons, 5% of twins) the vessels ramify over the membranes from the marginal cord insertion toward the placenta. If they pass over the internal os of the uterus, then the possibilty of rupture of such "vasa previa" has to be considered, an event more common in multiple pregnancy. In addition to acute exsanguination during labor when such vasa previa rupture, the membranous vessels predispose to thrombosis and are more readily compressed by the fetal head during labor. Thrombosis can be widespread in such vessels and is, on occasion, associated with signs of disseminated intravascular coagulation in the neonate (Chapter 34). Calcification also may occur in such vessels. The etiology of velamentous insertion is in dispute. However, there is ultrasonographic evidence that it results from a wandering away of the placenta in the course of development from its original site of implantation.

With the increased use of amniocentesis as a diagnostic tool (Chapters 9 and 16), placentas may be observed with holes in the surface, at times in fetal vessels, from which the fetus may exsanguinate. Often the amnion and chorion are discolored because of hemosiderin deposition subsequent to bleeding. Even with ultrasonic verification of placental site, the placenta cannot always be avoided by the needle. At times the tip of the needle has injured the placental fetal surface vessels on the opposite side of the uterus (Fig. 11-6). The defects in the fetal vessels may be very small, but they are very distinctive and may be recognized by careful inspection of the surface. Occasional spontaneous fetus-to-mother hemorrhage has no recognizable placental lesion (Chapter 32).

THE PLACENTA PROPER

The weight of this portion of the placenta alone, membranes and cord trimmed off, is of limited use in assessing fetal/placental ratio. It is usually between 5:1 and 6:1, but major deviations from this ratio occur with normal neonates. The fetal surface may suggest several diagnoses. The opacity referred to previously allows one to suspect infection. An unusually blue surface, mottled with less than normal patches of subchorial fibrin, suggests maternal diabetes. There may be associated placental congestion, thickness, and an unusual spongy consistency. Conversely, unusual pallor, particularly on cut sections, is indicative of fetal anemia, since the color of this organ is imparted primarily by its content of fetal blood. Thus it is very pale in erythroblastosis, α-thalassemia, and in the donor of the transfusion syndrome. When erythroblastosis is not the obvious cause of marked placental anemia, a careful study is warranted. Fetal blood should be obtained for electrophoresis, and placental tissue samples should be taken to rule out such conditions as syphilis, viral infections, and storage diseases.

The surface also displays *cysts* on occasion (Fig. 11-7). They are usually in a subchorial position, have a mucinous content, and may be blood tinged. These cysts arise in placental septa and are formed by the secretory activity of the so-called X cells, trophoblastic derivatives without known function. The presence of cysts in septa or under the surface, in general, connotes maturity, as does the presence of fine, yellow calcium stippling on the maternal surface. On very rare occasions a surface cyst exists that represents a twin pregnancy with a minute fetus papyraceus inside.

Inspection of the surface also may identify the *circumvallate placenta*. This is produced when chronic circumferential hemorrhages detach the membranes from the edge. It may recur in successive pregnancies and is responsible for some premature terminations. A direct correlation with low birth weight infants has not been substantiated. Other abnormal outlines of the placenta, such as elongate, bilobed, or succenturiate lobed, may reflect some abnormality of implantation or uterine shape, but they have no known influence on fetal growth.

Chorangiomas occur perhaps once in 1,000 placentas. Some bulge on the fetal surface and weigh up to 600 gm, whereas others are small and multiple, detectable only on sectioning or palpation. They are fleshy, congested, and often septated masses of sinusoids or capillaries and have a tendency to infarct. They are fetal vascular anomalies—hamartomas—and are associated with a higher incidence of fetal angiomas and other anomalies. Chorangiomas are always benign, but their presence often leads to prematurity, abruptio placentae, hydramnios, and other complications. Because they represent a peripheral mass of high resistance or arteriovenous fistulas, the fetal heart may be hypertrophied or the fetus may be in heart failure. They also may bleed during pregnancy, resulting in fetomaternal blood loss.

The maternal surface should be freed from its loosely attached postpartum clot, and the lighter color from oxygen exposure should not be mistaken for pathologic

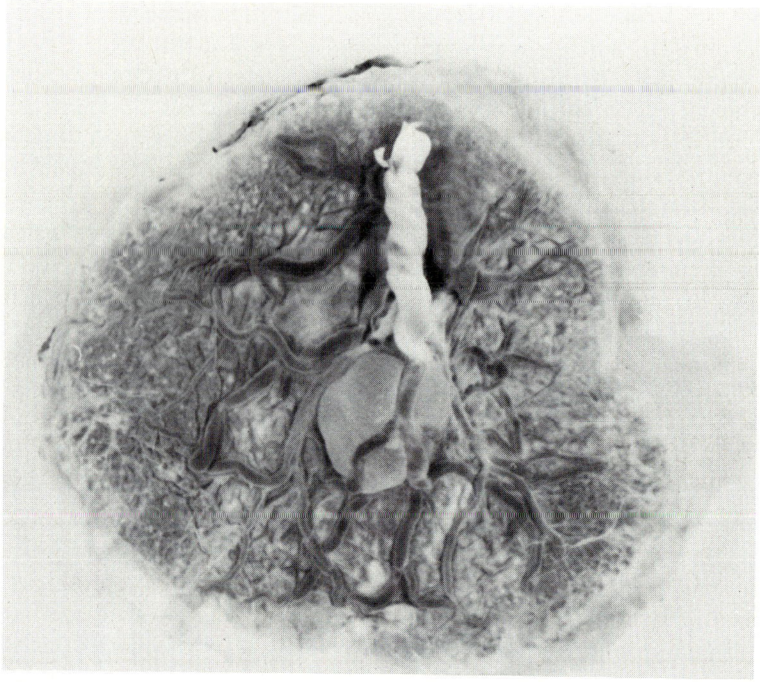

Fig. 11-7. Fetal surface of a mature placenta displaying a subchorionic cyst without pathologic significance.

events. The only important lesion identified on examination of the maternal surface is *abruptio placentae*. In its classic form abruptio placentae is a retroplacental hemorrhage associated with abdominal pain and often stillbirth and is followed by many maternal problems. In such patients there is a large, somewhat firm retroplacental blood clot compressing the placenta; it may cause subjacent villous infarction. More often, *retroplacental hematomas* are found on examination of the placenta of patients who do not have classic symptoms or have no clinical syndrome. Their recognition is important in the assessment of growth retardation. Blood undergoes hemolysis relatively rapidly in vivo. Consequently, retroplacental hematomas discolor within a day or more. They become dry, flaky, brown-yellow, and then green. Sometimes they are very large and, because the blood interposes between the supplying maternal vessels and the intervillous space, the placental tissue is often infarcted and necrotic.

Infarcts are the result of deficient intervillous perfusion and are most often secondary to decidual vascular occlusion or interposing hemorrhage. They are at first red but firmer than the adjacent normal tissue. Later they lose fetal blood color and become yellow and then white, firm, and contracted. They never "organize" but only shrink with time. They are readily felt on palpation, and the estimation of their total mass reflects in some measure the total transfer membrane available. The maternal vascular lesions that are the cause of the retroplacental hemorrhages or infarcts are often not identifiable by placental examination. They are destroyed in the infarctive process or are more proximal in the uterine bed. Curettage (placental bed biopsy) discloses thrombosis or the atherosis of preeclampsia and other complex vascular changes. Maternal vascular lesions may exist in the absence of clinical symptoms and signs of toxemia. Sectioning of infarcts or intervillous thrombi is usually useless for diagnostic purposes. Their quantitation and the documentation of vascular changes are relevant to the diagnosis of fetal growth retardation (Chapter 7).

Few additional lesions are recognized when the fresh placenta is sectioned with a long knife. It is probably more important to save a complete cross section in an appropriate fixative (Bouin's solution; formalin) so that the structures can be studied if the infant has an abnormal course. This practice is of particular importance in growth-retarded newborns, when the placenta has unusual color or consistency.

Chronic villitis is a condition of varied etiology that has no precise macroscopic counterpart. Villi are infiltrated with lymphocytes, macrophages, and particularly with plasma cells (Fig. 11-8). It may be confined to only a few terminal villi or be scattered throughout the villous tissue. At times it is associated either with small hemorrhages and hemosiderin or with fetal vascular thrombosis, while at other times it leads to dissolution or fi-

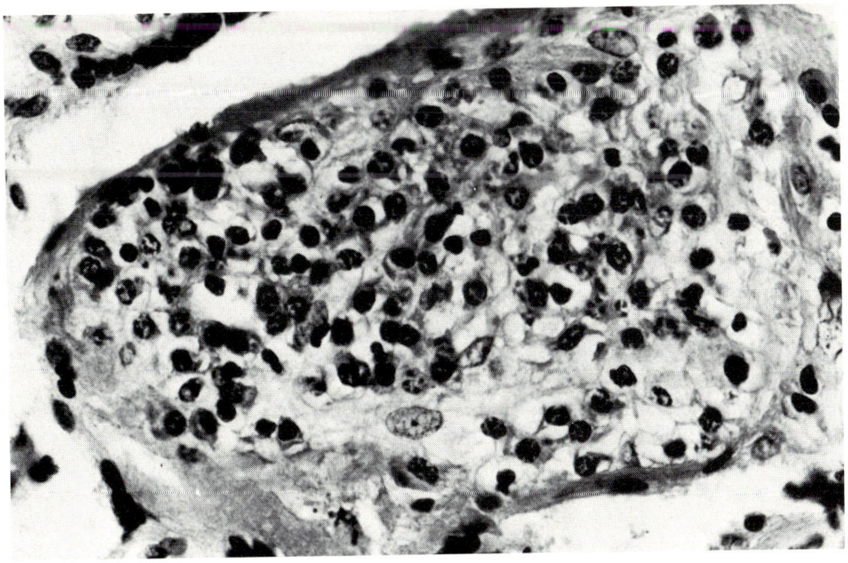

Fig. 11-8. Chronic villitis in the placenta of a premature infant with cytomegalovirus hepatitis and nephritis. This unusually dense infiltrate is composed largely of plasma cells and lymphocytes. Some are degenerating; fetal vessels are occluded, and thus the placenta is pale. Inclusion bodies, fibrosis, and hemosiderin were present in other villi. The infant survived with defects. The placenta was examined only because of maternal "porphyria." (From Benirschke, K., and others: Virchows Arch. [Cell Pathol.] **16:**121, 1974.) (H & E, ×650.)

brosis of many villi. Up to 3% of placentas are affected. Known causes include the TORCH complex, syphilis, and Chagas' disease. Cytomegalovirus is the most common etiologic agent. Villitis might also be an expression of an immune response against normal cellular proteins and it might trigger maternal rejection of the fetal allograft. Some cases of recurrent villitis may have an immunologic basis, accounting for the high perinatal mortality that has been attributed to this disorder.

A microscopic evaluation of the placenta is indicated in evaluating small for dates infants to diagnose chronic villitis (Chapter 7). It is important to recognize that the severity of fetal disease is not necessarily reflected in the extent of villitis. In the placenta, scarring of villi after previous villitis may lead to an underestimation of the extent of disease. Finally, massive and at times recurrent destructive villitis has been observed with fetal death or intrauterine growth retardation in patients in whom no etiologic agent has been identified. The impact and pathogenesis of this varied lesion are not yet fully understood, but it must be considered in the differential diagnosis of the small for date infant.

Listeriosis (Chapter 31) may require rapid diagnosis and therapy. The placenta acquires typical features in this transplacental infection. Aside from funisitis and chorioamnionitis, the fetal septicemic process leads to placental villous abscesses that have been interpreted as granulomas. In contrast to the more common chronic villitis, in listeriosis the villi contain polymorphonuclear exudate in which the gram-positive rods are readily seen. Occasional macroscopic nodules are found, representing a more chronic state of infection.

Some storage diseases (Chapter 36) can be diagnosed by the histology of their placental lesions. GM_1-gangliosidosis causes a recognizable trophoblastic vacuolization. Powell and colleagues have studied five stillborn infants in whose pale placentas masses of stored products produced diffuse vacuolization. In at least one patient, I cell disease could be identified as the causative defect. This suggests that placental study should become an integral part of all newborn examinations and perinatal autopsies. It also should be recognized that a tissue culture from the placenta can be established that represents the fetal genome. This technique is possible even with macerated stillbirths. The ideal tissue to sample sterilely is the chorionic membrane, after the amnion has been stripped off the surface. Villous tissue also can be established in culture but grows less rapidly.

In *trisomies* (Chapter 16) no specific placental anomalies exist, but small, malformed placentas and single umbilical artery are more common.

MULTIPLE PREGNANCY

See also Chapter 10.

Examination *and* recording of the appearance of the placenta should be done for all multiple births. *Monozy-*

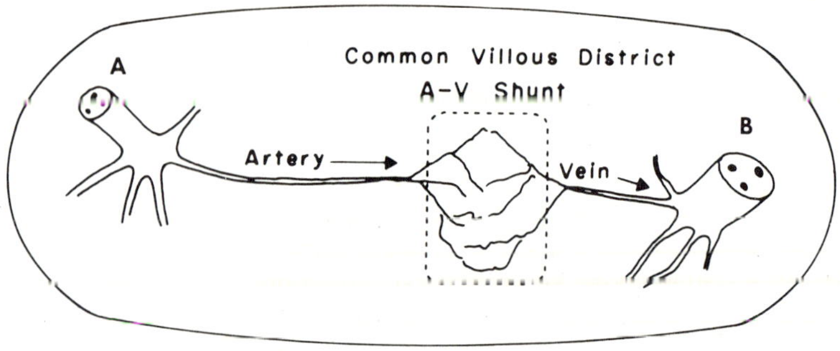

Fig. 11-9. Diagrammatic relationship of arteriovenous shunt in the transfusion syndrome of monochorial, monozygotic twins. The donor *A* delivers blood to a cotyledon, which in turn is drained through a vein into twin *B*. The latter (recipient) becomes plethoric and hypertrophied. The twins may differ by between 10 gm of hemoglobin and over 1,000 gm and still be "identical." (From Benirschke, K., and Driscoll, S.G.: The pathology of the human placenta, New York, 1967, Springer-Verlag New York, Inc.)

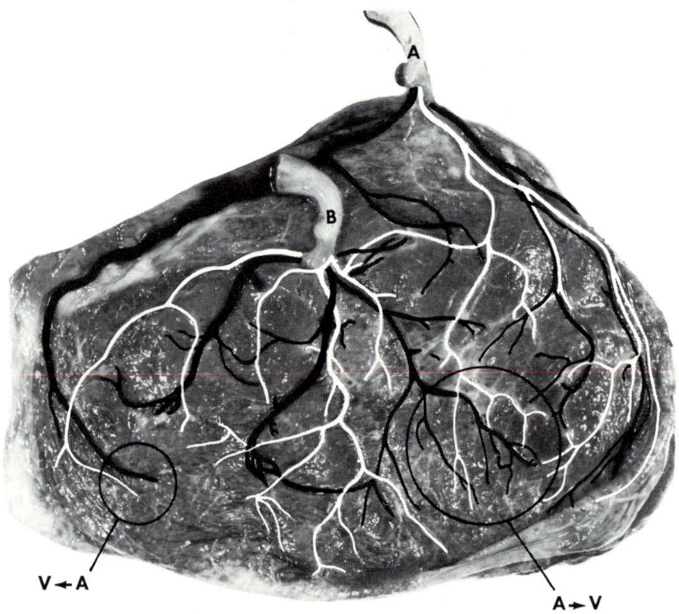

Fig. 11-10. These premature twins (26 weeks) delivered with severe hydramnios and had the prenatal transfusion syndrome. The diamnionic membranes of this placenta have been stripped; a single chorion remains. The placental area of the donor *(A)* is much smaller than that of the recipient *(B)*. Several arteriovenous shunts from *A* to *B* are present in the central right portion, whereas only one arteriovenous shunt (lower left) compensates partly for this transfusion.

gosity can be firmly established by inspection of the membranes in the majority of identical twins. Also, the markedly increased perinatal mortality in twin pregnancies can be understood only by placental examination of the twins; such study may have therapeutic implications. It should begin with identification of the cords of each infant, A and B. This is best accomplished at the time of delivery, with appropriate ties around the cut ends. The sacs are reconstructed and the dividing membranes examined. They may be composed of two amnions or of two amnions plus two chorions. Rarely, no dividing membrane exists (monoamnionic), in which case the monozygotic twins suffer a 50% mortality from entangling of the cords. Monochorionic placentation (two amnions only) is diagnostic of identical twins, and almost invariably the placenta is a single mass. Dichorionic, diamnionic placentation is usually the mode of fraternal twin placentation. Nevertheless, one third of monozygotic (like-sex) twins also have this membrane relationship, and their zygosity can be ascertained only by blood grouping, conveniently and harmlessly from umbilical cord blood, or more detailed immunologic study.

Twins have a higher incidence of velamentous cords, ruptured vasa previa, single umbilical artery, and other anomalies. A study of their vascular relationships is most important. Anastomoses exist, for all intents and purposes, only in monochorionic placentas. They are studied most easily after careful stripping of the amnion and with the placental tissue kept intact. In monochorionic placentas the fetal vasculature is almost invariably joined, sometimes in a very complex manner. Artery-to-artery communications cross *over* placental veins and, when anastomoses are present, blood can readily be stroked from one side into the other fetal vascular bed. Such vessels have the least significance. Vein-to-vein communications are less common and similarly recognized. Artery-to-artery plus vein-to-vein anastomoses form the basis for the development of an *acardiac fetus*. Single umbilical artery is nearly always present, and the normal twin may have cardiac hypertrophy and other problems. A monozygotic twin, differing in karyotype through postmeiotic chromosomal nondisjunction (the so-called heterokaryotic twin), also may be a lymphocyte mosaic because the blood passes through such anastomoses and establishes clones.

More important are arteriovenous shunts in the twin placenta that take the course diagrammatically shown in Fig. 11-9. In essence, these twins share one cotyledon. An artery from one delivers blood that is drained through the vein of the other. The latter becomes plethoric, large, and often has accompanying hydramnios, whereas oligohydramnios, anemia, and smaller size characterize the donor in this transfusion syndrome (Chapters 7 and 32). It is now well recognized in neonatology, but the recognition of the causal placental shunt is rarely accomplished. Injection with milk may facilitate identification of the causal placental shunt. Several types of anastomoses may coexist in the same placenta, whose sum flow determines the disparity of fetal development and blood content. The complexity of the vascular relationship may be appreciated from Fig. 11-10.

Recognition of the placental abnormalities in multiple birth placentas is important not only for immediate therapy of newborns; their record is also needed for the future care of the child. For instance, it is now recognized that congenital anomalies are more common in monozygotic twins than in fraternal sets. Moreover, one of the monozygotic twins may be abnormal (discordant), and this has a bearing for future genetic counseling.

Kurt Benirschke

BIBLIOGRAPHY

Altshuler, G., and Russell, P.: The human placental villitides: a review of chronic intrauterine infection, Curr. Top. Pathol. **60**:63, 1975.

Altshuler, G., Russell, P., and Ermocilla, R.: The placental pathology of small-for-gestational age infants, Am. J. Obstet. Gynecol. **121**:351, 1975.

Altshuler, G., Tsang, R.C., and Ermocilla, R.: Single umbilical artery: correlation of clinical status and umbilical cord histology, Am. J. Dis. Child. **129**:697, 1975.

Benirschke, K.: Diseases of the placenta. In Gluck, L., editor: Modern perinatal medicine, Chicago, 1974, Year Book Medical Publishers, Inc.

Bernirschke, K.: Placental causes of maldevelopment. In Berry, C.L., and Poswillo, D.E., editors: Teratology, trends and application, New York, 1975, Springer-Verlag New York, Inc.

Benirschke, K., and Driscoll, S.G.: The pathology of the human placenta, New York, 1967, Springer-Verlag New York, Inc.

Benirschke, K., Mendoza, G.R., and Bazeley, P.L.: Placental and fetal manifestations of cytomegalovirus infection, Virchows Arch. (Cell Pathol.) **16**:121, 1974.

The Collaborative Perinatal Study of the National Institute of Neurological Diseases and Stroke; the women and their pregnancies, DHEW Publ. No. (NIH) 73-379, Washington, D.C., 1972, Department of Health, Education, and Welfare.

Froehlich, L.A., and Fujikura, T.: Follow-up of infants with single umbilical artery, Pediatrics **52**:6, 1973.

Gruenwald, P.: Pathology of the deprived fetus and its supply line. In Size at birth (Ciba Foundation Symposium 27), Amsterdam, 1974, Elsevier Publishing Co., p. 3.

Kellogg, S.G., Davis, C., and Benirschke, K.: *Candida parapsilosis:* previously unknown cause of fetal infection; a report of two cases, J. Reprod. Med. **12**:159, 1974.

King, D.L.: Placental migration demonstrated by ultrasonography: a hypothesis of dynamic placentation, Radiology **109**:167, 1973.

Lowden, J.A., and others: Prenatal diagnosis of GM_1-gangliosidosis, N. Engl. J. Med. **288**:225, 1973.

Perrin, E., editor: Pathology of the placenta, New York, 1984, Churchill Livingstone.

Poswillo, D.: Fetal posture and causal mechanisms of deformity of palate, jaws and limbs, J. Dent. Res. **45**:584, 1966.

Powell, H.C., and others: Foamy changes of placental cells in fetal storage disorders, Virchows Arch. (Pathol. Anat.) **369**:191, 1976.

Redline, R.W., and Abramowsky, C.R.: Clinical and pathologic aspects of recurrent placental villitis, Hum. Pathol. **16**:727, 1985.

Schirar, A., and others: Congenital mycosis *(Candida albicans)*, Biol. Neonate **24**:273, 1974.

Sieracki, J.C., and others: Chorangiomas, Obstet. Gynecol. **46**:155, 1975.

Shanklin, D.R.: The influence of placental lesions on the newborn infant, Pediatr. Clin. North Am. **15**:25, 1970.

Soma, H., and others: Fetal abnormalities associated with twin placentation, Teratology **12**:211, 1975.

Torpin, R.: The human placenta: its shape, form, origin and development, Springfield, Ill., 1969, Charles C Thomas, Publisher.

CHAPTER 12

Perlnatal ultrasound

The use of ultrasound in evaluation of the pregnant uterus was first described by Donald in 1958. Since then ultrasound has replaced all other imaging modalities, including radiography and radionuclide scanning, in the evaluation of the uterus and fetus. The development of gray-scale instrumentation in the mid-1970s provided greatly improved visualization of fetal anatomic structures. More recently the use of high-resolution real-time scanners has made possible the routine evaluation of fetal anatomy in great detail.

In addition to its accuracy, ultrasound has the major advantage of safety. In contrast to x rays, ultrasound is nonionizing. Although very high-intensity sound is known to produce definite biologic effects, such as heat production, cavitation, shearing stresses, changes in cell membrane permeability, and chromosomal damage, the intensity at which these effects occur is many times greater than that used in diagnostic ultrasound. Average intensity in most commercial ultrasound instruments is less than 10 mW/cm^2; no biologic ill effect has been comfirmed at these low intensities.

PRINCIPLES OF ULTRASONOGRAPHY

Ultrasound is defined as sound above the human hearing range, that is, 20,000 cycles per second (cps). In obstetric ultrasonography the frequency used is usually in the region of 2 to 5 million cps (2 to 5 MHz). Ultrasound is a form of mechanical energy produced by applying a voltage across a crystal that has what is known as a piezoelectric property, which can convert the electrical energy of the applied voltage to mechanical energy in the form of ultrasound. The ultrasound beam is propagated through tissue mainly as a longitudinal waveform. The velocity of sound varies in different tissues, with the average velocity being about 1,540 m/second. Different tissues also have varying densities. The product of the density of the tissue and the velocity of sound in the tissue is referred to as its acoustic impedance. When sound encounters an interface between two tissues of different acoustic impedances, it behaves very much like light in that a portion of the sound is reflected at the interface. If the interface is large in relation to the wavelength of the sound beam, that is, the surface of an organ, it acts as a specular reflector, and the angle of reflection is equal to the angle of incidence. Reflected echoes will return to the transducer only if the angle of incidence is within a few degrees of perpendicular to that interface. Ultrasound is also scattered by interfaces that are small in relation to the wavelength of the beam, such as the microarchitecture of tissues. Sound is then scattered in every direction, and the resultant echoes are very much weaker than those from specular reflectors. These weak, scattered echoes give the characteristic tissue texture echoes seen in a gray-scale display.

Since the velocity of sound in a given tissue is constant, the wavelength is inversely proportional to the frequency. The lower the frequency (i.e., the longer the wavelength) the greater distance the sound beam will penetrate because it will interact with fewer interfaces within tissue. Conversely, high-frequency sound with very short wavelengths has much less penetration, but because of the short wavelengths, the resolution improves as frequency increases. The frequency actually employed for any given application is a trade-off between the desirability of getting high resolution with increased frequency and the necessity to penetrate to a sufficient depth, which may require a lower frequency. In practice, the highest frequency that will provide adequate penetration should always be used, and this will vary in obstetric applications, usually between 3 and 5 MHz. The higher frequency can be used in thin patients and in the evaluation of early pregnancy, whereas obese people will require a lower frequency, perhaps even as low as 2 MHz, to provide adequate penetration.

Two basic types of ultrasonic equipment are used in obstetric ultrasonography. The traditional static B-scanner is still widely used and has the advantage of providing a complete cross section of the uterus and its contents on a single scan. This can be particularly useful in showing the exact position of the fetus and placenta in the uterus. The other main type of ultrasonic instrument used in obstetrics is the real-time scanner, which provides a dynamic image of the fetus at a frame rate of 15 to 30 frames per second. With a real-time scanner it is possible to continuously scan the fetus without interruption and also to observe fetal movements. One can obtain much more detailed information in a very short time with real-time scanning and, in our opinion, it should always be the primary method used in evaluating the pregnant uterus and fetus. Two general designs of real-time scanners are available. One is a so-called sector scanner, which produces a diverging scanning field, narrower near the surface and becoming wider with depth. Such a sector scanner can use a single oscillating crystal or multiple rotating crystals, or, in a somewhat more sophisticated design, a phased array of crystals can be electronically steered to produce the beam pattern. The other main type of real-time scanner is the linear array, which produces a rectangular scan. In general, the linear array scan produces better resolution in the near field and the sector scanner is superior for deep structures. Overall, the linear array scanners are probably preferable for obstetric examinations from the second trimester onward, whereas sector scanners are superior in early pregnancy and for gynecologic examinations.

For examination of the uterus, the bladder should be moderately distended with urine. This is particularly crucial in early pregnancy because the distended bladder displaces bowel out of the pelvis and provides an acoustic window to the posteriorly situated uterus. In later pregnancy, bladder distension is also desirable but not quite as crucial. It is important, however, that the bladder is not overdistended, since this can compress the lower uterine segment and cause a false impression of a low-lying placenta.

DIAGNOSIS OF EARLY PREGNANCY AND ESTIMATION OF GESTATIONAL AGE

Pregnancy can be diagnosed sonographically as early as 5 weeks after the last menstrual period. A gestational sac is seen within the uterus. The actual embryo can be seen at 6 to 7 weeks, and cardiac movement can be documented by real-time scanning (Fig. 12-1).

A blighted ovum will be seen as an empty gestational sac, which is inappropriately small for the duration of amenorrhea. The gestational sac may be distorted and collapsed and may also be situated unusually low in the uterine cavity. The diagnosis of blighted ovum can be confirmed by repeating the study after 7 to 10 days and documenting no interval growth or appearance of an embryo.

The most accurate method of estimating gestational age is by measuring the crown-rump length in the first trimester. This has an accuracy of ±3 days. Measurement of gestational sac diameter also can be used for estimating gestational age during the first trimester, although it is not as accurate as the crown-rump length, since its shape can be quite variable.

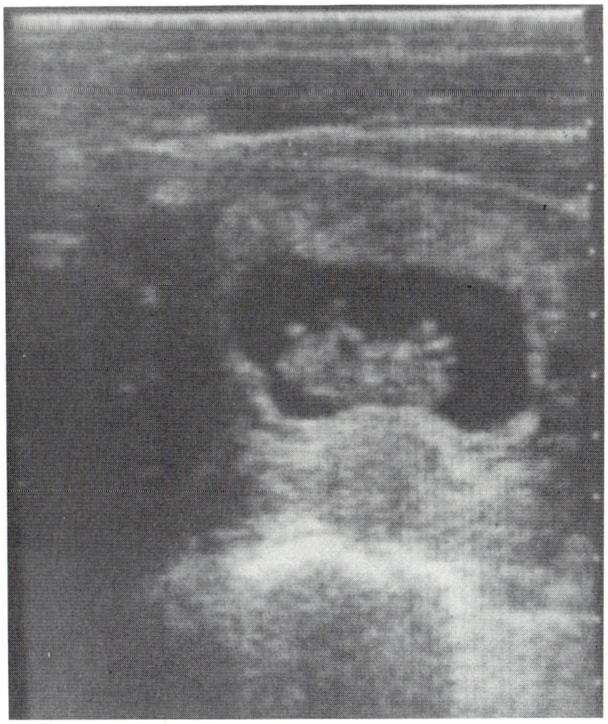

Fig. 12-1. First trimester pregnancy. The embryo is seen within the gestational sac. The crown-rump length can be measured on this image for estimation of gestational age.

Cephalometry

From the beginning of the second trimester onward, the most widely used method of estimating gestational age is the biparietal diameter (BPD). Campbell described a technique for obtaining accurate BPDs using static B-scanners in 1968, and his method became universally adopted. Since the advent of high-resolution real-time scanners, it has become possible to obtain reliable and reproducible BPDs quickly and easily. Details of intracranial anatomy should be seen routinely from the second trimester onward (Figs. 12-2 and 12-3). The midbrain and cerebral peduncles can almost always be identified as relatively echo-free structures, and the basilar artery can be seen pulsating on the anterior aspect of the midbrain. The thalami can be seen also as relatively hypoechoic structures on either side of the third ventricle, but the third ventricle itself is sometimes not seen as a discrete structure due to its small size. The pulsations of the internal carotid arteries can be seen in the region

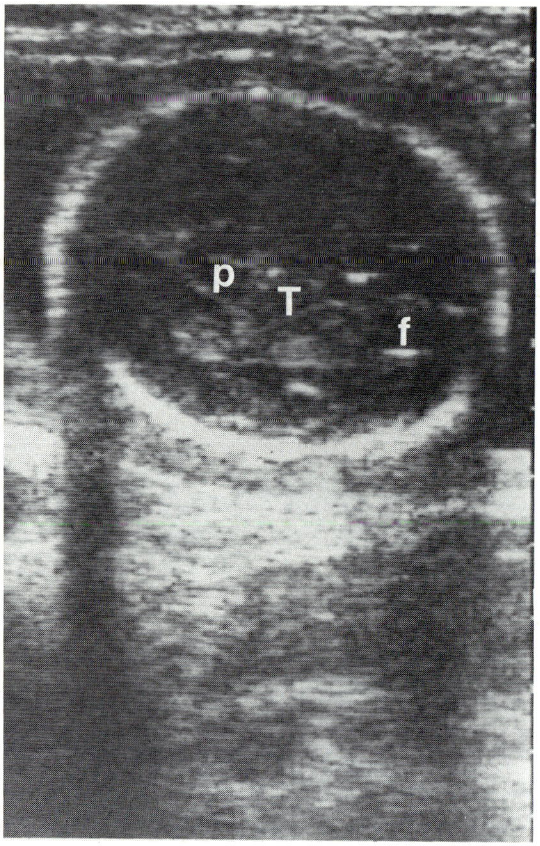

Fig. 12-2. Normal intracranial structures. *p*, Cerebral peduncles; *T*, thalamus; *f*, frontal horn of lateral ventricle.

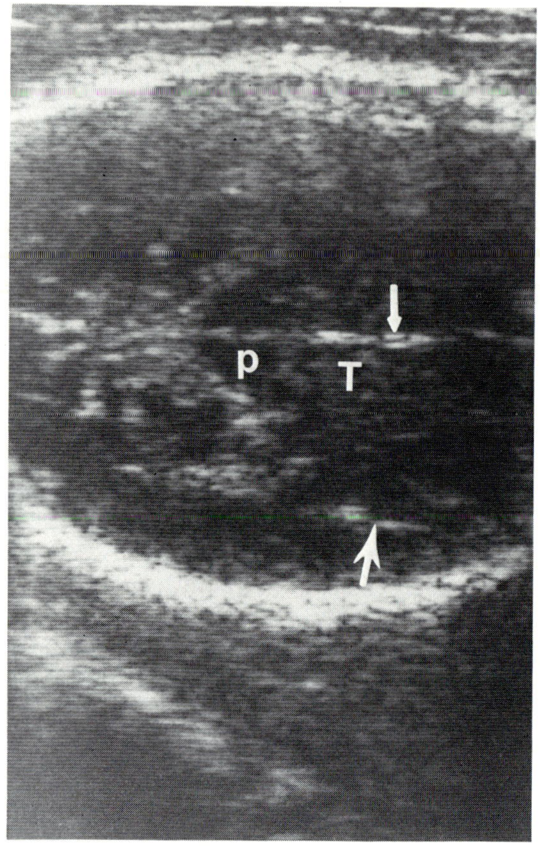

Fig. 12-3. Normal anatomy. Small arrow shows third ventricle; large arrow shows sylvian fissure. *p*, Cerebral peduncle; *T*, thalamus.

of the circle of Willis, and branches of the middle cerebral artery can be seen producing pulsations in the sylvian fissures, which appear as linear echogenic structures parallel to the skull vault and approximately two thirds of the distance from the midline to the periphery. A strong midline echo is routinely seen; it represents the interhemispheric fissure and falx at more superior levels and the septum pellucidum and third ventricle at more caudal levels. The lateral ventricles can be seen routinely from the beginning of the second trimester onward. In the second trimester the lateral ventricles are relatively large compared with the size of the brain and may extend as far as two thirds of the way from the midline to the periphery at 15 weeks' gestation. As pregnancy progresses toward term, the brain grows at a relatively faster rate than the lateral ventricles, and at term the ratio should be less than 35%. The measurement done from the midline echo to the lateral margin of the lateral ventricle does not represent the true size of the lateral ventricle but also includes a portion of the corpus callosum medially. The medial wall of the normal lateral ventricle is frequently not seen, since it is not perpendicular to the sound beam. When the ventricle becomes dilated, the medial wall frequently does become perpendicular to the beam, and the true size of the lateral ventricle can then be measured. It should never exceed 13 mm. The normal choroid plexus is seen as a strongly echogenic structure within the lateral ventricle. In the presence of hydrocephalus, the ventricle can be seen to contain predominantly clear fluid and, as mentioned previously, both walls of the ventricle can be seen when it is dilated. The occipital horn is frequently the first portion of the ventricle to dilate.

To consistently obtain BPDs in a reproducible fashion and at the maximum levels, the structures around the region of the thalamus should be included in the plane of measurement. The cross section of the head will then be ovoid when it is scanned in the axial plane. If the head is measured at the level of the interhemispheric fissure, the diameter will usually not be maximal and the measurement derived may underestimate the gestational age by several weeks. The accuracy of BPD estimations is ±10 days up to about 34 weeks, and thereafter, due to a falling off in the rate of growth, the accuracy dimin-

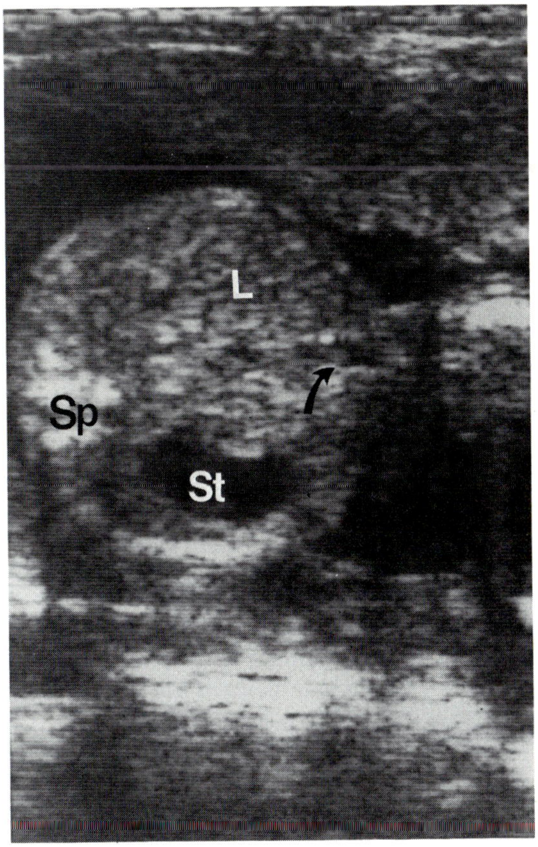

Fig. 12-4. Cross section of abdomen at level of umbilical vein *(arrow)*, *L*, Liver; *St*, stomach; *Sp*, spine.

ishes to ±3 weeks. Measuring the head circumference can be more helpful than the BPD when there is an unusual head shape, for example, dolichocephaly.

Other methods of estimating gestational age

In addition to the BPD, the fetal abdominal diameter should be measured. This is conventionally done at the level of the liver, and the umbilical vein is used as a reproducible landmark to indicate the appropriate level (Fig. 12-4). Either average fetal body diameter (average of anteroposterior and lateral diameters) or abdominal circumference can be used. We have found that using the average diameter is simpler and just as useful as measuring the circumference. In the presence of intrauterine growth retardation, head growth tends to be preserved at the expense of body growth, and the abdominal diameter will lag behind the BPD (Chapter 7). They should normally be within 5 mm of each other, with the head being larger up to about 34 weeks and the body becoming larger thereafter.

The length of the fetal femur can easily be measured, particularly using real-time scanning, and this also proves to be a reliable indicator of gestational age. It is particularly useful if an adequate BPD measurement cannot be obtained due to fetal position. Some workers use estimates of total intrauterine volume both to estimate gestational age and to assess the presence of intrauterine growth retardation. Accurate measurements of total intrauterine volume are difficult to obtain and have a wide normal variation. We have not found them to be sufficiently useful to warrant the time it takes to perform such estimates on a routine basis.

DIAGNOSIS OF FETAL ANOMALIES

Ultrasonography now offers the opportunity to evaluate selected high-risk pregnancies for the presence of fetal malformations that are amenable to corrective measures as well as those that are incompatible with life. Although radiography has been applied with some success in detection of fetal malformations involving osseous structures, invasive amniography has heretofore usually been required for the diagnosis of soft tissue or gastrointestinal abnormalities. Ultrasonography has now virtually replaced x-ray examinations for the diagnosis of fetal anomalies, since, in addition to its being safe and noninvasive, it also provides vastly superior detail of fetal anatomy. During a 7-year period, we observed major fetal malformations in approximately 1% of 22,000 cases that underwent antenatal ultrasonographic evaluation. Statistics from this study follow:

Number of patients examined	22,200
Structurally abnormal fetuses	197
Multiple abnormalities	25
Organ systems involved	
Central nervous	75
Gastrointestinal	24
Genitourinary	42
Skeletal	6
Cardiopulmonary	7
Other	38

This incidence is probably higher than that to be expected in the general population, since the series included high-risk patients referred from a population of about 5 million. Hobbins and co-workers found an approximately equal incidence of fetal anomalies in a series of 2,548 scans on high-risk patients. The major fetal anomalies can be diagnosed as early as 15 to 16 weeks' gestational age. Indications for antenatal ultrasound follow.

A. Dating pregnancy
   1. No accurate dates
   2. Uterine size/dates discrepancy
      a. Suspected growth retardation
      b. Suspected large for dates; rule out
         (1) Multiple gestation
         (2) Polyhydramnios

(3) Macrosomia
(4) Uterine abnormality, e.g., fibroid
(5) Molar pregnancy

B. Fetal/placental localization
1. Confirm pregnancy
2. Suspected missed abortion
3. Suspected ectopic pregnancy
4. Suspected placenta previa
5. Prior to amniocentesis
6. Prior to fetal transfusion/surgery

C. Survey of fetal anatomy; rule out congenital malformation, especially with:
1. History of previous malformation
2. Elderly mother
3. Diabetic pregnancy
3. Polyhydramnios/oligohydramnios
5. Abnormal presentation
6. Exposure to teratogens
7. Elevated serum alpha-fetoprotein levels

Normal fetal anatomy

In addition to the normal intracranial structures previously described, many other fetal organs can be routinely visualized (Figs. 12-4 and 12-5). Structures that should always be identified include the heart, liver, gallbladder, kidneys, stomach, umbilical vein, urinary bladder, spine, and extremities. Organs that are usually seen but can sometimes be obscured by an unfavorable fetal position include the individual cardiac chambers, aorta, vena cava, and external genitalia (Figs. 12-6 and 12-7).

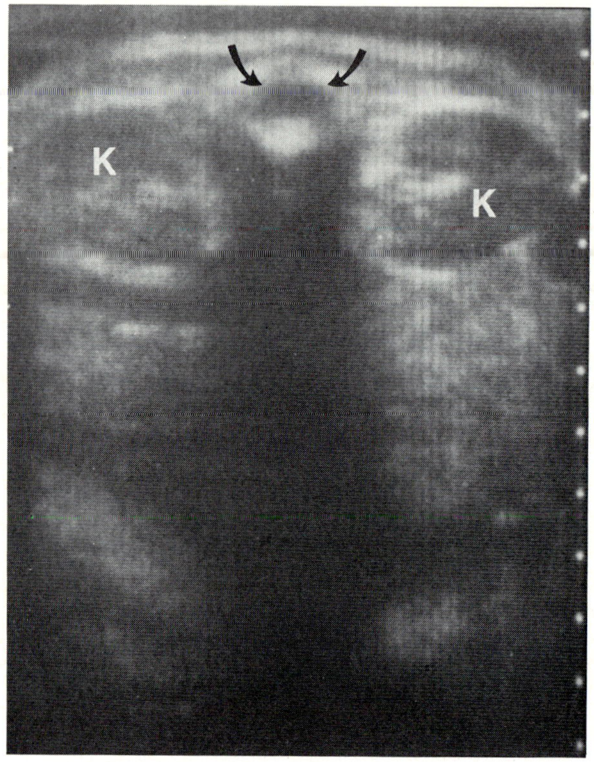

Fig. 12-5. Normal fetal kidneys *(K)* and spinal canal *(arrows)*.

Genitourinary abnormalities

The kidneys can be identified as early as 14 weeks' gestation as two circular structures situated on either side of the fetal spine (Fig. 12-5). The bladder can be seen as early as 14 or 15 weeks' gestation. If serious renal malfunction such as severe obstruction or renal agenesis is present, the absence of fetal urine production causes severe oligohydramnios. Thus, whenever oligohydramnios is encountered on an ultrasound examination, particular attention should be paid to the fetal urinary tract. The fetal bladder should always be visualized after about 15 weeks, and if it is not seen at the first attempt, the patient should be rescanned at 30-minute intervals in case the failure to visualize it on the first attempt is due to recent voiding. Unfortunately, the lack of surrounding amniotic fluid makes it much more difficult to see details of fetal anatomy. Nevertheless, if the bladder and kidneys cannot be seen in the presence of oligohydramnios, this is strongly suggestive of renal agenesis. The fetal adrenals are relatively much larger than they are in later life, and sometimes the adrenals can be seen and misinterpreted as kidneys in cases of renal agenesis.

Hydronephrosis may be unilateral due to pelviureteric junction obstruction or bilateral due to lower urinary tract obstruction, such as posterior urethral valves. In mild cases only a dilated pelvis will be seen, and the renal parenchymal thickness will be normal. However, if the degree of hydronephrosis is severe, a markedly dilated pelvis and calyces can be seen with thinning of the renal parenchyma (Fig. 12-8). Minimal dilation of the renal pelvis can sometimes be seen in normal kidneys, and the presence of minimal dilation does not necessarily indicate obstruction.

In posterior urethral valves a distended bladder will usually be seen in addition to hydronephrosis, which is most often bilateral but may be unilateral. Dilation of the posterior urethra and of the ureters may also be identified (Fig. 12-9).

Multicystic renal dysplasia is the most common cause of an abdominal mass in the newborn and is readily diagnosable in the fetus. It appears as a multicystic mass in the renal fossa alongside the spine with cysts of varying size that lack any apparent organization (Fig. 12-10). This is in contrast to the findings in severe hydronephrosis, in which there is an orderly arrangement of a large renal pelvis surrounded by smaller calyces (Fig. 12-8). (See Chapter 35.)

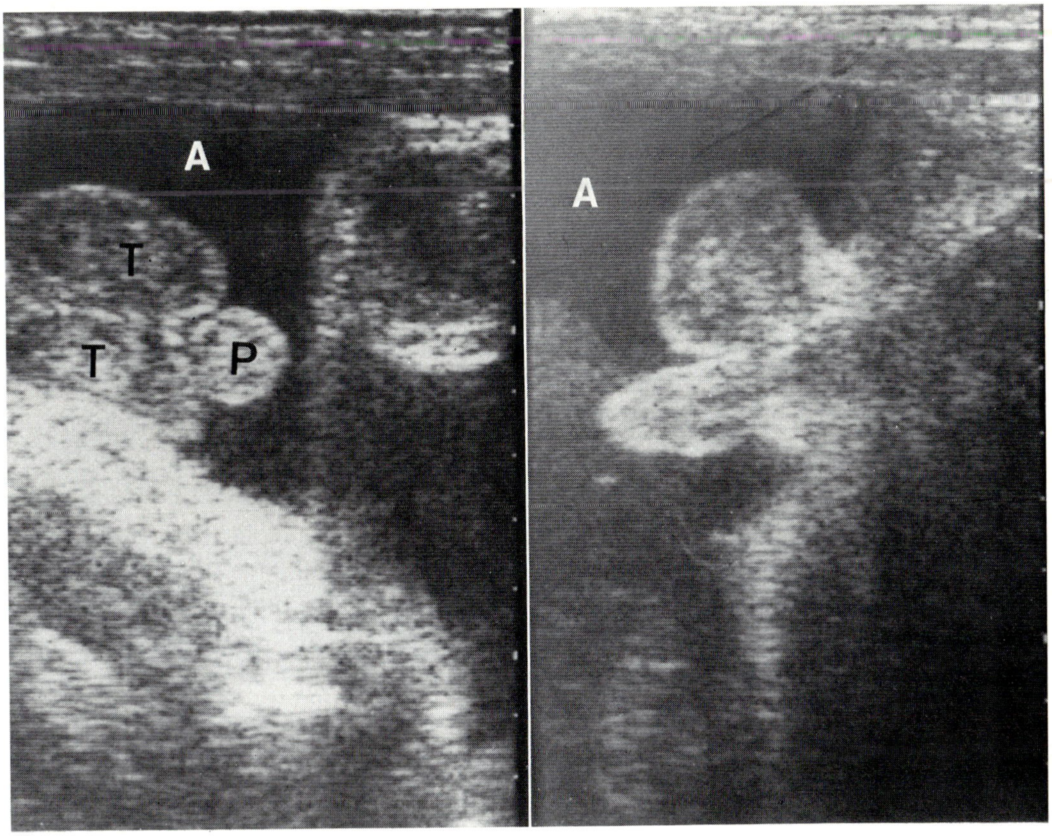

Fig. 12-6. Two scans showing external genitalia of a male fetus. *T*, Testis; *P*, penis; *A*, amniotic fluid.

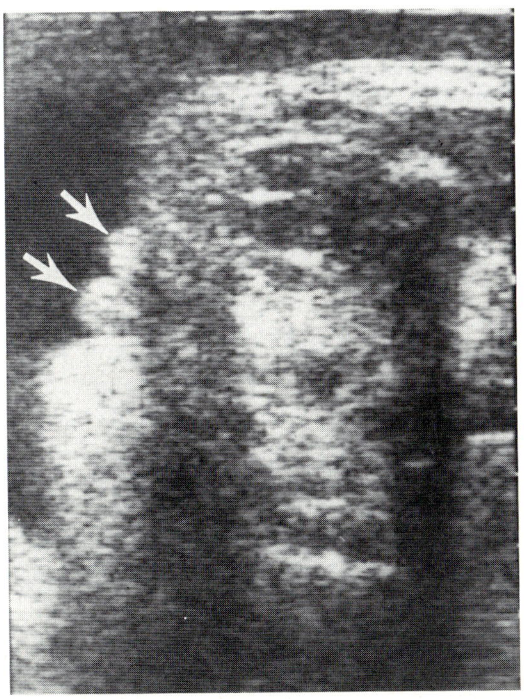

Fig. 12-7. Labia majora *(arrows)* of a female fetus.

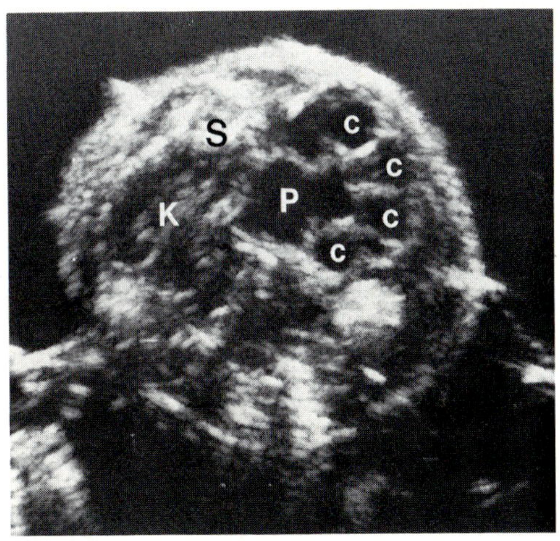

Fig. 12-8. Unilateral hydronephrosis in a newborn. Note the orderly arrangement of dilated pelvis *(P)* and calyces *(c)*. The contralateral kidney *(K)* appears normal. *S*, Spine.

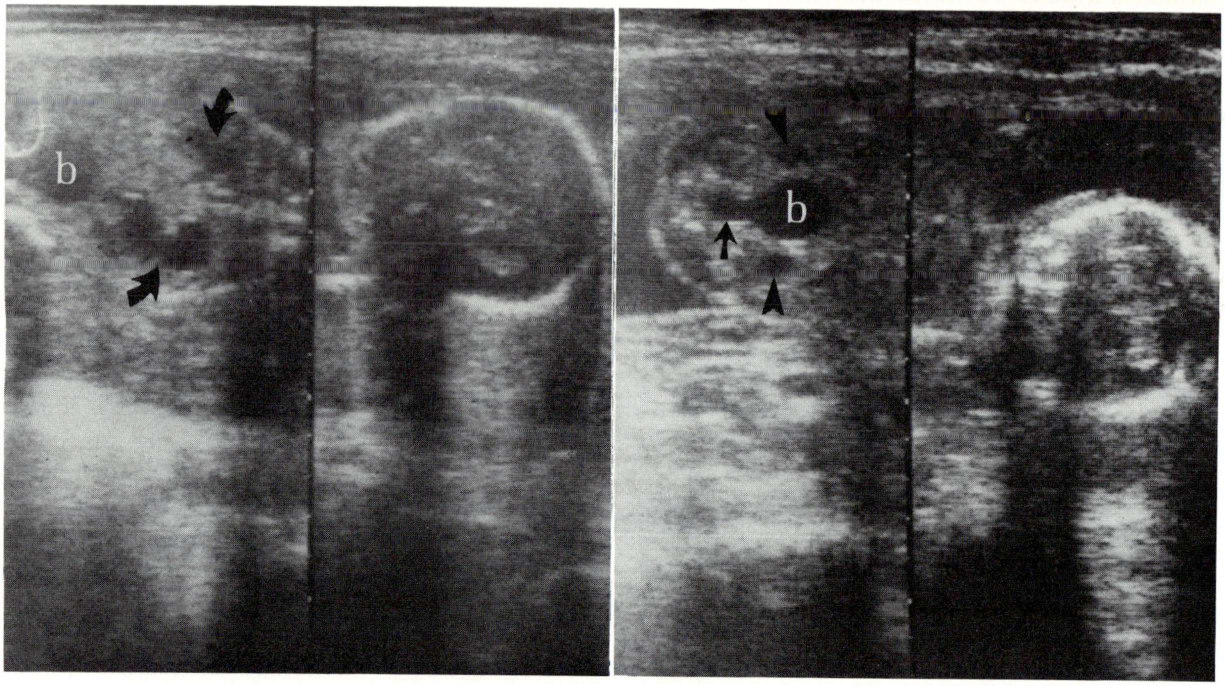

Fig. 12-9. Posterior urethral valves. **A,** Longitudinal scan through the fetus shows severe bilateral hydronephrosis *(curved arrows)*. **B,** Scan in a slightly different plane shows dilation of the posterior urethra *(straight arrow)* and of both ureters *(arrowheads)*. *b,* Bladder.

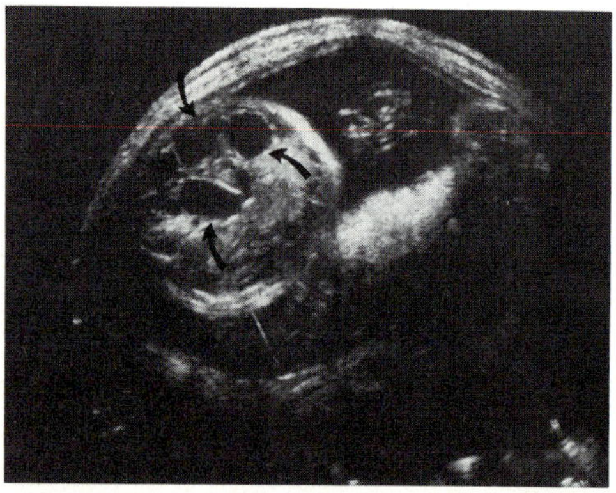

Fig. 12-10. Multicystic dysplastic kidney *(arrows)*. The cysts appear as echo-free structures of varying sizes without apparent organization.

Gastrointestinal malformations

Obstruction at various levels of the gastrointestinal tract can be easily diagnosed by ultrasound. Obstruction of the proximal alimentary canal interferes with the normal process of amniotic fluid turnover, which involves swallowing and absorption of the amniotic fluid by the fetus. Thus, in proximal bowel obstruction, polyhydramnios is an invariable finding (Chapter 6).

In esophageal atresia, absence of the stomach and bowel loops in association with polyhydramnios should alert the examiner to the diagnosis. In duodenal atresia, the presence of a distended stomach and duodenum provides a so-called double-bubble sign and makes the diagnosis almost certain (Fig. 12-11). Similarly, ileal atresia can be diagnosed by the presence of multiple dilated loops of bowel (Fig. 12-12). The same pattern can be seen in meconium ileus and anal atresia.

Abdominal wall defects are among the more common abnormalities detected in the neonate with an approximate incidence of 1 in 2,500 births. The presence of the abdominal viscera in the base of the umbilical cord is an ultrasonic characteristic of omphalocele (Fig. 12-13), whereas in gastroschisis (Fig. 12-14) free bowel loops and liver are seen floating in the amniotic cavity, and the defect is usually lateral to the cord insertion (Chapter 33).

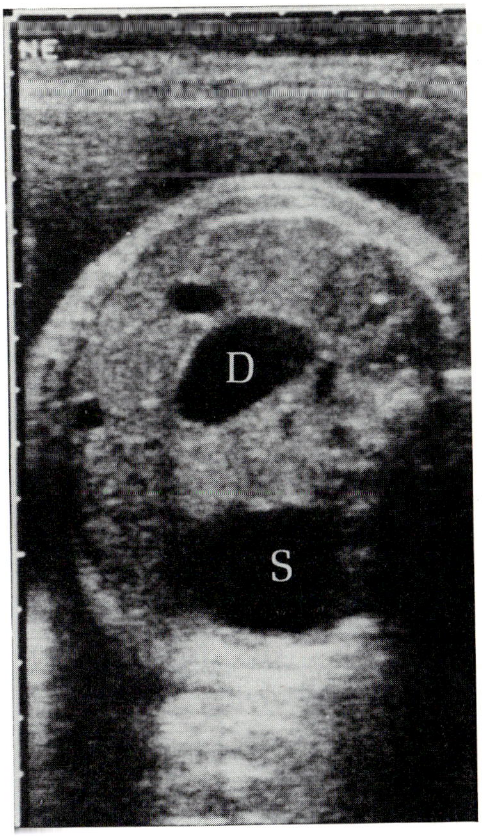

Fig. 12-11. Duodenal atresia. The dilated stomach *(S)* and proximal duodenum *(D)* produce the "double-bubble" sign. Duodenal obstruction can also be caused by an annular pancreas or malrotation of the bowel.

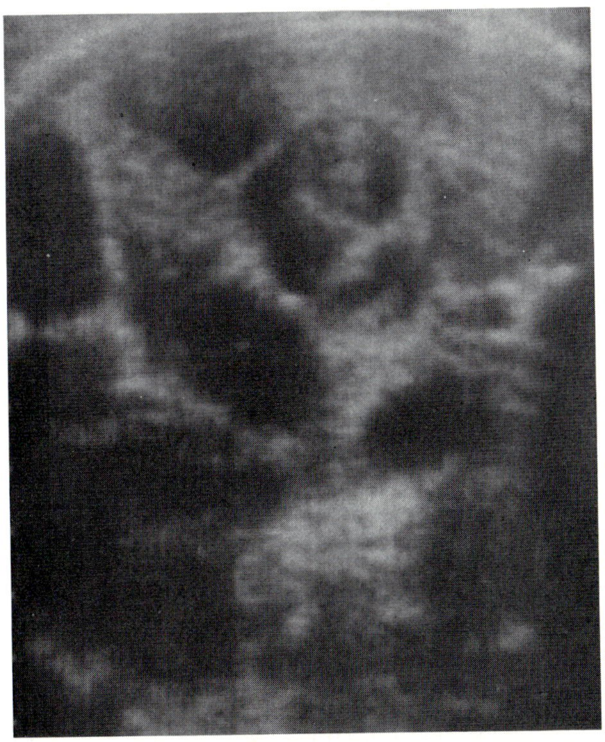

Fig. 12-12. Ileal atresia. Multiple dilated fluid-filled loops of bowel are seen in the fetal abdomen.

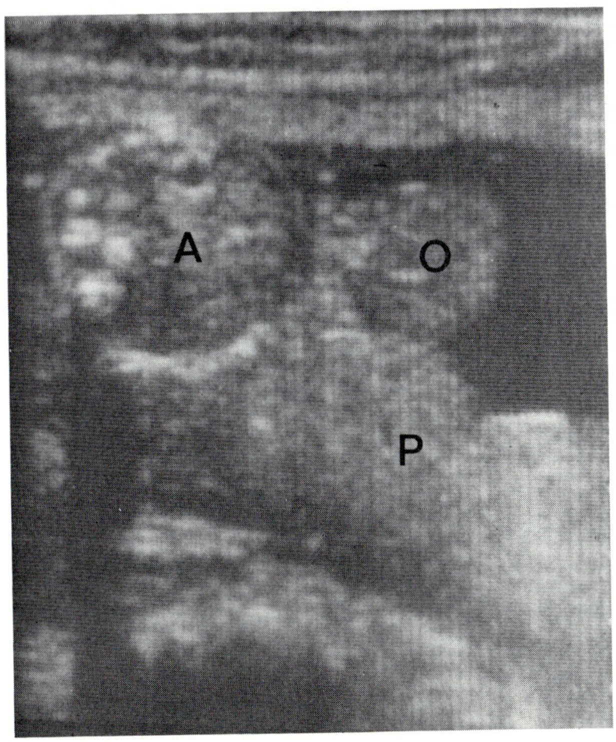

Fig. 12-13. An omphalocele *(O)* is seen adjacent to the fetal abdomen *(A)*. *P*, Placenta.

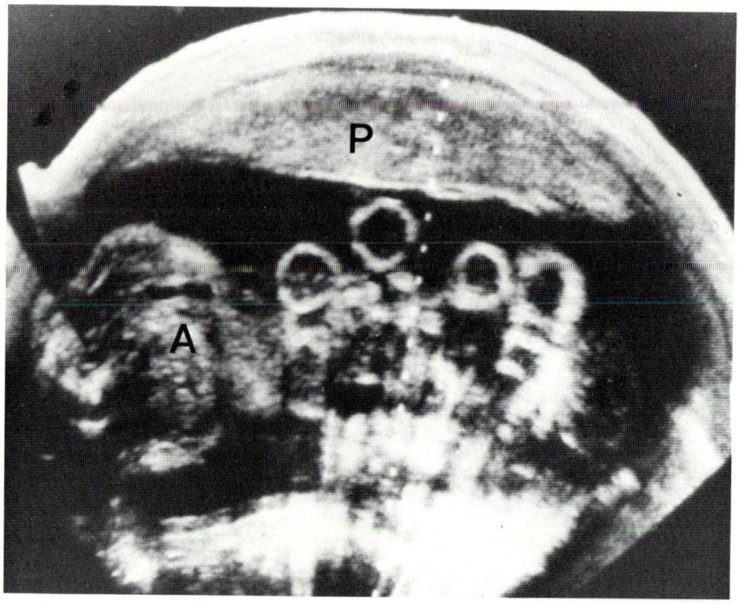

Fig. 12-14. Gastroschisis. Multiple loops of bowel are seen floating freely in the amniotic fluid. The fetal abdomen *(A)* is relatively small, and polyhydramnios exists. *P,* Placenta.

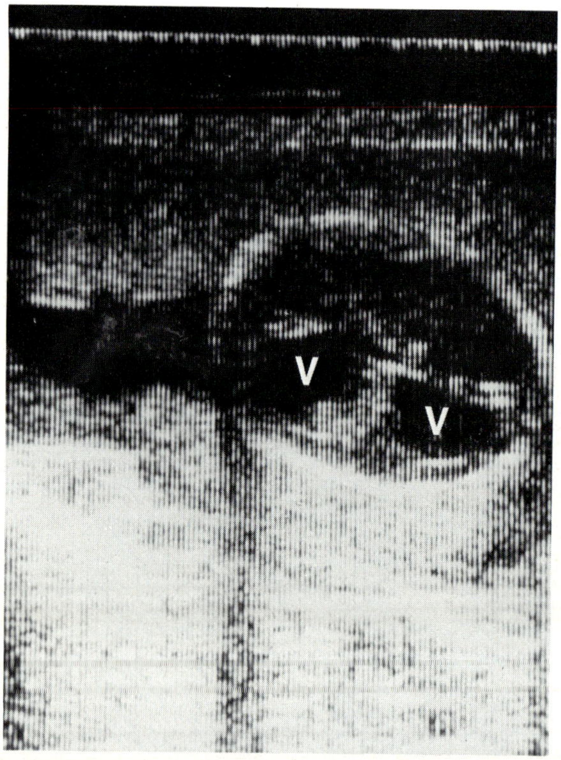

Fig. 12-15. Hydrocephalus. The occipital and frontal horns of the lateral ventricles *(V)* are seen to be dilated, and there is thinning of the cerebral mantle.

Central nervous system

As described previously, the lateral ventricles can be visualized from 15 weeks' gestation. Hydrocephalus can be diagnosed as early as 17 weeks by dilation of the lateral ventricles (Fig. 12-15). The dilation usually occurs before any change in the BPD.

Meningoencephaloceles can be identified as a defect in the calvaria with projection of a membrane containing cerebrospinal fluid or brain tissue outside the skull (Fig. 12-16).

Spina bifida

The spine can be examined by ultrasound in both longitudinal and transverse planes. Longitudinally the spine appears as two parallel lines, and in transverse sections the spinal canal is seen as a circular structure (Fig. 12-5). In the presence of spina bifida, increased separation of the two lines will be noted longitudinally, and a V-shaped or U-shaped defect will be seen in the transverse section (Fig. 12-17). With meningomyelocele a membrane can be seen bulging from the spine (Fig. 12-18).

Anencephaly

Absence of the normal cranium can be detected by approximately 14 to 15 weeks' gestation (Fig. 12-19). There is usually associated polyhydramnios.

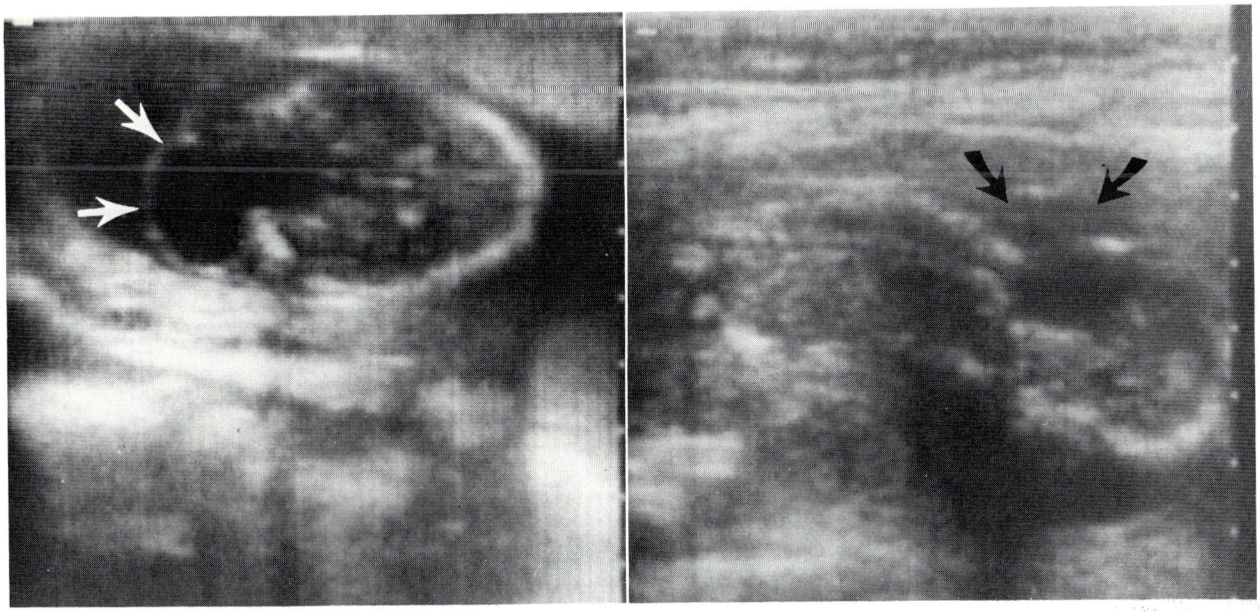

Fig. 12-16. Occipital meningocele. A transverse axial scan **(A)** shows the defect in the calvaria with the membrane *(arrows)* projecting out into the amniotic fluid. A longitudinal scan **(B)** shows the meningocele *(arrows)* at the base of the occiput.

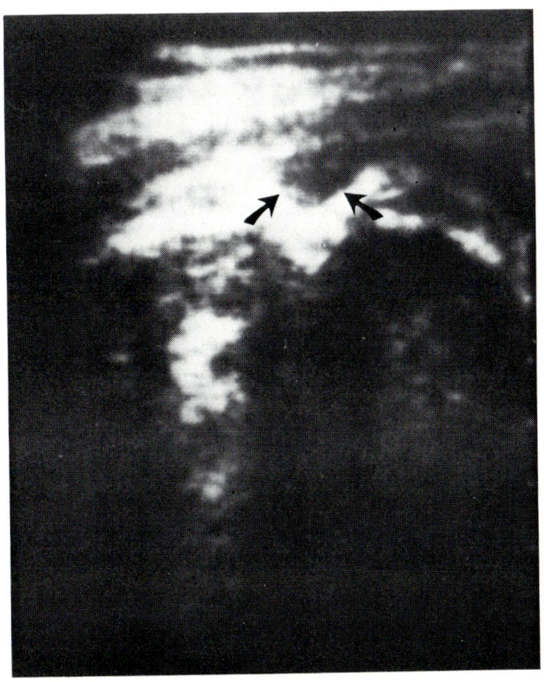

Fig. 12-17. Spina bifida. A V-shaped defect is seen on this transverse scan *(arrows)*.

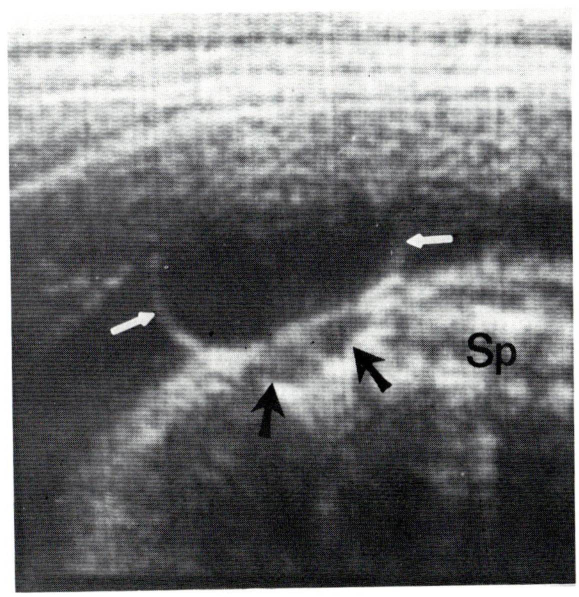

Fig. 12-18. Longitudinal scan of fetus showing spina bifida with meningocele *(small arrows)*. The normal spina *(Sp,* superior to the defect) is seen as parallel lines. The posterior line is interrupted at the level of the spina bifida *(large arrows)*.

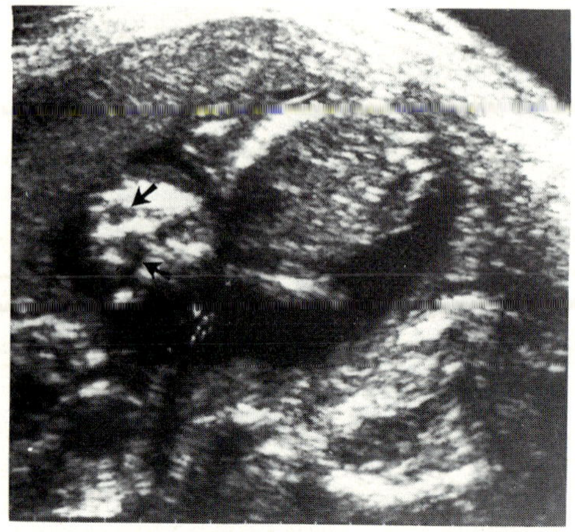

Fig. 12-19. Anencephaly. The fetal body and facial bones are seen, but there is no cranial vault. Arrows point to the orbits.

Microcephaly

Microcephaly can be diagnosed by ultrasound as early as 19 weeks' gestation by the presence of a small head relative to the size of the body. We have had one case in which we made the diagnosis at approximately 21 weeks' gestation after repeating the examination three times. We noted that the abdominal diameter was larger than the head, which in itself is abnormal at that stage of gestation. In addition, we noted a decrease in the rate of the growth of the BPD in the 3-week period during which we repeated the study. Postmortem examination of the fetus confirmed the diagnosis.

Skeletal system

A variety of congenital malformations of the fetal limbs can be detected by ultrasound after 16 weeks' gestation. Both upper and lower extremities can be measured by real-time ultrasonography from 16 weeks' gestation, and the length can be ascertained and compared with O'Brien and associates' data.

We have diagnosed several cases of dwarfism and one case of osteogenesis imperfecta (Fig. 12-20).

Abnormalities of the chest, such as hydrothorax (Fig. 12-21), microthorax due to hypoplastic lungs (Fig. 12-22), diaphragmatic hernia, and major cardiac abnormalities, can be diagnosed by ultrasound.

Fetal tumors

Various benign and malignant tumors of the fetus, including those of the kidneys, adrenals, liver, lungs, soft tissues, and central nervous sytem can be identified antenatally by sonography (Figs. 12-23 and 12-24). As would be expected, the likelihood of detection is related to the size of the tumor.

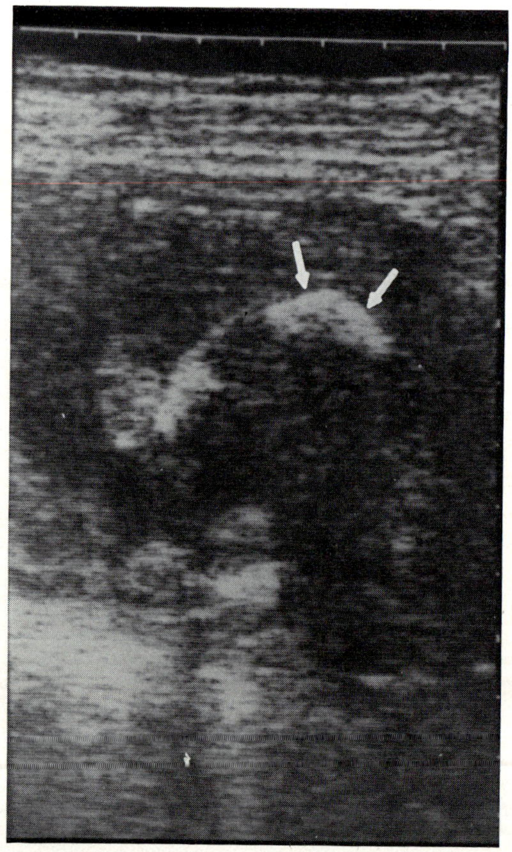

Fig. 12-20. Osteogenesis imperfecta. Sonogram of the fetal femur *(arrows)* shows that the femur is bent, indicating an in utero fracture.

A
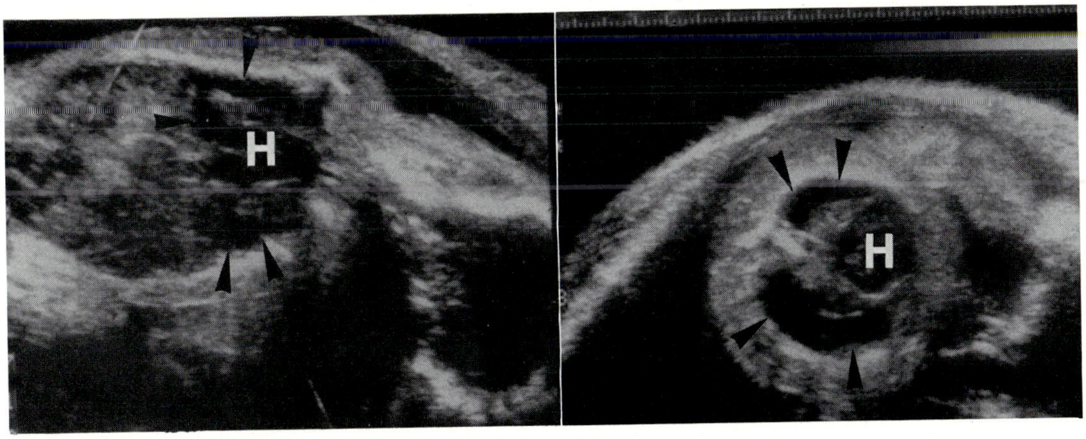

B

Fig. 12-21. Bilateral fetal hydrothorax with severe subcutaneous edema and polyhydramnios. The coronal **(A)** and transverse **(B)** scans show bilateral fetal hydrothorax *(arrowheads)*. The lungs are compressed against the heart *(H)* by the pleural fluid. Note marked thickening of the thoracic wall caused by fetal edema.

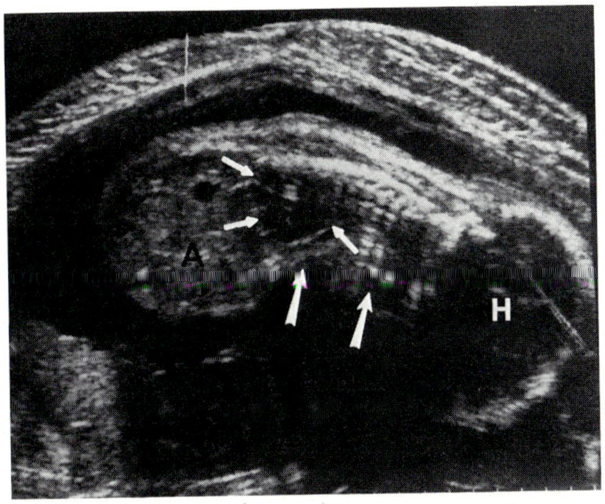

Fig. 12-22. Small thorax in a thanatophoric dwarf, secondary to hypoplasia of the lungs. Note the small diameter of the thorax relative to the abdomen *(A)*. Large arrows show the thorax; small arrows show the fetal heart. *H,* Head.

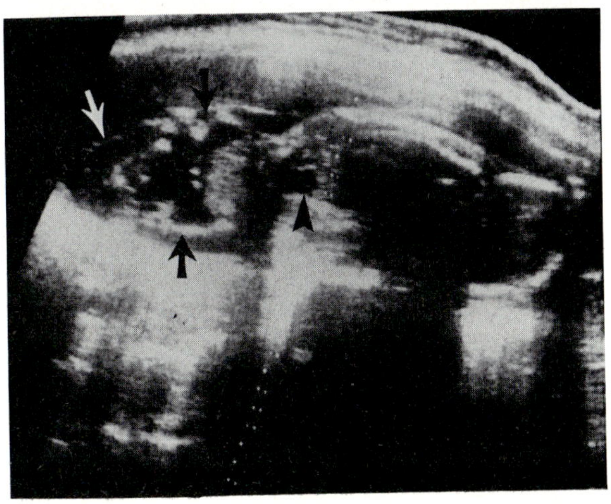

Fig. 12-23. Sacrococcygeal teratoma. A large complex mass with both solid and cystic components *(arrows)* is seen projecting from the region of the sacrum. *Arrowhead,* Fetal bladder.

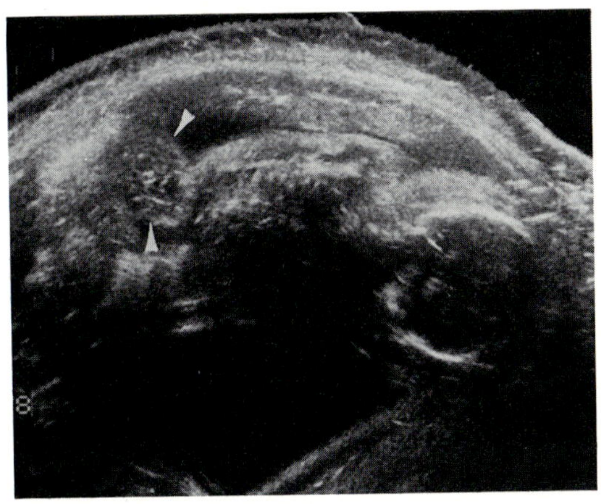

Fig. 12-24. Malignant melanoma of fetus. Longitudinal scan of the fetus shows a predominantly solid echogenic mass *(arrowheads)* in the region of the sacrum. The antenatal diagnosis was probable teratoma, but the mass proved histologically to be a malignant melanoma.

Diagnosis of fetal death

Absence of the visible fetal heartbeat by real-time imaging is the most reliable method of diagnosing intrauterine fetal death. Other signs include absence of fetal limb movement and collapse of the bones of the calvaria. The latter occurs about a week after fetal demise and was a valuable sign before the availability of good real-time equipment.

USE OF ULTRASOUND IN HIGH-RISK PREGNANCY

Intrauterine growth retardation is associated with a significantly increased rate of perinatal mortality and long-term morbidity (Chapter 7). Improved perinatal outcome is contingent on accurate early identification. Confirmation of the diagnosis of intrauterine growth retardation (IUGR) by hormonal studies is inadequate. Campbell assessed the value of urinary estrogen in 85 "small for dates" infants and found that only 53% had abnormal estrogens; a similar finding was reported by Martin and associates. Therefore considerable attention has been focused recently on the use of ultrasonography in the diagnosis of growth retardation.

Campbell and Dewhurst used serial BPD measurements to predict intrauterine growth retardation complicated by intrauterine growth retardation and found that in 82% the BPD growth was below normal. They reported two different patterns of abnormal BPD growth. In the first pattern there is normal growth until the third trimester, with flattening of the growth rate thereafter. In the second pattern the BPD shows steady but abnormally low growth rate, usually very early in pregnancy, and this is the so-called low-profile growth. However, other investigators using BPD measurements alone could predict growth retardation in only 50% of cases.

Another method used for detection of growth retardation is the head/body ratio. This is of value because in growth retardation the brain is relatively spared and the body diameter or circumference will lag behind the head, reflecting reduced growth of the fetal liver. Normally the average fetal body diameter measured at the level of the umbilical vein should be within 5 mm of the BPD, and in late pregnancy it is usually greater than the BPD. A body diameter in excess of 5 mm less than the BPD indicates probable growth retardation.

Hobbins used total intrauterine volume measurements for diagnosis of growth retardation and found that when the volume was more than 1.5 standard deviations below the mean for the gestational age most of the fetuses were growth retarded. However, other investigators could not confirm those findings. Other methods of diagnosing growth retardation include using combined head/body ratio, placental appearance, and amniotic fluid volume. Many authorities agree that there is no single placental abnormality that is common to small for gestational age (SGA) fetuses. However, there are certain lesions that occur with high frequency in the placentae of such neonates, including infarction, villous vascularity, fibrosis, and a nonspecific villous inflammation. With advances in ultrasound techniques it is possible to study the placental structure in detail prior to delivery. Calcification and fibrous maturity rings are found in most placentae near term. However, excessive calcification prior to 36 weeks' gestation indicates possible fetal compromise. Amniotic fluid volume also tends to be reduced in IUGR. Once identification of possible growth retardation has been made, hospitalization is imperative.

Ultrasound is of particular value in following the growth of twin gestations. In early pregnancy the BPDs of twins are always identical. In later stages of pregnancy the abdominal circumference or abdominal diameter is more helpful in diagnosis of growth retardation in twin gestations than is the BPD. Because of increased pressure, the BPD may be altered due to variations in the shape of the baby's head, such as dolichocephaly.

Rh incompatibility

Hobbins described the sequence of events in Rh disease observed on ultrasonography (Chapter 5). The first sign of fetal compromise is excessive accumulation of amniotic fluid, followed by increase in the placental thickness to more than 5 cm. The next change is in the fetal liver with development of hepatomegaly. Usually the abdominal diameter or the abdominal circumference is larger than normal in relation to the head. The last sign is the appearance of fetal ascites (Fig. 12-25). Ultrasound is valuable not only in localizing for amniocentesis but also to follow the progress of the fetus in conjunction with the ΔOD. Once the decision is made for intrauterine transfusion, the procedure nowadays is usually performed under direct real-time ultrasound guidance, with the needle tip being monitored into the fetal abdomen or, more recently, into the umbilical vein. Its presence in the peritoneal cavity can be confirmed by injecting a small amount of contrast material and obtaining a radiograph (Fig. 12-26). The success of the procedure is confirmed by seeing the transfused blood in the peritoneal cavity.

Diabetes

The ultrasound findings in diabetes vary according to the class. From classes A to C the general picture is that of an abdominal diameter that is large relative to that of the head, increase in amniotic fluid volume, and a placenta that is thicker than normal. The degree of macrosomia of the fetus can be followed by the rate of growth of the fetal head and by the head/abdomen ratio. In classes D to F diabetes there is an increased incidence of growth retardation due to vascular involvement, and the patient should be followed for possible intrauterine growth retardation (Chapter 3).

Antepartum hemorrhage

Antepartum hemorrhage occurs in about 3% of pregnancies. Placenta previa and abruption account for less than half of all cases. The remainder are caused by many other factors including polyps, ascites, varicosities, laceration, and carcinoma.

Placenta previa

Sonographic placental localization has replaced all other methods of diagnosis such as soft tissue placentography and radionuclide scintigraphy. The placenta first becomes visible as a focal thickening along the periphery of the gestational sac at approximately 8 weeks' gestation. By the end of the first trimester it can be identified as a fine granular disklike structure occupying a major part of the endometrial surface. As pregnancy progresses, the proportion of the endometrial surface occupied by the placenta diminishes. Apparent change in placental location with advancing gestational age has been noted, and low lying placenta is a common occurrence in midgestation. More than 90% of these early low implantations convert to normal position at term. The overall risk

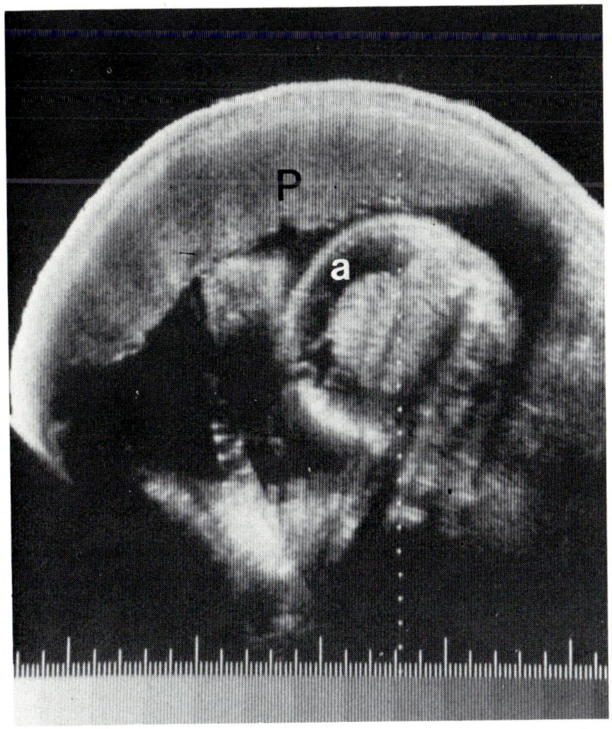

Fig. 12-25. Rh incompatibility with fetal ascites *(a)*. The placenta *(P)* is thickened.

A

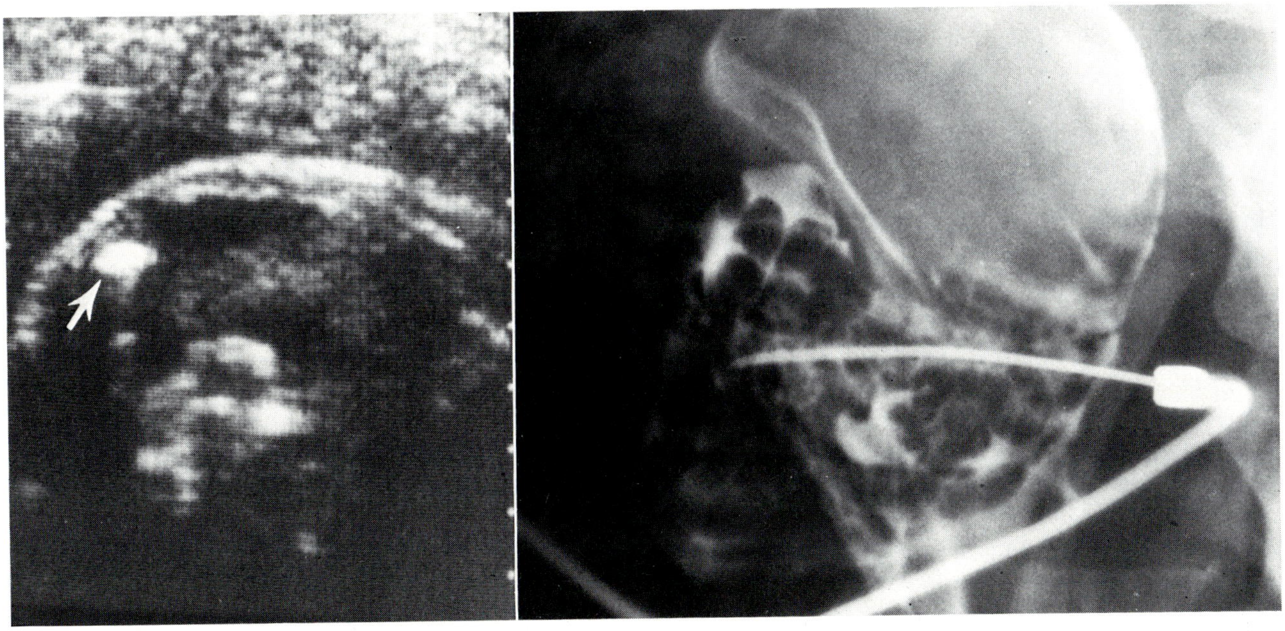

B

Fig. 12-26. Intrauterine transfusion for Rh incompatibility. **A,** The needle produces a strong echo *(arrow)* in the fetal abdomen. **B,** Radiograph obtained after injection of a small amount of contrast through the needle shows loops of bowel and liver outlined by the contrast. This confirms the intraperitoneal location of the needle tip.

of placenta previa in the third trimester is approximately 5% to 6% if the placenta covers any of the cervix earlier in gestation. Infrequently there is an adverse sequel later in gestation. Despite the return to normal position, an increased risk of abortion, bleeding, and intrauterine growth retardation has been suggested by European and Australian centers. There have been reports of an increase in midtrimester abortion and cases of threatened abortion in which the placenta is low but the scan is otherwise normal.

Sonographic recognition of placenta previa depends on identifying the inferior margin of the placenta in relation to the cervix. Central placenta previa is present when the placenta completely covers the internal os. Partial previa indicates that a portion of the internal os is covered. When the placental edge reaches the margin of the internal os, it is called a marginal placenta previa. During the examination, the patient's bladder should be full, but not overdistended. An overdistended bladder can compress the lower segment of the uterus and cause a false appearance of a low-lying placenta. Anterior placenta previa is easier to visualize and diagnose. The posteriorly located placenta is more difficult to identify sonographically because there is considerable attenuation of the sound as it passes through the fetal parts. Placenta previa should be suspected when the presenting part is placed outside the pelvis or when the distance between the presenting part and the sacral promontory is greater than 1.5 cm.

The accuracy of ultrasonography in diagnosing placenta previa is 90% to 97% depending on the experience of the examiner. The etiology of low implantation remains controversial. The major theories focus on endometrial damage and defective placentation. Prior cesarean section, therapeutic abortion, and increased age and parity have been shown to increase the risk of placenta previa.

Abruptio placentae

Abruptio placentae is defined as separation of the normally implanted placenta after the twentieth week of gestation and before the third stage of labor. It is probably initiated by hemorrhage into the decidua basalis. The incidence varies between 0.2% and 2%. Conditions that may be associated with abruptio placentae include a short umbilical cord, external trauma, sudden decompression of the uterus, polyhydramnios, maternal hypertension, folate deficiency, and uterine tumors. Bleeding from abruption may appear through the vagina externally or remain retroplacental and concealed.

Clinical diagnosis of abruptio placentae is usually based on the clinical triad of abdominal uterine rigidity, tenderness, and vaginal bleeding. Sonographically, retroplacental hematoma may be visualized as an anechoic or a complex collection between the uterine wall and the placenta. The echogenicity of the hematoma depends on the degree of organization of the blood clot. The diagnosis of retroplacental hemorrhage is often difficult to establish. Diagnosis is usually confirmed at delivery with microscopic examination of the placenta. Occasionally a retroplacental hematoma does not form and blood may dissect beneath the chorionic membrane, resulting in subchorionic hematoma. This may be seen sonographically as an echo-free complex collection behind the chorionic plate causing elevation of the plate. The differential diagnosis includes uterine fibroids posterior to the placenta and endometrial veins along the base of the placenta, which can simulate hematoma. Physiologic thickening of the uterine wall may also occasionally simulate hematoma.

AMNIOCENTESIS

Amniocentesis for the analysis of amniotic fluid has contributed greatly to the evaluation of the fetus in utero. Although the procedure was used before the twentieth century for aspiration of amniotic fluid to relieve hydramnios, in early 1950 Bevis used the procedure for evaluation of Rh-sensitized pregnancies. Since that time there have been several expanded uses of the technique. The most common indications for amniocentesis are:

1. Genetic studies
2. Evaluation of fetal maturity
3. Follow-up of Rh sensitized patients

Less important indications include:

1. Detection of fetal meconium in high-risk pregnancies
2. Confirmation of premature rupture of the membrane by injection of dye such as indigo carmine
3. Detection of bacteria and white cells in suspected amnionitis

Midtrimester genetic amniocentesis is usually performed between 16 and 18 weeks' gestation so sufficient time is allowed for culture of the cells and for the parent to exercise her options concerning the outcome of the pregnancy. For those infants with a serious congenital malformation detected by ultrasound during the procedure, the information obtained may provide life-saving early detection, so that before the birth, appropriate advance preparation may be made for medical and surgical care of the sick neonate. For those abnormalities that are incompatible with life, heroic interventions will be avoided, thus lessening the psychologic trauma to the parents.

A complete real-time ultrasound examination is performed prior to the amniocentesis to determine fetal age, placental location, and complete evaluation of fetal anatomy before selection of a suitable puncture site. Almost all centers that perform amniocentesis use ultrasound routinely prior to the procedure. The principal justifications for routine use of ultrasound prior to genetic studies are for detection of twin gestation, determination of fetal viability, exclusion of major structural abnormalities, and determination of gestational age. However, controversy still exists over whether the routine use of ultrasound prior to amniocentesis lowers the incidence of multiple needle insertions or influences the frequency of bloody taps. Golbus and associates found no such benefit, although other investigators have found a definite decrease in the incidence of complications related to the amniocentesis and of bloody taps when the procedure utilized ultrasound.

Our usual technique is as follows: the insertion point is identified on the maternal abdomen by real-time ultrasonography, and the angle of approach and depth are determined. If possible, the placenta should be avoided, especially the thick portion of the placenta near the insertion of the umbilical cord. It is also important to avoid hitting the fetus with the needle, particularly in the head and chest. The maternal bladder may be full or empty depending on the preference of the operator. The skin is prepared with a Betadine solution, draped, and a 20- or 22-gauge needle is inserted into the identified pocket of fluid. Local anesthesia is not necessary with such fine needles, and we do not use it.

An alternative technique is to use a biopsy transducer for continuous visualization of the needle. The needle insertion can also be visualized with a simple (nonbiopsy) sector or linear array real-time scanner. We use this technique whenever the available pool of amniotic fluid is small or if we do not obtain fluid initially at the selected depth. We find this technique extremely useful in those circumstances. We also use it in third trimester amniocenteses and in Rh negative mothers in the late second trimester.

Risks of amniocentesis

The United States collaborative study on amniocentesis during the years 1969 to 1973 did not demonstrate an increased risk of spontaneous abortion, prematurity or other morbidity in the fetus after amniocentesis. A Canadian study also failed to demonstrate any ill effect from the procedure. However, the British collaborative study suggested a higher risk of fetal loss after amniocentesis, that is, 2.6% compared to 1.1% in a control population, and an increase of 1% to 1.5% in certain types of infant morbidity, namely unexplained respiratory difficulty at birth and also orthopedic postural abnormalities. However, the British study has drawn considerable criticism because of the manner in which the control group was selected. Also, 30% of the patients in that study had amniocentesis because of elevated serum alpha-fetoprotein, a condition associated with higher perinatal mortality. During the last few years, other investigators reported various morbidity and mortality rates. For example, Philip and Bang reported an incidence of fetal death after amniocentesis in the range of 0.3% to 0.7%. Park reported fetal loss of 2.4%, and the majority of these resulted from fetal infection. Fetal complications recorded include pneumothorax and skin lesions. During amniocentesis fetal to maternal bleeding can occur; therefore all Rh negative unsensitized patients should receive a full dose of Rh immunoglobulin (Rho gam) in a dose of 300 mg.

CONCLUSION

With recent improvements in technology, ultrasound has become the most important modality for evaluating the pregnant uterus and the fetus. The growth and well-being of the fetus can be evaluated and several major fetal anomalies diagnosed antenatally. This may be crucial because it alerts the pediatricians and pediatric surgeons to the need for immediate corrective therapy or surgery after birth.

Patrick J. Bryan
Majida N. Jassani

BIBLIOGRAPHY

Adam, A.H., and Robinson, H.P.: An evaluation of real-time scanning in the first trimester of pregnancy. In Bennett, M.J., and Campbell, S., editors: Real-time ultrasound in obstetrics, Boston, 1980, Blackwell Scientific Publications.

Azimi, F., Bryan, P.J., and Marangola, J.P.: Ultrasonography in obstetrics and gynecology: historical notes, basic principles, safety considerations, and clinical applications, CRC Crit. Rev. Clin. Radiol. Nucl. Med., 1976.

Bennett, M.J.: Real-time ultrasound in the second and third trimesters of pregnancy. In Bennett, M.J., and Campbell, S., editors: Real-time ultrasound in obstetrics, Boston, 1980, Blackwell Scientific Publications.

Bevis, D.C.A.: The antenatal prediction of haemolytic disease of the newborn, Lancet **1**:395, 1952.

Bryan, P.J., and Champlin, F.M.: Apparent placental migration caused by uterine rotation. In White, D., and Brown, R.E., editors: Ultrasound in medicine, vol. 3A, New York, 1977, Plenum Publishing Corp.

Campbell, S.: An improved method of fetal cephalometry by ultrasound, J. Obstet. Gynaecol. Br. Commonw. **75**:568, 1968.

Campbell, S.: The prediction of fetal maturity by ultrasonic measurement of the biparietal diameter, J. Obstet. Gynaecol. B. Commonw. **76**:603, 1969.

Campbell, S., and Dewhurst, C.J.: Diagnosis of small-for-dates fetus by serial ultrasonic cephalometry, Lancet **2**:1002, 1971.

Campbell, S., and Little, D.J.: Clinical potential of real-time ultrasound. In Bennett, M.J., and Campbell, S., editors: Real-time ultrasound in obstetrics, Boston, 1980, Blackwell Scientific Publications.

Chayen, S.: An assessment of the hazards of amniocentesis: report to the medical research council by their working party on amniocentesis, Br. J. Obstet. Gynecol. **85**(suppl. 2), 1978.

Deter, R.L., and others: The use of ultrasound in the assessment of normal fetal growth: a review, J. Clin. Ultrasound **9**:481, 1981.

DeVore, G.R., and Hobbins, J.C.: Fetal growth and development: the diagnosis of intrauterine growth retardation. In Hobbins, J.C., editor: Diagnostic ultrasound in obstetrics, New York, 1979. Churchill Livingstone.

Donald, I.: Sonar: a new diagnostic echo-sounding technique in obstetrics and gynaecology, Proc. R. Soc. Med. **55**:637, 1962.

Donald I., and Brown, T.G.: Demonstration of tissue interfaces within the body of ultrasonic echo sounding, Br. J. Radiol. **34**:539, 1961.

Donald, I., MacVicar, J., and Brown, T.G.: Investigation of abdominal masses by pulsed ultrasound, Lancet **1**:1188, 1958.

Fadel, H.E., and Martin, S.: Realtime sonographic diagnosis of fetal dysplastic kidney, Int. J. Gynaecol. Obstet. **18**:140, 1980.

Finnegan, J.K.: Amniotic fluid and midtrimester amniocentesis: a review, Br. J. Obstet. Gynaecol. **91**:745, 1984.

Golbus, M.S., and others: Prenatal genetic diagnosis in 3000 amniocenteses, N. Engl. J. Med. **300**:157, 1979.

Grannum, P., Berkowitz, R.L., and Hobbins, J.C.: The ultrasonic changes in the maturing placenta and their relation to fetal pulmonic maturity, Am. J. Obstet. Gynecol. **133**:915, 1979.

Grannum, P., and others: Assessment of fetal kidney size in normal gestation by comparison of ratio of kidney circumference to abdominal circumferences, Am. J. Obstet. Gynecol. **136**:249, 1980.

Grossman, M., and others: Pitfalls in ultrasonic determination of total intrauterine volume, J. Clin. Ultrasound **10**:17, 1982.

Hadlock, F.P., Deter, R.L., and Park, S.K.: Real-time sonography: ventricular and vascular anatomy of the fetal brain in utero, Am. J. Roentgenol. **136**:133, 1981.

Hobbins, J.C., and Venus, I.: Congenital anomalies. In Hobbins, J.C., editor: Diagnostic ultrasound in obstetrics, New York, 1979, Churchill Livingstone.

Hobbins, J.C., and others: Ultrasound in the diagnosis of congenital anomalies, Am. J. Obstet. Gynecol. **134**:331, 1979.

Hobbins, J.C.: Use of ultrasound in complicated pregnancies. In Berkowitz, R.L., editor: Clinics in perinatology, vol. 7, Philadelphia, 1980, W.B. Saunders Co.

Jassani, M.N., and others: Twin pregnancy with discordancy for Down's syndrome, Obstet. Gynecol. **55**(3):45S, 1980.

Jassani, M.N., and others: A perinatal approach to the diagnosis and management of gastrointestinal malformations, Obstet. Gynecol. **59**(1):33, 1982.

Johnson, M.L., and others: Evaluation of fetal intracranial anatomy by static and real-time ultrasound, J. Clin. Ultrasound **8**:311, 1980.

Keirse, M., Meerman, D., and Meerman, R.H.: Antenatal diagnosis of Potter syndrome, Obstet. Gynecol. **52**(1):64S, 1978.

King, D.L.: Placental migration demonstrated by ultrasonography, Radiology **109**:167, 1973.

Kossoff, G., and Garrett, W.J.: Intracranial detail in fetal echograms, Invest. Radiol. **7**:159, 1972.

Martin, J.D., and others: Urinary oestrogen excretion in women with intra-uterine fetal growth retardation, Aust. NZ J. Obstet. Gynaecol. **12**:102, 1972.

McGahan, J.P., and others: Sonographic spectrum of retroplacental hemorrhage, Radiology **142**:481, 1982.

Meire, H.B.: Diagnosis of renal agenesis using ultrasonography, Br. J. Radiol. **53**:381, 1980.

NICHD National Registry for Amniocentesis Study Group: Midtrimester amniocentesis for prenatal diagnosis, JAMA **236**:1471, 1976.

O'Brien, G.D., Queenan, J.T., and Campbell, S.: Assessment of gestational age in the second trimester by real-time ultrasound measurement of the femur length, Am. J. Obstet. Gynecol. **139**:540, 1981.

O'Brien, W.F. Midtrimester genetic amniocentesis: a review of the fetal risks, J. Reprod. Med. **29**:59, 1984.

Park, I.J., and others: Spontaneous abortion after midtrimester amniocentesis, Obstet. Gynecol. **53**:190, 1976.

Philip, J., and Bang, J.: Outcome of pregnancy after amniocentesis for chromosomal analysis, Br. Med. J. **2**:1183, 1978.

Platt, L.D., and Manning, F.A.: Real-time ultrasound in special procedures. In Hobbins J.C., editor: Diagnostic ultrasound in obstetrics, New York, 1979, Churchill Livingstone.

Queenan, J.T., and Kubarych, S.F.: Detecting and managing polyhydramnios, Contemp. Obstet. Gynecol. **16**:113, 1980.

Simpson, N.E., and others: Prenatal diagnosis of genetic disease in Canada: report of a collaborative study, Can. Med. Assoc. J. **115**:739, 1976.

Spirt, B.A., Cohen, W.N., and Weinstein, HM.: The incidence of placental calcification in normal pregnancies, Radiology **142**:707, 1982.

Tabsh, K.M.A., Lbeherz, T.B., and Crandall, B.F.: Risks of prophylactic anti-D immunoglobulin after second-trimester amniocentesis, Am. J. Obstet. Gynecol. **149**:225, 1984.

CHAPTER 13

Diagnostic imaging

In attempting to present a subject as comprehensive as neonatal imaging within the confines of a single chapter, many important aspects of the discipline must be omitted and others mentioned only briefly. It is not our intention to cover in detail the imaging of specific disorders that affect the neonate, since these are dealt with elsewhere in this book; rather it is our purpose to discuss the indications and the basic methodology of commonly used imaging methods. In addition, a roentgenologic approach to diagnosis based on frequently occurring roentgenographic findings is presented.

PATIENT PROTECTION

Prolonged survival of premature infants has resulted in larger numbers of roentgenograms being taken, thus increasing radiation exposure. Consequently, radiologists have become more concerned with the possible long-term effects of low-dosage diagnostic roentgenograms. These effects are extremely difficult to measure, since most data must be obtained from laboratory experiments or following accidental human exposure to high doses of radiation. Investigations such as those showing an apparent increased risk for development of leukemia in children exposed to diagnostic x rays in utero might imply a similar effect on the preterm neonate. A long latent period between low-dose exposure and development of a radiation effect is an additional difficulty in studying current intensive care nursery populations. However, certain practical steps can be taken to prevent unnecessary radiation. These include careful collimation of the x-ray beam to the field of interest, gonadal shielding, avoidance of overexposure and repeat examinations by meticulous attention to technical detail, and a thorough evaluation of the indications for the examination on the part of the attending physician.

High-speed radiographic film combined with rare earth intensifying screens can markedly decrease radiation exposure and reduce the likelihood of motion artifacts. When such equipment is used in the nursery, however, state of-the-art portable x-ray units are necessary to realize these benefits.

CHEST

Chest roentgenograms account for the majority of roentgenographic studies in newborn infants. Most of these are required because of problems of respiratory distress in premature infants. Roentgenographic techniques for the neonate differ from those used in older infants and children because of the small size and rapid respiratory rates of the newborn. Radiologists, neonatologists, and nursery personnel must understand the special requirements for proper roentgenographic examination of these patients.

Assessment of an optimum examination

A simple check of several technical aspects of the film greatly increases the likelihood of proper interpretation of suspected abnormalities. The following points should be considered:

1. *Exposure*. This is a subjective evaluation and is represented by the degree of blackening of the film. In general, details of the thoracic spine should be visible through the cardiothymic silhouette.
2. *Motion*. This will cause obvious blurring of the images and will result in decreased definition of structures such as the pulmonary vessels and diaphragm.
3. *Positioning*. Rotation will increase magnification of the structures closest to the beam. For example, in the supine position, rotation of the patient to the right will cause magnification of the left ribs and the left hilum. Also, the heart will be projected within the right hemithorax. A simple method of assessing rotation is to compare the relative positions of the anterior ends of a pair of ribs.
4. *Extraneous objects*. A large portion of the chest of a small premature infant can be completely obscured by electrocardiogram electrodes, cutaneous oxygen monitors, and other equipment. When possible, these as well

as other opaque densities such as warming mattresses and respirator tubing should be removed prior to roentgenography.

5. *Inspiration*. The roentgenogram should be exposed at the end of inspiration, a difficult task in neonates with rapid respiratory rates. In some the tidal volume is so small that there is little difference in the degree of lung aeration during the respiratory cycle. In others it is difficult to determine whether the resultant increase in lung opacity is due to expiration or a pathologic decrease in lung volume. As a general rule, on a good inspiratory film the right diaphragmatic dome should be projected at about the level of the anterior end of the sixth rib.

Methods of examination

Except for special studies, most roentgenography of the chest can be accomplished in the newborn nursery using modern portable roentgenographic equipment. These units employ a single-phase generator capable of exposure times of less than 5 msec at the relatively low kilovoltage required for these infants. In almost every case, blurring due to respiratory motion can be prevented. Recently, further decreases in exposure time have been achieved by using rare earth screens, although there is some resultant loss of detail with an increase in graininess or mottle because of increased quantum "noise."

Within the radiology department, most chest roentgenography is done at a distance of 72 inches. This must be reduced to approximately 40 inches when using portable equipment. Although in the larger patient this results in considerable distortion of structures due to magnification, no important degradation of the image occurs with small infants.

Portable roentgenographic examinations of the chest consist of an anteroposterior (AP) view made with a vertical beam and, frequently, a lateral view made with a horizontal beam. Careful positioning, which is often undertaken by the nursery personnel, is of extreme importance in obtaining a high quality roentgenogram. The AP view is made with the patient lying supine, and proper positioning is facilitated by extending the patient's arms above the head and immobilizing the thighs. For the lateral view the x-ray tube can then be moved so that the x-ray beam is directed horizontally. The patient, therefore, need not be turned as would be the case with a vertical beam lateral view. Occasionally a lateral decubitus view is necessary, particularly for evaluation of a pneumothorax. This also is made with a horizontal x-ray beam. The patient is turned so that the unaffected side is dependent.

It is debatable whether a lateral as well as an AP view need be done for each examination. The increased radiation dose and the necessity of further handling of a fragile infant must be weighed against the possibility of significant gain in diagnostic information from the lateral view. In a recent study the addition of a lateral view did not increase the diagnostic accuracy of initial chest roentgenograms made in the nursery. Whether this would hold true for subsequent roentgenographic examinations is not known, but in our nursery we no longer do lateral views routinely.

Other useful roentgenographic techniques in newborn chest disease include magnification radiography, which is done with a small focal spot (0.2 to 0.3 mm) that approximates a point source. The patient is no longer in contact with the film; thus divergence of the x-ray beam projects a magnified image onto the film. This usually requires removal of the infant from the incubator. Also, high-kilovoltage films may be made to assess the airways and mediastinal structures. These are done in the radiology department using extra filtration of the x-ray beam. The rationale for this technique is to increase the relative absorption of x rays in bone and soft tissue by using a higher energy beam, thus enhancing the radiolucency of the air-containing structures. This technique also may be combined with magnification roentgenography.

Fluoroscopy, tomography, bronchography, angiography, computed tomography, and radionuclide lung scan-

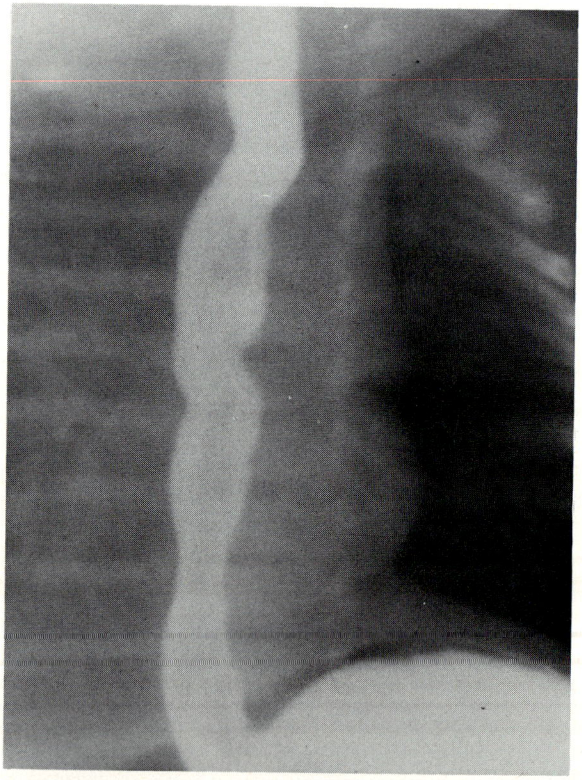

Fig. 13-1. Massive gastroesophageal reflux and abnormal esophageal peristalsis in a 3-week-old infant with apnea.

ning are other roentgenologic techniques that are available for specific diagnostic problems.

Barium esophagrams frequently are indicated in neonates with feeding problems, signs of airway obstruction and apnea. During this examination, swallowing function and esophageal peristalsis are monitored. Extrinsic lesions compressing the trachea and esophagus, such as vascular rings due to aortic arch anomalies, vascular slings (aberrant left pulmonary artery), and bronchogenic cysts, may be identified. Gastroesophageal reflux frequently is observed in patients being investigated for "near-miss" sudden infant death syndrome (Fig. 13-1).

Ultrasonography is less useful for chest diagnosis than in the abdomen because of reduced transmission of sound waves in air. However, if an appropriate "window" can be found, it can be very useful in further characterization of intrathoracic masses and fluid collections. This modality is particularly helpful in differentiating cystic from solid masses (Fig. 13-2).

Ultrasound is also a useful method of evaluating diaphragmatic motion and diagnosing pleural effusions. A wide variety of abnormalities can be diagnosed prenatally (Chapter 12).

Computed tomography (CT) with image acquisition times of 5 seconds or less is capable of producing exquisite anatomic detail of intrathoracic structures even in rapidly breathing newborn infants (Fig. 13-2). The indications for computed tomography in newborn chest diagnosis are usually limited to the evaluation of masses and air- or fluid-containing cysts. The CT scan is also an excellent method of evaluating choanal atresia.

An obvious disadvantage of this method of examination is the need to transport the infant to the scanner and to remove the patient from the protective environment during the scan.

These disadvantages also apply to the newest diagnostic modality, magnetic resonance imaging (MRI). Although MRI is capable of producing excellent images

A

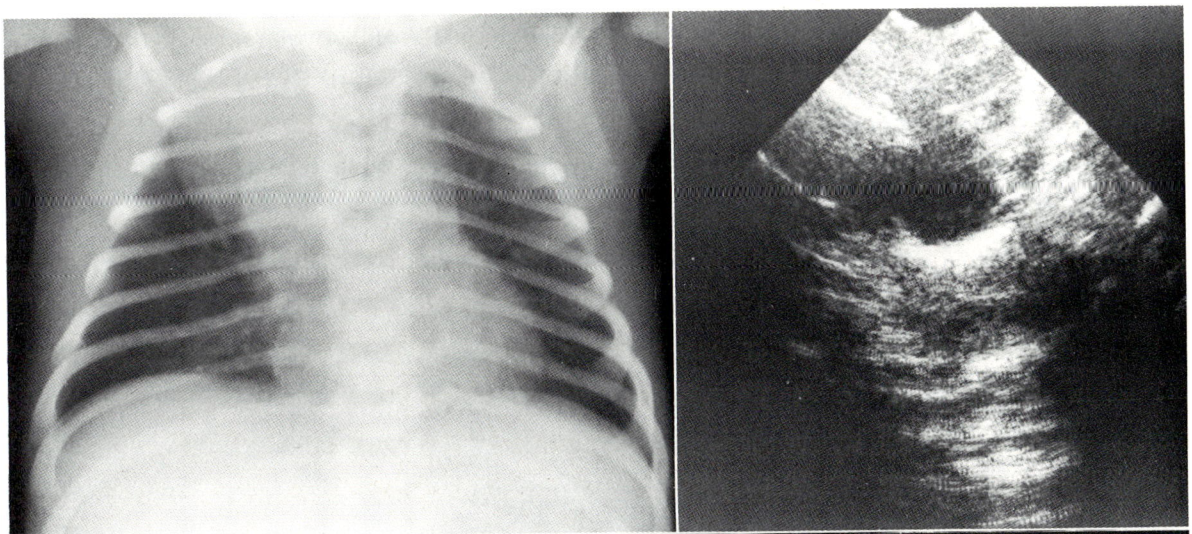

B

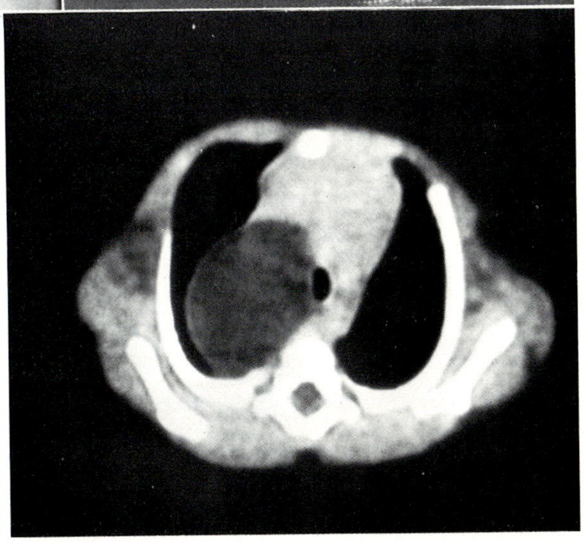

C

Fig. 13-2. Comparison between conventional radiography, ultrasonography, and computed tomography in a patient with a large right upper mediastinal mass. **A,** The chest radiograph shows a well-defined mediastinal tumor compressing the trachea. There is no indication as to whether the mass is solid (e.g., neurogenic tumor) or cystic. **B,** Ultrasound shows the cystic nature of the lesion. **C,** Computed tomography shows that the cyst has a well-defined, thin wall and contains material of homogeneously decreased attenuation. Note the compression of the right wall of the trachea. The adjacent vertebra is not involved. The lesion was a bronchogenic cyst.

with a wider range of contrast than CT and exposure to ionizing radiation is avoided, imaging time is longer. In neonates, MRI has found its greatest use in evaluating development of the brain, since it is capable of tracking myelinization. Using ECG-gated techniques, MRI is capable of imaging the neonatal cardiovascular structures (Fig. 13-3).

Normal chest

The appearance of the normal chest varies throughout the first few days of life. The lungs may be slightly opaque due to retained lung liquid in the early newborn period. The lungs eventually become radiolucent except for well-defined pulmonary vessels branching from the hila. The minor fissure of the right lung is frequently seen as a fine horizontal line in the midportion of the lung field. The cardiophrenic and costophrenic angles should be clear. The heart borders, except for the portions adjacent to the hila, should be distinct, and the diaphragmatic pleura should be clearly outlined against the lungs except for that portion of the left hemidiaphragm that is contiguous to the heart.

The cardiothoracic ratio should be no greater than 0.60. In the first few days of life a rounded opacity may be seen in the left upper mediastinum due to a normal "ductus bump" associated with the closing ductus arteriosus. The tracheal air shadow should curve gently to the right around the aortic arch. Displacement of the trachea to the left is abnormal and suggests a mediastinal mass or right aortic arch. The descending thoracic aorta is rarely visible in the newborn.

The thymus is frequently prominent in the newborn, and because of its variable configuration, its appearance causes frequent confusion. The thymus overlies the anterior aspect of the pericardium, obscuring much of the cardiac silhouette; thus it may simulate a large heart. It is frequently asymmetric and more prominent on the right, sometimes producing a sail-like appearance. Wave-like undulations of its lateral border may be seen due to pressure of the costal cartilages. Aside from these fairly characteristic normal features, the thymus can generally be identified by its homogenous density, anterior location, lack of associated compression of the trachea, and sharp definition of its edges. A lateral view will often exclude cardiomegaly by demonstrating an absence of posterior enlargement of the heart. The ratio between the transverse diameter of the cardiothymic image and that of the thoracic cage tends to be slightly larger in babies with respiratory distress syndrome (RDS) than in those with normal lungs.

Roentgenologic signs of pulmonary abnormalities

Pulmonary consolidation and pneumonia

The term *consolidation* indicates a process that causes the alveoli to be filled with a substance having the density of water. The most frequent cause is pneumonia, but hemorrhage, pus, and edema also are included under this term. Varying degrees of opacification of the lungs are the result of consolidation. The densities may be localized or diffuse and are frequently "patchy." The edges of the consolidation are indistinct, and there is frequently an "air bronchogram," with visualization of the relatively radiolucent bronchi within the involved area of the lung.

As opposed to a process in which the air spaces are opacified, involvement of the interstitial tissues of the lung may predominate. In this case a diffuse reticular or

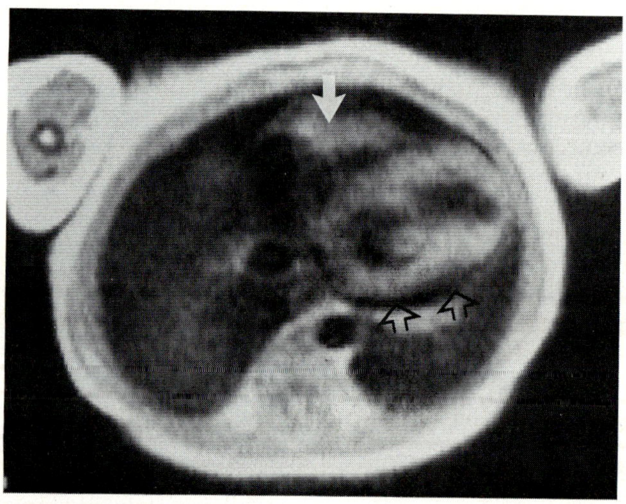

Fig. 13-3. Axial MR image of the chest of a newborn infant. There is a small pericardial effusion *(open arrows).* Note the normal thymus *(solid arrow).*

nodular pattern results. Peribronchial disease results in small ring shadows when the smaller, more peripheral bronchi are seen in cross-sections, but air bronchograms are not seen.

Generalized pulmonary hyperinflation also frequently accompanies diffuse pneumonia and is particularly apparent in meconium aspiration pneumonitis. Completely airless, consolidated lobes and segments of lung tend to be less voluminous than when they are filled with air.

Group B streptococcal pneumonia deserves special mention, since some small premature infants may have a lung pattern which closely resembles that seen in RDS. This pattern, once thought to be specific for RDS, consists of diffuse bilateral reticulogranularity with exaggerated air bronchograms. We have also noted this pattern in neonatal pneumonias of other causes (Fig. 13-4).

Chlamydia pneumonia typically results in coarse bilateral interstitial infiltrates in afebrile infants 2 weeks to 3 months of age (Fig. 13-5). Pulmonary candidiasis should be considered in small premature infants with bronchopulmonary dysplasia who develop extensive air-space consolidation.

Atelectasis

Like consolidation, atelectasis also causes an increase in lung density. Furthermore, until the gas is completely resorbed from the bronchi, an air bronchogram may be present. Lobar atelectasis is primarily manifested as changes in position of the fissures. For example, with lower lobe collapse the major fissure moves posteromedially. In middle lobe collapse the minor fissure is depressed, whereas right upper lobe collapse causes elevation of this fissure.

Atelectasis also results in a shift of the mediastinum toward the side of the collapse (Fig. 13-6). This is most notable in lower lobe atelectasis, but in newborn infants the compliant mediastinal structures will also shift slightly toward the side of an upper lobe collapse. In

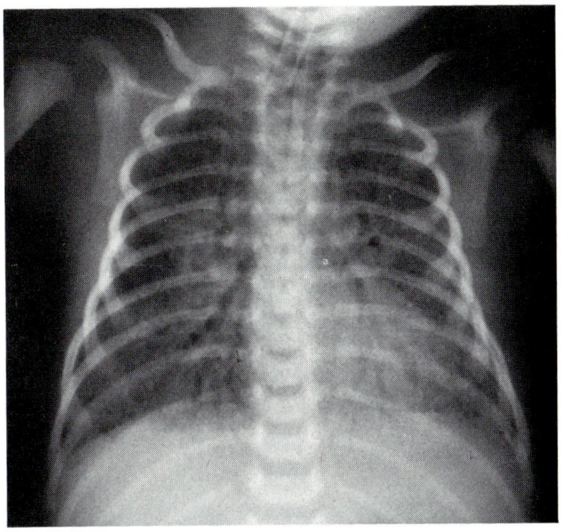

Fig. 13-4. Diffuse bilateral pulmonary consolidation due to pneumococcal pneumonia in the newborn. Note the prominent "air bronchograms" and reticular pattern resembling respiratory distress syndrome. The lungs have increased in volume, an uncommon finding in RDS.

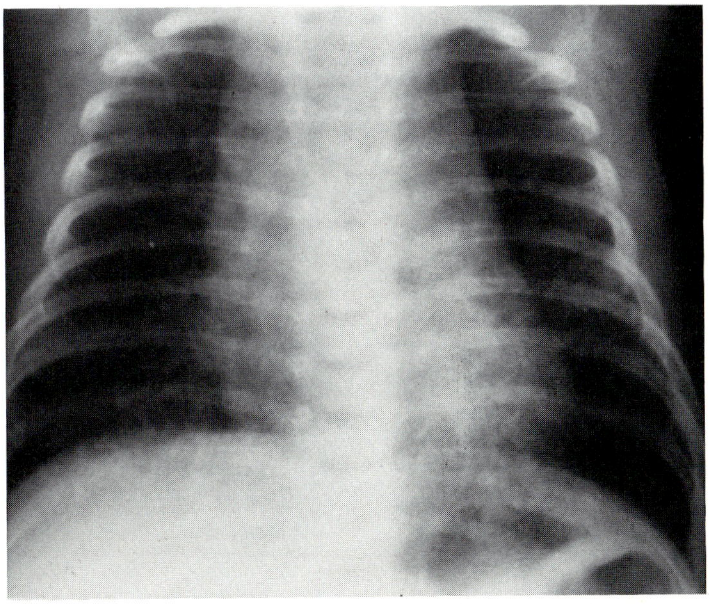

Fig. 13-5. Bilateral streaky, interstitial markings resulting from *Chlamydia* pneumonia.

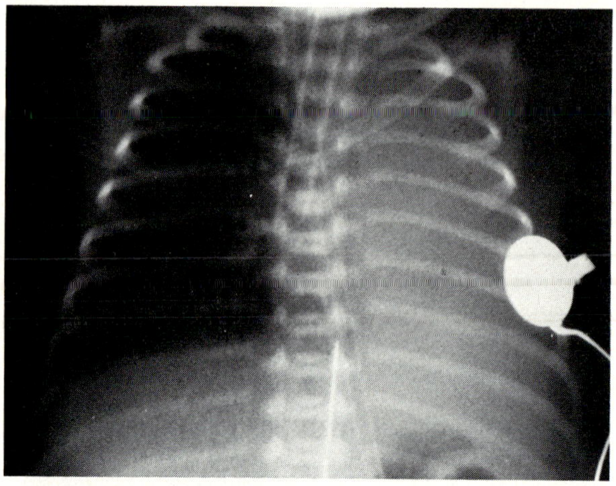

Fig. 13-6. Atelectasis of the entire left lung. The mediastinum has shifted into the left hemithorax. The atelectasis is due to the aberrant position of the endotracheal tube in the right main bronchus.

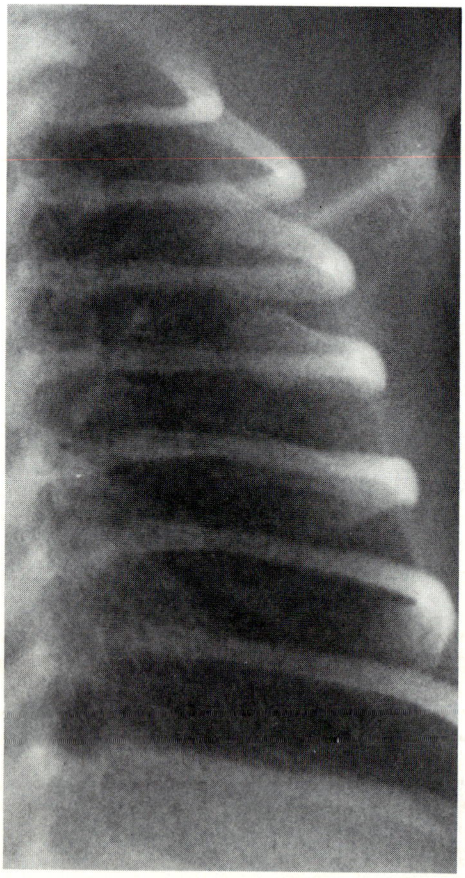

Fig. 13-7. Typical reticulogranular pattern of mild RDS.

addition, lower lobe atelectasis results in elevation of the ipsilateral hemidiaphragm. Narrowing of the intercostal spaces is a frequent secondary sign. Compensatory hyperinflation of uninvolved portions of lung or of the opposite lung will also occur and must be differentiated from a primary increase in lung volume, such as that which occurs in congenital lobar emphysema.

In neonates the most frequent site of lobar atelectasis is the right upper lobe. This may be due to occlusion of the right upper lobe bronchus associated with faulty position of an endotracheal tube, but it is also a frequent finding following extubation, probably because of mucus accumulation and decreased ciliary activity.

Diffuse atelectasis occurs in premature infants who have unstable alveoli due to surfactant deficiency. The roentgenographic hallmark of RDS is a diffuse reticulogranular pattern (Fig. 13-7). This is the result of microatelectases interspersed with dilated air spaces. In more severe RDS a roentgenologic "white-out" may result from generalized atelectasis. A similar appearance may also result from sudden collapse of both lungs in babies who have been breathing high concentrations of oxygen, if they become apneic or develop airway obstruction.

Distinguishing between diffuse bilateral consolidation and increased lung density due to expiration is sometimes difficult. In general, however, expiration results in constricted, centralized air bronchograms whereas airspace disease is associated with peripheral extension of air bronchograms.

Pulmonary hypoplasia and agenesis

In the absence of a diaphragmatic hernia, unilateral agenesis or pulmonary hypoplasia may be indistinguishable from atelectasis on neonatal chest radiographs. The presence of associated vertebral anomalies or esophageal atresia, however, suggests a pulmonary malformation rather than atelectasis, and pulmonary angiography may be indicated. Bilateral pulmonary hypoplasia is suggested by a small, bell-shaped thorax and the presence of an air leak such as pneumothorax or pneumomediastinum (Fig. 13-8). These findings often are associated with maternal oligohydramnios, in which case ultrasonographic investigation of possible renal malformations is recommended. The thorax may also appear bell-shaped in the presence of various neuromuscular abnormalities, as well as in infants requiring therapeutic neuromuscular paralysis for assisted ventilation. In the latter situation, there is often decreased bowel gas and soft tissue edema.

Air leak

See Chapter 28.

Extravasation of alveolar air is a frequent complication of ventilatory assistance for respiratory failure. The ex-

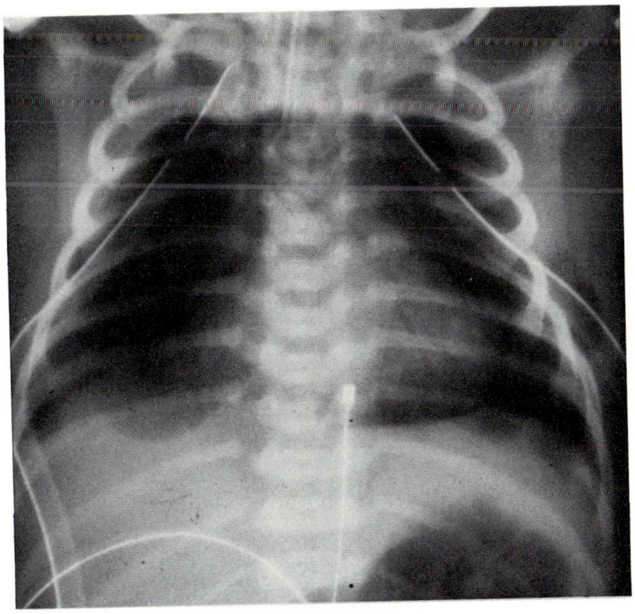

Fig. 13-8. Infant's small, somewhat bell-shaped chest caused by severe renal malformations and maternal oligohydramnios. Bilateral thoracostomy tubes were inserted for treatment of pneumothoraces. There is still a large pneumomediastinum.

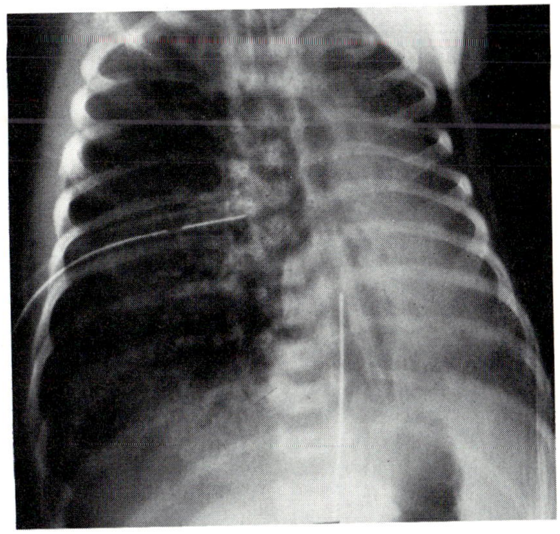

Fig. 13-9. Lateral decubitus film made with the left side down shows a residual right pneumothorax in spite of the presence of a chest tube. Part of the intrapleural gas also is trapped medial to the right lung. The increased right lung volume and streaky lucencies are caused by interstitial emphysema.

travasated air travels from the alveolus, dissects through the interstitium of the lung, and enters the mediastinum. The air may then enter the pleural space and result in a pneumothorax. Alternatively, air dissecting via the pulmonary lymphatics may perforate the visceral pleura and cause a pneumothorax. Pneumopericardium and pneumoperitoneum are less common manifestations of extraventilatory air.

Pneumothorax in a newborn infant is usually readily recognizable when the gas in the pleural space clearly outlines the visceral pleura. In addition, there is usually considerable mediastinal shift toward the contralateral side and a varying amount of collapse of both lungs. Occasionally, even fairly large pneumothoraces may not be obvious. This is because the air in the supine neonate's thorax tends to assume a position anterior and medial to the lung. The only sign may be enlargement and increased lucency of the affected hemithorax (Fig. 13-9). In this case a lateral decubitus film, made with the normal side dependent, will demonstrate air adjacent to the visceral pleura of the costal surface of the involved lung.

In pneumomediastinum a halo of air may be recognizable on either side of the mediastinum. The hallmark, however, is displacement of the thymus away from the parietal pericardium, the so-called spinnaker sail sign (Fig. 13-10). Air less commonly dissects into the soft

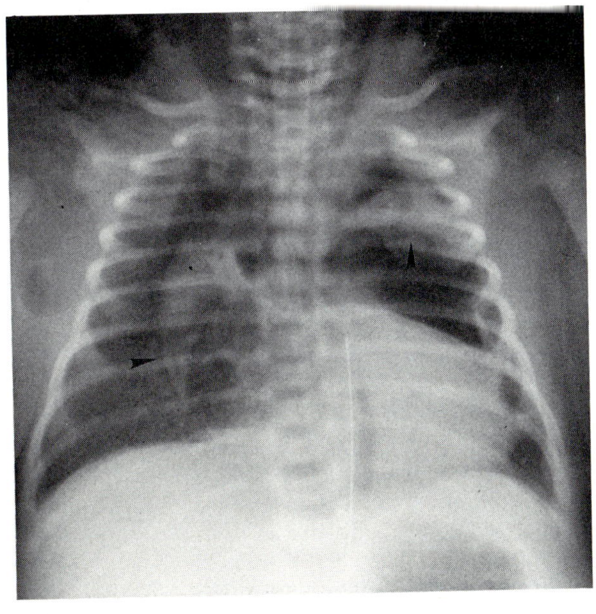

Fig. 13-10. Separation of the thymic lobes *(arrowheads)* from the pericardial surface due to a large pneumomediastinum. There is also a large amount of air in the neck and soft tissues of the chest wall, which occurs less commonly in the newborn than in the older child.

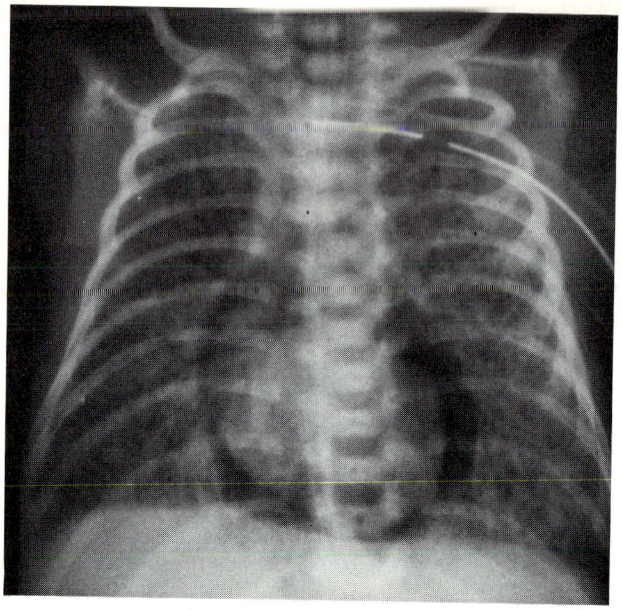

Fig. 13-11. A pneumopericardium completely surrounds the heart.

tissues of the neck in neonates than it does when pneumomediastinum occurs in older infants and children. Unlike mediastinal emphysema, which is limited inferiorly by the central tendon of the diaphragm, a pneumopericardium completely surrounds the heart and origins of the great vessels (Fig. 13-11).

Interstitial emphysema may be diffuse, bilateral, or localized to a single lung or lobe (Fig. 13-9). The interstitial gas appears as multiple well-defined circular or elongated lucencies contrasted against the collapsed lung parenchyma. In addition, there is a marked increase in volume of the involved portion of lung. The "bubbly" pattern of diffuse interstitial emphysema can usually be distinguished from focal emphysema associated with stage 3 bronchopulmonary emphysema by its rapid onset and the uniform appearance of the bubbles, which typically radiate from the hila. Occasionally continued expansion of the interstitial gas collections results in localized pulmonary overdistension resembling congenital lobar emphysema.

Cardiovascular abnormalities

Congestive heart failure

Infants with congestive heart failure exhibit varying degrees of cardiomegaly as demonstrated on AP chest roentgenograms. In a mature infant the heart is considered to be enlarged when the cardiothymic-thoracic ratio is greater than 0.6. In preterm infants the normal ratio is smaller, and cardiomegaly often less obvious. Pulmonary venous congestion is manifested by engorgement and increase in size of the pulmonary veins. As pulmonary venous pressure rises, interstitial edema occurs. This is observed as a decrease in the definition of the lung vasculature and by Kerley lines, which are produced by leakage of fluid into the interlobular septa. Kerley B-lines are seen as short horizontal linear densities in the lung extending to the pleural surface. They are typically found above the costophrenic angles but may be seen to better advantage, in infants, in the retrosternal portion of the lungs on lateral views. Kerley A-lines are longer linear densities radiating from the hila. Edema of the subpleural areolar tissue and pleural effusions are more easily seen in small infants than are Kerley lines (Fig. 13-12).

Extravasation of edema fluid into the air spaces results in more diffuse opacification of the lungs, typically involving the perihilar regions. Identical pulmonary changes without cardiomegaly can be observed during resorption of normal alveolar lung liquid.

Left-to-right shunts

An increase in caliber of the pulmonary arteries can be detected when there is a moderate increase in blood flow to the lungs through a left-to-right shunt. The size of the hila, as well as the intrapulmonary vessels, is increased, and the main pulmonary artery is frequently enlarged. Enlargement of tiny peripheral vessels results in a reticular appearance that superficially resembles interstitial edema. Frank pulmonary edema may then occur due to overload of the pulmonary circulation. This event occurs rapidly in preterm infants with persistent patent ductus arteriosus.

Cyanotic congenital heart disease

The size of the heart may range from relatively normal, as in transposition of the great arteries, to huge, as in Ebstein's anomaly. In most cases the caliber of the pulmonary vessels is reduced. The hila are consequently small, and the lungs appear relatively lucent. Also, the thymus tends to be involuted due to stress, and the lungs are often hyperinflated. Pulmonary vascular engorgement, rather than oligemia, accompanies cyanosis in patients with d-transposition of the great arteries due to incomplete mixing of systemic and pulmonary blood. Cyanosis with congestive heart failure and roentgenographic signs of pulmonary edema with a relatively small cardiothymic silhouette suggest the diagnosis of subdiaphragmatic total anomalous pulmonary venous drainage.

Persistence of the fetal circulation may also, on occasion, mimic cyanotic congenital heart disease on chest roentgenograms, since there may be cardiomegaly and pulmonary oligemia (Fig. 13-13). In other cases congestive heart failure or pulmonary disease may also be present.

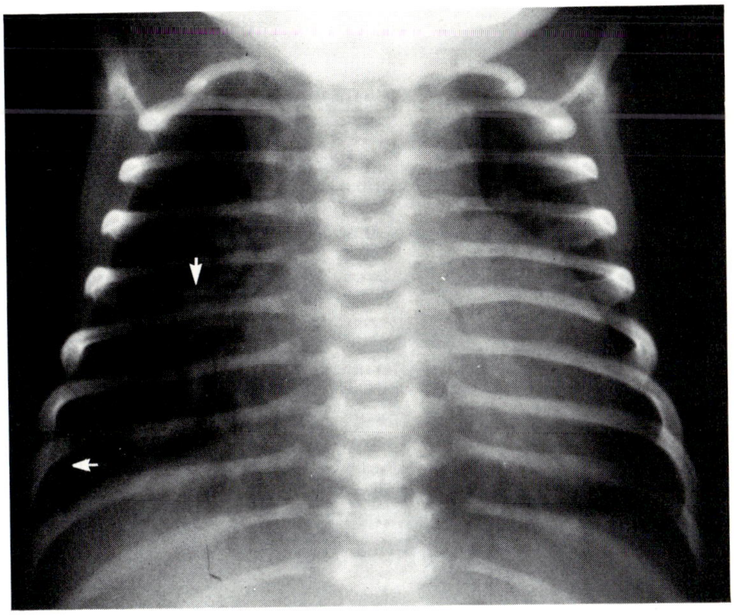

Fig. 13-12. Cardiomegaly and pulmonary vascular engorgement in an infant with coarctation of the aorta and a left-to-right interatrial shunt. Fluid adjacent to or within the minor fissures makes it appear "thickened," and there is a faint vertical density in the right costophrenic angle due to similar involvement of the inferior portion of the major fissure *(arrowhead)*.

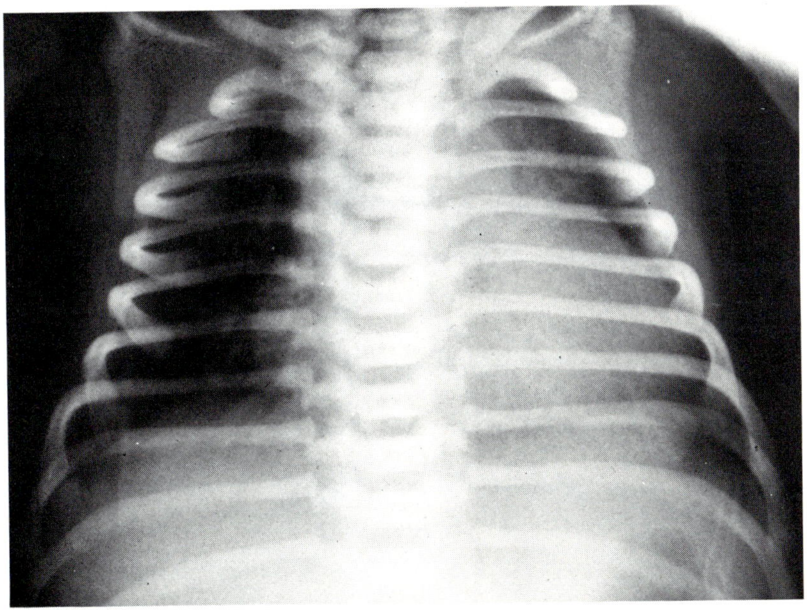

Fig. 13-13. Marked enlargement of the cardiothymic silhouette and diminished caliber of the pulmonary vessels in a patient with the syndrome of persistent fetal circulation, simulating cyanotic congenital heart disease.

GASTROINTESTINAL TRACT

See Chapter 33.

Roentgenologic evaluation of the gastrointestinal tract has become more common, particularly in premature infants, because of the emergence of necrotizing enterocolitis as a serious cause of morbidity and mortality. Acute surgical emergencies constitute another major group of disorders that require roentgenologic diagnosis. In addition, roentgenograms taken to localize umbilical catheters have provided incidental experience with the normal plain film appearance of the gut.

Methods of examination

Initial plain film examination usually consists of an AP supine film made with a vertical beam and includes both the chest and the abdomen. As with chest roentgenography, additional lateral and decubitus views are made with a horizontally directed x-ray beam. These films can be made without removing the infant from the incubator and allow visualization of air-fluid levels and permit more precise demonstration of free intraperitoneal air (Fig. 13-21). A horizontal beam lateral view of the abdomen with the infant prone is an aid in demonstrating gas in the rectum and sigmoid colon when obstruction is suspected. Roentgenograms made with the infant erect or inverted are not recommended, since they are stressful to the patient and present considerable technical difficulties.

Ultrasonography is now an accepted method of diagnosing hypertrophic pyloric stenosis. The elongated and narrowed pyloric channel can be seen surrounded by hypoechogenic muscle layers (Fig. 13-14). Ultrasonography has the advantage of being noninvasive, but it is technically demanding. If the characteristic ultrasonographic findings of hypertrophic pyloric stenosis are not demonstrated, a fluoroscopic procedure may be required to identify other possible causes of vomiting.

Contrast media

Air is a very satisfactory contrast medium that frequently can be used to demonstrate the site of bowel obstruction. When it is necessary to opacify the stomach or bowel, barium sulfate is usually the medium of choice, since it is relatively inert. Water-soluble, iodine-containing contrast media are useful when perforation of the gut is suspected, since they are readily absorbed from the peritoneal surface but if aspirated, they may produce pulmonary edema.

The most frequently used water-soluble contrast medium is Gastrografin, a 76% solution of sodium methylglucamine diatrizoate containing 37% bound iodine. The major disadvantage of this product is its high osmolarity (1,900 mOsm/L), which causes a shift of water and electrolytes into the lumen of the bowel. Furthermore, absorption occurs through the bowel wall, enhancing the resultant systemic dehydration. The problem of dehydration due to hypertonicity of conventional water-soluble contrast agents can be avoided by using them in an isotonic (1:5) dilution.

Another problem with water-soluble contrast media is possible mucosal damage of the intact bowel, especially if the bowel is overdistended with the contrast media. In addition, further compromise of an already tenuous mesenteric vascular supply may occur in the distended loops proximal to a bowel obstruction.

A contrast enema is indicated in neonates with suspected Hirschsprung's disease, which may be the cause of meconium plug syndrome. A transition zone, usually involving the sigmoid, between the distal aganglionic bowel and the proximal ganglionic bowel, may not always be apparent in neonates. In fact, retention of barium over a period of 24 hours may be the only finding of aganglionosis in this age group.

Water-soluble contrast media are indicated for therapeutic enemas to relieve meconium plugs or meconium ileus. For these purposes they are usually used in higher concentrations than for diagnosis. The therapeutic benefits are due to osmosis of water into the lumen of the bowel and resultant softening of the meconium, as well as the surface-active properties of a polysorbate wetting agent and emulsifier contained in Gastrografin. Other similar substances, such as Hypaque and Renografin, also have been used therapeutically.

Contrast enemas must be carried out under fluoroscopic control in the radiology department. They are performed using a flexible infant feeding tube that is

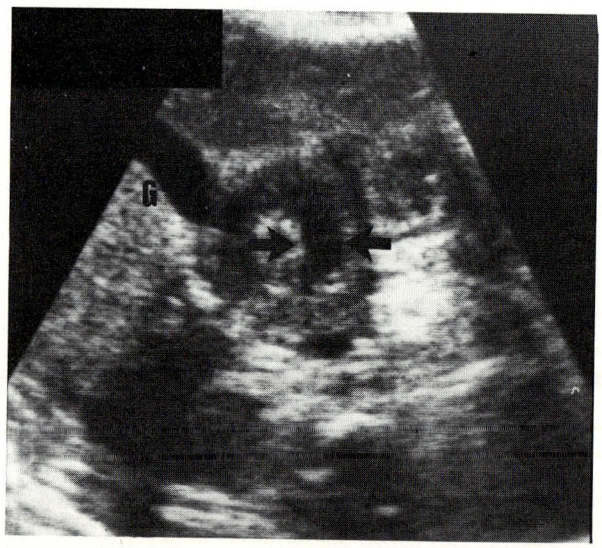

Fig. 13-14. Anechoic hypertrophic muscle *(arrows)* surrounds the pylorus in an infant with hypertrophic pyloric stenosis. The gallbladder *(G)* is also shown.

taped in place. Inflation of a balloon catheter in the rectum should be avoided because of the risk of perforation. Preparation of the bowel is not necessary and is especially contraindicated when there is suspicion of Hirschsprung's disease. Upper gastrointestinal studies also are preferably done fluoroscopically, but if this is contraindicated because of the clinical condition of the infant, the contrast medium can be monitored during its course through the gastrointestinal tract using portable roentgenologic equipment. In this situation the opaque media may be administered through a nasogastric tube after removal of residual gastric contents.

Recently developed nonionic contrast materials are expected to afford a greater degree of safety because they can be prepared in an isotonic solution. They permit more prolonged visualization of the gut than do ionic agents and are rapidly absorbed from the peritoneum of patients with gastrointestinal perforation. Preliminary experience with these relatively expensive materials suggests that they will provide greater safety than ionic contrast media and will be useful for diagnosis of esophageal abnormalities, intestinal obstruction, necrotizing enterocolitis, and lesions of the colon.

Normal findings

Air is swallowed immediately after birth and reaches the small bowel at about 3 hours of postnatal life. After approximately 6 to 8 hours of age, gas is present throughout the large and small bowel, although rectal gas may not be visible if the bladder is distended. Mild generalized gaseous distension often occurs due to air-swallowing.

Newborn infants present a special diagnostic problem because of the similarity in appearance and caliber of the large and small bowel. However, the colon sometimes can be distinguished by its anatomic position and the presence of haustra.

The liver often appears prominent in normal infants, and roentgenograms are not an accurate index of hepatomegaly. On roentgenograms taken with the infant supine, the spleen is usually obscured by overlying gas in the stomach and splenic flexure.

Gastrointestinal distension and obstruction

An increase in the amount of intestinal gas does not necessarily indicate obstruction, since it may occur in a variety of conditions, including tracheoesophageal fistula, necrotizing enterocolitis, maternal drug therapy, hypothyroidism, septicemia, and hypermagnesemia. In these disorders the gas is distributed throughout the small and large bowel. Obstruction also may be mimicked by excess air-swallowing due to respiratory distress. Furthermore, as in mechanical obstruction, air-fluid levels may be present. Mild generalized gastrointestinal distension is a frequent finding on films obtained to check umbilical catheter placement.

Mechanical bowel obstruction produces gaseous intestinal distension, and air fluid levels are seen proximal to the site of obstruction. Distal to the obstruction the intraluminal gas may be diminished or absent. A different pattern is often seen, however, in obstruction due to meconium ileus. In this disorder the bowel loops vary in size, are unevenly distributed, and contain few air-fluid levels. The inspissated meconium in the small bowel becomes mixed with air, producing a bubbly appearance (Fig. 13-15).

Duodenal obstruction is usually easily recognizable on plain films because of distension of the stomach and duodenal bulb, which produces the classic "double-bubble" appearance. These structures often contain air-fluid levels, and the amount of gas distal to the obstruction varies with the degree of obstruction. The most common entities that produce this finding are duodenal stenosis or atresia, annular pancreas, and malrotation with peritoneal bands and midgut volvulus (Fig. 13-16).

Contrast examinations are often indicated when duodenal obstruction is suspected clinically or is demonstrated on plain films. These studies are particularly urgent because of the importance of recognition and

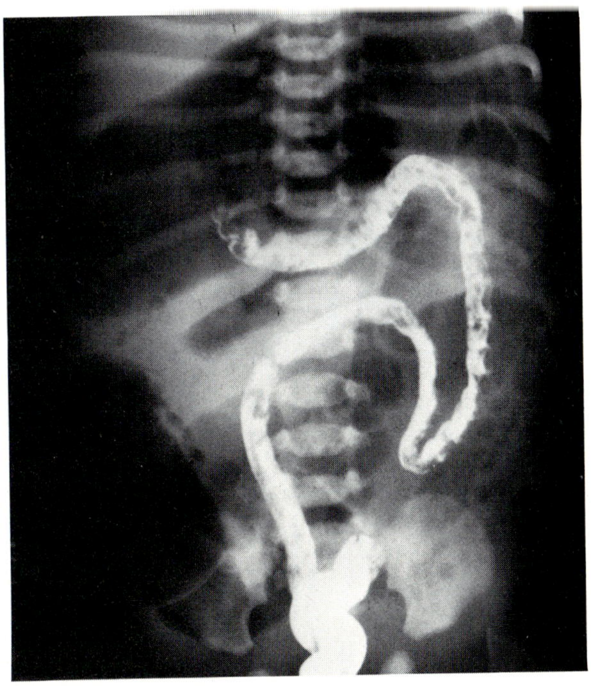

Fig. 13-15. AP recumbent film of the abdomen in an infant with meconium ileus. Note the distended bowel loops of varying sizes and the bubbly appearance of the intestinal contents, particularly in the left flank (compare with Fig. 13-22). The distal ileal obstruction is reflected by the marked diminution in caliber of the colon (microcolon).

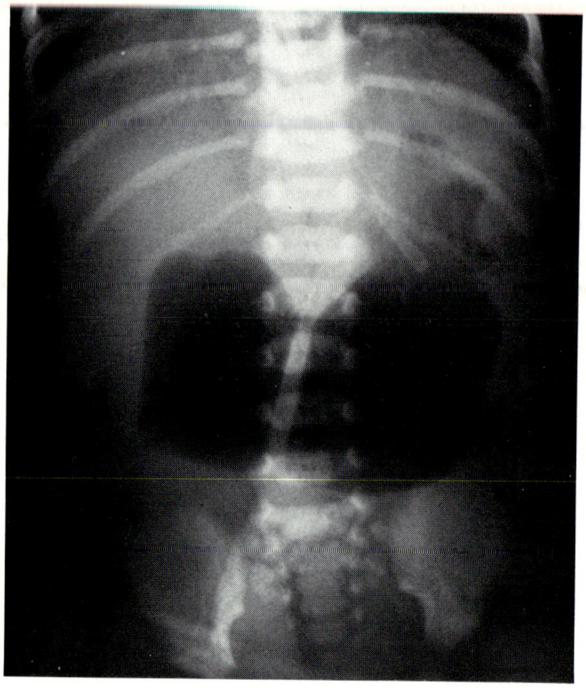

Fig. 13-16. AP recumbent film of the abdomen demonstrating the "double-bubble" due to gaseous distension of the stomach and first portion of the duodenum caused by duodenal atresia. Note the complete absence of gas distal to the duodenum.

prompt surgical treatment of malrotation and midgut volvulus with associated mesenteric vascular insufficiency. When the degree of obstruction appears to be incomplete, the volvulus can be diagnosed by introducing barium into the stomach. If there is an associated malrotation of the midgut, the duodenojejunal junction is displaced medially and inferiorly from its normal position in the left upper abdominal quadrant, and the duodenum and proximal jejunum have a corkscrew or Z-shaped configuration (Fig. 13-17). Evidence of malrotation also can be obtained by a barium enema, which will demonstrate the cecum in an unusually superior or medial position (Fig. 13-18). The cecum also may be abnormally mobile. If there is nonrotation of the bowel, the cecum and most of the colon are seen to the left of the midline. A barium enema is especially useful when upper gastrointestinal examination is not feasible because of complete duodenal obstruction. Malrotation of the small bowel may, however, occasionally coexist with a normally positioned colon.

The caliber of the colon is another important observation made on contrast enemas. A ribbonlike microcolon occurs when there is lack of normal distension by intestinal contents due to exclusion of succus entericus from the colon during fetal life (Fig. 13-15). The diminished colonic caliber usually indicates some type of distal ileal obstruction such as meconium ileus or ileal atresia.

A

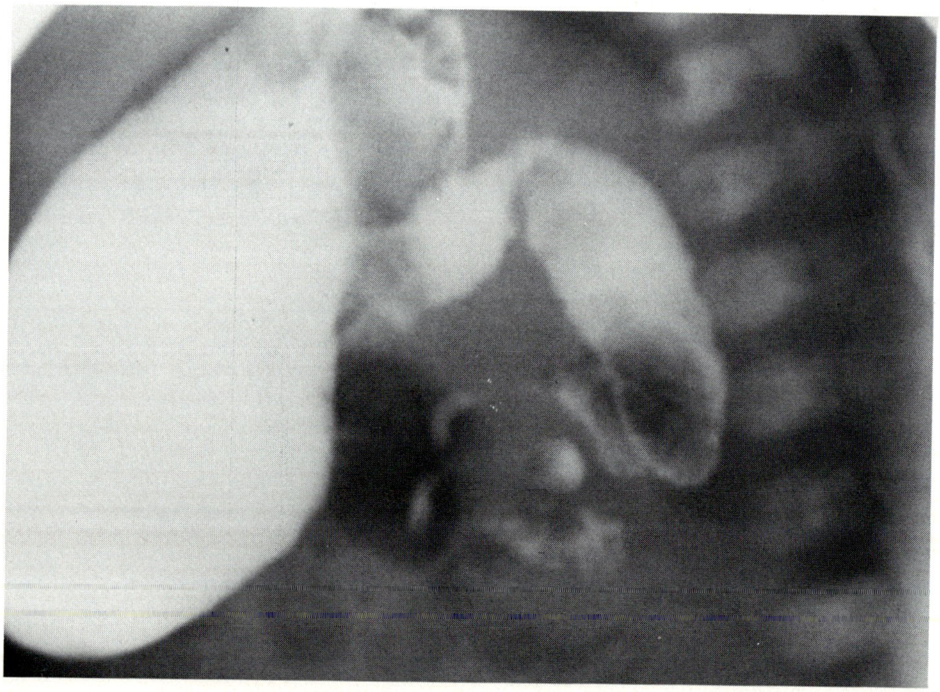

Fig. 13-17. Partial duodenal obstruction due to midgut malrotation with volvulus. **A,** With the patient in a steep oblique position, the distal duodenum and proximal jejunum have a "corkscrew" appearance and the duodenojejunal junction is not identifiable.

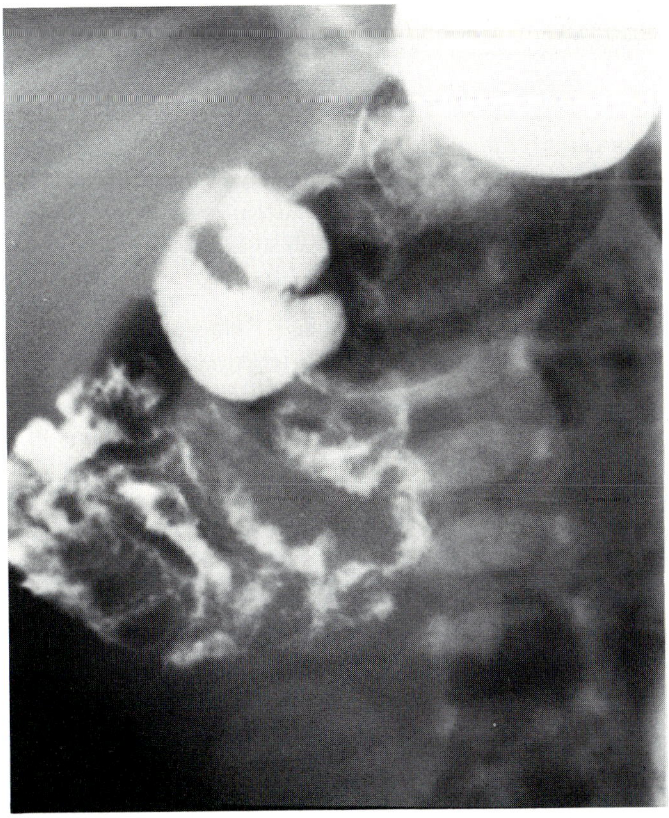

B

Fig. 13-17, cont'd. B, The proximal small bowel is to the right of the midline.

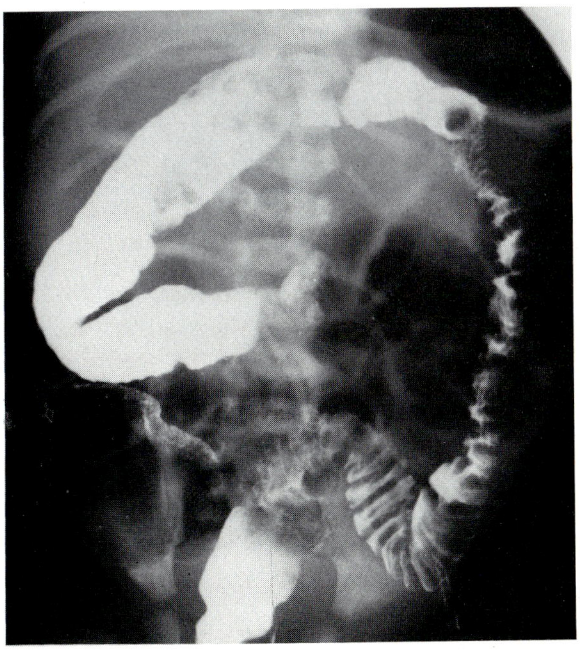

Fig. 13-18. Barium enema demonstrates an abnormally high and medially positioned cecum in a patient with small intestinal obstruction due to malrotation and midgut volvulus.

On the other hand, the caliber of the colon is predicted to be normal in the presence of duodenal or high jejunal obstruction.

Exceptions to this rule may occur, however. If the distal ileal atresia occurs late in fetal life, the caliber of the colon may be normal. On the other hand, the caliber of the colon is decreased in nearly 40% of patients with total colonic aganglionosis, presumably due to functional small intestine obstruction. We have also noted decreased colonic caliber in premature infants with obstruction alone, and a microcolon may be seen in premature infants with functional small bowel obstruction. Localized decrease in caliber of the left colon occurs in Hirschsprung's disease, meconium plug syndrome, and the neonatal small left colon syndrome (Fig. 13-19).

Pneumoperitoneum

Early diagnosis of pneumoperitoneum often depends on its recognition on routine AP supine views. Since the air rises anteriorly, a lucency will be seen overlying the liver adjacent to the inferior surface of the diaphragm. A large collection of air causes generalized abdominal distension, and structures not usually visible, such as the falciform ligament, umbilical vein, or a persistent urachus, may be outlined by the air (Fig. 13-20). Perhaps the most valuable indicator of small amounts of free air is the double-wall sign, in which the mucosal surface of the bowel is outlined by intraluminal air and the serosal surface by intraperitoneal air. The intraperitoneal air is best demonstrated on films made with a horizontal beam in supine or decubitus positions, which show collections

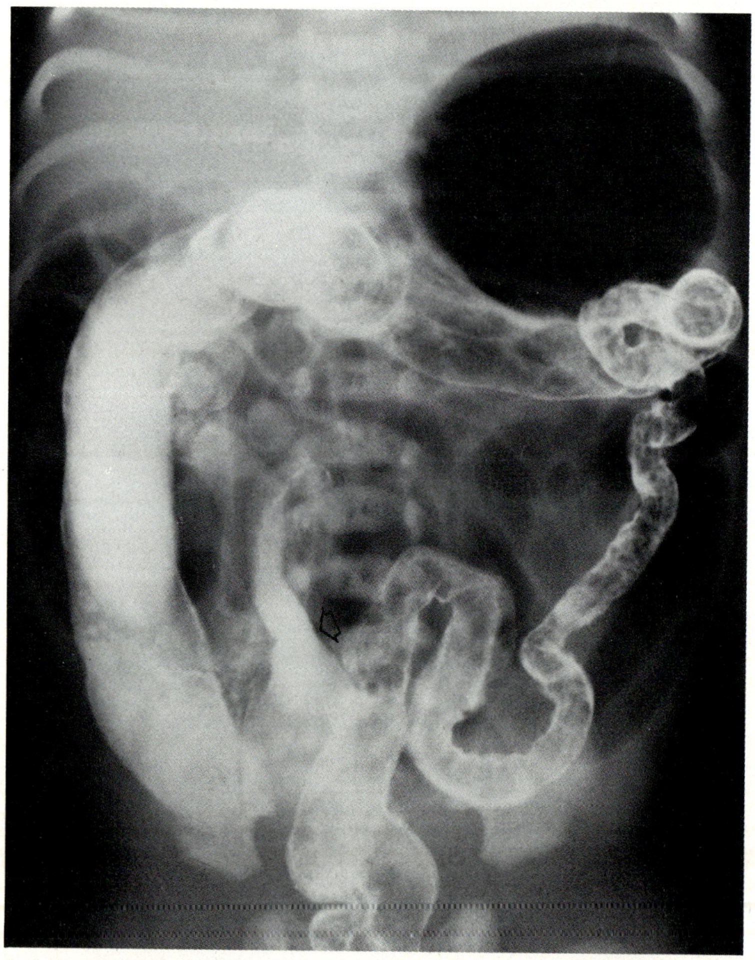

Fig. 13-19. Barium enema demonstrates decreased caliber of the left side of the colon with an apparent transition zone at the splenic flexure. The bowel contains a moderate amount of meconium. Besides Hirschsprung's disease, these findings can occur in infants of diabetic mothers with the neonatal small left colon syndrome and in meconium plug syndrome. Note the large "fetal" appendix *(arrowhead)*.

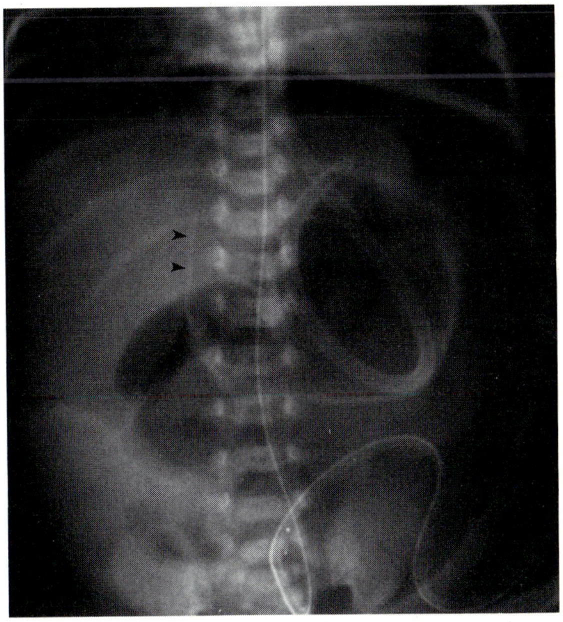

Fig. 13-20. AP recumbent film of the abdomen demonstrates a large pneumoperitoneum, with free air inferior to the diaphragm and outlining the falciform ligament *(arrowheads)*.

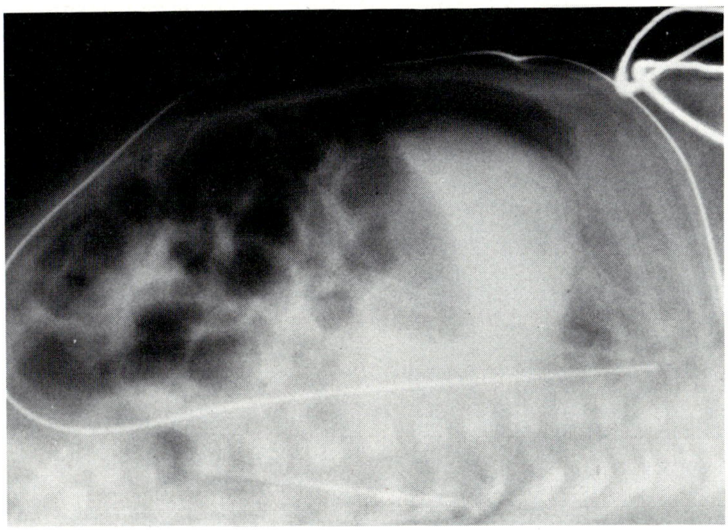

Fig. 13-21. Horizontal-beam lateral view of the abdomen made with the infant supine demonstrates intraperitoneal gas anterior to the liver and adjacent to the anterior abdominal wall. Several examples of the double-wall sign, with the inner wall of the bowel outlined by intraluminal air and the outer wall outlined by intraperitoneal air, also are visible anteriorly. There is no intraperitoneal air fluid level to suggest peritonitis.

of gas adjacent to the anterior abdominal wall or flanks (Fig. 13-21).

Although the most important cause of pneumoperitoneum is perforation of the bowel, the possibility of extension of gas from a pneumomediastinum into the peritoneal cavity must be considered in infants with respiratory distress. An air-fluid level in the peritoneal cavity almost certainly indicates bowel perforation, but absence of an air-fluid level is not a completely reliable sign of an intact gastrointestinal tract. The presence of perforation can be demonstrated by instilling a small amount of water-soluble contrast medium through a nasogastric tube and observing its passage into the peritoneal cavity.

Pneumatosis intestinalis

The most common etiology of pneumatosis intestinalis is necrotizing enterocolitis, although bowel ischemia secondary to intestinal obstruction is also an occasional cause. The intramural gas that collects beneath the serosa or in the submucosa of the intestine may be either localized or diffusely distributed throughout the bowel and appears as small linear or bubbly lucencies (Fig. 13-22). In patients with necrotizing enterocolitis, intestinal distension with air-fluid levels, portal venous gas, inflammatory masses, pneumoperitoneum, or intraperitoneal fluid also may be present.

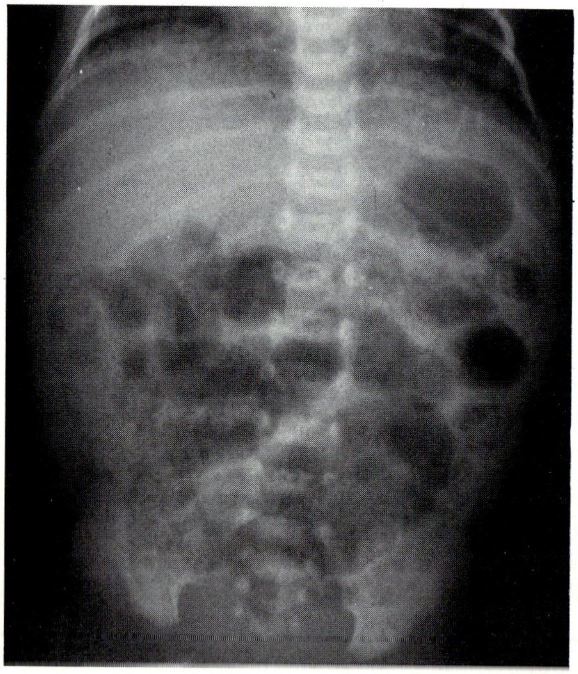

Fig. 13-22. Numerous linear and bubbly lucencies caused by intramural gas associated with necrotizing enterocolitis. The bubbly pattern is difficult to distinguish from the intraluminal bubbles shown in Fig. 13-15.

It is also important to emphasize that necrotizing enterocolitis may occur in the absence of pneumatosis. In these patients, a disturbed bowel gas pattern consisting of elongation, dilation, and separation of bowel loops may be seen. A persistently distended loop of bowel suggests impending perforation even in the absence of pneumatosis intestinalis. Air trapped in a normal, redundant sigmoid loop may, however, mimic abnormal dilation. Sequential supine and prone radiographs may help to distinguish normal from pathologic bowel loops. Pneumoperitoneum is an absolute indication for surgical intervention.

Intravascular gas

In necrotizing enterocolitis the intramural gas may dissect into the portal venous system and is seen radiating into the liver from the hilus. Ultrasonography may demonstrate portal venous gas in infants with necrotizing enterocolitis before abnormalities are apparent on roentgenograms. In the absence of necrotizing enterocolitis, portal vein gas also may be introduced through umbilical venous catheters.

Pulmonary gas embolism is another cause of intravascular gas and is unrelated to gastrointestinal disease. The embolism occurs when alveolar gas ruptures into the pulmonary vascular bed. The gas is then rapidly distributed throughout the systemic vessels, usually resulting in sudden death. The gas is often particularly prominent within the hepatic veins. The roentgenologic findings may be mimicked by postmortem accumulations of gas.

Decreased intraabdominal gas

Since most intestinal gas is produced by ingested air, any mechanism that reduces the infant's ability to swallow causes diminished bowel gas. Thus a reduction in the amount of bowel gas may occur due to central nervous system depression and can indicate deterioration of the infant's condition. Pharyngeal obstruction due to an orotracheal tube has a similar effect. If the swallowed gas contains a high concentration of oxygen, it can be absorbed very rapidly. Curariform drugs are a more recently observed iatrogenic cause of gasless abdomen. Gas also may be expelled by severe vomiting and diarrhea.

Bowel gas is also absent in esophageal atresia without distal tracheoesophageal fistula. In diaphragmatic hernias the intestinal gas is contained within the thorax, and the abdomen is markedly scaphoid.

Ascites

Neonatal ascites is often associated with intrauterine perforation of the bowel. Other causes include obstruction of the portal circulation, urine ascites associated with anomalies of the lower urinary tract, chylous ascites, erythroblastosis, and intrauterine infections such as syphilis. Massive neonatal ascites is accompanied by a relatively gasless abdomen, which is also markedly distended (Fig. 13-23). If any gas-containing loops of bowel are present, they tend to be localized centrally within the abdomen. Separation of the right lateral border of the liver from the adjacent abdominal wall is a helpful sign that can be frequently observed in infants. This has been ascribed to a relatively greater radiodensity of the liver as compared with that of the intraperitoneal fluid. This difference in densities can be enhanced by total body opacification. The presence of even small amounts of intraperitoneal fluid can be well demonstrated by ultrasonography.

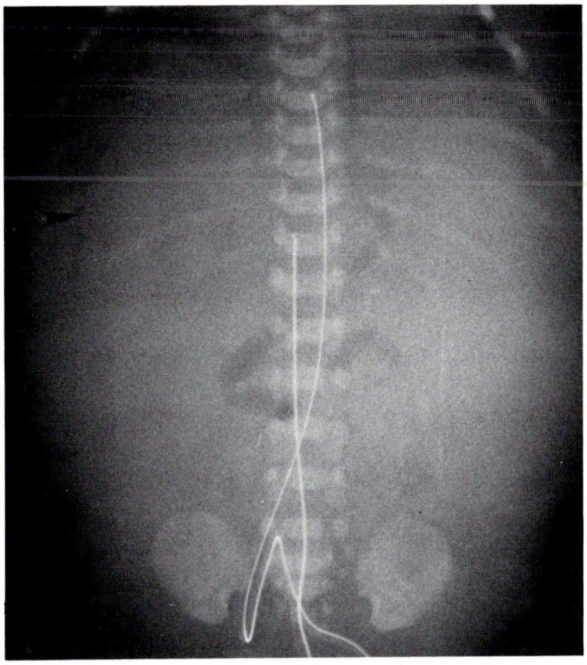

Fig. 13-23. Massive neonatal ascites associated with erythroblastosis. The abdomen is distended and contains little intestinal gas. The lateral liver edge *(arrowhead;* retouched) could be readily seen on the original film because of the difference in radiodensities of the liver and ascitic fluid. An umbilical venous catheter is present. The umbilical arterial catheter is to the left of the midline, extending to the level of T8.

Intraabdominal calcifications

In the fetus and the newborn, intraabdominal calcifications can occur within a few days. Calcifications of the peritoneum, intestinal wall, or even intraluminal contents are occasional but important clues to intestinal disorders.

The most frequently recognized calcifications involve the peritoneum and are caused by sterile meconium peritonitis due to intrauterine bowel perforation associated with meconium ileus or vascular occlusion. The calcifications are usually streaky or plaquelike and often occur over the liver, abdominal surface of the diaphragm, or along the flanks (Fig. 13-24).

Calcifications of intraluminal meconium appear as small rounded densities that follow the course of the small or large bowel. Within the colon they have been seen in association with imperforate anus. Small intestinal calcifications have been documented in cases of ileal stenosis, atresia, and total colonic aganglionosis. Rarely, calcification of the bowel wall may occur in patients with intestinal volvulus or atresia. Neuroblastomas and retroperitoneal teratomas commonly contain calcium, and intrahepatic calcifications have been observed in the neonate due to transplacental infections and neoplastic lesions.

Cholelithiasis is occasionally seen in newborn infants and may be related to parenteral alimentation or furosemide therapy. Spontaneous resolution of gallstones in this age group also has been reported.

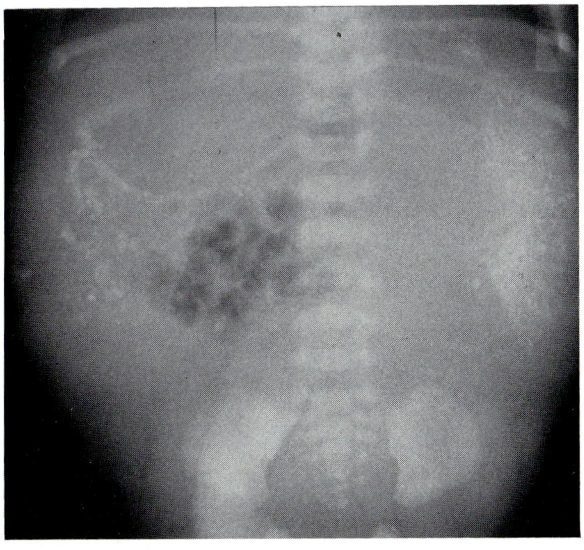

Fig. 13-24. Ascites and peritoneal calcification due to meconium peritonitis.

Biliary abnormalities

The biliary tract in the neonate is best imaged by a combination of ultrasound, which may detect a congenital lesion such as a choledochal cyst, and biliary scintigraphy using technetium-labeled iminodiacetic acid (IDA) derivatives (Fig. 13-25). Oral phenobarbital, used

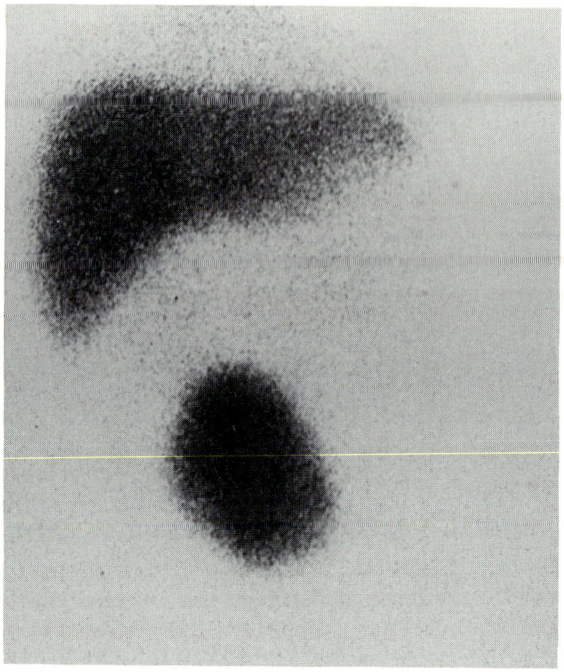

Fig. 13-25. Tc-IDA radionuclide study in a patient with biliary atresia. No activity is noted in the gut 90 minutes after injection of the radiopharmaceutical agent. Renal excretion has resulted in radioactivity within the urinary bladder.

as a chloretic, increases the sensitivity of IDA scans. These procedures are most frequently employed in the evaluation of jaundice. Passage of the radionuclide from the liver to the gut indicates patency of the biliary tree, and ultrasonographic demonstration of a normal gallbladder strongly suggests neonatal hepatitis. Biliary atresia is more likely in the absence of these two findings, and surgical exploration is recommended.

THE URINARY TRACT

See also Chapter 35.

A number of roentgenologic examinations are used to image the urinary tract and retroperitoneum. Selection of the most effective diagnostic modality and the sequence in which it may optimally be employed requires individual consideration of each case and a close dialogue between the referring physician and the radiologist. In this section we outline some of the important indications and diagnostic signs pertaining to the various examinations.

Traditionally the excretory urogram has been the primary mode of examination of the urinary tract. More recently, ultrasound has been recognized as an effective diagnostic tool. Under many circumstances, particularly when anatomic information is required, sonographic examination is now the method of choice. In comparison with sonography, which is noninvasive, computed tomography gives similar but slightly more detailed images, although this is achieved at a higher cost and radiation dosage. The relatively long exposures required, however, make it less practical for use in the neonate. Umbilical aortography is used to delineate the renal arteries. Radioisotope renograms are more valuable indicators of renal function than of renal structure. The lower urinary tract and vesicoureteral reflux are best evaluated by means of voiding cystourethrography. Micturating radionuclide studies also are used to identify vesicoureteral reflux.

Excretory urography

In today's practice, indications for a neonatal urogram rarely exist. Anatomic structures can be visualized by ultrasound, and physiologic information is provided by nuclear imaging. Because reactions to the injection of contrast materials and other complications, including pulmonary edema and hemorrhage, have been reported even in the usual doses, this study should not be performed in low birth weight infants (under 1,500 gm) or in infants who are sick or hypotensive. If the study is thought to be essential, then waiting until the child is older and bigger is prudent, at which time more satisfactory urograms can be performed.

Voiding cystourethrography

In neonates, voiding cystourethrography is useful in the evaluation of vesicoureteral reflux, posterior urethral valves in the male urethra, ambiguous genitalia, and anorectal malformations.

A small plastic feeding tube serves as an ideal catheter. The water-soluble contrast medium is instilled with a syringe or as a drip infusion. The bladder is filled until the patient voids, during which rapid serial imaging is carried out. A steep oblique position is necessary for visualization of the bladder neck and the entire length of the urethra (Fig. 13-26).

Normally the contour of the bladder is symmetrical and smooth. Slight irregularity appears during voiding. Trabeculation and diverticula suggest outlet obstruction or neurogenic bladder. An ectopic ureterocele may cause a smooth, rounded intraluminal filling defect. This may be missed if the contrast medium is too dense.

Roentgenographic evaluation of the urethra in females is usually unrewarding. During micturition, contrast medium normally may reflux into the vagina. Roentgenographic evaluation of the male urethra, however, is essential to demonstrate anatomic abnormalities such as posterior ureteral valves.

The presence or absence of vesicoureteral reflux is an extremely important observation. Since reflux may be identified only during voiding, careful filming must be

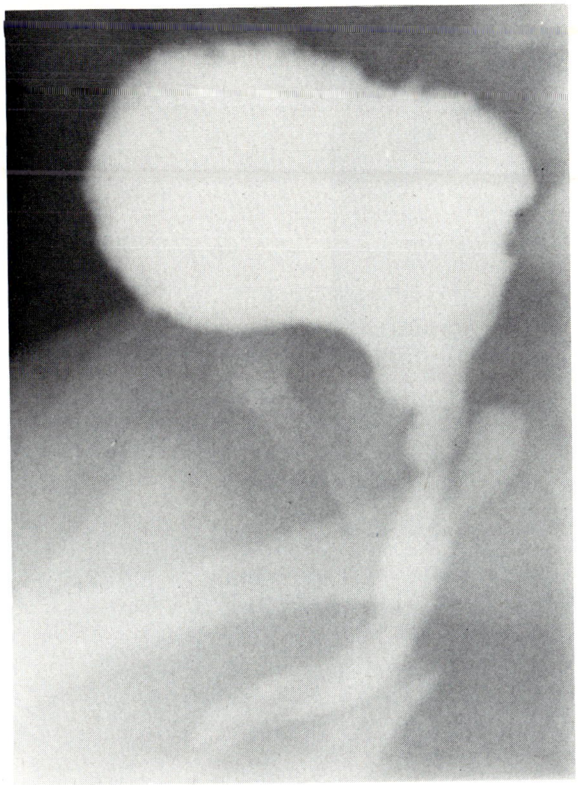

Fig 13-26 Cystourethrogram done for evaluation of ambiguous genitalia shows a short penile urethra and demonstrates a prostatic utricle, which is prevalent in males with hypospadias. Note the normal irregularity of the dome of the partially emptied bladder.

carried out during this time. Vesicoureteral reflux also allows morphologic assessment of the ureters and collecting systems in infants with reduced or absent renal function.

Nuclear imaging

Renal scintigraphy provides important functional information about the kidneys that cannot be obtained by other imaging modalities. Renal blood flow and function can be estimated by employing intravenous injections of technetium-tagged diethylenetriamine pentaacetic acid (DTPA). This radiopharmaceutical is excreted purely by glomerular filtration, and images of the collecting systems can be subsequently obtained. Unfortunately, nuclear imaging of neonatal kidneys is limited by their small size, which approaches the limits of resolution of the gamma camera.

Ultrasonography

Sound waves are produced by a transducer which, employing the piezoelectric effect, changes electrical energy to mechanical sound waves. Typical frequencies used for these transducers would be 5 MHz and 7.5 MHz. Sound waves travel from the transducer, which is in contact with the infant's skin, and are reflected at interfaces where differences in acoustical properties are present. The reflected sound waves, or echoes are "heard" by the transducer and converted into electrical signals that produce the image. Since interfaces between soft tissues and bone and between soft tissues and air produce virtually no echoes, the bony skeleton, lungs, and gas-filled loops of bowel are not usually appreciated by ultrasound. Ultrasound does not produce ionization and, as far as we are aware, is biologically safe at the energy levels used. Moreover, no contrast material or intravenous injections are used. Sedation and preparation are not necessary, and portable ultrasound equipment can easily be transferred to the nursery.

Examination of the neonatal genitourinary system should include identification of both kidneys, both adrenals, and the bladder. Fluid in the peritoneal cavity, such as urinary ascites, can easily be identified by ultrasound, and the position of catheters inserted into the umbilical artery and vein should also be checked for a complete study.

The normal neonatal kidney

On a sonogram, normal neonatal kidneys differ from those of the older child and adult in three important ways. They display an echogenic renal cortex, a relatively sonolucent and slightly enlarged pyramid, and a lack of renal sinus fat (Fig. 13-27).

The increased cortical echo pattern of the renal cortex approaches that of the adjacent liver. This is a normal neonatal pattern and should not be mistaken for renal parenchymal disease. It is found in all full-term and premature infants. By 17 weeks of age, this pattern is usually replaced by one with decreased echoes that persists throughout life. Approximately 50% of infants will have already changed to this adult-type pattern by 8 weeks. Explanations for the increased echogenicity of the normal neonatal kidney include a greater number of glomeruli, greater cellular content of the glomerular tuft, and the presence of loops of Henle within the cortex. These histologic variations result in numerous cellular interfaces in the renal cortex and therefore greater echogenicity. The lack of perirenal fat is a normal finding in neonates and is one reason why CT scanning, which relies on the natural contrast material provided by fat around abdominal organs, is often unsatisfactory in these infants.

The neonatal adrenal glands are relatively large, and both can usually be identified. The adrenal cortex is sonolucent or anechoic, whereas the adrenal medulla is echogenic. The adrenal gland can be identified as a V- or Y-shaped structure, with the right adrenal usually easier to identify than the left one.

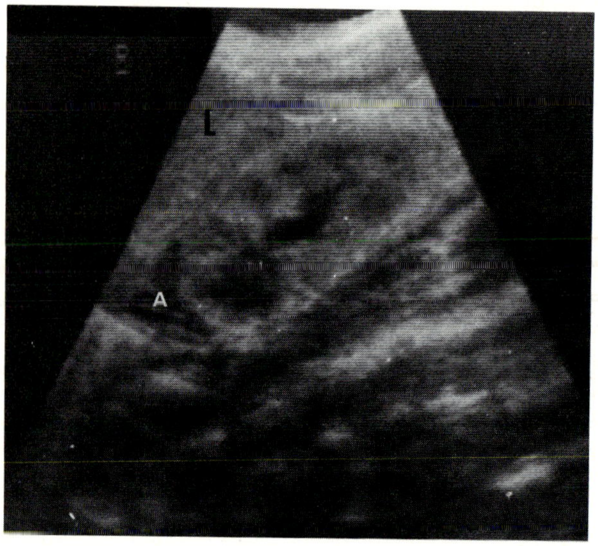

Fig. 13-27. Normal neonatal kidney and adrenal. Longitudinal view of the right upper quadrant shows the liver *(L)*, kidney and normal right adrenal *(A)*. The adrenal shows a normal echogenic (white) medulla and sonolucent (black) cortex. Note the normal echogenic renal parenchyma, which is almost the same density as that of the adjacent liver. By contrast, the pyramids appear sonolucent (black).

The renal arteries can be identified because of pulsations, and the renal veins are often seen. Identification of thrombi within them, however, is more difficult, although such pathologic processes within the adjacent aorta and inferior vena cava usually are easily seen.

Renal masses

The most common renal masses in the newborn period are caused by multicystic dysplasia and hydronephrosis. These can be identified and differentiated by ultrasound, which should be the initial examination of choice (Fig. 13-28). For confirmation, nuclear imaging will demonstrate lack of perfusion in multicystic kidneys, and delayed function will be noted in hydronephrosis (Fig. 13-29).

On ultrasound, a multicystic dysplastic kidney shows many noncommunicating cysts of various size. Hydronephrosis also appears multicystic but is usually bilateral, and the "cysts" communicate with the enlarged renal pelves. Renal parenchyma is usually identifiable in hydronephrosis but not in multicystic dysplastic kidney. Occasionally, a kidney may show features of multicystic kidney and hydronephrosis.

Autosomal recessive infantile polycystic disease produces bilaterally large kidneys that are very echogenic (Fig. 13-30). There is also a loss of the normal distinction between cortex and medulla. Increased echogenicity of the cysts seems paradoxic but can be explained by the small size of the cysts, which cannot be identified separately. The many tiny cysts produce a multitude of interfaces, each of which produces echoes.

Other renal masses are rare in the newborn period. A solitary solid mass of the kidney often indicates a benign mesoblastic nephroma. Wilm's tumor is less common in this age group and cannot be distinguished from mesoblastic nephroma by ultrasound alone.

Ultrasound is also helpful in the diagnosis of pelvic masses. Hydrocolpos and hydrometrocolpos can be identified and distinguished from other pelvic masses such as a distended bladder, anterior meningocele, presacral teratoma, neuroblastoma, and ovarian cyst. Finally, renal calculi in neonates receiving long-term furosemide therapy are becoming more common and can often be identified on ultrasound.

Adrenal hemorrhage

Adrenal hemorrhage can be identified on ultrasound as a mass that replaces the normal adrenal gland (Fig. 13-31). Usually the mass has a mixed echo pattern that will be observed to change as the hemorrhage resolves. Follow-up ultrasound studies are recommended to show a decrease in size of the mass and to exclude a rare adrenal abscess or incidental finding of a neuroblastoma. Occasionally, on follow-up abdominal roentgenograms, calcifications can be identified in the region of an earlier adrenal hemorrhage.

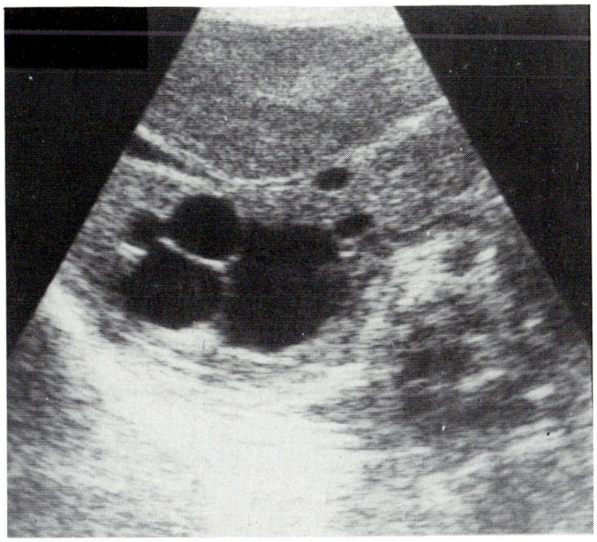

Fig. 13-28. Multicystic dysplastic kidney: ultrasound. Transverse view of the upper abdomen shows several cystic collections in the region of the right renal fossa. These do not communicate and are of various sizes.

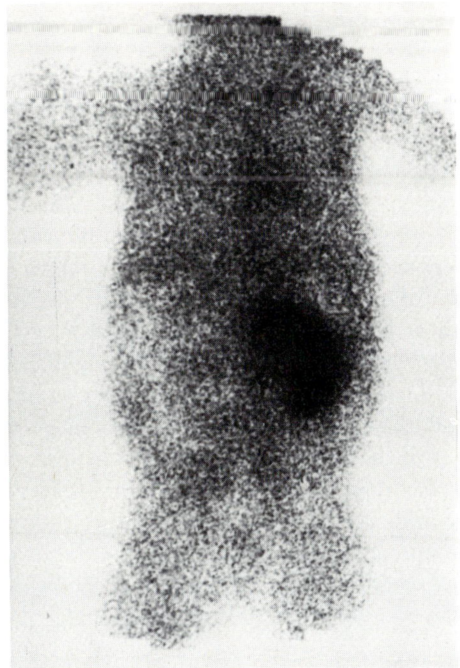

Fig. 13-29. Multicystic dysplastic kidney; radionuclide study. The right multicystic dysplastic kidney shows up as an area of decreased function. Normal functioning kidney is identified on the left side.

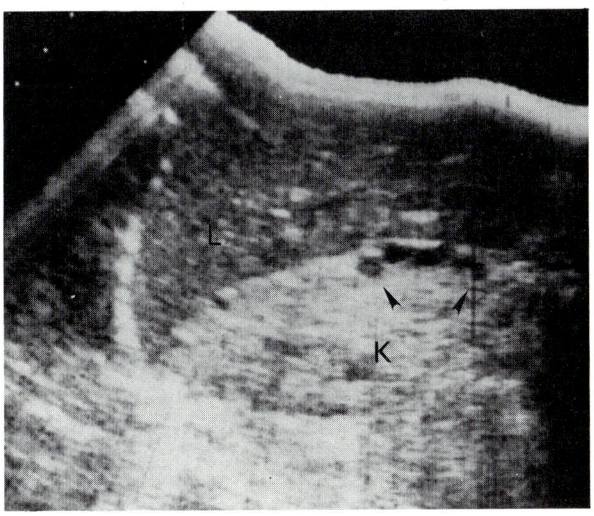

Fig. 13-30. Sagittal supine sonogram in the plane of the right kidney in a patient with typical sonographic findings of infantile polycystic kidney disease. The kidney *(K)* is seen posterior to the liver *(L)* and demonstrates increased echogenicity relative to the liver, multiple cortical cysts *(arrowheads),* and no demonstrable pelvicalyceal complex.

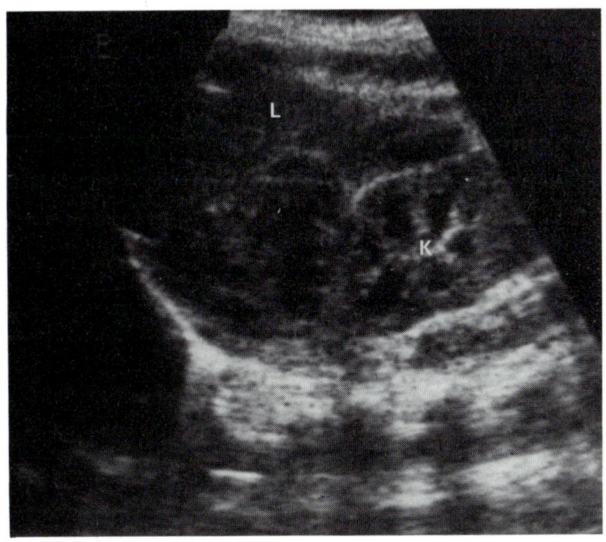

Fig. 13-31. Adrenal hemorrhage: ultrasound. Longitudinal view of the right upper quadrant shows a mass of variable echogenicity above the right kidney *(K)* and beneath the liver *(L)*. This represents an adrenal hemorrhage.

SKELETAL SYSTEM

No attempt is made to describe all of the numerous bone abnormalities that can exist in the neonate. However, important observations can be made from the bones visible on films of the chest and abdomen, which reflect physiologic and pathologic changes.

The bones of a gestationally mature infant are normally dense. During the first 4 to 6 weeks of life this density diminishes as bone growth accelerates. By approximately 2 months of age, physiologic periosteal new bone formation may be seen along the shafts of long bones in rapidly growing healthy infants. This usually can be differentiated from abnormal periosteal reaction by its symmetry and lack of underlying osseous lesions. In contrast, the bones of the premature infant appear less well mineralized than normal, and the cortices are relatively thin.

On roentgenograms of the chest and abdomen the proximal metaphyses of the humeri or femurs almost always are visible. Abnormalities of these bony structures may reflect either intrauterine or postnatal disorders.

Antenatal disorders

Intrauterine infections frequently cause metaphyseal abnormalities. In rubella and cytomegalovirus infections the metaphyses typically are rarefied and contain dense, vertical striations that resemble a celery stalk (Fig. 13-32). Syphilis also causes metaphyseal irregularity, proximal to which is a zone of radiolucency. Intrauterine insults, such as meconium peritonitis, produce a horizontal band of increased density in the metaphysis due to growth arrest.

Postnatal disorders

Osteomyelitis in the newborn is usually due to *Staphylococcus*, *Streptococcus*, or *Candida* organisms. These organisms produce focal lucent metaphyseal areas of bone destruction with or without associated septic arthritis (Fig. 13-33).

The efficacy of bone scans in the diagnosis of osteomyelitis is less firmly established in neonates than in older children. Although such scans may not offer additional information when radiographs are positive, they may reveal lesions when radiographs are normal. These lesions may be silent and found incidentally on films done for other purposes. Since they are often multifocal, a complete skeletal survey should be done when one lesion is discovered.

Serial films of chronically ill premature infants, even those receiving intravenous alimentation, should be observed closely for signs of rickets. In this disorder the metaphysis is abnormally lucent, and there is a loss of the zone of provisional calcification, which is the dense line at the metaphyseal end of the bone adjacent to the epiphyseal cartilage plate. This abnormality is accompanied by metaphyseal fraying and cupping. The metaphyses of the knees and wrists are particularly sensitive indicators of rickets as are the anterior rib ends, which may show a rachitic rosary (Fig. 13-34). Rib fractures also are common in these infants.

Spine, pelvis, and hips

These portions of the skeleton also are visible on many routine chest and abdominal films of the neonate. Common anomalies of vertebral segmentation, such as sagittally cleft (butterfly) vertebrae and hemivertebrae, may be incidental roentgenologic findings or accompany other congenital anomalies such as esophageal atresia, imperforate anus, agenesis of the lung, and bronchopulmonary foregut malformations. Spinal dysraphism is manifested on AP views as an increase in the interpediculate distance of the involved portion of the vertebral column, which indicates a widening of the spinal canal (Fig. 13-35). Although this finding is commonly associated with me-

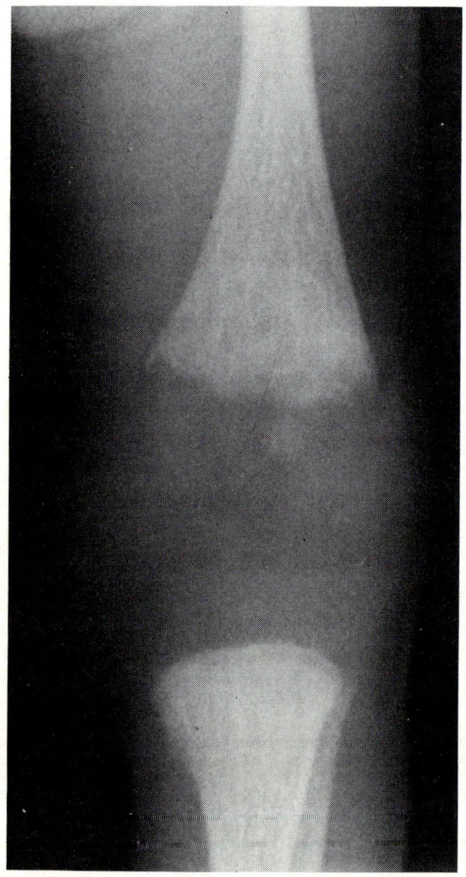

Fig. 13-32. Radiograph of the knee of a full-term infant was prompted by suspicious findings in the proximal humeri on the chest film. There are numerous vertical metaphyseal striations due to intrauterine rubella infection. Note the delayed ossification of the epiphyses.

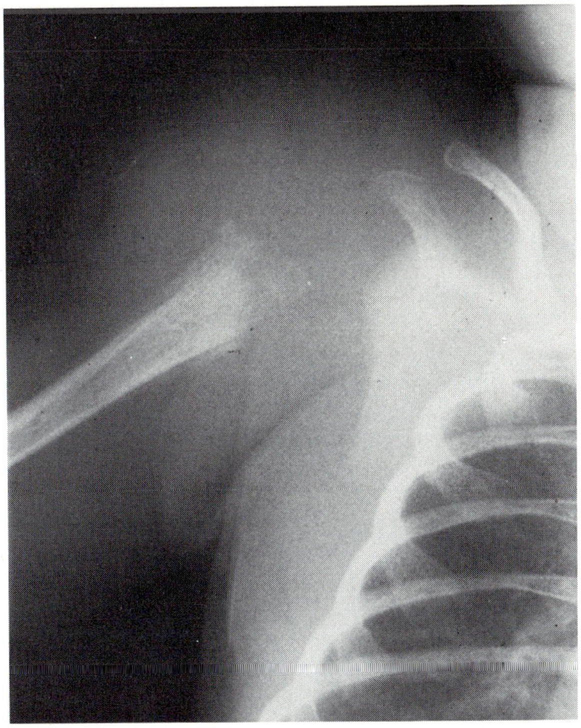

Fig. 13-33. Osteomyelitis with septic arthritis. Note the severe soft tissue swelling, metaphyseal destruction and periosteal new bone formation of the proximal humerus.

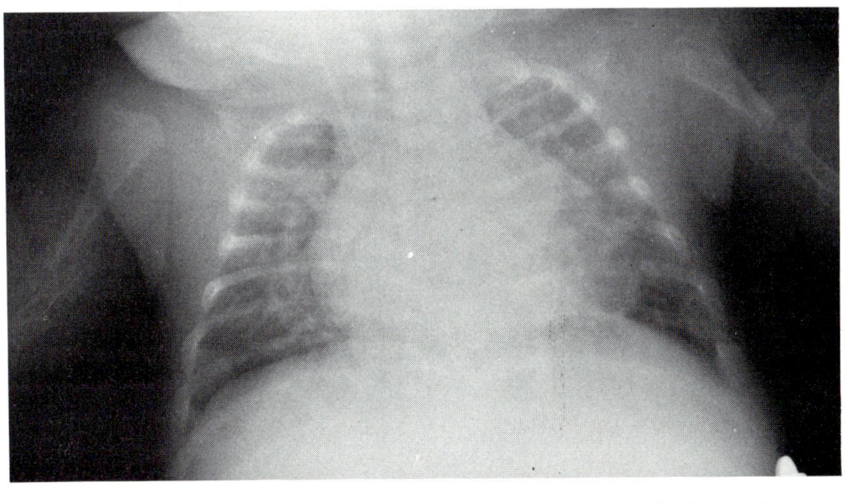

Fig. 13-34. Infant with chronic lung disease has severe osteopenia, flaring and rarefaction of the metaphyses, and expansion of the anterior ends of the lower ribs due to rickets. There also were multiple long bone fractures. An alimentation catheter extends into the superior vena cava.

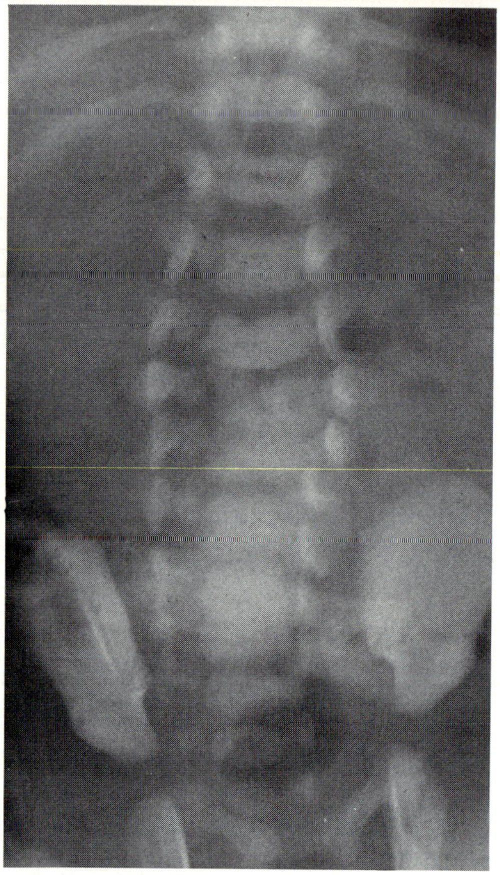

Fig. 13-35. Supine view of the lumbosacral spine shows widening of the interpediculate distances and dysplasia of the neural arch characteristic of spinal dysraphism. A meningomyelocele has been repaired surgically.

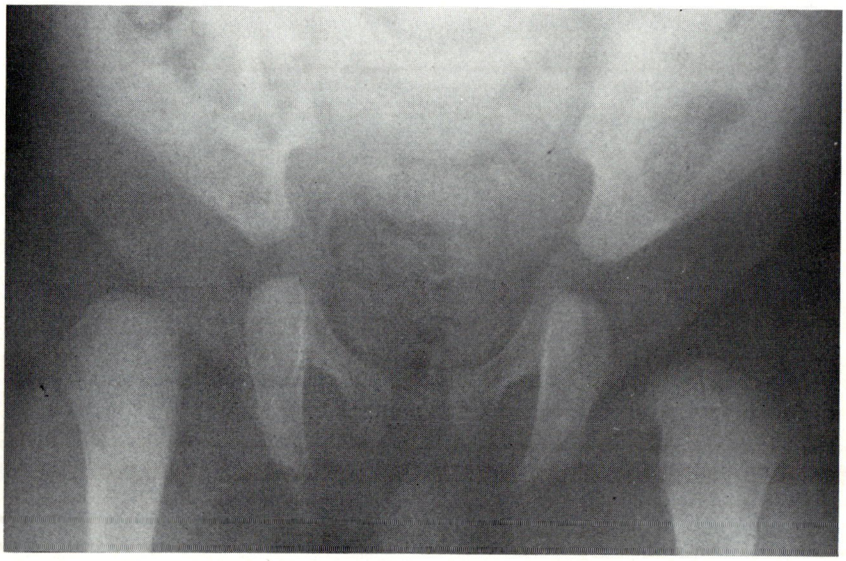

Fig. 13-36. AP view of the hips and pelvis demonstrates superolateral displacement of the right femur in a male with congenital dislocation of the hip. There is an associated dysplasia of the ipsilateral acetabulum manifested by an increased acetabular angle. The left acetabulum is also slightly dysplastic, but there is no subluxation.

ningomyelocele, lesser degrees of widening of the interpediculate distance may indicate the presence of an occult intraspinal lesion. Varying degrees of caudal regression with agenesis of the lumbosacral spine may be found in infants of diabetic mothers. A thorough evaluation of the genitourinary tract should be performed in all patients with spinal anomalies.

The femoral heads are rarely ossified in the early newborn period. This is unfortunate, since they are important landmarks in the diagnosis of congenital hip dislocation. In the absence of femoral head ossification, this diagnosis is recognized by superolateral displacement of the proximal femoral metaphyses and associated acetabular dysplasia (Fig. 13-36). Septic arthritis causes rapid subluxation or dislocation of the hips in the absence of acetabular dysplasia.

Congenital hip dislocation can also be diagnosed sonographically. Computed tomography and, more recently, magnetic resonance imaging have been advocated as methods of determining the anatomic relationship of the femoral head and acetabulum following reduction.

Estimation of gestational age

Traditionally, ossification of the epiphyseal centers of the knee has been used for roentgenologic assessment of gestational age, although the appearance of these centers is quite variable. In addition, the humeral heads are readily visible on chest roentgenograms, They are rarely ossified before 38 weeks of age and, if visible, indicate gestational maturity. Although their presence is not diagnostic of postmaturity, infants with respiratory distress in whom these centers are ossified have a statistically high chance of having meconium aspiration syndrome (Fig. 13-37).

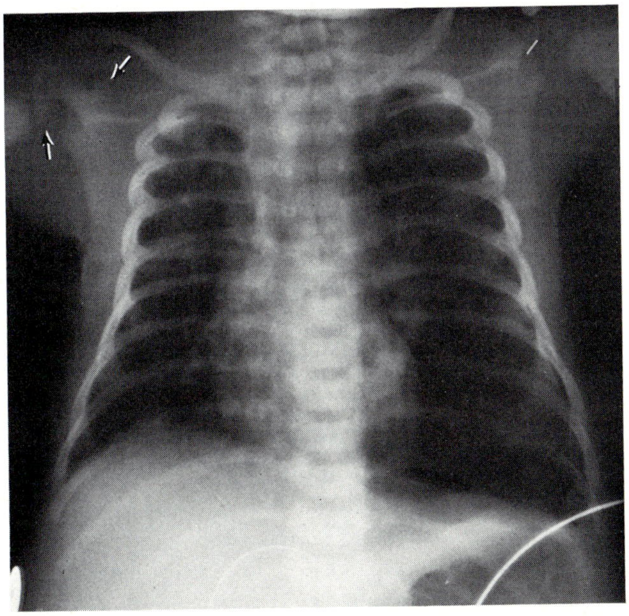

Fig. 13-37. Ill-defined streaky lung densities caused by meconium aspiration pneumonia. Note the ossification of the humeral heads and coracoid apophyses *(arrowheads)*. The barely discernible left pneumothorax can be suspected by the increased volume and lucency of the left hemithorax.

A delay in ossification of the epiphyses may occur in a small for gestational age fetus. Ossification also may be retarded by severe intrauterine infection such as rubella (Fig. 13-32). However, the lower deciduous molar teeth are more reliable indicators of gestational age and are frequently included on chest roentgenograms. Mineralization of the first deciduous molar indicates at least 33 weeks of gestation, whereas mineralization of the second molar indicates at least 36 weeks.

SKULL AND BRAIN

Although computerized tomography is now established as the primary diagnostic modality for suspected intracranial abnormalities, skull roentgenography is more useful for examination of the calvarium. Other diagnostic modalities, such as nuclear scintigraphy and angiography, have more limited applications in the neonate.

Roentgenographic evaluation of the neonatal skull requires three basic views: frontal, lateral, and Townes. Submental-vertex, tangential, and other views may be obtained for specific indications.

Soft tissues

Soft tissue swelling is common in neonates as a result of caput succedaneum and cephalhematoma. Cephalhematomas are caused by subperiosteal hemorrhage and are confined by the periosteal attachment at the sutural edges. They are most frequent over the parietal bones and eventually ossify and become incorporated into the outer table of the skull. Approximately 5% of cephalhematomas are accompanied by skull fractures.

Calvarium

Considerable experience is required in interpreting skull roentgenograms of infants because of the ongoing changes in craniofacial proportions. Craniofacial proportions are assessed on lateral roentgenograms by comparison of the relative areas of the face and calvarium. At birth the ratio of the cranial area to the facial area is normally about 4:1. A higher ratio indicates macrocrania, which is most often secondary to hydrocephalus. Microcrania reflects micrencephaly (Fig. 13-38).

In the immediate postnatal period the skull may be misshapen due to molding. Later, asymmetry and other abnormal skull configurations may indicate underlying abnormalities of the developing brain due to cerebral atrophy and also may be caused by sutural synostoses.

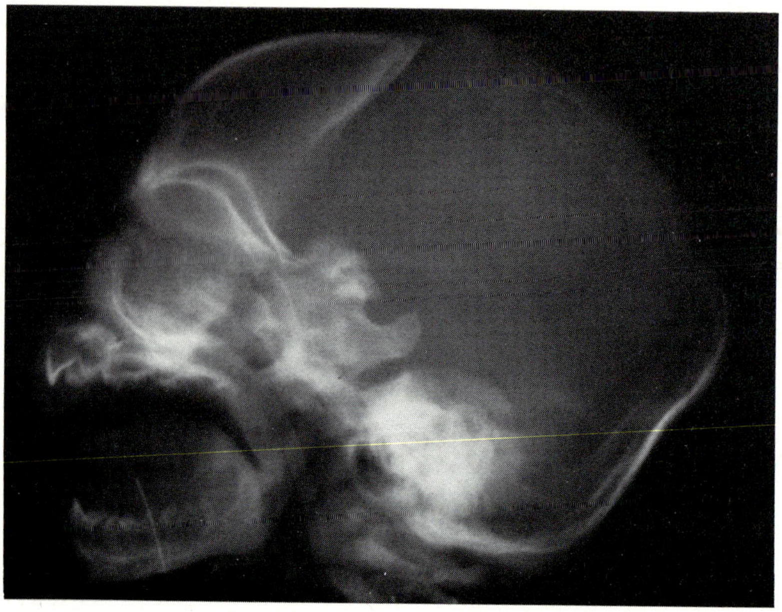

Fig. 13-38. Lateral film of the skull of a micrencephalic infant demonstrates a severely reduced craniofacial proportion of approximately 1.5:1. The sutures are markedly narrowed.

Minor degrees of calvarial asymmetry are, however, fairly common in normal infants, and parietooccipital flattening due to prolonged dependency of this portion of the skull is frequent, especially in debilitated infants. Convolutional markings are not usually prominent until the anterior fontanel closes but may be seen posteriorly with parietooccipital flattening or asymmetrically with premature synostosis or cerebral atrophy. They must be differentiated from the rounded dysplastic lucencies seen in craniolacunia and meningomyelocele.

Sutures

There is a wide range of normal suture widths in neonates because of molding, skeletal maturation, and gestational age. The size of the fontanels also is quite variable. During the first few days of life, sutural overriding is usually due to molding, after which the sutures appear relatively wide. The more premature the infant, the smaller the ossification centers of the various membranous bones and the greater the apparent widening of the sutures. With postnatal growth and subsequent ossification, the sutures decrease in width. In premature infants the sutures are often difficult to visualize because of lack of mineralization of the adjacent calvarium. Intrasutural (wormian) bones may be normal but also may indicate an alteration of normal membranous ossification due to osteogenesis imperfecta, cleidocranial dysostosis, or hypothyroidism.

Early closure of a suture may be either an isolated primary abnormality or, less commonly, secondary to generalized bone diseases such as hypophosphatasia and rickets, or it may be associated with congenital anomalies, as in Apert's or Crouzon's syndrome. Associated abnormalities of the shape of the cranium due to limitation of directional growth of the brain may precede anatomic closure of the suture. Lack of normal brain growth is an important cause of generalized sutural narrowing (Fig. 13-38).

Calcifications

Artifacts on the scalp, such as bandages, tape, iodoform gauze, electrode paste, blood, and matted hair, may appear as focal areas of increased density suggesting intracranial calcifications. Calcification or ossification of the scalp occurs within soft tissue lesions such as hemangioma or an organizing cephalhematoma. Intracranial calcifications in neonates are usually secondary to intrauterine infections such as herpes, cytomegalovirus, and toxoplasmosis.

Computed tomography scanning

Computed tomography of the head is far more expensive than ultrasound, and infants usually need to be restrained and often sedated for this study. However, contrast material is rarely needed in young infants. The advantages of CT scanning are that it can identify subarachnoid and subdural bleeds that may not be demonstrated on ultrasound, and it is capable of detecting calcification not visible on conventional roentgenograms.

The neonatal brain differs from that of the adult in several important respects. The normal white matter of a premature infant is of much lower density, especially

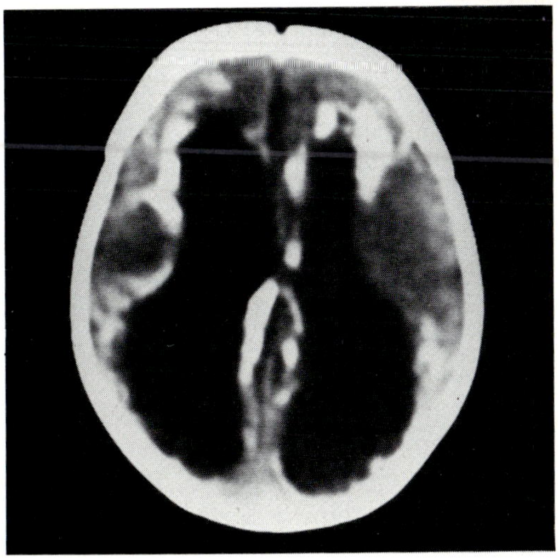

Fig. 13-39. In utero cytomegaloviral infection: head CT scan. Dilated lateral ventricles with periventricular calcification.

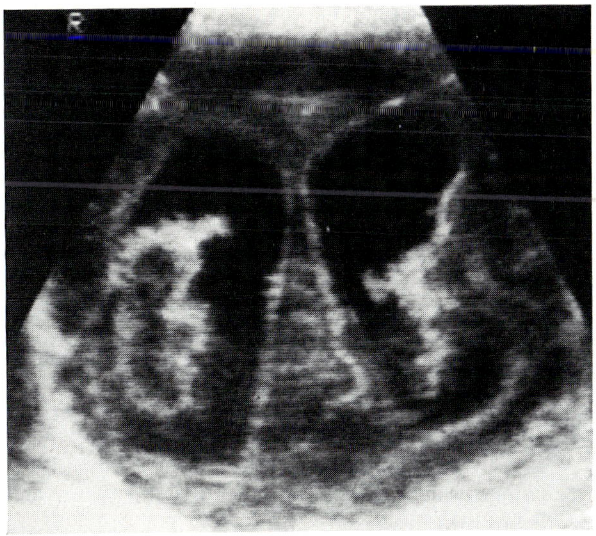

Fig. 13-40. Head ultrasound of premature infant shows dilated lateral ventricles together with blood clot within the enlarged lateral ventricles.

in the frontal, parietal, and occipital regions, and consequently it may be misinterpreted as representing white matter edema. These symmetric areas of low density slowly increase in density, presumably because of myelination. In full-term infants, the areas of low density in the white matter are usually present only in the frontal lobes. In addition, intracranial calcifications can be detected by CT scanning before they become apparent on roentgenograms (Fig. 13-39).

Ultrasonography

Although bone is usually a barrier to the transmission of ultrasound waves, the infant brain can be studied by placing a transducer on the anterior fontanel. By varying the angle of the transducer, the brain can be scanned in any projection. Standard views include the coronal, sagittal, and axial projections. The study can be performed with portable equipment at the cribside. The entire procedure can be stored on videotape and copied on film for a permanent record. No sedation, contrast material, or ionizing radiation are required.

Pulsations of the normal intracranial arteries can be identified, and Doppler ultrasound can be performed to assess flow. Ultrasound, however, cannot distinguish between gray and white matter.

Because the neural arches of the neonatal and infant spine are not ossified, ultrasonography employing high-frequency transducers is capable of demonstrating the spinal cord and subarachnoid space. The position of the spinal cord can be identified with respect to the adjacent bony structures, as can anomalies such as a tethered cord, lipoma, or other evidence of spinal dysraphism.

Intracranial hemorrhage in the premature infant

See Chapter 27.

Intracranial hemorrhage occurs in approximately two thirds of infants of 28 to 32 weeks' gestational age. Most hemorrhages occur within the first week of life, with the majority occurring within 3 days. Since clinical predictions of intracranial bleeding are unreliable, all infants under 32 weeks' gestational age or weighing less than 1,500 gm should be routinely scanned by ultrasound (Fig. 13-40).

Most hemorrhages originate from the germinal matrix in the groove between the thalamus and the head of the caudate nucleus; they are identified on ultrasound as an echogenic area with no shadowing. This subependymal bleeding may be confined to the germinal matrix or may extend further into the adjacent lateral ventricle. Enlargement of the lateral ventricle may then occur, and hemorrhage may extend further into the brain parenchyma. The blood remains echogenic for weeks and, occasionally, even months. A central sonolucency eventually develops because of the change in the physical properties of the blood, and the clots also will often retract in size. Intraparenchymal bleeding commonly results in porencephalic cysts communicating with the lateral ventricles. A commonly used grading system that has some prognostic value is described here:

- Grade 1: subependymal germinal matrix hemorrhage
- Grade 2: hemorrhage extending into the lateral ventricles, in which the lateral ventricles are of normal size
- Grade 3: hemorrhage extending into the lateral ventricles, which are now enlarged

Grade 4: intraparenchymal hemorrhage

Infants with grades 1 and 2 hemorrhages have a good prognosis with no difference in outcome compared to other infants of similar gestational age. Patients with grades 3 and 4 hemorrhages however, do poorly, and approximately 50% of infants with grade 4 hemorrhages die.

Intracranial hemorrhage in the full-term infant

Bleeding from the brain parenchyma is very rare in full-term infants. Full-term infants who are asphyxiated or have traumatic deliveries may have subarachnoid bleeding or, occasionally, subdural hemorrhage. Computed tomography scanning is often the best modality for diagnosis of hemorrhage in full-term infants, since subarachnoid, and some subdural hemorrhages, are not identifiable on ultrasound.

Congenital malformations and hydrocephalus

Ultrasound offers the best imaging technique for the diagnosis and follow-up of cases of ventriculomegaly and hydrocephalus. Ultrasound is also the imaging modality of choice for the many congenital anomalies that occur in the developing brain due to failures of diverticulation or failures of segmentation.

MONITORING AND TREATMENT DEVICES

An important aspect of the roentgenologic examination of the newborn infant is the assessment of the position of various devices, such as endotracheal tubes, nasogastric tubes, umbilical catheters, and intravenous alimentation catheters. For obvious reasons these devices must be radiopaque (see Fig. 13-23).

The endotracheal tube is visible on most chest roentgenograms. Its tip should be approximately halfway between the vocal cords and the carina, at approximately the level of the first ribs. In small premature infants, even slight alterations in the degree of flexion of the neck will cause a remarkable difference between the position of the tube as seen on AP and lateral roentgenograms.

The position of the nasogastric tube also should be noted on the chest roentgenogram. Its tip may be displaced inadvertently from the stomach into the lower esophagus. On occasion the tube will be found curled above a previously unsuspected esophageal atresia.

To assess umbilical arterial and venous catheters, a film should be done that includes both the chest and the abdomen. The umbilical arterial catheter can be seen in the aorta, to the left of the midline. Proper position of its tip is either in the thoracic aorta between T6 and T10 or in the abdominal aorta just above the aortic bifurcation. The umbilical vein catheter ascends toward the porta hepatis to the right of the midline and bypasses the portal system by entering the ductus venosus, which leads to the inferior vena cava. The optimum position of this catheter tip is in the intrathoracic portion of the inferior vena cava.

Catheter position also can be determined by ultrasound. Although this method requires greater technical expertise, it avoids the use of ionizing radiation and is capable of detecting catheter-related complications, such as thrombi (Fig. 13-41).

Intravenous alimentation catheters are usually inserted via the internal or external jugular vein into the superior vena cava so that the tip comes to lie immediately superior to the right atrium.

Numerous complications of intravenous alimentation have been reported, including hydrothorax due to per-

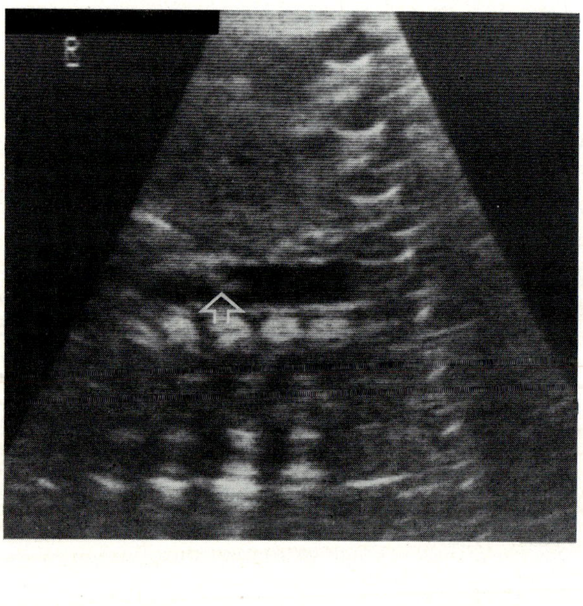

Fig. 13-41. Abdominal ultrasound shows an echogenic thrombus *(arrow)* within the lumen of the aorta, immediately anterior to the spine.

foration of the catheter into the pleural space and chylothoraces due to superior vena caval thrombosis. Venous alimentation and arterial catheters may be responsible for septic or aseptic emboli, which may disturb growth at the physes of the long bones.

Barry D. Fletcher
Stuart C. Morrison
Barry S. Yulish

BIBLIOGRAPHY

General

Avery, M.E., Fletcher, B.D., and Williams, R.G.: The lung and its disorders in the newborn infant, ed. 4, Philadelphia, 1981, W.B. Saunders Co.

Caffey, J.: Pediatric x-ray diagnosis, ed. 8, Chicago, 1984, Year Book Medical Publishers, Inc.

Dunn, V., and others: Infants of diabetic mothers: radiographic manifestations, Am. J. Roentgenol. **137**:123, 1981.

Franken, E.A., and Smith, W.L.: Gastrointestinal imaging in pediatrics, ed. 2, Philadelphia, 1982, Harper & Row.

Poznanski, A.K.: Practical approaches to pediatric radiology, Chicago, 1976, Year Book Medical Publishers, Inc.

Rumack, C.M., and Johnson, M.L.: Perinatal and infant brain imaging: role of ultrasound and computed tomography, Chicago, 1984, Year Book Medical Publishers, Inc.

Methods and contrast media

Clarke, E., and Siegle, R.L.: Effect of oral metrizamide on hematocrit and serum osmolality in the neonate, Invest. Radiol. **19**:599, 1984.

Cohen, M.D.: Prolonged visualization of the gastrointestinal tract with metrizamide, Radiology **144**:327, 1982.

Davis, L.A.: Standard roentgen examination in newborns, infants, and children: techniques, "portable" films, immobilization devices, and fluoroscopy, Progr. Pediatr. Radiol. **1**:3, 1967.

Franken, E.W., and others: Initial chest radiography in the neonatal intensive care unit: value of the lateral view. Am. J. Roentgenol. **133**:43, 1979.

Haller, J.O., and others: Sonographic evaluation of the chest in infants and children, Am. J. Roentgenol. **134**:1019, 1980.

Haney, P.J.: Infant apnea: findings on the barium esophagram, Radiology **148**:425, 1983.

Harris, P.D., Neuhauser, E.B.D., and Gerth, R.: The osmotic effect of water-soluble contrast media on circulating plasma volume, Am. J. Roentgenol. Radium. Ther. Nucl. Med. **991**:694, 1964.

Hope, J.W., and O'Hara, A.E.: Use of air as a contrast medium in the diagnosis of intestinal obstruction of the newborn, Radiology **70**:349, 1958.

Joseph, P.M., and others: Upper airway obstruction in infants and small children: improved radiographic diagnosis by combining filtration, high kilovoltage and magnification, Radiology **121**:143, 1976.

Keller, M.S., and Chawla, H.S.: Neonatal metrizamide gastrointestinal series in suspected necrotizing enterocolitis, Am. J. Dis. Child. **139**:713, 1985.

Leonidas, J.C., and others: Possible adverse effect of methylglucamine diatrizoate compounds on the bowel of newborn infants with meconium ileus, Radiology **121**:693, 1976.

Lorenzo, R.L., and Harolds, J.A.: The use of prone films for suspected bowel obstruction in infants and children, Am. J. Roentgenol. **129**:617, 1977.

Lutzger, L.G., and Factor, S.M.: Effects of some water-soluble contrast media on the colonic mucosa, Radiology **118**:545, 1976.

MacEwan, D.W., and others: Pneumothorax in young infants—recognition and evaluation, J. Can. Assoc. Radiol. **22**:264, 1971.

McAlister, W.H., and Askin, F.B.: The effect of some contrast agents in the lung: an experimental study in the rat and dog, Am. J. Roentgenol. **140**:245, 1983.

Noblett, H.R.: Treatment of uncomplicated meconium ileus by Gastrografin enema: a preliminary report, J. Pediatr. Surg. **4**:190, 1969.

Ratcliffe, J.F.: The use of low osmolality water soluble (LOWS) contrast media in the pediatric gastro-intestinal tract: a report of 115 examinations, Pediatr. Radiol. **16**:47, 1986.

Schey, W.L., and others: Esophageal dysmotility and the sudden infant death syndrome: clinical experience, Radiology **140**:67, 1981.

Shopfner, C.E.: Genitography in intersex problems, Progr. Pediatr. Radiol. **3**:97, 1970.

Slovis, T.L., and others: Choanal atresia: precise CT evaluation, Radiology **155**:345, 1985.

Wood, B.P., and others: Diatrizoate enemas: facts and fallacies of colonic toxicity, Radiology **126**:441, 1978.

Patient protection

Margulis, A.R.: The lessons of radiobiology for diagnostic radiology, Am. J. Roentgenol. Radium Ther. Nucl. Med. **117**:741, 1973.

Mazzi, E., Herrera, A.J., and Linton, H.: Neonatal intensive care and radiation, Johns Hopkins Med. J. **142**:15, 1978.

Smathers, R.L., and others: Radiation dose reduction in the neonatal intensive care unit: comparison of three gadolinium oxysulfide screen-film combinations, Invest. Radiol. **19**:578, 1984.

Smith, W.L., and others: Selection of optimal screen-film combination for use in the neonatal intensive care unit, Am. J. Roentgenol. **139**:1051, 1982.

Normal findings

Berdon, W.E., Baker, D.H., and James, L: The ductus bump: a transient physiologic mass in chest roentgenograms of newborn infants, Am. J. Roentgenol. Radium Ther. Nucl. Med. **95**:91, 1965.

Fletcher, B.D., and others: Thymic response to endogenous and exogenous steroids in premature newborn infants, J. Pediatr. **95**:111, 1979.

Kemp, F.H., Morley, H.M.C., and Emrys-Roberts, E.: A sail-like triangular projection from the mediastinum: a radiographic appearance of the thymus gland, Br. J. Radiol. **21**:618, 1948.

Kleinman, P.K., and others: The neonatal colon: an anatomic approach to plain films, Am. J. Roentgenol. **128**:61, 1977.

Podolsky, M.L., and Jester, A.W.: The distribution of air in the intestinal tract of infants during the first twelve hours as determined by serial roentgenograms, J. Pediatr. **45**:633, 1954.

Taybi, H.: Roentgen evaluation of cardiomegaly in the newborn period and early infancy, Pediatr. Clin. North Am. **18**:1031, 1971.

Pulmonary abnormalities

Ablow, R.C., and others: The radiographic features of early onset group B streptococcal neonatal sepsis, Radiology **124**:771, 1977.

Clarke, T.A., and Edwards, D.K.: Pulmonary pseudocysts in newborn infants with respiratory distress syndrome, Am. J. Roentgenol. **133**:417, 1979.

Fletcher, B.D.: Medial herniation of the parietal pleura: a useful sign of pneumothorax in supine neonates, Am. J. Roentgenol. **130**:469, 1978.

Fletcher, B.D., and Avery, M.E.: The effects of airway occlusion after oxygen breathing on the lungs of newborn infants: radiologic demonstration in the experimental animal, Radiology **109**:665, 1973.

Fletcher, B.D., and others: Pulmonary interstitial emphysema in a newborn infant treated by lobectomy, Pediatrics **54**:808, 1974.

Johnson, J.F., and Dean, B.L.: The expiratory film in hyaline membrane disease: preliminary observations, Am. J. Roentgenol. **139**:31, 1982.

Kassner, E.G., and others: Pulmonary candidiasis in infants: clinical radiologic, and pathologic features, Am. J. Roentgenol. **137**:707, 1981.

Kopecky, K., Cohen, M., and Schreiner, R.: Therapeutic neuromuscular paralysis in neonates: characteristic radiographic features, Am. J. Roentgenol. **139**:25, 1982.

Leonidas, J.C., Bhan, I., and Beatty, E.C.: Radiographic chest contour and pulmonary air leaks in oligohydramnios-related pulmonary hypoplasia (Potter's syndrome), Invest. Radiol. **17**:6, 1982.

Macklin, M.T., and Macklin, C.G.: Malignant interstitial emphysema of the lungs and mediastinum as an important occult complication in many respiratory diseases and other conditions: an interpretation of the clinical literature in the light of laboratory experiment, Medicine **23**:281, 1944.

Moseley, J.E.: Loculated pneumomediastinum in the newborn: a thymic "spinnaker sail" sign, Radiology **75**:788, 1960.

Moskowitz, P.S., and Griscom, N.T.: The medial pneumothorax, Radiology **120**:143, 1976.

Radkowski, M.A., and others: Chlamydia pneumonia in infants: radiography in 125 cases, Am. J. Roentgenol. **137**:703, 1981.

Recavarren, S., Benton, C., and Gall, E.A.: The pathology of acute alveolar diseases of the lung, Semin. Roentgenol. **2**:22, 1967.

Wood, B.P., and others: Pulmonary lymphatic air: locating "pulmonary interstitial emphysema" of the premature infant, Am. J. Roentgenol. **138**:809, 1982.

Wyman, M.L., and Kuhns, L.R.: Lobar opacification of the lung after tracheal extubation in neonates, J. Pediatr. **91**:109, 1977.

Yeh, T.F., Vidyasagar, D., and Pildes, R.S.: Neonatal pneumopericardium, Pediatrics **54**:429, 1974.

Cardiovascular abnormalities

Bauer, C.R., Tsipuras, D., and Fletcher, B.D.: Syndrome of persistent pulmonary vascular obstruction of the newborn: roentgen findings, Am. J. Roentgenol. Radium Ther. Nucl. Med. **120**:285, 1974.

Higgins, C.B., and others: Patent ductus arteriosus in preterm infants with idiopathic respiratory distress syndrome: radiographic and echocardiographic evaluation, Radiology **124**:189, 1977.

Kuhn, J.P., Fletcher, B.D., and deLemos, R.A.: Roentgen findings in transient tachypnea of the newborn, Radiology **92**:751, 1969.

Gastrointestinal tract

Ablow, R.C., and others: Z-shaped duodenojejunal loop: sign of mesenteric fixation anomaly and congenital bands, Am. J. Roentgenol. **141**:461, 1983.

Abramson, S.J., Treves, S., and Teele, R.L.: The infant with possible biliary atresia: evaluation by ultrasound and nuclear medicine, Pediatr. Radiol. **12**:1, 1982.

Berdon, W.E., and others: Necrotizing enterocolitis in the premature infant, Radiology **83**:879, 1964.

Berdon, W.E., and others: Midgut malrotation and volvulus, Radiology **96**:375, 1970.

Blumhagen, J.D., and Noble, H.G.S.: Muscle thickness in hypertrophic pyloric stenosis: sonographic determination, Am. J. Roentgenol. **140**:221, 1983.

Burko, H.: Toxic depression of the newborn causing deficient intestinal gas pattern, Am. J. Roentgenol. Radium Ther. Nucl. Med. **88**:575, 1962.

Callahan, J., and others: Cholelithiasis in infants: association with total parenteral nutrition and furosemide, Radiology **143**:437, 1982.

Davis, W.S., and others: Neonatal small left colon syndrome, Am. J. Roentgenol. Radium Ther. Nucl. Med. **120**:322, 1974.

Fletcher, B.D., and Yulish, B.S.: Intraluminal calcifications in the small bowel of newborn infants with total colonic aganglionosis, Radiology **126**:451, 1978.

Franken, E.A.: Ascites in infants and children: roentgen diagnosis, Radiology **102**:393, 1972.

Griscom, N.T., and others: Diagnostic aspects of neonatal ascites: report of 27 cases, Am. J. Roentgenol. **128**:961, 1977.

Johnson, J.F., and Robinson, L.H.: Localized bowel distension in the newborn: a review of the plain film analysis and differential diagnosis, Pediatrics **73**:206, 1984.

Kassner, E.G., and others: Gasless abdomen in neonates with orotracheal tubes, Radiology **112**:659, 1974.

Leonard, T., Jr., Johnson, J.F., and Pettett, P.G.: Critical evaluation of the persistent loop sign in necrotizing enterocolitis, Radiology **142**:385, 1982.

Leonidas, J.C., and others: Meconium ileus and its complications, Am. J. Roentgenol. Radium Ther. Nucl. Med. **108**:598, 1970.

Leonidas, J.C., and others: Pneumoperitoneum in ventilated newborns, Am. J. Dis. Child. **128**:677, 1974.

Leonidas, J.C.: Neonatal necrotizing enterocolitis, Am. J. Dis. Child. **136**:1097, 1982.

Merritt, C.R.B., Goldsmith, J.P., and Sharp, M.J.: Sonographic detection of portal venous gas in infants with necrotizing enterocolitis, Am. J. Roentgenol. **143**:1059, 1984.

Miller, R.E.: Perforated viscus in infants: a new roentgen sign, Radiology **74**:65, 1960.

Neuhauser, E.B.D.: The roentgen diagnosis of fetal meconium peritonitis, Am. J. Roentgenol. Radium Ther. Nucl. Med. **51**:421, 1944.

Pochaczevsky, R., and Kassner, E.G.: Necrotizing enterocolitis in infancy, Am. J. Roentgenol. Radium Ther. Nucl. Med. **113**:283, 1971.

Pochaczevsky, R., and Leonidas, J.D.: The meconium plug syndrome, Am. J. Roentgenol. Radium Ther. Nucl. Med. **120**:342, 1974.

Robinson, A., Grossman, H., and Brumley, G.: Pneumatosis intestinalis in the neonate, Am. J. Roentgenol. Radium Ther. Nucl. Med. **120**:333, 1974.

Rosenfield, N.S., and others: Hirschsprung disease: accuracy of the barium enema examination, Radiology **150**:393, 1984.

Sane, S.M., and Girdany, B.R.: Total aganglionosis coli, Radiology **107**:397, 1973.

Schey, W.L., Vesely, J.J., and Radkowski, M.A.: Shard-like calcifications in retroperitoneal teratomas, Pediatr. Radiol. **16**:82, 1986.

Siegle, R.L.: Neonatal gasless abdomen: another cause, Am. J. Roentgenol. **133**:522, 1979.

Urinary tract

Alton, D.J., and McDonald, P.: Urinary obstruction in the neonatal infant, Rad. Clin. North Am. **13**:343, 1975.

Berdon, W.E., and others: Tamm-Horsfall proteinuria: its relationship to prolonged nephrogram in infants and children and to renal failure following intravenous urography in adults with multiple myeloma, Radiology **92**:714, 1969.

Ultrasonography

Atkinson, G.O., Jr., and others: Adrenal abscess in the neonate, Radiology **155**:101, 1985.

Berdon, W.E.: Pulmonary edema in infants who receive contrast material, Radiology **139**:507, 1981.

Haller, J.O., Berdon, W.E., and Friedman, A.P.: Increased renal cortical echogenicity: a normal finding in neonates and infants, Radiology **142**:173, 1982.

Hayden, C.K., Jr., and others: Ultrasonographic evaluation of the renal parenchyma in infancy and childhood, Radiology **152**:413, 1984.

Hricak, H., and others: Neonatal kidneys: sonographic anatomic correlation, Radiology **147**:699, 1983.

Oppenheimer, D.A., Carroll, B.A., and Yousem, S.: Sonography of the normal neonatal adrenal gland, Radiology **146**:157, 1983.

Sanders, R.C., and Hartman, D.S.: The sonographic distinction between neonatal multicystic kidney and hydronephrosis, Radiology **151**:621, 1984.

Skeletal system

Binstadt, D.H., and L'Heureux, P.R.: Rickets as a complication of intravenous hyperalimentation in infants, Pediatr. Radiol. **7**:211, 1978.

Brill, P.W., and others: Osteomyelitis in a neonatal intensive care unit, Radiology **131**:83, 1979.

Hernandez, R.J., Tachdjian, M.O., and Dias, L.S.: Hip CT in congenital dislocation: appearance of tight iliopsoas tendon and pulvinar hypertrophy, Am. J. Roentgenol. **139**:335, 1982.

Kuhns, L.R., and Poznanski, A.K.: Radiological assessment of maturity and size of the newborn infant, CRC Crit. Rev. Diagn. Imaging **13**:245, 1980.

Lachman, R.S., Yamauchi, T., and Klein, J.: Neonatal systemic candidiasis and arthritis, Radiology **105**:631, 1972.

McCook, T.A., Felman, A.H., and Ayoub, E.: Streptococcal skeletal infections: observations in four infants, Am. J. Roentgenol. **130**:465, 1978.

Merten, D.F., and Gooding, C.A.: Skeletal manifestations of congenital cytomegalic inclusion disease, Radiology **95**:333, 1970.

Mok, P.M., Reilly, B.J., and Ash, J.M.: Osteomyelitis in the neonate: clinical aspects and the role of radiography and scintigraphy in diagnosis and management, Radiology **145**:677, 1982.

Novick, G., Ghelman, B., and Schneider, M.: Sonography of the neonatal and infant hip, Am. J. Roentgenol. **141**:639, 1983.

Poznanski, A.K.: Bone dysplasias: not so rare, definitely important, Am. J. Roentgenol. **142**:427, 1984.

Singleton, E.B., and others: The roentgenographic manifestations of the rubella syndrome in newborn infants, Am. J. Roentgenol. Radium Ther. Nucl. Med. **97**:82, 1966.

Wolfson, J.J., and Engel, R.R.: Anticipating meconium peritonitis from metaphyseal bands, Radiology **92**:1055, 1969.

Skull and brain

Burstein, J., Papile, L., and Burstein, R.: Subependymal germinal matrix and intraventricular hemorrhage in premature infants: diagnosis by CT, Am. J. Roentgenol. **128**:971, 1977.

Dorst, J.P.: Functional craniology: an aid in interpreting roentgenograms of the skull, Rad. Clin. North Am. **2**:347, 1964.

Fiske, C.E., Filly, R.A., and Callen, P.W.: The normal choroid plexus: ultrasonographic appearance of the neonatal head, Radiology **141**:467, 1981.

Grant, E.G., and others: Evolution of porencephalic cysts from intraparenchymal hemorrhage in neonates: sonographic evidence, Am. J. Roentgenol. **138**:467, 1982.

Shinnar, S., and others: Intraventricular hemorrhage in the premature infant: a changing outlook, N. Engl. J. Med. **306**:1464, 1982.

Siegel, M.J., and others: Cranial computed tomography and real-time sonography in full-term neonates and infants, Radiology **149**:111, 1983.

Swischuk, L.E.: The normal newborn skull, Semin. Roentgenol. **9**:101, 1974.

Volpe, J.J.: Neonatal intraventricular hemorrhage, N. Engl. J. Med. **304**:886, 1981.

Zelson, C., Lee, S.J., and Pearl, M.: The incidence of skull fractures underlying cephalhematomas in newborn infants, J. Pediatr. **85**:371, 1974.

Monitoring and treatment

Campbell, R.E.: Roentgenologic features of umbilical vascular catheterization in the newborn, Am. J. Roentgenol. Radium Ther. Nucl. Med. **112**:68, 1971.

Knight, L., Tobin, J., Jr., and L'Heureux, P.: Hydrothorax: a complication of hyperalimentation with radiologic manifestations, Radiology **111**:693, 1974.

Kramer, S.S., and others: Lethal chylothoraces due to superior vena caval thrombosis in infants, Am. J. Roentgenol. **137**:559, 1981.

Kuhns, L.R., and Poznanski, A.K.: Endotracheal tube position in the infant, J. Pediatr. **78**:991, 1971.

Oppenheimer, D.A., Carroll, B.A., and Garth, K.E.: Ultrasonic detection of complications following umbilical arterial catheterization in the neonate, Radiology **145**:667, 1982.

Oppenheimer, D.A., and others: Sonographic localization of neonatal umbilical catheters, Am. J. Roentgenol. **138**:1025, 1982.

Seibert, J.J., and others: Acquired bone dysplasia secondary to catheter-related complications in the neonate, Pediatr. Radiol. **16**:43, 1986.

CHAPTER 14

Anesthesia for labor and delivery

The close cooperation among obstetricians, pediatricians, and anesthesiologists over the past decade has given birth to the field of neonatal-perinatal medicine. Anesthesiologists may be left out of this all-important triad, however, by omission, by error, or even by their possible refusal to care for the special needs of the obstetric patient. This omission is unacceptable in terms of medical ethics and patient safety. Neonatal-perinatal medicine depends on a team concept, with the obstetrician coordinating efforts during a high-risk gestation with colleagues in the fields of neonatal medicine and anesthesiology. The result is protection for the mother and child at delivery through the composite skills of the three team members. With careful consideration, coordination, cooperation, and respect for one another's capabilities, these three provide a continuum of care.

This chapter deals with the specific skills of the anesthesiologist as a team member whose careful and considered management can further the effort to reduce perinatal mortality and morbidity. Both normal and abnormal gestations are discussed.

ANALGESIA FOR NORMAL LABOR AND DELIVERY

Psychologic methods

The three most common techniques used during labor and delivery for pain relief without medication are natural childbirth, psychoprophylaxis, and hypnosis.

The natural childbirth method became popular in the 1930s. It emphasizes the importance of physical training, health, and stamina to develop conditioning skills and embraces the concept of the birth process as a contest between the pregnant woman and the forces of parturition. For many patients this is an effective tool to combat pain and a sense of loss of control. Furthermore, the mother who is conditioned and in optimum physical condition obviously fares better in the labor and delivery process than her unprepared counterpart who is in poor physical shape.

The second technique was popularized in the 1950s by the Russians as the "psychotherapeutic analgesic method." It became widely accepted throughout that country over the next decade and eventually spread to parts of Europe, where it was referred to as "psychoprophylaxis" and "childbirth without pain." Successfully introduced to the United States in the early 1970s, it has been widely accepted. One of the most impressive aspects of the method is the enthusiasm and dedication of the teachers, who have a quieting effect on the mother. The patient is taught to enjoy, not fear, contractions and to view the labor and delivery process as a stimulating, pleasing experience, not a painful one. Finally, she is taught vigorous ventilation exercises to compete physically with the effacement and dilation process.

The last method of nonmedical pain relief is hypnosis. To be effective, this method requires a strong physician-patient relationship, in which the teacher relieves pain by repeating suggestions in a calm, authoritative voice in a quiet, controlled environment. Hypnosis necessitates training by practitioner and client in repeated sessions in the third trimester, during which the patient is motivated to succeed in her birth-without-medication experience. The power of suggestion, as well as belief in her own inner strengths and in her physician, helps to make this technique successful. Many participants develop vigorous zeal and enthusiasm for the method.

Systemic drug methods

In general, systemic drugs used in the first stage of labor should be injected intravenously in small increments to minimize total fetal drug exposure and to adjust the dose more effectively to counteract maternal discomfort as cervical dilation progresses. The intramuscular route may also be used, but larger doses are required to obtain relief comparable to the intravenous method. The most frequently used analgesic drugs are meperidine hydrochloride (Demerol), fentanyl (Sublimaze), and alphaprodine (Nisentil); hydroxyzine hydrochloride (Atarax, Vistaril) or promethazine hydrochloride (Phenergan) is often administered as a tranquilizer. Meperidine has attained its prominence in obstetric analgesia because of its relatively short duration of effect in the mother and relatively low central nervous system penetrance in the fetus and neonate as compared to morphine. Nonetheless, neonatal depression can occur and appears to be related to the amount of unmetabolized meperidine that has been transferred from mother to fetus rather than to the presence of the active metabolite normeperidine. Potential neonatal depression correlates best with the injection-delivery interval. Intervals of less than 1 hour are associated with essentially no negative effects. Neonatal depression occurs most often when meperidine is administered 2 to 3 hours before delivery. Alphaprodine is structurally similar to meperidine with a shorter duration of effect; however, fewer pharmacologic data are available for this drug than for meperidine.

Fentanyl, which has become one of the most popular narcotic drugs used in operating room anesthesiology over the last decade, also has begun to gain some acceptance in obstetric anesthesia. Generally, it is used more as an adjunctive agent with a local anesthetic in the epidural space; recent studies confirm that its use as a solitary agent in the systemic compartment is not adequately impressive. It appears, however, that in the future, use of both the dilute narcotic and possibly even enkephalins administered in the epidural space may prove favorable. Single-agent opiate therapy can provide good analgesia with the possibility of essentially complete pharmacologic reversibility.

Nerve block methods

The *paracervical block* was viewed as an effective first-stage analgesic method, but occasionally it did have untoward effects on the fetus because of fetal local anesthetic toxicity. This was usually the result of an unexpected vascular spill into the fetal compartment, which elicited bradycardia of varying degrees of severity and duration. Bradycardia of an extended duration caused fetal acidosis in utero, for which the fetus often could not compensate. At worst it resulted in intrauterine demise and, at best, the delivery of severely depressed neonate. It became a popular analgesic technique in the 1950s, 1960s, and early 1970s because its simplicity demanded little skill. It was also a highly effective analgesic method that, in most cases, provided complete pain relief at a time when fetal monitoring and an understanding of the cause-and-effect relationship of drug depression was not appreciated. The most popular local anesthetics, administered exclusively by obstetricians, were 1% lidocaine and 1.5% mepivacaine given in 10 ml doses on each side of the cervix. This technique is extremely restricted now because of the potential lethal fetal effect.

The *pudendal block* is another technique the obstetrician mastered because it is similar to the local infiltration block of the perineum. It is important to note that the pudendal nerve block necessitates the careful deposition of local anesthetic in a narrowly circumscribed area of the pudendal nerve where it closely approaches the ischial spines in its course through the pelvis and out the perineum. In skilled hands it produces an impressive perineal block for complete pain relief for the second stage of labor. Most often 10 ml of 2% lidocaine or 10 ml of 0.25% bupivacaine is injected on each side to obtain an adequate block. It is usually administered only by the obstetrician. Although this technique is usually safe, there have been reports of maternal toxic responses and even maternal infection and abscess formation.

The *local infiltration block,* also administered by the obstetrician, is used primarily for the relief of discomfort of episiotomy. It is given late in the phase of perineal dilation, usually just at maximum distension of the perineum. Usually 5 to 10 ml of 0.5% lidocaine is the local anesthetic agent of choice.

Regional methods

In the late 1950s it was identified that babies born of mothers who received regional anesthesia were more active and vigorous at delivery than those delivered with general anesthesia. This is understandable, since general anesthesia at that time meant deep planes of depression with such agents as cyclopropane, ether, and halothane. Today general anesthesia for cesarean section means maternal muscle paralysis with short-acting muscle relaxants and mental obtundation with miniscule amounts of thiopental and a 50% concentration of nitrous oxide. Because the mother is minimally exposed to drugs, the fetus is more active and vigorous. The smaller maternal drug dosage, whether administered via the tissue, epidural, or pulmonary routes, has made the difference.

Subarachnoid block

The subarachnoid block is a technique begun by the obstetrician for terminal second-stage pain relief at a time when anesthesiology did not provide adequate relief. The block is popular for primiparas; when administered in the sitting position in small amounts of tetracaine (0.2 mg to 0.4 mg,) it usually evokes a very low lumbar or even lower sacral block. The sacral block, referred to as a *saddle block,* was popular because of its effectiveness for perineal pain relief and its low incidence of complications. It is difficult to name a more rapid-acting, dependable, or safer technique. If these are the primary determinants, it could in fact be identified as the "ideal" obstetric anesthetic.

The subarachnoid block is also safe and effective for cesarean section delivery if certain hazards are avoided. The following steps are necessary: first, reducing the possibility of hypotension by administration of rapid intravenous hydration just before maternal sympathectomy; second, using maternal displacement of the uterus off the vena cava; third, minimizing the time between onset of the anesthetic and delivery of the fetus; and fourth, monitoring maternal blood pressure repeatedly every 30 seconds for the first 5 minutes to detect a fall in maternal blood pressure early so that immediate and effective countermeasures can be initiated. At present, the technique is performed exclusively by anesthesiologists at most larger centers. The most popular drugs are tetracaine and lidocaine. Although the technique is often deemed simple and safe, it has lethal consequences if attention to detail is not maintained. This includes close, constant attention to the effective level of the anesthetic, alveolar ventilation, and maternal blood pressure.

Lumbar epidural block

The significant pioneer work of Dr. John G. P. Cleland, published in 1933, formed the foundation on which pain relief via the lumbar epidural and caudal epidural blocks began. With only minor modifications, his work still provides the basis of regional pain relief in obstetrics.

Over the years the lumbar epidural method of pain relief for labor and cesarean section has been modified. Today the segmental lumbar epidural block is the most useful and popular technique that provides excellent first- and second-stage pain relief. It also minimizes the complications formerly associated with the larger-volume sympathetic block. An alternative approach is the use of the lumbar epidural block for first stage and the caudal epidural block for the second stage of labor. This difficult technique allows the physician to insert the epidural catheters when the patient is relatively pain free and to administer less medication subsequently, when the patient's discomfort demands pain relief. Even though the effects of epidural block are complex, its effects on the cardiovascular system are much more predictable; the incidence of hypotension is low when compared to that produced by subarachnoid block. Spinal anesthesia predictably produces a greater depression of the heart rate, cardiac output, and mean arterial pressure than does the lumbar epidural block.

Sometimes these regional blocks are not fully effective in relief of pain in the second stage of labor. In such cases, inhalation analgesia with nitrous oxide–oxygen (50% concentration) or subanesthetic concentrations of enflurane or isoflurane can be used to manage an extremely uncomfortable or uncooperative patient. Psychoprophylaxis, with a competent staff dedicated to the technique and a motivated patient, also may be effective in relieving the discomfort of the second stage. The combination of psychoprophylaxis for early labor and the lumbar epidural or the lumbar epidural–caudal epidural technique for later added relief is best for the normal patient.

Inhalation methods

Inhalation analgesia refers to the pain relief for a brief period during the expulsion phase of the second stage of labor. This method has a long history and was used primarily in the 1940s, 1950s, and 1960s for the mother when no regional technique was available. Nurse anesthetists or nurses who could apply a mask to a patient and administer nitrous oxide-oxygen for a brief time during expulsion of the child usually performed this method. Nitrous oxide and oxygen were the preferred inhalation drugs to use together. At one time, however, methoxyflurane became popular as an agent to combine with pure oxygen, although it is no longer used. Before this, cyclopropane and oxygen were used almost exclusively for this type of second-stage analgesia.

A major difference exists between anesthesia with loss of consciousness and analgesia only with full awareness. Analgesia allows patient cooperation and alertness and, because of the small concentrations of drug being administered, offers benefits of pain relief. The technique of inhalation is still popular in dental anesthesia, where nitrous oxide and oxygen in 20% to 40% concentrations are used to ameliorate pain. Primary concerns in use of this technique include careful maintenance of the airway and maintenance of a light plane of analgesia. It can also be used today to supplement inadequate blocks for perineal discomfort during second-stage expulsion. A major concern is ensuring the patient does not enter the second stage, in which unwanted reflexes such as vomiting occur. Although all obstetric patients are asked to refrain from oral intake when they go into labor, personnel in obstetric anesthesia know their first concern is always to prevent vomiting. When they are used properly, inhalation methods can provide an important adjunct for pain relief for the mother and present little or no threat to the fetus.

ANESTHESIA FOR SPECIAL CIRCUMSTANCES

Diabetes mellitus

See also Chapter 3.

Diabetes mellitus is an unique endocrine abnormality that affects fetal size, promotes placental deterioration, and threatens the fetus and neonate with hyperglycemia and hypoglycemia. Anesthesia for the diabetic obstetric patient necessitates close cooperation and coordination between the obstetrician and anesthesiologist. The fetus of diabetic women is at risk because of the loss of an unknown degree of placental reserve. Since oxygen supply to and carbon dioxide removal from the fetus are the primary determinants of fetal safety, these must be protected in the fetus of a diabetic mother, who already has only a margin of placental reserve. Since both oxygen supply and carbon dioxide removal depend on blood supply to the intervillous space, which in turn depends on maternal blood pressure, the latter must be maintained regardless of the analgesic technique chosen. The primary concern or complication secondary to the regional techniques is maternal hypotension and a resultant reduction in regional blood flow to the intervillous space, which can jeopardize the fetus already at risk. No mother wants pain relief at the risk of possible harm to her unborn fetus. The obstetric anesthesiologist must be concerned about the safety of the fetus before pain relief for the mother and satisfactory surgical conditions for the obstetrician.

Analgesia for labor and delivery in diabetes can best be provided by adherence to two important tenets of anesthesia: minimizing the amount of drug exposure to mother and fetus and the threat of extensive sympathetic block. Fortunately, both of these can be satisfied with the use of continuous lumbar epidural infusion with 0.125% bupivacaine. After lumbar epidural catheter placement, an infusion by pump of 0.125% bupivacaine is begun at a rate of 8 to 10 ml/hour. This usually provides excellent pain relief throughout the earlier phase of cervical dilation (4 to 8 cm). Because of intensification of pain and spread of referred pain to the lower lumbar area, a single dose of 3 to 5 ml of 0.5% bupivacaine may be necessary to alleviate pain between 8 to 10 cm of cervical dilation.

Dysmaturity

See also Chapters 7 and 10.

The dysmature fetus is at risk similar to the fetus of a diabetic mother. The organ at risk is again the placenta; in this case, instead of undergoing vascular change that embarrasses gas exchange, the placenta undergoes degenerative change with the same result. The fetus may be at great risk in utero, but does well in extrauterine life. Because of diminished placental perfusion, the anesthesiologist once again must be careful to maintain maximum blood flow to the fetus, who may have essentially no placental reserve. Therefore, any method of analgesia that lowers maternal blood pressure will compromise fetal oxygenation and ventilation. The duration of embarrassment will determine the result. For example, a brief period of hypotension that is quickly diagnosed and successfully treated may not affect the fetus, but a longer period may cause dire consequences.

A secondary concern in dysmaturity is excessive fetal entrapment of respiratory depressant drugs administered to the mother when the fetus is acidotic in utero. The neonatologist must be alerted to this possibility, since a vigorous infant at birth may give a false sense of security only to give way to a subsequent hypotonia, hypotension, and respiratory depression in the nursery, which may go unnoticed. This situation demands close communication and coordination between anesthesiologist, obstetrician, and neonatologist.

Analgesia for labor and delivery is difficult in dysmature infants and may tax the imagination of the obstetric anesthesiologist. A combination of first-stage psychoprophylaxis with a carefully administered segmental epidural block may seem logical; the catheter may be placed early in labor and a small amount of local anesthetic administered only when discomfort occurs later in the cervical dilation process. With 4 to 6 ml of either 0.125% bupivacaine or 1% lidocaine without epinephrine administered in the epidural space, there is really no threat of maternal hypotension. For the second stage of labor, one can use either 15 ml of 2% lidocaine via the epidural catheter, pull the epidural catheter and administer a "saddle block spinal," or administer analgesic concentrations of nitrous oxide in oxygen during the expulsion phase for analgesia. Cesarean section is probably best done under general anesthesia if definite evidence of fetal compromise exists. This obviates any threat of hypotension to the already embarrassed fetus during the induction or delivery process. On the other hand, if the fetus is dysmature but otherwise healthy and not compromised and if the mother insists on being awake for delivery, then one can consider a modified epidural block. The anesthesiologist must carefully describe this process and its risks to the mother and father for their complete understanding and agreement. Such a procedure can be carried out with minimal risk to the fetus, but once again, any risk superimposed on already existent fetal compromise may be too great.

Prematurity

See also Chapter 9.

The premature infant is at an increased risk of central nervous system depression from anesthesia and analgesia. Therefore narcotic analgesics for discomfort in the first stage of labor should be severely restricted. Relief of pain during the first stage of labor can be effected by use of selective regional analgesia while maintaining maternal and fetal homeostasis. Segmental lumbar epidural analgesia is recommended with a minimal amount of a longer-lasting local anesthetic, 8 ml of 0.25% bupivacaine, to reduce maternal and fetal drug accumulation. The technique of lumbar epidural analgesia for first-stage labor and caudal epidural analgesia for second-stage labor may also be used. The use of paracervical block during labor with a premature fetus should be avoided because of the hazard of inadvertently elevated fetal anesthetic drug levels due to fetal injection or even inadvertent intravascular injection. Several alternative forms of analgesia are available for the second stage of labor. A subarachnoid block may be restricted to the sacral area by manipulating the patient's position. A bilateral pudendal block or local infiltration may also be used for restricted perineal analgesia. Psychoprophylaxis may also be an important adjunct to the management of premature labor because of high maternal motivation. The combination of psychoprophylaxis for the early first stage of labor followed by segmental lumbar epidural analgesia alone or with the segmental caudal epidural analgesia may be best for mothers delivering a premature infant.

Toxemia

See also Chapter 4.

Toxemia of pregnancy is also referred to as the syndrome of preeclampsia or eclampsia. The syndrome is manifest by salient hypertension, edema, and proteinuria. For purposes of classification, it is subdivided into mild, moderate, and severe categories. As in diabetes and dysmaturity, the placenta also is the affected target organ because generalized arterial spasm is the primary problem. Once again, special considerations must be made for analgesia and anesthesia, since the use of regional blockade may result in serious sequelae for both mother and fetus. Management of toxemic patients must include a careful evaluation by the anesthesiologist. Special attention should be given to fluid balance, electrolyte stability, and urinary output. This section divides management of anesthesia into two categories: the patient with mild toxemia and the patient with either moderate or severe toxemia.

Patients with mild toxemia have blood pressures in the range of 140 to 160 mm Hg systolic and 90 mm Hg diastolic, a trace amount of proteinuria, and only slight edema. Usually there is no fetal embarrassment before delivery or during the intrapartum period unless precipitated by some event such as hypotension or by uterine stimulation. This patient may obtain relief of discomfort in the first stage of labor through psychoprophylaxis or a mild narcotic analgesic. However, if the mother wants the benefits of regional anesthesia, a segmental lumbar epidural block for the first stage of labor and a sacral block for the second stage should be considered. This technique is preferred in preeclampsia, not only because there is minimal effect on blood pressure after adequate fluid replacement, but also because it can be instituted with minimal agitation to the patient; once given, it also provides stable and controlled blood pressure during contractions. An ineffective block for delivery may also be supplemented with nitrous oxide–oxygen, a spinal block, or even an infiltrative local anesthetic.

Management of moderate or severe toxemia is considered together because fetal compromise often is associated with a blood pressure greater than 160 mm Hg systolic and 110 mm Hg diastolic and more placental dysfunction. The primary problems are hypertension and associated cerebral complications, including hemorrhage; hypotension following regional block because of reduced intravascular volume; and muscle fatigue and a tendency toward extended phases of muscle paralysis following administration of muscle relaxants due to high doses of magnesium sulfate.

In severe toxemia physiologic changes are exaggerated. Regional blockade, in the presence of a restricted intravascular volume, may result in a considerable depression of blood pressure. Profound reductions in maternal systemic pressure may occur when standard epidural or low subarachnoid blocks are given, for example, a large volume (usually 12 to 15 ml) deposition of local anesthetic in the epidural space. The restricted segmental lumbar epidural block has been safely used in patients with toxemia when careful attention is paid to management of intravascular blood volume and the use of small doses of local anesthetics (not greater than 5 ml of drug, with restriction of the analgesic block to the T10 to L2 levels). All patients are kept on their sides to offset the effect of the vena cava syndrome. For the second stage of labor modified caudal analgesia, with only an S2 to S5 block, or a true saddle block may also be the anesthetic technique of choice.

When the obstetrician notifies the anesthesiologist that fetal compromise and a significantly elevated maternal blood pressure are present, there is really little choice except general anesthesia for what usually is an anticipated cesearean section delivery. One maternal complication of concern is marked elevation of the mother's blood pressure under light anesthesia during delivery. Significant pressure elevations may be managed by a potent intravenous vasodepressor. Elevated blood pressure must not be taken lightly, since some patients with eclampsia die from cerebral hemorrhage.

Forceps and vacuum-assisted delivery

Continued critical appraisal of fetal and maternal trauma subsequent to midforceps deliveries has severely restricted the use of this procedure. In midforceps maneuvers, the obstetrician must use an additional space-occupying instrument in a restricted pelvic area. Therefore both profound vaginal tract and perineal analgesia and muscular relaxation are indicated before starting the procedure. Since timing and certain specific requirements for rotation may differ, the obstetrician should determine these factors and, with the anesthesiologist, decide on the most suitable technique and agent for each patient. During the induction of anesthesia, the patient should not be stimulated by forceps application or attempted rotation until the anesthesiologist is ready to proceed. Vigorous suprafundic pressure should be avoided during the expulsion phase.

Regional anesthesia is the preferred method of pain relief, since it provides complete analgesia and relaxation without significant maternal or fetal depression. The subarachnoid block is the ideal choice because of minimal drug dose, rapid onset, and intense muscular relaxation of the entire lumbar and sacral plexus. Lumbar epidural or combined lumbar epidural and caudal analgesia also will provide sensory analgesia and motor relaxation adequate for these procedures by obtunding thoracic segments T10 or T12 and L1 and sacral segments S2, S3, and S4. Pudendal block is not adequate for midforceps rotational maneuvers and, even when combined with light inhalation analgesia, usually will not provide sufficient relaxation to protect the mother and fetus. Similarly, inhalation analgesia with intubation and administration of a muscle relaxant could be used, but this would be highly unusual and only a last resort if a suitable regional method was not effective.

Elective or prophylactic forceps deliveries require minimal analgesia restricted to the perineum and lower portion of the vagina. In addition, relaxation is not always necessary; a cooperative patient may often aid the descent and delivery with moderate Valsalva maneuvers. The duration of required perineal analgesia is short, since no manipulation is necessary and the time of traction is minimal. Local analgesia by infiltration and supplemental nitrous oxide–oxygen inhalation analgesia or pudendal block may be sufficient in a cooperative patient. Saddle block, low caudal epidural, and lumbar epidural analgesia also may be used in low forceps deliveries with good results.

Vacuum extraction may be useful when the fetal position is not easily ascertained or use of a space-occupying instrument in tight pelvic conditions is contraindicated. It has occasionally been associated with reports of scalp lacerations, cephalohematomas, and intracranial hemorrhage. Analgesic requirements for vacuum extraction are not demanding. Some relief of discomfort and adequate vaginal relaxation during the introduction of the examiner's hand and manipulation of the extraction cup are sufficient. If the patient is cooperative and has a sufficiently relaxed vagina, this may be performed without analgesia or an anesthetic. When the mother is not cooperative and the obstetrician has difficulty in placing the extraction cup, a saddle block may be performed to provide adequate vaginal analgesia and relaxation. This denervates only sacral fibers and is compatible with continued uterine contractions and good Valsalva maneuvers when required for descent and rotation of the fetal head. Lumbar epidural, caudal epidural, and pudendal analgesia also suffice to reduce pelvic muscle tension and may be used successfully to aid in ease of application.

Breech delivery

Breech presentations (frank, complete, incomplete, footling) may occur in 3% to 5% of all mothers in labor. The perinatal mortality in breech delivery is significantly greater than that associated with vertex delivery. In many centers all breech presentations, except frank breech, are considered best managed by cesarean section. Frank breech presentation may provide a wedge to the cervix of sufficient diameter to produce cervical dilation and simultaneously protect the fetal umbilical cord from prolapse during dilation, descent, and rotation. In the frank breech presentation during vaginal delivery the obstetrician and anesthesiologist should be prepared for the necessity of immediate inhalation anesthesia and profound uterine relaxation to deliver an entrapped fetal head.

The primary life-threatening situation to the fetus is entrapment of the head after delivery of the smaller-diameter pelvic girdle and shoulders. This is a special threat in a premature infant, whose head is proportionately larger than the shoulder or pelvic girdle. The midpelvis may also present a secondary threat to delivery of the fetal head; the cervix cannot be relaxed and dilated with a suitable uterine relaxant, since its lower portion is primarily connective tissue. Normally 1 hour is needed for each 2 cm of cervical dilation; this process cannot be accelerated even when profound myometrial relaxation results from inhalation anesthesia. Persistent forceful attempts at dilation will only produce maternal trauma, possible rupture of the lower uterine segment, and fetal injury. In contrast, many breech deliveries involve only increased tone of the lower uterine segment, which traps the fetal head, and of the levator ani and coccygeal muscles, which hinder manipulation. The use of the inhalation anesthetic technique for emergency vaginal delivery may be the indicated treatment under these circumstances. The two phases of general anesthesia for emergency vaginal delivery include the preparatory and induction phases:

A. Preparatory
   1. Antacid, 30 ml
   2. Denitrogenation
   3. Glycopyrrolate, 0.2 mg IV
   4. *d*-Tubocurarine chloride, 3 mg IV
B. Induction
   1. Thiopental sodium, 2.t mg/kg IV
   2. Cricoid pressure

3. Succinylcholine chloride, 80 to 100 mg IV
4. Avoidance of positive pressure
5. Endotracheal intubation
6. Halothane, 2% to 3%

A pudendal block may be used during the descent of the breech to the introitus. When decent is adequate, as shown by delivery of the umbilicus to the perineum, induction is started. This gives the anesthesiologist adequate time to place an endotracheal tube and begin administration of 2% halothane with 50% oxygen while the obstetrician is delivering the lower extremities and then the upper extremities and thorax. By this time both lower uterine segment and pelvic relaxation should be adequate for manipulation of the fetal head by either Piper forceps or the Mauriceau maneuver. When halothane is administered and the anesthesiologist increases alveolar ventilation to effect rapid myometrial relaxation, endotracheal intubation and blood pressure monitoring are essential to be prepared for possible hypotension. It cannot be stressed too emphatically that, if an anesthesiologist is called only at the time an obstetrician encounters difficulty with entrapment of the fetal head, it will be almost impossible to anesthetize the mother safely and effectively and provide optimum conditions for a nontraumatic delivery.

Twin gestation

See also Chapter 10.

Internal podalic version and extraction is principally of historic significance. It has been associated with uterine rupture, cervical and perineal laceration, hemorrhage, and puerperal sepsis. A high incidence of maternal death has been associated with the procedure. Nevertheless, under optimum conditions of uterine relaxation and full cervical dilation, internal podalic version and extraction may be useful to a second twin in fetal distress immediately after extraction of the first twin. Maternal and fetal safety depend on an experienced obstetrician working with a competent obstetric anesthesiologist. Unless conditions are ideal, cesarean section delivery is the procedure of choice.

Success with version and extraction depends on adequate uterine relaxation. Before the procedure the patient is prepared for routine general anesthesia. In emergencies some steps may be shortened, such as elimination of the curare and reduction of the preoxygenation period to 15 seconds of hyperventilation. Once the endotracheal tube is inserted, halothane and oxygen are administered in an appropriate concentration and duration to rapidly achieve the uterine relaxation necessary for more complete version and extraction without excessive postpartum atony. This requires close communication and interaction between obstetrician and anesthesiologist during delivery. If at any time the obstetrician believes that manipulation is too difficult, a cesarean section should be performed.

Cesarean section

Ideally, without jeopardizing the fetus and neonate, general anesthesia for cesarean section should permit the mother to be unconscious and analgesic and to have no bad memories of the procedure. The nitrous oxide relaxant technique for cesarean section has gained substantial popularity in the United States because the gas is not explosive, the procedure reduces the need for more potent inhalation anesthetics that cause myometrial and neonatal depression, and it should involve no risk of maternal hypotension. Thiobarbiturates, muscle relaxants, nitrous oxide, and oxygen are typically used during the interval between induction and delivery. As noted, this approach is unlikely to produce hypotension; in skilled hands, it should produce ideal fetal and neonatal conditions even in cases of known maternal, fetal, or uteroplacental compromise. The technique consists of:

1. Antacid, 30 ml
2. Glycopyrrolate, 0.2 mg IV
3. *d*-Tubocurarine, 3 mg
4. Thiopental sodium, 2.5 mg/kg IV
5. No positive airway pressure
6. Cricoid pressure
7. Succinylcholine, 80 to 100 mg IV for intubation
8. Nitrous oxide and oxygen, 50% mixture

The antacid regimen before induction is intended to elevate the gastric pH. The *d*-tubocurarine prevents fasciculations from succinylcholine chloride and subsequent increased intragastric pressure, which may release gastric air and acid into the esophagus. Misdirected positive pressure in the esophagus could worsen this problem. Cricoid pressure against the vertebral body of the upper cervical spine effectively closes the esophagus and reduces the incidence of gastric fluid escape into the upper airway. For maternal amnesia and fetal protection, 2.5 mg/kg of thiopental sodium is best. If fetal distress occurs, increased maternal ventilation with oxygen is indicated despite the possibility of greater maternal recall. All deliveries should be done with left uterine displacement by a wedge under the mother's right hip. A maternal inspired oxygen concentration of 50% is adequate for the inhalation technique during cesarean section; fetal oxygenation does not significantly improve when values for maternal arterial oxygen pressure rise above 300 mm Hg.

John S. McDonald

BIBLIOGRAPHY

Abboud, T.K., and others: Comparison of the effects of general and regional anesthesia for cesarean section on neonatal neurologic and adaptive capacity scores, Anesth. Analg. **64**:996, 1985.

Arozenius, S., and others: A comparison of the analgesic effects of methoxyfluranenitrous oxide and nitrous oxide alone during labour related to the Eysenck personality inventory test, Acta Obstet. Gynecol. Scand. **59**:203, 1980.

Bailey, P.W., and Howard, F.A.: Forum: epidural analgesia and forceps delivery: laying a bogey, Anaesthesia **38**:282, 1983.

Baraka, A., Noueihid, R., and Hajj, S.: Intrathecal injection of morphine for obstetric analgesia, Anesthesiology **54**:136, 1981.

Beck, N.C., and Siegel, L.J.: Preparation for childbirth and contemporary research on pain, anxiety, and stress reduction: a review and critique, Psychosom. Med. **42**:429, 1980.

Belfrage, P., and Floberg, J.: Obstetrical paracervical block with chloroprocaine or bupivacaine: a comparison, Acta Obstet. Gynecol. Scand. **62**:245, 1983.

Brownridge, P.: Spinal anaesthesia revisited: an evaluation of subarachnoid block in obstetrics, Anaesth. Intensive Care **12**:334, 1984.

Chandler, C.J., and Davidson, B.A.: The influence of lumbar epidural analgesia in labor on mode of delivery, Int. J. Gynaecol. Obstet. **20**:353, 1982.

Concepcion, M., and Covino, B.G.: Rational use of local anaesthetics, Drugs **27**:256, 1984.

Confino, E., and others: Extradural analgesia in the management of singleton breech delivery, Br. J. Anaesth. **57**:892, 1985.

Danforth, D.N.: Cesarean section, JAMA **253**:811, 1985.

Dobrovits, H., and others: Theory and practice in the care of diabetic pregnancy—a timely concept, Wien. Wochenschr. **95**:728, 1983.

Dondi, A., and others: The mother-child relationship and the pregnancy experience in mothers delivered under autohypnosis, Pediatrics **35**:921, 1983.

Gibbs, C.E.: Report of Committee on Maternal and Child Health: a maternal death associated with toxemia and an anesthetic, Tex. Med. **79**:50, 1983.

Greis, J.B., Bieniarz, J., and Scommegna, A.: Comparison of maternal and fetal effects of vacuum extraction with forceps or cesarean deliveries, Obstet. Gynecol. **57**:571, 1981.

Hecht, C.: An answer to childbirth educator burn-out, **9**:35, 1982.

Hollingsworth, D.R., Jones, O.W., and Resnik, R.: Expanded care in obstetrics for the 1980s: preconception and early postconception counseling, Am. J. Obstet. Gynecol. **149**:811, 1984.

Howie, P.W., and Patel, N.B.: Obstetric management of preterm labour, Clin. Obstet. Gynaecol. **11**:373, 1984.

Jimenez, S.L.: Education for the childbearing year: comprehensive application of psychoprophylaxis, JOGN Nurs. **9**:97, 1980.

Johnson, J.M.: Teaching self-hypnosis in pregnancy, labor, and delivery, Matern. Child Nurs. J. **5**:98, 1980.

King, J.C., and Sherline, D.M.: Paracervical and pudendal block, Clin. Obstet. Gynecol. **24**:587, 1981.

Kofinas, G.D., Kofinas, A.D., and Tavakoli, F.M.: Maternal and fetal beta-endorphin release in response to the stress of labor and delivery, Am. J. Obstet. Gynecol. **152**:56, 1985.

Krasznai, P., and others: Patterns of frequency of use of peridural analgesia in surgical deliveries, Orv. Hetil. **125**:3107, 1984.

Langhoff-Roos, J., and Lindmark, G.: Analgesia and maternal side effects of pudendal block at delivery: a comparison of three local anesthetics, Acta Obstet. Gynecol. Scand. **64**:269, 1985.

Maresh, M., Choong, K., and Beard, R.: Delayed pushing with lumbar epidural analgesia in labour, Br. J. Obstet. Gynaecol. **90**:623, 1983.

Marx, G.F., Luykx, W.M., and Cohen, S.: Fetal-neonatal status following caesarean section for fetal distress, Br. J. Anaesth. **56**:10,009, 1984.

McCaffery, M.: Problems with IM meperidine (Demerol), PRN Forum **3**:1, 1984.

Merkow, A.J., and others: The neonatal neurobehavioral effects of bupivacaine, mepivacaine, and 2-chloroprocaine used for pudendal block, Anesthesiology **52**:309, 1980.

Moore, T.R., and others: Evaluation of the use of continuous lumbar epidural anesthesia for hypertensive pregnant women in labor, Am. J. Obstet. Gynecol. **152**:404, 1985.

Moquin, T.F.: The anesthetic management of uncomplicated labor and delivery using the segmental technique of continuous lumbar epidural analgesia, AANA J. **50**:372, 1982.

Okasha, A.S., Motaweh, M.M., and Bali, A.: Maternal and fetal effects of continuous lumbar epidural analgesia for labour and delivery in pre-eclamptic patients, Middle East J. Anaesthesiol. **7**:203, 1983.

Philipson, E.H., and others: Intrapartum paracervical block anesthesia with 2-chloroprocaine, Am. J. Obstet. Gynecol. **146**:16, 1983.

Philips, K.C., and Thomas, T.A.: Second stage of labour with or without extradural analgesia, Anaesthesia **38**:972, 1983.

Puolakka, J., and others: Maternal and fetal effects of low-dosage bupivacaine paracervical block, J. Perinat. Med. **12**:75, 1984.

Rafferty, T.D., and Berkowitz, R.L.: Hemodynamics in patients with severe toxemia during labor and delivery, Am. J. Obstet. Gynecol. **138**:263, 1980.

Richardson, D.K., Gabbe, S.G., and Wind, Y.: Decision analysis of high-risk patient referral, Obstet. Gynecol. **63**:496, 1984.

Rudick, V., and others: Epidural analgesia for planned vaginal delivery following previous cesarean section, Obstet. Gynecol. **64**:621, 1984.

Schnider, S.M., and others: Maternal catecholamines decrease during labor after lumbar epidural anesthesia, Am. J. Obstet. Gynecol. **147**:13, 1983.

Sheerin, S.P.: Kiellands forceps delivery, Br. Med. J. (Clin. Res.) **288**:769, 1984.

Shime, J., and others: Prolonged pregnancy: surveillance of the fetus and the neonate and the course of labor and delivery, Am. J. Obstet. Gynecol. **148**:547, 1984.

Swanstrom, S., and Bratteby, L.E.: Metabolic effects of obstetric regional analgesia and of asphyxia in the newborn infant during the first two hours after birth, Acta Paediatr. Scand. **70**:801, 1981.

Widstrom, A.M., Wahlberg, V., and Matthiesen, A.S.: Increased incidence of tissue rupture in pudendal block in delivery? Jordemodern **96**:24, 1983.

Worthington, E.L., Jr., Martin, G.A., and Shumate, M.: Which prepared-childbirth coping strategies are effective? JOGN Nurs. **11**:45, 1982.

Yurth, D.A.: Placental transfer of local anesthetics, Clin. Perinatol. **9**:13, 1982.

CHAPTER 15

Anesthesia for premature infants

During the past 15 years, survival of premature infants has increased markedly. Associated with this increase has been a rise in the number of complications (patent ductus arteriosus, retrolental fibroplasia, necrotizing enterocolitis) that require surgery and anesthesia, often while the patient is still very premature and still very ill. Lack of understanding on the part of anesthesiologists and neonatologists of the effects of anesthesia on preterm neonates has led to heated discussions (and occasionally something resembling warfare) between these two groups of physicians. This chapter provides information that will enable both groups to improve their care of premature neonates who require surgery.

Anesthesia should be administered by an experienced pediatric anesthesiologist when possible, because those who only occasionally anesthetize infants cannot be fully familiar with the myriad of problems that can and do occur in these patients. However, this ideal cannot always be achieved. Occasionally, for one reason or another, it is necessary for a nonpediatric anesthesiologist to anesthetize premature neonates. When this occurs, it is useful for the anesthesiologist to obtain consultation from a pediatric anesthesiologist, if possible, before proceeding with anesthesia.

Anesthetizing premature neonates is more difficult than anesthetizing older patients because prematures often have both multisystem disease and immature organs; they respond differently to anesthetics than older children, and small changes in arterial pressure, blood volume, and ventilation may cause greater changes in the condition of prematures than in older patients. To reduce the number of problems that occur, the anesthesiologist must gather as much information as possible about the patient before inducing anesthesia. This information comes from the chart, from discussions with the nurses and neonatologists caring for the patient, and from a thorough examination of the patient. It is neither appropriate nor sensible for the anesthesiologist to alter the plan of care for a patient without discussing the proposed changes with the neonatologists. It is likewise not sensible for the neonatologists to attempt to force a plan of anesthesia on the anesthesiologist that is inconsistent with the surgery. For example, it is inappropriate to insist on tight fluid restriction during anesthesia in patients who will have large third space losses during surgery. Doing so will make the patient hypotensive, hypoxic, and acidotic, and may cause him or her to die if this plan is followed. Only by discussing problems preoperatively can we prevent significant problems for the patient.

PREOPERATIVE PREPARATION

History

The preoperative evaluation of preterm neonates, like that of any other patient, is directed toward developing an understanding of the patient's previous history, physical examination, and hospital course. A review of the nursing notes and a discussion with the nurse caring for the patient are obligatory. Nurses who stand at the bedside all day and give the minute-to-minute care consequently know the quirks of each particular patient, which physicians may not know. For example, the nurse may know that briefly disconnecting the endotracheal tube from oxygen or stopping ventilation for a few seconds causes hypoxemia and cyanosis, or that the patient's perfusion decreases when the blood glucose level falls below 40 mg/dl or when the calcium is below 7.0 mg/dl. The nurse also may report that the patient becomes hypoxic when turned on one side or the other, which is very important information if the patient must be turned on that side and the other lung must be collapsed to perform surgery.

The birth history is extremely important when planning anesthesia. If the patient was asphyxiated at birth, the effects of asphyxia may remain. Cerebral vascular autoregulation may still be absent. Allowing sudden increases in arterial pressure may cause intracranial hemorrhage. Myocardial function may still be depressed, and gut blood flow may still be reduced. The hemoglobin concentration and blood volume may be low. Clotting abnormalities may be present. Since some anesthetics affect cerebral vascular autoregulation and all of them affect myocardial function and peripheral vascular tone, the anesthesiologist needs as much information as possible to enable the choice of an anesthetic that least affects the abnormalities in the particular patient.

SYSTEMS REVIEW AND EXAMINATION

Head, eyes, ears, nose, and throat

Congenital anomalies of the face and mouth are common, either as part of a syndrome or as a single entity. A cleft palate often is missed in infants who require tracheal intubation and mechanical ventilation from birth. This poses no problems for the anesthesiologist unless tracheal reintubation is necessary. Then a cleft palate may create problems by making it difficult to move the tongue out of the line of vision. Each time the tongue is moved to the left, it tends to ooze over the top of the laryngoscope blade and obstruct the laryngoscopist's view of the larynx. The small mouth of premature neonates allows their relatively large tongue to obstruct breathing, especially if pressure is applied to the submental triangle while a mask is held on the face. Even slight pressure in this area can cause fatal obstruction of the airway.

A nasogastric tube will obstruct half of the upper airway of most neonates because they are predominantly nose breathers. This obstruction increases respiratory work and in some cases causes apnea or hypoventilation, especially if the anesthetic used inhibits the muscles of respiration. Anesthetized premature neonates, like lambs, may not increase their ventilation to compensate for the increased work. Consequently, their arterial carbon dioxide pressure ($PaCO_2$) rises.

Evidence should be sought for the presence of retrolental fibroplasia, glaucoma, or cataracts. Giving atropine to patients with glaucoma can increase their intraocular pressure to dangerous levels.

Pulmonary system

Inhaled anesthetics are commonly used to anesthetize premature neonates because the drug concentration can be adjusted easily and because the anesthetic can be turned off and withdrawn quickly if a problem arises. However, inhaled anesthetics can have undesirable effects on both ventilation and perfusion. They reduce functional residual capacity (FRC), which delays the onset of and awaking from anesthesia. Inhaled anesthetics reduce the FRC of adults by 15% to 20%; they reduce the FRC of preterm neonates by 40% or more unless ventilation is controlled and a positive end-expiratory pressure (PEEP) of 3 or more cm H_2O is maintained during anesthesia. Usually ventilation is accomplished with an anesthesia bag and enough pressure to expand the chest during inspiration. A pressure gauge and underwater pressure pop-off valve make it easier for the anesthesiologist to avoid excessive airway pressures. Neonatal ventilators are usually ineffective in the operating room because they cannot compensate for the effects of sponges, retractors, or the surgeon's hands on lung compliance. Nor can they be adapted easily to administer inhaled anesthetics safely.

The anesthesiologist should obtain the answers to several questions about the patient's ventilation before inducing anesthesia. How much ventilation was required to maintain normal blood gases and pH in this particular patient? What were the last blood gases and pH? How labile have the blood gases and pH been? Do the blood gases change when the patient is turned on one side or the other? Does the patient have pneumonia or pulmonary hemorrhage? How is the endotracheal tube fixed in place? Is it secure? What was the nature of the tracheal secretions in the past 24 hours? How often does the trachea have to be suctioned? All of this information is important for the anesthesiologist and should be acquired during the preoperative visit. The fraction of inspired oxygen (FiO_2) will probably have to be higher to maintain a normal arterial oxygen pressure (PaO_2) during surgery than it was in the nursery. Therefore the neonatologist and anesthesiologist should decide on the appropriate range of oxygenation for each patient, and the anesthesiologist should adjust ventilation and FIO_2 to keep the PaO_2 in this range during surgery. Commonly, anesthesiologists use air as the carrier gas and add enough oxygen to keep oxygen saturation between 85% and 92% or the transcutaneous oxygen pressure ($tcPO_2$) between 50 and 70 mm Hg. The latter is affected by anesthetics; oxygen saturation is not. Therefore oxygen saturation is generally preferred over $tcPO_2$. Oxygen saturation is affected, however, by pH and temperature. Transcutaneous PCO_2 is usually unaffected by hypotension, hypothermia, or peripheral perfusion (Chapter 28, part three).

Cardiovascular system

Preterm neonates frequently have cardiovascular problems but infrequently have congenital heart disease. Because they have less muscle in their pulmonary arteries and ductus arteriosus, blood is more likely to shunt left to right through a ductus arteriosus or ventricular septal defect (if one exists) than it is in term neonates. Left-to-right shunting occurs earlier in preterm neonates (3 to 5 days) than it does in term neonates (7 to 14 days). Consequently, many premature neonates have pulmonary edema at the time of surgery or can easily be put into pulmonary edema by reducing pulmonary vascular resistance (hyperventilation) or by administering too much fluid. The excessive pulmonary blood flow caused by left-to-right shunting produces pulmonary edema, congestive heart failure, reduced lung compliance, and delayed induction of and awakening from anesthesia (Chapter 29). Most anesthetics reduce myocardial function, which can worsen preexisting heart failure.

Since mild congestive heart failure is less commonly heralded in premature neonates by tachycardia, as it is in older patients, mechanically ventilated premature infants can be in congestive heart failure without it being obvious, especially to those who have not cared for the patient continuously. Evidence of congestive failure (pulmonary edema and myocardial enlargement on x-ray film, abnormal chamber and vessel size on echocardiogram, and enlarged liver) should be discussed with the anesthesiologist during the preoperative visit. People not used to listening to the heart of premature neonates may miss third heart sounds and quiet murmurs, especially when the heart rate is rapid or there is a lot of environmental noise (ventilators, monitors, voices). If these cardiac abnormalities exist, they should be pointed out to the anesthesiologist. Eyelid edema and abnormal weight gain are important clues to the presence of congestive heart failure in prematures.

It is often difficult for those who infrequently look at chest radiographs of premature neonates to determine whether the radiograph is indicative of congestive heart failure or the respiratory distress syndrome. The increased central vascular and coarse lung markings of congestive failure may be overlooked.

Abdomen

Information about the gastrointestinal tract is also important for the anesthesiologist. Preoperative vomiting increases the likelihood of aspirating gastric contents into the lung during the induction of anesthesia if anesthesia is induced by mask. Ascites may interfere with breathing and delay the onset of anesthesia. On occasion it is necessary to remove some of the ascitic fluid preoperatively. Ascites also may reduce blood return to the heart. Sudden release of the abdominal pressure during surgery may cause hypotension or, in some cases, sudden right heart failure.

The presence of necrotizing enterocolitis is especially dangerous. If the bowel is distended with gas or fluid, gastric contents may be aspirated during the induction of anesthesia. The volume of gas in the bowel wall (pneumatosis intestinalis) or gut lumen will increase if nitrous oxide is administered, because nitrous oxide may cause rapid expansion of gas pockets. Nitrous oxide diffuses into pockets of gas about 30 times faster than nitrogen diffuses out of them. The resultant increase in pressure may cause bowel ischemia. Abdominal wall edema is usually a sign of peritonitis.

An imperforate anus may go undetected for days in sick premature neonates if not carefully looked for. Anal patency must always be ensured before patients go to the operating room.

Central nervous system

It is difficult for someone other than a neonatologist or pediatrician to detect subtle abnormalities of the central nervous system of premature neonates. What appears to be normal tone to a neonatologist may look like flaccidity to someone else. The false belief that the patient has central nervous system damage may subtly affect the care the patient receives. Meningomyeloceles, especially small ones, may be missed in sick preterm neonates unless their back is examined carefully. The anesthesiologist needs to know whether the patient has had seizures or an intracranial hemorrhage so that an anesthetic is used that does not increase cerebral blood flow or oxygen consumption or lower the seizure threshold (hyperventilation). If the patient has had an intracranial hemorrhage, the surgeon and anesthesiologist probably will want to avoid administering heparin.

Laboratory findings

Most sick preterm neonates have had many laboratory tests performed. The anesthesiologist must be aware of all abnormalities before beginning the anesthetic because they may affect the choice of anesthetic or cause delay of surgery until the abnormalities are corrected. For instance, induction of anesthesia in patients with abnormal serum electrolyte levels may lead to cardiac arrest.

Hematology. The hemoglobin concentration should exceed 10 g/dl in sick premature neonates to ensure adequate oxygen-carrying capacity and to provide some leeway for blood loss. If hemoglobin concentration is low, the patient should be transfused with packed cells before anesthesia is induced, if possible. If the patient has been transfused extensively, adult, not fetal, hemoglobin predominates. This alters the shape of the oxygen dissociation curve and changes the level of oxygenation acceptable for Sa_{O_2} and Pa_{O_2}. With adult hemoglobin, blood having a Pa_{O_2} of 50 mm Hg is 82% saturated with oxygen at normal pH and body temperature. With fetal hemoglobin, the same Pa_{O_2} causes blood to be 92% saturated with oxygen. At a given Pa_{O_2}, adult hemoglobin gives up more oxygen to the tissues than fetal hemoglobin (Chapter 28, part two).

Electrolytes. The electrolyte levels in the blood of preterm neonates vary more than those of older patients because prematures are more easily affected by small changes in fluid and electrolyte intake and by evaporation. A rise in serum sodium may occur with excessive sodium administration, renal failure, or dehydration. Fluid administration during surgery will vary depending on which pathology is responsible for the hypernatremia.

Hyperkalemia and hypokalemia are especially common in patients treated with potent diuretics. Both hyperkalemia and hypokalemia can cause dysrhythmias and cardiac arrest when certain anesthetics (e.g., halothane) are used. Hypocalcemia also is common in premature neonates, and it can cause severe hypotension and reduced cardiac output in anesthetized neonates. Hyperventilation further reduces the concentration of ionized calcium, exacerbating the problem of hypocalcemia.

Glucose. Sick premature neonates tolerate glucose administration less well during anesthesia than adults. Prematures often become hyperglycemic during surgery despite receiving the same quantity of glucose they received preoperatively. This is probably related to the 40% to 50% reduction in oxygen consumption that occurs with anesthesia. Thus it may be necessary to reduce the intake of glucose during anesthesia and surgery. How much it should be reduced can be determined only by measuring serum glucose levels intermittently during surgery, usually with Dextrostix. Glucose intake should be adjusted to maintain a normal blood glucose concentration (40 to 90 mg/dl). Hyperglycemia will almost certainly occur when glucose-containing solutions are used to replace third space fluid losses during surgery. Therefore the anesthesiologist should administer enough glucose to maintain normoglycemia, usually 3 to 5 mg/kg/minute, and use plain Ringer's lactate for any additional fluid requirements. Ringer's lactate most closely approximates the electrolytes in third space fluid losses. Premature neonates can easily excrete this fluid when their extracellular fluid volume is repleted. *Third space fluid losses should never be repleted with intravenous alimentation fluids*.

Clotting status. Neonates who suffer intrapartum asphyxia often have a bleeding diathesis. Factors V, VII, VIII, and the concentration of platelets are low when this occurs. Neonates who are resuscitated quickly have normal clotting factors and platelets in 3 to 4 days, whereas those who are resuscitated more slowly may require 7 to 10 days for these values to return to normal. Although most asphyxiated babies do not bleed abnormally when in the newborn intensive care unit (NICU), they commonly bleed during surgery if these abnormalities are still present. Vitamin K should be given preoperatively to patients who have not eaten or who have received antibiotics during the previous 72 hours and have not received vitamin D during that time. Fresh frozen plasma and platelets or fresh whole blood may be needed to correct clotting abnormalities if immediate surgery is required. If the patient is in congestive heart failure, an exchange transfusion may be required to correct the clotting abnormalities preoperatively. Diffuse intravascular coagulation should be corrected by giving fresh frozen plasma and platelets preoperatively.

Preoperative plan

When all the data have been collected, an anesthetic plan can be formulated and the anesthetic equipment needed can be obtained. It is useful to have a second person in the operating room to help with the myriad of tasks that must be performed while anesthetizing a premature neonate. It is difficult for one person to ventilate the lungs, give fluid and blood, watch the surgical field and monitors, and keep the anesthesia record at the same time. Before the patient enters the room, it should be warmed to 35° to 37° C. A servo-controlled infrared heater should be placed over the operating table (if used) and turned on, and a water-circulated heating blanket should be placed on the table and turned to 37° C. Placing a thermometer between the heating blanket and the sheet that covers the blanket permits continuous monitoring of the blanket temperature. Rather than use the operating table, we use specially modified neonatal intensive care unit (NICU) beds that serve both as the patient's NICU bed and an operating table. The patients' monitors accompany them from the NICU. By using this bed and the patient's monitors, we avoid having to move the patient from one bed to another and having to disconnect and reconnect monitors. We also dislodge fewer intravascular lines and shorten the time out of the NICU. If the patient must be moved to the operating table, monitors should be set up and calibrated *before* the patient comes to the operating room. Intravenous solutions should be set up if they differ from those being infused in the nursery. When possible, all fluids should be delivered through an infusion pump. Drip chambers should contain no more than 1 hour's worth of fluid to prevent fluid overload from occurring if the intravenous line inadvertently runs wide open. If the intravenous tubing is placed between the heating blanket and the mattress of the operating table (patient's bed), the fluids will be near body temperature when they enter the vein.

Transporting premature neonates to and from the operating room can be dangerous. The anesthesiologist should always accompany the patient and should monitor heart rate, arterial blood pressure, and oxygen saturation during transport if possible. Infusion pumps should continue to infuse fluids, especially vasopressors. If ventilation was controlled in the NICU, ventilation should be controlled during transport, usually with a Jackson-Reese-type device. During transport, the anesthesiologist should give only enough oxygen to keep the oxygen saturation normal. Thus the transport bed *must* have both air and oxygen and a means of blending them. Keeping the patient warm during transport is often difficult. Table 15-1 shows the changes in body temperature of preterm neonates being transported to and from the operating room for ligation of a patent ductus arteriosus. Note that the patients have lost nearly a degree of body

Table 15-1. Changes in body temperature during transportation of preterm infants from the neonatal intensive care unit to the operating room*

Location	Temperature (degrees Celsius)	
	Without Saran Wrap	Covered with Saran Wrap
Nursery	36.4 ± 0.5	36.6 ± 0.4
Upon arrival in operating room	35.7 ± 0.7	36.5 ± 0.6
Before leaving operating room	36.4 ± 1.0	36.5 ± 0.9
Upon arrival in nursery	35.9 ± 1.9	36.5 ± 0.8

*All infants were covered with warm blankets. Those covered with Saran Wrap in addition had less change in temperature.

temperature during this short period (less than 10 minutes). This loss can be reduced if the patient's head is covered with a cloth cap, the entire body is covered with Saran Wrap, and a warm blanket is placed over the top of the Saran Wrap. Arterial or venous lines must be visible at all times because they can become disconnected during transport. The elevator should be waiting for the patient, not the other way around. As soon as the patient enters the operating room, he or she should be placed under a radiant warmer and kept there until prepared and draped for surgery.

Induction of anesthesia

Premature neonates require anesthesia, albeit less than is required by neonates born at term. Failure to provide adequate anesthesia for premature neonates is not only immoral, but it increases the potential for intracranial hemorrhage, especially if cerebral vascular autoregulation is abnormal. Providing adequate anesthesia attenuates or prevents these changes. Deep anesthesia, on the other hand, reduces arterial blood pressure and cerebral blood flow more in neonates than it does in adults and can cause death or central nervous system damage. Thus the anesthesiologist usually uses that amount of anesthetic that provides loss of consciousness and prevents increases in heart rate and arterial blood pressure with surgery. Heart rate is usually relatively constant during surgery and anesthesia if the level of anesthesia is adequate, because even light levels of anesthesia almost totally obliterate the baroresponses. Even 70% nitrous oxide obliterates most of the baroresponse in term animals.

If the patient's trachea is not intubated before surgery, it must be intubated before surgery begins. Except in special circumstances (e.g., full stomach, moribund state), anesthesia should be induced before the trachea is intubated. Once the patient has lost consciousness, it is usually necessary to control ventilation.

Anesthesia is usually induced with an inhaled anesthetic (isoflurane or halothane). An alternative method of inducing anesthesia is to administer 1 to 2 mg/kg of thiopental sodium (Pentothal) as a bolus or 20 to 30 μg/kg of fentanyl (Sublimaze) over 1 to 2 minutes and to control ventilation. Once the trachea is intubated, a low dose of inhaled anesthetic can be added to the inspired gas mixture. Usually muscle relaxants are not needed to intubate the trachea of premature neonates. The likelihood of an endobronchial intubation can be reduced by having an assistant place a finger in the suprasternal notch and tell the person doing the intubation when the tip of the tube strikes the finger. When this occurs, the tube should be fixed in place and taped securely to the patient's face. Although this method of determining tube position reduces the incidence of inadvertent endobronchial intubation, it does not totally eliminate it. Therefore it may on occasion be necessary to obtain a chest radiograph to determine the position of the endotracheal tube tip. If muscle relaxants are required, the patient can be given pancuronium (Pavulon 0.1 mg/kg), curare (0.3 mg/kg), or metacurine (Metubine 0.2 mg/kg). Muscle paralysis should *not* be used as a substitute for anesthesia, except in those rare instances when patients are moribund and any anesthetic will cause cardiac arrest (see the following discussion).

Monitoring during anesthesia

See also Chapter 24, part three.

Monitoring frequently makes the difference between survival and nonsurvival of premature neonates. Therefore these patients deserve at least as much monitoring as sick adults. The type of monitoring depends on the procedure being done and how sick the patient was preoperatively. As a minimum, monitoring should include a precordial or esophageal stethoscope, electrocardiogram, arterial blood pressure cuff, temperature thermistor, and pulse oximeter.

Arterial blood pressure can be measured with a Doppler blood pressure device in most instances. The cuff bladder must be placed directly over the brachial artery and should not cover the olecranon process because repeated pressure in this area may damage the ulnar nerve. Placing a Doppler transducer over the radial artery makes it easier to measure arterial pressure and allows constant monitoring of blood flow in the artery. The latter allows early detection of changes in peripheral blood flow, which often occur before the arterial blood pressure falls. In neonates whose condition is unstable, or in those who have the potential for significant blood loss or fluid shifts between intravascular and extravascular spaces, the arterial blood pressure should be monitored continuously. This can be done through an umbilical artery catheter in very young neonates or through a radial, ulnar, dorsalis pedis, or posterior tibial arterial catheter in older patients. Arterial pressure is an important indicator of hypovolemia. It also gives an early warning of anesthetic overdose, especially in sick neonates. The ECG, on the other hand, is often not affected by hypotension. It continues to be normal even during severe hypotension.

Measurement of skin surface oxygen tension ($tcPo_2$) is a useful indicator of reduced peripheral blood flow; $tcPo_2$ also is affected by halothane, nitrous oxide, and some other inhaled anesthetics because they are oxidized in the electrode. This causes falsely high $tcPo_2$ readings and can be eliminated or reduced by choosing the appropriate membrane for the electrode and by polishing the electrode frequently. Oxygen saturation and $tcPo_2$ are similar to arterial values, even when the patient is hypothermic, acidotic, or hypotensive.

Pulse oximetery is now the standard method of monitoring oxygenation during anesthesia and surgery. It is not affected by arterial blood pressure or anesthetics. However, oxygen saturation is affected by the type of hemoglobin, the amount of 2,3-diphosphoglycerate in red blood cells, and by body temperature and pH. All of these variables affect the position of the oxygen dissociation curve and must be taken into account when deciding whether the oxygen saturation is normal, too high, or too low. If the pH is normal, oxygen saturation can be maintained between 85% and 92% in premature neonates who have fetal hemoglobin. This level of oxygenation is adequate for the patient's needs, but it is not high enough to cause retrolental fibroplasia in most instances. If the patient has adult hemoglobin, the saturation should be kept between 90% and 95%. Measuring oxygen saturation does not eliminate the need to intermittently measure blood gases and pH.

There is no effective way to monitor pulmonary function during anesthesia except by measuring blood gases. Lung compliance and resistance change during anesthesia and surgery, which is why the anesthesiologist should ventilate the lungs of neonates with an anesthesia bag and not with a mechanical ventilator. The machine may deliver the same tidal volume with each breath, but, because of changes in the lung compliance and resistance and changes in the compression volume of the breathing circuit and humidifier, varying amounts of gas will be delivered to the lungs.

Body temperature should be measured in all patients, especially premature infants, who have a large surface to volume ratio that allows them to lose large quantities of heat to the environment. Heat loss is greater with thoracic or abdominal surgery because the surface area is markedly increased. Rectal temperatures should seldom be measured in premature neonates, even in the operating room, because it is easy to perforate the sigmoid colon with a thermistor or thermometer, especially if the patient's position must be changed during surgery. It is much easier and safer to measure axillary or esophageal temperatures. If the surgical incision does not include the right upper quadrant of the abdomen, the skin temperature above the liver also can be measured. The difference between the skin and esophageal or axillary temperature should not exceed 1° C.

MAINTENANCE OF ANESTHESIA

There are few data on the anesthetic requirements of preterm neonates. However, experience suggests that they require less anesthesia than healthy neonates born at term, who in turn require less anesthesia than 1- to 6-month-old infants. The anesthetic requirement of term lambs just before birth is about one third of the requirement 12 hours after birth. Lerman and others recently showed that the mean alveolar concentration for isoflurane (Forane) is lower in preterm neonates than it is in neonates born at term. The halothane requirement of preterm neonates undergoing patent ductus arteriosus ligation is considerably lower than that of healthy, term neonates. It also appears that preterm neonates require less fentanyl and other fixed agents than older patients. The reasons for these differences are unknown.

There are still some people who believe that neonates, especially preterm neonates, do not feel pain and therefore do not require anesthesia. That is clearly not the case. They feel and respond to pain the same as adults. In addition, inadequate anesthesia during surgery increases acidosis and volume depletion and may increase the likelihood of an intracranial hemorrhage. Even if these things were not true, it would still be morally unacceptable to operate on most premature neonates without anesthetizing them. There are *rare* instances when patients are so ill that any amount of anesthetic may kill them. However, once they have been resuscitated and their blood volume and arterial blood pressure have stabilized at a normal level, it is usually possible to carefully add some anesthetic. In such cases, muscle relaxants may be required to permit surgery.

Inhaled anesthetics are more likely to cause hypotension in premature than in mature neonates, probably because their peripheral vessels are less responsive to catecholamines and because they have more myocardial depression and less baroresponse than older patients. Since preterm neonates depend primarily on a rise in heart rate to increase cardiac output, loss of baroresponse can have detrimental effects. Table 15-2 shows the heart rates and arterial pressures of preterm neonates anesthetized with halothane for ligation of their patent ductus arteriosus. Note the lack of heart rate variation with blood pressure changes.

Table 15-2. The relationship between heart rate and systolic blood pressure in preterm infants anesthetized with halothane who were undergoing patent ductus arteriosus ligation

Condition	Heart rate (beats/min)	Systolic pressure (mm Hg)
Preinduction	146 ± 20	62 ± 16
Preductal ligation	143 ± 17	48 ± 16
Postductal ligation	145 ± 16	66 ± 15

Fentanyl is commonly used in place of inhaled anesthetics to try to avoid the cardiovascular effects of inhaled anesthetics. Twenty to 30 μg of fentanyl per kilogram of body weight prevents the tachycardia and hypertension associated with light or absent anesthesia in most preterm neonates, suggesting that this amount of drug is sufficient to anesthetize these patients. Hypotension is uncommon with fentanyl anesthesia in normovolemic preterm neonates. However, hypovolemic neonates still become hypotensive with this drug. The disadvantage of fentanyl, like other intravenous drugs, is that it cannot be removed from the system if adverse effects occur. Inhaled anesthetics, on the other hand, can usually be removed quickly. Whatever anesthetic is given, it should be one that the anesthesiologist is comfortable with. This is not the time to test a new agent.

For surgery on the lower half of the body, spinal or caudal anesthesia may be appropriate, especially if the patient had apneic spells in the neonatal period and is still less than 50 weeks' gestation. Even if a spinal or caudal anesthetic is used, it is almost always necessary to control ventilation throughout the procedure. Care must be taken to prevent surgeons from resting their hands or surgical instruments on the patient's abdomen, because this will reduce ventilation. The level of anesthesia is usually at or below the T10 dermatome. If the patient normally uses abdominal muscles to exhale (as occurs when there is gas trapping within the lung), a spinal or caudal anesthetic may seriously interfere with breathing. The primary use of spinal and caudal anesthesia is to try to prevent postoperative apnea in infants who were premature. However, this does not guarantee that the patient will not develop apnea postoperatively. Therefore patients who receive spinal anesthesia must be observed and monitored in the hospital for 24 hours postoperatively; they should not be discharged the day of surgery. If they have not developed apnea by 24 hours, it is unlikely that they will.

Muscle relaxants often are used to prevent movement during surgery, especially in neonates who are very sick and will tolerate only small amounts of anesthetic. Muscle relaxants also are given when narcotics are used as the primary anesthetic. Adding nitrous oxide to the inspired gases significantly increases the depth of anesthesia, even though nitrous oxide is an incomplete anesthetic in and of itself (70% nitrous oxide provides only about 50% of a minimum alveolar concentration in term neonates and probably 80% in preterm neonates). Although nitrous oxide alone is inadequate in most cases, its addition to narcotic or low-dose potent inhaled anesthetics provides adequate anesthesia. Nitrous oxide, however, like all anesthetics, depresses the cardiovascular system of preterm neonates, that is, it decreases the arterial blood pressure and inhibits the baroresponses, and in some cases causes cardiac arrest.

As already stated, ventilation must be controlled when preterm neonates are anesthetized, because anesthetics reduce the functional residual capacity and interfere with the muscles of respiration. Ventilation is usually controlled with a Jackson-Reese device, which is easy to use, valveless, can deliver up to 100% oxygen, and permits instantaneous compensation for changes in compliance and resistance of the lungs and airways. It is also easy to apply and maintain a positive end-expiratory pressure with this device.

Appropriate fluid replacement is crucial during anesthesia and surgery. Since the blood volume of preterm neonates is 85 to 100 ml/kg of body weight, 8 to 10 ml of blood loss is equal to 10% of the blood volume in a 1 kg neonate. Blood loss should be replaced as it occurs if it is anticipated that blood loss will reduce the hematocrit to 30% or less.

Many premature neonates are hypovolemic when they come to the operating room because they were dehydrated preoperatively to prevent or treat congestive heart failure. Their blood volume must be increased (usually with at least 10 ml/kg of Ringer's lactate) before anesthesia is induced, or the patient will become hypotensive and can develop cardiac arrest with the induction of anesthesia. It is dangerous to replace the fluid deficit or intraoperative fluid losses with anything other than a balanced salt solution. Doing so may cause hyponatremia, seizures, and death.

It is difficult to accurately determine blood loss during surgery. Weighing the used sponges is the most accurate method available. A 1 mg increase in dry sponge weight equals 1 ml of blood loss. Blood suctioned from the wound should be collected in a small calibrated bottle. Blood loss into the sponges and suction is relatively easy to quantitate, but blood loss into the drapes and tissues is difficult to estimate. Thus it is common to automatically add 25% to 30% to the measured blood loss. One must use the best estimate of blood loss plus arterial and central venous pressure measurements, hematocrit, and frequent examinations of the patient to determine the adequacy of blood and fluid replacement. If the hematocrit

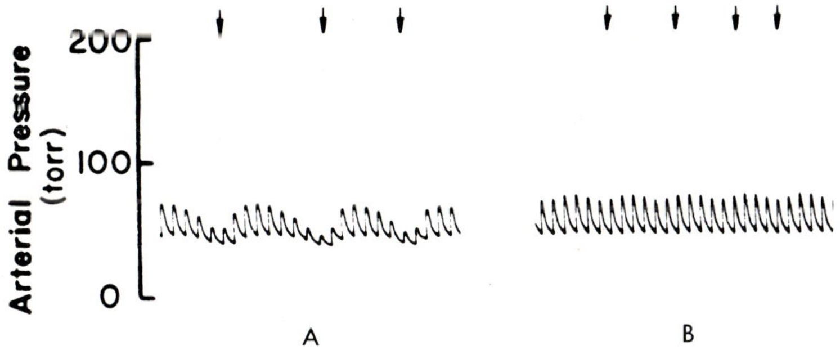

Fig. 15-1. The effects of positive pressure ventilation on the arterial pressure tracing before **(A)** and after **(B)** administering 15 ml/kg of whole blood to a hypovolemic infant. The arrows mark inspiration. Note the marked fall in pressure **(A)** when the patient was hypovolemic. The fall in arterial pressure with each breath was considerably less after the blood transfusion **(B).**

is low preoperatively, blood loss should be replaced with packed red blood cells. However, the hematocrit should not be raised above 55%, or sudden extracellular fluid loss may raise the hematocrit to levels that can reduce organ blood flow.

The amount of extracellular fluid loss during surgery depends on the amount of surgically induced tissue trauma and cannot be arbitrarily defined. Abdominal and thoracic surgery is more traumatic than extremity surgery and requires replacement with at least 10 to 15 ml/kg/hour of Ringer's lactate in addition to the 0.3 to 0.5 g/kg/hour of glucose (see previous discussion).

The adequacy of fluid and blood replacement can be determined by measuring arterial pressure, central venous pressure, and urine output. Arterial blood pressure is a good indicator of intravascular volume in preterm neonates. If the mean arterial pressure is more than two standard deviations below normal for that age group or if there is a greater than 5 mm Hg change in systolic pressure with each inspiration, the neonate is probably hypovolemic (Fig. 15-1). Infusing fluids returns the pressure to normal and eliminates all but a small variation in pressure with each inspiration. Second, a central venous pressure (measured from percutaneously inserted subclavian or internal jugular catheters) of less than 3 cm H_2O is indicative of hypovolemia. Third, an adequate urine output (>0.7 ml/kg/hour) is indicative of adequate intravascular volume unless the urine glucose concentration exceeds 2+. The urine specific gravity is usually under 1.005 in well-hydrated preterm neonates. A specific gravity of more than 1.009 generally indicates volume depletion and will usually be associated with hypotension when anesthesia is induced. A urinary catheter is required to measure urine output during surgery. Fourth, a fontanel that is below the inner table of the skull also indicates volume depletion.

Recovery from anesthesia

Emergence from anesthesia can be just as dangerous as the induction of anesthesia. There is usually pressure to remove the patient from the operating room and to proceed to the next case. This pressure must be resisted. Before the patient leaves the operating room, the NICU nurses must be informed that the patient is returning from surgery. Confusion results if the patient arrives in the NICU while the nurse is at lunch. It is better to wait in the operating room where the situation is controllable than to stand in the nursery or hall waiting for the nurse to return.

The patient should be ventilated on the way to the nursery. Surgery does not necessarily ensure immediate improvement. On return to the NICU the decision can be made as to whether the endotracheal tube should be removed immediately, which is rare. Once the NICU staff understands what occurred during anesthesia and surgery, care of the patient can be turned over to them.

George A. Gregory

BIBLIOGRAPHY

Systems review and examination

Head, eyes, ears, nose, and throat

Hansen, T.N., and Tooley, W.H.: Skin surface carbon dioxide tensions in sick infants, Pediatrics **64**:942, 1979.

Payne, J.P., and Severinghaus, J.W.: Pulse oximetry, Berlin, 1986, Springer-Verlag.

Robinson, S.L., and others: Halothane anesthesia reduces pulmonary function in the newborn lamb, Anesthesiology **62**:578, 1985.

Pulmonary system and cardiovascular system

Levin, D.L., and others: Congenital heart disease in low birth weight infants, Circulation **52**:500, 1975.

Stevenson, J.G.: Fluid administration in the association of patent ductus arteriosus in premature infants by inhibition of prostaglandin synthesis, N. Engl. J. Med. **295**:530, 1976.

Laboratory findings

Glucose

Gregory, G.A.: Monitoring during anesthesia. In Pediatric anesthesia, New York, 1983, Churchill-Livingstone.

Robinson, S., and Gregory, G.A.: Circulatory effects of anesthesia in the developing sheep. I. Halothane, Anesthesiology **53**:S330, 1980.

Clotting status

Hartman, J.R., and Howell, D.A.: Disorder of blood coagulation during the first week of life, Am. J. Dis. Child. **90**:594, 1966.

Hemmingway, W.E.: The bleeding newborn, Semin. Hematol. **12**:175, 1975.

Preoperative plan

Bain, J.A., and Sparrel, W.E.: A streamlined anaesthetic system, Can. Anaesth. Soc. J. **19**:426, 1972.

Inkster, J.S.: The T-piece technique in anesthesia: an investigation into the inspired gas concentrations, Br. J. Anaesth. **28**:512, 1956.

Induction of anesthesia

Bednarek, F.J., and Kuhns, L.R.: Endotracheal tube placement in infants determined by suprasternal palpation: a new technique, Pediatrics **56**:224, 1975.

Cameron, C.B., and others: The cardiovascular and metabolic effects of halothane in normoxic and hypoxic newborn lambs, Anesthesiology **62**:732, 1985.

Duncan, P., Gregory, G.A., and Wade, J.: The effect of nitrous oxide on the baroreceptor response of newborn and adult rabbits, Can. Anaesth. Soc. J. **28**:339, 1981.

Gregory, G.A.: The baroresponses of preterm infants during halothane anesthesia, Can. Anaesth. Soc. J. **29**:105, 1982.

Gregory, G.A., and others: Fetal anesthetic requirement (MAC) for halothane, Anesth. Analg. (Cleveland) **62**:9, 1983.

Lou, H.C., Lassen, N.A., and Friis-Hansen, B.: Impaired autoregulation of cerebral blood flow in the distressed newborn infant, Lancet **1**:1215, 1979.

Lou, H.C., Lassen, N.A., and Friis-Hansen, B.: Is arterial hypertension crucial for the development of cerebral hemorrhage in premature infants. Lancet, **1**:1215, 1979.

Robinson, S.R., and Gregory, G.A.: Fentanyl-air-oxygen anesthesia for ligation of patent ductus arteriosus in preterm infants, Anesth. Analg. (Cleveland) **60**:504, 1981.

Wear, R., Robinson, S., and Gregory, G.A.: Effect of halothane on the baroresponses of adult and baby rabbits, Anesthesiology **56**:188, 1982.

Monitoring during anesthesia

Gregory, G.A.: The baroresponses of preterm infants during halothane anesthesia, Can. Anaesth. Soc. J. **29**:105, 1982.

Gregory, G.A.: Transcutaneous oxygen measurements, Clin. Crit. Care. Med. **4**:74, 1982.

Hill, G.E., and Machin, R.H.: Doppler determined blood pressure recordings: the effects of varying cuff size in children, Can. Anaesth. Soc. J. **23**:323, 1976.

Peabody, J.L., and others: The Huch transcutaneous Po_2 electrode in sick infants, Pediatr. Res. **10**:775, 1976.

Tremper, K.K., Waxman, K., and Shoemaker, W.C.: Effect of hypoxia and shock on transcutaneous Po_2 values in dogs, Crit. Care. Med. **7**:526, 1979.

Wilkinson, A.R., and others: In vivo oxygen dissociation curves in transfused and untransfused newborns with cardiopulmonary disease, Am. Rev. Respir. Dis. **122**:629, 1980.

Maintenance of anesthesia

Abajian, J.C., and others: Spinal anesthesia for surgery in the high-risk infant, Anesth. Analg. **63**:359, 1984.

Cameron, C.B., Robinson, S., and Gregory, G.A.: The minimum anesthetic concentration of isoflurane in children, Anesth. Analg. **63**:418, 1984.

Duncan, P., Gregory, G.A., and Wade, J.: The effect of nitrous oxide on the baroreceptor response of newborn and adult rabbits, Can. Anaesth. Soc. J. **28**:339, 1981.

Gregory, G.A.: The baroresponse of preterm infants during halothane anesthesia, Can. Anaesth. Soc. J. **29**:105, 1982.

Gregory, G.A., and Steward, D.J.: Life-threatening perioperative apnea in the ex-"premie," Anesthesiology **59**:495, 1983.

Gregory, G.A., and others: Fetal anesthetic requirement (MAC) for halothane, Anesth. Analg. **62**:9, 1983.

LeDez, K.M., and Lerman, J.: Minimum alveolar concentration (MAC) of isoflurane in premature infants, Anesthesiology **65**:A453, 1986.

Lerman, J., and others: Anesthetic requirements for halothane in young children 0-1 months and 1-6 months of age, Anesthesiology **83**:421, 1983.

Liu, L.M.P., and others: Life threatening apnea in infants recovering from anesthesia, Anesthesiology **59**:506, 1983.

Robinson, S., and Gregory, G.A.: Circulatory effects of anesthesia in developing sheep. I. Enflurane, Anesthesiology **53**:S331, 1980.

Robinson, S.R., and Gregory, G.A.: Fentanyl-air-oxygen anesthesia for ligation of patent ductus arteriosus in preterm infants, Anesth. Analg. **60**:504, 1981.

Robinson, S., and Gregory, G.A.: Urine specific gravity as a predictor of hypotensive response to anesthesia in newborn infants, Manuscript submitted for publication, 1986.

Robinson, S.L., and others: Halothane anesthesia reduces pulmonary function in the newborn lamb, Anesthesiology **62**:578, 1985.

Rudolph, A.M.R.: Congenital diseases of the heart, Chicago, 1974, Year Book Medical Publishers.

Versmold, H.T., and others: Aortic blood pressure during the first twelve hours of life in infants with birth weights 610 to 4,220 grams, Pediatrics **67**:607, 1981.

CHAPTER 16

Genetic disease and chromosomal abnormalities

Genetic disease and congenital malformations cause approximately 10% of deaths during the first 28 days of life and have been noted as incidental findings at autopsy in more than 20% of infants dying from other causes and in 33% of stillbirths. Children with one or more congenital anomalies make up approximately 25% of pediatric admissions to university hospitals. The National Foundation–March of Dimes of New York estimates that genetic errors afflict more than 15 million Americans with mental retardation, diabetes, complete or partial blindness, impaired hearing, defects in specific organ systems, and congenital bone, muscle, or joint disease.

Much of the neonatal morbidity and mortality of genetic disease is the result of major malformations, that is, structural defects with potentially clinically significant consequences. The incidence of major anomalies varies according to definition and ascertainment methods but is estimated to occur in from 1% to 7% of all live births (Chapter 17). Minor malformations are detected much more frequently. In a survey of 5,000 consecutive deliveries Marden noted minor malformations in over 10% of newborns (Table 16-1). The clinical significance of minor defects lies in their frequent association with more serious anomalies. When two minor abnormalities are present, an infant's chance of having a major anomaly rises to 90%. Half of all malformations are not recognized at birth, becoming apparent as the child grows and develops.

Table 16-1. Common minor malformations in newborns (frequency greater than 1:1,000)

Minor malformation	Percentage of newborns
Craniofacial	
Borderline micrognathia	0.32
Eye	
Inner epicanthal folds	0.42
Ear	
Lack of helical fold	3.52
Posteriorly rotated pinna	0.25
Preauricular and/or auricular skin tags	0.23
Small pinna	0.14
Auricular sinus	0.12
Skin	
Capillary hemangioma other than on face or posterior aspect of neck	1.06
Pigmented nevi	0.49
Mongoloid spots in white infants	0.21
Hand	
Simian creases	2.74
Bridged upper palmar creases	1.04
Bilateral combinations of above	0.51
Other unusual crease patterns	0.28
Clinodactyly of fifth finger	0.99
Foot	
Partial syndactyly of second and third toes	0.016
Total	12.34

Data from Marden, P.M., Smith, D.W., and McDonald, M.J.: J. Pediatr. **64:**357, 1964. Courtesy Thaddeus Kurczynski, M.D.

The causes of birth defects or genetic disorders are most easily considered in terms of chromosomal abnormalities: single gene disorders with or without a known biochemical defect, multifactorial defects, environmental disorders, or those of unknown cause. Of 317 serious malformations identified among 18,355 neonates at Boston Hospital for Women, 9% were secondary to recognized chromosomal aberrations, 21% were caused by single mutant genes with mendelian inheritance, and 40% were of multifactorial origin. The remaining malformations were unclassified and probably caused in part by environmental agents. For many of the malformations encountered during the neonatal period no cause will be immediately apparent.

EVALUATION OF THE NEONATE WITH MULTIPLE MALFORMATIONS

See also Chapter 17.

An organized plan for evaluation of each neonate with multiple malformations should be developed at the time the infant is initially examined and should include a detailed pedigree and pregnancy history, physical examination, laboratory evaluation of the affected infant and parents if indicated, determination of the genetic mechanism and risk, and counseling and psychologic support for the family.

The family pedigree and pregnancy history are important sources of information in separating genetic disorders from nongenetic disease. The age, sex, and past and present health of parents, siblings, and other closely related family members should be determined. Parents may not mention stillbirths or spontaneous abortions unless specifically questioned about these events. It is also important to determine if there is consanguinity, since this increases the likelihood that an infant's disorder is caused by an autosomal recessive gene. Offspring of first-cousin marriages will have identical genes at one sixteenth of their loci. Parent-child and brother-sister matings result in children who have identical genes at 25% of their loci. Offspring of these marriages may be homozygous for a deleterious gene and therefore manifest a debilitating genetic disorder. Consanguineous marriages have the greatest effect on the incidence of recessive conditions that have a low frequency in the population. For example, if the frequency of a recessive gene in the population is 0.2, then the expected ratio of affected individuals among children of first-cousin marriages to the number of affected individuals in the general population will be 1.25:1. However, if the frequency of the recessive gene is 0.002, then this ratio will increase to 32.25:1.

The ethnic background of the infant's family and the geographic area from which they originate may be important information. Many genetic disorders occur with increased frequency among certain ethnic populations. For example, Tay-Sachs disease is noted once in every 3,600 births among Ashkenazi Jews and only once in 360,000 births in the general population. Similarly, tyrosinemia is especially common among French Canadians in the Lac St. Jean–Chicoutimi region of Quebec and extremely rare elsewhere in the world.

A history of maternal disease, notably diabetes is associated with an increased frequency of malformations (Chapter 3) and should be specifically sought. Intrauterine growth retardation often is associated with congenital malformations. The relationship between birth weight and gestational age and the incidence of congenital malformations have been studied by Van Den Berg and Yerushalmy. These investigators have demonstrated that the severest anomalies are found in term newborns with intrauterine growth retardation, whereas the highest incidence of both minor anomalies and congenital malformations has been noted in preterm SGA infants (27%). This frequency is more than four times the incidence of anomalies seen in appropriate for gestational age preterm infants. Term infants with intrauterine growth retardation have a 9% incidence of malformations.

Polyhydramnios frequently is observed in mothers delivering infants with malformations (Chapter 6). The excessive amniotic fluid in cases with malformations often is attributed to decreased fetal swallowing; however, other factors may be important in the fluid accumulation. Malformations associated with a high frequency of polyhydramnios include Down's syndrome, trisomy 18, esophageal atresia, obstruction of the gastrointestinal tract proximal to the ileum, intrathoracic cysts, and central nervous system anomalies. Approximately 20% of infants with a history of polyhydramnios will have congenital anomalies. Thus an excess of amniotic fluid should alert the physician to search for gastrointestinal anomalies if there are no other apparent major malformations.

A detailed description of drug exposures and illnesses (especially viral syndromes) during the pregnancy should be obtained in a manner that precludes potential reinforcement of maternal guilt. Most women will recall having used several medications and having a viral syndrome at some time during pregnancy. The vast majority of illnesses will involve the upper respiratory or gastrointestinal tract and resolve spontaneously without affecting the fetus. Only rubella virus and cytomegalovirus have strong proven associations with structural malformations. It is important that a causal relationship between malformations and either drug exposure or maternal viral illnesses not be made or suggested in the process of eliciting this history. Although retrospective epidemiologic studies at times have suggested an association of an increased frequency of birth defects with many commonly used drugs (e.g., aspirin), the number of proven human teratogens is relatively small. The drug history is taken to reveal the few known teratogenic agents and to identify new teratogens. It should be clearly emphasized to both parents that the maternal drug history is most likely to be unrelated to the congenital malformations of the infant (Chapter 19).

During physical examination of the infant with multiple malformations particular attention should be directed to describing and categorizing the anomalies, examining the infant's eyes, and evaluating the patterns of ridged skin (dermatoglyphics) (Chapter 17). Every infant with multiple malformations should have the eyes examined by an experienced ophthalmologist. Numerous syndromes, including those secondary to chromosomal aberrations, have eye findings that are readily detectable. With some abnormalities (e.g., glaucoma or chorioretinitis) the findings are so characteristic that they may suggest specific diagnoses. The evaluation of dermatoglyphics on the palms, fingers, and soles also should be performed as part of the physical examination of these infants (Chapter 17). Characteristic dermatoglyphics have been described in a number of disorders and are particularly helpful in diagnosing chromosomal syndromes.

Evaluation of the infant with multiple malformations or suspected genetic disease often includes roentgenographic studies (bone films, computed axial tomography, and intravenous pyelography), ultrasonography, cytogenetic studies, and metabolic screening or testing to diagnose inborn errors of metabolism. An orderly sequence of diagnostic testing should be based on the differential diagnosis suggested by the history and findings on physical examination. Photographs and a skeletal survey may be useful in monitoring changes in appearance or progression of roentgenographic findings suggestive of certain diagnoses.

Counseling the parents

See also Chapter 17.

It should be remembered that formal genetic counseling is only one step in a long process of informing a family about their child's illness. Before delivery most parents expect their children to be normal. During the initial meeting with the physician, an appraisal of the severity of the infant's problems may be overwhelming. Although many parents will accept the information and respond appropriately, some will deny that the illness is serious. In spite of the information transmitted, they may selectively remember the positive aspects of the conversation. To help counteract this denial, it is important that both parents be given the same information and, when possible, that both parents be present at all meetings. There is often a tendency for the father to want to protect the mother from the anguish that he is experiencing. When both parents continually deny the severity of the illness, it may be useful to suggest that other close family members or clergy be brought into the counseling session.

Couples may be so overwhelmed by the extent of their child's illness that they will not visit the intensive care nursery or communicate with anyone in the hospital. They may only request notification of the infant's death. This refusal to make an emotional commitment may be an attempt to protect themselves from further emotional suffering or at times reflect their inability to accept the concept of caring for an infant with a congenital defect. This approach may compound their guilt if the infant dies or may result in psychologic abandonment of a child with nonfatal disease (occasionally an infant with only a cosmetic problem). All families should be strongly encouraged to become involved with the decisions concerning the care of their infants. The stimulus for continuing involvement should come from physicians, nurses, and social service personnel.

At the time of the first meeting it is inadvisable to give the parents a list of all possible diagnoses and the outcome for each disorder. If too much information is communicated, the family may be overwhelmed and confused. The extent of the illness should be described in realistic terms and be reiterated and expanded at subsequent meetings. Any decision regarding withdrawal of intensive care should be made with the family. In doing so, the parents should not be made to feel that they are responsible for letting their child die. When a child with multiple malformations dies, autopsy permission should be sought. Even when this is denied, specific arrangements must be made with the family to continue the counseling. Details of counseling for specific genetic problems are discussed after the relevant sections in this chapter.

CHROMOSOMAL ABNORMALITIES

Chromosomal abnormalities occur in approximately 1 in every 200 newborns, in 5% to 10% of perinatal deaths, and in as many as 50% of early spontaneous abortions. These disorders may be classified as numeric abnormalities of either the autosomes or sex chromosomes and structural chromosomal abnormalities that may be balanced or unbalanced. Clinically it is the autosomal trisomies and unbalanced structural chromosomal abnormalities that most often result in major developmental defects apparent during the neonatal period. Additional autosome material (e.g., trisomy) is somewhat better tolerated than deficiency of an autosome. Nevertheless, the majority of autosomal abnormalities, either duplication or deficiency, that occur in human conceptions are lost by early abortion. The amount of material that is duplicated or deficient, the particular genes within these segments, and perhaps other factors (e.g., maternal factors) influence the likelihood of live birth. Abnormalities of the sex chromosomes and balanced structural rearrangements have their greatest impact on reproductive function. The former generally are associated with gonadal dysgenesis, and the latter may result in reproductive wastage from conception of pregnancies with chromosome imbalance secondary to the parental chromosome rearrangement.

Numeric chromosomal abnormalities (aneuploidy) most often arise by *nondisjunction* (uneven distribution of chromatids or chromosomes in meiosis or mitosis) (Fig. 16-1). Nondisjunction during meiosis will result in gametes and consequently conceptions with an extra (tri-

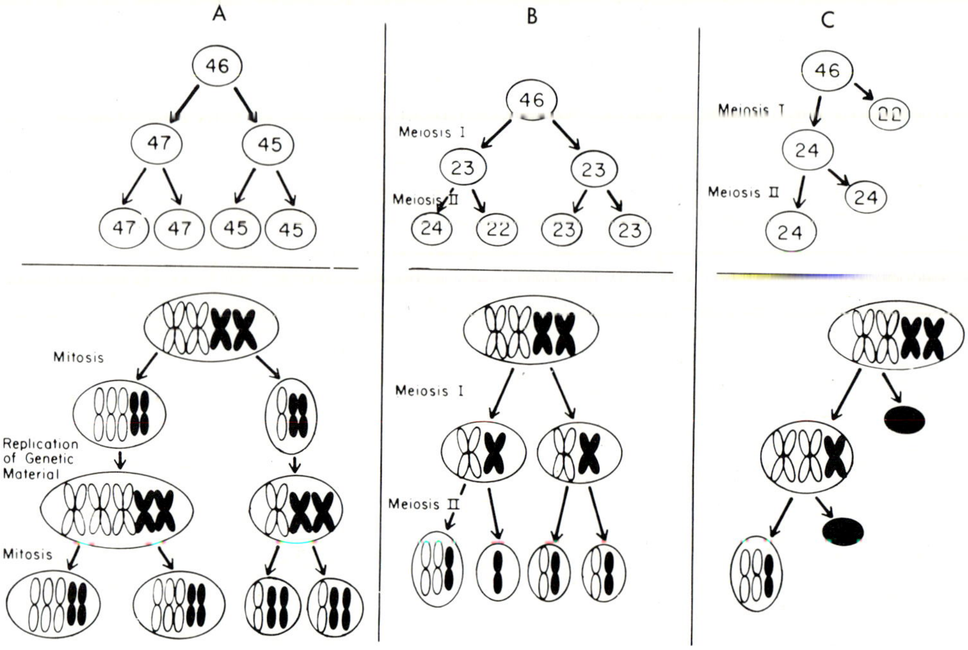

Fig. 16-1. A, Nondisjunction in mitosis demonstrating development of mosaicism with one cell line having 45 chromosomes and the other cell line having 47 chromosomes. **B,** Nondisjunction in male meiosis II resulting in spermatozoa having 22, 23, and 24 chromosomes. **C,** Nondisjunction in female meiosis I resulting in ovum with 24 chromosomes. Blackened circles represent the first and second polar bodies.

somy) or missing (monosomy) chromosome. Conceptions with autosomal monosomy resulting from nondisjunction are presumably lost by abortion, before recognition of pregnancy. On the other hand, approximately 40% of the chromosomal abnormalities found in recognized early abortuses are autosomal trisomies. Nondisjunction occurring after normal gametogenesis and fertilization will result in a fetus or newborn having two or more cell lines that have differing chromosomal constitutions (mosaicism) (Fig. 16-1, A). Mosaicism is relatively more frequent in individuals with sex chromosome aneuploidy, but it also occurs with autosomal abnormalities.

Anaphase lag, a mechanism resulting in loss of a chromosome, occurs when homologous chromosomes fail to pair or segregate correctly on the spindle during cell division. The loss of one member of the chromosome pair during anaphase by this mechanism results in a monosomy and is believed to be the mechanism that accounts for a large proportion of Turner's syndrome (45,X) conceptions. X chromosome monosomy constitutes 20% of the chromosomal abnormalities in spontaneous abortion. Based on the low frequency of this abnormality in liveborn infants, it is apparent that the vast majority of Turner's syndrome conceptions are lost during early pregnancy. Anaphase lag during mitotic division following conception may give rise to mosaicism.

The autosomal trisomies (trisomy 21, 18, and 13) account for the majority of numeric chromosomal abnormalities that are diagnosed during the neonatal period. It has long been considered that nondisjunction in meiosis resulting in trisomies occurs most often during oogenesis. This is supported by the well-established association of Down's syndrome births and advancing maternal age. The identification of normal variants using banding methods, especially Q-banding (quinacrine fluorescence), permits determination of the parental origin of trisomies in a proportion of families. Such testing in informative matings indicates that the paternal origin of Down's syndrome (20% to 30% of cases) is much more frequent than previously estimated. Studies associating nondisjunction with paternal age have shown conflicting results but suggest that there may be an effect, especially after the age of 55 years. The frequency of Down's syndrome at specific paternal ages has not been defined for clinical counseling as it has for maternal age but probably does not reach the same level of clinical significance.

Causes of nondisjunction in humans, other than the association with advanced maternal age, have not been established. Familial clustering of numeric chromosomal abnormalities in isolated cases and the occurrence of children with double aneuploidies (e.g., 48,XXY, +21) suggests that there may be a genetic influence to nondisjunction in some families or individuals. Association of numeric chromosomal abnormalities with autoimmune thyroid disease, previous radiation exposure, or certain otherwise normal chromosomal variants has been suggested but not well substantiated. Because of the high frequency of spontaneous abortion and the large proportion of early abortuses who are chromosomally abnormal, studies to determine genetic or environmental factors that may cause nondisjunction must necessarily be approached through surveillance of early pregnancy wastage.

Chromosomal constitutions in which there are multiples of the haploid number ($n = 23$) of chromosomes other than diploid ($2n = 46$) are known as polyploidy (for example, triploidy, $3n = 69$, tetraploidy, $4n = 92$). Polyploidy may arise by a number of theoretic mechanisms, such as failure of segregation of chromosomes in meiosis, fertilization of an ovum by two sperm (dispermy), and failure of division and cleavage after fertilization. Triploidy and tetraploidy account for approximately 20% to 25% of the chromosomal aberrations observed in early abortuses. Of these two abnormalities, only triploidy occurs very rarely in late stillborns or liveborn infants.

Structural chromosomal abnormalities result from breakage and reunion of chromosomes. These are considered balanced if all the genetic material is conserved (e.g., balanced translocations or inversions). Unequal crossing over within a rearrangement of abnormal segregation of members of pairs involved in a translocation during gametogenesis may result in an unbalanced chromosome constitution of the gamete and conception.

After a single break and loss of the chromosome fragment without a centromere (acentric fragment), the subsequent cell division will result in deletion (Fig. 16-2, *A*). This is most commonly exemplified by the cri du chat syndrome caused by deletion of the short arm of chromosome 5(5p–). Two or more breaks within the same chromosome with rearrangement of material and reunion result in more complex structural abnormalities, such as ring chromosomes or inversions (Fig. 16-2, *B* and *C*). To form a ring chromosome, terminal segments of both the long arm and the short arm of the chromosome are lost as acentric fragments (Fig. 16-2, *C*). Inversion of material within one arm of a chromosome is kown as a *paracentric inversion*. Inversions involving the centromere and the adjacent segments of each arm of the chromosome are termed *pericentric inversions*. Balanced inversions are observed quite frequently as incidental findings. For example, pericentric inversion of chromosome 9 has been observed to occur in 1% of some populations studied with seemingly no clinical consequence. To pair with an inverted homologue during meiosis, the normal chromosome must form a loop. An odd number of cross-

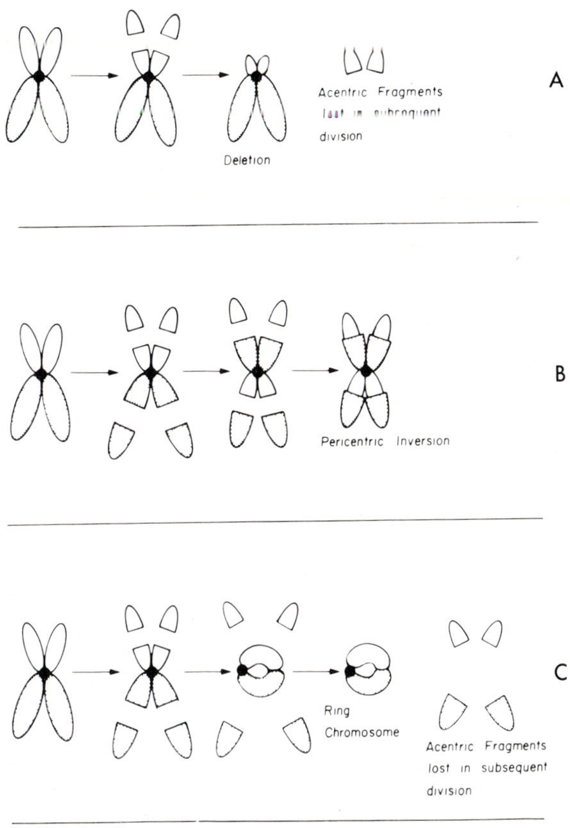

Fig. 16-2. A, Single break in the short arm of a metaphase chromosome resulting in deletion of short-arm material. **B,** Breaks in both the short arm and long arm of metaphase chromosome. **C,** Union of short arm and long arm segments adjacent to centromere results in formation of ring chromosomes.

overs with the inversion loop will result in a derivative chromosome having duplication and deficiency of the terminal segments of the chromosome. In this way balanced carriers of an inversion may produce unbalanced gametes, which result in children with a chromosomal abnormality.

Abnormal separation of the centromere during cell division with separation of the replicated arms of the chromosomes, rather than separation of the chromatids, results in a structurally abnormal chromosome known as an *isochromosome* (Fig. 16-3). When examined during the metaphase of subsequent divisions, these derivative chromosomes appear as mirror images of the short arms or long arms of the original chromosome, the net affect being duplication of one set of arms and deficiency of the other. When observed clinically, isochromosomes most often involve the X chromosome and only very rarely an autosome or the Y chromosome.

Translocations result when there is breakage and exchange of material between two different chromosome

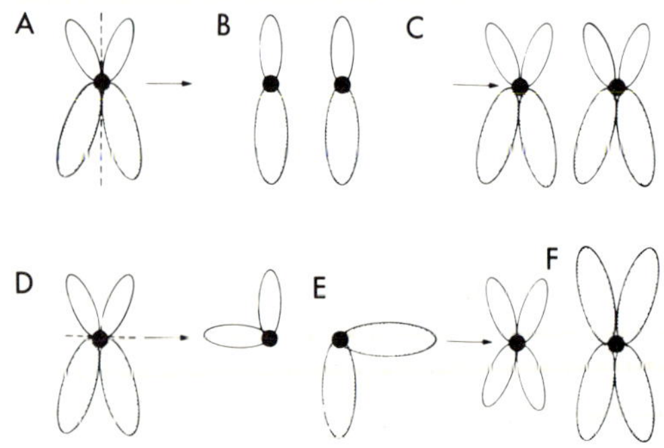

Fig. 16-3. A, Metaphase chromosome replicated for division. Dotted line depicts normal longitudinal division of centromere. **B,** Normally separated chromatids. **C,** Replicated chromosomes as seen in daughter cells during subsequent metaphase. **D,** Metaphase chromosome. Dotted line depicts abnormal division of centromere. **E,** Separated chromatids that result are "mirror image" of short arm (on left) and mirror image of long arm (on right). **F,** Replicated isochromosomes as seen in daughter cells during subsequent metaphase. The chromosome on left is an isochromosome of short arms, and the chromosome on right is an isochromosome of the long arm.

pairs. Translocations are classified as balanced reciprocal when there is exchange of material between arms of two chromosomes or robertsonian when there is centric fusion (fusion at the centromere) of two acrocentric chromosomes. In the latter situation there is loss of short arms, stalks, and satellites with fusion of the long arm of one acrocentric chromosome to the long arm of another. The carrier of such a translocation has only 45 chromosomes by count, that is, missing two acrocentric and having a derivative chromosome composed of the long arms of each chromosome. For example, balanced robertsonian fusion of chromosomes 13 and 14, which is the most common translocation found in humans (1 in 800), would be expressed karyotypically as 45,XY, −13, −14, +t (13q; 14q). The loss of repetitive DNA in the short arms of the acrocentric chromosomes does not have clinical consequences. By definition, balanced translocations do not have phenotypic expression except those related to reproductive problems associated with conception of pregnancies with an unbalanced chromosome.

The occurrence of a balanced structural rearrangement of chromosomes in a newborn is most often a result of familial transmission of the rearrangement. Familial transmission of a balanced translocation or inversion can be expected in approximately 50% of normal offspring of parents who are carriers of one of these rearrangements. Abnormal phenotypic features should not be ascribed to a familial structural rearrangement or other normal variants unless it can be clearly demonstrated that there is duplication or deficiency of chromosome material in the child that is not present in the parent with the rearrangement.

Although certain mutant genes and a number of environmental agents (e.g., ionizing radiation, drugs, chemicals, and viruses) may cause breakage of chromosomes, the cause of a de novo (nonfamilial) structural abnormality cannot be determined in an individual case. A de novo structural rearrangement with duplication and/or deficiency of a chromosome segment can be considered the cause of multiple malformations in a child. As opposed to familial transmission of balanced rearrangements, the presence of a de novo structural rearrangement without apparent duplication or deficiency of chromosome segments, even by high-resolution banding techniques, should be regarded with some suspicion when the child has malformations. In such cases the possibility of duplication or deficiency of genetic material that is not within the limits of detection by currently available laboratory techniques still must be considered.

Clinical features

A chromosomal abnormality should be considered in all stillborn or live-born infants with multiple malformations. Certain clinical findings in a neonate or child that increase the likelihood of a chromosomal abnormality being present include the following:

1. General: low birth weight, failure to thrive, short stature, developmental delay, mental retardation
2. Head: microcephaly, central nervous system malformation, dysmorphic facies, micrognathia, facial clefts, eye anomalies, malposition or malformation of the ears
3. Multisystem involvement: skeletal, cardiovascular, gastrointestinal or genitourinary malformations

4. Dermatoglyphics: abnormal or atypical patterns (Chapter 17).

The striking facial resemblance and relative consistency of certain phenotypic features among infants with the same trisomy permit clinical diagnosis in a large proportion of cases. Confidence in the clinical diagnosis of trisomies in the very premature infant is less likely because assessment of facial features and dysmorphic characteristics (e.g., dermatoglyphics) is more difficult. The finding of a single dysmorphic feature (e.g., transverse palmar crease or abnormal ear) in a newborn without other phenotypic features or malformations associated with a trisomy generally should be regarded as a normal variant. At times suspicious but isolated features in young children or newborns may be determined to be normal familial variations by examination of the parents or siblings.

The diagnosis of a specific chromosomal syndrome will provide the basis for searching for other malformations known to be associated with the disorder and also to formulate with the parents an approach to treatment or surgical correction of defects. In some instances diagnosis may allow reasonable prediction of the prognosis for survival and development. In cases where there is a relatively unique chromosomal disorder or one with variable phenotypic expression, caution must be exercised in predicting the prognosis.

Principal features of the three autosomal trisomies are listed in Fig. 16-4 (see also Figs. 17-1, 17-2, 17-4, 17-7, 17-21, 17-22, 17-24, 17-26, 17-28, and 17-30). Other autosomal trisomies in live-born infants are almost exclusively observed as mosaic (e.g., trisomy 8 mosaicism). It should be recognized that with mosaicism the percentage of abnormal cells observed in peripheral lymphocytes of the adult or newborn may not reflect the chromosome constitution of other tissues or organs and, more important, may not accurately reflect the fetal situation during early development. Thus, although a phenotypic syndrome may be described from review of a small number of reported cases, more variability may be expected with mosaicism than is seen in the trisomies. Clinical management and counseling in such cases must be based on phenotype rather than the relative percentage of normal and abnormal cells in peripheral lymphocyte cultures.

Structural abnormalities with duplicated or deficient chromosome segments are more reliably detected since the development of banding methods (Fig. 16-5). These methods enable identification of each member of the chromosome groups, small subsegments of the individual chromosomes, and a number of normal variants of chromosome structure. Before the development of chromosome banding, infants with duplicated or deficient segments often were not diagnosed, or the origin of segments involved was not identified by conventional staining methods. As more newborns with duplication or deficiency of specific chromosome segments are diagnosed, new phenotypes are being described (such as 5p–). Caution often must be exercised in directly applying reported case history comparisons to clinical counseling of the parents. This is true not only because of the small number of similar cases that may have been reported, but particularly because many cases are relatively unique in that they involve both duplication of a segment of one chromosome and deficiency of a segment of the same or another chromosome.

With the observation of a large number of infants with a duplication or deficiency of a particular chromosome segment, phenotypic features are able to be "mapped" to specific regions or bands. In the future this experience may permit more reliable prediction of associated malformations as well as confidence in determining prognosis for survival and development. For certain types of abnormalities, such as ring chromosomes, experience only serves to underscore the variability of the phenotype.

Laboratory diagnosis

In most instances chromosomal diagnosis can be established by short-term (72 hours) culture of peripheral blood lymphocytes collected in heparin. The addition of a mitogen (phytohemagglutinin) to the culture medium promotes cell division, which is arrested in metaphase by an agent such as colchicine. After exposure to a hypotonic solution, used to cause swelling of the cells, the metaphases are preserved by fixative, spread on a slide, and stained for microscopic examination and photography. Pretreatment with particular chemical agents (e.g., trypsin) or stains will reveal the different characteristic banding patterns. In the event that more rapid diagnosis is required, 48-hour cultures may be performed, or direct preparation of dividing cells from the bone marrow may be used. The latter procedure is particularly helpful when a lethal trisomy such as trisomy 18 or trisomy 13 is suspected in an infant, necessitating heroic life-support measures. In this situation the analysis of a limited number of cells by conventional stain, all of which are abnormal, may confirm the clinical diagnosis.

With the use of trypsin G-banding, deletions of chromosome material are readily identified. Duplicated segments may not be readily identifiable as to their chromosome of origin. In such cases the finding of a balanced parental rearrangement may provide identification of the source of the extra material. When extra material is present as a de novo event, use of several different forms of banding may identify the segment involved or narrow the possibilities.

When there is stillbirth or perinatal death of an infant suspected of having a chromosomal abnormality, tissue

A

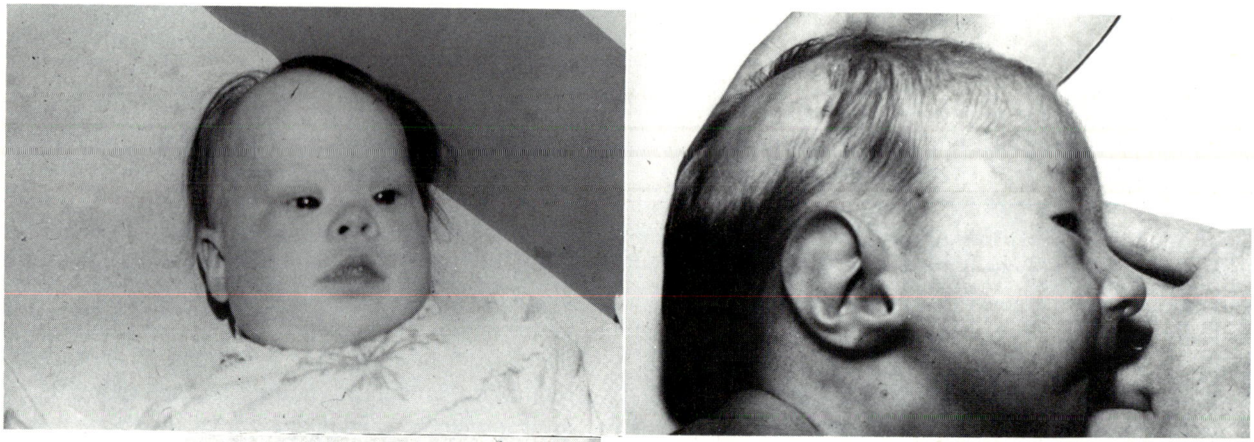

B

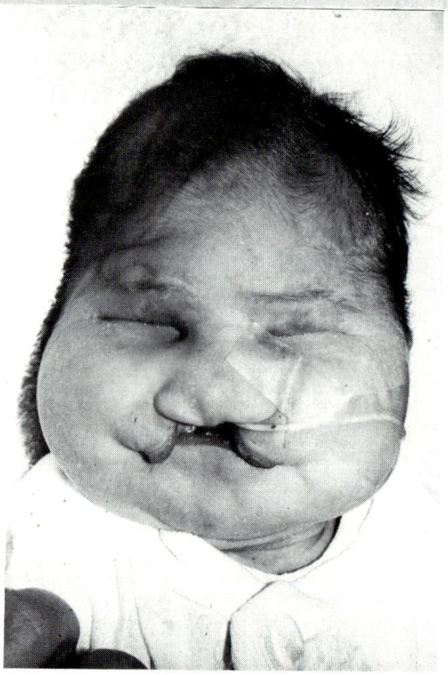

Fig. 16-4. A, Trisomy 21. Prominent features of the syndrome noted during the neonatal period are listed, along with the system or organ involved. CNS: abnormal neurologic examination (hypotonia); head: mild microcephaly, flat occiput, midfacial hypoplasia; eyes: Brushfield spots, epicanthal folds, upslanting, palpebral fissures; mouth: protuberant tongue; ears: anomalous auricles; hands: simian crease, distal triradius, increased ulnar loops, short metacarpals and phalanges; fingers: dysplasia of midphalanx of fifth finger; cardiac: cardiac defects (approximately 40%); genitalia: hypogonadism; pelvis: hypoplasia, shallow acetabular angle; other: redundant skin at nape of neck, wide space between first and second toe. **B,** Trisomy 13. Prominent features of the syndrome noted during the neonatal period are listed, along with the system or organ involved. CNS: severe malformations, holoprosencephaly; head: microcephaly, sloping forehead; eyes: microphthalmia, colobomata; mouth: cleft lip/cleft palate; ears: abnormal auricles, low-set ears; hands: distal triradius, simian crease; fingers: polydactyly; chest wall: thin and/or missing ribs; cardiac: cardiac defects (over 80%); genitalia: cryptorchidism, abnormal scrotum; pelvis: hypoplasia; other: apneic spells, seizures, persistence of fetal hemoglobin, increased nuclear projection in neutrophils. **C,** Trisomy 18. Prominent features of the syndrome noted during the neonatal period are listed, along with the system or organ involved. CNS: malformations; head: narrow biparietal diameter, occipital prominence; eyes: short palpebral fissures; mouth: micrognathia, small mouth; ears: malformed auricles, low-set ears; hands: increased arches, hypoplastic nails; fingers: overlapping fingers; chest wall: short sternum; cardiac: cardiac defects (over 50%); genitalia: cryptorchidism; pelvis: small pelvis, limited hip abduction; other: growth deficiency, thrombocytopenia.

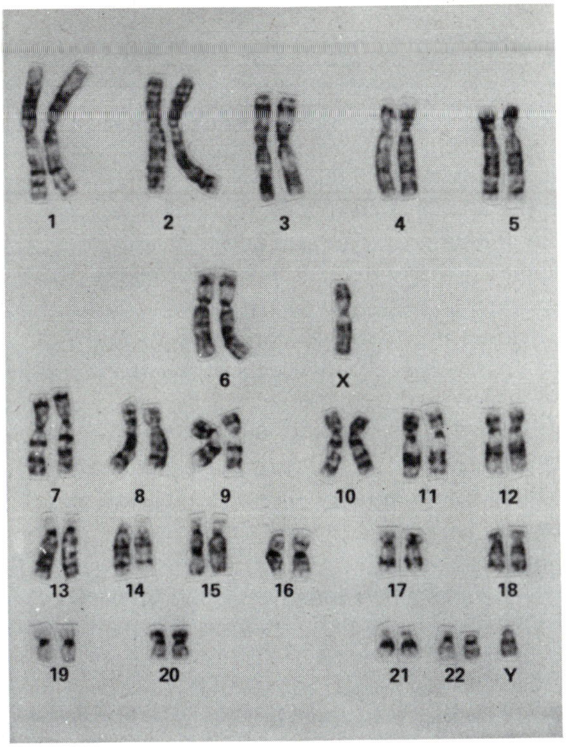

Fig. 16-5. Trypsin G-banded karyotype from normal male cell (46,XY).

biopsy (e.g., skin or amnion) should be obtained in the event that lymphocytes are not viable for study. Skin fibroblast chromosome analysis also may be required when recent blood transfusion renders lymphocyte chromosome analysis inaccurate. When an unusual chromosomal abnormality is observed, skin biopsy provides the opportunity for permanent cell lines to be established that can be used for application of methods of chromosome study that may be developed in the future and also for research studies, such as gene mapping to specific chromosome bands. Fibroblast cultures also may be needed for confirmation or exclusion of the diagnosis of mosaicism.

Counseling the parents

Parents having a child with a chromosomal abnormality most frequently express the view that, in retrospect, they would have wished to have known the diagnosis as soon as it was suspected by the physician. Often, however, clinical diagnosis alone cannot be relied on for counseling. In most cases the parents will be aware of the malformations that the infant has. Although counseling should be individualized, it is reasonable to inform parents that these malformations suggest that the cause may be a chromosomal disorder; the normal constitution of 46 chromosomes in each cell of the body carrying all the genes also is explained at this time. The potential effect of an extra chromosome on fetal development as reflected by multisystem involvement is thus understandable. Often parents may inquire about the specific features that arouse the suspicion that there is chromosomal abnormality. If these are demonstrated to the parents, it is important to point out that many of these features in themselves are not deleterious and are often present as isolated findings in normal individuals. It should be emphasized that it is the presence of several of these features that suggests that a chromosomal abnormality may be present. This will help the parents understand the reasons for a chromosome study but prevent them from focusing on subtle dysmorphic features at a later time. To dispel guilt, but not to overstate the case with a complex explanation that may be irrelevant later, it is usual to explain that the presence of a chromosomal abnormality cannot be related to something the parents did or neglected to do at the time of conception or during pregnancy.

When a chromosomal abnormality is diagnosed unequivocally by the laboratory, the parents should be informed of the results. A counseling session should be arranged with both parents whenever possible. It is often useful to have a normal karyotype and the infant's karyotype available to show the parents in an effort to have them accept and understand the diagnosis. Reviewing the features of the syndrome that the child has in common with other infants having the same abnormality is also useful.

A discussion of the mechanism by which the abnormality occurs often is requested. This should be explained in terms that the parents can understand. Ultimately, for sporadic events, the parents must be told that, although we understand "how this happens," we do not understand "why this happened." When the infant has a trisomy, the parents are told that either the egg or the sperm may have contributed the extra chromosome and that in most cases it is not possible to identify the parental origin of the extra chromosome. The goal of the initial counseling session should be to promote understanding and acceptance of the diagnosis as the underlying cause of the widely dispersed malformations and problems of the infant and to alleviate parental guilt and anger.

During subsequent counseling a more detailed description of the disorder and the prognosis should be given when this is well defined. For disorders that are unique or in which the additional chromosome segment cannot be identified with confidence, giving the parents generalizations regarding chromosomal abnormalities may be subject to serious pitfalls. Rather, the child's malformations or problems should be discussed, and the prognosis for survival and development, although necessarily guarded, must be individualized or approached from a "wait and see" position.

For some parents the question of "will this happen again" comes up at this time. In a few families with recurrence of trisomy 21, mosaicism (i.e., a low-percentage cell line with 47 +21) has been demonstrated in one parent. In such cases this provides a reasonable explanation for the occurrence of the chromosomal abnormality in the offspring and identifies the family to be at increased risk for recurrence. In the vast majority of cases parental chromosomes will be normal, and no reasonable explanation can be provided other than a sporadic occurrence of nondisjunction. In these cases the recurrence risk for trisomy 21 is estimated to be 1% to 2%. This is based on empiric data from studies of families with Down's syndrome children and is supported by experience with prenatal diagnosis. The availability of prenatal cytogenetic diagnosis for future pregnancies should be mentioned, but details regarding amniocentesis usually are reserved for a later counseling session. The knowledge that prenatal monitoring is available is often of great consolation to the parents and may also forestall premature but permanent reproductive decisions such as sterilization during this difficult adjustment period.

Empiric data establishing the risks of recurrence for trisomy 18 or trisomy 13 are not available. Based on current experience it seems reasonable to consider that this is certainly no greater than that determined for trisomy 21 and in fact may not be increased over that of the general population. Nevertheless, one can expect that many of these families will elect to have prenatal cytogenetic diagnosis performed during future pregnancies for reassurance.

The guidelines for counseling a family having a child with mosaicism for autosomal trisomy are more difficult to establish. Even though mosaicism develops as a postconceptual event, it has not been determined whether this arises from a trisomic conception by anaphase lag as a secondary event or more often represents a primary error in an otherwise normal fetus. Studies of chromosomal abnormalities in abortuses suggest that the former mechanism may be more common than previously considered. Thus recurrence counseling must include the possibility that the primary abnormality was a trisomic conception.

The finding of a structural chromosomal abnormality in an infant always should be investigated by parental chromosome analysis. Balanced or unbalanced chromosome rearrangements in the child that are not inherited from either parent are considered random events. Attempts to explain isolated instances of otherwise unexplained recurrence of chromosomal abnormalities in families as being caused by gonadal mosaicism in a parent or balanced structural rearrangements below the limits of detection by current methods are somewhat speculative when counseling a family having a single child with a de novo chromosomal abnormality. Thus parents should be told that the likelihood of recurrence appears to be the same as that of the general population.

The finding of a parental balanced structural rearrangement (most often a translocation or inversion) as the cause of an unbalanced chromosome constitution in the offspring is important information for future reproduction by the parent and for other family members who may be identified as heterozygous for the same rearrangement. For translocation carriers, theoretically one might predict that a sixth of pregnancies conceived would have the normal chromosome pattern, a sixth would result in balanced carrier conceptions, and the remaining two thirds of conceptions would be one of the four different unbalanced combinations (Fig. 16-6). This presumes that, after pairing in meiosis, segregation of the chromosomes involved in the translocation is random. This, however, is not necessarily the case. Diminished viability of unbalanced gametes also may be operative. Most important, the possibility of having a live-born child with an unbalanced chromosome constitution would depend on the specific chromosome segments that might be duplicated or deficient in the offspring based on the parental karyotype. Thus prediction of the likelihood of recurrence is difficult, because empiric risk figures have only been determined for the most common translocations. For example, the risk of having a child with Down's syndrome is estimated to be 10% to 15% if a woman carries a D/G translocation of the robertsonian type involving chromosome 21, or 3% to 8% if the father is the carrier of the same translocation. On the other hand, the risk of having a child with trisomy 13 syndrome if either parent carries a 13/14 translocation appears to be quite low (less than 1%). When a translocation or inversion has resulted in a malformed live-born or late stillborn infant for whom no empiric data are available it has been suggested that a reasonable estimate of recurrence risk is about 10% or less, or one substantial enough to justify consideration of prenatal cytogenetic diagnosis for future pregnancies.

MENDELIAN DISORDERS

Physical traits of every individual (the phenotype) are determined by multiple sets of gene pairs (alleles), with one member of each pair donated by each parent. In *recessive* traits the gene is expressed only when paired with an identical gene (homozygous state). An allele that is expressed whether homozygous or heterozygous is a *dominant* gene. Four basic patterns of inheritance have been identified: autosomal recessive, autosomal domi-

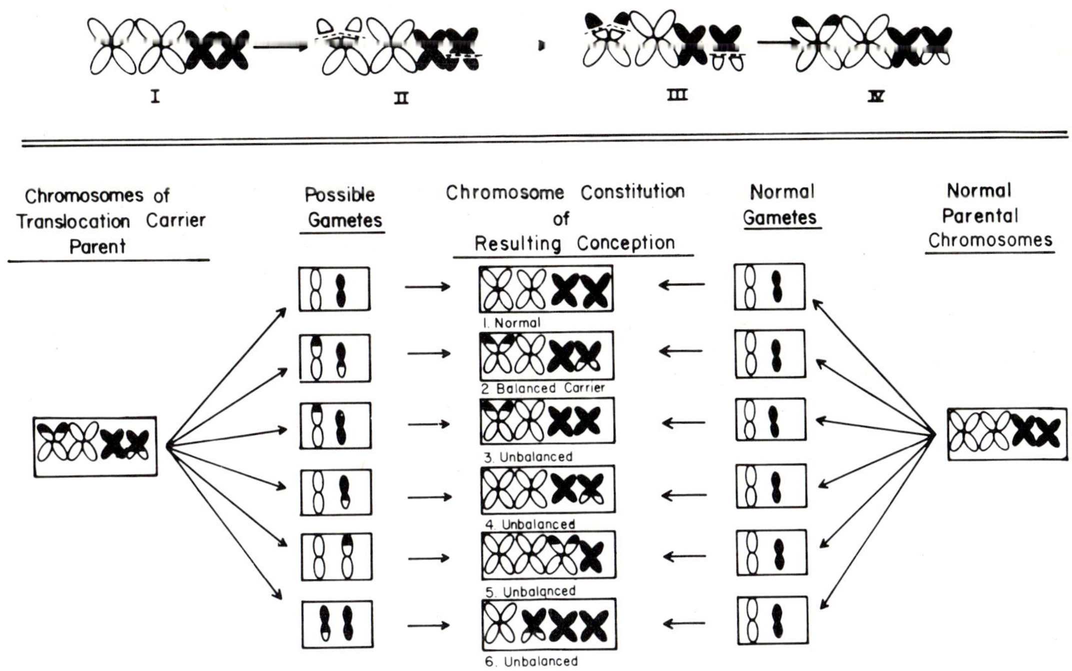

Fig. 16-6. *Upper portion; I,* Two normal chromosome pairs. *II,* Chromosome breaks occurring in one member of each chromosome pair. *III,* Exchange of broken fragments between members of each chromosome pair. *IV,* Reunion of broken fragments resulting in balanced reciprocal translocation. *Lower portion,* Possible gametic contributions from parent with balanced reciprocal translocation, and chromosome constitution of resulting conceptions after union with normal gametes from parent not carrying a translocation.

nant, X-linked recessive, and X-linked dominant. The diagnostic criteria for each of these patterns are the following:

A. Autosomal recessive inheritance
   1. The trait appears in siblings and not in parents or other relatives.
   2. The recurrence risk is one in four for each birth.
   3. Males and females are equally affected.
B. Autosomal dominant inheritance
   1. The trait it noted in the parents and frequently in other siblings.
   2. The trait appears in every generation.
   3. The recurrence risk is one in two for each birth.
   4. Males and females are equally affected.
C. X-linked recessive inheritance
   1. The trait is more frequently expressed in males than in females.
   2. An affected male can only transmit the defective gene to his daughter.
   3. Mothers of affected males will transmit the defective gene to half the sons and daughters. In general, only the sons will manifest the trait.
D. X-linked dominant inheritance
   1. Affected males will transmit the trait to all daughters and no sons.
   2. Affected females who are heterozygous for the defective gene will transmit the trait to half the sons and daughters.
   3. Affected females who are homozygous for the defective gene will transmit the trait to all sons and daughters.
   4. Affected females are twice as common as affected males.

There are several factors that may interfere with the ability to determine inheritance patterns. Certain phenotypes may be etiologically heterogeneous, that is, the same or similar physical characteristics may result from different genetic mechanisms. For example, Marfan's syndrome is an autosomal dominant condition whose phenotype is very similar to that observed in homocystinuria, an autosomal recessive disorder caused by a defined biochemical defect. Unless care is taken in the examination of the patient with features of Marfan's syndrome and appropriate biochemical tests are ordered, the diagnoses may be confused, and erroneous information may be given to the parents regarding the prognosis and risk of recurrence. Genetic deafness is another example of genetic heterogeneity. There are at least 16 to 18 different types of autosomal recessive deafness and numerous other autosomal dominant syndromes in which hearing may be severely impaired.

A second factor that can interfere with the ability to determine inheritance patterns is that mutations may result in multiple phenotypic abnormalities even though the primary alteration resides in a single gene. This phenomenon has been labeled *pleiotropy*. The diversity of phenotype expression from a single gene defect results in the clinical findings designated as a syndrome. Not every feature of a syndrome is detected in all individuals with the same genetic defect; environmental factors also may influence the signs or symptoms that appear. For example, voluntary or prescribed dietary restriction of a substrate when there is impaired metabolism is one approach to alleviation of symptoms of genetic treatment.

Some mutant genes are not expressed in every individual with the defect (reduced penetrance), or the expression of the trait may differ from individual to individual (variable expressivity). Both phenomena will influence the ability to distinguish genetic from nongenetic disease and inheritance of a genetic disorder from new mutations. Clinically, penetrance is the percentage of individuals with the genotype who manifest the trait, and expressivity is a reflection of disease severity. Reduced penetrance and variable expressivity are more frequently observed in autosomal dominant conditions than in recessive disorders. Variation in the severity of a defect at a single locus is thought to represent heterogeneity of the mutation, the effects of modifying genes, or the influence of environmental conditions. Neurofibromatosis and cystic fibrosis are examples of inherited disorders that may demonstrate variable expressivity.

The age of the affected individual also may interfere with diagnosis of disease or determination of its inheritance pattern. Although the diagnosis of Huntington's chorea is made easily in the affected adult, manifestations of the disease are not evident in infancy or childhood. Many other inherited disorders, especially dominant diseases, become apparent only as the infant develops, and some may be detected biochemically before physical abnormalities are in evidence. Other disorders may be limited in their expression by the sex of the individual (sex-limited or sex-influenced disease). An example of a sex-limited disease is autosomal dominant precocious puberty, which occurs only in males. On the other hand, adrenogenital syndrome has been classified as a sex-influenced trait because the ratio of affected females to males is greater than 1:1. Neither of these disorders is carried on either the X or Y chromosome; however, the ability of the gene to exert its effect is influenced by the sex of the affected individual.

The Lyon hypothesis

Disorders that are carried on the X chromosome, such as hemophilia or color blindness, are rarely noted in females, even though female infants may inherit the X-linked mutant gene. The explanation for this observation is based on the random inactivation of one X chromosome in cells of the female. This theory is known as the Lyon hypothesis. One X chromosome is inactivated early in embryonic life and may be observed as a Barr body with light miscroscopy. The particular X chromosome that becomes inactivated (maternal or paternal) in any cell is randomly determined. The Lyon hypothesis explains clinical observations concerning X-linked disorders. Phenotypic females may manifest an X-linked recessive disorder when there is only a single X chromosome or there is nonrandom inactivation of one of the two X chromosomes. Nonrandom inactivation is more likely to occur in females with a structurally abnormal X chromosome and suggests that all female infants with X-linked recessive diseases should have a chromosomal analysis. The second observation explained by the Lyon hypothesis is that in a population of women carrying a defective X chromosome there will be marked variability of expression. Although most women will not manifest the abnormal trait, a small percentage of women will be affected because in a majority of their cells the abnormal X chromosome will be active as a chance phenomenon. This variability in X chromosome inactivation may make it difficult to identify female carriers of X-linked recessive disorders even when a biochemical defect or marker is available for testing (e.g., factor VIII levels for hemophilia or creatinine phosphokinase for Duchenne's muscular dystrophy). When the mother of an affected male does not have other affected sons, brothers, or uncles, the determination of new mutations from an inherited defect can be difficult. The theoretic likelihood of each possibility has been suggested for certain disorders; however, recent evidence seems to indicate that the frequency of a new mutation in the affected male is less than had been previously estimated.

Counseling the parents

For a few families with a dominant disorder it will have been clear that there was a substantial risk for an affected child. In many cases the factors previously discussed (such as variable expressivity, reduced penetrance, pleiotropy, genetic heterogeneity, and sex limitation) will result in families having interpreted for themselves some mechanism or risk other than dominant inheritance. This may give rise to the false reassurance that a particular generation of the family will be "skipped." Diagnosis of a more severely affected newborn, with subtle findings in an affected parent and no history of the disorder in grandparents, may lead to the misconception that the manifestations of the disease are worsening with each successive generation. Diagnosis of familial transmission of a dominant gene may require clinical or laboratory examination of parents, grandparents, or other family members suspected of having the gene. Identification of individuals with the gene can have important implications for their health as well as reproductive expectations. In some instances failure to establish inheritance of the gene suggests that the infant has a new mutation. This is particularly true for severe dominant diseases, which have diminished reproductive fitness.

An association between fresh dominant mutation and advanced paternal age has been defined. Because of the very low frequency of this type of event, prospective clinical counseling regarding this observation is not generally given. The diagnosis of a new mutation in a newborn carries a recurrence risk, which is presumably no greater than that of the general population. If familial inheritance is established or cannot be excluded, then the mode of inheritance and the 50% risk of transmission of the gene are explained to the parents. The risk then may be modified by empiric data regarding the penetrance and expression of the gene. Recently it has been observed that in infants with early onset or more severe manifestations of certain dominant disorders (e.g., myotonic dystrophy) there is more frequently maternal transmission of the gene. This interesting phenomenon remains unexplained. It has been suggested that the disease in the mother may adversely modify expression of the gene in the fetus.

A history of consanguinity suggests that the disorder in the newborn may be inherited as an autosomal recessive trait. It is important to explain to parents having a child with an autosomal recessive condition that every individual carries several deleterious recessive genes. By definition, the carrier state for a recessive gene does not have clinical consequences. The birth of a child with a recessive disorder confirms that the parents are both heterozygous for the same, often rare, disorder. In addition to counseling families about future pregnancy risks (25% recurrence), it is important to give them information regarding carrier detection of unaffected siblings and relatives who may be heterozygous for the mutant gene. For many autosomal recessive conditions biochemical testing can detect unaffected heterozygotes.

Previously affected sons, brothers, or maternal uncles may identify a disorder as X-linked recessive. Women who are carriers will transmit the gene to half their sons and daughters. With rare exceptions female heterozygotes will be unaffected because of random X chromosome inactivation. Affected males will transmit the gene to all their daughters (who will be carriers) and none of their sons. For some X-linked recessive disorders it is possible to detect unaffected female carriers using biochemical assays; however, lyonization may limit the accuracy of such testing. The possibility of a new mutation versus the probability that a woman is a carrier for an X-linked recessive disorder once she has an affected son can be calculated using formulas developed by population geneticists and the risk modified by the number of unaffected maternal male relatives. Early neonatal diagnosis of X-linked recessive disorders should be considered for males at risk. In some instances (e.g., hemophilia) this will have important implications for neonatal care. In other cases neonatal diagnosis of a disorder with delayed onset (e.g., cord blood creatinine phosphokinase for Duchenne's muscular dystrophy) may be important information to the parents for future reproduction.

MULTIFACTORIAL DEFECTS

The most common birth defects that occur as a single major malformation in an affected child have population and familial distributions that cannot be explained on the basis of a single gene or chromosomal abnormality. These are considered to occur on a continuous variability basis with an increased liability (i.e., lowered threshold in embryogenesis for the defect) because of several genes (i.e., polygenic) and also environmental factors. The combination of polygenic liability and environmental factors, which may be either maternally derived or transmitted from the maternal environment, has led to the use of the term *multifactorial* for classification of these defects.

Many of the defects in embryogenesis that are considered multifactorial also are observed as one of several or multiple malformations in infants with chromosomal disorders or single gene disorders. For example, isolated neural tube defects are considered to be multifactorial but also are observed as one of multiple malformations caused by a single gene (Meckel's syndrome, a recessive disorder) or trisomy 18, trisomy 13, triploidy, etc. Cleft lip is most often multifactorial in origin but is seen as an autosomal dominant trait when associated with lower lip pits or may be present in infants with a trisomy. Thus infants with a single obvious malformation (e.g., congenital heart defect, spina bifida, or cleft lip and palate) should be evaluated for other malformations that may indicate a chromosomal disorder, mendelian disorder, or a specific multiple malformation syndrome.

The most common multifactorial defects and their frequencies are listed in Tables 17-2 and 17-5. The relative importance of the genetic versus the environmental factors in the development of these varied defects has not been defined. Family history, epidemiologic data, and environmental exposure of the pregnancy should be ascertained and recorded for potential use in retrospective studies.

Table 16-2. Recurrence risk (percent) for the second in a sibship to be affected given that the first is born with various common congenital malformations with no other family history of such

Congenital malformation	Male (%)	Female (%)
Cleft lip and/or palate (England)	2.6	3.1
Talipes equinovarus (England)	1.4	1.6
Pyloric stenosis (England)	3.2	4.6
Hip dislocation (England)	4.8	3.2
Hirschsprung's disease (United States)	1.3	1.7
Atrial septal defect (England)	2.2	1.9
Ventricular septal defect (United States)	3.6	3.6
Aortic stenosis (Germany)	1.3	1.5
Anencephaly-myelomeningocele (Wales)	5.0	4.0
Anencephaly-myelomeningocele (England)	4.2	3.6

Data from Bonaiti-Pellie, C., and Smith, C.: J. Med. Genet. **11:**374, 1974; Computer Program RISKMF. Courtesy Thaddeus Kurczynski, M.D.

When counseling parents of a child with a multifactorial defect, it is important to point out that these are not "classically genetic" in the mendelian sense. The familial nature of the occurrence of the defects should be described (Table 16-2). The empiric data that are most applicable (e.g., geographic and ethnic) are used to determine the risk of recurrence. It is also important to define the risk for other close relatives so that the parents may suggest counseling to them if they feel that this is appropriate. This is particularly of value when the disorder is able to be diagnosed prenatally and may be severely handicapping, as is the case with spina bifida.

ENVIRONMENTAL DISORDERS

General considerations

Congenital infections, drugs, and toxic chemicals are three classes of environmental agents accounting for approximately 7% of congenital malformations. Each is responsible for 2% to 3% of developmental defects, and radiation for less than 1%. The spectrum of congenital malformations that results will depend on the time in gestation when the embryo or fetus is exposed to the agent. Although such agents may produce detrimental effects from gametogenesis until the infant is born, periods of development during which toxic effects are most likely to occur (critical periods) have been defined.

During gametogenesis (a process that takes about 64 days in males and until the time of ovulation in females), agents that exert toxic effects probably result in death of the egg or sperm or perhaps preclinical abortion. In experimental animals LSD administration produces chromosomal breaks in meiotic cells; however, LSD has been shown to cause malformations in humans or to increase the frequency of chromosomal disorders in offspring. As yet, preconceptual drug therapy has not been shown to have a teratogenic effect on subsequent conceptions. Several drugs, including thalidomide, methadone, and phenytoin, have been demonstrated in the semen of humans and experimental animals. In addition, two children with malformations have been reported whose fathers, but not their mothers, received thalidomide. Similarly, infants with congenital malformations have been born to women whose husbands received phenytoin for epilepsy but who never took the drug themselves. The possibility that some drugs exert teratogenic effects by binding to sperm is an important area for investigation (Chapter 19).

Early embryonic development (first 3 weeks of pregnancy) begins with fertilization and ends with formation of the primitive streak. This period of development is thought to be relatively insensitive to embryotoxic influences. In some experimental animals administration of actinomycin D or cyclophosphamide during this time results in death of the embryo and structural abnormalities. Such effects may exist in human infants but have not yet been demonstrated. It is during the embryonic period (fourth to ninth week of gestation) that many adverse environmental agents exert their teratogenic effect. Such agents include drugs and toxic chemicals, radiation, and infections caused by viruses and other microorganisms. Those drugs for which a cause and effect relationship with malformations has been suggested include thalidomide, methyl mercury (Minamata disease), hydantoin, trimethadione, warfarin, aminopterin, alcohol, estrogens, and androgens (Chapter 19). Exposure to high levels of radiation during the embryonic period may produce microcephaly. Viral infections during the embryonic period generally result in widespread damage to multiple organ systems. The fetal period (ninth week of gestation until birth) may be adversely affected by numerous environmental agents; however, the outcome is usually organ damage or growth disturbance rather than malformation.

For each organ system a critical period of development may be identified during which specific malformations will result if there is interference with development. For example, myelomeningocele occurs during closure of a portion of the posterior neural tube (before 28 days). Cleft lip forms before closure of the lip at 38 days and cleft maxillary palate before fusion of the palatine ridges at 10 weeks. Table 16-3 lists the critical period of development for some common congenital malformations.

Table 16-3. Time of development of common congenital malformations

Site of malformation	Malformation	Time of development
Face	Cleft lip	5-7 weeks
	Posterior cleft palate	8-12 weeks
Gastrointestinal tract	Esophageal atresia plus tracheoesophageal fistula	4 weeks
	Rectal atresia (with fistula)	6 weeks
	Malrotation	10 weeks
	Omphalocele	10 weeks
	Duodenal atresia	7-8 weeks
Central nervous system	Anencephaly	3-4 weeks
	Meningomyelocele	4 weeks
Cardiovascular system	Transposition of great vessels	5 weeks
	Ventricular septal defect	5-6 weeks
Genitourinary system	Agenesis of kidney	30 days
	Extroversion of bladder	4 weeks
	Bicornuate uterus	10 weeks
	Retained testis (cryptorchidism)	36-40 weeks
	Hypospadias	12 weeks
Limb	Aplasia of radius	38 days
	Syndactyly	6 weeks

Radiation

Much of the information on the adverse effects of radiation comes from research on experimental animals and data accumulated on survivors of the atomic bomb at Hiroshima. The central nervous system is the organ system most frequently affected. An increased incidence of microcephaly has been demonstrated in the offspring of pregnant women who were within 1,200 m of the hypocenter of the atomic bombing. Beyond this distance the frequency of microcephaly was not increased. Three factors appear to determine the extent of the radiation effect on the embryo or fetus: the dose of radiation, the time period over which this dose was administered, and the stage of gestation. The peak incidence of gross malformation occurs when the embryo is irradiated during the early organogenetic period, whereas growth retardation can result from irradiation at any stage after implantation. The preimplantation state is more sensitive to the lethal effects of radiation, and those embryos who survive irradiation at this stage rarely show malformations. A threshold or minimum dose of radiation considered to be important for induction of congenital defects in humans has not been established. For clinical counseling purposes some have suggested that less than 10 rad is a reasonable limit for reassuring patients. In general, the earlier the stage of gestation, the more sensitive is the developing organism to the effects of radiation.

The dose of natural background radiation to which every human is exposed varies from 80 mrad per year to almost 1,000 mrad per year in some parts of India and Brazil. In the United States most residents receive 100 to 400 mrad per year (40 mrad from cosmic x-rays, 60 mrad from terrestrial sources, and 25 mrad from radionuclides). The human embryo and fetus are exposed to a background radiation rate of about 90 mrad for the entire gestational period. The total amount of background and fallout radiation is so low it is not thought to influence the incidence of congenital malformations.

Radionuclides administered to pregnant women for diagnostic or therapeutic purposes provide another source of radiation for the fetus. The clinical effect will depend on the type and dose of radiation and the period of gestation during which it was administered. Pathologic effects, including thyroid destruction, have been reported in the human fetus when ablative doses of radioactive iodine 131 have been given to pregnant women. If iodine 131 *must* be given, it should be used during the first 5 to 7 weeks of pregnancy before the fetal thyroid has formed. The radiation dose to the embryo or fetus should be calculated whenever radioactive material is to be administered to a pregnant woman. Once the radiation dose is calculated, rational decisions may be reached regarding the potential risk. In general, the embryo and fetus will receive much less radiation than the mother when the radioactive material does not cross the placenta in appreciable quantities. Because diagnostic roentgenograms would not be expected to exceed 10 rad, and because of concerns regarding preconceptual ovarian radiation (e.g., a possible associated increased risk of trisomic conceptions), the concept of a "safe time" in the menstrual cycle for diagnostic roentgenograms has been abandoned. Rather it seems reasonable to suggest that all unnecessary roentgenologic studies be avoided in women during the reproductive years, and whenever feasible the ovaries should be shielded.

Counseling the parents

Counseling regarding malformations potentially caused by environmental agents must be done with caution. The parental guilt generated can be overwhelming, and the medicolegal consequences should not be overlooked. Before a firm association is made between the infant's defects and a particular agent, the evidence must be reviewed with care. Nevertheless, if a causal agent can be established, immunity to a viral infection or the ability to avoid a particular drug during a subsequent pregnancy provides reassurance for future reproduction.

Counseling parents during pregnancy regarding the

possible effects of an environmental exposure often presents considerable difficulty. The temptation to glibly recommend abortion simply on the basis of diagnostic roentgenogram or multiple drug exposure should be avoided. It is quite clear that counseling regarding pregnancy termination should be nondirective. When proven or suspected viral or teratogenic exposure has occurred, the most reliable and up-to-date information regarding the risk should be presented to the couple along with the available options. Routine or specialized laboratory testing for viral infections must be expertly performed and interpreted. Frequently questions regarding drug exposure arise because of warnings in the lay press, an obstetrician's reluctance to offer reassurance for medicolegal reasons, or ambivalence on the part of the patient regarding the pregnancy. For most drug exposure, clear information regarding safety or possible low-level teratogenic effects has not been established. This is particularly true of new drugs or those that are likely to be used only infrequently during pregnancy. Extrapolation from animal studies or definition of risk using isolated case reports is fraught with pitfalls.

When data are not available but the drug is one that has been marketed for some time and is likely to be taken during pregnancy, counseling may be approached in a general way. Defining the population frequency of birth defects, the potential contribution of drug exposure to this, and the fact that the particular drug has not been established as a potent or possible teratogen may serve to reassure the patient. Nevertheless, the inability to guarantee the safety of any specific drug for a particular pregnancy may lead to a decision on the part of the patient to terminate the pregnancy if this is an available option.

PRENATAL GENETIC DIAGNOSIS

Prenatal diagnosis of genetic disease has developed rapidly and become widely available during the past decade. The perinatologist is in a unique position to identify families who may wish to use these services during subsequent pregnancies, either because of recurrence risk or simply for reassurance that a particular sporadic event has not recurred. Methods of prenatal diagnosis may be considered in two categories: phenotypic studies and genotypic studies. Those methods that determine the phenotype or anatomy of the fetus with regard to a particular defect or defects hold the most promise for diagnosing disorders that are multifactorial, the skeletal dysplasias, and multiple malformation syndromes for which no clear genetic cause has been defined. Methods that determine the genotype of the fetus require fetal cells for study and are used for detection of chromosomal disorders and certain mendelian diseases.

Roentgenography offers the potential for diagnosis of many of the skeletal dysplasias. The major limitation of roentgenograms for early prenatal diagnosis is the poor visualization of the fetal skeleton until beyond 20 weeks' gestation. Enhancement of visualization is achieved by amniography (injection of water-soluble contrast dye into the amniotic fluid) with maternal positioning for roentgenograms determined by fluoroscopic guidance. This procedure is useful for diagnosis of disorders having severe and characteristic skeletal findings that are detectable as early as 20 weeks of pregnancy (e.g., thrombocytopenia–absent radius [TAR] syndrome or achondrogenesis). Because of limited experience and the difficulties of visualization, inadequate or false negative testing is a concern. By outlining soft tissue, amniography provides the opportunity for diagnosis of large soft tissue masses and facilitates orientation of the fetal structures for skeletal examination. Omphalocele, sacral teratoma, encephalocele, and meningomyelocele are potentially diagnosable by this method. The diagnostic potential is limited by the ability to visualize small lesions or, in the case of spina bifida, those that are open but have flat surfaces contiguous with the fetal back. Fetal swallowing and concentration of the contrast dye in the intestinal tract are useful for diagnosis of bowel atresia or obstruction.

Ultrasound has proved to be a far more versatile method for definition of fetal anatomy than the roentgenogram (Chapter 12). The utility of ultrasound for diagnosis of birth defects first became apparent when it was recognized that consistent definition of the fetal head by 16 weeks' gestation virtually excluded the diagnosis of anencephaly. The diagnosis of early hydrocephalus, renal agenesis, polycystic kidney disease, omphalocele, encephalocele, spina bifida, and a variety of cystic or solid masses has been reported. Fetal echocardiography has been used for diagnosis of many congenital heart defects. Definition of fetal limbs and the appendicular skeleton is useful for diagnosis of reduction deformities, disorders characterized by absence of a bone (e.g., TAR) or even polydactyly. Standards for length of long bones as measured ultrasonically permit diagnosis of skeletal dysplasias characterized by shortening and/or bowing of the limbs. Defective mineralization (such as hypophosphatasia) also may be observed ultrasonically.

Direct fetal visualization is possible by percutaneous introduction of a fine-caliber endoscope, known as the fetoscope. This technique is limited by the narrow field of vision and by difficulty that may be encountered in maneuvering to a specific area of the fetal anatomy, even with ultrasonic guidance (as described later).

Amniocentesis provides a source of desquamated fetal cells, of which a proportion are viable. These cells originate from the amnion, fetal skin, and gastrointestinal and urogenital tracts. In addition to the cellular element, supernatant amniotic fluid has a number of other constituents (such as hormones and proteins) that are potentially useful for diagnosis of birth defects or genetic disease. Percutaneous amniocentesis is technically feasible as early as 14 weeks' menstrual age. The procedure is generally performed on an outpatient basis; however, strict aseptic technique is required. Local anesthesia in skin may be administered prior to insertion of a spinal needle into the amniotic cavity to withdraw the fluid. The amount of fluid required varies with the study to be performed but generally ranges from a few to as much as 30 to 40 ml. The fluid that is removed rapidly reaccumulates. Patients most often return to full activity immediately after the procedure with only minimal discomfort.

The rate of successfully obtaining an adequate sample of amniotic fluid increases with advancing gestation such that generally it is recommended that the procedure be performed at 16 weeks' gestation. At this gestational age fluid usually can be obtained in 90% or more of cases by a single needle insertion. Although measurement of a constituent in supernatant fluid (e.g., alpha-fetoprotein) or direct assay of the cell pellet for enzyme activity is at times useful for diagnosis, tissue culture of the amniotic fluid cells is required in most cases. Success in establishing tissue culture of amniotic fluid cells will vary with the laboratory but can be expected in more than 95% of cases. Because of the relatively small number of viable cells collected at amniocentesis, completion of testing usually requires 2 to 3 weeks or longer.

Although regarded as safe, midtrimester amniocentesis carries important risks. Several collaborative studies have been conducted to determine the frequency of pregnancy loss attributable to this procedure. A matched control study of 1,040 patients in the United States and a similar number of patients in Canada demonstrated a fetal loss rate of 3.5% in the study group without a significant difference from control subjects. A British collaborative study showed an excess fetal loss rate among amniocentesis patients of about 1%, but the rate in control subjects was somewhat lower than expected. The reason for the differences in the findings of the British study compared with those of other studies remains unclear. Nevertheless, it is generally believed that the rate of fetal loss attributable to the procedure is probably less than 0.5%. Ultrasonic placental localization is recommended before the procedure. A number of studies have demonstrated a reduction in the frequency of bloody fluids and particularly fetal red cells when preliminary ultrasound has been used.

Chorioamnionitis occasionally has been observed shortly after amniocentesis and inevitably results in septic abortion. The actual frequency of this complication has not been defined but is perhaps 1 or 2 in 1,000 cases. Fetal injury during midtrimester amniocentesis is almost exclusively limited to superficial scars, which may be seen as dimpling of the skin. The frequency of fetal injury varies considerably from no injuries in a number of large series to more than 1% in several smaller series. The difference in these observations is difficult to explain but may be related to experience with the procedure as well as bias of ascertainment. Interestingly, "amniocentesis injury" was reported as frequently in control newborns as in study patients in the British collaborative study. Thus it seems that the neonatal diagnosis of needle injury secondary to midtrimester amniocentesis should be made with caution. Fetomaternal bleeding occurs in about 10% of cases following midtrimester amniocentesis. Studies have shown an excess sensitization rate of 5% when Rh immunoglobulin is not administered to unsensitized Rh-negative women carrying an Rh-positive fetus who undergo early amniocentesis. This complication is avoidable by the administration of Rh immunoglobulin to these patients at the time of amniocentesis.

An increased risk of chromosomal disorders continues to be the most frequent indication for prenatal genetic diagnosis. Maternal age greater than 35 years at the time of anticipated delivery is the most common factor that enables identification of a risk that is appreciably greater than that of the general population. Although the risk for trisomy 21 increases gradually throughout the reproductive years, the rapid upswing at about age 35 years generally is taken as an indication for this testing (Table 16-4). There is a significant discrepancy between the age-related risk determined from live-born infant studies and the frequency of positive diagnosis of trisomy 21 from prenatal diagnosis experience. This may in large part be a result of the likelihood of fetal loss in these pregnancies after 16 weeks' gestation. Thus it seems most reasonable to counsel patients that their risk for having a child with a trisomy is most accurately defined from surveys of live-born children but that the chance of positive prenatal diagnosis is somewhat higher.

Others who elect to have chromosome study by amniocentesis include couples with a previous trisomic child or those in which one parent carries a balanced structural rearrangement. Sex determination when the fetus is at risk of an X-linked recessive disease is another indication for karyotyping. Although fetal sex may be determined by hormone measurement in amniotic fluid (testosterone and follicle-stimulating hormone) or nuclear sex chromatin (Barr body or Y-fluorescent bodies), the accuracy of diagnosis required is such that a standard chromosome analysis is performed.

Chromosome analysis of amniotic fluid cells may be performed for fully informed patients at no identifiable increased risk for having a child with one of these disorders. Often these couples have increased anxiety about

Table 16-4. Incidence of Down's syndrome at birth and of fetal chromosomal abnormalities at amniocentesis, by maternal age

Maternal age	Down's syndrome at birth*	Down's syndrome at second trimester		Total aneuploidies at second trimester	
		Hook's study†	Golbus' study‡	Hook's study†	Golbus' study‡
15-19	1/1,682				
20-24	1/1,352				
25-29	1/1,133				
30	1/885				
31	1/826				
32	1/725				
33	1/592				
34	1/465				
35	1/365				
35-36					
36	1/287	0	1/143	1/104	1/66
37	1/225				
37-38					
38	1/176	1/128	1/100	1/48	1/54
39	1/139				
39-40					
40	1/109	1/149	1/45	1/75	1/35
41	1/85				
41-42					
42	1/67	1/32	1/41	1/23	1/31
43	1/53				
43-44					
44	1/41	1/18	1/18	1/14	1/10
45	1/32				
46	1/25				

From Amniocentesis for prenatal chromosomal diagnosis, Atlanta, Centers for Disease Control, U.S. Department of Health, Education, and Welfare.
*Data from Hook, E.B., and Lindsjo, A.: Am. J. Hum. Genet. **30**:19, 1978.
†Data from Hook, E.B.: Birth Defects **14**:249, 1978.
‡Data from Golbus, M., and others: N. Engl. J. Med. **300**:157, 1979.

the possibility of having a child with Down's syndrome on the basis of a family member with this disorder, occupational contact with affected individuals, etc. Chromosome testing also is generally offered to patients who have amniocentesis primarily to detect other disorders (e.g., neural tube defects or inborn errors of metabolism).

The accuracy of chromosome analysis on cultured amniotic fluid cells is estimated to approach 99%. This is dependent on the ability to establish a pure culture of fetal cells without maternal cell contamination and the potential for laboratory error. Maternal cell contamination probably occurs in less than 1% of cases. When this is suspected, fetal sex confirmation by hormone measurement or comparison of parental chromosome variants with those of the amniotic cell culture by banding techniques (usually Q-banding) may clarify the origin of the cells. Polyploidy is quite frequent in amniotic cells and may be disregarded unless consistent triploidy is observed. Single aberrant cells on the basis of an in vitro phenomenon are observed from time to time and are of no apparent consequence. The diagnosis of true fetal mosaicism, however, continues to be a difficult dilemma. A consistent abnormality observed in a proportion of cells from separate cultures or in more than one patch of cells from the same culture raises the suspicion of true fetal mosaicism. Thus far, in those cases in which true fetal mosaicism has been confirmed, the abnormality has been one that also has been observed in live-born infants (e.g., trisomy 21, trisomy 18, trisomy 13, trisomy 8, or sex chromosome abnormalities). Although these observations have assisted in the clinical delineation of true fetal mosaicism from pseudomosaicism in cultured amniotic fluid cells, this distinction is not possible in every case in which this problem arises. The finding of mosaicism or of a sex chromosome abnormality can present a significant dilemma for the parents in terms of a decision to continue or to terminate the pregnancy.

A large number of inborn errors of metabolism are diagnosable by study of cultured amniotic fluid cells (Table 16-5). The majority of these are rare autosomal recessive disorders, and a few are X-linked recessive (i.e., Hunter's syndrome, Fabry's disease, and Lesch-Nyhan syndrome).

Table 16-5. Prenatal diagnosis of metabolic diseases

Disease	Diagnostic test
Lipid metabolism	
Tay-Sachs	Hexosaminidase A
Sandhoff	Hexosaminidase A and B
Gaucher	β-Glucosidase
GM_1 gangliosidosis	β-Galactosidase
Niemann-Pick	Sphingomyelinase
Fabry	α-Galactosidase
Metachromatic leukodystrophy	Arylsulfatase A
Krabbe	Galactosylceramide-galactosidase
Wolman	Acid esterase
Farber	Ceramidase
Familial hypercholesterolemia	Low-density lipoprotein cell–surface receptor
Mucopolysaccharidoses (MPS) and related disorders	
Hurler (MPS IH)	α-Iduronidase
Scheie (MPS IS)	α-Iduronidase
Hunter (MPS II)	Sulfoiduronate sulfatase
Sanfilippo A (MPS IIIA)	Heparin sulfate sulfamidase
Sanfilippo B (MPS IIIB)	α-*N*-Acetylglucosaminidase
Maroteaux-Lamy (MPS IV)	Arylsulfatase B
Mucolipidosis II (I cell disease)	Lysosomal hydrolases
Mucolipidosis III	Lysosomal hydrolases
Mucolipidosis IV	EM ultrastructure
Fucosidosis	α-Fucosidase
Mannosidosis	α-Mannosidase
Sialidosis (variant)	Neuraminidase + β-galactosidase
Amino acid metabolism	
Phenylketonuria	Molecular genetics
Ornithinetranscarbamylase	Molecular genetics
Argininosuccinicaciduria	Argininosuccinate
Cystinosis	Cystine ^{35}S uptake
Citrullinemia	Argininosuccinate synthetase
Homocystinuria	Cystathionine synthetase
Maple syrup urine disease	α-Keto acid decarboxylase
Methylmalonic acidemia	
B_{12}-responsive	Deoxyadenosyl-B_{12} synthesis
B_{12}-nonresponsive	Methylmalonyl-CoA mutase
Propionic acidemia	Propionyl-CoA decarboxylase
Carbohydrate metabolism	
Glycogen storage type II	α-Glucosidase
Glycogen storage type IV	Amylo(1,4→1,6)transglucosidase
Galactosemia	Galactose-1-phosphate uridylyltransferase
Pyruvate decarboxylase deficiency	Pyruvate decarboxylase
Blood	
Hemophilia A	Molecular genetics
Sickle cell	Molecular genetics
Homozygous β-thalassemia	Molecular genetics
Homozygous α-thalassemia	Molecular genetics
βδ-Thalassemia	Molecular genetics
Chronic granulomatous disease	NBT/superoxide formation
Miscellaneous	
Combined immunodeficiency	Adenosine deaminase
Lesch-Nyhan syndrome	Hypoxanthine-guanine phosphoribosyltransferase
Menkes syndrome	Copper uptake
Zellweger syndrome	Long chain fatty acid synthesis
Cystic fibrosis	DNA probes and/or intestinal alkaline phosphatase using molecular genetics
Xeroderma pigmentosum	DNA repair
Hypophosphatasia	Alkaline phosphatase isoenzymes
Acute intermittent porphyria	Uroporphyrinogen I synthesis
Congenital adrenal hyperplasia (21-hydroxylase)	HLA-B linkage
Lysosomal acid phosphatase deficiency	Acid phosphatase
Congenital nephrosis	Alpha-fetoprotein

Occasionally identification of a couple at risk may be on the basis of carrier testing done because there is a close relative with one of these disorders. Measurement of an enzyme in supernatant fluid or uncultured cells is useful for diagnosis of only a few disorders. Most testing for inborn errors of metabolism must be conducted on cultured cells, and the number of cells required often necessitates greater delay from amniocentesis to diagnosis (4 to 6 weeks) when compared with what is required for chromosome analysis (2 to 4 weeks).

The accuracy of biochemical testing also depends on the limitations of the particular assay method used. For autosomal recessive disorders it is imperative that the affected pregnancies be clearly distinguished from those with heterozygous (maternal) carriers, since the latter group will constitute two thirds of the normal pregnancies of these parents. At times confidence in this testing is limited by the relatively small experience with the methods of prenatal diagnosis. For this reason referral of these couples or their amniotic fluid samples to centers having the greatest expertise with diagnosis of the particular disorder is recommended.

For other single gene disorders, especially many of those that are autosomal dominant, the defect is not known at the biochemical level. One approach to prenatal diagnosis is the study of a linked gene that would serve as a marker for the disease. This is only useful if there is close linkage of a marker to the gene for the disease, and this marker is detectable by amniocentesis. In addition, variability of the marker (e.g., isoenzymes) is necessary for a large proportion of matings to be informative for study. Until recently the best example of using such a system for prenatal diagnosis has been the linkage between secretor status and the gene for myotonic dystrophy. Although this is of limited use at present, rapidly accumulating information about linkages and further mapping of the human genome make this a promising direction for development of methods for prenatal diagnosis of other diseases.

The availability of an increasing number of DNA probes for the human genome has dramatically advanced prenatal genetic diagnosis. Using the technique of Southern blotting, prenatal diagnosis of a much greater number of genetic diseases is possible by analysis of the fetal DNA. In some instances, when the genetic defect is understood at the molecular level, diagnostic studies can be performed to search for point mutation within the gene or for a deletion of a portion of the gene that causes disease. For diagnosis of many other diseases, we are limited to tracking an abnormal gene through a family by study of a closely linked marker known as a restriction fragment length polymorphism (RFLP). As mentioned above, the linked marker must be polymorphic for the mating to be informative. The accuracy of testing is limited by proximity of the marker, in this instance the RFLP, and the gene. Thus the opportunity for recombination (crossing over) in meiosis necessarily limits the predictive value of these tests. Such studies often require the availability of DNA from the proband as well as several generations of the family. Neonatologists and pediatricians need to be aware of the increasing number of diseases in which obtaining and saving samples of DNA from a dying child may be a prerequisite for future diagnostic studies for the family. Molecular genetic methods have added many diseases to those listed in Table 16-5, including disorders of the collagen genes, Huntington's chorea, hemoglobinopathies, coagulopathies, cystic fibrosis, and a number of diseases caused by mutant genes on the X chromosome. It is expected that the diagnosis of many more diseases will be possible in the near future using these methods.

Measurement of *alpha-fetoprotein* concentration in amniotic fluid has become established as a reliable method for diagnosis of open neural tube defects and certain other disorders. This protein is the major serum protein of early fetal life and reaches peak concentration (3 to 4 mg/ml) in the fetal serum at about 14 weeks' gestation. Low-level amounts of alpha-fetoprotein are present in amniotic fluid. The concentration of alpha-fetoprotein in fetal serum declines with advancing gestational age, as does that in amniotic fluid. On the other hand, the very low concentration of alpha-fetoprotein in maternal serum (nanogram amounts) rises as pregnancy advances, with peak levels being reached at about 34 weeks' gestation.

When the fetus has an open neural tube defect, leakage of alpha-fetoprotein from the fetal blood into the amniotic fluid will cause diagnostic elevation of alpha-fetoprotein (more than 5 SD above the mean) in most cases. Because of the declining concentration of amniotic fluid alpha-fetoprotein during the second trimester, interpretation of this test is dependent on accurate gestational dating by ultrasound. It is now well recognized that intraamniotic fetal bleeding secondary to amniocentesis, fetal death, or a number of other defects may be associated with leakage of alpha-fetoprotein from the fetal circulation into the amniotic fluid. Other defects that have been associated with elevated amniotic fluid alpha-fetoprotein include omphalocele, sacral teratoma, cystic hygroma (most commonly associated with Turner's syndrome), and fetal nephrosis.

A practical false positive rate with measurement of amniotic fluid alpha-fetoprotein that excludes fetal death, intraamniotic bleeding, or other serious fetal abnormalities is quite low (0.25% or less). Nevertheless, because of the problems inherent in the interpretation of a quantitative test that reflects a heterogeneous group of defects, other methods for diagnosis of neural tube defects have been sought. A number of other markers in amniotic fluid have been investigated as more specific confirmatory tests for neural tube defects. Of these, the most promising is measurement of acetylcholinesterase in amniotic fluid. Reliable anatomic definition of neural tube defects is highly desirable in establishing the diagnosis. This can be done by ultrasonographers highly experienced in evaluating fetal anatomy.

Maternal serum alpha-fetoprotein also is increased in a large portion of pregnancies in which the fetus has a neural tube defect. Measurement of maternal serum alpha-fetoprotein serves as a useful screening test for neural tube defects. As with amniotic fluid alpha-fetoprotein, interpretation of the test is gestational-age dependent. Thus false positive or false negative results may occur on the basis of errors in gestational dating and require ultrasound confirmation of dates. Elevated maternal serum alpha-fetoprotein also is observed in a proportion of cases in which there are twins, other defects resulting in elevated amniotic fluid alpha-fetoprotein, fetal death, and fetal to maternal bleeding. As with amniotic fluid alpha-fetoprotein, elevation of concentration of alpha-fetoprotein in maternal serum is not seen with closed neural tube defects. The degree of overlap of maternal serum alpha-fetoprotein between women carrying fetuses with an open neural tube defect and those with unaffected fetuses is somewhat greater than with amniotic fluid alpha-fetoprotein measurement. At cutoff levels that detect 80% of open spina bifida and 90% of anencephaly, the false positive rate with serum alpha-fetoprotein is quite high (3%). Often an explanation for the false positive elevation can be found by ultrasound. In the remaining cases the risk of a neural tube defect is dependent on the prior risk of a defect, which will vary with the geographic population risk. Even in low-risk populations such as the United States, the risk of a neural tube defect after two elevated maternal serum alpha-fetoprotein concentrations between 16 and 18 weeks' gestation is high enough (5%) to warrant consideration of diagnostic testing by amniocentesis.

A major limitation of amniocentesis for prenatal genetic diagnosis has been the late gestational age at which the results of testing are available. In response to the need for earlier or more rapid diagnosis, techniques have been developed for first trimester sampling of fetal tissues. This procedure is commonly known as *chorionic villi sampling or CVS*. A number of different methods for obtaining small fragments of the developing placenta have been developed. In some centers transcervical endoscopic biopsy and in others transabdominal needle biopsy of the placenta are being evaluated. However, the most commonly used method for CVS is a transcervical technique in which a fine plastic catheter is ultrasonically guided to the developing placenta. Small fragments of chorionic villi are aspirated using suction applied by a syringe. The procedure is relatively painless for the patient and can be performed in an ambulatory setting. The optimum time for CVS from a technical point of view and also from preliminary data evaluating the safety seems to be about 9 to 11 weeks' gestation from the last menstrual period.

Samples of approximately 10 to 50 mg. wet weight of tissue are adequate for most diagnostic studies. Virtually all of the laboratory techniques used to study amniotic fluid cells can be applied to chorionic villi samples. Thus all of the diseases diagnosed by amniocentesis also can be diagnosed by CVS with the exception of the neural tube defects. Diagnosis of the latter is usually based on measurement of amniotic fluid alpha-fetoprotein. Because the rapidly growing placental tissue fragments contain many spontaneous cell divisions, laboratory techniques were developed for direct metaphase chromosome analysis. Thus a cytogenetic study of chorionic villi may be completed within a few days rather than the several weeks required for amniotic cell culture.

The advantages for the couple of earlier and more rapid diagnosis have led to considerable enthusiasm for this method of prenatal diagnosis. The safety, accuracy, and limitations of transcervical CVS using a plastic catheter and other similar procedures are the subject of active investigation. Early reports indicate that the rate of pregnancy loss following this procedure is approximately 4%. This is surprisingly low when one considers the background rate for late first trimester abortion. It should be noted, however, that these are usually pregnancies that have been deemed normal by both ultrasound exam and chromosome study. Other important risks include septic abortion, puncture of the amniotic sac, and Rh sensitization. The frequency of these complications has not been defined; however, the latter may be avoided by administration of Rh immune globulin (Chapter 5). Chorionic villi samples sufficient for diagnostic studies can be obtained in the majority of cases with a maximum of three passes of the catheter. The diagnostic accuracy appears to be very high. As with amniocentesis, considerable experience will be needed to interpret unusual results such as chromosomal mosaicism, marker chromosomes, etc. The rate of maternal cell contamination in tissue cultures of chorionic villi samples appears to be much higher than with amniocentesis. Further experience with the processing of these samples may reduce the frequency of this problem. At present, follow-up amniocentesis seems the most reasonable option when the result of a study from CVS is unclear or when an error caused by maternal cell contamination is suspected.

In addition to amniocentesis, a number of other methods are used to obtain fetal cells for study. Fetoscopy has been used to obtain blood samples from a fetal vessel on the placental surface, most commonly near the cord insertion. These samples have been used in cases at risk for disorders of the blood elements that are not amenable to diagnosis by studying amniotic fluid cells, and also to verify diagnoses made from amniotic fluid cells. Biopsy of the fetal skin and fetal liver also have been used for diagnosis of diseases requiring tissue-specific tests, including histologic or metabolic studies. Although experience with this technique is relatively limited compared to amniocentesis, the risk of fetal loss following this procedure is approximately 5%, and the risk of prematurity is approximately 10%. Most recently, fetal blood samples have been obtained by ultrasonically guided percutaneous umbilical vessel puncture. This procedure, known as *percutaneous umbilical cord sampling (PUBS)*, promises to be less invasive than fetoscopic sampling, although the actual risks of the procedure have not been well defined. The potential ease and availability of fetal blood samples using the PUBS technique have led to more diverse application of this test (e.g., evaluation of fetal chromosome mosaicism, Rh isoimmunization, and isoimmune fetal thrombocytopenia).

Counseling the parents

It is important that the neonatologist recognize families who are at risk for recurrence of diagnosable defects in future pregnancies and advise the parents of the availability of testing. Complete genetic counseling should be given to all couples considering prenatal genetic diagnosis. In addition, the risks, accuracy, and limitations of the studies to be performed must be described in detail. A decision regarding prenatal genetic diagnosis is tempered by the couple's moral, ethical, and religious beliefs, in addition to their perceptions of the risks and benefits of the testing. In most instances the benefit of prenatal diagnosis will be a high degree of assurance that the fetus is not affected by a particular genetic disease. Nevertheless, studies must be initiated and completed in a time sequence that will permit an abortion should there be a positive diagnosis. Clearly, counseling for prenatal diagnosis and selection of reproductive options must be comprehensive but *nondirective*.

Richard A. Polin
Michael T. Mennuti

BIBLIOGRAPHY

Bergsma, D., editor: Birth defects compendium, ed. 2, The National Foundation-March of Dimes, New York, 1977, Alan R. Liss, Inc.

Berkowitz, R.L., and Coustan, D.R., editors: The handbook for drugs in pregnancy, Boston, 1981, Little, Brown & Co.

Chayen, S., editor: An assessment of the hazards of amniocentesis, Br. J. Obstet. Gynecol. **85**(Supp. 2):1, 1978.

Elias, S., and others: Chorionic villus sampling in continuing pregnancies. I. Low fetal loss rates in initial 109 cases, Am. J. Obstet. Gynecol. **154**:1349-52, 1986.

Heinonen, O.P., Sloane, D., and Shapiro, S., editors: Birth defects and drugs in pregnancy, Littleton, Mass., 1977, Publishing Sciences Group, Inc.

Hogge, W.A., Schonberg, S.A., and Golbus, M.S.: Chorionic villus sampling: experience of the first 1000 cases, Am. J. Obstet. Gynecol. **154**:1249-52, 1986.

Lilford, R.J.: Chorionic villus biopsy, Matern. Child Health **10**:198-202, 1985.

Martin, A.O., and others: Chorionic villus sampling in continuing pregnancies. II. Cytogenetic reliability, Am. J. Obstet. Gynecol. **154**:1353-62, 1986.

McKusick, V., editor: Mendelian inheritance in man: catalogs of autosomal dominant, autosomal recessive and X-linked phenotypes, Baltimore, 1978, Johns Hopkins University Press.

NICHD National Registry for Amniocentesis Study Group: Midtrimester amniocentesis for prenatal diagnosis: safety and accuracy, JAMA **236**:1471, 1976.

Prevention of embryonic, fetal and perinatal disease, Fogarty International Center Series on Preventative Medicine, vol. 3, Pub. No. 76-853, Washington, D.C., Department of Health, Education, and Welfare (National Institute of Health).

Shepard, T.H., editor: Catalog of teratogenic agents, Baltimore, 1973, Johns Hopkins University Press.

Simpson, N.E., and others: Prenatal diagnosis of genetic disease in Canada: report of a collaborative study, Can. Med. Assoc. J. **115**:739, 1976.

Smith, D.W., editor: Recognizable patterns of human malformation, ed. 2, Philadelphia, 1976, W.B. Saunders Co.

Thompson, J.S., and Thompson, M.W., editors: Genetics in medicine, ed. 3, Philadelphia, 1980, W.B. Saunders Co.

U.K. Collaborative Study on Alpha-fetoprotein in Relation to Neural-tube Defects: Maternal serum-alpha-fetoprotein measurement in antenatal screening for anencephaly and spina bifida in early pregnancy, Lancet **1**:1323, 1977.

Van der Berg, B.J., and Yerushalmy, J.: The relationship of the rate of intrauterine growth of infants of low birth weight to mortality, morbidity, and congenital anomalies, J. Pediatr. **69**:531, 1966.

Warkany, J., editor: Congenital malformations, Chicago, 1971, Year Book Medical Publishers, Inc.

CHAPTER 17

Congenital malformations

Congenital malformations are a common cause of illness, long-term disability, and death in children. Their incidence varies with the age of the patient being evaluated. Although many malformations are detectable at birth, internal anomalies involving organs such as the kidneys, heart, and brain may become apparent only in succeeding years. This chapter reviews some of the significant epidemiologic and genetic aspects of congenital malformations and provides a framework for the evaluation of the dysmorphic infant. (See also Chapter 16.)

TERMINOLOGY

A number of terms used in the description of malformations require definition. A structural abnormality may be referred to as either an *anomaly* or *malformation*, both terms being synonymous. A major malformation has significant surgical and/or cosmetic consequences for the patient, whereas a minor anomaly has neither surgical nor cosmetic importance. Minor anomalies overlap with normal phenotypic variation and are arbitrarily defined as occurring in 4% or less of infants of the same racial group. A localized malformation consists of an isolated or single abnormality, such as a myelomeningocele. Multiple malformations involve more than one discrete structure or organ system.

A newer term used to describe certain anomalies is a *sequence*, defined as a pattern of multiple abnormalities derived from a single known or presumed cause. An example is sirenomelia, which consists of multiple anomalies involving variable fusion of the lower extremities, abnormalities in the urogenital system, and defects of the lower intestinal tract and spine, all presumably the result of a primary disturbance in the posterior midaxis mesoderm at the primitive streak stage of development. The term *association* refers to a nonrandom occurrence of multiple malformations for which no specific or common etiology has been identified. An example is the VATER association, an acronym for a pattern of anomalies consisting of vertebral abnormalities, anal atresia, tracheoesophageal fistula with esophageal atresia, and radial and renal dysplasia. The various anomalies may occur in different combinations with no known etiology, and the patterns of malformation overlap but contrast with sirenomelia, in which the different abnormalities are structurally derived from an early localized mesodermal defect. Finally, the term *syndrome* refers to a recognized pattern of malformations with a single, specific etiology, such as the Holt-Oram syndrome, in which radial dysplasia and cardiac defects occur as a consequence of an autosomal dominant gene.

EPIDEMIOLOGY AND GENETICS

Frequency and etiology of major malformations

As indicated by the data in Tables 17-1 and 17-2, about 2% of newborn infants have a serious malformation that has surgical or cosmetic importance. This figure is a minimum estimate, since it is based on examination of newborn infants only, and additional anomalies are detected with increasing age. The largest number (86%) of congenital malformations are localized, and of this group the majority, constituting 0.58% of all newborns, are the consequence of multifactorial inheritance involving the interaction of multiple genetic and environmental factors. The most common and familiar congenital malformations fall into this category and include congenital heart disease, neural tube defects, cleft lip and/or palate, clubfoot, and congenital hip dislocation. The timing of some common developmental malformations is summarized in Table 17-3.

Approximately 20% of serious malformations are inherited in a mendelian manner in which one locus exerts a predominant effect on the formation of a particular structure. The most common mode of mendelian inheritance for major malformations is autosomal dominant, with a minority due to autosomal recessive or, rarely, X-linked recessive genes. X-linked dominant inheritance is the least common mendelian pattern. Limb anomalies, including postaxial polydactyly, syndactyly, and brachy-

Table 17-1. Malformations in 12,000 consecutive newborns

Type of malformation	Number of newborns		Percent of total malformations		Percent of total newborns	
Localized		161		85.6		1.34
Multifactorial inheritance	70		37.2		0.58	
Mendelian inheritance	41		21.8		0.34	
Unknown	50		26.6		0.42	
Multiple		27		14.4		0.22
Chromosomal	11		5.9		0.09	
Mendelian inheritance	6		3.2		0.05	
Unknown	10		5.3		0.08	
Total		188		100		1.56

Data from Holmes, L.B.: N. Engl. J. Med. **192:**763, 1974.

Table 17-2. Type and etiology of major malformations in 18,155 newborns

Malformation		Number
Multifactorial inheritance		128 (0.7%)
Anencephaly-myelomeningocele-encephalocele	25	
Cardiac anomalies	45	
Cleft lip and/or palate	14	
Clubfoot	21	
Congenital hip dislocation	12	
Hypospadias	8	
Omphalocele	2	
Bilateral renal agenesis	1	
Mendelian inheritance		67 (0.4%)
Autosomal dominant disorders (excluding polydactyly)	57	
Autosomal recessive disorders	9	
X-linked recessive disorders	1	
Chromosome abnormalities		27 (0.2%)
Down's syndrome	21	
Trisomy 13	3	
Other	3	
Teratogenic conditions		15 (0.1%)
Infants of diabetic mothers	14	
Effects of warfarin	1	
Unknown		107 (0.6%)
Total number affected		344 (2%)

Data from Holmes, L.B.: N. Engl. J. Med. **195:**204, 1976.

dactyly, constitute the most prevalent major localized malformations and are frequently the result of a dominant gene. Any type of malformation, however, may be under the control of a single locus, including multiple anomalies arising in different structures or organ systems. Altogether, single major genes are responsible for 0.4% of newborns having major malformations. Inborn errors of amino acid metabolism, on the other hand, are one tenth as prevalent, occurring in 0.04% of newborns. In contrast to the amino acid disorders, relatively little is understood about the biochemical defects underlying the production of malformations by mutant genes. As a result, their specific diagnosis relies heavily on the family history and clinical evaluation.

About 0.2% of newborns have a major malformation secondary to a chromosomal disorder, and this amounts to 10% of all the major congenital malformations. It is important to note, however, that approximately 0.6% of newborns have a noteworthy chromosomal anomaly, but two thirds of these infants do not have any abnormalities detectable by physical examination at birth. Included among these early phenotypically undetectable chromosomal anomalies are common disorders of the sex chromosomes, such as 47,XXY; 47,XYY; and 47,XXX. The most prevalent malformation syndrome due to an abnormal chromosomal constitution is Down's syndrome, or trisomy 21, which occurs in about one in 1,000 births. The other common trisomies are trisomy 18 and trisomy 13, each occurring approximately once in 10,000 births. All three trisomies are more frequent with increased maternal age. Other well-known chromosomal syndromes are Kleinfelter's syndrome, due to 47,XXY, occurring in one in 1,000 male births, and Turner's syndrome, due to 45,X present in one in 5,000 female births. Many other types of chromosomal aberrations have been identified, including translocations, inversions, ring chromosomes, and deletions using chromosome banding techniques.

Known teratogenic factors are rare causes of congenital malformations in spite of the ever-expanding list of potential teratogens in our increasingly chemical environment. As shown in Table 17-2, in studying more than 18,000 newborns, 0.1% were found to have major malformations thought to be related to teratogenic conditions. The most frequently identified were infants of diabetic mothers. Such infants appear to be at increased risk for the development of congenital heart disease, particularly transposition of the great vessels, ventricular septal defect, and coarctation of the aorta, as well as limb

Table 17-3. Prevalence of localized malformations in spontaneously aborted fetuses and newborns (per 1,000)

Malformation	Spontaneous abortions*			Newborns†
	2 to 8 weeks	9 to 18 weeks	19 weeks	
Anencephaly-myelomeningocele-encephalocele	31	10	116	1.4
Cleft lip/palate	3	14.5	0	0.8
Cloacal exstrophy	0	7.3	10.6	0.1
Polydactyly	0	7.3	0	0.1

*Data from Nelson, T., Oakley, G.P., Jr. and Shephard, T.H.: Collection of human embryos and fetuses. In Hook, E.B., Javevick, D.T., and Porter, I.A., editors: Monitoring birth defects and environment: the problem of surveillance, New York, 1971, Academic Press, Inc.
†Data from Holmes, L.B.: N. Engl. J. Med. **195:**204, 1976.

anomalies and sacral agenesis. The total risk of congenital anomalies is about 6% and represents a threefold increase over the normal risk. The specific factors responsible for this greater risk of malformations are not exactly clear, but labile control of the blood glucose during pregnancy does not appear to be one of them. Diabetic women with vascular complications, however, are particularly at risk of having infants with congenital malformations. (See Chapter 3.)

The relatively low risk of congenital malformations in the offspring of diabetic women may be contrasted with the high teratogenic risk in untreated maternal phenylketonuria. The success of newborn screening programs for phenylketonuria has led to an increasing number of successfully treated affected female infants who are now reaching their reproductive years. Mental retardation, microcephaly, congenital heart disease, and other anomalies are common in the offspring of such mothers, and the risk of these abnormalities is correlated with the maternal blood phenylalanine level. The risk of mental retardation in the offspring is over 90% if the mother's phenylalanine blood level is 20 mg/100 ml or higher. Pre-conception dietary restriction of phenylalanine may diminish the risks for the offspring, but this requires recognition of women who are at risk. Follow-up of these women and appropriate counseling and obstetric care are essential.

The occurrence of certain maternal infections during early pregnancy is well known to be associated with various congenital malformations. The most common and best understood infections are represented by the acronym TORCH, for toxoplasmosis, rubella, cytomegalic virus, and herpes hominis (Chapter 31). Herpes hominis results in a severe systemic illness in newborns that is often fatal, and survivors may have residual neurologic defects and chorioretinitis. The other congenital infections likewise may result in an encephalopathy with various anomalies, including microcephaly, chorioretinitis, intracranial calcifications, microphthalmia, and cataracts. To a certain extent the varied clinical manifestations of these infections overlap, but a specific diagnosis can be made by the constellation of clinical findings, as well as specific antibody studies.

Although many drugs may have teratogenic potential, several commonly used ones are worthy of some discussion. Ethanol carries serious risks when used during pregnancy. Chronic maternal ethanol use during pregnancy is associated with increased perinatal mortality and the risk of congenital anomalies such as intrauterine growth retardation, microcephaly, short palpebral fissures, maxillary hypoplasia, and other anomalies. The entire pattern of malformations has been termed the *fetal alcohol syndrome*, but the full syndrome is uncommon even in the offspring of alcoholic mothers. The risk of occasional or low ethanol use during pregnancy remains unclear, but some argue the safest course may be abstinence. (See Chapter 37, part four.)

The use of anticonvulsants during pregnancy, particularly phenytoin, also is associated with an increased incidence of anomalies, including intrauterine growth retardation, large anterior fontanel, ocular hypertelorism, depressed nasal bridge, low set abnormal ears, cleft lip and palate, hypoplasia of distal phalanges with nail hypoplasia, hirsutism, mental retardation, and other anomalies. (See Chapter 19.) The broad spectrum of abnormalities has been termed the *fetal hydantoin syndrome*, but similar anomalies occur from maternal use of barbiturates. As with the fetal alcohol syndrome, the full spectrum of anomalies is uncommon and many of the individual features are nonspecific. The overall risk of congenital malformations in the offspring of epileptic women who are treated with phenytoin alone or in combination with other anticonvulsants is 200% to 300% higher than the general population risk. Whether this increased risk is due to the medications per se or is confounded by the effects of the epilepsy, genetic predisposition, or environmental factors is unclear. Unfortunately, many limited or poorly controlled studies have failed to resolve the effects of the various interacting variables, and a specific cause and effect relationship between phenytoin and congenital malformations remains to be proved. Similar considerations apply to ethanol abuse when there may also be a specific genetic predisposition, as well as poor nutrition and prenatal care affecting the pregnancy. The hazards of anticonvulsants during pregnancy, however, must be weighed with the danger to both mother and fetus of uncontrolled seizures, and such pregnancies require careful follow-up.

In contrast to the relatively low teratogenic risk of phenytoin and ethanol, vitamin A derivatives are potent teratogens in experimental animals. The inadvertent use during pregnancy of one such derivative, isotretinoin (Accutane) for the treatment of acne, has led to multiple reports of adverse pregnancy outcomes, including spontaneous abortions, stillbirths, and multiple congenital malformations. The anomalies are similar to those reported in experimental animals and involve the central nervous system, cranial-facial structures, the heart, and the thymus. The most frequent specific malformations are hydrocephalus, microtia or anotia, micrognathia, thymic dysgenesis, aortic arch abnormalities, and conotruncal heart defects. The risk of such anomalies after the use of isotretinoin early in pregnancy is at least 15% and comparable to the risk of malformations associated with thalidomide.

Somewhat less than one out of three major malformations have no known etiology, and as a group they are more frequent than severe anomalies due to either major gene or chromosome abnormalities. It is likely that, as our understanding of congenital malformations increases, specific genetic and/or environmental causes will be identified.

Malformations in aborted fetuses

Fetuses that are aborted spontaneously or therapeutically have a higher incidence of malformations than liveborn infants, and this presumably represents a natural selection process. Data on spontaneously aborted fetuses in the United States are given in Table 17-3. The common major newborn malformations, such as neural tube defects and cleft lip and palate, are also frequent in abortuses but are much more severe. Other malformations, such as cloacal exstrophy, are relatively rare in newborns but comparatively frequent in the aborted fetus. In addition to these rather localized anomalies, more severe generalized abnormalities commonly occur, manifested by marked growth retardation and gross malformations with few recognizable anatomic details.

Chromosome studies in abortuses likewise demonstrate a much higher prevalence of chromosomal anomalies with an overall frequency of about 50% in fetuses aborted by 20 weeks' gestation. The most common single chromosome abnormality is 45,X, occurring in 18% of the chromosomally abnormal fetuses. This is followed by triploidy in 17% of those with an abnormal karyotypes. Both X and triploidy are much more common in abortuses than in newborns.

As a group, the trisomies account for 50% of all chromosome anomalies among aborted fetuses. The most frequent, accounting for almost one third of the trisomies, is trisomy 16, which does not occur in newborns. Trisomy 21, the most common trisomy in newborns, occurs in less than 10% of all trisomic fetuses.

Unbalanced products of translocations account for 2% to 4% of all chromosomally abnormal fetuses and are three to six times more frequent than in newborns. In stillborn infants the frequency of chromosomal anomalies is much lower, about 5%.

The total prevalence of chromosomal abnormalities in aborted fetuses, like the overall frequency of malformations, is much increased over that in newborns. In addition, specific anomalies in each category markedly diminish the chance of fetal survival to term.

Minor malformations and phenotypic variants

Major malformations often are not difficult to identify. Minor anomalies, however, by their nature are more subtle and may not be appreciated unless specifically looked for. They are nevertheless significant for several reasons. First, they may be important as part of a characteristic pattern of malformations and thus may provide the basis for a diagnosis. Second, they are more likely associated with a remarkable pregnancy outcome such as low birth weight, postmaturity, and stillbirths. Third, their occurrence may be an indication of the presence of a more serious anomaly. Table 16-1 shows the frequencies of the more common minor malformations. Approximately 12% of newborns will have a single minor anomaly. Multiple minor anomalies, however, are uncommon. About 0.8% of newborns will have two minor malformations; three or more occur in only 0.5%. In those infants with three or more minor anomalies, however, the probability of at least one major malformation is 90%. A single minor anomaly, on the other hand, is associated with a major malformation in only 1.4% of cases.

Minor malformations are most frequent in areas of complex and variable features, such as the face and distal extremities. Among the most common are a lack of a helical fold of the pinna and complete or incomplete simian crease patterns. Typical simian creases occur in almost 3% of normal newborns, as indicated in Table 16-1. There is a natural overlap between minor anomalies and normal variants, and the latter are arbitrarily distinguished by a prevalence greater than 4%. As shown in Table 17-4, capillary hemangioma on the face or posterior

Table 17-4 Common phenotypic variants

Phenotypic variant	Percent of newborns
Craniofacial	
Flat nasal bridge	7.3
Ear	
Folding-over of upper helix	43.0
Darwinian tubercle	11.0
Skin	
Capillary hemangioma on face and/or posterior aspect of neck	14.3
Mongolian spots in blacks and Orientals	45.8
Hand	
Hyperextensibility of thumbs	12.3
Foot	
Mild calcaneovalgus	4.7
Genital	
Hydrocele	4.4

Data from Marden, P.M., Smith, D.W., and McDonald, M.J.: J. Pediatr. **64:**357, 1964.

aspect of the neck are common, occurring in 14% of newborns. In other locations, however, they are present in only 1% and constitute a minor anomaly. Among the most frequent phenotypic variants are a folded-over helix of the pinna and mongolian spots in blacks and Orientals. Before attributing medical significance to an apparent minor anomaly or phenotypic variation, it is useful to determine whether it is present in other family members or whether it is common in that particular racial or ethnic group. It is common for isolated minor anomalies to be familial.

Racial differences in the prevalence of congenital malformation

The prevalence of congenital malformations varies significantly between racial groups. This may be partly the consequence of differing genetic predispositions, as well as variable environmental factors operating in diverse areas. Table 17-5 shows the prevalence of common major congenital malformations in American whites and blacks and in Chinese. It is of interest that certain anomalies are especially common in a particular race, such as polydactyly in blacks and hypospadias and clubfoot in whites. Minor malformations may show an equally striking racial predisposition, as shown in Table 17-6. Brushfield spots are common in whites but rare in blacks. Umbilical hernias, on the other hand, are common in black infants but relatively infrequent in whites. The widely varying frequencies of various traits in different races demonstrate that whether any given characteristic is considered a minor malformation or a phenotypic variant may be strongly dependent on the race of the patient being studied. One of the best examples is mongolian spots, which occur in almost 50% of black or Oriental infants but in only 0.2% of white infants.

Table 17-5. Frequency of common congenital malformations in various racial groups (per 1,000)

Malformation	U.S. whites*	U.S. blacks*	Chinese†
Anencephaly-myelomeningocele-encephalocele	2.4	0.9	1.5
Cleft lip and palate	1.1	0.6	1.3
Cleft palate	.6	.4	
Clubfoot (talipes equinovarus)	3.9	2.3	0.1
Polydactyly	1.2	11.0	1.5
Hypospadias	2.4	1.2	0.6

*Data from Erickson, J.D.: Ann. Hum. Genet. **39:**315, 1976.
†Data from Emanuel, I., and others: Teratology **5:**159, 1972.

Table 17-6. Racial differences in the frequencies of some minor malformations (per 100)

Malformation	White	Black
Third sagittal fontanel	3.8	11.7
Metopic suture open to bregma	0.7	2.4
Brushfield spots	9.4	0.3
Flat nasal bridge	0.8	5.4
Prominent nasal bridge	2.4	0.4
Preauricular sinus	0.3	2.9
Accessory nipple	0.2	1.6
Umbilical hernia	0.9	6.9
Sacral dimple	4.9	0.4
Scrotum up on penis	4.4	1.0
Prominent heel	3.7	8.8

Data from Holmes, L.B.: N. Engl. J. Med. **195:**204, 1976.

EVALUATION OF THE INFANT WITH CONGENITAL MALFORMATIONS

History

Every infant with a congenital malformation deserves a thorough diagnostic evaluation, which always begins with a detailed history. The important goal is to attempt to identify a possible etiology in terms of genetic predisposition and environmental factors. It is useful to begin with the pregnancy and document complications, illnesses, maternal use of any medications, or possible exposure to teratogens (Chapter 19). The extent of smoking and alcohol consumption should be determined. A careful family history charted in a concise manner, using squares for males and circles for females, should be drawn up. Horizontal lines are used to indicate genetic union and vertical lines for genetic descent. All abortions and stillbirths must be noted. A question should always be specifically asked in regard to possible consanguinity. A simple way to inquire is to ask if the families of the parents are related. If so, then the charting should indicate the exact relationship. The presence of other relatives with congenital anomalies of any type should be recorded along with other pertinent information, such as the maternal and paternal ages and the nature of the anomaly. Family photographs are often very useful in clarifying questions of possible unusual phenotypic features. The pedigree should, at a minimum, include all siblings and parents of the proband as well as aunts, uncles, cousins, and grandparents. In the case of dominant or X-linked disorders a more extensive pedigree may be needed if many relatives are affected.

Physical examination

The goal of the examination of an infant with congenital anomalies is to detect a recognizable pattern of malformations so that a specific etiologic diagnosis can be made. The usual physical examination forms the foundation for this assessment (Chapter 24). In addition, careful attention must be directed not only to an exact description of the major malformation but also to apparent minor anomalies or variations. For the most part this involves detailed inspection and measurement of various features of external anatomy wherever appropriate. In this section an outline of this external examination will be presented by region or structure and certain helpful points, as well as aspects of the differential diagnosis, will be discussed. Greater detail in regard to examination and abnormalities of various organ systems is given in other relevant chapters in this book.

Skin

The normal infant skin, particularly when exposed to cold, shows a marbling pattern termed cutis marmorata or livido reticularis. In rare instances this may be unusually prominent and familial, inherited as an autosomal dominant trait. A similar prominent pattern may occur in the Cornelia de Lange syndrome, hypothyroidism, trisomy 21, and homocystinuria.

A variety of lesions with altered pigmentation may provide useful clues to a diagnosis. Cafe au lait spots are characteristic of neurofibromatosis but also occur in the McCune-Albright syndrome, Bloom's syndrome, and the Russell-Silver syndrome. Hypopigmented macules may be the earliest manifestation of tuberous sclerosis in the young infant. Multiple irregular pigmented lesions arranged in whorls is very suggestive of incontinentia pigmenti. An angiomatous patch over one side of the face may be an isolated anomaly or part of the Sturge-Weber or Klippel-Weber-Trenaunay syndrome.

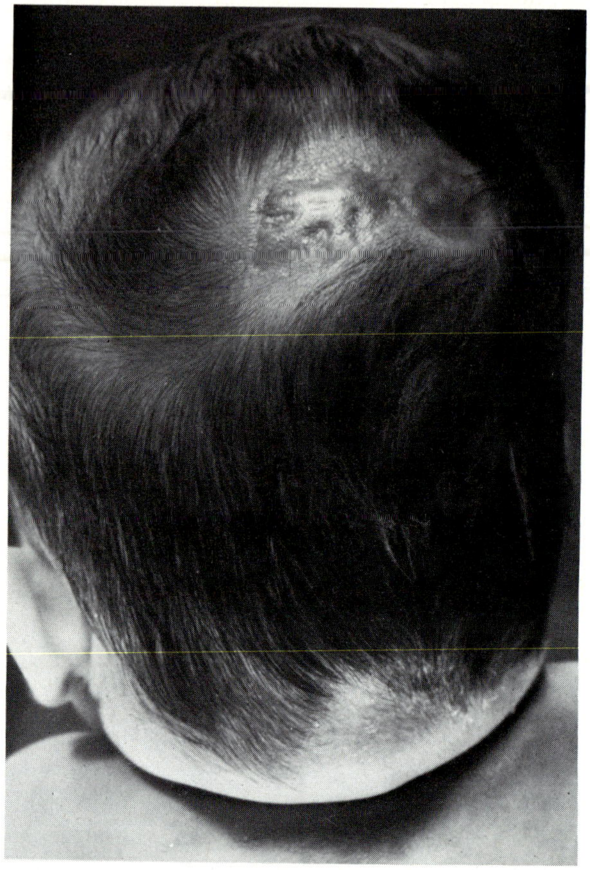

Fig. 17-1. Scalp lesions in trisomy 13.

Hair

The relative sparseness or prominence of body hair should be noted. Sparse hair is characteristic of an ectodermal dysplasia but occurs in other syndromes, such as cartilage hair hypoplasia and oculodentodigital syndrome. Hirsutism is typical of Cornelia de Lange syndrome and the fetal hydantoin and alcohol syndromes but may occur in trisomy 18. It also may be a racial or familial characteristic.

Abnormal scalp hair patterns may reflect underlying brain abnormalities. In microcephaly there may be a lack of the normal parietal whorl, or it may be displaced more centrally or posteriorly. In addition, the frontal hair may show a prominent upsweep. A low posterior hairline occurs with a short neck or webbed neck, as in Noonan's syndrome. Punched-out scalp lesions in the parietal occipital area are typical of trisomy 13 (Fig. 17-1).

Head

The size of the head, measured by the maximum head circumference, and the sizes of the anterior and other fontanels should be compared with appropriate standards

A 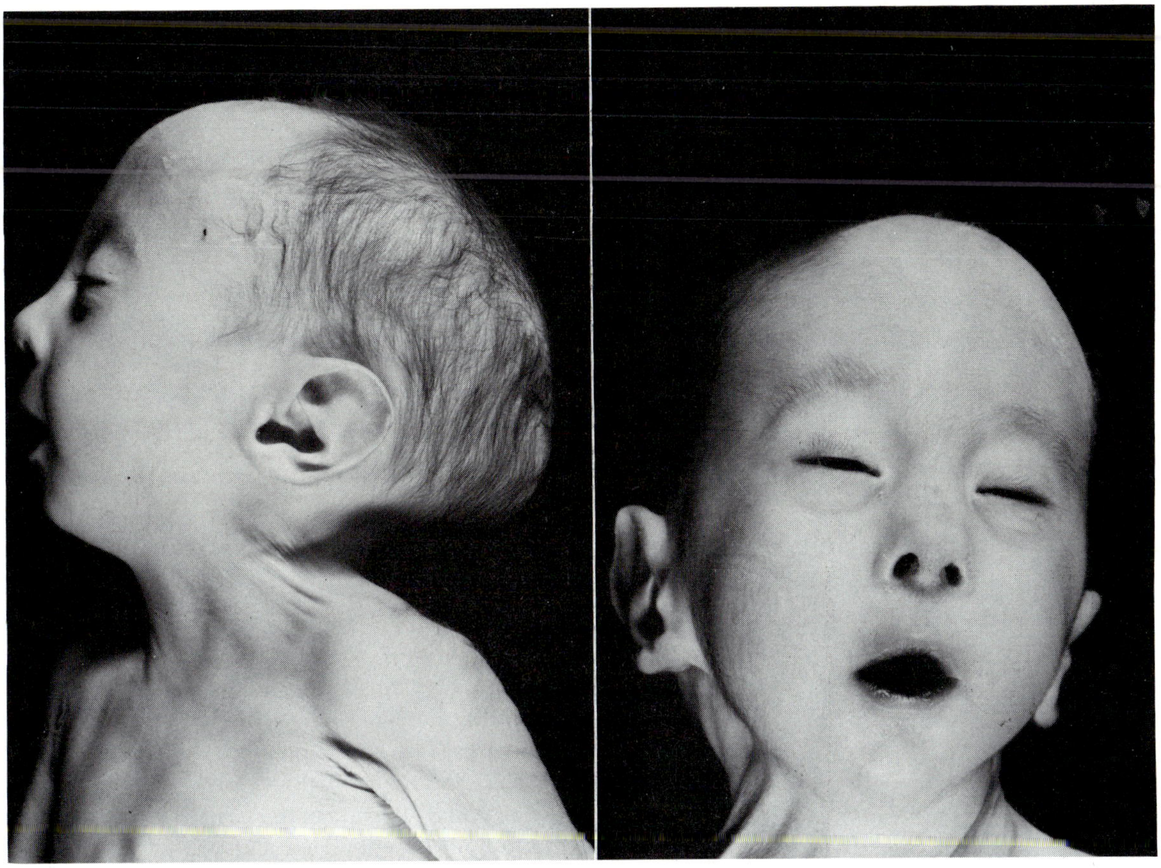 B

Fig. 17-2. Trisomy 18. **A,** Note dolicocephaly. **B,** Note small mouth and anomalous ears.

(see Chapter 27). Head size will vary with age, sex, and racial group and has a general correlation with body size. Macrocephaly as an isolated anomaly is often familial and inherited in an autosomal dominant fashion. Determining the head circumferences of the parents may be diagnostic. Macrocephaly, however, also may be a manifestation of a number of disorders, including hydrocephalus and various diseases affecting bones and/or growth, such as achondroplasia. Microcephaly also can be familial, either autosomal dominant or recessive, but it is more commonly a manifestation of many syndromes that result in mental retardation. Large fontanels occur in hypothyroidism, trisomies 21, 18, and 13, and many bone disorders, such as hypophosphatasia and cleidocranial dysostosis. A small anterior fontanel may be a sign of failure of normal brain growth.

The normal shape of the head may vary from long-headedness, or dolicocephaly, to short-headedness, or brachycephaly. These terms are precisely defined by the cephalic index (CI), which is the maximum breadth over the maximum length times 100. A CI less than 76 indicates dolichocephaly, and brachycephaly is present when the CI is greater than 80. Intermediate values of CI denote mesocephaly. Premature infants and those with trisomy 18 characteristically have dolicocephaly (Fig. 17-2), but either type of head shape may be familial or racial. Many Oriental infants, for example, have striking brachycephalic heads.

Premature fusion of cranial sutures results in an abnormal alteration in head shape. Various types occur depending on the sutures involved and are discussed further (Chapter 27).

A common anomaly in head shape is frontal bossing, which is frequent in many syndromes involving the skeletal system, including achondroplasia, osteopetrosis, I cell disease, and GM_1 gangliosidosis.

Face

The face is composed of a series of structures, each of which demonstrates considerable normal variation and which in toto provide a distinctive and particularly unique appearance to every human being. Since examination of the face is both complex and important, a systematic approach is necessary. It is never sufficient

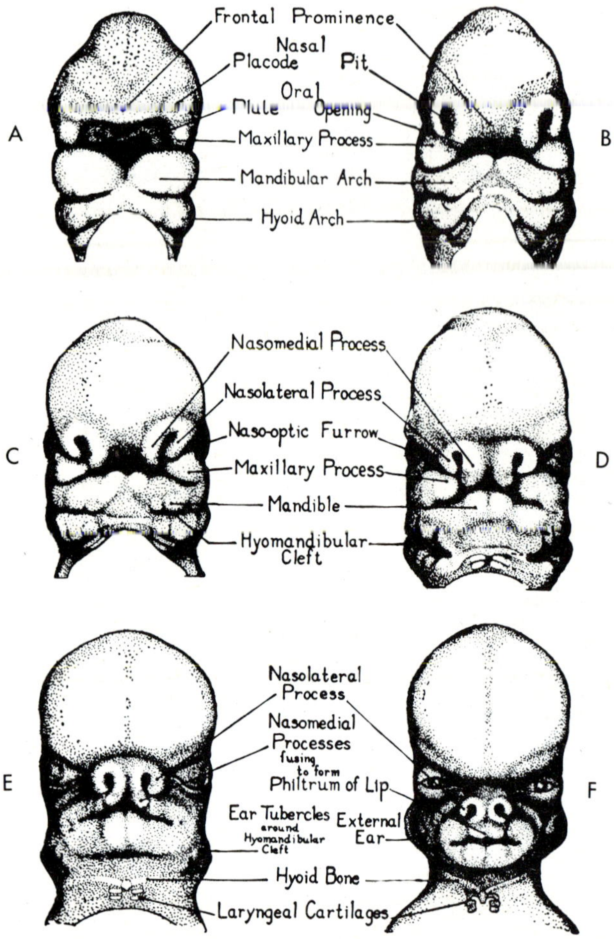

Fig. 17-3. Development of the face, **A,** 4 weeks (3.5 mm). **B,** 5 weeks (6.5 mm). **C,** 5½ weeks (9 mm). **D,** 6 weeks (12 mm). **E,** 7 weeks (19 mm). **F,** 8 weeks (28 mm). (From Patten, B.M.: Human embryology, New York, 1953, McGraw-Hill Book Co., Inc. Copyright © 1953 by McGraw-Hill Book Co. Used with permission of McGraw-Hill Book Co.)

Table 17-7. Natural development junctions of the face along which clefts and other anomalies occur

Junction	Cleft or anomaly
Nasomedial processes with each other	Median notch or cleft of upper lip
Nasomedial process with maxillary process	Common lateral cleft lip
Nasolateral process with maxillary process along line of nasooptic furrow	Oblique facial cleft
Maxillary and mandibular processes	Horizontal cleft/macrostomia
Mandibular and hyoid arch	Pits, sinus tracts, clefts, and ear anomalies
Maxillary process and frontonasal prominence at lateral aspect of lower eyelid	Colobomas of lower eyelid
Mandibular processes with each other	Clefts or pits of lower lip and median cleft mandible

to merely describe the face as "funny looking" or unusual. Specific abnormalities must be analyzed, even though an overall gestalt impression may suggest a diagnosis in some cases. Before considering individual features of the face in detail, it is helpful to review some aspects of facial embryology.

The face has basically a dual embryologic origin, and its development is illustrated in Fig. 17-3. Upper and medial facial structures arise from the frontonasal process. Lateral facial structures develop from the branchial arches. In the embryo of 4 weeks the primitive face consists of an upper frontal prominence, a mouth or stomodeum bordered laterally by maxillary processes, and the mandibular and hyoid arches. Subsequently nasal placodes, which are thickenings of the ectoderm, develop above the stomodeum to either side of the frontal prominence. During the fifth week ridges appear on each side of the nasal placode—the nasolateral and nasomedial processes. The lateral processes eventually form the nasal alae, and the medial processes result in the formation of the middle portion of the nose, the philtrum or middle portion of the upper lip, and that part of the maxilla in which the incisor teeth develop. The nasomedial processes fuse during the seventh week, and failure of this fusion leads to a midline cleft. Each nasomedial process also fuses laterally with the corresponding maxillary process, and failure of this fusion results in the common lateral cleft lip. In addition, the maxillary process fuses with the nasolateral process, eventually forming the nasolacrimal duct. An oblique facial cleft results from failure of this fusion. The nasolateral maxillary processes form the medial orbital regions. The maxillary processes, which are derived from the first branchial arch, ultimately give rise to the maxilla, the lateral aspects of the upper lip and gum, and the upper cheek regions. The mandibular processes of the first branchial arch eventuate in the lower lip and gum, the chin, and the lower cheek region. The junction between the mandibular process of the first branchial arch and the hyoid arch derived from the second branchial arch results in the hyoid-mandibular cleft, around which the external ear eventually forms. Defects in this developmental field result in abnormalities of the mandible and ear. As the mandible develops and grows, the relative position of the ears ascends to the level of the eyes. During the tenth week the palatal shelves from the maxillary process fuse with each other and the nasal septum, and a cleft palate results from failure of this fusion. The final adult facial structures and their origins follow:

A. Frontonasal prominence
   1. Frontal bones
   2. Crista galli
   3. Ethmoid bone
   4. Nasal bone
   5. Vomer bone and cartilaginous septum
   6. Premaxillary bone
   7. Anterior palatine triangle
B. Branchial arches
   1. Temporal bones in part and ossicles
   2. Zygomatic arch
   3. Maxillary bone
   4. Mandible
   5. Hard palate

The consequences of various failures of fusion are given in Table 17-7.

Eyes

See also Chapter 39.

The orbits originate partly from the frontonasal prominence, and thus their development is intimately related to the formation of midline structures such as the nose and interorbital region. Hypotelorism occurs when the eyes are unusually close together; when they are too far apart there is hypertelorism. Clinically, hypotelorism and hypertelorism are defined by the interpupillary distance, which may be estimated in a relaxed patient by approximating a tape measure between the midpoints of the pupils. Two other relevant measures that are useful and relatively easier to obtain are the inner canthal distance and the outer canthal distance. Telecanthus is an increase in the inner canthal distance and may occur in the absence of hypertelorism, such as in Waardenburg's syndrome (Chapter 39). Other factors that also can cause an illusion of hypertelorism follow:

1. Blepharophimosis
2. Cryptophthalmos
3. Epicanthal folds
4. Exotropia
5. Flat nasal bridge
6. Microphthalmos
7. Small face with normally spaced eyes
8. Small nose
9. Symblepharon
10. Telecanthus
11. Widely spaced eyebrows

For this reason a subjective impression always should be confirmed by measurement of all three distances. From a prognostic and diagnostic point of view it is important to identify hypotelorism, since it is often associated with holoprosencephaly, as in trisomy 13. Examples are shown in Fig. 17-4. Hypertelorism, on the other hand, occurs in a number of syndromes, such as frontonasal dysplasia, and even if it is severe it is less likely to be

Fig. 17-4. A, Trisomy 13; note anomalous midline facial development with hypotelorism, a midline cleft lip, and lack of a nose. **B,** Trisomy 13; note hypotelorism and an abnormal nose.

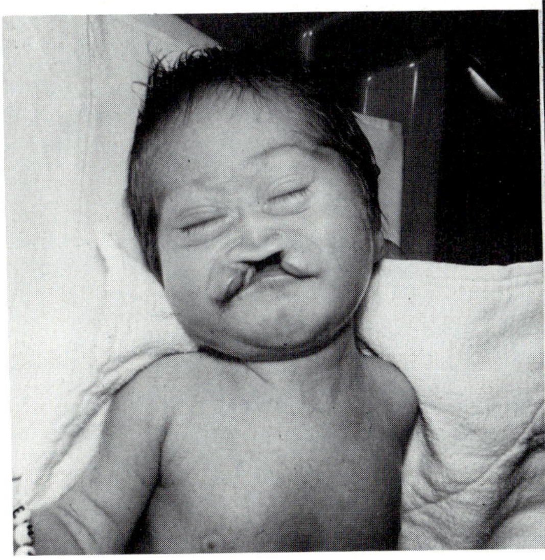

A

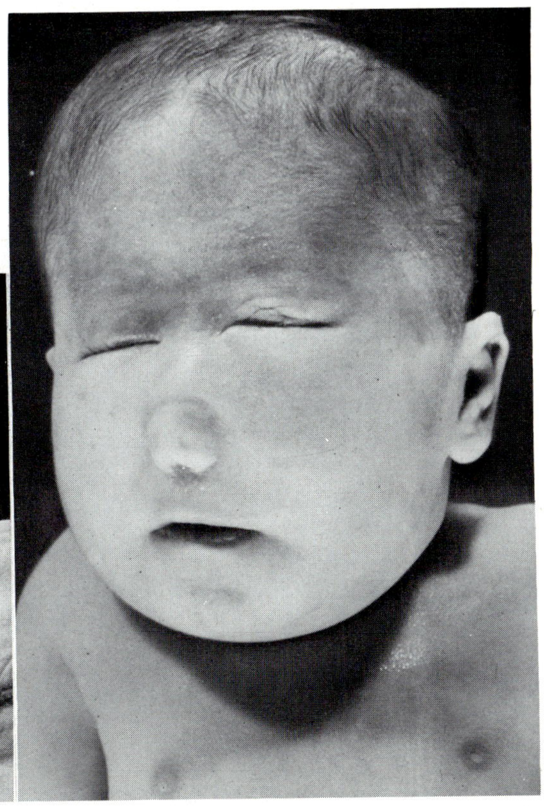

B

related to an underlying brain malformation. Figs. 17-5 and 17-6 illustrate hypertelorism with midline facial anomalies.

Epicanthal folds are a feature of normal fetal development but after birth are prominent in less than 1% of normal infants. They are characteristic in trisomy 21 (Fig. 17-7, *A* and *B*) but occur in many other malformation syndromes.

Normally an imaginary line through the inner and outer canthi should be perpendicular to the sagittal plane of the face. When the line slopes upward laterally, there is a mongoloid or upward slant (Fig. 17-7, *A*), and an antimongoloid or downward slant occurs when the line deviates downward laterally in a patient with mandibulofacial dysostosis (Fig. 17-7, *C*). As the term implies, a mongoloid slant is common in trisomy 21, but either type of slant is present in a number of syndromes.

Palpebral fissure length is measured from the inner to the outer canthus. A short palpebral fissure may occur in association with other ocular anomalies, such as microophthalmia, and is characteristic of syndromes such as fetal alcohol and trisomy 18 (Fig. 17-2, *B*).

Colobomas are developmental defects in the normal continuity of a structure and may occur in the eyelid border resulting in a notch or angulation of the eyelid margin. Such defects are characteristic in the Goldenhar and Treacher Collins syndromes (see Fig. 17-7, *C*).

Synophrys, or fusion of the eyebrows in the midline, is common in hirsute infants and usually occurs in the Cornelia de Lange syndrome.

Other types of anomalies involving the internal structure of the eyes are discussed in Chapter 39.

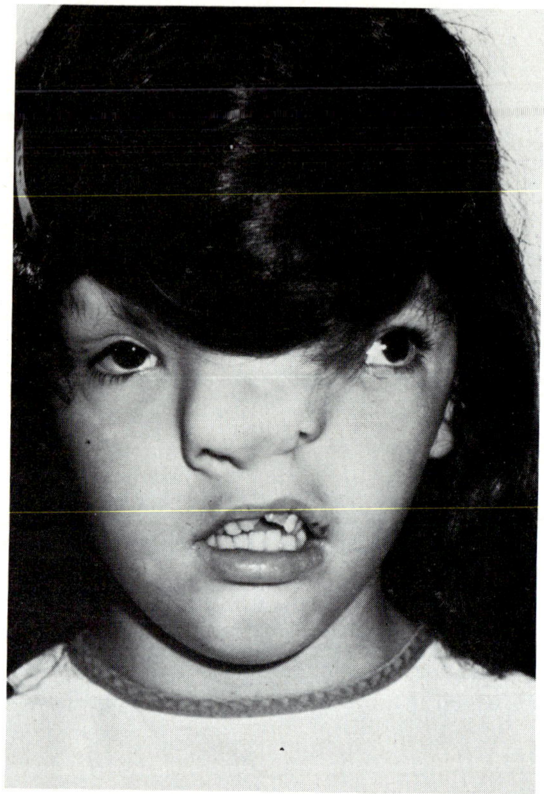

Fig. 17-5. Frontonasal dysplasia with hypertelorism and bifid nose.

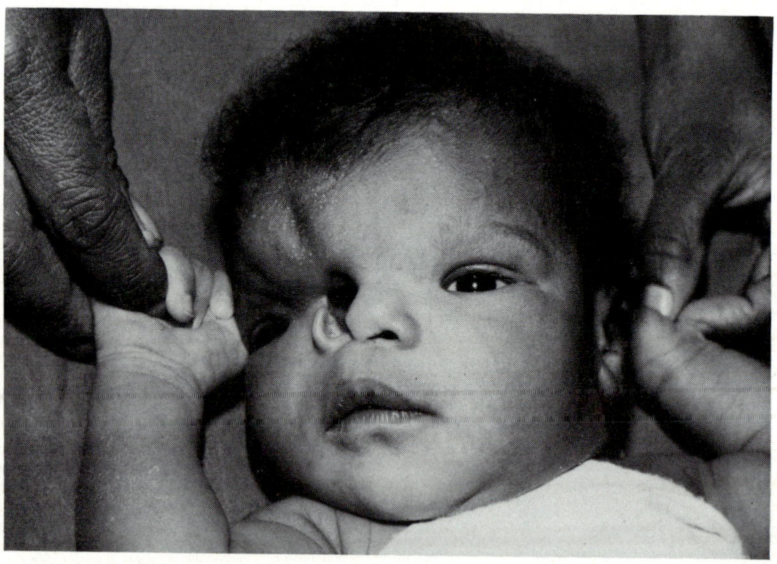

Fig. 17-6. Frontonasal dysplasia with a nasal cleft.

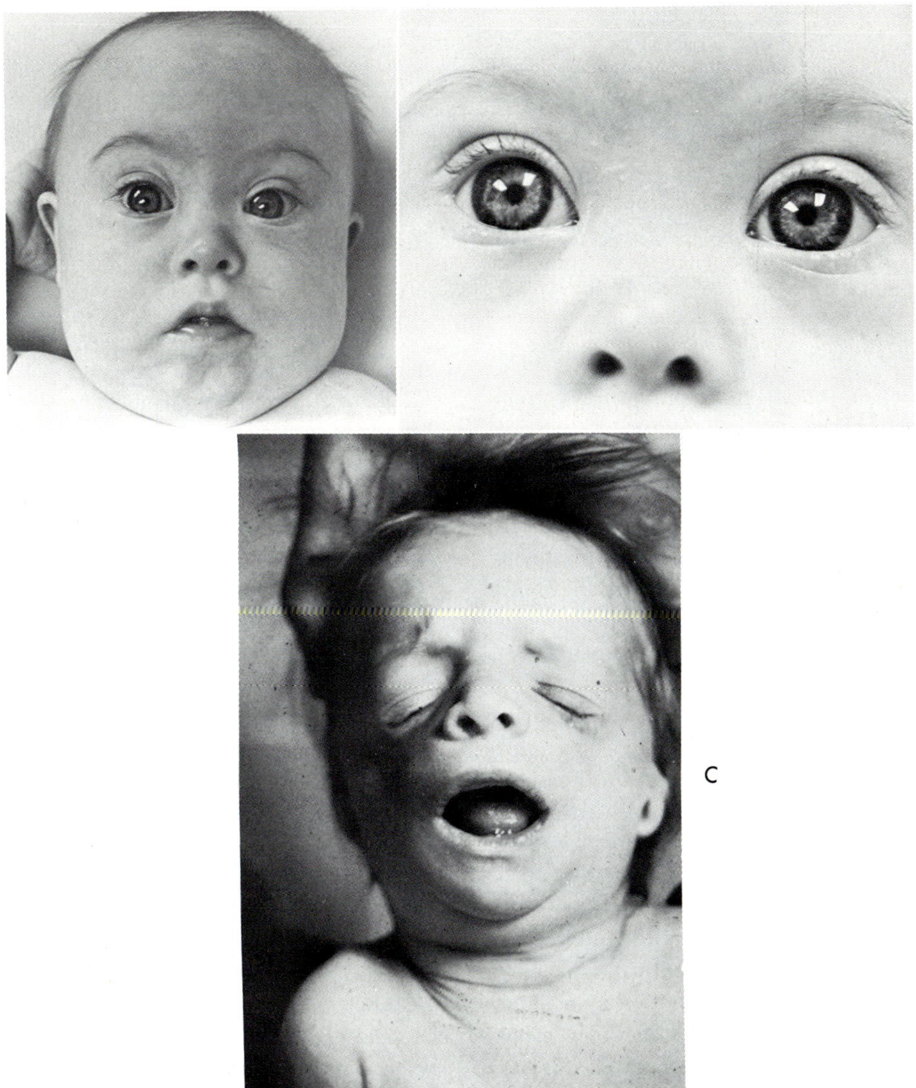

Fig. 17-7. A, Trisomy 21; note epicanthal folds and a mongoloid slant of the eyes. **B,** Enlargement of the eyes of the patient in **A.** Note the Brushfield spots on the irides. **C,** Mandibulofacial dysostosis (Treacher Collins syndrome) with an antimongoloid slant of the eyes. Note the coloboma, or notch, in the left lower eyelid.

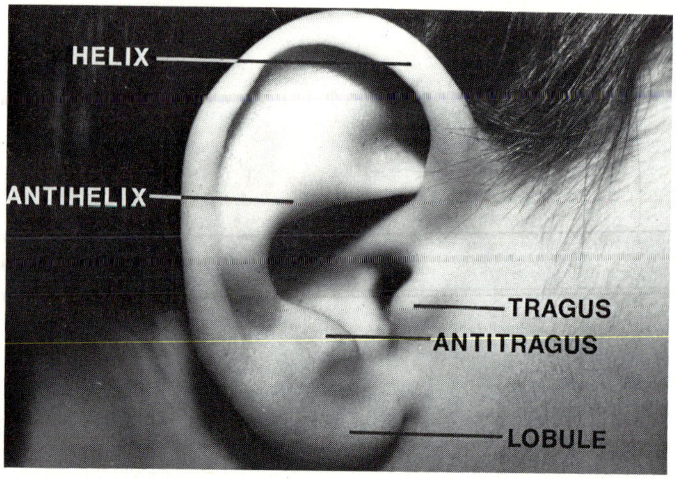

Fig. 17-8. Normal pinna and its landmarks.

Ear

The external ear, or pinna, commonly shows great variation, but a number of anatomic landmarks can be identified and should be evaluated in the anomalous ear. These include the helix, antihelix, tragus, antitragus, external meatus, and lobule (Figs. 17-8 and 17-10). Microtia or macrotia should be determined by measuring the maximum length of the pinna from the lobule to the superior margin of the helix. Preauricular tags or pits may be isolated or associated with other abnormalities of the pinna (Fig. 17-9).

Low-set ears are designated when the helix joins the head below a horizontal plane passing through the outer canthi perpendicular to the vertical axis of the head. It is critical that this condition be assessed with the head in vertical alignment with the body, since any posterior rotation of the head can easily create an illusion of low-set ears.

When the vertical axis of the ear deviates more than 10 degrees from the vertical axis of the head, the ears are posteriorly rotated. This anomaly is often associated with low-set ears and represents a lag in the normal ascent of the ear during development (Figs. 17-11 and 17-12).

It is important to note that any abnormality of the external ear may be an indication of additional anomalies of the middle or inner ear and associated hearing loss. Therefore an early hearing assessment may be needed in such cases (Chapter 27). Fig. 17-13 illustrates a patient with hemifacial microsomia, a severely malformed pinna, and absent external auditory meatus.

Nose

The nose, like the external ear, shows great individual variation, but certain alterations in shape are frequent in malformation syndromes involving the face. The nose may be unusually thin with hypoplastic alae nasi, as in Hallerman-Streiff syndrome; or it may be unusually broad, as in the cranial metaphyseal dysplasias and frontonasal dysplasia, or prominent, as in the trichorhinophalangeal syndrome. A depressed nasal bridge with an upturned nose occurs in many skeletal dysplasias, such as achondroplasia. When the depression is severe, the nostrils may appear anteverted and the nose shortened with a high philtrum.

Mouth

The mouth is a complex structure with component parts, each requiring separate evaluation. The lower portion of the mouth is formed by the mandible, which in young infants is relatively small. An excessively small mandible is termed *micrognathia,* which is a feature of many syndromes. It is characteristic in the Pierre Robin malformation complex, which consists of the triad of micrognathia, glossoptosis, and a U-shaped cleft palate, as opposed to the common V-shaped cleft. A typical patient is shown in Fig. 17-14. The Pierre Robin complex may be part of a syndrome, and thus other anomalies must be searched for. In other syndromes the maxilla likewise may be hypoplastic, decreasing the prominence of the upper cheeks.

The size and shape of the mouth may be altered; a small mouth, or *microstomia,* occurs in trisomy 18; severe macrostomia may result in association with a lateral facial cleft. The common cupid's bow configuration of the lips may be exaggerated, leading to a highly tented upper lip, a characteristic of myotonic dystrophy. The corners of the mouth may be downturned, as in the Russell-Silver syndrome. An asymmetric face during crying occurs with congenital deficiency in the depressor anguli oris muscle on one side, and this may be associated with congenital heart defects and other abnormalities.

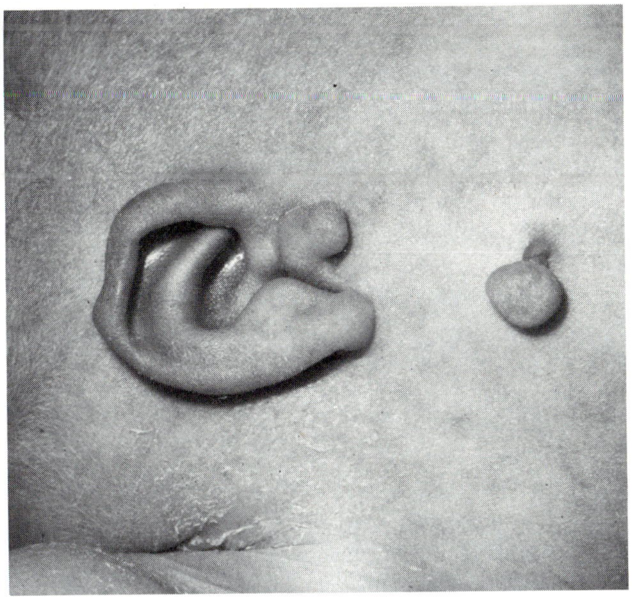

Fig. 17-9. Preauricular tags with a malformed pinna.

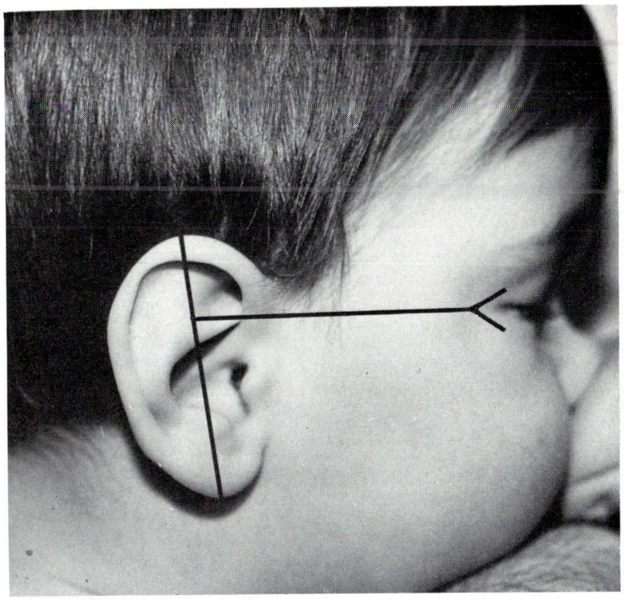

Fig. 17-10. Normal pinna and its orientation with respect to the eyes.

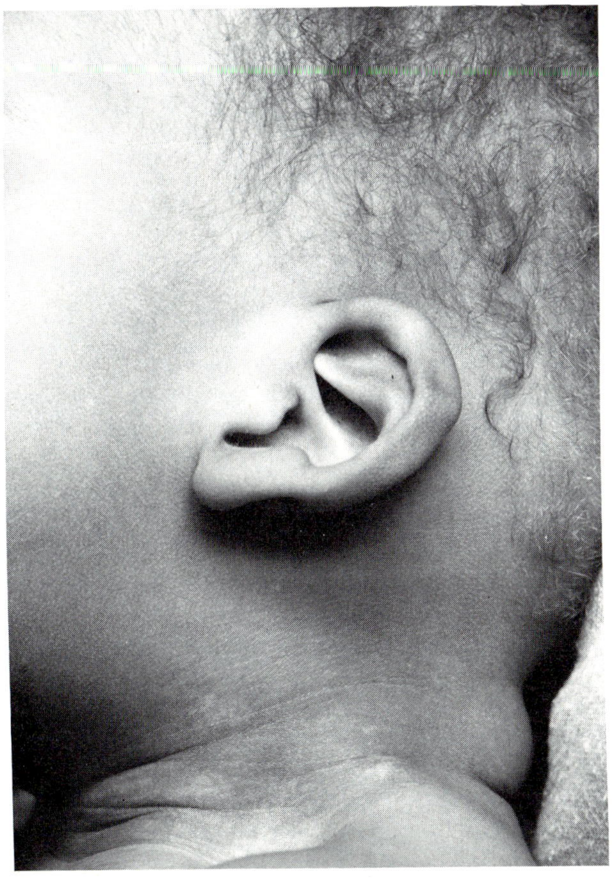

Fig. 17-11. Abnormal pinna that is low set and posteriorly rotated in a patient with the Smith-Lemli-Opitz syndrome.

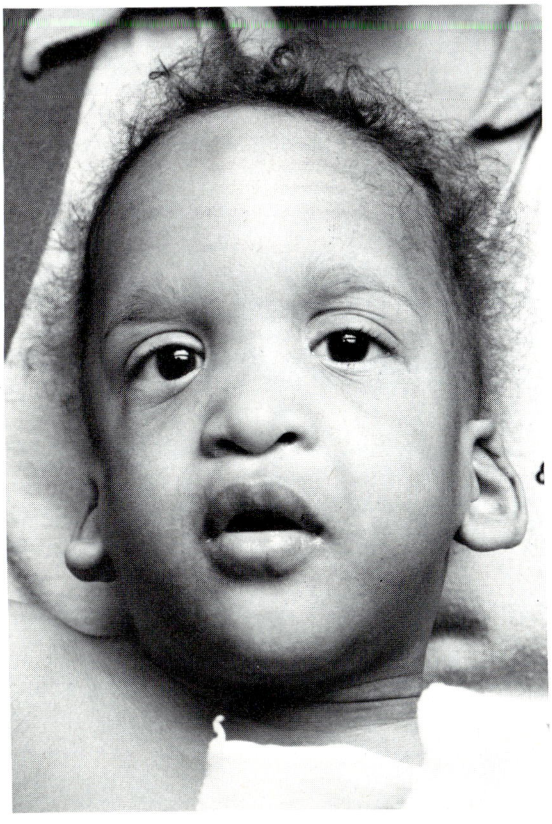

Fig. 17-12. Facial view of the patient in Fig. 17-11.

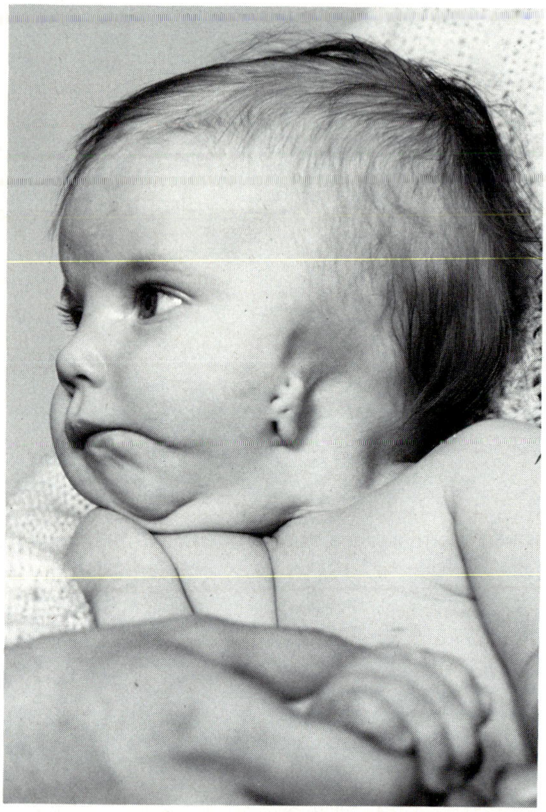

Fig. 17-13. Hemifacial microsomia showing mandibular hypoplasia and a severely malformed pinna and absent ear canal.

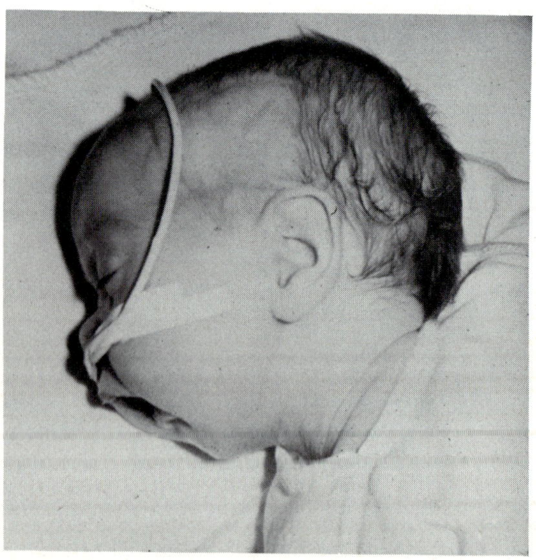

Fig. 17-14. Micrognathia in the Pierre Robin malformation complex.

Prominent full lips occur in various syndromes characterized by coarse facies, such as Hurler's disease (Fig. 17-15). A cleft upper lip is commonly median, as in trisomy 13, or lateral, as in the common multifactorial cleft lip and/or palate anomaly. The presence of pits in the lower lip associated with a cleft lip or palate, however, is suggestive of a different malformation syndrome inherited in an autosomal dominant manner. In fact, there are diverse syndromes with cleft lip and/or palate that are important to identify, since they may have relatively high genetic risks of recurrence. Following is an outline of the common cleft lip and/or palate syndromes.

A. Autosomal dominant
    1. Lip pits
    2. Filiform fusion of eyelids
    3. Ectrodactyly-ectodermal dysplasia (EEC)
    4. Popliteal pterygium
    5. Rapp-Hodgkin ectodermal dysplasia
    6. Acrocephalosyndactyly
    7. Arthroophthalmopathy (Stickler's syndrome)
    8. Mandibulofacial dysostosis
    9. Spondyloepiphyseal dysplasia congenita
    10. Brachial plexus neuritis
    11. Lateral synechial CKSP
    12. Metatropic dysplasia (Kniest's syndrome)
    13. Ectrodactyly
    14. Micrognathia, dysplastic ears, ectrosyndactyly
    15. Joint dislocations, unusual facies (Larsen's syndrome)
    16. Microcephaly, large ears, short stature, proximal thumbs, hypoplastic distal phalanges
B. Autosomal recessive
    1. Encephalocele, polydactyly, polycystic kidneys (Meckel's syndrome)
    2. Ablepharon
    3. Tetraphocomelia (Robert's syndrome)
    4. Hypertelorism, microtia, ectopic kidney, congenital heart disease, growth deficiency
    5. Orocraniodigital
    6. Diastrophic dwarfism
    7. Multiple pterygium
    8. Stapes fixation and oligodontia
    9. Cerebrocostomandibular
    10. Branchioskeletogenital
    11. Craniostenosis, microcephaly, arthrogryposis, adducted thumbs
    12. Short stature, mental retardation
    13. Joint dislocations, unusual facies (Larsen's syndrome)
    14. Truncus arteriosus, abnormal right pulmonary artery
    15. Micromelic dwarfism
    16. Microcephaly, mental retardation, bulbous nasal tip, clinodactyly of toes (Palint's syndrome)

17. Growth retardation, flexion contractures of hands, small fingers, and nails, ureteral stenosis, coarse facies (Rudiger's syndrome)

C. X-linked syndromes
1. Orofaciodigital
2. Otopalatodigital
3. Nephritis, deafness (Alport's syndrome)
4. Micrognathia, talipes equinovarus, atrial septal defect, and persistence of left superior vena cava
5. Short stature
6. Submucous connective tissue dysplasia

D. Multifactorial or unknown etiology
1. Median cleft face
2. Thoracopagus
3. Anencephaly
4. Congenital oral teratoma
5. Clefting ectropian
6. Premaxillary agenesis
7. Short rib, polydactyly (Majewski's sydnrome)
8. Coarse facies, hirsutism, absent fifth finger and toenails (Coffin-Sires syndrome)
9. Aglossia-adactyly (Hanhart's syndrome)
10. Buccopharyngeal membrane
11. Oral duplication

E. Chromosome defects
1. 1q+
2. 3p+
3. 3p−, q+
4. 4p−
5. Trisomy 13
6. 14q+
7. Trisomy 18
8. 18q−
9. Trisomy 22
10. 49,XXXXY
11. Triploidy
12. Many translocations

Isolated cleft palate has a different genetic predisposition than that associated with cleft lip. Mild forms of cleft palate are represented by submucosal clefts, pharyngeal incompetence with nasal speech, and bifid uvula. Occasionally a palatine torus is noted as a midline swelling of the hard palate. It has no particular medical significance but is more common in Orientals and was described in *Homo erectus* from China. A high arched palate may occur normally but is also a feature of many syndromes.

Hypertrophied alveolar ridges are apparent in the palate along the inner margin of the teeth and are suggestive of a mucopolysaccharidosis or mucolipidosis, such as I cell disease. They are also present in the Smith-Lemli-Opitz syndrome (Fig. 17-16).

Macroglossia may be relative, as in the Pierre Robin malformation complex, where the primary abnormality is mandibular hypoplasia. In other cases, such as cretinism, the mucopolysaccharidoses, or a mucolipidosis such as GM_1 gangliosidosis, the tongue appears protruding and enlarged. A cleft or irregular tongue or oral frenula occur in various syndromes such as the orofaciodigital syndrome.

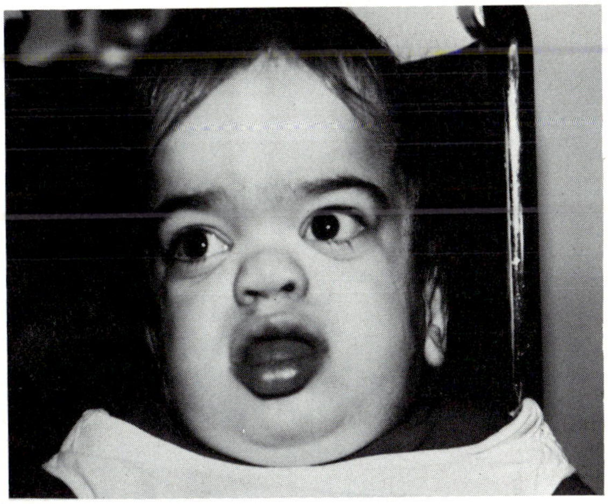

Fig. 17-15. Hurler's disease; note coarse facies, prominent lips, and large tongue.

Neck

The neck may be short with limitation of rotation, as in a Klippel-Feil anomaly, with fusion of cervical vertebrae. Excessive skinfolds are characteristic of Turner's or Noonan's syndrome (Fig. 17-17).

Chest

The thoracic cage may be unusually small as part of a skeletal dysplasia, such as thoracic asphyxiating dystrophy (Fig. 17-18). A relative increase in the anteroposterior diameter occurs in Turner's or Noonan's syndrome, but the apparent increase in internipple distance is illusionary, since it is normal relative to the chest width.

The sternum itself may be unusually short, as is typical in trisomy 18, or it may be altered in shape, as in pectus excavatum or pectus carinatum. The latter anomalies are common with a variety of skeletal dysplasias. (See Chapter 28, part five.)

Abdomen

Hypoplasia of the abdominal musculature may occur associated with in utero obstruction and other anomalies of the urogenital system resulting in a characteristic prune belly appearance (Chapter 35). An omphalocele may be part of the Beckwith-Wiedemann syndrome (Chapter 37, part one). Anomalies of a more minor na-

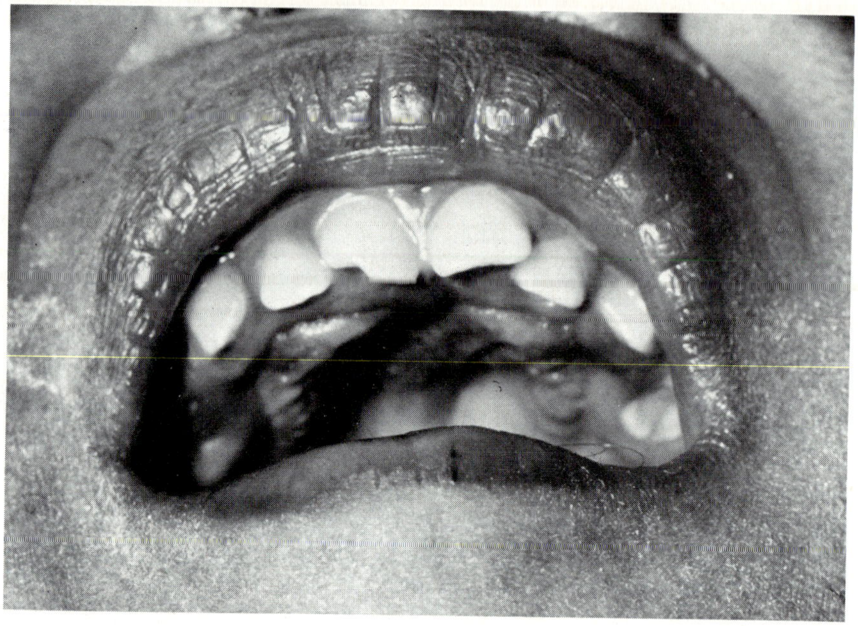

Fig. 17-16. Prominent alveolar ridges in a patient with the Smith-Lemli-Opitz syndrome.

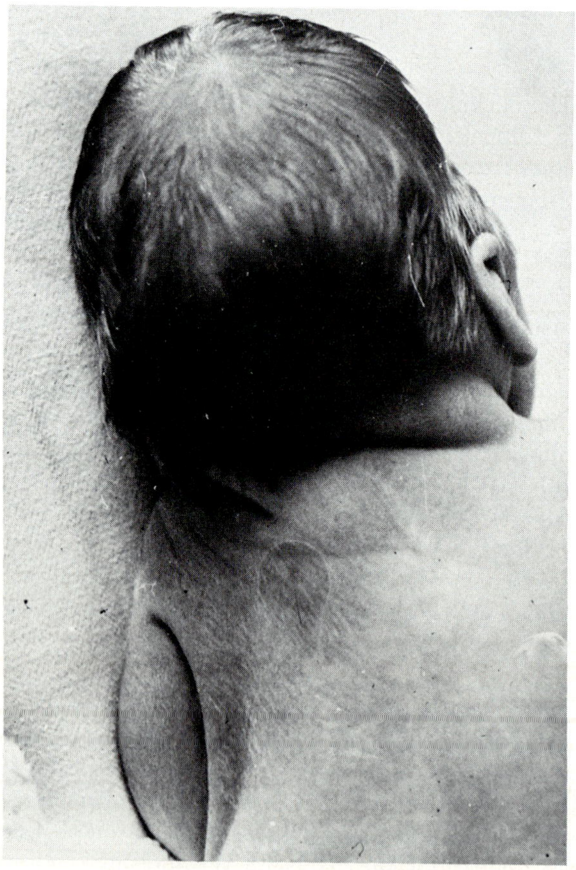

Fig. 17-17. Excess skinfolds of the neck in a patient with Turner's syndrome.

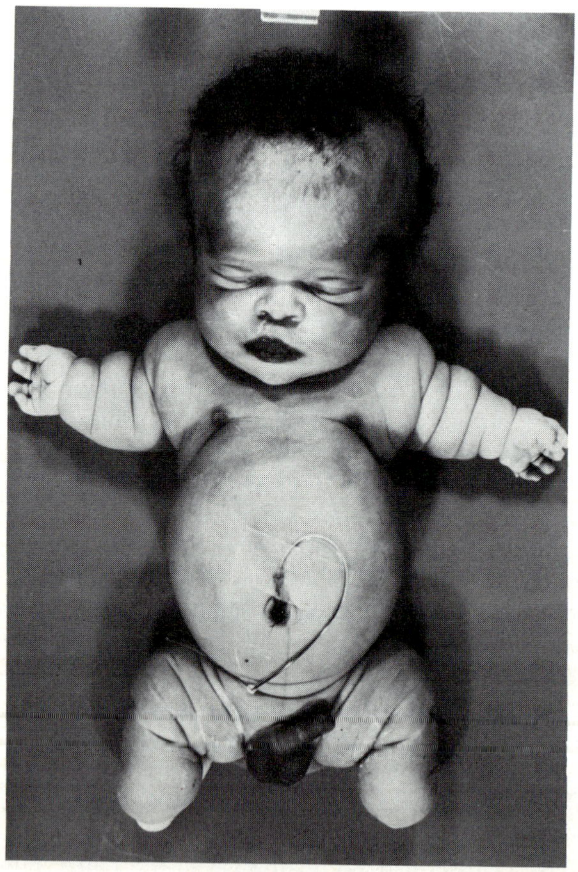

Fig. 17-18. Thanatophoric dwarf. Note the short limbs and narrow thoracic cage.

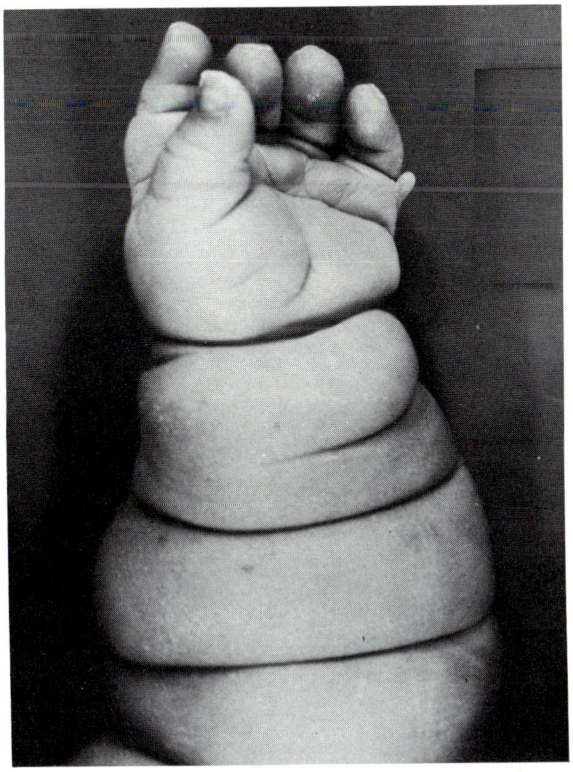

Fig. 17-19. Forearm and hand of the patient in Fig. 17-18. Note the rudimentary postaxial polydactyly.

ture, such as inguinal or umbilical hernias, occur in normal infants but are more frequent in various syndromes, particularly connective tissue disorders such as the mucopolysaccharidoses.

Anus

Imperforate anus may occur as the mildest expression of a caudal regression malformation complex, which in severe cases has extensive lower-body abnormalities (Chapter 37, part one). It also may be part of a constellation of malformations, such as the VATER association or the VACTERL association, which consists of VATER plus congenital heart and limb anomalies.

Genitalia

Abnormalities in the development of the genitalia and the associated hormonal influences are discussed in Chapter 37, part five.

Spine

Among the most common congenital anomalies are the neural tube defects, which involve abnormalities of the central nervous system along with defects in the associated bony structures. These lesions are discussed in detail in Chapter 27. Minor external anomalies, particularly of the lower spine, include unusual pigmentary lesions or hair tufts, sacral dimples and sinuses, and pilonidal sinuses. Some of these changes, such as hair tufts, may be an indication of a more significant deeper anomaly, such as diastematomyelia.

Extremities

Abnormalities of length. Extremities may be either relatively long, as occurs in Marfan's syndrome or homocystinuria, or unusually short, as occurs in a diverse number of skeletal dysplasias, the prototype and most common being achondroplasia. A simple guide to evaluating relative extremity length is to determine where the fingertips are in relation to the thighs when the upper extremities are adducted alongside the body. In the normal infant the fingertips fall below the hip joint in the midthigh region. When the upper extremities are short, they align with the hip joint or above (Fig. 17-18), and when they are relatively long, they may reach the knees. A more precise and useful measurement is to determine the upper-to-lower segment ratio. The upper segment is measured from the vertex to the pubic symphysis, and the distance from the pubis to the heel constitutes the lower segment. In normal newborns this ratio is about 1.75 and decreases with age to 0.85 in the adult. A high ratio suggests relative shortening of the extremities, and a low ratio implies either unusually long extremities or a foreshortened trunk, as may occur in spondyloepiphyseal dysplasia.

Paired extremities may be asymmetric in either length or overall size, suggesting either atrophy of one or hypertrophy of the other. The distinction may be difficult to make at times, although it is often evident if an extremity is unusually large or excessively small. Hypertrophy of limbs more often occurs on the right side and may be a manifestation of neurofibromatosis, the Beckwith-Wiedemann syndrome, or the Klippel-Weber-Trenaunay syndrome. There is also an association with Wilms' tumor as well as other tumors of the adrenal glands and liver. Isolated hemiatrophy is more common on the left side and may occur with long-standing corticospinal tract damage as well as in the Russell-Silver syndrome.

Foreshortening of long bones will lead to various limb abnormalities, depending on the segments involved. A number of terms have been used to describe such anomalies. *Amelia* refers to complete absence of a limb. *Peromelia* and *hemimelia* are both used to describe limb defects with shortened or deformed long bones. *Rhizomelia* denotes proximal shortening of the limbs, such as occurs in achondroplasia. *Phocomelia* refers to seal-like limbs in which distal segments such as the hands appear attached to the trunk as a result of marked foreshortening of the intervening segments. Such defects among other limb anomalies occurred as a consequence of maternal use of thalidomide. A shortened forearm with secondary prominence of skinfolds is shown in Fig. 17-19.

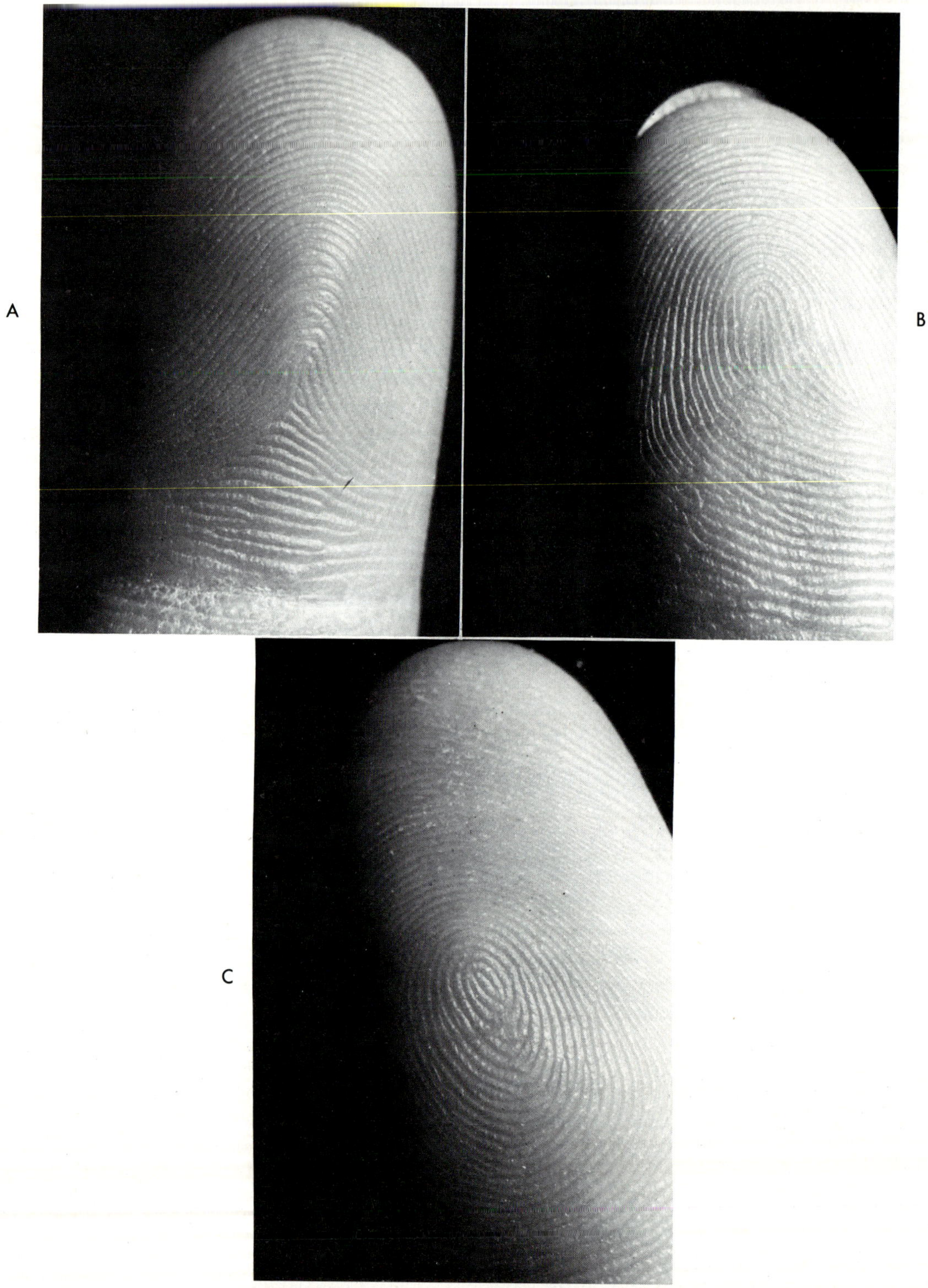

Fig. 17-20. A, Arch dermal ridge pattern. **B,** Loop dermal ridge pattern. **C,** Whorl dermal ridge pattern.

Abnormalities of hands and feet

Dermatoglyphics. The hands and feet have epidermal ridges and creases forming a variety of configurations. These dermatoglyphic patterns may be altered in various malformation syndromes and, although the changes are rarely pathognomonic of a particular condition, they provide useful additional diagnostic information. A permanent record may be obtained by using special pads and paper, or examination can be done with a magnifying glass. Epidermal ridge patterns and creases are well developed by the fourth month of gestation and are under multifactorial genetic control.

The finger patterns are divided into arches, loops, and whorls (Fig. 17-20). Triradii occur at the juncture of three sets of converging ridges. In the arch pattern, ridges enter from one side and flow to the other in an arch shape. A loop pattern has one triradius and may be open toward either the radial or ulnar side of the hand forming radial or ulnar loops, respectively. Whorls have at least two triradii and may consist of a spiral or ellipse pattern or two interlocking loops in the double whorl. Ridge count is obtained from the total number of ridges crossed by a line from the triradii up to the pattern core. The total finger ridge count averages 145 in males and 127 in females.

Palmar patterns shown in Fig. 17-21 include the distal triradii *a*, *b*, *c*, and *d* found beneath each finger from the index finger to the little finger, respectively. The axial triradius, called *t*, occurs in the axial line of the palm and is usually not more than 10% of the distance from the distal creases of the wrist to the proximal crease of the third finger. It may be displaced distally or to either side in various malformation syndromes. Normally there are two deep transverse palmar creases that do not completely cross the palm. In various conditions, such as trisomy 21, there may instead be a single transverse palmar crease, termed a *simian crease*. Simian creases may be completely transverse across the palm or may

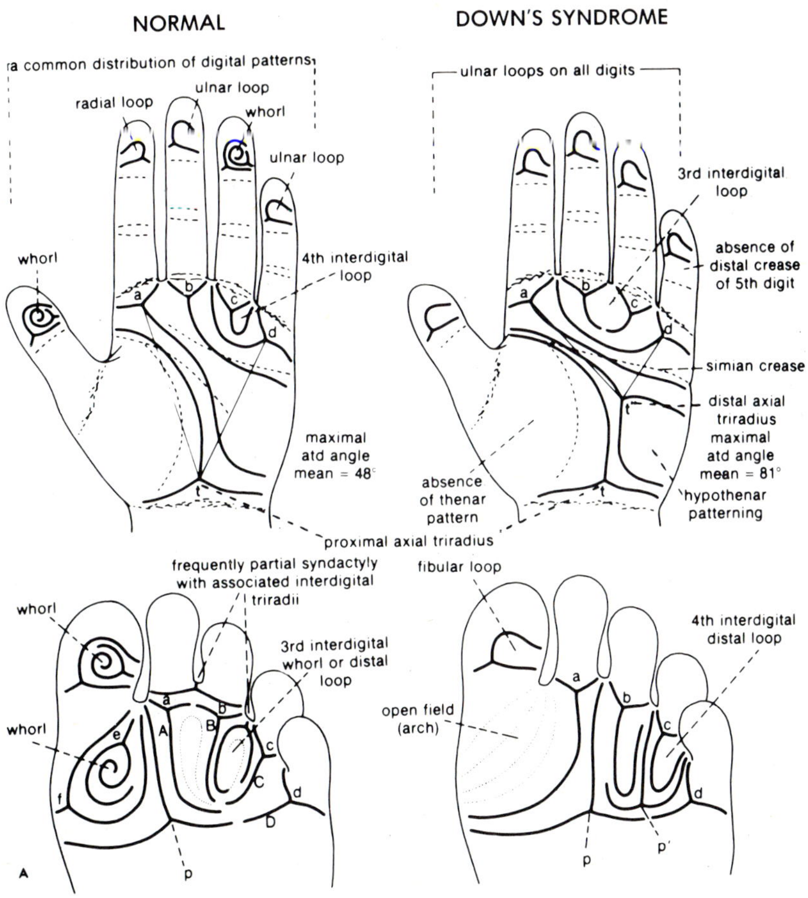

Fig. 17-21. Dermal ridge patterns of the palm and foot: normal and Down's syndrome. (From Smith, D.W.: Recognizable patterns of human malformation, Philadelphia, 1981, W.B. Saunders Co.)

A

B

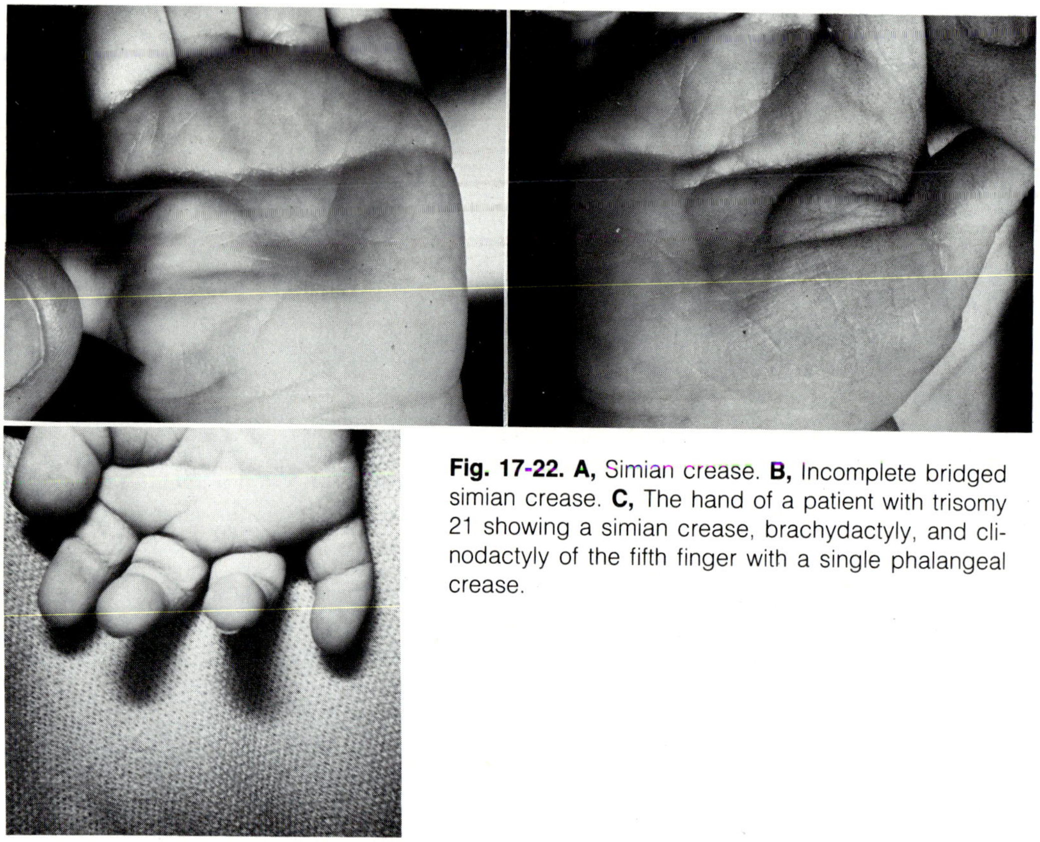

C

Fig. 17-22. A, Simian crease. **B,** Incomplete bridged simian crease. **C,** The hand of a patient with trisomy 21 showing a simian crease, brachydactyly, and clinodactyly of the fifth finger with a single phalangeal crease.

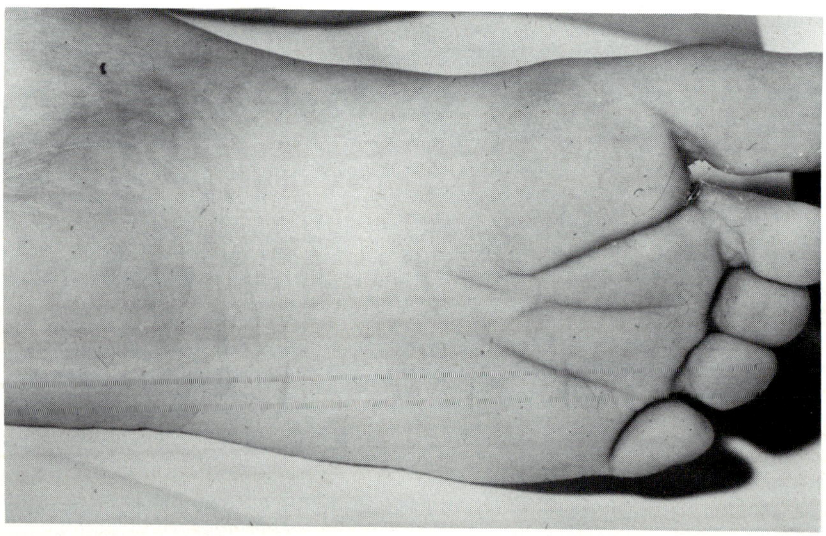

Fig. 17-23. Sandal line furrows in trisomy 8.

be incomplete (Fig. 17-22). They may become more apparent when the palm is slightly flexed. A single phalangeal crease on the fifth finger instead of the normal two also occurs commonly in trisomy 21 (Fig. 17-22).

The foot also has ridge patterns (Fig. 17-21). The great toe may have arches, loops, and whorls, and the hallucal area of the sole usually has a loop or whorl. The absence of the latter pattern, termed an open field, is frequent in trisomy 21 and other disorders. A sandal pattern of furrows is typical of trisomy 8 (Fig. 17-23). Fig 17-24 illustrates the increased separation of the first and second toes and a prominent interdigital furrow in trisomy 21.

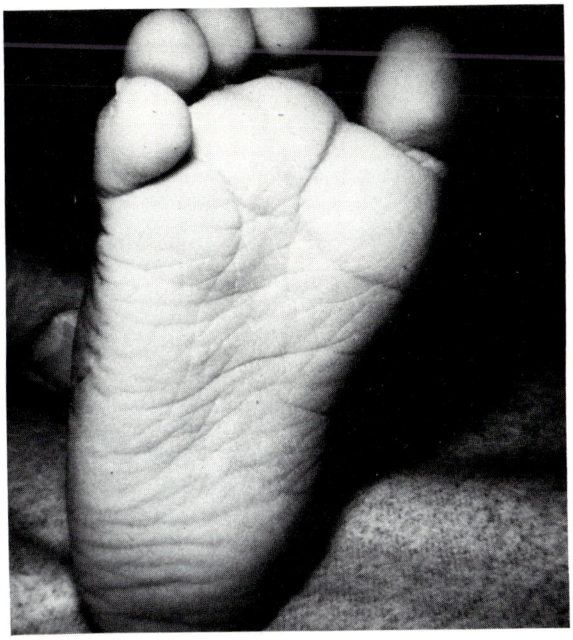

Fig. 17-24. Trisomy 21; note increased separation of the first and second toes.

Abnormalities in size and shape. The hands and feet may be enlarged as a result of lymphedema. This can be a generalized process and is characteristic of infants with Turner's or Noonan's syndrome in which the dorsum of the hands and feet may have a puffy appearance (Fig. 17-25). Congenital lymphedema can also be an autosomal dominantly inherited condition with variable expressivity.

Rocker-bottom feet (Fig. 17-26) are manifested by a prominent heel and a loss of the normal concave longitudinal arch of the sole. They are common in trisomy 18 and other syndromes.

Enlargement of the hands and feet may occur as part of a generalized growth disturbance such as cerebral gigantism or the Soto syndrome or may be a manifestation

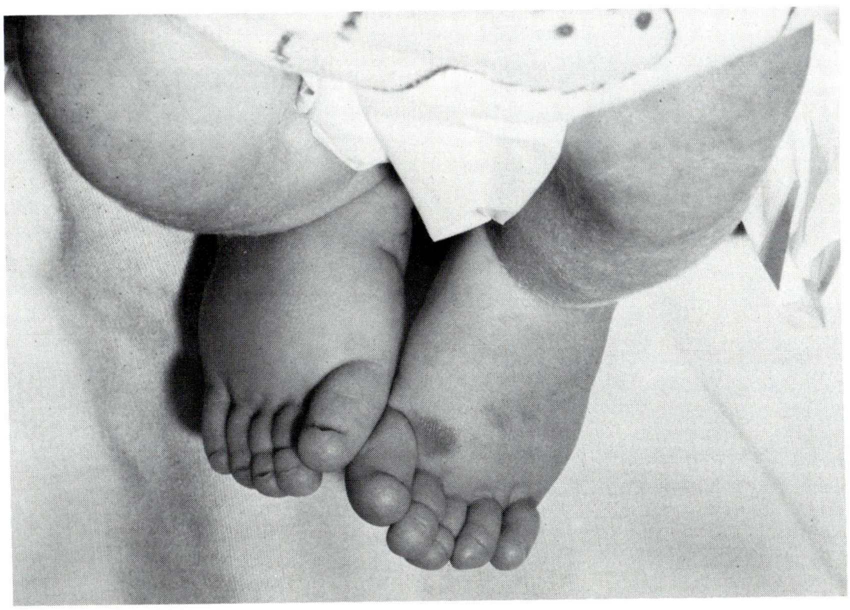

Fig. 17-25. Dorsal edema of the feet in a patient with Turner's syndrome.

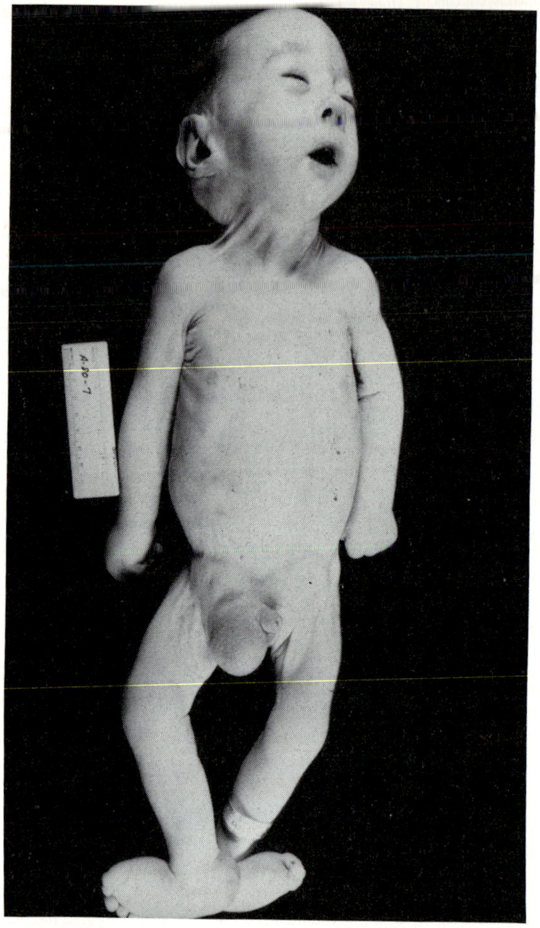

Fig. 17-26. Trisomy 18; note right hydrocele and rocker-bottom feet.

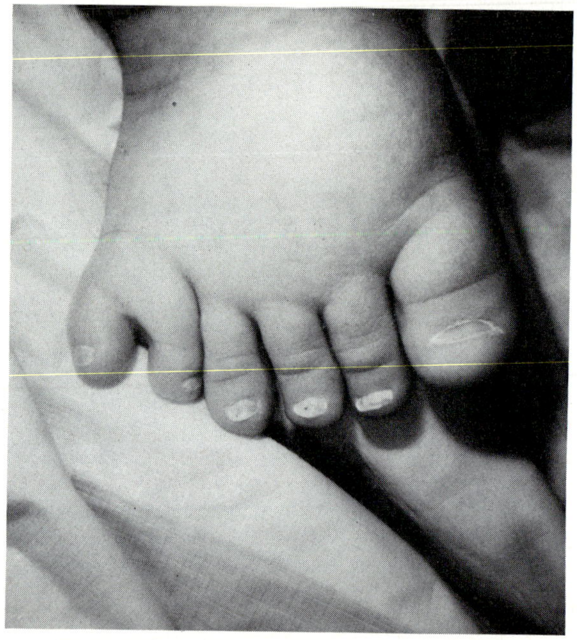

Fig. 17-27. Postaxial polydactyly.

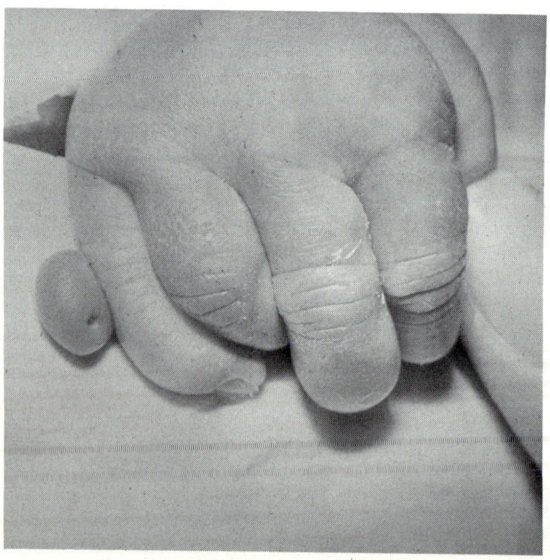

Fig. 17-28. Postaxial polydactyly in trisomy 13.

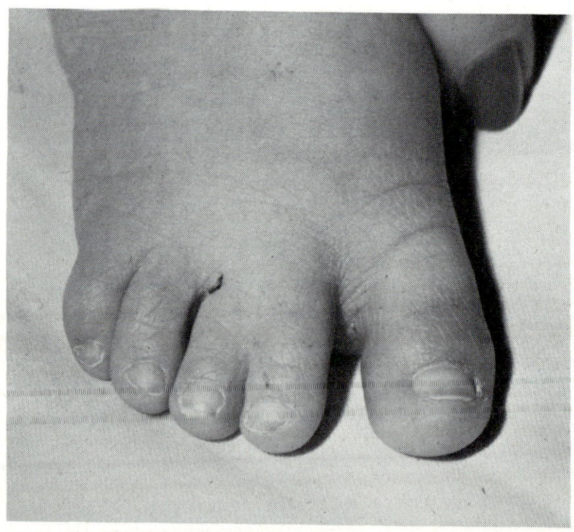

Fig. 17-29. Syndactyly between the second and third toes.

of a partial macrosomia such as in congenital hemihypertrophy, discussed previously.

Significant anomalies of the underlying bony structure will produce alterations in the normal form of the hands and feet. Such abnormalities may be classified into the following categories: absence deformities, polydactyly, syndactyly, brachydactyly, arachnodactyly, and contracture deformities. These types of anomalies are briefly discussed (Chapter 40).

The congenital absence of an entire hand is termed *acheria*, whereas absence of both hands and feet is *acheiropody*.

Ectrodactyly refers to a partial or total absence of the distal segments of a hand or foot with the proximal segments of the limbs more or less normal. All such anomalies are examples of terminal transverse defects and may occur sporadically or as part of a syndrome. It is useful to determine whether the defects involve primarily the radial or preaxial side of the limb or the ulnar or postaxial side. For example, blood dyscrasias such as the Fanconi pancytopenia syndrome, the Blackfan-Diamond syndrome, and the thrombocytopenia–absent radius (TAR) syndrome commonly involve radial defects (Chapter 32). Ulnar defects of a limb are frequent in the Cornelia de Lange syndrome.

Polydactyly refers to partial or complete supernumerary digits and is one of the most common hand malformations. Postaxial polydactyly is more frequent than preaxial, particularly in blacks; two types, A and B, can be distinguished. In type A there are fully developed extra digits (Fig. 17-27); in type B there are rudimentary digits. As an isolated anomaly, polydactyly may be inherited as an autosomal dominant trait. It also may be a manifestation of multiple malformations. Postaxial polydactyly may occur in a variety of syndromes, including trisomy 13 (Fig. 17-28), chondroectodermal dysplasia, asphyxiating thoracic dystrophy (Fig. 17-19), Noonan's syndrome, the Meckel-Gruber syndrome, and the Laurence-Moon-Bardet-Biedl syndrome. Preaxial polydactyly is characteristic of the Carpenter type of acrocephalosyndactyly and the Majewski short rib polydactyly syndrome.

Syndactyly refers to a fusion of digits, which may be solely cutaneous or involve bone as well. It is the most common congenital malformation of the hand and is a normal characteristic in some marsupials, rodents, and various primates. Minimal syndactyly of the second and third toes is common in normal newborns. An excessive amount is shown in Fig. 17-29. As an isolated anomaly, different clinical types may be distinguished, but each of them is inherited as an autosomal dominant trait with variable expressivity and incomplete penetrance.

Syndactyly also may be part of a syndrome, and typical examples include the various forms of acrocephalosyndactyly, such as the Apert, Saethre-Chotzen, and Pfeiffer syndromes.

Brachydactyly is a shortening of the digits due to anomalous development of any of the phalanges, metacarpals, or metatarsals. Various clinical types may be distinguished, but most isolated forms of brachydactyly are inherited in an autosomal dominant fashion. It is also a component of numerous skeletal dysplasias such as achondroplasia.

Arachnodactyly refers to unusually long, spiderlike digits and is characteristic but not invariable in the Marfan syndrome and homocystinuria. These may be distinguished on various clinical grounds, including the congenital occurrence of ectopia lentis in Marfan's syndrome but not in homocystinuria. Arachnodactyly and associated dolichostenomelia also occur in the Marfanoid hypermobility syndrome, congenital contractural arachnodactyly and the Achard syndrome.

Joint deformities. A variety of congenital joint deformities involving the limbs may occur. *Arthrogryposis* refers to multiple congenital contractures that are most often sporadic and may be associated with oligohydramnios or be the result of some underlying neuromuscular abnormality. Talipes equinovarus or calcaneovalgus deformities of the ankle are common isolated joint contractures (Chapter 40). Limitation of movement of joints or contractures occur in numerous syndromes. Joint hypermobility is frequent in various connective tissue disorders, such as the Marfan and Ehlers-Danlos syndromes.

Cubitus valgus refers to an increase in the angle formed by the arm and forearm with the elbow extended. This angle is more acute in normal females and those with the Turner or Noonan syndrome.

Camptodactyly is a flexion contracture involving the proximal interphalangeal joints. In the hand it practically always involves the fifth finger but may affect other fingers as well. *Dupuytren's contracture* is a flexion deformity of the digits at their proximal interphalangeal joints due to thickening and shortening of the palmar fascia. Both isolated camptodactyly and Dupuytren's contracture may be inherited as autosomal dominant traits, but they can be distinguished because the latter does not usually appear until middle age. Camptodactyly also may be part of a syndrome such as trisomy 8, trisomy 10q, the cerebrohepatorenal syndrome of Zellweger, and the whistling face syndrome of Freeman-Sheldon.

Camptodactyly should be distinguished from clinodactyly, which designates an incurving of a digit, most often the fifth finger. This is common in trisomy 21 and other syndromes. A characteristic clinodactyly involving the fourth and fifth fingers radially and second finger in an ulnar direction occurs in trisomy 18, or less often trisomy 13 (Fig. 17-30).

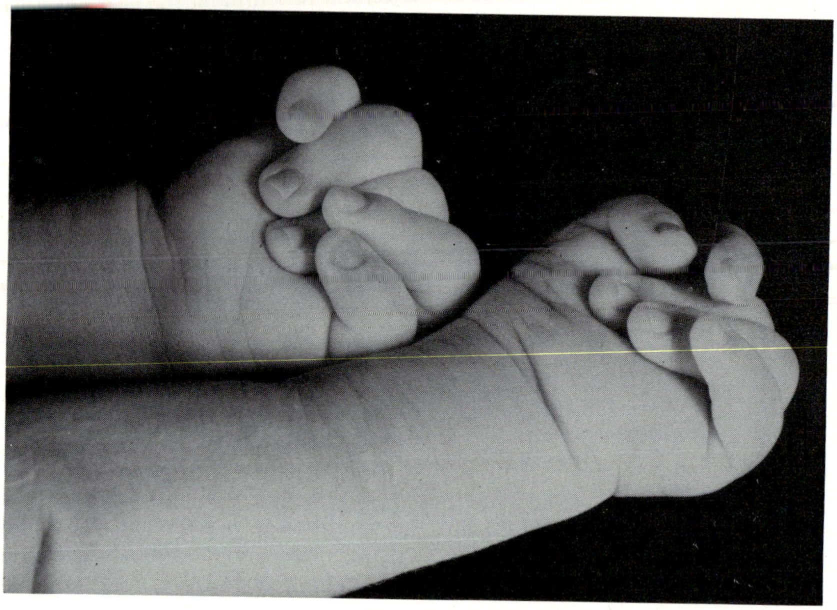

Fig. 17-30. Trisomy 18; note characteristic clinodactyly of the second, fourth, and fifth fingers.

After the clinical examination

Once the history and clinical findings are noted, various laboratory studies may be indicated to confirm or establish a diagnosis. TORCH titers and chromosome analyses are frequently obtained from blood specimens. Chromosome studies are essential in every case of multiple minor or major malformations of unclear etiology. It must be remembered, however, that multiple malformations also can be the consequence of a single mutant gene. Chromosome studies are therefore only part of the appropriate diagnostic evaluation. They are also indicated in known chromosome syndromes such as Down's syndrome, since the chromosomal aberration may be sporadic or hereditary, and clinical evaluation alone cannot make the distinction. If a structural chromosomal rearrangment is detected, such as an inversion, deletion, or translocation, then additional chromosome studies will usually be necessary in both parents to determine if either is a carrier for an abnormal chromosome. The malformed infant who is stillborn or dies soon after birth also should have a thorough evaluation, including photographs, radiographs, chromosome studies, and complete postmortem examination. A common error is failure to obtain tissue for chromosome studies. Although a blood sample may not be adequate in a dying or dead infant, tissue such as amnion, skin, thymus, lung, or gonad can be obtained sterilely after death for tissue culture and subsequent chromosome analysis. Failure to do so may forever obscure a diagnosis and a significant genetic recurrence risk for the family.

The physician who evaluates infants with congenital anomalies should be familiar with standard references on teratogens and malformation syndromes. These are listed in the bibliography. Puzzling cases may require referral to various specialists, particularly when there are multiple organ system malformations. Ultimately the patient may be seen by a clinical geneticist, who may be involved not only in the initial diagnostic evaluation but also in continued follow-up and treatment, as well as providing genetic counseling for the family.

GENETIC COUNSELING

See also Chapter 16.

The goals of genetic counseling are to provide information in meaningful fashion to an individual or family in regard to a hereditary or potentially teratogenic condition and to provide emotional support in the adjustment to a serious birth defect. It is equally as important to state that a problem is not of genetic origin as it is to explain a specific genetic abnormality. Since many malformations have a relatively low risk of recurrence, a negative family history is common. The family may assume, however, that the absence of affected relatives means that the problem is not a genetic disorder. Furthermore, they may blame themselves or implicate some other unrelated factor as a cause for the condition. It is important to clarify these misconceptions and to relieve the individual and family of any unwarranted guilt for a problem over which they had no control. Malformations that lead to serious disability or death cause a grief reaction in the parents, which may require more extensive supportive counseling.

The basis for an accurate assessment of the risk of recurrence of a birth defect is a specific diagnosis. Abnormalities that are the consequence of a single mutant gene will have a probability of recurrence that depends on the mendelian pattern of inheritance. Thus an autosomal dominant condition will have a 50% recurrence risk for an affected parent. The risk of recurrence for an autosomal recessive trait is 25%, and in this case both parents are usually asymptomatic carriers of the mutant allele. Dominantly inherited conditions may occasionally arise for the first time in a family as a new mutation, and in this situation limited data may make it difficult to differentiate them from an autosomal recessive disorder. The latter is not likely to originate in one individual as a consequence of mutation, since two rare mutational events would be necessary. In X-linked recessive disorders the risk in most cases is confined to male offspring of asymptomatic carrier mothers. For such males the risk is 50%, whereas the female sibs have a 50% chance of being carriers like their mother. In an X-linked recessive disorder, females can be affected if their mothers are carriers or are affected and their fathers are affected also, an unlikely combination. However, the normal random inactivation of one of the X chromosomes in females can occasionally result in a predominance of cells expressing the mutant allele, resulting in some clinical expression in carrier females. X-linked dominant disorders are the least common single gene traits, and in this case male and female offspring have a 50% risk when the mother is affected. When the father is affected, all the daughters, but none of the sons, will be affected by an X-linked dominant disorder.

Chromosome disorders have variable risks of recurrence depending on the specific abnormality and condition. The common form of trisomy 21 due to nondisjunction has a 1% empirically determined recurrence risk. The general risk also increases particularly with maternal age over 35. Trisomy 21 due to translocation has a risk of recurrence dependent on the nature of the translocation and which parent is the carrier of the abnormal chromosome. It can be as high as 100% in a 21 to 21 translocation.

Many of the common major malformations are inherited in a multifactorial manner, and the risks of recurrence are based on empirical data from large numbers of families. Generally the recurrence risk for a second affected offspring will be approximately 2% to 5%. Unlike mendelian inheritance, the risk increases with the number of affected relatives and decreases with decreasing genetic relationship to the affected proband. Table 17-2 summarizes some empirical risk figures for various common malformations.

In addition to informing the family about recurrence risks, genetic counseling also must consider the possibility of prenatal diagnosis (Chapter 16). The standard procedures include ultrasonography for evaluation of fetal growth and structural defects, and amniocentesis to obtain fluid and cells for various studies. The amniotic fluid is routinely assayed for *alpha-fetoprotein*, which may be significantly elevated if the fetus has a neural tube defect, an abdominal wall abnormality, or certain other malformations. The cells are cultured for chromosome studies. Various biochemical tests may be performed on either the fluid or the cells for specific disorders. The DNA may be extracted from the cells and examined for the presence of a specific mutant gene by using recombinant DNA methodology.

These newer molecular genetic approaches make possible a direct determination of the genotype and have simplified the prenatal diagnosis of hemoglobin disorders such as sickle cell anemia. Before the application of recombinant DNA techniques, the prenatal diagnosis of such disorders required fetal blood sampling by fetoscopy, a procedure associated with significant risks and performed only in a few centers. The continued development of DNA probes for specific mutant genes will play an important role in expanding the prenatal diagnosis of mendelian disorders.

Amniocentesis is usually performed at 15 to 18 weeks' gestation, but earlier prenatal diagnosis may be accomplished by chorionic villus sampling, a newer technique being evaluated in various centers. This procedure is done at 9 to 10 weeks and utilizes a suction tube to withdraw chorionic villi for chromosomal and biochemical studies.

Maternal serum alpha-fetoprotein screening at 15 to 18 weeks' pregnancy is increasingly used to detect pregnancies at risk for an adverse outcome, including congenital anomalies in the fetus. This simple blood test may detect an affected fetus in the absence of any positive family history. High values are associated with multiple gestations, neural tube defects, omphalocoeles, congenital nephrosis, and other problems. Low values may indicate a chromosome disorder such as trisomy 21. Routine maternal serum alpha-fetoprotein screening programs require coordination with genetic counseling and prenatal diagnostic services; they are a significant development in obstetric care and the prevention of birth defects.

Thaddeus W. Kurczynski

Acknowledgment

Various photographs of patients were graciously provided by Drs. Haynes B. Robinson, Avroy Fanaroff, and Samuel J. Horwitz.

BIBLIOGRAPHY

General

Beighton, P.: Inherited disorders of the skeleton, New York, 1978, Churchill Livingstone, Inc.

Bergsma, D.: Birth defects compendium, New York, 1979, Alan R. Liss, Inc.

de Grouchy, J., and Turleau, C.: Clinical atlas of human chromosomes, New York, 1984, John Wiley and Sons, Inc.

Dyken, P.R., and Miller, M.D.: Facial features of neurologic syndromes, St. Louis, 1980, The C.V. Mosby Co.

Gellis, S.S., and Feingold, M.: Atlas of mental retardation syndromes, Washington, D.C., 1968, U.S. Government Printing Office.

Goodman, R.M., and Gorlin, R.J.: Atlas of the face in genetic disorders, St. Louis, 1977, The C.V. Mosby Co.

Goodman, R.M., and Gorlin, R.J.: The malformed infant and child, New York, 1983, Oxford University Press.

Gorlin, R.J., Cohen, M.M., Jr., and Pindborg, J.J.: Syndromes of the head and neck, New York, 1975, McGraw-Hill Book Co., Inc.

McKusick, V.A.: Mendelian inheritance in man: catalog of autosomal dominant, autosomal recessive, and X-linked phenotypes, Baltimore, 1986, The Johns Hopkins University Press.

Myrianthopoulos, N.C.: Malformations in children from one to seven years, a report from the collaborative perinatal project, New York, 1985, Alan R. Liss, Inc.

Nyhan, W.L., and Sakati, N.O.: Genetic and malformation syndromes in clinical medicine, Chicago, 1973, Year Book Medical Publishers, Inc.

Patten, B.M.: Human embryology, New York, 1953, McGraw-Hill Book Co., Inc.

Smith, D.W.: Recognizable patterns of human malformation, Philadelphia, 1981, W.B. Saunders Co.

Spanger, J.W., Langer, L.O., and Wiedemann, H.R.: Bone dysplasias: an atlas of constitutional disorders of skeletal development, Philadelphia, 1974, W.B. Saunders Co.

Temtamy, S.A., and McKusick, V.A.: The genetics of hand malformations, Birth Defects **4**(3), 1978.

Warkany, J.: Congenital malformations, Chicago, 1971, Year Book Medical Publishers, Inc.

Warkany, J., Lemire, R.J., and Cohen, M.M.: Mental retardation and congenital malformations of the nervous system, Chicago, 1981, Year Book Medical Publishers, Inc.

Wynne-Davies, R.: Heritable disorders in orthopedic practice, Oxford, 1973, Blackwell Scientific Publications, Ltd.

Terminology

Freire-Maia, N.: Congenital skeletal limb deficiencies—a general review, Birth Defects **5**(3):7, 1969.

Holmes, L.B.: Inborn errors of morphogenesis: a review of localized hereditary malformations, N. Engl. J. Med. **192**:763, 1974.

Holmes, L.B.: Current concepts in genetics: congenital malformations, N. Engl. J. Med. **195**:204, 1976.

Merboli, P., Swan, Y., and Reisner, S.H.: Anthropometric measurements of the newborn infant, Birth Defects **20**(7), 1984.

Montagu, M.F.A.: A handbook of anthropometry, Springfield, Ill., 1960, Charles C Thomas, Publisher.

O'Rahilly, R.: The nomenclature and classification of limb anomalies, Birth Defects **5**(3):14, 1969.

Spranger, J., and others: Errors of morphogenesis: concepts and terms, J. Pediatr. **100**:160, 1982.

Epidemiology and genetics

Carr, D.H., and Gedeon, M.: Population cytogenetics of human abortuses. In Hook, E.B., and Porter, I.H., editors: Population cytogenetics, New York, 1977, Academic Press, Inc.

Emanuel, I., and others: The incidence of congenital malformations in a Chinese population: the Taipei collaborative study, Teratology **5**:159, 1972.

Erickson, J.D.: Racial variations in the incidence of congenital malformations, Ann. Hum. Genet. **39**:315, 1976.

Holmes, L.B.: Congenital malformations: incidence, racial differences and recognized etiologies. In Biologic and clinical aspects of malformations, Mead Johnson Symposium on Perinatal and Developmental Medicine, no. 7, Evansville, Ind., 1976, Mead Johnson.

Hook, E.B., and others: Some aspects of the epidemiology of human minor birth defects and morphological variants in a completely ascertained newborns population (Madison study), Teratology **13**:47, 1976.

Jacobs, D.A., Melville, M., and Ratcliff, S.: A cytogenetic survey of 11,680 newborn infants, Ann. Hum. Genet. **37**:359, 1974.

Marden, P.M., Smith, D.W., and McDonald, M.J.: Congenital anomalies in the newborn infant, including minor variations, J. Pediatr. **64**:357, 1964.

Nelson, T., Oakley, G.P., Jr., and Shepard, T.H.: Collection of human embryos and fetuses. In Hook, E.B., Javevick, D.T., and Porter, I.A., editors: Monitoring birth defects and environment: the problem of surveillance, New York, 1971, Academic Press, Inc.

Nishimura, H.: Incidence of malformations in abortions. In Fraser, F.C., and McKusick, V.A., editors: Proceedings of the Third International Conference on Birth Defects, New York, 1969, Excerpta Medica.

Warshaw, J.B., and Holmes, L.B.: Congenital malformations—some genetics, embryological and environmental considerations. In Genetics and the perinatal patient, Mead Johnson Symposium on Perinatal and Developmental Medicine, no. 1, Evansville, Ind., 1973, Mead Johnson.

Teratogenic states

Clarren, S.K., and Smith, D.W.: The fetal alcohol syndrome, N. Engl. J. Med. **298**:1063, 1978.

Committee on Drugs, American Academy of Pediatrics: Anticonvulsants and pregnancy, Pediatrics **63**:331, 1979.

Council on Scientific Affairs: Fetal effects of maternal alcohol use, JAMA **249**:2517, 1983.

Dalessio, D.J.: Seizure disorders and pregnancy, N. Engl. J. Med. **312**:559, 1985.

Day, R.E., and Insley, J.: Maternal diabetes mellitus and congenital malformation, Arch. Dis. Child **51**:935, 1976.

DeLa Cruz, E., and others: Multiple congenital malformations associated with maternal isotretinoin therapy, Pediatrics **74**:428, 1984.

Dudgeon, J.A.: Infective causes of human malformations, Br. Med. Bull. **32**:77, 1976.

Hanshaw, J.B., and Dudgeon, N.A.: Viral diseases of the fetus and newborn, Philadelphia, 1978, W.B. Saunders Co.

Heinonen, O.P., Slone, D., and Shapiro, S.: Birth defects and drugs in pregnancy, Boston, 1982, Wright-PSG, Inc.

Kelly, T.E.: Teratogenicity of anticonvulsant drugs. I. Review of the literature, Am. J. Med. Gen. **19**:413, 1984.

Kelly, T.E.: Teratogenicity of anticonvulsant drugs. III. Radiographic hand analysis of children exposed in utero to diphenylhydantoin, Am. J. Med. Gen. **19**:445, 1984.

Kelly, T.E., Rein, M., and Edwards, P.: Teratogenicity of anticonvulsant drugs. IV. The association of clefting and epilepsy, Am. J. Med. Gen. **19**:451, 1984.

Kelly, T.E., and others: Teratogenicity of anticonvulsant drugs. II. A prospective study, Am. J. Med. Gen. **19**:435, 1984.

Lammer, R.J., and others: Retinotic acid embryopathy, N. Engl. Med. **313**:837, 1985.

Lenke, R., and Levy, H.L.: Maternal phenylketonuria and hyperphenylalaninemia, N. Engl. J. Med. **303**:1202, 1980.

Levy, H.L., and Waisbren, S.E.: Effects of untreated maternal phenylketonuria and hyperphenylalaninemia on the fetus, N. Engl. J. Med. **309**:1269, 1983.

Monson, R.R., and others: Diphenylhydantoin and selected congenital malformations, N. Engl. J. Med. **289**:1049, 1973.

Nishimura, H., and Tanimura, T.: Clinical aspects of the teratogenicity of drugs, Amsterdam, 1976, Excerpta Medica, American Elsevier—North Holland.

Passage, E.: Congenital malformations and maternal diabetics, Lancet **1**:324, 1965.

Pedersen, L.M., Tygstrup, I., and Pedersen, J.: Congenital malformations in newborn infants of diabetic women, Lancet **1**:1124, 1964.

Rosett, H.L., and others: Patterns of alcohol consumption and fetal development, Obstet. Gynecol. **61**:539, 1983.

Rowland, T.W., Hubbell, J.P., Jr., and Nadas, A.S.: Congenital heart disease in infants of diabetic mothers, J. Pediatr. **83**:815, 1973.

Rutsteins, D.D., and Veech, R.L.: Genetics and addictions to alcohol, N. Engl. J. Med. **298**:1140, 1978.

Shephard, T.H.: Catalog of teratogenic agents, Baltimore, 1980. The Johns Hopkins University Press.

Simpson, J.L.: Genetics of diabetes mellitus and anomalies in offspring of diabetic mothers. In Merkatz, I.R., and Adam., P.A.J., editors: The diabetic pregnancy: a perinatal perspective, New York, 1979, Grune and Stratton, Inc.

Stumpf, D.A.: Anticonvulsant use during pregnancy, Clin. Therapeutics **7**:258, 1985.

Selected malformations

Alexious, D., and others: Frequency of other malformations in congenital hypoplasia of depressor anguli oris muscle syndrome, Arch. Dis. Child. **51**:891, 1976.

Banks, H.H.: Birth defects and the orthopedic surgeon, Orthopedic Clinics of North America, vol. 7, no. 2, Philadelphia, 1976, W.B. Saunders Co.

Bergoma, D., and Lenz, W., editors: Morphogenesis and malformations of the limb, Birth Defects, vol. 13, no. 1, 1977.

Collins, E.: The illusion of widely spaced nipples in the Noonan and Turner syndromes, J. Pediatr. **83**:557, 1973.

DeMyer, W.: The median cleft face syndrome, Neurology **17**:961, 1967.

DeMyer, W.: Median facial malformations and their implications for brain malformations, Birth Defects **11**(7):155, 1975.

Gorlin, R.J., Cervenka, J., and Pruzansky, S.: Facial clefting and its syndromes, Birth Defects **12**(7):3, 1971.

Hanson, J.W., and Smith, D.W.: U-shaped palatal defect in the Robin anomalad: developmental and clinical relevance, J. Pediatr. **87**:30, 1975.

Hanson, J.W., Smith, D.W., and Cohen, N.N., Jr.: Prominent lateral palatine ridges: developmental and clinical relevance, J. Pediatr. **89**:54, 1976.

Heyn, R., Kurczynski, E., and Schmickel, R.: The association of Blackfan-Diamond syndrome, physical abnormalities, and an abnormality of chromosome 1, J. Pediatr. **85**:531, 1974.

Jaffe, B.F.: Pinna anomalies associated with congenital conductive hearing loss, Pediatrics **57**:332, 1976.

Jones, K.L., Hanson, J.W., and Smith, D.A.: Palpebral fissure size in newborn infants, J. Pediatr. **92**:787, 1978.

King, C.R., and Prescott, G.: Pathogenesis of the prune belly anomalad, J. Pediatr. **93**:273, 1978.

Noveh, Y., and Friedman, A.: Familial imperforate anus, Am. J. Dis. Child. **130**:441, 1976.

Paradice, B.A., and Poland, B.J.: A 94 mm human fetus with the VACTERL association of anomalies, Teratology **13**:21, 1976.

Popich, G.A., and Smith, D.W.: The genesis and significance of digital and palmar hand creases: preliminary report, J. Pediatr. **77**:1917, 1970.

Quan, L., and Smith, D.W.: The VATER association: vertebral defects, anal atresia, tracheo-esophageal fistula with esophageal atresia, radial dysplasia, Birth Defects 8(2):75, 1972.

Rapin, I., and Ruben, R.J.: Patterns of anomalies in children with malformed ears, Laryngoscope **86**:1469, 1976.

Ross, R.B.: Lateral facial dysplasia, Birth Defects **11**(7):51, 1975.

Schaumann, B., and Alter, M.: Dermatoglyphics in medical disorders, New York, 1976, Springer-Verlag.

Schnall, B.S., and Smith, D.W.: Normandom laterality of malformations in paired structures, J. Pediatr. **85**:509, 1974.

Sedano, H.O., and others: Frontonasal dysplasia, J. Pediatr. **76**:906, 1970.

Smith, D.W., and Greely, M.J.: Unruly scalp hair in infancy: its nature and relevance to problems of brain morphogenesis, Pediatrics **61**:783, 1978.

Woodard, J.R.: The prune belly syndrome, Urol. Clin. North Am. **5**:75, 1978.

Wilkens, L.: The diagnosis and treatment of endocrine disorders in childhood and adolescence, Springfield, Ill., 1966, Charles C Thomas, Publisher.

Wynne-Davis, R., and Lloyd-Roberts, G.C.: Arthrogryposis multiplex congenita, Arch. Dis. Child. **51**:618, 1976.

Human genetics, genetic counseling, and prenatal diagnosis

Bonaiti-Pellie, C., and Smith, C.: Risk tables for genetic counseling in some common congenital malformations, J. Med. Genet. **11**:374, 1974.

Ferguson-Smith, M.A.: Early prenatal diagnosis, Brit. Med. Bull. **39**(4), Oct. 1983.

Fuhrman, W., and Vogel, F.: Genetic counseling, New York, 1986, Springer-Verlag.

Galton, D.J.: Molecular genetics of common metabolic disease, New York, 1985, John Wiley & Sons, Inc.

Garver, K.L., and Marchese, S.G.: Genetic counseling for clinicians, Chicago, 1986, Year Book Medical Publishers, Inc.

Golbus, M.S., and others: Prenatal diagnosis in 3,000 amniocenteses, N. Engl. J. Med. **300**:157, 1979.

Kelly, T.E.: Clinical genetics and genetic counseling, Chicago, 1980, Year Book Medical Publishers, Inc.

Milunsky, A.: Genetic disorders and the fetus, New York, 1979, Plenum Publishing Corp.

The NICHD National Registry for Amniocentesis Study Group: Midtrimester amniocentesis for prenatal diagnosis, JAMA **236**:1471, 1976.

Nora, J.J., and Fraser, F.C.: Medical genetics: principles and practice, Philadelphia, 1974, Lea & Febiger.

Thompson, J.S., and Thompson, M.W.: Genetics in medicine, Philadelphia, 1986, W.B. Saunders Co.

Vogel, F., and Molulsky, A.G.: Human genetics, New York, 1979, Springer-Verlag.

CHAPTER 18

Bioethics of the mother, fetus, and newborn

Bioethics is the synthesis of the traditional principles of ethics with the goals of medical practice. Bioethics provides a basis for both good medical behavior and a guide for appropriate decision making. Good clinical medicine is ethical medicine with the overall intent of a satisfactory outcome for the patient with the physician acting as a patient advocate.

The goals of good clinical medicine are based on the assumption that medicine is engaged on behalf of the patient. These goals include the cure or prevention of disease, the care of suffering and relief of symptoms, the restoration of impaired function, and the alleviation of pain. Additional goals include patient education, counseling, and avoiding harm. Although these goals are sound and just, there are often difficulties interpreting what action is in the best interest of a patient who has a complicated clinical problem. Inherent in the dilemma of interpretation is the additional important concern of who should decide what is in the best interest for a particular patient. Previous arbitrary decisions of nontreatment of handicapped infants have resulted in a need for clear procedural (who is to decide) and substantive (by what criteria) principles for future decision making.

Traditional principles of bioethical decision making

Patient preferences	Autonomy
Medical indications	Beneficence/nonmaleficence
Quality of life	Beneficence/utilitarianism
External factors	Justice/utilitarianism

Modified from Jonsen, A., Siegler, M., and Winslade, W.: Clinical ethics: a practical approach to ethical decisions in clinical medicine, New York, 1982, Macmillan Publishing Company.

These principles must be morally defensible and not based on ad hoc biased opinions.

Bioethical problems are usually very complex and associated with conflicts, disagreements among family or caretakers, or uncertainty about the patient's treatment or outcome. Physicians have very organized systems concerning how to approach medical problems, such as the review of systems, history and physical examination, and laboratory tests. However, there is also a need to analyze ethical problems in the same organized systematic approach. The ethical approach to a clinical problem must take into consideration the risks and the benefits of therapy, but more important the ethical assessment must include a detailed analysis of the principles of autonomy, beneficence/nonmaleficence (doing good/not doing harm), and justice. (See box below). The physician's moral obligations to the patient are interpreted in terms of these three ethical principles. Traditionally, these principles have been applied to the competent adult patient. Ethics that involves the pregnant woman, the fetus, and the newborn needs to be adapted to the perinatal period to avoid applying adult standards or criteria of decision making to these patients. Applying adult standards may potentially discriminate against the fetus or newborn infant.

AUTONOMY (PATIENT PREFERENCES)

Autonomy, both as a legal and an ethical principle, pertains to a competent adult patient. Autonomy is synonymous with freedom of choice and the right of self-rule or self-determination. A competent patient should have the wisdom to determine what is right for the patient based on the patient's values, principles, and rational beliefs. The physician's respect for the patient's autonomy and preferences is a moral obligation based on the concept that competent individuals are the best judges of their own best interests. A competent patient has the best understanding and perspective of what is in that individual's own best interests. Whether or not the patient's choice appears to be in his or her own best interest, the physician must respect the patient's rights.

The principle of informed consent provides guidelines for honoring the patient's autonomy in medical decision making. Important information is given to the patient out of respect for his or her autonomy to achieve an action that will be in the patient's best interests. Only after this information is explained can a patient give informed consent. Truthful disclosure, with informed consent, is good ethical medicine and not just a legal defense. One of the goals of informed consent is patient education. Informed consent will enhance patient autonomy and permit more educated decision making. The new information can be combined with the patient's prior values and beliefs and permit the patient to make an appropriate medical decision.

Informed consent may be defined as the amount of information that a reasonable person would require to make an appropriate medical decision. Full disclosure of all the pertinent information is essential to understand the risk-to-benefit ratio and thus be able to make an informed autonomous decision. The patient needs to know whatever is necessary to make such decisions. Therapeutic privilege or withholding of information to "protect" the patient is not justifiable in the vast majority of clinical situations. Withholding of information is justified only if the patient refuses to know the information or in the very unusual circumstance when this knowledge will severely upset the patient, making the patient incapable of decision making. Physician paternalism, often falsely justified in an attempt to do good, is in direct conflict with the physician's obligation to respect the patient's autonomy. It is morally wrong to think that patients are incapable of understanding medical facts, thus causing them to be incapable of making educated decisions.

Why patients refuse treatment

- Anger
- Fear of treatment
- Denial
- Depression
- Misunderstanding of severity of illness
- Religious belief
- Unusual belief
- Irrational belief
- Wish for control
- True incapacity due to acute or chronic dementia

It is also incorrect to think that paternalistic decision making by physicians avoids guilt on the part of the patients or parents. Parents will experience guilt even though the decision to withdraw support was made by the physician. It is far better for the patient to make decisions voluntarily—without coercion, duress, deceit, or manipulation. If physicians ignore the competent patient's preferences, distrust may develop in the patient-physician relationship. Absence of informed consent may constitute battery. Not giving information to the pregnant patient who is at risk for fetal chromosomal disorders has resulted in successful litigation, specifically related to "wrongful life" for the birth of an infant with Down's syndrome. In each legal case medical negligence was cited as the physician's error in not offering information about the risk of genetic disorders.

Once the essential information is given by the physician, the competent patient should make a decision that will enhance his or her best interests according to that patient's values. If the patient is competent but does not choose the appropriate action, the physician should continue repeated educational discussions with vigorous persuasion. There are many reasons why a competent patient might refuse appropriate treatment (see box below). The physician should be aware of these conflicts and deeply explore these potential reasons for refusing medically beneficial treatment.

Complicated situations of informed consent with or without refusal of medically indicated therapy involve (1) patients with true incapacity, (2) emanicipated minors, and (3) legal minors such as younger children, the newborn, and the fetus.

SURROGATE OR PROXY CONSENT

Only a competent patient can make an informed autonomous decision about his or her medical care. The ability to make medical decisions requires the intellectual and emotional capacity to understand the risks and benefits involved in the planned medical action. This involves the ability to reason and to appreciate the nature and consequences of the choice. If a person is 18 years of age or older and can understand the risks and benefits involved in treatment, the individual can make an educated autonomous decision. Patients under 18 years of age are often emotionally and intellectually mature enough to make such decisions. These children should be included in the decision-making process despite the legal requirement of a chronologic age of 18 years.

The emancipated minor is a common clinical situation in perinatology, and it is most problematic with adolescent pregnancies. The emancipated minor, by definition, is an individual who is physically and financially independent of his or her parents. The emanicipated minor is further defined as being over 14 years of age. Furthermore, the emancipated minor must also be judged to be emotionally and intellectually capable of making decisions. In many states consent for treatment of the emancipated minor or the mature minor (over 14 years old but dependent) can be given by the minor for the therapy of drug abuse, venereal disease, abortion, and contraception. Furthermore, the mature minor can give consent for other medical problems, if (1) the minor can understand the risks associated with therapy, (2) the treatment is directly beneficial to the minor, (3) the care is standard medical care, and (4) there is a good reason for lack of parental consent.

Neonatologists often are faced with obtaining consent for the treatment of the child of the emancipated minor. In many circumstances teenage mothers still live in the home of their own mother (infant's grandmother); thus they are not truly emancipated. Legally one must therefore obtain consent from the infant's grandmother, but morally it is advisable to obtain consent from both the infant's mother and grandmother.

The determination of legal incapacity of an adult to give informed consent and make medical decisions must be made by the courts. If legal incompetence is determined, a guardian or conservator is appointed as a surrogate to give proxy consent. The courts usually appoint the closest family member to serve as surrogate for an incompetent adult. This is a logical choice, because the family is a central social unit and family members are those most concerned about the best interest of the patient.

Substitute judgment is the surrogate's attempt to reach a decision that the patient would have made based on prior direct knowledge of the patient's wishes and values, or an understanding of the history of the patient's wishes. The surrogate can thus continue to represent the autonomy of the patient. If the patient's wishes are unknown, the surrogate can make decisions based on how a "reasonable person" would choose to act.

Surrogate proxy decision making is also the mechanism used for infants and young children. It is impossible to determine the desires or to make decisions based on the infant's autonomy. Therefore the overriding bioethical principle to use in making decisions about newborn infants is to act in the patient's best interests. This implies beneficence and nonmaleficence, discussed later.

The parents are the logical surrogates to give proxy consent for the medical care of their infant, because parents have a moral responsibility for their child's care. Parents should be in a position to judge what is best for their infant, assuming the parents act unselfishly. To be able to act in the best interest of their child the parents need unbiased, full disclosure of information, so they can understand the risks and benefits of the proposed medical plan. The parents need the best available medical information to help understand the child's condition. Therefore the autonomous decision of the parents should result in an action that is in the best interest of the child. The parents also need empathy to help overcome the unexpected shock of a serious medical problem.

The parent's right to decision making must be taken seriously as part of the physician's obligation to respect parental autonomy. The parents' right is not unlimited, however, because surrogate consent by parents must benefit the well-being of the child. If the medical action chosen by the parents does not promote the infant's welfare, the rights of the parents can be overruled for a medical action that is in the best interest of the child.

An example of such a situation is the infant born to Jehovah's Witness parents who denied a blood transfusion for the infant based on the parents' beliefs. This child is too young to have established beliefs and cannot have an autonomous opinion. The parents' decision opposes the best interests of the child according to society. The transfusion should be given and is justified on both moral and legal principles of promoting the child's best interests or welfare. However, in this situation the courts would respect the autonomy of a competent adult who refuses treatment because of a sincere personal belief and who also understands the consequences of the chosen action. Nonetheless, the courts have not allowed the pregnant Jehovah's Witness or parent to jeopardize the fetus or newborn infant's well-being by refusing to permit a needed blood transfusion to the pregnant woman or newborn infant.

BENEFICENCE/NONMALEFICENCE

The bioethical principles of beneficence (to do good) and nonmaleficence (to do no harm) best exemplify the physician's obligation to act in the patient's best interests. Taken literally these principles reflect the pledge of the Hippocratic oath to help the patient or at least to do no harm. These principles make the physician assess the options for the care of the patient and to choose actions that promote and protect the patient's best interests. Together they work to ensure that the benefits are greater than the risks. Because of these basic ethical principles, the physician must do good for his or her patients. The utilitarian goals to have greater pleasure than pain and to improve the quality of life by doing good are basic to beneficent and nonmaleficent medical decision making. Nonetheless, the best interest of the patient is not to be subordinated to the interests of others, such as to the parents for their burden of caring for an ill infant or to society for the financial burden of health care.

The concept of quality of life has been used in a utilitarian way to interpret the principle of beneficence. Conversely, beneficence has been used to justify decision making on the basis of quality of life. The ability to define poor quality of life is subjective and judgmental. The American Academy of Pediatrics takes issue with the use of quality-of-life decisions and states that the consideration of anticipated poor potential or the future availability of care is irrelevant for medical decision making. Judgment of poor quality of life by an individual observer is often biased and vague, and the decisions are often not unequivocal. Quality of life may potentially be influenced by biases to certain life-styles such as drug addiction or to intellectual incapacity such as mental retardation.

However, the American Medical Association supports the concept of quality of life, because it is believed that there is a minimum quality of life that would be unacceptable for all observers. This poor quality of life is believed to be defensible and not subject to observer bias. It does not include patients with mental retardation or usual physical handicaps. Rather the minimum quality of life would refer to medical conditions such as persistent vegetative states where there is an absence of cognition and communication. The total absence of higher brain functions would be considered an unacceptable quality of life. Nevertheless, because quality of life is subjective, vaguely defined, and possibly influenced by biases against groups of people, the principles of beneficence and nonmaleficence should be employed without invoking quality-of-life issues. To act in the best interest of the patient by weighing the benefits and the risks and to relieve suffering without introducing excessive pain are paramount to the principles of beneficence and nonmaleficence.

JUSTICE AND EXTERNAL FACTORS

The physician's obligation of justice involves consideration of equality of care and possibly external factors related to a patient's illness. Justice is the principle that is exemplified by the desire to give every patient his or her just due. Justice entails a sense of fairness. It would be unjust to deny benefits based on characteristics for which a patient has no responsibility; thus race, sex, and socioeconomic status are irrelevant for medical decision making in terms of justice. Justice involves equality of care (e.g., a handicapped person with pneumonia should receive the same care as a nonhandicapped person). Similar cases should receive equivalent treatment, thus assuring a consistent medical approach or standards of medical care. This does not imply that a child with anencephaly needs to be treated in a similar manner as a normal child. The best interest of the patient and weighing the risk-to-benefit ratio remain pertinent. Justice, as a principle, states there should be an equal distribution or balance of the benefits and harms of those involved. This concern primarily reflects on what is to happen to the patient, but it also reflects on external factors outside the patient such as the family and society.

External factors in which justice also needs to be considered are the risks and benefits to the family and society. Both financial and emotional burdens may be accrued by the family, while financial and public health concerns are potentially accrued by society. The family has no legal authority for the adult competent patient, but it does have a moral obligation to the care of that patient. Furthermore, whether the patient is an adult or a minor with the family acting as a surrogate, conflicts may develop between the intents of the family and those of the patient. The family may be forced to weigh the burdens and the benefits to the family against those to the patient.

Although justice calls for a fair distribution of benefits, the principles of autonomy and beneficence are stronger factors that place the best interests of the patient above the interests of the family. The obligation to the patient's best interest is utmost above all other factors. If the outcome of medical treatment is uncertain or doubtful—thus the patient's best interests are impossible to determine—or if the patient's preferences are unknown, the family's decision should be respected.

External factors may also be relevant to the safety of health care workers and to those of society. (For example, futile transfusions in a patient with fulminant and terminal hepatitis place undue risk on the health care workers.) Additional relevant concerns of society relate to public health problems and those of criminal acts. These concerns often create a conflict between the concept of autonomy, the associated obligation of confidentiality, and the principle of justice as they apply to the risks to the patient and the risks to society. Weighing an equal distribution of risks in an attempt to protect the public, the physician now has an obligation to break confidentiality in certain circumstances. These include various contagious diseases such as venereal disease, gunshot wounds, rape, and child abuse, or if the patient is a danger to self or to others.

Another external variable is the allocation of limited resources. This is becoming a critical issue (e.g., a request for transfer of a sick neonate to an already full neonatal intensive care unit). The concept of medical justice, the equality of care of similar cases, must be weighed against the obligation to care for the patients already in the neonatal unit. Thus, if the neonatal intensive care unit is full, if there are infants less ill than the patient to be transferred, and if there is another treatment area for the less ill patient who is already in the unit, it is justified to send the less ill patient to another treatment area and accept the more seriously ill patient from another hospital. However, if all the patients in the intensive care unit are equally ill and none can be moved to another area, the obligation to treat the patients who are presently in your care supersedes any obligation for a patient in an outlying hospital. Arrangements must be made to transfer this patient to another neonatal unit.

PERINATAL ETHICS

Bioethics of pregnancy

During pregnancy the physician has many ethical obligations both to the mother and to the fetus. There is the moral obligation to respect the autonomy of the competent mother and to act in a beneficial manner to the mother. Because the wishes of a fetus cannot be determined, autonomy is not an issue with respect to the fetus; rather the physician has the moral obligation to act in the best interest of the fetus: to act with beneficence and nonmaleficence. The mother also has an ethical obligation to promote and protect the well-being of her fetus. When the fetus becomes a patient, the physician must act as a fetal advocate and ensure safe and optimal health care. This includes prevention and/or treatment of potentially life-threatening or damaging (handicapping) situations, such as preterm birth or birth asphyxia.

For the most part the physician's obligation to respect maternal autonomy and the maternal and physician obligation to the beneficence of the fetus are harmonious. However, occasionally the obligation to respect maternal autonomy and fetal beneficence may conflict. In these situations the mother may refuse treatment, such as ritodrine to prevent preterm labor, close control of maternal diabetes with insulin therapy, or transfusion for severe maternal anemia. The usual assumption is that a competent adult can determine what is in their own best interest. However, because of self-interest a pregnant woman may not be able to determine what is in the best interest of her fetus. Refusal of medically beneficial treatment during pregnancy may endanger the fetus, whereas forcing such therapy to protect the fetus may violate maternal autonomy.

It is clear that the mother is not merely an incubator for fetal growth. The mother has a moral obligation to ensure fetal well-being. The time at which this becomes most significant is after the point in gestation when the fetus would be considered viable. The Supreme Court decision of *Roe v. Wade* established the right of women over the right of being born for the first trimester and first half of the second trimester of pregnancy. However, once the time in gestation passes where neonatal viability has been achieved, the fetus has the right to be "wellborn." Some philosophies state that, if a mother chooses not to have an abortion (since these are freely available), the woman has a moral obligation to continue the pregnancy to term and to ensure a good outcome for the fetus. This right of the mature fetus may supersede the mother's autonomy and the potential risks to the mother that may be encountered in treatment of both pregnancy complications and those of the fetus. Physicians have obtained court orders to perform cesarean sections on nonconsenting mothers to treat the fetus who has signs of severe distress. The hazard of maternal surgery was considered less than the risk of fetal distress to the future infant. The individual rights of self-determination of the mother were superseded by the obligations to do good or to do no harm to the distressed fetus. Furthermore, children have sued parents for birth defects that may have been preventable or treated during pregnancy or labor.

Many perinatal conflicts can be analyzed and managed with the same ethical framework as discussed for the competent nonpregnant adult. A conflict between the physician's obligation of beneficence to the mother and the physician's obligations to respect the autonomy of the mother could be resolved with a traditional approach as long as potential fetal harm is not expected. The mother's autonomy must be respected after she has been given all the pertinent information to enable her to make an educated autonomous decision. The physician should be aware of and respect the values and beliefs of the mother. The reproductive self-determination of a competent woman assures that she is capable of determining what is in her *own* best interest. Coercion would be an assault on the woman's personal freedom. However, if the mother is incapable of making a decision or to understand the medical treatment choices, the physician's obligation of beneficence to the mother becomes more important.

Another possible conflict may be between the physician's obligation of beneficence to the fetus and the mother's obligation of beneficence to the fetus. This may involve conflict as to what is in the best interest of the fetus and whose interpretation of this interest is to be primary. One must weigh the risks and benefits of a given medical action such as in utero therapy of nonlethal congenital anomalies. In these circumstances if there are two equally risky choices, both with uncertain outcomes, the physician should defer to the mother, who may be in a better position to determine the best interests of the fetus.

A potentially more common ethical conflict during pregnancy is that between the physician's obligation to respect maternal autonomy and the physician's obligation of beneficence to the fetus. Persuasive educational efforts may help the mother become informed of the risks to the fetus of various maternal behavioral actions such as alcohol, cigarette, or drug abuse. Efforts to explain the benefits of bed rest, tocolysis, or good diabetic control with insulin and diet may persuade a dissenting woman to understand the risks to her fetus and consent to such treatment. The greater the actual benefit to the fetus for a newborn infant (see box below). Furthermore, recent federal guidelines have also echoed these principles, although the government's rulings are more specific than previous recommendations by physicians and ethicists (see boxes below and on facing page). Nonetheless, the governmental regulations do not condone futile therapy or therapy with inhumane risks and harms.

Despite medical advances in the neonatal intensive care unit, it must be emphasized that every newborn infant cannot be cured (see box on p. 288). Because we can sustain cardiopulmonary function does not mean that we should do so in every case. It has been estimated that as many as 15% to 30% of deaths in neonatal intensive care units are the result of terminating life support. Further treatment was thought to be futile in such cases. This must not be considered a negative effect. Indeed, over the last decade survival without neurodevelopmental sequelae has improved substantially for all weight-group categories.

There are times when the medical treatment either inflicts pain or cannot alleviate it and cannot alter an irreversible medical problem. It is morally unjustifiable to prolong life manifested by cardiopulmonary function alone. When such treatment is not effective it is no longer beneficial to the patient and can be stopped.

Prolonging life in these circumstances is no longer in the best interest of the patient. In these futile clinical situations the right to die needs to be respected by the physician. Under these tragic circumstances life is not necessarily an absolute good and death is not an absolute evil.

Criteria to withhold a treatment should not be based on the "ordinary/extraordinary" treatment argument. Extraordinary treatment is often ill-defined and only obscures the real issues of benefit and risks. Furthermore, ordinary care is not always universally warranted and is not obligatory in futile situations. Whenever a decision is made to withdraw or withhold medical treatment the physician must continue to care for the patient's needs. The patient is entitled to continued treatment with respect and dignity and should continue to receive medication to treat pain and discomfort. Patients should not be medically or emotionally abandoned.

Another important principle is that there is no moral distinction between withholding or withdrawing a treatment that is not beneficial to a patient. Withdrawing or withholding of medical treatment differs from active euthanasia. Euthanasia means "good death" and active euthanasia implies mercy killing to many observers. If this principle were applied to the newborn, it would cause

Government regulations*

Withholding of medically indicated treatment is defined as:

Failure to respond to disabled infant's life-threatening condition

Failure to provide appropriate nutrition, hydration, or medication that, in reasonable medical judgment, would effectively ameliorate or correct all conditions

Medical neglect or child abuse

Withholding treatment when with reasonable medical judgment:

The infant is chronically and irreversibly comatose

Treatment would prolong dying, would not be effective in ameliorating or correcting all life-threatening conditions, or would be futile for survival

Treatment would be futile for survival and would be inhumane

*Prior regulations were based on discrimination to the handicapped; the present are based on child-abuse legislation.

Summary of President's Commission report on seriously ill newborns

I. Parents to be surrogates for infant unless:
   A. They are incapable of decision-making
   B. Parental disagreement exists.
   C. Choice of action is not infants best interest.
II. Futile therapy is not needed.
III. Infants comfort must be ensured.
IV. Beneficial therapies should not be withheld.
V. Decision makers must have access to all essential and accurate information.
VI. Institutions will have policies for review of such decisions.
   These policies should state:
   A. Decisions on withdrawal of futile therapy need not be reviewed.
   B. Best interests of child will be of the only consideration if these interests are clear.
   C. Parental discretion will be permitted if child's interests are ambiguous.
   D. Courts will intervene if best interests of child are not followed.
VII. Legal system has a limited role.
   A. Civil courts will intervene if parents are to be disqualified as surrogates.
   B. Special laws requiring reporting of all cases are not warranted.
   C. The ability of criminal penalities to ensure good decision-making is limited.
   D. Using governmental financial sanctions to punish hospitals' "incorrect" decision is likely to be ineffective and harm "innocent" patients.
VIII. Current laws do not preclude good decision making.

Summarized from the President's Commission for the Study of Ethical Problems in Medicine and Biomedical and Behavioral Research, March 1983, U.S. Government Printing Office..

Conditions associated with neonatal ethical issues

Birth weight less than 700 gm
Life-threatening congenital anomalies
Serious inborn errors of metabolism
Severe birth asphyxia
Severe intraventricular hemorrhage
Hyperalimentation-dependent short bowel syndrome
Ventilator-dependent severe bronchopulmonary dysplasia

nonvoluntary euthanasia because there would be no decision making by the infant. Withholding or withdrawing medical treatment allows a patient to die when there is no further beneficial treatment available and the patient or the patient proxy agrees to such a plan. Withholding or withdrawing treatment under such circumstances is passive and an act of omission. Such medical action is possible only after the duty to treat has been exhausted or in an attempt to respect a competent patient's request. Active euthanasia is prohibited by most moral, religious, medical, secular, and legal standards. Active euthanasia is considered by some experts to be outside the bounds of medical practice; it could place too much power in one person or group and may take away the patient's basic trust of the medical profession. Thus withdrawing or withholding of medically nonbeneficial treatment in the best interest of a patient may be distinct from actively taking a patient's life.

"Do not resuscitate" orders

Another component of withdrawing or withholding therapy is the "do not resuscitate" order. Such an order is in anticipation of an event, cardiopulmonary arrest, that will occur in all patients before death. Furthermore, dying is a process and not necessarily an event, although medical practice usually approaches dying as an acute event. If the patient has suffered from an incurable disease and has accrued no benefit from treatment, or if there is a very poor prognosis (severe brain injury, extreme suffering and pain or the patient is terminally ill), resuscitative efforts will prolong the unrelievable pain or prolong the process of dying. Indeed, the purpose of cardiopulmonary resuscitation is to treat patients with sudden unexplained cardiac arrest. Cardiopulmonary resuscitation should not be employed when death is imminent and treatment is futile or when the competent patient refuses resuscitation.

"Do not resuscitate" orders need prior communication with the patient and the family (although the wishes of the family do not supersede the wishes of a competent adult). This decision must be medically and morally justified, and both the justification and communication with the patient and/or family must be documented in the patient's chart. Furthermore, there should be careful documentation and review of the contents of the medical diagnosis and seriousness of the prognosis. Specific orders should be written in the chart defining what is and is not to be done in the event of a cardiac arrest. Such notes as slow codes and chemical codes are vague and confuse the nurses and house staff. The written note and specified orders help improve communication and the understanding of the nurses and other physicians. Specific levels of care should be documented in the order book. These include (1) no CPR, which means no chest compression and ventilation; (2) no drugs for cardiac arrest, arrythmias, or hypotension; (3) no ancillary care such as dialysis, defibrillation, laboratory studies (e.g., blood gases, hematocrit, blood cultures), antibiotics for suspected infection, or transfusion for suspected anemia; (4) a provision to withdraw treatments such as ventilators, drugs, and dialysis. This order should be reviewed daily to ascertain the appropriateness of the plan. Under no circumstances should the patient be abandoned, because pain and suffering must be alleviated and the patient must be treated with respect and dignity.

Brain death

Brain death is an important criterion that often results in determining whether to write a "do not resuscitate" order or whether treatment is to be withdrawn or withheld. Death is defined as either the permanent cessation of circulatory or respiratory function or the irreversible loss of all functions of the entire brain, including the brainstem. The most severe brain damage compatible with cardiopulmonary life is brain death, which must be determined with appropriate medical tests. The physical examination reveals a comatose unresponsive patient without brainstem reflexes (pupillary, oculocephalic, corneal, gag, vestibulo-ocular or auriculo-ocular and respiration) and no body movement other than spinal reflexes. Laboratory tests include an isoelective electroencephalogram (EEG) during continuous monitoring for 30 minutes and absent cerebral blood flow determined by radionucleotide scans. A flat EEG may be influenced by drugs and prematurity, whereas EEG activity (albeit minimal) has been detected in clinically brain-dead patients without cerebral blood flow.

Brain damage severe enough to irreversibly damage the cortex but below the threshold for brainstem injury may be seen as a persistent vegetative state. Cortical or cerebral death has occurred, but the patient's brainstem maintains respiration. Neocortical brain death in the permanently unconscious person is traditionally not recognized as true brain death, but it has been recommended by many—including the federal government—as a reason to withdraw or withhold treatment in patients, including newborn infants (see boxes on p. 287).

Criteria for brain death apply only if there are no unusual circumstances. These qualifying conditions include drugs, metabolic toxins (uremia, inborn errors of metabolism), hypothermia, and age less than 5 years. More specifically, the criteria to document brain death among preterm infants are very vague. Such immature infants may have discontinuous EEG activity and may recover after temporary but complete suppression of brainstem reflexes. Thus the physician should be careful when assessing the newborn infant for brain death. In addition, criteria other than brain death should be considered when contemplating withdrawal or withholding of treatment because of the uncertainty of the diagnosis of brain death in newborn infants.

PROCEDURAL PRINCIPLES OF DECISION MAKING

Procedural aspects of bioethical decision making are concerned with who decides which medical action is in the best interest of the patient. The question of who decides is closely coupled with whose interpretation of what is in the best interest of the patient. For the adult competent patient, autonomy-based decisions are to be respected by the physician. There is a moral and legal obligation to respect the values, beliefs, and wishes of a competent adult's medical decisions. An educated adult knows what is in his or her own best interest. If disagreement develops between the physician's understanding of the best interests of the patient (physician's obligations of beneficence) and the patient's medical preferences (autonomy), the physician may continue to educate the patient but should not use coercive means to force the patient into a medical action the patient does not desire. Furthermore, family members have no legal or moral right to supersede the decision of a competent adult.

When the patient is a legal minor, more specifically when the patient is a newborn infant, autonomy-based decision making is impossible because the wishes of the patient cannot be ascertained. The people who make decisions for the newborn infant must then serve the best interests of the child. The priority of decision making for newborn infants depends on closeness to the infant. Thus, the parents, by nature of the family's obligation to protect and promote the well being of their child, are the most logical and traditional choice.

The physician also has a role in decision making by the nature of the professional relationship and the goals of medicine, including the role as the patient advocate with the obligation of beneficence. Usually the relationship between the parents and physician permits a collaborative arrangement (see box). Shared decision making between parents and physicians, although not necessarily able to relieve parental guilt, helps to ensure that the best interests of the child are taken into consideration. Surrogate decision making by proxy consent by parents is morally and legally justifiable as long as the parents act in the best interests of the child. The parents' surrogate proxy consent is not an absolute right, and the decision should only be respected if the choice of action will result in a clear benefit to the infant. If parents refuse medically beneficial treatment, the physician has a responsibility to promote the child's best interests and take other measures, such as court action, to assure appropriate treatment. This proposed treatment must be available, recognized as being successful, and able to alleviate the condition without ambiguity. If bad decisions are made by the parents, the physician has the duty to be an advocate for the infant; this obligation supersedes the physician's obligation to respect the autonomy of the family. The usual process for the resolution of disagreement of treatment plans for newborn infants begins with the parents and physician and may end with the courts (see box above). The further the decision-making process is extended away from the patient the greater the loss of confidentiality and possible diffusion of responsibility.

Decision making in neonatal intensive care units

Parents—family
Physician
Parent—physician
Medical—nursing team
Ethics committees
Child protective services
Courts

Ethics committees are another mechanism that may be used to resolve disagreement between parents and the physician. Even when there is no disagreement between parents and physicians, ethics committees may provide a broader forum to discuss a patient's difficult ethical problems or to reinforce a decision agreed on by the parents and the physician. Ethics committees facilitate consensus and usually function in an advisory capacity. Although most view the use of the hospital ethics committee as voluntary or optional, others believe that certain patient situations must be reviewed on a mandatory basis. Cases that have been suggested for mandatory review include (1) when life support is to be withheld or withdrawn and death is not imminent; (2) when there is disagreement between the parents and physicians; (3) when life support is to be withdrawn or withheld (because this is an irreversible act and committee review may reduce the risks of a mistake in judgment), and (4) when it is necessary to ensure that the parents understand the consequences of the medical action and that reasonable medical judgment has been used. Furthermore, some believe the decision of the committee should also be mandatory and binding, rather than advisory. Nonetheless, most authorities view ethics committees as a consensus-development forum to be used as any consultation on an optimal rather than mandatory basis.

To function as an ideal observer or group of observers, the ethics committee members need to have *omniscience* or access to all the important facts; *omnipercipience*, or an ability to understand the feelings of others; *disinterest*, or impartiality; *dispassion*, or the ability to form a judgment without being influenced by emotion; and *consistency* of judgment, having the same recommendations for similar cases.

Ethics committees should function by observing the traditional obligations to respect autonomy, promote beneficence and nonmaleficence, and assure justice. Competent patients' preferences are to be respected. If the patient is not competent, the patient's best interests are the supervening moral consideration. When the best interests of the child are impossible to be determined, the family's interpretation of these interests is to be respected (see boxes on pp. 286 and 287). However, the family's own interests, preferences, or burdens are secondary to the best interests of the patient. Confidentiality is to be respected as long as it does not jeopardize the interests of the patient. Finally, the committee's recommendations should be based on moral rather than economic or legal issues.

Ethics committees can be convened by any member of the committee after being consulted or, more likely, by any professional person (and/or family member) involved with the patient. For prospective review of a life-or-death case, the committee should be available to meet within hours after a meeting is needed. Life support should continue. The person to present the ethical question to the committee should ascertain the current and future expectations and possibilities for the patient. The parents should be allowed to come to at least part of the meeting. If time permits, it may be appropriate to delay a meeting briefly to permit the parents sufficient time to overcome the immediate denial, shock, and depression associated with the birth of an ill newborn.

At the actual meeting all the relevant medical and psychosocial facts are presented, in addition to risks, benefits, alternate modes of treatment, and eventual prognosis. Subspecialists, such as neurologists, should be in attendance if relevant. Questions and answers and open discussion follow the presentation. If unanimity and/or a consensus develops, no further discussion is needed and the results are reported to the physicians and parents. If no consensus develops, a majority and minority opinion or consensus with dissenting opinion should be stated and reported to the involved persons. If the parents' or physician's plan of action is not in the patient's best interests and the committee agrees that another plan of medical action should be taken, the committee's opinion is reported to the medical team and the director of the department. At this time the committee has fulfilled its advisory function.

Although prospective review is the most urgent function of the committee, the committee has a responsibility to be educational as well. The primary educational task is to inform and familiarize the committee members with the principles of bioethics. Self-education will enable the committee to function as ideal observers and to serve the best interests of the patient. Retrospective discussion of ethically important questions could also serve an educational function. Additional educational tasks include informing the hospital and later the community of the role of the ethics committee and to instruct these groups in the field of bioethics. In addition to its educational role, the committee could also help to develop responses to bioethical issues such as "do not resuscitate" orders, organ transplants, and the rights of the incompetent patient.

Ideally, only after the educational and policy functions of the committee are fulfilled should a committee engage in a prospective review. Unfortunately, the pressing nature of these urgent patient situations may require a committee to meet before completing these other important goals.

Ethics committees inherently have potential risks (see box below). The committee may exert undue social pressure and undermine or usurp the physician's role with a family. Responsibility may be diffused, while there is no direct accountability of ethics committees. Further-

Potential problems of ethics committees

- Diffusion of responsibility
- Absence of direct accountability
- Loss of confidentiality
- Coercion
- Protection of hospital's interests
- Emphasis on legal rather than moral issues
- Need to adequately educate all members
- Litigation against committee
- Physician resistance to use committee

more, one must be careful not to be involved in a conflict between the interests of a patient and the interests of the hospital.

The legal status of such committees is also unknown. Although not likely, committees may be subject to litigation for homicide or conspiracy to commit homicide and the minutes of the committee may be admissible evidence in court. Nonetheless, the careful and critical process of facilitated decision making by an ethics committee may actually reduce the risk of litigation for medical negligence. Furthermore, careful and sensitive guidance, with particular awareness of the potential problems of the committee, should prevent these risks from interfering with the positive functions of the group. Finally, success of ethics committees should not be measured by the number of consultations per year, but by the number of ethically difficult situations that are successfully resolved. Indeed, with a successful ethics committee and effective bioethical education fewer moral problems will need to be resolved in a formal meeting, because more and more ethical dilemmas will now be resolved on the patient wards by ethically trained health care workers, patients, and families.

Robert M. Kliegman

BIBLIOGRAPHY

Abrams, F.: Bioethical considerations for high risk pregnancy. In Abrams, R., and Wexler, P., editors: Medical care of the pregnant patient, Boston, 1983, Little, Brown & Co.

American Academy of Pediatrics Infant Bioethics Task Force: guidelines for infant bioethics committees, Pediatrics **74**:306, 1984.

American College of Physicians Ethics Manual: Part II: Research, other ethical issues, Ad Hoc Committee on Medical Ethics, American College of Physicians, Ann. Intern. Med. **101**:263, 1984.

Beauchamp, T., and Childress, J.: Principles of biomedical ethics, ed. 2, London, 1983, Oxford University Press, Inc.

Beauchamp, T., and McCullough, L.: Medical ethics, New York, 1984, Prentice-Hall, Inc.

Bernat, J.L., Culver, C.M., and Gert, B.: On the definition and criterion of death, Ann. Intern. Med. **94**:389, 1981.

Billings, J.A.: Comfort measures for the terminally ill: is dehydration painful? J. Am. Geriatr. Soc. **33**:808, 1985.

Cassel, E.J.: The nature of suffering and the goals of medicine, N. Engl. J. Med. **306**:639, 1982.

Chervenak, F.A., and McCullough, L.B.: Perinatal ethics: a practical method of analysis of obligations to mother and fetus, Obstet. Gynecol. **66**:3, 1985.

Drake, B., Ashwal, S., and Schneider, S.: Determination of cerebral death in the pediatric intensive care unit, Pediatrics **78**:107, 1986.

Duff, R.S., and Campbell, A.G.: Moral and ethical dilemmas in the special care nursery, N. Engl. J. Med. **289**:890, 1973.

Dworkin, G.: Legality of consent to nontherapeutic medical research on infants and young children, Arch. Dis. Child. **53**:443, 1978.

Engelhardt, H.T.: Current controversies in obstetrics: wrongful life and forced fetal surgical procedures, Am. J. Obstet. Gynecol. **151**:313, 1985.

Engelhardt, H.: The foundations of bioethics, New York, 1986, Oxford University Press, Inc.

Firth, R.: Ethical absolutism and the ideal observer, Philosophy Phenom. Res. **12**:317, 1952.

Fleischman, A.R., and Murray, T.H.: Ethics committee for infants Doe? Hastings Cent. Rep. **13**:5, 1983.

Fletcher, J.C., and Schulman, J.D.: Fetal research: the state of the question, Hastings Cent. Rep. April, 1985.

Fost, N.: Ethical problems in pediatrics, Curr. Probl. Pediatr. **64**:10, 1976.

Fost, N.: Counselling families who have a child with a severe congenital anomaly, Pediatrics **67**:321, 1981.

Fost, N., and Cranford, R.E.: Hospital ethics committees: administrative aspects, JAMA **253**:2687, 1985.

Gillespie, C.: Letting die severely handicapped children, J. Med. Ethics **9**:231, 1983.

Green, H.G.: Caring and communication: observations on 19 baby Doe patients, Am. J. Dis. Child. **139**:1082, 1985.

Gustaitis, R., and Young, E.: A time to be born, a time to die: conflicts and ethics in an intensive care nursery, Reading, Mass., 1986, Addison Wesley Publishing Co., Inc.

The Hasting Center Report (Overview), Ethics committees: how are they doing? June, 1986.

Infant Bioethics Task Force and consultants, Guidelines for infant bioethics committees, Pediatrics **74**:306, 1984.

Johnson, D.E., and Thompson, T.R.: The baby Doe rule: is it all bad? Pediatrics **73**:729, 1984.

Jonsen, A., Siegler, M., and Winslade, W.: Clinical ethics: a practical approach to ethical decisions in clinical medicine, New York, 1982, Macmillan Publishing Company.

Kliegman, R., Mahowald, M., and Younger, S.: In our best interest: experience and working of an ethics review committee, J. Pediatr. **108**:178, 1986.

Leikin, S.: Minor's assent or dissent to medical treatment, J. Pediatr. **102**:169, 1983.

Lenke, R.R., and Nemes, J.M.: Wrongful birth, wrongful life: the doctor between a rock and a hard place, Obstet. Gynecol. **66**(5):719, 1985.

Levine, C.: Questions and answers about hospital ethics committees, Hastings Cent. Rep. **14**:9, 1984.

Lidz, C., and others: Barriers to informed consent, Ann. Intern. Med. **99**:539, 1983.

Lo, B., and Jonsen, A.: Clinical decisions to limit treatment, Ann. Intern. Med. **93**:764, 1980.

Mackenzie, T.B., and Nagel, T.C.: When a pregnant woman endangers her fetus, Hastings Cent. Rep. Feb., 1986.

Micetich, K.C., Steinecker, P.H., and Thomasma, D.C.: Are intravenous fluids morally required for a dying patient? Arch. Intern. Med. **143**:975, 1983.

Miles, S.H., Cranford, R., and Schultz, A.L.: The do-not-resuscitate order in a teaching hospital, Ann. Intern. Med. **96**:660, 1982.

Outwater, K.M., and Rockoff, M.A.: Apnea testing to confirm brain death in children, Crit. Care Med. **12**:357, 1984.

Paris, J.J.: Terminating treatment for newborns: a theological perspective, Law Med. Health Care, **10**:206, 1982.

President's Commission for the Study of Ethical Problems in Medicine and Biomedical and Behavioral Research, Deciding to forego life-sustaining treatment, Bethesda, Md., 1983, U.S. Government Printing Office.

Purtilo, R.: Ethics consultations in the hospital, N. Engl. J. Med. **311**:983, 1984.

Rachels, J.: Active and passive euthanasia, N. Engl. J. Med. **292**:78, 1975.

Report of the medical consultants on the diagnosis of death to the President's Commission for the Study of Ethical Problems in Medicine and Biomedical and Behavioral Research, JAMA **246**:2184, 1981.

Robertson, J.A.: Committees as decision makers: alternative structures and responsibilities. In Cranford, R.E., and Doudera, A.E., editors: Institutional ethics committees and health care decision making, Ann Arbor, Mich., 1984, Health Administration Press.

Rowland, T.W., Donnelly, J.H., and Jackson, A.H.: Apnea documentation for determination of brain death in children, Pediatrics **74**:505, 1984.

Shaw, A.: Dilemmas of "informed consent" in children, N. Eng. J. Med. **17**:885, 1973.

Silverman, W.: Human experimentation, a guided step into the unknown, New York, 1985, Oxford University Press, Inc.

Sims, D.G., Wynn, J., and Chiswick, M.L.: Outcome for newborn babies declined admission to a regional neonatal intensive care unit, Arch. Dis. Child. **57**:334, 1982.

Strong, C.: The neonatologist's duty to patient and parents, Hastings Cent. Rep. Aug., 1984.

Swinyard, C., editor: Decision making and the defective newborn, Springfield, Ill., 1978, Charles C Thomas, Publisher.

Terminal dehydration (editorial), Lancet **1**:306, 1986.

Tooley, M.: Decisions to terminate life and the concepts of person. In Ladd, J., editor: Ethical issues relating to life and death, New York, 1979, Oxford University Press, Inc.

Veatch, R.M.: DRG's and the ethical reallocation of resources, Hastings Cent. Rep. June, 1986.

Wanzer, S.H., and others: The physician's responsibility toward hopelessly ill patients, N. Engl. J. Med. **310**:955, 1984.

Watchko, J.F.: Decision making on critically ill infants by parents, Am. J. Dis. Child. **137**:795, 1983.

Weir, R.: Selective nontreatment of handicapped newborns, New York, 1984, Oxford University Press, Inc.

Whitelaw, A.: Death as an option in neonatal intensive care, Lancet **ii**:328, 1986.

Youngner, S.L., and others: Patients' attitudes towards hospital ethics committees, Law Med. Health Care **12**:21, 1984.

Zawacki, B.E.: ICU physician's ethical role in distributing scarce resources, Crit. Care Med. **13**:57, 1985.

CHAPTER 19

Developmental pharmacology

DRUGS AND THE FETUS

Exposure of the fetus to drugs

Although advances in prenatal diagnosis may soon permit physicians to consider the fetus as the primary patient, currently the fetus is only the passive recipient of drugs, and consequently any drug effects are undesirable. Such effects on the fetus may vary from transient behavioral changes to irreversible consequences. Concern has increased over the potentially harmful effects on the fetus from drugs taken during pregnancy. The catastrophic teratogenic effects of thalidomide were discovered in the early 1960s. This drug, thought to be harmless, illustrated the totally unpredictable nature of drug toxicity in the fetus during the first trimester; thalidomide doses that induced analgesia in the mother with no demonstrable undesirable side effects produced major structural defects in the fetus.

Although several drugs are possible teratogens in human beings, at present only a few have been positively identified. Probably the best known teratogen is thalidomide. Drugs increasing the incidence of abnormalities that occur quite often in the population may not alert the physician to a direct causal relationship between exposure of the fetus to the drug and the adverse effect. It has been estimated that to establish that a given drug changes the naturally occurring frequency of a congenital deformity by 1% would require a sequential trial involving approximately 35,000 patients. The discovery that thalidomide caused congenital malformations was possible because this drug was widely used, induced dramatic and rare congenital defects, and had a high probability (an estimated 20% to 35%) of producing a teratogenic effect after exposure between the third and eighth week after conception. Unfortunately, these three criteria are rarely met when attempting to assess the teratogenicity of any given drug. Thus much of the data in the biomedical literature concerning adverse effects of drugs on the fetus is circumstantial.

Maternal consumption of drugs

Drugs are usually administered for symptomatic relief of benign problems in the mother with little or no consideration given to the unintended recipient, the fetus. The magnitude of the problem can be appreciated by considering that in several studies the average number of drugs prescribed during pregnancy numbered about four. When self-prescribed drugs were included in these studies, the average number of drugs taken increased from four to between 8.7 and 11. From 92% to 100% of all obstetric patients took at least one physician-prescribed drug, and 65% to 80% also took self-prescribed drugs. Compounding this problem for women of childbearing age is their additional occupational or environmental exposure to potential teratogens. In a recent controlled study a significant association was found between fetal loss and the occupational exposure of nurses to antineoplastic drugs.

During the years 1959 to 1965 a large-scale epidemiologic study investigated the possible teratogenic role of drugs, using a cohort of over 50,000 mother-child pairs recruited in 12 centers in the United States. The rates of exposure of these mother-child pairs to different drug groups is presented in Table 19-1. The highest rate of exposure was to analgesic and antipyretic drugs (32% of patients in the first trimester). Based on other studies, exposure to alcohol and cigarette smoke would also be expected to be high. Most studies of drug use during pregnancy performed since 1965 have found that the number of drugs consumed has stayed constant or even increased.

Placental transfer of drugs

The physicochemical properties that allow most drugs to cross cell membranes also permit their passive transport across the placenta into the fetus. The factors involved in placental transfer of drugs include lipid solubility and degree of ionization, molecular weight, protein

Table 19-1. Percentages of drug exposure in mother-child pairs from the first day of the last menstrual period to 48 hours before delivery

	Mother-child pairs exposed (n = 50,282)	
Drug group	**Lunar months 1-4**	**Anytime during pregnancy**
Analgesics and antipyretic drugs	31.6	67.3
Immunizing agents	18.3	45.2
Antimicrobial and antiparasitic agents	16.1	34.9
Antinauseants, antihistamines, and phenothiazines	12.0	28.6
Caffeine and other xanthine derivatives	11.5	26.9
Drugs affecting the autonomic nervous system	9.3	24.9
Sedatives, tranquilizers, and antidepressants	6.2	28.4
Anesthetics, anticonvulsants, muscle relaxants, and stimulants	5.3	13.9
Inorganic compounds and certain vitamins	5.1	20.1
Hormones, hormone antagonists, and contraceptives	4.6	7.0
Cough medicines	1.9	15.8
Diuretics and drugs taken for vascular disorders	0.8	31.6

binding, placental circulation, fetal circulation, and placental maturation and metabolism of drugs. Most drugs administered to the mother will reach the fetus, and the extent of fetal exposure to a drug administered to the mother depends on these physicochemical properties, on the dose and duration of maternal treatment, and on the rate of maternal drug elimination. If the drug is readily diffusible, it will equilibrate between maternal and fetal compartments very rapidly (single or multiple doses) (Fig. 19-1). With fast transplacental equilibration and slow maternal elimination, the fetal pharmacokinetic profile will mimic the maternal pattern after either single or multiple drug doses. A drug that is polar or protein bound will diffuse more slowly into the fetus. However, high concentrations of drug may still accumulate in the fetal compartment if multiple doses are administered to the mother (Fig. 19-1).

Drug ingestion by the father

In the last 25 years, concern for the teratogenic effects of maternally ingested substances has grown. However, no such widespread concern surrounds possible paternally mediated teratogenic effects, and most physicians and researchers, on initial contact with this phenomenon, view it as implausible.

In animals, experimental evidence now available on the adverse effects of various agents on the progeny of male animals ingesting these chemicals, either chronically or acutely, before mating has revealed that decreased litter size and birth weights, malformations, and increased neonatal mortality may result. It is difficult to elucidate the mechanisms underlying this phenomenon. The drug itself may be present in semen and may cause alterations in development after fertilization; alternatively, drug exposure may directly alter the genetic material or its packaging in spermatozoa and consequently alter the developmental process of fertilized eggs.

Although many methodologic problems face the researcher investigating the relationship between paternal drug ingestion and perinatal outcome in human beings, physicians probably will become aware of paternally mediated teratogenic effects.

Effect of drugs on the fetus

The adverse effects of in utero exposure to drugs can vary from reversible effects such as transient changes in clotting time or fetal breathing movements to irreversible effects such as fetal death, intrauterine growth retardation, structural malformations, or mental retardation. The specific drug, the dosage, the route of administration, the timing of treatment, and the genotype of the mother or the fetus all may be critical determinants of the effect of a drug on the fetus. The disease being treated may be an important consideration. The factors that may combine to influence the outcome of drug administration include diet and coadministration of drugs. It is at best difficult to control these parameters in human beings, and thus the incontrovertible establishment of a drug as a teratogen in human beings requires the combination of extreme situations such as those previously outlined for thalidomide. Consequently it has been necessary to rely heavily on animal studies to assess the teratogenic potential of drugs.

The *timing* of drug exposure is frequently a critical determinant of the effect of the drug on the fetus (Fig. 19-2). The first week after fertilization is the "period of the zygote" (cleavage and gastrulation); during this time the most common adverse effect of drugs is termination of pregnancy, which may occur even before the woman knows she is pregnant. Exposure of the preimplantation embryo to embryotoxic drugs may also retard development, perhaps by decreasing cell number in the blastocyst. The second to the eighth weeks of gestation are the "period of the embryo." It is mainly during this period of organogenesis that drugs produce dramatic and catastrophic structural malformations. Other adverse effects during this phase may include fetal wastage, trans-

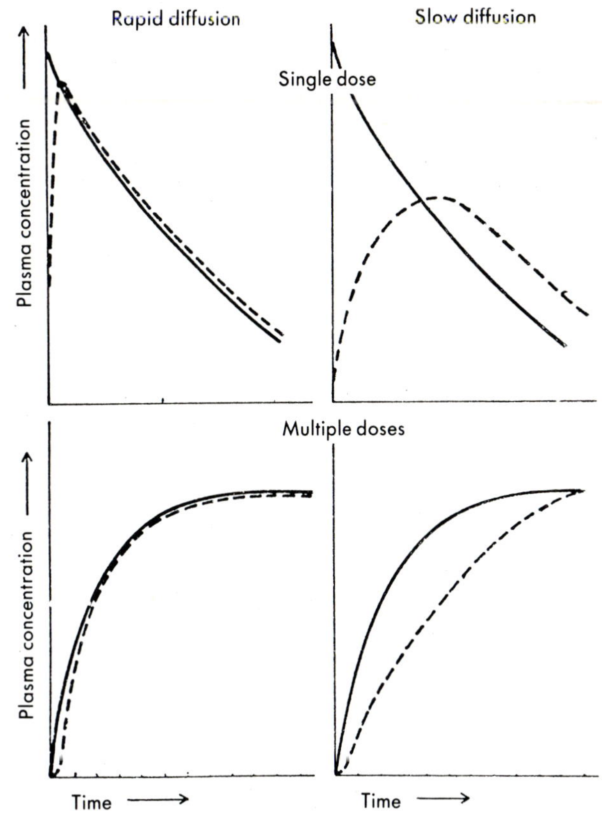

Fig. 19-1. Schematic representation of maternal *(solid line)* and fetal *(dotted line)* plasma concentrations of drug with time after single intravenous or multiple doses. Simple transplacental diffusion rates that are rapid *(left)* or slow *(right)* are hypothesized; it is assumed that the half-lives of the drugs diffusing rapidly or slowly are the same. (From Neims, A.H., and others: Principles of neonatal pharmacology. In Schaffer, A.J., and Avery, M.E., editors: Diseases of the newborn, ed. 4, Philadelphia, 1977, W.B. Saunders Co.)

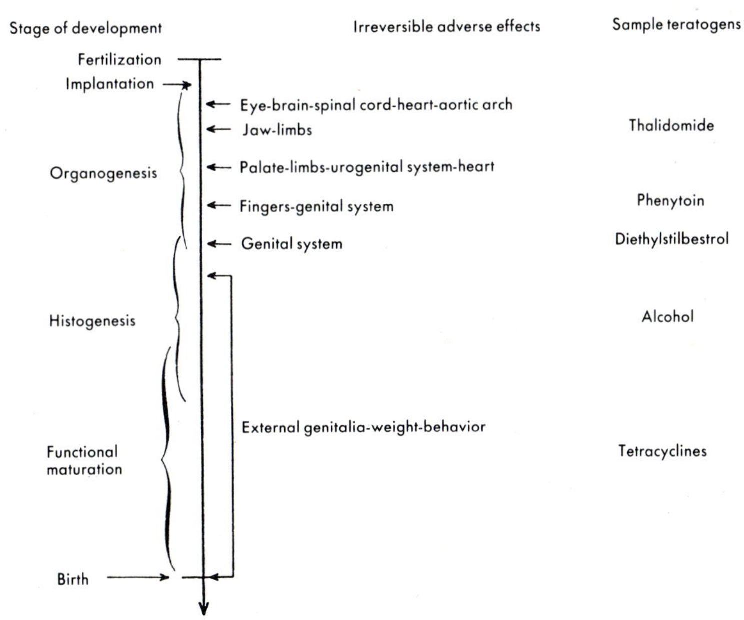

Fig. 19-2. Critical periods in human embryogenesis.

placental carcinogenesis (e.g., diethylstilbestrol), and intrauterine growth retardation. From the third to ninth months of gestation, the "period of the fetus," differentiation of the central nervous system and reproductive system continues. Drugs given during this time have been implicated as behavioral teratogens. In this period, drugs may cause disproportionate growth retardation (infants whose head growth has been spared, after 30 or more weeks) or may alter the external genitalia.

Consideration of irreversible adverse effects of drugs on development usually stops with birth. However, it is well known that sensory and other higher nervous system functions are not fully developed until well after birth. Thus birth is not really a termination point but only another milestone in development. Little is known about the long-term or delayed adverse effects of drugs administered to the mother during labor and delivery or directly to the neonate. When administered postnatally, antitumor agents such as cyclophosphamide can have long-term effects on the histogenesis of the cerebellum, on growth and development, and on reproductive function.

The effects of individual drugs on the fetus are highly dependent on the specific drug involved. There are no infallible means for predicting which drug will be "selectively toxic" to the fetus. Within some groups of drugs each individual drug can cause the same type of malformation. The anticonvulsants exemplify a family of drugs in which the core structure necessary for activity as an anticonvulsant appears also to fulfill the requirements for inducing characteristic malformations. In other instances, such as the sedative-hypnotics, individual drugs with common therapeutic effects differ greatly with respect to teratogenic potential. Thalidomide was withdrawn from the market because of its marked effect on the fetus. However, glutethimide, which has the same dioxopiperidine ring as thalidomide, is not teratogenic. It is obvious that more information on how drugs induce malformations is needed before knowledge of their molecular structure or pharmacologic action will permit prediction of teratogenicity. The decision as to whether to give a drug during pregnancy is difficult. Some of the information available on the potential adverse effects of pharmacologic classes of drugs often administered during pregnancy is summarized in Table 19-2.

Table 19-3 summarizes the results of studies on the teratogenicity of various frequently used therapeutic agents.

Self-administered nontherapeutic agents

Chronic alcohol intake during pregnancy is associated with a readily identifiable fetal alcohol syndrome (Chapter 37, part four) and has been cited as the most frequently documented cause of mental deficiency in the

Table 19-2. Drugs associated with congenital malformations in human beings

	Fetal factor, organ system involved								
Drugs	**Fetal growth**	**Growth retardation**	**Mental retardation**	**Central nervous system**	**Cardiovascular**	**Musculoskeletal**	**Urogenital**	**Eye and ear**	**Thyroid**
Antimicrobials									
Tetracycline						X			
Streptomycin							X		
Quinine?							X		
Antineoplastics									
Methotrexate	X	X		X		X			
Bisulfan, chlorambucil, cyclophosphamide				X		X	X	X	
Central nervous system drugs									
Morphine, methadone, heroin	X	X							
Thalidomide						X			
Anticonvulsants									
Phenytoin		X	X			X		X	
Barbiturates			X		X	X			
Trimethadione			X		X	X		X	
Valproic acid				X					
Steroid hormones									
Androgens							X		
Diethylstilbestrol							X		
Estrogen, progestins							X		
Iodine, propylthiouracil									X
Warfarin		X				X		X	
Propranolol		X							
Alcohol		X	X		X	X	X	X	
Tobacco smoking	X	X			X	X			
Isotretinoin			X	X		X		X	

Table 19-3. Teratogenicity of physician- or self-administered therapeutic agents

Specific agents	Studies reported	Results and recommendations
ANTINEOPLASTIC AGENTS		
(antimetabolites, alkylating agents, antitumor antibiotics, etc.)		As a group these are the most potent teratogens known. It is difficult to delineate one agent because of frequent combined uses in addition to irradiation.
Antimetabolites (purine analogs, pyrimidine analogs, folic acid antagonists)	Milunsky, Nicholson	Most potent teratogens of this group; they are associated with skeletal defects.
Alkylating agents (busulfan, chlorambucil, cyclophosphamide, nitrogen mustard)	Diamond, Garrett, Greenberg, Schardein, Shotton	Some reports have described drug-related defects; others have reported cases with no drug-related defects. Avoid use during first trimester; less critical after this time but may still result in intrauterine growth retardation (IUGR).
ANTIMICROBIALS		
Sulfonamides	Richards, Schardein	Conflicting reports on teratogenicity; avoid use in third trimester because of risk of kernicterus.
Tetracyclines	Colhan	Result in staining of dentition; avoid use in second and third trimesters and early childhood. Permanent teeth are unaffected.
Penicillins Cephalosporins	Nelson	These appear to be safe when administered at any phase of pregnancy.
Aminoglycosides Streptomycin, dihydrostreptomycin	Scheinhorn, Warkany, (1979)	Auditory nerve defects and ocular nerve damage occur in infants following prenatal exposure.
Antitubulars		
Isoniazid (INH)	Monnet	Five childern with severe encephalopathies were reported after prenatal exposure; prophylactic administration of vitamin B_6 to pregnant women receiving INH is often recommended.
Ethionamide, ethambutol, rifampin	Schardein	No clear relationship with abnormal fetal development has been noted.
Antiparasitics	Schardein	Quinidine has caused deafness; others, no definite teratogenicity.
ANTICONVULSANTS	Smith	Women requiring anticonvulsant therapy should be counseled before becoming pregnant as to the nature and magnitude of risk to the fetus; overall risk of having a malformed child is about 1 in 10.
Hydantoins Phenytoin	Hanson	Typical *fetal hydantoin syndrome* with mild to moderate growth and mental deficiencies, limb anomalies, and dysmorphic facies (low nasal bridge, short nose, mild ocular hypertelorism) have been reported.
Barbiturates, deoxybarbiturates Primidone, phenobarbital, secobarbital, amobarbital	Bethenod, Heinonen	Postnatal effects are similar to those in fetal hydantoin syndrome; associated cardiovascular malformations also may occur.
Oxazoladinediones Trimethadione	Goldman	Fetal trimethadione syndrome has been reported, with developmental delay, speech difficulty, V-shaped eyebrows, epicanthus, low-set ears, palatal anomaly, and irregular teeth.
Valproic acid		Neural tube defects have been found.
PSYCHOTROPIC AGENTS		The teratogenicity of most psychotropics is not established; caution is necessary in administering them during pregnancy; all minor tranquilizers should be avoided during pregnancy.
Thalidomide	Schardein	Teratogenic to human beings when administered in the first to eighth weeks of pregnancy; limb reduction anomalies.
Meprobromate Benzodiazepines Diazepam, chlordiazepoxide	Heinonen, Milkovich (1974), Rosenberg, Safra, Saxen	Greatly conflicting results; ingestion before parturition may cause hypotonia, apnea, and hypothermia.

Continued

Table 19-3. Teratogenicity of physician- or self-administered therapeutic agents—cont'd

Specific agents	Studies reported	Results and recommendations
PSYCHOTROPIC AGENTS—cont'd		
Tricyclic antidepressants	Schardein	Increased incidence of malformation is possible.
Monoamine oxidase inhibitors	Samojlik	Little data available for human beings; only phenelzine is reported as embryotoxic in rats.
ANTINAUSEANTS; ANTIHISTAMINES	Heinonen, Paterson, Shapiro, Smithells	No evidence of association to malformation in human beings; chlorcyclizine and meclizine are teratogenic in laboratory animals but not in human beings.
NONNARCOTIC ANALGESICS, ANTIINFLAMMATORY ANTIPYRETIC AGENTS	Eriksson	Little evidence exists to associate these with malformations (see specific exceptions following). As a group, considering wide usage, they are not considered to be teratogenic in human beings.
Salicylates	Shapiro, Turner	Conflicting results regarding perinatal mortality and birth weight; great concern exists regarding effects on platelet function that could cause hemorrhagic complications in a traumatic birth. Possible intrauterine closure of PDA, pulmonary hypertension.
p-Aminophenols Acetaminophen	Schardein	These may be related to development of cataracts, but a causal relationship has not been confirmed.
NARCOTIC ANALGESICS	Rothstein	These appear to be nonteratogenic to human beings; withdrawal symptoms may occur in infants of narcotic-addicted women.
HORMONES AND HORMONE ANTAGONISTS		
Androgens	Forsberg	Increased risk of masculinization or pseudohermaphroditism in human beings has been reported.
Antiandrogens Cyproterone acetate	Forsberg	These are associated with abnormal sexual development in male laboratory animals; effects in human beings unknown.
Progestins Ethisterone, norethindrone	Wilkins	Association with equivocal or frankly masculinized external genitalia of varying degrees related to the treatment period during pregnancy has been found.
Estrogens Diethylstilbestrol	Barnes, Henderson, Herbst, Ulfelder	These are associated with vaginal adenosis and adenocarcinoma in young women exposed in utero; in exposed males there was increased incidence of genitourinary tract disturbances but no increase in cancer incidence.
Antiestrogens Clomiphene	Oakley	Multiple pregnancy has been reported.
Oral contraceptive agents	Levy, Nora, Ortiz-Perez, Rothman, Yasuda	Conflicting reports of results; it seems reasonable to conclude that there are no large risks of malformation facing offspring born after exposure to oral contraceptives.
Corticosteroids (natural and synthetic mineralocorticoids and glucocorticoids)	Schardein	All are teratogens in animals and have possibly been associated with cleft palate, limb anomalies, and heart defects in human beings.
Antithyroid agents (iodides and propylthiouracil)		These may produce neonatal goiter and tracheal obstruction; also may be associated with hypospadias, aortic atresia, and developmental retardation.
HYPOGLYCEMIC DRUGS (tolbutamide, chlorpropamide)	Landauer (1972)	Generally, hypoglycemic drugs have little if any teratogenic potential in human beings; possible increased incidence of caudal dysplasia (agenesis of sacrum and coccyx).
Insulin	Schardein	Insulin is teratogenic to mice and rabbits but *not* to human beings.

Table 19-3. Teratogenicity of physician- or self-administered therapeutic agents—cont'd

Specific agents	Studies reported	Results and recommendations
VITAMINS AND IRON		These are used almost universally by pregnant women with only rare reports of associated malformations (see following).
Vitamin A	Bernhardt, Pilotti, Schardein	Hypervitaminosis appears to be teratogenic in animals, and two cases of related urinary malformations have been reported in human beings.
Isotretinoin	Lammer	Characteristic pattern of malformations involving craniofacial, cardiac, thymic, and central nervous system structures has been found.
Iron-containing drugs	McBride, Nelson	Association with congenital malformations has been reported but remains unconfirmed by other studies.
DIURETICS		In general, these are not associated with congenital malformations.
Benzothiadiazides	Rodriguez, Torilla	Thrombocytopenia, altered carbohydrate metabolism, and hyperbilirubinemia have been reported in infants exposed late in gestation.
CARDIOVASCULAR DRUGS (antiarrhythmics, digitalis, glycosides, antihypertensives)		Very few reports relate these to malformations in human beings.
Propranolol	Oakes, Pruyn	Associations with decreased uterine blood flow and IUGR have been reported; bradycardia and hypoglycemia in the newborn.
ANTICOAGULANTS Warfarin	Schardein, Warkany (1976)	Of this group, only warfarin has shown teratogenicity in human beings. Exposure during the first trimester has been related to chondrodysplasia punctata and nasal hypoplasia associated with roentgenographic stippling of the epiphyses (Conradi's disease). Exposure in the third trimester is known to cause fetal or placental hemorrhage; thus it is recommended that patients requiring anticoagulant therapy be treated with an agent that will not cross the placenta.
COUGH AND COLD MEDICINES		
Bronchodilators, centrally acting antitussive agents, decongestants, expectorants	Schardein	Of these, only the iodide expectorants have been associated with adverse effects (fetal hypothyroidism and goiter).
Sympathomimetic amines (phenylephrine, phenylpropanolamine, ephedrine, dextroamphetamine)	Heinonen	These have been associated with facial malformations, inguinal hernia, and clubfoot; it is difficult to determine if these malformations were caused by these agents or by the viral infection being treated.

Western world. Prenatal and postnatal growth retardation, mental deficiency, persistent microcephaly, and minor anomalies of the face, eyes, heart, joints, and genitalia have been identified. The Collaborative Perinatal study reported a mortality of 17% and mental retardation in 44% of infants of alcoholic mothers.

A dose-response relationship may exist between the severity of fetal alcohol syndrome and the alcohol consumption by the mother. Among babies born to mothers who drank 1.5 ounces or more of absolute alcohol daily, 63% demonstrated neurologic impairment, 16% were born prematurely, and 28% were small for gestational age; 32% of the infants born to heavy drinkers had congenital malformations, and 16% had major malformations. The mechanisms whereby alcohol produces teratogenic effects on the fetus are unknown.

There now seems to be no question that maternal smoking substantially reduces the birth weight of offspring (Chapter 7). There is a significant dose-response relationship, and early cessation of smoking can result in birth weights similar to those among offspring of nonsmoking mothers. The largest studies also document a 30% to 35% increase in mortality resulting from abruptio placentae, placenta previa, prematurity, and respiratory disease. Some studies also report an increased incidence of spontaneous abortion in smoking mothers.

Data concerning an association between smoking during pregnancy and congenital defects in the infant are conflicting. There may be important functional consequences for the fetus of exposure to cigarette smoke, such as decreased fetal breathing movements and increased fetal heart rate. Several studies have reported a significant relationship between maternal smoking during pregnancy and low achievement, increased hyperactivity, and "minimal cerebral dysfunction" in the offspring.

Exactly which ingredient(s) in cigarette smoke causes the effects is not known; nicotine, carbon dioxide, and thiocyanate have all been implicated. There does not seem to be a significant beneficial effect on birth weight or perinatal mortality from reduction in nicotine and tar content or filtering of cigarettes. Prevention of the harmful effects of tobacco on the fetus can apparently only come from the cessation of smoking.

Although caffeine has been found to be teratogenic in high doses in animal experiments, reports suggest little teratogenic danger to human beings. Administration of caffeine does alter ovine fetal respiratory activity, however, and the presence of caffeine in most cord plasma samples suggests that it may alter human fetal respiratory activity or even neonatal breathing patterns.

Smoking and consumption of alcohol and caffeine are highly correlated. The potential interaction of these influences plus other drug and environmental factors is presently being systematically considered.

Environmental chemicals

Many chemicals are present in the environment. Fortunately, few of these chemicals have shown teratogenic potential in animals or human beings. In Ireland the prevalence of anencephaly and spina bifida has been related to heavy dietary consumption of blighted potatoes, although this has not been confirmed. Intrauterine methylmercury poisoning (Minamata disease) was characterized by severe neurologic symptoms and convulsions.

It has been suggested that the abuse of gasoline by inhalation could cause congenital malformations characterized by profound retardation, initial hypotonia progressing to hypertonia, scaphocephaly, a prominent occiput, poor postnatal head growth, and additional minor abnormalities. Polycyclic aromatic hydrocarbons and halogenated aromatic hydrocarbons (insecticides) are embryotoxic in animals; future studies may demonstrate that these environmental chemicals are also fetotoxic in human beings.

In summary, it is interesting to consider the specificity of the adverse effects of various drug groups. Exposure to hormones and antimicrobials during gestation produces fetal effects involving only one or two organ systems. In contrast, the antineoplastics, anticonvulsants, alcohol, and cigarette smoke have adverse effects on the fetus encompassing diverse organ systems.

Factors modifying the fetal response to drugs

Genetic background

In addition to the drug itself, the dosage, timing during gestation, and genetic background of the individual fetus and mother may play an important role in determining susceptibility to the teratogenic effects of a drug.

Experiments in mice differing at one allele demonstrated the importance of both the maternal and the fetal genotype in determining the outcome of exposure to a toxic drug. Fraser demonstrated genetic (strain) differences in the susceptibility of inbred mice to development of a cortisone-induced cleft palate. Also, a genetic defect in arene oxide detoxification may increase the risk of

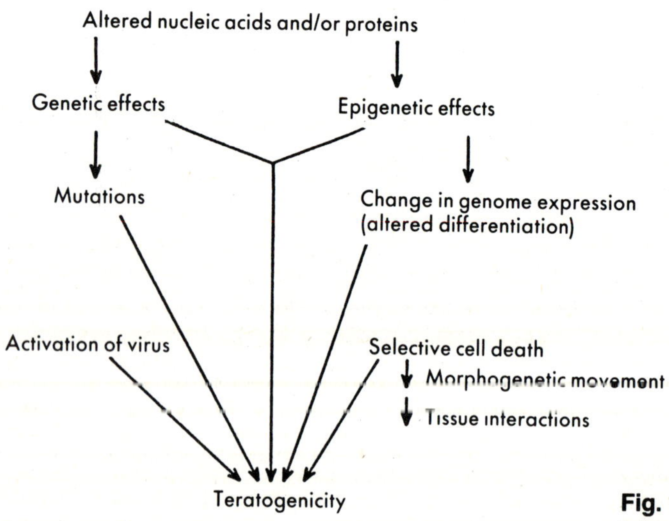

Fig. 19-3. Potential mechanisms of drug-induced teratogenicity.

epileptic women treated with phenytoin having a baby with major birth defects. Thus congenital malformations may be under multifactorial control.

Drug-drug interactions

Individuals taking drugs rarely consume a single drug; rather, they use various combinations. Animal experiments have provided examples of instances where the administration of one drug can modify the teratogenicity of another. For example, treatment of rats with phenobarbital increased the teratogenicity of the antitumor drug cyclophosphamide. It is thought that phenobarbital pretreatment induced maternal hepatic cytochrome P_{450}, increasing the activation of cyclophosphamide to mutagenic and/or teratogenic metabolites.

Mechanisms of drug toxicity in the fetus

Various mechanisms have been postulated for the adverse effects of drugs on the fetus. These include mutations, altered differentiation, inhibition of the biosynthesis of structural proteins (e.g., collagen), inhibition of tissue interactions, and altered morphogenetic movements caused by selective cell death (Fig. 19-3).

We now know that many chemical carcinogens (or mutagens) are *precarcinogens* (or premutagens) and must be metabolically activated to reactive electrophilic metabolites or "ultimate" carcinogens to initiate the cell damage leading to cancer. Experiments with limb bud and whole embryo culture techniques suggest that at least one teratogen, cyclophosphamide, also requires activation to its ultimate teratogen. Some evidence also suggests that thalidomide, phenytoin, chlorcyclizine, and diethylstilbestrol require metabolic activation to be teratogenic. The mechanisms whereby active metabolites produce their effects are thought to involve reactions with DNA (causing base substitution or frame shift mutations), with proteins (blocking crucial steps in cell metabolism), or with structural lipids (promoting lipid peroxidation). We know that many active metabolites, because of their instability, react with any available cell nucleophile. Thus a combination of these mechanisms may be involved.

Such reactive electrophilic metabolites can be detoxified by conjugation with nucleophiles such as glutathione, catalyzed by the glutathione S transferases. Animal experiments have revealed the presence of enzymes during development that may result in other deactivation processes, including hydration, glucuronidation, acetylation, or sulfation.

Determination of adverse drug effects in the fetus

Human studies of the effects of drugs during pregnancy are often retrospective. Amniocentesis and ultrasound can be used to screen for some birth defects, but pregnancy is already well advanced by the time these can be used. An alternative has been developed, *chorionic villi sampling*, which permits detection of genetic abnormalities in the first trimester.

Epidemiologic studies can, after the fact, correlate a drug with a defect and thus prevent exposure of future fetuses. However, to delineate the effects of drugs, taken either alone or in combination, on unidentified multiple factors in development is difficult in human beings, even in large epidemiologic studies.

Fortunately, animal models are now available to study the effects of drugs on the fetus. Such studies permit the definition of dosage of the drug, its timing during gestation, environment, and genotype and allow controls matched for weight and xenobiotic exposure. The definition of genotype and environment that these studies allow has increased understanding of the mechanisms of drug-induced teratogenicity. Rodents, specifically, mice and rats, are frequently chosen as animal models because they are easy to breed, inexpensive, and have short gestational periods. Although animal models are generally useful in identifying teratogens, certain limitations must be kept in mind. Thalidomide is an unfortunate example of a human teratogen that is not teratogenic in rodents. Aspirin (acetylsalicylic acid) is an example of a drug that is probably not a human teratogen but is teratogenic in rodents.

Further study of the mechanisms of drug-induced teratogenicity may permit the development of antiteratogens to prevent the fetotoxic effects of drugs essential for the mother during pregnancy. A variety of such compounds (e.g., nicotinamide, ascorbate, cysteine, vitamins) has been studied in laboratory experiments.

New, quick, and inexpensive screening tests for teratogens need to be developed. Preferably such tests should include metabolic routes of the drug similar to those in human beings. Perhaps whole embryo or organ culture techniques (limb bud, palate) will be accepted as screening systems to test teratogens in vitro. Such systems would have drug-metabolizing enzymes incorporated (in liposomes or intact liver parenchymal cells) to activate any preteratogen such as thalidomide or cyclophosphamide. Other studies have suggested that the inhibition of tumor cell attachment may be useful in the prediction of drug teratogenicity in vitro.

DRUG USE, DISPOSITION, AND METABOLISM IN THE NEWBORN

At birth a full-term infant in North America receives at least three types of drugs: an ophthalmic antimicrobial agent (e.g., silver nitrate), vitamin K, and triple dye for the cord. Low birth weight and sick infants in a neonatal

Table 19-4. Comparative plasma half-lives (in hours) of antimicrobial drugs excreted by the kidneys in newborns and adults

Drug	Birth weight (gm)	Newborn <7 days	Newborn >7 days	Adults*	Approximate relative prolongation <7 days	Approximate relative prolongation >7 days	References (first authors)
AMINOGLYCOSIDES							
Neomycin	Term	5.0	0-4	8	—	—	Axline (1964)
Streptomycin		7	—	2.5	2.5	—	Axline (1964), Sereni (1968)
Kanamycin	<2,000	7.7	5.2	3-4	2	1.4	Howard (1975)
	>2,000	5.3	3.8		1.5	—	
Gentamycin	<2,000	All infants	All infants	2	6	—	McCracken (1971)
	>2,000	5	3.2		2.5	1.6	
Tobramycin	<2,000	8.5	5.1	2	4	2.5	Kaplan, McCracken (1976)
	>2,000	6	4		3	2	
Amikacin	<2,000	6.6	5.5	2	3	2.5	Bodey, McCracken (1976)
	>2,000	5.8	4.9		2.5	2.4	
CEPHALOSPORINS							
Cephalothin	Term	1.5-2	—	0.5-0.8	2	—	Grossman
Cephazolin	Term	4.5-3	3	1.5	3	2	Nakasawa
PENICILLINS							
Penicillin G	<2,000	4.9	2.6	0.5	9	5	Braude, McCracken (1975)
	>2,000	2.6	2.1		5	4	
Ampicillin	<2,000	6.4	2.2	1.5	4	1.4	Eickoff, McCracken (1977)
	>2,000	4.9	2.3		3	1.5	
Carbenicillin	<2,000	5.7	3.6	1.5	6	4	Morehead
	>2,000	4.2	2.1		4	2	
Methicillin	<2,000	2.8	1.8	0.5	6	4	Howard (1975), McCracken (1977)
	>2,000	2.2	1.1		4	2	
Oxacillin	Premature	3	1.5	0.5	6	3	Axline (1967)
TETRACYCLINE		15-18 (1 day)†	6-8 (1 mo-11 yr)†	6.9	2	—	Sereni (1965)
SULFISOXAZOLE		12.4	7.8	5	2	1.3	Krauer (1975)

*Adult data derived from Weinstein, L.: Chemotherapy of microbial disease: antimicrobial therapy. In Goodman, L., and Gilman, A., editors: The pharmacological basis of therapeutics, ed. 5, New York, 1975, MacMillan Publishing Co., Inc.
†Age at study.

intensive care unit additionally receive an increasing number of drugs (Table 19-4), with the constant introduction of old drugs with new indications (e.g., caffeine and theophylline for apnea, indomethacin for closure of the ductus arteriosus) and new drugs (e.g., bumetanide) in the neonatal therapeutic armamentarium. Thus the overall xenobiotic exposure of the fetus and newborn exceeds current estimates, particularly when environmental agents (e.g., lead, methylmercury, volatile hydrocarbons) and drugs of habit (e.g., caffeine, alcohol) are taken into consideration. Since many of these agents are pharmacologically active, their effects may be significant if sufficient amounts reach the fetus or newborn. Besides the usual oral or parenteral routes, unintentional portals of drug entry include the transplacental route; inadvertent direct fetal injection; pulmonary, skin, or conjunctival entry; or via breast milk. Lack of awareness or underestimation of the degree of drug entry through these routes and of altered drug disposition and metabolism in the perinatal period have led to well-recognized therapeutic misadventures in neonatology. Possible prevention of drug toxicity and a rational and safe use of drugs require a thorough understanding of the various pharmacologic profiles of each drug used in the neonate.

Fig. 19-4 illustrates many of the interrelationships of the absorption, distribution, binding, biotransformation, and excretion of a drug and its concentration at the locus of action. To produce its characteristic effect, a drug must

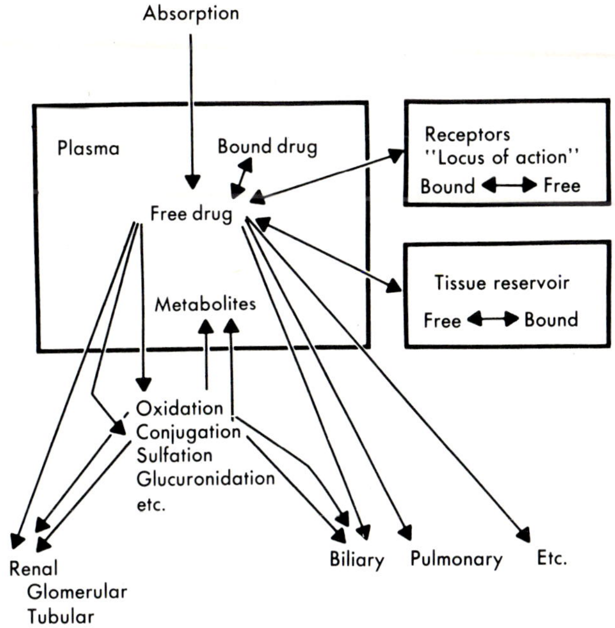

Fig. 19-4. Interrelationships of absorption, distribution, biotransformation, and excretion of a drug and its concentration at the receptor site.

be present in appropriate concentrations at its sites of action or the receptor sites. The concentration of drug at the receptor site depends not only on the amount of drug administered but also on the interrelationships listed. Those factors that have been evaluated in the newborn infant differ substantially from those in the adult and even in the young infant beyond the neonatal period.

Absorption of drugs in the newborn

Drug absorption is the passage of a drug from its site of administration into the circulation. In the sick neonate the intravenous route is preferred because of ease of delivery, accuracy of dosage, possible poor peripheral perfusion, and poor gastrointestinal function. In neonates who can tolerate gastric feedings, the oral route of drug administration is the most convenient and probably the safest. Absorption of a drug or substance through the gastrointestinal system may be comprehensively defined as the net movement of a drug from the gastrointestinal lumen into the systemic circulation draining this organ. This process entails the movement of drugs across the gastrointestinal epithelium, which behaves as a semipermeable lipid membrane and constitutes the main barrier to absorption. The various processes operating to induce transepithelial membrane movement of drug molecules include (1) simple diffusion through lipid membranes or through aqueous pores of the membrane, (2) filtration through aqueous channels or membrane pores, and (3) carrier-mediated transport such as active transport or facilitated diffusion and vesicular transport such as pinocytosis. Of these, the most important is the process of simple diffusion, since most drugs administered orally are absorbed via this route. This is evident from the direct proportionality between the concentration of the drug in the intestine and the amount of drug absorbed over a wide range of concentrations. Moreover, one drug does not compete with another for transfer, indicating that the process of absorption is a simple, nonsaturatable one.

The rate and extent of drug absorption are partly determined by the physical and chemical characteristics of the drug. Polarity, nonlipid solubility, and large molecular size tend to decrease absorption. In contrast, nonpolarity, lipid solubility, and small molecular size increase absorption. The degree of ionization, determined by the pK_a of the drug and the pH of the solution in which it exists, is an important determinant in drug absorption. The gastrointestinal epithelium is more permeable to the nonionized form, since this portion is usually lipid soluble and favors absorption. The degree of drug ionization will change as the pH increases from the stomach through the distal portion of the gut. The slow gastric emptying time in the newborn may retard drug absorption and could be rate limiting. This is because the major absorption occurs in the proximal bowel, which has the greatest absorptive surface area. On the other hand, a slow transit time or slow intestinal motility may facilitate the absorption of some drugs.

These physiologic processes do, however, undergo substantial changes during the neonatal period. Gastric acid production is generally low at birth, and the gastric pH is usually 6 to 8, decreasing within a few hours to pH values of 3 to 1. Acid secretion is low in the first 10 days of life; it tends to rise thereafter and approaches adult values around 6 to 8 months. Intestinal motility is slow in the newborn, and transit time from the stomach to the cecum is generally prolonged relative to that in the adult. The gastric emptying time after milk feeding is considerably prolonged in the neonate and approaches adult values at ages 6 to 8 months. The precise influence of milk feeding on neonatal drug absorption has not been studied.

Drug absorption requires an intact splanchnic vascular circulation. In sick neonates, especially those with hypotension, perfusion of the gut may decrease to maintain adequate perfusion of vital organs, resulting in decreased drug absorption.

Current evidence indicates that the amount of absorption of most drugs is independent of age, although the rate of absorption of certain drugs shows a nonlinear correlation with age. Heimann studied the enteral absorption of various drugs (i.e., sulfonamides, phenobarbital, digoxin, methyldigoxin. D[−]xylose and L[−]arabinose) and found reduced absorption rates in neonates relative to older children. There is very little specific information concerning other drugs; however, available information indicates that gastrointestinal absorption of drugs is relatively slow in the newborn and undergoes maturational changes similar to those found in drug distribution, metabolism, and disposition. Although the neonatal drug absorptive deficit may influence the achievement of a desired pharmacologic effect, it is very likely that its significance is minor relative to the age-related alterations in drug distribution, metabolism, and disposition.

Protein binding of drugs in the newborn

The unbound drug in the plasma is considered to be the pharmacologically active fraction of the drug. For some drugs, including theophylline, phenytoin, phenobarbital, penicillin, and salicylates, the binding to plasma protein in the newborn is decreased compared to that in the nonpregnant adult. This suggests that a more intense pharmacologic response may be obtained in the newborn than in the adult for the same total drug concentration. The developmental changes in protein-drug binding and the postnatal age at which adultlike binding is achieved have not been defined with confidence. Some drugs, such as phenytoin, may exhibit adultlike binding before the infant reaches 3 months.

The reasons underlying this deficient plasma protein binding of drugs at birth have not been definitely established. Possible explanations include decreased plasma albumin concentrations, possible qualitative differences in neonatal plasma proteins, and competitive binding by many endogenous substrates, such as hormones. Hyperbilirubinemia may accentuate this competition by displacing a drug, such as phenytoin, from its albumin-binding site. This contrasts to the well-known bilirubin drug-protein binding interaction, where drugs such as sulfonamides may displace bilirubin from its binding site.

Deficient plasma protein binding is not usually considered in calculating neonatal drug dosages. This factor must be considered in the application of adult therapeutic plasma concentrations to the neonatal patient. Moreover, decreased protein binding will influence calculations of apparent volumes of distribution based on plasma concentrations of total drug. In terms of therapeutic monitoring, drug concentrations obtained from saliva reflect the concentrations of the unbound fraction in plasma.

Drug metabolism and disposition in the newborn

Many drugs administered to the newborn infant need to undergo metabolism for efficient elimination from the body (Fig. 19-4). In the past decade, spurred by the chloramphenicol "gray baby" syndrome and the increased awareness of altered drug disposition in the newborn, the pharmacokinetic disposition and metabolism of some drugs have been studied in the neonate, and available data permit the following generalizations:

1. The rates of drug biotransformation and overall elimination are slow.
2. The rate of drug elimination from the body exhibits marked interpatient variability.
3. The maturational changes in drug metabolism and disposition as a function of postnatal age are extremely variable and depend on the substrate (or drug) being used.
4. Neonatal drug biotransformation and elimination are vulnerable to pathophysiologic states.
5. Neonates may exhibit activation of alternate biotransformation pathways.

The observation that drug elimination is slower in the neonate relative to adults is well recognized, although the magnitude and duration of this deficit as a function of specific drugs have not been adequately appreciated. Tables 19-4 and 19-5 shows the approximate prolongation of the plasma half-lives of certain drugs in the newborn relative to adults. Drugs that are closely related structurally, such as caffeine and theophylline, may even vary significantly. Thus application of dose rates for theophylline to caffeine in the treatment of neonatal apnea led to marked accumulation of caffeine in the blood. One apparent exception to this observed functional deficit is carbamazepine. Transplacentally acquired carbamazepine was eliminated in four of five infants in the immediate postnatal period as rapidly as in adults. In contrast, some drugs, such as indomethacin, caffeine, and theophylline, are eliminated much more slowly.

One possible basis for this difference in oxidative biotransformation and elimination capability relates to the existence of multiple forms of cytochrome P_{450}, each with its own distinctive substrate specificity. The cytochrome

Table 19-5. Comparative plasma half-lives of miscellaneous drugs in newborns and adults*

Drug	Plasma half-life (hours)		Approximate prolongation†	References (first authors)
	Newborn	Adult		
ANALGESICS-ANTIPYRETICS				
Acetaminophen	2.2-5.0 (3.5)	1.6-2.8 (2.2)	1.5-2	Levy
Aminopyrine	30-40	2-4	11	Reinecke
Phenylbutazone	21-34	12-30	1-1.5	Gladtke
Indomethacin	(7.5-51)	2-11 (6)	4	‡
Meperidine	22	3-4	5-6	Caldwell (1976)
ANESTHETICS				
Bupivacaine	25	1.3	19	Caldwell (1976)
Mepivacaine	8.7	3.2	2.5-3	Moore
ANTIEPILEPTICS				
Phenytoin				
Premature	(75)	—	3	Loughnan
Term	21	11-29	—	Rane (1974)
Carbamazepine	8-28	21-36	—	Rane (1975)
Phenobarbital	82-199	24-140	1.5-2	Boreus
				Harvey
OTHER DRUGS				
Amobarbitol	17-60	12-27	2	Krauer (1973)
Caffeine	40-231 (100)	(6)	17	Aranda (1979)
Theophylline	14-57 (30)	(6)	5	Aranda (1976)
Tolbutamide	10-40 (30)	4.4-9 (7)	4	Nitowsky (1966)
Chloramphenicol	14-24	2.5	5-9	Hodgman
				Weiss
Salicylates	4.5-11.5	2.7	1.3-4.5	Levy
Digoxin				
Premature	90	31-40	2.5-1.3	Wettrell
Term	52	—	1.3	Wettrell

*Values are expressed as ranges or individual values. Numbers in parentheses indicate mean.
†Approximate prolongation calculated from the mean values, if available.
‡Derived from several authors, as compiled from Aranda, J.V., and others: Ther. Drug Monit. **2**:39, 1980.

P_{450} monooxygenases are hemoproteins localized at the smooth endoplasmic reticulum of the liver microsomes that catalyze many oxidative drug biotransformation processes by the liver. Data on the comparative measurements of the hemoprotein cytochrome P_{450} in the human fetal, neonatal, and adult liver do not, however, fully explain the observed deficiency in drug biotransformation and elimination. Drugs that undergo conjugation may exhibit characteristics similar to those of drugs requiring oxidative biotransformation for elimination. Glucuronidation is virtually absent in midgestational human fetal liver, and this deficit persists at birth, whereas sulfation is active in the neonate. Acetylation and other synthetic or conjugative reactions, such as those with glutathione, are likely to be somewhat deficient at birth.

The time after birth at which adult rates of elimination are achieved and the rates at which these maturational changes occur vary with the drug used. Rapid increases in rate of elimination during the first week postnatally have been observed with phenytoin and phenobarbital (Figs. 19-5 and 19-6). Large interindividual variability in plasma half-lives was observed at birth but rapidly diminished with increasing postnatal age. This means that some neonates receiving a standard recommended dose may exhibit subtherapeutic drug concentrations in the plasma, whereas others may exceed the upper limit of the presumed therapeutic range. In neonates given phenobarbital for seizures, repeated doses of 5 mg/kg/day yielded mean plasma concentrations of about 40 mg/L during the first week, whereas a lower dosage (2.5 to 5 mg/kg/day) yielded plasma concentrations below 15 mg/L by the second and third weeks. The rapidity at which these developmental changes occur would warrant monitoring of plasma concentrations, since dose rates for many drugs usually held constant during the neonatal period may result in poor or exaggerated clinical re-

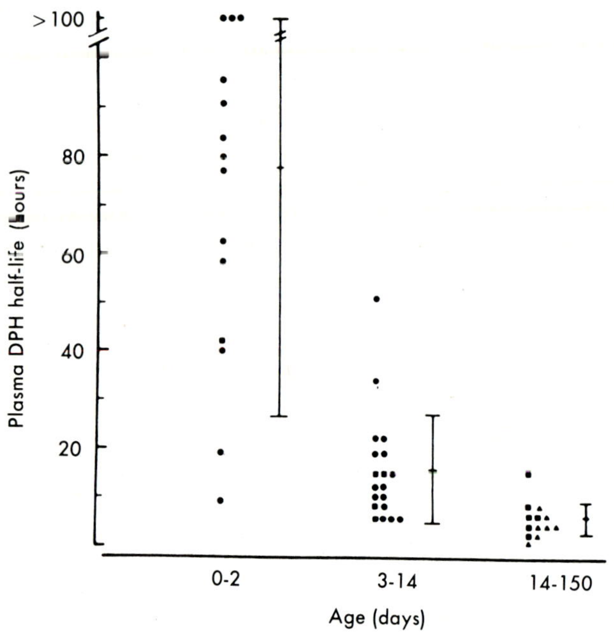

Fig. 19-5. Plasma phenytoin *(DPH)* half-lives measured in infants grouped according to postnatal age. Each infant received the drug via transplacental transfer (●) or as an initial therapeutic dose (■). Half-lives derived from steady-state plasma phenytoin as shown (▲). Bars indicate mean and standard deviations. Data were obtained from several published studies. (Reproduced, with permission, from Neims, A.H., and others: Annual Review of Pharmacology and Toxicology **16:**427, 1976. © 1976 by Annual Reviews Inc.)

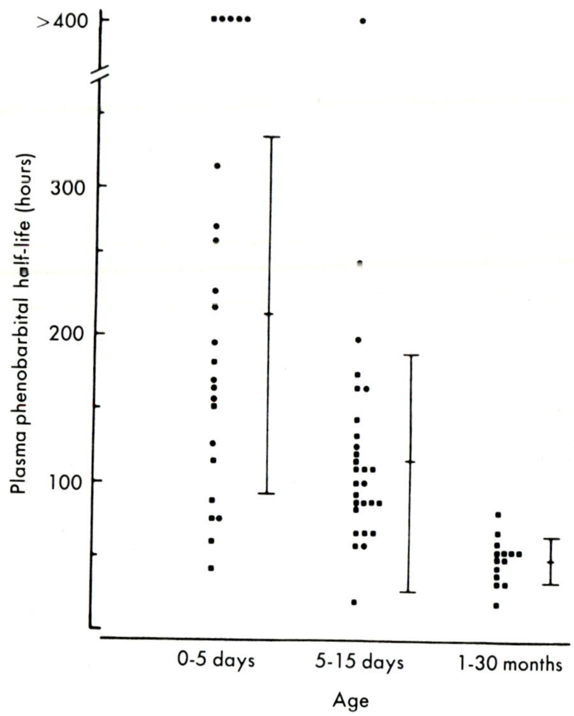

Fig. 19-6. Plasma half-lives of phenobarbital administered transplacentally (●) or postnatally (■) in infants, plotted as a function of postnatal age. Data were obtained from several published sources; means and standard deviation are shown. (Reproduced, with permission, from Neims, A.H., and others: Annual Review of Pharmacology and Toxicology **16:**427, 1976. © 1976 by Annual Reviews Inc.)

sponses that may be partly attributed to plasma drug concentrations below or above the presumed therapeutic range. Adjustment of dosage based on plasma concentrations of the drug and accounting for a rapid postnatal increase in drug clearance may result in maintenance of plasma concentrations of phenobarbital within the suggested therapeutic range (15 to 25 mg/L). In contrast, caffeine exhibits negligible maturational changes in the neonatal period. Adult rates of elimination are achieved at about 3 to 4 months and may be exceeded thereafter.

The need to eliminate xenobiotic compounds from the body in the face of decreased oxidative and conjugative pathways in the fetus and neonate may lead to activation and/or use of available biotransformation pathways. For example, premature neonates given theophylline may produce caffeine via methylation pathways, which are active as early as the first trimester, as shown in human hepatic organ culture studies. Since minimum oxidative function is present at this stage of gestation, the relative increase in activity of the methylase pathway leads to the production of caffeine as one of the major metabolites of theophylline in the human fetus and newborn. Both caffeine and theophylline exhibit similar phamacologic activity but of variable specific potency; therefore interpretation of clinical effect must account for both methylxanthines.

Disease states (e.g., congestive heart failure, liver disease) are well recognized in adults as factors that alter drug elimination. The presence of pathophysiologic states (e.g., hypoxia, asphyxia) in neonates can further diminish a deficient drug elimination capability, thus allowing the accumulation of drug in the plasma. For example, neonates with seizures who experienced perinatal asphyxia may have higher steady-state plasma concentrations of phenobarbital than those without asphyxia.

The dynamicity and variability in neonatal drug disposition and metabolism make generalization of dosage schedules and application of data obtained from one drug to another extremely difficult if not dangerous. Available data further reinforce the need for acquisition of specific

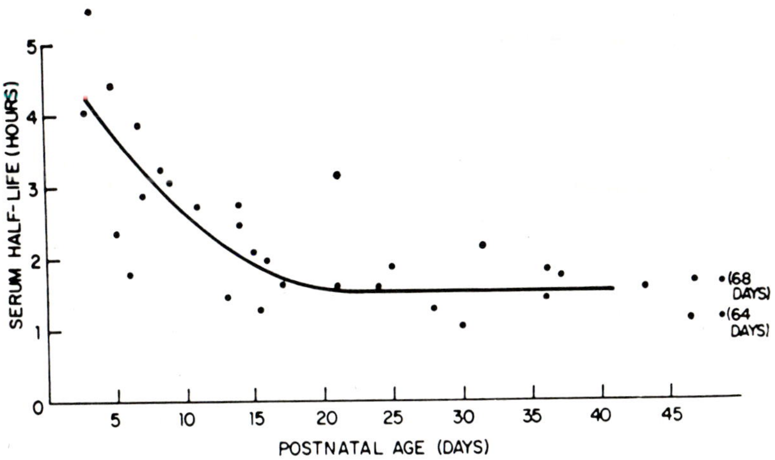

Fig. 19-7. Postnatal changes in the serum half-life of ampicillin. (From Axline, S.G., and others: Pediatrics **39:**97, 1967. Copyright American Academy of Pediatrics 1967.)

pharmacologic data for each drug used in the neonatal period.

Renal excretion of drugs

The kidneys are the most important organs for drug elimination in the newborn, since the most frequently used drugs, such as antimicrobial agents, are excreted via these organs. Renal elimination of these drugs reflects and depends on neonatal renal function, characterized by low glomerular filtration rate, low effective renal blood flow, and low tubular function compared to that in the adult (Chapter 35). Neonatal glomerular filtration rate is about 30% of the adult value and is greatly influenced by gestational age at birth. The most rapid changes occur during the first week of life, and these events are reflected by the plasma disappearance rates of aminoglycosides, which are eliminated mainly by glomerular filtration. These changes have been considered in the dosage regimen recommended by McCracken for these drugs and other antibiotics.

Effective renal blood flow may influence the rate at which drugs are presented to and eliminated by the kidneys. Effective renal blood flow, as measured by para-aminohippurate (PAH) clearance, is substantially lower in infants relative to adult values, even when PAH extraction values are correlated (i.e., PAH extraction is 60% in infants compared with greater than 92% in adults). Recent data suggest a low effective renal blood flow during the first 2 days of life (34 to 99 ml/minute/1.73 m^2), which increases to 54 to 166 ml/minute/1.73 m^2 by 14 to 21 days and further increases to adult values of about 600 ml/minute/1.73 m^2 by age 1 to 2 years.

The pharmacokinetic behavior of drugs eliminated via the neonatal kidneys exhibits characteristics similar to those underlying hepatic biotransformation. For instance, the half-life of many antimicrobials, such as ampicillin (Fig. 19-7), shows marked interindividual variability at birth, which narrows somewhat with advancing age. The plasma half-life also shortens progressively after birth, achieving adult rates of elimination within 1 month postnatally. The drug-dependent variability in the elimination process may reflect, in part, the major renal mechanism of drug excretion. Those drugs that undergo substantial elimination via glomerular filtration (e.g., aminoglycosides) may be excreted more rapidly than those requiring substantial tubular excretion (e.g., penicillins). These differences may reflect neonatal glomerular preponderance.

As with hepatic metabolism, renal excretion of certain drugs may be as efficient as in adults. For example, colistin, an antibiotic, is eliminated by neonates at rates similar to those in adults. However, as a rule, drug excretion via the neonatal kidneys is deficient relative to that in the adult. Pathophysiologic insults further compromise the inherent deficiency in drug elimination, thus complicating individual drug dosage regimens. Moreover, very small infants who receive the most drugs in the neonatal population exhibit the worst functional deficiency in drug elimination. This could result in overdosage, as in the case of digoxin. Neonates weighing less than 1,000 gm achieved steady-state plasma concentrations of digoxin three times higher than their full-term counterparts. Hypoxemia further decreases the slow glomerular and tubular function in the neonates, thus leading to slower renal excretion of drugs, as has been shown with amikacin. A linear relationship between oxygen tension and hepatic oxidation has been reported, so drugs that require hepatic biotransformation or renal excretion may be excreted much more slowly in the phase of hypoxemia. Determinations of plasma concentration of drugs, coupled with appropriate caution and clinical awareness, will help in optimum and safe drug therapy in the neonate.

PHARMACOKINETIC CONSIDERATIONS, DOSAGE GUIDELINES, AND THERAPEUTIC MONITORIING IN NEONATAL DRUG THERAPY

Knowledge of the kinetic profile of a drug allows manipulation of the dosage to achieve and maintain a given plasma concentration. Many drugs administered in the newborn period exhibit a plasma disappearance curve (Fig. 19-8). In this example the log of the plasma concentration decreases linearly as a function of time with a brief but fast distributive (α) phase and a slower elimination (β) phase. This exemplifies a two-compartment model and first-order kinetics, that is, a certain fraction (not amount) of the drug remaining in the body is eliminated with time, and after the distribution phase, the plasma concentration reflects or is proportional to the concentration of drug in other portions of the body. This model is applicable to a wide variety of drugs used in the neonatal period, although some drugs (e.g., gentamicin, diazepam, digoxin) fit a multicompartmental model; others (e.g., ethanol) exhibit saturation kinetics; that is, a certain amount (not fraction) of the drug is eliminated per unit time. In the newborn, where the elimination (or β phase is extremely prolonged relative to the distribution (α) phase, the relative contribution of the distributive phase to overall elimination and to dosage computations may not be significant. Thus the entire body may behave kinetically as though it were a single compartment.

The administration of a loading dose (mg/kg) to achieve quickly a given plasma drug concentration depends on the rapidity with which the onset of drug action is required. For many drugs used in neonates, loading doses would generally be greater relative to older children or adult subjects. The prolonged half-life warrants a substantially lower maintenance dosage given at longer intervals to prevent toxicity or overdosage. The rapid postnatal changes in drug elimination require adjustment of maintenance dosage rates (mg/kg/day) with advancing postnatal age; this adjustment may also be a function of the drug being used. Monitoring of drug concentrations is extremely useful if the desired pharmacologic effect is not attained or if adverse reactions occur. Moreover, therapeutic drug monitoring seems prudent, especially for drugs with a narrow therapeutic index used during a period in which there is rapid change in drug elimination.

DRUGS AND LACTATION

Until recently, investigations of drugs and other compounds in breast milk were hampered by the very small numbers of lactating women studied and the insensitivity of drug assay methods. Much of the earlier literature concerns isolated case reports and a small selection of drugs. Several recent papers review these data. At present a higher incidence of breast-feeding provides more situations in which lactating women are exposed to various medications, and an increasing number of useful studies of these drugs in milk can be expected.

In addition to pharmaceuticals, environmental pollutants and nontherapeutic or "social" chemicals find their way into human milk. Public awareness of these prob-

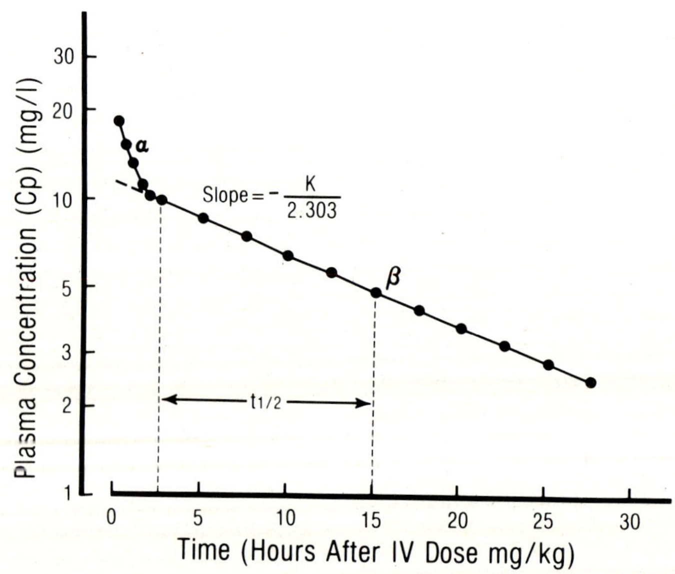

Fig. 19-8. Representative plasma disappearance curve of a drug given intravenously, plotted semilogarithmically as a function of time. A fast distribution phase (α) is followed by a slower elimination phase (β).

lems is high, and the physician is often called on for counseling.

Passage of exogenous compounds from maternal blood to milk

The presence and concentration of compounds in human milk depend on molecular weight, degree of ionization, protein binding in blood, lipid solubility, and specific uptake by mammary tissue. Drugs that are not absorbed after oral ingestion will obviously not appear in milk.

Small compounds with molecular weight of less than about 200 appear freely in milk and are presumed to have passed through pores in the mammary alveolar cell. Large compounds such as insulin or heparin do not pass into milk. Intermediate-size compounds must penetrate the lipoprotein cell membrane by diffusion or active transport.

In general, drugs that are not ionized at blood pH will traverse the alveolar cell membrane with greater ease than will highly ionized compounds. Since milk pH is about 7 or slightly less, milk will act as a trap for weak bases.

Drugs pass the cell membrane only in their free form; thus highly protein-bound drugs are less available for passage. Drugs or other chemicals that are very lipid soluble readily cross the alveolar cell, and, since milk contains a considerable amount of lipid, these compounds are also trapped in milk.

Finally, certain compounds are actively taken up by mammary tissue and are found in milk in concentrations substantially higher than in blood.

Modifications of passage of compounds into milk

Drugs may be metabolized by the maternal body to active or inactive metabolites. These derivatives may then be secreted into milk less readily than is the parent compound. The timing of maternal ingestion of a drug in relation to the time of milk synthesis may influence the concentration of the drug in any particular milk feeding.

In animals, changes in mammary gland blood flow control the amount of drug presented to sites of uptake. Mammary tissue itself can metabolize certain compounds. Drugs already secreted into milk may be secreted back into the alveolar cell and then into blood. Finally, the stage of lactation plays a role; drugs may be secreted more easily in the colostral phase.

Delivery of compounds to, and disposition by, the infant

The total volume of milk consumed in a known period of time determines the dosage to the infant. Since daily volume intake of breast milk is exceedingly variable and impractical to routinely measure, one could assume a *high average* daily milk consumption to be about 1 L.

To produce an effect, the drug in the milk must either act locally in the gut or be absorbed. It is possible that the proteins of milk will bind certain drugs and thereby impede absorption; it is also possible that the bowel of a very young infant may permit absorption of normally excluded large molecules.

The infant's disposition of the drug in milk will change with postnatal age; in addition, one must always be aware of the drug's potential for displacement of bilirubin from serum albumin.

Compounds in human milk

Anticoagulants

Heparin does not enter breast milk. Oral anticoagulants of the *inandione* group as well as *bishydroxycoumarin* and ethyl *biscoumacetate* are found in milk and have been associated with infant coagulopathies. *Warfarin* must be considered the drug of choice, since by virtue of its acidity as well as its high degree of protein binding it is undetectable in human milk.

Antiinflammatory and analgesic drugs

Acetylsalicylic acid (ASA) appears to be without danger when used occasionally. Older infants have been found to receive about 0.2% to 0.3% of a single dose of ASA administered to the mother. Although detailed studies do not exist, *acetaminophen* seems to be safe.

Antimicrobial drugs

Fortunately, most antimicrobial agents in human milk appear safe for the nursing infant. Drugs of the *penicillin* group may change the infant's intestinal flora and cause diarrhea and thrush; in theory they could also incite hypersensitivity. The *cephalosporins* appear to be secreted in insignificant amounts in milk. The passage of the various *sulfonamide derivatives* is influenced by their differing degrees of ionization and protein binding; all have the potential to displace bilirubin from albumin. Ingestion of *salicylazosulfapyridine* leads to the appearance of the metabolite sulfapyridine in milk; it has been estimated that the infant of a mother chronically using this drug will receive about 0.3% of the maternal dose per day. *Erythromycin* is present in milk in higher concentration than in maternal plasma, suggesting that the infant could receive a significant dose. The *tetracyclines* in milk have the theoretic potential to cause dental staining. Most authors recommend that *chloramphenicol* not be taken by lactating women, even though the drug levels in milk do not lead to a dose as large as those associated with the "gray baby" syndrome. The *aminoglycosides* are poorly absorbed from the infant's gastrointestinal tract. *Isoniazid* and *PAS* have not been associated with ill effects to the nursing infant. *Metronidazole* was considered contraindicated because of carcinogenicity in animals; however, recent human data suggest noncarcinogenicity. Also, metronidazole has been used in neonatal infections with no apparent immediate adverse effects.

Drugs affecting the cardiovascular system

The amount of *digoxin* present in milk depends on the maternal dose; infants whose mothers received 0.25 mg/day did not ingest enough digoxin in milk to have detectable blood levels. *Diuretics* in general seem to be harmless, although if a nursing woman were to become dehydrated because of diuretic use, lactation would be greatly depressed. The effects of diuretics on milk composition are unclear. *Spironolactone* and its less active metabolite are secreted in milk, and an estimated 0.2% of the mother's daily dose is received by the infant. *Chlorthalidone* appears in small amounts in milk but could potentially accumulate in the young infant. *Propranolol* seems to be safe. *Quinidine* is secreted in milk to a concentration about 60% that of maternal blood, but no ill effects have been observed.

Drugs affecting the central nervous system

Diazepam is converted in the body to an active metabolite, *desmethyldiazepam,* and both are excreted in milk. Both these compounds have a prolonged half-life in infants, and chronic use of diazepam by nursing women has been associated with lethargy and weight loss in their babies. The *barbiturates* appear in milk in concentrations that depend on their different degrees of ionization and lipid solubility. In anticonvulsant doses they seem to be safe. *Chlordiazepoxide* in breast milk has been linked to depression in the nursing infant. *Meprobamate* should probably be avoided, since the drug achieves milk concentrations several times greater than the maternal plasma levels.

Lithium is definitely contraindicated during lactation, since it has been found to cause significant cardiovascular and CNS signs in the infant. The *phenothiazines* and *tricyclic antidepressants* have been found in breast milk but appear to be safe in modest doses. The *amphetamines* also appear in milk and may cause jitteriness.

Phenytoin is found in milk in concentrations about one-fifth those of maternal blood. *Primidone* and *ethosuximide* both achieve milk levels near that of maternal blood, although significant symptoms in the infants have not been noted.

Drugs affecting the endocrine system

Drugs of the *thiouracil* family, *methimazole, carbimazole,* and *iodides,* are contraindicated during breast-feeding; they achieve a high milk concentration and can suppress the infant's thyroid function. Revision of this dogma was recently suggested, and *propylthiouracil* may be given to nursing mothers provided the infant's thyroid function is monitored.

Thyroxin and other thyroid hormone preparations seem to be safe; endogenous thyroid hormone naturally secreted in breast milk may mask congenital cretinism during breast-feeding. The long-term effects of exogenous *glucocorticoids* and their derivatives in milk are not known. Women receiving *prednisone* and *prednisolone* excrete very small amounts of these compounds in milk.

A common dilemma is the use of *oral contraceptives* during lactation. Little is known about the effects of long exposure to small doses of these compounds in milk. Contraceptives with a high concentration of estrogen and progestin will depress lactation, especially if they are begun soon after parturition. If their use is imperative, it would seem best to start treatment about 4 weeks after delivery, ensuring that lactation is already well established, and to use the lowest dosage possible. The infants should be followed with some care, since there have been reports of gynecomastia and changes in vaginal epithelium. A study of late effects in exposed infants is urgently needed.

Other drugs

Cimetidine, a histamine-H_2-receptor antagonist, has been reported in breast milk in concentrations 3 to 12 times greater than in maternal blood; this drug may be actively transported into milk. Until there is more information concerning its effects in infants, cimetidine should not be used during lactation. *Theobromine* from chocolate has been found in milk at a level of 80% of maternal serum. *Theophylline* ingestion by the mother has been associated with infant irritability. Extracts of *ergot* have been responsible for toxic reactions in nursing infants and should be avoided. The use of *isotopes* for diagnosis or therapy should be avoided during lactation. An acceptable level of an isotope in milk is not known. It has been suggested that women not nurse for 10 days after exposure to ^{131}I, for 3 days after ^{99m}Tc exposure, and for 2 weeks following ^{67}Ga exposure.

"Nontherapeutic" agents in human milk

Caffeine

One hour after the ingestion of an average cup of coffee, a peak milk caffeine level of about 1.5 μg/ml is obtained. Caffeine levels in milk are about half the corresponding maternal blood level. Although the daily amount of caffeine consumed by a nursing infant might be small, the long half-life of caffeine could cause symptoms such as wakefulness or jitteriness.

Ingredients of cigarettes

The *nicotine* content of breast milk from women smoking one pack per day has been found to be about 100 to 500 parts per billion. No symptoms have been ascribed to this degree of contamination. *Thiocyanate*, which is elevated in the blood of smoking women, does not appear in elevated amounts in their milk.

Ethanol

Ethanol, a small molecule, diffuses freely into milk and achieves levels equivalent to those in blood. The metabolite *acetaldehyde* does not appear in milk. Excessive ethanol intake by the mother may depress the infant's central nervous system.

Narcotics

Heroin, methadone, morphine, and other *opiate derivatives* have been found in milk and may be responsible for both addiction and withdrawal symptoms in the nursing infant. Opiates used briefly appear to have little clinical effect. It has been suggested that women receiving methadone maintenance doses take their daily dose after the last breast-feeding in the evening, since milk methadone levels are found to peak about 4 hours after administration of the drug by mouth.

Environmental pollutants in human milk

Lead

Lead has been found in both bovine and human milk, as well as in commercial infant formulas. The lead content of human milk has remained rather constant over the past 4 decades, in contrast to levels of some other pollutants. One study found the lead level in human milk in the United States to be about 0.03 μg/ml. There are no reports of signs and symptoms of lead toxicity from this source.

Mercury

Metallic or inorganic mercury poisoning in adults has usually be in association with occupational exposure. There are no reports of metallic mercury poisoning from human milk. Organic mercury, more specifically *methylmercury*, has been used industrially in fungicides, in pulp and paper factories, and in chlor-alkali plants. In the late 1950s Minamata Bay in Japan was contaminated with industrial wastes containing methylmercury; the compound found its way into human beings through contaminated fish. There was a high incidence of neurologic abnormalities in children born in this area, probably related to in utero exposure to the chemical rather than to exposure during lactation. Methylmercury was found in human milk in a concentration about 5% of that in blood; the half-life for disappearance of mercury from milk was estimated to be about 70 days.

Several epidemics in Iraq in the last 15 years were traceable to the contamination of grains with methylmercury fungicides. A number of nursing infants ingested enough methylmercury in milk to achieve blood levels above the toxic limit.

Pesticides

Organic pesticides are concentrated in body fat, and milk production, with its export of large quantities of lipid, is a very efficient way for the female to rid her body of these poisons. The nursing human infant thus becomes the highest animal in the "food chain." *DDT* (dichlorodiphenyltrichloroethane) was first identified in breast milk in 1951, and milk levels have been falling slowly since its use was restricted in North America in the early 1970s. Current levels of DDT in human milk vary geographically and are related to agricultural use of the compound. In Canada in 1979, average milk DDT was 44 ng/gm of human milk. A 5 kg infant ingesting 1 kg of breast milk each day would thus take in about 0.009 mg/kg/day. The FAO/WHO recommendations for maximum allowable intake by an adult is about 0.005 mg/kg/day. Nonetheless, there are no known harmful effects to the infant from the ingestion of human milk contaminated to this degree.

Many other pesticides have been found in human milk, and this reflects the current commercial use in the region or country. *Dieldrin*, for instance, which was banned in the United States after 1974, is decreasing in concentration in breast milk.

Industrial by-products

The extremely toxic dioxin *TCDD* (2,3,7,8-tetrachlorodibenzo-*p*-dioxin) caused environmental contamination in Seveso, Italy, in 1976. Children who were directly exposed developed chloracne; further effects remain to be determined. This toxin has been found in human milk.

There has been great public interest in the *polychlorinated biphenyls (PCBs)*. This class of compounds has had 50 years of industrial usage, primarily in the manufacture of electric apparatus (transformers, capacitors), although such usage seems to be declining. Because of contamination of rivers and lakes by industrial effluent, PCBs are widely distributed in fresh-water fish and in those animals that eat them. As with organic pesticides, PCBs remain in body fat stores and are excreted with the fat of breast milk. An epidemic of poisoning by PCBs (Yusho disease) occurred in 1968 in Japan, when a commercial rice oil product was inadvertently contaminated with PCBs. Fetuses exposed in utero suffered growth retardation both antenatally and postnatally. Several infants whose only exposure was via human milk developed weakness and apathy. It is of great concern that milk levels of PCBs in North America appear to be increasing. In Canada in 1979, the average PCB level in human milk was 12 ng/gm, whereas women who are exposed occupationally to PCBs or who consume game fish from contaminated waters may have much higher levels in milk.

The *polybrominated biphenyls (PBBs)* were brought to attention by an incident in Michigan in 1973 and 1974, in which several hundred pounds of PBBs, normally used as fire retardants in the plastics industry, accidently contaminated cattle feed; widespread intoxication of farm animals resulted. PBBs have the usual propensity to lodge in fat tissue and to persist in the body. To date, no ill effects have been noted in infants exposed to PBBs through their mother's milk. In Michigan, breast milk PBB surveillance has provided an accurate picture of the contamination of the general population. This method of epidemiologic analysis for fat-soluble poisons has much to recommend it, since the collection of milk samples is far easier than the collection of adipose tissue specimens. Breast milk PBB levels in the contaminated areas of Michigan averaged 0.07 parts per million.

Conclusion

As with the helpless fetus in utero, the nursing infant is exposed to nearly everything entering the body of its mother. The dangers, especially over the long term, are unclear. Environmental pollutants are almost impossible to avoid, and elimination of nontherapeutic (recreational) compounds involves changing life-styles. Drug administration is the easiest to control, but often a difficult choice must be made between maternal therapy and potential infant harm. The following are some simple guides to be observed:

1. A lactating woman should not receive a drug that one would be reluctant to give directly to her infant at that particular postnatal or gestational age.
2. Drug secretion into milk is so variable that one should not attempt to *treat* an infant by administering the drug to the lactating mother.
3. Milk that is donated to milk banks must be free from contamination.
4. When maternal drug administration is necessary, one may attempt to minimize the dosage to the infant by withholding nursing at the time of maximum secretion of the drug into milk.
5. Signs and symptoms in a nursing child should be correlated with drug ingestion by the mother. In investigations it is perhaps most useful to measure levels of the drug and its metabolites in the infant's body fluids, rather than at isolated times in maternal blood or milk.

Jacob V. Aranda
Barbara F. Hales
Judith Gibbs

BIBLIOGRAPHY
Drugs and the fetus

Barnes, A.B., and others: Fertility and outcome of pregnancy in women exposed in utero to diethylstilbestrol, N. Engl. J. Med. **302**:609, 1980.

Bernhardt, I.B., and Dorsey, D.J.: Hypervitaminosis A and congenital renal anomalies in a human infant, Obstet. Gynecol. **43**:750, 1974.

Bethenod, M., and Frederich, A.: Les enfants des antiepileptiques, Pediatrie **30**:227, 1975.

Bleyer, W.A., and others: Studies on the detection of adverse drug reactions in the newborn. I. Fetal exposure to maternal medication, JAMA **213**:2046, 1970.

Bongiovanni, A.M., and McFadden, A.J.: Steroids during pregnancy and possible fetal consequences, Fertil. Steril. **11**:181, 1960.

Braun, A.G., Emerson, D.J., and Nichinson, B.B.: Teratogenic drugs inhibit tumour cell attachment to lectin-coated surfaces, Nature **282**:507, 1979.

Butler, N.R., and Goldstein, H.: Smoking in pregnancy and subsequent child development, Br. Med. J. **4**:573, 1973.

Chung, L.W.K., and others: Perinatal toxicology: the question of delayed and residual effects. In Sellers, E.M., editor: Pharmacology of psychoactive drugs, Toronto, 1975, Alcohol and Addiction Foundation.

Clarren, S.K., and Smith, D.W.: The fetal alcohol syndrome, N. Engl. J. Med. **298**:1063, 1978.

Cohlan, S.Q.: Tetracycline staining of teeth, Teratology **15**:127, 1977.

Diamond, I., Anderson, M.M., and McCreadie, S.R.: Transplacental transmission of busulfan (Myleran) in a mother with leukemia: production of fetal malformation and cytomegaly, Pediatrics **25**:85, 1960.

Doering, P.L., and Stewart, R.B.: The extent and character of drug consumption during pregnancy, JAMA **239**:843, 1978.

Dunn, H.G., and others: Maternal cigarette smoking during pregnancy and the child's subsequent development. II. Neurological and intellectual maturation to the age of 6½ years, Can. J. Public Health **68**:43, 1977.

Ellenhorn, M.J.: The FDA and the prevention of drug embryopathy, J. New Drugs **4**:12, 1964.

Ericson, A., Kallen, B., and Westerholm, P.: Cigarette smoking as an etiologic factor in cleft lip and palate, Am. J. Obstet. Gynecol. **135**:348, 1979.

Eriksson, M., Catz, C.S., and Yaffe, S.J.: Drugs and pregnancy, Clin. Obstet. Gynecol. **16**:199, 1973.

Fantel, A.G., and others: Teratogenic bioactivation of cyclophosphamide in utero, Life Sci. **25**:67, 1979.

Fedrick, J., Alberman, E., and Goldstein, H.: Possible teratogenic effect of cigarette smoking, Nature **231**:529, 1971.

Forsberg, J.G., and Jacobsohn, D.: The reproductive tract of males delivered by rats given cyproterone acetate from days 7 to 21 of pregnancy, J. Endocrinol. **44**:461, 1969.

Fraser, F.C.: The multifactorial/threshold concept—uses and misuses, Teratology **14**:267, 1976.

Garrett, M.J.: Teratogenic effects of combination chemotherapy, Ann. Intern. Med. **80**:667, 1974.

Goldman, A.S., and Yaffe, S.J.: Fetal trimethadione syndrome, Teratology **17**:103, 1978.

Greenberg, L.H., and Tanaka, K.R.: Congenital anomalies probably induced by cyclophosphamide, JAMA **188**:423, 1964.

Hales, B.F.: Modification of the mutagenicity and teratogenicity of cyclophosphamide in rats with inducers of the cytochromes P-450, Teratology **24**:1, 1981.

Hales, B.F., and Jain, R.: Characteristics of the activation of cyclophosphamide to a mutagen by rat liver, Biochem. Pharmacol. **29**:256, 1980.

Hales, B.F., and Neims, A.H.: Developmental aspects of glutathione S-transferase B (ligandin) in rat liver, Biochem. J. **160**:231, 1976.

Hanson, J.W.: Fetal hydantoin syndrome, Teratology **13**:185, 1976.

Hanson, J.W., and others: Risks to the offspring of women treated with hydantoin anticonvulsants, with emphasis on the fetal hydantoin syndrome, J. Pediatr. **89**:662, 1976.

Hanson, J.W., Streissguth, A.P., and Smith, D.W.: The effects of moderate alcohol consumption during pregnancy on fetal growth and morphogenesis, J. Pediatr. **92**:457, 1978.

Harada, M.: Congenital Minamata disease: intrauterine methylmercury poisoning, Teratology **18**:285, 1978.

Heinonen, O.P., Slone, D., and Shapiro, S.: Birth defects and drugs in pregnancy, Littleton, Mass., 1977, Publishing Sciences Group, Inc.

Henderson, B.E., and others: Urogenital tract abnormalities in sons of women treated with diethylstilbestrol, Pediatrics **58**:505, 1976.

Herbst, A.L., and others: Prenatal exposure to stilbestrol: a prospective comparison of exposed female offspring with unexposed controls, N. Engl. J. Med. **292**:334, 1975.

Hill, R.M., Desmond, M.M., and Kay, J.L.: Extrapyramidal dysfunction in an infant of a schizophrenic mother, J. Pediatr. **69**:589, 1966.

Hunter, A.G.W., Thompson, D., and Evans, J.A.: Is there a fetal gasoline syndrome? Teratology **20**:75, 1979.

Joffe, J.M.: Influence of drug exposure of the father on perinatal outcome, Clin. Perinatol **6**:21, 1979.

Jones, K.L., and others: Pattern of malformation in offspring of chronic alcoholic mothers, Lancet **1**:7815, 1973.

Kline, J., and others: Smoking: a risk factor for spontaneous abortion, N. Engl. J. Med. **297**:793, 1977.

Lamba, P.A., and Sood, N.N.: Congenital microphthalmus and colobomata in maternal vitamin A deficiency, J. Pediatr. Ophthalmol. **5**:115, 1968.

Lambert, G.H., and Nebert, D.W.: Genetically mediated induction of drug-metabolizing enzymes associated with congenital defects in the mouse, Teratology **16**:147, 1977.

Lammer, E.J., and others: Retinoic acid embryopathy, N. Engl. J. Med. **313**:837, 1985.

Landauer, W.: Is insulin a teratogen? Teratology **5**:129, 1972.

Landauer, W.: Antiteratogens as analytical tools. In Persaud, T.V.N., editor: Teratogenic mechanisms: advances in the study of birth defects, Baltimore, 1979, University Park Press.

Landesman-Dwyer, S., and Emanuel, I.: Smoking during pregnancy, Teratology **19**:119, 1979.

Lenz, W.: Kindliche Missbildungen nach Medikamenteinnahme wahrend der graviditat? Dtsch. Med. Wochenschr. **86**:2555, 1961.

Levy, E.P., Cohen, A., and Fraser, F.C.: Hormone treatment during pregnancy and congenital heart defects, Lancet **1**:611, 1973.

Manning, F.A., and Feyerabend, C.: Cigarette smoking and fetal breathing movements, Br. J. Obstet. Gynaecol **83**:262, 1976.

Manson, J.M., and Simons, R.: In vitro metabolism of cyclophosphamide in limb bud culture, Teratology **19**:149, 1979.

Maren, T.H.: Teratology and carbonic anhydrase inhibition, Arch. Ophthalmol. **85**:1, 1971.

Martz, F., Failinger, C., III, and Blake, D.A.: Phenytoin teratogenesis: correlation between embryopathic effect and covalent binding of putative arene oxide metabolite in gestational tissue, J. Pharmacol. Exp. Ther. **203**:231, 1977.

McBride, W.G.: Thalidomide and congenital abnormalities, Lancet **2**:1358, 1961.

McBride, W.G.: The teratogenic action of drugs, Med. J. Aust. **2**:689, 1963.

Metzler, M., and McLachlan, J.A.: Oxidative metabolites of diethylstilbestrol in the fetal, neonatal, and adult mouse, Biochem. Pharmacol. **27**:1087, 1978.

Milkovich, L., and van den Berg, B.J.: Effects of prenatal meprobamate and chlordiazepoxide hydrochloride on human embryonic and fetal development, N. Engl. J. Med. **291**:1268, 1974.

Milkovich, L., and van den Berg, B.J.: An evaluation of the teratogenicity of certain antinauseant drugs, Am. J. Obstet. Gynecol. **125**:244, 1976.

Milunsky, A., Graef, J.W., and Gaynor, M.F.: Methotrexate-induced congenital malformations, J. Pediatr. **72**:790, 1968.

Monnet, P., Kalb, J.C., and Pujol, M.: Doit on craindre une influence teratogene eventuelle de l'isoniazide? Rev. Tuberc. (Paris) **31**:845, 1967.

Mulvihill, J.J.: Caffeine as teratogen and mutagen, Teratology **8**:69, 1973.

Naeye, R.L.: Relationship of cigarette smoking to congenital anomalies and perinatal death, Am. J. Pathol. **90**:289, 1978.

Nelson, M.M., and Forfar, J.O.: Associations between drugs administered during pregnancy and congenital abnormalities of the fetus, Br. Med. J. **1**:523, 1971.

Newcombe, R.G.: Cigarette smoking in pregnancy (letter), Br. Med. J. **2**:755, 1976.

Nicholson, H.O.: Cytotoxic drugs in pregnancy, J. Obstet. Gynaecol. Br. Cowlt. **75**:307, 1968.

Nishimura, H., and Nakai, K.: Congenital malformations in offspring of mice treated with caffeine, Proc. Soc. Exp. Biol. Med. **104**:140, 1960.

Nora, J.J., and Nora, A.H.: Birth defects and oral contraceptives, Lancet **1**:941, 1973.

Nora, J.J., and others: Maternal exposure to potential teratogens, JAMA **202**:1065, 1967.

Nora, J.J., Nora, A.H., and Toews, W.H.: Lithium, Ebstein's anomaly, and other congenital heart defects, Lancet **2**:594, 1974.

Oakes, G.K., and others: Effect of propranolol infusion in the umbilical and uterine circulations of pregnant sheep, Am. J. Obstet. Gynecol. **126**:1038, 1976.

Oakley, G.P., and Flynt, J.W.: Increased prevalence of Down's syndrome (mongolism) among the offspring of women treated with ovulation-inducing agents, Teratology **5**:264, 1972.

Ortiz-Perez, H.E., and others: Abnormalities among offspring of oral and non-oral contraceptive users, Am. J. Obstet. Gynecol. **134**:512, 1979.

Paterson, D.C.: Congenital deformities associated with Bendectin, Can. Med. Assoc. J. **116**:1348, 1977.

Poor, J. A., Bernhard, W.G., and Gordon, H.W.: Vitamin deficiency as a cause for birth deformities, Acad. Med. N.J. Bull. **10**:140, 1964.

Phelan, J.P.: Diminished fetal reactivity with smoking, Am. J. Obstet. Gynecol. **136**:230, 1980.

Piercy, W.N., and others: Alteration of ovine fetal respiratory-like activity by diazepam, caffeine and doxapram, Am. J. Obstet. Gynecol. **127**:43, 1977.

Pilotti, G., and Scorta, A.: Hypervitaminosis A during pregnancy and neonatal malformations of the urinary apparatus, Minerva Ginecol. **17**:1103, 1965.

Poland, A., and Glover, E.: 2,3,7,8-Tetrachlorodibenzo-p-dioxin: segregation of toxicity with the Ah locus, Mol. Pharmacol. **17**:86, 1980.

Posner, H.S., and others: Experimental alteration of the metabolism of chlorcyclizine and the incidence of cleft palate in rats, J. Pharmacol. Exp. Ther. **155**:494, 1967.

Pruyn, S.C., Phelan, J.P., and Buchanan, G.C.: Long-term propranolol therapy in pregnancy: maternal and fetal outcome, Am. J. Obstet. Gynecol. **135**:485, 1979.

Renwick, J.H.: Spina bifida, anencephaly, and potato blight, Lancet **2**:967, 1972.

Rhead, W.J.: Smoking and SIDS (letter), Pediatrics **59**:791, 1977.

Richards, I.D.G.: A retrospective inquiry into possible teratogenic effects of drugs in pregnancy. In Klingberg, M.A., Abramovici, A., and Chemke, J., editors: Drugs and fetal development, New York, 1972, Plenum Press.

Robaire, B., and others: Consequences to the progeny of paternal drug exposure. In Lobl, T.J., and Hafez, E.S.E., editors: Male fertility and its regulation, 1985, MTP Press.

Rodriguez, S.O., Leikin, S.L., and Hiller, M.C.: Neonatal thrombocytopenia associated with ante-partum administration of thiazide drugs, N. Engl. J. Med. **270**:881, 1964.

Rosenberg, L., and others: Lack of relation of oral clefts to diazepam use during pregnancy, N. Engl. J. Med. **309**:1282, 1983.

Rothman, K.J., and Louik, C.: Oral contraceptives and birth defects, N. Engl. J. Med. **299**:522, 1978.

Rothstein, P., and Gould, J.B.: Born with a habit: infants of drug-addicted mothers, Pediatr. Clin. North Am. **21**:307, 1974.

Safra, M.J., and Oakley, G.P.: Association between cleft lip with or without cleft palate and prenatal exposure to diazepam, Lancet **11**:478, 1975.

Samojlik, E.: Effect of monoamine oxidase inhibition on fertility, fetuses, and reproductive organs of rats. I. Effect of monoamine oxidase inhibition on fertility, fetuses and sexual cycle, Endokrynol. Pol. **16**:60, 1965.

Sarma, V.: Maternal vitamin deficiency and fetal microcephaly and anophthalmia, Obstet. Gynecol. **13**:299, 1959.

Saxen, I., and Saxen, L.: Association between maternal intake of diazepam and oral clefts, Lancet **11**:498, 1975.

Schardein, J.L.: Drugs as teratogens, Cleveland, Ohio, 1976, CRC Press, Inc.

Scheinhorn, D.J., and Angelillo, V.A.: Antituberculous therapy during pregnancy, West. J. Med. **127**:195, 1977.

Scott, J.R.: Fetal growth retardation associated with maternal administration of immunosuppressive drugs, Am. J. Obstet. Gynecol. **128**:668, 1977.

Selevan, S.G., and others: A study of occupational exposure to antineoplastic drugs and fetal loss in nurses, N. Engl. J. Med. **313**:1173, 1985.

Shapiro, S., and others: Antenatal exposure to doxylamine succinate and dicyclomine hydrochloride (Bendectin) in relation to congenital malformations, perinatal mortality rate, birth weight and intelligence quotient score, Am. J. Obstet. Gynecol. **128**:480, 1977.

Shapiro, S., and others: Perinatal mortality and birth weight in relation to aspirin taken during pregnancy, Lancet **1**:375, 1976.

Short, R.D., and Gibson, J.E.: Development of cyclophosphamide activation and its implications in perinatal toxicity to mice, Toxicol. Appl. Pharmacol. **19**:103, 1971.

Shotton, D., and Monie, I.W.: Possible teratogenic effect of chlorambucil on a human fetus, JAMA **186**:74, 1963.

Sieber, S.M., and Adamson, R.H.: Toxicity of antineoplastic agents in man: chromosomal aberrations, antifertility effects, congenital malformations, and carcinogenic potential, Adv. Cancer Res. **22**:57, 1975.

Smith, D.J., and Joffe, J.M.: Increased neonatal mortality in offspring of male rats treated with methadone or morphine before mating, Nature **253**:202, 1975.

Smith, D.W.: Teratogenicity of anticonvulsive medications, Am. J. Dis. Child. **131**:1337, 1977.

Smithells, R.W., and Sheppard, S.: Teratogenicity testing in humans: a method demonstrating safety of Bendectin, Teratology **17**:31, 1978.

Sobel, D.E.: Fetal damage due to ECT, insulin coma, chlorpromazine, or reserpine, Arch. Gen. Psychiatry **2**:606, 1960.

Soyka, L.F., Peterson, J.M., and Joffe, J.M.: Lethal and sublethal effects on the progeny of male rats treated with methadone, Toxicol. Appl. Pharmacol. **45**:797, 1978.

Spiers, P.S., and others: Human potato consumption and neural-tube malformation, Teratology **10**:125, 1974.

Strickler, S.M., and others: Genetic predisposition to phenytoin-induced birth defects, Lancet **2**:746, 1985.

Terrila, L., and Vartieinen, E.: The effects and side-effects of diuretics in the prophylaxis for toxaemia of pregnancy, Acta Obstet. Gynecol Scand. **50**:351, 1971.

Trasler, J., and others: Paternal cyclophosphamide treatment of rats causes fetal loss and malformations without affecting male fertility, Nature **316**:144, 1985.

Turner, G., and Collins, E.: Fetal effects of regular salicylate ingestion in pregnancy, Lancet **2**:338, 1975.

Ulfelder, H.: DES—Transplacental teratogen—and possibly also carcinogen, Teratology **13**:101, 1976.

Underwood, P.B., and others: Parental smoking empirically related to pregnancy outcome, Obstet. Gynecol. **29**:1, 1967.

Van Waes, A., and Van de Veldi, E.: Safety evaluation of haloperidol in the treatment of hyperemesis gravidarum, J. Clin. Pharmacol **9**:224, 1969.

Warkany, J.: Warfarin embryopathy, Teratology **14**:205, 1976.

Warkany, J.: Antituberculosis drugs, Teratology **20**:133, 1979.

Wilkins, L.: Masculinization of female fetus due to use of orally given progestins, JAMA **172**:1028, 1960.

Wilson, J.G.: Teratogenic effects of environmental chemicals, Fed. Proc. **36**:1698, 1977.

Drug use, disposition, and metabolism in the newborn

Agunod, M., and others: Correlative study of hydrochloric acid, pepsin, and intrinsic secretion in newborns and infants, Am. J. Dig. Dis. **14**:400, 1969.

Aranda, J.V., and Turmen, T.: Methylxanthines in apnea of prematurity, Clin. Perinatol. **6**:87, 1979.

Aranda, J.V., and others: Pharmacokinetic aspects of theophylline in premature newborns, N. Engl. J. Med. **295**:413, 1976.

Aranda, J.V., and others: Pharmacokinetic profile of caffeine in the premature newborn with apnea, J. Pediatr. **94**:665, 1979.

Axline, S.G., and Simon, J.G.: Clinical pharmacology of antimicrobials in premature infants. I. Kanamycin, streptomycin and neomycin, Antimicrob. Agents Chemother. **135**:141, 1964.

Axline, S.G., Yaffe, S.J., and Simon, H.J.: Clinical pharmacology of antimicrobials in premature infants. II. Ampicillin, methicillin, oxacillin, neomycin, and colistin, Pediatrics **39**:97, 1967.

Bada, H.S., and others: Interconversion of theophylline and caffeine in newborn infants, J. Pediatr. **94**:993, 1979.

Bodey, G., and others: Pharmacology of amikacin in humans, Antimicrob. Agents Chemother. **5**:508, 1974.

Boreus, L.O., Jalling, B., and Walling, A.: Plasma concentrations of phenobarbital in mother and child after combined prenatal and postnatal administration for prophylaxis of hyperbilirubinemia, J. Pediatr. **93**:695, 1978.

Bory, C., and others: Metabolism of theophylline to caffeine in the premature newborn infant, J. Pediatr. **94**:988, 1979.

Braude, A.I.: Antimicrobial drug therapy. In Smith, L.H., Jr., editor: Major problems in internal medicine, vol. 8, Philadelphia, 1976, W.B. Saunders Co.

Caldwell, J., and others: Pharmacokinetics of bupivacaine administered epidurally during childbirth, Br. J. Clin. Pharmacol. **3**:956P, 1976.

Caldwell, J., and others: Maternal and neonatal disposition of pethidine in childbirth—a study using quantitating gas chromatography mass spectrometry, Life Sci **22**:589, 1978.

Cumming, J.F., and Manngering, G.J.: Effect of phenobarbital administration on the oxygen requirement for hexobarbital metabolism in the isolated perfused rat liver and in the intact rat, Biochem. Pharmacol. **19**:973, 1970.

Dauber, I.M., and others: Renal failure following perinatal anoxia, J. Pediatr. **88**:851, 1976.

Ehrnebo, M., and others: Age differences in drug binding by plasma proteins: studies on human fetuses, neonates, and adults, Eur. J. Clin. Pharmacol. **3**:189, 1971.

Eickhoff, T.C., Kislak, J.W., and Finland, M.: Sodium ampicillin—absorption and secretion of intramuscular and intravenous doses in normal young men, Am. J. Med. Sci. **249**:163, 1965.

Faucett, D.W.: Surface specialization of absorbing cells, J. Histochem. Cytochem. **13**:75, 1965.

Gladtke, E.: Pharmacokinetic studies on phenylbutazone in children, Farmaco (Sci) **23**:897, 1968.

Grossman, M., and Tichnor, W.: Serum levels of ampicillin, cephalothin, cloxacillin, and nafcillin in the newborn infant, Antimicrob. Agents Chemother. **5**:214, 1965.

Guignard, J.P., and others: Glomerular filtration rate in the first three weeks of life, J. Pediatr. **87**:268, 1975.

Guignard, J.P., and others: Renal function in respiratory distress syndrome, J. Pediatr. **88**:845, 1976.

Harvey, S.C.: Hypnotics and sedatives. In Goodman, L., and Gilman, A., editors: Pharmacologic basis of therapeutics, ed. 5, New York, 1975, Mcmillan Publishing Co., Inc.

Heimann, G.: Enteral absorption and bioavailability in children in relation to age, Eur. J. Clin. Pharmacol. **18**:43, 1980.

Hodgman, J.E., and Burns, L.E.: Safe and effective chloramphenicol dosages for premature infants, Am. J. Dis. Child. **101**:140, 1961.

Howard, J.B., and McCracken, G.H.: Pharmacologic evaluation of amikacin in neonates, Antimicrob. Agents Chemother. **8**:86, 1975.

Howard, J.B., and McCracken, G.H.: Reappraisal of kanamycin usage in neonates, J. Pediatr. **86**:949, 1975.

Jalling, B.: Plasma concentrations of phenobarbital in treatment of seizures in newborns, Acta Paediatr. Scand. **64**:514, 1975.

Kaplan, J.M., and others: Clinical pharmacology of tobramycin in newborns, Am. J. Dis. Child. **125**:656, 1973.

Krauer, B.: The development of diurnal variation in drug kinetics in the human infant. In Morselli, P.L., Garattini, S., and Sereni, F., editors: Basic and therapeutic aspects of perinatal pharmacology, New York, 1975, Raven Press.

Krauer, B., and others: Elimination kinetics of amobarbital in mothers and their newborn infants, Clin. Pharmacol. Ther. **14**:442, 1973.

Levy, G., and others: Pharmacokinetics of acetaminophen in the human neonate: formation of acetaminophen glucuronide and sulfate in relation to plasma bilirubin concentration and D, glucaric acid excretion, Pediatrics **55**:818, 1975.

Loughnan, P.M., and others: Pharmacokinetic observations of phenytoin disposition in the newborn and young infant, Arch. Dis. Child **52**:302, 1977.

McCracken, G.H., West, N.R., and Horton, L.F.: Urinary excretion of gentamicin in the neonatal period, J. Infect. Dis. **123**:257, 1971.

McCracken, G.H., Jr., and others: Clinical pharmacology of penicillin in newborn infants, J. Pediatr. **82**:692, 1973.

McCracken, G.H., Jr., and Nelson, J.D.: Commentary: an appraisal of tobramycin usage in pediatrics, J. Pediatr. **88**:314, 1976.

McCracken, G.H., Jr., and Nelson, J.D.: Antimicrobial therapy for newborns, Monogr. Neonatol., New York, 1977, Grune & Stratton, Inc.

Mirhig, N., Reeves, M.D., and Roberts, R.J.: Effects of hypoxia on amikacin pharmacokinetics, (Abstr.) Pediatr. Res. **10**:192A, 1976.

Moore, R.G., and others: The pharmacokinetics and metabolism of the anilide local anesthetics in neonates. III. Mepivacaine, Eur. J. Clin. Pharmacol. **14**:203, 1978.

Morehead, C.D., and others: Pharmacokinetics of carbenicillin in neonates of normal and low birth weights, Antimicrob. Agents Chemother. **2**:267, 1972.

Morselli, P.L., and Ronel, V.: Placental transfer of pethidine and norpethidine and their pharmacokinetics in the newborn, Eur. J. Clin. Pharmacol. **18**:25, 1980.

Morselli, P.L., and others: Diazepam elimination in premature and full term infants and children, J. Perinat. Med. **1**:133, 1973.

Nakazawa, S., and others: Studies on cefazolin in the pediatric field, Chemotherapy **18**:659, 1970.

Neims, A.H., and others: Developmental aspects of the hepatic cytochrome P450 monooxygenase system, Annu. Rev. Pharmacol. Toxicol. **16**:427, 1976.

Nitowsky, H.M., Matz, L., and Berzofsky, J.A.: Studies on oxidative drug metabolism in the full term newborn infant, J. Pediatr. **69**:1139, 1966.

Odell, G.B.: The dissociation of bilirubin from albumin and its clinical implications, J. Pediatr. **55**:268, 1959.

Painter, M.J., and others: Phenobarbital and diphenylhydantoin levels in neonates with seizures, J. Pediatr. **92**:315, 1978.

Pinsky, W.W., and others: Serum digoxin levels in premature infants, Pediatr. Res. **10**:196A, 1976.

Rane, A., Bertillson, L., and Palmer, L.: Disposition of placentally transferred carbamazepine in the newborn, Eur. J. Clin. Pharmacol. **8**:283, 1975.

Rane, A., and others: Plasma protein binding of diphenylhydantoin in normal and hyperbilirubinemic infants, J. Pediatr. **78**:877, 1971.

Rane, A., and others: Plasma disappearance of transplacentally transferred diphenylhydantoin in the newborn studied by mass fragmentography, Clin. Pharmacol. Ther. **15**:39, 1974.

Reinecke, C., and others: Die Wirkung von phenylbutazon and phenobarbital auf die amidopyrin-elimination, die bilirubin-gisamtkonzentration im serum und eimige Blutgerin-nungsfatoren bie neugeborenen kinderm, Pharmacol. Clin. **2**:167, 1970.

Schanker, L.S., and others: Absorption of drug from the rat small intestine, J. Pharmacol. Exp. Ther. **123**:81, 1958.

Schedl, H.D., and Clifton, J.A.: Small intestinal absorption of steroids, Gastroenterol. **41**:491, 1961.

Seigel, S.R., and Oh, W.: Renal function as a marker of human fetal maturation, Acta Paediatr. Scand. **65**:481, 1976.

Sereni, F., and Principi, N.: Developmental pharmacology, Annu. Rev. Pharmacol. Toxicol. **8**:453, 1968.

Sereni, F., and others: Tissue distribution and urinary excretion of a tetracycline derivative in newborn and older infants, J. Pediatr. **67**:299, 1965.

Sertel, H., and Scopes, J.: Rates of creatinine clearance in babies less than one week of age, Arch. Dis. Child. **48**:717, 1973.

Sjoqvist, F., and others: Plasma disappearance of nortriptyline in a newborn infant following placental transfer from an intoxicated mother: evidence for drug metabolism, J. Pediatr. **80**:495, 1972.

Weinstein, L.: Chemotherapy of microbial diseases: antimicrobial therapy. In Goodman, L., and Gilman, A., editors: Pharmacologic basis of therapeutics, ed. 5, New York, 1975, Macmillan Publishing Co., Inc.

Weiss, C.F., Glazko, A.J., and Weston, J.K.: Chloramphenicol in the newborn infant: a physiologic explanation of its toxicity when given in excessive doses, N. Engl. J. Med. **262**:787, 1960.

Welbrandt, W., and Rosenberg, T.: The concept of carrier transport and its corollaries in pharmacology, Pharmacol. Rev. **13**:109, 1961.

Wettrel, G., and Anderson, K.W.: Clinical pharmacokinetics of digoxin in infants, Clin. Pharmacokinet. **2**:17, 1977.

Drugs and lactation

Ananth, J.: Side effects in neonates from psychotropic agents excreted through breast-feeding, Am. J. Psychiatry **135**:801, 1978.

Anderson, P.O.: Drugs and breast-feeding, Semin. Perinatol. **3**:271, 1979.

Bagnell, P.C., and Ellenberger, H.A.: Obstructive jaundice due to a chlorinated hydrocarbon in breast milk, Can. Med. Assoc. J. **117**:1047, 1977.

Berlin, C.M., and Yaffe, S.J.: Disposition of salicylazosulfapyridine (Azulfidine) and metabolites in human breast milk, Dev. Pharmacol. Ther. **1**:31, 1980.

Binkiewica, A., Robinson, M.J., and Senior, B.: Pseudo-Cushing syndrome caused by alcohol in breast milk, J. Pediatr. **93**:965, 1978.

Brillant, L.B., and others: Breast-milk monitoring to measure Michigan's contamination with polybrominated biphenyls, Lancet **2**:643, 1978.

Chan, V., Tse, T.F., and Wong, V.: Transfer of digoxin across the placenta and into breast milk, Br. J. Obstet. Gynaecol. **85**:605, 1978.

Committee on Drugs, American Academy of Pediatrics: The transfer of drugs and other chemicals into human breast milk, Pediatrics **72**:375, 1983.

DeSwiet, M., and Lewis, P.J.: Excretion of anticoagulants in human milk, N. Engl. J. Med. **297**:1471, 1977.

Dickey, R.P.: Drugs affecting lactation, Semin. Perinatol. **3**:279, 1979.

Dickinson, R.G., and others: Transmission of valproic acid (Depakene) across the placenta: half-life of the drug in mother and baby, J. Pediatr. **94**:832, 1979.

Eeg-Olofsson, O., and others: Convulsions in a breast-fed infant after maternal indomethacin, Lancet **2**:215, 1978.

Erickson, S.H., and Oppenheim, G.L.: Aspirin in breast milk, J. Fam. Prac. **8**:189, 1979.

Erickson, S.H., Smith, G.H., and Heidrich, F.: Tricyclics and breast feeding, Am. J. Psychiatry **136**:1483, 1979.

Erkkola, R., and others: Excretion of methylergometrine (methylergonovine) into the human breast milk, Int. J. Clin. Pharmacol. **16**:579, 1978.

Finely, J.P., and others: Digoxin excretion in human milk, J. Pediatr. **94**:339, 1979.

Fumita, M., and Takabatake, E.: Mercury levels in human maternal and neonatal blood, hair and milk, Bull. Environ. Contam. Toxicol. **18**:205, 1977.

Gelenberg, A.J.: Amoxapine, a new antidepressant, appears in human milk, J. Nerv. Ment. Dis. **167**:635, 1979.

Ghodse, A.H., Reed, J.L., and Mack, J.W.: The effect of maternal narcotic addiction on the newborn infant, Psychol. Med. **7**:667, 1977.

Giacoia, G.P., and Catz, C.S.: Drugs and pollutants in breast milk, Clin. Perinatol. **6**:181, 1979.

Hill, L.M., and Malkasian, G.D.: The use of quinidine sulfate throughout pregnancy, Obstet. Gynecol. **54**:366, 1979.

Jonsson, V., and others: Chlorohydrocarbon pesticide residues in human milk in Greater St. Louis, Missouri, 1977, Am. J. Clin. Nutr. **30**:1106, 1977.

Kaneko, S., Sato, T., and Suzuki, K.: The levels of anticonvulsants in breast milk, Br. J. Clin. Pharmacol. **7**:624, 1979.

Karim, A.: Spironolactone: disposition, metabolism, pharmacodynamics, and bioavailability, Drug Metab. Rev. **8**:151, 1978.

Karpow, S., Gotz, V., and Lauper, R.D.: Cimetidine, JAMA **239**:402, 1978.

Koup, J.R., Rose, J.Q., and Cohen, M.E.: Ethosuximide pharmacokinetics in a pregnant patient and new newborn, Epilepsia **19**:535, 1978.

Kuwabara, K., and others: Levels of polychlorinated biphenyls in blood of breast-fed children whose mothers are non-occupationally exposed to PCB's, Bull. Environ. Contam. Toxicol. **21**:458, 1979.

Lawrence, R.A.: Breast-feeding: a guide for the medical profession, St. Louis, 1980, The C.V. Mosby Co.

Levy, M., Granit, I., and Lanfer, N.: Excretion of drugs in human milk, N. Engl. J. Med. **297**:789, 1977.

Loughnan, P.M.: Digoxin excreted in human breast milk, J. Pediatr. **22**:1010, 1979.

Mandelli, M., Tognoni, G., and Garattini, S.: Clinical pharmacokinetics of diazepam, Clin. Pharmacokinet. **3**:72, 1978.

Meberg, A., and others: Smoking during pregnancy: effects on the fetus and on thiocyanate levels in mother and baby, Acta Paediatr. Scand. **68**:547, 1979.

Mes, J., and Davids, D.J.: Presence of polychlorinated biphenyl and organochlorine pesticide residues and the absence of polychlorinated terphenyls in Canadian human milk samples, Bull. Environ. Contam. Toxicol. **21**:381, 1979.

Mischler, T.W., and others: Cephradine and epicillin in body fluids of lactating and pregnant women, J. Reprod. Med. **21**:130, 1978.

Mulley, B.A., and others: Placental transfer of chlorthalidone and its elimination in maternal milk, Eur. J. Clin. Pharmacol. **13**:329, 1978.

Niebyl, J.R., and others: Carbamazepine levels in pregnancy and lactation, Obstet. Gynecol. **53**:139, 1979.

Nilsson, S., Nygren, K., and Johansson, E.D.B.: d-Norgestrel concentrations in maternal plasma, milk, and child plasma during administration of oral contraceptives to nursing women, Am. J. Gynecol. Obstet. **129**:178, 1977.

Nilsson, S., Nygren, K., and Johansson, E.D.B.: Transfer of estradiol to human milk, Am. J. Obstet. Gynecol. **132**:653, 1978.

Olszyna-Marzys, A.E.: Contaminants in human milk, Acta Paediatr. Scand. **67**:571, 1978.

Orme, M.L., and others: May mothers given warfarin breast-feed their infants? Br. Med. J. **1**:1564, 1977.

Pagliaro, L.A., and Levin, R.H., editors: Problems in pediatric drug therapy, Hamilton, Ill., 1979, Drug Intelligence Publications.

Phelps, D.L., and Karim, A.: Spironolactone: relationship between concentrations of dethioacetylated metabolite in human serum and milk, J. Pharm. Sci. **66**:1203, 1977.

Pynnonen, S., and others: Carbamazepine: placental transport, tissue concentrations in fetus and newborn, and level in milk, Acta Pharmacol. Toxicol. **41**:244, 1977.

Resman, B.H., Blumenthal, H.P., and Jusko, W.J.: Breast milk distribution of theobromine from chocolate, J. Pediatr. **91**:477, 1977.

Somogyi, A., and Gugler, R.: Cimetidine excretion into breast milk, Br. J. Clin. Pharmacol. **7**:627, 1979.

Sovner, R., and Orsulak, P.J.: Excretion of imipramine and desipramine in human breast milk, Am. J. Psychiatry **136**:451, 1979.

Tyrala, E.E., and Dodson, W.E.: Caffeine secretion into breast milk, Arch. Dis. Child. **54**:787, 1979.

Update: drugs in breast milk, Med. Lett. Drugs Ther. **21**:21, 1979.

Vuori, E., and others: The occurrence and origin of DDT in human milk, Acta Paediatr. Scand. **66**:761, 1977.

Wiles, D.H., Orr, M.W., and Kolakowska, T.: Chlorpromazine levels in plasma and milk of nursing mothers, Br. J. Clin. Pharmacol. **5**:272, 1978.

Yoshida, S., and Nakamura, A.: Residual status after parturition of methylsulfone metabolites of polychlorinated biphenyls in the breast milk of a former employee in a capacitor factory, Bull. Environ. Contam. Toxicol. **21**:111, 1979.

Yoshioka, H., and others: Transfer of cefazolin into human milk, J. Pediatr. **94**:151, 1979.

CHAPTER 20

Birth injuries

Birth injuries are those sustained during the birth process, which includes labor and delivery. They may be avoidable, or they may be unavoidable and occur despite skilled and competent obstetric care, as in an especially hard or prolonged labor or with an abnormal presentation. Fetal injuries related to amniocentesis (Chapter 16) and intrauterine transfusions (Chapter 5) and neonatal injuries following resuscitation procedures (Chapter 22) are not considered birth injuries. However, injuries related to the use of intrapartum monitoring of fetal heart rate (FHR) and collection of fetal scalp blood for acid-base assessment are discussed here. Factors predisposing the infant to birth injury include macrosomia, prematurity, cephalopelvic disproportion, dystocia, prolonged labor, and abnormal presentation.

The significance of birth injuries is most accurately assessed by review of mortality data. In recent years these data have demonstrated a steady decline in birth injuries as a cause of neonatal mortality. In 1981 birth injuries ranked sixth among major causes of neonatal mortality, resulting in 23.8 deaths per 100,000 live births. In 1984 birth injuries caused 8.9 deaths per 100,000 live births, falling to eighth among leading causes. This apparent improvement has been attributed to refinements in obstetric techniques, the increased use of cesarean section over difficult vaginal deliveries, and elimination or decreased use of vacuum extractors and version and extraction.

Despite this decrease, birth injuries still represent an important source of neonatal morbidity. In fact, Cyr and associates have demonstrated an increase in fractures and paralyses. They attribute this to more liberal use of midforceps to expedite deliveries in which the second stage is slowed.

Therefore, the clinician should consider the broad spectrum of birth injuries in the differential diagnosis of neonatal clinical disorders. Although many injuries are mild and self-limited, others are serious and potentially lethal. This chapter describes lesions that can be managed by observation only, as well as those that require more aggressive intervention.

INJURIES TO SOFT TISSUES

Erythema and abrasions

Erythema and abrasions frequently occur when dystocia has occurred during labor secondary to cephalopelvic disproportion or when forceps have been used during delivery. Injuries secondary to dystocia occur over the presenting part; forceps injury occurs at the site of application of the instrument. Forceps injury frequently has a linear configuration across both sides of the face outlining the position of the forceps. The affected areas should be kept clean to minimize the risk of secondary infection. These lesions usually resolve spontaneously within several days with no specific therapy. The recent use of padded forceps blades promises to reduce the incidence of these lesions significantly.

Petechiae

Occasionally, petechiae are present over the head, neck, upper chest, and lower back at birth following a difficult delivery; they are more frequently observed after breech deliveries.

Etiology.

Petechiae are probably caused by a sudden increase in intrathoracic and venous pressures during passage of the chest through the birth canal. An infant born with the cord tightly wound around the neck may have petechiae only above the neck.

Differential diagnosis

Petechiae may be a manifestation of an underlying hemorrhagic disorder. The birth history, early appearance of the petechiae, and absence of bleeding from other sites help to differentiate petechiae secondary to increased tissue pressure or trauma from petechiae caused by hemorrhagic disorders (Chapter 32). The localized distribution of the petechiae, the absence of subsequent crops of new lesions, and a normal platelet count exclude neonatal thrombocytopenia. The platelet count may also be low secondary to infections or disseminated intravascular coagulation (DIC). Infections may be clinically distinguished from traumatic petechiae by the presence of other signs and symptoms. DIC is usually associated with excessive and persistent bleeding from a variety of sites. Petechiae are usually distributed over the entire body when associated with systemic disease.

Treatment

If the petechiae are caused by trauma, neither steroids nor heparin should be used. No specific treatment is necessary.

Prognosis

Traumatic petechiae usually fade within 2 or 3 days.

Ecchymoses

Ecchymoses may occur after traumatic or breech deliveries. The incidence is increased in premature infants, especially after a rapid labor and poorly controlled delivery. When extensive, ecchymoses may reflect blood loss severe enough to cause anemia and, rarely, shock. The reabsorption of blood from an ecchymotic area may result in significant hyperbilirubinemia (Fig. 20-1).

Treatment

No local therapy is necessary. The rise in serum bilirubin that follows severe bruising may be decreased by the use of phototherapy (Chapter 34). Ecchymoses rarely result in significant anemia.

Prognosis

The ecchymoses usually resolve spontaneously within 1 week.

Subcutaneous fat necrosis

See also Chapter 37, part two. Subcutaneous fat necrosis is characterized by well-circumscribed indurated lesions of the skin and underlying tissue.

Etiology

The etiology is uncertain, although obstetric trauma is considered a possible cause. Many affected infants are large and have been delivered by forceps or after a prolonged, difficult labor involving vigorous fetal manipulation. The distribution of the lesions is usually related to the site of trauma, thereby explaining frequent involvement of shoulders and buttocks. Other etiologic factors that have been implicated include hypothermia, local ischemia, and intrauterine asphyxia. One suggested mechanism of pathogenesis proposes that diminished in utero circulation and mechanical pressure during labor and delivery result in vascular compromise to specific areas, which eventually causes localized fat necrosis.

Pathology

Initially, histopathologic studies reveal endothelial swelling and perivascular inflammation in the subcutaneous tissues. This is followed by necrosis of fat and a dense granulomatous inflammatory infiltrate containing foreign body–type giant cells with needle-shaped crystals resembling cholesterol.

Clinical manifestations

Necrotic areas usually appear between 6 and 10 days of age but may be noted as early as the second day or as late as the sixth week. They occur on the cheeks, neck, back, shoulders, arms, buttocks, thighs, and feet, with relative sparing of the chest and abdomen. The lesions vary in size from 1 to 10 cm; rarely they may be more extensive. They are irregularly shaped, hard, plaquelike, and nonpitting (Fig. 20-2). The overlying skin may be colorless, red, or purple. The affected areas may be slightly elevated above the adjacent skin; small lesions may be easily movable in all directions. There is no local tenderness or increase in skin temperature.

Differential diagnosis

This includes lipogranulomatosis and sclerema neonatorum, which present a serious prognosis, and nodular nonsuppurative panniculitis, which is usually associated with fever, hepatosplenomegaly, and tender skin nodules.

Treatment

These lesions require only observation. Surgical excision is not indicated.

Prognosis

The lesions slowly soften after 6 to 8 weeks and completely regress within several months. Occasionally minimal residual atrophy, with or without small calcified areas, is observed.

Lacerations

Accidental lacerations may be inflicted with a scalpel during cesarean section. They usually occur on the scalp, buttocks, and thighs but may occur on any part of the body. If the wound is superficial, the edges may be held in apposition with butterfly adhesive strips. Deeper, more freely bleeding wounds should be sutured with the finest material available, preferably 7-0 nylon. Rarely the amount of blood loss and depth of wound require suturing in the delivery room. After repair, the wound should be left uncovered unless it is in an area of potential

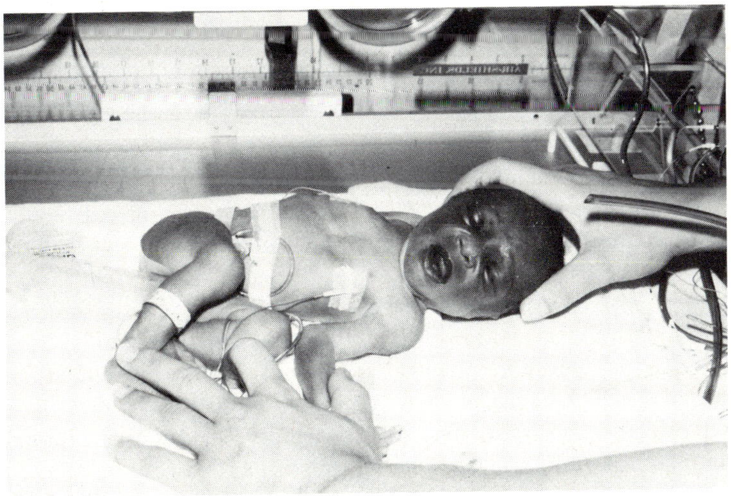

Fig. 20-1. Marked bruising of the entire face of a 1,490 gm female born vaginally after face presentation. Less severe ecchymoses were present on the extremities. Despite use of phototherapy from the first day, icterus was noted on the third day, and exchange transfusions were required on the fifth and sixth days.

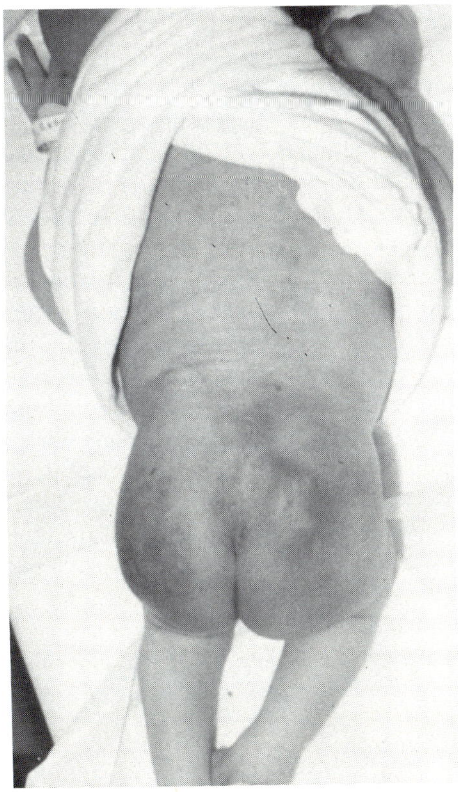

Fig. 20-2. Subcutaneous fat necrosis in a 2,900 gm, full-term infant delivered vaginally; pregnancy, labor, and delivery were completely uncomplicated. Note nodular raised lesion over the right buttock that is surrounded by erythema (darkened area). (Courtesy Dr. Rajam Ramamurthy, Cook County Hospital, Chicago.)

soiling such as the perineal area; in such locations the wound should be sprayed with protective plastic. Healing is usually rapid, and the sutures may be removed after 5 days.

INJURIES TO THE HEAD

Skull

Caput succedaneum

Caput succedaneum, a frequently observed lesion, is characterized by a vaguely demarcated area of edema over that portion of the scalp that was the presenting part during a vertex delivery.

Etiology. Serum or blood or both accumulate above the periosteum in the presenting part during labor. This extravasation results from the higher pressure of the uterus or vaginal wall on those areas of the fetal head that border the caput. Thus, in a left occiput–transverse presentation the caput succedaneum occurs over the upper and posterior aspect of the right parietal bone; in a right-sided presentation it occurs over the corresponding area of the left parietal bone.

Clinical manifestations. The soft swelling is usually a few millimeters thick and may be associated with overlying petechiae, purpura, or ecchymoses. Because of its location external to the periosteum, a caput succedaneum may extend across the midline of the skull and across suture lines. After especially difficult labors an extensive caput may obscure various sutures and fontanels.

Differential diagnosis. Occasionally a caput succedaneum may be difficult to distinguish from a cephalhematoma, particularly when the latter occurs bilaterally. Careful palpation usually indicates whether the bleeding is external to the periosteum (a caput) or beneath the periosteum (a cephalhematoma).

Treatment. Usually no specific treatment is indicated. Rarely a hemorrhagic caput may result in shock and require blood transfusion.

Prognosis. A caput succedaneum usually resolves within several days.

Cephalhematoma

Cephalhematoma is an infrequently seen subperiosteal collection of blood overlying a cranial bone. The incidence is 0.4% to 2.5% of live births; the frequency is higher in male infants and in infants born to primiparous mothers.

Etiology. A cephalhematoma is caused during labor or delivery by a rupture of blood vessels that traverse from skull to periosteum. Repeated buffeting of the fetal skull against the maternal pelvis during a prolonged or difficult labor and mechanical trauma caused by use of forceps in delivery have been implicated.

Clinical manifestations. The bleeding is sharply limited by periosteal attachments to the surface of one cranial bone; there is no extension across suture lines. The bleeding usually occurs over one or both parietal bones. Less often it involves the occipital bones and, very rarely, the frontal bones. The overlying scalp is not discolored. Because subperiosteal bleeding is slow, the swelling may not be apparent for several hours or days after birth. The swelling is often larger on the second or third day, when sharply demarcated boundaries are palpable. The cephalhematoma may feel fluctuant and is often bordered by a slightly elevated ridge of organizing tissue that gives the false sensation of a central bony depression. In 1952 Kendall and Woloshin noted an underlying skull fracture in 25% of cephalhematomas; a subsequent study by Zelson and associates indicated an incidence of 5.4%. These fractures are almost always linear and nondepressed.

Roentgenographic manifestations. These vary with the age of the cephalhematoma. During the first 2 weeks bloody fluid results in a shadow of water density. At the end of the second week bone begins to form under the elevated pericranium at the margins of the hematoma; the entire lesion is progressively overlaid with a complete shell of bone.

Differential diagnosis. A cephalhematoma may be differentiated from caput succedaneum by (1) its sharp periosteal limitations to one bone, (2) the absence of overlying discoloration, (3) the later initial appearance of the swelling, and (4) the longer time before resolution. Cranial meningocele is differentiated from cephalhematoma by pulsations, increase in pressure during crying, and the demonstration of a bony defect by roentgenogram. An occipital cephalhematoma may be confused initially with an occipital meningocele and with cranium bifidum because all occupy the midline position.

Treatment. Therapy is not indicated for the uncomplicated cephalhematoma. Rarely a massive cephalhematoma may result in blood loss severe enough to require transfusion. Significant hyperbilirubinemia may also result, necessitating phototherapy or other treatment of jaundice (Chapter 34).

The most common associated complications are skull fracture and intracranial hemorrhage. Linear fractures do not require specific therapy, but roentgenograms shoud be taken at 4 to 6 weeks to ensure closure and to exclude formation of leptomeningeal cysts; depressed fractures require immediate neurosurgical consultation. Specific treatment for blood loss or hyperbilirubinemia or both may be indicated if there has been an intracranial hemorrhage. Incision or aspiration of a cephalhematoma is contraindicated because of the risk of introducing infection. Rarely bacterial infections of cephalhematomas occur, usually in association with septicemia and meningitis. Focal infection should be suspected when a sudden enlargement of a static cephalhematoma occurs during the course of a systemic infection, a relapse of meningitis or sepsis after treatment with antibiotics, or the development of local signs of infection over the cephalhematoma (Fig. 20-3). Diagnostic aspiration may be indicated. If a local infection is present, surgical drainage and specific antibiotic therapy should be instituted.

Prognosis. Most cephalhematomas are resorbed within 2 weeks to 3 months, depending on their size; most are resorbed by 6 weeks. In a few patients, calcium is deposited (Fig. 20-4), causing a bony swelling that may persist for several months and, rarely, up to 1½ years.

Roentgenographic findings persist after disappearance of clinical signs. The outer table remains thickened as a flat, irregular hyperostosis for several months. Widening of the space between the new shell of bone and the inner table may persist for years; the space originally occupied by hematoma usually develops into normal diploic bone, but cystlike defects may persist at the sites of the hematoma for months or years. Rarely a neonatal cephalhematoma may persist into adult life as a symptomless mass, the *cephalhematoma deformans of Schüller*.

Skull fractures

Fracture of the neonatal skull is uncommon, since the bones of the skull are less mineralized at birth and thus more compressible. In addition, the separation of the bones by membranous sutures usually permits enough alteration in the contour of the head to allow its passage through the birth canal without injury.

Etiology. Skull fractures usually follow a forceps deliv-

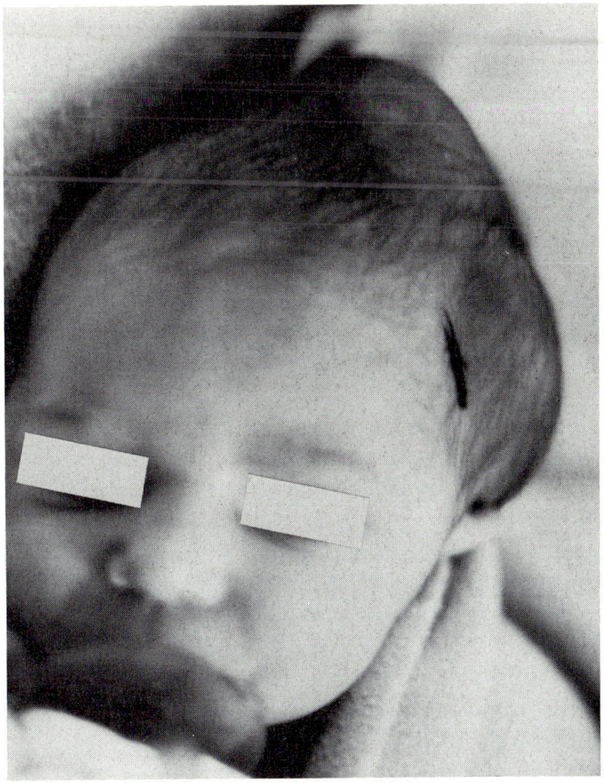

Fig. 20-3. Massive, persistently enlarging cephalhematoma in a 13-day-old female, who had been delivered by midforceps after occiput-posterior presentation. Surgical drainage revealed 300 ml of yellowish material that cultured *Escherichia coli.*

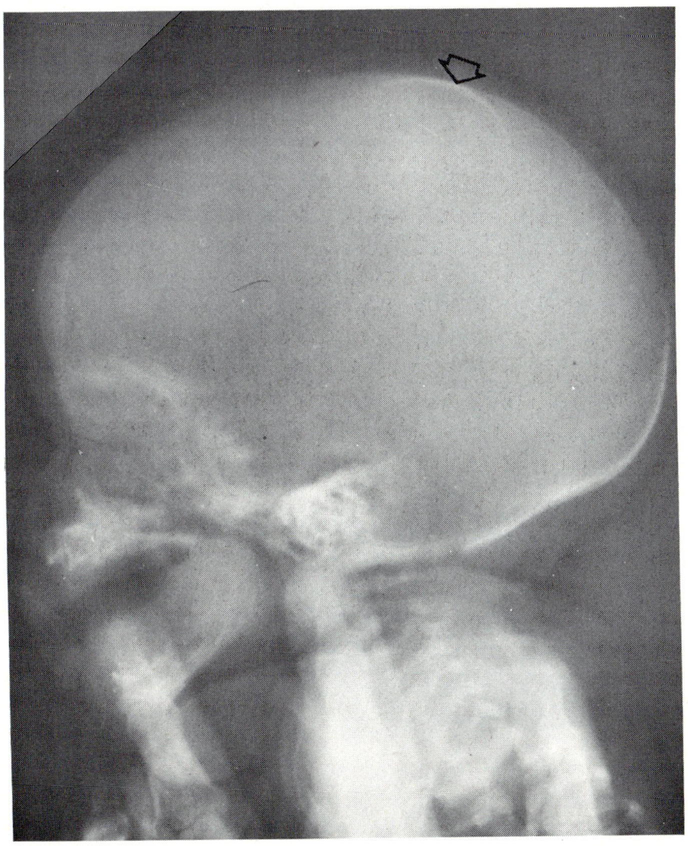

Fig. 20-4. Calcified cephalhematoma in left parietal region of a 5-week-old female. Infant weighed 1,410 gm at birth and was delivered rapidly because of prolapsed cord. Hard left parietal swelling was detected at 5 weeks by nurses while feeding the infant.

ery or a prolonged, difficult labor with repeated forceful contact of the fetal skull against the maternal symphysis pubis, sacral promontory, or ischial spine. Most of the fractures are linear. Depressed fractures almost always result from forceps application. However, they may occur spontaneously following cesarean section or vaginal delivery without forceps. Factors that have been implicated include pressure on the fetal skull by a maternal bony prominence (e.g., sacral promontory) or uterine fibroid, a fetal hand or foot, or the body part of a twin. Occipital bone fractures usually occur in breech deliveries as a consequence of traction on the hyperextended spine of the infant when the head is fixed in the maternal pelvis.

Clinical manifestations. Linear fractures over the convexity of the skull are frequently accompanied by soft tissue changes and cephalhematoma. Usually the infant's behavior is normal unless there is an associated concussion or hemorrhage into the subdural or subarachnoid space. Fractures at the base of the skull with separation of the basal and squamous portions of the occipital bone almost always result in severe hemorrhage caused by disruption of the underlying venous sinuses. The infant may develop shock, neurologic abnormalities, and drainage of bloody cerebrospinal fluid from the ears or nose.

Depressed fractures are visible and palpable indentations in the smooth contour of the skull, similar to dents in a Ping-Pong ball (Fig. 20-5). The infant may be entirely asymptomatic unless there is associated intracranial injury.

Roentgenographic manifestations. The diagnosis of a simple linear or fissure fracture is seldom made without roentgenograms, where fractures appear as lines and strips of decreased density. Depressed fractures appear as lines of increased density. On some views they are manifested by an inward buckling of bone with or without an actual break in continuity. Either type of fracture may be seen on only one view.

Differential diagnosis. Occasionally the fragments of a linear fracture may be widely separated and simulate an open suture. Conversely, parietal foramina, the interparietal fontanel, mendosal sutures, and innominate synchondroses may be mistaken for fractures. In addition, normal vascular grooves, "ripple lines" that represent soft tissue folds of the scalp, and lacunar skull may be mistaken for fractures.

Treatment. Uncomplicated linear fractures over the convexity of the skull usually do not require treatment. Fractures at the base of the skull often necessitate blood replacement for severe hemorrhage and shock, in addition to other supportive measures. If cerebrospinal fluid rhinorrhea or otorrhea is present, antimicrobial coverage is indicated to prevent secondary infection of the meninges.

Small (less than 2 cm) "Ping-Pong" fractures may be observed without surgical treatment. Loeser and associates reported three infants with depressed skull frac-

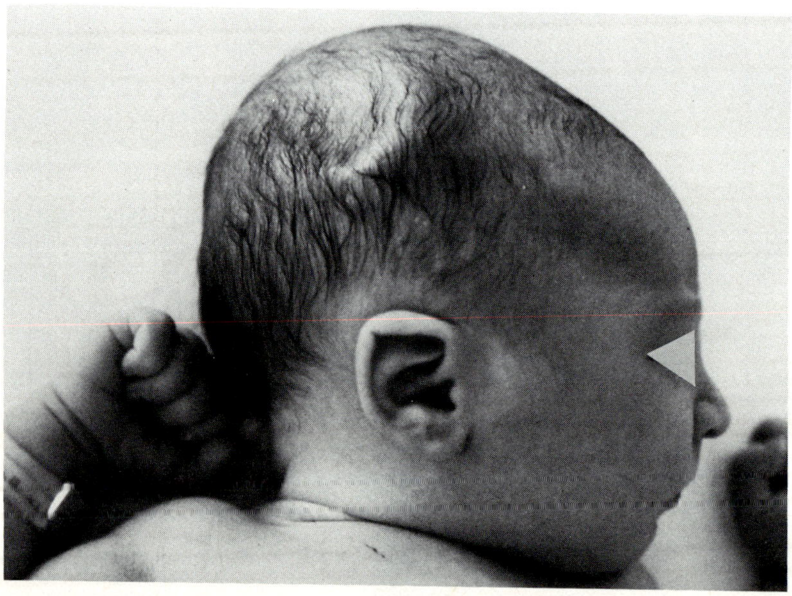

Fig. 20-5. Depressed skull fracture in a full-term male delivered after rapid (1 hour) labor. The infant was delivered by occiput-anterior presentation after rotation from occiput-posterior position.

tures in whom spontaneous elevation of the fractures occurred within 1 day to 3½ months of age. Follow-up at 1 to 2½ years revealed normal neurologic development in all three.

Several nonsurgical methods have been described for elevation of depressed skull fractures in certain infants:

1. A thumb is placed on opposite margins of the depression and gentle, firm pressure exerted toward the middle. After several minutes of continuous pressure the area of depression gradually disappears.
2. A hand breast pump is applied to the depressed area. Petroleum jelly placed on the pump edges ensures a tighter seal, and gentle suction for several minutes results in elevation of the depressed bone.
3. A vacuum extractor is placed over the depression, and a negative pressure of approximately 0.2 to 0.5 kg/cm^2 is maintained for approximately 4 minutes.

Since these methods are technically easier and less traumatic, they may be preferable to surgical intervention in an asymptomatic infant with an isolated lesion.

Comminuted or large fractures associated with neurologic signs or symptoms should be treated by immediate surgical elevation of the indented segment to prevent underlying cortical injury from pressure. Other indications for surgical elevation include manifestations of cerebrospinal fluid beneath the galea and failure to elevate the fracture by nonsurgical manipulation.

Prognosis. Simple linear fractures usually heal within several months without sequelae. Rarely a leptomeningeal cyst may develop from an associated dural tear, and meninges or part of the brain may protrude through the fracture. The fracture line may widen rapidly within weeks, or a large defect in the skull may be noted many months later. If detected early, the cyst may be excised successfully and brain atrophy prevented. It is therefore advisable to repeat skull roentgenograms within 2 to 3 months to detect early widening of the fracture line.

Basal fractures carry a poor prognosis. When separation of the basal and squamous portions of the occipital bone occurs, the outcome is almost always fatal; surviving infants have an extremely high incidence of neurologic sequelae.

The prognosis for a depressed fracture is usually good when treatment is early and adequate. When therapy is delayed, especially with a large depression, death may occur from pressure on vital areas of the brain. Since the natural history of depressed skull fractures in neonates has not been clearly elucidated, the outcome is uncertain for infants with smaller lesions that have been treated either by simple observation or by surgery after significant delays. Despite the apparently normal outcome in the three infants reported by Loeser and associates, one cannot completely exclude the possibility of subtle neurologic sequelae developing years later.

Intracranial hemorrhage

See Chapter 27.

Face

Facial nerve palsy

Facial nerve palsy in the neonate may follow birth injury or rarely may result from agenesis of the facial nerve nucleus. The latter condition is occasionally hereditary but is usually sporadic.

Etiology. Traumatic facial nerve palsy most often follows compression of the peripheral portion of the nerve, either near the stylomastoid foramen through which it emerges or where the nerve traverses the ramus of the mandible. The nerve may be compressed by forceps, especially when the fetal head has been grasped obliquely. The condition also occurs after spontaneous deliveries following prolonged pressure by the maternal sacral promontory. Less frequently injury is sustained in utero, often in association with a mandibular deformity, by the persistent position of the fetal foot against the superior ramus of the mandible. An extremely rare cause is the pressure of a uterine tumor on the nerve.

A traumatic facial nerve palsy may follow a contralateral injury to the central nervous system (CNS), such as a temporal bone fracture or hemorrhage, tissue destruction, or both to structures within the posterior fossa. This central nerve injury is less frequent than a peripheral nerve injury.

Clinical manifestations. Paralysis is usually apparent on the first or second day but may be present at birth. It usually does not increase in severity unless considerable edema occurs over the area of nerve trauma. The type and distribution of paralysis are different for central facial paralysis compared with peripheral paralysis.

Central paralysis is a spastic paralysis limited to the lower half or two thirds of the contralateral side of the face. The paralyzed side is smooth and full and often appears swollen. The nasolabial fold is obliterated, and the corner of the mouth droops. When the infant cries, the mouth is drawn to the normal side, the wrinkles are deeper on the normal side, and movement of the forehead and eyelid is unaffected. Usually other manifestations of intracranial injury appear, most often a sixth nerve palsy.

Peripheral paralysis is flaccid and, when complete, involves the entire side of the face. When the infant is at rest, the only sign may be a persistently open eye on the affected side caused by paralysis of the orbicular muscle of the eye. With crying the findings are the same as those in a central facial nerve injury, with the addition of a smooth forehead on the involved side. Since the tongue is not involved, feeding is not affected.

A small branch of the nerve may be injured with involvement of only one group of facial muscles. Paralysis is then limited to the forehead, eyelid, or mouth. Peripheral paralysis secondary to nerve injury distal to the geniculate ganglion may be accompanied by a hematotympanum on the same side.

Differential diagnosis. Central and peripheral facial nerve palsies must be distinguished from *nuclear agenesis (Möbius' syndrome)*. The latter frequently results in bilateral facial nerve palsy; the face is expressionless and immobile, suggesting muscle fibrosis. Other cranial nerve palsies and deformities of the ear, palate, tongue, mandible, and other bones may be associated with *Möbius' syndrome*. Congenital absence or hypoplasia of the depressor muscle of the angle of the mouth may also simulate congenital facial palsy and has been associated with an increased incidence of other congenital anomalies.

Treatment. No specific therapy is indicated for most facial palsies. If the paralysis is peripheral and complete, initial treatment should be directed at protecting the cornea with an eye pad and 1% methylcellulose drops instilled every 4 hours. The functional state of the nerve should be followed closely. If no evidence of improvement occurs within 7 to 10 days, electrodiagnostic tests should be performed to determine whether there is neuropraxia or degeneration with interruption of the anatomic continuity of the nerve. If the latter condition is present, surgical intervention should be considered. The best surgical results are obtained with decompression or neuroplasty or both. The ideal time for surgery is not known. Occasionally facial tone may be improved after anastomosis of the facial nerve to the hypoglossal or accessory nerves. Adrenocorticotropic hormone (ACTH) is not indicated.

Prognosis. Most facial palsies resolve spontaneously within several days; total recovery may require several weeks or months. Electrodiagnostic testing is beneficial in predicting recovery; repeatedly normal nerve excitability indicates a good prognosis, but decreased or absent excitability early in the course suggests a poor outlook. The subsequent appearance of muscle fibrillation potentials indicates nerve degeneration. The prognosis in surgically treated infants worsens with increasing age at treatment.

Fractures and dislocations of facial bones

Facial bone fractures may occur during passage through the birth canal, during forceps application and delivery, and during obstetric manipulation (most often the Mauriceau maneuver for delivery of the fetal head in a breech presentation). Manipulation may result in mandibular fractures and mandibular joint damage but is rarely severe enough to cause separation of the symphysis of the mandible. Fracture of the nose may result in early respiratory distress and feeding difficulties. The most frequent nasal injury is dislocation of the cartilaginous part of the septum from the vomerine groove and columella. This may result from intrauterine factors, such as a uterine tumor or persistent pressure on the nose by fetal small parts, or during delivery from pressure on the nose by the symphysis pubis, sacral promontory, or perineum. The presence of nasal septal dislocation may be differentiated from the more common normal variant of misshapen nose by a simple compression test, in which the tip of the nose is compressed (Fig. 20-6). In the presence of septal dislocation the nostrils collapse and the deviated septum becomes more apparent; in the normal nose no nasal deviation occurs with compression.

Treatment. Early reduction and immobilization are advised for fracture of the mandible because rapid, firm union may occur as early as 10 to 14 days. Fractures of the maxilla, lacrimal bones, and nose unite even faster, with fixation in 7 to 10 days. Therefore nasal fractures should be treated even sooner. Since nasal trauma frequently requires extensive surgery, the pediatrician should request immediate consultation with a physician with expertise in nasal surgery. While waiting, the pediatrician should provide an oral airway to relieve respiratory distress. Often the surgeon can grasp the traumatized nose and elevate and remold it manually, resulting in relief of respiratory distress. Fractures of the septal cartilage may also be reduced by simple manual

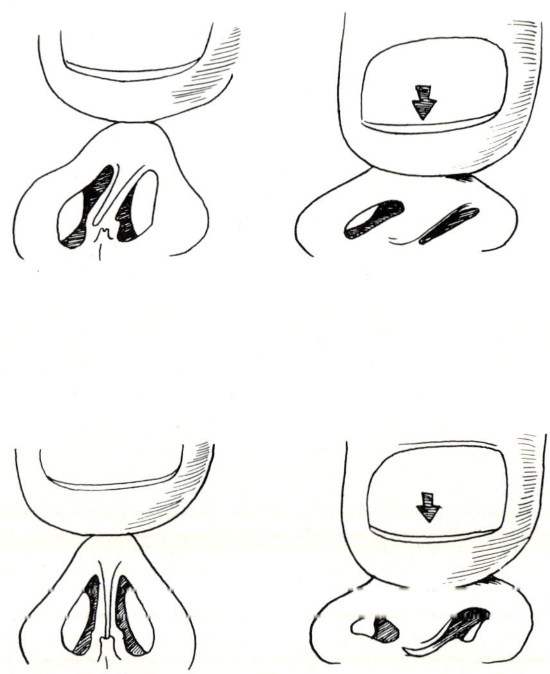

Fig. 20-6. Result of finger compression **(A)** when nasal septum is dislocated. Normal septal relationship **(B)** results in no nasal deviation with pressure. (Modified from Daily, W., and Davis, W.E.: Mo. Med. **74:**381, 1977.)

remolding, but most are associated with hematomas that should be promptly incised and drained. The surgeon can visualize the deformity with an infant nasal speculum, place a septal elevator in the nose, and guide the septal cartilage into the vomerine groove; an audible and palpable click indicates return of the septum into position.

Prognosis. If the fracture is reduced and fixated within a few days, rapid healing without complication is the usual course. If treatment is inadequate, missed, or delayed, subsequent developmental deformities are common. Ankylosis of the mandible in the second year of life is thought to result from birth trauma to the temporomandibular joint. Recently a young child was described with unilateral mandibular hypoplasia, which was thought to be a result of fibrous ankylosis secondary to perinatal trauma to the condylar cartilage of the ipsilateral temporomandibular joint. Other deformities may not become apparent until adolescence or young adulthood.

Eyes

See also Chapter 39.

Mechanical trauma to various regions of the neonatal eye usually occurs during abnormal presentation, in dystocia from cephalopelvic disproportion, or as a result of inappropriate forceps placement in normal deliveries. Most of the injuries are self-limited, mild, and require no specific treatment.

Eyelids

Edema, suffusion, and ecchymoses of the eyelids are common, especially after face and brow presentations or forceps deliveries. Severely swollen lids should be forced open by an ophthalmologist for examination of the eyeball; retractors may be necessary. These findings usually resolve within a week without treatment, although an infant was reported with totally everted upper eyelids that required suturing for 4 days before remaining in the normal position. Some believe that these injuries represent a possible cause of congenital ptosis.

Lagophthalmos, the inability to close an eye, is an occasional finding thought to result from facial nerve injury by forceps pressure. It usually is unilateral. The exposed cornea should be protected by an eye pad and methylcellulose drops instilled every 4 hours. The condition usually resolves within a week.

Orbit

Orbital hemorrhage and fracture may follow direct pressure by the apex of one forceps blade, most often in high forceps extractions. In most instances immediate death occurs. Surviving infants demonstrate traumatic eyelid changes, disturbances of extraocular muscle movements, and exophthalmos. The presence of the latter two findings warrants immediate ophthalmologic consultation. Subsequent management may also require neurosurgical and plastic surgery consultations.

Sympathetic nervous system

Horner's syndrome, resulting from cervical sympathetic nerve trauma, frequently accompanies lower brachial plexus injury (see later in this chapter). The syndrome consists of miosis, partial ptosis, slight enophthalmos, and anhidrosis of the ipsilateral side of the face. Although small, the pupil reacts to light. The presence of neurologic signs indicating brachial plexus injury helps to distinguish this syndrome from intracranial hemorrhage as a cause of anisocoria. Pigmentation of the ipsilateral iris is frequently delayed to several months of age; occasionally pigmentation never occurs. Resolution of other signs of the syndrome depends on whether the injury to the nerve is transient or permanent.

Subconjunctival hemorrhage

Subconjunctival hemorrhage, characterized by bright red patches on the bulbar conjunctiva, is a relatively common finding in the neonate. It may be found after a difficult delivery but often is noted after easy, completely uncomplicated deliveries. If the baby is otherwise well, treatment consists of reassuring the parents. The blood is usually absorbed within 1 to 2 weeks. As the blood pigments break down and are absorbed, the color changes from bright red to orange and yellow.

External ocular muscles

Injury involving the external ocular muscles may result from direct trauma to the cranial nerve (in the form of compression or surrounding hemorrhages) or from hemorrhage into the muscle sheath, with subsequent fibrosis. The sixth nerve (abducens) is the most frequently injured cranial nerve because of its long intracranial course; the result is paralysis of the lateral rectus muscle. This injury may follow a tentorial laceration with extravasation of a small amount of blood around the intracranial portion of the nerve. The involvement may be mild and transient; internal strabismus noted at birth may resolve gradually within 1 to 2 months. The seventh cranial nerve may be injured simultaneously with the sixth nerve by compression with forceps. Improvement in lateral gaze of the affected eye may appear within 1 to 2 months. Alternate patching of either eye in the severely affected infant maintains visual acuity until, with time, maximum improvement has occurred. At 6 months the degree of nerve regeneration may be evaluated. Some infants subsequently require surgical repair of their strabismus.

Fourth cranial nerve (trochlear) palsy occurs infrequently. It may follow small brainstem hemorrhages with nuclear damage. The affected muscle is the superior oblique, which mainly turns the eye inferiorly and medially. This is difficult to identify in the newborn. Surgical correction may be necessary later.

Third cranial nerve (oculomotor) palsy, when complete, causes paralysis of the inferior oblique and medial, superior, and inferior rectus muscles. This results in ptosis, a dilated fixed pupil, and outward and downward deviation of the eye, with inability to adduct or elevate up and in or up and out or to depress down and out. This palsy may also occur in partial form, with or without pupillary involvement. Partial palsies may recover function spontaneously within several months, whereas complete palsies usually require surgical intervention.

Optic nerve

The optic nerve may be directly injured by a fracture in the region of the optic canal or from a shearing force on the nerve, with resultant hemorrhage into the nerve sheath. The latter injury is seldom recognized because of the more apparent and severe changes in the sensorium. Occasionally a fracture through the optic foramen results in formation of callus, which slowly compresses the nerve. A difficult forceps delivery is a frequent preceding event. If optic nerve injury is not diagnosed within several hours with prompt surgical intervention, irreversible damage is likely. The result is optic atrophy and blindness. This is characterized by a blue-white optic disc, in contrast to the grayish disc of the normal newborn. In primary optic atrophy (e.g., that caused by birth trauma), the disc margin is well defined, and fine vessels are rarely present in the disc tissue. In secondary atrophy the disc margin is blurred; a central gray area and evidence of intraocular disease are present.

Cornea

A diffuse or streaky haziness of the cornea is relatively common. This is usually caused by edema related to the birth process but may also follow use of a silver nitrate solution more concentrated than 1%. The haziness usually disappears in 7 to 10 days. When it persists, a rupture of Descemet's membrane has probably occurred; usually this results from malpositioning of forceps at delivery. The consequence of a ruptured Descemet's membrane is a leukoma or diffuse white opacity of the cornea. This results from interstitial damage of the substantia propria by fluids entering through the tear in the membrane. These leukomas are often permanent and are accompanied by a high incidence of amblyopia and strabismus (Chapter 39).

Intraocular hemorrhage

Trauma at birth may result in retinal hemorrhage, hyphema, or vitreous hemorrhage. Retinal hemorrhage is the most common, with a reported incidence of 2.6% to 50% of all births. The extreme variability in incidence is probably related to the infant's age when first examined; the incidence is higher with earlier observations. The cause is most likely compression of the fetal head, resulting in venous congestion. The fetal head has been shown to be compressed two to four times more forcefully than other fetal parts during the second stage of labor. Retinal hemorrhage is more common in primiparous deliveries and after forceps or vacuum extraction; it is rare after cesarean section. It may occur in normal deliveries. The most common lesion is the flame-shaped or streak hemorrhage found mainly near the disc and sparing the macula and extreme periphery; it usually disappears within 1 to 3 days (occasionally 5 days) with no residual effects. Rarely hemorrhages may take up to 21 days to resolve. Retinal hemorrhages may reduce the resolving power of the macula, either bilaterally to produce nystagmus or unilaterally to produce amblyopia, which may not always respond to prolonged covering of the fixing eye with improvement of the amblyopic eye.

Hyphemas and vitreous hemorrhages, usually result from misplaced forceps and are often associated with ruptures of Descemet's membrane. One infant was reported in whom a hyphema developed in one eye following spontaneous delivery. The hyphema usually is clear of gross blood within 5 days; during this time the infant should be handled gently and fed frequently to minimize crying and agitation. If blood persists or secondary hemorrhage occurs, systemic administration of acetazolamide (Diamox) and surgical removal of blood may be necessary.

Vitreous hemorrhage is manifested by large vitreous floaters, blood pigment seen with the slit lamp, and an absent red reflex. The prognosis is guarded; if resolution does not occur in 6 to 12 months, surgical correction should be considered.

Ears

The proximity of ears to the site of application of forceps make them susceptible to injury at birth. Most of the injuries are mild and self-limited, but serious injuries may occur because of slipping or misplacement of forceps (Fig. 20-7).

Abrasions and ecchymoses

Abrasions must be cleansed gently to minimize the risk of secondary infection. Ecchymoses, if extensive and involving other areas of the body, may result in hyperbilirubinemia.

Hematomas

Hematomas of the external ear, if not treated promptly, liquefy slowly, followed by early organization and

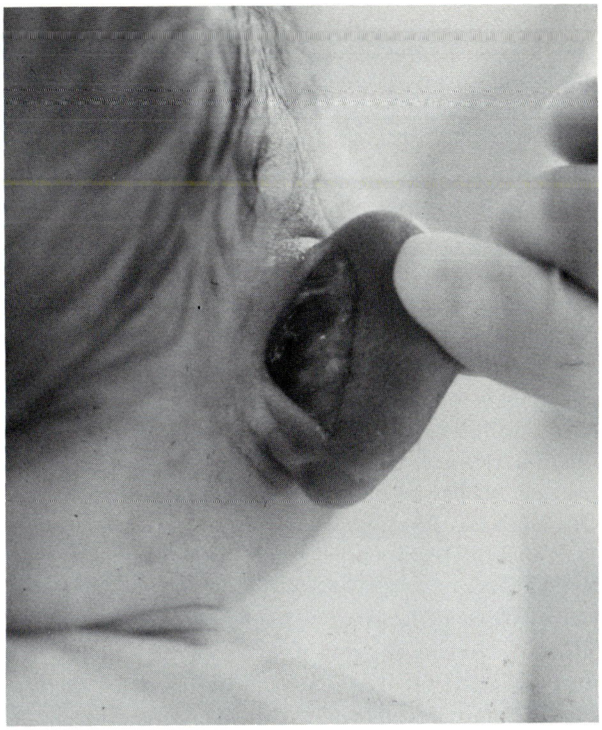

Fig. 20-7. Extensive avulsion and laceration of auricle in full-term infant, resulting from forceful traction of misplaced forceps. (Courtesy Dr. Bhagya Puppala.)

development of cauliflower ear. Wide incision and evacuation of the hematoma may be indicated.

Lacerations

Lacerations of the auricle may be repaired by the pediatrician if they are superficial and involve only skin. After thorough cleansing and draping, the wound edges are sutured with interrupted 6-0 or 7-0 nylon sutures, with exact edge-to-edge approximation. If the laceration involves cartilage, surgical consultation should be obtained because of the tendency for postoperative perichondritis, which is refractory to treatment and leads to subsequent deformities. A sterile field and more meticulous presurgical preparation are essential. A contour pressure dressing is applied postoperatively.

Vocal cord paralysis

Unilateral or bilateral paralysis of the vocal cords is uncommon in the neonate.

Etiology

Unilateral paralysis may be a consequence of excessive traction on the head during a breech delivery or lateral traction with forceps in a cephalic presentation. The recurrent laryngeal branch of the vagus nerve in the neck is injured. The left side is more often involved because of this nerve's lower origin and longer course in the neck. Bilateral paralysis may be caused by peripheral trauma involving both recurrent laryngeal nerves, but more frequrently it is caused by a CNS insult, such as hypoxia or hemorrhage involving the brainstem.

Clinical manifestations

An infant with a unilateral paralysis may be completely asymptomatic when resting quietly, but crying is usually accompanied by hoarseness and mild inspiratory stridor. Bilateral paralysis results in more severe respiratory symptoms. At birth the infant may have difficulty in establishing and maintaining spontaneous respiration; later dyspnea, retractions, stridor, cyanosis, or aphonia may develop.

Differential diagnosis

Unilateral paralysis of the vocal cords must be distinguished from congenital laryngeal malformations that produce neonatal stridor (Chapter 22). A history of difficult delivery, especially involving excessive traction on the fetus, may suggest laryngeal paralysis; the diagnosis can be confirmed only by direct laryngoscopic examination. Bilateral paralysis also must be distinguished from a number of causes of respiratory distress in the neonate (Chapter 28); stridor should suggest the larynx as the site of disturbance. Direct laryngoscopy is necessary to establish the diagnosis.

Treatment

Infants with unilateral paralysis should be closely observed until there is evidence of improvement. Gentle handling and frequent small feedings will aid in keeping the infant quiet and minimizing the risk of aspiration. Bilateral paralysis necessitates immediate tracheal intubation to establish an airway. Tracheostomy is required subsequently in most patients. Laryngoscopic examinations then should be performed at intervals to look for evidence of return of vocal cord function; early extubation may be attempted if complete return occurs within a short time.

Prognosis

The infant with unilateral paralysis usually improves rapidly without treatment, and complete resolution occurs within 4 to 6 weeks. The prognosis of bilateral paralysis is more variable. If untreated, the infant may develop a funnel deformity in the lower sternal area; this may appear as early as the fifteenth day of life. After tracheostomy a decrease in the severity of the deformity may occur within several weeks. Some of the affected infants subsequently regain normally shaped chests; others may have residual fixed depressions, occasionally severe enough to require surgical correction. The recovery of vocal cord function varies in time and degree. Some infants may show partial recovery within a few months, with several years elapsing before complete movement of the cords is restored. Other infants who have been followed for years show no improvement. Bilateral paralysis of central origin may improve completely if it is caused by cerebral edema or hemorrhage that rapidly resolves.

INJURIES TO THE NECK AND SHOULDER GIRDLE

Fracture of the clavicle

The clavicle is the most frequently fractured bone during labor and delivery. Most clavicular fractures are of the greenstick type, but occasionally the fracture is complete.

Etiology

The major causes of clavicular fractures are difficult delivery of the shoulders in vertex presentations and extended arms in breech deliveries. Vigorous, forceful manipulation of the arm and shoulder usually has occurred.

Clinical manifestations

Most often a greenstick fracture is not associated with any signs or symptoms but is first detected after the appearance of an obvious callus at 7 to 10 days of life. Complete fractures and some greenstick fractures may be apparent shortly after birth; movement of the arm on the affected side is decreased or absent. Deformity and, occasionally, discoloration may be visible over the fracture site with obliteration of the adjacent supraclavicular depression as a result of sternocleidomastoid muscle spasm. Passive movement of the arm elicits cries of pain from the infant. Palpation reveals tenderness, crepitus, and irregularity along the clavicle. Moro's reflex on the involved side is characteristically absent. Roentgenograms confirm the diagnosis of fracture.

Differential diagnosis

A similar clinical picture of impaired movement of an arm with an absent Moro's reflex may follow fracture of the humerus or brachial palsy. The fracture is confirmed by roentgenograms; palsy is accompanied by additional clinical findings.

Treatment

Therapy is directed toward minimizing the infant's pain. The affected arm and shoulder should be immobilized with the arm abducted above 60 degrees and the elbow flexed above 90 degrees. A callus forms, and pain usually subsides by 7 to 10 days, when immobilization may be discontinued.

Prognosis

Prognosis is excellent, with growth resulting in restoration of normal bone contour after several months.

Brachial palsy

Brachial palsy is a paralysis involving the muscles of the upper extremity that follows mechanical trauma to the spinal roots of the fifth cervical through the first thoracic nerves (the brachial plexus) during birth. Three main forms occur, depending on the site of injury: (1) Duchenne-Erb, or upper arm, paralysis, which results from injury of the fifth and sixth cervical roots and is by far the most common; (2) Klumpke's, or lower arm, paralysis, which results from injury of the eighth cervical and first thoracic roots and is extremely rare; and (3) paralysis of the entire arm, which occurs slightly more often than the Klumpke type.

Etiology

Most cases of brachial palsy follow a prolonged and difficult labor culminating in a traumatic delivery. The affected infant is frequently large, relaxed, and asphyxiated and thereby vulnerable to excessive separation of bony segments, overstretching, and injury to soft tissues. Injury of the fifth and sixth cervical roots may follow a breech presentation with the arms extended over the head; excessive traction on the shoulder in the delivery of the head may result in stretching of the plexus. The same injury may follow lateral traction of the head and neck away from one of the shoulders while attempting to deliver the shoulders in a vertex presentation. More vigorous traction of the same nature will result in paralysis of the entire arm. The mechanism for isolated lower arm paralysis is uncertain; it is thought to result from stretching of lower plexus nerves under and against the coracoid process of the scapula during forceful elevation and abduction of the arm. Excessive traction on the trunk during a breech delivery may result in avulsion of the lower roots from the cervical cord. In most patients the nerve sheath is torn and the nerve fibers are compressed by the resultant hemorrhage and edema. Less often the nerves are completely ruptured and the ends severed, or the roots are avulsed from the spinal cord with injury to the spinal gray matter.

Clinical manifestations

The infant with upper arm paralysis holds the affected arm in a characteristic position, reflecting involvement of the shoulder abductors and external rotators, forearm flexors and supinators, and wrist extensors. The arm is adducted and internally rotated, with extension at the elbow, pronation of the forearm, and flexion of the wrist. When the arm is passively abducted, it falls limply to the side of the body. Moro's, biceps, and radial reflexes are absent on the affected side. There may be some sensory deficit on the radial aspect of the arm, but this is difficult to evaluate in the neonate. The grasp reflex is intact. Any signs of respiratory distress may indicate an accompanying ipsilateral phrenic nerve root injury (see following section).

Lower arm paralysis involves the intrinsic muscles of the hand and the long flexors of the wrist and fingers. The hand is paralyzed, and voluntary movements of the wrist cannot be made. The grasp reflex is absent; the deep tendon reflexes are intact. Sensory impairment may be demonstrated along the ulnar side of the forearm and hand. Frequently, dependent edema and cyanosis of the hand and trophic changes in the fingernails develop. After some time there may be flattening and atrophy of the intrinsic hand muscles. Usually an ipsilateral *Horner's syndrome* (ptosis, miosis, and enophthalmos) is also present because of injury involving the cervical sympathetic fibers of the first thoracic root. Often this is associated with delayed pigmentation of the iris, sometimes of more than 1 year's duration.

When the entire arm is paralyzed, it is usually completely motionless, flaccid, and powerless, hanging limply to the side. All reflexes are absent. The sensory deficit may extend almost up to the shoulder.

Differential diagnosis

The presence of a flail arm in a neonate may be caused by cerebral injury or by a number of injuries about the shoulder. The former is usually associated with other manifestations of CNS injury. A careful roentgenographic study of the shoulder, including lower cervical spine, clavicle, and upper humerus, should be made to exclude tearing of the joint capsule, fracture of the clavicle, and fracture, dislocation, or upper epiphyseal detachment of the humerus.

Treatment

The basic principle of treatment is prevention of contractures while awaiting recovery of the brachial plexus. This is accomplished by partial immobilization during the first 1 to 2 weeks, appropriate positioning, and an exercise program. Active physical therapy should be avoided initially because of a painful traumatic neuritis that usually affects the brachial plexus. By 7 to 10 days of age gentle range of motion exercises may be started.

In upper arm paralysis the arm should be abducted 90 degrees with external rotation at the shoulder, 90 degrees flexion at the elbow, full supination of the forearm, and slight extension at the wrist so that the palm of the hand is turned toward the face. This may be done with cautious use of a splint or brace during the first 1 to 2 weeks, until the traumatic neuritis has resolved. Current authorities warn against the potential risk of abduction contractures occurring following prolonged or persistent splinting. Many question whether splinting results in any beneficial effects other than decreasing the pain that would accompany movement of the affected limb. Accordingly, splinting should only be administered intermittently throughout the day; a useful routine is to immobilize the affected limb while the infant is asleep, between feedings, followed by removal of the splint during the feeding. After the first 1 to 2 weeks gentle massage and passive range of motion exercises are indicated to prevent development of contractures. If the infant is otherwise stable, the parents may be easily instructed in the exercise procedures, thereby permitting discharge of the infant. The infant must be followed closely and active and passive corrective exercises continued until normal scapulohumeral rhythm has been reestablished. Patients who demonstrate persistent lack of abduction and external rotation may benefit from a teres major tendon transfer to the rotator cuff. Most authorities recommend delaying this procedure until the child is approximately 3 or 4 years of age to permit a valid preoperative muscle assessment.

In lower arm paralysis the forearm and wrist should be splinted in a neutral position, and padding should be placed in the fist. Passive range of motion exercises of the wrist, hand, and fingers should be gently performed. When the entire arm is paralyzed, the same treatment principles should be followed; immobilization in a neutral position, padding of the fist, massage, and range of motion exercises.

Routine neurosurgical exploration and repair of the injury are not indicated. Mild injuries are self-limited, and severe injuries usually involve avulsion of the roots from the cord, making suture of the nerves impossible. Dissection of the plexus is so difficult that more damage may be inflicted, resulting in formation of additional scar tissue and symptoms years after surgery. Matson has explored the brachial plexus and performed neurolysis on infants who showed no improvement after 3 to 6 months and in whom there was palpable thickening in the supraclavicular fossa or swelling or ecchymosis over the plexus during the acute phase of injury. Although the results have been generally discouraging, several infants have shown a greater degree of improvement following surgery than would have been expected to occur spontaneously.

Prognosis

If the nerve roots are intact, return of function may appear within several days as the local hemorrhage and edema resolve. The rate of recovery varies with the degree of injury. In some infants recovery is complete within a few weeks. Most appropriately treated infants will recover completely within 3 to 6 months. An occasional infant with severe injury may show continued improvement over a period of up to 2 years. Even if recovery of function appears complete, close examination will usually reveal peculiar posturing of the arm in abduction at the shoulder, tightness in internal rotation, difficulty in forearm supination, and minimal winging of the scapula.

Lower arm paralysis is associated with a relatively poor prognosis; a claw deformity may develop. Paralysis of the entire arm may show recovery of some function eventually.

Electrodiagnosis is helpful in distinguishing a neuropraxis lesion from a root avulsion. An infant with a severe lesion of the former type may be predicted to have partial, and possibly total, return of function, whereas an infant with an avulsion injury may be predicted to have permanent paralysis. In avulsion injuries and untreated stretch injuries, residual contractures and bony deformities develop. Contractures may be treated with gentle stretching in the infant and by tenotomies in the older patient. Bony deformities may be treated by osteotomies or tendon transfers. These procedures produce no increase in muscle power but may make motion of the arm less awkward.

Phrenic nerve paralysis

See also Chapters 27 and 28.

Phrenic nerve paralysis results in diaphragmatic paralysis and rarely occurs as an isolated injury in the neonate. Most injuries are unilateral and are associated with an ipsilateral upper brachial plexus palsy.

Etiology

The most common cause is a difficult breech delivery. Lateral hyperextension of the neck results in overstretching or avulsion of the third, fourth, and fifth cervical roots, which supply the phrenic nerve.

Clinical manifestations

The first sign may be recurrent episodes of cyanosis, usually accompanied by irregular and labored respirations. The respiratory excursions of the involved side of the diaphragm are largely ineffectual, and the breathing is therefore almost completely thoracic so that no bulging of the abdomen occurs with inspiration (Fig. 20-8, *A* and *B*). The thrust of the diaphragm, which often may be felt just under the costal margin on the normal side, is absent on the affected side. Dullness and diminished breath sounds are found over the affected side. In a severe injury, tachypnea, weak cry, and apneic spells may occur.

Roentgenographic manifestations

Roentgenograms taken during the first few days may show only slight elevation of the affected diaphragm, occasionally so subtle that it may be considered normal. Repeated films will show the more apparent elevation of the diaphragm, with displacement of the heart and mediastinum to the opposite side (Fig. 20-8, *C*). Frequently areas of atelectasis appear bilaterally. Early diagnosis can be confirmed only by fluoroscopy, which reveals an abnormal elevation of the affected hemidiaphragm and seesaw movements of the two hemidiaphragms with respiration (elevation of the affected side and descent of the normal side during inspiration); opposite movements occur during expiration. Fluoroscopy reveals a shift of the mediastinum toward the normal side during inspiration. In questionable cases diagnosis can be further enhanced by transvenous electric stimulation of the phrenic nerve.

Differential diagnosis

Careful physical examination should allow differentiation between CNS, cardiac, and pulmonary causes of neonatal respiratory distress. The diagnosis can be confirmed by fluoroscopy and electric stimulation of the phrenic nerve.

Treatment

Most infants require only nonspecific medical treatment. The infant should be positioned on the involved side, and oxygen should be administered for cyanosis or hypoxemia. Intravenous fluids may be necessary the first few days. If the infant begins to show improvement, progressive oral or gavage feedings may be started. Antibiotics are indicated if pneumonia occurs.

Infants with more severe respiratory distress, particularly those with bilateral phrenic nerve palsy, may require assisted ventilation shortly after delivery. Other modes of therapy that have been successfully used include continuous positive airway pressure (CPAP) by nasal cannula and continuous negative pressure via a negative-pressure respirator. These forms of therapy may be used either primarily or secondarily to facilitate weaning the infant off the respirator. Electric diaphragmatic pacing may also be used as an adjunct to assisted ventilation if the diaphragm shows significant contraction following electric stimulation of the phrenic nerve.

Haller and associates have developed a treatment protocol that uses mechanical ventilation followed by weaning with CPAP. If extubation is unsuccessful after 4 to 6 weeks, surgical plication is recommended. Others consider surgery for the infant with severe or increasing respiratory distress despite medical management or for the infant who, after 3 or 4 months, is only mildly symptomatic but has shown no roentgenographic evidence of functional recovery of the affected hemidiaphragm. Electric stimulation of the phrenic nerve is helpful in deciding on the advisability of surgical treatment. The infant who demonstrates absence of diaphragmatic contraction following phrenic nerve stimulation has probably incurred nerve damage below the level of stimulation or diaphragmatic muscle atrophy and should be considered for sur-

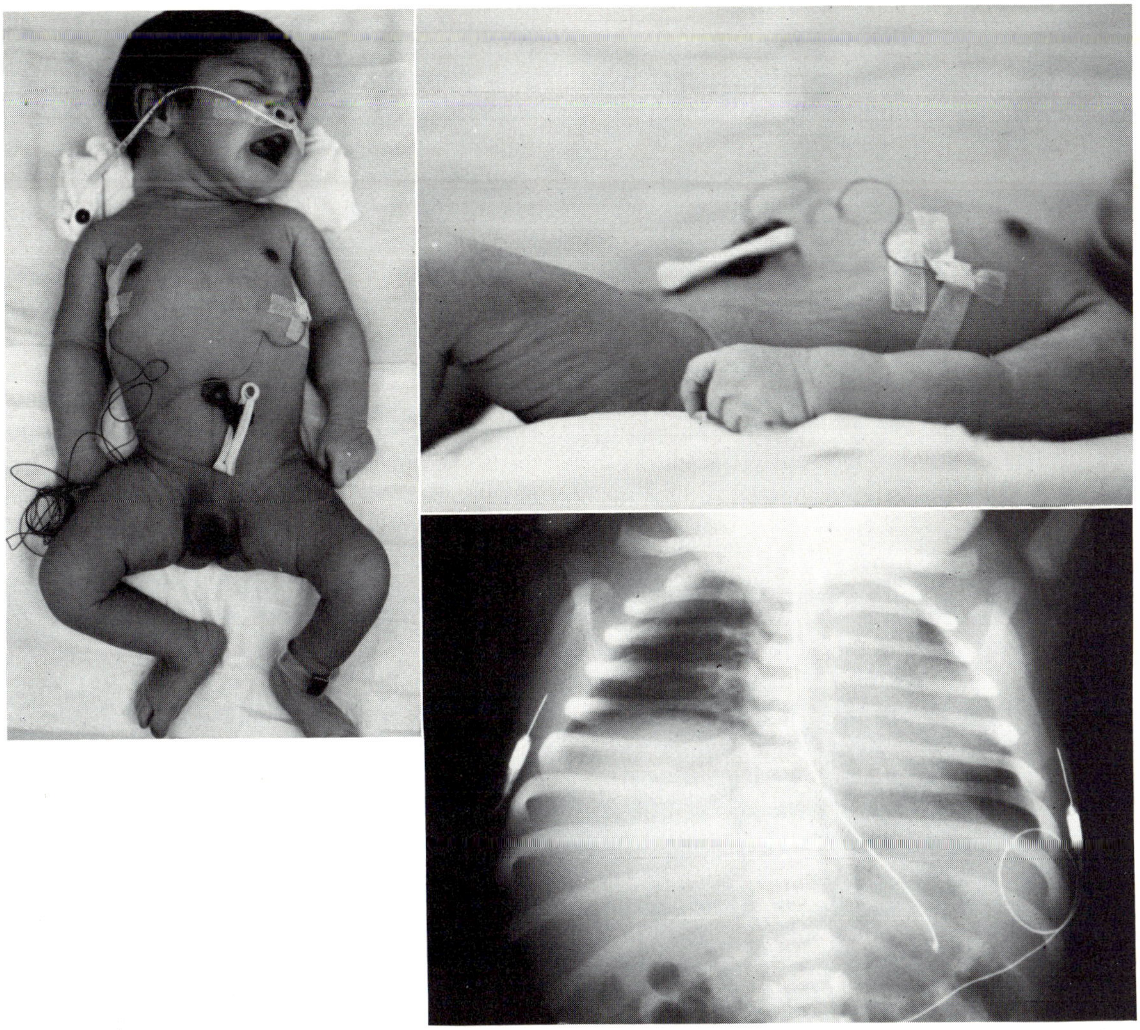

Fig. 20-8. A, A 9-hour-old 3,190 gm female born after difficult total breech extraction; during delivery cervix clamped down on head, necessitating extensive tugging and pulling on both arms. Note markedly hyperexpanded chest and classic appearance of both upper extremities in Erb's palsy positions. **B,** Lateral view of same infant, demonstrating increased anteroposterior diameter of chest as well as close-up of left upper extremity adducted at shoulder, extended at elbow, and pronated and flexed at wrist. **C,** Significant elevation of right hemidiaphragm to T5 level in same infant, compatible with paralysis of the right hemidiaphragm. Note significant shifting of the heart and mediastinum to the left.

gery. The procedure of choice is either plication or excision of part of the paralyzed diaphragm. This results in a tightening of the diaphragm and brings the dome of the diaphragm down to a normal level, allowing the mediastinum to return to its normal position.

Prognosis

Most infants recover spontaneously. This may be complete by 6 weeks but usually takes several months. If avulsion of the cervical nerves has occurred, spontaneous recovery is not possible, and in the absence of surgery the infant is susceptible to pneumonia in the atelectatic lung. Many of these infants die before 3 months of age. Infants treated surgically do well, with no recurrence of pneumonia and no late pulmonary or chest wall complications. The repaired hemidiaphragm remains in a satisfactory position despite permanent paralysis of the phrenic nerve. The accuracy of prognosis may be improved by electric phrenic nerve stimulation. If the stimulation results in adequate diaphragmatic contraction, nerve injury below the level of stimulation is unlikely and diaphragmatic muscle fibers are intact. If diaphragmatic contraction does not occur, nerve damage has probably occurred below the level of stimulation.

Injury to the sternocleidomastoid muscle

This injury is designated muscular torticollis, congenital torticollis, or sternocleidomastoid fibroma. Its cause and pathology have been controversial.

Etiology

The birth trauma theory suggests that the muscle or fascial sheath is ruptured during a breech or difficult delivery involving hyperextension of the muscle. A hematoma develops and is subsequently invaded by fibrin and fibroblasts with progressive formation of scar tissue and shortening of the muscle. The intrauterine theory postulates abnormal pressure, position, or trauma to the muscle during intrauterine life. Another theory suggests a hereditary defect in the development of the muscle. Still others have noted pathologic findings resembling infectious myositis, suggesting an infection in utero or a muscle injured at delivery.

Clinical manifestations

A mass in the midportion of the sternocleidomastoid muscle may be evident at birth, although usually it is first noted 10 to 14 days after birth. It is 1 to 2 cm in diameter, hard, immobile, fusiform, and well circumscribed; there is no inflammation or overlying discoloration. The mass enlarges during the following 2 to 4 weeks and then gradually regresses and disappears by age 5 to 8 months.

A transient torticollis produced by contracture of the involved muscle appears soon after birth. The head tilts toward the involved side, and the chin is somewhat elevated and rotated toward the opposite shoulder. The head cannot be moved passively into normal position. If the deformity persists beyond 3 or 4 years, the skull becomes foreshortened. Flattening of the frontal bone and bulging of the occipital bone occur on the involved side, whereas the contralateral frontal bone bulges and the occiput is flattened. The ipsilateral eyebrow is slanted; the clavicle and shoulder become elevated compared with the opposite normal side, and the ipsilateral mastoid process becomes more prominent. If treatment is not instituted, a lower cervical, upper thoracic scoliosis subsequently develops. Rarely calcification develops in the affected muscles.

Differential diagnosis

Careful roentgenographic examination should be made of the cervical spine and shoulders to rule out Sprengel's deformity or Klippel-Feil syndrome, cervical myelodysplasia, and occipitalization of the atlas.

Treatment

Treatment should be instituted as early as possible. The involved muscle should be stretched to an overcorrected position by gentle, even, and persistent motion with the baby supine. The head is flexed forward and away from the affected side, and the chin is rotated toward the affected side. The mother can be instructed to repeat this maneuver several times a day. The infant should also be stimulated to turn the head spontaneously toward the affected side; the crib may be positioned so that the infant must turn to the desired position of overcorrection in looking for window light or at a mobile or favorite rattle. During sleep the baby should be placed on the side of the torticollis; in this position sandbags should be placed on each side of his body for fixation. An alternative approach recently described involves a helmet that is custom made for the infant. Rubber straps made of surgical drain tubing attached to the helmet are in turn fixed to the side rails of the crib at night, with appropriate adjustments made to force the infant to sleep on the prominent side of the head. This results in stretching of the shortened sternocleidomastoid muscle.

Conservative therapy should be continued for 6 months. If the deformity has not been fully corrected, surgery should be considered to prevent permanent skull and cervical spine deformities. Removal of the tumor is not necessary and will needlessly deform the outline of the neck. The procedure of choice is lengthening and division of the sternal portion of the muscle from the mastoid process at its origin; the neck outline is preserved. After surgery the head should be immobilized in an overcorrected position for several weeks, followed by an exercise program.

Prognosis

Most infants treated conservatively show complete recovery within 2 to 3 months. If surgery is necessary and if it is performed early, the facial asymmetry will disappear almost entirely. Infants treated before their first birthday have a better outcome than those treated later, regardless of the type of treatment. Nonsurgical treatment after 1 year is rarely successful.

INJURIES TO THE SPINE AND SPINAL CORD

See also Chapter 27.

Birth injuries to the vertebral spine and spinal cord are rarely diagnosed. It is not certain whether the low incidence is real, reflecting improved obstetric techniques, or represents a tendency for postmortem examination to overlook spine and spinal cord lesions.

Etiology

These injuries almost always result from breech deliveries, especially difficult ones where version and extraction were used. Other predisposing factors include brow and face presentations, dystocia (especially shoulder), prematurity, primiparity, and precipitous delivery.

The injuries are usually caused by stretching of the cord and not by compression. The most common mechanism responsible is probably forceful longitudinal traction on the trunk while the head is still firmly engaged in the pelvis. When combined with flexion and torsion of the vertebral axis, this becomes a more significant problem. Occasionally a snap is felt by the obstetrician while exerting traction. Although cesarean section has been recommended as the optimum delivery for infants in breech presentation with a hyperextended head, several reports have appeared documenting vertebral or spinal cord injury following cesarean section. Maekawa and co-workers reported a patient who demonstrated weak fetal movements during the third trimester, suggesting that injury was occurring before delivery. Difficulty in delivery of the shoulders in cephalic presentations may result in a similar mechanism of injury. The spinal cord is very delicate and inelastic. Its attachments are the cauda equina below and the roots of the brachial plexus and medulla above. Because the ligaments are elastic and the muscles delicate, the infant's vertebral column may be stretched quite easily. In addition, the dura is more elastic in the infant than in the adult. Consequently, strong longitudinal traction may be expected to cause elongation of the spinal column and to stretch the spinal cord and its membranes. The possible result is vertebral fracture or dislocation or both and cord transection. Most often, hemorrhage and edema produce a physiologic transection. The lower cervical and upper thoracic regions are most often involved, but occasionally the entire length of the spinal canal contains a heavy accumulation of blood.

Clinical manifestations

Affected infants may follow one of four clinical patterns. Those in the first group are either stillborn or in poor condition from birth, with respiratory depression, shock, and hypothermia. They deteriorate rapidly; death occurs within several hours, often before neurologic signs are obvious. These infants are usually victims of a high cervical or brainstem lesion.

The second group consists of infants who at birth may appear normal or show signs similar to group one; these infants die after several days. Cardiac function is usually relatively strong. Within hours or days the central type of respiratory depression, which is initially present, may be complicated by respiratory distress of pulmonary origin, usually pneumonia. The spinal lesion, usually in the upper or midcervical region, frequently is not recognized for several days, when flaccidity and immobility of the legs are noted. Occasionally urinary retention may be the first symptom. Paralysis of the abdominal wall is manifested by a relaxation of the abdominal wall and bulging at the flanks when the baby is held upright. The intercostal muscles may be affected if the lesion is high enough. Sensation is absent over the lower half of the body. Deep tendon reflexes and spontaneous reflex movements are absent. The infant is constipated. The brachial plexus is involved in about 20% of all cases. The spinal column is usually clinically and roentgenographically normal.

The third group, with lesions at C8 to T1 or lower, is composed of infants who survive for long periods, some for years. Paraplegia noted at birth may be transient. The lesion in the cord may be mild and reversible, or it may result in permanent neurologic sequelae with no return of function in the lower cord segments. The skin over the involved part of the body is dry and scaly, predisposing the infant to bedsores and ulcers. Muscle atrophy, severe contractures, and bony deformities follow. Bladder distension and constant dribbling persist, and recurring urinary tract infections and pneumonia are common. Within several weeks or months this clinical picture is replaced by a stage of reflex activity or paraplegia-inflexion. This is characterized by return of tone and rigid flexion of the involved extremities, improvement in skin condition with healing of decubiti, and periodic mass reflex responses composed of tonic spasms of the extremities, spontaneous micturition, and profuse sweating over the involved part of the body.

Infants in the fourth group have subtle neurologic signs of spasticity thought to represent cerebral palsy. These patients have incurred partial spinal cord injuries and occasional cerebrovascular accidents.

Differential diagnosis

During the first few weeks of life, injuries to the spinal cord may be confused with amyotonia congenita or myelodysplasia associated with spina bifida occulta (Chapter 27). The former may be differentiated by the generalized distribution of the weakness and hypotonia and by the presence of normal sensation and sphincter control. The latter is usually associated with some cutaneous lesions over the sacral region such as dimples, angiomas, or abnormal tufts of hair; it is always associated with defects in the spinal lamina. Other conditions less often considered include transverse myelitis and spinal cord tumors, particularly in infants who demonstrate paralysis following an apparently normal labor and delivery. Cerebral hypotonia should be considered in infants who also demonstrate cranial nerve abnormalities, persistent primitive reflexes, and a dull facial appearance, contrasting with the bright, alert facies of the spinal cord trauma victim. However, the concomitant occurrence of cerebral damage in an infant with spinal cord injury may confound the diagnosis. A final consideration is the infant with bilateral brachial plexus palsy with associated motor and sensory loss, or Horner's syndrome; the demonstration of normal lower extremity function should rule out spinal cord injury. Recently somatosensory-evoked potential was demonstrated to be useful in establishing a diagnosis of spinal cord injury.

Treatment

Therapy is supportive and usually unsatisfactory. The infant affected at birth requires basic resuscitative and supportive measures. Infants who survive present a therapeutic challenge that can be met only by the combined and interested efforts of the pediatrician, neurologist, neurosurgeon, urologist, psychiatrist, orthopedist, nurse, physical therapist, and occupational therapist.

While the infant is reasonably stable, cervical and thoracic spine roentgenograms should be obtained. In the rare occurrence of vertebral fracture or dislocation or both, immediate neurosurgical consultation is necessary for reduction of the deformity and relief of cord compression, followed by appropriate immobilization. Lumbar puncture in the acute period is of little practical value and may aggravate existing cord damage if the infant is excessively manipulated during the procedure. After several days, however, a persistent spinal fluid block may be demonstrated and may be an indication for exploratory laminectomy at the site of trauma. This possibility should be suspected in an infant with partial paraplegia and normal roentgenograms.

Prompt and meticulous attention must be given to skin, bladder, and bowel care. The position of paralyzed parts should be changed every 2 hours. Areas of anesthetic skin should be washed, dried, and gently massaged daily. Lamb's-wool covers are helpful in preventing pressure necrosis of skin. Benzoin tincture applications help protect the skin in pressure areas. A decubitus ulcer is treated by scrupulous cleansing and complete freedom from weight bearing and friction. An indwelling urethral catheter should be inserted within several hours after severe cord trauma at any level. In the smaller infant a no. 3 feeding tube may be used. Repeated instrumentation should be avoided. Cultures of urine should be obtained at least weekly and antibiotic therapy employed only in the presence of infection. After several weeks the infant reaches the stage of paraplegia-in-flexion, and urinary retention is usually replaced by regular episodes of spontaneous voiding. If this is accompanied by a decrease in bladder size to normal, the catheter is removed. When prompt return of bladder function does not occur, intermittent catheterization has proved valuable. Periodic renal ultrasound and nuclear cystogram may be necessary. Renal function should also be monitored.

The first infection should be treated with the appropriate antibiotic for 2 weeks. After the neonatal period, this should be followed by suppressive therapy with trimethoprim and sulfamethoxazole (Bactrim, Septra), 2 mg/kg/day in one daily dose; nitrofurantoin (Furadantin), 2 mg/kg/day in two divided doses, or cephalexin (Keflex), 25 mg/kg/day in two divided doses. This therapy should be continued for 6 to 12 months or longer, depending on the reversibility of the lesion. Cultures of urine should be obtained at 1 week, monthly for 3 months, then every 3 months for 1 year or until recovery.

Fecal retention is also a common problem, especially after total cord transection. Appropriate dietary balance should aid in keeping the stools soft. Early use of glycerin suppositories at regular intervals will encourage automatic defecation. Digital manipulation may be necessary to relieve fecal impactions.

Finally, physical rehabilitation should be instituted early in an attempt to minimize deformity. After several years orthopedic procedures may still be necessary to correct contractures and bony deformities.

Prognosis

The prognosis varies with the severity of the injury. Most severe injuries result in death shortly after birth. Infants with cord compression from vertebral fractures or dislocations or both may recover with reasonable return of function if prompt neurosurgical removal of the compression is performed. Infants with mild injuries or partial transections may recover with minimal sequelae. Infants who exhibit complete physiologic cord transection shortly after birth without vertebral fracture or dislocation have an extremely poor outlook for recovery of function. Many die in infancy of ascending urinary tract infection and sepsis. Long-term survivors have been reported to live into their third decade. These are extremely rare, and although they may have normal intelligence and learn to walk with special appliances, these children face the late complications of pain, spasms, autonomic dysfunction, bony deformities, and genitourinary, psychiatric, and school problems.

INJURIES TO INTRAABDOMINAL ORGANS

Although birth trauma involving intraabdominal organs is uncommon, it frequently must be considered by the physician who manages neonates because deterioration can be fulminant in an undetected lesion, and therapy can be very effective when a lesion is diagnosed early. Intraabdominal trauma should be suspected in any newborn infant with shock and abdominal distension or pallor, anemia, and irritability without evidence of external blood loss.

Rupture of the liver

The liver is the most frequently injured abdominal organ during the birth process. The autopsy incidence varies from 0.9% to 9.6%.

Etiology

Birth trauma is the most significant contributing factor. The condition usually occurs in large infants, infants with hepatomegaly (e.g., erythroblastosis fetalis and infants of diabetic mothers), and breech deliveries. Manual pressure on the liver during delivery of the head in a breech presentation is probably a typical mechanism of injury. Prematurity and postmaturity also are thought to predispose the infant to this injury. Other contributing factors include asphyxia and coagulation disorders. Trauma to the liver more often results in subcapsular hematoma than actual laceration of the liver.

Clinical manifestations

The infant usually appears normal the first 1 to 3 days and rarely for as long as 7 days. Nonspecific signs related to loss of blood into the hematoma may appear early; these include poor feeding, listlessness, pallor, jaundice, tachypnea, and tachycardia. A mass may be palpable in the right upper quadrant. The hematocrit and hemoglobin values may be stable early in the course, but serial determinations will suggest blood loss. These manifestations are followed by sudden circulatory collapse, usually coincident with rupture of the hematoma through the capsule and extravasation of blood into the peritoneal cavity. The abdomen then may be distended, rigid, and dull to percussion, occasionally with a bluish discoloration of the overlying skin, which may extend over the scrotum. Abdominal roentgenograms may reveal uniform opacity of the abdomen, indicating free intraperitoneal fluid. Paracentesis confirms the presence of free blood in the peritoneal cavity. Computed tomography (CT) scan of the abdomen may assist in establishing a diagnosis of subcapsular hemorrhage without rupture.

Differential diagnosis

This lesion is one of several that can result in hemoperitoneum; others include trauma to the adrenals, kidneys, gastrointestinal tract, and spleen. Presence of a right upper quadrant mass suggests trauma to the liver, but absence of a mass does not rule it out. Abdominal roentgenograms, ultrasonography, and intravenous pyelography may assist in pinpointing the site of trauma, but ultimately a definite diagnosis can be made only by laparotomy.

Treatment

Immediate management consists of prompt transfusion with whole blood to restore the blood volume and of recognition and correction of any coagulation disorder. This should be followed by laparotomy with evacuation of the hematoma and repair of any laceration with sutures placed over a hemostatic agent. Any fragmented, devitalized liver tissue should be removed to prevent subsequent fatal secondary hemorrhage. Because of the successful treatment of two infants with blood transfusion only and because of hemostatic difficulty in one infant at surgery, it has been suggested that blood transfusion and the tamponade of intraabdominal pressure might be adequate therapy in some infants.

Prognosis

In unrecognized liver trauma with formation of a subcapsular hematoma, shock and death may result if the hematoma ruptures through the capsule, reducing the pressure tamponade and resulting in new bleeding from the liver. Recognition of the possibility of liver rupture in infants with a predisposing birth history, followed by early diagnosis and prompt therapy, should improve the prognosis. Early diagnosis and correction of any existing coagulation disorder will also improve the prognosis.

Rupture of the spleen

Rupture of the spleen in the newborn occurs much less often than rupture of the liver. However, recognition of this condition is equally important because of its similar potential for fulminant shock and death if the diagnosis is delayed.

Etiology

The condition is most common in large babies, babies delivered in breech position, and babies with erythroblastosis fetalis or congenital syphilis, in whom the spleen is enlarged and more friable and thereby susceptible to rupture either spontaneously or after minor trauma. An underlying clotting defect has also been implicated. Rupture of the spleen has occurred in normal-sized infants with uneventful deliveries and no underlying disease.

Clinical manifestations

Clinical signs indicating blood loss and hemoperitoneum are similar to those described for hepatic rupture. The hemoglobin and hematocrit values decrease, and abdominal paracentesis may reveal free blood. Several infants have been described in whom the blood was circumscribed within the leaves of the phrenicolineal ligament and therefore not clinically detectable. Occasionally a left upper quadrant mass may be palpable, and roentgenograms of the abdomen may show medial displacement of the gastric air bubble.

Differential diagnosis

Rupture of the liver and trauma to the adrenals, kidneys, and gastrointestinal tract must be distinguished.

Treatment

Whole blood should be transfused promptly, and any coexisting clotting defect should be corrected. This should be followed by immediate exploratory laparotomy. In contrast to earlier recommendations in favor of splenectomy, the current philosophy is to attempt repair and preservation of the spleen to prevent the subsequent increased risk of infection. Matsuyama and associates reported an infant in whom the almost transected spleen was successfully repaired surgically.

Prognosis

With early recognition and emergency surgery, survival should approach 100%.

Adrenal hemorrhage

Neonatal adrenal hemorrhage is more common than previously suspected; some autopsy studies have revealed a high incidence of subclinical hemorrhage. Massive hemorrhage is much less common, and the incidence is difficult to determine, since the diagnosis is often unsuspected and only considered retrospectively years later when calcified adrenals are unexpectedly found on roentgenograms or at autopsy.

Etiology

The most likely cause is birth trauma; risk factors include macrosomia, diabetic mothers, breech presentation, congenital syphilis, and dystocia. Placental hemorrhage, anoxia, hemorrhagic disease of the newborn, prematurity, and more recently neuroblastoma have been implicated. Pathologic findings vary from unilateral minute areas of bleeding to massive bilateral hemorrhage. The increased size and vascularity of the adrenal gland at birth may predispose it to hemorrhage.

Clinical manifestations

Signs vary with the degree and extent of hemorrhage. The classic findings are fever, tachypnea out of proportion to the degree of fever, yellowish pallor, cyanosis of the lips and fingertips, a mass in either flank with overlying skin discoloration, and purpura. Findings suggesting adrenal insufficiency include poor feeding, vomiting, diarrhea, obstipation, dehydration, abdominal distension, irritability, hypoglycemia, uremia, skin rash, listlessness, coma, convulsions, and shock.

Roentgenographic manifestations

Initial roentgenographic manifestations may be limited to widening of the retroperitoneal space with forward displacement of stomach and duodenum or downward displacement of intestines or kidneys. In time, calcification may appear. Typically this is rimlike and has been observed as early as the twelfth day of life. After several weeks the calcification becomes denser and retracted and assumes the configuration of the adrenal gland (Fig. 20-9). The increased experience with ultrasound in the neonate provides another adjunctive method of diagnosis. Abdominal ultrasound performed during the first several days may reveal a solid lesion in the location of the adrenal hemorrhage; this is thought to represent either clot fragmentation or diffuse clotted blood throughout the adrenal gland. If adrenal hemorrhage is suspected, ultrasound should be repeated at 3- to 5-day intervals. If adrenal hemorrhage has occurred, the lesion will change from a solid to a cystic appearance, coincident with liquefaction, degeneration, and lysis of the clot.

Differential diagnosis

Adrenal hemorrhage must be distinguished from other causes of abdominal hemorrhage. In addition, when a mass is palpable, the differential diagnosis must include the multiple causes of flank masses in the newborn infant, such as genitourinary anomaly, Wilms' tumor, and neuroblastoma. If the infant is large or the delivery is traumatic or breech, an adrenal hemorrhage is most likely. Neuroblastoma may be distinguished by persistent demonstration of a solid lesion on serial ultrasound examinations, as well as by increased excretion of vanillylmandelic acid (VMA) and other urinary catecholamines in 85% to 90% of affected infants. Blood pressure measurements and roentgenograms may also help to evaluate this possibility.

Treatment

Significant blood loss should be replaced with whole blood transfusion. Suspicion of adrenal insufficiency may warrant use of intravenous fluids and steroids. The decision for surgical intervention is dictated by the location and degree of hemorrhage. If it appears to be retroperitoneal and limited by the perinephric fascia, some authors recommend blood replacement and careful observation in the hope of spontaneous control by tamponade; often this approach is successful and surgery is not necessary. If paracentesis reveals blood or if blood loss exceeds replacement, exploratory laparotomy is indicated. Surgery may involve evacuation of hematoma, vessel ligation, and adrenalectomy with or without nephrectomy. When the hemorrhagic process extends to the peritoneal cavity, peritoneal exploration and evacuation of clots are indicated.

Prognosis

Small hemorrhages are probably often asymptomatic and have no associated significant morbidity, judging from the unexpected discovery of calcified adrenals on abdominal roentgenograms taken for other reasons later in infancy and childhood. If hemoperitoneum or adrenal insufficiency or both develop, the outlook depends on the speed with which diagnosis is made and appropriate therapy instituted. Surviving infants should be followed

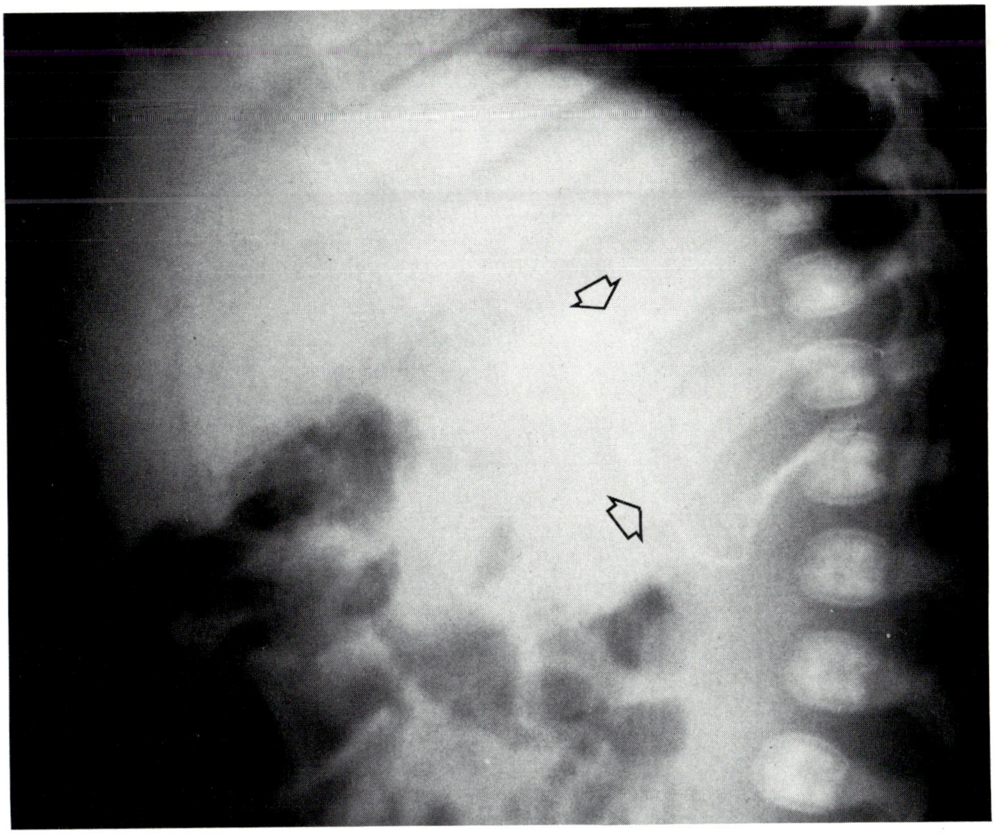

Fig. 20-9. Lateral abdominal roentgenogram of a 5,312 gm male delivered vaginally, with difficulty after shoulder dystocia. At 48 hours fever, icterus, and slow feeding were noted, and a mass was palpable above the left kidney. At 31 days there was dense, retracted calcification, assuming the configuration of the adrenal gland.

closely after discharge from the hospital. Adrenal function should be tested with ACTH stimulation at a later date to determine whether a normal response occurs in the urinary excretion of 17-hydroxycorticosterone.

INJURIES TO THE EXTREMITIES

Fracture of the humerus

After the clavicle, the humerus is the bone most often fractured during the birth process.

Etiology

The most common mechanisms responsible are difficult delivery of extended arms in breech presentations and of the shoulders in vertex presentations. Besides traction with simultaneous rotation of the arm, direct pressure on the humerus is also a factor. This may account for the occurrence of fracture of the humerus in spontaneous vertex deliveries. The fractures are usually in the diaphysis. They are often greenstick, although complete fracture with overriding of the fragments occasionally occurs.

Clinical manifestations

A greenstick fracture may be overlooked until a callus is noted. A complete fracture with marked displacement of fragments presents an obvious deformity that calls attention to the injury. Often the initial manifestation of the fracture is immobility of the affected arm. Palpation reveals tenderness, crepitation, and hypermobility of the fragments. The ipsilateral Moro's response is absent. Roentgenograms confirm the diagnosis.

Differential diagnosis

This includes all the previously noted lesions that cause immobility of the arm. An associated brachial plexus injury occasionally occurs.

Treatment

The affected arm should be immobilized in adduction for 2 to 4 weeks. This may be accomplished by maintaining the arm in a hand-on-hip position with a triangular splint and a Velpeau bandage, by strapping the arm to the chest, or by application of a cast.

Prognosis

The prognosis is excellent. Healing is associated with marked callus formation. Moderate overriding and angulation disappear with time because of the excellent remodeling power of infants. Complete union of the fracture fragments usually occurs by 3 weeks. Fair alignment and shortening of less than 1 inch indicate satisfactory closed reduction. Long bone fractures in infants always result in epiphyseal stimulation; the closer the fracture to the epiphyseal cartilage, the greater the degree of subsequent overgrowth.

Fracture of the femur

Although a relatively infrequent injury, fracture of the femur is by far the most common fracture of the lower extremity in the newborn.

Etiology

This injury usually follows a breech delivery, when the leg is pulled down after the breech is already partially fixed in the pelvic inlet or when the infant is improperly held by one thigh during delivery of the shoulders and arms.

Clinical manifestations

Usually an obvious deformity of the thigh is seen; as a rule the bone breaks transversely in the upper half or third, where it is relatively thin. Less often the injury may not be appreciated until several days after delivery when swelling of the thigh is noted; this may be caused by hemorrhage into adjacent muscle. The infant refuses to move the affected leg or cries in pain during passive movement or with palpation over the fracture site. Roentgenograms almost always show overriding of the fracture fragments.

Treatment

Optimum treatment is traction-suspension of both lower extremities, even if the fracture is unilateral. The legs are immobilized in a spica cast; and with Bryant's traction the infant is suspended by the legs from an overhead frame with the buttocks and lower back just raised off the crib. The legs are extended and the thighs flexed on the abdomen. The weight of the infant's body is enough to overcome the pull of the thigh muscles and thereby reduce the deformity. The infant is maintained in this position for 3 to 4 weeks until adequate callus has formed and new bone growth has started. During the treatment period, special attention should be given to careful feeding and protection of bandages and casts from soiling with urine and feces.

Prognosis

The prognosis is excellent; complete union and restoration without shortening are expected. Extensive calcification may develop in the areas of surrounding hemorrhage; this is resorbed subsequently.

Dislocations

Dislocations caused by birth trauma are rare. Often an apparent dislocation is actually a displaced fracture through an epiphyseal plate. Since the epiphyseal plate is radiolucent, a fracture occurring adjacent to an unmineralized epiphysis will give a radiographic picture simulating a dislocation of the neighboring joint. This type of injury has been termed *pseudodislocation*. Since the humeral and proximal femoral epiphyses are usually not visible on roentgenograms at birth, a pseudodislocation can occur at the shoulder, elbow, or hip.

Of the true dislocations, those involving the hip and knee are probably not caused by the trauma of the birth process. Most likely they are either intrauterine positional deformities or true congenital malformations. A true dislocation resulting from birth trauma is that involving the radial head. This has been asociated with traumatic breech delivery. Examination reveals adduction and internal rotation of the affected arm, with pronation of the forearm; Moro's response is poor, and palpation reveals lateral and posterior displacement of the radial head. This is confirmed by roentgenograms. With supination and extension the radial head can be readily reduced. This should be done promptly, followed by immobilization of the arm in this position in a circular cast for 2 to 3 weeks. Early recognition and treatment should result in normal growth and function of the elbow.

Bayne and Rang recently illustrated the importance of establishing an early diagnosis when they described a full-term infant with a swollen, tender elbow following breech delivery. Movement produced obvious pain. Roentgenograms at that time and again at 8 months of age were misinterpreted as normal. At 1 year an orthopedist diagnosed anteromedial dislocation. Because of several unsuccessful attempts at closed reduction, future osteotomy was required to treat this now permanent deformity.

Epiphyseal separations

As with dislocations, epiphyseal separations are rare. They occur mostly in primiparity, dystocic deliveries, and breech presentations, especially those requiring manual extraction or version and extraction. Any delivery associated with vigorous pulling may predispose the infant to this injury. The upper femoral and humeral epiphyses are most often involved. Usually on the second day the soft tissue over the affected epiphysis develops a firm swelling with reddening, crepitus, and tenderness. Active motion is limited, and passive motion is painful. If the injury is in the upper femoral epiphysis, the infant assumes the frog position with external rotation of the leg.

Early roentgenograms will show only soft tissue swelling, with occasional superolateral displacement of the proximal femoral metaphysis. Since the neonatal femoral capital epiphysis is not ossified, this can be interpreted mistakenly as congenital hip dislocation. However, the presence of pain and tenderness would make dislocation unlikely. Besides plain roentgenograms of the hips, an infant with a history and physical examination compatible with traumatic epiphysiolysis should also be studied by arthrography before attempting manipulation. Hip arthrography in such an infant would demonstrate a normal femoroacetabular relationship, in contrast to abnormal findings in septic arthritis and congenital hip dislocation. In addition, in the presence of traumatic epiphysiolysis, the femoral head and neck would not be continuous, in contrast to the findings of septic arthritis and congenital hip dislocation. Further differentiation between traumatic epiphysiolysis and septic arthritis can be provided by arthrocentesis; in epiphysiolysis the joint does not contain excess fluid and what is obtained may be serosanguineous, whereas in septic arthritis, purulent fluid is obtained. After 1 to 2 weeks extensive callus appears, confirming the nature of the injury; during the third week subperiosteal calcification appears.

If possible, treatment should be conservative. Closed reduction and immobilization are indicated within the first few days before rapidly forming fibrous callus prevents mobilization of the epiphysis. The hip is immobilized in the frog-leg position as in congenital dislocation. Poorly immobilized fragments may require temporary fixation with a Kirschner wire. Union usually occurs within 10 to 15 days. Untreated or poorly treated epiphyseal injuries may result in subsequent growth distortion and permanent deformities such as coxa vara. Mild injuries carry a good prognosis.

Other peripheral nerve injuries

In contrast to the brachial plexus and phrenic and facial nerves, other peripheral nerves are injured less often at birth, and usually in association with trauma to the extremity. Radial palsy has occurred following difficult forceps extractions, both from pressure of incorrectly applied forceps and in association with fracture of the arm. Occasionally the palsy occurs later when the radial nerve is enmeshed within the callus of the healing fracture. Frequently, associated subcutaneous fat necrosis overlies the course of the radial nerve along the lateral aspects of the upper arm. The presence of isolated wrist-drop with weakness of the wrist, finger, and thumb extensors; skin changes overlying the course of the nerve; and absence of weakness above the elbow serve to distinguish this from brachial plexus injury. Palsies of the femoral and sciatic nerves have occurred after breech extractions; the sciatic palsy has followed extraction by the foot. Passive range of motion exercises are usually the only therapy required. Complete recovery usually occurs within several weeks or months.

TRAUMA TO THE GENITALIA

Soft tissue injuries involving the external genitalia sometimes occur, especially after breech deliveries and in large babies.

Scrotum and labia majora

Edema, ecchymoses, and hematomas can occur in the scrotum and labia majora, especially when these are the presenting parts in a breech presentation. Since the newborn male has a pendulous urethra that is vulnerable to compression or injury, it is possible for significant trauma to occur following a protracted labor in the breech position; the mechanism is believed to be compression of the urethra against a firm structure in the maternal bony pelvis. Cromie managed four male infants who developed marked temporary hydronephrosis following delivery in the breech position. The hydronephrosis resolved within 3 days. Because of laxity of the tissues, the degree of swelling and discoloration occasionally is extreme enough (Fig. 20-10) to evoke considerable concern among the medical and nursing staff, especially regarding deeper involvement (e.g., periuretheral hemorrhage and edema), which might hinder normal micturition. However, generally this has not been a problem, and frequently these babies void shortly after arriving in the nursery. Spontaneous resolution of edema occurs within 24 to 48 hours and of discoloration within 4 to 5 days. Treatment is not necessary. Secondary ulceration, necrosis, or eschar formation is rare unless an associated underlying condition such as herpes simplex infection is present.

Deeper structures

Much less often birth trauma may involve the deeper structures of the genitalia. If the tunica vaginalis is injured and blood fills its cavity, a hematocele is formed. Absence of transillumination distinguishes this from a hydrocele. If the infant appears to be in pain, the scrotum may be elevated and cold packs applied. Spontaneous resolution is the usual course.

The testes may be injured, often in association with injury to the epididymis. Usually the involvement is bilateral. The testes may be enlarged, smoothly rounded, and insensitive. The infant may be irritable, with vomiting and poor feeding. Urologic consultation is indicated; occasionally exploration and evacuation of blood are necessary, especially with increasing size of the testes. Severe trauma may result in atrophy or failure of the testes to grow. The occasional finding in older children of a circumscribed fibrous area within the testicular tissue is thought to represent past birth trauma to the gland.

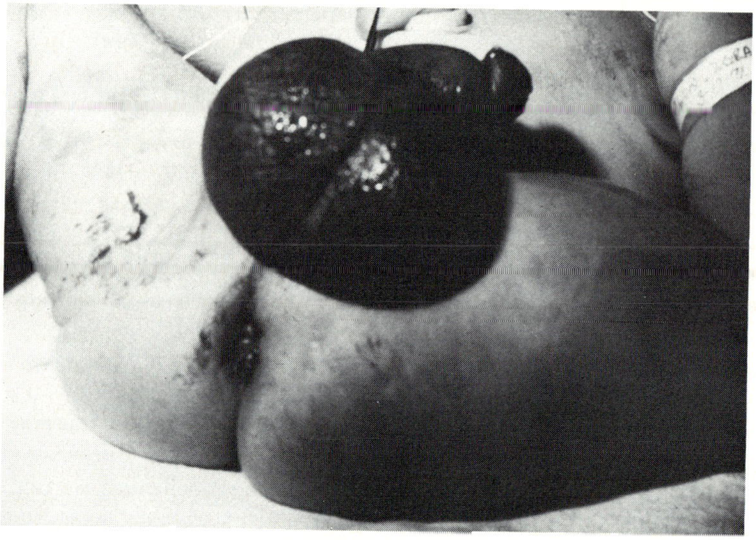

Fig. 20-10. Hematoma of scrotum and penis in a 3,895 gm male delivered vaginally after frank breech presentation. The infant voided at 22 hours and regularly thereafter. Swelling diminished appreciably within 5 hours and was gone by the third day. Discoloration was greatly diminished by the second day.

INJURIES RELATED TO INTRAPARTUM FETAL MONITORING

Continuous monitoring of the FHR and the intermittent sampling of fetal scalp blood for determination of acid-base status are often employed to monitor the fetus during labor. Thousands of patients have now been monitored by these methods (Chapters 8 and 22). The relative infrequency of complications indicates that in experienced hands these procedures are generally safe. However, certain specific complications have occurred.

Injuries related to direct FHR monitoring

Direct monitoring of the FHR during labor depends on application of an electrode to the fetal scalp or other presenting part. Superficial abrasions, lacerations, and hematomas have occurred at the site of application of the electrode. These complications require no specific therapy beyond local treatment.

Several investigators have reported abscesses of the scalp associated with application of scalp electrodes. These usually have been sterile and have required only local treatment. Systemic signs or symptoms require evaluation for possible septicemia.

Thomas and Blackwell reported a potentially more serious complication related to use of a spiral fetal scalp electrode. At delivery this electrode was noted to have penetrated the substance of an eyelid, with considerable secondary local edema and minimal scleral hematoma. The complication was believed to have resulted from movement of the fetus before application of the electrode. The electrode was removed, and the infant recovered without sequelae.

Injuries related to fetal scalp blood sampling

Fetal biochemical monitoring requires puncture of the presenting part, usually the scalp, with a 2 mm blade and the collection of blood under direct visualization in a heparinized tube. The major complications that have occurred are excessive bleeding and accidental breakage of the blades. The bleeding can be stopped by pressure, but on occasion may require sutures. Several infants have required blood replacement. It is important to obtain a detailed family history of bleeding disorders before initiation of this procedure.

The second major complication has been breakage of the blade within the fetal scalp. Removal soon after delivery has been recommended to prevent secondary infection. This has been accomplished by use of a magnet attached to a small forceps that probes the puncture site and elicits a click as the blade is attracted to the magnet. On occasion radiographic localization followed by a small incision is necessary for withdrawal of the blade.

Henry H. Mangurten

BIBLIOGRAPHY

General

Cyr, R.M., Usher, R.H., and McLean, F.H.: Changing patterns of birth asphyxia and trauma over 20 years, Am. J. Obstet. Gynecol. **148**:490, 1984.

Wegman, M.E.: Annual summary of vital statistics—1981, Pediatrics **70**:835, 1982.

Wegman, M.E.: Annual summary of vital statistics—1984, Pediatrics **76**:861, 1985.

Injuries to soft tissues

Chen, T.H., and others: Subcutaneous fat necrosis of the newborn, Arch. Dermatol. **117**:36, 1981.

Davis, J.A., and Schiff, D.: Bruising as a cause of neonatal jaundice, Lancet **1**:636, 1966.

Hebertson, R.M., and others: Obstetric forceps pad designed to reduce infant trauma, Obstet. Gynecol. **65**:275, 1985.

Injuries to the head

Berger, S.S., and Stewart, R.E.: Mandibular hypoplasia secondary to perinatal trauma: report of case, J. Oral Surg. **35**:578, 1977.

Besio, R., and others: Neonatal retinal hemorrhages and influence of perinatal factors, Am. J. Ophthalmol. **87**:74, 1979.

Birrell, J.F.: The ear, nose, and throat diseases of children, London, 1960, Cassell & Co., Ltd.

Cavanagh, F.: Vocal palsies in children, J. Laryngol. Otolaryngol. **69**:399, 1955.

Chasler, C.N.: The newborn skull (the diagnosis of fracture), Am. J. Roentgenol. Radium Ther. Nucl. Med. **100**:92, 1967.

Daily, W., and Davis, W.E.: Nasal septal dislocation in the newborn, Mo. Med. **74**:381, 1977.

Eisenberg, D., Kirchner, S.G., and Perrin, E.C.: Neonatal skull depression unassociated with birth trauma, AJR **143**:1063, 1984.

Ferguson, C.F.: Congenital abnormalities of the infant larynx, Otolaryngol. Clin. North Am. **3**:185, 1970.

Garza-Mercado, R.: Intrauterine depressed skull fractures of the newborn, Neurosurgery **10**:694, 1982.

Hepner, W.R., Jr.: Some observations on facial paresis in the newborn infant: etiology and incidence, Pediatrics **8**:494, 1951.

Jaworski, S., and Dudkiewicz, Z.: Mandibular fractures in the course of labor in a newborn infant, Pediatr. Pol. **48**:1501, 1973.

Jeppesen, F., and Windfeld, I.: Dislocation of the nasal septal cartilage in the newborn, Acta Obstet. Gynecol. Scand. **51**:5, 1972.

Kendall, N., and Woloshin, H.: Cephalhematoma associated with fracture of the skull, J. Pediatr. **41**:125, 1952.

Lee, Y., and Berg, R.B.: Cephalhematoma infected with *Bacteroides*, Am. J. Dis. Child. **121**:77, 1971.

Loeser, J.D., Kilburn, H.L., and Jolley, T.: Management of depressed skull fracture in the newborn, J. Neurosurg. **44**:62, 1976.

McHugh, H.E.: Facial paralysis in birth injury and skull fractures, Arch. Otolaryngol. **78**:443, 1963.

Pohjanpelto, P., Niemi, K., and Sarmela, T.: Anterior chamber haemorrhage in the newborn after spontaneous delivery: a case report, Acta Ophthalmol. **57**:443, 1979.

Rainin, E.A.: Eversion of upper lids secondary to birth trauma, Arch. Ophthalmol. **94**:330, 1976.

Raynor, R., and Parsa, M.: Nonsurgical elevation of depressed skull fracture in an infant, J. Pediatr. **72**:262, 1968.

Saunders, B.S., and others: Depressed skull fracture in the neonate: report of three cases, J. Neurosurg. **50**:512, 1979.

Schrager, G.O.: Elevation of depressed skull fracture with a breast pump, J. Pediatr. **77**:300, 1970.

Sezen, F.: Retinal haemorrhages in newborn infants, Br. J. Ophthalmol. **55**:248, 1971.

Silverman, S.H., and Leibow, S.G.: Dislocation of the triangular cartilage of the nasal septum, J. Pediatr. **87**:456, 1975.

Tan, K.L.: Elevation of congenital depressed fracture of the skull by the vacuum extractor, Acta Paediatr. Scand. **63**:562, 1974.

Zelson, C., Lee, S.J., and Pearl, M.: The incidence of skull fractures underlying cephalhematomas in newborn infants, J. Pediatr. **85**:371, 1974.

Injuries to the neck and shoulder girdle

Bennet, G.C., and Harrold, A.J.: Prognosis and early management of birth injuries to the brachial plexus, Br. Med. J. **1**:1520, 1976.

Bingham, J.A.W.: Two cases of unilateral paralysis of the diaphragm in the newborn treated surgically. Thorax **9**:248, 1954.

Bishop, H.C., and Koop, C.E.: Acquired eventration of the diaphragm in infancy, Pediatrics **22**:1088, 1958.

Claren, S.K., Smith, D.W., and Hanson, J.W.: Helmet treatment for plagiocephaly and congenital muscular torticollis, J. Pediatr. **94**:43, 1979.

Eng, G.D.: Brachial plexus palsy in newborn infants, Pediatrics **43**:18, 1971.

Greenwald, A.G., Schute, P.C., and Shiveley, J.L.: Brachial plexus birth palsy: a 10-year report on the incidence and prognosis, J. Pediatr. Orthop. **4**:689, 1984.

Haller, J.A., and others: Management of diaphragmatic paralysis in infants with special emphasis on selection of patients for operative plication, J. Pediatr. Surg. **14**:779, 1979.

Harris, G.B.C.: Unilateral paralysis of the diaphragm in the newborn, Postgrad. Med. **50**:51, 1971.

Hoffer, M.M., Wickenden, R., and Roper, B.: Brachial plexus birth palsies: results of tendon transfers to the rotator cuff, J. Bone Joint Surg. **60-A**:691, 1978.

Matson, D.D.: Neurosurgery of infancy and childhood, ed. 2, Spingfield, Ill., 1969, Charles C Thomas, Publisher.

Sanerkin, N.G., and Edwards, P.: Birth injury to the sternomastoid muscle, J. Bone Joint Surg. **48-B**:441, 1966.

Vassalos, E., Prevedourakis, C., and Paraschopoulou-Prevedouraki, P.: Brachial plexus paralysis in the newborn, Am. J. Obstet. Gynecol. **101**:554, 1968.

Weisman, L., Woodall, J., and Merenstein, G.: Constant negative pressure in the treatment of diaphragmatic paralysis secondary to birth injury, Birth Defects: Original Article Series **XII**:297, 1976.

Yasuda, R., and others: Bilateral phrenic nerve palsy in the newborn infant: a case report, J. Pediatr. **89**:986, 1976.

Zajkowski, E.J., and Kravath, R.E.: Bilateral diaphragmatic paralysis in the newborn infant: treatment with nasal continuous positive airway pressure, Chest **75**:392, 1979.

Injuries to the spine and spinal cord

Bell, H.J., and Dykstra, D.D.: Somatosensory evoked potentials as an adjunct to diagnosis of neonatal spinal cord injury, J. Pediatr. **106**:298, 1985.

Brans, Y.W., and Cassady, G.: Neonatal spinal cord injuries, Am. J. Obstet. Gynecol. **123**:918, 1975.

Koch, B.M., and Eng, G.M.: Neonatal spinal cord injury, Arch. Phys. Med. Rehabil. **60**:378, 1979.

Maekawa, K., Masaki, T., and Kokubun, Y.: Fetal spinal-cord injury secondary to hyperextension of the neck: no effect of cesarean section, Dev. Med. Child. Neurol. **18**:229, 1976.

Towbin, A.: Latent spinal cord and brain stem injury in newborn infants, Dev. Med. Child. Neurol. **11**:54, 1969.

Walter, C.E., and Tedeschi, L.G.: Spinal injury and neonatal death, Am. J. Obstet. Gynecol. **106**:272, 1970.

Injuries to intraabdominal organs

Drucker, V., and Rodriguez, C.E.: Extensive bilateral calcification within adrenal hemorrhage, Radiology **64**:258, 1955.

Eraklis, A.J.: Abdominal injury related to trauma of birth, Pediatrics **39**:421, 1967.

French, C.E., and Waldstein, G.: Subcapsular hemorrhage of the liver in the newborn, Pediatrics **69**:204, 1982.

Gross, M., Kottmeier, P.K., and Waterhouse, K.: Diagnosis and treatment of neonatal adrenal hemorrhage, J. Pediatr. Surg. **2**:308, 1967.

Holder, T.M., and Leape, L.L.: The acute surgical abdomen in the neonate, N. Engl. J. Med. **278**:605, 1968.

Leape, L.L., and Bordy, M.D.: Neonatal rupture of the spleen, Pediatrics **47**:101, 1971.

Matsuyama, S., Suzuki, N., and Nagamachi, Y.: Rupture of the spleen in the newborn: treatment without splenectomy, J. Pediatr. Surg. **11**:115, 1976.

Mineau, D.E., and Koehler, P.R.: Ultrasound diagnosis of neonatal adrenal hemorrhage, Am. J. Roentgenol. **132**:443, 1979.

Monson, D.O., and Raffensperger, J.G.: Intraperitoneal hemorrhage secondary to liver laceration in a newborn, J. Pediatr. Surg. **2**:464, 1967.

Injuries to the extremities

Bayne, O., and Rang, M.: Medial dislocation of the radial head following breech delivery: a case report and review of the literature, J. Pediatr. Orthop. **4**:485, 1984.

Haliburton, R.A., Barber, J.R., and Fraser, R.L.: Pseudodislocation: an unusual birth injury, Can. J. Surg. **10**:455, 1967.

Labelle, P.: Orthopedic anxieties in the newborn, Appl. Ther. **8**:226, 1966.

Mortens, J., and Christensen, P.: Traumatic separation of the upper femoral epiphysis as an obstetrical lesion, Acta Orthop. Scand. **34**:239, 1964.

Schubert, J.J.: Dislocation of the radial head in the newborn infant, J. Bone Joint Surg. **47**:1019, 1965.

Towbin, R., and Crawford, A.H.: Neonatal traumatic proximal femoral epiphysiolysis, Pediatrics **63**:456, 1979.

Wilson, J.C., Jr.: Fractures and dislocations in childhood, Pediatr. Clin. North Am. **14**:659, 1967.

Trauma to the genitalia

Cromie, W.J.: Genitourinary injuries in the neonate, Clin. Pediatr. **18**:292, 1979.

Hodgman, J.E., Friedman, R.I., and Levan, N.E.: Neonatal dermatology, Pediatr. Clin. North Am. **18**:713, 1971.

Injuries related to intrapartum fetal monitoring

Chan, W.H., Paul, R.H., and Toews, J.: Intrapartum fetal monitoring: maternal and fetal morbidity and perinatal mortality, Obstet. Gynecol. **41**:7, 1973.

Cordero, L., and Hon, E.H.: Scalp abscess: a rare complication of fetal monitoring, J. Pediatr. **78**:533, 1971.

Modanlou, H., and others: Complications of fetal blood sampling during labor, Clin. Pediatr. **12**:603, 1973.

Paul, R.H., and Hon, E.H.: Clinical fetal monitoring: a survey of current usage, Obstet. Gynecol. **37**:779, 1971.

Thomas, G., and Blackwell, R.J.: A hazard associated with the use of spiral fetal scalp electrodes, Am. J. Obstet. Gynecol. **121**:1118, 1975.

Chapter 21

Neonatal clinical cardiopulmonary monitoring

Monitoring of biophysical and biochemical parameters is an integral part of neonatal intensive care (Chapter 24, part three). When monitoring a patient, it is important to determine what parameter must be followed and to understand the characteristics of the parameter being measured. Knowledge of principles and techniques by which instruments operate should be shared by all members of the team responsible for patient care. Furthermore, review of monitoring records is a valuable teaching tool and an objective method for quality control.

NEONATAL HEART RATE MONITORING

The clinical evaluation of the neonatal heart rate (NHR) has traditionally been based on stethoscopic auscultation or analysis of electrocardiographic (ECG) tracings. These techniques average the counted heart beats and, in addition to the loss of large amounts of data, detect only tachycardia or bradycardia, not transient changes. Figure 21-1 shows the comparison of instantaneous and average heart rate counting techniques and illustrates the increased detail of the instantaneous heart rate. This is obtained using a cardiotachometer that displays beat-to-beat heart rate after each cardiac cycle. The bioengineering aspects of neonatal heart rate monitoring are further discussed in Chapter 24.

Normal heart rate

The baseline NHR is related to gestational age, postnatal age, race, and state of sleep or wakefulness. Variations in this baseline level reflect differences in the degree of neurocirculatory control exerted at specific times and in different sleep states. The heart rate can be properly interpreted only when sleep state is taken into account because variability is greatly increased during active as compared with quiet sleep. From the first minute of life the NHR appears to be a good indicator of the infant's tolerance for the stresses of labor and delivery and reflects the adequacy of adaptation to extrauterine life. Following delivery of a vigorous infant, the NHR will change rapidly, with a higher baseline observed at this time than during labor. The mean NHR of healthy term infants is 175 beats per minute at 1 minute; within 2 minutes the NHR rises to a mean of 189 beats per minute and then declines, falling by 20 beats at 5 minutes and by 40 beats at 20 minutes. The NHR of healthy preterm infants follows a similar pattern after birth but shows a significantly lower peak and a slower rate of decline.

The baseline NHR for healthy and sick preterm infants as a function of postnatal age during the first week of life is shown in Fig. 21-2. After the first week of life the heart rate reaches a maximum of 148 and 132 beats per minute for preterm and term infants between 4 and 8 weeks of age. Thereafter it rapidly decreases for approximately 2 months and then stabilizes during the remainder of the first 6 months. Although the changes in NHR of small for gestational age (SGA) infants follow a similar pattern to those of appropriate for gestational age (AGA) neonates, during the fourth to the sixteenth hours of life the heart rate of SGA infants with birth weight less than 1,000 gm is significantly lower than that of AGA infants (Fig. 21-3). This difference may result from advanced maturity of autonomic control of heart rate or from the decreased incidence of patent ductus arteriosus found in SGA infants.

Baseline changes

The interpretation of NHR recordings requires a classification of changes in heart rate levels. Four alterations of the baseline heart rate have been described according to the direction and duration of the changes. *Tachycardia* and *bradycardia* are defined as baseline levels above or below the normal limits for the patient's age and maturity. More transient rises or falls from baseline levels are referred to as *accelerations* or *decelerations*. Continuous beat-to-beat NHR recordings show rapid alterations in the NHR associated with changes in respiratory rate and pattern of respiration, with procedures, as a response

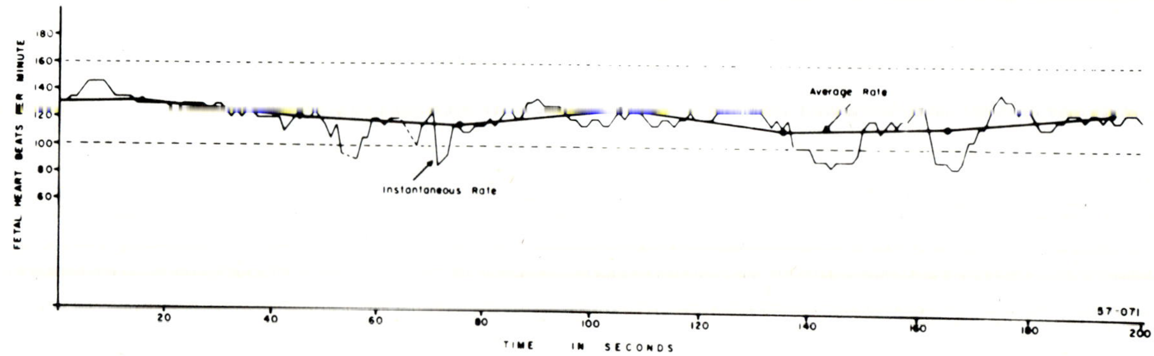

Fig. 21-1. Comparison of instantaneous and average heart rates. (From Hon, E., Cabal, L., and Zanini, B.: An introduction to neonatal heart rate monitoring, North Haven, Conn., 1975, W. Mack Publishing Co.)

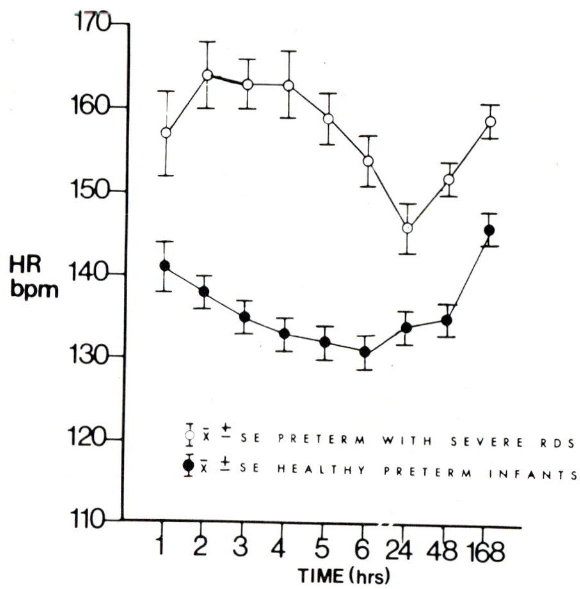

Fig. 21-2. Mean (± SEM) heart rate levels as a function of postnatal age in healthy preterm infants (n = 38) and sick preterm infants with severe respiratory distress syndrome (n = 19).

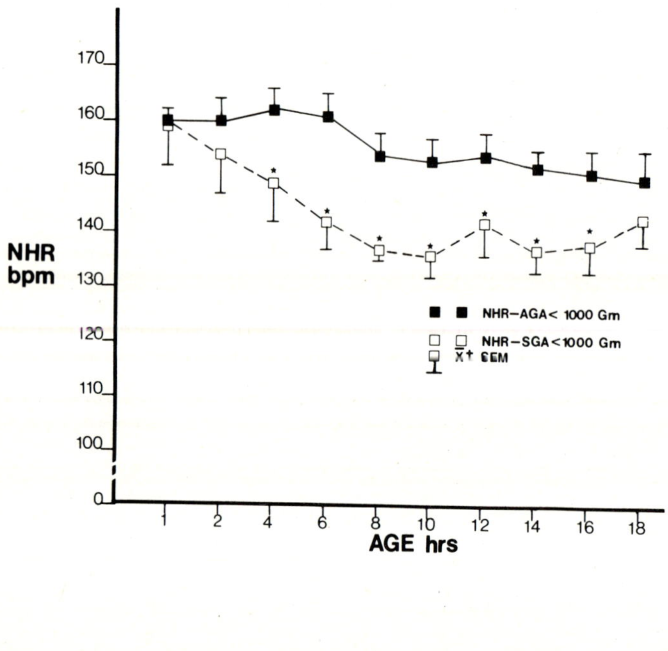

Fig. 21-3. Heart rates (mean ± SEM) of 19 appropriate (AGA) and nine small for gestational age (SGA) infants, with birth weights less than or equal to 1,000 gm during the first 18 hours of life. Values marked by asterisks indicate statistically significant difference (p < 0.01).

to medications, and as a manifestation of various clinical entities. Following is an outline of entities or procedures that may elicit such alterations. Neonatal cardiac arrhythmias are discussed in Chapter 29.

A. Causes of neonatal tachycardia
   1. Physiologic reactions
      a. Somatic activity (prolonged)
      b. Following delivery
   2. Maneuvers and procedures
      a. Hyperventilation
      b. Heat stress
      c. Cold stress
      d. Pain stimuli
   3. Drugs
      a. Isoproterenol
      b. Tolazoline
      c. Atropine
      d. Pancuronium bromide
      e. Epinephrine
      f. Aminophylline
      g. Glucagon (IV)
      h. Atracurium
   4. Pathologic conditions
      a. Hypoxia
      b. Shock
      c. Hypercapnia
      d. Fever
      e. Anemia
      f. Sepsis
      g. Patent ductus arteriosus
      h. Congestive heart failure
      i. Cardiac arrhythmias
      j. Postasphyxic states
      k. Metabolic disorders
      l. Hyperammonemia
      m. Hyperthyroidism
      n. Pheochromocytoma
B. Causes of neonatal bradycardia
   1. Physiologic reactions
      a. Swallowing
      b. Micturition
      c. Defecation
      d. Vomiting
      e. Head compression
      f. Carotid compression
      g. Ocular compression
   2. Maneuvers and procedures
      a. Pharyngeal stimulation
      b. Tracheal stimulation
      c. Gavage feedings
      d. Airway suction
      e. Abdominal compression
      f. Visceral manipulation during surgery
      g. Excessive transpulmonary pressure
   3. Drugs
      a. Propranolol
      b. Digitalis
      c. Atropine (during hypoxia)
      d. Local anesthetics
      e. Calcium infusions
   4. Pathologic conditions
      a. Hypoxia
      b. Acidosis (severe)
      c. Hypothermia (severe)
      d. Shock (late)
      e. Apnea
      f. Congestive heart failure
      g. Pneumothorax, pneumopericardium
      h. Airway obstruction
      i. Hyperkalemia
      j. Cardiac arrhythmias
      k. Pulmonary hemorrhage
      l. Hydrocephalus
      m. Intracranial bleeding
      n. Convulsions
      o. Diaphragmatic hernia
      p. Hypothyroidism
      q. Bile pigments

Cardiac output in newborn infants depends on changes in heart rate, since the neonatal heart works at near maximal capacity and is unable to compensate for bradycardia by increasing stroke volume. A direct relationship between oxygen consumption and heart rate levels has been demonstrated in neonates. Furthermore, the clinical importance of NHR monitoring has been emphasized by recent work demonstrating a decrease in cerebral blood flow velocity during apnea and bradycardia, particularly severe bradycardia, in the preterm infant. These data suggest that repeated episodes of severe cardiac deceleration or bradycardia may cause or exacerbate hypoxic and ischemic brain injury.

Heart rate variability

In normal subjects, heart rate is determined by the intrinsic rhythm of the sinoatrial node pacemaker modified by the interaction of the different physiologic control systems. Fig. 21-4 illustrates the heart rate control by the autonomic nervous system through the cardioinhibitor (parasympathetic) and the cardioaccelerator (sympathetic) components. The sympathetic and parasympathetic systems are physiologic antagonists in their controlling action over the sinoatrial node and, because of their changing tone and different time constants, the result of their interaction is the beat-to-beat variability of heart rate.

Heart rate variability has been shown to have at least two components: (1) long-term variability (LTV), defined as the difference between the minimum and maximum oscillations of heart rate within a time period, and (2) short-term variability (STV), obtained from the mean of

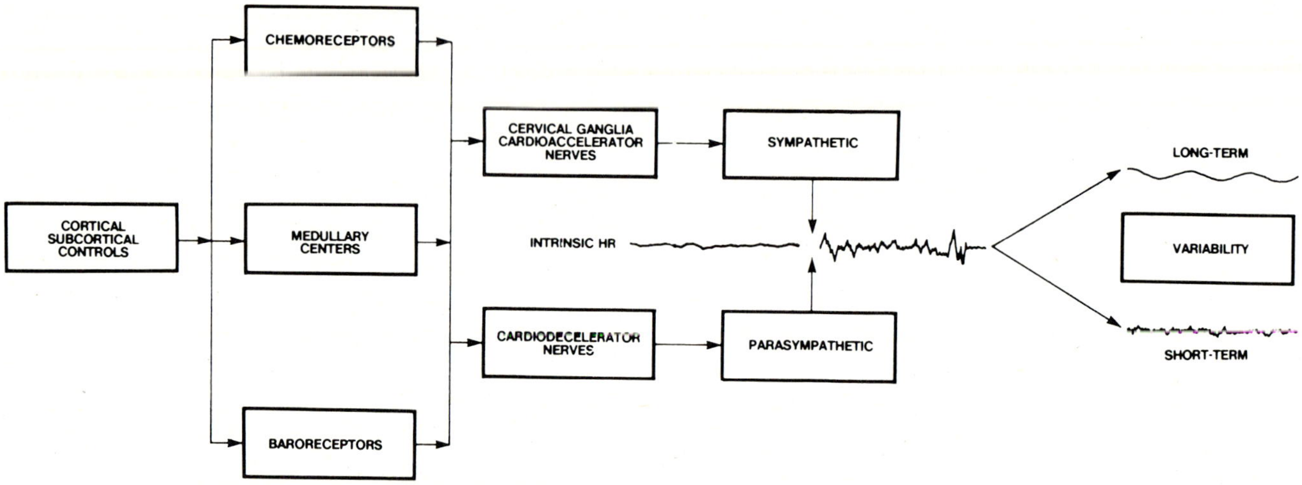

Fig. 21-4. Control of the heart rate by the autonomic nervous system through the cardioinhibitor (parasympathetic) and the cardioaccelerator (sympathetic) components. The result of their interaction is the beat-to-beat variability of the heart rate.

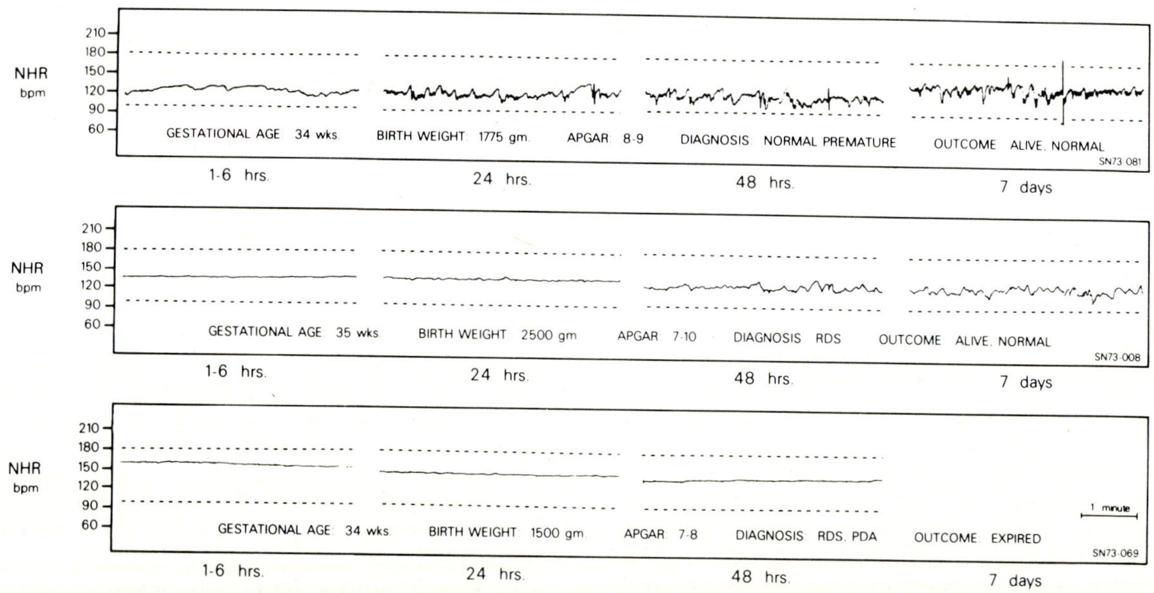

Fig. 21-5. Recordings illustrating the baseline neonatal heart rate (NHR) variability of three infants with different clinical conditions at varying ages of life.

successive R-R interval length differences. LTV is thought to result from the dynamic balance between the sympathetic and parasympathetic divisions of the autonomic nervous system, whereas STV is generated by the oscillations of vagal tone controlling the heart rate. Variability is an integral part of the NHR, and its absence may reflect damage, obtundation, or immaturity of the autonomic nervous system control over the heart. Furthermore, since the mechanisms of heart rate control include the reflex interaction with other higher centers and peripheral receptors, the quantification of variability thereby provides a technique for evaluating pathophysiologic and pharmacologic fetal and neonatal responses. Most studies dealing with NHR variability have been performed in healthy term infants, and only a few are available in preterm infants.

Recent studies have provided quantitative data of NHR variability. They show that in healthy preterm infants the baseline heart rate variability is stable during the first 48 hours of life and increases between 5 and 7 days. An inverse relationship exists between NHR variability and baseline heart rate levels. Heart rate variability can be interpreted only when the heart rate levels, in beats per minute or as R-R intervals, are taken into account. NHR variability, corrected for heart rate levels, increases with advancing postnatal age in healthy infants, suggesting maturation and stabilization of the autonomic nervous system.

Our studies, as well as those of others, have demonstrated that heart rate variability corrected for heart rate levels is decreased in preterm infants with respiratory distress syndrome (RDS). The decrease in heart rate variability is proportional to the increasing severity of RDS. The lack of variability is reversible in infants who recover from RDS and persists in infants dying from this disorder (Fig. 21-5). In infants recovering from RDS the return of variability heralds a good prognosis. Decreased heart rate variability found in infants with RDS may reflect functional or anatomic suppression of the cardioregulatory centers. In addition, changes in heart rate variability have been associated with neonatal intraventricular hemorrhage. Recently it has been suggested that absence of heart rate variability could be used as one of the clinical criteria of brain death.

RESPIRATION

Respiration can be monitored by direct and indirect methods (Table 21-1). Direct methods sense the air ex-

Table 21-1 Techniques for monitoring respiration

System	Elements	Operation
Thermistor	Thermistor in face mask, nasal prongs, or under nose	Resistance of thermistor changes as it is warmed or cooled by inhaled air
Pneumotachograph	Fine mesh screen placed across patient's airway	Detects air flow by measurement of pressure drop across screen
Spirometer	Reservoir connected to patient's airway	Measures volume of air breathed by patient
Phonopneumograph	Microphone under nose or on skin over upper airway	Detects airflow by sensing inspiratory and expiratory breath sounds
Capnograph	Infrared light connected to patient's airway	Detects carbon dioxide (percentage or tension) change during inspiration and expiration by sensing changes in infrared light absorption
Impedance pneumograph	A 10 to 100 kHz electric current of about 50 μA is passed through two chest electrodes placed across thorax	Change in chest air and blood volume with each breath causes impedance that generates voltage change
Body plethysmograph	Infant placed in airtight box with face exposed to outside; box is connected with string gauge or with pneumotachometer	Volume of air displaced with each breath is sensed by pneumotachometer or pressure transducer
Air-filled tubing	Two small, hollow, corrugated rubber tubes strapped around chest and/or thorax and connected to an air tambour	Air tambour senses air displacement caused by thoracoabdominal motion during breathing
Air mattress	Tubing connected to heated thermistor	Breathing movements displace air in coiled air-filled tubing; displaced air cools heated thermistor
Capacitive mattress	Two capacitors in mattress interspaced with fine wire mesh	Vertical components of breathing movements induce changes in capacitance, which are interpreted as breathing
Pressure transducer mattress	Pressure transducer	Respiratory movements alter pressure on mattress; these pressure changes are interpreted as breathing
Airway pressure	Tap between endotracheal tube and ventilator circuits is connected to pressure transducer	Detects pressure changes occurring with patient's spontaneous respiration and with cycling of ventilator
Central venous and esophageal pressures	Central venous and water-filled esophageal catheter or balloon placed at lower third of esophagus and connected to strain gauges	Detect changes in pleural pressures caused during inspiration, expiration, and cycling of ventilator

change between the infant's airway and an outside source. Indirect methods detect body motion or measure changes in physical properties of the body caused by breathing. Some direct methods not only sense a change occurring with breathing but also may add information regarding the effectiveness of respiration, that is, the volume exchanged or the degree to which carbon dioxide is removed from the lungs.

Pneumotachographs are often used to study pulmonary changes in infants and neonates, and these devices are found in pulmonary function laboratories and in some intensive care units. A low mechanical resistance is placed in the gas flow. The pressure difference across the resistance is proportional to flow and is transduced electronically by integration against time, then a volume measurement is derived. Expired carbon dioxide monitoring has become a widely used method to evaluate respiration and ventilation in neonates and older infants. Its use has acquired prestige as being reliable, especially in the operating room. The instruments employed in this method, called capnometers or capnographs, are significantly more reliable than similar instruments used in the past. Most infrared carbon dioxide absorption analyzers have been modified to make them linear. Drift is almost negligible; the analyzers are not affected by electrocautery apparatus; and interference from nitrous oxide and other anesthetics has been adequately compensated. Table 21-2 summarizes the advantages and disadvantages of the various methods used for respiratory monitoring; the bioengineering aspects of the commonly employed techniques are discussed in Chapter 24, part three.

Patterns of breathing

The description of the various patterns of breathing is based on the relationship between the rate and depth of breathing, either from one respiratory cycle to another or over longer periods. The patterns of breathing found in newborn infants are (1) regular breathing, (2) irregular breathing, (3) periodic breathing, (4) paradoxic (disorganized) breathing, (5) oscillatory breathing, and (6) apnea (Fig. 21-6).

Table 21-2. Advantages and disadvantages of respiratory monitoring methods

	Impedance	Thermistor	Capnograph	Phonopneumograph	Mattress	Magnets
DISADVANTAGES						
Easily damaged, deteriorated, or lost		X			X	X
Sensitive to noise, humidity, air currents, or magnetic materials		X	X	X		X
Sensitive to cardiovascular artifacts	X		X			
Sensitive to vibration					X	X
Sensitive to body movements	X				X	X
Others	Skin trauma; possibility of electric shock	May increase airway resistance; difficult to clean	Changes with circulation		Displacement of infant or sensor	Radiopaque
ADVANTAGES						
Easy setup				X	X	X
Easy to operate	X	X	X	X	X	X
No electric contact with infant			X	X	X	X
No direct contact with infant			X		X	
Others	Uses ECG electrodes; reflects chest volume changes			Identifies inspiratory and expiratory phases	Radiolucent	

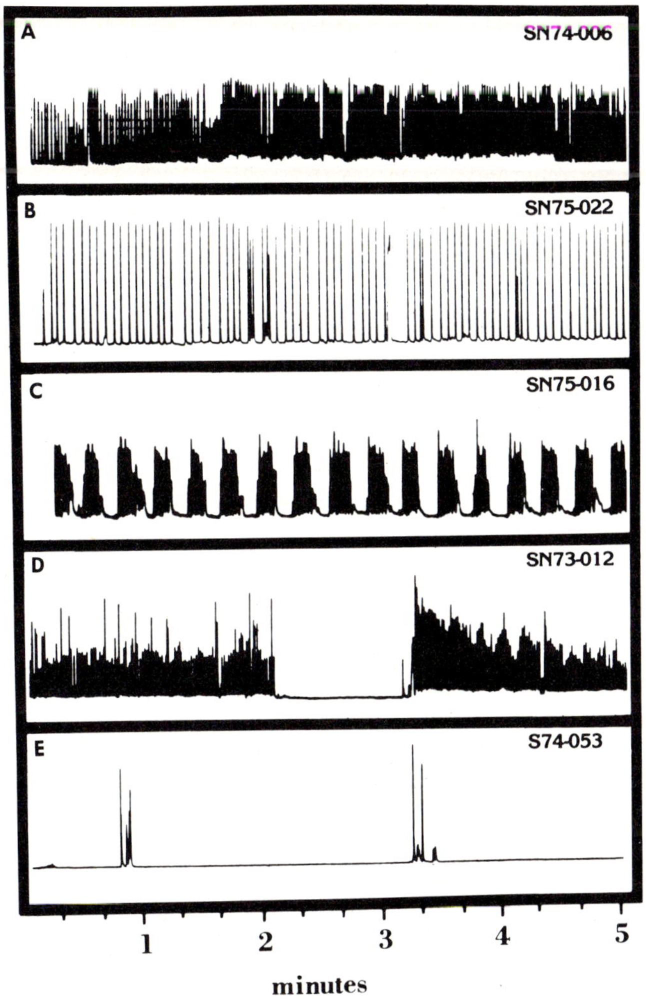

Fig. 21-6. Various patterns of breathing found in newborn infants. **A,** Fast and regular; **B,** slow and regular; **C,** periodic; **D,** apnea; **E,** terminal gasping.

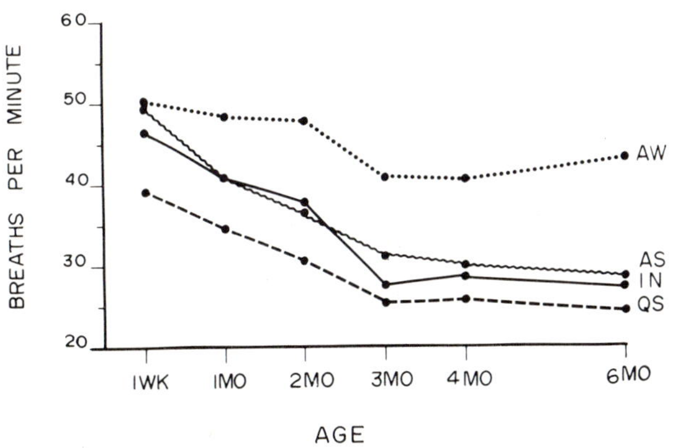

Fig. 21-7. Average median respiratory rate obtained from eight healthy term infants at various ages while awake *(AW)* and in active *(AS)*, quiet *(QS)*, and indeterminate *(IN)* sleep states. (From Hoppenbrouwers, T., and others: Pediatr. Res. **12:**120, 1978.)

Regular breathing is the pattern during which breath-to-breath intervals are nearly equal and individual breaths are of similar depth. This pattern is typically found in mature infants during quiet (non–rapid eye movement [NREM]) sleep. Irregular breathing is characterized by marked variability of the depth and timing of respiration; it is typically found in preterm infants during active (REM) sleep (Chapter 28, part five). Short, repeated cessations of air exchange for 3 seconds or longer, occurring at regular intervals, are defined as periodic breathing. The breathing pattern of preterm infants is usually periodic and irregular; as gestation advances, the pattern becomes less periodic and more regular. The rate of respiration decreases greatly in all sleep states from the first week to the third month of life (Fig. 21-7).

The literature does not agree on the duration of nonbreathing periods that can be either defined as apnea or classified as pathologic (Chapter 28, part five). For sleep studies, respiratory pauses of longer than 2 seconds have been measured; however, the clinical definitions of significant apnea range from greater than 10 up to 20 seconds. Apnea has been considered more significant when it is associated with heart rate decelerations, bradycardia, or evidence of impaired oxygenation.

PULSE OXIMETRY

See also Chapter 28, part three.

Pulse oximetry is a noninvasive technique that measures transcutaneously the arterial hemoglobin-oxygen saturation. The transcutaneous pulse oximeter consists of an oxygen sensor placed over the patient's skin and a microprocessor-controlled oximeter. The oxygen sensor has a two-wavelength light source and a photodetector; the intensity of the light passing through the skin and tissue is measured by the photodetector. The techniques involved are spectrophotometric oximetry and plethysmography. The two wavelengths that are used vary. The most common practice is to select one wavelength where the absorbance difference between the reduced and oxygenated hemoglobin is maximal and the other where this difference approaches zero. The innovative concept of pulse oximetry is that only the pulsatile component, which is entirely in synchrony with the arterial pulse and arises mostly from the changing volume of arterial blood, is in the field of view. The intensity of the light emitted by the diodes reaching the photodetector depends on the color and thickness of the skin, the capillary perfusion, and the absorption of light by arterial and venous blood. The outputs indicate primarily the percentage of oxygen saturation and the pulse rate per minute. The sensors are small and light, do not require heating or a stabilization period, and may be used on a finger, toe, ear, palm, or sole.

Pulse oximetry is particularly useful in neonates with an arterial oxygen tension (PaO_2) in the 40 to 50 mm Hg range; in these patients the saturation could vary from as low as 75% to greater than 85%. In our nursery pulse oximetry is used primarily in infants with chronic lung disease lasting more than 8 weeks, whereas infants with acute lung disease are monitored with transcutaneous oxygen and carbon dioxide electrodes.

The limitations for pulse oximetry have not been defined because of the lack of extensive clinical experience. Pulse oximetry does not pick up an adequate signal in patients with severe cardiovascular shock and in infants with cardiac arrhythmias, that is, supraventricular tachycardia with heart rate greater than 195 beats per minute. In addition, it is important to know that, in the presence of excessive ambient light, as occurs during phototherapy, the pulse oximeter records higher oxygen saturations than those obtained simultaneously from arterial blood and measured by a co-oximeter. This fact has led to recommendations to cover the oximeter sensor with a clip or similar device.

The following factors may interfere with the measurements of oxyhemoglobin saturation:

1. High fetal hemoglobin concentration
2. High bilirubin (>20 mg/dl) levels
3. High methemoglobin levels
4. Lipid particles in blood
5. Interfering dyes, such as indocyanine, cardiogeen, methylene blue, Evans blue
6. Phototherapy lights
7. Cardiovascular shock
8. Motion artifacts

ARTERIAL BLOOD PRESSURE

Close attention to the technical details of measurement and cautious interpretation of the pressure values are essential in monitoring arterial blood pressure in the newborn infant. The clinician should remember that the so-called normal blood pressure values reported for small premature infants may be influenced by the abnormal transitional circulation. Also, the temptation to equate low arterial blood pressure with hypovolemia should be avoided, and arterial blood pressure should be interpreted in the context of the infant's clinical condition.

The pressure pulse is generated in the arterial system as a result of cardiac ejection. The maximum pressure reached in the arterial system during cardiac ejection is the systolic pressure. During the diastolic phase of the cardiac cycle, the arterial pressure falls progressively, reaching the minimum or diastolic pressure. Mean blood pressure is determined by integration of pulse contour during the interval of the cardiac cycle. The pulse pressure is the difference between systolic and diastolic pressure. A crude estimate of the mean blood pressure may be obtained by adding one-third the pulse pressure to the diastolic pressure.

Mean blood pressure is equal to the cardiac output times the total peripheral resistance. The systolic pressure depends on the stroke volume, cardiac contractility, and arterial distensibility; the diastolic pressure depends on the level of systolic pressure, peripheral resistance, heart rate, and arterial elastic recoil.

Methods of measurement

With the exception of the intraarterial pressure measurement, all other methods use a blood pressure cuff that interrupts blood flow on inflation; the pressure may be detected at or beyond the cuff during deflation. The width of the pressure cuff should be 25% greater than the diameter of the arm or leg where blood pressure is being measured. Several methods for determining blood pressure are in use. The biophysical aspects of various techniques for pressure measurement are discussed in Chapter 24.

1. *Auscultation*. This is based on the detection of Korotkoff sounds during cuff deflation. The systolic pressure corresponds to the point at which the initial Korotkoff sounds are heard. Muffling of the sound is the best index of the diastolic pressure.
2. *Palpation*. This technique is not particularly useful in the neonatal period, since the pulse may be difficult to feel in either the arm or the leg beyond the cuff.
3. *Flush technique*. This method consists of placing a suitable cuff around the forearm of the calf, raising and squeezing the limb while quickly inflating the cuff, and on deflation detecting the earliest appearance of cutaneous flush in the blanched area. This pressure reading is more likely to be a mean pressure.
4. *Oscillometry*. Pressure changes are transmitted through the arterial wall to the pressure cuff, and the oscillations are detected by a sensitive pressure indicator.
5. *Doppler ultrasound technique*. A Doppler ultrasound transducer detects arterial wall oscillations that produce the major components of Korotkoff sounds. The frequency analysis of these oscillations accurately indicates the systolic pressure and, with a lesser degree of accuracy, the diastolic pressure.
6. *Direct measurement of arterial blood pressure*. A saline-filled catheter connected to the arterial line is attached to a strain gauge pressure transducer. The strain gauge is zeroed at the level of the midaxillary line while the infant is lying supine in a horizontal position. In this manner it is possible to record the arterial pressure and the pressure wave.

Analysis of aortic pulse wave

An undamped aortic pressure pulse recorded through an umbilical arterial catheter can be analyzed for pulse

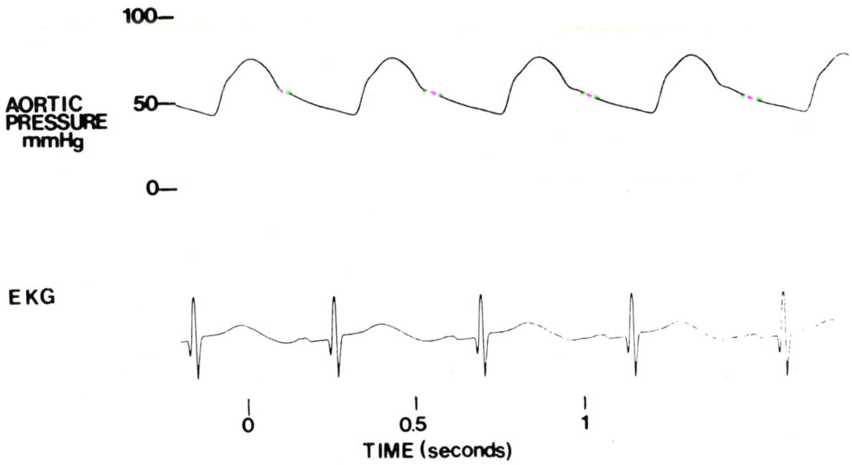

Fig. 21-8. Aortic pressure pulse. Note rapid upstroke during early systole interrupted by an anacrotic shoulder. The end of systole is heralded by a dicrotic notch followed by the diastolic phase.

wave characteristics providing potentially useful information. The pulse contour in the aorta shows a rapid upstroke during systole, interrupted by the anachrotic notch and a slower rise to peak pressure. The end of systole with the sudden closure of the aortic valve is indicated by the dicrotic notch. During diastole, as the blood flows out of the aorta into the peripheral vessels, initially the diastolic pressure decreases more rapidly and then more slowly (Fig. 21-8).

In the absence of aortic stenosis, the rate of aortic systolic pressure rise gives an indication of the state of contractility of the left ventricle. In the presence of valvular aortic stenosis, the upstroke of the aortic pressure is decreased. The rate of aortic diastolic pressure decay gives an indication of systemic vascular resistance. A rapid aortic diastolic pressure drop may be present in infants with left-to-right shunt through the ductus arteriosus.

Pitfalls in the measurement and interpretation of arterial blood pressure

The indirect methods of arterial blood pressure measurement should be considered an approximation of the true arterial pressure in the neonate. Most indirect techniques are reasonably reliable in determining the systolic pressure, whereas the diastolic pressure is measured less accurately. The indirect methods of pressure measurements are less reliable in neonates in shock. The Doppler ultrasound and oscillometric techniques are generally considered to give the most reliable noninvasive systolic pressure measurements.

Direct arterial pressure recording provides the most accurate technique for determining the arterial pressure, provided that (1) the catheter and the connecting tube systems are free of leaks; (2) clots and air bubbles are excluded; (3) the lumen of the indwelling catheter and needle is large enough; (4) the connecting tube is nondistensible; and (5) the transducer is free of defects, properly calibrated, and zeroed accurately. If the indwelling catheter's lumen is of small caliber or is decreased by fibrin deposition or if an air bubble is present in the pressure system, a damped pressure will be recorded. Under these circumstances the systolic pressure will be decreased and the diastolic pressure will be altered (increased, decreased, or unchanged). Therefore the mean pressure will be either unaltered or decreased, and the pulse wave will be diminished with disappearance of the dicrotic notch. Furthermore, intraarterial pressure obtained from small distal arteries (radial, temporal, dorsalis pedis) will diminish or even disappear in circulatory shock and other conditions with peripheral vasoconstriction.

Arterial blood pressure of neonates is best correlated with body weight in infants with birth weight greater than 1,000 gm (Fig. 21-9) (Chapter 29 and Appendix C). Arterial blood pressure values obtained in infants with birth weights equal to or less than 1,000 gm and without cardiopulmonary pathology appear in Fig. 21-10. In general, a neonatal diastolic pressure lower than 25 mm Hg and a mean pressure less than 30 mm Hg should cause concern. Conversely, a diastolic pressure greater than 50 mm Hg in preterm and 60 mm Hg in term infants, or a mean pressure greater than 60 mm Hg in preterm and 70 mm Hg in term infants, should be considered beyond normal range and investigated, with the pathophysiology kept in mind. A national study recently found that infants with birth weights less than 1,500 gm accounted for 25% of the hypertensive patients admitted to neonatal intensive care units. The same group of investigators reported a significantly higher incidence of hypertension in neonates with arterial catheters in place for 7 days or longer as compared to those with catheters for less than 3 days. Furthermore, some of the commonly accepted clinical manipulations, such as physician examination, may have a profound transient effect on arterial pressure. Following is an outline of some of the disease states that can alter arterial blood pressure.

A. Systolic and diastolic hypertension
   1. Renal
      a. Renal parenchymal disease: acute renal failure, hydronephrosis, polycystic kidneys
      b. Renovascular hypertension
   2. Neurogenic
      a. Increased intracranial pressure: intracranial hemorrhage, hydrocephalus, meningitis, hyperammonemia
   3. Endocrine
      a. Hyperthyroidism
      b. Pheochromocytoma
      c. Congenital adrenal hyperplasia
   4. Coarctation of the aorta
   5. After cardiac surgery
      a. Patent ductus arteriosus ligation
      b. Ligation of arteriovenous fistula
      c. Miscellaneous
   6. After abdominal surgery (omphalocele, gastroschisis)
   7. Idiopathic (essential hypertension?)
   8. Drugs: phenylephrine, epinephrine, dopamine, pancuronium bromide, atracurium, doxapram
B. Systolic hypertension
   1. Patent ductus arteriosus
   2. Anemia
   3. Fever
   4. Aortic regurgitation
   5. Arteriovenous fistula
   6. Thyrotoxicosis
   7. Drugs: isoproterenol
C. Systolic and diastolic hypotension
   1. Cardiogenic shock
      a. Myocardial dysfunction: asphyxia, hypoglycemia, hypocalcemia
      b. Severe cardiac arrhythmias, heart block, tachyarrhythmia

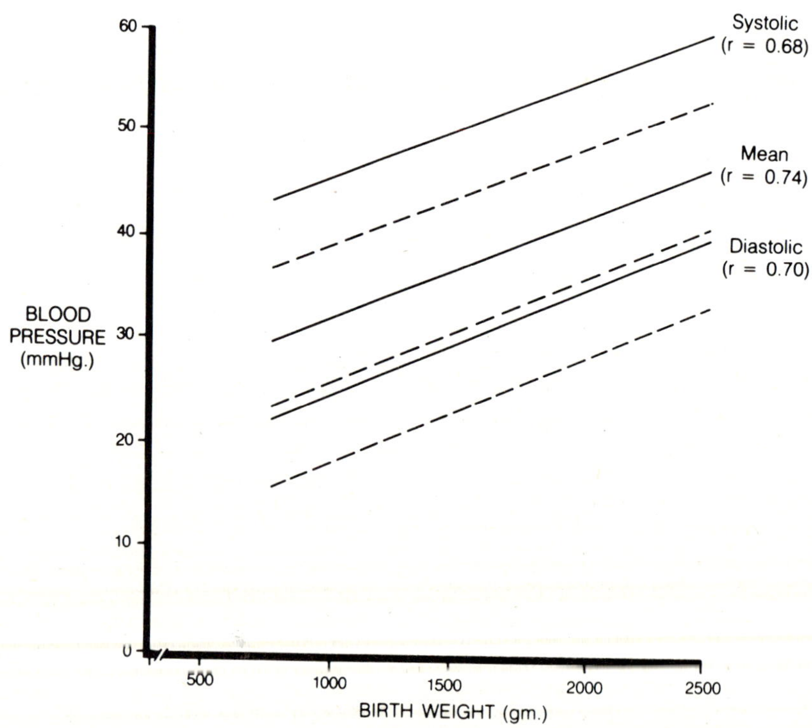

Fig. 21-9. Linear regression of systolic, mean, and diastolic blood pressure versus birth weights during the first 24 hours of life in 59 premature infants (n = 120). The dashed lines represent lowest systolic, diastolic, and mean pressure at 90% confidence level.

c. Mechanical restrictions of cardiac function or venous return: tension pneumothorax, diaphragmatic hernia, cardiac tamponade
d. Congenital cardiac defects: hypoplastic left side of the heart, coarctation of the aorta, critical aortic stenosis, patent ductus with left ventricular failure, arteriovenous fistula, critical pulmonary stenosis, cor triatriatum

2. Hypovolemic shock
   a. Antepartum blood loss: placenta previa, abruptio placentae, fetomaternal and twin-to-twin transfusions, birth injuries
   b. Postpartum blood loss: vitamin K deficiency, disseminated intravascular coagulation, iatrogenic
   c. Fluid and electrolyte loss: heat stress, gastrointestinal abnormalities, iatrogenic causes
3. Neurogenic shock
   a. Massive intracranial hemorrhage
   b. Severe hypoxic damage
4. Septic shock
   a. Gram positive: group B *Streptococcus, Staphylococcus, Listeria* infections
   b. Gram negative: *Escherichia coli, Pseudomonas, Klebsiella, Proteus* infections
5. Drug toxicity: digitalis, barbiturates, phenothiazines, diuretics, vasodilators, calcium channel blockers, anesthetic agents

D. Diastolic hypotension
   1. Patent ductus arteriosus
   2. Bradycardia
   3. Early sepsis
   4. Arteriovenous fistula
   5. Vasodilators

CENTRAL VENOUS PRESSURE (CVP)

The value of central venous or right atrial pressure measurement in the critically ill child and adult is well established. It has been useful mainly as an aid for fluid replacement, in postoperative management of patients undergoing cardiac surgery, and in the management of shock. Less agreement surrounds the value of CVP monitoring during infancy; however, it is now generally agreed that factors affecting CVP in older children and adults are operative during infancy. In general, right atrial pressure is affected by the pumping effectiveness of the right ventricle, the systemic venous return, and the pressure surrounding the heart. Acute left ventricular failure is usually not associated with right-sided heart failure. Accordingly, premature infants with patent ductus arteriosus and left ventricular failure often have normal right atrial pressures, except during terminal stages when combined ventricular failure with cardiogenic shock supervenes. In contrast, in severe right ventricular failure, such as in hypoplastic left ventricle, CVP is almost invariably increased. Changes in venous return as a determinant of right atrial pressure are the basis for the use of CVP to determine adequacy of fluid replacement. Large intravascular volume expansion is required to affect the CVP in patients with normal cardiopulmo-

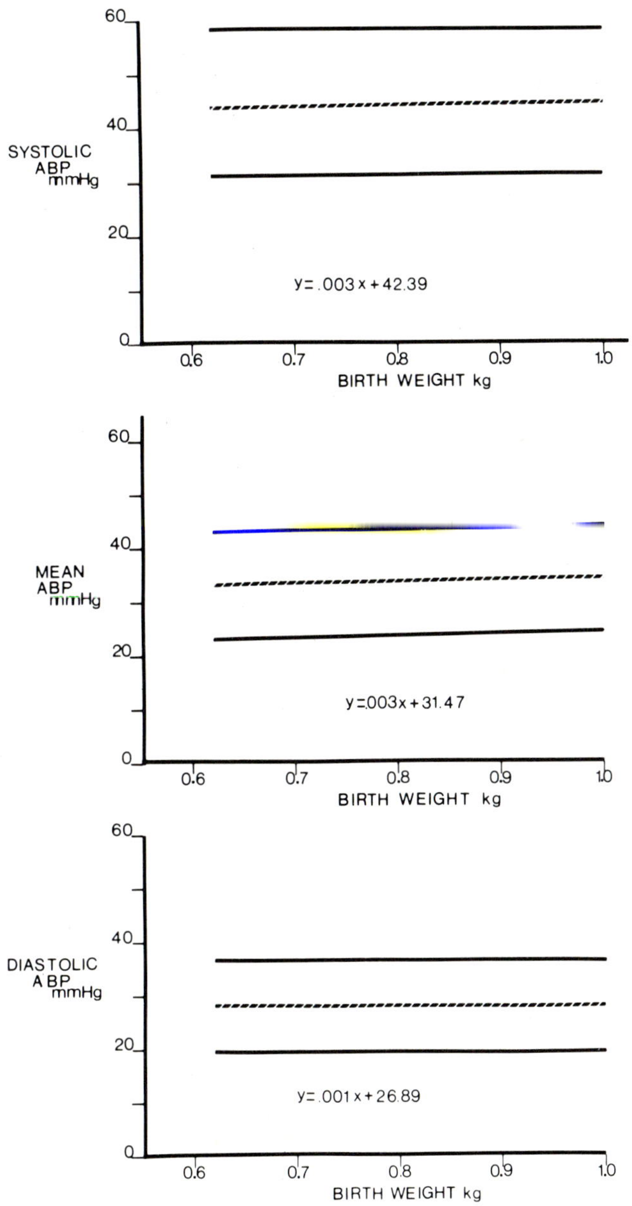

Fig. 21-10. Linear regressions *(broken lines)* and 95% confidence limits *(continuous lines)* of systolic, mean, and diastolic aortic blood pressures during the first 18 hours of life in 28 stable newborn infants with birth weights less than or equal to 1,000 gm.

nary systems. Neonates with borderline right ventricular failure, however, may show significant changes in CVP after moderate intravascular volume expansion. The changes in pressure surrounding the heart have the most dramatic effect on the right atrial pressure. Thus development of tension pneumothorax or cardiac tamponade is associated with immediate rise in CVP in newborn infants.

Method of measurement

Since central venous or right atrial pressures fluctuate within a few millimeters of mercury, an accurately calibrated and zeroed strain gauge transducer should be employed for their measurement. The catheter tip should be located in the right atrium, inferior vena cava, or superior vena cava close to the right atrium. Special care should be taken when measuring CVP through the umbilical vein, ductus venosus, interior vena cava, right atrium, superior vena cava, or left atrium. The location of the tip of the catheter can be determined from the length inserted, pressure wave analysis, and oxygen saturation measurements and should be confirmed by a chest roentgenogram. The transducer should be zeroed to the midaxillary line while the infant is resting in a supine horizontal position.

Pressure wave analysis (Table 21-3)

Central venous and atrial pressures are influenced by cardiac action and respiration. Two major pressure waves are generated as the result of cardiac actions: the *a* wave is generated by atrial contraction, whereas the *v* waves are produced by atrial filling against a closed atrioven-

Table 21-3. Venous pressure: site, characteristics, and normal range

Site	Pressure level	Venous waves	Changes with respiration	Average range	
Portal system	High	Absent	Slight ↑ with inspiration		6.5 (2.5 to 10.5) mm Hg
Right atrium	Low	Present; $a > v$ wave	Prominent ↓ with inspiration	*a* Wave	4.9 (+2 to +8) mm Hg
				Inspiratory wave	−3.2 (0 to −8) mm Hg
				Mean pressure	1.4 (−3 to +4) mm Hg
Left atrium	Low	$v > a$ wave	Prominent ↓ with inspiration	*a* Wave	6.5 (+3 to +10) mm Hg
				v Wave	8.5 (+5 to +12) mm Hg
				Mean pressure	3.5 (+1 to +6) mm Hg

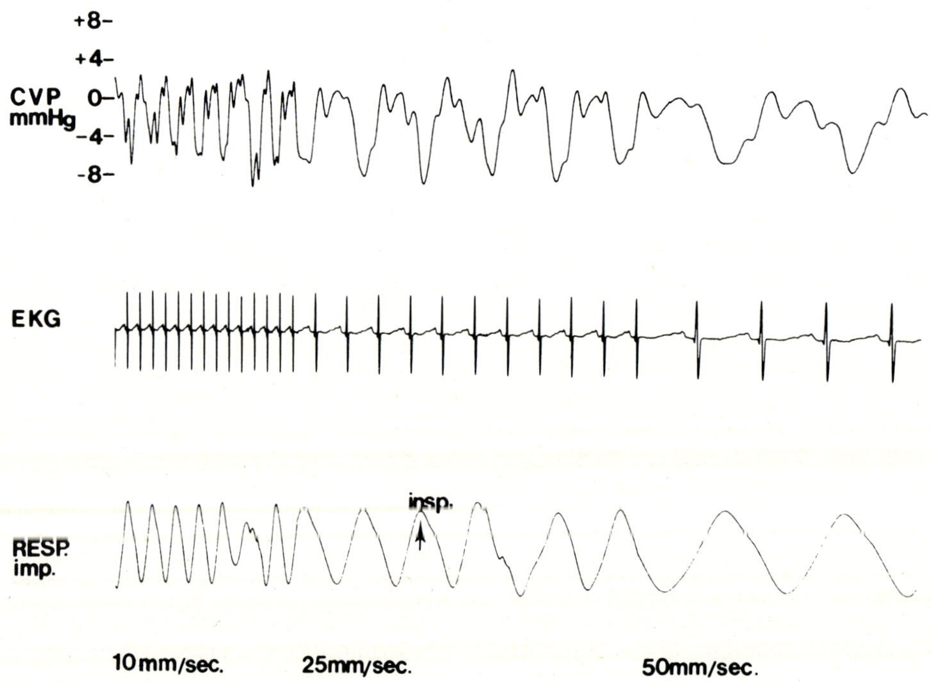

Fig. 21-11. Right atrial pressure measurement in a premature infant with RDS. Note *a, v,* and inspiratory waves

tricular valve. During spontaneous respiration the negative intrathoracic pressure generated during inspiration is transmitted to the central veins and atria and is inscribed as a negative pressure wave, whereas during intermittent positive pressure respiration a positive pressure wave is transmitted during mechanical respiration. The pressure waves are minimal or absent in peripheral veins, portal vein, and ductus venosus and are prominent in central veins and the atria. Normally the right atrial *a* wave is higher than *v* wave, whereas in the left atrium both *a* and *v* waves are prominent (Fig. 21-11).

During the early neonatal period the central venous and atrial pressures are not correlated with birth weights. Infants with atrioventricular valve insufficiency have prominent *v* waves in the corresponding atrial tracings. Prominent *a* waves are seen with nodal beats, and giant *a* waves are seen in atrial tracings due to superimposition of atrial and ventricular contractions.

Risk of central venous pressure monitoring

The benefit of CVP monitoring should be weighed against risks of prolonged right atrial or central venous catheterization. Indwelling central venous or right atrial catheterization carries an increased risk for thromboembolism, infection, and vascular perforation. This could be minimized by shortening the duration of catheterization and adhering strictly to aseptic catheter maintenance techniques. The central venous line should be closed off to the patient to prevent the possibility of air embolism during the negative pressure created by the infant's inspiratory efforts.

PULMONARY ARTERY PRESSURE

The most crucial change that occurs during the transition from a fetal to a neonatal circulation is the sharp decrease in pulmonary vascular resistance and pressure below systemic levels. Except occasionally during the first hour of life, pulmonary artery pressure in healthy newborn infants remains lower than systemic arterial pressure and should be below 50% of systemic pressure by 24 hours of life. If pulmonary vascular resistance remains higher than systemic vascular resistance, right-to-left shunting may persist across the fetal channels, leading to neonatal cyanosis. The persistence of pulmonary hypertension, or persistence of the fetal circulation (Chapter 29), may be primary or occur in several entities involving diseases or abnormalities of the heart and lungs. Some of the factors that affect pulmonary artery pressure are:

Increased pressure

1. Hypoxemia
2. Acidosis
3. Polycythemia
4. Primary increase in pulmonary artery smooth muscle
5. Chronic intrauterine stress
6. Fetal systemic hypertension
7. Perinatal asphyxia
8. Decreased cross-sectional area of pulmonary vascular bed: diaphragmatic hernia, pulmonary hypoplasia, lobar emphysema
9. Congenital cardiac defect with left-to-right shunts: ventricular septal defect, patent ductus arteriosus, transposition of great vessels
10. Left-sided heart failure: myocardial dysfunction, congenital cardiac defects
11. Obstruction to pulmonary venous return: diaphragmatic hernia, tension pneumothorax, congenital lobar emphysema, total anomalous pulmonary venous return, cor triatriatum
12. Pulmonary parenchymal disease: meconium aspiration, RDS, pneumonia
13. Mechanical ventilation with high mean airway pressure
14. Pulmonary edema
15. Drugs: norepinephrine, dopamine (high dose), epinephrine

Decreased pressure

1. Hyperoxia
2. Decrease in pulmonary arterial smooth muscle
3. Drugs: isoproterenol, chloropromazine, tolazoline, acetylcholine

Continuous direct monitoring of pulmonary artery pressure through an indwelling catheter has become an accepted practice in critically ill adults. Recent experience with indwelling pulmonary artery catheters in critically ill neonates suggests the potential usefulness of such a technique in selected cases.

Methods of measurement

Pulmonary artery catheters can be inserted percutaneously through the umbilical or femoral veins and by a cutdown technique through the external jugular or femoral veins. Usually a no. 5F catheter, with or without ballooned tip, is manipulated under fluoroscopic control through the right ventricle and is left with its tip in the right or the left pulmonary arteries. Although balloon flotation catheters are placed routinely without fluoroscopy in older children and adults, we believe it is safer to place the catheter under direct vision in newborn infants. The pulmonary arterial pressure is measured using a strain gauge transducer, similar to the technique of direct arterial pressure monitoring (Fig. 21-12).

Risk of direct pulmonary arterial pressure monitoring

Perforation of the pulmonary artery, pulmonary embolism, infection, and massive pulmonary hemorrhage have been reported in adult patients with prolonged indwelling pulmonary arterial catheters. In view of the

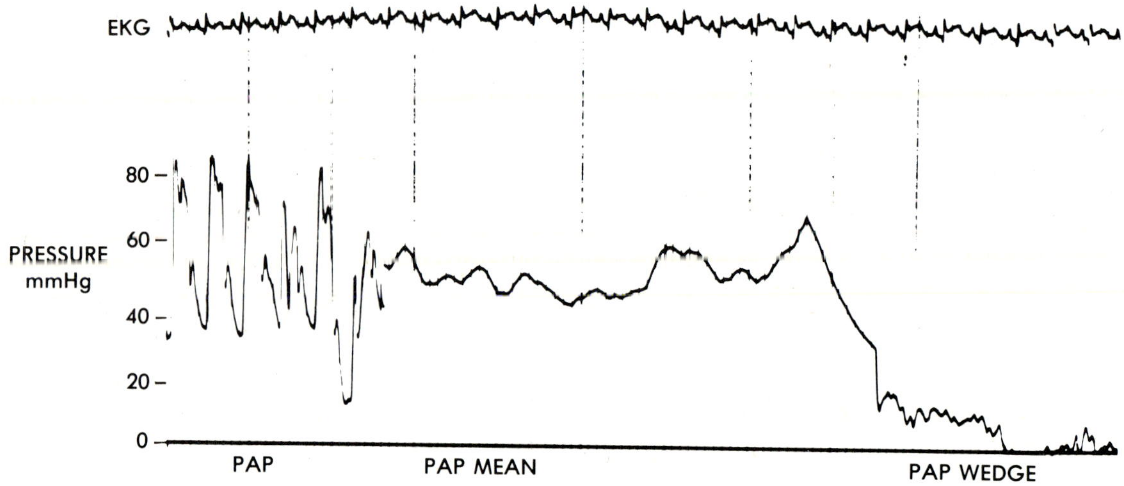

Fig. 21-12. Pulmonary artery pressure *(PAP)* in a 3-day-old, full-term infant with meconium aspiration and persistent pulmonary hypertension. Note elevated pulmonary artery pressure and normal wedge pressure. In this case pulmonary artery pressure was monitored through a no. 5F Swan-Ganz balloon catheter; the wedge pressure was obtained after inflation of the balloon to occlude the right pulmonary artery.

Table 21-4. RPEP/RVET* during first week of life: mean (5th-95th percentile range)

	Birth weight (gm)	
Age	**<2,000**	**>2,000**
<8 hours	0.40 (0.25-0.62)	0.38 (0.21-0.50)
At 24 hours	0.26 (0.17-0.35)	0.31 (0.18-0.42)
>48 hours	0.27 (0.16-0.35)	0.29 (0.17-0.38)

*Right-sided preejection period/ventricular ejection time.

Table 21-5. Left ventricular (LV) parameters in 100 healthy neonates weighing 760-4,700 gm during first week of life*

Parameter*	Mean	5th-95th percentile
LPEP/LVET	0.36	0.28-0.42
LV shortening fraction	0.33	0.27-0.46
LA/AO	1.18	0.9-1.40

*LPEP/LVET, Left-sided preejection time/ventricular ejection time; LA/AO, left atrial/aortic root diameter.

limited experience in the neonate, the risks of such procedures are not well evaluated. It is reasonable, however, to assume that the dangers are similar to those of prolonged central venous catheterization. To minimize such risks, we restrict direct pulmonary arterial pressure monitoring to critically ill full-term infants and limit the duration to less than 72 hours. Further experience will define the relative risk/benefit ratio for this procedure.

NONINVASIVE EVALUATION OF CARDIAC PERFORMANCE

See also Chapter 29.

Echocardiography has been established as the main noninvasive technique for evaluation of cardiac structure and function in the fetus and the neonate. It is now possible to identify congenital cardiac defects accurately in the fetus and the neonate by this technique. The use of echocardiography for evaluation of cardiac performance has been extensively studied in pediatric and adult populations and is being rapidly expanded to include the fetus and the neonate. M-mode, two-dimensional, and Doppler echocardiography are used to evaluate cardiac performance.

M-mode echocardiography

Indirect evidence for pulmonary hypertension may be obtained from M-mode echocardiographic measurement of the right ventricular (RV) systolic time intervals (Table 21-4). An accurate prediction of pulmonary pressure and resistance is not possible; however, an elevated RV systolic time interval ratio, right-sided preejection period/ventricular ejection time (RPEP/RVET), is usually associated with persistent pulmonary hypertension. Serial measurements of RV systolic time intervals may be used to follow changes in clinical condition or response to therapy in the neonate.

Table 21-6. Left ventricular parameters in 100 healthy neonates weighing 760-4,700 gm during first week of life: mean (5th-95th percentile range)

	Weight (gm)			
Parameter*	**760-1,500**	**1,501-2,500**	**2,501-3,500**	**3,501-6,700**
LAd	0.72 (0.50-0.90)	0.93 (0.65-1.10)	1.11 (0.90-1.30)	1.30 (1.10-1.55)
LVEDd	1.23 (1.05-1.35)	1.57 (1.20-1.95)	1.83 (1.60-2.05)	1.99 (1.80-2.45)
AO	0.66 (0.60-0.80)	0.83 (0.75-0.95)	0.95 (0.83-1.05)	1.04 (0.95-1.10)

*LAd, Left atrial dimension at end of systole; LVEDd, left ventricular end-diastolic dimension; AO, aortic root dimension.

M-mode echocardiographic measurements can also be used to evaluate left ventricular (LV) function in the neonate. An accurate estimation of left atrial and LV sizes and LV contractility may be obtained from these measurements (Tables 21-5 and 21-6). Decreased LV performance in neonates with structural heart disease is discussed in Chapter 29. In the neonate with functional cardiac disorders resulting from adverse perinatal factors, the following abnormalities indicate decreased LV performance:

1. *Increased LPEP/LVET*. LV systolic time interval ratio is influenced by (a) preload, which is determined by the LV end-diastolic volume; (b) afterload, which is related to the arterial diastolic pressure; (c) LV contractility; and (d) abnormalities in LV conduction. However, in the presence of normal or decreased aortic pressure, increased LPEP/LVET is a sensitive indicator of decreased LV performance.
2. *Reduced LV shortening fraction*. The shortening fraction is the percentage change in the LV minor axis. This is measured directly from an M-mode echocardiogram and correlates closely with the LV ejection fraction.
3. *Left atrial and ventricular enlargement*. The dimensions of left atrium and ventricle are enlarged in congestive heart failure or left-to-right shunts.
4. *Decreased wall thickness*. Thickness of the intraventricular septum and the LV posterior wall is reduced in neonates with decreased LV performance.
5. *Other measurements*. Other functional parameters such as the ejection fraction and the velocity of circumferential shortening may be derived indirectly from the echocardiogram; however, such measurements add little information to the parameters just listed.

Contrast M-mode echocardiography can be used to demonstrate left-to-right shunt in premature neonates with patent ductus arteriosus. It also can indicate right-to-left shunt through a patent foramen ovale in most neonates with persistent pulmonary hypertension and in some neonates with myocardial dysfunction resulting from perinatal asphyxia.

Two-dimensional echocardiography

Although two-dimensional echocardiography has been established as an invaluable technique for detection of congenital cardiac defects in the neonate, its potential as a tool for evaluation of cardiac performance is less developed. Although dilation of chamber sizes and decreased contractility are readily visualized by this technique, normative values for quantitative measurements are lacking. Contrast two-dimensional echocardiography will readily demonstrate left-to-right shunt through a patent ductus arteriosus and right-to-left shunt through a patent foramen ovale.

Doppler echocardiography

Both continuous wave and pulsed Doppler echocardiography have been used to evaluate changes in flow velocity, as encountered in stenotic lesions; to detect regurgitant flow through insufficient valves; and to measure quantitatively blood flow through the aorta and pulmonary artery and across the atrioventricular valves. Directional Doppler echocardiography has also been used in detection of left-to-right shunt through a patent ductus arteriosus in the neonate.

Both continuous wave and pulsed Doppler echocardiography can be used to measure *cardiac output*. LV output is calculated from mean aortic flow velocity and measurements of aortic root diameter. Flow velocity is detected by a suprasternal notch transducer, and the aortic diameter is measured by M-mode or two-dimensional echocardiography. Preliminary data indicate close correlation between Doppler echocardiography and direct methods of cardiac output measurement. LV output measured by pulsed Doppler ultrasound technique in healthy neonates is shown in Fig. 21-13. Serial noninvasive measurements of cardiac output aid in detection and appropriate management of neonates in low cardiac output states (Fig. 21-14). Similarly, RV output can be calculated from main pulmonary artery flow measurements.

Luis A. Cabal
Bijan Siassi
Joan E. Hodgman

rapidly from moment to moment. This is extremely valuable on a busy obstetric service where there may not be time for detailed notation of the changing clinical state.

Defining infants at high risk

A further advantage of the Apgar scoring system is to identify the infants at high risk with regard to both mortality and morbidity. The mortality in low-score infants is nearly 15 times that in the high-score group, and respiratory distress syndrome (RDS) occurs significantly more frequently in low-score than high-score infants.

Time to assign the score

A simple alarm timer should be firmly fixed on the delivery room wall and set for 60 seconds. When the head and feet of the infant are visible, the timer is started, and when the alarm sounds at 60 seconds, the score is assigned.

Person to score

The person delivering the infant should not be the one to assign the score. He or she is usually emotionally involved with the outcome of the delivery and with the family and may not make an objective evaluation. Ideally a specially trained observer should be present (physician or nurse), but this situation is seldom possible. If a pediatrically oriented person is not routinely present for all deliveries, the anesthesiologist should assign the score, and the infant should be placed in a bassinet near the head of the delivery table.

Five-minute score

The 5-minute score is more predictive of survival or neurologic abnormality at 1 year of age than the 1-minute score. This is not surprising, since the longer asphyxia exists, the more likely death or permanent damage will occur. Furthermore, if the first observation is made as late at 5 minutes, some asphyxiated infants will remain untreated, with subsequent higher mortality and morbidity.

Scoring the very low birth weight infant

The Apgar scoring system is equally useful for the immature infant, and the same principles are applied for making this evaluation. The only necessary adjustment relates to muscle tone. This is normally reduced in the very low birth weight (VLBW) infant, and the scorer should take this reduction into account when evaluating the degree of flexion of the extremities.

Scoring and the pH

A significant association has been found between the acid-base states of low-score infants (0 to 3) and those who are vigorous (7 to 10). Recently, however, the significance of this relationship has been questioned. Failure to find a strong correlation appears to result from the combination of all infants scoring below 7 into a single group. This results in the inclusion of mildly asphyxiated infants scoring 4 to 6 with those who are more severely affected. This will clearly reduce the significance of the correlation.

Limitations

Although the Apgar score is useful, it is no substitute for a careful physical examination or for serial observations over the first few hours of life. It is useful in estimating the probability of survival and morbidity in groups of infants, but it will not predict neonatal survival of individual infants or their long-term prognoses.

RESUSCITATION SITE: DELIVERY ROOM OR TRANSITIONAL NURSERY?

The immediate resuscitation should be performed in the delivery room, since time will be lost if the severely depressed infant is first transported to another room. Once the initial emergency has been dealt with and respiration has been established, further procedures can be undertaken in the transitional nursery (TN).

We have found the TN to be invaluable in the initial institution of intensive care and recommend that it be located adjacent to the cesarean section room or high-risk delivery room. It should be organized so that all aspects of intensive care, including artificial ventilation and exchange transfusions, can be carried out. This permits proper evaluation and stabilization of the infant before being transported to the neonatal intensive care unit (NICU). It also gives the NICU time to prepare for the admission of a sick infant. Such preparation can take place in an orderly fashion when no other emergencies exist; it also avoids the need for an admission unit. The TN should be staffed by nurses and physicians from the NICU.

TREATMENT OF MODERATELY DEPRESSED INFANTS

If initial resuscitative measures have produced no response by 1 1/2 minutes after delivery, the progressing asphyxia usually leads to diminished muscular tone and a fall in the heart rate. A small plastic oropharyngeal airway should then be inserted into the mouth and oxygen applied under pressure of 16 to 20 cm water for 1 or 2 seconds. Although this pressure is insufficient to expand the alveoli, some oxygen will reach the respiratory bronchioles. The rise in intrabronchial pressure stimulates pulmonary stretch receptors. This stimulus, added to that of the chemoreceptors, initiates a gasp in about 85% of infants.

If no respiratory effort occurs and the heart rate continues to fall, with the infant becoming completely flaccid, the larynx should be visualized with the laryngoscope and the infant intubated. This is not a difficult procedure, but skill should be obtained by practice on stillborn infants.

Intubation is best accomplished with the infant lying supine on a flat surface. A folded towel under the head and slight extension of the neck will place the infant in a position resembling a sniffing posture. The head should be steadied with the right hand and kept in line with the body. The laryngoscope is held in the left hand, and the blade is introduced at the right corner of the mouth and advanced between tongue and palate for about 2 cm. As it is advanced, the blade is swung to the midline. This moves the tongue to the left of the blade. The operator looks along the blade for the rim of the epiglottis. The laryngoscope is gently advanced into the space between the base of the tongue and the epiglottis. Slight elevation of the tip of the blade will expose the glottis as a vertical dark slit bordered posteriorly by pink arytenoid cartilages.

If foreign material such as small blood clots, meconium-stained mucus, or vernix obstructs the larynx, quick brief suction is indicated. When the glottis is seen to be patent, a curved endotracheal tube is introduced at the right corner of the mouth and inserted through the cords until the flange of the tube rests at the glottis. Care must be taken not to intubate the esophagus. The laryngoscope is then withdrawn. Rarely, the glottis is obstructed by a laryngeal web. If the web is partial or thin, it may be perforated, or the opening may be enlarged with an endotracheal tube. The presence of a thick membrane requires immediate tracheostomy.

If stimuli from these procedures have not initiated a spontaneous gasp, positive pressure should be applied to the endotracheal tube. Brief puffs of air blown through the tube by means of an Ambu bag with enough force to cause the lower chest to rise gently will usually start spontaneous respiration. If the stomach rises, however, the esophagus has been intubated instead of the trachea, and the position of the tube must be corrected. Pressures between 25 and 35 cm water are necessary to expand normal alveoli initially and can be applied safely for 1 or 2 seconds. Experience in applying such pressures should be gained by puffing into a spring manometer. Oxygen-enriched gas may be delivered to the infant by attaching a tube carrying oxygen to the Ambu apparatus. The endotracheal tube, however, should be fitted with appropriate-sized adapters that can be connected to the Ambu bag. The pressure may also be applied by the operator blowing through the endotracheal tube.

Artificial expansion of the lungs can initiate a spontaneous gasp. With the first or second application of positive pressure, the infant usually makes an effort to breathe. The endotracheal tube may be withdrawn after the infant has established sustained spontaneous ventilation.

TREATMENT OF SEVERELY DEPRESSED INFANTS

No time should be lost in establishing ventilation in severely depressed infants. The glottis should be inspected immediately with the laryngoscope. If meconium or thick meconium-stained mucus has been aspirated into the trachea, it must be suctioned out at once before inflation of the lungs. It is usually possible to accomplish this within 1 minute after delivery. These severely depressed infants may require 3 to 8 minutes of artificial ventilation before a spontaneous gasp is taken. The endotracheal tube can be removed as soon as quiet and sustained respiration is established.

PROCEDURE FOR INFANT RESUSCITATION

During resuscitation, heat loss should be prevented or minimized by placing the infant under a radiant heat lamp. Three persons should be available for optimum emergency resuscitation: one for establishing an airway and ventilating the infant, one for cardiac massage and monitoring the heart rate, and one for umbilical catheterization and the administration of alkali. When possible, the procedure should be carried out under sterile conditions, including sterile gowns and gloves. All equipment, including laryngoscope, endotracheal tubes, and stethoscope, should be sterile. The resuscitation area should be covered with a sterile sheet previously warmed from an overhead heat lamp.

Attention must first be directed to establishing pulmonary ventilation in resuscitating the severely asphyxiated newborn. The steps should be as follows: establishment and maintenance of a clear airway, expansion of the lungs, and continuation of ventilation with up to 100% oxygen at a rate of 30 to 40 inflations per minute. Ventilation should be interrupted every six or seven breaths and alternated with periods of cardiac massage as needed to maintain a rate of 120 beats per minute. Both ventilation and cardiac massage may be carried out by one person; if two are involved, it is important that they coordinate their actions so that cardiac massage and artificial ventilation are not given simultaneously. This can result in a pneumomediastinum or a pneumothorax, since ventilation will be done against a compressed and distorted tracheobronchial tree. While these measures are being initiated, another physician should insert a catheter into the umbilical vein.

Aspiration syndrome

The importance of suctioning meconium from the trachea and bronchi deserves special emphasis. Meconium is passed following an asphyxial episode in utero. If the asphyxial episode is accompanied by prolonged gasping, meconium will be drawn deeply into the lungs. The fetus may recover from this episode with regard to acid-base state and CNS responsiveness but may be born with the lungs full of meconium (Chapter 28). Such infants initially may be responsive and vigorously attempt to breathe. It is essential that the larynx be observed in all infants who have passed meconium during labor or whose amniotic fluid is heavily stained with meconium, as soon as they are born, irrespective of their initial responsiveness. If thick meconium appears at the back of the pharynx, it should be suctioned out under direct vision and the larynx intubated with an endotracheal tube. Suction then should be applied directly to this tube, which is gradually withdrawn while suction is applied. Occasionally a large piece of meconium, too thick to pass up the endotracheal tube, is observed clinging to the tip of the tube. If this occurs, the trachea should be reintubated immediately and the procedure repeated until only watery mucus is obtained. The fluid normally produced by the fetal lung continues to form and washes out meconium from the deeper radicals of the lung. If this procedure is followed in all cases of meconium aspiration, many subsequent complications can be avoided.

Four conditions exist in which lung expansion is impossible despite proper intubation: (1) massive aspiration of meconium that cannot be removed by suctioning, (2) intrauterine pneumonia with organization of exudate, (3) large bilateral diaphragmatic hernias with hypoplastic lungs, and (4) congenital adenomatous cysts of the lung. Infants with the first two conditions are usually severely depressed at birth. However, those with hypoplastic lungs may be vigorous initially and score as high as 7 on the Apgar scale at 1 minute of age, making strenuous but ineffective respiratory efforts. Congenital adenomatous cysts of the lung are usually associated with hydrops fetalis, and the condition is usually fatal.

Cardiac massage

Blood pressure and heart rate fall during prolonged asphyxia. If the blood pressure is very low at the beginning of resuscitation, positive pressure ventilation is unlikely to be successful unless cardiac massage is employed. Cardiac massage should not be initiated until after the lungs have been well expanded by two or three inflations. If the heartbeat cannot be heard or if a slow heartbeat has not increased in rate, cardiac massage should be commenced. External manual compression of the heart between the chest wall and vertebral column forces blood into the aorta. Relaxation of pressure allows the heart to fill with venous blood.

The technique consists of intermittent compression of the middle and lower third of the sternum 100 to 200 times per minute with the index and middle fingers. Initially massage is interrupted every 5 seconds to permit two or three inflations of the lung; subsequently, if the heart is responding, six or seven breaths should be alternated with massage. Cardiopulmonary resuscitation is most successful when there has been no clinical evidence of fetal distress and when a normal FHR has been heard between contractions up to the moment of birth.

Administration of alkali

The rationale for rapid correction of an acid pH from asphyxia is based in part on experiments in newborn monkeys. The maintenance of a normal pH during asphyxia by rapid intravenous infusions of alkali together with glucose prolongs gasping and delays cardiovascular collapse. Resuscitation is also facilitated if alkali and glucose are infused at the same time as artificial ventilation is started; oxygen consumption is greater, and the time for establishing spontaneous breathing is shorter. In addition, there is a significant decrease in cardiac output in fetal lambs in the presence of hypoxemia plus acidosis. Pulmonary vascular resistance has been shown to vary directly with pH; a sudden rise in arterial pH improves pulmonary blood flow and Pa_{O_2}. Mortality from RDS was reduced with early administration of intravenous glucose and sodium bicarbonate, and the early treatment of neonatal acidosis in low birth weight infants was found to be associated with a reduced morbidity. Furthermore, the synthesis of lecithin is greatly reduced in the presence of acidosis. It has been proposed that the beneficial effects of pH correction are derived from a prolongation and acceleration of anaerobic glycolysis, a restitution of the oxygen-carrying capacity of hemoglobin, the increased response of cardiovascular muscle to sympathomimetic amines, and a fall in pulmonary vascular resistance.

The most severely asphyxiated infants—those with an arterial pH below 7.0—will have a base deficit of 26 mEq/L or greater in addition to a marked elevation in P_{CO_2}. By means of artificial ventilation alone, the base deficit can be reduced by approximately 10 mEq/L in a matter of 5 to 10 minutes, provided good alveolar ventilation is achieved and the infant does not remain in circulatory collapse. This change occurs as a result of a significant bicarbonate shift at a P_{CO_2} greater than 70 mm Hg, which should be taken into consideration in calculations for the initial base administration to prevent overcorrection. It is advisable initially to attempt to correct half the residual metabolic component of the mixed acidosis. Thus a 3 kg infant would receive 8 mEq of base:

$$\frac{\text{Base deficit } (26 - 10)}{2} \times \frac{\text{Body weight (3 kg)}}{\text{ECV (3)}}$$

This working formula is only an approximation and assumes the extracellular volume (ECV) to be one third of the body weight (Chapter 25).

Sodium bicarbonate rather than tris(hydroxymethyl) aminomethane (THAM) is recommended because THAM is able to enter the cell and occasionally cause depression of the respiratory center and arrest of breathing. Sodium bicarbonate, as obtained from the commercial ampule, contains nearly 1 mEq/ml (44.7 mEq in 50 ml, 0.9 M solution.) This solution has an osmolality of 1,400 and a pH of 7.8. It should be diluted in equal parts with distilled water to reduce its osmolality to 700 and infused at a rate not greater than 2 to 3 ml/minute. If the heart rate is slow and irregular, the infusion should be accompanied by intermittent cardiac massage. The alkali may be infused into either the umbilical vein or artery.

Subsequent alkali administration

The infant's response to alkali administration will vary according to the degree of asphyxia, the effectiveness of ventilation, and the responsiveness of the cardiovascular system. It is important, therefore, to have a measurement of the acid-base state as soon as the initial dose of sodium bicarbonate has been given. This can usually be made by 15 minutes of age. The required amount of sodium bicarbonate for subsequent correction to a pH of 7.3 may then be calculated.

Controversy and risk

Considerable concern has arisen following the demonstration of a significant association between intracranial hemorrhage, hypernatremia, and alkali administration in a retrospective study. In a controlled prospective trial, the finding of intracranial hemorrhage in 4 of 26 infants who received alkali by rapid intravenous infusion has raised further doubts about this therapy. However, another retrospective study has failed to confirm the association between alkali therapy and intracranial hemorrhage, and in our experience the incidence of intracranial hemorrhage was acutally higher in those infants who did not receive alkali. Examination of the effect of alkali administration in the presence of elevated Pa_{CO_2} revealed that a further rise in Pa_{CO_2} was transient, and bicarbonate appeared to be effective as a base for correcting acidosis.

From experimental work there seems little doubt that infusion of hypertonic solutions containing sodium can cause intracranial hemorrhage and may also cause hypocalcemia. When bicarbonate is administered in a "closed" system, the P_{CO_2} may rise and pH actually fall. Rapid infusion of bicarbonate to newborn puppies with mechanically fixed hypoventilation resulted in a rise in both Pa_{CO_2} and osmolality.

Administration of alkali therefore is not without risk and will outweigh the benefits if it is given in too high a concentration, in too great a quantity, and in the presence of severely impaired ventilation. Apparently the adverse effects of alkali have resulted from injudicious use, particularly in the presence of impaired carbon dioxide elimination. Sodium bicarbonate will be ineffective in correcting acidosis if a prompt increase in carbon dioxide excretion cannot be ensured.

In summary, the beneficial effects of alkali would appear to outweigh the risks in the immediate resuscitation of the newborn, provided that the lungs can be expanded promptly and pulmonary ventilation established.

Technique for catheterization of umbilical vein

A standard umbilical catheter, if advanced to a distance of 7 to 10 cm from the skin surface of the umbilical vein, will lie just beyond the ductus venosus in the inferior vena cava in a mature, term weight infant. If the catheter is even slightly curved, it may be deflected into one of the radicals in the portal system. Any tendency for the catheter to bounce back as it is advanced should suggest that it is not passing through the ductus venosus. Rapid verification of the correct site can be obtained if the catheter has been previously attached to a strain gauge and a recording polygraph. The moment the ductus venosus is passed, the venous pulsations (*a*, *c*, and *v* waves) can be readily seen, unless there is cardiac arrest. This means of verification of catheter position is more rapid and suitable for delivery room treatment than the use of an image-intensified roentgenogram (Chapter 21).

Technique for catheterization of umbilical artery

Only fine catheters should be used (3 1/2 or 5, French). They should be nonrigid and pliable, with a hole in the softly rounded tip. They should also be radiopaque for radiologic localization. The lumen of the artery should be carefully identified after cutting of the cord close to the abdominal wall with sharp scissors. Fine, curved, nontoothed forceps should be gently placed in the pinpoint clot that usually marks the vessel opening. Pressure on the forceps is then gradually released to allow the natural spring to open the vessel. This procedure is repeated four or five times, with the forceps gently advanced to a depth of 1/4 to 1/2 inch. The catheter then may be introduced and will usually pass readily down to the region of the iliac artery. Occasionally, some obstruction is met 1/2 inch from the skin, but this rarely causes any difficulty. If resistance is felt at the entrance into the internal iliac artery, only moderate pressure should be applied. If the catheter will not advance, 0.5 ml of 0.5% procain hydrochloride (Novocain) may be slowly infused. This may be sufficient to release any spasm and permit further advancement of the catheter. If this maneuver is unsuccessful and resistance persists, the second umbilical artery should be catheterized. If damage to the vessels is to be avoided, resistance in the region of the internal iliac artery should not be responded to aggressively; efforts to catheterize should be discontinued if unsuccessful after three attempts.

Once the venous or arterial catheter is in place, a lateral roentgenogram should be taken to verify position. In the posteroanterior view the catheter cannot be distinguished from the maze of wires attached to the thermistors (Fig. 22-2). A catheter introduced into the umbilical vein may reach a variety of positions. If advanced far enough, it will pass directly through the ductus venosus and foramen ovale into the left atrium. It may also pass into the right or left branches of the portal vein, the superior or inferior mesenteric veins, or even the splenic vein. Lodged in these areas, catheters can occlude blood flow and serve to localize any solutions infused. The ideal position for the umbilical vein catheter is just beyond the ductus venosus in the inferior vena cava.

A catheter introduced into the umbilical artery will usually pass into the aorta from the internal iliac artery. Occasionally it will pass down the femoral artery or into the gluteal artery. The two latter sites are unsuitable for sampling and pressure measurements or for the infusion of alkali. Either of two positions in the aorta is recommended for the catheter placement: in the lower abdomen below the renal arteries and inferior mesenteric artery or just above the diaphragm. If left in the internal iliac or the region of the aortic bifurcation, the chances of arterial spasm are increased.

The status of the infant's circulation is obviously of great importance when hypertonic or strongly alkaline solutions are administered. From a clinical point of view, blood flow can be fairly reasonably assessed from blood pressure, and if the pressure is low, cardiac massage is indicated during injection. If the umbilical vein is used for infusion, the catheter should be just beyond the ductus venosus and the alkali administered into the inferior vena cava.

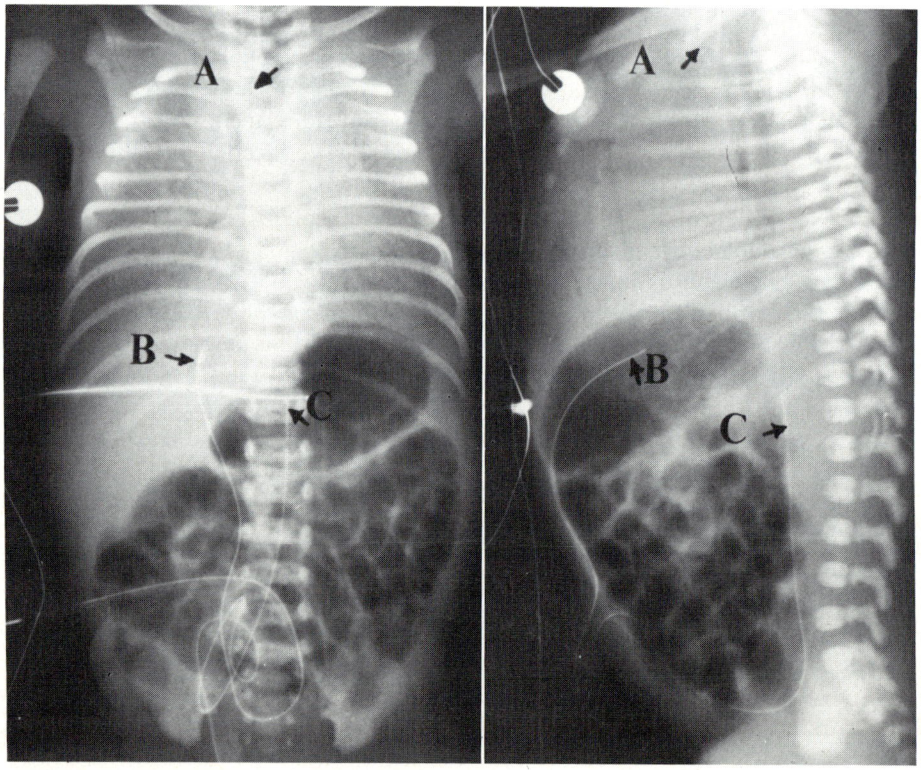

Fig. 22-2. Anteroposterior roentgenogram of infant with thermistors and an umbilical catheter in place; note that maze of wires prevents identification of catheter position in this view. The lateral view clearly identifies that catheter has been inserted into an umbilical vein and is lying in the portal system of the liver. *A*, Endotracheal tube; *B*, umbilical venous catheter at the juncture of the umbilical vein, ductus venosus, and portal vein; *C*, umbilical artery catheter passed up the aorta to T12. (Courtesy Walter E. Berdon, Babies Hospital: Infant with RDS. Note granular lungs, air bronchogram, and air-filled esophagus.)

Complications from umbilical catheterization

See also Chapter 24, part four and Chapter 28, part three.

Although catheterization of the umbilical vein and artery are relatively simple maneuvers and allow easy infusion of fluids or blood sampling, the procedures are not without hazard. Complications relate to trauma during insertion, the duration of catheterization, the size of the catheters used, the state of the circulation when solutions are being infused, and the pH or tonicity of the solutions infused. Although the incidence of complications is relatively low, the procedure is not recommended as the usual route for fluid or drug therapy and should be used only in very ill infants or those at high risk when monitoring is essential for diagnosis and therapeutic management.

False lumen and perforation. If the lumen of the constricted artery is not localized accurately, it is possible to create a false lumen in the wall of the vessel. This may be erroneously interpreted as spasm when obstruction is met in the region of the internal iliac artery. If the catheter being inserted is rigid, the vessels may be perforated at this point, with the catheter passing into the abdominal cavity. If undue force is exerted, even with a soft catheter, it may track extraperitoneally and result in retroperitoneal hemorrhage.

Blanching of the limb or alteration in pulse. This complication occurs in approximately 5% of infants. It is directly related to the relative size of the catheter in the aorta. It also has been seen when a cold solution is rapidly infused into the aorta. The signs will usually disappear after removal of the catheter. If the limb blanches, the catheter should be removed promptly. We do not advocate warming the contralateral limb as the initial procedure to cause vasodilation of the affected limb because of the higher risk with such delay.

Accidental hemorrhage. This is associated with inexperience. The incidence is negligible when physicians and nursing personnel are accustomed to the use of stopcocks and connections and are experienced in the placement of catheters.

Infection. The incidence of infection is related to the sterility conditions at the time of catheter placement and to maintenance procedures and the experience of the personnel.

Serious complications at necropsy. The incidence of serious complications at necropsy ranges from 1.5% to 7% and appears as a significant cause of death in less than 2% of cases. The lesions include embolization, thrombosis of hepatic vein, liver necrosis, aortic thrombi, and infarcts. Aortic thrombi are common, and their occurrence usually increases the longer the duration of the catheterization. A serious complication is thrombosis of the renal arteries and renal shutdown, leading to death. A recent increase in the incidence of neonatal hypertension may be related in whole or part to renal vascular complications of umbilical arterial catheters. In newborn monkeys where the aorta is relatively small, occlusion of the inferior mesenteric arteries by the catheter with infarction of the bowel has been observed; the presenting sign was bloody stool.

Hemorrhagic necrosis of the liver has been observed in asphyxiated newborn infants and newborn monkeys treated with strong alkalis (sodium bicarbonate or THAM). In relating liver necrosis to catheterization and the infusion of hypertonic solutions, it should be recalled that this complication also occurs following severe asphyxia alone. The incidence of intracranial hemorrhage also may be associated with hyperosmolar infusions causing hypernatremia, hypervolemia, or hypertension.

CARE OF THE UMBILICAL CORD

The umbilical cord is clamped approximately 2 inches from the skin as soon as the infant is born. After initial resuscitation and care are complete, a plastic clamp replaces the forceps. For healthy infants, the cord is painted with triple dye and allowed to dry as soon as they have been admitted to the regular nursery. For sick infants, the cord and surrounding skin are cleansed with Betadine and alcohol before catheterization. For those not being catheterized immediately, the cord is kept moist with saline after the Betadine and alcohol treatment.

DEPRESSION FROM DRUGS VERSUS ASPHYXIA

An infant depressed primarily as a result of maternal analgesics or anesthetics can usually be distinguished by clinical signs from one depressed from asphyxia. The infant depressed from medication will not have passed meconium before birth: the skin may be cyanotic rather than pale, since the infant has not received an asphyxial stimulus to cause peripheral vasoconstriction; the heart rate may be slow but the pulse strong and full; the cord will be filled with blood, since the cardiovascular system has not been depressed by asphyxia; and the infant will usually not be completely hypotonic. In contrast, the infant depressed primarily as a result of asphyxia may be meconium stained and pale as a result of intense peripheral vasoconstriction; the heart rate will be slow and the sounds soft, distant, and occasionally irregular; the umbilical cord will be limp and contain little blood.

The Apgar score does not distinguish between depression from these two causes. Differentiation is useful, since the medicated infant will frequently respond quite promptly to simple resuscitative procedures, that is, stimulation and positive pressure ventilation applied with a mask. Intubation and artificial inflation of the lungs are rarely necessary. Recognition of the infant depressed by medication is also important if drug antagonists are to be administered. On the other hand, the severely asphyxiated infant may require not only intubation, artificial ventilation, and cardiac massage, but also correction of a severe metabolic acidosis by infusion of alkali.

Use of analeptics, drug antagonists, and cardiovascular stimulants

Analeptics and drug antagonists should never be administered before the lungs have been expanded and the infant oxygenated by artificial ventilation. Analeptics, such as nikethamide, are not indicated in resuscitation of the newborn. Although they may shorten primary apnea, they are ineffective in secondary apnea and may cause hypotension and convulsions even if given in the recommended dosage. The morphine antagonist naloxone may be of value (Appendix B).

However, with the decreasing use of meperidine (Demerol) in obstetrics, the occasions when naloxone would be beneficial are infrequent. We recommend its use only when the infant remains depressed after effective lung expansion and oxygenation. Furthermore, the possibility that naloxone could interfere with the normal process of adaptation through its antagonism of endorphins should also be considered.

In general, the use of various cardiovascular stimulants that are administered in cardiopulmonary resuscitation, particularly in adults and older children, are not recommended for resuscitation at birth. Unlike the adult and older child, cardiac arrest in the neonate occurs very late in the course of asphyxiation. Consequently the severely asphyxiated infant who does not respond to cardiac massage and effective lung expansion is likely to have already suffered damage to the brain and other vital organs.

Toxicity from local anesthetics

Rarely, local anesthetics may be injected accidentally into the fetus during an attempted caudal anesthesia or paracervical block. The infant may be profoundly depressed at birth. However, as soon as the neonate is oxygenated during the course of resuscitation and the responsiveness of the CNS is partially restored, generalized convulsions may occur. The presenting part of the infant should be carefully examined for a needle puncture if accidental injection is suspected and the convulsion treated promptly with intravenous phenobarbital, 10 to 15 mg/kg body weight. It may be necessary to repeat the barbiturate and maintain the infant on a ventilator. As soon as possible, a 2- to 3-volume exchange transfusion should be performed.

Delayed depression from maternally administered analgesia and anesthesia

Drugs that cross the placenta enter the fetus through the umbilical vein and the ductus venosus. A significant but variable portion of the umbilical vein flow also passes to the inferior vena cava through the liver and hepatic veins and not through the ductus venosus. This places the liver in a strategic position for uptake of drugs, particularly those with a high fat solubility. From the liver they can be released slowly over a period of hours. Thus infants delivered soon after the mother has been given a drug may initially appear vigorous but develop a marked CNS depression 2 to 4 hours later. Therefore, when relatively large doses of sedatives or narcotics have been given to the mother and the infant breathes well at birth, the infant should nevertheless be carefully observed for delayed secondary depression.

Drug-addicted newborn infant

See Chapter 37, part four.

Signs of drug withdrawal are not usually seen for 12 to 24 hours after birth. However, if the mother has not taken a dose of narcotic recently, both mother and infant may be in a state of withdrawal at the time of delivery.

ACUTE HEMORRHAGE

Acute blood loss may occur under several circumstances: placenta previa, as a complication of fetal blood sampling, in multiple pregnancy, with cord occlusion, or at cesarean section (Chapter 32). If the blood loss has occurred during the final stages of delivery, the infant will appear pale, but the onset of respiration will not be inhibited. If it has occurred at a longer interval before delivery and the fetus has become hypotensive, severe asphyxia will be superimposed, and the infant will be depressed and unresponsive at birth. The mechanism of blood loss in placenta previa is obvious. A description of its occurrence as a complication of fetal blood sampling follows. However, in the other three conditions hemorrhage may not be immediately apparent or suspected.

In multiple pregnancy one fetus may bleed into another, or partial placental separation with hemorrhage may occur with delivery of the first infant (Chapter 11). Mild cord occlusion sufficient to constrict the vein but not arteries is occasionally seen; under these circumstances the fetus literally bleeds into the placenta. Such blood loss is usually not severe, being limited by the capacity of the placental vascular bed. Blood loss at cesarean section also occurs into the placenta. When the infant is removed from the uterus, he is usually held up by the feet while the cord is clamped. In a few seconds a considerable volume of blood can flow into the placenta from the arteries, and venous blood can be prevented from returning from the placenta to the infant as a result of the hydrostatic pressure caused by the infant being held in the air. The venous blood loss by this mechanism is usually not severe. Nevertheless, unless special precautions are taken to prevent this occurrence, such as placing the infant on the mother's abdomen and milking the umbilical cord once or twice toward the infant before clamping the cord, the hematocrit value of the infant at 3 hours of age will be 6% to 12% lower than that in healthy infants delivered vaginally. Blood "loss" or redistribution into the placenta does not occur in infants delivered normally, since they are usually held at the level of their mother's perineum, and the uterus, having expelled the infant, is firmly clamped on the placenta.

The hemoglobin and hematocrit values should be measured in all circumstances where blood loss may have occurred if there is any abnormality, such as low Apgar score; slow, delayed, or difficult breathing; pallor; or cyanosis. If there is pallor and peripheral vasoconstriction, a hematocrit reading from the peripheral capillaries will not be reliable, and a venous sample should be taken as soon as is practical after delivery. If blood loss has occurred acutely at delivery, it will not be reflected in the hematocrit value of central circulating blood during the first minutes of life. Therefore measurement should be repeated at 3 hours, the time usually necessary for readjustment of blood volume and circulating red blood cells after birth. In normal infants the mean hematocrit value usually increases from 48% to 52% during this time (Chapter 32). If the hematocrit value is below 40% at birth or if a significant fall occurs in the first 3 hours of life accompanied by pallor and respiratory distress, the infant should be given a transfusion of blood.

Monitoring of arterial and venous pressure

See also Chapter 21.

Monitoring blood pressure or central venous pressure is helpful in assessing the need for volume replacement in acute hemorrhage. Blood pressure may be obtained from a central arterial line, if in place, or from a blood pressure cuff and Doppler detector. Central venous pressure is obtained from a catheter inserted into the umbilical vein. This catheter should be inserted only as far as the portal sinus from 4 to 7 cm, depending on the size of the infant. The pressure here is normally 5 to 8 cm water. Care must be taken not to advance the catheter beyond the ductus venosus and into the inferior vena cava, where the pressure is normally 0 to 3 cm water; this could be interpreted erroneously as indicating hypovolemia.

Except when severe blood loss is known to have occurred, as in placenta previa, arterial or central venous pressure should not be used as a measure of hypovolemia until after the infant has been well ventilated and oxygenated. Correction of hypoxia and acidosis will frequently be sufficient to restore the blood pressure. Unnecessary volume replacement in a severely asphyxiated infant can have an adverse effect on cardiopulmonary performance.

In a high-risk obstetric service we have found the need for fluid replacement occurs relatively infrequently, in only one of every 300 to 400 deliveries.

Fluid replacement

Fluid for replacement is ideally blood. If O negative blood is immediately available, this should be used; otherwise initial replacement is carried out using normal saline. This may be followed by crossmatched blood if the infant's hematocrit level indicates the need. The initial volume administered should be calculated on the basis of 10 ml/kg.

PNEUMOTHORAX AND PNEUMOMEDIASTINUM

See also Chapter 28.

Pneumothorax and pneumomediastinum usually occur spontaneously and in association with aspiration syndromes. Occasionally they may be a result of incorrect or injudicious resuscitative procedures. If mild, they will not be recognized clinically and may only be discovered accidently when a roentgenogram is taken of the infant for another reason.

Pneumomediastinum should be suspected if heart sounds become distant or suddenly cannot be heard in an infant who otherwise appears normal. It should also be suspected if the anteroposterior diameter is increased. No treatment is necessary. The infant should be observed carefully after a chest roentgenogram has been taken, since this complication may progress to pneumothorax.

A tension pneumothorax is a serious complication that requires immediate treatment (Chapter 28). It appears as respiratory distress that becomes progressively more severe. The respirations are often rapid rather than labored. The heart will be shifted away from the affected side, which will move little and may appear hyperinflated. The infant usually appears pale rather than cyanotic. Since a diaphragmatic hernia may be similar, particularly when the stomach and small bowel become filled with air, it is important first to pass a catheter into the stomach and attempt to suck out any air (Chapter 33). If symptoms are not relieved by this procedure, transillumination of the chest should be performed and, if positive in an infant with severe respiratory distress, a needle may need to be inserted into the thoracic cavity in the midaxillary line at about the level of the sixth rib and the air pressure released. Following this, a tube should be inserted surgically and connected to underwater drainage. If the pneumothorax is not under tension, it is usually possible to obtain a roentgenogram of the chest to confirm the clinical diagnosis and aid in deciding on the management, which may require oxygen administration, placement of a chest tube, or a combination of these therapies.

SEVERE ERYTHROBLASTOSIS

See also Chapter 5.

In severe cases of erythroblastosis with hydrops (Chapter 32) certain emergency procedures in the delivery room may be indicated. These all focus on promptly establishing good cardiopulmonary function and ensuring that the oxygen-carrying capacity of the blood is satisfactory. If the infant is born by vagina, a blood sample should be obtained from the cord or from a peripheral venous site for Coombs' test, for determination of hemoglobin or hematocrit value, and for crossmatching with compatible blood. It is also possible to obtain a sample of capillary blood from the presenting part before delivery. If delivery is by cesarean section, O negative blood compatible with the mother's should be available before delivery. The red blood cells should be partially packed. The blood should be in readiness on the resuscitation table together with umbilical catheters, a laryngoscope, an endotracheal tube, and a 20-gauge needle.

As soon as the infant is delivered, he or she should be intubated, the lungs expanded, and positive pressure ventilation initiated. This is necessary because these infants are prone to develop pulmonary edema, since lung capillary permeability is increased and serum proteins are usually low. If there is marked abdominal distension from ascites or a recent intrauterine infusion of blood, a 20-gauge needle may need to be inserted in the lateral flank to remove fluid and relieve pressure on the diaphragm. Although fluid is usually present in the thoracic cavity of such infants, we do not recommend removal as a blind emergency procedure. Positive pressure ventilation should be continued until the infant is stabilized in the neonatal intensive care unit and can be closely observed for the development of pulmonary edema.

During the initial resuscitation, blood should be withdrawn from a clamped segment of the cord for measurement of the central hematocrit value and from the umbilical artery for a pH measurement. These results should be available to the physician within 5 to 6 minutes of delivery. If the infant is severely anemic, both umbilical vein and artery should be quickly catheterized and the blood administered through the vein, approximately 20 ml/kg, while an equal quantity is slowly withdrawn from the artery if there are signs of congestive cardiac failure. The speed of infusion and withdrawal should be about 10 ml/minute to prevent any sudden change in hemodynamics. If a hematocrit reading has been obtained from fetal capillary blood during labor, catheterization and administration of blood can proceed while the infant is being intubated and ventilated. Freshly drawn heparinized blood is desirable but is rarely available in the delivery room. This will have a pH in the range of 7.3. Citrate phosphate dextrose (CPD) blood that has a pH of about 7.25 is an adequate substitute for heparinized blood. If only citrated blood is available, the pH will be 6.9 or less (Chapter 32, part two). This pH should be corrected with sodium bicarbonate. Citrated blood also has a high potassium content.

During these procedures every effort should be made to prevent heat loss by having an overhead radiant heat source turned on well in advance of delivery. Prompt oxygenation and restoration of the oxygen-carrying capacity of the blood are essential if these infants are to be given an optimum chance to survive.

IMMATURE INFANT

Immature infants require the application of all the principles of resuscitation just described. Because of their relatively large surface area, particular attention should be paid to preventing heat loss by drying the infant promptly and ensuring that the resuscitation area is warmed with a radiant heater and is as draft free as possible. This is sometimes difficult in modern air-conditioned delivery rooms. The small size of the infant and the delicacy of immature tissues demand greater manual dexterity and gentleness if intubation is to be performed rapidly and without trauma. Intubation, if necessary, is facilitated by the physician placing the fifth finger of the left hand, which holds the laryngoscope, over the larynx. Gentle pressure on the larynx as the blade is tilted will bring the glottis into view.

We do not recommend routine intubation and umbilical catheterization of the VLBW infant, since many are vigorous and can be managed conservatively. Only those with a low Apgar score or those who fail to respond promptly with effective respiratory efforts are intubated. If the infant shows evidence of respiratory difficulty with retraction or tachypnea, continuous positive airway pressure (CPAP) will be instituted using nasal prongs. This mode of supporting respiration is instituted even if the infant does not require supplemental oxygen.

Cord blood should be routinely analyzed for acid-base composition, and an arterial sample should be obtained within the first 15 to 20 minutes if evidence of respiratory difficulty is present. Blood pressure (indirect or direct) is monitored, together with heart rate, respiration, and body temperature. Oxygen should be administered if necessary to maintain the infant's PaO_2 between 50 and 70 mm Hg. A metabolic acidosis with a base excess (BE) greater than 13 mg/L is treated with bicarbonate.

If the infant cannot be maintained on CPAP, as evidenced by severe retraction and apneic spells, a PaO_2 less than 50 mm Hg on a fractional inspired oxygen concentration (FIO_2) of 1.0 and a $PaCO_2$ greater than 65 mm Hg, artificial ventilation is instituted at our center.

Every effort should be made to minimize barotrauma to the lungs. The intermittent mandatory ventilation (IMV) mode is employed. This allows the patient to breathe spontaneously, in addition to being supplied with mechanical ventilation, permitting a lower rate of IMV, reducing the damage of barotrauma, and facilitating weaning. The rate of IMV is usually started at a rate of between 20 and 30. This rate provides sufficient expiration time for the patient to breathe spontaneously and maintain a $PaCO_2$ in the range of 50 mm Hg. The patient soon adjusts to this and synchronizes with the respirator. A flow rate of 5 to 7 L/minute is used, and an FIO_2 between 40% and 100% is selected, depending on the clinical condition or the previous FIO_2. It should be quickly adjusted to maintain the PaO_2 between 50 and 70 mm Hg.

Inspiratory time is set at 0.6 seconds, and inspiratory pressure is adjusted so that chest excursion is visible. This pressure is usually in the range of 20 to 30 cm water. Lower pressures are used for the less severely ill infant. Positive end expiratory pressure (PEEP) is initially set at 5 cm water. A Bennett Cascade humidifier is used in the circuit. This humidifier has been shown to give a relative humidity of 100% at whatever water temperature is inside the cascade. Water temperature is kept at 32° to 38° C (90° to 100° F); higher temperatures are used for thick secretions. Maintenance of adequate humidity is essential to keep secretions thin and easy to suction. Collapse of a lung or a lobe during mechanical ventilation is rare with this technique.

The endotracheal tube is suctioned at least every 2 to 3 hours; more frequent suctioning is done for copious secretions. The suction catheter is advanced 3 to 5 cm beyond the tip of the endotracheal tube, depending on the size of the infant.

The process of weaning from mechanical ventilation is begun immediately. The FIO_2 is lowered in decrements of 5% to 10% to maintain a PaO_2 between 50 and 70 mm Hg and IMV rate lowered to maintain a $PaCO_2$ less than or equal to 50 mm Hg in decrements of 2 to 5 breaths per minute depending on the blood gas measurement. Inspiratory pressure is lowered to prevent excessive chest excursion and avoid barotrauma as the patient's clinical state improves.

Extubation is undertaken when the rate of IMV is down to 6 per minute. At this stage the patient usually requires an FIO_2 of less than or equal to 40% and the general condition is stable.

COMPLICATIONS OF FETAL BLOOD SAMPLING

Two major complications following fetal blood sampling have been observed: (1) abscess formation in the area of the sampling incision and (2) hemorrhage from the incision itself. These complications have occurred in about 1% of cases (Chapter 8).

Abscess formation has been seen where the incision was made in an area that had been previously traumatized, with the subsequent formation of a cephalhematoma, or where the tissue had become traumatized during delivery from the application of either forceps or a vacuum extractor at the incision site. Risk of infection following sampling in the breech presentation also increases, since healing of incisions in the sacral region is poor. The fact that abscesses do occur underscores the importance of careful aseptic techniques in the fetal blood sampling procedure.

Hemorrhage may occur if the incision is made over a small artery. It will usually stop when firm pressure is applied, but occasionally the incision may have to be sutured. This is a potentially lethal complication. It is important that the incision area be observed directly for two or three contractions after a blood sample has been taken to ensure that hemostasis is present. Clotting studies have been abnormal in several infants who have bled from the scalp sampling site. Most infants reported to have bled following fetal scalp sampling have suffered from chronic intrauterine asphyxiation, and this is sometimes associated with depletion or deficiency in certain clotting factors, particularly the labile factors V and VII. It is therefore important that neonates who bleed readily from sampling incisions have a screening coagulation study (Chapter 32). Postnatal bleeding from a sampling incision may be the first manifestation of a severe neonatal coagulation disorder.

If the scalp appears pale when visualized through the amnioscope and does not blanch when compressed by the instrument, severe peripheral vasoconstriction and hypotension are likely to be present. Under these circumstances it may be difficult to obtain blood when an incision is made. If blood does not flow readily from the first incision, the temptation is to make multiple incisions. However, after delivery and alleviation of asphyxia, the peripheral circulation will improve; the infant then may bleed from several sites and sustain substantial blood loss.

Maternal intrapartum or postpartum infection has been seen more frequently in mothers of infants who develop complications from fetal blood sampling. Therefore infants whose mothers develop infections should be observed very closely for infection and hemorrhage at the site of a sampling incision.

IMMEDIATE COMPLICATIONS OF ASPHYXIA

Major signs of dysfunction of the central nervous system in the full-term infant following intrauterine asphyxia include abnormal respiratory pattern, stereotyped movements, fixed posturing, poor suck and feeding, reduced oculovestibular response, abnormal pupillary response, and fullness of the anterior fontanel. The sign that appears to be the most indicative of the degree of insult to the nervous system is the loss of tone. Loss of tone in the infant is the last of the components of the Apgar score to return following recovery from asphyxia. For this reason it appears to be one of the best and earliest clinical indicators of the severity of the intrauterine insult. If the tone returns to normal within 1 or 2 hours, the infant has a good chance of surviving with an intact nervous system. However, if the infant remains significantly hypotonic during the first 4 to 5 days of life, there is an increased chance that the child will not survive the neonatal period, or if the child survives, there will be severe cerebral damage. If hypotonia is replaced with marked hypertonia and increased activity during the first 24 hours, chances of survival increase greatly, but there is an increased incidence of cerebral damage (Chapter 27).

Pathologic features

In the full-term infant pathologic features depend on the length and severity of the intrauterine asphyxial episode, the care of the patient in the neonatal period, and the length of survival of the patient. Patients who die in the first few hours after birth may show no gross or microscopic changes. Those patients dying after the first 24 hours of age frequently have brain swelling and cerebral necrosis. Full-term infants who survive the intrauterine asphyxial episode and the neonatal period have been described as having two primary neuropathologic conditions: ulegyria and status marmoratus of the basal ganglia. The principal focus of damage is in the cortical mantle and not in the paraventricular region of brain, as in the premature infant.

There has been much discussion regarding the issue of whether brain swelling occurs before or after cerebral necrosis. It is likely that the initial swelling is intracellular, occurring first at the depths of the sulci. The extent and pattern of ulegyria obviously depend on the degree and location of the cerebral ischemia and subsequent cerebral necrosis. The presence of gross brain swelling is simply the result of the increasing focal areas of cerebral swelling and ischemia, leading not only to the generalized brain swelling but also to generalized cerebral necrosis. If the infant survives, the existing areas of cerebral necrosis, through the reparative process of brain gliosis, are converted into areas of ulegyria.

In the preterm infant the most common brain lesion at autopsy is subependymal hemorrhage/intraventricular hemorrhage (SEH/IVH) (Chapter 27). Most observations regarding SEH/IVH, before the advent of computed tomography and cranial ultrasonography, have come from autopsy studies indicating that the incidence of SEH/IVH in the neonate varies from 25% to 75%, with a higher incidence of hemorrhage occurring in the more immature infant.

Clinical signs that are statistically related to severe SEH/IVH are the following:

1. Fall in hematocrit level
2. Failure of rise in hematocrit level when transfusion of packed red cells is given
3. Tight anterior fontanel
4. Decrease in spontaneous activity
5. Decrease in tone
6. Abnormal eye signs
7. Seizures

Milder degrees of SEH/IVH may be completely asymptomatic. The quantity of blood appears to be prognostically significant with regard to survival.

Two areas of concern regarding the outcome of neonates who survive SEH/IVH are progressive posthemorrhagic hydrocephalus and long-term neurobehavioral abnormalities. Contrary to previous belief, progressive hydrocephalus is not always an invariable outcome in patients with documented significant hydrocephalus. There is spontaneous resolution of hydrocephalus in a significant number of patients without any therapy.

Effect of hypoxia on other organ systems

Other organs, which can be dispensed with functionally by the fetus, are likely to be more severely compromised than is the brain. Blood flow to the gut, kidneys, and lungs is decreased with redistribution to the myocardium and CNS during asphyxia (Chapter 1). The blood flow to the adrenals is also maintained during asphyxia in experimental animals, but the role of the adrenals and their hormone products has been incompletely studied. Thus, if evidence of brain damage in an asphyxiated infant is found, there is almost always evidence of more profound damage to other organs. The degree of damage and the extent of the interaction between compromised gut, lungs, and kidneys will depend on many factors, including gestational age.

The effect of intrauterine asphyxia on the lungs is reflected in the development of RDS in immature infants and in persistence of the fetal circulation and meconium aspiration in the more mature infants. There is a significant relationship both to the development of RDS and its severity with intrapartum and neonatal asphyxia. The reduction in blood flow to the lungs of the fetus leads to damage to the cells lining the tracheobronchial tree, resulting in loss of function and in the severest cases cellular destruction. In the liver, despite preferred perfusion, processes that cause compromise of oxygen delivery from the placenta can result in anything from extremes of necrosis to subtle hepatic functional changes related to problems of hypoglycemia and hyperbilirubinemia. The importance of the alteration in hepatic enzyme function that occurs with perinatal asphyxia and hypoxia is incompletely defined but may play a critical role in the handling of maternal drugs and endogenous metabolic products. The gut is a target organ for profound cellular damage in the presence of any compromise to blood flow or oxygenation. Evidence suggests that hypoxia plays a leading role in preparing the neonatal gut for necrotizing enterocolitis.

Particularly wide variation in renal function is incurred during and following perinatal hypoxia. As yet there has been no systematic investigation of the neonatal kidney's ability to maintain homeostatic adjustments of water and electrolytes and thus body composition in the presence of perinatal asphyxia. Active research in fetal and neonatal animals has begun to elucidate the mechansims by which hypoxia may cause alterations in renal function or varying degrees and patterns of renal failure. The derangements in function related to hypoxia and acidosis have been shown to depend not only on the duration and degree of insult, but also on the actions of vasopressin, angiotensin, and catecholamines. High concentrations of these hormones are found in fetal plasma during and subsequent to asphyxial insult.

DIAGNOSIS OF CONGENITAL ANOMALIES

Incidence

The incidence of congenital defects has been estimated to occur in 1% to 7% of all live births (Chapter 17). This incidence will depend on the kind of conditions that are included, but probably 2% to 3% of all live-born infants show one or more significant congenital malformations that may require medical attention soon after birth. Disorders of the skeleton are the most common of these malformations and comprise approximately one third of all defects. Most of these can be seen or felt and can be verified by roentgenography. However, several defects are not immediately apparent on visual examination. About 20% of deaths in the third trimester of gestation and about 15% in the neonatal period may be attributed to gross congenital malformations. Prompt diagnosis of the anomalies as soon as the patient is born may enable life-saving medical and surgical treatment to be instituted.

Polyhydramnios

See also Chapter 6.

A congenital anomaly should be suspected if the mother has either polyhydramnios or oligohydramnios. Congenital anomalies associated with hydramnios follow:

A. Anencephaly
B. Hydrocephaly
C. Microcephaly
D. Spina bifida
E. Mongolism
F. Volvulus
   1. With atretic upper jejunum
   2. With congenital bands of upper jejunum
   3. With common mesentery and herniation of liver
G. Tracheoesophageal fistula with atretic esophagus
H. Imperforate anus
I. Cleft palate
J. Congenital heart disease
K. Pyloric stenosis
L. Genitourinary disease
M. Deformed extremities
N. Agenesis of ears (Oligohydramnios is frequently associated with renal agenesis or other anomalies of the genitourinary tract. See later in this section.)
O. Neuromuscular disorders

Choanal atresia and laryngeal stenosis

During the initial appraisal of the newborn particular attention should be paid to the evenness and ease of respiration. If respiratory difficulty is present and persists after pharyngeal suctioning, choanal atresia or laryngeal stenosis should be suspected. Although rare, these anomalies are emergencies. Choanal atresia is a bony or membranous obstruction between the nose and pharynx (Chapter 28). Clinically, although the airway from the mouth to the larynx is patent, this anomaly may result in complete respiratory obstruction, since infants are obligatory nose breathers. Respiratory difficulty at birth may require intubation and artificial ventilation. However, this anomaly usually presents as respiratory distress or apnea after the onset of breathing at 5 to 10 minutes of age. Once breathing is established, choanal atresia is diagnosed by occluding the mouth and the right or left nostril. It may also be diagnosed by inserting a catheter first into one nostril and then into the other, passing it ventromedially along the floor of the nose. The catheter should pass with ease for 3 to 4 cm. If an obstruction is detected, a temporary airway should be promptly provided. This is best achieved by inserting a small plastic infant airway between the tongue and the palate. Once ventilation is established, the infant will then breathe through the mouth while awake. During sleep, however, the infant will attempt to revert to obligatory nose breathing. If laryngeal stenosis is present, it will be recognized immediately when the glottis is visualized with the laryngoscope. Immediate tracheostomy is imperative.

Diaphragmatic hernia and congenital adenomatous lung cysts

A diaphragmatic hernia with abdominal viscera (Chapter 33) in the chest or congenital cysts of the lungs (Chapter 28) may cause immediate respiratory difficulty. The lungs may be hypoplastic if the diaphragmatic hernia is large and bilateral. These two congenital anomalies are likely to be diagnosed during the course of resuscitation. Following intubation for respiratory difficulty, strong resistance is felt when an attempt is made to expand the lungs by positive pressure. Two other conditions must be considered in the differential diagnosis of this type of respiratory obstruction: massive aspiration of meconium that cannot be removed by suctioning and intrauterine pneumonia with organization of exudate. Infants with hypoplastic lungs or congenital adenomatous cysts of the lungs may be vigorous initially and score as high as 7 on the Apgar scale at 1 minute of age, making strenuous but ineffective respiratory efforts. In contrast, infants with meconium aspiration or intrauterine pneumonia are usually severely depressed at birth. Congenital adenomatous cysts of the lungs may be associated with hydrops.

A small or unilateral diaphragmatic hernia may not be apparent initially. However, this is usually manifested in the first 10 to 15 minutes of life as respiratory difficulty and may be verified by observing asymmetry of chest movements and diminution or absence of air sounds on the affected side. In some circumstances the diaphragmatic hernia is not apparent for the first 30 to 60 minutes of life or even later. Manifestation of the anomaly in these instances appears to depend on the infant's swallowing air and the gradual distension of gut in the thorax by this swallowed air.

Tracheoesophageal fistula

Atresia of the esophagus with tracheoesophageal fistula should be investigated in every baby (Chapter 33). As soon as good ventilation is established, a catheter should be introduced into the mouth on either the left or right side of the tongue and advanced down into the esophagus and stomach. The outline of the tip of the catheter is usually seen in the left half of the abdomen as it is gently advanced. If not, the examiner's hand is placed over the upper quadrant, and a puff of air is blown into the catheter. A bubble is immediately felt. It may also be detected by listening over the stomach with a stethoscope. If the catheter does not enter the stomach, the esophagus probably ends in a blind pouch. The longer this anomaly remains undiagnosed, the greater is the risk of aspiration pneumonia. In rare instances a fistula occurs with a patent esophagus. This condition is difficult to diagnose. The anomaly should be suspected if the infant coughs during feeding. It may be verified using a barium swallow and cineradiography.

Anomalies of the upper gastrointestinal tract

If complete intestinal obstruction is above the midjejunum, the stomach may contain a large volume of fluid (Chapter 33). The average volume of fluid found in healthy infants delivered by the vaginal route is 5.7 ml (range, 1 to 20 ml); for those delivered in breech position, 4.3 ml; and for those delivered by cesarean section, 7.2 ml (range, 0 to 50 ml). The smallest amount of fluid that has been associated with a high gastrointestinal obstruction is 38 ml. A catheter should be passed into the newborn's stomach and the contents removed. If more than 15 ml of fluid are present in the stomach, a roentgenogram of the abdomen should be obtained during the first 3 hours of life to detect the presence of gas. The absence of gas below the pylorus may indicate obstruction and necessitate early exploration. Under normal circumstances the upper intestine is filled with air within 3 hours. When obstruction is present, the roentgenogram has an even, flat, opaque appearance. A small amount of contrast air is seen only in the stomach and duodenum. Duodenal or jejunal atresia, malrotation of the gut, or an annular pancreas may be the cause.

High gastrointestinal obstructions should be suspected if the mother has polyhydramnios. Normally there is a constant equilibrium of amniotic fluid between the mother and baby. Swallowing of fluid by the fetus and subsequent absorption from its intestinal tract into the circulation is one of the principal modes by which fluid returns to the placenta and finally to the mother. Any anomaly of the gastrointestinal tract that interferes with this process may cause amniotic fluid to accumulate and produce polyhydramnios. CNS anomalies that interfere with swallowing may also produce polyhydramnios. In these cases as much as 170 ml of fluid has been aspirated from the baby's stomach.

Perforation of the stomach by a catheter may occur in the newborn period, but this is rare (Chapter 33) provided that the catheter used for gastric aspiration is soft and flexible.

Anal atresia

A catheter should be used to rule out anal atresia (Chapter 33). With the infant's thighs flexed, the catheter should be introduced through the anal opening as far as it can be easily passed. If it passes for 3 cm, obstruction is unlikely.

Skeletal anomalies

Anomalies of the skeleton are usually readily verified visually or by palpation. The association between chromosomal abnormalities and congenital defects particularly relates to the skeletal system. The anterior fontanel is normally open and should be palpated for size and tension. Bulging is diagnostic of increased intracranial pressure and may indicate hydrocephalus and intracranial hemorrhage. The posterior fontanel is normally closed and is frequently difficult to outline because of scalp edema and molding of the sutures. A small or closed anterior fontanel occurs in craniosynostosis (Chapter 27) and is not infrequently accompanied by microcephaly or an abnormally shaped head. Soft spots in the skull (craniotabes), usually located in the parietal areas, are present in about one third of all newborns. Rarely, a cranial bone may be absent, indicating osteogenesis imperfecta. The sacral region should be examined for pigmentation and abnormal hair, which is typically associated with occult spina bifida.

Cleft palate

The mouth should be carefully examined for the presence of a cleft palate. This may occur even if the upper lip is normal. A small-sized laryngoscope with a premature blade is an ideal instrument with which to visualize both the hard and soft palate. The extent of the defects may vary from a small round hole to a large triangular opening with the base at the site of the uvula. Although treatment for this anomaly is not an emergency, feeding problems and an increased risk of aspiration may be anticipated.

Anomalies of the genitourinary system

Malformations of the external ear are associated with renal anomalies. If the ears are low set or the configuration is deformed, the infant should be closely observed for the passage of urine. The abdomen should be carefully palpated, both for the verification of normal position of the liver and spleen and for the presence of abnormal masses. In the first few minutes of life, before the infant has swallowed sufficient gas to distend the gut and while the tone of the abdominal wall is somewhat reduced, the kidneys may be readily felt for verification of their normal position, size, and shape. Congenital obstruction of the bladder outlet or urethra will usually be associated with a distended bladder, readily palpable as a firm, central, dome-shaped structure in the lower abdomen. Finally the umbilical, inguinal, and femoral regions should be examined for hernias. The presence of both testes in the scrotum should be determined and the possibility of hypospadias evaluated.

PROGNOSIS

The outcome of a difficult and complex resuscitation is not always a happy one. With the introduction of new life-saving techniques that include more effective and efficient artificial ventilation, cardiac massage, and correction of pH, we now have the means of saving infants with brain damage who would otherwise have died. The decision not to resuscitate a severely brain-damaged infant is extremely difficult. The answer to this dilemma undoubtedly lies in the development of better means of diagnosing congenital anomalies, assessing the fetal condition before the onset of labor, measuring the capacity of the placenta to support the infant during labor, and evaluating the fetus as labor progresses. These measures will provide the obstetrician with more information from which to make the best judgment and deliver the infant in optimum condition. When these advances in preventive medicine are achieved and introduced into obstetric practice, the birth of severely asphyxiated infants requiring a complex resuscitation should become a rare occurrence.

L. Stanley James

BIBLIOGRAPHY

Adamsons, K., Gandy, G., and James, L.S.: The influence of thermal factors upon oxygen consumption of the newborn infant, J. Pediatr. **66**:495, 1965.

Adamsons, K., and others: The treatment of acidosis with alkali and glucose during asphyxia in fetal rhesus monkeys, J. Physiol. (Lond.) **169**:679, 1963.

Adamsons, K., and others: Resuscitation by positive pressure ventilation and tris-hydroxymethyl-aminomethane of rhesus monkeys asphyxiated at birth, J. Pediatr. **65**:807, 1964.

Apgar, V., and James, L.S.: Further observations on the newborn scoring system, Am. J. Dis. Child. **104**:419, 1962.

Baker, D.H., Berdon, W.E., and James, L.S.: Proper localization of umbilical, arterial and venous catheters by lateral roentgenograms, Pediatrics **43**:34, 1969.

Banker, B.Q., and Larroche, J.: Periventricular leucomalacia of infancy, Arch. Neurol. **7**:386, 1962.

Bland, R.D., Clark, T.I., and Harden, L.B.: Rapid infusion of sodium bicarbonate and albumin into high-risk premature infants soon after birth: a controlled, prospective trial, Am. J. Obstet. Gynecol. **124**:263, 1976.

Cockburn, F., and others: The effect of pentobarbital anesthesia on resuscitation and brain damage in fetal rhesus monkeys asphyxiated on delivery, J. Pediatr. **75**:281, 1969.

Cohn, H.E., and others: Cardiovascular responses to hypoxemia and acidemia in fetal lambs, Am. J. Obstet. Gynecol. **120**:817, 1974.

Cole, V.A., and others: Pathogenesis of intraventricular haemorrhage in newborn infants, Arch. Dis. Child. **49**:772, 1974.

Corbet, A.J., and others: Controlled trial of bicarbonate therapy in high-risk premature newborn infants, J. Pediatr. **91**:771, 1977.

Daniel, S.S., and James, L.S.: Abnormal renal function in the newborn, J. Pediatr. **38**:856, 1976.

Daniel, S.S., and others: Analeptics and resuscitation of asphyxiated monkeys, Br. Med. J. **2**:562, 1966.

D'Souza, S.W., and others: Umbilical venous blood pH: a useful aid in the diagnosis of asphyxia at birth, Arch. Dis. Child. **58**:15, 1983.

Dweck, H.S., and others: Developmental sequelae in infants having suffered severe perinatal asphyxia, Am. J. Obstet. Gynecol. **119**:811, 1974.

Finberg, L., Luttrell, C., and Redd, H.: Pathogenesis of lesions in the nervous system in hypernatremic states. II. Experimental studies of gross anatomic changes and alterations of chemical composition of the tissues, Pediatrics **33**:46, 1959.

Gandy, G.M., and others: Thermal environment and acid-base homeostasis in human infants during the first few hours of life, J. Clin. Invest. **43**:751, 1964.

Goldstein, G.W.: Pathogenesis of brain edema and hemorrhage: role of the brain capillary, Pediatrics **96**:357, 1979.

Hagberg, B., and others: Incidence of cerebral palsy according to cause, Acta Paediatr. Scand. **64**:187, 1975.

Haglund, U., and others: The intestinal mucosal lesions in shock (2 parts), Eur. Surg. Res. **8**:435, 448, 1976.

Harding, R., and others: Cardiovascular changes in new-born lambs during apnoea induced by stimulation of the laryngeal receptors with water, J. Physiol. (Lond.) **256**:35P, 1975.

Hobel, C.J., and others: Early versus late treatment of neonatal acidosis in low birth weight infants: relation to respiratory distress syndrome, J. Pediatr. **81**:1178, 1972.

James, L.S.: Acidosis of the newborn and its relation to birth asphyxia, Acta Paediatr. (Upps) **49**(suppl. 122):17, 1960.

James, L.S.: Physiology of respiration in newborn infants and in the respiratory distress syndrome, Pediatrics **24**:1969, 1969.

James, L.S., and Adamsons, K.: Respiratory physiology of the fetus and newborn infant, N. Engl. J. Med. **271**:1403, 1964.

Leuenberger, P.J., and others: Decrease in angiotensin I conversion by acute hypoxia in dogs, Proc. Soc. Exp. Biol. Med. **158**:586, 1978.

Merritt, T.A., and Farrell, P.M.: Diminished pulmonary lecithin synthesis in acidosis: experimental findings related to RDS, J. Pediatr. **57**:132, 1976.

Moya, F., and others: Hydramnios and congenital anomalies, JAMA **173**:1552, 1960.

Moya, F., and others: Cardiac massage in the newborn infant through the intact chest, Am. J. Obstet. Gynecol. **84**:798, 1962.

Ostrea, E.M., Jr., and Odell, G.B.: The influence of bicarbonate administration on blood pH in a "closed system": clinical implications, J. Pediatr. **80**:671, 1972.

Rudolph, A.M., and Yuan, D.: Response of the pulmonary vasculature to hypoxia and H^+ ion concentration changes, J. Clin. Invest. **43**:399, 1966.

Russell, G., and Cotton, E.K.: Effects of sodium bicarbonate by rapid injection and of oxygen in high concentration in respiratory distress syndrome of the newborn, Pediatrics **41**:1063, 1968.

Silverman, F., and others: The Apgar score: is it enough? Obstet. Gynecol. **66**:331, 1985.

Simmons, M.A., and others: Hypernatremia and intracranial hemorrhage in neonates, N. Engl. J. Med. **291**:6, 1974.

Stalcup, S.A., and others: Inhibition of converting enzyme activity by acute hypoxia in dogs, J. Appl. Physiol. **46**:227, 1979.

Steichen, J.J., and Kleinman, L.I.: Effect of HCO_3 therapy on acid-base homeostasis in newborn dogs with and without ventilatory restriction, Pediatr. Res. **11**:543, 1977.

Sykes, G.S., and others: Do Apgar scores indicate asphyxia? Lancet **1**:494, 1982.

Thorne, I.: Cerebral symptoms in the newborn, Acta Paediatr. Scand. **58**(suppl.):915, 1969.

Usher, R.: Reduction of mortality from respiratory distress syndrome of prematurity with early administration of intravenous glucose and sodium bicarbonate, Pediatrics **32**:966, 1963.

CHAPTER 23

Care of the mother, father, and infant

The tribulations and struggles of parents of premature infants in learning to cope with their infants provided the stimulus to explore how normal parents develop a close attachment to their infants. As investigators began to study the ways in which the parent of a premature infant manages to meet the needs of this immature, sleepy, fragile infant, they noted many common adaptations and problems. During the last 15 to 20 years, research on parent-infant attachment has mainly focused on the parents of full-term infants. However, in recent years several investigators have looked closely at the complex and confusing ecology parents encounter when the birth of a premature, sick, or malformed infant brings them into an intensive care nursery.

This chapter attempts to place in perspective the creative work of the investigators who have ventured into this arena. Research in these intensive care units is not easy or straightforward but rather is frequently confounded by harassed, overworked nurses and physicians, overwhelmed parents, and critically sick infants. Recent observations based on the completed studies suggest several interventions that appear to have merit and deserve further investigation in the traditional hospital environment. A few investigators have been refreshingly innovative and have broken down the walls of the intensive care unit to create a new and more positive environment for parents of sick infants.

In an attempt to determine what triggers, fosters, or disturbs a mother's attachment to her infant, information has been gathered from clinical observations during medical care procedures; naturalistic observations of mothering; long-term, in-depth interviews of mothers, primarily by psychoanalysts; structured interviews of observations; and results from closely controlled studies on the parents of full-term infants. This chapter attempts to integrate these studies into a general framework from which to develop some clinical recommendations.

Events that are important to the formation of a mother's attachment to her infant include the following:

A. Before pregnancy
   1. Planning the pregnancy
B. During pregnancy
   1. Confirming the pregnancy
   2. Accepting the pregnancy
   3. Fetal movement
   4. Accepting the fetus as an individual
C. After birth
   1. Birth
   2. Seeing the baby
   3. Touching the baby
   4. Giving care to the baby

By observing and studying the human mother according to these periods, we can begin to fit together the interlocking pieces that lay the foundations of attachment.

BEFORE PREGNANCY

The literature on child development suggests that children are socialized by the powerful process of imitation or modeling. Their behavior is influenced by how they are mothered or what they observe. Long before a woman becomes a mother, she has obtained a repertoire of mothering behaviors through observation, play, and practice. She has already learned whether infants are picked up when they cry, how much they are carried, and whether they should be chubby or thin. It is an interesting phenomenon that these modes of conduct, absorbed when children are very young, become unquestioned imperatives for them throughout life. Unless adults consciously and painstakingly reexamine these learned behaviors, they will probably unconsciously repeat them when they become parents.

PREGNANCY

Caplan considers pregnancy to be a developmental crisis involving two particular adaptive tasks.

Acceptance of pregnancy

During the first stage of pregnancy a woman must come to terms with the knowledge that she will be a mother. When she first realizes that she is pregnant, a mother will often have mixed feelings. Many considerations, ranging from a change in her familiar patterns to more serious matters such as economic and housing hardships or interpersonal difficulties, all influence her acceptance of the pregnancy. This initial stage, as outlined by Bibring, is the mother's identification of the growing fetus as an "integral part of herself."

Perception of the fetus as a separate individual

The second stage involves a growing awareness of the baby in the uterus as a separate individual. It usually starts with the remarkably powerful event of *quickening*, the sensation of fetal movement. It appears to occur earlier for mothers who see their baby and its movements on the screen during ultrasonography. During this period the woman must begin to change her concept of the fetus from a being that is part of herself to a living baby who will soon be a separate individual. Bibring believes that this realization prepares the woman for birth and physical separation from her child. In turn, this preparedness lays the foundation for a relationship with the child.

After quickening, a woman will usually begin to have fantasies about what the baby will be like, attributing some personality characteristics and developing feelings of attachment. At this time she may further accept her pregnancy and show significant changes in attitude toward the fetus. Objectively, there will usually be some outward evidence of the mother's preparation. She may purchase clothes or a crib, select a name, and rearrange her home to accommodate a baby, a type of human "nesting."

The production of a normal child is a major goal of most women. Yet most pregnant women have hidden fears that the infant may be abnormal or reveal some of their own secret inner weaknesses. Brazelton has clarified the importance of these changes and turmoil that occur during pregnancy for the subsequent development of attachment to the new infant*:

> The prenatal interviews with normal primiparas, in a psychoanalytic interview setting, uncovered anxiety which often seemed to be of pathological proportions. The unconscious material was so loaded and distorted, so near the surface, that before delivery one felt an ominous direction for making a prediction about the woman's capacity to adjust to the role of mothering. And yet, when we saw her in action as a mother, this very anxiety and the distorted unconscious material could become a force for reorganization, for readjustment to her important new role. I began to feel that much of the prenatal anxiety and distortion of fantasy could be a healthy mechanism for bringing her out of the old homeostasis which she had achieved to a new level of adjustment. . . . I now see the shakeup in pregnancy as readying the circuits for new attachments, as preparation for the many choices which they must be ready to make in a very short critical period, as a method of freeing her circuits for a kind of sensitivity to the infant and his individual requirements which might not have been easily or otherwise available from her earlier adjustment. Thus, this very emotional turmoil of pregnancy and that in the neonatal period can be seen as a positive force for the mother's adjustment and for the possibility of providing a more individualized environment for the infant.

The caregiver's ability to help parents during this emotional turmoil probably has a strong influence in determining whether the pregnancy will be a positive or negative experience in the woman's life.

Cohen, however, emphasizes that any stress, such as moving to a new geographic area, marital infidelity, death of a close friend or relative, previous abortions, or loss of previous children, that leaves the mother feeling unloved or unsupported or that precipitates concern for the health and survival of either her infant or herself may delay preparation for the infant and retard bond formation. After the first trimester, behaviors that are a reaction to stress and suggest rejection of pregnancy include a preoccupation with physical appearance or negative self-perception, excessive emotional withdrawal or mood swings, excessive physical complaints, absence of any response to quickening, or lack of any preparatory behavior during the last trimester.

It is difficult to evaluate the many factors that determine the interactional and parenting behavior of an adult human who has lived for 20 to 30 years. A mother's and father's behavior toward their infant is derived from a complex combination of their own genetic endowments, the infant's responses to them, a long history of interpersonal relationships with their own families and with each other, experiences with this or previous pregnancies, the absorption of the practices and values of their cultures, and, probably most important, the way in which each was raised by his or her parents. The mothering and fathering behavior of each woman and man, the ability of each to tolerate stresses, and the needs each has for special attention differ greatly and depend on a mixture of these factors.

Fig. 23-1 is a schematic diagram of the major influences on parental behavior and the resulting disturbances that may arise from them. At the time the infant is conceived, some of these determinants, such as the mothering the father and mother received when they were infants, the practices of their culture, their endowments, and their relationships with their own families, are contributed by

*From Brazelton, T.B.: Early Child Dev. Care 2:259, 1973. Copyright © Gordon and Breach Science Publishers, Inc. Reprinted by permission of the author and publisher.

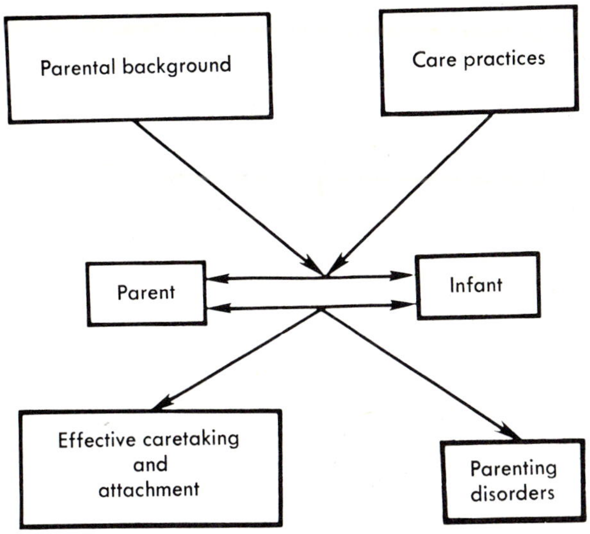

Fig. 23-1. Major influences on parent-infant attachment and the outcomes.

the parents. We originally believed these determinants fixed and unchangeable. However, other investigators have argued that the influence of some of these may be changed during the crisis of birth. Other determinants relate to the hospital culture. For example, the attitudes, statements, and practices of the nurses and physicians in the hospital; whether there is separation from the infant in the first days of life; the infant's temperament; and whether the infant is healthy, sick, or malformed obviously also affect the relationship. Most mothers and fathers develop warm and close attachments with their infants. However, a series of mothering disorders ranging from mild anxiety, such as persistent concerns about a baby after a minor problem that has been completely resolved in the nursery, to the most severe manifestation, the battered child syndrome, occur in a few parents. Some problems result in part from separation and other unusual circumstances that occur in the early newborn period as a consequence of present hospital care policies. Experiences during labor, parent-infant separation, and hospital practices during the first hours and days of life are the most easily manipulated variables in this scheme. Recent studies have partly clarified some of the steps in mother-infant attachment during this early period.

LABOR

Before childbirth moved from the home to the hospital, the practice in industrialized nations was for family members to support the mother in labor, often with the assistance of a trained or untrained midwife. In all but one of 150 cultures studied by anthropologists, a family member or friend, usually a woman, remained with the mother during labor and delivery. Although more fathers, relatives, and friends have been allowed into labor and delivery rooms in the past 10 years, a significant number of mothers still labor and deliver in some hospitals without the presence of family members or close friends. There has been little systematic study of this issue since the Newtons reported in 1962 that mothers who were quiet and relaxed and had better emotional relationships with their attendants during labor and delivery were more pleased at the first sight of their babies. Two recent studies in Guatemala were designed to investigate the effects of a supportive companion (Raphael termed such a person a *doula*) on perinatal complications and mother-infant interaction after delivery, in an obstetric setting in which mothers routinely labor alone.

Table 23-1. Mean length of labors in hours

	No doula	doula	p
First study	19	9	<0.001
Second study	14	8	<0.0001

From Klaus, M.H., and Kennell, J.H.: Parent-infant bonding, ed. 2, St. Louis, 1982, The C.V. Mosby Co.

Initial assignment of mothers to the experimental (doula) or control group was random, but controls showed a higher rate ($p < 0.001$) of subsequent perinatal problems (e.g., cesarean section, meconium staining) (Table 23-1). In both studies the time from admission to delivery was much shorter in the experimental group. Significantly more mothers who had a doula present during labor remained awake after delivery and were more interactive with their infants during the time they were awake. These observations suggest that major perinatal benefits result from constant human support during labor.

AFTER BIRTH

Immediately after the birth parents enter a unique period during which events may have many effects on the family. We have named this period, which lasts a short time and during which the parents' attachment to their infant sometimes begins to blossom, the *maternal sensitive period*. The first feelings of love for the infant are not necessarily instantaneous with the initial contact.

The relation between the time when a mother falls in love with her baby and the sensitive period is not clear at present. Several mothers have shared with us their distress and disappointment when they did not experience feelings of love for their baby in the first minutes or hours after birth. It should be reassuring for them and similar mothers to learn about two studies of normal, healthy mothers in England.

MacFarlane and associates asked 97 Oxford mothers, "When did you first feel love for your baby?" The replies were as follows: during pregnancy, 41%; at birth, 24%;

first week, 27%; and after the first weeks, 8%.

In a study of two groups of primiparous mothers, 40% recalled that their predominant emotional reaction when holding their babies for the first time was one of indifference. The same response was reported by 25% of 40 multiparous mothers. Forty percent of both groups felt immediate affection. Most mothers in both groups had developed affection for their babies within the first week. The onset of this maternal affection after childbirth was more likely to be delayed if the membranes were ruptured artificially, if the labor was painful, or if the mothers had been given meperidine (Demerol).

Donald Winnicott, who started as a pediatrician and became a distinguished psychoanalyst, has made remarkably perceptive observations that suggest he was describing the sensitive period. From these observations Winnicott proposed that a healthy mother goes through a period of *primary maternal preoccupation*. He found that the mother who developed this state provided a setting for the infant's constitution to begin to make itself evident. He believed that only if a mother was able to reach this state of heightened sensitivity could she feel her way into her infant's place and so meet the infant's needs.

Fig. 23-2 illustrates the time pattern of this special state or sensitivity. It rises during pregnancy, is maintained at a heightened level right after delivery, and then decreases in the early months following birth. It is interesting that the timing and course of primary maternal preoccupation are similar to those described for the maternal sensitive period. We suspect that endocrine changes play a significant role in starting and enhancing both these processes. Are they initiated by the rise in estradiol and drop in progesterone in the weeks before delivery? Interestingly, the heightened sensitivity of primary maternal preoccupation is sometimes misinterpreted by physicians and nurses as excessive anxiety. Studies of other cultures are important in this regard because in most societies the mother and baby are placed together with support, protection, and isolation for at least 7 days after birth. The provision of food, heat, and water and a private time for the mother and infant to get to know each other are common in most cultures.

The clinical observations of Rose and associates and Kennell and others suggested that affectional ties can be easily disturbed and may be permanently altered during the immediate postpartum period. Relatively mild illness in the newborn, such as slight elevations of bilirubin levels, slow feeding, additional oxygen for 1 to 2 hours, and the need for incubator care in the first 24 hours for mild respiratory distress, appear to affect the relationship between mother and infant. The mother's behavior is often disturbed during the first year or more of the infant's life, even though the infant's problems are completely resolved before discharge and often within a few hours. That early events have long-lasting effects is one of our principles of attachment. A mother's anxieties about her baby in the first few days after birth, even about a problem that is easily resolved, may affect her relationship with the child long afterward.

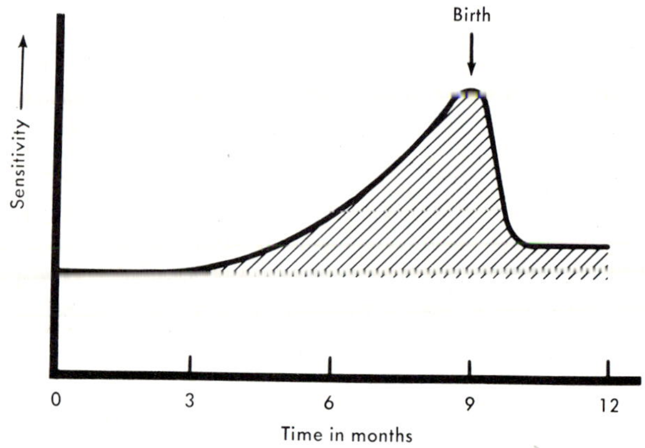

Fig. 23-2. Hypothesized change in maternal sensitivity during pregnancy and in the postnatal period.

In the past 15 years, 17 separate studies have focused on whether additional time for close contact of the mother and infant in the first minutes, hours, and days of life alters the quality of the attachment. Fig. 23-3 illustrates the timing of the contact in the 17 human studies. In three studies the extra time was added not only during the first 3 hours but also during the next 3 days of life. At 1 month the mothers in the group who had extra contact showed significantly more affectionate behavior toward their infants. They stood closer and watched over them more during the physical examination, soothed them more when they cried, engaged in more eye-to-eye contact and fondling during feeding, and were more reluctant to leave them with someone else. At 1 year the two groups of mothers were again significantly different, with extra-contact mothers spending more time assisting and soothing their infants during stressful office visits. At 2 years the linguistic behavior of the two groups was compared. Extra-contact mothers used longer sentences but fewer content words and imperatives than did the controls.

In 13 studies the additional mother-infant contact occurred only during the first hour of life. Ten of these studies noted significant differences in the behavior of the mothers. As an example, DeChateau and Wiberg investigated the effects on maternal behavior of skin-to-skin contact and suckling during the first 30 minutes after delivery in 40 primiparous middle-class Swedish mothers. The mothers with early contact received only an additional 15 minutes of extra contact in the first 30

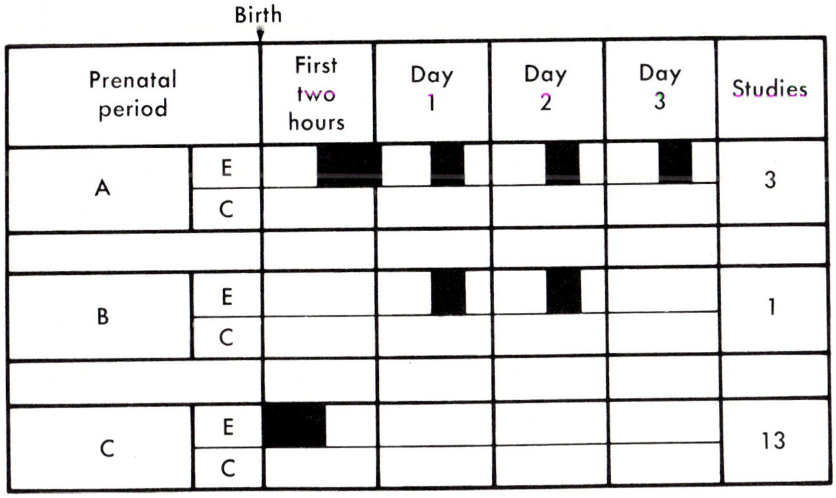

Fig. 23-3. Time patterns and number of three types of controlled studies in which one group of mothers has additional contact *(E)* with their infants compared with another group with routine contact *(C)*.

minutes of life. Following this both the control and the experimental groups had a similar amount of time with their babies. When the infants were 3 months old, detailed observations at home revealed that early-contact mothers spent significantly more time looking at their infants face to face and kissing them, whereas control mothers spent more time cleaning their babies. The infants of mothers with early contact cried significantly less and smiled significantly more than infants of control mothers. In seven of nine studies breast-feeding was significantly increased by permitting the mother additional time with her infant in the first hour.

When additional time is given for close mother-infant contact following the first 8 hours after delivery, differences in later mothering behavior also occur. In a study of 301 primiparous patients, O'Connor and others noted that increasing the time by 12 hours (6 hours on days 1 and 2) significantly decreased the number of mothering disorders with 10 such occurrences in the control group but only two in the group of mothers who received extra time with their infants (Table 23-2). Siegel and associates in a group composed of new and multiparous mothers did find differences in parenting at 4 and 12 months but no difference in mothering disorders. A woman was defined as having a mothering disorder if her infant was battered, had nonorganic failure to thrive, was abandoned, or was given up for an unplanned adoption.

Several questions come to mind. Is the time a mother spends with her newborn in the first hour as significant as a longer period together on the second or third day of life? Is the effect in the first hour due to the quiet, alert state of the infant, to the state of the mother, or to a combination of the two? In the first hour after birth

Table 23-2. Child abuse or neglect in the first year of life

Study	Total	Abuse or neglect
O'Connor and others, 1980		
Extended contact	134	2
Control	143	10*
Siegel and others, 1980		
Extended contact	97	7
Control	105	10

*$p < 0.05$.

the newborn infant is in a heightened state of alertness and responsivity. Interestingly, no matter when increased amounts of contact between mother and infant are added in the first 3 postpartum days, there appears to be improved mothering behavior. At present it is not known why such striking alterations in caretaking have been noted when mother-infant contact is increased for such a short time in the first hours of life.

Lamb has criticized the results of the controlled trials that suggest a sensitive period. Lamb noted that early contact may not necessarily have clear, enduring, universal, and clinically significant benefits. Some misinterpretations of studies in this area may have resulted from a too literal acceptance of the word *bonding*. Nonetheless, there is strong evidence that at least 30 to 60 minutes of early contact in privacy should be provided for every parent and infant to enhance the bonding experience. Studies have not clarified how much of the effect may be apportioned to the first hours and how much to the first days, but it would appear that additional contact in both periods will probably help mothers become attached to their babies. When we make it possible for parents to be together with their baby, in privacy, for the first hour and throughout the hospital stay, we establish the most beneficial and supportive environment for the beginning of the bonding process.

Talents of the infant

The recent accumulation of information in a closely related field has greatly augmented our understanding of parent-to-infant attachment. Detailed studies of the amazing behavioral capacities of the normal neonate have shown that the infant sees, hears, imitates facial gestures, and moves in rhythm to his mother's voice in the first minute and hours of life, resulting in a beautiful linking of the reactions of the two and a synchronized "dance" between the mother and infant. The infant's appearance coupled with this broad array of sensory and motor abilities evokes responses from the mother and father and provides several channels of communication that are most helpful in the process of attachment and the initiation of a series of reciprocal interactions.

Lang noted that, immediately after a home delivery, most mothers suckle their infants. The infants she observed did not suck but licked the area around the nipple. MacFarlane has shown that 6 days after birth infants will have the abililty to distinguish reliably by scent their mother's breast pad from the breast pads of other women. The mother has an intense interest in looking at her newborn baby's open eyes. In the first 45 minutes of life the infant is awake and alert and will visually follow the mother for 180 degrees. The licking of the nipple will induce a marked increase in prolactin secretion in the mother, and at the same time oxytocin, to contract the uterus and decrease bleeding. With the mother's strong desire to touch and see her child, nature has provided for the immediate and essential union of the two. The alert newborn rewards the mother for her efforts by following her with his or her eyes, thus maintaining their interaction and kindling the tired mother's fascination with her baby.

Lind and associates in Stockholm have shown that a surprising increase in blood flow to the breast occurs when a mother hears the cries of her infant. These intricate interactions have focused attention on the cascade of interlocking sensory patterns that quickly develop between mother and infant in the first hours of life.

Evidence suggests that many of these early interactions also take place between the father and his newborn child. Parke in particular has demonstrated that, when fathers are given the opportunity to be alone with their newborns, they spend almost exactly the same amount of time as mothers holding, touching, and looking at them.

In the triadic situation the father tends to hold the infant nearly twice as much as the mother, vocalizes more, touches the infant slightly more, and smiles at the infant significantly less than the mother. The father clearly plays the more active role when both parents are present in contrast to the cultural stereotype of the father as a passive participant. In fact, in this triadic interaction the mother's overall interaction declines. All but one of the fathers whom Parke studied had attended labor and birth, and this could be expected to produce an unusual degree of father-to-infant attachment. However, he conducted another study using a similar design but in which the fathers rarely participated in labor and birth. Despite these social and institutional differences, the fathers again played the more active and dominant role with increased holding, vocalizing, and touching.

In his work with a mother and her 3-month-old twins, Stern observed that the pattern of interaction between a mother and her child has a characteristic rhythm. Intricate interchanges occur within a few seconds. When these interactions are repeatedly out of phase—for example, if one partner looks away just as the other looks at him—many aspects of the relationship between the two individuals are disturbed. Our observations suggest that this dance of mother and infant, which may or may not be in rhythm, is first initiated in the immediate postpartum period. As Brazelton and his colleagues have stated, "This interdependency of rhythms seems to be at the root of their 'attachment' as well as communication." Thus it seems important that the family have privacy in the first hours of life, in which the new and older members may become attuned to each other.

On the basis of our observations and the reports of parents, we believe that every mother has a task to perform during the postpartum period. She must look and "take in" her real live baby and reconcile the fantasized image of the infant she anticipated with the one she actually delivered. Many cultures recognize this need by providing the mother with a doula, or "aunt," who mothers her and relieves her of other responsibilities so that she can devote herself completely to this task.

In an interesting and significant observation of fathers, Rödholm and Larsson noted that paternal caregiving greatly increased when the father was allowed to interact and establish eye-to-eye contact with his infant for 1 hour during the first hours of life. Keller and others have recently reported that the group of fathers who received extended postpartum hospital contact with their infants, compared to a traditional contact group, engaged in more en face behavior and vocalization with their infants and were more involved in infant caretaking responsibilities 6 weeks after the baby's birth. They also had higher self-esteem scores than the other group of fathers.

Parke believes that the father must have an extensive early exposure to the infant in the hospital where the parent-infant bond is initially formed: "There is a lot of learning that goes on between the mother and infant in the hospital from which the father is excluded and in which he must be included so he'll not only have the interest and a feeling of owning the baby, but also the kinds of skills that the mother develops." Parke interpreted his findings as indicating that the father is much more interested in and responsive toward his infant than U.S. culture has acknowledged.

PRACTICAL CONSIDERATIONS

In 1959 Bibring wrote, "What was once a crisis with carefully worked-out traditional customs of giving support to the woman passing through this crisis period has become at this time a crisis with no mechanisms within the society for helping the woman involved in this profound change of conflict-solutions and adjustive tasks." This deficiency accounts for the development of the many support systems in our society. The wide assortment of childbirth classes, which attempt to continue previous customs, are good examples. These groups help the mother through the delivery period as well as aiding her in later infant and child care. They also lessen the tensions, fears, and fantasies that occur during normal pregnancies. By joining a group of mothers with whom she can chat and share her feelings, a woman can alleviate many of the emotional upsets that occur during normal pregnancies. We therefore believe that these courses, particularly those in which mothers participate actively, have a valuable supportive role during pregnancy.

To minimize the number of unknowns for a mother while she is in the hospital, she and the father (or other supportive companion who will stay with her throughout labor and delivery) should visit the maternity unit to see where labor and delivery will take place. She should also learn about the anesthetic (if she is to receive one), delivery routines, and all the procedures and medication she will receive before, during, and after delivery. By reducing the possibility of surprise, such preparation will increase confidence during labor and delivery. For an adult, just as for a child entering the hospital for surgery, the more meticulously every step and event is detailed in advance, the less the subsequent anxiety. The less anxiety the mother experiences while delivering and becoming attached to her baby, the better will be her immediate relationship with the infant.

The mother must have continuing support and reassurance during her labor and delivery, whether from her husband, the father, her mother or other female family member or friend, a midwife, or a nurse. She also must be satisfied with the arrangements that have been made to maintain her home during her hospitalization.

In an effort to reduce the amount of tension on the mother, she should have a supportive companion with her and should labor and deliver in the same room, preventing the necessity of rushing to a delivery room in the last minutes of labor. Once the delivery is completed and the mother has quickly glanced at the infant, it is important for her to have a few seconds to regain her composure and, in a sense, catch her breath before she proceeds to the next task—taking on the infant. This breath-catching usually occurs during the period when the placenta is being delivered, while the mother is being cleansed and is having any necessary suturing. We have found that it is best not to give a mother her baby until she indicates that she is ready. It should be *her* decision.

In many hospitals it is customary to put the baby on the mother's chest for 1 or 2 minutes shortly after delivery. This is helpful, but the short time coupled with the lack of privacy and narrow table does not allow sufficient opportunity for the mother to touch and explore her baby. Even 5 or 10 minutes of contact, particularly without privacy, are probably not sufficient to optimize maternal attachment.

After delivery, the father, mother, and baby should have a period alone in either the delivery room or an adjacent room (i.e., a recovery room). Obviously this is only possible if the infant is normal and the mother is well. The mother should have and hold the infant with her on the bed. The infant should not be off in a bassinet where the face cannot be seen. She should be given the baby nude so that she can perform a complete inspection. We have found it valuable to encourage the mother to move over in her regular hospital bed, so that she only takes up about half of it, leaving the other half for her partially dressed or nude infant. A heat panel easily maintains or, if necessary, increases the body temperature of the infant. Several mothers have told us of the unforgettable experience of holding their nude baby against their bare chest, so we recommend skin-to-skin contact (Fig. 23-4). The father sits or stands at the side of the bed by the infant. This allows the parents and infant to become acquainted. Because the eyes are so important for both the parents and baby, we withhold the application of silver nitrate ($AgNO_3$) or erythromycin ophthalmic ointment to the eyes until after this rendezvous.

We also have found it valuable for the mother, father, and infant to be together for about 30 to 60 minutes. After 10 to 15 minutes the mother and baby often fall into a deep sleep. In Guatemalan hospitals, where drugs and anesthesia are used more sparingly, a study showed that most mothers were awake after 45 minutes of privacy with their infants. We must emphasize that up to 40% of normal mothers take a week or longer before they feel

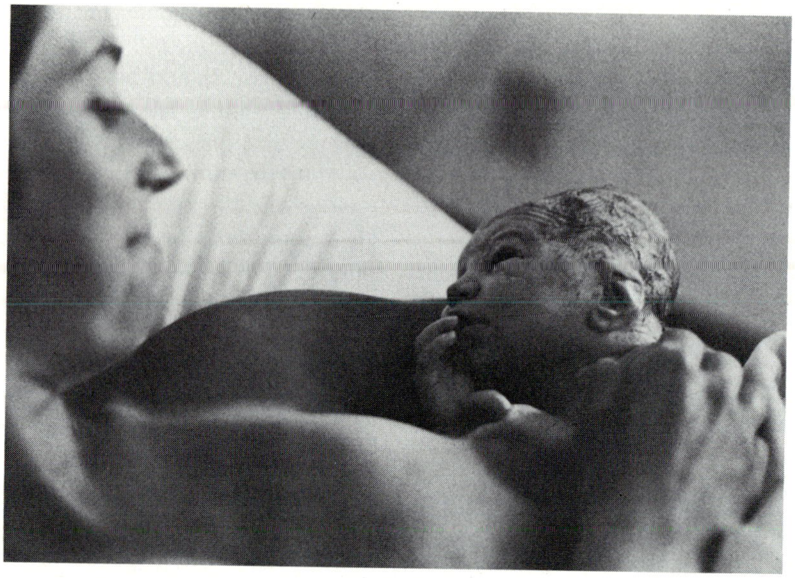

Fig. 23-4. A mother and her infant shortly after birth. (From Klaus, M.H., and Klaus, P.: Amazing newborn, Menlo Park, Calif. 1985, Addison-Wesley Publishing Co. with permission. Copyright Suzanne Arms Wimberley.)

the baby is really theirs. Obviously close contact with the husband is also important.

PREMATURE OR SICK INFANTS

In the years since parental visiting has been permitted in the intensive care nursery, studies have revealed that most parents continue to suffer severe emotional stress. Harper and others noted that this occurred even when parents had close contact with their infants. However, despite their anxiety, they believed the opportunity to have this contact was helpful, and over 90% of parents questioned were opposed to restricting their contact with their infants. Most parents thought that holding their infant made the infant feel more loved. Benfield and associates also noted that most parents experienced grief reactions. Interestingly, the level of their response was unrelated to the severity of the baby's problems. Green graphically described the parents' plight when he noted "geographically displaced, their work and lives disrupted, their biologic rhythms in disarray, bewildered, anxious and terribly tired, parents in the delirium of crisis are simply unable to comprehend what is happening."

From interviews and observations, researchers suggested that early parental reactions predicted how the mother would manage with her infant in the early weeks at home. From interviews, Mason found that if the mother expressed a fairly high level of anxiety, actively sought information about the condition of her baby, showed strong maternal feelings for the baby, and had strong support from the father, there was usually a favorable outcome. If the mother showed a low level of anxiety and activity, her relationship with her child probably would be poor.

Minde and associates noted that the most important variable was the mother's relationship with her mother, her relationship with her father, and whether or not the mother had a previous abortion. Highly interacting mothers in the nursery visited and telephoned the nursery more frequently while the infants were hospitalized and stimulated their infants more at home. However, the authors noted that mothers who touched and fondled their infants more in the nursery had infants who opened their eyes more. Minde noted the contingency between the infant's eyes being open and the mother's touching and also between gross motor stretches and the mother's smiling. He and his colleagues could not determine to what extent the sequence of touching and eye opening reflected the primary contribution of the mother or the infant.

Thus, from interviews and observations, these researchers noted that mothers who become involved, interested, and anxious about their infants will have an easier time when the infant is taken home.

In the last 15 years numerous studies have revealed that if small, premature infants are either touched, rocked, fondled, or cuddled daily during the stay in the nursery, they may have significantly fewer apneic periods, increased weight gain, fewer stools, and in some studies even advances in certain areas of higher central nervous system functioning that persist for a short time after discharge from the hospital. As a result, parents and caretakers have often begun additional stimulation of the preterm infant after she goes home.

Based on his observations of many normal mothers and their full-term infants, Winnicott noted that what the baby observes in the caretaker's face in the early months of life helps the baby develop a self-concept. He noted that some infants have mothers who do not imitate the baby, and thus the babies do not see themselves. In these situations he postulated that the infant's own creative capacity may be atrophied and that such an infant would look for other ways of getting to know themselves from the environment. The important observation that Winnicott noted was that in normal mother-infant dyads the mother was often following or imitating the infant.

Trevarthen confirmed these observations in mothers and infants using fast film technique and noted that mothers imitate their babies during spontaneous play. He also noted that the mother's imitation of her infant's behavior, rather than the reverse, sustained their interaction and communication. Detailed analysis revealed that mothers were studiously imitating the infant's expression with a lag of a few tenths of a second. Thus the infant was choosing the rhythm.

In a series of creative experimental manipulations of infant-mother face-to-face interactions, Field noted that the mother and the normal full-term infant were each interacting about 70% of the time in their spontaneous play. However, when the mother was asked to increase her attention-getting behavior (stimulation), her activity increased to 80% of the time, and strikingly, the infant's gaze decreased to 50%. When the mother imitated the movements of the infant, which greatly reduced her activity, the infant's gaze time greatly increased.

Field noted that in the spontaneous situation the mothers of high-risk preterm infants were interacting up to 90% of the time, whereas the infant was looking only 30% of the time. If the mother was told to use attention-getting gestures, her activity increased more than 90% of the time and the infant's gaze decreased further. If her interactions were decreased by asking her to imitate the baby's movements, the infant's gaze increased greatly. Although generally the parents' activity was aimed at encouraging more activity or responsiveness from the premature infant, the approach appeared to be counterproductive, leading to less instead of more infant reponsiveness. Thus by three separate and different techniques it appears that mothers of normal infants follow or mirror their infant's behavior for significant periods.

Interventions for parents of premature infants

To help parents deal with the stressful situation of having a sick or small infant, several interventions have been introduced. In some cases these have involved the parents and infant together, whereas others have focused on either the parent or the infant. The ecology of the intensive care nursery is a difficult environment in which to make detailed and definitive assessments. Nurseries not only differ in their physical environment but also in patient population and physician interests, background, training, and sensitivity. Despite this, sufficient data and measurements from several nurseries enable us to begin to make recommendations. However, in assessing the potential value of any intervention, it may be inappropriate to generalize to a much wider population from a study carried out in one premature unit. The following interventions have been adopted.

1. Opening the intensive care nursery to parents
2. Transporting the mother to be near her infant
3. Maternal day care for premature infants
4. Rooming-in for the parent of a premature infant
5. Nesting
6. Early discharge
7. Listening to parents (interviewing) during the infant's hospitalization
8. Parent groups
9. Programmed contact and reciprocal interaction
10. Transporting the healthy premature infant to the mother
11. Home-based intervention for young parents
12. Discussion with the parents after discharge

We recommend the following procedures.

1. It is useful and safe for the mother to have the baby placed in her bed in the first hour of life with a heat panel above them when a premature baby weighing 1.5 to 2.5 kg is delivered and appears to be doing well without grunting and retractions. We do not recommend this approach unless the physician is sure the infant is healthy.

2. A mother and her infant should be kept near each other in the same hospital, ideally on the same floor. When the long-term significance of early mother-infant contact is kept in mind, a modification of restrictions and territorial traditions can usually be arranged.

3. If the baby does have to be moved to a hospital with an intensive care unit, the mother should be given a chance to see and touch her infant, even if the baby has respiratory distress and is in an oxygen hood. The house officer or the attending physician stops in the mother's room with the transport incubator and encourages her to touch and look at her baby. A comment about the baby's strength and healthy features may be long remembered and appreciated.

4. We encourage the father to follow the transport team to the hospital so he can see what is happening with his baby. He uses his own transportation so that he can stay in the premature unit for 3 to 4 hours. This extra time allows him to get to know the nurses and physicians in the unit, to find out how the infant is being

treated, and to talk with the physician about what we expect will happen to the baby in the succeeding days. We allow him to come into the nursery and explain in detail everything that is going on with his infant. We ask him to help act as a link between us and his family by relaying information to his wife, and we request that he come to our unit before he visits his wife so that he can let her know how the baby is doing. We suggest that he take an instant photograph, even if the infant is on a respirator, so that he can describe the baby's care to his wife in detail.

5. In many communities the mother is transported from the community hospital before delivery to the maternity division of the medical center so she will be with her baby after birth. The mother is also being transported more often with the baby after delivery.

6. A mother should be permitted to enter the premature nursery as soon as she is able to maneuver easily. When she makes her first visit, it is important to anticipate that she may become faint or dizzy when she looks at her infant. We always have a stool nearby so that she can sit down, and a nurse stays at her side during most of the visit describing in detail the procedures being carried out, such as respiration and heart rate monitoring, the umbilical catheter and endotracheal tube placement, feeding through the various infusion lines, and the functioning of the incubator and ventilator.

7. We also encourage grandparents, brothers, sisters, and other relatives to view the infant through the glass window of the nursery so they will begin to know and to feel attached to the infant. We believe it is important to arrange for the grandparents and special close friends or relatives to enter the nursery and visit the baby, particularly when the baby is very ill or expected to die, so that they can provide firsthand support and understanding to the parents. We selectively allow siblings to enter the nursery when we believe it will truly relieve (and not aggravate) a child's confusion and anxiety.

8. It is necessary to find out what the mother believes is going to happen or what she has read about the problem if one has developed. We try to move at her pace during any discussion to ensure that she understands.

9. In discussing the infant's condition by telephone with the mother, who is still in the referring hospital, we ask the father to stand nearby so that we can talk to them both at the same time and they can hear the same message. This group communication reduces misunderstandings and usually is helpful in assuring the mother that we are telling her the whole story.

10. If the sick infant has any chance of survival, we are optimistic with the parents from the beginning. No evidence has shown that, if a favorable prediction proves to be incorrect and the baby expires, the parents will be harmed by early optimism. They can almost always be prepared before the baby actually dies. If the infant lives and the physician has been pessimistic, it is more difficult for parents to become closely attached. We recognize that this recommendation is contrary to many past customs and places a heavy burden on the physician. It is our belief that, if the infant does expire, we must continue to work with the mother and father and help them with their mourning reactions.

11. Once the possibility that a baby has brain damage has been mentioned, the parents will not forget it. Therefore, unless we are convinced that the baby is damaged, we do not mention the possibility of any brain damage or retardation to the parents.

12. It is important to emphasize that, if there is a clear objective finding such as a cardiac abnormality or a specific congenital malformation, we see no reason to hide it from the parents.

13. As soon as possible we describe to both the father and the mother the value of touching in helping them to get to know the infant, in reducing the apneic episodes (if this is a problem), and possibly increasing weight gain, thus hastening discharge from the unit.

14. It is important to remember that feelings of love for the baby are often elicited through eye-to-eye contact. Therefore, if an infant is under bilirubin lights, we turn them off and remove the eye patches so the mother and her infant can see each other.

15. From our previous observations we have found that keeping a book in which to record parental phone calls and visits is useful in determining which mothers are likely to require additional help from a social worker or extra discussions about the health of their infant. If a mother visits the nursery less than three times in 2 weeks, the chance of her developing a mothering disorder increases. Therefore, if her visiting pattern is less than that of most other mothers, she is given extra help in adapting to the hospitalization.

16. Minde and associates have shown that parent groups are especially effective in helping parents.

INFANTS WITH CONGENITAL MALFORMATIONS

The birth of an infant with a congenital malformation presents complex challenges to the physician in charge and the infant's family. Despite the relatively large number of infants with congenital anomalies, our understanding of how parents develop an attachment to a malformed child remains incomplete. Although previous investigators agree that the child's birth often precipitates major family stress, relatively few have described the process of family adaptation during the infant's first year of life. A major advance was Solnit and Stark's conceptualization of parental reactions. They emphasized that a significant aspect of adaptation is the necessity for parents to mourn the loss of the normal child they had expected. Other observers have noted the pathologic aspects of family reactions, including the chronic sorrow that envelops the

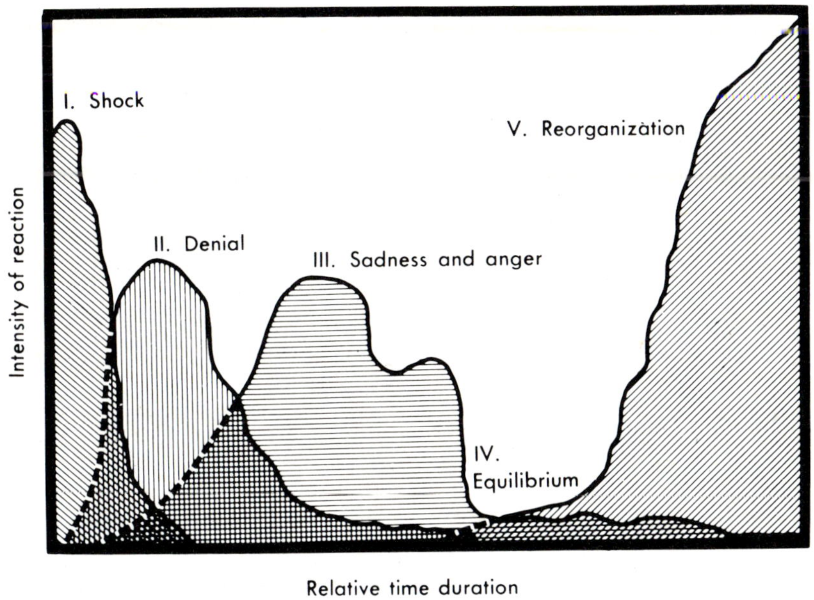

Fig. 23-5. Hypothetic model of a normal sequence of parental reactions to the birth of a malformed infant. (Modified from Drotar, D., and others: Pediatrics **56:**710, 1975. Copyright American Academy of Pediatrics, 1975. Reproduced by permission of Pediatrics.)

family of a defective child. Less attention has been given to the more adaptive aspects of parental attachment to children with malformations.

Parental reactions to the birth of a child with a congenital malformation appear to follow a predictable course. For most parents initial shock, disbelief, and a period of intense emotional upset, including sadness, anger, and anxiety, are followed by gradual adaptation marked by a lessening of intense anxiety and emotional reaction (Fig. 23-5). This adaptation is characterized by an increased satisfaction with and ability to care for the baby. These stages in parental reactions are similar to those reported in other crisis situations, such as with terminally ill children. The shock, disbelief, and denial reported by many parents seem to be an understandable attempt to escape the traumatic news of the baby's malformation, so discrepant with usual parental expectations for a normal newborn.

Solnit and Stark have likened the crisis of the birth of a child with a malformation to the emotional crisis following the death of a child, in that the mother must mourn the loss of her expected, normal infant. In addition, she must become attached to her living, damaged child. However, the sequence of parental reactions to the birth of a baby with a malformation differs from that following the death of a child in yet another respect. The mourning or grief work apparently does not occur in the usual manner because of the complex issues raised by continuation of the child's life and the demands of physical care. The parents' sadness, which is important initially in their relationship with their child, diminishes in most instances once the parents take over the physical care. Most parents reach a point at which they are able to care adequately for their children and cope effectively with disrupting feelings of sadness and anger. The mother's initiation of the relationship with her child is a major step in the reduction of anxiety and emotional upset associated with the trauma of the birth. As with normal children, the parents' initial experience with their infant seems to release positive feelings that aid the mother-child relationship following the stresses associated with the news of the child's anomaly and, in many instances, the separation of mother and child in the hospital.

Interventions for parents of malformed infants

1. We believe that the infant should be left with the mother for the first 2 or 3 days, if medically feasible. If the child is rushed to the hospital where special surgery will eventually be done, the mother will not have enough opportunity to become attached to the infant. Even if the surgery is required immediately, as for bowel obstruction, it is best to bring the baby to the mother first, allowing her to touch and handle the infant and point out to her how normal he or she is in all other respects.

2. The parents' mental picture of the anomaly is often far more alarming than the actual problem. Any delay during which the parents suspect that a problem may exist greatly heightens their anxiety, and they imagine the worst. Therefore we suggest that the baby be brought to both parents when they are together as soon after delivery as possible.

3. We have arranged for the father to stay with the

mother in her room on the maternity division on several occasions. We believe that this opportunity to support each other, to cry and curse and talk together, is highly beneficial. We use the process of early crisis intervention, meeting several times with the parents, whether the father lives in with the mother or not. During these discussions we ask the mother how she is doing, how she feels her husband is doing, and how he feels about the infant. We then reverse the questions and ask the father how he is doing and how he thinks his wife is progressing. The hope is that they will think not only about their own reactions but will begin to consider each other as well.

4. We believe that parents should not be given tranquilizers. These tend to blunt their responses and slow their adaptation to the problem. A small dose of secobarbital (Seconal) at night, however, is often helpful.

5. It has been our experience that parents who are initially adapting reasonably well often ask many questions and at times appear to be almost overinvolved in clinical care. In our unit we are pleased by this and more concerned about parents who ask few questions and who appear stunned and overwhelmed by the problem.

6. Many anomalies are very frustrating, not only to the parents but also to the physicians and nurses as well. The physician may be tempted to withdraw from the parents and their infant. The many questions asked by the parent who is trying to understand the problem are often very frustrating for the physician. The parent often appears to forget and asks the same questions repeatedly.

7. Each parent may move through the process of shock, denial, anger, guilt, and adaptation at a different pace, so the two parents may not be synchronized with one another. If they are unable to talk with each other about the baby, their relationship may be severely disrupted. We have found it best to move at the parents' pace. Moving too quickly runs the risk of losing the parents along the way. It is beneficial to ask the parents how they view their infant.

SUMMARY

Since the newborn baby completely depends on the parents for survival and optimum development, it is esential to understand the process of bonding as it develops from the first moments after the child is born. Although we have only begun to understand this complex phenomenon, those responsible for the care of mothers and infants should reevaluate hospital procedures that interfere with early, sustained mother-infant contact. They should consider measures that promote a mother's contact with her infant and help her appreciate the wide range of sensory and motor responses of her neonate.

Marshall H. Klaus
John H. Kennell

BIBLIOGRAPHY

Anisfeld, E., and Lipper, E.: Early contact, social support and mother-infant bonding, Pediatrics **72**:79, 1983.

Anisfeld, E., and others: Maternal-infant bonding: a joint rebuttal (editorial), Pediatrics **72**:569, 1983.

Barnett, C.R., and others: Neonatal separation: the maternal side of interactional deprivation, Pediatrics **45**:197, 1970.

Benfield, D.G., Leib, S.A., and Reutor, J.: Grief response of parents following referral of the critically ill newborn, N. Engl. J. Med. **194**:975, 1976.

Berg, R.B., and Salisbury, A.: Discharging infants of low birth weight: reconsiderations of current practice, Am. J. Dis. Child. **122**:414, 1971.

Bibring, C.: Some considerations of the psychological processes in pregnancy, Psychoanal. Study Child **14**:113, 1959.

Bloom, R.: Definitional concepts of the crisis concept, J. Consult. Clin. Psychol. **27**:42, 1963.

Bowlby, J.: Nature of a child's tie to his mother, Int. J. Psychoanal. **39**:350, 1958.

Brazelton, T.B.: Effect of maternal expectations on early infant behavior, Early Child Dev. Care **2**:259, 1973.

Brazelton, T.B., Koslowski, B., and Main, M.: In Lewis, M., and Rosenblum, L.A., editors: The effect of the infant on its caregiver, New York, 1974, John Wiley & Sons, Inc.

Brazelton, T.B., Scholl, M., and Robey, J.: Visual responses in the newborn, Pediatrics **37**:284, 1966.

Bronfenbrenner, U.: Early deprivation in mammals: a cross-species analysis. In Newton, G., and Levine, S., editors: Early experience and behavior, Springfield, Ill., 1968, Charles C Thomas, Publisher.

Caplan, H.: Patterns of parental response to the crisis of premature birth, Psychiatry **23**:365, 1960.

Cohen, R.L.: Some maladaptive syndromes of pregnancy and the puerperium, Obstet. Gynecol. **25**:562, 1966.

Condon, W.S., and Sander, L.W.: Neonate movement is synchronized with adult speech: interactional participation and language acquisition, Science **183**:99, 1974.

Davis, J.A., Richards, M.P.M., and Roberton, N.R.C., editors: Parent-baby attachment in premature infants, Kent, 1983, Croom Helm Ltd.

DeChateau, P., and Wiberg, B.: Long-term effect on mother-infant behaviour of extra contact during the first hour post partum. I. First observations at 36 hours, Acta Paediatr. Scand. **66**:137, 1977.

DeChateau, P., and Wiberg, B.: Long-term effect on mother-infant behaviour of extra contact during the first hour post partum. II. Follow-up at three months, Acta Paediatr. Scand. **66**:145, 1977.

Dillard, R.G., and Korones, S.B.: Lower discharge weight and shortened nursery stay for low birth-weight infants, N. Engl. J. Med. **288**:131, 1973.

Drotar, D., and others: The adaptation of parents to the birth of an infant with a congenital malformation: a hypothetical mode, Pediatrics **56**:710, 1975.

Emde, R.N., and Robinson, J.: The first two months: recent research in developmental psychobiology and the changing view of the newborn. In Noshpitz, J., and Call, J., editors: Basic handbook of child psychiatry, New York, 1979, Basic Books.

Evans, S., Reinhart, J., and Succop, R.: A study of 45 children and their families, J. Am. Acad. Child Psychiatry **11**:440, 1972.

Fanaroff, A.A., Kennell, J.H., and Klaus, M.H.: Follow-up of low birth-weight infants—the predictive value of maternal visiting patterns, Pediatrics **49**:288, 1972.

Field, T.M.: Effects of early separation, interactive deficits and experimental manipulations on infant-mother face-to-face interaction, Child Dev. **48**:763, 1977.

Field, T., and Sostek, A.: Infants born at risk: psychological perceptual, and cognitive processes, New York, 1983, Grune & Stratton, Inc.

Friedman, S.B., and others: Behavioral observations on parents anticipating the death of a child, Pediatrics **32**:610, 1963.

Garrow, D.: Personal communications, 1979.

Geleerd, E.R.: Two kinds of denial: neurotic denial and denial in the service of the need to survive. In Schur, M., editor: Drives, affects and behavior, vol. 2, New York, 1965, International Universities Press.

Gottfried, A.W., and Gaiter, J.L., editors: Infant stress under intensive care. In Environmental neonatology, Baltimore, 1985, University Park Press.

Green, M.: Parent care in the intensive care unit. Am. J. Dis. Child. **133**:1119, 1979.

Greenberg, M., Rosenberg, I., and Lind, J.: First mothers rooming-in with their newborns: its impact on the mother, Am. J. Orthopsychiatry **43**:783, 1973.

Hare, E.H., and others: Spina bifida cystica and family stress, Br. Med. J. **2**:757, 1966.

Harper, R.G., and others: Observations on unrestricted parental contact with infants in the neonatal intensive care unit, J. Pediatr. **89**:441, 1976.

Hersher, L., Richmond, J., and Moore, A.: Maternal behavior in sheep and goats, In Rheingold, H., editor: Maternal behavior in mammals, New York, 1963, John Wiley & Sons, Inc.

James, V.L., Jr., and Wheeler, W.E.: The care-by-parent unit, Pediatrics **43**:488, 1969.

Johns, N.: Family reactions to the birth of a child with a congenital abnormality, Med. J. Aust. **7**:277, 1960.

Kahn, E., Wayburne, S., and Fouche, M.: The Baragwanath premature baby unit—an analysis of the case records of 1000 consecutive admissions, S. Afr. Med. J. **28**:453, 1954.

Keller, W.D., Hildebrandt, K.A., and Richards, M.: Effects of extended father-infant contact during the newborn period, Infant Behav. Dev. **8**:337, 1985.

Kennell, J., and Rolnick, A.: Discussing problems in newborn babies with their parents, Pediatrics **27**:832, 1960.

Kennell, J.H., and others: Nesting in the human mother after mother-infant separation, Pediatr. Res. **7**:269, 1973.

Kennell, J.H., and others: Maternal behavior one year after early and extended post-partum contact, Dev. Med. Child Neurol. **16**:172, 1974.

Klaus, M., and Fanaroff, A.: Care of the high-risk neonate, Philadelphia, 1986, W.B. Saunders Co.

Klaus, M.H., and Kennell, J.H.: Parent-infant bonding, ed. 2, St. Louis, 1982, The C.V. Mosby Co.

Klaus, M.H., and others: Human maternal behavior at the first contact with her young, Pediatrics **46**:187, 1970.

Klaus, M.H., and others: Maternal attachment—importance of the first post-partum days, N. Engl. J. Med. **286**:460, 1972.

Klaus, M.H., and others: Effects of social support during parturition on maternal and infant morbidity, Br. Med. J. **293**:585, 1986.

Klopfer, P.: Mother love! What turns it on? Am. Sci. **49**:404, 1971.

Lamb, M.: The bonding phenomenon: misinterpretations and their implications, J. Pediatr. **101**:555, 1982.

Lang, R.: Birth book, Ben Lomond, Calif., 1972, Genesis Press.

Lind, J., Vuorenkoski, V., and Wasz-Hoeckert, O.: The effect of cry stimulus on the temperature of the lactating breast primipara: a thermagraphic study. In Morris, N., editor: Psychosomatic medicine in obstetrics and gynaecology, Basel, Switzerland, 1973, S. Karger.

MacFarlane, J.A.: Olfaction in the development of social preferences in the human neonate. In the parent-infant relationship, Ciba Foundation, Amsterdam, 1975, Elsevier Publishing Co.

MacFarlane, J.A., Smith, D.M., and Garrow, D.H.: The relationship between mother and neonate. In Kitzinger, S., and Davis, J.A., editors: The place of birth, New York, 1978, Oxford University Press.

Mason, E.A.: A method of predicting crisis outcome for mothers of premature babies, Public Health Rep. **78**:1031, 1963.

McBryde, A.: Compulsory rooming-in in the ward and private newborn service at Duke Hospital, JAMA **45**:625, 1951.

Meier, G.W.: Maternal behavior of fetal- and laboratory-reared monkeys following the surgical delivery of their infants, Nature **206**:492, 1965.

Michaels, J., and Shucman, H.: Observations on the psychodynamics of parents of retarded children, Am. J. Ment. Defic. **66**:568, 1962.

Minde, K., and others: Mother-child relationships in the premature nursery: an observational study, Pediatrics **61**:373, 1978.

Minde, K., and others: Self-help groups in a premature nursery—a controlled evaluation, J. Pediatr. **96**:933, 1980.

National Association for Mental Health Working Party: The birth of an abnormal child: telling the parents, Lancet **2**:1075, 1971.

Newman, L.F.: Parents' perceptions of their low birth weight infants, Paediatrician **9**:182, 1980.

Newton, N., and Newton, M.: Mother's reactions to their newborn babies, JAMA **181**:206, 1962.

O'Connor, S., and others: Reduced incidence of parenting inadequacy following rooming-in, Pediatrics **66**:176, 1980.

Olshansky, S.: Chronic sorrow: a response to having a mentally defective child, Soc. Casework, **43**:190, 1962.

Parke, R.: Father-infant interaction. In Klaus, M.H., Leger, T., and Trause, M.A., editors: Maternal attachment and mothering disorders: a round table, Sausalito, Calif., 1974, Johnson & Johnson Co.

Parke, R.D.: Perspectives on father-infant interaction. In Osofsky, J.D., editor: The handbook of infant development, New York, 1979, John Wiley & Sons, Inc.

Parke, R.D., and others: The father's role in the family system, Semin. Perinatol. **3**:25, 1979.

Parke, R.D., and others: Fathers and risk: a hospital based model of intervention. In Sawin, D.B., and others: editors: Psychosocial risks in infant-environment transactions, New York, 1980, Brunner/Mazel, Inc.

Raphael, D.: The tender gift: breastfeeding, Englewood Cliffs, N.J., 1973, Prentice-Hall, Inc.

Rappoport, L.: The state of crisis: some theoretical considerations. In Parad, H.J., editor: Crisis intervention, New York, 1965, Family Service Association.

Ringler, N.M., and others: Mother-to-child speech at two years: effects of early postnatal contacts, Behav. Pediatr. **86**:141, 1975.

Robson, K.: The role of eye-to-eye contact in maternal-infant attachment, J. Child Psychol. Psychiatry **8**:13, 1967.

Robson, K., and Kumar, R.: Delayed onset of maternal affection after childbirth, Br. J. Psychiatry **136**:347, 1980.

Rödholm, M.: Effects of father-infant postpartum contact on their interaction 3 months after birth, Early Hum. Dev. **5**:79, 1981.

Rödholm, M., and Larsson, K.: Father-infant interaction at the first contact after delivery, Early Hum. Dev. **3**:21, 1979.

Rödholm, M., and Larsson, K.: The behavior of human male adults at their first contact with a newborn (thesis), Goteborg, Sweden, 1980, University of Goteborg.

Rose, J., Boggs, T., Jr., and Alderstein, A.: The evidence for a syndrome of "mothering disability" consequent to threats to the survival of neonates: a design for hypothesis testing including prevention in a prospective study, Am. J. Dis. Child. **100**:776, 1960.

Roskies, E.: Abnormality and normality: the mothering of thalidomide children, New York, 1972, Cornell University Press.

Rubin, R.: Maternal touch, Nurs. Outlook, November 1963, p. 828.

Siegel, E., and others: Hospital and home support during infancy: impact on maternal attachment, child abuse and neglect, and health care utilization, Pediatrics **66**:183, 1980.

Solnit, A.J., and Stark, M.H.: Mourning and the birth of a defective child, Psychoanal. Study Child **16**:523, 1961.

Sosa, R., and others: The effect of a supportive companion on perinatal problems, length of labor, and mother-infant interaction, N. Engl. J. Med. **303**:597, 1980.

Spitz, R.: The first year of life, New York, 1965, International Universities Press.

Stern, D.: A micro-analysis of mother-infant interaction, J. Am. Acad. Child. Psychiatry **10**:510, 1971.

Trevarthen, C.: Descriptive analysis of infant communicative behavior. In Schaffer, H.R., editors: Studies in mother-infant interaction, New York, 1977, Academic Press, Inc.

Tronick, E.Z., editor: Social interchange in infancy affect, cognition and communication, Baltimore, 1982, University Park Press.

Waterman, J.H.: Psychogenic factors in parental acceptance of feebleminded children, Dis. Nerv. Syst. **9**:184, 1948.

Winnicott, D.W.: Playing and reality, London, 1971, Tavistock Publications, Ltd.

Winters, M.: The relationship of time of initial breastfeeding to success of breastfeeding (submitted nursing master's thesis), University of Washington, 1973.

Yarrow, L.J.: Maternal deprivation: toward an empirical and conceptual re-evaluation, Psychol. Bull. **58**:459, 1961.

Zuk, G.H.: Religious factor and the role of guilt in parental acceptance of the retarded child, Am. J. Ment. Defic. **64**:145, 1950.

CHAPTER 24

Routine and special care

PART ONE

Physical examination

The initial physical examination of the newborn should be done in the delivery room to detect significant anomalies, birth injuries, and cardiorespiratory disorders that may compromise a successful adaptation to extrauterine life. A more detailed examination should then take place in the nursery before parents are advised about their infant. The entire examination in the delivery room and nursery should be performed under a radiant heat source to prevent significant heat loss from the infant.

TRANSITION PERIOD

To detect disorders in adaptation soon after delivery, one must be aware of the normal features of the transitional stage. During labor there are a host of sensory inputs to the fetus, and at delivery a new set of stimuli influence fetal adaptation to the extrauterine environment. Both the intrapartum and the immediate neonatal events result in a sympathetic discharge that is reflected in changes in heart rate, color, respiration, motor activity, gastrointestinal function, and temperature of the infant.

During the late stages of labor, the infant's heart rate normally fluctuates with a certain degree of variability around a baseline of 120 to 140. After delivery there is a rapid increase in the heart rate to the range of 160 to 180, lasting 10 to 15 minutes, with a gradual fall by 30 minutes to a baseline rate of between 100 and 120. During the *first* 15 minutes of life, respirations are irregular; peak respiratory rates range between 60 and 80 per minute. During this period rales are also present on auscultation; grunting, flaring, and retractions may also be noted, and there may be brief periods of apnea. Coincident with these changes in heart rate and respiratory rate, the infant is alert and his behavior is marked by spontaneous startle reactions, gustatory movements, tremors, crying, and movements of the head from side to side. This characteristic exploratory behavior is accompanied by a decrease in body temperature and a generalized increase in motor activity with increase in muscle tone.

In healthy infants who have not been subjected to adverse factors during labor there are characteristic changes accompanying the normal adaptation to extrauterine existence. The initial period of reactivity, previously described, is followed by a period of unresponsiveness and a second period of reactivity. The initial period of reactivity generally lasts 15 to 30 minutes. The gastrointestinal manifestations of this initial period of reactivity include the appearance of bowel sounds, the passage of meconium, and the production of saliva, all a result of parasympathetic discharges occurring during this period. The duration of this first period of reactivity, although varying between 15 and 30 minutes in healthy infants, is prolonged in term infants who have had an abnormal labor or delivery and in sick infants and normal premature infants.

Following this first period of reactivity the infant either sleeps or has a marked decrease in motor activity. The heart rate falls into the range of 100 to 120, and the infant becomes relatively unresponsive. This period of unresponsiveness, frequently accompanied by sleep, lasts from 60 to 100 minutes and is followed by a second period of reactivity, which lasts from 10 minutes to several hours. Periods of tachycardia and tachypnea, associated with changes in tone, color, and mucus production, are noted. Meconium is frequently passed during the second period of time (Fig. 24-1). Foreknowledge of the normal changes occurring during the transitional period allows early recognition of the infant who is not making a normal extrauterine adaptation.

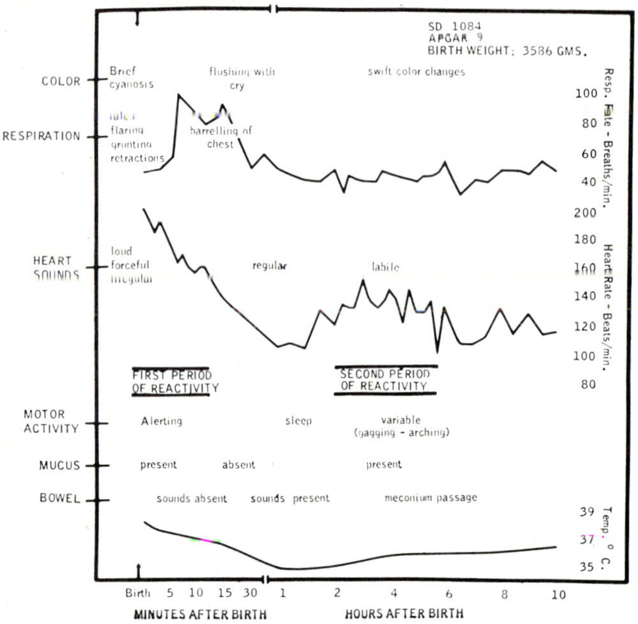

Fig. 24-1. Normal transition period. (From Desmond, M., Rudolph, A., and Phitakspharaiwan, P.: Pediatr. Clin. North Am. **13:**651, 1966.)

EXAMINATION IN THE DELIVERY ROOM

In the delivery room color is of immediate concern. Generalized cyanosis may indicate significant heart or lung disease or, rarely, the presence of methemoglobinemia. Differential cyanosis involving the lower extremities indicates persistence of a right-to-left shunt through the ductus, increased pulmonary vascular resistance, and, on occasion, a preductal coarctation (Chapter 29). Many normal infants have transient differential cyanosis that clears in the first minutes of life.

The pale infant either has been severely asphyxiated (asphyxia pallida) with the pallor caused by intense peripheral vasoconstriction or is severely anemic, secondary to acute blood loss from placenta previa, fetomaternal hemorrhage, or hemolysis from erythroblastosis fetalis (Chapters 5 and 32). An immediate decision regarding the cause is imperative if shock from acute blood loss is to be reversed by transfusion.

The meconium-stained infant should alert the examiner to the special risks of the acute or chronically asphyxiated infant (Chapter 22), who is often small for gestational age. Jaundice is seldom noted in the delivery room, even with severe erythroblastosis.

After determining the color of an infant, the examiner should evaluate the cardiopulmonary status. Initial inspection determines the respiratory rate. Tachypnea (a respiratory rate greater than 50 breaths per minute) should alert the examiner to possible pulmonary problems; bradypnea (less than 30 breaths per minute) or apnea or both should focus attention on the central nervous system and causes for central nervous system depression. Intercostal retractions, an audible grunt, and nasal flaring are additional signs of respiratory distress commonly present in the delivery room. Inspiratory or expiratory stridor should be noted and when present requires careful direct examination of the upper airway and magnification film of the airway if available.

Auscultation of the chest reveals the quality of breath sounds bilaterally, the presence or absence of rales, rhonchi, or expiratory wheezing, and the ease with which heart tones are heard. (Detailed examination of the cardiovascular system is covered in Chapter 29.) In the delivery room each infant's heart rate should be recorded as well as the quality of the heart tones; heart murmurs may be transient or may be indicative of significant heart disease. The absence, presence, and quality of peripheral pulses provide additional vital information.

The abdomen is inspected for protuberance, which may be secondary to abdominal masses, or concavity, which may be secondary to displacement of intestinal contents into the chest when there is a diaphragmatic hernia. Palpation and auscultation complete the initial examination of the abdomen. In the delivery room the relaxed muscle tone of the infant allows the best opportunity for abdominal examination; both kidneys should be palpated to exclude renal anomalies. The umbilical vessels should be counted to exclude the presence of a single umbilical artery, which correlates with an increased incidence of congenital anomalies.

The genitalia are examined to exclude the possibility of ambiguous genitalia before telling parents the sex of their infant (Chapter 37, part five).

The presence of significant choanal atresia should be excluded by manually occluding the mouth and each nostril and observing the infant for signs of respiratory distress or by passing a suction catheter through each naris into the stomach. The gastric contents should then be aspirated; the presence of more than 20 to 30 ml of gastric aspirate should raise the suspicion of upper intestinal obstruction. After the catheter has passed to a length that should be in the stomach, the instillation of 5 to 10 ml of air under direct gastric auscultation may be used to exclude the most common type of tracheoesophageal fistula. After exclusion of choanal atresia and upper intestinal anomalies, the same catheter can be used to establish the patency of the rectum.

The mental status and muscular tone of the infant should then be assessed. The neurologic examination is discussed in detail in Chapter 27 part one.

Before transfer of the infant from the delivery room, significant anomalies should be sought (for example, clubfeet, cleft lip or palate, or meningomyelocele).

EXAMINATION IN THE NURSERY

See also Chapter 17.

The initial examination should be followed by a more detailed evaluation within the first 12 hours of life. Measurements of head and chest circumference and length and recordings of temperature and heart and respiratory rate should be included.

Jaundice is the most likely change in skin color to be noted on subsequent examination. In addition, cyanosis and pallor should be reevaluated. The infant should also be carefully examined for the presence of hemangiomas, pigmented or depigmented nevi, and mongolian spots.

The skull should be checked for overlapping sutures, the patency of sutures, caput succedaneum with its poorly defined margins, and cephalhematoma with its clearly demarcated margins. The eyes should be examined (Chapter 39). Approximately 40% of all infants will have conjunctival or retinal hemorrhages noted in the initial examination. The presence of a red reflex should be established, pupil size and reaction to light recorded, and the lens checked for the presence of cataracts. The size of the globes should be examined for possible microphthalmia.

The face should be examined for evidence of disorders that may present with distinctive facies (for example, trisomies and cretinism) (Chapter 17). The symmetry of the face should be evaluated to exclude possible facial nerve injuries following traumatic deliveries or in infants delivered by forceps.

Malformation of the ears may provide evidence of associated renal anomalies but more often is familial and only of cosmetic concern. The presence or absence of cartilage aids in establishing gestational age.

With the use of both a finger and a light with good direct visualization, both the soft and hard palates should be checked to exclude a cleft palate. High-arched palates as isolated findings are generally of no significance. Epithelial inclusion cysts are frequently noted along the gum margins and are benign entities requiring only parental reassurance. The tongue should be an appropriate size for its cavity; an inappropriately large tongue should raise the suspicion of a hemangioma or lymphangioma. The large tongue of cretinism is accompanied by other stigmata. The association of macroglossia with Beckwith's syndrome and Pompe's disease (type II glycogen storage disease) is well established. In infants with micrognathia a normal tongue may seem large. The well-known association of micrognathia, glossoptosis, and cleft palate (Pierre Robin syndrome) often presents initially as an upper airway obstruction and later becomes a cosmetic problem (Chapter 17).

The skinfolds of the neck should be checked for webbing or fistulous openings associated with either branchial clefts or thyroglossal duct cysts. During examination of the neck, each clavicle should be palpated for possible fracture. An asymmetric Moro reflex will often confirm a suspicious clinical finding noted on palpation.

The chest is examined for its musculature, bony structure, and location of nipples. By feeling for the pectoralis major in the axilla, one excludes absence of this muscle. Pectus excavatum or carinatum is of genuine concern to parents but only rarely is of clinical or cosmetic significance. The areolar size provides additional evidence on the gestational age of each infant.

The lungs and heart are again examined, but with particular attention to questionable findings previously noted at birth, especially transient heart murmurs or adventitial sounds. Radial, brachial, and femoral pulses should all be palpated and compared. Poor or diminished quality of pulses is an indication of inadequate cardiac output, whatever the cause. Absent femoral pulses are associated with coarctation of the aorta; bounding femoral pulses may be equally grave indicators of congenital heart disease. If pulses are suspect, a blood pressure taken either by flush or by the Doppler technique (Chapter 21) should be recorded in the upper and lower extremities.

The abdominal examination is also repeated to exclude the presence of a mass. Examination of the genitalia provides additional evidence for establishing gestational age. Males should be checked for hypospadias, to determine the location of the testes, and to exclude either inguinal hernias or hydrocele, the latter being far more common. Most female infants have a mucoid vaginal discharge in the first week of life that occasionally becomes sanguinous secondary to hormonal withdrawal. Either a large penis or clitoris should raise the question of adrenogenital syndrome, and there should be appropriate evaluation to exclude or confirm the diagnosis with its life-threatening sequelae (Chapter 37, part five).

The extremities of each infant are examined for the presence of structural anomalies, such as congenital dislocation of hip, clubfeet, and neurologic disorders.

At the end of the initial examination in the delivery room or transitional or normal nursery, the gestational age of each infant should be estimated. There are four methods employed to assess gestational age: physical criteria, neurologic examination, combined physical and neurologic examination, and examination of the lens. Table 24-1 lists the physical criteria used to establish gestational age. The characteristics progress in an orderly fashion during gestation. Close examination of sole creases, breast nodule diameter, scalp hair, cartilage in the earlobe, and testes and scrotum provides a rough guide to age that becomes more exact when using neurologic assessment.

Although the physical criteria can be used to establish gestational age immediately following delivery, the neu-

Table 24-1. Estimation of gestational age

	Evaluation	Approximate week of gestation when findings appear								
		24	28	30	32	34	36	38	40	
	Head circumference in cm ±2 SD		**23 20.3**	**25-30.4**	**26.8-32.4**	**28.6-34**	**30.5-35.5**	**32-36.5**	**33-37**	**Based on 300 single live births—all Caucasian**
Clinical	Sole creases	Anterior transverse crease only →					Occasional creases anterior two thirds →		Sole covered with creases →	
Clinical	Breast nodule diameter	Not palpable—absent →					2 mm →	4 mm →	7 mm →	If small may represent fetal malnutrition
Clinical	Scalp hair	Fine and fuzzy → Hard to distinguish individual strands						Thick and silky → Appears as individual strands		
Clinical	Earlobe	Pliable—no cartilage →					Some cartilage →		Stiffened by thick cartilage →	
Clinical	Testes and scrotum	Testes in lower canal Scrotum small—few rugae →					Intermediate →	Testes pendulous, scrotum full, extensive rugae →		

From Behrman, R.E., Fisher, D., Paton, J.B., and Keller, J.: In utero disease and the newborn infant. In Schulman, I., editor: Advances in pediatrics, vol. 17, Chicago. Copyright © 1970 by Year Book Medical Publishers, Inc. Used by permission. (Modified from Amiel-Tison, Brett, Koenigsbergh, and Usher.)

rologic criteria used to determine gestational age require the infant to be in an alert, rested state. In some infants this may not occur during the initial or subsequent examinations on the first day; in many infants accurate assessment of gestational age by neurologic criteria is not possible until the second or third day of life. Infants who are asphyxiated at the time of delivery, have a primary neurologic disorder, or are transiently depressed related to maternal medication characteristically underscore during neurologic examination. For this reason neurologic assessment should not be done until the infant is fully recovered. The assessment of gestational age using neurologic criteria was originally described by the French school and simplified by Amiel Tison. The examination involves assessment of posture, passive and active tone, reflexes, and righting reactions (Chapter 26).

Using a system that combines the physical criteria and the neurologic assessment of gestational age, Dubowitz described and developed a combined scoring system. The scores from the physical and neurologic assessment are combined to give each infant a total score. The gestational age of the infant is calculated using the scores from the examination. The disadvantage of the Dubowitz scoring system is that it involves the assessment of 11 physical criteria and 10 neurologic findings. Although the physical criteria allow clear distinction of infants with varying gestational ages greater than 34 weeks, neurologic criteria are essential to differentiate infants between 26 and 34 weeks where the physical changes are less evident. Ballard and her colleagues abbreviated the Dubowitz scoring system to include six neurologic and seven physical criteria. These criteria are listed in Fig. 24-2. The accuracy and reliability of the abbreviated Ballard scoring system have been confirmed. The assessment can be performed in a significantly shorter period of time and thus facilitates accurate gestational age assessment, particularly of sick infants.

No matter what method of assessing gestational age is used, the infants should be examined in an optimum state of alertness and with strict adherence to the directions described by the original authors. Regardless of the method used, the assessment of gestational age using physical and neurologic criteria is accurate to ±2 weeks.

Hittner used the orderly disappearance of the anterior vascular capsule of the lens as a means of accurately assessing gestational age in premature infants between 26 and 34 weeks of gestation. She arbitrarily divided the disappearance of the anterior vascular capsule into four grades (Fig. 24-3). Examination requires observation with a direct ophthalmoscope following dilation of the pupils. The examination should be done within the first 24 to 48 hours, since the vascular system changes rapidly

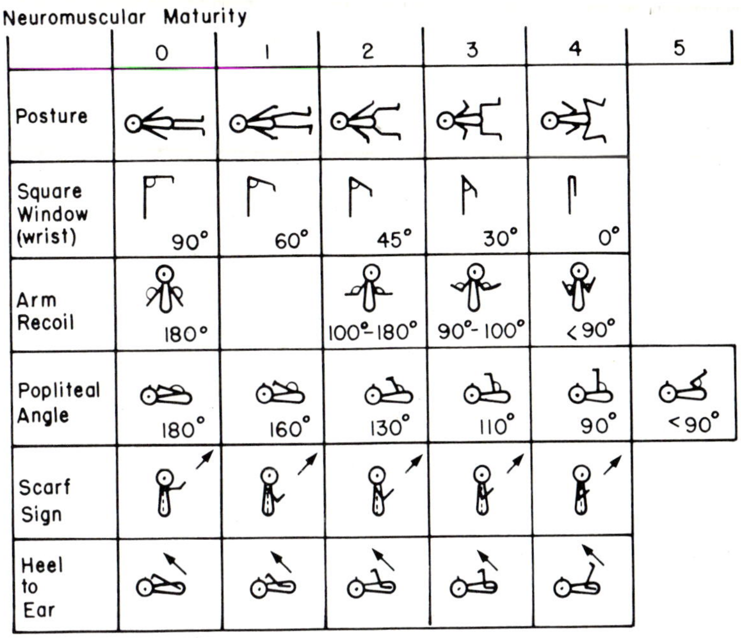

Apgars 1 min 5 min

Age at Exam hrs

Race Sex

B.D.

LMP

EDC

Gest. age by Dates wks

Gest. age by Exam wks

B.W. gm. %ile

Length cm. %ile

Head Circum. cm. %ile

Clin. Dist. None Mild

Mod. Severe

PHYSICAL MATURITY

Skin	gelatinous red, trans-parent	smooth pink, vis-ible veins	superficial peeling &/or rash few veins	cracking pale area rare veins	parchment deep cracking no vessels	leathery cracked wrinkled
Lanugo	none	abundant	thinning	bald areas	mostly bald	
Plantar Creases	no crease	faint red marks	anterior transverse crease only	creases ant. 2/3	creases cover entire sole	
Breast	barely percept.	flat areola no bud	stippled areola 1–2 mm bud	raised areola 3–4 mm bud	full areola 5–10 mm bud	
Ear	pinna flat, stays folded	sl. curved pinna; soft with slow recoil	well-curv. pinna; soft but ready recoil	formed & firm with instant recoil	thick cartilage ear stiff	
Genitals ♂	scrotum empty no rugae		testes descend-ing, few rugae	testes down good rugae	testes pendulous deep rugae	
Genitals ♀	prominent clitoris & labia minora		majora & minora equally prominent	majora large minora small	clitoris & minora completely covered	

MATURITY RATING

Score	Wks
5	26
10	28
15	30
20	32
25	34
30	36
35	38
40	40
45	42
50	44

Fig. 24-2. Assessment of gestational age using the Ballard method. (From Ballard, J.L., Novak, K.Z., and Driver, M.: J. Pediatr. **95:**769, 1979.)

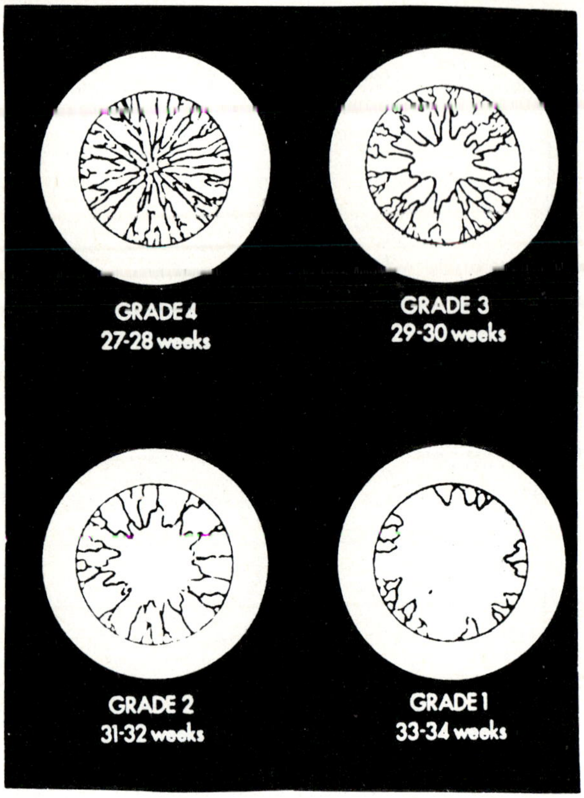

Fig. 24-3. Assessment of gestational age by examination of anterior vascular capsule of lens. (From Hittner, H.M., Hirsch, N.J., and Rudolph, A.J.: J. Pediatr. **91**:455, 1977.)

within the first several days. Using this method the correlation between gestational age and the vascularity is highly significant.

After completion of the gestational assessment and physical examination, the parents of the new infant should be advised as to the infant's general health. After the initial examination, the infant should be examined every 3 days during hospitalization. All infants should be examined within 24 hours of discharge.

John M. Driscoll, Jr.

BIBLIOGRAPHY

American Academy of Pediatrics and the American College of Obstetricians and Gynecologists: Guidelines for perinatal care, Evanston, Ill., 1983, The Academy.

Ballard, J.L., Novak, K.Z., and Driver, M.: A simplified score for assessment of fetal maturation of newly born infants, J. Pediatr. **95**:769, 1979.

Behrman, R.E., and others: In utero disease and the newborn infant, vol. 17, Advances in Pediatrics, Chicago, 1970, Year Book Medical Publishers, Inc.

Desmond, M., Rudolph, A., and Phitakspharaiwan, P.: The transitional care nursery, Pediatr. Clin. North Am. **13**:651, 1966.

Dubowitz, L., Dubowitz, V., and Goldberg, C.: Clinical assessment of gestational age in the newborn infant, J. Pediatr. **77**:1, 1970.

Hittner, H.M., Hirsch, N.J., and Rudolph, A.J.: Assessment of gestational age by examination of the anterior vascular capsule of the lens, J. Pediatr. **91**:455, 1977.

PART TWO

Physical environment

THE THERMAL ENVIRONMENT

Temperature and survival

Babies are protected against excessive heat loss because of published evidence demonstrating that such protection (1) improves their chances for survival (Table 24-2), (2) reduces their need to perform heat-producing metabolic work, and (3) eliminates dealing with the problems associated with the rewarming of an infant who becomes hypothermic. In 1957 Silverman and Blanc reported that premature infants housed in incubators humidified to more than 80% had higher survival rates than babies housed in incubators humidified to less than 60%. The conclusion that these results were related to thermal differences was reinforced in 1958, when Silverman reported that babies housed in humidified convectively heated incubators survived at a greater rate when the air temperature was controlled to 32° C as compared to 29° C. Premature sick infants largely contributed to the significant differences in mortality noted in these and subsequent studies. The degree to which thermal conditions affect the survival of full-term infants remains unknown.

In 1963 Agate and Silverman described an enclosed incubator warmed by a radiant heater controlled in servoresponse to the infant's skin temperature. The incubator control ensured that the infant had normal and stable body temperatures. Design of the incubator included an appreciation of the importance of radiant heat losses in simple convectively heated incubators (Fig. 24-4). The new incubator was used to compare survival rates of premature infants with similar skin temperatures but housed in two contrasting humidity settings. The results indicated that enhanced survival could not be credited to the nonthermal use of high humidity in an enclosed radiantly heated incubator. This report has been misinterpreted as providing proof that incubator environments do not have to be humidified but the results did not negate the earlier evidence that humidity may be important when warming infants in convectively heated incubators.

Subsequent studies demonstrated a thermal advantage for neonates housed in radiantly versus convectively heated enclosed incubators. Nonetheless, because of difficulties encountered in the fabrication of radiantly heated incubators, radiant heaters were replaced by convective heaters in the design of incubators for commercial distribution. Although elimination of the radiant heater did not compromise skin temperature stability, it did result in the production of an environment different from that produced in the radiantly heated incubator. In the radiantly heated enclosed incubator, the air temperature

Table 24-2. Mortality of premature infants maintained in environments providing more or less protection against heat loss

	More		Less	
	Number	Died (%)	Number	Died (%)
Silverman and co-workers (1985)	91	16	91	32
Beutow and co-workers (1964)	89	42	69	54
Day and co-workers (1964)	60	23	65	37
Perlstein and co-workers (1976)	105	22	105	35
Totals	345	26	330	40

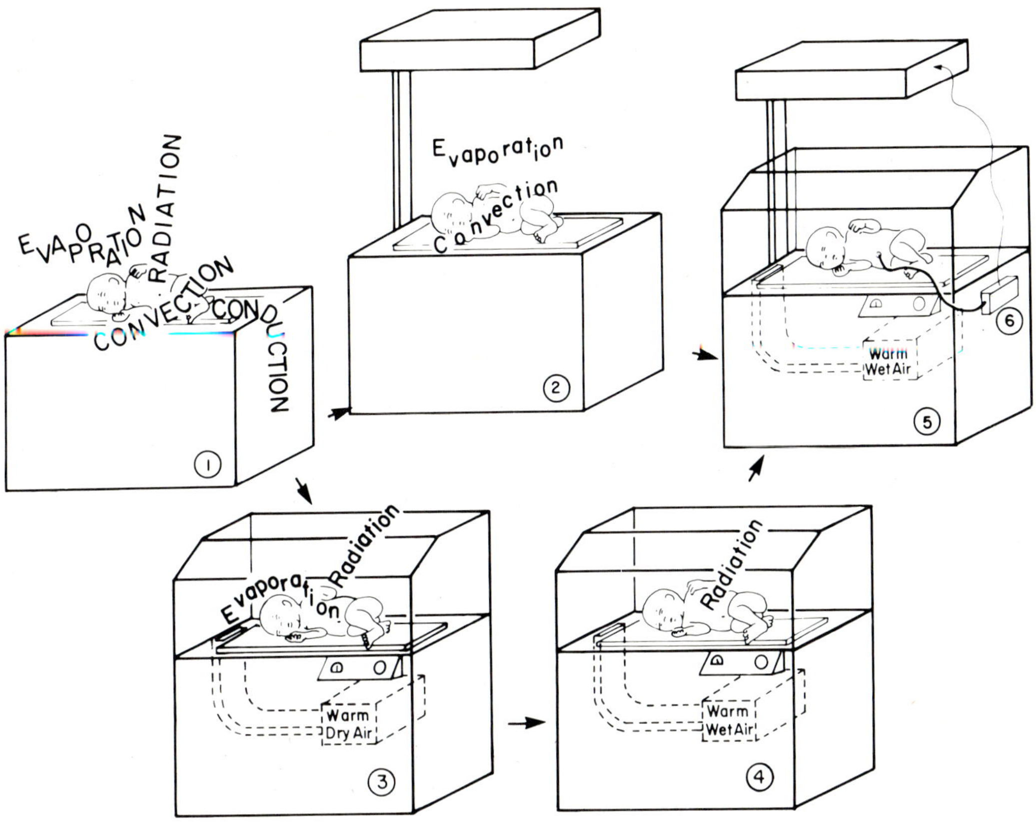

Fig. 24-4. Logic leading to development of skin servocontrolled radiantly heated convectively ventilated incubator. *1,* An unprotected baby loses body heat from skin surfaces by conduction, convection, evaporation, and radiation. *2,* A radiant heater eliminates radiant and conductive losses but not those caused by convection and evaporation. *3,* An unhumidified convectively heated incubator eliminates convective and conductive losses but not those caused by radiation and evaporation. *4,* Humidifying a convectively heated incubator eliminates all major heat losses except for the losses by radiation. *5,* Using a radiant heater to warm a convectively ventilated and humidified incubator should eliminate all sources of heat loss from the infant's skin. *6,* Normal infant temperature can be ensured by adding a controller to the incubator so that power is delivered to the radiant heater whenever the infant's skin temperature falls below a preset value.

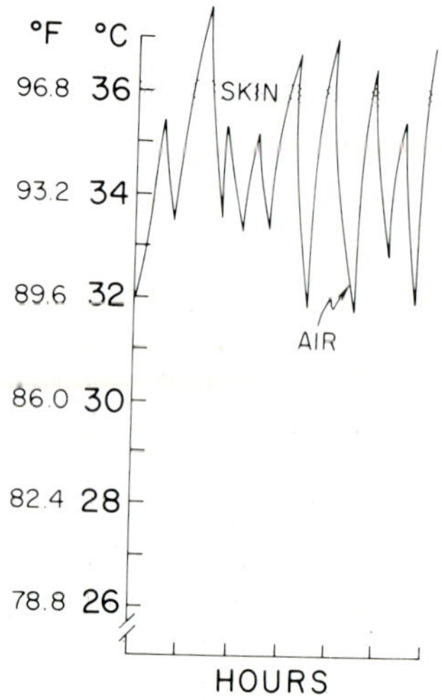

Fig. 24-5. Typical air temperatures in convectively heated incubator, servocontrolled to maintain infant's skin temperature at 36° C.

was stable, whereas in the convectively heated servocontrolled incubator air temperatures can vary over short periods by 3° to 4° C and after severe disruptions by as much as 5° to 10° C (Fig. 24-5). These rapid excursions in temperature have been correlated with apneic spells in some premature infants.

In 1976 Perlstein and associates reported improved survival of babies housed in computer-controlled incubators constrained to prevent wide thermal change in the environment. The stable thermal environment created by the computer-controlled system is similar to the environment created in the earlier radiantly heated enclosed incubators. The systems do differ in many details, however. For example, while stabilizing the environmental temperature, the computer-controlled system uses logic that allows skin temperature to vary freely within the range of 35.5° and 37° C. In contrast, the simpler radiantly heated system assumed abnormality if the infant's skin temperature varied by more than ±0.2° C. In any case, although documented to enhance survival, neither the radiantly heated nor the computer-controlled incubator systems are commercially available. Of the commercially available incubator systems, none has been documented to improve infant survival when compared with other available systems.

Temperature and homeothermy

As a rule, babies are treated as homeotherms who attempt to maintain their body temperatures within some narrow range. They respond to heat loss by generating more heat. The consequences of prolonged and maximum heat production include the conversion of life-sustaining substrates to acidic metabolic by-products (Fig. 24-6).

Infants are alerted to cold stress when thermal receptors in the skin are stimulated. The face is particularly sensitive, and even when the baby's body is warm, cooling of the face will cause a responsive rise in metabolic rate. Conversely, warming of the facial skin when the body is cold suppresses homeothermically induced hypermetabolism.

Measurement of body temperature alone is of limited value in assessing the probable metabolic state of an infant. An infant with a specific body temperature will become hypermetabolic if the environmental temperature drops sufficiently below the skin temperature to cause a rate of heat loss exceeding the rate of heat generated by the infant's basal metabolic activity. Even with a low body temperature, however, if the environmental temperature is rising or is close enough to the skin temperature to limit heat loss to a rate not exceeding the rate of basal heat production, a baby will not become hypermetabolic. High body temperatures also activate distress mechanisms that require an increase in metabolic work.

An infant can limit heat loss by changes in body posture that reduce the skin surface area exposed to the environment. This capability is compromised in premature, unconscious, sedated, and physically restrained babies. Infants also can reduce shunting of internal heat to body surfaces by vasoconstricting peripheral vessels. This mechanism can be defeated in shock and by some autonomic drugs (Fig. 24-6). An infant may generate heat by crying and becoming hyperactive when cold stressed to the point of jitteriness, although shivering does not appear to occur.

A cold-stressed baby primarily depends on mechanisms that cause chemical thermogenesis. When stimulated by cold, norepinephrine and thyroid hormones are released, inducing lipolysis in brown fat stores principally found in the interscapular, paraspinal, and perirenal areas. Although not all of the chemical pathways are known, triglycerides in the fat are broken down to fatty acids and glycerol. The former enter thermogenic metabolic paths that end in the common pool of metabolic acids. Glycolysis may be stimulated during severe stress when epinephrine, released from the adrenals, activates glycogen stores and may result in transient hyperglycemia. Lowered blood sugars have also been reported by Cornblath in cold-stressed infants, possibly due to inhibition of glycolysis by lipolysis or to exhaustion of glycogen stores.

The absolute maximum or "summit" amount of heat production is affected by gestational and postnatal age and is demonstrably less during the first days of life. An infant not exposed to periodic cold stress may adapt to the protective environment and lose the ability to respond homeothermically when exposed to an unfamiliar cold stimulus.

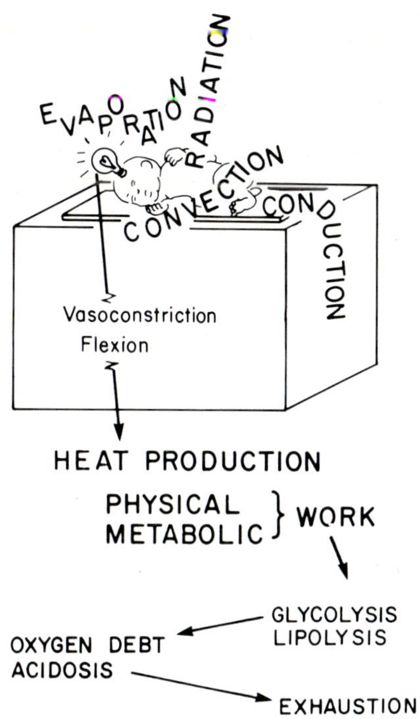

Fig. 24-6. Schematic of homeothermy in newborns. On sensing loss of body heat, the infant minimizes heat loss from the skin and increases metabolic rate. The increase in metabolism can produce acidosis and substrate depletion.

Central nervous system damage, sedation, shock, hypoxia, and drugs may all reduce the metabolic response to cold. This may represent a direct antimetabolic effect or be caused by a blunting of the sensory mechanisms that alert the intact baby to the stress stimuli. After prolonged stress, depletion of hormonal and energy stores may reduce the ability to further respond.

The concept of an optimum thermal environment for newborn babies evolved during the 1960s. This idealized setting, called the *neutral thermal environment*, is one in which a baby can maintain a normal body temperature while producing only the minimum amount of heat generated from basal life-sustaining metabolic processes. Maintenance of neutral thermal conditions is considered to be of greatest importance in the youngest, most immature infants, whose ability to generate additional heat in a heat-losing environment may be minimal. The ability to increase metabolic rate in these infants may be further hampered by impaired gas exchange in the lungs and/or restriction of caloric intake.

The physics of heat exchange

The temperature of an object is a measure of the balance between heat leaving and entering the object. Heat can only be lost from a substance that is warmer to one that is cooler. A baby, therefore, will lose heat only when the surrounding environment is colder than the infant. The rate of heat loss is directly proportional to the magnitude of the difference between the infant's skin temperature and the temperature of the environment. This proportionality can be expressed mathematically by introducing a constant called the thermal transfer coefficient (h), the value of which depends on the material of the substance transferring the heat:

Heat loss = h (Skin temperature − Environmental temperature) × (Surface area)

The exposed surface area of the infant is critical in the equation used to calculate heat loss. Thus a baby that is diapered or swaddled has less exposed surface than an unclothed infant.

The thermal transfer coefficient describes the rate at which heat leaves the body surface and is related to body shape, thickness of the boundary layer of air surrounding the body, and the characteristic way in which tissue absorbs or reflects radiant energy. Heat loss is also modified by the thermal conductance of an infant. The thermal conductance is computed using the difference between the baby's core and skin temperatures multiplied by a thermal coefficient describing the speed with which heat is transferred from the inferior to the exterior of the body. This variable coefficient depends on body size, tissue composition and thickness, skin blood flow, and vascular shunting.

The differences between body shapes and sizes and tissue thickness result in babies having thermal conduction and transfer coefficients that are much higher than in adults. Because of this difference in coefficients, babies lose more heat than adults in identical heat-losing environments.

Definition of normal body temperature

Silverman and Agate in 1964 defined body temperature as a weighted value in which a colonic measurement contributed 60% and a skin measurement 40%. For practical purposes, however, it is traditional to rely on a single-site measurement. There is no reason to believe that infants have a different normal temperature than adults. If an infant's internal temperature is within the range of 35.5° to 37.5° C, with a ±0.5° C diurnal variation, the infant's temperature can be considered normal. Since body temperature is a measure only of the balance between heat production and net heat loss, a normal body temperature should not be confused with a "normal" metabolic rate (Fig. 24-7).

Internal body temperature measurements

Although esophageal and tympanic membrane temperatures have been used in some physiologic studies, it is easier and traditional in a clinical setting to equate rectal temperature with the baby's internal body temperature.

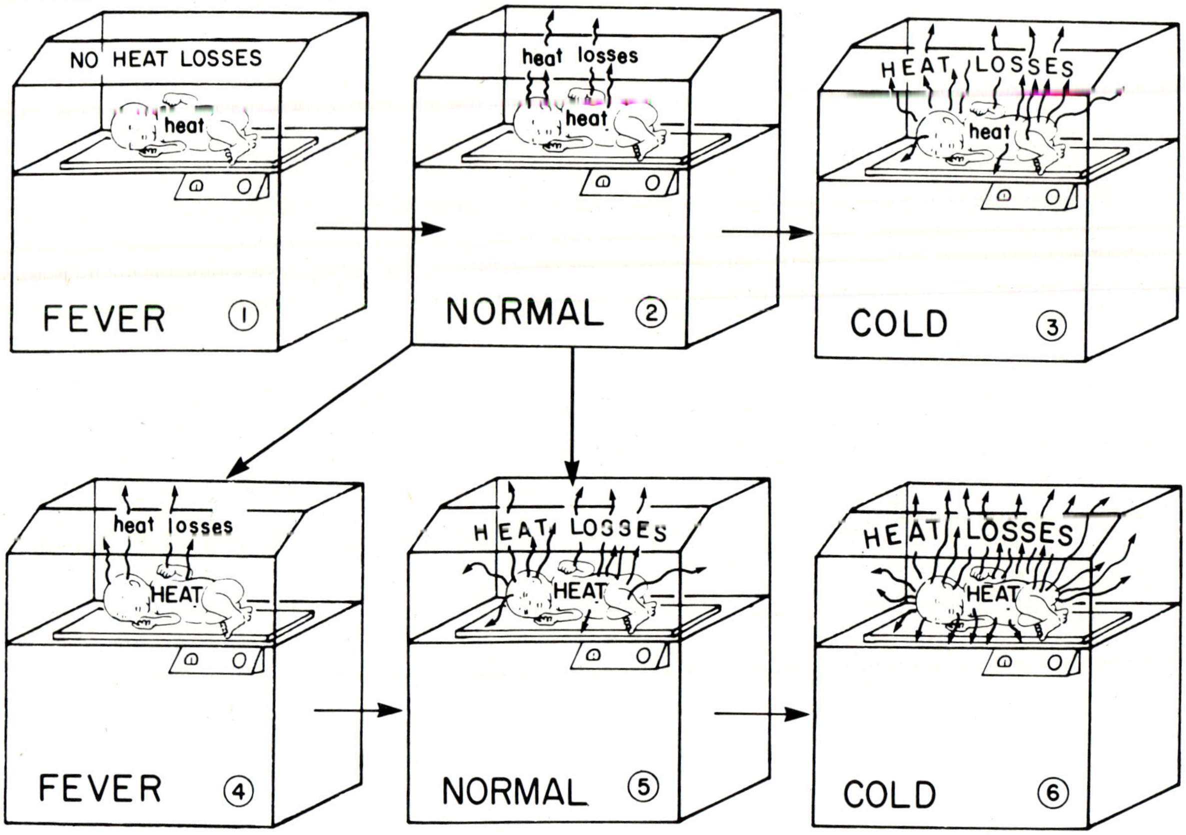

Fig. 24-7. *1,* Fever caused by total elimination of heat losses from minimally metabolic baby. *2,* Normal temperature when heat losses are minimized and equal to heat produced by minimally metabolic baby (neutral thermal conditions). *3,* Hypothermia caused by large heat losses from baby who is temporarily poikilothermic. *4,* "Fever" when heat losses are less than heat produced by hypermetabolic baby. *5,* Normal temperature when heat losses are large but equal to heat produced by hypermetabolic infant. *6,* Hypothermia caused by very large heat losses that exceed the heat produced by a hypermetabolic infant.
heat = minimal heat production.
HEAT = maximal heat production.
FEVER = internal temperature of more than 37.5° C.
NORMAL = internal temperature of 35.5° to 37.5° C.
COLD = internal temperature less than 35.5° C.

In measuring the rectal temperatures of newborn babies, the depth of insertion of the thermometer is very important. Karlberg documented that the difference between rectal temperature measured by a thermistor inserted 1 cm and then 5 cm into the rectum can exceed 1.5° C. Serial readings should be taken at a common depth. Thermometers used for temperature transduction in babies ideally should be accurate to ±0.1° C and have a range that spans 33° to 40° C.

Over the years some concern has been expressed about the danger of perforation or other injury when using rigid thermometers or thermistors to transduce rectal temperatures. Measurement of axillary temperature has been suggested as a safer alternative. Although axillary temperatures have been found variably comparable to simultaneous measurements of rectal temperature, both Torrance and Mayfield demonstrated that, if care is taken to place a thermometer firmly in the axilla with the infant's arm held against the body of the baby, accurate and comparable temperature readings can be obtained if a sufficient period of time is allowed for the transducer to reach its maximum reading.

Skin temperature measurements

Skin temperature is usually measured with thermocouples or thermistors attached to the skin. These three-dimensional temperature transducers sense the temperatures of their tops, sides, and bottoms. They are affected by the temperature of the transducing element and by the temperature of the wires used to connect the element

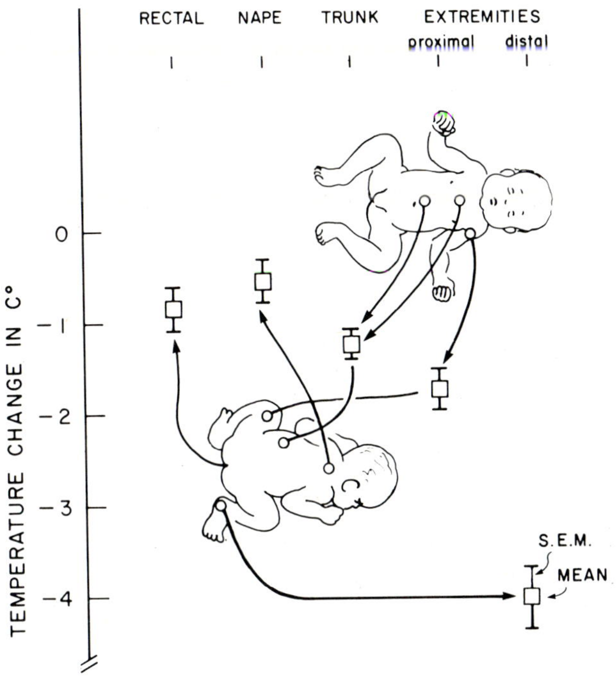

Fig. 24-8. Cooling of skin over different body surfaces after heat-losing exposure. Skin temperature changes measured in 16 infants of varying weights, gestations, and postnatal ages. Infants were exposed naked for 1 hour to room temperatures ranging between 23° and 29° C. (Modified from Silverman, W.A., and others: Pediatrics 33:984, 1964. Copyright American Academy of Pediatrics 1964.)

to an electronic thermometer. They actually transduce both skin temperature *and* environmental temperature. The relative contribution of each of these thermal sources to the final numerical readout of skin temperature is a function of the construction, insulation, location, and mode of attachment of the transducer. The attachment of a skin sensor also produces compression of underlying vessels, further causing a distortion of the true skin temperature value.

There is a very wide distribution of different temperatures over varying skin surface sites. These variations make interpretation of a single skin temperature difficult. It has been suggested that, when only a single skin temperature is to be sensed, the transducer be attached to the skin over the liver or between the umbilicus and the pubis. In a clinical setting, however, attachment sites sometimes need to be changed to prevent skin irritation. In addition, the rotation of babies into various positions requires attachment sites to be altered so that the infant's body does not cover the probe and cause a measurement of mattress instead of skin temperature.

In practice it is common to move single skin probes freely so that they are always on a skin surface exposed to the environment. In search of a "mean" surface temperature, the transducers are usually not attached over the least and most vasoreactive body regions. Bony prominences and the extremities, therefore, are the least favored attachment sites. It is also sensible to avoid placing probes on the skin overlying the metabolically reactive brown fat collections in the interscapular region (Fig. 24-8). Additionally, attachment near heat-producing transcutaneous gas-monitoring transducers or over areas of bruised or burned skin will result in false temperature measurements.

Environmental temperature measurements

The environment in which an object resides is defined as everything that surrounds the object. The components of the environment can be idealized by discussing the four simple mechanisms by which most heat is lost from the body: conduction, convection, radiation, and evaporation. This idealization is a useful way to emphasize the near independence of each of these mechanisms and the mistake in considering "air temperature" as a synonym for "environmental temperature." In fact, it has been suggested that an actual measurement of the true environmental temperature probably can only be idealized, and to avoid the implication of greater precision in this context the word "environment" should be modified to "operative environment."

Conductive and convective heat losses

Conduction is a term that describes the transfer of heat between contacting solid objects of different temperatures.

In ordinary circumstances, heat losses by conduction can be kept to a minimum by ensuring that an infant is lying on a warm mattress of very low conductivity, or if swaddled, that the infant is wrapped in prewarmed materials. If the mattress and swaddling materials are at the same temperature as the baby's skin, no heat loss or gain will occur by conduction. If, however, the baby is placed on a cold table or wrapped in a blanket at room temperature, these heat losses can become tremendous. Conversely, if placed close to a hot water bottle or heating pad that is warmer than the infant, the baby will gain heat at a rate directly proportional to the temperature difference between the conductive heat source and the baby's skin, and overheating may result.

Convection can be thought of as a special subset of conduction, referring to heat exchange between the dense material of a solid object and the solid but less dense material in the gaseous environment. Convective temperatures are usually equated with the simple measure of air temperature. Convective heat losses, however, are increased not only when the air cools but also with higher rates of airflow. The air temperature in an enclosed incubator must be thought of in terms of both its absolute value and the way this value is modified by an association wind chill factor introduced by a circulating fan.

The measured air temperature should be that perceived by the infant. Thus, ideally, the air temperature immediately adjacent to the infant's skin surface should be the temperature transduced. Measurement of air temperatures elsewhere in an incubator can introduce an error of up to 10° C, which is the span of temperature values that can coexist within an incubator chamber. Sometimes it is necessary to monitor multiple air temperatures influencing heat exchange over different body surfaces. When a baby is in a head hood flushed by air or oxygen, both incubator chamber and head hood temperature measurements are needed. Traditionally, convective losses were considered only as a heat transfer from the skin surfaces into the surrounding air, but consideration also must be given to heat exchanges that occur between the respiratory system and cooler gases delivered by respirators.

Radiant heat losses

Heat loss by radiation is heat loss at the speed of light. It is heat loss from a warmer object to a cooler one with which the warmer object is not in contact. Objects can be characterized by their ability to absorb or emit energy in the infrared range of the electromagnetic spectrum. The degree to which infrared rays are absorbed or emitted is called the emissivity of an object and can range from near 0 for a perfectly reflecting substance such as shiny silver to the value of almost 1 for a substance that, like carbon black, absorbs and reemits all infrared energy received. Human skin is more like carbon than silver and for practical purposes is considered to have an emissivity of 1. Emissivity is related more to the tissue's moisture content, texture, and porosity than to its color.

Walls, windows, chairs, light bulbs, and other people are examples of surfaces with which babies exchange radiant heat. This route of heat exchange is essentially independent of all other routes. A baby can get cold in a room containing air warmer than the infant's skin if the walls and windows are sufficiently cold. A baby in the warm air of an incubator can get cold if the incubator walls are cold, and a baby in an incubator with cold air can get overheated if the walls are too hot.

Because of the radiant "greenhouse" effect, a baby in an incubator can get too hot even if the incubator walls are not subjected to any obvious heating. Because the acrylic plastic walls of most incubators are opaque to infrared waves, they behave like the glass in a greenhouse, through which visible short-wave light rays pass easily. On absorption of the short electromagnetic waves by the housed plants, the short waves are converted into heat energy and reemitted as long infrared rays that, upon reaching the glass inner surface, are absorbed and not transmitted. The glass is heated by the infrared energy, and this energy is reemitted toward the plants. In this way visible light can be used to generate heat, which is trapped in the greenhouse whose contents become warmer.

It is not uncommon to find babies in incubators near windows become cold in the evening when incubator walls radiate their heat to the night-chilled glass panes. The same infants can be found febrile in the morning when the bright sun streams through glass and plastic to warm the incubator occupant. Such environmental changes can occur without causing changes in incubator air temperature.

To define environmental temperature requires at least a measurement of surrounding wall temperatures with which the baby lives in radiant harmony. Since radiant exchanges are quantitatively related not only to absolute temperature gradiants but also to the distance between the surfaces exchanging heat, to the angles subtended by electromagnetic rays traveling from one surface to the other, and to the emissivities of each of the radiant surfaces, no single measurement can provide any but a gross approximation of a baby's radiant world. When an infant is within the chamber of an enclosed incubator, however, the measurements are greatly simplified and the approximations more believable than those made when an infant is in an open crib.

Evaporative heat losses

With every milliliter of water that evaporates, approximately 0.58 Cal of body heat are lost. It is therefore theoretically possible to use insensible weight loss measurements to estimate the amount of heat that an infant has lost by this mechanism. Since accurate and continuous insensible weight loss measurements are somewhat difficult to obtain, this form of monitoring is reserved for research purposes.

To understand heat loss by evaporation is to appreciate the distinction that exists between humidity and vapor pressure. The vapor pressure of water is the specific atmospheric pressure of water vapor at any given temperature at which water can exist in both its liquid and vaporous states. The partial pressure of water vapor is the actual pressure being exerted by water vapor at any given temperature. If the partial pressure equals the vapor pressure, the vapor is saturated. If the partial pressure is less than the vapor pressure, the vapor is unsaturated. Relative humidity is a percentage expression of this degree of saturation and is computed using the following relationship:

$$\text{Relative humidity (\%)} = 100 \times \frac{\text{Partial pressure of water vapor}}{\text{Vapor pressure at same temperature}}$$

Although relative humidity is easy to quantitate, it is not the relative humidity but the difference between the partial pressure of the water vapor in the boundary layers around the baby's body and the vapor pressure of water in the environment outside this boundary layer that actually sets up the driving force causing evaporative water losses. The vapor pressure rises with higher temperature. Therefore, as long as the baby's skin is warmer than the environment, evaporative losses can occur even when the humidity is 100%.

How to keep a baby warm

Prevention of heat loss is often best achieved by simple methods applied with the knowledge born from common sense. Since heat loss requires the presence of a thermal gradient, it is important to avoid exposing the baby to a cold environment by either warming the environment or covering the baby.

The delivery room

In utero a fetus is warmer than the mother. Born wet, warm, and naked into the usual environment of a delivery room, the newborn infant loses heat rapidly. Even if the oxygen consumption of a homeothermic infant increases to the maximum summit of 15 ml/kg/minute, the 0.075 Cal/kg/minute of heat produced is still two or three times less than the approximate rate of loss of 0.2 Cal/kg/minute. The consequences of this heat loss depend on many factors, including the general condition of the baby at birth. Gandy and associates in 1964 reported that poorly protected infants tend to have a metabolic acidosis mixed with a compensatory respiratory alkalosis. Based on various methods used to protect infants, it would appear that elimination of heat loss in a clinical setting can be effective but is seldom complete (Table 24-3).

In the delivery room a large proportion of heat loss is caused by evaporation. The skin should be dried with warm towels and evaporative losses severely limited using plastic bags or other swaddling materials to insulate the skin from the dry room air. Attention should be directed toward drying the head and face, since a brief clean-up with a dry towel in the delivery room may prevent the subsequent cold exposure that accompanies a prolonged cosmetic cleansing bath in the nursery. Even with the most careful drying of the newborn, it is almost impossible to completely dry the hair. To keep the head warm it is necessary to use caps or hooded blankets.

The resuscitation of a newborn should not be allowed to interfere with thermal protection. If, during resuscitation, access is needed to some body surface, then only that body surface and no other should be exposed. If the umbilicus is to be tied or cannulated, there is no need to unswaddle the infant's head, arms, chest, or legs. Closed cardiac chest massage can be performed without exposing the lower half of the body. Only one leg requires exposure when applying an identification band to an ankle, when taking an identifying footprint, or for that matter when starting an intravenous infusion in the extremity. It is reasonable to back up the protection of swaddling by using a radiant heater to add extra warmth to the area assigned for infant care in the delivery room. Radiant heaters in the delivery room can provide excellent protection that is almost equal to that provided by careful swaddling, and when used together the protection can be superb (Table 24-3).

The control over heat loss must not be loosened during the transfer of a baby from the delivery room to another care area. Even within the delivery room, the baby

Table 24-3. Postnatal temperature fall within 30 minutes with various methods of limiting heat loss

Method	Source of data	30-Minute temperature (°C)*	30-Minute fall in temperature (°C)†
Infant placed in crib 30-40 cm under 60 W bulb covered with warm blanket; later dressed and put in incubator	Miller and Oliver	35.5 ± 0.16	2.6
Infant placed in preheated crib, covered loosely with warm blanket, and then bathed, dressed, and swaddled	Miller and Oliver	35.6 ± 0.14	2.5
Infant swaddled in warm, dry towel	Baum and Scopes	36.1 ± 0.59	2.0
Infant dried, placed in incubator (procedures through portholes)	Miller and Oliver	36.2 ± 0.15	1.9
Naked baby, 80 cm under 750 W radiant heater	Besch and associates	36.2 ± 0.10	1.9
Transparent swaddler without heat shield	Besch and associates	36.2 ± 0.11	1.9
Naked baby, 64 cm under 400 W radiant heater	Du and Oliver	36.4 ± 0.16	1.7
Silver swaddler	Baum and Scopes	36.6 ± 0.61	1.5
Transparent swaddler with head shield	Besch and associates	36.9 ± 0.09	1.2
Transparent swaddler with head shield and 750 W radiant heater at 80 cm	Besch and associates	37.3 ± 0.11	0.8

Modified from Besch, N.J., and others: N. Engl. J. Med. **284**:125, 1971.
*Mean ± SE.
†From fetal intrauterine temperature of 38.1° C.

should remain swaddled when carried to a weighing scale or for display to the parents. Weighing scales should be placed under a radiant heater, and if the mother desires skin-to-skin contact with her baby, they should be "swaddled" together under warm blankets.

The nursery

As nicely discussed by Hey (1971), swaddling may be ancient but it is not archaic. In fact, it is the simplest and most effective method for keeping babies warm who do not need to be unclothed for procedures or observation. Infants who are swaddled while lying in an open cot can be maintained in cooler ambient environments and can tolerate wider variations in environmental temperatures than can infants who are naked and in a warming device (see Fig. 24-11). Nonetheless, if swaddling is to be discontinued either in the delivery room or nursery, then alternatives to swaddling must be considered. These alternatives can be reduced to three common choices:

1. Warm up the room.
2. Place the baby in a warm enclosed incubator.
3. Place the baby under an open radiant heater.

The warm room. Heating a room to the 36° to 37° C needed to keep some small and sick babies warm may distress personnel working in the nursery. These conditions also may be unfavorable for larger and healthier infants in the same area. For long-term care, heating and humidifying nurseries to appropriate temperatures is probably the least desirable method for limiting heat losses from infants, although in short-term situations such as in radiology departments, operating rooms, and treatment rooms this method of protection can be the most applicable and effective. Raising the room temperature to meet the needs of a small baby is an important responsibility of those who deliver infants at home. Ambulances used in transporting between institutions should always be warmed before initiating the transfer.

Convectively heated incubators. These are the most common devices available for creating a microclimate in which to care for an individual baby. They all provide a single- or double-layered plastic-walled chamber into which a baby is placed on an insulating mattress. The plastic walls of the chamber have portals in various places to provide hand access to the enclosed infant. All convectively heated incubators use fans to force filtered room air at various rates of flow over relatively large heaters and pans that can be optimally filled with water. The heating of incubator air can be controlled variably by a thermostat referenced to the temperature within the chamber or the temperature under the incubator chamber base. The heating can also be controlled in a servo-loop that references the heater-on or heater-off decision to a narrow band of infant skin temperatures.

Different brands of incubators use differing techniques and thermal limits to prevent excessive heating within the incubator chamber. Only a few studies of the differences between various convectively heated incubators have been published, but they all confirm that general statements assuming homeogeneity in the environments produced are somewhat naive.

The differences become very clear when comparing how different incubators react when their control systems and environmental chambers are subjected to influences that potentially disrupt their integrity. As an example, Ahlgren demonstrated that, whereas incubators with solid acrylic plastic port doors cool rapidly when the doors are opened, incubators with flexible plastic sleeves as port covers can be entered with minimum change in incubator temperature. The first kind of incubator, however, probably provides the contained infant with more protection against radiant heat losses. In maintaining incubator air temperatures, positioning of the sensing thermistor may make it vulnerable to situations that might cause false temperature recordings. For example, the probe may be warmed by a covering of diapers and blankets lying in the incubator or artifactually cooled by a stream of cold oxygen from a resuscitation bag placed carelessly next to the infant.

In general, although incubator chambers can be cooled rapidly, they take a relatively long time to reach a stable thermal equilibrium during warming. Therefore, before placement of a baby within the chamber, the incubator should be prewarmed. A prewarmed incubator should always be ready and available in anticipation of the arrival of a sick infant. Prewarming an incubator so that the air is at 36° C will produce a thermal environment of about 35° C, which is sufficient to reduce heat loss from most infants. If oxygen is to be administered by head hood or respirator, the gas humidification chambers also should be prewarmed.

Since the initial care provided a sick baby ordinarily requires multiple entries into the incubator chamber, it is reasonable, especially when caring for very small babies, to provide the infant with some form of additional thermal protection. This protection can be provided by turning the incubator humidity control to a maximum setting, keeping the baby partially swaddled, or using a supplementary portable radiant heat source over the incubator top. The initial focus of thermal control should be the prevention of heat loss without excessive concern about optimizing the environment for long-term care.

There are various guidelines that can be used when adjusting incubator temperatures for infants of various sizes and ages. No available guidelines, however, negate the responsibility to measure and record the infant's core and skin temperatures along with incubator air temperatures periodically, if not continuously. Clear orders should specify the desired ranges for both incubator and baby temperatures, and the site of air temperature measurement should be that perceived by the baby. There are now many types of relatively inexpensive electronic thermometers commercially available for use in making these measurements. The incubator temperature should be increased and decreased in small stepwise degrees as frequently as needed to maintain the infant's temperature within the specified normal range. Because of the possible induction of apnea, rapid and large changes in temperature should be prevented, especially when the incubator houses a small, sick premature infant.

When thermostat control of the air temperature is not considered sufficiently exact, an incubator with skin servocontrol electronics can be used to control incubator air temperature more precisely. The skin probe need only be suspended in the airstream near the baby and the setpoint adjusted to the desired temperature. As with any system, however, frequent adjustments may need to be made in the air temperature setpoint. Servocontrolling a convective heater to automatically maintain an infant's skin temperature at a specified level is best reserved for healthier, more mature infants. Since body warming is offset by environmental cooling in a skin servocontrolled incubator, an infant who becomes hypermetabolic because of sepsis or other cause may not become febrile, and the problem remains unrecognized. It is imperative, therefore, that careful records of skin and environmental temperatures be maintained to diagnose when an infant becomes infected. When using skin servocontrol, the thermistor probe must be firmly attached to the skin and carefully protected against artifacts that might interfere with the accurate transduction of the infant's true temperature. Since very little data exist to help in selecting a single appropriate skin temperature as a control point in a servocontrolled system, any value in the range between 35.5° and 37° C could probably be defended. Daily and co-workers observed more apneic spells when premature infants were controlled to skin temperatures of 36.5°, as opposed to 36° C.

During the ongoing monitoring of incubators in a busy intensive care nursery, Perlstein and associates found incubators out of predictable control more than 10% of the time because of unrecognized events that interfered with the equipment's proper functioning. Alarm systems can and have been designed to warn of such disruptions, but until these designs become generally available, only an understanding of incubator frailty, constant awareness, and unflagging attentiveness can reduce the response of incubated babies to unintended hazards. It should also be obvious that enclosed incubators can be protective only when they are kept closed. If the limits of skill and requirements of care preclude keeping the incubator closed during care procedures, then use of open radiantly heated beds should be considered.

Convective heating and thermoneutrality. The only way to certify that an infant with a normal body temperature is in a neutral thermal environment is to monitor the infant's metabolic rate continuously. This is usually done by measuring the baby's oxygen consumption, which requires techniques unsuited for ongoing clinical care. To estimate an infant's metabolic status, it also is possible to compare measurements of an infant's incubator temperature to the infant's skin temperature.

From the data of Adamsons it is probable that an infant is in a minimal metabolic state if the incubator environment is less than 2.5° C cooler than the infant's skin temperature (Fig. 24-9). Several difficulties are encountered when using this guideline. True environmental temperature is difficult to transduce and different from the air temperature in an incubator. A way around this problem has been provided by Hey, who determined that the incubator environmental temperature is approximately 1° C cooler than the incubator air temperature for every 7° C gradient that exists between incubator and nursery air temperatures. An incubator environment is therefore approximately 1° to 2° C cooler than the measured chamber air tempertaures in the usual nursery environment.

Moreover, to believe that neutral thermal conditions always exist when the environment is no more than 2.5° C cooler than the infant's skin is to assume that an infant always has an oxygen consumption of less than 6 ml/kg/minute, and for each milliliter of oxygen used, 5 gram calories of heat are produced. Basal oxygen consumption rates actually vary with an infant's gestational and postnatal ages, body size and shape, and weight (Fig. 24-10). It is difficult to certify, therefore, that any gradient is really appropriate when the assumptions ignore that basal metabolic rates vary with dynamic growth and development. A 2.5° C gradient would be excessively large, for example, for a newborn 1,500 gm infant with a basal oxygen consumption rate of 4.5 ml/kg/minute, and may be excessively constraining for the same infant 2 weeks later when the basal rate may have risen to 7 ml/kg/minute. Scopes has provided the most complete data for helping to resolve this problem of changing requirements with age and has reduced his observations to guidelines for incubator temperature settings, which should at least be close to the lower limit of the neutral thermal range expected for the specific infant (Fig. 24-11).

Open radiantly heated beds. The use of overhead radiant heaters to keep infants warm has become popular because they provide unimpeded access to infants receiving intensive care. Overhead radiant heaters are usually high-energy heat sources that require the use of skin servocontrol to ensure that babies do not become over-

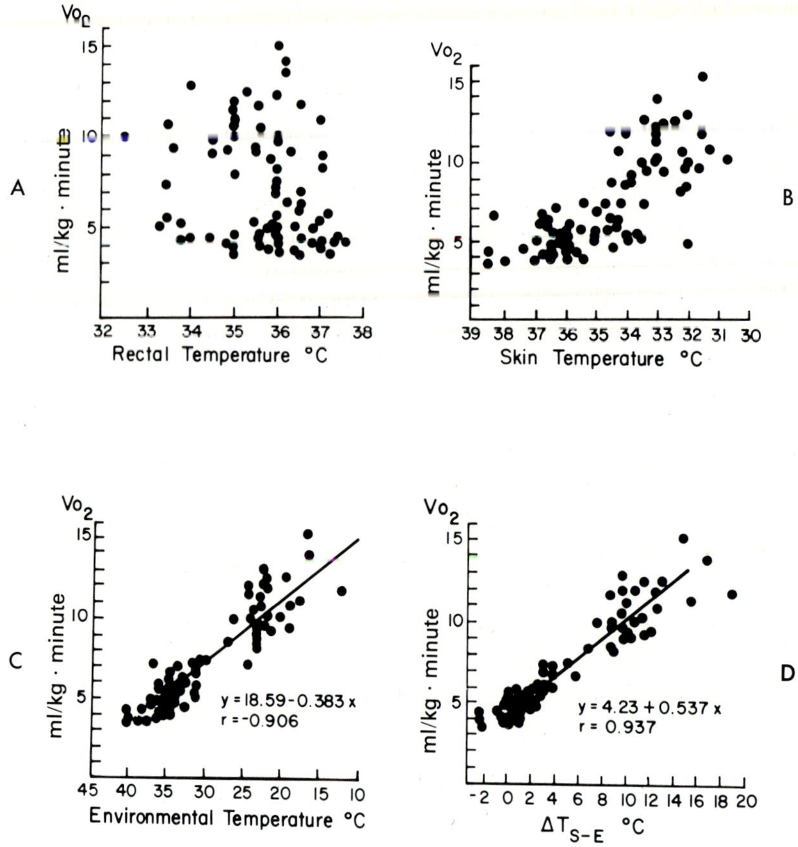

Fig. 24-9. A, Relationship between oxygen consumption and rectal temperature in various environments; **B,** skin temperature in various environments; **C,** environmental temperature when incubator walls and air are within ±2° C of each other; **D,** the difference between skin and environmental temperatures (ΔT_{S-E}) when incubator walls and air are within ±2° C of each other. (Modified from Adamsons, K., Jr., Gandy, G.M., and James, L.S.: J. Pediatr. **66:**495, 1965.)

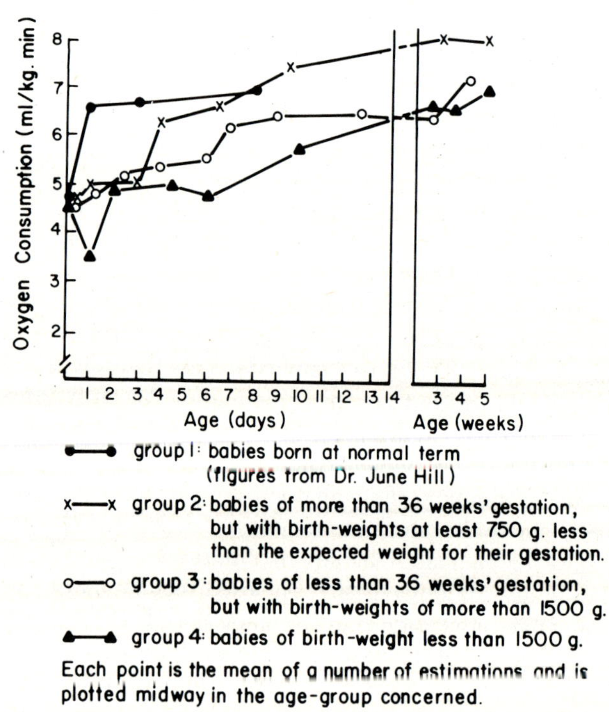

Fig. 24-10. Change in minimum oxygen consumption with age. (From Scopes, J.W.: Br. Med. Bull. **22:**88, 1966.)

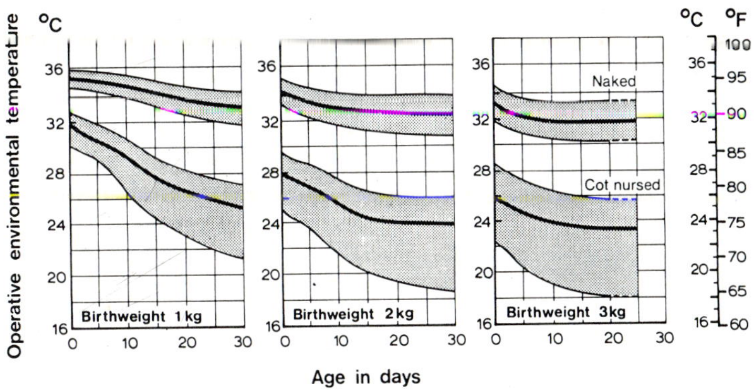

Fig. 24-11. Changes that usually occur with age in mean temperature to provide warmth for babies weighing 1-3 kg at birth, in draft-free, uniform temperature surroundings at 50% relative humidity; upper curves for naked infants, lower curves for swaddled, "cot nursed" babies. *Thick lines,* Usual "optimum" temperature; *shaded area,* range within which to maintain normal temperature without increasing heat production or evaporative water loss by more than 25%. The operative environmental temperature inside a single-walled incubator is *less* than the internal air temperature recorded by the thermometer; the effective environmental temperature provided by the incubator can, however, be estimated by subtracting 1° C from the air temperature for each 7° C by which incubator air temperature exceeds room temperature. (From Hey, E.N. In Gairdner and Hull: Recent advances in paediatrics, ed. 4, London, 1971, Churchill Livingstone.)

heated when under their influence. The only exception to this requirement is when radiant heaters are used to protect infants for short periods immediately after birth. The heat loss from the wet body of a freshly delivered newborn is sufficiently great to balance even the heat provided by the 800 W potential in the largest radiant heaters. It is good that this balance exists, since the attachment of a skin servocontrol probe to the amniotic fluid—covered skin of a baby can be very difficult, and temperatures recorded may be unreliable.

Because of the known risk of causing hyperthermia when using a radiant heater, manufacturers have been adding increasing amounts of logic to the heater control designs. There is usually a provision to cause an alarm to sound if the skin probe becomes unattached. Failure to reactivate silenced alarms may expose infants under radiant heaters to a subsequent risk of hyperthermia; thus the safe use of a radiant heater requires an informed awareness of the specific way that the alarms operate in the heater employed. The proper attachment of a thermistor probe to the skin of an infant under a radiant heater remains undefined. Various authoritative opinions have been expressed that support techniques of attachment that both maximally and minimally shield the probe from the infrared energy emitted by the heater element. Since insulated probes do provide different information than exposed probes, a consistent technique is recommended during the care of any individual baby.

The radiantly heated open bed is unquestionable more convenient and allows superior access to the infant when compared with the enclosed convectively heated incubator. Data exist, however, to suggest some special problems to consider when using a radiant heat source. Babies under radiant heaters are known to have higher insensible losses of water than do infants housed in enclosed incubators (Chapter 25, part three). Wu and Hodgman confirmed that infants in unhumidified enclosed incubators had age-dependent insensible losses ranging from means of 17.8 ml/kg/24 hours for infants weighing more than 1,500 gm to 37.4 ml/kg/24 hours for babies weighing less than 1,500 gm. In contrast, infants weighing more than 1,500 gm had insensible water losses (depending on the brand of heater) ranging between means of 32.4 and 51.6 ml/kg/24 hours when they were on open beds that were radiantly heated. Infants weighing less than 1,500 gm and under radiant heaters had insensible water losses that ranged between means of 55.2 and 88.9 ml/kg/24 hours. Although the metabolic implications of this increased evaporative loss are uncertain, at least the fluid and electrolyte management of babies under radiant heaters must be modified from that provided infants housed in enclosed incubators. Since the fluid and probably also electrolyte losses vary widely from infant to infant and from day to day, the specific replacement requirements can be determined only by carefully assessing the needs for each baby (Chapter 25, part three). Some amelioration of this fluid loss problem is possible by using plastic sheets or bags to swaddle infants when they are under radiant heaters. It has also been suggested that the use of an acrylic plastic heat shield reduces insensible water loss under a radiant heater.

In some cases large evaporative losses from infants can

be considered therapeutic. When dealing with an infant with decreased urinary output, the minimum amount of fluid required in administering drugs may exceed the usual fluid losses by insensible routes. Increasing these insensible losses by placing the infant under a radiant heater may diminish the danger of fluid overloading the baby. It is unclear whether the thermal cycling of an open radiant heater can induce apneic spells as has been observed when susceptible infants are housed in enclosed incubators.

The introduction of radiant heating has provided a valuable alternative way to keep babies warm. In some settings this is the only controllable way to protect babies against heat loss.

Radiant heating and thermoneutrality. Although it has been documented by several investigiators that babies under radiant heaters can have minimum oxygen consumption, these demonstrations have all been made using head hoods for collecting and sampling the infant's expired air. A plastic head hood becomes warm under a radiant heater, and by heating a baby's face a warm head hood might suppress a hypermetabolic state. The available data therefore do not answer the important question about whether the radiant heating of babies who are not in head hoods would be sufficient to prevent the possible homeothermic stimulation from cold and dry air-conditioned convective currents in the open nursery. Nonetheless, the use of a plastic hood to cover the head of an infant under a radiant heater may provide a way to produce conditions consistent with thermoneutrality.

Special note about very low birth weight infants. The smaller the infant and the lower the gestational age, the larger the evaporative heat losses. Supplemental humidification devices are often required to offset these losses and to add sufficient water to the environment. Very small immature infants also behave more like true poikilotherms than homeotherms and may require environmental temperatures equal to or even higher than their skin and core temperatures to remain warm.

Helping a cold infant rewarm

Because of a reduced responsiveness to bacterial pyrogens, a baby may not become hypermetabolic and febrile when septic. Sepsis does, however, frequently suppress an infant's normal homeothermic reactions, and such an infant, although previously able to maintain a warm body temperature in a cool environment, may now get cold in the same environment. The probable mechanism is that the sepsis resulted in shock, which inhibited homeothermy, although it was the cold environment that made the infant hypothermic. Since rewarming some infants may induce apnea, an infant should be constantly observed and the environment carefully analyzed and controlled during the rewarming process.

Debates over the comparative virtues of rapid versus slow rewarming procedures notwithstanding, there is no convincing argument available to certify any method as being better than another. Almost all of the published arguments are based on evidence from uncontrolled studies. Tafari found no difference when comparing rapid and slow techniques of rewarming. The approach presented here has been developed partly from a logical use of known physical and physiologic principles and partly from numerous observations of infants of all weights and gestations during the rewarming process. The approach is pragmatic and absolutely dependent on multiple adjustments in environmental heating as indicated by the responses of the baby as the environmental and body temperatures increase.

As a first step in rewarming, produce a heat-gaining environment that eliminates any further significant heat losses from the baby. Warm the incubator air to 36° C and do not let the baby get colder. The existence of a heat-gaining environment can be certified only if the infant begins to get warmer, and simply warming the air temperature to a level that is higher than the baby's temperature is inadequate. It should be remembered that the actual environmental temperature in a convectively heated incubator is probably 1° to 2° C less than the measured air temperature. Evaporative losses should be minimized by raising the incubator humidity. Radiant losses should be minimized by protecting the incubator walls from excessive cooling or, as described by Hey, an inner incubator shield wall or heat shield can be inserted. If evaporative and radiant losses are minimized, the absolute air temperature becomes more meaningful, which is important, since it is the only really controllable heating factor in a convectively heated incubator.

A temperature-monitoring thermistor or thermometer should be suspended directly in the air over the infant's body to measure actual incubator air temperature. The 36° C air temperature should provide a sufficient heat-gaining gradient for any infant with a skin temperature below 35° C. The gradient should also be suffficiently narrow to prevent too rapid transfer of heat from the environment to the infant. The goal is to produce an environment in which the infant is rewarmed by the heat actually generated by the infant. Excessive external warming of an infant tends to cause vasodilation of the skin vessels, which can result in the shunting and pooling of blood to a degree that produces sharp decreases in blood pressure. Continual monitoring of the rewarming infant's rectal temperature can be used to certify that heating of the skin temperature has not become excessive. The rate of warming should be such that the skin temperature never is more than 1° C warmer than the coexisting rectal temperature.

If in this initial environment the infant's temperature

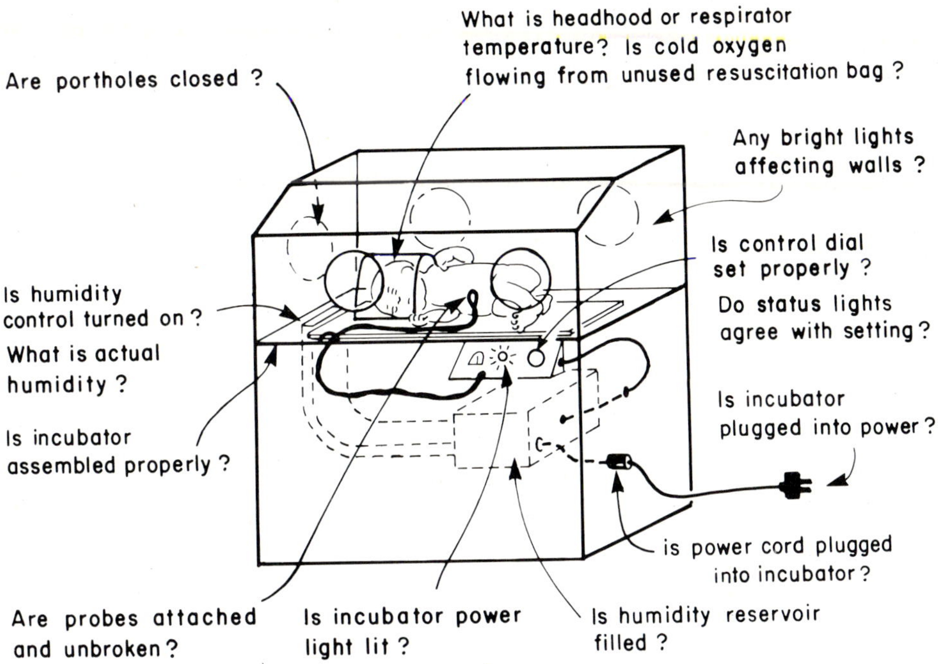

Fig. 24-12. Troubleshooting an incubator.

ceases to fall or slowly begins to rise, the settings should be maintained at that level and monitoring of all temperatures continued. If the temperature of the baby continues to fall, then raise the incubator temperature 1° to 37° C and carefully search for any previously undiscovered source of heat loss (Fig. 24-12). If within 15 minutes body temperature has not stabilized when the air temperature is 37° C, raise the air temperature to 38° C and, assuming that a heat sink still exists, look again for any further potential causes of the heat loss. In these searches, incubator humidity should be measured and certified to be at a level of more than 70%. If, in spite of all these attempts, the baby continues to cool, call for someone else to evaluate the environment, since sometimes the obvious can be seen only by an outside observer.

Heating an incubator to an air temperature of more than 38° C is sometimes difficult because of overriding safety thermostats built into most incubators. If the source of heat loss escapes discovery when the air temperature is at 38° C, this failure does not provide reason to allow an infant to continue to cool. The baby can be swaddled, or a radiant heater can be suspended over the incubator and, with the probe attached to the plastic chamber, servocontrolled to raise the incubator wall temperature by slow 1° C increments to higher levels until heat losses are completely offset. If a baby becomes apneic during rewarming, the rate of warming should be slowed. On occasion, it may be necessary to completely halt the warming process for a period to allow the infant to adjust to the new conditions, even though the infant may still be hypothermic.

The baby who is too hot

It has been nearly 30 years since DuBois wrote, "Fever is only a symptom, and we are not sure that it is an enemy. Perhaps it is a friend."

This fairly well summarizes what is known today about the febrile infant, although there is a new wave of scientific interest in the physiologic significance of fever. Most neonatal thermoregulatory studies have focused on the effects, prevention, and amelioration of hypothermia. Hyperthermia has been noted primarily as a sign of hypermetabolism when a baby is septic or otherwise stimulated. There is general agreement that it is probably beneficial to cool a baby who has become febrile because of exposure to an overheated environment. Whether it is good, however, to cool infants who are febrile because they are septic or otherwise stressed by internal conditions is less clear, although usually attempted.

An infant with a body temperature higher than 37.5° C may be considered abnormally warm. To determine whether the elevated temperature is caused by an increase in heat production, as might occur if the baby was septic, or by a decrease in heat loss, some simple presumptive clinical measures can be made.

A physiologically competent infant will respond to a hot environment by incorporating heat-losing mechanisms. The baby's skin vessels will dilate, the infant may appear to be flushed, and the hands and feet will be suffused and warm. Evaporative losses will increase and, although uncommonly observed in premature babies, active sweating may be noted in the full-term infant. If the heat stress is severe, the baby may begin to protest and complain, becoming hyperactive and irritable. The overheated skin of the infant will be warmer than the infant's core temperature.

An infant who is febrile because of an increase in endogenous heat production will reflect a state of stress. The baby will be vasoconstricted and, compared with the skin on the trunk, the extremities will appear pale and blue and feel cold. Unlike the gradients expected in overheated infants, the core temperature of the hypermetabolic infant will be warmer than the skin temperature.

Simultaneous measurements, of rectal, abdominal skin, and foot temperatures will therefore often help to distinguish the infant who is febrile because of iatrogenic overheating from the infant who is hypermetabolic because of sepsis or stimulating drugs. In the afebrile and minimally metabolic baby the abdominal skin temperature usually will be no more than 1° to 2° C cooler than the infant's rectal temperature. The normal infant's foot temperature will be no more than 2° to 3° C colder than the abdominal skin temperature. In the febrile and hypermetabolic infant the rectal temperature will be warmer than the skin temperature and the foot temperature will be more than 3° C colder than the abdominal skin temperature. In the overheated infant the rectal temperature will be colder than the skin temperature and the foot temperature will be less than 3° C cooler than the abdominal skin temperature.

THE NONTHERMAL SENSORY ENVIRONMENT

Babies in incubators are exposed to continuous noise levels of between 50 and 86 decibels (dB) with frequent peaks that can reach levels of 90 to 100 and beyond. The addition of each new piece of life-support equipment can add 15 to 20 dB to the background noise. The American Academy of Pediatrics (AAP) Committee on Environmental Hazards has recommended that efforts be directed toward reducing the known high level of noise in nurseries. The industrial standard that allows the exposure of workers to 90 dB for an 8-hour day is probably too generous when establishing criteria for infants. Young animals suffer auditory damage at lower sound levels than do adults of their species. Drugs commonly used in the nursery, such as ethacrynic acid, furosemide, and the animoglycosides streptomycin, kanamycin, neomycin, gentamicin, and tobramycin, are known from animal studies to potentiate noise-induced hearing loss.

Nurseries are too noisy, and the recommendation by the AAP committee to reduce these noise levels to less than 70 dB is sensible. Noise can be reduced simply by asking personnel to care for the babies more quietly. As a first step toward noise abatement, it is helpful to ask whether all the beeping sounds from heart rate monitors are really helpful.

With rare exception the lighting in nurseries, the colors used to paint walls, the decorations, and windows with a view are examples of environmental factors designed to suit the observational and psychologic needs of adults who provide infants with care. There is little question that daylight-simulating illumination enhances the ability to observe color and other changes that occur in sick babies. It is, however, unclear whether the illumination is otherwise beneficial or harmful to the infants, although the near constant illuminaton of most special care nurseries is almost certainly perceived by the babies. It is known that high-intensity lighting can cause retinal damage in newborn animals; and recent data suggests that a link exists between background nursery light levels and the occurrence of retrolental fibroplasia in premature human infants. More work is needed to sort out these effects and to arrive at meaningful recommendations for nursery illumination. The visual acuity and perception of infants are discussed in Chapter 26.

Along with the recent increase in the interest being paid to the social and educational development of babies, many programs are being introduced that use visual, auditory, tactile, and proprioceptive techniques to enhance the sensory stimulation of infants. There is nothing inherently wrong with the concept of socializing and educating newborns, but a critical stance must be maintained during the development of these programs. Babies respond to stimulation not only socially but also with a variety of autonomic responses, some of which may be detrimental to the sick neonate.

ENVIRONMENTAL POLLUTION

The questionable quality of the air we breathe is one of many environmental subjects generating debate in our society. It is rare to quantitatively analyze the composition of nursery or incubator air. The report by Waffarn in which 18 of 42 infant incubators were found to contain detectable concentrations of mercury vapor suggests that such quantitation may be appropriate.

Various combinations of metal pipes and plastic tubes are used to deliver gases to an incubator, into a head hood, or directly into a baby's lungs. Because of soldered and glued joints, protectively coated surfaces, and other sources of contamination, the air can contain oils, lead, cadmium, bismuth, mercury, and various other residues of organic and metallic salts. The gases also can contain bacteria and fungi. Many of these contaminants can be eliminated by appropriate filters, but the success of any filtering must be certified by laboratory testing.

As more studies are generated to evaluate the health impact of radiation, ultraviolet light, microwaves, radar, radioactivity, and other environmental components, it is to be hoped that the specific susceptibility of babies to these potential hazards will be considered in research designs. The lack of existing awareness that radiation may be a hazard is suggested every time a baby's pelvis is included in a roentgenographic field when only a chest film is ordered. (Chapter 13). It also is exemplified whenever a portable roentgenogram is taken in a nursery and the adults, concerned about their own exposure, run out of range of the x-ray unit or shield themselves with protective lead aprons while ignoring the exposure of the naked baby in the next incubator. At present insufficient data exist to express more than serious concern about potential environmental pollution in the nursery.

Paul H. Perlstein

BIBLIOGRAPHY

Thermoregulation

Subject reviews

Adamsons, K.: The role of thermal factors in fetal and neonatal life, Pediatr. Clin. North Am. **13**:599, 1966.

Ahlgren, E.W.: Environmental control of the neonate receiving intensive care, Int. Anesthesiol. Clin. **12**:173, 1974.

Bruck, K.: Heat production and temperature regulation. In Stave, U., editor: Perinatal physiology, New York, 1978, Plenum Publishing Corp.

Dawes, G.S.: Oxygen consumption and temperature regulation in the newborn. In Foetal and neonatal physiology, 1968, Year Book Medical Publishers, Inc.

DeLue, N.A.: Climate and environmental concepts, Clin. Perinatol. **3**:425, 1976.

Hey, E.N.: The care of babies in incubators. In Gairdner, D., and Hull, D., editors: Recent advances in paediatrics, ed. 4, London, 1971, Churchill Livingstone.

Hey, E.N., and Katz, G.: The optimum thermal environment for naked babies, Arch. Dis. Child. **45**:328, 1970.

Klaus, M., Fanaroff, A., and Martin, R.J.: The physical environment. In Klaus, M.H., and Fanaroff, A.A., editors: Care of the high risk neonate, Philadelphia, 1979, W.B. Saunders Co.

Lutz, L., and Perlstein, P.H.: Temperature control in newborn babies, Nurs. Clin. North Am. **6**:15, 1971.

Oliver, T.K.: Temperature regulation and heat production in the newborn, Pediatr. Clin. North Am. **12**:765, 1965.

Scopes, J.W.: Thermoregulation in the newborn. In Avery, G.B., editor: Neonatology, Philadelphia, 1975, J.B. Lippincott Co.

Sinclair, J.C.: The effect of the thermal environment on neonatal mortality and morbidity. In Adamsons, K., and Fox, H.A., editors: Preventability of perinatal injury, New York, 1975, Alan R. Liss, Inc.

Sinclair, J.C.: Metabolic rate and temperature control. In Smith, C.A., and Nelson, N.M., editors: The physiology of the newborn infant, Springfield, Ill., 1976, Charles C Thomas, Publisher.

General

Adamsons, K., Jr., Gandy, G.M., and James, L.S.: The influence of thermal factors upon oxygen consumption of newborn human infant, J. Pediatr. **66**:495, 1965.

Agate, F.J., and Silverman, W.A.: The control of body temperature in the human premature infant by low energy infrared radiation, Anat. Rec. **136**:152, 1960.

Aherne, W., and Hull, D.: Brown adipose tissue and heat production in the newborn infant, J. Pathol. **91**:223, 1966.

Aynsley-Green, A., Roberton, N.R.C., and Rolfe, P.: Air temperature recordings in infant incubators, Arch. Dis. Child. **50**:215, 1975.

Babak, E.: Ueber die Warmeregulation der Neugeborenen, Pfleugers Arch. **89**:154, 1902.

Baum, J.D., and Scopes, J.W.: The silver swaddler: device for preventing hypothermia in the newborn, Lancet **1**:672, 1968.

Baumgart, S.: Partitions of heat losses and gains in premature newborn infants under radiant warmers, Pediatrics **75**:89, 1985.

Belgaumkar, T.K., and Scott, K.E.: Effects of low humidity on small premature infants in servocontrol incubators. I. Decrease in rectal temperatures, Biol. Neonate **26**:337, 1975.

Belgaumkar, T.K., and Scott, K.E.: Effects of low humidity on small premature infants in servocontrol incubators. II. Increased severity of apnea, Biol. Neonate **26**:348, 1975.

Bell, E.F., and Rios, G.R.: Air versus skin temperature servo control of infant incubators, J. Pediatr. **103**:954, 1983. (See also: Reply to editorial correspondence, J. Pediatr. **104**:958, 1984.)

Bell, E.F., Weinstein, M.R., and Oh, W.: Heat balance in premature infants: comparative effects of convectively heated incubator and radiant warmers, with and without plastic heat shield, J. Pediatr. **96**:460, 1980.

Benedict, F.G., and Talbot, F.B.: The physiology of the newborn infant: character and amount of catabolism, Washington, D.C., Carnegie Institute, Publication No. 233, 1915.

Besch, N.J., and others: The transparent baby bag: a shield against heat loss, N. Engl. J. Med. **284**:121, 1971.

Blackfan, K.D., and Yaglou, C.P.: The premature infant, Am. J. Dis. Child. **46**:1175, 1933.

Bolton, D.R., Fox, A.M., and Kennaird, D.L.: Preliminary observations on the application of thermography to the study of brown adipose tissue in the human newborn, J. Physiol. (Lond.) **208**:23p, 1970.

Bruck, K.: Temperature regulation in the newborn infant, Biol. Neonate **3**:65, 1961.

Bruck, K.: Which environmental temperature does the premature infant prefer? Pediatrics **41**:1027, 1968.

Bruck, K., Parmalee, A.H., Jr., and Bruck, M.: Neutral temperature range and range of "thermal comfort" in premature infants, Biol. Neonate **4**:32, 1962.

Budin, P.: The feeding and hygiene of premature and fullterm infants. In Dion, O., editor: The nursling, London, 1907, Caxton Publishing, (Translated by W.J. Maloney.)

Buetow, K.C., and Klein, S.W.: Effect of maintenance of "normal" skin temperature on survival of infants of low birth weight, Pediatrics **34**:163, 1964.

Clark, R.P., and others: Neonatal natural forced convection, J. Physiol. (Lond.) **284**:22, 1978.

Cornblath, J., and Schwartz, R.: Disorders of carbohydrate metabolism in infancy. In Major problems in clinical pediatrics, vol. 3, Philadelphia, 1966, W.B. Saunders Co.

Cree, J.E., Meyer, J., and Hailey, D.M.: Diazepam in labour: its metabolism and effect on the clinical condition and thermogenesis of the newborn, Br. Med. J. **3**:251, 1973.

Cross, K., Dawes, G.S., and Karlberg, P. In Oliver, T.K., Jr., editor: Neonatal respiratory adaptation, Public Health Service Pub. No. 1432, Washington, D.C., 1966, p. 117.

Cross, K., Tizard, J.P.M., and Trythall, D.A.H.: The gaseous metabolism of the newborn infant, Acta Paediatr. Scand. **46**:265, 1957.

Cross, K., Tizard, J.P.M., and Trythall, D.A.H.: The gaseous metabolism of the newborn infant breathing 15 percent oxygen, Acta Paediatr. Scand. **47**:217, 1958.

Cross, K., and others: Lack of temperature control in infants with abnormalities of the central nervous system, Arch. Dis. Child. **46**:437, 1971.

Dahm, L.S., and James, L.S.: Newborn temperature and calculated heat loss in the delivery room, Pediatrics **49**:504, 1972.

Daily, W.J., Klaus, M., and Meyer, H.B.: Apnea in premature infants: monitoring, incidence, heart rate changes, and an effect of environmental temperature, Pediatrics **43**:510, 1969.

Dangman, B.C., and others: The variability of PO_2 in newborn infants in response to routine care, Pediatr. Res. **10**:422, 1976.

Daniel, S.S., and others: Hypothermia and the resuscitation of asphyxiated fetal rhesus monkeys, J. Pediatr. **68**:45, 1966.

Darnall, R.A., Jr., and Ariagno, R.L.: Minimal oxygen consumption in infants cared for under overhead radiant warmers compared with conventional incubators, J. Pediatr. **93**:283, 1978.

Darnall, R.A., Jr., and Ariagno, R.L.: Resting oxygen consumption of premature infants covered with a plastic thermal blanket, Pediatrics **63**:547, 1979.

Dawes, G.S.: Neonatal respiratory adaptation. In Proceedings of Interdisciplinary Conference on Neonatal Respiratory Adaptation, Public Health Service Pub. No. 1432, Washington, D.C., 1966. U.S. Government Printing Office.

Dawes, G.S., and Mott, J.C.: The increase in oxygen consumption of the lamb after birth, J. Physiol. **146**:295, 1959.

Dawkins, M.J.R., and Scopes, J.W.: Non-shivering thermogenesis and brown adipose tissue in the human newborn infant, Nature **206**:201, 1965.

Day, R.: Regulation of body temperature during sleep, Am. J. Dis. Child. **61**:734, 1941.

Day, R.: Respiratory metabolism in infancy and childhood, Am. J. Dis. Child. **65**:376, 1943.

Day, R.L., and others: Body temperature and survival of premature infants, Pediatrics **34**:171, 1964.

Du, J.N.H., and Oliver, T.K., Jr.: The baby in the delivery room: a suitable microenvironment, JAMA **207**:1502, 1969.

Eckstein, A.: Ueber die Warmregulierung der Fruhgeborenen, Z. Kindelh. **42**:5, 1926.

Edwards, N.K.: Radiant warmers. In Iatrogenic problems in neonatal intensive care, Report of the 69th Ross Conference on Pediatric Research, 1976, p. 79.

Emergency Care Research Institute: Evaluation: infant radiant warmers, Health Devices **3**:4, 1973.

Fanaroff, A.A., and others: Insensible water loss in low birth weight infants, Pediatrics **50**:236, 1972.

Fenner, A., and List, M.: Observations of body temperature regulation in young, premature and full term newborns while being connected to a servocontrol temperature unit, Biol. Neonate **18**:300, 1971.

Fisher, D.A., and Oddie, T.H.: Neonatal thyroidal hyperactivity, Am. J. Dis. Child. **107**:574, 1964.

Fisher, D.A., and Odell, W.D.: Acute release of thyrotropin in the newborn, J. Clin. Invest. **48**:1670, 1969.

Foster, K.G., Hey, E.N., and Katz, G.: The response of the sweat glands of the newborn baby to thermal stimuli and to intradermal acetylcholine, J. Physiol. **203**:13, 1969.

Gandy, G.M., and others: Thermal environment and acid-base homeostasis on human infants during the first few hours of life, J. Clin. Invest. **43**:751, 1964.

Glass, L., Silverman, W.A., and Sinclair, J.C.: Effect of the thermal environment on cold resistance and growth of small infants after the first week of life, Pediatrics **41**:1033, 1968.

Glass, L., Silverman, W.A., and Sinclair, J.C.: Relationship of thermal environment and caloric intake to growth and resting metabolism in the late neonatal period, Biol. Neonate **14**:324, 1969.

Gold, A.J., and Zornitzer, A.: Effect of partial body cooling on man exercising in a hot environment, Aerospace Med. **39**:944, 1968.

Gordon, H.H.: Inclusions of studies, mostly of premature infants, Pediatrics **8**:163, 1951.

Grausz, J.P.: The effects of environmental temperature changes on the metabolic rate of newborn babies, Acta Paediatr. Scand. **57**:98, 1968.

Haroy, J.D.: Physiology of temperature regulation, Physiol. Rev. **41**:521, 1961.

Heim, T., Kellenmayer, M., and Dani, M.: Thermal conditions and the mobilization of lipids from brown and white adipose tissue in the human neonate, Acta Paediatr. Acad. Sci. Hung. **9**:109, 1968.

Hess, J.H.: Premature and congenitally diseased infants, Philadelphia, 1922, Lea & Febiger.

Hey, E.N.: The relation between environmental temperature and oxygen consumption in the newborn baby, J. Physiol. **200**:589, 1969.

Hey, E.N., and Katz, G.: Evaporative water loss in the newborn baby, J. Physiol. **200**:605, 1969.

Hey, E.N., and Katz, G.: Temporary loss of a metabolic response to cold stress in infants of low birthweight, Arch. Dis. Child. **44**:323, 1969.

Hey, E.N., and Katz, G.: The optimum thermal environment for naked babies, Arch. Dis. Child. **45**:328, 1970.

Hey, E.N., Katz, G., and O'Connell, B.: The total thermal insulation of the newborn baby, J. Physiol. (Lond.) **207**:683, 1970.

Hey, E.N., Kohlinsky, S., and O'Connell, B.: Heat losses from babies during exchange transfusion, Lancet **1**:335, 1969.

Hey, E.N., and Maurice, N.P.: Effect of humidity on production and loss of heat in the newborn baby, Arch. Dis. Child. **43**:166, 1968.

Hey, E.N., and Mount, L.E.: Temperature control in incubators, Lancet **2**:202, 1966.

Hey, E.N., and Mount, L.E.: Heat losses from babies in incubators, Arch. Dis. Child. **42**:57, 1967.

Hey, E.N., and O'Connell, B.: Oxygen consumption and heat balance in the cot-nursed baby, Arch. Dis. Child. **45**:335, 1970.

Hill, J.R.: Oxygen consumption of newborn and adult mammals: its dependence on oxygen tension in inspired air and on environmental temperature, J. Physiol. (Lond.) **149**:346, 1959.

Hill, J.R., and Rahimtulla, K.A.: Heat balance and the metabolic rate of newborn babies in relation to environmental temperature; and the effect of age and of weight on basal metabolic rate, J. Physiol. **180**:239, 1965.

Holzman, I.R.: A method to maintain infant temperature, Am. J. Dis. Child. **139**:390, 1985.

Hull, D., and Segall, M.J.: The contribution of brown adipose tissue to heat production in the newborn rabbit, J. Physiol. (Lond.) **191**:449, 1965.

Indyk, L.: A dangerous situation encountered in the administration of oxygen to an infant in a baby warmer, Pediatrics **47**:503, 1971.

Jolly, H., Molyneux, P., and Newell, D.J.: A controlled study of the effect of temperature on premature babies, J. Pediatr. **60**:889, 1962.

Kaplan, M., and Eidelman, A.J.: Improved prognosis in severely hypothermic newborn infants treated by rapid rewarming, J. Pediatr. **105**:470, 1984.

Karlberg, P.: The significance of depth of insertion of the thermometer for recording rectal temperatures, Acta Paediatr. Scand. **38**:359, 1949.

Karlberg, P.: Determination of standard energy metabolism in normal infants, Acta Paediatr. Scand. (Suppl.) **41**: 1952.

Karlberg, P.: Proceedings of Interdisciplinary Conference on Neonatal Respiratory Adaptation, Public Health Service Pub. No. 1432, Washington, D.C., 1966, U.S. Government Printing Office.

Karlberg, P., Moore, R.E., and Oliver, T.K., Jr.: The thermogenic response of the newborn infant to noradrenalin, Acta Paediatr. Scand. **51**:284, 1962.

LeBlanc, M.H.: Oxygen consumption in premature infants in an incubator of proven clinical efficacy, Biol. Neonate **44**:76, 1983.

Levison, H., and Swyer, P.R.: Oxygen consumption and the thermal environment in newly born infants, Biol. Neonate **7**:305, 1964.

Lewis, H.E., and others: Aerodynamics of the human microenvironment, Lancet **50**:1273, 1969.

Mann, T.P., and Elliott, R.I.K.: Neonatal cold injury, Lancet **1**:229, 1957.

Marks, K.H., Friedman, Z., and Maisels, M.J.: A simple device for reducing insensible water in low birth weight infants, Pediatrics **60**:223, 1977.

Marks, K.H., and others: Intravenous alimentation and insensible water loss in low birth weight infants, Pediatrics **63**:54, 1979.

Marks, K.H., and others: Thermal head wrap for infants, J. Pediatr. **107**:956, 1985.

Mayfield, S.R., and others: Temperature measurement in term and preterm neonates, J. Pediatr. **104**:271, 1984.

Mestyan, J., Jarai, I., and Fekete, M.: The total energy expenditure and its components in premature infants maintained under different nursing and environmental conditions, Pediatr. Res. **2**:161, 1968.

Mestyan, J., and others: Surface temperature versus deep body temperature and the metabolic response to cold of hypothermic premature infants, Biol. Neonate **7**:230, 1964.

Mestyan, J., and others: The significance of facial skin temperature in the chemical heat regulation of premature infants, Biol. Neonate **7**:243, 1964.

Miller, D.L., and Oliver, T.K., Jr.: Body temperature in the immediate neonatal period: the effect of reducing thermal losses, Am. J. Obstet. Gynecol. **94**:964, 1966.

Miller, J.A., Jr., Miller, F.S., and Westin, B.: Hypothermia in treatment of asphyxia neonatorum, Biol. Neonate **6**:148, 1964.

Mordhorst, H.: Uber die chemische Warmeregulation fruhgeborener Sauglinge, Monatsschr. Kinderheilkd. **55**:174, 1932.

Motil, K.J., Blackburn, M.G., and Pleasure, J.R.: The effects of four different radiant warmer temperature set points used for rewarming neonates, J. Pediatr. **85**:546, 1974.

Mount, L.E.: The oxygen consumption of the newborn pig in relation to environmental temperature, J. Physiol. (Lond.) **142**:37p, 1958.

Nielsen, L., and others: Evaluation of the Porta-Warm mattress as a source of heat for neonatal transport, Pediatrics **58**:500, 1976.

Oh, W., and Karecki, H.: Phototherapy and insensible water loss in the newborn infant, Am. J. Dis. Child. **124**:230, 1972.

Oliver, T.K., Jr., and Karlberg, P.: Gaseous metabolism in newly born human infants—the effects of environmental temperature and 15 percent oxygen in the inspired air, Am. J. Dis. Child. **105**:427, 1963.

Perlstein, P.H.: Thermal control. In Iatrogenic problems in neonatal intensive care. Report of the 69th Ross Conference on Pediatric Research, 1976, p. 75.

Perlstein, P.H., Edwards, N.K., and Atherton, H.D.: Incubator control with computer assistance, Perinatol. Neonatal. **1**:16, 1977.

Perlstein, P.H., Edwards, N.K., and Sutherland, J.M.: Apnea in premature infants and incubator air temperature changes, N. Engl. J. Med. **282**:461, 1970.

Perlstein, P.H., Edwards, N.K., and Sutherland, J.M.: Age relationship to thermal patterns on the backs of cold stressed infants, Biol. Neonate **20**:127, 1972.

Perlstein, P.H., and others: Thermal patterns on the backs of cold stressed babies, Pediatr. Res. **4**:472, 1970.

Perlstein, P.H., and others: Adaptation to cold in the first three days of life, Pediatrics **54**:411, 1974.

Perlstein, P.H., and others: Computer-assisted newborn intensive care, Pediatrics **57**:494, 1976.

Pribylova, H., and Znamenacek, K.: The effect of body temperature on the level of carbohydrate metabolites and oxygen consumption in the newborn, Pediatrics **37**:743, 1966.

Schiff, D., Stern, L., and Leduc, J.: Chemical thermogenesis in newborn infants, Pediatrics **37**:577, 1966.

Schmitt, B.D.: Fever in childhood, Pediatricis **74**:929, 1984.

Scopes, J.W.: Metabolic rate and temperature control in the human body, Br. Med. Bull. **22**:88, 1966.

Scopes, J.W., and Ahmed, I.: Indirect assessment of oxygen requirements in newborn babies by monitoring deep rectal temperature, Arch. Dis. Child. **41**:25, 1966.

Scopes, J.W., and Ahmed, I.: Minimal rates of oxygen consumption in sick and premature newborn infants, Arch. Dis. Child. **41**:407, 1966.

Scopes, J.W., and Tizard, J.P.M.: The effect of intravenous noradrenaline on the oxygen consumption of newborn animals, J. Physiol. **165**:305, 1963.

Shvartz, E.: Effect of a cooling hood on physiological responses to work in a hot environment, J. Appl. Physiol. **29**:36, 1970.

Silverman, W.A.: Thermoregulation of the newly born. In Thompson, S.G., editor: Reports of Ross Conference on Pediatric Research, (Suppl. 2) Columbus, Ohio, 1964, Ross Laboratories.

Silverman, W.A.: Use and misuse of temperature and humidity in care of the newborn infant, Pediatrics **33**:276, 1964.

Silverman, W.A.: Incubator-baby side shows, Pediatrics **64**:127, 1979.

Silverman, W.A., and Agate, F.J.: Variations in cold resistance among small newborn infants, Biol. Neonate **6**:113, 1964.

Silverman, W.A., Agate, F.J., Jr., and Fertig, J.W.: A sequential trial of the nonthermal effect of atmospheric humidity on survival of newborn infants of low birth weight, Pediatrics **31**:719, 1963.

Silverman, W.A., and Blanc, W.A.: The effect of humidity on survival of newly born premature infants, Pediatrics **20**:477, 1957.

Silverman, W.A., Fertig, J.W., and Berger, A.P.: The influence of the thermal environment upon the survival of newly born premature infants, Pediatrics **22**:876, 1958.

Silverman, W.A., and Parke, P.C.: Keep him warm, Am. J. Nurs. **65**:81, 1965.

Silverman, W.A., Sinclair, J.C., and Agate, F.J.: The oxygen cost of minor changes in heat balance of small newborn infants, Acta Paediatr. Scand. **55**:294, 1966.

Silverman, W.A., and others: Warm nape of the newborn, Pediatrics **33**:984, 1964.

Sinclair, J.C., Scopes, J.W., and Silverman, W.A.: Metabolic reference standards for the neonate, Pediatrics **39**:724, 1967.

Sokal, M., and Sinclair, J.C.: Effect of temperature on growth of newborn rabbits, Biol. Neonate **28**:1, 1976.

Stephenson, J.M., Du, J.N., and Oliver, T.K., Jr.: The effect of cooling on blood gas tensions in newborn infants, J. Pediatr. **76**:848, 1970.

Stern, L., Lees, M.H., and Leduc, J.: Environmental temperature, oxygen consumption and catecholamine excretion in newborn infants, Pediatrics **36**:367, 1965.

Sulyok, E., Jequier, E., and Ryser, G.: Effect of relative humidity on thermal balance of the newborn infant, Biol. Neonate **21**:210, 1972.

Tafari, N., and Gentz, J.: Aspects on rewarming newborn infants with severe accidental hypothermia, Acta Paediatr. Scand. **63**:595, 1974.

Tahti, E., and others: Changes in skin temperature of the neonate at birth: a cine-thermographic study, Acta Paediatr. Scand. **61**:159, 1972.

Talbot, F.B., and others: The basal metabolism of prematurity. III. Metabolism findings in twenty-one premature infants, Am. J. Dis. Child. **26**:29, 1923.

Topper, W.H., and Stewart, T.P.: Thermal support for the very-low-birth-weight infant: role of supplemental conductive heat, J. Pediatr. **105**:810, 1984.

Torrance, J.T.: Temperature readings of premature infants, Nurs. Res. **17**:312, 1968.

Turnell, R.: The influence of different environmental temperatures on pulmonary gas exchange and blood gas changes after birth, Acta Paediatr. Scand. **64**:57, 1975.

Walker, D., Walker, A., and Wood, C.: Temperature of the human fetus, Br. J. Obstet. Gynaecol. **76**:503, 1969.

Williams, R.A., and Chambers, A.B.: Effect of neck warming and cooling on thermal comfort. In Proceedings of the second Conference of Portable Life Support Systems, NASA SP-**302**:289, 1971.

Winslow, C.E.A., Herrington, L.P., and Gagge, A.P.: Physiological reactions of the human body to varying environmental temperatures, Am. J. Physiol. **120**:1, 1937.

Wolf, H., and Stave, U.: Free fatty acids and glycerol in plasma and tissue of normal, hypothermic, and hypotrophic newborn rabbits, Biol. Neonate **19**:132, 1971.

Wood, C., and Beard, R.W.: Temperature of the human fetus, Br. J. Obstet. Gynaecol. **71**:768, 1964.

Wu, P.Y.K., and Hodgman, J.F.: Changes in insensible water loss in infants with and without phototherapy, Clin. Res. **20**:284, 1972.

Wu, P.Y.K., and Hodgman, J.E.: Insensible water loss in preterm infants: changes with postnatal development and non-iodizing radiant energy, Pediatrics **54**:704, 1974.

Yeh, T.F., and others: Reduction of insensible water loss in premature infants under the radiant warmer, J. Pediatr. **94**:651, 1979.

Ylppo, A.: Zur Physiologie, Klinik und zur Schicksal der Fruhgeborenen, Z. Kinderh, **24**:1, 1919.

Young, I.M.: Vasomotor tone in the skin blood vessels of the newborn infant, Clin. Sci. **22**:325, 1962.

Nonthermal sensory environment

Bergman, I., and others: Cause of hearing loss in the high-risk premature infant, J. Pediatr. **106**:95, 1985.

Bess, F.H., Peek, B.F., and Chapman, J.J.: Further observations on noise levels in infant incubators, Pediatrics **63**:100, 1979.

Blennow, G., Svenningsen, N.W., and Almquist, B.: Noise levels in infant incubators (adverse effects?), Pediatricis **53**:29, 1974.

Bower, T.G.R.: The object in the world of the infant, Sci. Am. **224**:30, 1971.

Dayal, V.S., Kokshanian, A., and Mitchell, D.P.: Combined effects of noise and kanamycin, Ann. Otol. Rhinol. Laryngol. **80**:897, 1971.

Dayton, G., and others: Developmental study of coordinated eye movements in the human infant. I. Visual acuity determined by electrooculography, Arch. Ophthalmol. **71**:865, 1964.

Doueck, E., and others: Effects of incubator noise on the cochlea of the newborn, Lancet **2**:1110, 1976.

Falk, S.A., and Farmer, J.C., Jr.: Incubator noise and possible deafness, Arch. Otolaryngol. **97**:385, 1973.

Falk, S.A., and Woods, N.F.: Hospital noise levels and potential health hazards, N. Engl. J. Med. **289**:774, 1973.

Falk, S.A., and others: Noise-induced inner ear damage in newborn and adult guinea pigs, Laryngoscope **84**:444, 1974.

Fantz, R.L.: Patterned vision in newborn infants, Science **140**:296, 1963.

Fitzgerald, H.E.: Autonomic pupillary reflex action during early infancy and its relation to social and non-social visual stimuli, J. Exp. Child. Psychol. **6**:470, 1968.

Gadeke, R., and others: The noise level in a children's hospital and the wake-up threshold in infants, Acta Paediatr. Scand. **58**:164, 1969.

Glass, P., and others: Effect of bright light in the hospital nursery on the incidence of retinopathy of prematurity, N. Engl. J. Med. **313**:401, 1985.

Goren, C.C., Sarty, M., and Wu, P.Y.: Visual following and pattern discrimination of face-like stimuli by newborn infants, Pediatrics **56**:544, 1975.

Gorman, J.J., Cogan, D.G., and Gellis, S.S.: An apparatus for grading the visual acuity of infants on the basis of optokinetic nystagmus, Pediatrics **19**:1088, 1957.

Kiff, R., and Lepard, E.: Visual response of premature infants, Arch. Opthalmol. **75**:631, 1966.

Kirner, A.,and others: Effects of waterbed flotation on premature infants: a pilot study, Pediatrics **56**:361, 1975.

Kramer, L., and Pierpont, M.: Rocking waterbed and auditory stimuli to enhance growth of preterm infants, J. Pediatr. **88**:207, 1076.

Long, J.G., Alistair, G.S., and Lucey, J.F.: Use of continuous $TcPO_2$ monitoring to avoid handling and pain as causes of hypoxemia, Pediatr. Res. **13**:499, 1979.

Long, J.G., Lucey, J.F., and Philip, A.G.S.: Noise and hypoxemia in the intensive care nursery, Pediatrics **65**:143, 1980.

Miller, R.W., and others: Noise pollution: neonatal aspects. Committee on Environmental Hazards, American Academy of Pediatrics, Pediatrics **54**:476, 1974.

Rosen, S.: Noise, hearing and cardiovascular function. In Welch, B., and Wesch, A.S., editors: Physiological effects of noise, New York, 1970, Plenum Press.

Scarr-Salapatek, S., and Williams, M.: The effects of early stimulation on low birth weight infants, Child. Dev. **44**:94, 1973.

Shenai, J.P.: Sound levels for neonates in transit, J. Pediatr. **90**:811, 1977.

Siqueland, E., and Lipsitt, L.: Learning ability and its enhancement. In Henkes, J., and Schein, R., editors: Learning disorders in children. Report of the 61st Ross Conference on Pediatric Research, Columbus, Ohio, 1971, Ross Laboratories.

Solkoff, N., and others: Effects of handling on the subsequent development of premature infants, J. Dev. Psych. **1**:765, 1969.

Vidyasagar, D., Joseph, M.E., and Hamilton, L.R.: Noise levels in the neonatal intensive care unit, J. Pediatr. **88**:115, 1976.

Welch, B.L., and Welch, A.S.: Physiological effects of noise, New York, 1970, Plenum Press.

Environmental pollution

Hamel, A.J., Deane, R.S., and Paquette, R.D.: Compressed air and oxygen supply lines as a source of contamination of respiratory therapy equipment, Items and Topics **22**:8, 1976.

Waffarn, F., aand Hodgman, J.E.: Mercury vapor contamination of infant incubators: a potential hazard, Pediatrics **64**:640, 1979.

PART THREE

Biomedical engineering aspects of neonatal monitoring

See also Chapter 21.

Electronic instrumentation is assuming an ever-expanding role in neonatal intensive care. Although it is perhaps ambitious to expect neonatologists to have the expertise of engineers, a basic understanding of the principles involved in neonatal electronic instrumentation is important. By being aware of the various electronic techniques of physiologic measurement, the neonatologist not only can know the strengths and limitations of the instrumentation but also can avoid many errors that result from either incorrect application of the instrumentation or minor malfunctions. Sometimes the manufacturers of neonatal electronic apparatuses design these as merely scaled-down versions of electronic monitoring devices for adults. The neonatologist, of course, is acutely aware that the neonate is certainly not a miniature adult but rather has unique characteristics and problems. Thus

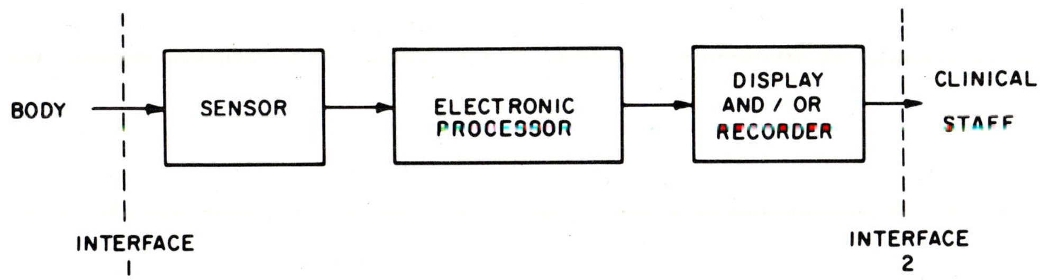

Fig. 24-13. Basic medical electronic instrumentation system. Interfaces *1* and *2* require special consideration for optimum clinical performance of the instrument.

it is important that instrumentation for neonatal monitoring be specifically designed by engineers and physicians together to meet the special requirements of the neonate and not to be just variations of adult monitors. The major requirements for neonatal monitoring equipment are as follows:

1. Safe for patients and personnel
2. Solid and resistant to wear
3. Small and space saving
4. Noninvasive and nonobstructive for patient care
5. Easy to use
6. Specific and sensitive

This section is devoted to cardiac, blood pressure, and respiration monitoring. Instrumentation for temperature and blood gas monitoring is covered in part four and in Chapter 28.

The basic arrangement of an electronic instrumentation system is shown in Fig. 24-13. For the physician the most important part is the interface between the instrumentation system and the patient. The sensor makes up the instrument side of this interface. It must detect accurately the physiologic variable being monitored but must not in itself provide constraints on the system that could change this variable. The portion of the instrumentation concerned with modifying and interpreting the signal from the sensor is known as the processor. It is in this block that most of the electronic manipulation of the data is carried out. The processor can be anything from a simple amplifier to a complex digital computer programmed to recognize and indicate normal and pathologic signs on the signal. The final block on the instrumentation system is again concerned with interface, but this time between the instrument and the clinical staff who uses it. This so-called display and recording section is concerned with indicating the variables being measured and providing a permanent record of them such as on a paper chart recorder, a magnetic tape recorder, or a computer disk. This section should be designed to minimize communication errors between the machine and the clinical staff.

CARDIAC MONITORING

Cardiac monitoring, as considered here, is only the monitoring of the heart rhythm through the electrocardiogram and the monitoring of heart rate. The sensor function of a neonatal cardiac monitor is carried out by the skin biopotential electrodes. Their function is to convert the electrical signal in the body to one that can be handled by the remainder of the instrumentation system. The carriers of electrical charge in the body are the electrolyte ions, whereas in an electronic device electrical charge is transferred by electrons. Thus the biopotential electrodes must convert an ionic type of electrical signal to one that is electronic in nature. This means that an oxidation-reduction reaction must occur at the electrode surface. In this chemical reaction electrons are transferred from ions to the electrode or vice versa. At the surface of the electrode there must be available ions for the reaction, and once the reaction occurs, the products of the reaction must be removed. In addition, chemical differences between the electrode material and the ions in the body also can cause an accumulation or depletion of specific ionic species at the electrode surface. Thus it is fair to say that the concentration of ions near the surface of the electrode in general will be different from that in the body away from the electrode. This phenomenon is known as polarization, and it is responsible for many of the problems encountered with biopotential-measuring electrodes. For the best results it is therefore desirable to find electrodes that will minimize polarization. Unfortunately ideal nonpolarizable electrodes do not exist in practice; however, electrochemists have developed electrodes that come close to behaving as though they were nonpolarizable.

The silver–silver chloride electrode is one of these sensors that receives widespread application in cardiac monitoring. In its simplest form this electrode can be thought off as a silver surface that is coated with the salt silver chloride. This electrode is found to have high electrical stability and low polarization in chloride-containing electrolytic solutions. Since chloride is the principal anion of extracellular fluid in the body, it is reasonable to apply the silver–silver chloride electrode in biology.

Electrodes attached to the skin surface may not have appropriate ionic solutions coupling the extracellular fluid to their surface, so it is necessary to provide such a coupling medium. This is the so-called electrolyte gel, which consists of an aqueous solution of ions in a gelatinous base to give it a high viscosity. Normally electrode gels are designed to have the same electrolyte content as that of the extracellular fluid; however, it is the belief of some neonatologists that the chloride content of the electrode gel causes excessive irritation of neonatal skin. For that reason electrode gels for use with neonates that contain low or even no chloride are available. When these gels are used with silver–silver chloride electrodes, however, the advantages of the electrode stability are no longer present because of absence or reduced concentration of chloride ions in the gel. Thus, in instrumentation systems where silver–silver chloride electrodes are required for best performance, the use of these special electrode gels may compromise the overall operation of the system.

Polarization effects on biopotential electrodes also can be minimized by making certain that only an absolute minimum of electrical current flows across the electrode-body interface. Although theoretically a measurement can be made with zero current across this interface, in practice there always has to be some current. Nevertheless, by using processor electronic blocks that provide a very high electrical resistance between the electrode input connections (technically referred to as a processor with a high electrical input resistance or input impedance), one can minimize these polarization effects. Modern electronics has made it possible to routinely have input resistance on the order of 10^7 ohms (Ω) on medical electronic equipment. In many cases this is sufficiently high to make it possible to use pure silver or even stainless steel electrodes without severe polarization problems. In these cases low-chloride electrolyte gel can be used much more effectively. The processor must not inject current into the electrodes either. Thus another important feature of the processor is that this current (sometimes referred to as bias current) be very small.

Some special considerations are necessary when dealing with neonatal skin electrodes. Because the neonate is much smaller than the adult, the radius of curvature and variations in the radius of curvature at different locations on the thorax will be much greater than they are for the adult. Thus, to effectively keep the neonatal skin electrodes in place and to maintain stable electrical operation, one must take into account some mechanical considerations as well as electrical ones. The electrodes must be small and flexible so that they conform to the skin surface. They must be attached in such a way that they are secure, but so that their method of attachment does not cause skin irritation. Finally, in addition to the electrolyte gel considerations previously described, one desires a gel material that will not rapidly dry out, requiring that the electrodes be frequently changed. Some of the problems related to the electrodes, their placement, or the adhesives are as follows:

1. Skin injury: erythema, vesiculation, ulceration, pigmentary changes
2. Infection
3. Pneumothorax (needle electrodes)
4. Poor contact (false alarms)
5. Size: interference with care

The remaining functions of the neonatal cardiac monitor are concerned with signal processing and display or recording (Fig. 24-14). The first stage of signal processing is concerned with providing electrical isolation between the patient and the monitor. The isolation stage is necessary to prevent interaction between the cardiac monitor and any other electrical device that might come in contact with the patient. Without isolation, electrical current from one device might flow through the patient to the other device, causing electrical shock.

The isolated electrocardiographic signal from the electrodes is now amplified to provide a strong enough signal to operate the remainder of the system. In the simplest cardiac monitors the display function is carried out by an oscilloscope that indiciates the electrocardiogram as it is taken. Generally, a 6- to 10-second segment of the most recent electrocardiogram is shown on the oscilloscope. Another means of displaying the electrocardiogram is through the use of a chart recorder. Here a permanent record is made on a paper strip. Obviously this cannot be used for continuous monitoring because of the impractical lengths of paper involved.

Most neonatal cardiac monitors determine heart rate. This is done by the functional blocks shown on the right side of Fig. 24-14. A cardiotachometer circuit determines the heart rate from the electrocardiogram in one of two ways. Instantaneous, or beat-to-beat, cardiotachometers measure the interval between each R wave, and a heart rate is calculated as though each and every RR interval of the electrocardiogram were the same. This process is updated at the completion of each RR interval, and the rate meter indicates heart rate as determined for the previously completed interval. Such a cardiotachometer is capable of determining the beat-to-beat variability in heart rate. In addition to the rate meter, some neonatal cardiac monitors have a chart recorder so that heart rate variability can be visualized as it is on a fetal monitor.

The other type of cardiotachometer determines an average heart rate. There are several ways in which this can be done, and the essence of each is that several RR intervals are averaged before a heart rate is determined.

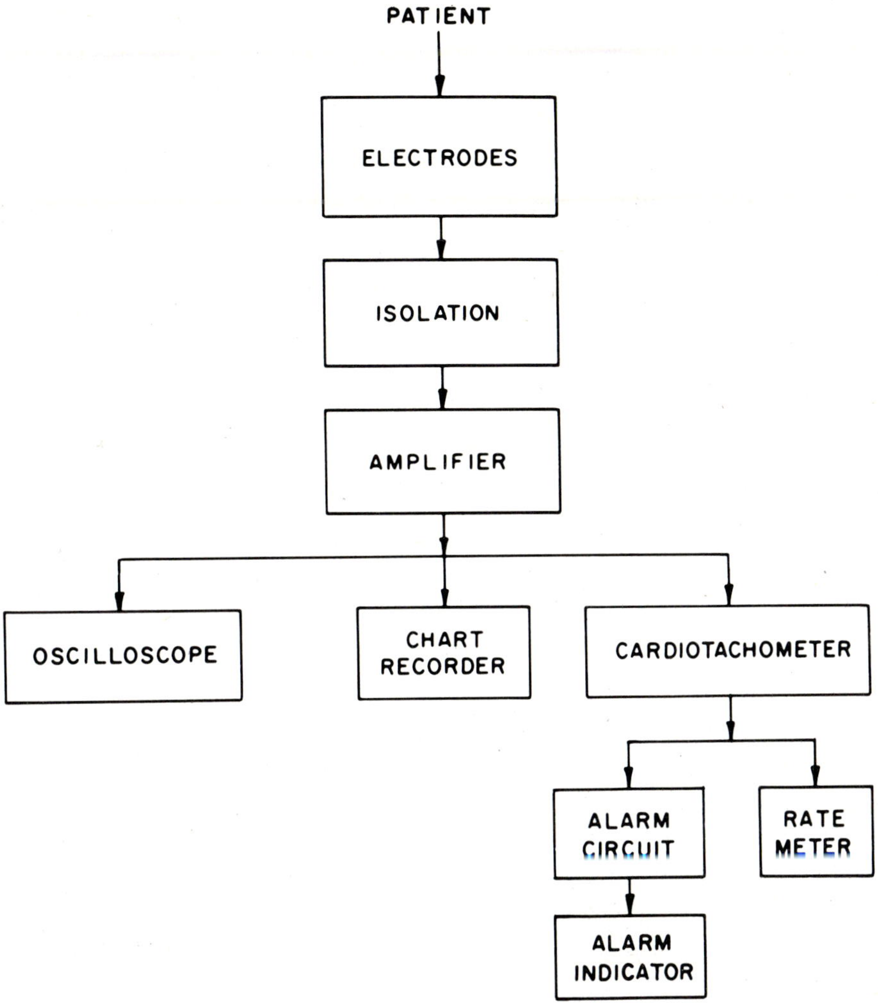

Fig. 24-14. Functional blocks of a typical neonatal cardiac monitor.

Thus the rate meter indicates the average heart rate as determined from several previous beats. This method cannot be used to determine beat-to-beat variability, since the averaging process eliminates some of that variability.

In addition to the oscilloscope and chart recorder, the clinician-machine interface is provided by the rate meter and the alarm system. Digital rate meters are becoming quite popular because they are easy to read. However, when they are used with beat-to-beat cardiotachometers, the new calculation of heart rate with each heart beat causes the meter to frequently change its indication. This can be confusing to the clinical staff and makes it difficult to read the indicator. Often this problem is avoided by having the digital meter display only averaged values of heart rate. An analog indicator such as a meter having a scale of heart rates and a pointer also is frequently used. A disadvantage of this system is that there can be errors introduced on reading the meter. The advantage of this type of indicator is the ease with which one can tell the relation of the present value to a predetermined limit.

The alarm system is used to indicate when the heart rate has fallen beneath or exceeded preset values. An alarm circuit compares the heart rate at the present time with the upper and lower limits, as determined by the operator; as long as the heart rate is between these limits, nothing happens. If this condition is not met, the alarm circuit activates the alarm indicator, which produces an audible and visible alarm.

A major concern in the application of neonatal electronic monitoring devices is the occurrence of false alarms. In some cases these occur so frequently that frustrated clinical staff members deactivate the alarm system altogether. False-positive tachycardiac alarms are the result of artifactual signals that the cardiotachometer interprets as R waves. Thus the cardiotachometer registers extra erroneous "heart beats," resulting in a falsely elevated heart rate. An artifact of this type can be the result of electrode polarization and motion. If a layer of electrolyte ions builds up adjacent to the electrode surface, motion of the electrode with respect to this polarization layer in the electrolyte gel will result in a relocation of electrical charge, which manifests itself as a signal on the electrode. There are two ways to minimize this problem. One is to use a nonpolarizable electrode such as a silver–silver chloride electrode, and the second is to eliminate relative motion between the electrode and the electrolyte gel. Neither technique in itself can completely eliminate the problem. Thus it is best to attempt both. No matter what one does, the motion-induced polarization artifact cannot be entirely eliminated.

Another source of artifact that produces false-positive tachycardiac alarms is interference from extraneous signals. These signals also have the possibility of fooling the cardiotachometer into interpreting them as R waves. Common sources of such signals are the electrical power lines, other pieces of electrical apparatus located near the patient and monitor, and other bioelectrical signals emanating from the patient. Power line interference often can be recognized on the oscilloscope or chart recorder of a cardiac monitor. A broad baseline on the electrocardiogram is the clue. Interference from other electrical devices is seen on the oscilloscope or the chart recorder as a sudden jumping in the baseline. The best way to eliminate this source of artifact is to remove or repair the offending device whenever possible. When trying to locate an extraneous source of artifact of this type, one should first suspect electrical apparatus employing motors and/or heaters. The major biologic source of extraneous signals is the electromyogram. The influence of the electromyogram on the cardiotachometer can be minimized by choosing electrode positions that maximize the amplitude of the QRS complex of the electrocardiogram while minimizing the magnitude of any electromyogram derived from muscle groups underneath and between the electrodes.

Since the false-positive tachycardiac alarms result from the misrecognition of artifact, the problem can be minimized by developing more sophisticated cardiotachometers that can differentiate between true signal and artifact. Biomedical engineers have described various techniques for doing this ranging from electronic filters to computer recognition of the QRS complex. It is important for clinicians to be aware of any of these techniques that might be used in their monitors, since they could also result in the modification of important data. For example, a cardiotachometer that is set to recognize only QRS complexes will miss ectopic ventricular beats because of their different wave shape. If a cardiotachometer uses extensive signal processing, it is desirable that the monitor incorporate a control to enable the clinician to turn off this processing if desired.

PRESSURE MONITORING

Physicists define pressure as the force exerted by a fluid on a surface of unit area; thus the measurement of pressure is really the measurement of a force. There are both direct and indirect methods to measure pressures. In the former the pressure sensor is in direct contact with the fluid being measured, whereas in the latter the fluid being measured is separated from the sensor.

The sensor function of pressure monitors is carried out by a pressure transducer. This device measures the force detected by a diaphragm in contact with the fluid being measured. The pressure in the fluid exerts a force on the diaphragm that deflects it, and this deflection is measured electrically to provide the signal for the processor portion of the instrument. Since pressure in the fluid being measured causes the diaphragm to deflect, some fluid must flow into the pressure transducer. It is thus possible to characterize a pressure transducer in terms of its compliance: the change in volume produced by a change in pressure divided by that change in pressure. It is noted that the definition of compliance of a pressure transducer is the same as that for the lungs, but, as is pointed out later, unlike the lungs, the pressure transducer should have a very low compliance for optimum performance.

Coupling the body to the sensor is an important problem in pressure-monitoring systems (interface *1*, Fig. 24-13). In direct pressure measurement the fluid being measured must be coupled to the pressure transducer itself. This can be done through a fluid-filled tube or catheter. The fluid in the catheter should have properties similar to those of the fluid being measured. For example, physiologic saline solution can be used as the coupling medium in the catheter when one desires to make a direct measurement of blood pressure. As long as the distal end of the catheter is at the same level as the pressure transducer, Pascal's law tells us that the pressure at the transducer will be the same as the pressure at the distal tip of the catheter. This only applies to static (constant) pressures. If the pressure at the distal tip of the catheter is varying, fluid must flow along the catheter to the pressure transducer because of its nonzero compliance. The catheter offers resistance to this fluid flow, and this introduces distortion in the pressure measurement. The amount of fluid that must flow through the catheter is determined by the compliance of the pressure transducer, and so a pressure transducer with low compliance will require less fluid to flow; therefore catheter resistance effects will be minimized.

The compliance of the pressure transducer, the mass of the fluid, and the resistance of the catheter are responsible for another type of distortion that can occur in time-varying pressure measurements. This distortion is a result of mechanical resonance in the system and can produce additional undulations in the pressure waveform, as seen at the transducer, that were not present in the waveform at the distal tip of the catheter. This type of distortion can result in overshoot, which causes the instrument to read a peak pressure that is greater than the actual peak of the pressure waveform.

Additional artifact from the catheter can be seen as the result of movement. Even though a steady pressure is maintained at the distal tip of the catheter and the transducer is at the same height as the distal tip of the catheter, moving the catheter will produce transient pressure changes at the transducer. This type of motion-induced distortion is generally short-lived but makes it difficult to make direct pressure measurements.

Thus, to measure neonatal arterial or venous blood pressure by the direct technique, a catheter must be placed in the appropriate umbilical vessel and advanced until it reaches the central circulation, that is, the aorta or the inferior vena cava. A pressure transducer should be attached to the proximal end of the catheter and positioned so that it is at the same height as the distal end of the catheter. In this way baseline errors are avoided. Even though these errors are small and not too damaging in the measurement of arterial blood pressure, they can be quite serious in the measurement of venous blood pressure. A 10 cm difference in height between the distal catheter and the pressure transducer results in an error of 7.7 mm Hg. The transducer and catheter also should be placed such that there is a minimum of motion so as to reduce artifact.

Until recently pressure transducers were expensive electronic components and had to be reused on different patients. This required the transducer to be sterilized between patient applications since there was a direct connection between it and the infant. The development of silicon microelectronic pressure transducers has changed this requirement. Inexpensive, disposable transducers packaged in a plastic chamber that can be attached to the catheter allow direct measurements of neonatal blood pressure. The cost of these sensors is generally less than 5% of the cost of the reusable sensors; thus the problem of cross-contamination can be reduced by using a transducer on only one patient. These transducers are also smaller than the reusable devices so that they can be located closer to the patient, thereby minimizing the length of the catheter and, hence, its resistance. Their small size also results in a lower compliance, which helps improve the fidelity of waveforms measured by the device.

Pressure can be measured indirectly by tonometry. The basic principle is illustrated in Fig. 24-15. Depicted are two fluid-filled chambers separated by an elastic membrane of finite thickness and under tension (*T*). The pressure in the chamber above the membrane (P_1) and that in the chamber below the membrane (P_2) are equal. Since the areas of the membrane surface facing P_1 and P_2 are equal, the force exerted by the fluid on each side of the membrane must be the same, or in other words: $F_1 = F_2$. The membrane tends to assume the position in which it is stretched the least, that is, where it is perpendicular to the sides of the container (Fig. 24-15, *A*).

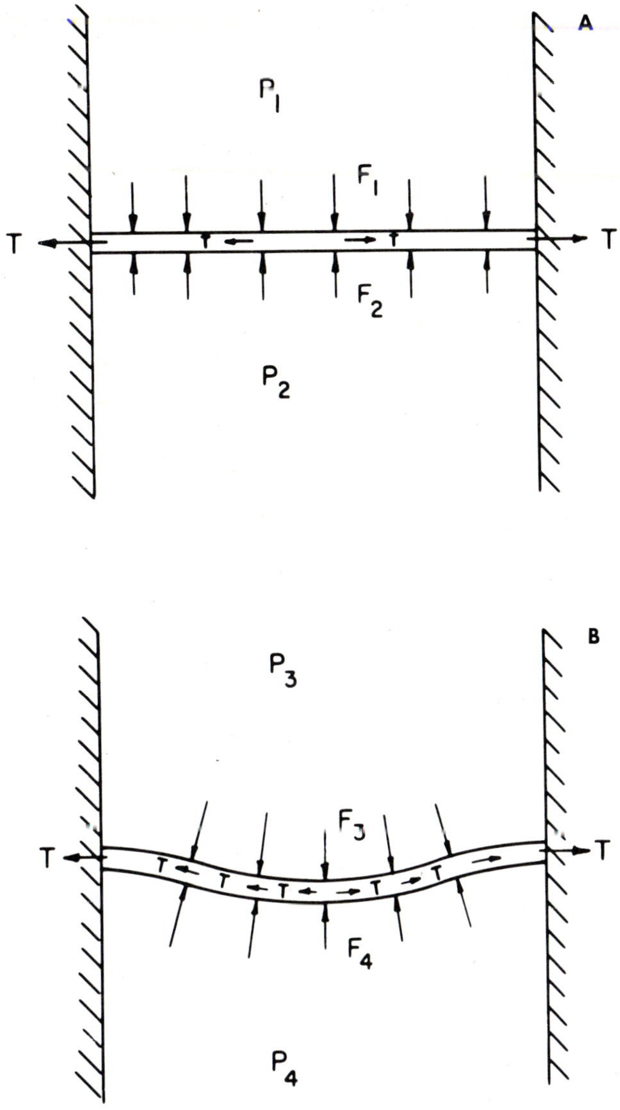

Fig. 24-15. Pressure difference across an elastic membrane under tension. **A,** Equal pressure on each side of the membrane. **B,** Pressure above the membrane is greater than that below the membrane.

In Fig. 24-15, *B*, where the pressure above the membrane is greater than the pressure beneath it, the force F_3 is greater than the force F_4. The membrane therefore will be stretched to the shape shown. The tension in the membrane (*T*) tends to flatten it out to a position where it is stretched the least. The membrane tension therefore exerts a force that aids F_4 and opposes F_3. This force is determined by the amount of curvature in the membrane and its tension. At equilibrium the sum of this force and F_4 will equal F_3. Since we do not know the membrane tension or curvature, it is not possible to determine pressure P_4 by measuring P_3. In the situation of Fig. 24-15, A, where the membrane is planar, it is possible to determine pressure P_2 by measuring pressure P_1. Thus, in general, one can measure the pressure on one side of an elastic membrane if one can determine the pressure on the other side and maintain the planarity of the membrane.

As seen in the preceding discussion, there are several possibilities for errors in pressure measurements by tonometry. Nevertheless there are some instances in which it is the only safe method available. For example, several investigators have shown that transdural and transfontanel *monitoring of intracranial pressure* can be efficacious (Chapter 27). In the former case the dura and part of the pressure sensor serve as the membrane between the two compartments, whereas in the latter the effective membrane includes the scalp as well as the dura and pressure transducer.

The functional block diagram of a typical pressure-monitoring system is shown in Fig. 24-16. As is the case with the cardiac monitor, effective electrical isolation of the pressure transducer and thus the patient from the rest of the machine is essential for safe operation in all types of clinical environments. The isolated electrical pressure signal is then amplified, and special circuits are employed to determine the systolic and diastolic pressures from the pressure waveforms when arterial blood pressure is monitored. The instrument also contains some circuitry for calculating mean pressures. The monitor can consist of only these blocks when it is used for watching pressures that vary slowly such as venous blood pressure or cerebral spinal fluid pressure. Often monitors intended for this purpose have the pressure indicator connected directly to the amplifier, since the variations are so slow that it is not necessary to calculate a mean.

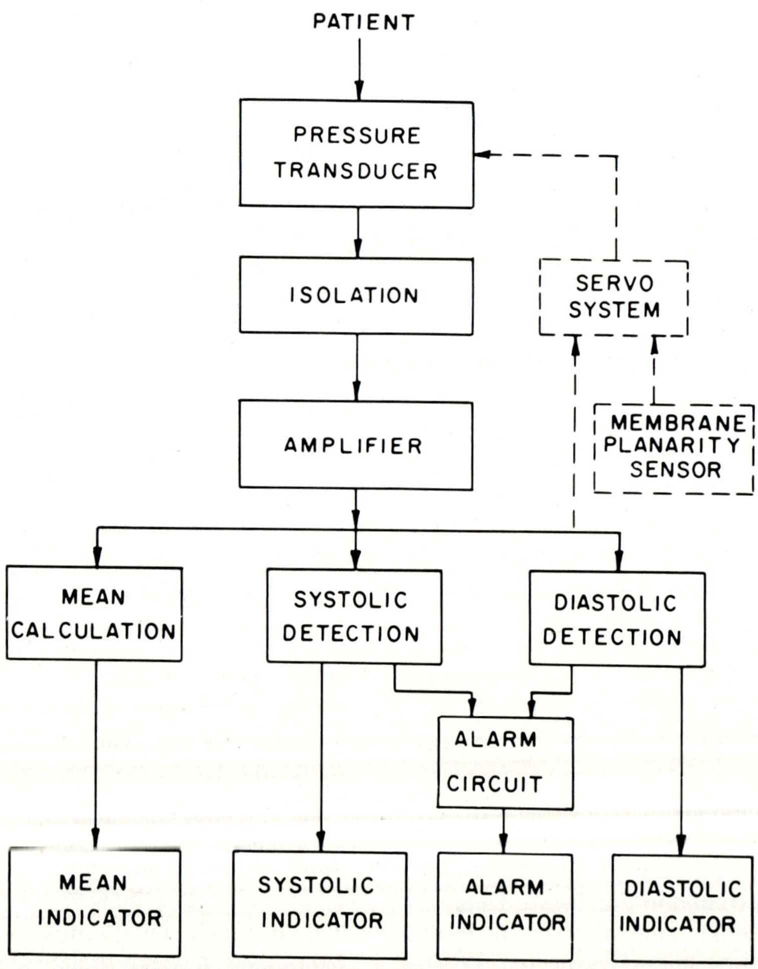

Fig. 24-16. Functional block diagram of a typical pressure monitor. The blocks indicated by dashed lines must be added when indirect tonometric monitoring is performed.

The alarm circuit in Fig. 24-16 is shown connected to the systolic and diastolic detectors for arterial blood pressure monitoring. This circuit compares systolic and diastolic pressures with preset limits, and, if either of the pressures is outside this predetermined range, an audible and visible alarm is activated. It is also possible to have the alarm circuit connected to the mean pressure channel.

In the indirect pressure-measurement system the signal processor must carry out additional functions. If the pressure below the membrane is to be measured, it is necessary to adjust the pressure above the membrane to produce membrane planarity. Thus a system must be included in the monitor that is capable of modifying the pressure above the membrane until membrane planarity is achieved. This system must sense the position of the membrane and adjust the pressure accordingly. Once the membrane is planar, the pressure above the membrane can be sensed, and the signal can be processed in the same way as the direct signal. The system for carrying out this function is known as a servo system, since it must adjust the pressure in the transducer to provide planarity of the membrane. The additional functional blocks in the instrumentation system are shown with dashed lines in Fig. 24-16.

As with the cardiac monitors, pressure monitors have several sources of error. Catheter artifact resulting in baseline and pressure transient errors already have been discussed. In addition, the catheter can become partially or fully obstructed, or an air bubble can form in the catheter. All these problems produce distortion of the pressure waveform. Leaks in the catheter system can result in abnormally low pressure readings or, when the leak is severe, can lead to rapid exsanguination of the patient when the catheter is placed in an artery. Thus it is extremely important that this problem be avoided. In the indirect method of measuring pressure, additional errors can be introduced by the "membrane." The thickness of the membrane in Fig. 24-15 is relatively small compared with dimensions of the area over which pressure is measured, and the membrane itself was assumed to be homogenous. When the pressure is measured across a neonatal fontanel, the membrane is no longer thin with respect to the dimensions of the sensor, nor is it homogenous. Materials of varying elastic properties and tensions are found between the pressure transducer and the neonatal cerebral spinal fluid. One cannot even be certain that there is only cerebral spinal fluid in contact with the inner surface of the "membrane." The process of establishing planarity of the membrane most likely presses the central portion of the dura under the transducer against the cortex and perhaps might even cause minor distension of the cortex. In this case the cortex will exert a force against the membrane that is added to the force produced by the cerebral spinal fluid pressure (F_2 in Fig. 24-15). So for the pressure in the transducer to overcome this force, it is necessary that P_1 be greater than P_2; therefore the measurement is in error. In the indirect method one also has problems in maintaining stable contact between the pressure sensor and the body, as well as in making certain that this contact does not modify the membrane and its tension. Therefore, when indirect pressure-measurement techniques must be used, great care must be employed in their application, and the results must be viewed critically.

A discussion of neonatal pressure monitoring would not be complete without mentioning the measurement of neonatal blood pressure using a sphygmomanometer cuff and ultrasonic or oscillometric detection of the systolic and diastolic pressures. Even though these are not methods of continuous monitoring, they are frequently used for measuring neonatal blood pressure.

Conventional sphygmomanometry and auscultation cannot be used with neonates because of the difficulty in detecting Korotkoff's sounds. By adding an ultrasonic Doppler detection system to a conventional sphygmomanometer cuff, systolic and diastolic pressures can be determined. Ultrasound kinetoarteriography determines the systolic and diastolic pressures by sensing the movement of the wall of the brachial artery that is in the portion of the arm surrounded by the occluding cuff. An ultrasonic transducer is centrally placed under the cuff so that it is approximately over the brachial artery. A portion of the ultrasound beam illuminating the artery is reflected back to the transducer from the arterial wall. If the arterial wall moves with respect to the transducer under the cuff, the frequency of the reflected sound will be shifted in relation to the incident sound. This frequency change, known as a Doppler shift, is a basic physical property of propagating waves and is the same effect that causes the pitch of an automobile horn to sound higher than normal when the vehicle is approaching the listener and lower than normal as it speeds away. Thus, by electronically sensing the shift in frequency of the reflected ultrasound and converting this to an audible signal, it is possible to indicate arterial wall movements under the pneumatic cuff.

The arterial wall will move only when the pressure surrounding the artery and, roughly, the pressure in the cuff lie between the systolic and diastolic pressure. When the cuff pressure is greater than systolic pressure, the artery is collapsed, and blood cannot flow through it. As the cuff pressure drops beneath systolic arterial pressure, the blood pressure is able to force the artery open during systole, but the artery once again collapses when the blood pressure drops below the cuff pressure. Such arterial expansion and collapse will cause two Doppler frequency shifts to occur during each cardiac cycle. The first is a result of the expanding of the artery during the rising phase of arterial pressure as it exceeds the cuff pressure. The second Doppler shift occurs as the arterial pressure falls below the cuff pressure and the artery collapses. When the cuff pressure is close to systolic blood pressure, the two Doppler shifts occur close together in time, and, when the cuff pressure is close to diastolic pressure, there is more time between the two Doppler shifts, since the artery is patent for a longer period.

Once the cuff pressure falls below the diastolic pressure, arterial pressure always will be higher than the cuff pressure; therefore there will be only slight changes in the arterial diameter, which result in only small Doppler shifts in the frequency of the reflected ultrasonic wave. Thus with ultrasonic kinetoarteriography it is possible to detect the systolic and diastolic pressures in a similar manner to the method of ausculation, but ultrasound rather than audible sound is used. The principal advantage of this method is the great ease with which blood pressures can be determined. Unlike auscultation, with which Korotkoff's sounds are especially difficult to hear in premature neonates, ultrasound kinetoarteriography is relatively easy to perform. The ultrasonic sensors are unaffected by ambient noise; and because the ultrasonic signal is processed electronically and converted to audible sound, if the device is used in a noisy environment or the neonate is crying, one need only increase the sound level of the instrument to be able to conveniently detect systolic and diastolic pressures. Automated instruments are even available that automatically determine these points and indicate them on a digital display or scale.

Although the ultrasonic Doppler system described in the previous paragraphs made the routine indirect measurement of neonatal blood pressure possible, the instrumentation was complex and expensive. A less expensive method with approximately the same accuracy is now widely used in neonatal intensive care units. This oscillometric blood pressure instrument is based on the fact that the volume of the tissue in a limb under a sphygmomanometer occlusion cuff changes in a similar way to the patency of the artery in the description of the ultrasonic Doppler technique. A cuff is placed around the infant's limb such that the outside circumference of the cuff remains fixed. When the cuff is inflated so that its inner surface is in good contact with the limb, the total volume of tissue and air in the cuff and under it remains constant. When the pressure in the cuff is well above systolic pressure, most of the blood has been squeezed from the tissue under the cuff, and the tissue volume remains constant. The air volume in the cuff will, therefore, also remain constant. As the cuff pressure slowly decreases, it will eventually approach systolic blood pressure. At a cuff pressure somewhat greater than this some blood will begin to enter the tissue under the cuff during systole. This happens because the cuff does not completely enclose the tissue, and the tissue under both sides of the cuff will be at a pressure somewhat lower than the cuff pressure. During systole, the tissue volume increases by the volume of blood entering the tissue. Because the total volume must remain constant, the volume of air in the cuff must decrease by the same amount as the tissue volume increased. The amount of air in the cuff is fixed (at least for a relatively short period, since the cuff is being slowly deflated), so the pressure in the cuff must increase slightly as a result of this tissue volume decrease according to Boyle's law. As the cuff pressure continues to drop, more and more blood is allowed into the tissue at systole. This causes the tissue volume to increase more and more with each heartbeat and, hence, causes the pressure in the cuff to oscillate at the heart frequency. This oscillation is caused by the increased blood volume in the tissue under the cuff during systole and the runoff or decrease in volume in the tissue under the cuff during diastole.

The cuff is connected to an electronic instrument that has a pressure sensor that detects the pressure oscillations. The pressure sensor also measures the absolute pressure in the cuff. The electronic system in many instruments controls the bleeding of air from the cuff so that once the cuff is pumped to a pressure well above systolic pressure, the cuff pressure is dropped until the instrument sees pressure oscillations beyond a preset amplitude. Once these occur, the instrument measures the absolute pressure in the cuff and displays this as systolic pressure. As the cuff pressure continues to drop the amplitude of the pressure oscillation increases until it reaches a maximum value. Investigators have shown that this maximum oscillation occurs at a cuff pressure equal to the mean arterial pressure. Most oscillometric blood pressure instruments for infants and adults take advantage of this fact and determine the mean arterial pressure and display it as well.

As cuff pressure continues to slowly drop, the amplitude of the oscillations decreases until the cuff pressure reaches diastolic pressure. As the cuff pressure drops below this point, the amplitude of the oscillations becomes independent of cuff pressure. The electronic system detects this and indicates the pressure in the cuff at the point where constant amplitude oscillations began to appear as the diastolic pressure. This latter determination is the most difficult for the oscillometric instrument, and one can see great variation in the diastolic pressure values measured with different instruments. Most manufacturers employ electronic microprocessor chips to make the necessary calculations for the determinations described in the previous paragraphs. Each instrument has a slightly different method of determining the three principal points, systolic, mean, and diastolic pressure, and so variations from one instrument to the next are frequently seen.

An important consideration in both the ultrasonic and the oscillometric methods of indirect blood pressure measurement is the rate at which the cuff pressure is dropped. Systole must occur for the instrument to determine each of the pressures described previously. Thus the precision of the instrument will be no greater than the pressure drop in the cuff from one heartbeat to the next. Although no standard has been established for neonatal blood pressure measuring instruments, the American Heart Association recommends that cuff pressure be dropped by no more than 3 mm Hg per heartbeat during indirect blood pressure measurement in adults, and this is a good rule of thumb for infants as well. The disadvantage of such a slow cuff deflation is that measurements take a relatively long time. When a human is controlling the deflation of a cuff in measuring adult blood pressures, the cuff pressure can be slowly decreased around the expected systolic and diastolic pressures and more rapidly decreased at other points to speed up the measurement. Unfortunately, machines cannot do this yet.

A second concern regarding indirect blood pressure measurement using cuff techniques on infants is that both the ultrasonic Doppler and the oscillometric techniques are exquisitely sensitive to motion. Thus the infant's limb must be relatively quiet during the measurement. Even though this is not always possible, one can frequently obtain a useful signal. However, a certain amount of caution is wise when making measurements on an active infant. Restraint of the limb during the measurement and a second check are always good ideas for best results.

RESPIRATION MONITORING

The monitoring of respiratory gas exchange also can be done by direct and indirect methods. As is the case with pressure monitoring, the direct method is more invasive than the indirect methods; however, it also is more accurate. In the direct method airway flow is sensed by instrumentation that has direct access to the airway. If the therapy applied to the neonate already requires a direct connection to the airway, such as an endotracheal cannula, direct instrumentation is no problem, but to make this connection for purposes of monitoring respiration usually is not justified.

Direct methods of sensing ventilation have been used in the pulmonary physiology and pulmonary function laboratories but for the most part are not suitable for patient monitoring. These methods, nevertheless, can serve as standards for calibrating and testing indirect methods that are suitable for monitoring. The pneumotachograph is one such device that can be placed in series with the airway and will quantitatively measure flow, which can then be integrated to determine volumes. The basic principle is that it is possible to measure the volume flow of a gas through a channel of known resistance by measuring the pressure drop across the resistance. The resistance can be made very small so as not to interfere with ventilation, and sensitive electronic pressure sensors can determine the pressure drop across this resistance. Although this method can yield quantitative flows and volumes, it requires a tight connection to the airway and often adds dead space.

If one is interested only in patterns of ventilation with only qualitative relationships between actual flows and volumes, tight connections to the airway are not required. Respiration monitors based on temperature or carbon dioxide sensors in the airway can be used for clinical monitoring and pneumogram studies. Temperature sensors in the airway may detect ventilation in two ways: by measuring the temperature differences between inspired and expired air, or by measuring the cooling of a heated probe as inspired or expired air is transported past it. In both cases, the temperature sensor of choice is a small, low-mass thermistor that changes its electrical resistance as a function of temperature. The low thermal mass of the sensor allows it to rapidly respond to temperature variations so that it can follow infant breathing patterns. An important consideration in using the nasal thermistor for respiration monitoring in infants is the placement of it in the flowing air. For young infants who are believed to be obligate nasal breathers, the sensor can be taped to the nose or face so that the thermistor itself is near the center of one nostril. If, however, the infant breathes through the mouth, a different sensor placement is required, such as placing a thermistor within a face mask that covers both the mouth and nose. This bulky structure may alter breathing patterns, however, and make the baby considerably more uncomfortable.

Expired air from the lungs has a higher carbon dioxide fraction than inspired air. This can be sampled by placing an open-ended tube at the nose and/or mouth so that suction on the tube causes a small amount of airway gases to flow into the tube. The sampled gases are transported along the tube to an instrument containing a rapidly responding sensor of carbon dioxide. An increase in carbon dioxide is noted when expired air is sampled, and a decrease is seen as air about to be inspired passes the tube. The distal end of the tube can be located beneath an infant's nose using a support attached to the face. This technique allows monitoring of infant respiration with little interference to the infant or the airway.

The indirect methods of measuring respiration involve detecting chest and abdominal wall movement, whole body movement, or changes in thoracic electrical impedance. Chest and abdominal wall movement can be sensed by several methods: by sensors attached to the neonate or by sensors not placed directly on the patient. A strain gauge—an electrical sensor that changes its electrical resistance when its dimensions are changed—can be taped on the neonate to detect dimensional changes in the chest and/or abdominal wall with breathing. When such a sensor is used, it is important that it not be stiff and that it does not alter the normal movement of the part of the body on which it is placed. A small permanent magnet (magnetometer) also can be taped on the anterior aspect of the chest or abdominal wall when the infant is supine. A magnetic field sensor, such as an electrical coil, then can be placed under the infant; it produces an electrical signal that is related to the position of the magnet. In this way an electrical signal is produced that is related to chest or abdominal wall movement when the infant breathes.

Neonatal body movements also can be detected by placing the patient on a special mattress that is sensitive to patient movement. When the infant moves, electrical signals are produced by the sensor, and these can be related to respiratory motion. The problem with this method is that the sensors are also sensitive to nonrespiratory movements of the neonate, and it may be difficult to obtain an accurate respiration signal. Body movements during apneic periods may be interpreted erroneously as breaths.

One of the most frequently used methods of sensing respiration is to measure changes in the transthoracic electrical impedance. Electrical impedance relates the current through a circuit to the voltage across the circuit for an AC signal in much the same way that electrical resistance describes the relationship for DC signals. Transthoracic electrical impedance is determined by placing biopotential electrodes on the thorax and measuring the electrical impedance between them. This is done by passing a very low-level current, usually less than 100 μA, through the electrodes and measuring the voltage drop across them. This voltage will be proportional to the impedance between the electrodes. Since there is an impedance associated with the polarization layer in the electrodes, it is important to minimize this impedance so that the signal will be dominated by the actual impedance in the body. This can best be done by passing a high-frequency current through the electrodes. At a frequency of 50 kHz, electrode impedance is minimal and is independent of the excitation current frequency.

The change in transthoracic electrical impedance with respiration is small, with typical changes being approximately 0.5% of the baseline over the tidal volume. Thus, even at elevated frequencies where electrode impedances are minimal, they must be constant to avoid introduction of artifact. Not only this but also other sources of impedance variation in the thorax must be minimized for stable operation. Neither of these requirements can be optimally achieved in practice. Electrode impedances vary with electrode motion, and transthoracic impedance also varies with movement of the neonate. In addition, thoracic blood volume can change transthoracic electrical impedance. Indeed this can be applied to estimating cardiac output noninvasively while a subject holds his breath so that respiratory impedance variations are eliminated. Thus the typical neonatal respiration signals seen from transthoracic-impedance sensing contain three components: the respiratory component, the cardiac component, and artifact. Since only the first component is being measured, the other two can cause significant errors, especially by giving false-negative apnea alarms.

Cardiogenic artifact is frequently seen in the respiration signal. It is most prevalent when the transthoracic-impedance sensing method is used, but it can be seen with other indirect sensors of respiration as well. A typical example of respiration signals during a brief apnea is shown in Fig. 24-17. Simultaneous recordings were made from the same infant using the transthoracic impedance, abdominal strain gauge, and nasal thermistor techniques. Note that during the apnea one sees small excursions in the impedance signal that correspond to each heartbeat indicated by the electrocardiogram. This cardiogenic artifact can confuse the breath-detecting circuits of transthoracic-impedance types of apnea monitors, causing them to detect a breath when one does not occur. To minimize this problem manufacturers of apnea monitors have incorporated special signal processing into their systems. Unfortunately, this signal processing limits somewhat the monitor's ability to detect breaths and apnea, and errors can still occur. In some cases cardiogenic artifact is still detected as a breath, while in other cases the signal processing of the monitor causes actual breaths to be missed. In prescribing a transthoracic-impedance apnea monitor for a patient, the physician must understand the method of breath detection and cardiac artifact rejection used in the monitor, so that a method that minimizes false-positive and false-negative alarms can be used.

It is shown in Fig. 24-17 that the shape of the respiration waveform is somewhat different from different sensors. Thus it is important to understand which technique was used to obtain the data when viewing a respiration recording. In general, the most frequently used technique of transthoracic electrical impedance suffers from the greatest discrepancies when compared to a pneumotachograph. In addition to increased cardiogenic artifact, the impedance signal can vary in apparent breath amplitude even though tidal volume remains unchanged.

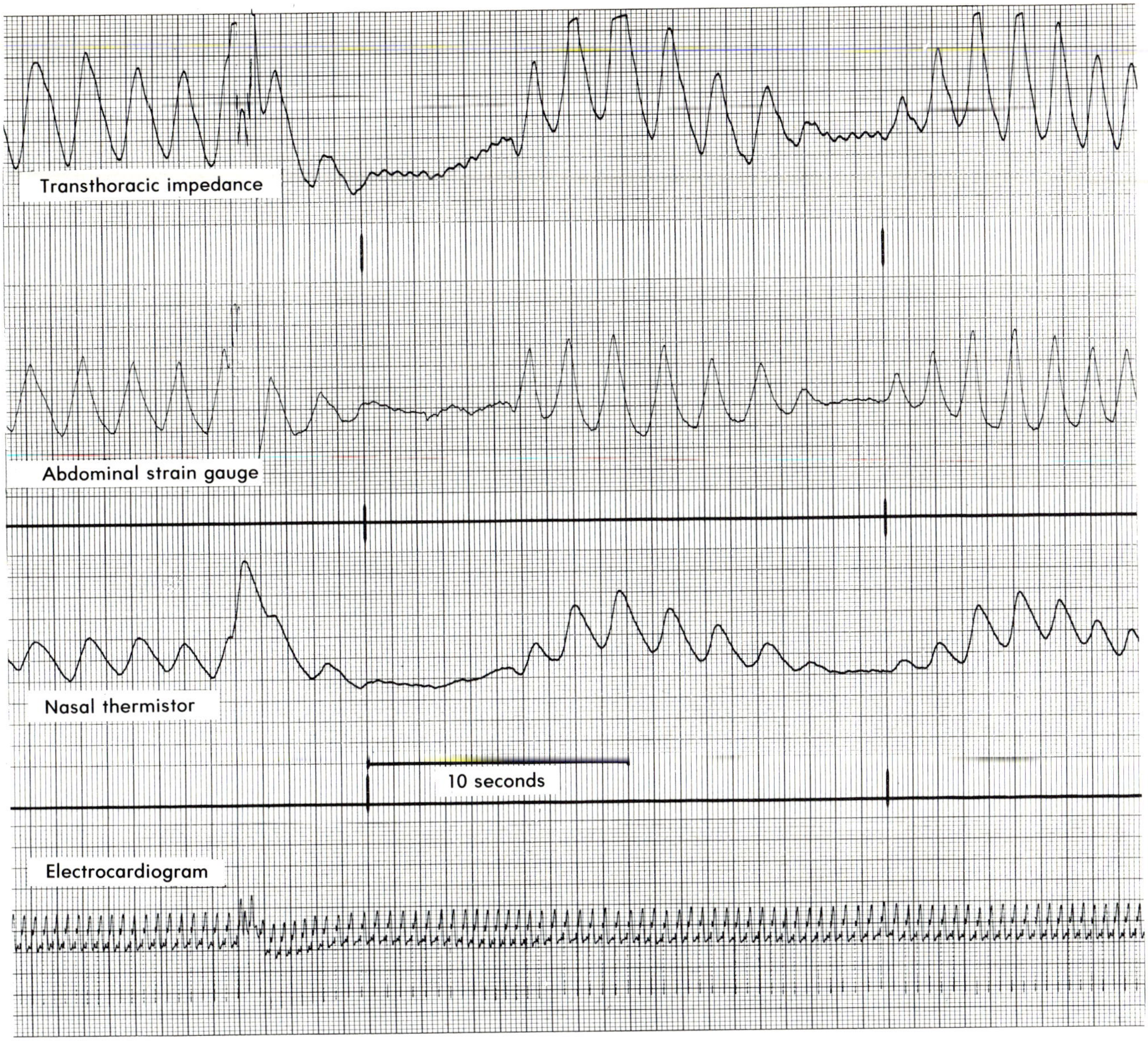

Fig. 24-17. Tracing of an infant's respiratory signals, obtained by different techniques.

The impedance signal can also be more susceptible to motion artifact than signals from an abdominal strain gauge.

The signal processing aspect of apnea monitors can greatly differ from one brand of monitor to the next. The availability of modern microcomputer electronic technology to medical monitors has allowed complex signal-processing algorithms to be carried out in bedside monitors. However, when processing algorithms are not 100% efficacious, as is the case with all methods in use for respiration monitoring, errors are likely to occur. Tests comparing three different commercially available apnea monitors in my laboratory demonstrated this point. A recording of an infant respiration signal containing a 14-second apnea was played into each monitor, and apneas ranging from 9 to 17 seconds were detected and indicated by the different machines. Again, understanding the method of signal processing used in a monitor is important in monitor choice.

The anatomy of a typical neonatal respiration monitor is shown in Fig. 24-18. These devices are primarily designed to detect apnea, and they are frequently referred to as apnea monitors. The respiration signal is sensed by one of the techniques described previously. When the electrical impedance technique is used, the same electrodes usually are employed to obtain the electrocardiogram as well, and the respiration monitor also includes a cardiac monitor such as the one shown in Fig. 24-14.

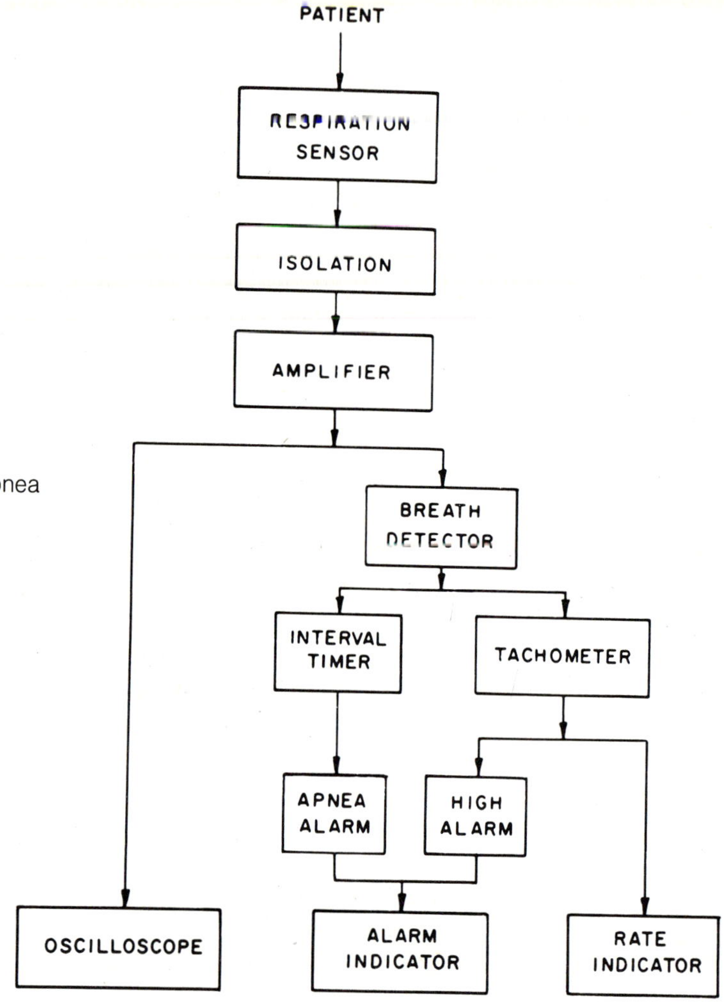

Fig. 24-18. Functional block diagram of a typical apnea monitor.

As with all the other electronic monitoring equipment described in this chapter, it is important to electrically isolate the sensor from the rest of the electronic system. The signal is then amplified and may be displayed directly on an oscilloscope. In monitors that carry out combined functions, all the signals can be shown on different channels of the same oscilloscope. The amplified signal also is fed to a breath detector, a circuit designed to indicate when the neonate takes a breath. This function is not easy to carry out electronically, since the neonatal respiration waveform can be quite complex. The presence of artifact makes the detection even more difficult. Once a breath is detected, a tachometer circuit is used to determine the respiration rate that is displayed on the rate indicator. These circuits are similar to the ones used in the cardiac monitor, and most respiration monitors use an averaging tachometer. An alarm circuit can be employed to indicate when the respiration rate falls outside the preset limits. The breath detector also signals an interval timer that determines the interval between breaths. In newer monitors this function is carried out as a part of the tachometer, but it is shown separately in Fig. 24-18 for clarity. The apnea alarm circuit determines when the interval between breaths reaches a preset time, for example, 20 seconds, and then activates the alarm indicator to give a visible and audible alarm.

The overall problem with neonatal apnea monitors is the frequency of false-positive and false-negative alarms. As was pointed out in the discussion of respiration sensors, motion and cardiac artifacts frequently interfere with the respiration signal. If the monitor misinterprets these artifacts as respiration, an abnormally high respiration rate will be calculated by the tachometer, and the interval timer will not measure the true interval between breaths. This, as pointed out earlier, can disable the apnea alarm when apnea is occurring, giving a false-negative alarm condition.

There also can be problems with the breath detector

sensing true breaths. In cases involving large excursions in tidal volume from one breath to the next, the amplitude of the respiration signal will show similar variations. Often the smaller breaths are missed by the respiratory monitor, and this will give erroneously low values for the respiration rate and may trigger false-positive apnea alarms.

A problem with all the types of indirect respiration sensors is that they are unable to detect obstructive apnea. In this case the neonate goes through respiratory efforts even though no air is exchanged, and there are chest wall movements, whole body movements, and thoracic electrical impedance changes. Only direct measurement from the airway can reliably detect this type of apnea.

In general, currently available methods for indirect respiration and apnea monitoring are not ideal. False alarms do exist in all the different types of monitors, and the clinician should be aware of conditions that produce these false alarms. Nevertheless, respiration and apnea monitors have been of considerable help in neonatal intensive care, and although not currently ideal, they are certainly the best alternative.

Apnea monitors used at home can alert parents to life-threatening episodes of apnea or bradycardia so that resuscitative measures can be taken. In these cases false alarms can be very disruptive to the family.

SAFETY CONSIDERATIONS

Neonatal intensive care involves the use of many electrical, electronic, and other types of devices that have been shown to benefit the patient, yet their use also introduces a small amount of risk. Thus, to effectively apply these devices and systems in the care of the neonate, it is necessary to understand the threat they present to the patient and the clinical personnel along with their benefits. In this way necessary safety precautions can be understood and practiced when these devices are used in patient care.

A major consideration in using electrical and electronic devices in the nursery is the electrical shock hazard. Unfortunately, when safety considerations in intensive care units are discussed, it is implied that the electrical problem is the only safety problem. This is certainly not the case. In neonatology there are many examples of hazards to the neonate from the use of monitoring and therapeutic devices in the nursery. For example, small air emboli introduced into the neonatal circulation through intravenous lines can severely compromise cardiac output; leaks in arterial catheter lines can result in serious bleeding; and overheating of the incubator can expose the neonate to dangerous thermal environments. These potential hazards are discussed in other sections of this text and therefore are not described in detail here, but the reader is reminded that they represent safety hazards every bit as severe as the electrical shock hazard.

The electrical shock problem is a result of the fact that the 120 V electrical power system is connected in such a way that one side of the power line is attached to the earth, or "ground." This means that if anything capable of conducting electrical current comes in contact with the other side of the power line and the earth or an electrical conductor connected to the earth, an electrical current can flow. An extreme example of this is a person taking a bath and reaching for an electrical appliance in the bathroom. The water in the bathtub is connected to the earth (or ground) through the metal water pipes; if in touching the electrical appliance this person inadvertently comes in direct or indirect contact with the ungrounded side of the power line because of a defective appliance, the person could experience electrical currents sufficiently high to cause cardiac arrest.

This example of a bather reaching for an electrical appliance is not so far removed from the situation of neonates and for that matter sometimes the clinical staff in the intensive care nursery. Even though these individuals are not lounging in a bathtub, often they are still connected to ground. In the case of the infant in an incubator the incubator itself is connected to the electrical power system, and its metal parts are grounded through the electrical power plug. The infant is surrounded by these metal parts, and thus it is very easy to become connected to ground either by direct contact with a metal interior part in the incubator or by having the connection made by an electrolytic solution such as spilled intravenous fluids, urine, and formula. Similarly, clinical staff members also can be grounded by touching the metal parts of devices that are grounded, such as an incubator, or by contact through the floor of the nursery itself in cases where a conductive floor and shoes are employed.

This situation is represented in Fig. 24-19. Here the neonate is connected to ground. When electronic monitoring devices are used, the neonate can be electrically connected to them through various transducers such as surface biopotential electrodes or a pressure transducer connected to an indwelling catheter. Since the electronic monitoring device is connected to the power line, it is possible for electrical leakage pathways to exist between the ungrounded side of the power line and the transducer on the patient. Thus it is possible for an electrical current to flow from the power line through the electronic circuit, the transducer, and the neonate to ground. Such a current leakage pathway usually will result in a negligibly small current. However, in circumstances in which the connection of the electronic monitoring device to ground

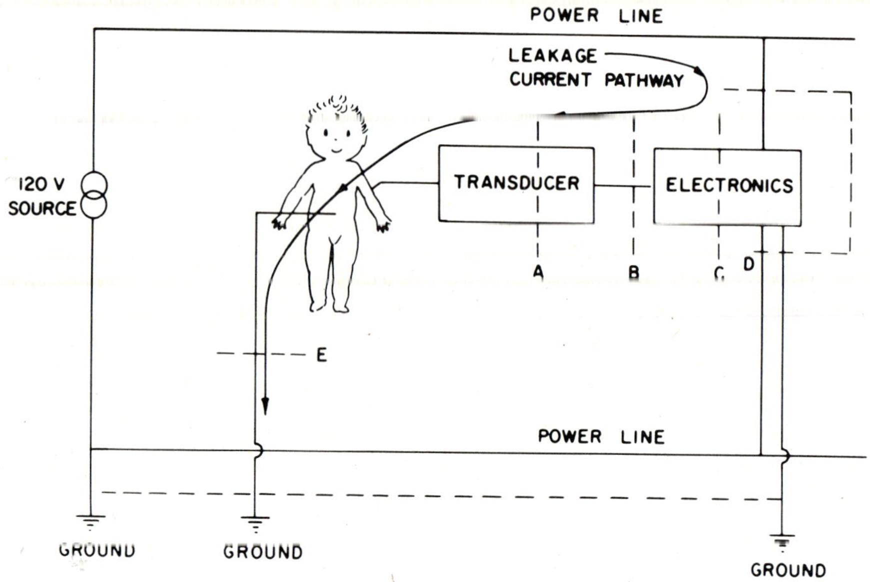

Fig. 24-19. Connection of an electronic monitor to a neonate showing a possible leakage current pathway from the power line to ground through the patient.

through its power source is interrupted, such as with a defective power cord, plug, or electrical outlet, the electrical current leakage pathway through the neonate is the only ground connection to the instrument, and relatively high and potentially lethal current through the patient can exist.

The possibility that an electrical current will follow the path through the patient shown in Fig. 24-19 can be greatly reduced by taking special precautions. Electrical isolation circuits incorporated into the monitors can maintain leakage currents below a critical maximum point for safe operation of the system. Such isolation can be applied to the monitoring device at any of the points indicated by dashed lines in Fig. 24-19. For example, specially designed transducers with built-in electrical isolation, such as pressure transducers used for direct monitoring of arterial blood pressure, can be used, resulting in isolation at line *A* in the figure. An electronic isolation circuit also can be placed between the transducer and the monitor of the electronic circuit, as indicated by the dashed line *B*. Similarly, isolation circuitry can be incorporated into the electronic circuit itself so that all portions of this circuitry that are connected to the power supply and hence the power line will be isolated from those portions of the circuit that are connected to the transducer and hence the patient. This isolation would interrupt the leakage current pathway at dashed line *C*.

Isolation can be introduced between the main power line and the power connection to the medical instrument, as indicated by the dashed line *D*. In this case the goal of isolation is to provide a power source to the monitoring instrument that no longer has one side connected to the ground. In this way the possibility of currents returning to ground through the patient is eliminated. Isolation transformers between the power line and the monitoring instrument are used to achieve this independence from ground. Some neonatal intensive care units have built-in isolation transformers at each patient location so that the electrical outlets are already electrically isolated from ground and from the power sources at other patient locations in the nursery.

The final method to eliminate the shock hazard is to isolate the patient from ground, as indicated by the dashed line *E* in Fig. 24-19. Since the neonate connection to ground is most likely to be through the incubator, the incubator itself can be disconnected from ground so that its interior metal surfaces are no longer sources of ground connections for the neonate. Of course any other piece of electrical apparatus or personnel that the neonate is likely to contact also must be isolated from ground for this system to work. This is difficult to achieve, and thus this last approach is not recommended.

THE FUTURE

Electronic instrumentation for intensive care monitoring of neonates will continue to be important in their care. Improved technology and experience in applying the technology will bring about more reliable instruments, and new sensors will allow additional physiologic variables to be monitored. Computer technology and the microcomputer will make it possible to have monitors that can critically evaluate the quality of a signal and be better able to differentiate true alarm conditions from false alarms. Computer technology also will make it possible to have automated data-recording and charting functions on the monitors, as well as to combine monitored data with other clinical data from the patient. This chapter has examined electronic neonatal monitors that for the most part have enjoyed widespread clinical application. There is a wide range of other more specialized monitoring devices that have been developed for clinical research. Although most of these will never be used for routine patient care, the scientific results that they will make available will certainly affect our understanding and care of the neonate in the future.

Michael R. Neuman

BIBLIOGRAPHY

General

Hill, D.W., and Dolan, A.M.: Intensive care instrumentation, New York, 1976, Grune & Stratton, Inc.

Neuman, M.R.: The biophysical and bioengineering bases of perinatal monitoring. V. Neonatal cardiac and respiratory monitoring, Perinatol. Neonatol. **3**:17, 1979.

Neuman, M.R.: The biophysical and bioengineering bases of perinatal monitoring. VI. Neonatal temperature, blood pressure and blood gas instrumentation, Perinatol. Neonatol. **3**:25, 1979.

Rolfe, P.: Monitoring in newborn intensive care, Biomed. Eng. **10**:399, 1975.

Rolfe, P.: Monitoring equipment for the neonate, Br. J. Hosp. Med. **1**:69, 1970.

Webster, J.G., editor: Medical instrumentation—application and design, Boston, 1978, Houghton Mifflin Co.

Cardiac monitoring

Cobbold, R.S.C.: Transducers for biomedical measurements: principles and applications, New York, 1974, John Wiley & Sons, Inc.

Delgado, J.M.R.: Electrodes for extracellular recording and stimulation. In Nastuk, W.L., editor: Physical techniques in medical research, vol. 5A, New York, 1964, Academic Press, Inc.

Ferris, C.D.: Introduction to bioelectrodes, New York, 1974, Plenum Press.

Geddes, L.A.: Electrodes and the measurement of bioelectric events, New York, 1972, John Wiley & Sons, Inc.

Miller, H.A., and Harrison, D.C., editors: Biomedical electrode technology, New York, 1974, Academic Press, Inc.

Webster, J.G.: Interference and motion artifact in biopotentials, Region 6 Conference Record, IEEE Trans. Biomed. Eng. p. 53, 1977.

Pressure measurement

Fleming, D.G., Ko, W.H., and Neuman, M.R.: Indwelling and implantable pressure transducers, Cleveland, 1977, CRC Press, Inc.

Geddes, L.A.: The direct and indirect measurement of blood pressure, Chicago, 1970, Year Book Medical Publishers, Inc.

Greatorex, C.A.: Indirect methods of blood pressure measurement. In Watson, B.W., editor: IEE medical electronics monographs 1 to 6, London, 1971, Peter Peregrinus.

Hill, A.: Intracranial pressure measurements in the newborn. In Phillip, A.G., editor: Symposium on noninvasive neonatal diagnosis, Clin. Perinatal. **12**(1):161, 1985.

Hugh, A., and others: A new device for non-invasive measurement of intracranial pressure (ICP) in newborns, Med. Prog. Technol. **6**:185, 1979.

Salmon, J.H., Hajjar, W., and Bada, H.S.: The fontogram: a noninvasive intracranial pressure monitor, Pediatrics **60**:721, 1977.

Stegall, H.F., Kardon, M.B., and Kemmerer, W.T.: Indirect measurement of arterial blood pressure by Doppler sphygmomanometry, J. Appl. Physiol. **25**:793, 1968.

Vidyasagar, D., and Raju, T.N.K.: Non-invasive technique of measuring intracranial pressure in the newborn, Pediatrics (Suppl.) **59**:957, 1977.

Respiration monitoring

Baker, L.E.: Electrical impedance pneumography. In Rolfe, P., editor: Non-invasive physiological measurements, vol. 1, London, 1979, Academic Press, Inc.

Nyboer, J.: Electrical impedance plethysmography, ed. 2, Springfield, Ill., 1970, Charles C Thomas, Publisher.

Olsson, T., and others: Transthoracic impedance with special reference to newborn infants and the ratio of air-to-fluid in the lungs, Acta Paediatr. Scand. (Suppl.) **207**:1, 1970.

Rolfe, P.: A magnetometer respiration monitor for use with premature babies, Biomed. Eng. **6**:402, 1971.

PART FOUR

Care of the newborn

Newborn intensive care units (NICUs) are now considered necessities in university or large community hospitals; a need for a transitional care area has been established, as has the value of special transportation vehicles that permit care of sick infants in transit. Each hospital must realistically assess its particular needs and capabilities on the basis of regional population, staff, services, and facilities. Regionalization of care for the newborn has been implemented in many areas, but when regional centers are not yet functional, existing services and facilities for the newborn must be continually and critically reassessed to ensure that they deliver the best care possible with the available resources. The American Academy of Pediatrics Guidelines for Perinatal Care should be used as a guide in implementing and reviewing regional service.

Review of the different facilities established to care for the newborn provides a basic understanding of the role of each unit as it relates to the general care of the infant, as well as an appreciation of the specific medical needs for infants requiring a wide range of medical services. Following the definition of each unit and its facilities and staff, aspects of care common to all units are discussed. These suggestions are offered as *minimum standards*. Application of principles of care and definition of the physical location for the delivery of care remains the prerogative and responsibility of each hospital and its medical staff. In areas that have been regionalized, the role of each unit in the region should be reviewed on a regular basis by regional directors to assure the most effective use of facilities within that network.

NORMAL NEWBORN NURSERY—TYPE I CARE

Characteristics of patients

Infants admitted to this area may include:

1. Well full term newborns who are in the lowest mortality group by weight and gestational age. They will be 38 through 41 weeks of gestational age and 2,000 to 4,000 gm in weight.
2. Well preterm newborns who weigh 2,000 to 2,500 gm and who are at least 36 weeks' gestational age. The capacity to adequately care for these infants depends on the presence of personnel skilled in feeding.
3. Other newborns who are at a comparably low mortality and morbidity risk (once this fact has been firmly established), who do not qualify under type II care and who are well at the time of admission.

Personnel

Registered nurses

One nurse per shift is required but does not necessarily have to be in constant attendance and may share responsibilities in an adjacent obstetric area. The nurse *must* be responsible for maintenance of all emergency equipment and know the appropriate physician to call for emergencies.

Paramedical personnel (practical nurses, aides, and others)

One individual must be attending the infants at all times (regardless of census), with a ratio of between 1:6 and 1:8 required (3-4 hours of care every 24 hours). These individuals should be trained in routine care, pharyngeal suction, oxygen administration by mask and bag, and routine feeding. They also must understand principles of hemostasis and be able to tie an umbilical cord as an emergency measure. If rooming-in is used, at least one person trained in these procedures must be available in an adjacent area at all times.

Physicians

A specific pediatrician should be designated as the physician responsible for general, medical, and administrative policies and routines affecting these infants and should regularly review all such matters. Each infant should have a particular physician responsible for his medical care.

Facilities and services

1. Infants should be cared for in a unit near the maternity ward or in rooming-in accommodations.
2. Care may be rendered centrally in one large room with a minimum of 2 feet in all directions between bassinets and approximately 20 square feet per infant.
3. The number of bassinets should at least equal the number of postpartum beds plus 20% to 30% to allow for multiple births, prolonged maternal or infant hospitalizations, and variation in the census. Because the area requires one caretaker for each 6 to 8 infants, the rooms should be designed to accommodate 6 to 8, 12 to 16, or 18 to 24 infants.
4. The hospital's laboratory must be able to provide on a 24-hour basis standard bacteriologic studies, urinalyses, hematocrit determinations, white blood cell counts with differentials, blood typing and cross matching, direct and indirect Coombs' tests, and microdeterminations of direct and indirect bilirubin, blood glucose, calcium, sodium, potassium, and chloride concentrations. Serology testing for phenylketonuria also should be regularly available during the day shift.
5. Roentgenologic services for the nursery should include the capability of taking portable films on a 24-hour basis.
6. Equipment should include foot-controlled sinks and soap dispensers, stethoscopes, sterile umbilical tape, examining equipment, and emergency resuscitation equipment.

Medical policy and administration

1. Hospitals in which 500 or more infants are delivered each year should provide this type of care. Hospitals with fewer than 500 deliveries should be encouraged to discontinue their obstetric services and concentrate these services in one regional facility.
2. Special protocols should be established for observation of infants during the first 12 to 24 hours of life.
3. Any infant who becomes ill, in whom a presumptive diagnosis of sepsis is made, or whose course requires other than routine care should be transferred to an area where type II care is available.
4. Infants who underwent unsterile or unregistered deliveries, or both, not otherwise included under type II care may be admitted to this unit and maintained in an incubator with the special observation protocols used for the first 12 to 24 hours applied throughout their hospitalization.
5. All infants should be examined by a physician within 24 hours of birth and within the 24 hours before discharge. In nurseries where babies are discharged within 3 days of birth, two examinations should be required within 72 hours.
6. Caps and masks should not be required in the nursery. Short-sleeved gowns and hand-to-elbow washing techniques should be used by all visiting personnel. Scrub gowns or freshly laundered uniforms should be worn by nurses.
7. Regular monthly bacteriologic monitoring protocols should be instituted.
8. An area for emergency resuscitation with appropriate

equipment, suction equipment, and oxygen must be available in each nursery and available on a portable basis for rooming-in arrangements.

TRANSITIONAL OR INTERMEDIATE CARE NURSERY—TYPE II CARE

Characteristics of patients

Unless also qualifying for type III care, patients admitted to this unit should include:

A. Infants of high-risk mothers
   1. Maternal toxemia, preeclampsia, and eclampsia
   2. Maternal diabetes
   3. Maternal cardiac or pulmonary disease
   4. Maternal hypertension
   5. Maternal drug addiction
   6. Prepartum mothers with fever or evidence of infection
   7. Rh-negative mothers with positive history and present evidence of sensitization
   8. Mothers under 15 or over 40 years of age
   9. Mothers whose infants were delivered by cesarean section
   10. Grand multiparas
   11. Mothers with evidence of polyhydramnios or oligohydramnios
   12. Mothers with any other major medical or surgical complication (for example, thyrotoxicosis, hepatitis, or sickle cell disease)

B. Infants with birth weights from 750 to 2,250 gm

C. Infants with birth weights over 4,000 gm

D. Infants with gestational age by last menstrual period over 42 weeks

E. Infants with birth weight below the tenth percentile or above the ninetieth percentile for gestational age

Personnel

Registered nurses

At least one registered nurse must be in attendance on each shift and should be part of the pediatric nursing service and have no nursing responsibilities other than those related to care of these infants. The overall responsibilities should include the availability and continued maintenance of all emergency equipment.

Paramedical personnel (practical nurses, aides, and others)

These additional personnel must be available to provide a final total personnel-to-patient ratio of 1:3-4 (6-8 hours of care every 24 hours). The nurses working in this unit must have special training in cardiopulmonary resuscitation, be proficient in cardiac and respiratory monitoring, and be able to assist with procedures, including intubation, umbilical vessel catheterization, decompression of a pneumothorax, and lumbar punctures. The nurses also must be trained to care for infants requiring assisted ventilation for 2 to 3 hours. Nurses in these units should be able to initiate or change therapy, even when a physician is not present, using established protocols. The nursing staff may serve in an expanded role and should be trained, when appropriate, to intubate, to decompress a pneumothorax, and to initiate mechanical ventilation.

Pediatrician

The board-certified pediatrician in charge should have additional training in the management of high-risk infants. In some instances, the director should have subspecialty certification in neonatal medicine. In coordination with the senior nursing staff, the pediatrician should establish guidelines that will determine the ultimate location of most patients admitted to this unit and review the admissions daily to monitor the appropriateness of the previous day's transfers. When questions arise about particular patients, the physician or a designee should evaluate the patient before a final disposition.

Facilities and services

1. Infants can be cared for in an area either completely separated or contiguous to the well baby nursery or the NICU. This area may be located in the delivery suite.
2. Care in this area requires 50 square feet per infant. There should be 4 feet on all sides between bassinets and/or incubators in this area. Infants requiring intermediate care can be located in a single large room or smaller rooms with sufficient space to house three infants, since this level of care requires a nurse for every three patients.
3. Since approximately 3 to 4.5 infants per 100 deliveries require the services of such a unit, a specific hospital's needs should be based on annual delivery rate and the short duration of admission. Maximum capacity should rarely exceed four beds even in the largest perinatal centers.
4. Basic equipment for this area should include all the items required for type I care, as well as incubators, appropriate monitoring equipment, and respirators. All equipment and supplies for resuscitation can be conveniently stored in an emergency cart.
5. Infusion pumps should be used to control administration of fluids.
6. There should be eight electrical outlets, two oxygen outlets, two compressed air outlets, and two suction outlets per patient care area.
7. The hospital's laboratory should provide the same support as that for type I care. In addition, it should provide acid-base measurement and blood gas determination on a 24-hour basis.

8. A portable roentgen unit with trained technicians must be available to provide radiologic studies in the unit.
9. The laboratory, radiology, and ultrasound technicians should either be in the hospital or on-call 24 hours to guarantee their availability to the nursery. Respiratory therapists with expertise in the newborn should be in the hospital at all times.

Medical policy and administration

1. Hospitals with more than 1,000 deliveries per year should provide this level of care.
2. Administrative policies for type I care are applicable.
3. The duration of stay depends on the functional capability of the unit. Some type II nurseries provide care only slightly more complex than a type I nursery; the duration of stay in this type of unit should be limited to less than 6 to 8 hours with subsequent transfer to type I or type III care. In other type II nurseries with capabilities approaching type III care the duration of stay may have no limitations, but guidelines should be established by the unit in conjunction with its supporting type III nursery. Written contracts with regional tertiary units should guarantee availability of transport when required. Premature infants with birth weights of 1,500 to 2,500 gm should be cared for in a specific area located adjacent to either the NICU or the regular nursery.
4. A transport module that provides oxygen, maintains temperature, and allows easy access to the infant should be available for transfer of infants between areas.

NEONATAL INTENSIVE CARE NURSERY: TYPE III CARE

Characteristics of patients

Infants admitted to this area should include:

1. Any infant 4 weeks or less of age who requires intensive care. Occasionally older infants who are small and have special nursing needs (for example, intravenous alimentation of a 3-month-old baby with a short bowel syndrome) may be admitted to this area and cared for in an incubator.
2. All infants with birth weights less than 1,500 gm. If such infants are otherwise normal after 24 to 48 hours, they may require less intensive observation. However, they must be cared for by a staff with skill and experience in feeding and observing low birth weight or premature infants. It may be convenient to group these infants in the intermediate care nursery.
3. Any infant less than 4 weeks of age who requires surgery (exclusive of circumcision).
4. Infants with sepsis, meningitis, pneumonia, syphilis, or other infections may remain in this area at the discretion of the director of the nursery with institution of appropriate isolation procedures.

Personnel

Registered nurses

There should be a 2:1 patient-to-nurse ratio with 1:1 ratio for the sickest infants (for example, an infant requiring mechanical ventilation). Nurses in this area should have no other assignments outside this nursery unless it is on regular rotation to a type II nursery. All nurses in this area should have a closely supervised, well-controlled orientation program with its duration suited to the needs of the particular nurse; nurses without this orientation should not work in this area.

Paramedical personnel (practical nurses and aides)

These personnel should assist in the routine aspects of care, freeing the registered nurses for more technical duties and for more intensive care of the sickest infants.

Physician

The director of this unit should be a full-time neonatologist. Twenty-four hour in-hospital coverage by a pediatric resident staff, a pediatrician, or specially trained neonatal nurses is essential, and consultants must be available in all medical and surgical specialities.

Facilities and services

1. Infants must be cared for in an area that is separated from the well baby nursery, but the area may be contiguous to the transitional care nursery. In designing new units this area should be adjacent to the delivery suites if possible. Older hospitals may be unable to rearrange existing facilities to provide this access at reasonable costs.
2. A minimum of 80 to 100 square feet per infant is needed to provide this care.
3. Approximately 1 to 1.5 infants per 100 deliveries will need intensive care.
4. This area should have all the equipment required for type II care, as well as more extensive monitoring facilities; the question of using open versus closed (incubator) care for sick infants should be resolved by the physician in charge.
5. There should be 12 to 16 electrical outlets, three to four oxygen and compressed air outlets, and three suction sources for each infant. All electrical outlets should be on both regular and emergency power.
6. The hospital laboratory must provide all the determinations needed for type I and type II care. In addition to 24-hour service for the aforementioned, platelet counts and coagulation studies should be available. Where delays in acid-base determinations

and particularly Pa_{O_2} are unavoidable because of location of the laboratories or limitation of personnel, a unit to measure pH, P_{O_2}, and P_{CO_2} should be available within the nursery.

7. Roentgenographic and ultrasonographic facilities and trained personnel should be provided for the unit on a 24-hour basis.

Medical policy and administration

1. Hospitals with more than 3,000 deliveries per year should establish intensive care nurseries or have regularized means of transfer to a nearby unit.
2. Administration and medical care of patients in this area should be the responsibility of the director of the unit.
3. Provisions should be made to ensure admission for sick infants transferred from smaller services; interhospital transportation of sick infants should be done to provide regional coverage and should be closely supervised by the director of this unit.

TRANSPORT UNITS

See also Chapter 2.

The goal of an effective transport system is to guarantee a continuum of care from the moment a problem is identified until it is resolved. To assure accomplishment of this task, all type I and II units must have an ongoing relationship with a regional intensive care unit. Ideally, infants at high risk should be delivered in institutions capable of providing intensive care from the moment of delivery. Nonetheless, it is estimated that 40% of neonatal problems are at present unpredictable. To provide for such emergencies, an effective transport system with specially trained nursing and medical personnel is essential. The early transfer of unexpected high-risk infants to a special care unit significantly alters neonatal morbidity and mortality. Much can be done to protect the infant from the risks involved in such a transfer. Transport facilities capable of initiating therapy in a critically ill infant before effecting transfer to a regional special care unit may be required.

An alternate and more effective solution to this problem is the establishment of an acute treatment area in each hospital in the region. This facility allows treatment and stabilization of sick infants before transport. It also provides an educational and training opportunity for the tertiary transport team.

HOSPITAL UNITS

Physical facilities

Lighting

Lighting should allow easy detection of both cyanosis and jaundice and is best provided by deluxe, cool white fluorescent bulbs emitting 100 to 150 foot-candles' illuminance at the infant's bedside. This intensity also will alleviate the problem of shadows within the nursery. Spotlights may be provided in selected locations with either portable lamps containing two 150-W fluorescent bulbs or by ceiling- or wall-mounted spotlights. Such white infrared lamps provide warmth as well as light; ceiling mounting of these lamps permits procedures to be done outside the icubator without the infant losing heat to the environment. The use of blue lighting in nurseries has been limited because of frequent complaints of nausea and dizziness from personnel working in these units. (See Chapter 34 for discussion of phototherapy.)

Walls

True skin color is best seen in nurseries with walls that are beige or white; brighter tones of blue and yellow interfere with the ability to evaluate jaundice and cyanosis.

Because of problems with temperature regulation in sick infants and reports of heat loss or overwarming in selected infants, some authorities have suggested elimination of outside windows for neonatal intensive care areas. However, nurseries without windows create an additional mental strain on personnel that may negate the thermal advantages. Air insulation between two glass panes will reduce severe variations in temperature and is a compromise when windows are present. Outside awnings in parts of the country where radiant heat gain is a problem also reduce the chance of overheating.

Storage

Nursing efficiency is increased in a unit where easy accessibility to disposable supplies is guaranteed by design of the unit; modular storage walls can be effectively used to this end. Storage areas for bulky equipment, such as respirators, incubators, and phototherapy lamps, should be available near the nursery.

Temperature control and ventilation

The air temperature in nurseries should be maintained between 72° and 76° F (22° and 26° C) with the relative humidity between 35% and 60%. These temperature and humidity ranges prevent excessive heat loss or gain for the infant and ensure personnel comfort.

The American Academy of Pediatrics suggests a minimum of 12 changes of room air per hour for control of infection. The fresh air input should be located either on or near the ceiling, with the exhaust outlet near the floor; the ventilation unit for the NICU should be separated from the remainder of the hospital system. A slight positive pressure differential between the unit and adjacent hallways should exist within the ventilation system. Most nurseries also incorporate an air-conditioning system within the ventilation system. Attention to filtering outside air with adherence to established standards is particularly important in urban nurseries where polluted air is an increasing ecologic problem.

Laminar flow provides direct vertical, sterile air flow more efficiently than currently used ventilation systems. Recently constructed newborn centers have successfully incorporated laminar flow systems into their units without any reported changes in the incidence of nosocomial infections.

Oxygen and compressed air

Oxygen and compressed air are generally supplied to the intensive care unit from a central source. The capability to provide mixtures of air and oxygen producing concentrations from 21% to 100% must be available. These mixtures should be available at atmospheric pressure and pressures up to 50 psi in units where positive pressure ventilators are used. Warning devices to alert personnel to falls in pressure should be part of each system. Compressed air systems require detailed planning and meticulous care once they are operational. Air should be washed, filtered, and then dehumidified before delivery into the system. All intakes must be closely checked to minimize the introduction of contaminated air. Small compressor units are unreliable and should be avoided; also, compressor units should be operated pneumatically and not electrically, because of an increasing number of power failures in some urban areas.

Acoustics

Design of intensive care units should use available methods of sound dampening. Monitors, respirators, ventilation systems, and incubators all create noise, and at the present time no safe level of noise has been established. By restricting the noise level within the nursery and within the incubator to less than 75 dB, the hearing of both personnel and patients may be protected.

Electricity

See also Chapter 24, part three.

The medical profession is often uninformed about electrical hazards (cardiac arrests, burns, and so on) related to the use of monitors, and hospitals used to have no routine safety testing procedures appropriate for patient safety. In an attempt to minimize electrical hazards, certain recommendations can be made. The use of a single ground of low-resistance wire is particularly effective when connected to all outlets in the nursery. Frequent checking of the integrity of this ground and all wiring will prevent the hazard of stray electrical currents. When more than one piece of eletrical equipment is used, there must be enough outlets at each incubator to accommodate the equipment, with all units connected to a common ground. Before installation and at regular monthly intervals subsequently all electrical equipment should be tested and maintained by a qualified engineer to detect defective equipment and current leakage and to specify appropriate safety precautions. Plugs on all equipment should be hospital grade, and extension cords, adapters, and junction boxes must not be used. No piece of equipment should exceed a leakage of more than 10 μA, and a leakage of 100 μA for a combination of devices must be avoided. The amount of leakage that is safe for the newborn remains unknown.

An appropriate number of the electrical outlets in the nursery must be on the hospital's emergency circuit to maintain life support systems. In-service training programs should be maintained to educate all nursery personnel in the proper use of equipment and recognition of potential electrical hazards. All new equipment should be checked for proper insulation and approved by a qualified engineer *before* use in a clinical area, regardless of previous approvals by the manufacturer.

Wash basins

There should be a wash basin adjacent to the door in each area and one basin for each four to six incubators. All basins should have foot, knee, or remote controls for hot and cold water and soap. Scrub brushes and paper towels should be conveniently placed near each basin.

Equipment

Apnea monitors

See also Chapters 21 and 24, part three.

The availability of an increasing array of monitors has improved the care of the high-risk infant but has placed additional responsibilities on all personnel. The concept of a central nursing area with centralized monitoring, although quite useful in adult coronary units, has not been generally accepted in newborn units.

Most apnea monitors use the principle of impedance pneumography and present problems in proper application and maintenance of leads. The size of the electrodes, the irritation of the electrode paste or tape or both, and the lack of flat areas on the infant for application are recurrent problems for the nursery staff. The technique of applying electrodes to the arm of the sick infant provides a solution to this problem.

Cardiac monitor

See also Chapters 21 and 24, part three.

Cardiac monitors either record the heart rate on an established scale or display the eletrocardiographic figure on an oscilloscope. Rate changes indicate both ventilation problems and cardiovascular instability. The technical problems of electrode placement and grounding are common to all cardiac monitors. The proper application of the electrode ensures conductivity at the interfaces and minimizes false alarms or alarm failures; with currently available systems, proper application of leads on the small infant is less of a problem for the nursing staff.

Blood pressure recorders

See also Chapter 21

Continuous blood pressure monitoring by direct recording with arterial catheters through a transducer is commonly used in NICUs. This mode of monitoring demands an awareness of the increased hazard of blood loss, infections, and electrocution and of the need for adequate safeguards. The transcutaneous Doppler method for measuring blood pressure provides a simple, noninvasive method for monitoring blood pressure. The Doppler method detects very weak impulses that the sphygmomanometer would be unable to detect. Correlations with the direct measurement of blood pressure are firmly established, but the determinations are intermittent, which is a disadvantage in acute situations.

Incubators

See also Chapter 24, part two.

Thermal protection, reverse isolation, and complete visual observation of high-risk infants are possible with the use of incubators. The inspired air in such units is filtered, protecting the infant from airborne infections; but the infant, if infected, can still expire contaminated air into the incubator and nursery, placing infants outside incubators in jeopardy.

Ideally incubators should permit easy access to the infant; thus the open-front incubator with a movable patient tray is superior to a unit with a back hinge and front posts in allowing immediate access to the infant. Access holes for intravenous lines, monitor wires, suction tubing, and respirator apparatus also are required.

Monitors and infusion pumps often are placed on the top of an incubator; this may damage them, impair visual observation of the infant, and cause delays in gaining access to the infant in emergencies. A shelf attached to the incubator itself or mounted on the wall above each unit should be used to avoid accidentally dislodging equipment from the hood of the incubator.

Oxygen or humidity or both may be provided by the incubator itself or by means of a head box placed within it. The hazard of waterborne organisms and the cost of nursing time to clean water traps should be carefully weighed against the benefits of and need for additional humidity. Each nursery should have a clean, warm incubator on standby at all times for unexpected admissions and emergencies. There also should be a regular check of all incubators to safeguard against electrical hazards.

Bassinets

Bassinets should allow examination and care for the infant and be easy to clean; each unit should provide a storage area beneath the bassinet for disposable items used in the routine care of infants. A complete, functional unit for each infant provides an additional safeguard against cross-infection within the nursery.

Laboratory support

Intensive care units require responsive and rapid chemistry, bacteriology, and radiology laboratory support; the closer such facilities are to the intensive care area, the more efficient and responsive they are. Continuous communication between the intensive care unit and paramedical laboratory personnel regarding the exact nature of the clinical problems ensures a more responsive laboratory and minimizes the problems associated with a heavy demand on the laboratory staff. Regular conferences with laboratory personnel to explain the common problems of the newborn have proved very useful in many nurseries.

Microchemical techniques should be available 24 hours a day in the intensive care facility. The availability of a blood gas analyzer within the intensive care area ensures immediate results as a basis for prompt changes in therapy. The obvious disadvantages of blood gas services provided by nonlaboratory personnel is poor quality control. Because of the legitimate need for this capability within intensive care units, clinical pathology services have assumed responsibility in some units with their own laboratory personnel.

The bacteriology laboratory should employ culture and sensitivity techniques that allow rapid identification of pathogens and their antibiotic sensitivities. If the bacteriology laboratory is not near the unit, the provision of a microscope, appropriate stains, and a small incubator will facilitate diagnostic evaluations and improve the efficiency of the staff.

A portable roentgen unit in the intensive care area ensures immediate roentgenologic support while simultaneously avoiding the hazards of hypothermia and hypoxia, which may be involved in the transport of a sick infant to the radiology department (Chapter 13). Newer magnification techniques promise improved quality of roentgenograms and more exact definition of radiologic signs. Proper shielding of patients and personnel is vital. With modern portable collimated roentgen units, light localizers, and proper technique there should be little radiation scatter beyond the light field. Ultrasonographic facilities must be available to the unit each 24 hours.

Control of environment

The establishment of stringent microbiologic environmental control has been the most significant factor in reduction of nosocomial infections in nurseries. Critical evaluation of these controls should be continued, although recent studies permit some modification of previously established standards. Before altering existing procedures and techniques, personnel must realistically compare the type of hospital (for example, university) where the study was conducted with their own institution. Many smaller hospitals have very wisely demanded the continuation of established environmental controls, acknowledging inherent differences between their own facilities and those where innovations have been initiated.

Growing procedures in nurseries are either strict or modified. The strict version requires physicians and paramedical personnel other than the nursing staff to remove outer coats and jewelry, to scrub hand to elbow, and to gown before entering the unit; nurses change from nursing uniforms to scrub gowns. When the nursing staff leaves the unit for other parts of the hospital, they should wear long-sleeved gowns over their scrub dress and discard them on return to the nursery.

In modified gowning, personnel may enter the unit without changing their outer garments but before examination of an infant must remove their coats and vigorously scrub to the elbow. If an infant is to be removed from the incubator (his own microenvironment), the person must wear a surgical gown that is discarded after completion of the examination. Many authorities still believe that incubators should be employed if the modified gowning procedure is used, but there is disagreement on this point. However, it is mandatory that nurseries adopting modified gowning procedures supervise and strictly enforce other basic environmental controls.

Thorough hand washing eliminates the most common route of cross-infection within nurseries. It requires accessible antiseptic agents and a sufficient number and proper location of washbasins. A diluted (less than 3%) solution of hexachlorophene is frequently used for personnel, even though the iodophors are superior because of their additional effectiveness against gram-negative organisms. Proper technique for washing calls for rolling sleeves above the elbow, initially washing hand to elbow for 2 minutes and repeating the wash a second time for 15 to 30 seconds. Because of cutaneous sensitizing effects of the iodine-containing compounds, nurseries that use these compounds as the primary agent always should have a second solution readily available.

In addition to gowning and thorough hand washing, random periodic bacteriologic surveillance of intensive care units and personnel offers an additional safeguard against nursery epidemics. However, a survey that is too extensive not only overtaxes the laboratory but also provides little useful information for personnel. Spot checks, unannounced to the staff, serve as an effective method for checking efficacy of disinfectant procedures.

The cleaning of equipment requires establishment of specific, detailed guidelines that are well known to all personnel. The aim of cleaning most equipment is disinfection (killing or decreasing the number of organisms known to be the potential cause of infection), but sterilization (killing of all organisms) is mandatory for certain items, such as surgical instruments. Gas sterilization has been recommended as the ideal solution to the problems of cleaning and disinfection, but such a gas system is unavailable in most hospitals at the present time. The most commonly used disinfectants are iodophors, chlorine compounds, phenolic compounds, and glutaraldehyde. Caution must be exercised to follow directions with certain phenolic disinfectants. A previous report of an increased incidence of hyperbilirubinemia in a hospital nursery was traced to excessive use of a phenolic disinfectant in greater concentrations than recommended. In addition, the nursery was inadequately ventilated; this promoted atmospheric contamination with the detergent. When ventilation defects were corrected and the disinfectant was used properly, the epidemic ceased. Before disinfection of equipment, thorough cleaning is necessary to remove dust particles and grease that may partially inactivate the disinfectant. Supervisory personnel should check the disinfectant procedure itself as well as periodically culture recently disinfected equipment. Specific guidelines for cleaning various equipment used in intensive care units are available in a manual of the American Academy of Pediatrics on hospital care of newborns. Meticulous attention to details and supervision of the technique of all personnel are critical for safe, effective microbiologic controls.

Temperature control

See also Chapter 24, part two.

Appropriate temperature regulation reduces infant mortality, particularly in premature infants. Most incubators control temperature by using a fan to circulate warm air (forced convection). The air temperature in the incubator should approximate the neutral thermal state. In these units the temperature is controlled by a cutaneous thermistor, usually secured over the liver, which regulates a fan within the incubator. Careful placement of the thermistor is essential to ensure proper recording of the abdominal skin temperature and to avoid errors introduced by loose placement. Improper placement results in artifacts produced by changes in posture or introduction of moisture through bathing or urination.

There is generally some warming beyond the set point, and previous reports indicated an increased incidence of apnea during the warming phase of the incubator. For this reason some investigators have suggested a radiant heat source rather than forced convection, since the former generally provides more sustained, less oscillating heat. The predominance of the forced convection units represents the manufacturers' decisions apparently based on technical and commercial considerations.

The use of the servocontrolled incubator alters the normal changes in body temperature that occur with infection. Fever interrupts the feedback loop in the servocontrolled unit so that high skin temperature causes incubator cooling. For this reason incubator air temperature must be monitored carefully.

The introduction into many units of open radiant warmers demands meticulous attention to control infection, the increased insensible water losses, and possible cooling effects of convective air currents within the nursery. Servomechanisms must be used with these units to minimize fluctuations in body temperature.

Whether cots or incubators are used, it is possible to calculate the air temperature that provides each infant adequate warmth and simultaneously limits the caloric expenditure. Tables 24-4 and 24-5 present the recommendations of the American Academy of Pediatrics of useful guidelines for this often neglected aspect of newborn care.

Generally, the relative humidifity in the incubator should be kept in the range of 30% to 60%. In many units the ambient humidity is sufficient to maintain the desired humidity within the incubator without use of the water reservoir. This arrangement avoids the risk of contaminating the incubator with waterborne organisms. Attention to this detail is particularly important with the very low birth weight infant. Because low humidity increases heat loss, the addition of humidity may result in

Table 24-4. Incubator air temperatures—first 24 hours

Birth weight		Temperatures			
		°C		°F	
Grams	Pounds	Median ± range		Median ± range	
	1	35.5	0.5	96.0	0.9
500		35.5	0.5	96.0	0.9
	2	35.0	0.5	95.0	0.9
1,000		34.9	0.5	94.9	0.9
	3	34.2	0.5	93.6	0.9
1,500		34.0	0.5	93.2	0.9
	4	33.7	0.5	92.7	0.9
2,000		33.5	0.5	92.3	0.9
	5	33.3	0.7	92.0	1.3
2,500		33.2	0.8	91.8	1.4
	6	33.1	0.9	91.6	1.6
3,000		33.0	1.0	91.4	1.8
	7	32.9	1.1	91.2	1.9
3,500		32.8	1.2	91.0	2.1
	8	32.8	1.3	91.0	2.3
4,000		32.6	1.4	90.7	2.5
	9	32.5	1.4	90.5	2.5

From Standards and recommendations for hospital care of new infants, ed. 6, Evanston, Ill., 1977, American Academy of Pediatrics, p. 90.
These tables are recommended for use as a guide when relative humidity is approximately 50%. Temperature should be higher than that in the table for lower humidity and altered in either direction, depending on various factors in the thermal environment and the individual infant's requirements.
Modified from data published by Scopes and Ahmed and Oliver.

Table 24-5. Incubator air temperatures according to age

	Birth weight											
	Under 1,500 gm (3 lb, 5 oz)				1,501 to 2,500 gm (3 lb, 5 oz, to 5 lb, 8 oz)				Over 36 weeks' gestation and over 2,500 gm (5 lb, 8 oz)			
Age	°C Median ± range		°F Median ± range		°C Median ± range		°F Median ± range		°C Median ± range		°F Median ± range	
1 day	34.3	0.4	93.8	0.7	33.4	0.6	92.1	1.1	33.0	1.0	91.4	1.8
2 days	33.7	0.5	92.7	0.9	32.7	0.9	90.9	1.6	32.4	1.3	90.4	2.3
3 days	33.5	0.5	92.3	0.9	32.4	0.9	90.4	1.6	31.9	1.3	89.4	2.3
4 days	33.5	0.5	92.3	0.9	32.3	0.9	90.2	1.6	31.5	1.3	88.6	2.3
5 days	33.5	0.5	92.3	0.9	32.2	0.9	90.0	1.6	31.2	1.3	88.1	2.3
6 days	33.5	0.5	92.3	0.9	32.1	0.9	89.8	1.6	30.9	1.3	87.6	2.3
7 days	33.5	0.5	92.3	0.9	32.1	0.9	89.8	1.6	30.8	1.4	87.4	2.5
8 days	33.5	0.5	92.3	0.9	32.1	0.9	89.8	1.6	30.6	1.4	87.0	2.5
9 days	33.5	0.5	92.3	0.9	32.1	0.9	89.8	1.6	30.4	1.4	86.7	2.5
10 days	33.5	0.5	92.3	0.9	32.1	0.9	89.8	1.6	30.2	1.5	86.4	2.7
11 days	33.5	0.5	92.3	0.9	32.1	0.9	89.8	1.6	29.9	1.5	85.8	2.7
12 days	33.5	0.5	92.3	0.9	32.1	0.9	89.8	1.6	29.5	1.6	85.1	2.8
13 days	33.5	0.5	92.3	0.9	32.1	0.9	89.8	1.6	29.2	1.6	84.6	2.8
14 days	33.4	0.6	92.1	1.1	32.1	0.9	89.8	1.6				
15 days	33.3	0.7	92.0	1.3	32.0	0.9	89.6	1.6				
4 weeks	32.9	0.8	91.2	1.4	31.7	1.1	89.0	1.9				
5 weeks	32.1	0.7	89.3	1.3	31.1	1.1	87.9	1.9				
6 weeks	31.8	0.6	89.2	1.1	30.6	1.1	87.1	1.9				
7 weeks	31.1	0.6	87.9	1.1	30.1	1.1	86.2	1.9				

From Standards and recommendations for hospital care of newborn infants, ed. 6, Evanston, Ill., 1977, American Academy of Pediatrics.
See footnotes to Table 24-4.

easier control of air temperature within the incubator and better control of infant temperature.

Oxygen therapy

The administration of oxygen to newborns requires clinical judgment supported by laboratory determinations. The use of cyanosis alone as a guide to the amount of oxygen that should be administered is potentially hazardous both in terms of underestimating (hypoxic brain injury) and exceeding (retrolental fibroplasia) the oxygen demands of a sick infant. The potential complications of oxygen therapy must be weighed aginst the risks involved in arterial catheterization. In institutions where physicians and nurses are inexperienced with technique, where laboratory support is inadequate, and where transfer to a special care center is impossible, clinical judgment of physical signs alone must be an acceptable compromise. In such cases, by gradually lowering the ambient oxygen concentration to a point where cyanosis is clinically detectable and then increasing the concentration by 10%, the physician has a rough guideline for both preventing hypoxia and avoiding hyperoxia. Regardless of existent institutional limitations, a general knowledge of the physiologic principle governing oxygen therapy is essential for any physician caring for sick infants.

When laboratory service and technical skill with umbilical and peripheral artery catheterization are available, more exact determination of the oxygenation of a sick infant is possible. The transport and delivery of oxygen to the tissues is a complex process involving many factors: Pao_2, hemoglobin concentration, oxygen content, tissue perfusion, and affinity of hemoglobin for oxygen. Periodic measurement of Pao_2, hemoglobin, and pH, in addition to close clinical observation, is the most reasonable and accurate approach to minimizing the risk of both hyperoxic and hypoxic insults to a sick infant. When arterial catheterization is contraindicated, radial or brachial artery puncture can be used, but repeated sampling from these sites requires skill and experience. In infants with mild respiratory distress not requiring arterial catheterization and in infants suspected of having significant right-to-left shunts, these sites for sampling are particularly useful.

Recent advances in noninvasive techniques to monitor arterial blood oxygen tension should decrease the need for umbilical and peripheral artery catheterization. Studies have demonstrated that, with adequate skin perfusion, the correlation between arterial oxygen tension and transcutaneous oxygen tension is very close (Chapter 28, part three). The obvious immediate advantage of the transcutaneous measurement is that it provides a continuous recording of oxygen tension as opposed to the intermittent values provided by the other methods. The transcutaneous method has been particularly helpful in weaning infants from ventilation and avoiding recurrent hypoxia during care. However, sick infants still require accurate monitoring of blood pressure as part of their care, thus necessitating umbilical artery catheterization. But in less acutely ill infants transcutaneous measurement of oxygen tension or oxygen saturation will prevent the risks of arterial catheterization while providing accurate recording of oxygen levels.

When it is determined that an infant requires supplemental oxygen in spite of its potential hazards, the delivery of oxygen should be carefully controlled and monitored. When small increases in ambient oxygen are required, direct delivery into the incubator often suffices. With concentrations exceeding 30% a head box within the incubator more accurately provides the correct concentration, while simultaneously limiting significant fluctuations in oxygen, especially when the incubator ports are opened. Some incubators have cut-off mechanisms to prevent administration of oxygen exceeding a preset concentration. In general, these controls cannot be relied on independently, and the ambient oxygen concentration should be checked at regular intervals by a paramagnetic oxygen analyzer or continuously monitored by means of an oxygen electrode. Orders for oxygen therapy should never be written in terms of flow (that is, liters per minute) but rather in terms of the desired ambient concentration with indicated intervals for routinely checking the concentration.

Oxygen should be humidified and warmed before delivery to a sick infant. If dry gas is administered to a patient, it will be humidified by evaporation from the respiratory mucosa. Under normal circumstances this process presents no problems; but in a sick infant, particularly with respiratory distress, difficulties arise. By drying the respiratory mucosa, the viscosity of pulmonary secretions is increased, and effective ciliary action is impaired. With these changes in major airways, airway resistance, already increased in most infants, may be further increased. Such therapy also may aggravate problems of water balance by significantly increasing insensible water losses from the respiratory tract. Oxygen that is not warmed presents significant cold stress to the premature infant. There is a marked increase in oxygen consumption with the delivery of cold air to the face.

Oxygen may be humidified and warmed through the use of humidifiers and, on occasion, nebulizers. Humidifiers are designed to produce a maximum amount of water vapor, whereas nebulizers produce water particles of a particular size. Infants requiring nasotracheal intubation need humidifiers for their ventilators, whereas babies who are breathing spontaneously in head boxes and who have copious secretions often are treated with nebulizers. With nebulizers exact control of humidity, condensation of water in the tubing, and difficulty of sterilization are common problems. The latter problem and the small droplet size produced by nebulizers have been suggested as possible explanations for the increased incidence of pulmonary infections in patients on respirators. Humidifiers are not difficult to sterilize and therefore are less likely to promote pulmonary infections, but they too are plagued with problems of condensation of water within gas lines and difficulty in controlling the temperature of the gas as it is delivered to the patient. Recent engineering improvements have alleviated the latter problem, but condensation remains a nuisance and demands nursing attention and time for observing and removing partial obstructions caused by condensed water.

FEEDING

The advantage of early feedings in maintaining normal metabolism and growth during the transition from fetal to extrauterine life is clear (Chapter 25, part one). As soon as an infant can safely tolerate enteral nutrition, feedings should be initiated. This approach may decrease the incidence of problems such as hypoglycemia, hyperkalemia, hyperbilirubinemia, and azotemia. In the regular nursery most infants are left without feedings for the first 6 hours of life. At this time an initial feeding of sterile water is offered, and, if tolerated, the breast or formula of choice is offered subsequently. Animal studies of the pulmonary findings after aspiration have demonstrated equally severe tissue reaction to glucose water and milk formula. When there is any question about tolerance of feeding because of physical or neurologic status of the infant, feeding should be withheld and parenteral fluids substituted.

Most term infants will rapidly progress from 30 ml every 3 to 4 hours to 75 to 90 ml before discharge at 4 to 5 days of life. Vigorous premature infants may require smaller (5 to 10 ml) feedings at more frequent intervals (every 2 hours) before progressing to larger, less frequent feedings. Very low birth weight infants may only tolerate 1 ml every hour. Caution and judgment must be continuously exercised in advancing the feedings of a premature infant. Rigid feeding schedules should be avoided, and the initial small volume should be fed gradually and cautiously increased. The rate of increase that is well tolerated varies considerably from infant to infant.

Parenteral fluids

Regardless of birth weight, if the neurologic or physical status of the infant prohibits early feeding, parenteral fluid therapy, rather than starvation, is indicated (Chapter 25, part one). The physician must select the intravenous route that minimizes complications and allows the infusate to be delivered with maximum efficiency. In the newborn the sites routinely used include peripheral veins on the hand or foot, scalp veins, the antecubital veins, and the umbilical vessels. If these sites have been exhausted, a venous cutdown may be performed; most frequently the saphenous vein is used. The technical expertise and previous experience of the individual physician usually determine the infusion site.

Hypodermoclysis should be abandoned as a route of parenteral therapy. If a saline-glucose solution is infused under the skin, it must enter the functional extracellular fluid to be effective. In dehydration, blood flow is reduced, and thus the rate at which the subcutaneous fluid can enter the circulation is decreased. Furthermore, in some patients not only does the fluid remain in the extravascular tissue but also sodium and water leave the blood volume and enter the clysis fluid, increasing the likelihood of circulatory collapse.

Peripheral veins on the dorsal aspect of the hand or the foot, antecubital veins, and scalp veins are readily available in most newborns for routine parenteral therapy. However, veins on the flexor surfaces of the wrist and dorsum of the foot should be avoided, if possible, when peripheral alimentation solutions are used. Infiltration with these solutions, if not immediately noted, may cause cutaneous sloughing and damage to underlying tendons.

The care used in starting the infusion, the subsequent nursing care, and the contents of the infusate are factors in determining how long each infusion site will be used. The administration of hypertonic alkaline or acid solutions through a peripheral vein shortens the amount of time that particular site can be effectively used. The use of percutaneous catheters in most units has limited the need for butterfly peripheral needles. These catheters require meticulous care to ensure their longevity and keep complications to a minimum. Careful scrutiny of the catheter tip is only possible when tape does not obscure the site. With attention to detail, peripheral catheters can simplify the care of sick infants. However, when a percutaneous catheter cannot be inserted or when the unit staff has had no experience with it, peripheral veins, including scalp veins, are used. Because the scalp generally has an abundant supply of superficial veins, these veins are often the most popular route for intravenous delivery of fluids in most nurseries. When approaching these vessels, the physician should be careful to avoid the fontanels, bony prominences, and small arteries. Nursery personnel should scrutinize each infusion site frequently to ensure its maximum longevity. If extravasation of acid, alkaline, hypertonic, or calcium-containing solution goes undetected, necrosis and sloughing of the involved area may occur, with a greater risk of infection.

Broviac catheters are used in critically ill infants requiring long-term parenteral therapy. In some infants receiving central intravenous alimentation, Dudrick's method for placing a catheter in the superior vena cava is still used and has demonstrated that aseptic technique during insertion of the catheter and meticulous care thereafter will allow constant, long-term infusion of a hypertonic, acidic (pH 5.5) solution with minimum risk of infection.

Umbilical vessels

See also Chapter 28, part three.

The sick neonate receiving supportive oxygen therapy as an intrinsic part of treatment requires careful, continuous monitoring of the PaO_2. Even though peripheral arteries (brachial, radial, and temporal) are available, the umbilical artery allows simple insertion of a catheter for continuous monitoring of blood gases. Employing the standards of Dunn (Fig. 24-20), the physician threads the catheter to a position 1 cm above the diaphragm (or at the level of L3 below the renal arteries) and carefully secures it with suture or tape. More recent criteria by Shukla for length of arterial catheter placement have employed regression equations using body weight. The position then is verified radiologically. Umbilical artery catheterization demands constant observation of the umbilicus for bleeding, meticulous care of the catheter to prevent propagation of thrombus or air embolism, continuous scrutiny of the lower extremities for evidence of arterial spasm (cyanosis or blanching), and limitation of the catheterization to a period as short as the clinical course allows.

The catheter should be removed cautiously to allow proximal arterial spasm for hemostasis. The acute and chronic risks of using the umbilical artery catheter should be carefully considered and weighed against the advantages for each individual patient; this route should not be used for routine parenteral therapy.

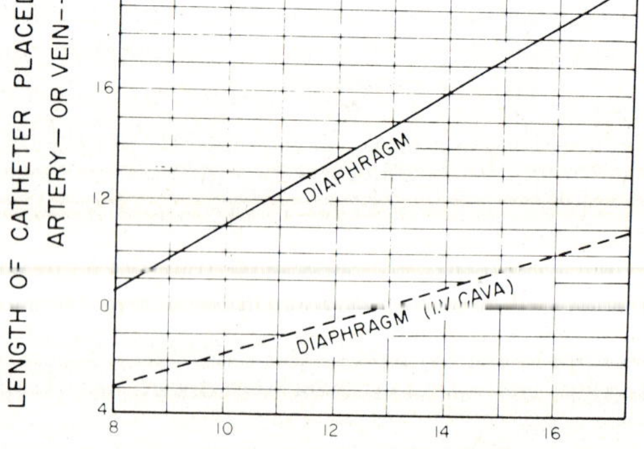

Fig. 24-20. Guide for placement of umbilical catheters.

Realizing the potential complications of the umbilical artery catheter and assuming that there is little risk in using the umbilical vein, many physicians have adopted the latter route for parenteral therapy. Accessibility, technical ease of inserting the catheter, and longevity of the umbilical vein catheter are obvious advantages to this site. However, the umbilical vein catheter may easily pass into the portal vein, and the administration of sodium bicarbonate through the catheter creates the risk of infusing a hypertonic and strongly alkaline solution directly into the liver. One necropsy series reported a significant incidence (33%) of hemorrhagic liver necrosis in patients receiving tromethamine via the umbilical vein. Umbilical vein phlebitis, pyemia, and pulmonary embolus were noted by Scott in infants whose therapy was delivered via umbilical vein catheters. Colonic perforation and peritonitis in infants following exchange transfusion via the umbilical vein have been noted. Thus this route of intravascular therapy should be used only when no other is available.

Regardless of the route selected for therapy, certain recommendations are generally applicable. The advantages of the selected route must be weighed against its risks; there must be use of the proper technique in starting the infusion to minimize hazards, to safeguard its continuation, and to promote its longevity; proper nursing observation is required during the infusion, including maintenance of intravenous flow records and frequent inspection of the infusion site; and peristaltic pumps should be used to ensure constant flow and to minimize the chance of overhydration of a sick infant.

Gavage feeding

See also Chapter 25, part one.

Many debilitated infants who are unable to suck and swallow adequately have evidence of active peristalsis (stools and bowel sounds). Various temporizing measures have been attempted to avoid the complications of parenteral fluid therapy and to take advantage of the infant's functioning intestinal tract. Gavage feeding is the oldest and most established of these techniques but is not entirely free of hazards. In addition to changes in heart rate and blood pressure during passage of the gavage tube, the tube itself may be an obstruction to respiration, particularly in the premature infant. The practice of passing a gavage tube before each feeding as opposed to an indwelling tube changed daily depends on the capability and experience of the nursing staff; with an experienced nurse the indwelling tube is not essential. When nasogastric fedings are used, the residual gastric aspirate should be noted before each feeding and recorded as a guide to the infant's likely tolerance of the volume of food offered.

A gastrostomy may be helpful in the postoperative period after gastrointestinal surgery. However, a controlled study has demonstrated increased mortality in premature infants routinely fed through a gastrostomy. A *Murphy drip*, an adaptation of the gastrostomy or the gavage feeding, allows slow, controlled introduction of formula into the stomach by partially occluding the feeding tube. In infants this method has been helpful primarily postoperatively. The introduction of a *nasojejunal feeding* tube allows slow infusion of formula into the jejunum and circumvents the problems of vomiting, distension, and the dumping syndrome, which may be encountered with the gastrostomy or gavage tube. The variety of complications reported to be associated with nasojejunal feedings using polyvinyl catheters has not been encountered with Silastic catheters, although nasojejunal feeding has not gained wide acceptance.

Total intravenous alimentation

See Chapter 25, part one.

SKIN CARE

In selecting a skin care technique for the newborn, the physician must weigh the benefit to the infant against the potential risk of the agent used. Hexachlorophene, which was widely used in the 1950s and 1960s, has been restricted because of its cutaneous absorption and potential neurotoxicity. Judicious use of dilute hexachlorophene (3%) may be indicated for skin infection and such use has been approved by the Food and Drug Administration. Use of iodophors, another commonly used agent, has not been proved to be safe or to effectively control skin colonization. Because of the current lack of a suitable agent, the American Academy of Pediatrics currently recommends dry skin care. The benefits of this approach are reduction of heat loss by exposure, decrease in skin trauma, limitation of exposure to agents with unknown toxicity, and reduction in nursing time. With this technique cleaning is delayed until an infant's temperature has stabilized. Then fresh water or a nonmedicated soap is used to remove blood and meconium from the face and head. The rest of the infant's skin may be left untouched, leaving the vernix caseosa in place. For the duration of hospitalization, the buttocks and perianal region can be cleaned with fresh water or a mild soap at diaper changes or as often as necessary.

There is no single method of cord care that is recommended to prevent colonization and subsequent disease. Currently acceptable agents include triple dye, bacitracin, or silver sulfadiazine. Alcohol may be used to dry the cord, but it is ineffective in preventing cord colonization.

Nursery personnel may continue to use hexachlorophene in hand washing, although other superior iodine-containing preparations currently are available. Skin irritation or allergic reaction may result from the use of these iodine preparations. A rigid requirement of washing from hand to elbow for 2 minutes in the initial wash and for 15 to 30 seconds in the second wash is needed to minimize infection and cross-contamination. Shorter but equally careful washes between handling of each infant also should be mandatory.

CHARTING

Charts should be organized in an orderly fashion so that the clinical problems, therapy, and progress of the patient are obvious to all personnel. In intensive care facilities nurses' notes, laboratory flow sheets, respirator and oxygen therapy logs, and intravenous therapy sheets should be kept at the infant's bedside. Organization of these records, allowing minimum reduplication and easy recording for the nursing staff, leads to development of concise record keeping and exact documentation of each infant's course. All too often reconstruction of a significant change in an infant's course is impossible through review of the records. Although continuous electronic recording of vital parameters is increasing, many factors require human observation and demand careful record keeping to avoid loss of valuable time when there is an urgent need to document the exact nature of the infant's course. Alternatively the value of detailed charting must be weighed against the nursing time required to complete flow sheets. The proper balance will increase the efficiency of care and will allow optimum use of time and effort by all personnel involved in delivery of care to sick infants.

PARENTS

The role of parents in any intensive care unit must be a serious concern for the team caring for each infant (Chapter 23). Maintaining strict environmental control, allaying parental anxiety, and preventing interference with patient care are no longer acceptable reasons for denying parents access to their critically ill infants. Unlimited visiting privileges for parents should be allowed in every unit, with obvious restrictions of visiting during procedures or medical emergencies; grandparents also should be allowed to see infants. More recently sibling visitation has been implemented in nurseries without increasing the risk of infection when appropriate screening for contagion is used. This change in visiting to include siblings has been particularly beneficial to families during long hospitalizations and when death of an infant is likely.

Before a policy of increased parent-child interaction is defined in a particular nursery, there should be a preliminary discussion of each person's role (the attending physician, resident, and nurses) in supporting the parents. There also should be a free exchange of ideas among the staff after implementation of such a program. Involvement of parents in the intensive care unit offers a means for personalizing what is often a stark, impersonal setting and for providing greater personal and professional motivation for the entire staff. Furthermore, without adequate access of parents to their infants, early parent-infant bonding is adversely affected with possible long-term untoward results (Chapter 23).

Under such policies the physician partially shares with paramedical personnel the previously exclusive right of talking to parents. This requires a greater degree of open communication with the nursing staff, which participates in communicating medical facts to parents. In any unit the parents' major contact is with the nurses, to whom they look for information; ideally this relationship should facilitate the care of the patient and the understanding of the parents. In such a setting the nursing staff may provide emotional support for a mother, supplementing that supplied by the physician; this support assumes significant proportions in the context of delivery of total care. The death of an infant is made more bearable to parents when the personnel consider this support a vital part of their responsibility.

Premature infants who survive a serious illness but who undergo prolonged hospitalizations should be in a nursery where parents are actively involved in routine care. Tasks that are often tedious and meaningless to paramedical personnel (such as diaper changing and washing) are cherished moments for parents who previously were separated from their infants. At the time of discharge the anxiety of parents who have been significantly involved in the care of their child, even at the worst moments, is significantly less than in those parents who have been anxious bystanders for 2 months.

John M. Driscoll, Jr.

BIBLIOGRAPHY

American Academy of Pediatrics: Hospital care of newborn infants, ed. 6, Evanston, Ill., 1977, The Academy.

American Academy of Pediatrics and the American College of Obstetricians and Gynecologists: Guidelines for perinatal care, Evanston, Ill., 1983, The Academies.

Babson, S.G.: Feeding the low birth weight infant, J. Pediatr. **79**:694, 1971.

Babson, S.G.: Peripheral intravenous alimentation of the small premature infant, J. Pediatr. **79**:494, 1971.

Canadian Pediatric Society, Committee on the Fetus and Newborn: Oxygen therapy in the preterm infant, Can. Med. Assoc. J. **99**:564, 1968.

Centers for Disease Control: Guidelines for the prevention and control of nosocomial infections, Washington, D.C., 1981, U.S. Government Printing Office.

Cheek, J.A., Jr., and Staub, G.F.: Nasojejunal alimentation for premature and full-term newborn infants, J. Pediatr. **82**:955, 1973.

Chernick, V., and Raber, M.B.: Electrical hazards in the newborn nursery, J. Pediatr. **77**:143, 1970.

Desmond, M., Rudolph, A., and Phitaksphraiwan, P.: The transitional care nursery, Pediatr. Clin. North Am. **13**:651, 1966.

Duc, G.: Assessment of hypoxia in the newborn: suggestions for a practical approach, Pediatrics **48**:469, 1971.

Dunn, P.M.: Localization of the umbilical catheter by postmortem measurement, Arch. Dis. Child. **41**:69, 1966.

Gluck, L.: Design of a perinatal center, Pediatr. Clin. North Am. **17**:777, 1970.

Goldenberg, V.E., Wiegenstein, L., and Hopkins, G.B.: Hepatic injury associated with tromethamine, JAMA **205**:71, 1968.

Heird, W.C.: Nasojejunal feedings: a commentary, J. Pediatr. **85**:111, 1974.

Heird, W.C., and others: Metabolic acidosis after intravenous alimentation with amino acids, N. Engl. J. Med. **287**:943, 1972.

Heird, W.C., and others: Intravenous alimentation in pediatric patients, J. Pediatr. **80**:351, 1972.

Hey, E.: The care of babies in incubators: recent advances in pediatrics, ed. 4, London, 1971. J. & A. Churchill.

Huch, A., and Huch, R.: Transcutaneous, noninvasive monitoring of PO_2, Hosp. Pract. **11**:43, 1976.

Kitterman, J.A., Phibbs, R.H., and Tooley, W.H.: Catheterization of umbilical vessels in newborn infants, Pediatr. Clin. North Am. **17**:895, 1970.

Klaus, M.H., and Kennel, J.H.: Mothers separated from their newborn infants, Pediatr. Clin. North Am. **17**:1015, 1970.

Klaus, M.H., and others: Maternal attachment: importance of the first postpartum days, N. Engl. J. Med. **286**:460, 1972.

Oliver, T.K., Jr.: Temperature regulation and heat production in the newborn, Pediatr. Clin. North Am. **12**:765, 1965.

Peabody, J., and others: Failure of conventional monitoring to detect hypoxia, Clin. Res. **25**:1902, 1977.

Perlstein, H., Edwards, N.K., and Sutherland, J.M.: Apnea in premature infants and incubator air temperature changes, N. Engl. J. Med. **282**:461, 1970.

Rhea, J.W., Ghazzawi, O., and Weidman, W.: Nasojejunal feeding: an improved device and intubation technique, J. Pediatr. **82**:951, 1973.

Rhea, J.W., and Kirby, J.O.: A nasojejunal tube for infant feeding, Pediatrics **46**:36, 1970.

Scott, J.M.: Iatrogenic lesions in babies following umbilical vein catherization, Arch. Dis. Child. **40**:426, 1965.

Segal, S.: Transportation of high risk infants, Vancouver, B.C., 1972, Canadian Pediatric Society.

Segal, S., and Pirie, G.E.: Equipment and personnel for neonatal special care, Pediatr. Clin. North Am. **17**:793, 1970.

Shukla, H., and Ferrara, A.: Rapid estimation of insertional length of umbilical catheters in newborns, Am. J. Dis. Child. **140**:786, 1986.

Sinclair, J.C., and others: Supportive management of the sick neonate: parenteral calories, water and electrolytes, Pediatr. Clin. North Am. **17**:863, 1970.

Spaulding, E.H.: Chemical disinfection in the hospital, J. Hosp. Res. **3**:25, 1965.

Swyer, P.R.: The regional organization of special care for the neonate, Pediatr. Clin. North Am. **17**:761, 1970.

Vengusamy, S., and others: A controlled study of feeding gastrostomy in low birth weight infants, Pediatrics **43**:815, 1969.

CHAPTER 25

Nutrition, body fluids, and acid-base homeostasis

PART ONE

Nutrition in the high-risk newborn

Because of major advances in respiratory and other life support, nutrition and the absorptive function of the gut have largely replaced the lungs as the major limiting factors in intact survival of the sick, premature, or low birth weight newborn. Mortality rates of 85% for infants weighing less than 1500 gm at birth were common 25 years ago but are now of the order of 10% to 15%. Hence these premature and sick infants are surviving to offer an unprecedented nutritional challenge in securing survival and normal growth. Nonetheless, even for well term infants there are still controversies surrounding desirable nutritional goals in growth and development.

OBJECTIVES IN GROWTH AND DEVELOPMENT

The general objective of a nutritional regimen for the normal or sick newborn is to support life and a rate of growth sufficient to fulfill the individual's genetic potential. We still, however, do not know the ideal nutritional goal, especially in terms of body composition. Should we aim for intrauterine rates of accretion of macronutrients and micronutrients as suggested by the Nutrition Committee of the American Academy of Pediatrics (1977) or are different accretion rates (e.g., the enhanced postnatal rate for fat) more suitable to the extrauterine environment? Is human milk appropriate for an infant who should still be fed placentally for the next 6 to 12 weeks? Should we feed by the enteral or parenteral route and continuously or intermittently? What is the optimal quantity and quality of nutritional support, and how soon after birth should it begin?

The aim of this chapter is to provide the theoretic background and practical answers to these questions insofar as present knowledge permits and in the face of intense research in this new area of "infant" or "quasi-fetal" nutrition.

THE CONCEPT OF "CRITICAL EPOCHS" IN GROWTH AND DEVELOPMENT

Widdowson and McCance have discussed the important concept of "critical epochs" in development "when the size of the animal arising from its previous plane of nutrition, determines its appetite thereafter and hence its rate of growth and dimensions at maturity. A small size at this critical time brought about by undernutrition, is not followed by catch-up growth, however liberal the diet."

This concept of critical epochs in growth applies not only to the organism as a whole but also to individual organs and, most significantly, to the brain. Dobbing has shown that this sensitivity extends to individual cellular populations within the brain that develop on different time schedules and that can be selectively compromised by nutritional or other insult sustained during a particular period of development. In the premature infant, for example, Purpura has shown that glial proliferation and cerebellar development along with general myelination and dendritic arborization are still proceeding during the last trimester of fetal life and into the neonatal period (Chapter 27, part one). If an infant is born prematurely the neonatologist has perforce to become the nutritional surrogate for the placenta, without, unfortunately, being endowed with all the subtle transfer and feedback mechanisms of that remarkable organ.

An example that dramatizes the effect of undernutrition in one of two individuals with identical genetic potentials is that of parabiotic twins for whom the vascular arrangement of the placenta has seriously deprived one of the pair. Such an infant may never catch up to the well-nourished sibling, despite our best postnatal nutritional efforts. In the same way, failure to adequately nourish a premature infant postnatally may result in a similar nonrecuperable shortfall. It behooves the neonatologist to nutritionally support the neonate in this sensitive epoch of development until the individual's appetite can safely be left to determine food intake and growth according to genetic programming.

OBSTACLES TO OPTIMAL NUTRITION

See also Chapter 33, part one.

Frequently the infant may be too sick to absorb nutrients from the gastrointestinal tract because of immaturity, ileus, cardiorespiratory failure, infection, or serious gastrointestinal or other anomaly. Severe illness also compromises the ability of the organism to adequately metabolize intravenously administered nutrients, as evidenced by the frequent occurrence of hyperglycemia, azotemia, and inability to clear intravenously administered lipids. The liver is one of the key organs in this respect and is important in the causation of the major macronutrient biochemical intolerance to carbohydrate (hyperglycemia), lipids (hyperlipidemia), and amino acids (abnormal serum levels, raised blood urea nitrogen). In addition there may be technical difficulties in administration, malabsorption, defective utilization, or inappropriate dosage of dietary components.

THE RELEVANCE OF FETAL NUTRITIONAL STATE TO NEONATAL CONDITION

Fetal macronutrient metabolism

Most of our knowledge of fetal nutrition is inferential from animal experimentation and from carcass analysis of human abortuses and stillbirths, which may not represent human normality. By analogy with animal (mostly ovine) fetal observation about 70% of the fetal energy substrate is derived from maternal glucose, 5% to 20% from lactate synthesized in the placenta, and up to 20% from maternally supplied amino acids. Small amounts of fatty acids, especially long-chain polyunsaturates, also pass to the fetus through the placenta, but the bulk of fetal fat is synthesized from the carbon of carbohydrate by the fetus during the third trimester.

Neonatal body composition compared with the adult

Table 25-1 shows the body composition of the infant at birth weights of 1, 2, and 3.5 kg, corresponding to postconceptional ages of 28, 35, and 40 weeks, respec-

Table 25-1. Body composition of infants weighing 1, 2, and 3.5 kg compared with the adult

	28 wks	35 wks	40 wks	Adult
Weight (gm) (comprised of):	1,000	2,000	3,500	70,000
Water (gm)	860	1,620	2,400	42,000
Protein (gm)	85	230	390	12,000
Fat (gm)	10	100	560	15,300
Carbohydrate (gm)	4.5	9	34	700
Energy content (total Cal)	460	1,900	6,950	188,500
Nonprotein Cal	110	970	5,350	140,500
MMR Cal	50	106	186	1,400
MMR/nonprotein Cal	1:2	1:9	1:29	1:100

Modified from Widdowson, E.M., and Spray, C.M.: Chemical development in utero, Arch. Dis. Child. **26:**205, 1951; Widdowson, E.M.: Growth and composition of the fetus and neonate. In Assali, N.S., editor: Biology of gestation, vol. 2, The fetus and neonate, New York, 1968, Academic Press, Inc.
MMR, Minimal metabolic rate.

Table 25-2. Heat production from energy conversion and deposition of the principal nutrients

Biochemical transformations involved in energy deposition*	Energy cost of conversions Cal/gm end product	% Initial energy lost during transformation
Fat into fat†: triglyceride → free fatty acids → triglyceride	0.095	1
Carbohydrate into fat‡: 14 glucose + 12 O_2 → tripalmitylglycerate + 33 CO_2 + 21 ATP	1.419	15
Protein into fat§: 21 amino acids + 48.3 O_2 → tripalmitylglycerate + 36 CO_2 + 14.4 urea	2.933	31
Protein into protein: 1 amino acid + 5 ATP → 1 peptide	0.648	15
Glucose into glycogen‖	0.376	9

From Heim, T.: Homeothermy and its metabolic cost. In Davis, J.A., and Dobbing, J., editors: Scientific foundations of pediatrics, ed. 2, London, 1981, Heinemann, pp. 91-128. Modified from Millward, D.G., and Garlick, P.J.: Proc. Nutr. Soc. **35:**339, 1976.
*Calculations based on molecular weights of 806, 162, and 110 and the heat content of 9.46, 4.18, and 4.32 kcal/gm for triglyceride, carbohydrate, and protein. Adenosine triphosphate (ATP) is assumed to be formed from dietary carbohydrate at a rate of 37 mol/mol glucose.
†Assuming a requirement of 6 ATP/mol triglyceride.
‡Assuming conversion as described in McGilvery (1970); respiratory quotient = 2.75.
§Assuming conversion via glucose and ketones as described in McGilvery (1970); respiratory quotient = 0.75.
‖Assuming a requirement of 3 ATP/mol glycogen.

tively, in comparison with the adult. The fetus of 1 kg is little more than a bag of water (86%) with a smattering of protein (8%), is virtually devoid of fat (1%), and has even less carbohydrate. The total energy content is 460 kcal, mostly proteinaceous. Table 25-1 shows that there is considerable accretion in the last trimester, but by comparison with the adult, energy reserves are minimal, particularly for the 1 kg infant, whose ratio of minimal metabolic rate to nonprotein energy reserve is only 1:2 compared with 1:29 for the term infant and 1:100 for the adult. Thus the urgency of supplying energy to the very low birth weight (VLBW) infant within a few hours of delivery can be appreciated.

Metabolic rates and energy reserves

The caloric consumption of the fetus is a function of body mass and not of surface area/body weight ratio as in the extra uterine homeothermic newborn; this consumption is about 35 Cal/kg/day. The immediate neonatal resting heat production is similar at 35 to 40 Cal/kg/day, but then it almost doubles during the next 2 or 3 weeks to 50 to 65 Cal/kg/day as a consequence of increasing macronutrient intake and weight gain. The increase in metabolic rate is closely related to the thermic effect of food (specific dynamic action), a manifestation of the exothermic reactions involved in the reorganization of the ingested food molecules into new tissue, notably protein (Table 25-2); this increase is 0.67 Cal for each gram of weight gain (Fig. 25-1), although the exact amount will depend on the composition of that weight gain.

The need to support growth by proper nutrition, especially for the sick neonate, introduces a completely new dimension to their intensive care compared to the sick adult. Undernutrition adds the future menace of stunted mental and physical development to the immediate threat of compromised physiologic function and death. In the adult (70 kg man) there are 6 kg of available protein (8.6% of body weight, 24,000 Cal). Since death occurs when the body protein is 40% to 50% depleted and the metabolic rate is approximately 1,500 to 2,000 Cal/kg/day, survival in starvation would only be 6 days if it were not prolonged to >60 days by catabolism of body fat (15 kg or 135,000 Cal). The term infant is also protected to a limited extent by a body fat content of approximately 600 gm, which explains the recovery after several days of some infants in viable condition from collapsed hospital buildings in the 1985 earthquake in Mexico City. In the low birth weight (LBW) newborn, however, fat reserves are almost nonexistent (Table 25-1) and carbohydrate reserves are very low (10 gm/kg). Therefore this infant has to rely on the 8% body weight of protein, thus theoretically survival could be only a few days before energy stores run out and cardiorespiratory function is halted through depletion of tissue protein.

NUTRITIONAL REQUIREMENT

Fetal and neonatal macronutrient accretion rates

The usual reference for designing the diet of the term infant is the postnatal accretion rates of macro- and micronutrients. For the LBW infant both the fetal accretion

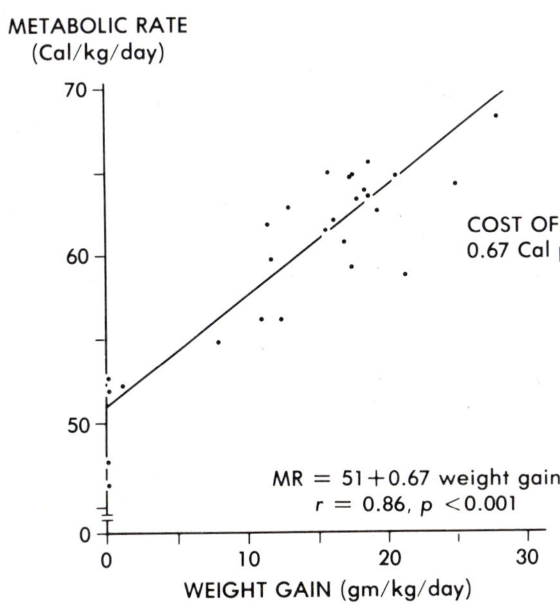

Fig. 25-1. Relationship between metabolic rate (*MR*, Cal/kg/day) and weight gain (gm/kg/day) in 28 studies. (From Chessex, P., and others: J. Pediatr. **99:**761, 1981.)

rates and required maintenance energy expenditures are relevant. For the term suckled infant an adequate milk supply, genetic programming, and appetite ensure, by definition, normal growth and development. For formula-fed infants some choices have to be made, mainly in regard to composition, since appetite can generally be relied upon to limit volume intake. For the premature infant who cannot go to the breast, absolute control over volume (either enteral or parenteral) and content exists and must be exercised with discretion. Several guidelines are available to aid in the necessary choices.

Desirable body composition

In general, metabolizable intake controls accretion of energy, fat, and protein (Fig. 25-2), although the form and composition of the enteral intake determine its metabolizable fraction, as documented by Reichman. In theory and probably largely in practice it is possible to control weight gain and body composition by manipulating the volume and composition of enteral and parenteral feeds. However, we have no clear idea of the desirable body composition or the rate at which it should be achieved, especially for the premature infant. There is no certainty that intrauterine accretion rates are necessarily suitable for the extrauterine "fetus." Although it is possible to deduce the composition of weight gain by nutrient balance studies combined with indirect calorimetry (Fig. 25-3), the measurement of body composition in vivo has hitherto been impossible in neonates. There is now some promise that this can be attained, at least on a research basis, by an ingenious application of Boyle's law to the measurement of body volume as devised by Taylor, permitting an estimate of body density from which body composition can be derived. Desirable body composition therefore remains to be defined but clearly can be influenced by diet, both qualitatively and quantitatively. For example, the composition of body fat reflects that of the dietary fat and its amount that of the metabolizable energy and fat intake being stored from intestinally derived chylomicrons. Some fat can be synthesized from carbohydrate, although the process is usually masked by simultaneous endogenous fat oxidation. When high carbohydrate loads are given there is net fat synthesis and storage.

At all levels of glucose intake above the usual resting oxidation rate of approximately 7.2 gm/kg/day, a proportion (approximately 15%) of carbohydrate intake cannot be accounted for by oxidation or storage as fat. The potential for storage as glycogen is limited, because total body stores are only of the order of 10 gm/kg. Incorporation of the glucose carbon skeleton into new tissue components in these growing infants seems the only reasonable alternative metabolic fate to explain the positive nonprotein carbon balance that can be demonstrated.

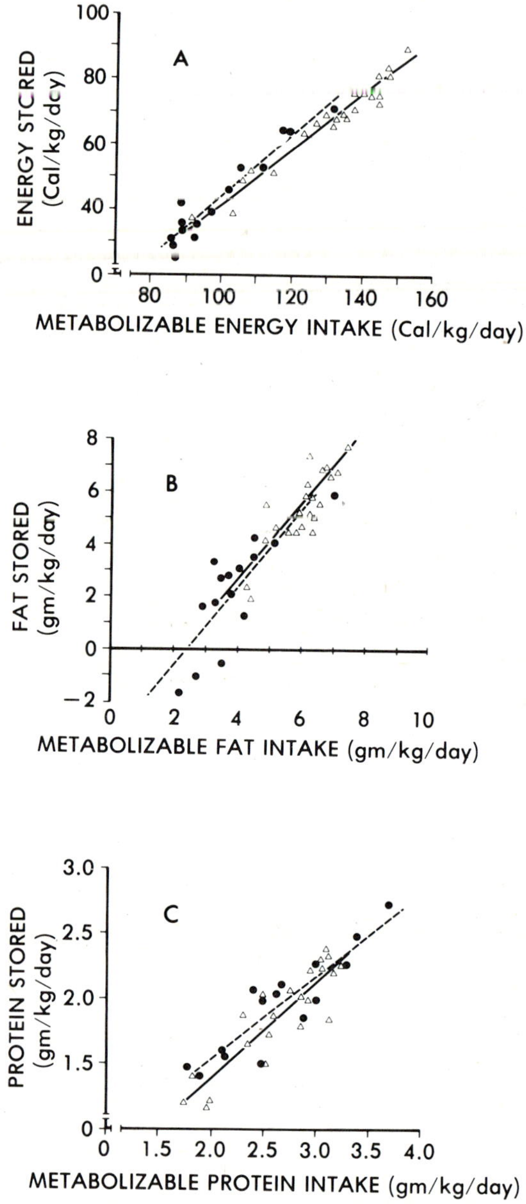

Fig. 25-2. Linear regression of metabolizable intake on storage from *(A)* energy, *(B)* fat, and *(C)* protein in own mother's milk–fed *(solid circle, broken line)* and formula-fed *(open triangle, solid line)* infants. Note similarity of regressions for two groups. Correlation coefficients ranged from 0.81 to 0.98 ($p < 0.001$). (From Reichman, B.L., and others: Pediatrics **72**:322, 1983. Reproduced by permission of Pediatrics.)

Relative levels of individual macronutrient intake

It is necessary to attend to the balance of macronutrients in the diet as well as to their absolute amounts, as a deficient energy supply may limit protein retention despite an adequate metabolizable protein intake. Balance between fat and carbohydrate components of the diet is also important to gas exchange and respiratory

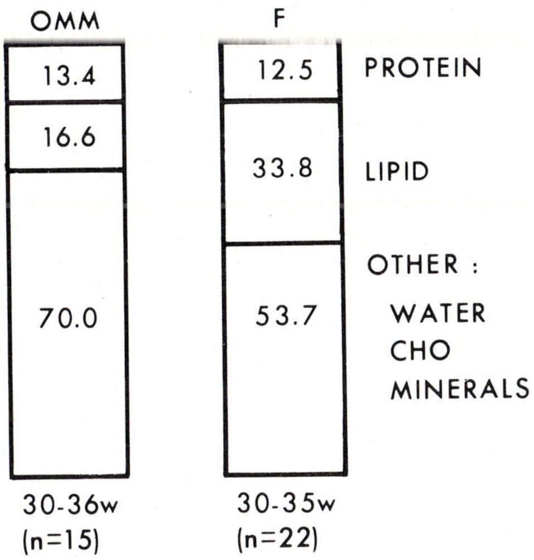

Fig. 25-3. Comparison of percentage composition of weight gain for infants fed their own mothers' milk (*OMM,* 30 to 36 weeks' postconceptional age) or formula (*F,* 30 to 35 weeks' postconceptional age). (From Reichman, B.L., and others: Pediatrics **72:**322, 1983. Reproduced by permission of Pediatrics.)

Table 25-3. Daily water, macronutrient, and metabolizable energy requirement for the newborn*

	Total intake (gm/kg/day)	Metabolizable intake (per kg/day)	Cal (metabolizable)
Water		150-200 ml	
Protein/ amino acid	3.5-4	3 gm	14
Lipid	3.5-4.6	3-4 gm	36
Carbohydrate	12-14	12-14 gm	50
Total			100

*Metabolizable energy is usually 80% to 85% of the ingested energy.

function, especially when high carbohydrate loads are given. For example, when 10% glucose and 2% amino acid solution is infused without lipid, increasing the intravenous glucose intake from 7.2 gm/kg/day (the resting rate of glucose utilization) to 24 gm/kg/day almost doubles carbon dioxide production and increases oxygen consumption by 33%. Alveolar ventilation increases directly and linearly with carbon dioxide production and therefore would also double, with a parallel increase in the work of breathing. Although the work of breathing in the normal neonate is only in the order of 2% to 3% of resting metabolism, premature infants with very compliant chest walls and poorly compliant lungs or those with chronic lung disease may have a considerably increased work of breathing. Administration of high carbohydrate loads to

Table 25-4. Protein and nonprotein composition of human milk

	Human milk (gm/dl)	%
Protein (gm/dl)		
Total proteins	0.89	100
Caseins	0.25	35
Total whey proteins	0.64	65
α-Lactalbumin	0.25	17
β-Lactoglobulin	—	—
Lactoferrin	0.17	17
Serum albumin	0.05	6
Lysozyme	0.05	6
Immunoglobulins		
IgA	0.10	11
IgG	0.003	
IgM	0.002	
Others	0.07	8
Nonprotein nitrogen (mg/100 ml)		
Total	50.0	
Urea	25.0	
Creatine nitrogen	3.7	
Creatinine nitrogen	3.5	
Uric acid nitrogen	0.5	
Glucosamine	4.7	
α-Amino nitrogen	13.0	
Ammonia nitrogen	0.2	
Other nitrogen components	?	

From Hambreus, L. Forsum, E., and Lonnerdal, B.: Nutritional aspects of breast milk versus cow's milk formula. In McFarlane, H., Hambreus, L., and Hanson, L.A., editors: Food and immunology: symposia of the Swedish Nutrition Foundation XIII, Stockholm, 1976, Almquist and Wiksell.

such an infant could induce respiratory failure, as has been reported in adults. Replacement of a proportion of the intravenous glucose by fat results in a reduction in energy expenditure, carbon dioxide production, and oxygen consumption. About 40% to 45% of the kilocalorie intake should be carbohydrate, 40% to 50% fat, and 10% protein. The absolute amounts of each macronutrient advised for a reasonable balance are summarized in Table 25-3, but their qualities are also important.

NATURE OF NITROGENOUS INTAKE

Table 25-4 shows the protein and other nitrogenous content of mature human milk. The whey/casein ratio is 60:40, in contrast to the 20:80 ratio for bovine milk. Lysozyme and the immunoglobulins are resistant to digestion and have an antiinfectious protective function rather than a nutritive function. Lactoferrin is also not digested and aids the absorption of iron as well as having an antibacterial role. Human milk also has a relatively high content of metabolizable nonprotein nitrogen in comparison to bovine milk (Table 25-4), including 30 mmol/L taurine, possibly important to neurologic and retinal function and to bile salt production.

The amino acid content of human milk protein is high

in cysteine and threonine and low in phenylalanine and tyrosine.

Human milk also contains carnitine, important in fatty acid metabolism.

About 88% of ingested human milk protein and 83% of a modified bovine protein premature formula are absorbed from the gut. Milk protein has a kilocalorie value of 5.65/gm.

NATURE OF THE FAT INTAKE

In human milk fat the beta position of the triglyceride molecule is filled by palmitic rather than stearic acid, as in bovine milk, rendering it more digestible. Medium-chain fatty acids are also easily hydrolyzed by lingual and gastric lipases in the stomach and upper intestine and hence are rapidly absorbed. They constitute about 17% of fatty acids in early human milk and 10% in mature milk. Unsaturated fatty acids are also better absorbed than saturated and they form 57% of the total fatty acid content, compared with 42% for saturated fatty acids. Essential fatty acids (linoleic 18:2, and higher series) form about 17% and amply satisfy the requirement of 3% of the daily kilocalories in this form.

Polyunsaturated fatty acids (PUFA) are important constituents of cell membranes, including those of the red cell, which are prone to oxidative damage in the presence of oxidizing agents such as iron, with the result being hemolytic anemia. Vitamin E is an antioxidant that has a specific protective action. Accordingly, the American Academy of Pediatrics recommends a ratio (in milligrams per gram) of >0.6 *d*-α-tocopherol/PUFA in the presence of an iron intake of about 2 mg/kg/day. The vitamin E intake and the E/PUFA ratios provided by human milk and current premature formulas containing vegetable oils are adequate for infants receiving up to 2 mg iron/kg/day (Chapter 32, part one). Table 25-5 shows that there is apparently little difference in the percent absorption of fat for preterm infants fed human milk (82.4%) compared with those fed a preterm formula (79.6%) with a similar fatty acid profile. Infants small for gestational age have a lower absorption (69%).

Almost 99% of the lipids in human milk are in the form of triglycerides, with 0.6% cholesterol and 0.4% phospholipids. Although the fat composition of human milk is constant, its concentration is variable. It increases from 2% in the colostral phase to 3% (transitional) to 4.5% in mature milk. There are also diurnal morning-to-evening and within-feed increases in concentration. The kilocalorie value of milk fat is 9.25/gm.

NATURE OF THE CARBOHYDRATE INTAKE

The carbohydrate in human milk is lactose (3.95 Cal/gm) and varies in concentration from 5.96 gm/dl at 3 days after delivery to 6.95 gm/dl at 28 days for preterm mothers and from 6.16 to 7.26 gm/dl for term mothers.

The LBW infant's gut mucosa is low in lactase, resulting in deficient hydrolysis, potential bacterial overgrowth, fermentation to absorbable ketones and hydrogen (detectable in the breath), and abdominal distension from its osmotic effect. However, incomplete lactose absorption, while common in both preterm and term infants, rarely gives rise to nutritional disadvantage or other symptoms, presumably because of bacterial transformation to absorbable ketones and short-chain fatty acids.

Table 25-5. Partition of energy and macronutrient metabolism

	Energy (Cal/kg/day)		Fat (gm/kg/day)		Carbohydrate (gm/kg/day)		Protein (gm/kg/day)	
	OMM	F	OMM	F	OMM	F	OMM	F
Gross intake	110.8* ±4.0	148.6 ±3.8	4.7* ±0.3	7.5 ±0.2	12.6* ±0.4	15.2 ±0.4	3.02 ±0.15	3.19 ±0.08
Losses in excreta	11.2† ±2.2	18.2 ±1.5	0.8† ±0.2	1.5 ±0.1	0.1 ±0.02	0.1 ±0.02	0.37‡ ±0.05	0.55 ±0.05
% Intake absorbed	90.2 ±1.8	87.9 ±1.8	82.4 ±3.6	79.6 ±1.8	99.3 ±0.2	99.7 ±0.2	87.9† ±1.6	83.4 ±1.5
Metabolizable intake	99.6* ±3.7	130.4 ±3.5	3.9* ±0.3	6.0 ±0.2	12.4* ±0.4	15.1 ±0.4	2.65 ±0.14	2.64 ±0.14
Oxidation	56.0* ±0.9	62.6 ±0.9	1.6† ±0.3	0.6 ±0.3	9.5* ±0.7	13.3 ±0.5	0.68 ±0.07	0.73 ±0.03
Storage	43.6* ±3.7	67.8 ±3.0	2.3* ±0.5	5.4 ±0.3	2.9 ±0.9	1.8 ±0.4	1.97 ±0.1	1.92 ±0.08

From Reichman, B.L., and others: Pediatrics **72:**322, 1983. Reproduced by permission of Pediatrics.
Results expressed as mean ± standard error of 15 studies in 11 infants fed own mother's milk (OMM) and 22 studies in 13 infants fed formula (F). Statistical significance of differences between means for OMM- and F-fed infants: *$p < 0.001$; †$p < 0.025$; ‡$p < 0.05$.

On the other hand the LBW infant's gut mucosa is well endowed with maltase, sucrase, and other glycosidases. Consequently preterm formulas usually have lactose replaced partially by glucose polymers (3.9 Cal/gm), commonly 40% to 50% lactose and 50% to 60% glucose polymers. The polymers have the advantage of reducing bowel content osmolality. The replacement of lactose may, however, reduce absorption of fat, calcium, and magnesium, and the desirability of such replacement is questionable.

The requirement for carbohydrate depends on a number of factors: the need to balance energy sources between carbohydrate and fat, energy requirement to cover metabolic rate, the thermal environment, and the levels of muscular activity and protein intake. A reasonable intake under average conditions is 12 to 14 gm/kg/day (Table 25-3).

ENERGY REQUIREMENT

The partition of energy utilization for formula- and human milk–fed infants

The partition of ingested energy for premature infants fed a high-energy (84.2 Cal/dl) formula between the ages of 2 to 6 weeks is shown in Fig. 25-4. For a gross energy intake of 149 Cal/kg/day, 18 Cal (or 12%) are lost in the excreta, 51 Cal are used in maintenance (4 for muscular activity, 11 for tissue synthesis), and 68 Cal/kg/day are stored in the components of new tissue. Note that more than half (53%) of the energy ingested is used to support growth in these formula-fed infants.

By contrast comparable infants fed their own mothers' milk by gavage in approximately similar volume, although at a lower kilocalorie intake of 111 Cal/kg/day, oxidized half their nonprotein energy intake, lost 10% in excreta, and accreted only 40% (Table 25-5). The differences are accounted for by the higher fat content and caloric density of the formula compared with milk from the infant's own mother and the consequent higher fat accretion of the formula-fed infant (5.4 versus 2.3 gm/kg/day). The rates of weight gain were similar, 16.8 gm/kg/day in the formula-fed compared with 15.2 gm/kg/day in the human milk–fed infants. These findings raise once again the question of the desirable body composition of the growing infant and the possibilities for modification of body composition by differing dietary regimens. Fig. 25-3 shows the percent composition of the weight gain in the high-calorie formula–fed infants compared with that of the infants fed their own mothers' milk. Except in special circumstances there seems little justification for feeding calorie-dense formulas (84 Cal/dl). There are now "special care" premature formulas available with a normal 68 to 70 Cal/dl density, and their use would seem preferable to the high-density formulas in order to avoid excessive fat accretion.

Macronutrient accretion rates and body composition

While the Nutrition Committee of the American Academy of Pediatrics (1985) has reaffirmed that fetal accretion rates are reasonable targets for postnatal growth in the LBW infant, there is no certainty that this is necessarily a desirable standard (Canadian Pediatric Society

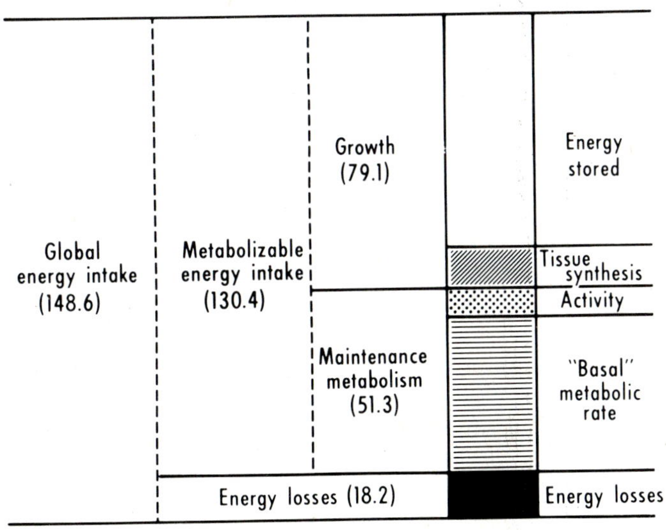

Fig. 25-4. Partition of energy metabolism in VLBW infants under thermoneutral conditions. These infants were fed high-calorie formula (84.2 Cal/dl) at 148.6 Cal/kg/day between ages 2 and 6 weeks. (From Reichman, B.L., and others: Pediatrics **69:**446, 1982. Reproduced by permission of Pediatrics © 1982.)

Nutrition Committee, 1981). The aquatic, undisturbed, thermoneutral, placentally maintained environment of the fetus differs markedly from the independent, stimulatory, gravity laden, intermittently cold-stressed extrauterine life. Fomon has shown a tendency for greater fat accretion after delivery in term infants; and prematures removed from thermoneutral incubators to bassinets apparently accelerate the acquisition of their subcutaneous fat layer. It cannot therefore be assumed necessarily that intrauterine accretion rates are the correct standard for extrauterine life.

Also relevant is the influence of the early over-acquisition of fat on the subsequent development of obesity. The evidence is conflicting, but during the period from 30 weeks of gestation to 9 months of postnatal age, there may be a sensitive period in adipocyte replication such that exceeding a certain adipocyte fat load constitutes a stimulus to divide, thereby increasing adipocyte number, perhaps setting the stage for subsequent refractory obesity. This possibility seems to be denied by a Danish study of 540 adoptees in whom eventual body mass correlated more strongly with that of the biologic parents than the adoptive parents. Genetically programmed appetite apparently controls body mass outside the early critical growth epoch. There nevertheless seems no advantage to oversupplying energy in early infancy.

Table 25-6. Usual water losses (ml/kg/24 hr)

	Body weight (gm)		
	<1,500	1,500-2,500	2,500-3,500
Basal IWL*	30-60	15-35	21-30
Urine	50-100	50-100	25-62
Stool	5-10	5-10	2-5
Total	85-170	70-145	48-97

From Perlman, M., and others. Guidelines for neonatal treatment, ed. 3, Toronto, 1986, The Hospital for Sick Children.
*IWL, Insensible water loss.

Table 25-7. Average daily water requirements (ml/kg/day)* for newborn infants (see part two)

	Day					
	1	2	3	4	5	>5
500-800 gm	150	140	130	130	150	150-200
800-1,000 gm	125	115	120	130	150	150-200
1,000-1,500 gm	80	70	100	120	150	150-200
1,500-2,000 gm	60	75	100	120	140	150-180
>2,000 gm	60	70	90	120	140	160-180

From Perlman, M., and others: Guidelines for neonatal treatment, ed. 3, Toronto, 1985, The Hospital for Sick Children.
*Add 30% for radiant warmer. Add 10% for phototherapy. Subtract 10% for plastic wrap.

WATER REQUIREMENT

See also Part two.

Factors that influence neonatal water requirement are maturity, thermal environment, rate of growth, nature of the diet, and illness.

Premature infants have imperfectly developed or absent sweat glands but extremely water-permeable skin, resulting in transepidermal water losses up to 170 ml/kg/day. The term infant can triple normal water loss by sweating from heat stress. The newborn and especially the premature infant's kidney has limited abilities to concentrate urine (to 600 to 700 mOsm) as compared with 1,200 mOsm in adults, resulting in high obligatory renal water excretion. Term and preterm infants lose 10% to 15% of body weight in the first week of life because of a diminution in extracellular water. Usual daily water losses are shown in Table 25-6. Thus the water requirements for the neonate are much higher per kilogram of body weight than for the adult. In fact an adult would need to take 14 L fluid daily rather than the usual 1.5 to 2 L to match the neonatal intake on a proportional weight basis!

Since 75% to 80% of the infant's body is composed of water, there is a requirement of 10 to 24 gm water for each daily weight increment of 15 to 30 gm/kg, but this is largely offset by the approximate 12 gm/kg of water derived from the metabolism of nutrients. Incorporation of nitrogen and other elements into tissue reduces the renal solute load and hence obligatory water for excretion. However, a catabolic state, fever, and changes in blood volume, body water, and electrolyte content consequent on disease will all, by various mechanisms, alter the daily water requirement. Average daily water requirements are shown in Table 25-7. Monitoring to ensure adequate water balance should include:

1. Intake/output
2. Weight, once to twice daily
3. Serum electrolytes, once to twice daily
4. Urine specific gravity, twice to three times daily
5. Urine electrolytes
6. Urine glucose, twice to three times daily; infants <1,250 gm

ELECTROLYTE AND MINERAL REQUIREMENTS

See also Parts two and three.

Third-trimester intrauterine accretion rates for the major minerals are shown in Table 25-8, along with average mineral content for mature human milk, recommended daily intakes with supplement if necessary, and

Table 25-8. Mineral content of human milk compared with average intrauterine accretion rate during the last trimester; recommended oral intake and expected retention for infants of low birth weight

Element	Human milk content (mmol/100 ml)	mmol intake/kg/day (150 ml milk/kg/day)	Intrauterine accretion (mmol/kg/day)	Oral intake with supplement (mmol/kg/day)	Net retention (mmol/kg/day)
Na^+	0.7	1.05	1.2	3.0	2
K^+	1.4	2.1	0.77	3-4	3
Ca^{++}	0.85	1.25	3.1-3.75	5.5*	3.5
Mg^{++}	0.15	0.22	0.2	0.2	0.2
P	0.5	0.75	2.3-2.8	2.3-2.8	1.1
Fe	0.0027	0.004	0.036	0.036	0.036
	(0.15 mg)	(0.22 mg)	(2 mg)	(2 mg)	(2 mg)

From Swyer, P.R.: The intensive care of the newly born, Basel, Switzerland, 1975, S. Karger AG.
*Caution: No more than 2.5 mmol Ca (5 mEq)/kg/day may be given intravenously.

net retention rates. The enhanced mineral content of human preterm milk tends to disappear during the third or fourth week after birth. Therefore it is probably advisable to feed the preterm infant supplements of sodium, calcium, and phosphorus.

The sodium supplements to human milk may be given orally as sodium bicarbonate 8.4%: 0.2 ml (0.2 mEq) every 4 hours with feeds (1.2 mEq/day) until the infant reaches a weight of 1,500 gm; then 0.4 ml (0.4 mEq) every 4 hours (2.4 mEq/day) until the infant reaches a weight of 1,800 gm, after which the sodium content of the oral milk suffices. A practical alternative is the use of commercially available human milk fortifiers designed for the premature infant. These contain additional calories, as well as minerals and vitamins, although the additional calories may be unnecessary.

Subsequent to recent studies of calcium and phosphorus metabolism, Salle and associates recommend the addition of disodium phosphate equivalent to 24.5 mg phosphorus followed by 27 mg calcium (glubionate) to 100 ml pooled mature human milk, in this sequence, to avoid precipitation of calcium. The calcium intake is increased from 47 mg/kg/day for unsupplemented human milk to 90 mg/kg/day for the milk supplemented in this way; they reported net calcium retentions of 63 mg/kg/day in supplemented preterm infants compared with 21 mg/kg/day for the unsupplemented infants. For the phosphorus supplemented milk, phosphorus intake was 62 mg/kg/day and retention was 53 mg/kg/day versus 21 mg/kg/day for the unsupplemented milk. A daily dose of 30 μg vitamin D (1,200 IU) was given concurrently.

During the third trimester the fetus accumulates 120 to 140 mg/kg/day of calcium and 70 to 75 mg/kg/day of phosphorus. The retentions attained by the recommended supplementations therefore fall short of the intrauterine ideal, but they represent a considerable improvement on retentions from unsupplemented mature human milk and appear to be sufficient to prevent significant bone demineralization. Higher levels of calcium supplementation may reduce fat and calcium absorption by the formation of insoluble calcium soaps in the intestine, while further increases in phosphorus intake may result in increased urinary losses. In general the special care formulas developed commercially for low birth weight premature infants contain adequate mineral supplements (American Academy of Pediatrics Committee on Nutrition, 1985).

Table 25-9. Suggested daily intravenous intake of essential trace elements

Trace element	Intake (μg/kg/day)
Zinc	
Premature infants (<3 kg)	300
Term infants	100
Copper	20
Chromium	0.14-0.2
Manganese	2-10

From American Medical Association Department of Foods and Nutrition, JAMA **241**:2053, 1979.

TRACE ELEMENTS

The recommended allowances are shown in Table 25-9. These needs are satisfied by the usual content in human milk and by commercial formulas, as well as by the content of the recommended intravenous feeding solutions.

VITAMIN REQUIREMENTS

The recommended oral intakes for term infants are shown in Table 25-10, and intravenous vitamin solutions are available to complement total parenteral nutrition, as discussed later (Table 25-11).

Table 25-10. Recommended daily intakes of vitamins

	NAS-NRC*	Ziegler et al.
Vitamin A (IU)	1,400	500
Vitamin D (IU)	400	600
Vitamin E (IU)	3	30
Vitamin K (μg)	12	15
Vitamin C (mg)	35	60
Vitamin B_1 (mg)	0.3	0.20
Vitamin B_2 (mg)	0.4	0.40
Niacin (mg)	6	5.0
Pantothenic acid (mg)	2	2.0
Vitamin B_6 (mg)	0.3	0.4
Vitamin B_{12} (μg)	0.5	1.5
Folic acid (μg)	30	60
Biotin (μg)	35	12
Choline (mg)	8.4	—
Inositol (mg)	4.8	—

*In most cases value given is recommended dietary allowance for term infants (0 to 6 months) suggested by the National Academy of Sciences–National Research Council (1980). For pantothenic acid, biotin, and vitamin K, values are the estimated safe and adequate daily intakes suggested by the same Council. Values for choline and inositol are minimum recommended intakes suggested by the Committee on Nutrition of the American Academy of Pediatrics (1979).

Table 25-11. Pediatric multivitamins for infusion (5 ml for dilution in intravenous infusion only)*

Ascorbic acid	80 mg
Vitamin A	2,300 IU
Vitamin D	400 IU
Thiamine (as HCl)	1.2 mg
Riboflavin (as phosphate)	1.4 mg
Pyridoxine HCl	1.0 mg
Niacinamide	17.0 mg
d-Pantothenic acid	5.0 mg
Vitamin E	7.0 IU
Biotin	20 μg
Folic acid	0.14 mg
Vitamin B_{12}	1 μg
Vitamin K_1	0.2 mg

*With 375 mg mannitol, 50 mg polysorbate 80, 0.8 mg polysorbate 20, 58 μgm butylated hydroxytoluene, 14 μgm butylated hydroxyanisole, and sodium hydroxide for pH adjustment. The daily dose is 65% of the above amount for infants <3 kg and 100% for infants >3 kg, given daily. The preparation is from USV Canada Inc., Mississauga, Ontario, Canada.

NUTRITIONAL STRATEGY

Choices for enteral feeding

Fresh human milk offers major psychologic benefit to mother and infant and protective advantages in supplying humoral (antibody) and cellular (macrophage and lymphocyte) defense against infection to the hypoimmune infant (Chapter 30). It also contains lipases to improve fat digestion and growth factors (e.g., epidermal growth factor). Mature milk (3 to 4 week postnatal milk) is, however, too low in protein (0.9 to 1.1 gm/dl) and in calcium, phosphate, and sodium to satisfy the enhanced requirements for growth of LBW infants, and supplementation may be necessary, as described above. The colostral phase of milk secretion, which is prolonged in mothers giving birth prematurely, provides enhanced concentrations of protein and electrolytes that render it more suitable for the LBW infant with increased needs for these nutrients. Thus fresh human milk is the first preference, followed by bank human milk supplemented with human milk protein and minerals, suitably screened for infection and heat treated to ensure sterility.

It has been the practice in human milk banks to modify the content of mature milk so called milk engineering, especially in regard to protein and fat, to make it more suitable for the premature infant. The technique of ultrafiltration is also now being applied to the fractionation of human milk in much the same way as it has been applied to blood products, raising new perspectives for special applications in infant feeding.

Special formulas for premature infants have mineral supplementation and additional bovine β-lactoglobulin as the whey protein to match the 60:40 whey/casein ratio of human milk. This provides extra high-quality protein, although the whey protein of human milk is α-lactalbumin. The fats in formulas are derived from vegetable oils and have relatively high contents of unsaturated fatty acids, which are better absorbed than bovine milk fat (Table 25-12).

There are many practical obstacles to adequate enteral nutrition for the newborn, especially the LBW or sick infant. These are: inability to coordinate sucking, swallowing, and breathing because of immaturity, tachypnea, or altered states of consciousness; a restricted stomach capacity at birth; ileus from immaturity or illness; or bowel obstruction from malformation or disease. Distension of the gastrointestinal tract with milk may, by raising intraabdominal pressure, embarrass respiration and cause a fall in resting lung volume, presumably as a result of airway closure and atelectasis with resultant hypoxemia and possibly apnea. Furthermore, "overloading" of the gut has been implicated in the causation of necrotizing enterocolitis (Chapter 33).

Table 25-12. Premature formulas comparison chart

	"preemie" SMA 24 Cal (per 100 ml)	Similac Special Care (per 100 ml)	Enfamil Premature (per 100 ml)
PROTEIN			
TOTAL (grams)	2.0	2.2	2.4
Whey protein: casein ratio	60:40	60:40	60:40
FAT			
TOTAL (grams)	4.4	4.41	4.1
MCT (medium chain triglycerides)	10%	50%	40%
Oleo oil	20%	0%	0%
Corn oil	0%	0%	0%
Oleic oil	25%	0%	0%
Coconut oil	27%	20%	20%
Soy oil	18%	30%	40%
CARBOHYDRATE			
TOTAL (grams)	8.6	8.61	8.9
Lactose	50%	50%	40%
Glucose polymers	50%	50%	60%
MINERALS (ash)			
TOTAL (mg)	400	650	500
Calcium (mg)	75	146	95
Phosphorus (mg)	40	73	48
Sodium (mg)	32	41	32
Potassium (mg)	75	114	90
Chloride (mg)	53	73	69
Magnesium (mg)	7	10	4
Zinc (mg)	0.8	1.22	0.8
Iron (mg)	0.3	0.3	0.2
Copper (μg)	70	203	130
Manganese (μg)	20	10	11
Iodine (μg)	8.3	16	6
VITAMINS (per liter)			
A (IU)	2400	5520	9720
D (IU)	480	1220	2640
E (IU)	15	32	37
K_1 (μg)	70	100	106
C (ascorbic acid) (mg)	70	300	285
B_1 (thiamine) (μg)	800	2030	2030
B_2 (riboflavin) (μg)	1300	5030	2850
B_6 (μg)	500	2030	2030
B_{12} (μg)	2.0	4.5	2.4
Niacin (mg)	6.3	40.6	33
Folic acid (μg)	100	300	285
Pantothenic acid (μg)	3600	15430	9720
Biotin (μg)	18	300	16
Choline (mg)	127	80	62
Inositol (mg)	32	45	38
SUMMARY			
Calories per liter	810	812	810
Calories per fluid ounce	24	24	24
Osmolality mOsm/kg H_2O	280	300	300
Potential renal solute load (PRSL) mOsm/L	175.0	197.0	220.0
Ca to P ratio	1.9:1	2:1	2:1
$\frac{Na + K}{Cl}$ ratio (mEq)	2:2	2:2	1:9

Courtesy of Wyeth Laboratories, Inc., Philadelphia, PA 19101.

Techniques of enteral feeding

See also Chapter 24, part four.

In the absence of an absolute contraindication it is generally advisable to start early oral-enteral feeding in healthy preterm infants, if necessary by gavage tube, not only on nutritional grounds but to expand stomach capacity, promote bowel development, enzyme induction in the brush border, and gut hormonal release, which may be important to normal function. Intestinal stasis is avoided and bile stasis with excessive enterohepatic recirculation and clinical jaundice reduced. Suitable feeding volumes, increments, and total daily volumes according to weight and postnatal age are shown in Table 25-7. Although tube stabilization is perhaps more difficult, some prefer peroral rather than pernasal placement because of presumed additional upper airway resistance to breathing associated with nasal tubes. Intragastric tube placement is preferable to jejunal, because it is easier to place, less liable to cause perforation, and apparently of equal or greater efficacy for absorption. Intermittent rather than continuous drip feeding seems more physiologic, although occasionally a continuous gravity drip may be more effective than bolus feeding in securing weight gain. In either case supervision must be close to detect abdominal distension or regurgitation. The smallest infants (<1000 gm) require intermittent gavage feeding at 1- to 2-hour intervals. Once weight gain has been established the interval may be increased to 2 to 3 hours, depending on gastric emptying time as judged by stomach aspiration before the next feed. A residue of more than 2 to 3 ml should prompt a review of volumes and feeding intervals and a check for the presence of abdominal distension and absence of bowel sounds signifying ileus caused by immaturity or some pathologic process such as sepsis or necrotizing enterocolitis.

Nonnutritive sucking by the use of a pacifier during tube feeding results in earlier effective nutritive sucking and may produce better weight gain and earlier discharge from the hospital.

Parenteral feeding for low birth weight premature infants

In the VLBW infant, neonatal feeding intolerance caused by ileus, or immaturity in enzyme systems and swallowing reflexes, mandates intravenous alimentation for at least the first 24 to 48 hours.

Techniques of intravenous nutrition

There are considerable technical problems associated with parenteral infusion in neonates, particularly in the VLBW infant.

The method of infusion through percutaneously placed scalp needles or through other peripheral veins requires skill, is short-lived, and may terminate in tissue infiltration and local necrosis depending on the volume and nature of the fluid extravasated. Teflon peripheral catheters have been found to have more than three times longer effective life and a lower infiltration rate then scalp needles.

Many of the difficulties associated with peripheral intravenous sites stem from the small and fragile nature of the veins, the minimal- or no-flow condition at the injection site, and the irritant chemical or hyperosmolar nature of the injected fluid. In order to overcome these disadvantages larger central veins, the umbilical vessels, venae cavae, and right atrium have all been cannulated. Umbilical venous catheterization has well-recognized hazards and is consequently seldom used except for short-term cannulation at birth. However, the placement of central venous silicone rubber catheters in the superior vena cava either percutaneously or by surgical incision and subcutaneous tunneling to exit at a remote easy-to-manage site has increasingly been refined. An 88% success rate has been reported for basilic or external jugular venous percutaneous placement to a central site in infants <1,000 gm in weight. These 0.64 mm external diameter, silicone rubber catheters remained functional for a mean of 24.8 ± 15.9 days, and there was no associated thrombosis or infection. This has now become the preferred technique for long-term intravenous therapy in newborns. Some centers are reporting similar success with the use of silicone rubber catheters advanced centrally from peripheral venous access.

Management of intravenous nutrition

Initially 5 to 7.5 gm/dl glucose water is given at the rates shown in Table 25-7, thus supplying 5 to 10 gm/kg/day (19 to 37.5 Cal) of glucose, covering immediate neonatal energy requirements.

At 12 to 24 hours of age sodium should be added by changing the infusion to 0.2% sodium chloride with 5% to 7.5% glucose, which supplies 3.4 mEq sodium/100 ml solution.

Premature and growth-retarded infants <1,250 gm are frequently intolerant of glucose and become hyperglycemic because of a poor insulinemic response and a consequent low glucose disappearance rate of less than the normal 1.4%/min. Fortunately, in most cases the insulin response becomes normal after 48 hours, but it is essential to monitor blood glucose levels and to adjust the amount of glucose infused accordingly. The normal glucose utilization rate of 5 to 6 mg/kg/min should not be exceeded if the infant is normoglycemic (blood glucose of 40 to 100 mg/dl). Even in hypoglycemia, rates of infusion in excess of 10 mg/kg/min are usually self-defeating in that they may provoke reactive hyperinsulinism. It is in fact difficult to satisfy energy requirements entirely from glucose during the newborn period. Infusion of 5 gm/dl at 100 ml/kg/day supplies only 18.75 Cal of an estimated minimal metabolic requirement of 35 to 40 Cal/kg/day. (See Chapter 7.)

The blood glucose should therefore be checked every 4 to 6 hours during the first 48 hours, and after stabilization every 12 to 24 hours. Urine output should be measured and tested for glycosuria. After 24 to 48 hours the glucose concentration infused may be increased.

Because of the sudden cessation of the calcium ion influx from the placenta and the immaturity of the calciostat hormonal control (parathormone/calcitonin balance), hypocalcemia is common (Chapter 37, part two). Thus calcium may need to be added as calcium gluconate to the infusion fluid at a rate of 2 mEq/kg/day. The serum calcium level should be monitored daily for at least the first 3 days.

After 36 to 48 hours, if intravenous alimentation needs to be continued a glucose (7.5 gm/dl) amino acid (1.5 gm/dl) solution is introduced. If intragastric feeding is occurring simultaneously the total volumes by both routes should approximate the daily totals shown in Table 25-7. The urine output should be monitored and should be about 2 ml/kg/hr. The total fluid intake should be adjusted for abnormal conditions (e.g., phototherapy, +10% to 25%; radiant heat, +25% to 30%) or decreased for pathologic circumstances (e.g., urinary suppression from asphyxial renal damage [acute tubular necrosis] or heart failure). Restrictions to fluid intake should not be allowed to impair nutritional supply for a prolonged period.

A particularly difficult problem is presented by the premature infant who develops a large left-to-right shunt through a persistently patent ductus anteriosus within a few days of birth. Under these circumstances fluid restriction may be necessary to treat impending or actual heart failure, thereby reducing energy and nutrient intake. (See Chapter 29.)

Depending on size and maturity intravenous supplementation of enteral feeding may last from 1 to 4 or more weeks. The compositions of solutions commonly used at Rainbow Babies and Childrens Hospital are shown in Table 25-13. They differ in their energy, amino acid, and electrolyte contents; the higher energy and amino acid concentrations are introduced as the infant's tolerance improves with maturity and as the high urinary sodium losses of the immediate neonatal period recede, usually in the second week. The multitude of potential complications associated with parenteral hyperalimentation are listed in Table 25-14.

Provided contraindications do not exist, a 10% lipid emulsion (e.g., Nutralipid; Pharmacia: 54% linoleic acid, 8% linolenic acid, 26% oleic acid, 9% palmitic acid, 1.2% egg lecithin, 2.5% glycerol) of 1.1 Cal/ml is then piggybacked in at a rate of 0.5 to 1 gm/kg/day, increasing gradually to 3 to 4 gm/kg/day over the succeeding 7 to 14 days, as indicated by monitoring serum triglyceride levels, daily at first and then twice weekly as tolerance is established. The serum tryglyceride level should be below 100 mg/dl.

There are decreased plasma levels of linoleic, linolenic, and arachidonic acids as early as 3 to 4 days of life in VLBW infants. Therefore the early introduction of lipids containing essential fatty acids is particularly important in the VLBW infant, whose virtual total lack of body fat stores renders him/her extremely susceptible to the clinical syndrome of essential fatty acid deficiency—desquamating skin rash, loss of hair, growth retardation, susceptibility to infection, delayed wound healing, and thrombocytopenia. There may be a lack of

Table 25-13. Progression of representative hyperalimentation solutions*

	Neonate formula I (dextrose 10%)	Neonate formula II (dextrose 12.5%)	Neonate formula III (dextrose 12.5%)
Nitrogen	1.6 gm/L	2.2 gm/L	2.7 gm/L
Protein	10 gm/L	14 gm/L	17 gm/L
Total calories	380 Cal/L	481 Cal/L	493 Cal/L
Electrolytes	mEq/L	mEq/L	mEq/L
Sodium	26	26	26
Potassium	20	20	20
Magnesium	4	4	4
Calcium	7	7	7
Acetate	30	43	47
Chloride	20	19	20
Phosphate	12 (6 mmol)	12 (6 mmol)	12 (6 mmol)
Heparin	500 units/L	500 units/L	500 units/L
Trace minerals	+	+	+
Multivitamins	+	+	+

*Infants are typically started with formula I and may progress to solutions containing greater amounts of protein and dextrose, depending on fluid requirements and external intake.

Table 25-14. Complications associated with parenteral alimentation

Metabolic
Hypo- and hyperglycemia
Electrolyte imbalance
Hypo- and hypercalcemia
Hypophosphatemia
Lower red blood cell content of adenosine triphosphate and 2,3-diphosphoglycerate
Acquired phagocyte dysfunction
Metabolic acidosis
Hyperammonemia
Isoosmolar coma
Cholestasis
Abnormal liver function
Fatty acid deficiency
Trace element deficiency
Infection
Candida sepsis is potentially the most dangerous
Bacterial sepsis
Fungal sepsis
(If sepsis develops, the line must be removed)
Catheter complications
Improper placement of catheter may lead to extravasation, hemorrhage, pneumothorax, and hydrothorax
Superior vena caval thrombosis
Pulmonary embolism
Local irritation or slough

From Fanaroff, A.A., and Klaus, M.H.: Feeding and selected disorders of the gastrointestinal tract. In Klaus, M.H., and Fanaroff, A.A.: Care of the high risk infant, ed. 3, Philadelphia, 1986, W.B. Saunders.

prostaglandin precursors and defects in membrane function.

While most newborns readily metabolize fat as shown by a fall in respiratory quotient to about 0.7 soon after birth and by indirect calorimetric studies during infusion of lipid emulsion, the VLBW infant is deficient in the key enzyme lipoprotein lipase and moreover lacks a developed fat organ in which to store lipid influx. As a consequence plasma clearance of chylomicrons and other lipids may be impaired. Intolerance to intravenous fat may also occur in association with infection. Sequelae may include reduced pulmonary diffusing capacity and arterial oxygen tension with pulmonary capillary lipid deposition, potential displacement of bilirubin from serum albumin binding sites by free fatty acids, and interference with photometric measurement of serum bilirubin levels. There may be lipid deposition in the lungs, liver, kidneys, and reticuloendothelial system and in leukocytes and macrophages, resulting in impaired defense against infection. Prolonged hyperlipidemia has been implicated as a cause of premature arteriosclerosis in infants. Unfortunately it is extremely difficult to predict intolerance to intravenous lipid infusion. Therefore it is mandatory to monitor serum levels. The use of lipid emulsions in infants with acute pulmonary disease, with hyperbilirubinemia or hepatic injury, with infection, or with extreme prematurity or intrauterine growth retardation may be hazardous, and the advantages should be carefully weighed against the risks.

TOTAL PARENTERAL NUTRITION FOR THE SURGICAL NEONATE

The availability of total parenteral nutrition has completely transformed the prognosis for infants with major anomalies and conditions affecting the gastrointestinal tract such as volvulus, atresia, malrotation, omphalocele, and gastroschisis (Chapter 33), especially when major resections have to be undertaken. Although it is possible to maintain infants almost indefinitely on total parenteral nutrition with an afunctional gut, the prospects for normal life and growth are remote when a major resection has removed the ileocecal valve and left <40 cm of small bowel to support alimentation and life. In such cases most would reject prolonged total parenteral nutrition. In all others total parenteral nutrition has been shown to support normal life and growth over many weeks, even months, until the remaining gut can adapt.

There is potential for liver damage to occur with long-term total parenteral nutrition, often accompanied by severe jaundice. The cause of this is currently uncertain but may be related to cholangitis from absorption of bacterial toxins from the gut that have accumulated during prolonged bowel stasis. Thus techniques of enteral and parenteral feeding now exist for the preterm or sick neonate that are adequate to preserve life and function, while the primary condition of immaturity or disease is managed. There are, however, still major uncertainties about the nutritional goals to optimize body composition and long-term growth and development.

Paul R. Swyer
Tibor Heim

BIBLIOGRAPHY

Nutritional requirements

Adam, P.A.J.: Control of glucose metabolism in the human fetus and newborn infant, Adv. Metab. Disord. **5**:183, 1971.

American Academy of Pediatrics Committee on Nutrition: Nutritional needs of low birthweight infants, Pediatrics **60**:519, 1977.

American Academy of Pediatrics Committee on Nutrition: Nutritional needs of low birthweight infants, Pediatrics **75**:976, 1985.

Avery, G.B., and Fletcher, A.B.: Nutrition. In Avery, G.B., editor: Neonatology, ed. 2, Philadelphia/Toronto, 1981, J.B. Lippincott Co., pp. 1038-1060.

Baker, J.P.: Metabolic aspects of starvation, Ann. R. Coll. Phys. Surg. Can. **15**:642, 1982.

Boersma, E.R.: Changes in fatty acid composition of body fat before and after birth in Tanzania: an international comparative study, Br. Med. J. **1**:850, 1979.

Brooke, C.G.D.: Evidence for a sensitive period in adipose cell replication in man, Lancet **11**:624, 1972.

Catzeflis, C., and others: Whole body protein synthesis and energy expenditure in very low birthweight infants, Pediatr. Res. **19**:679, 1985.

Chessex, P., and others: Influence of postnatal age, energy intake, and weight gain on energy metabolism in the very low birthweight infant, J. Pediatr. **99**:761, 1981.

Chessex, P., and others: Metabolic consequences of intrauterine growth retardation in very low birthweight infants, Pediatr. Res. **18**:709, 1984.

Cross, K.W., Tizard, J.P.M., and Trythall, D.A.H.: The gaseous metabolism of the newborn infant, Acta Paediatr. Scand. **46**:265, 1957.

Dark, D.S., Pingleton, S., and Kerby, G.R.: Hypercapnia during weaning—a complication of nutritional support, Chest **88**:141, 1985.

Dobbing, J.: The later development of the central nervous system and its vulnerability. In Davis, J.A., and Dobbing, J., editors: Scientific foundations of paediatrics, Philadelphia, 1974, W.B. Saunders Co., p. 565.

Editorial: Infants and adult obesity, Lancet **1**:17, 1974.

Fanaroff, A.A., and others: Insensible water loss in low birth weight infants, Pediatrics **50**:236, 1972.

Fomon, J.S.: Body composition of the male reference infant during the first year of life, Pediatrics **40**:863, 1967.

Gall, G.: Gastrointestinal development and neonatal nutrition. In Proceedings of the 72nd Ross Conference on Pediatric Research, Columbus, Ohio, 1977, Ross Laboratories, p. 175.

Heim, T.: Homeothermy and its metabolic cost. In Davis, J.A. and Dobbing, J., editors: London, 1981, Medical Books Ltd., pp. 91-128.

Heimler, R., and others: Thermal environment change in growing premature infants: Effects on general somatic growth and subcutaneous fat accumulation, Pediatrics **68**:82, 1981.

Hey, E.N., and Katz, G.: Evaporative water loss in the new-born baby, J. Physiol. (Lond.) **200**:605, 1969.

Katzman, G.H.: Insensible water loss by small infants in radiant heater, J. Pediatr. **83**:1094, 1973.

Maclean, Jr., W.C., and Fink, B.B.: Lactose malabsorption by premature infants: magnitude and clinical significance, J. Pediatr. **97**:383, 1980.

McGilvery, R.W.: Storage of the major fuels. In McGilvery, R.W., editor: Biochemistry, a functional approach, III, Philadelphia, 1970, W.B. Saunders Co., pp. 287-459.

Millward, D.G., and Garlick, P.J.: The energy cost of growth, Proc. Nutr. Soc. **35**:339, 1976.

Myres, A.Q.: Obesity: is it preventable in infancy and childhood? Can. Fam. Phys. **21**:73, 1975.

Nachman, R.L., and Esterly, N.B.: Increased skin permeability in preterm infants, J. Pediatr. **79**:628, 1971.

Purpura, D.P.: Dendritic differentiation in human cerebral cortex: normal and aberrant development patterns. In Kreutzberg, G.W., editor: Physiology and pathology of dendrites. Advances in neurology, vol. 12, New York, 1975, Raven Press, p. 91.

Radde, I.C., and others: Calcium ion activity in the sick neonate: effect of bicarbonate administration and exchange transfusions, Pediatr. Res. **6**:43, 1972.

Recommended dietary allowances, ed. 9, Washington, D.C., 1980, National Academy of Sciences.

Reichman, B., and others: Diet, fat accretion and growth in premature infants, N. Engl. J. Med. **305**:1495, 1981.

Reichman, B.L., and others: Partition of energy metabolism and energy cost of growth in the very low birthweight infants, Pediatrics **69**:446, 1982.

Reichman, B.L., and others: Dietary composition and macronutrient storage in preterm infants, Pediatrics **72**:322, 1983.

Salle, B., Chance, G.W., and Ruiton-Ugliengo, M.: Glucose assimilation in neonates. In Stetson, J.B., and Swyer, P.R., editors: Neonatal intensive care, St. Louis, 1976, Warren H. Green, pp. 165-181.

Sauer, P.J.J., and others: Glucose oxidation rates in newborn infants measured with indirect calorimetry and [U-^{13}C] glucose, Clin. Sci. **70**:587, 1986.

Shaw, J.C.L.: Evidence for the depletion of skeletal mineralisation in the low birthweight infant: the absorption of calcium and fat, Pediatrics **57**:16, 1976.

Stunkard, A.J., and others: An adoption study of human obesity, N. Engl. J. Med. **314**:193, 1986.

Swyer, P.R.: The intensive care of the newly born, Basel, Switzerland, 1975, Karger AG.

Swyer, P.R., Heim, T., and Reichman, B.L.: Letter to the editor regarding paper by Heimler et al., Pediatrics **68**:82, 1981.

Swyer, P.R., Reiman, R.C., and Wright, J.J.: Ventilation and ventilatory mechanics in the newborn, J. Pediatr. **56**:612, 1960.

Taylor, A., and others: Development of an air displacement method for whole body volume measurement of infants, J. Biomed. Eng. **7**:9, 1985.

Widdowson, E.M.: Growth and composition of the fetus and newborn. In Assali, N.S., editor: biology of gestation II. The fetus and neonate, New York, 1968, Academy Press.

Widdowson, E.M., and McCance, R.A.: A review: new thoughts on growth, Pediatr. Res. **9**:154, 1975.

Widdowson, E.M., and Spray, C.M.: Chemical development in utero, Arch. Dis. Child. **26**:205, 1951.

Wu, P.Y., and Hodgman, J.E.: Insensible water loss in preterm infants: changes with postnatal development and non-ionizing radiant energy, Pediatrics **54**:704, 1974.

Ziegler, E.E., Biga, R.L., and Fomon, S.J.: Nutritional requirements of the premature infant. In Suskind, R.M., editor: Textbook of pediatric nutrition, New York, 1981, Raven Press, pp. 29-39.

Ziegler, E.E., and others: Body composition of the reference fetus, Growth **40**:329, 1976.

Nutritional strategies

American Academy of Pediatrics Committee on Nutrition: Commentary on breast feeding and infant formulas, including proposed standards for formulas. In Pediatric nutrition handbook, Evanston, Ill., 1979, American Academy of Pediatrics, pp. 119-138.

Anderson, G.H., and Bryan, M.H.: Is the premature infant's own mother's milk best? (editorial) J. Pediatr. Gastroenterol. **1**:157, 1982.

Askanazi, J., and others: Respiratory distress secondary to a high carbohydrate load: a case report, Surgery **87**:596, 1980.

Atkinson, S.A., Bryan, M.H., and Anderson, G.H.: Human milk: difference in nitrogen concentration in milk from mothers of term and premature infants, J. Pediatr. **93**:67, 1978.

Atkinson, S.A., and others: Macromineral content of milk obtained during early lactation from mothers of premature infants, Early Hum. Dev. **4**:5, 1980.

Battaglia, F., Meschia, M.J., and Appelbaum, P.: Peripheral intravenous catheters in premature infants: a controlled study, Pediatrics **70**:487, 1982.

Batton, D.G., Maisels, M.J., and Appelbaum, P.: Peripheral intravenous catheters in premature infants: a controlled study, Pediatrics **70**:487, 1982.

Bitman, J., and others: Comparison of the lipid composition of breast milk from mothers of term and preterm infants, Am. J. Clin. Nutr. **38**:300, 1983.

Black, D.D., and others: The effect of short term total parenteral nutrition on hepatic function in the human neonate. A prospective randomised study demonstrating alteration of hepatic canalicular function, J. Pediatr. **99**:445, 1981.

Brady, M.S., and others: Formulas and human milk for premature infants: a review and update, J. Am. Diet. Assoc. **81**:547, 1982.

Broviac, J.W., Cole, J.J., and Scribner, B.H.: A silicone rubber catheter for prolonged parenteral alimentation, Surg. Gynecol. Obstet. **136**:602, 1973.

Bryan, M.H., and others: Intralipid—its rational use in parenteral nutrition of the newborn, Pediatrics **58**:787, 1976.

Canadian Paediatric Society Nutrition Committee: Feeding the low birthweight infant, Can. Med. Assoc. J. **124**:1545, 1981.

Chance, G.W., and others: Postnatal growth of infants of less than 1.3 kg birth weight: effects of metabolic acidosis, calorie intake and of calcium, sodium and phosphate supplementation, J. Pediatr. **91**:787, 1977.

Chappell, J.E., and others: Fatty acid balance studies in premature infants fed human milk or formula: effect of calcium supplementation, J. Pediatr. **108**:439, 1986.

Chessex, P., and others: The quality of growth in premature infants fed own mother's milk, J. Pediatr. **102**:107, 1983.

Covelli, H., and others: Respiratory failure precipitated by high carbohydrate loads, Ann. Intern. Med. **95**:579, 1981.

David, L., and Anast, C.S.: Calcium metabolism in newborn infants: the interrelationship of parathyroid function and calcium, magnesium and phosphorus metabolism in normal, sick and hypocalcemic newborns, J. Clin. Invest. **54**:287, 1974.

David, L., and others: Serum immunoreactive calcitonin in low birthweight infants. Description of early changes: effect of intravenous calcium infusion; relationships with early changes in serum calcium, phosphorus, magnesium, parathyroid hormone and gastrin levels, Pediatr. Res. **15**:803, 1981.

Day, G.M., and others: Growth and mineral metabolism in very low birth weight infants: effects of calcium supplementation on growth and divalent cations, Pediatr. Res. **9**:568, 1975.

Dolcourt, J.L., and Bose, C.L.: Percutaneous insertion of Silastic central venous catheters in newborn infants, Pediatrics **70**:484, 1982.

Field, T., and others: Non-nutritive sucking during tube feedings, Pediatrics **70**:381, 1982.

Filler, R.M., and others: Serum intralipid levels in neonates during parenteral nutrition: the relation to gestational age, J. Pediatr. Surg. **15**:4, 1980.

Forget, P.P., Fernandes, J., and Haverkampbegman, P.: Utilisation of fat emulsion during total parenteral nutrition, Acta Paediatr. Scand. **64**:377, 1975.

Friedman, Z., and others: Rapid onset of essential fatty acid deficiency in the newborn, Pediatrics **58**:640, 1976.

Friedman, Z., and others: Effect of parenteral fat emulsion on the pulmonary and reticuloendothelial systems in the newborn infant, Pediatrics **61**:694, 1978.

Gaull, G.E., Wright, C.E., and Isaacs, C.E.: Significance of growth modulators in human milk, Pediatrics **142**(suppl.): 1985.

Greene, J.C., Hazlett, D., and Demarec, R.: Relationships between intralipid induced hyperlipemia and pulmonary function, Am. J. Clin. Nutr. **29**:127, 1976.

Gross, S.J., and others: Nutritional composition of milk produced by mothers delivering preterm, J. Pediatr. **96**:641, 1980.

Hambreus, L., Forsum, E., and Lonnerdal, B.: Nutritional aspects of breast milk versus cow's milk formula. In McFarlane, H., Hambreus, L., and Hanson, L.A., editors: Food and immunology: symposia of the Swedish Nutrition Foundation XIII, Stockholm, 1976, Almquist and Wiksell.

Hamosh, M., and others: Lipids in milk and the first steps in their digestion, Pediatrics **75**(suppl.):146, 1985.

Herve, P., and others: Hypercapnic acidosis induced by nutrition in mechanically ventilated patients: glucose versus fat, Crit. Care Med. **13**:537, 1985.

Holman, R.T.: Atherosclerosis—a pediatric nutrition problem, Am. J. Clin. Nutr. **9**:565, 1961.

Jensen, R.G., Clark, R.M., and Ferris, A.M.: Composition of the lipids in human milk: a review, Lipids **15**:345, 1980.

Kwitterovich, Jr., P.O.: Neonatal screening for hyperlipidaemia, Pediatrics **53**:455, 1974.

Lemons, J.A., and others: Considerations in feeding the very-low-birthweight infant, Perinatol. Neonatol. **6**:75, 1982.

Lucas, A., and others: A human milk formula, Early Hum. Dev. **4**:15, 1980.

Morgan, W.W., and Heillen, G.W.: Percutaneous introduction of long-term indwelling vascular catheters in infants, J. Pediatr. Surg. **7**:538, 1972.

Perlman, M., and others: Guidelines for neonatal treatment, ed. 3, Toronto, 1986, The Hospital for Sick Children.

Pitcher-Wilmott, R., Shutack, J.G., and Fox, W.W.: Decreased lung volume after nasogastric feeding of neonates recovering from respiratory disease, J. Pediatr. **95**:119, 1979.

Roy, R.N., and others: Impaired assimilation of nasojejunal feeds in very low birth weight infants, J. Pediatr. **70**:487, 1982.

Salle, B., Barrois-Larouze, V., and Charlas, J.: The future of milk banks in 1985, Perinatal Medicine, Proceedings of the fifteenth National Seminar, Paris, 1985, Librairie Arnette.

Salle, B., and others: Effects of calcium and phosphorus supplementation on calcium retention and fat absorption in preterm infants fed pooled human milk, J. Pediatr. Gastroenterol. Nutr. **6**:638, 1986.

Shennan, A.L., Bryan, M.H., and Angel, A.: The effect of gestational age on intralipid tolerance in newborn infants, J. Pediatr. **91**:134, 1977.

Shulman, R.J., and others: Comparison of percutaneous and surgical placement of central venous catheters in neonates, J. Pediatr. Surg. **21**:348, 1986.

Smigura, F.C., Bryan, M.H., and Angel, A.: Postheparin lipase activity in newborn infants. In Halm, P., Segal, S., and Israels, S., editors: The role of fat in intravenous feeding of the newborn, Dorval, P.Q., 1974, Pharmacia (Can.) Ltd., p. 129.

Van Aerde, J., and others: Effect of increasing glucose loads on respiratory gas exchange in the newborn infant, Pediatr. Res. **20**:420A, 1986.

Watkins, J.B.: Lipid digestion and absorption, Pediatrics **151**(suppl.): 1985.

Weinstein, M.R., and Oh, W.: Oxygen consumption in infants with BPD, J. Pediatr. **99**:958, 1981.

Widdowson, E.M.: Gastrointestinal development and neonatal nutrition. In Proceedings of the 72nd Ross Conference on Pediatric Research, Columbus, Ohio, 1977, Ross Laboratories.

Widdowson, E.M., Colombo, V.E., and Artravius, C.A.: Changes in the organs of pigs in response to feeding for the first 24 hours after birth. II. The digestive tract, Biol. Neonate **28**:272, 1976.

PART TWO

Provision of water and electrolytes

During delivery the infant is moved from the sea of the amniotic fluid to terrestrial life. The constant water loss in this new environment with its threat of dehydration necessitates the exogenous provision of water and electrolytes to replace those lost. This section is concerned with the physician's formulation of this provision.

VOLUME AND COMPOSITION OF BODY FLUIDS

At birth the percentage of body weight represented by water is approximately 75% in term infants and greater in those born prematurely (Fig. 25-5). The sharp decrease in this percentage over the first year of life is due to the accumulation of body fat, representing only 12% of body weight at birth in full-term infants but 30% by age 1 year. In addition, the relative distribution of water between the intracellular and extracellular spaces changes during this period. In an infant born at term the intracellular volume occupies 35% of body weight and the extracellular volume 40%. By age 3 months these volumes are equal, each occupying 35% of body weight. In contrast, in the older infant and child the intracellular volume represents 45% of body weight and the extracellular volume 20%.

The composition of body fluid varies with the compartment in which it is contained, the primary cation of extracellular fluid being sodium and that of intracellular fluid potassium. The vascular membrane and cell membrane separating the major body fluid subdivisions are freely permeable to water. Therefore, although the electrolyte composition varies, osmotic equilibrium is obtained between these compartments. The size of the compartments then depends primarily on the number of osmoles within, which in turn is dependent on the cellular pump for the intracellular space and on the kidney for the extracellular space. Within the extracellular space the relative distribution between the intravascular and interstitial compartments is dependent on the oncotic pressure exerted by plasma proteins, which favors expansion of vascular volume at the expense of interstitial volume, and the counteracting influence of capillary hydrostatic pressure. Osmolality of serum can be measured easily by freezing-point depression (normally 285 to 295 mOsm/L), and a close approximation can be obtained by doubling the serum sodium concentration. Approximation by this method is reasonable, since sodium and an equal number of anions are nearly the sole determinants of osmolality in extracellular fluid. The osmolality of interstitial and intracellular compartments can be inferred from plasma osmolality, since osmotic equilibrium is present.

Real or apparent alterations in plasma osmolality, as estimated from the serum sodium concentration, may occur in several situations. Electrolytes are dissolved in body water (except for small amounts bound to plasma proteins). As measured in the clinical laboratory, however, the concentrations are determined not just in water but in plasma or serum, consisting of water plus the volume occupied by protein. The apparent volume in which these substances are dissolved (plasma) is greater than the actual volume of plasma water. In 1 L of plasma there are only 940 ml water; the remainder consists of 60 gm of protein. Concentrations in plasma water thus exceed those in plasma by 1,000/940, or 1.06. Although these differences in sodium concentration related to plasma protein are of little clinical significance, the differences due to elevation of plasma *lipids* may be important. A marked hyponatremia may be present when sodium is measured on a lactescent sample but disappears when lipid is extracted and the sodium concentration is measured in plasma water. Such elevation of lipids are only rarely encountered in the neonatal period. Increased concentrations of glucose and urea are more often observed, however, and may lead to erroneous es-

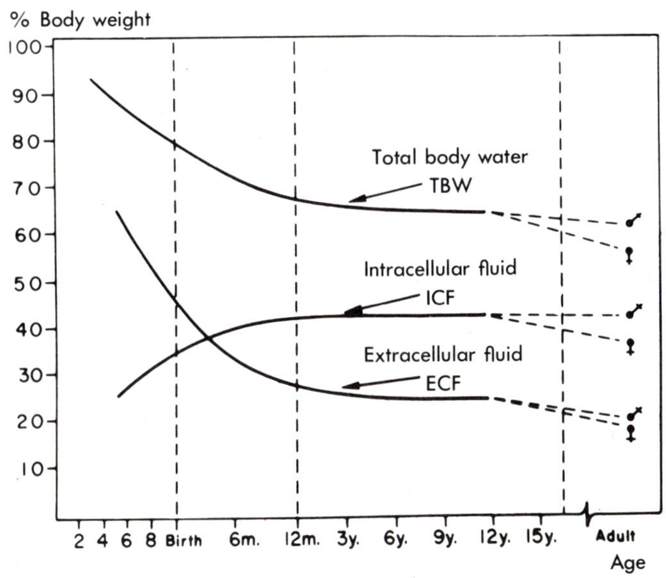

Fig. 25-5. Change with age in total body water and its major subdivisions. (Data from Friis-Hansen. From Winters, R.W., editor: The body fluids in pediatrics, Boston, 1973, Little, Brown & Co., p. 100.)

timation of osmolality if calculated only from serum sodium concentration.

The molecular weight of glucose is 180. At a plasma concentration of 90 mg/dl, glucose would contribute 5 mOsm/L of plasma. With marked elevation of plasma glucose levels, as in an infant of low birth weight given a parenteral infusion containing a high concentration of glucose, this substance may contribute 40 mOsm/L or more (representing plasma glucose levels of 800 mg/dl or greater). If a normal plasma osmolality were to be maintained in the presence of a plasma glucose concentration of 800 mg/dl, only 240 mOsm would be contributed by sodium and an equal number of anions, resulting in a serum sodium concentration of 120 mEq/L. The addition of glucose, which is osmotically active, to the extracellular fluid at a rate greater than maximal cellular metabolism of glucose causes water to move from the intracellular to the extracellular compartment to achieve osmotic equilibrium. The result is an expanded extracellular volume with increased osmolality and dilutional hyponatremia. This relationship has been quantified by Katz in an idealized fashion for the adult such that a decrease in serum sodium concentration of 1.6 mEq/L would be expected for each 100 mg/dl increase in serum glucose concentrataion over the baseline of 100 mg/dl. In the LBW infant the contraction of intracellular volume involves the potential danger of cerebral hemorrhage.

Urea readily diffuses across the cell membrane, and no osmotic gradient exists (except in acute elevations of serum urea levels). Each 28 mg of serum urea nitrogen (blood urea nitrogen) represents 1 mmol of urea. (Each millimole of urea contains two nitrogens with an atomic weight of 14 each.) A blood urea nitrogen concentration of 15 mg/dl is equivalent to 5.4 mmol of urea per liter. This would contribute only 5.4 mOsm to each liter of body water. However, an infant with acute renal failure may have a blood urea nitrogen concentration of 100 mg/dl, which would contribute 35.7 mOsm/L. If a normal plasma osmolality of 280 mOsm/L were maintained in this setting, serum sodium concentration must be 122 mEq/L, $\frac{280\text{-}36}{2}$.

DETERMINATION OF ADEQUATE FLUID AND ELECTROLYTE PROVISIONS

In the older infant and child the goal of parenteral fluid therapy is the maintenance of zero balance for water and electrolytes, assuming that there are no preexisting deficits or excesses. Over the short term the positive balances necessary for growth are neglected. In the neonate the volume of body fluids that is physiologically appropriate, and thus desirable to maintain, is not entirely clear. Some weight loss over the first few postnatal days has been called "physiologic." This decrease in weight is due largely to the loss of water and sodium from the extracellular space. A reasonable goal of fluid therapy during this period would be the prevention of dehydration, although not necessarily maintenance of zero balance for water and electrolytes. Weight loss should not be greater than 10% of birth weight (or 15% of birth weight for infants weighing less than 1,500 gm). Beyond the first 3 days of life therapy should be designed to maintain zero balance. Over the short term it is not necessary to provide sufficient calories for growth but only enough to retard catabolism. Oral or tube feedings should be instituted and progressed in volume as quickly as is feasible.

Zero balance for fluid and electrolytes occurs when the intake of these substances is exactly equal to the output from all sources. (Intake − output = 0.) The formulation of a reasonable plan for the intake of fluid and electrolytes thus requires the accurate determination of the output of these substances. Since fluid losses are related most closely to caloric expenditure, this is the most useful and most uniformly applicable frame of reference. During the neonatal period nongrowing infants (those receiving parenteral fluids only) expend about 75 Cal/kg/day. Over the first 2 days of life, however, metabolic rate is approximately 25% lower. The infant receiving oral feedings may expend 120 Cal/kg/day if intake is insufficient to allow growth. Those who are small for gestational age have higher metabolic rates than those with the same weight but appropriate for gestational age. Although calculation of fluid requirements based on caloric expenditure is more appropriate physiologically, it is recognized that computation of fluid administration based on body weight simplifies these calculations in a busy nursery. Since beyond the first 2 days of life the relationship between caloric expenditure and body weight is linear, this simplification is justifiable.

There are four normal sources of water loss: insensible loss, urine, sweat, and fecal water. *Insensible loss* is the loss of water through the lungs during respiration and through evaporation from skin. Of the total insensible loss, about 30% is pulmonary. An average insensible loss is 12 to 15 ml/kg/day during the first 2 days of life, increasing to 20 ml/kg/day by the third postnatal day for a term infant in an environment of moderate humidity (40% to 60%). In LBW infants, particularly those with weights less than 1,250 gm, insensible loss may be up to 300% higher than that predicted for term infants. The causes of this inverse relationship between insensible water loss and gestational age are several and include increased permeability of skin to water, greater surface area per unit of body weight, and a relative increase in the vascularity of skin in infants of lower birth weight. Transepidermal water loss in infants born at 25 weeks' gestation may be up to 15 times greater than that in term infants. This difference gradually narrows with postnatal age, but even at 4 weeks of age the loss is twice as great in the most premature infant as in the term baby.

Wide variations in *urine output* are possible because of the concentrating and diluting features of the kidney. The primary determinants of urine volume and osmolality in the neonatal period are water and solute intake and the presence or absence of growth. The minimum and maximum volume of urine is determined by the amount of solute for excretion and the maximal renal concentrating and diluting ability. The newborn is able to dilute urine maximally to osmolalities of 30 to 50 mOsm/L and to concentrate urine maximally to 700 to 800 mOsm/L (less than the 1,200 mOsm/L seen in children and adults). Thus, if 40 mOsm must be excreted per day and the maximal concentrating ability is 700 mOsm/L, the minimum volume of urine would be 57 ml; and the maximum volume, if the diluting capacity is 50 mOsm/L, would be 800 ml. The renal solute load in infants may vary from 10 to 30 mOsm/100 Cal metabolized; the lower values are characteristic of rapidly growing infants receiving breast milk or similar commercial formulas, and the higher values are for starved infants or those fed formulas with high protein and electrolyte content. A parenteral fluid regimen that is not electrolyte free should provide a solute load between these extremes. An average load for an infant on a parenteral fluid regimen containing glucose with no oral feeding would be 20 mOsm/100 Cal, approximately half from metabolism and half from added electrolyte. Using this range of values for solute excretion, one can calculate a water allowance for urine that will permit the excretion of this load within the middle range of urinary osmolalities, stressing neither the concentrating nor diluting capacities of the kidney. If 80 ml water are provided per 100 Cal (55 ml/kg), such urinary osmolalities should result (Table 25-15).

Sweat losses are generally negligible or nonexistent. LBW infants exhibit a limited or absent response to the stress of warmth; term infants, who are able to respond,

Table 25-15. Urinary osmolality at varying solute loads when 92 ml water/100 Cal is available for urine formation*

Renal solute load (mOsm/100 Cal)	Urinary osmolality (mOsm/L)
10	110
20	220
30	330

*92 ml water = 80 ml provided exogenously + 12 ml endogenously from water of oxidation. (At 70 Cal/kg = 56 ml/kg supplied exogenously.)

are generally in a temperature-controlled environment in the modern nursery. If sweating should occur term infants may increase evaporative loss threefold. *Fecal losses* are 0 to 10 ml/kg; infants on a parenteral feeding regimen alone have the lower values.

Based on a consideration of these losses, an average parenteral fluid plan for a term infant receiving no oral feeding should provide about 15 ml water/kg for insensible loss and 55 ml/kg for urine, resulting in a total volume of 70 ml/kg/day over the first 2 days of life. On day 3 the volume may be increased to 85 ml/kg/day and further increased to 100 to 125 ml/kg/day by the end of the first week. This volume is a first approximation and may need adjustment based on continuing clinical and laboratory evaluation and special modifying considerations discussed later.

Water allowances are calculated to avoid extremes of concentration or dilution, and electrolytes should be provided similarly to avoid maximal renal sodium reabsorption or excretion. Upper and lower levels of tolerance are not known. However, since babies historically have thrived on both human milk and cow's milk, it seems reasonable to provide an electrolyte intake somewhere between the two. Providing 2 mEq/kg each of sodium and potassium and 4 mEq/kg of chloride will accomplish this. Thus the electrolytes contained in the infusion (10 mOsm/100 Cal) plus endogenous solute from energy metabolism (10 mOsm/100 Cal) result in a calculated renal solute load of 20 mOsm/100 Cal. Potassium should be omitted during the first 24 hours.

VLBW infants may not be able to maintain zero sodium balance on this quantity of electrolyte because of increased renal excretion of sodium (decreased tubular reabsorption of sodium). These infants, particularly those weighing less than 1,250 gm, may sometimes require up to 6 mEq sodium/kg during the first 1 or 2 weeks of life to maintain zero or slightly negative balance during the period of "physiologic" weight loss, followed by decreasing requirement thereafter.

These calculations apply to a mature infant who is fairly inactive, is in a thermoneutral environment with a relative humidity of 40% to 60%, and has adequate renal function. Metabolic rate increases with activity, illness, or decrease in ambient temperature. Additional calories are expended if the infant is fed orally or is growing. Given this number of variables, it should be clear that repeated assessment of the adequacy of any parenteral therapy plan is essential. Accurate body weight should be determined as an index of hydration, daily or more frequently. Tissue turgor is often difficult to interpret, particularly in LBW infants with little subcutaneous fat, but nonetheless it should be examined. Edema should be sought in the pretibial, presacral, and facial areas as a sign of overhydration. Oral mucous membranes in a well-hydrated infant should be moist, as assessed by an examiner's clean finger. The measurement of urine and plasma osmolality or urine specific gravity is most valuable in judging hydration. In the absence of renal disease urinary osmolalities should be between 150 and 400 mOsm/L (specific gravity, 1.006 to 1.013). Plasma osmolality is estimated from the serum sodium concentration. Variations in serum sodium more often reflect changes in water balance than in sodium balance, and in the absence of very large sodium loads hypernatremia suggests an increased need for water. Modest hyponatremia is frequent in VLBW infants, but values under 130 mEq/L may reflect overhydration. The rate of excretion of sodium in urine (not sodium concentration) may be useful in distinguishing true sodium depletion from dilutional hyponatremia if the intake of sodium is known. Changes in the hematocrit value and in serum concentrations of urea and proteins are more dependent on variables other than hydration and therefore are of only ancillary value in assessing states of hydration.

MODIFIERS OF WATER AND ELECTROLYTE PROVISIONS

Since the quantitative recommendations mentioned above are predicated on a specific physiologic state, it is apparent that alterations in any of these physiologic components must change the parenteral fluid plan. Many factors influence insensible loss (Table 25-16). An *increase in insensible water loss* over the average values just discussed is encountered in infants of low birth weight. LBW infants, particularly those less than 1,250 gm, may have relatively enormous water requirements because of increased insensible loss. Average values compiled from several studies are given in Table 25-17. In such infants water allowances for the first day of life should be raised to 85 to 100 ml/kg and rapidly increased as necessary based on new clinical data to 140 ml/kg or more. Although the necessity for increasing parenteral fluid allowances in LBW infants to maintain water balance has been emphasized, it should also be stressed that overestimation of the rate of fluid administration in these infants may have undesirable consequences as well. The incidence of patent ductus arteriosus and necrotizing enterocolitis appears to be higher in premature infants receiving a high rate of fluid administration than in those receiving a volume 20 ml/kg/day less. Nonetheless, Lorenz and others found that considerable flexibility is possible in the rate of fluid administration in LBW infants. Whether receiving 80 or 140 ml/kg/day by day 5, there was no difference in the incidence of patent ductus arteriosus, intracranial hemorrhage, bronchopulmonary dysplasia, enterocolitis, duration of respiratory support, mortality, or duration of hospitalization. Suggested rates of fluid administration for different groups of LBW infants, based on the low-volume group in the study of Bell and others, are given in Table 25-18. *Phototherapy* increases both insensible water loss and stool water. The mechanism of the increased insensible loss is not known but is related most probably to elevated skin blood flow. The stool loss may be due to decreased gastrointestinal transit time secondary to photodecomposition products. An additional water increment of 10 to 20 ml/kg/day is a reasonable first approximation for infants undergoing phototherapy. The use of a *radiant warmer* will increase insensible loss. The magnitude of this increase depends on the type of warmer used, the maturity of the infant, and whether or not a heat shield is used. Allowances for insensible loss should be increased by 50% to 100% or more depending on feedback data. Elevated insensible loss is particularly marked in sick, very LBW infants under radiant warmers (Chapter 24, part two). *Elevation of ambient temperature* by 1° or 2° within the thermo-

Table 25-16. Factors modifying insensible water loss

	Direction of change in water loss (ml/kg)
Prematurity	↑
Activity	↑
High humidity	↓
Fever	↑
Radiant warmer	↑
Phototherapy	↑
Mechanical ventilation	↓

Table 25-17. Insensible water loss in preterm infants

Birth weight (gm)	ml/kg/day
>750-1,000	64
1,001-1,250	56
1,251-1,500	38
1,501-1,750	23
1,751-2,000	20
2,001-3,250	20

Table 25-18. Fluid requirement (ml/kg/day)

Birth weight (gm)	Days 1-2	Day 3	Days 15-30
>750-1,000	105	140	150
1,001-1,250	100	130	140
1,251-1,500	90	120	130
1,501-1,750	80	110	130
1,751-2,000	80	110	130

Modified from data of Bell, E.F., and others: Lancet **2**:90, 1979.

neutral zone will increase insensible water loss by about 50% (in infants weighing less than 1,250 gm by 70%). Elevation of ambient temperature outside this neutral zone will triple or quadruple the insensible loss.

Decreased insensible water loss occurs in infants on mechanical ventilation with highly humidified air or in those exposed to a high environmental humidity. Pulmonary loss of water is often zero in infants on respirators, and water allotment should be decreased by the 6 to 7 ml/kg/day normally lost through this route. The use of a plastic heat shield can reduce insensible loss by 25% in infants weighing less than 1,250 gm.

Alterations in water allotment for urine may be necessitated by obligatory increases or decreases in urine volume. An *increase in urine volume* may be due to defective concentrating ability or may result from an osmotic diuresis. Central diabetes insipidus is a potential but rare problem in neonates. Hydration is best maintained in these situations by measurement of urine volume and sodium and replacement of these losses in addition to 20 ml/kg provided for insensible loss. With marked polyuria extreme changes in hydration can occur rapidly. Careful and frequent monitoring of body weight and serum sodium concentration (every 8 to 12 hours) is therefore important.

An obligatory *decrease in urine volume* occurs with *renal failure;* in the neonatal period this is most often secondary to hypoxia or septic shock. The maintenance of zero balance for water in this situation requires replacement of the output from insensible loss (20 ml/kg) as 10% glucose in water. Since there is an endogenous input of water from oxidation, this allowance for net insensible loss may be too high. Urine volume, if any, can be replaced if one desires to maintain the present state of hydration. If there is preexisting expansion of extracellular volume, it may be preferable to allow a negative balance by not replacing urine volume until a normal state of hydration is achieved. Potassium should not be administered and sodium should be given only if there is sodium loss in urine and no expansion of extracellular volume. In states of *low cardiac output* often associated with congenital heart disease in the neonatal period, there may be an obligatory decrease in urine output, necessitating the same modification in fluid administration as for renal failure. In heart failure the urine has a moderately high specific gravity and osmolality and a low concentration of sodium (less than 20 mEq/L). This is due to increased proximal tubular reabsorption of sodium and water and to the action of elevated aldosterone and antidiuretic hormone. There may be other clinical situations with an *elevated level of antidiuretic hormone* and therefore an obligatory decrease in urine output. This situation is suggested by a low urine flow rate with osmolarity greater than 100 mOsm/L in the presence of hyponatremia. There is often an elevated urinary concentration of sodium caused by the presence of volume expansion. One must be certain that these findings are not due to decreased renal tubular reabsorption of sodium from prematurity or to the presence of adrenal insufficiency. It appears that such inappropriate secretion of antidiuretic hormone can occur after birth asphyxia, in some infants with severe pulmonary disease, and in those with intracranial disease.

Increased loss of stool water occurs in diarrhea. The best gauge of diarrheal losses is change in body weight. In general, these losses are isotonic and should be replaced with isotonic saline plus an additional 2 mEq of potassium per kilogram of body weight.

Ongoing losses from chest tubes and fistulas must not be overlooked. Even though losses may be small in daily volume, cumulative losses by these routes may cause serious dehydration and electrolyte imbalance. Drainage from chest tubes should be measured, and sodium and potassium content should be determined and then replaced by water and the appropriate electrolytes. Fistulous losses may be determined by weighing overlying bandages.

CONCLUSIONS

The most common error in fluid and electrolyte therapy is the failure to continually reevaluate clinical and laboratory data as a basis for quantitative alterations in the original plan. The specific recommendations given above are estimates, and their appropriateness for a given infant must be reassessed frequently during therapy. Since these infusions do not provide sufficient calories for growth, enteral feedings should be instituted as soon as possible.

Martin A. Nash

BIBLIOGRAPHY

Baumgart, S.: Radiant energy and insensible water loss in the premature newborn infant nursed under a radiant warmer, Clin. Perinatol. **9**:483, 1982.

Bell, E.F., and others: High volume fluid intake predisposes premature infants to necrotising enterocolitis (letter to editor), Lancet **2**:90, 1979.

Bell, E.F., and others: Effect of fluid administration on the development of symptomatic patent ductus arteriosus and congestive heart failure in premature infants, N. Engl. J. Med. **302**:598, 1980.

Bell, E.F., and others: The effects of thermal environment on heat balance and insensible water loss in low-birth-weight infants, J. Pediatr. **96**:452, 1980.

Doyle, L.W., and others: Insensible water loss in newborn infants, Clin. Perinatol. **9**:453, 1982.

Engelke, S.C., and others: Sodium balance in very low-birth-weight infants, J. Pediatr. **93**:837, 1978.

Fanaroff, A.A., and others: Insensible water loss in low birth weight infants, Pediatrics **50**:236, 1972.

Friis-Hansen, B.: Body water compartments in children: changes during growth and related changes in body composition, Pediatrics **28**:169, 1961.

Hey, E.N., and others: Evaporative water loss in the newborn baby, J. Physiol. **200**:605, 1969.

Katz, M.A.: Hyperglycemia-induced hyponatremia—calculation of expected serum sodium depression, N. Engl. J. Med. **289**:843, 1973.

Lorenz, J.M., and others: Water balance in very low-birth-weight infants: relationship to water and sodium intake and effect on outcome, J. Pediatr. **101**:423, 1982.

Okken, A., and others: Insensible water loss and metabolic rate in low birth weight newborn infants, Pediatr. Res. **13**:1072, 1979.

Rees, L., and others: Hyponatremia in the first week of life in preterm infants. Part I. arginine vasopressin secretion, Arch. Dis. Child. **59**:414, 1984.

Sedin, G., and others: Measurement of transepidermal water loss in newborn infants, Clin. Perinatol. **12**:79, 1985.

Sulyok, E., and others: On the mechanism of renal sodium handling in newborn infants, Biol. Neonate **37**:75, 1980.

Wu, P.Y.K., and Hodgman, J.E.: Insensible water loss in preterm infants: changes with postnatal development and non-ionizing radiant energy, Pediatrics **54**:704, 1974.

PART THREE

Acid-base physiology and disorders in the neonate

As in the adult the hydrogen ion concentration in the extracellular fluid of the newborn is strictly maintained within a narrow range of concentration. Growth and development, and even survival, are critically dependent on this homeostasis. Under basal conditions the pH of the blood ranges from 7.35 to 7.43, corresponding to a hydrogen ion concentration range of 44.7 to 37.2 nmol/L. The newborn, especially when premature and potentially ill, is subject to multiple stresses that may threaten this tight control. Immaturity may limit the homeostatic response of the neonate to these stresses. A careful understanding of the control systems involved and, in particular, of the maturation of these systems is a valuable aid in understanding acid-base balance in the newborn.

MAINTENANCE OF ACID-BASE BALANCE

It is convenient to consider the maintenance of the hydrogen ion concentration in terms of (1) compensatory mechanisms that respond rapidly to acute change and (2) systems that chronically maintain the overall balance between acid-base production and intake and between metabolism and excretion.

Acute compensation: body buffer systems

The effects of acute addition of either acid or base to the body are initially minimized through the actions of cellular and extracellular buffers. Bicarbonate, phosphates, and plasma proteins are the major extracellular buffers, whereas proteins such as hemoglobin, organic phosphates, and bone apatite are the major cellular buffers. To gain access to these cellular buffers, H^+ crosses the cell membrane via Na^+/H^+, K^+/H^+, or HCO_3^-/Cl^- exchange. Acute acidosis may therefore result in hyperkalemia, whereas alkalosis can significantly lower extracellular potassium. Intracellular buffering accounts for about 47% of an acute acid load and can reach even higher levels given continued acidosis. Much of this buffering capacity is in bone, and chronic acidosis results in increased bone resorption and loss of bone sodium, potassium, calcium, and carbonate. These effects on bone partially explain the invariable association of growth failure with acidosis, a factor of major importance in the neonate.

The major extracellular buffer system is the carbonic acid–bicarbonate pair. The buffer equation is:

$$H^+ + HCO_3^{-1} \Leftarrow\Rightarrow H_2CO_3 \Leftarrow\Rightarrow H_2O + CO_2\Uparrow$$

The efficiency of the carbonic acid–bicarbonate buffer is markedly improved by the respiratory system. In the presence of the enzyme carbonic anhydrase, H_2CO_3 is in equilibrium with CO_2 in plasma. Thus excretion or retention of CO_2 by the lung greatly increases the capacity of the bicarbonate system to buffer either acid or base. Addition or increased production of acid results in consumption of HCO_3^- and increased H_2CO_3 and CO_2. Stimulation of respiration by the acidosis leads to decreased CO_2 concentration and thereby blunts the fall in pH. This respiratory compensation occurs over 12 to 24 hours and is most likely due to central nervous system chemoreceptors sensitive to pH. Similar respiratory compensation occurs in most cases in response to alkali, with increased HCO_3^- concentration resulting in hypoventilation and accumulation of CO_2. The relationship of pH, P_{CO_2}, and HCO_3^- is expressed by the Henderson-Hasselbalch equation:

$$pH = 6.1 + \log \frac{[HCO_3^-]}{0.03 \times P_{CO_2}}$$

where 6.1 is the pK_a of the carbonic acid/bicarbonate buffer. It is important to note that although respiratory compensation minimizes changes, pH is not completely normalized. In acidosis, for each 1 mEq/L decrease in HCO_3^-, P_{CO_2} decreases by 1.25 mm Hg, limiting the decrease in pH to 0.012 units; with alkalosis a 1 mEq/L increase in HCO_3^- results in an increase of 0.2 to 0.9 mm Hg in P_{CO_2}, limiting the pH change to 0.003 to 0.008 units.

Chronic maintenance of acid-base balance

Chronic maintenance of acid-base balance depends on the balance between acid production and intake and between metabolism and excretion. Although a small amount of preformed acid may be ingested with foodstuffs, the majority of the daily acid load is a product of metabolism. A large proportion consists of CO_2, which is carried to the lung as bicarbonate and carbamino

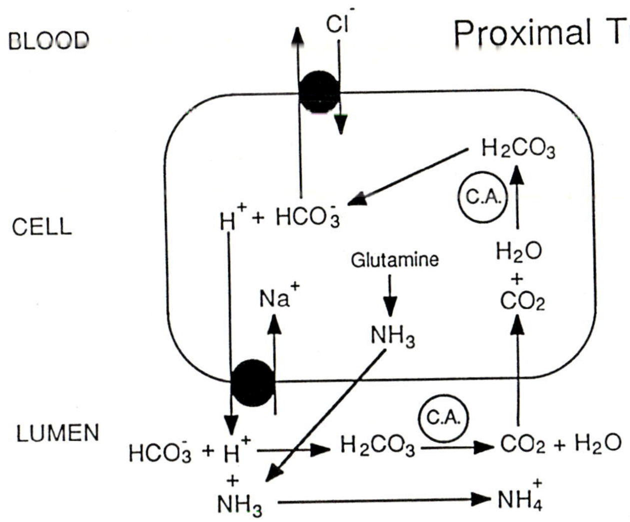

Fig. 25-6. Schematic drawing of proximal tubular HCO_3^- reabsorption and ammonia generation. See text for explanation.

groups bound to hemoglobin and is ultimately excreted through respiration. Abnormalities of respiration, either hypo- or hyperventilation, lead to either retention or increased excretion of CO_2, resulting in acidosis or alkalosis. In addition to CO_2 approximately 1 mEq/kg/day of *nonvolatile* acid is produced as a by-product of metabolism. Most of this consists of sulfuric acid, which results from the metabolism of the sulfur-containing amino acids methionine and cysteine. The remainder consists primarily of incompletely oxidized organic acids, with a small contribution from phosphoric acid and hydrochloric acid. Successful maintenance of acid-base balance depends on renal excretion of this nonvolatile acid.

The role of the kidney in acid-base balance is threefold:

1. Excretion of the daily production of nonvolatile acid
2. Reabsorption of the total amount of filtered HCO_3^-
3. Compensation for changes in P_{CO_2} as a result of respiratory aberrations by increases or decreases in HCO_3^- excretion, thereby minimizing changes in pH

All these are dependent on urinary acidification, which can be considered on an anatomic basis. From 60% to 85% of the filtered bicarbonate is reabsorbed in the proximal tubule. This reabsorption is dependent on Na^+ reabsorption and occurs through the action of a Na^+/H^+ exchange mechanism in the luminal membrane of the proximal tubular cells. The mechanism is schematically depicted in Fig. 25-6. As shown, excreted H^+ titrates filtered HCO_3^-, producing H_2CO_3, which is then dehydrated rapidly to CO_2 through the actions of carbonic anhydrase in the cellular brush border. CO_2 crosses into the cell, where HCO_3^- is regenerated and reabsorbed across the basal cell membrane, probably in exchange for Cl^-. By the end of the proximal convoluted tubule the pH of the tubular fluid has been reduced to 6.7. A second function of the proximal tubule is production of ammonia by deamination of glutamine. This NH_3 is secreted into the lumen, where it is "trapped" as NH_4^+ because of the decreased pH.

The loop of Henle and the distal tubule play little role in urinary acidification. HCO_3^- is concentrated in the loop via water extraction, thereby increasing the pH of the tubular fluid to 7.39. At this pH, NH_4^+ loses its proton and, as NH_3 crosses into the interstitium, where it is available to the medullary collecting duct.

The remainder of urinary acidification occurs in the cortical and medullary collecting tubule and is sufficient to titrate the residual HCO_3^- and filtered buffer anions, such as sulfate, thereby producing *titratable acid*. A schematic of the pathways involved is shown in Fig. 25-7. The primary mechanism is electrogenic secretion of H^+. This occurs against an increasing pH gradient, with minimal urinary pH values of 4.5 to 5. Ammonia is also taken up from the medullary interstitium and secreted, where it is again trapped as NH_4^+. This is important, as at minimal urinary pH some anions such as Cl^- and $SO_4^=$ will not be protonated. Urinary NH_4^+ is excreted with these anions, thereby preventing loss of cations such as Na^+, Ca^{++}, and K^+. Distal nephron H^+ secretion is controlled by several factors, among them luminal and peritubular pH and distal salt delivery. Aldosterone also stimulates proton secretion, both directly and through its actions on sodium and potassium.

Total acid excretion by the kidney then can be measured in the urine as:

$$\text{Titratable acid (TA)} + NH_4^+ - HCO_3^-$$

and, during steady state, will equal the production of acid from diet and metabolism. In addition to this basal

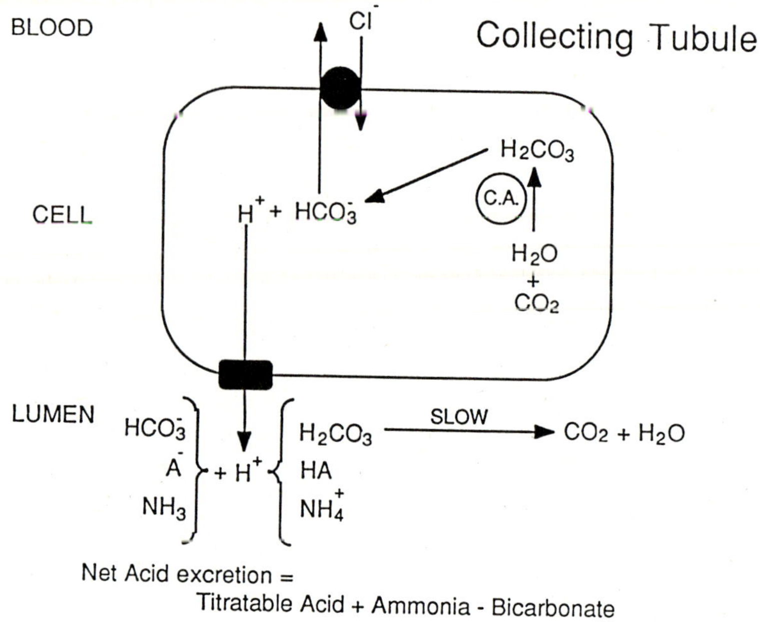

Fig. 25-7. Schematic drawing of distal methods of urinary acidification, with definition of net acid excretion. See text for explanation.

control, in response to respiratory changes in P_{CO_2} the kidney has the capacity to alter HCO_3^- reabsorption, affecting blood HCO_3^- and minimizing changes in pH. After an acute rise in P_{CO_2}, HCO_3^- increases 0.1 mEq/L for each 1 mm Hg rise in P_{CO_2} as a result of buffering of H_2CO_3 by HCO_3^-. Similarly, with a 1 mm Hg decrease in P_{CO_2} there is an acute decrease in HCO_3^- of 0.25 mEq/L owing to buffering. Renal compensation then occurs slowly over the next few days through changes in HCO_3^- reabsorption. In acidosis or alkalosis HCO_3^- increases or decreases a total of 0.5 mEq/L for each 1 mm Hg change in P_{CO_2}, limiting the change in pH to about 0.0025 units. As with respiratory compensation for metabolic changes, compensation does not fully correct pH.

DEVELOPMENTAL ASPECTS OF ACID-BASE PHYSIOLOGY

Immaturity of the kidney in the neonate, and particularly the preterm neonate, affects both the basal acid-base status and the response to additional acid and alkali loads. The fetal kidney is fully formed by 34 weeks' gestation; however, maturation and functional changes continue over the first year of life.

The blood HCO_3^- concentration in the neonate is typically lower than in the adult, ranging from 18 to 21 mEq/L, owing to a decrease in the proximal tubular T_m, or tubular maximum for reabsorption of HCO_3^-. The cause of this decrease is uncertain. Carbonic anhydrase activity is normal, as is the intrinsic reabsorptive capacity of the proximal tubule in neonates. With maturation over the first years of life, the length of the proximal tubule increases by approximately twentyfold; thus a smaller surface area for reabsorption might be one explanation. In addition, proximal tubular H^+ secretion is closely linked to Na^+ reabsorption. Volume expansion and diminished Na^+ reabsorption are the norm in neonates. This may contribute to diminished proximal tubular H^+ secretion. In support, volume contraction has been shown to raise the T_m of HCO_3^- in neonatal puppies. The blood pH of the neonate is only marginally decreased, as an increased respiratory rate in the infant results in a decreased P_{CO_2}, in the range of 34 torr, thereby partially compensating for the low HCO_3^-.

Distal acidification is also immature, especially in preterm infants. At birth the minimal urine pH is 6, in contrast to 4.5 to 5 in adults. Ammonia production and excretion are diminished in preterm infants, as is the amount of titratable acid. Although there is some evidence of decreased glutaminase activity in neonates, diet also may play an important role. Ammonia production was increased in infants fed cow's milk, in comparison to a group of breast-fed infants. This appears to be due to increased availability of substrate for ammonia production. Similarly, titratable anions are primarily diet derived and are increased in infants on cow's milk because of higher phosphate and protein levels.

In summary, both HCO_3^- conservation and net acid excretion are diminished in neonates owing to immaturity of the kidney. This is particularly true of premature infants, especially before 34 weeks' gestation, owing to

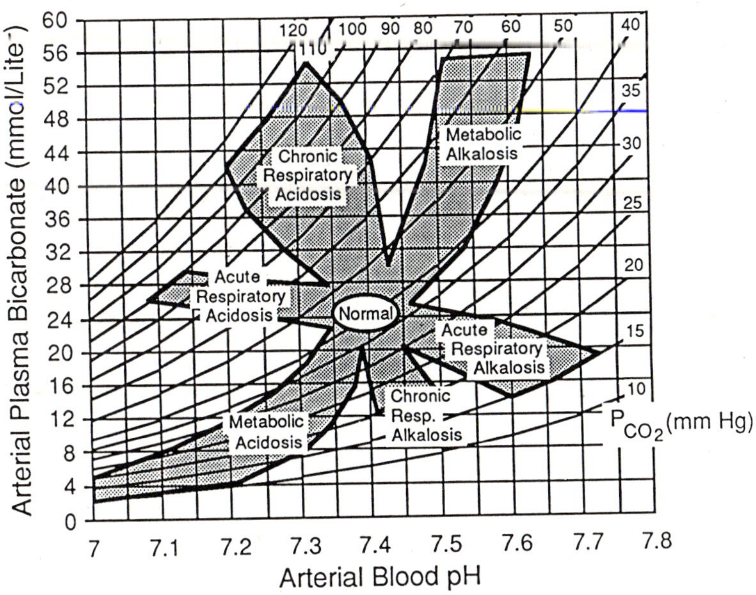

Fig. 25-8. Acid-base map showing 95% confidence limits for compensatory responses. (From Cogan, M.G., and Rector, Jr., F.C.: Acid-base disorders. In Brenner, B.M., and Rector, Jr., F.C.: The kidney, Philadelphia, 1986, W.B. Saunders, p. 473.)

Table 25-19. Acid-base parameters in neonates and adults (mean ± SD)

	Preterm	Term	Adult
pH	7.40 ± 0.08	7.40 ± 0.06	7.40 ± 0.03
P_{CO_2}	34.0 ± 9.0	33.5 ± 3.6	39.0 ± 2.6
Total CO_2	21.0 ± 2.0	21.0 ± 1.8	25.2 ± 2.8

Data from Chan, J.C.M.: Acid-base disorders and the kidney, Adv. Pediatr. **30:**401, 1983.

incomplete nephronogenesis. These limitations not only are responsible for decreased basal blood HCO_3^- but also limit the ability of the neonate to respond to additional stresses, particularly acid loading. Table 25-19 summarizes normal acid-base parameters in the newborn, in comparison to the adult.

DIAGNOSTIC APPROACH TO DISORDER OF ACID-BASE BALANCE

Disorders of acid-base balance can result from altered respiration, leading to abnormal retention or excretion of CO_2, or from metabolic causes, that is, either increased production or excretion of nonvolatile acid or base. Simple acid-base disorders consist of respiratory acidosis and alkalosis, with primary changes in P_{CO_2} and secondary changes in HCO_3^- affected by renal compensation, and metabolic acidosis and alkalosis, with primary changes in HCO_3^- and secondary respiratory changes in P_{CO_2}. In addition, respiratory and metabolic disorders can coexist, producing combined disorders. Many nomograms, similar to that shown in Fig. 25-8, have been developed to aid in diagnosis of these disorders. In general, these describe the 95% confidence limits of the expected compensatory response to a primary abnormality in either P_{CO_2} or HCO_3^-. A combined disorder can be readily detected when the compensatory change in either P_{CO_2} or HCO_3^- falls beyond these limits. A diagnosis can also be made by use of values for the expected compensatory response presented in Table 25-20. For example, consider a newborn with pH of 7.17, P_{CO_2} of 34 mm Hg, and HCO_3^- of 12 mEq/L. This is clearly an acidosis with a metabolic component, as demonstrated by the low HCO_3^-. If a normal neonate can be expected to have an HCO_3^- of ≈22, this represents a decrease in HCO_3^- of 10 mEq/L. Normal respiratory compensation should result in a decrease in P_{CO_2} of 12.5 mm Hg (i.e., to ≈21.5). This patient then has a respiratory acidosis superimposed on a metabolic acidosis; that is, the P_{CO_2} is elevated above the expected value. Compensation, either renal or respiratory, is the norm. Absence of compensation either is due to temporal factors, as in acute respiratory acidosis preceding the development of significant renal compensation, or is due to a superimposed disorder. In most cases the cause is apparent from the history, and most combined acid-base disorders can be readily evaluated with these principles.

BASIC PRINCIPLES OF THERAPY

Metabolic acidosis

Metabolic acidosis is a common problem, particularly in the critically ill neonate, and can result from either

Table 25-20. Expected compensation in acid-base disorders

Respiratory	ΔPco_2		ΔHCO_3^-
Acute acidosis	1 mm Hg ↑	→	↑ 0.1 mEq/L
Acute alkalosis	1 mm Hg ↓	→	↓ 0.25 mEq/L
Chronic acidosis	1 mm Hg ↑	→	↑ 0.5 mEq/L
Chronic alkalosis	1 mm Hg ↓	→	↓ 0.5 mEq/L
Metabolic	ΔHCO_3^-		ΔPco_2
Acidosis	1.0 mEq/L ↓	→	↓ 1.25 mm Hg
Alkalosis	1.0 mEq/L ↑	→	↑ 0.2-0.9 mm Hg

Table 25-21. Common causes of metabolic acidosis

Increased anion gap	Normal anion gap
Lactic acidosis: hypoxemia, shock, sepsis	Bicarbonate loss: acute diarrhea, ileal drainage
Renal failure	Renal tubular acidosis: distal and proximal
Ketoacidosis, organic acidosis: inborn errors of metabolism	Hypoaldosteronism
	Administration of acid i.e., arginine Cl, HCl, etc.
	Increased acid production: hyperalimentation, high-protein formula, ?late metabolic acidosis of prematurity

acid production greater than excretion, as in lactic acidosis caused by hypoxia, or increased loss of base. Loss of base can occur either renally or extrarenally as, for example, from the gastrointestinal tract with acute diarrhea. Common causes of metabolic acidosis in the neonate are listed in Table 25-21. A useful distinction can be made based on the presence of an increased anion gap. Acidoses that result from the addition, increased production, or retention of strong acid, as in lactic acidosis, or the acidosis of severe renal failure will be characterized by an increased anion gap owing to the unmeasured acidic anions. In contrast, acidoses resulting from bicarbonate loss, such as renal tubular acidosis, are characterized by a normal anion gap and elevated chloride. Therapy depends of course on the cause but will include administraton of alkali and correction of the underlying abnormality, if possible. The most common form of alkali used is sodium bicarbonate; when used intravenously in large doses, however, it can cause hypernatremia and hyperosmolality and may contribute to the incidence of intraventricular hemorrhage. In general, bicarbonate should be used at a concentration of 0.5 mEq/ml. A reasonable starting dose in an acidotic neonate is 1 to 2 mEq given slowly as a bolus over 30 minutes. Persistent acidoses can be treated with a continuous drip of 0.25 to 1 mEq/kg/hr. Progress of therapy should of course be monitored closely, with frequent electrolyte and blood gas measurements. Although attempts have been made to gauge therapy according to "base deficit," this is often difficult owing to uncertainty with respect to the distribution volume of administered bicarbonate.

Other forms of alkali may be of use in certain situations. Tris(hydroxymethyl)aminoethane (THAM) has been used and offers the advantages of no sodium load, direct lowering of Pco_2, and rapid cellular penetration. Negative factors, however, are 50% less base activity mole for mole compared to bicarbonate, the potential for respiratory depression after THAM infusion, and a possible effect of increasing the oxygen affinity of hemoglobin.

With severe acidosis, and particularly in situations where alkali administration is limited because of volume constraints such as renal failure, dialysis may be of benefit. Peritoneal dialysis provides base in the form of lactate, which forms bicarbonate when metabolized. In the presence of liver failure or impaired aerobic metabolism, as in severe hypoxia, lactate conversion is limited, and peritoneal dialysis may actually worsen the acidosis. Dialysis may, however, be effective in managing volume status and can allow additional administration of alkali. New techniques such as continuous arteriovenous hemofiltration may also be effective in controlling volume in appropriate patients and can allow administration of adequate amounts of alkali.

Metabolic alkalosis

Metabolic alkalosis results from loss of body acid, as in pernicious vomiting, from ingestion of base, and from increased renal acid excretion. The kidney usually is very effective in excreting excess alkali; however, two situations tend to interfere with this excretion and maintain an alkalosis:

1. Volume contraction and potassium deficiency combine to directly stimulate H^+ loss by increased reabsorption of Na^+ proximally and indirectly by stimulation of renin and aldosterone. In these patients the alkalosis responds to saline administration and potassium repletion.
2. Increased mineralocorticoid production directly stimulates distal H^+ secretion. This is most commonly seen in association with hypertension in primary hyperaldosteronism. In a normotensive individual this may indicate a rare cause, such as Bartter's syndrome.

Common causes of metabolic alkalosis in the neonate are listed in Table 25-22.

Therapy, especially in contraction alkalosis, consists of correction of the underlying disorder and repletion of volume and potassium. In disorders characterized by autonomous mineralocorticoid production, administration of volume is ineffective, and therapy must be directed toward removal of the source of increased hor-

Table 25-22. Common causes of metabolic alkalosis

Acid loss: vomiting, nasogastric suction
Diuretics
Chloride deficiency: chronic chloride-losing diarrhea, Bartter's syndrome, low-chloride formula
Administration of alkali: bicarbonate, lactate, acetate, citrate

mone. In rare situations acute correction of severe alkalosis may require administration of acid. This is most commonly done with arginine hydrochloride, which liberates hydrochloric acid in the body, with ammonium chloride, or with dilute hydrochloric acid. These agents must be used cautiously to prevent acidosis. A possible starting dosage is 2 mEq/kg given slowly over 6 to 12 hours, with careful attention to acid-base status.

Respiratory acidosis and alkalosis

Respiratory acidosis results from any disorder with decreased alveolar ventilation resulting in retention of CO_2. In the neonate this most commonly results from either the neonatal respiratory distress syndrome, meconium aspiration syndrome, congenital diaphragmatic hernia, or pulmonary infections. In general, therapy should be directed toward correction of the underlying disorder. For example, in respiratory distress syndrome diminished alveolar ventilation and retention of CO_2 may well require assisted ventilation. Some authors have advocated use of alkali acutely. This is generally a temporizing measure and should not be used in place of assisted ventilation. Additionally, alkali administration may increase P_{CO_2} and may be detrimental. Respiratory alkalosis is rare in the neonate (except when iatrogenically produced via assisted ventilation) but may occur as a result of central hyperventilation. In general, the alkalosis is not severe and does not require specific therapy. (See Chapter 28.)

BRIEF CONSIDERATION OF SPECIFIC DISORDERS

Renal tubular acidosis (RTA)

See also Chapter 35.

These disorders are a common cause of normal anion gap metabolic acidosis and result from deficient renal tubular H^+ secretion or HCO_3^- reabsorption. Several types have been described based on the involved region of the renal tubule. Type II, or proximal RTA, is a result of decreased proximal tubular HCO_3^- reabsorption. As 60% to 85% of the filtered HCO_3^- is reabsorbed in the proximal tubule, this results in large losses of HCO_3^- Distal urinary acidification is normal, and at the low plasma HCO_3^- levels that result from this HCO_3^- wastage, the patient will excrete a normally acid urine (i.e., ≤ 5.3). An increase in plasma HCO_3^- after alkali is administered results in an increase in filtered HCO_3^- beyond the capacity of the proximal tubule, HCO_3^- wastage, and an alkaline urine (i.e., > 7.6). Proximal RTA often presents in combination with Fanconi's syndrome and is associated with several recessive disorders, including cystinosis, Lowe's syndrome, tyrosinosis, and others. These children often present at age 1 to 2 years with failure to thrive. Treatment consists of alkali supplementation and can result in normal growth, although large quantities of alkali may be required owing to massive HCO_3^- wastage. As previously discussed, a mild proximal RTA is the norm in neonates because of immaturity of proximal tubular HCO_3^- reabsorption, with maintenance of plasma HCO_3^- in the range of 17 to 21 mEq/L. Over the first year of life the T_m for HCO_3^- increases to adult levels as the proximal tubule elongates and matures. Delayed maturation has been reported in some infants, resulting in a persistent proximal RTA.

Type I RTA, or distal RTA (classic RTA), results from diminished distal H^+ secretion and is less common in neonates. It may be inherited as an autosomal dominant trait. Patients with distal RTA are unable to fully acidify their urine and commonly have urinary pH >6.2. Failure to thrive is again the most common presentation in infants; the child may also have severe hypokalemia. Therapy consists of alkali; in this case the dose of alkali is governed by the endogenous acid production, which averages 3 mEq/kg/day.

Type IV RTA, or hyperkalemic RTA, is due to abnormalities in aldosterone production or to altered tubular sensitivity to aldosterone. Five subtypes have been described. Of these, subtypes 1, 4, and 5 may occur in infants. Subtype 1, seen in Addison's disease and congenital adrenal hyperplasia, is caused by deficiency of aldosterone, resulting in salt wasting, increased plasma renin activity, decreased urinary aldosterone, acidosis, and hyperkalemia. In subtype 4, or pseudohypoaldosteronism, urinary aldosterone is increased, but the tubule is insensitive to its effects. Thus symptoms are similar to those of subtype 1 and include salt wasting, acidosis, and hyperkalemia. This subtype is very rare. The most common type IV RTA in infants is subtype 5, or "early childhood" RTA. In this case the tubule is insensitive to the effects of aldosterone on potassium and H^+ secretion, although salt reabsorption is normal. Therapy for subtype 1 of course consists of mineralocorticoid supplementation, while subtypes 4 and 5 respond to alkali supplementation. The need for such supplementation seems to diminish by age 5 years, possibly as a result of further maturation of the kidney.

Type III RTA was originally described in infants (1972) as a distal defect in combination with marked HCO_3^- wastage. Rather than a separate disorder, this represents a variant of type I RTA seen in infants, with transient HCO_3^- wastage owing to immaturity of the proximal tubule.

Late metabolic acidosis of prematurity

In 1964 Kildeberg first used the term *late metabolic acidosis of prematurity* to describe a group of otherwise healthy premature infants between 1 and 3 weeks of age characterized by mild to moderate acidosis (base excess of −7 to −24.8 mEq/L) and decreased growth. All infants were receiving cow's milk formula that provided between 3 to 4 gm protein/kg body weight/day. Interestingly, net acid excretion in these infants was increased compared to that in a normal control group, leading to the conclusion that the excessive protein content of the cow's milk formula resulted in endogenous acid production beyond the excretory capacity of the premature kidney. More recently, the existence of late metabolic acidosis as a separate acid-base disorder has been questioned. As previously noted, basal plasma bicarbonate in the neonate is low compared to that in the adult (Table 25-18) as a result of diminished proximal tubular bicarbonate reabsorption. Many of the cases previously classified as late metabolic acidosis clearly fall within 2 standard deviations of the norm. In addition, other authors have been unable to demonstrate a separate group of otherwise normal, LBW infants with acidosis and poor growth. Over the last several years the recurrence of interest in breast-feeding and the development of special premature formulas have limited the use of high-protein formula in premature infants. This probably accounts for the disappearance of *late metabolic acidosis* as a separate entity.

Hypochloremic alkalosis

About 1980 a number of articles were published describing a severe hypochloremic metabolic alkalosis with failure to thrive in infants receiving most of their nutrition from a soybean formula deficient in chloride (Neo-Mull-Soy; Syntex Laboratories). In some of the cases renal tubular function was studied, revealing normal distal reabsorption of sodium and chloride. Urinary chloride was absent, confirming the ability of the infants to conserve chloride and establishing dietary chloride deficiency as the cause of the metabolic alkalosis. Metabolic alkalosis also occurs with increased loss of chloride. Examples include intractable vomiting, as in pyloric stenosis; increased loss through the skin, as in cystic fibrosis; and increased renal loss, as with diuretic therapy. Hypochloremic alkalosis also occurs in Bartter's syndrome. Infants with this syndrome generally present with failure to thrive. In addition to the alkalosis, hypokalemia, hyperreninemia, and increased urinary prostaglandins are hallmarks. Despite the high renin levels the children are normotensive and do not exhibit a pressor response to angiotensin II, probably owing to the increased levels of vasodilatory prostaglandins. Although many theories have been proposed to explain the primary defect in Bartter's syndrome, in at least some of the cases it appears to be the result of increased urinary chloride loss caused by a distal reabsorptive defect. Interestingly, infants with alkalosis resulting from chloride-deficient formula closely resemble those with Bartter's syndrome, and some of these cases were initially misdiagnosed as Bartter's, lending further support to chloride deficiency as a likely cause. Therapy for Bartter's is aimed toward correcting the hypokalemia and consists primarily of indomethacin, which by inhibition of prostaglandin production also decreases renin and aldosterone production. In many cases this is insufficient to correct the potassium, and potassium supplements must be added. There is no specific therapy to correct the abnormalities in chloride reabsorption.

Eileen K. Stork
John E. Stork

BIBLIOGRAPHY

Bartter, F.C., and others: Hyperplasia of the juxtaglomerular complex with hyperaldosteronism and hypokalemic alkalosis: a new syndrome, Am. J.Med. **33**:811, 1962.

Baum, J.D., and Robertson, N.R.C.: Immediate effects of alkaline infusion in infants with respiratory distress syndrome, J. Pediatr. **87**:255, 1975.

Chan, J.C.M.: Acid-base disorders and the kidney, Adv. Pediatr. **30**:401, 1983.

Chan, J.C.M.: Renal tubular acidosis, J. Pediatr. **102**:327, 1983.

Corbet, A.J., and others: Controlled trial of bicarbonate therapy in high-risk premature newborn infants, J. Pediatr. **91**:771, 1977.

Ekblad, H., Kero, P., and Takala, J.: Slow sodium acetate infusion in the correction of metabolic acidosis in premature infants, Am. J. Dis. Child. **139**:708, 1985.

Garin, E.H., Geary, D., and Richard, G.A.: Soybean formula (Neo-Mull-Soy) metabolic alkalosis in infancy, J. Pediatr. **95**:985, 1979.

Gill, Jr., J.R.: The role of chloride transport in the thick ascending limb in the pathogenesis of Bartter's syndrome, Klin. Wochenschr. **60**:1212, 1982.

Gill, J.R., and Bartter, F.C.: Evidence for a prostaglandin independent defect in chloride reabsorption in the loop of Henle as a proximal cause of Bartter's syndrome, Am. J. Med. **65**:766, 1978.

Greenberg, F., Cordero, J.F., and Erickson, J.D.: Withdrawal of two soy-based infant formulae (letter), Lancet **1**:462, 1979.

Grossman, H., and others: The dietary chloride deficiency syndrome, Pediatrics **66**:366, 1980.

Kildeberg, P.: Disturbances of hydrogen ion balance occurring in premature infants. II. Late metabolic acidosis, Acta Paediatr. Scand. **53**:517, 1964.

Kildeberg, P., Engel, K., and Winters, R.W.: Balance of net acid in growing infants, Acta Paediatr. Scand. **58**:321, 1969.

Kildeberg, P., and Winters, R.W.: Balance of net acid: concept, measurement and applications, Adv. Pediatr. **25**:349, 1978.

Linshaw, M.A., and others: Hypochloremic alkalosis in infants associated with soy protein formula, J. Pediatr. **96**:635, 1980.

McSherry, E.: Renal tubular acidosis in childhood, Kidney Int. **20**:799, 1981.

Nash, M.A., and Russo, J.C.: Neonatal lactic acidosis and renal failure: the role of peritoneal dialysis, J. Pediatr. **91**:101, 1977.

Reznik, V.M., Griswold, W.R., and Mendoza, S.A.: Neo-Mull-Soy alkalosis: a model of Bartter's syndrome? Pediatrics **66**:784, 1980.

Schwartz, G.J., and others: Late metabolic acidosis: a reassessment of the definition, J. Pediatr. **95**:102, 1979.

CHAPTER 26

The sensorimotor development of the preterm infant

He who sees things from their beginnings will have the finest view of them.

Aristotle

The progressive decrease in neonatal and infant mortality during the latter half of this century has been accompanied by a surge of interest in the behavioral capabilities of the newborn infant. Until the late 1950s the human neonate was considered to be immature and disorganized and to function mainly at a brainstem level. Neurobehavioral assessment of the neonate thus was based mainly on evaluation of muscle tone and primitive reflexes. More recent studies have recognized the full-term newborn at birth to be a very responsive and reactive being with remarkable sensory development and an ability for self-organization and social interaction. The major breakthrough came with the descriptions by both Wolff and Prechtl of the behavioral states of arousal in the newborn, leading to an understanding that physiologic and neurosensory responses may vary according to the infant's state of awakeness or sleep. Of equal importance was the documentation by Fantz of the newborn's ability to fixate and visually differentiate between patterns. Additional research has documented the neonate's ability to respond selectively to sound, to mimic, to move in rhythm to the human voice, and to exhibit visual and auditory habituation. Brazelton and later Dubowitz combined many of these measures to develop a neurobehavioral method for evaluation of the newborn, which has become very useful clinically to both evaluate and demonstrate newborn behaviors.

The improved outcomes for preterm infants have led to an extension of neonatal behavioral research to this less mature population of infants.

This chapter reviews the current knowledge of preterm neurobehavioral development, including state organization, visual and auditory responsiveness, sucking, and the development of active and passive muscle tone. The development of the full-term infant is referred to as a basis for describing preterm behavior.

Historically there has always been a fascination with the "tiny infant." Early reports of preterm behavior are difficult to evaluate, since gestational age seldom was noted. Also very few tiny infants survived prior to the 1960s so that most behavioral descriptions were of infants born weighing more than 1,500 gm. Gesell and, later, Saint-Anne Dargassies were the first to consider gestational age in their classical naturalistic observations of preterm infants. Gesell used the appropriate term *fetal infant* for infants born in the fetal period.

The earliest descriptions of spontaneous movement and reflex responses in previable infants were by Humphrey and Hooker in 1930, who filmed fetal aborti placed in saline after birth and documented a central nervous system already functional at 7 weeks' gestation. Fetal monitoring and real-time ultrasonography more recently have provided a totally new dimension to the observations of fetal sensorimotor maturation under normal physiologic conditions in utero. Since technical advances and improvements in perinatal care have extended the period of potential viability to some weeks before the previously defined limit of 28 weeks' gestation, both fetal and preterm behaviors are reviewed. Gestational age is defined as the age from the first day of the mother's last menstrual period until birth, and postmenstrual age is the sum of gestational and postnatal ages.

STATES OF AROUSAL

The sleep and awake states of arousal influence every physiologic and neurosensory function and must be considered in both the assessment and clinical care of the neonate.

The full-term infant

The observation by Aserinsky and Kleitman in 1953 of a relationship between rapid eye movement (REM) sleep and dreaming led to an explosion of research into the ontogenic development of the human awake-sleep cycles. Wolff introduced the concept of "state of arousal" and designed the first descriptive rating scale for the full-term infant. A state is defined as a clustering of recognizable physiologic and behavioral variables that repeat themselves.

Description and definition of states

Wolff noted that the infant has six organized patterns of behavior: two sleep states (quiet and active sleep), drowsiness, and three awake states (quiet awakeness, active awakeness, and crying).

In quiet sleep the infant is at full rest, respiration is very regular, and body movements are absent except for occasional startles or fine mouth movements. The eyelids are closed, and no eye movements are seen under the lids. In active sleep there is body activity ranging from gentle limb movements to an occasional stirring of the body, arms, and legs. Spontaneous erections occur in boys. Respiration is irregular, and facial grimaces are frequent, including smiling, frowning, mouthing, or bursts of sucking. The eyelids are closed, and occasionally rolling or rapid eye movements can be seen through the closed eye lids. The term *rapid eye movement*, or *REM sleep* originated from these movements in active sleep.

In drowsiness, which usually occurs while waking or falling asleep, the baby may be still or moving, and smiles, frowns, or mouthing sometimes can be seen. The eyes have a dull glazed appearance and usually do not fixate, the lids are droopy, and just before closing, the eyes may roll upward. In the quiet awake state the infant is fully alert but relatively inactive. The eyes are wide open with a bright shiny appearance (Fig. 26-1). The quiet awake state is considered to be qualitatively similar to conscious attention in the adult. In this state the infant is able to fixate and focus on visual objects, to orient to sound, and to respond to social cues such as a voice, a face, cuddling, and holding. During the active awake state there is frequent motor activity of the arms, legs, trunk, and head. The eyes are open and moving, and there may be vocalization. During crying there is vigorous motor activity with the eyes open or tightly closed.

Prechtl's definitions of the various states are similar to those of Wolff; however, he thought that the behaviors constituting a state should be present for at least 3 minutes. In addition, he omitted the drowsy state, regarding it as a transition between states, and defined only five states.

Although the states seem like a continuous spectrum ranging from quiet sleep to active awakeness, they are qualitatively highly specific with a distinct type of internal organization and brain center control. These states constitute the basic rest-activity cycles of sleep and wakefulness. They are relatively stable, and with the exception of short transitional periods repeat in regular cycles during the day and night. The central nervous system control of the various states originates at different levels of the reticular-activating system. Quiet sleep requires complex cortical integration and control and is regarded as the more mature sleep state. Active sleep is considered to be an ontogenically primitive sleep state in which dreaming occurs. Awakeness, like quiet sleep, is regulated by higher cortical centers.

The states can be described either clinically or by continuous polygraph recordings of various combinations of respiration, heart rate, eye movements, brain electrical activity, and muscle tone. These recordings provide objective quantitative information on sleep and awake states (Table 26-1). A sleep profile thus can be constructed according to the percentage of time spent in each state, the degree of organization of these states, the cycling regularity, and the number of transitions between states.

Temporal distribution of state

During the first week of life the full-term infant spends only 8% to 16% of the day in a state of quiet awakeness. The rest of the time is spent mainly in quiet or active sleep. A sleep cycle that includes a period of quiet and active sleep is 60 minutes long in full-term infants (range, 50 to 70 minutes), compared with 90 minutes in the adult. At full-term, active sleep constitutes 50% of the sleep cycle, and awakening usually follows active sleep, in contrast to adults, who waken from quiet sleep or drowsiness. Periods of awakeness usually occur at 4-hour intervals around feeding times. With increasing age there are longer periods of awakeness during the day with sleep throughout the night. The relative amount of quiet sleep also increases, so that by adulthood active sleep constitutes only 20% of total sleep, whereas the rest is quiet sleep (Fig. 26-2).

The state cycles are disrupted immediately after birth so that the infant stays awake longer with periods of quiet alertness alternating with activity. This results in increased alertness during the first 24 hours after birth. This is at the expense of active sleep, whereas the proportion of quiet sleep remains unchanged. By the fifth day the state cycles have stabilized.

Importance of state

Practically every physiologic body function and behavior in the newborn is dependent on state. For example, heart rate, blood pressure, and oxygen consumption are lower and transcutaneous PO_2 higher in quiet sleep.

Many external or environmental changes have a modifying effect on state. The kinesthetic and vestibular effects of picking up a crying baby, soothing him, and placing him up to the shoulder can induce increased quiet awakeness and attention, as can an interesting face

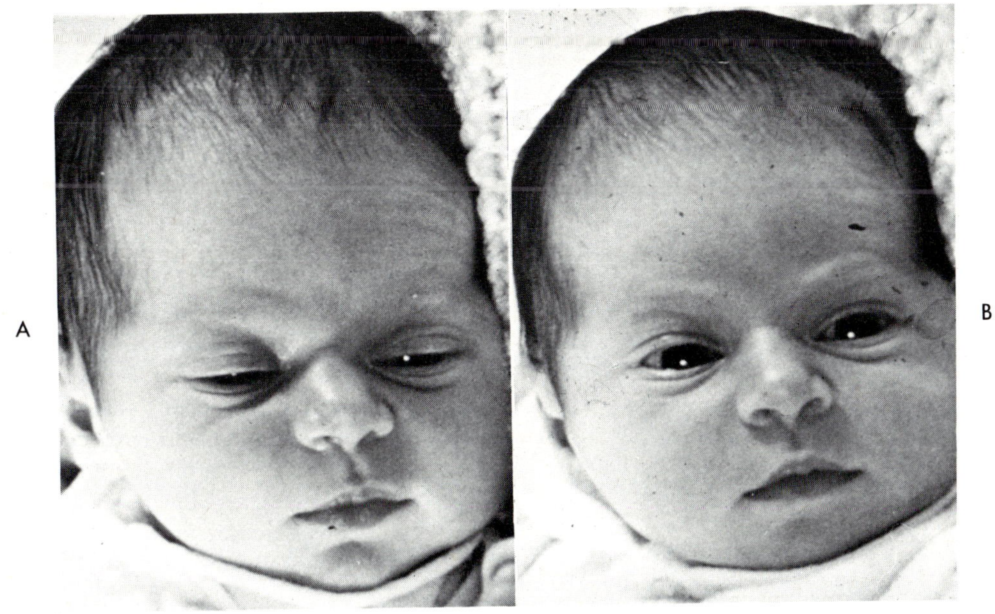

Fig. 26-1. Term infant in the drowsy **(A)** and quiet awake **(B)** states of alertness. (From The Amazing Newborn, Case Western Reserve University. [Film.])

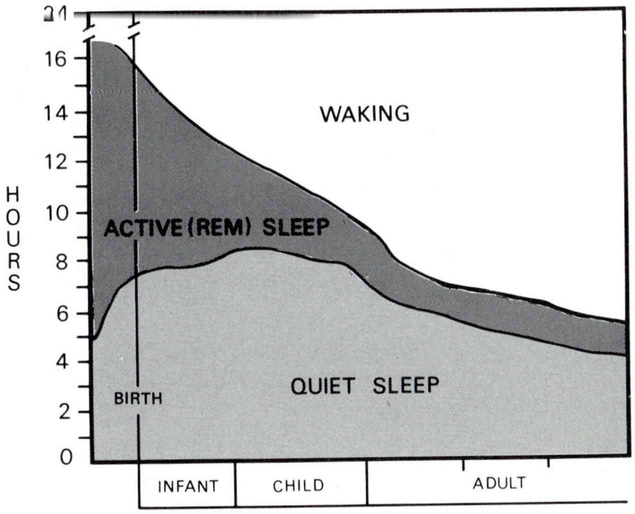

Fig. 26-2. Development of sleep and waking from infancy to adulthood. (Adapted from Roffwarg, H.P.: Science **152:**604, 1966. Copyright 1966 by the American Association for the Advancement of Science.)

Table 26-1. Polygraph documentation of states

	Quiet sleep	Active sleep	Awakeness
Heart rate	Regular, slower	Irregular, faster	Irregular
Respiration	Regular, slower	Irregular, faster	Irregular
Electromyogram activity	Present (tonic)	Absent (tonic)	Present
Eye movements (electrooculogram)	Absent	Frequent	Scanning or rapid
Electroencephalogram	Discontinuous, episodic activity	Low voltage, arrhythmic	Low voltage, slow waves

Table 26-2. Effects of state on intensity of responses to sensory stimulation

	Quiet sleep	Active sleep	Quiet awake
Proprioceptive reflexes			
Knee jerk	+ + +	±	+ +
Biceps jerk	+ + +	±	+ +
Ankle clonus	+ + +	–	–
Moro	+ + +	–	+ +
Exteroceptive reflexes			
Tactile			
Rooting	–	–	+ +
Palmar grasp	–	+	+ +
Plantar grasp	–	+	+ +
Nociceptive			
Babinski	+ +	+ + +	+ + +
Abdominal	+ +	+ + +	+ + +
Inguinal	+ + +	+ + +	+ + +
Visual attention	–	–	+ + +
Auditory (hearing)	±	+ +	+ + +

Modified from Prechtl, H.F.R.: In Clemente, C.D., and Purpura, D., editors: Sleep and the maturing nervous system, New York, 1972, Acadmic Press, Inc.

or change of tone of voice. State also can be affected by internal needs such as hunger or stooling and by various pathologic conditions including asphyxia, perinatal complications, and drugs given to the mother before birth.

The modifying effect of state on the various reflex responses is shown in Table 26-2. The following outline describes other important links between state, physiologic function, and the environment.

A. The influence of state on physiologic functions
   1. Heart rate: regular in quiet sleep; irregular and faster in active sleep and awake states (Chapter 21)
   2. Respiration: regular in quiet sleep; irregular and faster in active sleep and awake states; apnea and periodic breathing occur mainly in active sleep (Chapter 28)
   3. Oxygen consumption: lowest in quiet sleep; higher in crying
   4. Transcutaneous Po_2: lower in active sleep than in quiet sleep
   5. Blood pressure: lowest in quiet sleep; greater variability in active sleep; higher in awake activity and crying
   6. Cerebral blood flow: higher in active (REM) sleep than in nonREM sleep
   7. Endocrine: cortisol secretion increases with increasing arousal
   8. Neurophysiologic function
      a. Visual fixation: optimal in quiet awakeness; less in drowsiness and active awakeness
      b. Habituation: state changes act as dishabituating stimuli
         (1) Heart rate response to auditory stimulation: masked by state changes
         (2) Blink reflex to light: only in quiet sleep
      c. Conditioning: masked by state changes
B. Effects of environmental factors and external stimuli on state
   1. Touch
      a. Soothing and swaddling: reduces activity during active awakeness and crying
      b. Handling (rubbing, stroking, maternal holding, etc.): induces awakeness and activity
      c. Pain and tickling: increases awakeness and activity; inactive infants most sensitive to pain
   2. Visual (pictures, objects, or faces): induces quiet awakeness in drowsy, active, or crying infants; quiet awake state prolonged by interesting visual stimuli
   3. Light
      a. Light: active sleep reduced; quiet sleep increased; reduces level of activity in fussy or crying babies
      b. Darkness: increases level of activity; shift from quiet sleep to active sleep
   4. Auditory (sound)
      a. Variations in sound: increases activity
      b. Rhythmic sound (e.g., heartbeat): reduces activity; more sleep, less crying
      c. Continuous sound: reduces activity in crying and fussy babies; less active sleep and more quiet sleep
   5. Vestibular (proprioceptive—putting to shoulder and rocking in upright position): induces quiet awakeness in sleeping, active awake, fussy, and crying babies
   6. Temperature
      a. Decrease: increases motor activity; decreases quiet sleep
      b. Increase: reduces activity (induces apnea?)
   7. Sucking (pacifier or finger in mouth): induces quiet awakeness in active awake and crying infants; inhibits head movements and peripheral vision
   8. Stress
      a. Circumcision: increases fussy crying; shorter latency to sleep; increases quiet sleep
      b. Laboratory conditions: decreases alertness during awake states; more drowsiness, fussiness, and crying
      c. Repeated awakening: longer awakeness; more sleep after the deprivation period
   9. Body position: increased crying and active sleep in supine position; increased quiet sleep and higher Po_2 in prone position

C. Influence of internal physiologic needs on state
   1. Hunger: increases activity, active awakeness, and crying
   2. Satiety: quietens, increases sleep
   3. Full bladder: more erections in active sleep
   4. Need to stool: waking activity

D. Effects of pathologic conditions on state
   1. Coma: complete absence of state cycles and definable sleep
   2. Asphyxia: poor sleep cycle organization; decrease in active sleep; increase in quiet sleep
   3. Drugs
      a. Meperidine (Demerol) and barbiturates: decrease in awakeness, visual alertness, and active (REM) sleep spontaneous behavior
      b. Diazepam and barbiturates: increase in a state that looks like quiet sleep; active sleep decreases
      c. Heroin: quiet sleep reduced; sleep cycles longer
   4. Jaundice: decrease in quiet awake periods; increase in sleep cycle duration and active sleep; decreased alertness: poorer visual and auditory orientation
   5. Maternal diabetes: increases in active sleep
   6. Toxemia causing intrauterine growth retardation: poor organization of sleep states; disorganized quiet sleep with irregular respirations
   7. Malformation of brain
      a. Hydrocephalus and microcephaly syndromes: increases amounts of awakeness with less sleep; poor or absent sleep organization
      b. Down's syndrome: increase in awakeness; decrease in active sleep
   8. Biochemical disturbances (hypocalcemia, hypoglycemia, hypernatremia): hyperirritability or decreased awakeness

Fetal rest-activity cycles and behavioral states

Until real-time ultrasonography was developed there was doubt about whether true states of behavior existed in utero. Sterman, by recording fetal movements, had documented a periodicity to fetal activity from as early as 21 weeks' gestation. He described two motility cycles: a shorter cycle of 30 to 50 minutes' duration, which seemed to be intrinsic to the fetus, and a longer cycle of 80 to 110 minutes, which was related to the maternal sleep cycle. Dierker described similar activity cycles by monitoring fetal movements, heart rate, respiration, and EEG activity. He noted that these cycles occurred less frequently and were of longer duration with increasing gestation. By 1982, Nijhuis and Prechtl could observe fetal body and eye movements using real-time ultrasonographic imaging. By combining these observations with fetal heart rate monitor patterns they were able to document, for the first time, true behavioral states of 3 minutes' duration at 38 to 40 weeks' gestation. These fetal states are numbered 1F to 4F (quiet sleep, active sleep, awakeness, and active awakeness). They are less well organized prior to 36 weeks' gestation and difficult to classify as true states.

The preterm infant

Description and definitions

In the very young preterm infant, sleep and wakefulness or even periods of activity and inactivity are extremely difficult to classify. Nonetheless in 1945 Gesell and Amatruda gave a marvelous description of the observable behaviors associated with developing sleep and wakefulness in maturing preterm infants. Although Gesell documented many naturalistic behaviors, he made little attempt to quantify them. More recently Parmelee and also Emde classified multiple behavioral variations of state that can be used to describe the preterm infant, although many of the states, or clusters of behaviors, are so transient that they do not meet Prechtl's requirement of 3-minutes' duration to call them true states.

The development of the sleep states

To describe the many physiologic and behavioral components of the developing sleep states, both Dreyfus-Brisac and Parmelee used polygraphic recordings of electrophysiologic measures in addition to behavioral observations. For these studies sleep was defined as whenever the infant's eyes were closed without crying or gross body activity. Dreyfus-Brisac described an atypical type of sleep between 24 and 27 weeks' postmenstrual age. At this time there are constant small body movements, a fairly regular heart and respiratory rate, and very few REMs, and the EEG shows a discontinuous type of activity. With increasing gestational age there is increasing inhibition of these behaviors. Brief quiet periods without body movement appear at between 28 and 30 weeks gestation. By 32 weeks 53% of sleep time is spent without motion, and this increases to 60% by term. The near absence of REMs at 24 to 27 weeks is followed by infrequent sparse eye movements at 28 to 30 weeks. These increase and appear in clusters by 32 weeks' gestation and then decrease again by term. Birnholz has recently confirmed this description of the ontogeny of eye-movement patterns by ultrasonic visualization of eye movements in utero. Respiration, which is initially mainly irregular, becomes increasingly regular by term. The discontinuous EEG seen at 24 weeks gradually differentiates into patterns characteristic of active and quiet sleep from about 32 weeks.

Parmelee defined three types of sleep in preterm infants: quiet, active, and transitional sleep (Fig. 26-3). Using these definitions, Parmelee found a gradual increase in quiet sleep with a decrease in transitional and

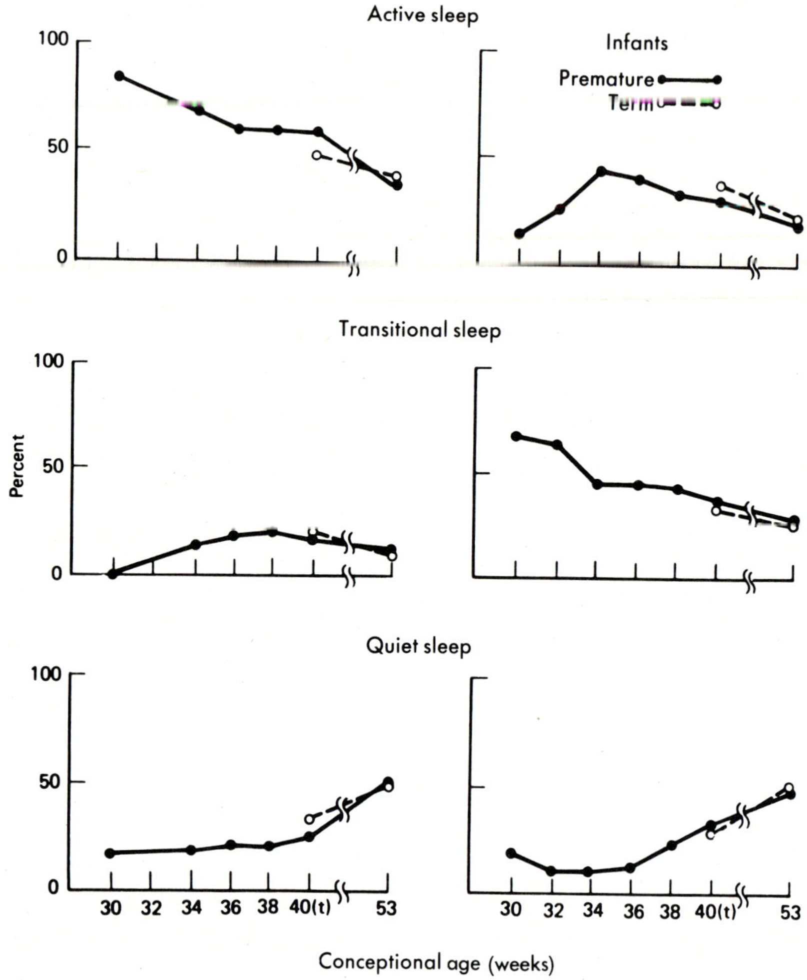

Fig. 26-3. Percentage of sleep states at each gestational age using two methods of state classification. (From Parmelee, A.H.: Dev. Med. Child Neurol. **9:**70, 1967.)

REM sleep with age. When the behaviors were classified into only quiet or active sleep, Parmelee found that most of the sleep time was spent in active sleep at 30 weeks. Thereafter there was a gradual increase in quiet sleep and a decrease in active sleep.

A primitive cycling of the sleep states appears at about 32 weeks' gestation; however, the respective periods for each state are shorter than at term. A cycle that includes active and quiet sleep is 40 minutes long at 36 weeks (range, 36 to 50 minutes) in comparison to 60 minutes at term. Most researchers report a fairly good correlation of all the behavioral parameters of active sleep by 34 to 36 weeks and of quiet sleep by 36 to 38 weeks.

There has been speculation about the reason for the increased amount of REM activity in immature infants. Roffwarg postulated that REM sleep provides a source of endogenous stimulation needed for central nervous system growth. This is supported by the fact that cerebral circulation and brain temperature are increased in active sleep. Active sleep is also accompanied by growth and increased protein synthesis in the brain.

The development of preterm awakeness

The development of awakeness has been far more difficult to classify than that of sleep. This is in part because of the short periods the infant spends with eyes open, and also because clinically and polygraphically it is often difficult to decide whether an immature infant with eyes open is awake or in active sleep. Awakeness, especially in the preterm infant, is best defined by behavioral observation because polygraphically many of the measures such as heart rate and respiration are similar in active sleep, as pointed out earlier. Also the EEG of the awake state can only be differentiated from that of active sleep by 36 weeks' gestation.

Saint-Anne Dargasies described "waking" with short

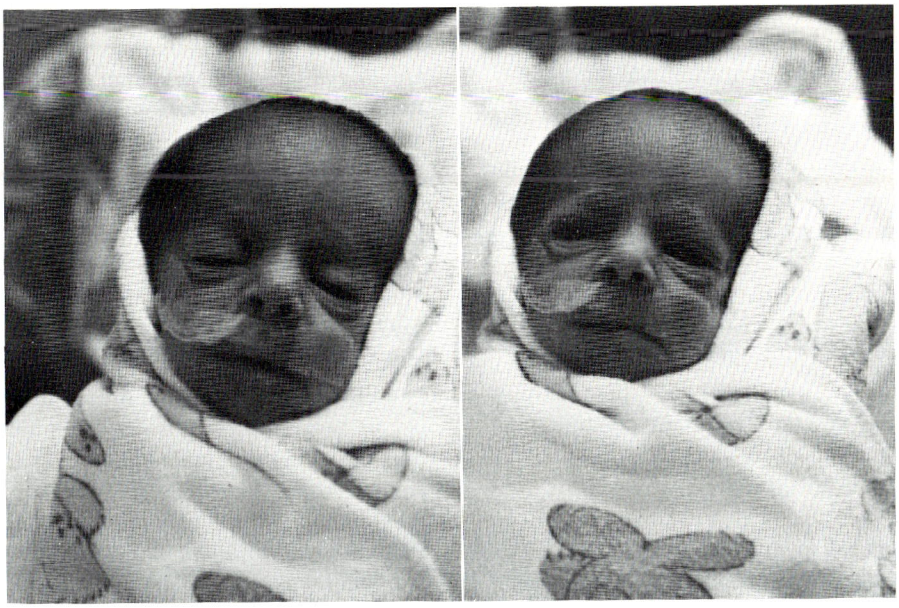

Fig. 26-4. Preterm infant (34 weeks postmenstrual age) in drowsy **(A)** and quiet awake **(B)** states of alertness. (From Hack, M.: Pediatrics **68:**87, 1981. Copyright American Academy of Pediatrics 1981.)

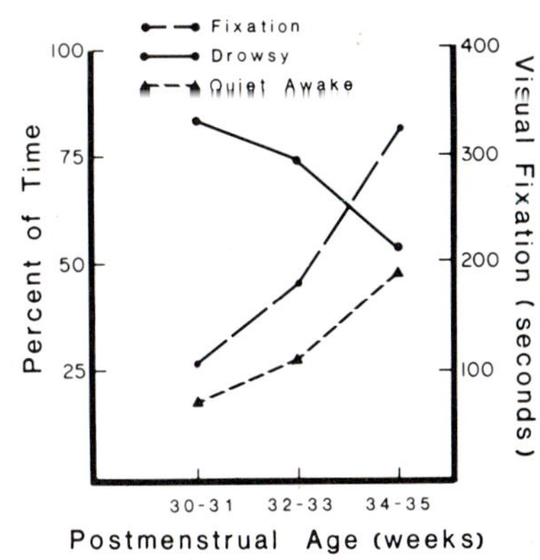

Fig. 26-5. Percent of time spent quiet awake or drowsy and mean total fixation time in preterm infants from 30 to 35 weeks postmenstrual age. (From Hack, M.: Pediatrics **68:**87, 1981. Copyright American Academy of Pediatrics 1981.)

eye-open periods from 30 weeks' postmenstrual age. By 32 weeks these periods occur spontaneously and are of longer duration. To define and describe the gradual progression of developing awakeness from 30 to 36 weeks, Hack used a rating of facial behaviors while the infant fixated on a black and white pattern. The less mature infants demonstrated mostly drowsiness, whereas quiet awakeness increased with age (Figs. 26-4 and 26-5). Uncoordinated and rolling eye movements and mouthing activity were observed in both quiet awakeness and drowsiness. These are rarely seen in awake term infants and probably indicate the lability and poor organization of awakeness in the preterm infant. It is interesting to note that the gradual increase in the ability to sustain quiet awakeness with the concomitant decrease in drowsiness parallels the relative increase in quiet sleep and decrease in active sleep during the same age period described by Parmelee (Fig. 26-3). The progressive organization of awake state control also coincided with an increase in visual attention and alertness. These developmental changes are probably dependent on the rapidly increasing complexity of dendritic interactions occurring at all levels of the maturing central nervous system at this time. They also may indicate increasing control of arousal at the reticular activating center and at higher cortical levels.

Although both the awake and sleep states reach a level of maturity close to that of the term infant by 36 to 37 weeks, there remain differences between infants born at term and preterm infants who have reached term after many weeks of extrauterine life. These include less organization and stability of the various parameters of state, less regular respiration, and also subtle EEG differences.

Modifying effects on preterm state

There is little information as to the effects of external and internal stimuli on the developing states of the preterm infant. It is known, however, that:

1. Preterm infants have more quiet sleep when they are cared for in a neutral thermal environment than in a cooler environment.
2. Infants older than 29 weeks' postmenstrual age have more awake periods when touched by their parents.
3. Preterm infants placed in the prone position have more quiet sleep, less active sleep, and higher Po_2 levels than infants in the supine position.
4. Kinesthetic and auditory stimulation provided by rocking incubators and recordings of heart beats induce quiet sleep and decrease active sleep and awakeness.
5. Stress associated with severe respiratory distress causes less quiet sleep and more active sleep in infants with respiratory distress syndrome (RDS) than in control infants without RDS. After recovery, these differences disappear.
6. Painful conditions such as necrotizing enterocolitis may result in open-eye periods with a vacant type of awake staring.
7. Preterm infants of 35 to 36 weeks' gestation are more likely to be awake and to have significantly more quiet sleep and less active sleep under low light levels than infants exposed to bright continuous illumination.
8. Preterm infants receiving aminophylline for apnea of prematurity demonstrate more awake and less sleep periods. The use of waterbeds may decrease this effect.
9. Sucking on a pacifier decreases body activity and increases cutaneous Po_2.

Although further information still is lacking, the many additional effects on state listed earlier in the outline probably affect preterm awakeness and sleep and should be considered when providing clinical care for immature infants.

FACIAL EXPRESSION AND SOCIAL BEHAVIORS

The preterm infant lacks many of the social signals and expressions of emotion necessary for eliciting early attachment and caretaking. Despite the multitude of facial movements seen in active sleep, there is very little expression of early affect seen before 30 to 32 weeks. Preterm behaviors suggestive of social expression that could potentially elicit social responses include eye opening, grimacing, smiling, yawning, and crying. Minde rated these behaviors from 32 to 34 weeks' postmenstrual age and found no changes during this period that could be related to age or maternal caretaking. Hack similarly documented the occurrence of behaviors such as smiling, yawning, chewing, tonguing, sucking, sneezing, or mouthing during 30-second epochs of visual fixation. No consistent patterns or coincidence of behaviors were noted.

Crying and other vocalizations

Aborti of 23 to 24 weeks' gestation may cry at birth, and infants as young as 26 weeks' gestation respond to painful stimuli by crying. Very little spontaneous crying occurs before 30 to 32 weeks' gestation. From this time the infant may demonstrate hunger by crying before feeding time. Crying is not elicited during the Moro reflex before 32 weeks' gestation, whereas after 34 weeks 80% or more of infants will cry.

Michelsson examined the pain-induced cry of preterm and term infants spectrographically and found a higher pitch in the less mature infants.

Other vocalizations occur such as grunts and squeaks. Grunting sometimes denotes fussiness and may occur instead of crying in infants from 32 to 36 weeks of age. Yawning tends to reflect well-being and has been found to occur later and at a lower frequency in sick as compared to healthy preterm infants.

Smiling

Two patterns of smiling are seen during infancy: endogenous, or spontaneous, smiling, which is present at birth, and exogenous, or elicited, smiling, which occurs in response to external stimuli from about 3 to 4 weeks after term birth.

Endogenous smiling is seen only in active sleep or drowsiness. It appears as a side stretching and upturning of the corners of the mouth with the rest of the face remaining relaxed and relatively undisturbed. It is subcortical and probably mediated along with frowning, mouth movements, and other spontaneous REM-associated behaviors such as sneezes, yawns, and stretching. It usually occurs in clusters during a mid-REM period and has no relationship to feeding. It also can be elicited by auditory or tactile stimuli during the first week of life. During the first months after birth endogenous smiling diminishes in frequency and disappears by about 6 months of age.

Exogenous smiling begins gradually during the first 4 weeks after term birth and occurs mainly during quiet awakeness and sometimes during drowsiness. This type of smiling looks more like a social responsive smile. The mouth stretches further and may open, the superficial muscles of the cheeks and eyes contract, and the skin at the corners of the eyes tends to wrinkle, giving the

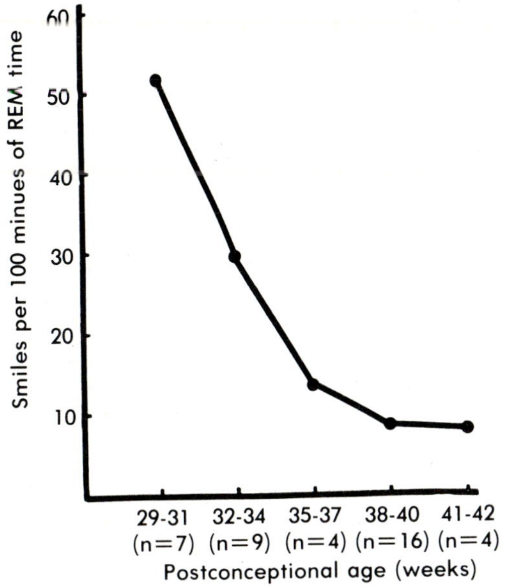

Fig. 26-6. Incidence of smiling during active (REM) sleep from 20 to 42 weeks. (From Emde, R.N., Gaesenbauer, T., and Harmon, R.: Emotional expression in infancy: a biobehavioral study. In Psychological issues, vol. 10, no. 1, monograph 37, New York, 1976, International University Press, Inc.)

impression that the whole face rather than the mouth alone is smiling. Exogenous smiling initially can be elicited by auditory, tactile, and nonsocial visual stimuli, but these are replaced by true social stimuli by 8 to 12 weeks of age. At this time the awake infant can respond to the caretaker's voice or moving face with an alert smile, brightening of the eyes, and a grin.

The ontogeny of smiling in preterm infants has been studied by Emde who observed facial behaviors during REM periods in preterm infants ranging from 29 to 37 weeks' postmenstrual age and compared them with term infants. The preterm infants smiled more (34 smiles per 100 minutes of REM sleep versus 8.8 smiles in the term infants). The preterm smiles also tended to occur more in bursts or clusters. In preterm infants 66% of smiling occurred in clusters compared with 33% in the term infants. The increased incidence of smiling in the preterm infants tended to decrease with maturity (Fig. 26-6).

SUCKING

The sucking reflex is one of the earliest coordinated behaviors in human fetal life. It is also one of the most important means of interaction between the infant and caretaker and is essential for biologic survival. Physiologically the process of sucking involves complicated integrations of oral, respiratory, and swallowing responses, whereas psychologically sucking is gratifying in itself and tends to soothe the infant.

For the effective accomplishment of sucking several sequential coordinated behaviors need to be completed. These include rooting, opening of the mouth, grasping of the nipple, sucking, and swallowing. The sucking reflex has two components: an expression component by which the tongue applies positive pressure to the nipple by pressing it up against the hard palate and moving backward, and a suction component whereby negative intraoral pressure is produced by lowering the floor of the mouth. Sucking precedes swallowing, which inhibits respiration. These functions must all be coordinated before effective, safe oral feeding can be achieved.

The term infant

All animals have a species-specific sucking rhythm with bursts of sucking interspersed with pauses. The human sucking reflex differs from that of other mammals in that humans have both a nutritive and a nonnutritive mode of sucking, whereas animals demonstrate only nutritive sucking.

In nonnutritive sucking, which can be induced by placing a nipple in the mouth without providing nutrient, there is a regularity to the burst-pause pattern. Rhythmic mouthing seen in infants in quiet sleep has the same temporal organization as that seen with nonnutritive sucking on a nipple. Term infants have an overall rate of two sucks per second per burst (range, 1.9 to 2.4), with a mean of eight sucks per burst (range, 4 to 13) and an interburst interval of about 6 seconds (range, 3 to 11 seconds). In nutritive sucking there are long bursts of sucks with a slower rate of sucking (about one suck per second). The burst-pause pattern appears mainly toward the end of the feeding period.

Nonnutritive sucking occurs in all the sleep and awake states, although less during quiet sleep and crying. Nutritive sucking is seen mainly in an awake hungry infant. Although long periods of sucking have been described in the immediate period after birth, effective sucking seems to develop gradually during the first few days of life, and many normal term infants only develop regular sucking rhythms by 4 days of age. This is probably related to perinatal factors that might affect the infant's early behavioral responses. Rooting is elicited mainly in a hungry awake infant and is less active on the first day of life.

Although sucking is a basal brain function it can be modified by higher brain centers. Its temporal organization (rhythmicity) and plasticity of response, (i.e., the ability to adapt to changes in the environment) make it an ideal research tool for evaluating early conditioning and learning. The sucking response can be modified by multiple factors, although the basic burst-pause pattern usually is maintained.

Intraoral factors affecting sucking include the shape and size of the nipple, the amount of nutrient and rapidity with which it is given, as well as the taste of the fluid. (Sweeter fluids tend to increase the total amount of sucking.) Extraoral stimuli such as presenting a visual or auditory stimulus may affect the rhythmicity of sucking. Perinatally stressed and abnormal newborns also demonstrate changes in nonnutritive sucking patterns.

The fetus and preterm infant

Most of the components of sucking are noted very early in life and were originally described in detail by Hooker. Mouth opening first appears at about 7 to 8 weeks' postmenstrual age. Only at 12 to 13 weeks do the oral reflexes first appear as isolated, separate reflex responses to trigeminal nerve stimulation. Other related reflexes (protrusion of the lips, mouth opening, and tongue movements) are noted at 16 weeks, and a gag reflex can be elicited at about 18 weeks. Lip puckering has been reported at 22 weeks and sucking at 24 weeks. More recently, ultrasonic imaging of the fetus in utero has revealed tongue protrusion at 13 weeks and sucking at 15 weeks' gestation. Fetal postural changes sometimes bring the hand in contact with the mouth, and reflex finger sucking can occur (Fig. 26-7). Swallowing of amniotic fluid, noted as early as 10 to 14 weeks' gestation, plays a role in amniotic fluid turnover and is essential for normal fetal-placental development.

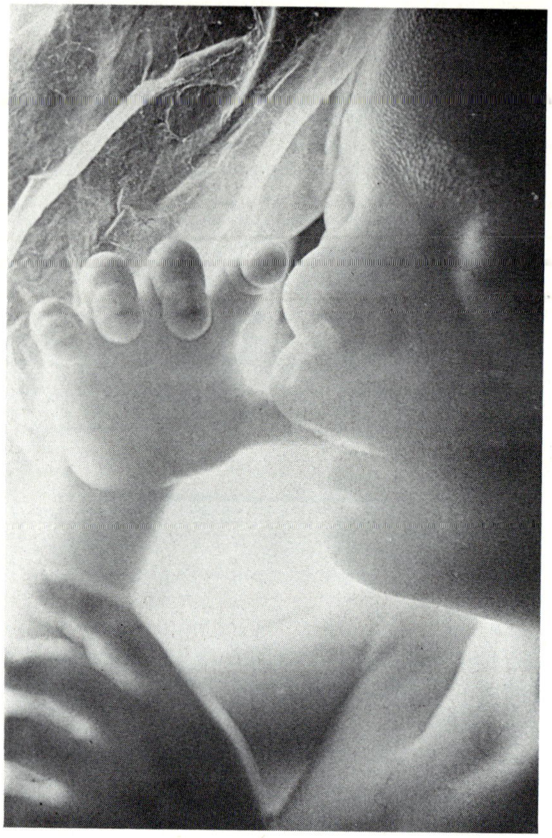

Fig. 26-7. Reflex sucking in utero. (From A CHILD IS BORN by Lennart Nilsson. English translation copyright © 1966, 1977 by Dell Publishing Co., Inc. Originally published in Swedish under the title ETT BARN BLIR TILL by Albert Bonniers Forlag. Copyright 1965 by Albert Bonniers Forlag, Stockholm. Revised edition copyright © 1976 by Lennart Nilsson, Mirjam Furuhjelm, Axel Ingerlman-Sunberg, Cales Wirson. Used by permission of DELACORTE PRESS/SEYMOUR LAWRENCE. A Merloyd Lawrence book.)

Although the isolated components of sucking and swallowing are all present before 28 weeks' gestation, they do not seem to be effectively coordinated for oral nipple feeding before 32 to 34 weeks, and even at this time they are immature.

Crump evaluated the sucking ability of low birth weight infants by measuring sucking rate. This was defined as the volume (milliliters) of fluid taken per second. Term infants had a sucking rate of 0.6 ml per second during the first 3 days of life, whereas low birth weight infants (mean birth weight, 2,109 gm) sucked at a rate of 0.24 ml per second. An increase in sucking rate is observed with increasing birth weight and postnatal age. Infants born after 37 weeks' gestation had a sucking rate and rhythm similar to those of term infants.

Gryboski observed nonnutritive sucking patterns and esophageal peristalsis from birth in groups of preterm infants. The infants showed irregular mouthing during the first few days after birth, the younger infants for up to 5 days and the older infants for 1 to 2 days. Thereafter an immature or a mature suck-swallow pattern was documented. The immature pattern, consisting of short sucking bursts preceded or followed by swallowing, occurred for 6 to 8 weeks in infants less than 35 weeks' gestation and only for a few days in older infants. The more mature suck-swallow pattern seen thereafter was characterized by longer bursts of sucking with multiple swallows occurring simultaneously with sucking.

Hack studied the development of the nonnutritional sucking rhythm of 6 preterm infants from 26 to 36 weeks' gestation. At less than 30 weeks' gestation, she noted mainly mouthing activity with infrequent sucks. Recognizable rhythmic bursts of sucking were recorded at 28 weeks' gestation in one infant and by 31 to 33 weeks in the other infants. Fig. 26-8 demonstrates an example of the progression of sucking and its rhythmicity in a typical infant. At 28 weeks' gestation there is mostly mouthing with single sucks not in bursts and long variable pauses. By 31 weeks sucking bursts are clearly identifiable with a rhythmic burst-pause pattern. Mouthing and single sucks are still seen. By 34 weeks the pace and rhythm within bursts has become remarkably stable. The interburst rhythm is less regular. Fig. 26-9 presents a

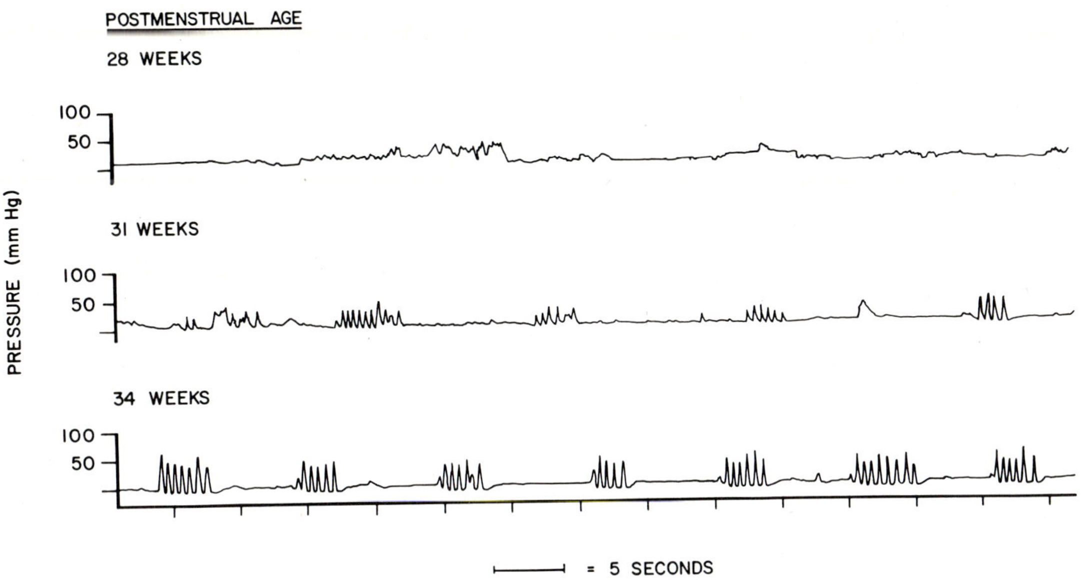

Fig. 26-8. The progressive development of nonnutritive sucking during active sleep followed from 28 through 34 postmenstrual weeks of age. (From Hack, M.: Early Hum. Dev. **11:**133, 1985.)

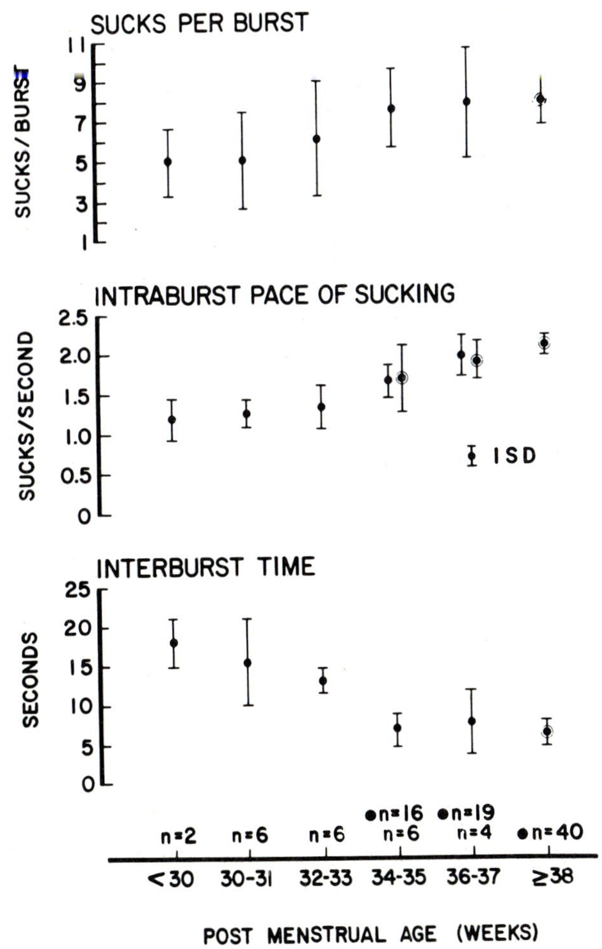

Fig. 26-9. The development of the parameters of nonnutritive sucking. Number of sucks per minute, intraburst pace of sucking, and interburst time from 30 postmenstrual weeks of age until term. Results based on Hack and Wolff. (From Hack, M.: Early Hum. Dev. **11:**133, 1985.)

description of the development of sucking until term.

In summary, although extrauterine fetal infants are able to "mouth" on a pacifier and suck repeatedly from 20 weeks' gestation, nonnutritive sucking may only assume a recognizable rhythmic pattern after 33 weeks' gestation. At this time the sucking rates per burst are slower (1.7 sucks per second per burst) and the interburst variability greater than those of term infants. A mature sucking rate and pattern are achieved by 37 weeks' gestation. Information is lacking as to whether postnatal oral experiences can accelerate this maturity.

ATTENTION AND PERCEPTION

Most information on neonatal attention and perception is based on observations of responses to visual and auditory stimuli. Attention during the neonatal period is defined as a selective orientation toward some part of the stimulus environment. Measures of visual attention include orientation to and following of a visual stimulus and the duration of fixation on the stimulus. Other indices of visual or auditory attention are decreasing body movements, cessation of sucking, heart rate deceleration, and increased skin potential reactivity. Measures of perceptual ability in infancy include testing for visual preferences, measuring differential attention to familiar versus novel stimuli for early recognition memory, measuring a progressive decline in attention to a given stimulus (habituation), and measuring increased or renewed attention when a different stimulus is presented (dishabituation). These perceptual abilities in the newborn, especially the preterm infant, are difficult to evaluate, since changes in the state of arousal during testing may alter or mask responses and confuse results: a quiet awake infant's attention may wane if he becomes drowsy or actively awake; similarly, responses to auditory stimuli in active sleep may decrease if the infant goes into quiet sleep and increase if he wakes up.

VISUAL ATTENTION

The term infant

Before the 1950s it generally was not believed that the term neonate could see much. Observations of visual following and attention by Wolff, Stechler, Brazelton, and others together with Fantz's objective recordings of neonatal visual fixation dramatically changed this view. A normal healthy term infant in the quiet alert state will respond to a visual stimulus such as a red ball by alerting with facial awakening and eye brightening. He might also decrease body movements and change his rate of sucking while he fixates and scans the stimulus. If the ball is moved slowly, the infant will turn his eyes and head and track horizontally or vertically with conjugate eye movements. This attention increases initially but gradually decreases with either a change of state or by the infant's turning away from the stimulus. Some infants may show an obligatory type of attention during the first week or two after birth with prolonged fixation of 10 minutes or more. The newborn also blinks much less than the adult, resulting in a staring type of gaze.

The method developed by Fantz for recording visual fixation is called the corneal reflection technique. The criterion for fixation is when the corneal reflection of the stimulus overlaps the pupil and presumably also is reflected on the retina. Using this method, Fantz documented the newborn's ability to fixate on a single pattern and to show preferences between patterns, preferring patterned over plain stimuli, curved over straight contours, and patterns of a larger size over patterns with an increased number of smaller details (i.e., simple rather than complex patterns). With infrared cameras it has been shown that infants tend to scan mainly the outer contours of patterns while looking less at inner details. When looking at human faces, they tend to scan the external features such as the eyes, side of the head, or hair outline. Only by about 2 months of age do they examine more the internal features of a face or pattern.

Visual attention in the neonate has been considered to be cortically mediated and thus reflect higher brain function. However, a recent report of visual tracking and pattern fixation in neonates who have complete destruction of the occipital cortex, and who later become cortically blind, suggests that neonatal visual responses might be subcortically mediated.

There has also been some discussion in the literature as to whether the newborn has an innate ability to recognize the human face. There is, however, very little definite evidence that the infant prefers a face over other geometric patterns when they are equal in contour, density, and number and size of details.

Factors affecting visual attention

Visual fixation and following are optimum in the quiet alert state but may occur to a lesser degree during drowsiness. Lifting an infant to an upright position may facilitate the ability to attend visually, and providing a pacifier tends to inhibit diffuse body activity and improve fixation. Combined auditory and visual social cues especially draw the attention of the newborn infant. Factors that disturb the state of quiet awakeness such as asphyxia, maternal drugs, or jaundice may affect the ability to fixate and attend visually (see outline earlier in this chapter). Prophylactic eye drops also may inhibit vision by causing periorbital edema and conjunctival irritation and are best postponed beyond the initial period of parent/infant contact.

Visual acuity

An acuity ranging from 10/400 to 10/820 Snellen equivalent has been documented in term neonates using the optokinetic response, with a best result of 10/150. With the visual preference method, acuity ranging from 20/300 to 20/1600 is described in term newborns. This poor acuity may explain the infants' preference for simple rather than more complex patterns. Furthermore the infant has a fixed focal length of approximately 19 cm and cannot accommodate to closer or more distant objects.

The preterm infant

Anatomically all the retinal layers are present by 22 weeks' gestation. Immature rods and cones can be distinguished at 23 weeks, myelinization of the optic nerve begins at 24 weeks, and all the neurons of the visual cortex are present by 25 to 26 weeks' gestation. Between 28 and 34 weeks there is a phase of rapid dendritic differentiation and synaptogenesis, with the cortical neurons undergoing changes in cell size, axonal length, and dendritic branching and synapses. Physiologically it has been shown that visual evoked potentials can transmit impulses from the cornea to the visual cortex by 26 weeks' gestation. These are initially very immature with long latencies that decrease somewhat consistently with age.

Although the preterm infant has a pupillary light response and can react to light by blinking at 29 weeks' gestation, there does not seem to be any awake visual attention before 30 to 32 weeks.

Using the corneal reflection technique, Hack demonstrated fixation on a single pattern from 30 weeks' postmenstrual age and visual preference to a patterned versus a plain surface from 31 weeks. Indices of alertness and attentiveness during fixation such as widening and brightening of the eyes, visual scanning, and cessation of sucking increase progressively from 30 weeks, so that an immature drowsy look is replaced by an awake, expressive visual alertness and active scanning of the stimulus by 36 weeks' postmenstrual age.

The time spent looking at a single pattern increases with age, with more fixation occurring during quiet awakeness than during drowsiness (Fig. 21-5).

In a separate study paired stimuli were presented to infants ranging in age from 31 to 34 weeks' postmenstrual age. The infants showed strong preferences for patterns of larger size or with greater details; however, no preferences for increasing detail were found when the amount of contrast in the pattern was held constant. These preferences did not differ from those of infants born at term or who had reached term after 8 to 10 weeks' postnatal experience.

Dubowitz recently studied both visual following and pattern preferences in preterm infants and found that under 30 weeks' gestation only 1 of 10 infants studied was capable of fixating on a moving red ball; between 30 and 32 weeks 20 of 25 infants fixated or followed, and after 32 weeks 11 of 12 infants demonstrated this ability. Pattern preferences were found in very few infants less than 32 weeks' gestation and in all infants over 32 weeks.

An orienting or attentional type of sucking response to visual stimuli has been documented by Barrett in preterm infants ranging in age from 33 to 37 weeks' gestation. Evidence of visual memory in preterm infants also has been documented by Sequeland. He presented a pattern continuously until infants showed familiarity by decreasing their rate of sucking. When a different stimulus was shown, the infants increased their rate of sucking, indicating recognition or memory of differences in the two patterns shown.

Visual acuity

Kiff and Lepard found a Snellen visual acuity of 20/820, and Miranda found that preterm infants (mean postmenstrual age, 35 weeks) could discriminate a ¼-inch line corresponding to a Snellen fraction of approximately 20/1280.

The term versus the preterm infant

Gesell noted an advanced attentiveness in preterm infants who had reached term when compared with term infants; however, this was only temporary and passed by 4 weeks after term. Kurtzberg, however, demonstrated decreased visual following in preterm infants at term. Kopp, Sigman, and Parmelee found that preterm infants at term spent more time looking at visual stimuli than did term infants. Friedman could not confirm these results but found that preterm infants took longer to fixate on a stimulus and also longer to decrease their response, indicating a possible inability to inhibit looking or a slower processing of information in the preterm infant. These studies suggest that preterm infants gain no benefit from the early visual stimulation they receive in the nursery. In fact, it is questionable how much visual stimulation these infants actually receive, since they have very short periods of awakeness and, considering their poor visual acuity and inability to accommodate, are exposed to very few appropriate visual stimuli in the incubator.

AUDITORY ATTENTION

The term infant

The specific behavioral response depends on the infant's state of arousal and on the tone, frequency, and repetitiveness of the auditory stimulus. When asleep, the infant responds by eye blinking, startling, and other body movements and with changes in respiration and heart rate. This response is greater in active than in quiet sleep. The awake infant responds to sound by an alerting of facial expression, by turning of eyes and sometimes head in the direction of the sound, and by a decrease in heart rate and change in respiration. These indices of attention are noted especially when the sound is in the range of human speech (500 to 900 cycles per second). Lower and higher frequency sounds have different effects. Low-frequency sounds, especially when continuous, tend to soothe the infant and induce sleep, whereas high-frequency sounds may cause distress with cardiac acceleration and crying. Infants tend to decrease responses (habituate) to repetitive auditory stimuli and respond again (dishabituate) when the frequency of sound is changed. Cairns and Butterfield showed that the term infant has different sucking responses to human and nonhuman auditory stimuli and that infants can be conditioned to modify their sucking rate to bring on the sound of a human voice. There is also some evidence that the newborn can differentiate between maternal and other voices within a few days of birth.

Fetal responses

There have been isolated reports of fetal movement and heart rate acceleration in response to auditory stimuli from as early as 26 weeks' gestation. The human auditory apparatus is structurally complete and physiologically functional at 24 weeks' gestation, so that this is feasible. There are, however, many factors that confound the evaluation of hearing in utero. The fetus is already exposed to high levels of background noise from the maternal circulatory and digestive systems, so that any additional auditory stimuli may not be heard. In addition, there is no air in utero so that sound can be conducted only through fluid or bone. Any documented fetal responses may in part be a result of the maternal response to the auditory stimulus or the vibration associated with giving the stimulus.

Parmelee reviewed the literature on fetal auditory responsivity and concluded that there is still uncertainty as to whether the fetus can respond to external auditory stimuli presented before 34 weeks' gestation. After 34 weeks the fetus responds clearly with body movements or heart rate acceleration. It may be possible to use these auditory responses as a measure of fetal well-being in utero.

The preterm infant

The extrauterine preterm infant responds to auditory stimuli from as early as 28 weeks' gestation. Gesell reported responses to sound at 28 to 30 weeks with a decrease in response after repeated stimulation. Monod and Garma measured preterm responses to auditory click stimuli and documented motor responses 29% of the time at 30 to 31 weeks' gestation and eye blink responses only 5% of the time. With increasing age the motor responses tended to decrease in quiet sleep, whereas in active sleep the percentage of motor responses did not change. Eye blink responses to sound increased in active sleep with increasing age.

Cortical evoked auditory responses have been documented from 25 weeks' gestation. With increasing age the complexity of the wave responses increase and their latency decreases.

Auditory brainstem evoked potentials (ABR) have been studied longitudinally from 26 weeks' gestation. The ABR consists of a series of waves evoked by an auditory stimulus such as a click, and gives information on the threshold sensitivity of the peripheral auditory system (cochlea and auditory nerve) and on the velocity of conduction along the auditory fibers ascending the brain stem en route to the cortex. The latencies (conduction times) of these waves decrease with increasing gestational age and are not dependent on the state of the infant. Infants born at term have latencies similar to those of preterm infants who have reached term. The ABR has been used to assess early hearing and to document the effects of neonatal risk factors on auditory and brainstem function. The only individual risk factors that have been found to correlate with increased latencies are intraventricular hemorrhage and prolonged acidosis secondary to asphyxia, although multiple risk factors may prolong latency periods.

In summary, cortical and base of brain evoked potentials show that the auditory system is functional from 26 weeks' gestation. Inconsistent behavioral auditory responses can be obtained from 28 weeks' gestation with more consistent responses from 32 to 34 weeks' gestation. There is no evidence that the noise environment of the nursery has a measurable effect on the ontogeny of auditory perception.

RESPONSE TO PAIN

Crying responses to pain result in a decrease in Po_2, an increase in blood pressure, an increase in cerebral blood flow, and an increase in cortisol secretion, as well as changes in state organization.

Circumcision has been used as the model for research on the effects of pain in term infants. (See effects on state earlier in this chapter.) There have been no systematic studies related to the preterm infant's response to pain. There has, however, been an increased awareness of both the term and preterm infants suffering related to pain and both local anesthesia and systemic analgesics are now widely used in the intensive care nursery.

MOTOR BEHAVIOR

This section reviews the development of resting posture, active and passive muscle tone, and spontaneous movement.

Fetal movements

Hooker described reflex fetal movement from 7 weeks' gestation. Initially there is a total body reflex movement

	6 months 28 weeks	6½ months 30 weeks	7 months 32 weeks	7½ months 34 weeks	8 months 36 weeks	8½ months 38 weeks	9 months 40 weeks
1. LOWER EXTREMITY	—	Beginning of extension of lower leg on thigh upon stimulation of soles in lying position	Good support when standing up but very briefly (see illustration below)	Excellent righting reaction of leg --→	--------→	--------→	
2. TRUNK	—	—	—	± transitory	Good righting of trunk with infant held in vertical suspension (see illustration below)	Good righting of trunk with infant held in walking position (see illustration below)	
3. NECK EXTENSORS Baby pulled backward from sitting position	—	—	Head begins to right itself with great difficulty	Still difficult and incomplete	Good righting but cannot hold it	Begins to maintain head which doesn't fall back for few seconds	Keeps head in line with trunk for more than a few seconds
4. NECK FLEXORS Baby pulled to sitting position from supine	— Head pendulant	— Head pendulant	Contraction of muscles is visible but no movement of head	Head begins to right itself but still hanging back at end of movement	At first head is hanging back, then with sudden movement head goes forward onto chest	Head begins to follow trunk, keeps in line for few seconds in upright position	Difference between Extensors and Flexors has diminished (see illustration below)
			Straightening of legs 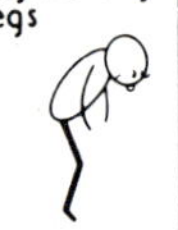		Straightening of trunk 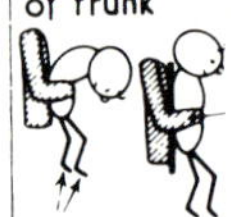 arm support; Stimulation		Straightening of head and trunk together 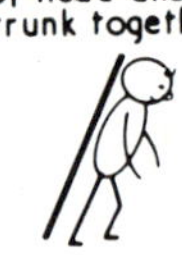

Fig. 26-12. Development of active muscle tone from 28 weeks' gestation until term. (From Amiel Tison, C.: Arch. Dis. Child. **43:**89, 1968.)

nancies (toxemia, premature rupture of membranes, and antepartum bleeding). Such infants also may have accelerated pulmonary maturity.

The term versus the preterm infant

In general, there are minimal differences in preferred posture and motor behavior between preterm infants who have reached term and those born at term. Subtle differences in motor behavior, however, do distinguish these two groups. The preterm infant has not been confined to a flexed position in utero and is less hypertonic and exhibits easier passive movement of limbs and more active and varied spontaneous movements. High-risk preterm infants tend to have a decrease in muscle tone at term as compared to low-risk preterm infants, who are neurologically more similar to the term-born neonate.

THE BRAZELTON NEONATAL BEHAVIORAL ASSESSMENT SCALE AND THE DUBOWITZ METHOD OF NEUROLOGIC EXAMINATION

The Brazelton neonatal behavioral assessment scale incorporates most of the behaviors described in this chapter. By using this method of assessment it is possible to evaluate the term newborn's behavioral capabilities and to see how the infant responds to the immediate environment. Although the full Brazelton examination seldom is used clinically by neonatologists, many of the responses are useful for evaluating an infant's interactive abilities and for demonstrating individual differences to parents. During the course of the examination, 26 behavioral responses are tested and rated on a nine-point scale, and 20 neurologic responses derived from the Prechtl method of neurologic examination are rated on a three-point scale.

Behavioral items

Response decrement to repeated visual stimuli
Response decrement to rattle
Response decrement to bell
Response decrement to pinprick
Orienting response to inanimate visual stimuli
Orienting response to inanimate auditory stimuli
Orienting response to animate visual stimuli: examiner's face
Orienting response to animate auditory stimuli: examiner's voice

Orienting responses to animate visual and auditory stimuli
Quality and duration of alert periods
General muscle tone, in resting and in response to being handled (passive and active)
Motor maturity
Traction responses as infant is pulled to sitting position
Cuddliness: responses to being cuddled by the examiner
Defensive movements: reactions to a cloth over face
Consolability with intervention by examiner
Peak of excitement and capacity to control self
Rapidity of buildup to crying state
Irritability during the examination
General assessment of kind and degree of activity
Tremulousness
Amount of startling
Lability of skin color (measuring autonomic lability)
Lability of states during entire examination
Self-quieting activity: attempts to console self and control state
Hand-to-mouth activity

Neurologic responses

Plantar grasp
Hand grasp
Ankle clonus
Babinski sign
Standing
Automatic walking
Placing
Incurvation
Crawling
Glabella
Tonic deviation of head and eyes
Nystagmus
Tonic neck reflex
Moro reflex
Rooting (intensity)
Sucking (intensity)
Passive movement
  Arms (R, L)
  Legs (R, L)

The best performance of every response is recorded. In addition, state changes are noted throughout the examination to assess the infant's capacity for self-organization. The examination starts with a sleeping baby and gradually works through the various responses as the infant awakens. Responses to visual, auditory, and tactile stimuli are tested, as well as the ability to habituate to repeated stimuli. During the course of the examination responses to aversive stimuli such as uncovering, undressing, a pinprick, and a cloth placed over the face also are tested together with the ability for self-quieting and the ability to respond to soothing and cuddling.

The Brazelton scale has been used to evaluate the effects on neonatal behavior of maternal obstetric drugs, narcotic addiction, and various neonatal conditions such as intrauterine growth retardation, jaundice, and asphyxia.

The Brazelton scale has also been extended to evaluate preterm behavior. Als has hypothesized that initially the main task for the preterm infant is to stabilize and integrate physiologic functions such as respiration, heart rate, temperature, digestion, and elimination. The motor system then gradually develops with active postural adjustments and movement. Later the awake and sleep states emerge with organization of state, and finally the alert state becomes available for social interaction.

It is thus possible to evaluate the infant's current status of behavioral organization along five subsystems of func-

Table 26-3. Items included in Dubowitz protocol

Habituation	Movement and tone	Reflexes	Neurobehavioral
Light	Posture	Tendon	(Eye appearances)
Sound	Arm recoil	Palmar grasp	Auditory orientation
	Arm traction	Rooting	Visual orientation
	Leg recoil	Sucking	Alertness
	Leg traction	Walking	Defensive reaction
	Popliteal angle	Moro	Peak of excitement
	Head control		Irritability
	post. neck muscles		Consolability
	ant. neck muscles		(Cry)
	Head lag		
	Ventral suspension		
	Head raising in prone		
	Arm release in prone		
	Spontaneous body movement		
	Tremors/startles		
	Abnormal movements		

tioning: physiologic, motor organization, state organization, interactive, and self-regulation. Studies on preterm infants have shown them to be variable in their behavior. In general they are poorer in orientation, motor performance, state regulation, and autonomic function. This test is not readily applicable for clinical use; however, it is of great importance because it compels the caretaker to view the preterm infant as part of an environmental system rather than as an isolated organism. The effects of various medical procedures always need to be viewed in this context.

Dubowitz more recently developed a method of neurologic examination for preterm and term infants based on Prechtl, Dargassies, and Brazelton methods. This method is shorter and thus more practical for clinical use. It can be used serially to follow the neurobehavioral maturation of preterm infants and can be used for sick as well as healthy infants (Table 26-3).

CONCLUSION

The improved survival rates and greater accessibility of neonatal intensive care units to developmental psychologists have resulted in a surge of interest and research in preterm behavioral development. The various studies reported in this chapter have focused mainly on the ontogeny of isolated sensory behaviors. As yet there have been very few studies on the interrelationship between the various sensory abilities and very little attention given to viewing the preterm infant as part of an interactional system between the infant, caretaker, and nursery environment. It has been shown, however, that infants in intensive care nurseries are seldom left to rest, are subjected to multiple medical caretaking procedures, and are exposed to continuous light and auditory stimuli. It is thus surprising that despite this unnatural and disturbing type of environment, the preterm infant who has reached term shows only minimal behavioral differences when compared with the term newborn. This may in part be caused by the preterm infant's relative lack of responsiveness, which protects him from the excessive stimuli of the outer world. It seems that the inherent program of biologic and structural development continues despite environmental changes and disease processes.

Maureen Hack

BIBLIOGRAPHY

General

Brazelton, B., Parker, W., and Zuckerman, B.: Importance of behavioral assessment of the neonate. In Gluck, L., editor: Curr. Probl. Pediatr. **7**(2), 1976.

Condon, W.S., and Sander, L.W.: Neonatal movement is synchronized with adult speech: interactional participation and language acquisition, Science **183**:99, 1974.

Dargassies, S. S.-A.: Neurological development in the full-term and premature neonate, Amsterdam, 1977, Exerpta Medica.

Dreyfus-Brisac, C.: Neurophysiological studies in human premature and full-term newborns, Biol. Psychiatry **10**:485, 1975.

Friedman, S., and Sigman, M., editors: Preterm birth and psychological development, New York, 1981, Academic Press.

Gesell, A., and Amatruda, C.S.: The embryology of behavior—the beginnings of the human mind, New York, 1945, Harper.

Gottfried, A., and Cornell, E.: Intervention with premature human infants, Child Dev. **47**:32, 1976.

Humphrey, T.: Some correlations between the appearance of human fetal reflexes and the development of the nervous system, Prog. Brain Res. **4**:93, 1964.

Hutt, S.G., Lenard, H.G., and Prechtl, H.F.: Psychophysiological studies in newborn infants, Adv. Child Dev. Behav. **4**:128, 1969.

Lawson, K., Daum, C., and Turkewitz, G.: Environmental characteristics of a neonatal intensive-care unit, Child. Dev. **48**:1633, 1977.

Lipsitt, L.P.: The study of sensory and learning processes of the newborn, Clin. Perinatol. **4**:163, 1977.

Meltzoff, A.N., and Moore, M.K.: Imitation of facial and manual gestures by human neonates, Science **198**:75, 1977.

Osofsky, J., editor: A handbook of infant development, New York, 1979, John Wiley and Sons.

Peiper, A.: Cerebral function in infancy and childhood, New York, 1963, Consultants Bureau.

Prechtl, H.F.R.: The behavioral states of the newborn infant: a review, Brain Res. **76**:185, 1974.

Wolff, P.: The causes, controls, and organization of behavior in the newborn, Psychol. Issues **5**:17, 1966.

Wolff, P.H., and Ferber, R.: The development of behavior in human infants, premature and newborns, Annu. Rev. Neurosci. **2**:291, 1979.

States of arousal

The term infant

Anders, T., Emde, R., and Parmelee, A., editors: Manual of standardized terminology, techniques, and for scoring of states of sleep and wakefulness in newborn infants, Los Angeles, 1971, Brain Information Service, School of Health Sciences, UCLA.

Anders, T.F., and Hoffman, E.: The sleep polygram: a potentially useful tool for clinical assessment in human infants, Am. J. Ment. Defic. **77**:506, 1973.

Anders, T.F., and Roffwarg, H.P.: The effects of selective interruption and deprivation of sleep in the human newborn, Dev. Psychobiol. **6**:79, 1973.

Anders, T.F., and Chalemian, R.J.: The effects of circumcision on sleep-wake states in human neonates, Psychosom. Med. **36**:174, 1974.

Aserinsky, E., and Kleitman, N.: Regularly occurring periods of eye motility and concomitant phenomena, during sleep, Science **118**:273, 1953.

Biosmier, J.D.: Visual stimulation and wake-sleep behavior in human neonates, Dev. Psychobiol. **10**(3):219, 1977.

Brackbill, Y.: Cumulative effects of continuous stimulation on arousal level in infants, Child Dev. **42**:17, 1971.

Brackbill, Y., Douthitt, T.C., and West, H.: Psychophysiologic effects in the neonate of prone versus supine placement, J. Pediatr. **82**:82, 1973.

Brazelton, T.: Psychophysiologic reactions in the neonate. I. The value of observation of the neonate, Pediatrics **58**:508, 1961.

Desmond, M.M., and others: The clinical behavior of the newly born, J. Pediatr. **62**:307, 1963.

Gaensbauer, T.H., and Emde, R.N.: Wakefulness and feeding in human newborns, Arch. Gen. Psychiatry **28**:894, 1973.

Emde, R.N., and others: Stress and neonatal sleep, Psychosom. Med. 33:491, 1971.

Emde, R.H., Swedberg, J., and Suzuki, B.: Human wakefulness and biological rhythms after birth, Arch. Gen. Psychiatry **32**:780, 1975.

Korner, A.F., and Thoman, E.B.: Visual alertness in neonates as evoked by maternal care, J. Exp. Child Psychol. **10**:67, 1970.

Long, J.G., Philip, A.G.S., and Lucey, J.F.: Excessive handling as a cause of hypoxemia, Pediatrics **65**:203, 1980.

Martin, R.J., Okken, A., and Rubin, D.: Changes in arterial oxygen tension during active and quiet sleep in the neonate, Birth Defects **15**:493, 1979.

Paludetto, R., and others: Effects of different ways of covering the eyes on behavior of jaundiced infants treated with phototherapy, Biol. Neonate **47**:1, 1985.

Prechtl, H.: Patterns of reflex behavior related to sleep in the human infant. In Clemente, C.D., and Purpura, D., editors: Sleep and the maturing nervous system, New York, 1972, Academic Press, Inc.

Rahilly, P.: Effects of sleep state and feeding on cranial blood flow of the human neonate, Arch. Dis. Child. **55**:265, 1980.

Roffwarg, H.P., Muzio, J.N., and Dement, W.C.: Ontogenetic development of the human sleep-dream cycle, Science **152**:604, 1966.

Schmidt, K.: The effect of continuous stimulation on the behavioral sleep of infants, Merrill-Palmer Quarterly **21**:77, 1975.

Theorell, K., Prechtl, H.F.R., and Vos, J.E.: A polygraphic study of normal and abnormal newborn infants, Neuropaediatrie **5**:279, 1974.

Wolff, P.H.: Observations on newborn infants, Psychosom. Med. **21**:110, 1959.

Fetal rest activity cycles and behavioral states

Griffin, R.L., Caron, F.J.M., and van Geijn, H.P.: Behavioral states in the human fetus during labor, Am. J. Obstet. Gynecol. **152**:828, 1985.

Nijhuis, J.G., and others: Are there behavioral states in the human fetus? Early Hum. Dev. **6**:177, 1982.

Sterman, M.B., and Hoppenbrouwers, T.: The development of sleep-waking and rest-activity patterns from fetus to adult in man. In Clemente, C.D., and Purpura, D., editors: Sleep and the maturing nervous system, New York, 1973, Academic Press.

Timor-Tritsch, I.E., and others: Studies of antepartum behavioral state in the human fetus at term, Am. J. Obstet. Gynecol. **132**:524, 1978.

The preterm infant

Birnholz, J.C.: The development of human fetal eye movement patterns, Science **213**:679, 1981.

Dreyfus-Brisac, C.: Sleep ontogenesis in early human prematurity from 24 to 27 weeks of conceptional age, Dev. Psychobiol. **1**:162, 1968.

Dreyfus-Brisac, C.: Ontogenesis of sleep in human prematures after 32 weeks of conceptional age, Dev. Psychobiol. **8**:91, 1970.

Eisengart, M., Gluckx, L., and Kessen, W.: Early feeding of premature infants effect on blood sugar and gross motor activity, Biol. Neonate **17**:151, 1971.

Emde, R.N., and Koenig, K.L.: Neonatal smiling and rapid eye movement states, J. Am. Acad. Child Psychiatr. **8**:57, 1969.

Emde, R.N., and Koenig, K.L.: Neonatal smiling, frowning, and rapid eye movement states. II. Sleep-cycle study, J. Am. Acad. Child Psychiatr. **8**:637, 1969.

Emde, R., and Metcalf, D.: An electroencephalographic study of behavioral rapid eye movement states in the human newborn, J. Nerv. Ment. Dis. **150**:376, 1970.

Hack, M., Muszynski, S., and Miranda, S.: State of awakeness during visual fixation in preterm intants, Pediatrics **68**:87, 1981.

Holmes, G., and others: Central nervous system maturation in the stressed premature, Ann. Neurol. **6**(6):518, 1979.

Korner, A.F., Ruppert, E.M., and Rho, J.M.: Effects of waterbeds on the sleep and motility of theophylline-treated preterm infants, Pediatrics **70**:864, 1982.

Minde, K., and others: Mother-child relationships in the premature nursery: an observational study, Pediatrics **61**:373, 1978.

Parmelee, A.H., Bruck, K., and Bruck, M.: Activity and inactivity cycles during the sleep of premature infants exposed to neutral temperatures, Biol. Neonate **4**:317, 1962.

Parmelee, A.H., Jr., and others: Sleep states in premature infants, Dev. Med. Child Neurol. **9**:70, 1967.

Parmelee, A.H.: Neurophysiological and behavioral organization of premature infants in the first months of life, Biol. Psychiatry **10**:501, 1975.

Stern, E., Parmelee, A.H., and Harris, M.A.: Sleep state periodicity in prematures and young infants, Dev. Psychobiol. **6**:357, 1973.

Facial expressions and social behaviors

Emde, R.N., McCartney, R.D., and Harmon, R.J.: Neonatal smiling in REM states. IV. Premature study, Child Dev. **42**:1657, 1971.

Emde, R.N., and Harmon, R.J.: Endogenous and exogenous smiling systems in early infancy, J. Am. Acad. Child. Psychiatr. **11**:177, 1972.

Emde, R., Gaensbauer, T., and Harmon, R.: Emotional expression in infancy: a biobehavioral study, Psychol. Issues Vol. X, No. 1, Monograph No. 37, 1976.

Foley, H.: When do pre-term and light-for-dates babies smile? Dev. Med. Child. Neurol. **19**:757, 1977.

Hines, R., and others: Behavioral development of premature infants: an ethological approach, Dev. Med. Child Neurol. **22**:623, 1980.

Michaelis, R., and others: Activity states in premature and term infants, Dev. Psychobiol. **6**:209, 1973.

Michelsson, K.: Cry analyses of symptomless low birth weight neonates and of asphyxiated newborn infants, Acta Paediatr. Scand. (suppl.) **216**:1, 1971.

Patel, D.A., and others: Yawning (stretch reflex) behavior in neonates, Perinatal Nurs. July-August, p. 56, 1984.

Sroufe, L.A., and Waters, E.: The ontogenesis of smiling and laughter: a perspective on the organization of development in infancy, Psychol. Rev. **83**:173, 1976.

Wolff, P.H.: Observations on the early development of smiling. In Foss, B.M., editor: Determinants of infant behavior, vol. II. London, 1963, Methuen.

Sucking

Anderson, G.C., and Vidyasagar, D.: Development of sucking in premature infants from one to seven days post birth, Birth Defects **15**:145, 1979.

Crook, C.K.: The organization and control of infant sucking, Adv. Child Dev. Behav. **14**:209, 1979.

Crump, E.P., Gore, P.M., and Horton, C.P.: The sucking behavior in premature infants, Hum. Biol. **30**:128, 1958.

Dubignon, J.M., Campbell, D., and Partington, M.W.: The development of non-nutritive sucking in premature infants, Biol. Neonat. **14**:270, 1969.

Gryboski, J.: Suck and swallow in the premature infant, Pediatrics **43**:96, 1969.

Hack, M., Estabrook, M.M., and Robertson, S.: Development of sucking rhythm in preterm infants, Early Hum. Dev. **11**:133, 1985.

Wolff, P.H.: The serial organization of sucking in the young infant, Pediatrics **42**:943, 1968.

Wolff, P.H.: The interaction of state and non-nutritive sucking. In Bosma, J., editor: Third symposium on oral sensation and perception, Springfield, 1972, Charles C Thomas, Publisher.

Pain responses

Gunnar, M.R., and others: Coping with aversive stimulation in the neonatal period: quiet sleep and plasma cortisol levels during recovery from circumcision, Child Dev. **56**:824, 1985.

Marshal, R., and others: Circumcision. I. effects upon newborn behavior, Inf. Behav. Dev. **3**:11, 1980.

Visual attention

The term infant

Brazelton, T.B., Scholl, M.L., and Robey, J.S.: Visual responses in the newborn, Pediatrics **37**:284, 1966.

Bruner, J.S.: Pacifier-produced visual buffering in human infants, Dev. Psychobiol. **6**:45, 1973.

Cohen, L.: Infant perception: from sensation to cognition. In Salapetek, P., editor: Basic visual processes, vol. 1, New York, 1975, Academic Press.

Cohen, L., DeLoache, J., and Strauss, M.: Infant visual perception. In Osofsky, J., editor: A handbook of infant development, New York, 1979, Wiley-Interscience Publication.

Dubowitz, L.M.S., and others: Visual function in the newborn: is it cortically mediated? Lancet **1**:1139, 1986.

Fantz, R.: Pattern vision in newborn infants, Science **140**:296, 1963.

Fredrickson, W., and Brown, J.: Posture as a determinant of visual behavior in newborns, Child Dev. **46**:579, 1975.

Friedman, S.: Newborn visual attention to repeated exposure of redundant vs "novel" targets, Perception Psychophysica **12**(3):291, 1972.

Gregg, C.L., Haffner, M.H., and Korner, F.: The relative efficacy of vestibular-proprioceptive stimulation and the upright position in enhancing visual pursuit in neonates, Child Dev. **47**:309, 1976.

Haynes, H., White, B., and Held, R.: Visual accommodation in human infants, Science **148**:528, 1965.

Kopp, C., Sigman, M., and Parmelee, A.: Neurological organization and visual fixation in infants at 40 weeks conceptional age, Dev. Psychobiol. 8(2):165, 1975.

Linksz, A.: Visual acuity in the newborn with notes on some objective methods to determine visual acuity, Doc. Ophthalmol. **34**:259, 1973.

Salapatek, P., and Kessen, W.: Visual scanning of triangles by the human newborn, J. Exp. Child Psychol. **3**:155, 1966.

Sigman, M., and others: Visual attention and neurological organization in neonates, Child Dev. **44**:461, 1973.

Sigman, M., and others: Infant visual attentiveness in relation to birth condition, Dev. Psychobiol. **13**:431, 1977.

Stechler, G.: Newborn attention as affected by medication during labor, Science **14**:315, 1964.

Stechler, G.: Attention in the newborn: its effects on motility and skin potential reactivity, Science **151**:1246, 1966.

Stechler, G., and Latz, E.: Some observations on attention and arousal in the human infant, J. Am. Acad. Child Psychiatry **5**:517, 1966.

Wolff, P.H.: The development of attention in young infants, Ann. NY Acad. Sci. **118**:815, 1965.

The preterm infant

Barrett, T.E., and Miller, L.K.: The organization of non-nutritive sucking in the premature infant, J. Exp. Child Psychol. **16**:472, 1973.

Dubowitz, L.M.S., and others: Visual function in the preterm and fullterm newborn infant, Dev. Med. Child Neurol. **22**:465, 1980.

Friedman, S., Jacobs, B., and Werthmann, M.: Sensory processing in pre- and full-term infants in the neonatal period. In Friedman, S., and Sigman, M., editors: Preterm birth and psychological development, New York, 1981, Academic Press.

Hack, M., Mostow, A., and Miranda, S.: Development of attention in preterm infants, Pediatrics **58**:669, 1976.

Hittner, H., Hirsch, J., and Rudolph, A.: Assessment of gestational age by examination of the anterior vascular capsule of the lens, Pediatrics **91**:455, 1977.

Kiff, R., and Lepard, C.: Visual response of premature infants: use of the optokinetic nystagmus to estimate visual development, Arch. Ophthalmol. **75**:631, 1966.

Miranda, S.: Visual abilities and pattern preferences of premature infants and full-term neonates, J. Exp. Child Psychol. **10**:189, 1970.

Purpura, D.P.: Morphogenesis of visual cortex in the preterm infant. In Brazier, M.A.B., editor: Growth and development of the brain, New York, 1975, Raven Press.

Robinson, R.: Assessment of gestational age by neurological examination, Arch. Dis. Child. **41**:437, 1966.

Schulte, F., and others: The ontogeny of sensory perception in preterm infants, Eur. J. Pediatr. **126**:211, 1977.

Sequeland, E.: Studies of visual recognition memory in preterm infants: differences in development as a function of perinatal morbidity factors. In Friedman, S., and Sigman, M., editors: Preterm birth and psychological development, New York, 1981, Academic Press.

Auditory function

Fetal

Bradley, R., and Mistretta, C.: Fetal sensory receptors, Physiol. Rev. **55**:352, 1975.

Luz, N., and others: Auditory evoked responses of the human fetus: behavior during progress of labor, Acta Obstet. Gynecol. Scand. **59**:395, 1980.

Read, J., and Miller, F.: Fetal heart rate acceleration in response to acoustic stimulation as a measure of fetal well-being, Am. J. Obstet. Gynecol. **129**:512, 1977.

Term and preterm infant

Cairns, G., and Butterfield, E.: Assessing infant's auditory functioning. In Friedlander, B., Sterritt, G., and Kirk, G., editors: Exceptional infant, New York, 1975, Brunner/Mazel, Inc.

Despland, P., and Galambos, R.: The auditory brainstem response (ABR) is a useful diagnostic tool in the intensive care nursery, Pediatr. Res. **14**:154, 1980.

Eisenberg, R.: Auditory behavior in the human neonate: methodologic problems, J. Aud. Res. **5**:159, 1965.

Hammond, J.: Hearing and response in the newborn, Dev. Med. Child Neurol. **12**:3, 1970.

Hutt, S., and others: Auditory responsivity in the human neonate, Nature **218**:888, 1968.

Marshall, R., and others: Auditory function in newborn intensive care unit patients revealed by auditory brain-stem potentials, J. Pediatr. **96**:731, 1980.

Monod, N., and Garma, L.: Auditory responsivity in the human premature, Biol. Neonate **17**:292, 1971.

Parmelee, A.H.: Auditory function and neurological maturation in preterm infants. In Friedman, S.L., and Sigman, M., editors: Preterm birth and psychological development, New York, 1981, Academic Press, Inc.

Schulman, C.: Effects of auditory stimulation on heart rate in premature infants as a function of level of arousal, probability of CNS damage, and conceptional age, Dev. Psychobiol. 2(3):172, 1969.

Schulman-Galambos, C., and Galambos, R.: Brain stem auditory evoked response in premature infants, J. Speech Hear. Res. **18**:456, 1975.

Starr, A., and others: Development of auditory function in newborn infants revealed by auditory brainstem potentials, Pediatrics **60**:831, 1977.

Motor behavior

Fetal movement

Birnholz, J., Stephen, J., and Faria, M.: Fetal movement patterns: a possible means of defining neurologic developmental milestones in utero, Am. J. Roentgenol. **130**:537, 1978.

Timor-Tritsch, I., and others: Classification of human fetal movement, Am. J. Obstet. Gynecol. **126**:70, 1976.

The preterm and term infant

Amiel-Tison, C.: Neurological evaluation of the maturity of newborn infants, Arch. Dis. Child. **43**:89, 1968.

Brandt, I.: Patterns of early neurological development. In Falkner, F., and Tanner, J., editors: Human growth, vol. 3, New York, 1979, Plenum Publishing Corp.

Condon, W.S., and Sander, L.W.: Neonate movement is synchronized with adult sleep, Science **183**:99, 1974.

Dubowitz, L., Dubowitz, V., and Goldberg, C.: Clinical assessment of gestational age in the newborn infant, Pediatrics **77**:1, 1970.

Forsland, M., and Bjerre, I.: Neurological assessment of preterm infants at term conceptual age in comparison with normal full term infants, Early Hum. Dev. **8**:195, 1983.

Gould, J., Gluck, L., and Kulovich, M.: The relationship between accelerated pulmonary maturity and accelerated neurological maturity in certain chronically stressed pregnancies, Am. J. Obstet. Gynecol. **127**:181, 1977.

Howard, J., and others: A neurologic comparison of pre-term and full-term infants at term conceptional age, J. Pediatr. **88**:995, 1976.

Kurtzberg, D., and others: Neurobehavioral performance of low birthweight infants at 40 weeks conceptional age: comparison with normal full-term infants, Dev. Med. Child Neurol. **21**:590, 1979.

Prechtl, H.F.R., and others: Postures, motility, and respiration of low-risk pre-term infants, Dev. Med. Child Neurol. **21**:3, 1979.

Robertson, S.S.: Human cyclic motility: fetal-newborn continuity and newborn state differences, Dev. Psychobiol. (In press.)

Saint-Anne Dargassies, S.: Neurological maturation of the preterm infant of 28 to 41 weeks' gestational age. In Falkner, F., editor: Human development, Philadelphia, 1966, W.B. Saunders Co.

Von Hofstein, C.: Eye-hand coordination in the newborn, Dev. Psychol. **18**:450, 1982.

Brazelton neonatal behavioral assessment scale and Dubowitz method of neurologic assessment

Als, H., Lester, B., and Brazelton, T.: Dynamics of the behavioral organization of the premature infant: a theoretical perspective. In Field, T., editor: Infants born at risk, New York, 1979, SP Medical & Scientific Books.

Als, H., and others: Towards a research instrument for the assessment of preterm infants' behavior (A.P.I.B.). In Fitzgerald, H., Lester, B., and Yogman, M., editors: Theory and research in behavioral pediatrics, New York, 1980, Plenum Publishing Corp.

Als, H., and others: Manual for the assessment of preterm infant behavior (A.P.I.B.). In Fitzgerald, H., Leater, B., and Yogman, M., editors: Theory and research in behavioral pediatrics, New York, 1980, Plenum Publishing Corp.

Brazelton, T.: Neonatal behavioral assessment scale, Clin. Dev. Med., Spastics International Medical Publications, No. 50, London, 1973.

Dubowitz, L., and Dubowitz, V.: The neurological assessment of the preterm and full-term newborn infant, Clin. Dev. Med., Spastic International Medical Publications, No. 79, Philadelphia, J.B. Lippincott, 1981.

Paludetto, R., and others: Early behavioral development of preterm infants, Dev. Med. Child Neurol. **26**:347, 1984.

Prechtl, H.F.R.: The neurological examination of the full-term newborn infant, Clin. Dev. Med., Spastic International Medical Publications, No. 63, London, Heineman Medical, 1977.

Conclusion

Parmelee, A.H.: Sensory stimulation in the nursery: how much and when? Dev. Behav. Pediatr. **6**:242, 1985.

Turkewitz, G., and Kenny, P.A.: The role of developmental limitations of sensory input on sensory/perceptual organization, Dev. Behav. Pediatr. **6**:302, 1985.

CHAPTER 27

Central nervous system disturbances

PART ONE

Assessment of neonatal neurologic function

THE IMMATURE BRAIN

The stage of brain development in the newborn is dependent on gestational age. The birth process or extrauterine life does not appear to significantly influence the rate of growth of the developing brain. Thus determination of the level of neurologic function must be made in relation to both gestational and chronologic age.

The nervous system is a heterogeneous organ with differing regional rates of growth and development. Differentiation and development of the brain are continuing at the time of birth. Myelination shows striking regional differences in rates of development and is still far from complete at 40 weeks' gestation. It is, however, much more advanced in the temporal lobes, midbrain, brainstem, spinal cord, and peripheral nerves than in the cerebral hemispheres. In the term neonate, dendritic sprouting and arborization are continuing, with the ongoing formation of interneuronal excitatory and inhibitory synaptic connections. The inhibitory synaptic connections are more numerous at this time than the excitatory ones.

The pluripotential cells originate in the germinal matrix of the developing brain, a very active cellular area located along the ventricular system, and migrate outward to populate the six layers of the cortex. The developing fetus has most of its neurons by 18 to 20 weeks' gestation. After this time reabsorption of this very vascular germinal area begins. This is usually completed by 35 to 36 weeks' gestation.

The brain capillaries are unique because of the presence of tight junctions; decreased numbers of pinocytotic vesicles; specific plasma membrane carriers; increased numbers of mitochondria, which can oxidize several different fuels, producing large amounts of ATP; and a tough basement membrane for protection of the capillaries during various types of stress. Although more information is being acquired about these unique characteristics, it is known that the basement membrane from isolated capillaries of developing animal brain is one fourth the thickness of that from capillaries of adult brain. The minimum capillary basement membrane may be one of the factors contributing to the occurrence of subependymal and intraventricular hemorrhage in the preterm infant.

The physiology of neuronal membranes in the newborn indicates that the neuronal pumps are less efficient and the cell membranes more leaky than later in development. Cerebral metabolism of the newborn differs from that of the older child. The newborn is far more resistant to anoxia than the older infant and seems better able to use both ketone bodies and anaerobic glycolysis as energy sources.

Since subcortical structures of the nervous system have a higher state of development both morphologically and neurophysiologically than cortical structures, information derived from the neonatal neurologic examination reflects primarily the functional status of subcortical structures. There is, however, increasing evidence of the neonate's cortical function as manifested by rudimentary learning ability and ability to integrate sensory stimuli (Chapter 26).

NEUROLOGIC ASSESSMENT

An optimum clinical neonatal neurologic assessment includes the following.

A. History
   1. Parental history
   2. Obstetric history
      a. Past pregnancy outcome
      b. Present obstetric history
         (1) Prenatal
         (2) Intrapartum
      c. Neonatal history

B. General pediatric examination
  1. Gestational age
  2. Head size and shape
  3. Cranial sutures
  4. Fontanels
  5. Transillumination of skull
  6. Bruit
  7. Facies
  8. Minor anomalies
  9. Eye
  10. Hepatosplenomegaly
  11. Skin lesions
  12. Back
  13. Odor
  14. Contractures

C. Neurologic examination
  1. Level of consciousness
  2. Motor system
    a. Posture
    b. Tone
    c. Strength
    d. Movements
  3. Reflexes
  4. Sensory system
  5. Cranial nerve tests
    a. Fix and follow: II, III, IV, VI, cortex
    b. Pupillary response: II, III
    c. Doll's eye: III, IV, VI, medial longitudinal fasciculus, VIII
    d. Suck: V, VII, XII
    e. Swallow: IX, X

D. Interpretation
  1. Low risk
  2. High risk
  3. Suspect

The general mechanics of performing this assessment are explained in the following section.

History

A detailed account of the parental, obstetric, and neonatal histories is necessary for a systematic evaluation of the neonatal nervous system. Parental history should include both parents' age, race, and familial diseases, as well as the mother's medical history.

A complete obstetric history should include information regarding the present pregnancy and details of all previous pregnancies and their outcome. The present obstetric history should include details of both the prenatal and intrapartum course, with complete information regarding any bleeding, infections during pregnancy, or maternal drug exposure.

Knowledge of the length of time the Apgar score was less than 3, along with information about methods of resuscitation, is essential. Data of particular note following resuscitation are the times elapsed until return of heart rate, onset of respiration, and reappearance of normal tone.

The neonatal history should include detailed information of the nursery course. Particularly relevant clinical events include seizures, cyanotic spells, apneic episodes, diminished or absent crying, distinct or prolonged episodes of hypotonia, and/or decreased activity, poor suck, and prolonged requirement for gavage feedings. The length and severity of any of these findings during a neonate's hospital course should be documented because they could be important in identifying an infant who may be at risk for subsequent abnormal development or who may require special follow-up.

General pediatric examination

The general pediatric examination is described in Chapter 24, part one. Particular findings in the general examination are of special importance from the neurologic standpoint. The head should be examined for size, shape, status of anterior fontanel, and evidence of any trauma such as cephalhematoma or fractures. Cranial bruits should be listened for, especially in a newborn with congestive heart failure in the first 24 hours of life. Peculiar facies, associated with over 300 specific syndromes or other designated minor anomalies, should be identified, since the central nervous system frequently is involved with a generalized malformation. If three or more minor anomalies are identified, the chances of a major internal anomaly occurring is approximately 90% (Chapter 17). The examination of the eyes is described in the discussion of cranial nerve II (Chapter 39). Of particular importance from the neurologic standpoint is evidence of skin lesions, such as the vesicles of congenital herpes, petechiae, cutaneous lesions of other TORCH agents, hemangioma of Sturge-Weber disease, pigmented lesions of neurofibromatosis, the pale nevi of tuberous sclerosis, or the vesicles of incontinentia pigmenti (Chapter 38). Hepatosplenomegaly may occur in diseases that also involve the nervous system, such as encephalitis secondary to infection with one of the TORCH agents. Abnormalities of the back should be identified, including the appearance of a small dermal sinus or tuft of hair, which may indicate either a direct channel to the subarachnoid space from the skin or a significant abnormality of the lumbosacral spinal column. Abnormalities in hair texture and swirls may be associated with underlying neurologic disorders. The particular smell of a neonate or his urine may lead to suspicion of aminoaciduria. The location and extent of joint contractures present at birth are important to document. Fixed contractures of joints at birth, known specifically as arthrogryposis multiplex congenita, indicate a syndrome that is usually secondary to disease of the nervous system at some level but in some patients may be secondary to joint disease.

Neurologic examination

Since the functional state of the neonatal nervous system is influenced by both exogenous and endogenous factors unrelated to disease, these must be considered if an accurate neurologic assessment is to be obtained. An infant examined in the immediate postprandial state is usually sleepy, with decreased responsiveness, and may be hypotonic as well as hyporeflexic. That same infant examined just before a feeding may be crying, irritable, hypertonic, hyperreflexic, and jittery. The optimum time to examine an infant in relation to feedings is approximately 1 to 2 hours afterward. A second major factor that can affect the functional state of the neonate's nervous system is the ambient temperature of the examining room or the temperature of the neonate. Since hypothermia can cause depression and hyperthermia can result in irritability, the infant is best examined in thermal neutrality. The third factor that may alter reflexes and responsiveness is the infant's state of consciousness. The infant is best examined in the quiet alert state (Chapter 26). The fourth factor is the gestational age of the infant, which is best documented by maternal history and a combination of physical and neurologic criteria during the first days of life. It is important to grade the functional status of the neonate's nervous system in relation to the gestational age, not the chronologic age of the neonate. The fifth factor that can influence the findings of the neurologic examination is the degree of illness of the infant. In severely ill neonates a generalized depression of the nervous system may be present. In addition, there may be limitations on examining sick infants when they are in incubators, when they are being mechanically ventilated, or when they are connected to multiple monitors with several catheters in place. One must be willing to examine and reexamine a neonate to confirm the presence of significant abnormalities.

Level of consciousness

An altered state of consciousness is a major sign of neonatal neurologic impairment. The level of consciousness is determined by an evaluation of spontaneous activity and response to stimulation. Since this is affected by sleep state, it is best to test the infant in the quiet alert state for documentation of optimum function of the central nervous system (Chapter 26). The neonate's level of consciousness can be divided into five levels ranging from normal to abnormal. The neonate is said to be normal when, in the quiet alert state, the arms and legs are flexed and nonstereotyped symmetric spontaneous activity is exhibited. The second level is the hyperalert state, identified in a neonate who does not sleep for extended periods of time during the first 24 hours. The eyes are wide open, possibly with a decreased blinking response and a decreased ability to fixate and follow. Although the activity level may be normal or decreased, it may appear increased because of the increased threshold to all types of tactile, auditory, visual, and proprioceptive stimuli. The third level is lethargy, which can be of variable degree. There is a decrease in spontaneous activity, although the threshold for responsiveness may be increased as just mentioned. Even though responses are delayed, a complete repertoire of responses to stimulation occurs. The fourth level is stupor, when the infant's responses are limited to withdrawal of an extremity or decerebrate posturing in response only to strong noxious stimuli. Corneal and gag reflexes are absent, and respiratory rhythm may be abnormal. The fifth level is coma, with no respone to external stimuli. In the neonate this is a relatively rare state, since the spinal withdrawal reflexes are almost never abolished. This state may be observed in infants on respirators who have had severe intraventricular hemorrhage.

Motor system

Posture. Observation of posture should be performed both before and after removing the neonates from the crib or incubator and undressing them (Fig. 27-1). Even if the neonate cannot be moved, such as when on a ventilator, much can be gained from observation of posture. When posture is evaluated, it is imperative to recognize the changes that occur with gestational age. With increasing age the infant's extremities normally begin to assume a much more flexed position (Chapter 26).

Abnormalities of posture at rest include asymmetry between sides, as seen in the infant with a brachial plexus lesion; asymmetries between arms and legs, as seen with a spinal cord lesion; the frog-leg position with hips completely abducted and knees flexed, following severe asphyxia, with severe systemic disease, or with neuromuscular disease producing hypotonia or paralysis; and head retraction and extensor posturing, which may occur with intracranial hemorrhage, hypoxic ischemic encephalopathy, or meningitis. The cortical thumb (a closed hand with the thumb inside the fingers) can be a normal position of the neonate's hand (Fig. 27-2). This position, however, is not obligatory, and the neonate will periodically open the hand and extend the thumb. An obligatory cortical thumb is an early sign of abnormal corticospinal tract function in the infant.

Tone. Muscle tone can be assessed by using the same maneuvers used in the gestational age assessment of the Dubowitz examination, including arm and leg recoil, popliteal angle, wrist-arm angle, foot dorsiflexion, hip flexion, shoulder adduction (scarf sign), head lag, and position in ventral suspension (Chapter 24, part one).

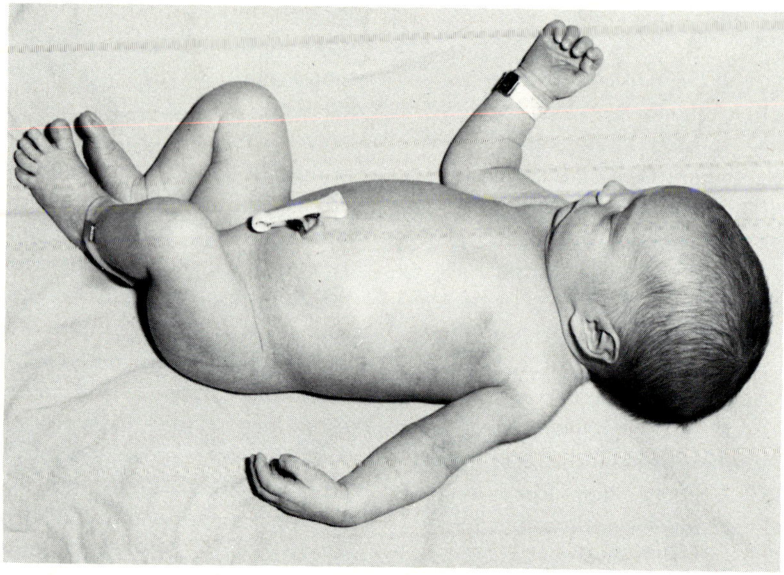

Fig. 27-1. Normal term newborn at rest. Note that the posture of the arms and legs is asymmetric. The arms are usually partially flexed; the legs are flexed at the knees and hips. Contrast this with the hypotonic infant, Fig. 27-20.

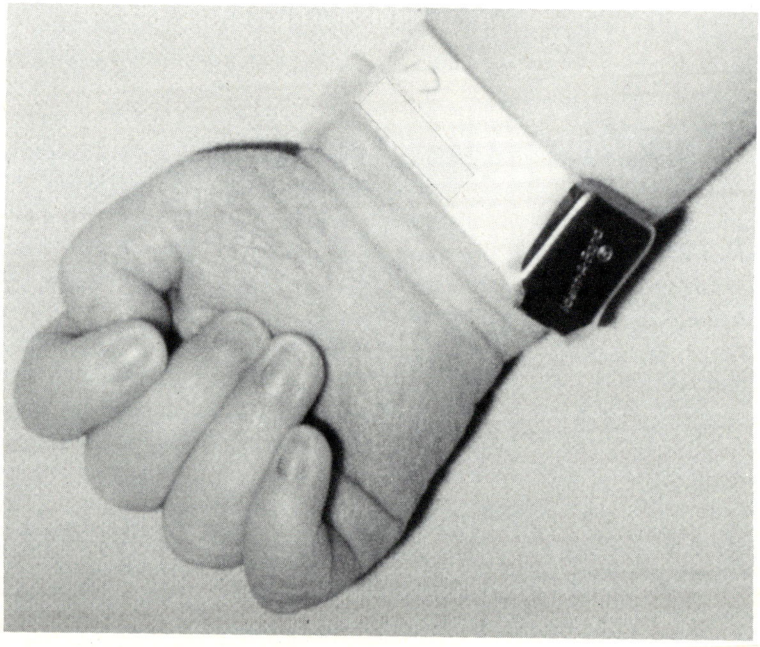

Fig. 27-2. The cortical thumb (fisting) in which the thumb is tightly enclosed within the clenched fingers. This is a common finding in the newborn but should not be present persistently. The infant should open his hand periodically (see Fig. 27-1 of the same infant). *Persistent* symmetric or asymmetric fisting is abnormal at any age and often is the earliest sign of cortical spinal tract damage.

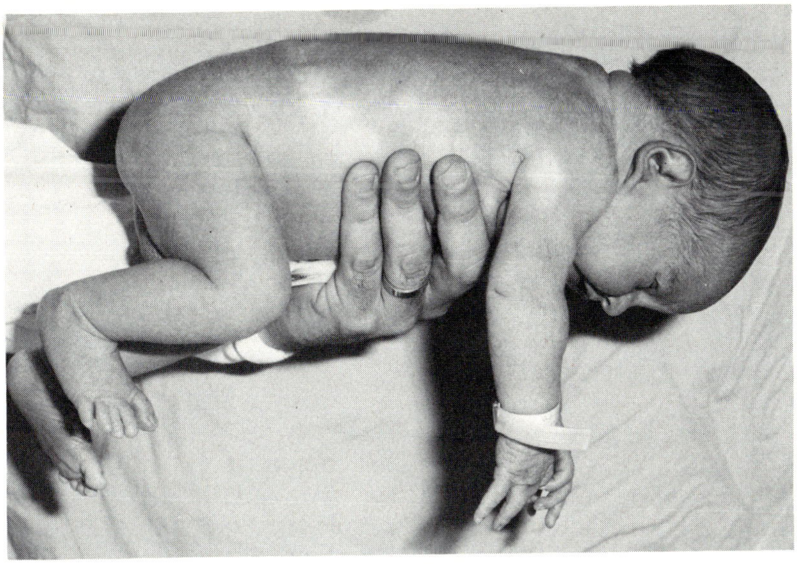

Fig. 27-3. Ventral suspension of the normal term newborn. Note the flexion of the hip and knee, the slight dorsiflexion of the back, and the momentary ability to support the head. Contrast this with the hypotonic infant in Fig. 27-19.

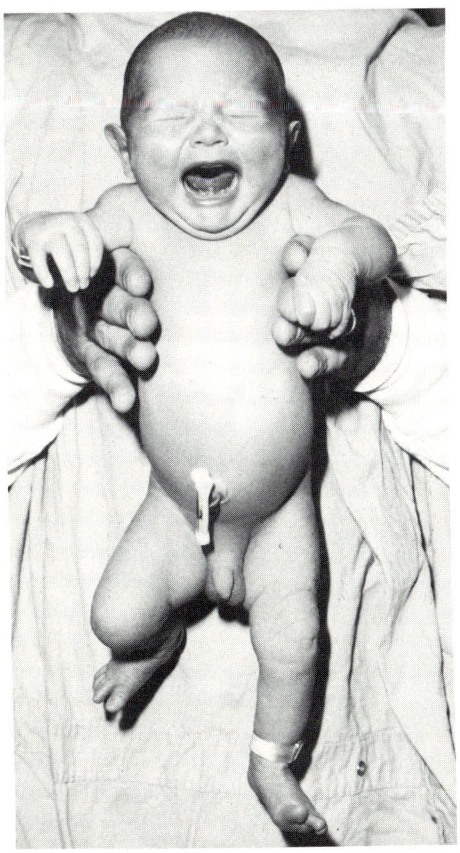

Fig. 27-4. Normal term newborn in upright suspension. Most of the baby's weight is supported by the resistance of the infant's arms. There is no tendency to slide through the examiner's fingers. The examiner is not holding the child around the chest.

The examiner must consider the gestational age of the infant when attempting to determine whether the tone is reduced, normal, or increased. A neonate with poor head control may be considered normal, for example, if the baby is a preterm infant rather than a small for gestational age term infant.

An example of ventral suspension is seen in Fig. 27-3. The baby of 40 to 42 weeks should dorsiflex the back with some elevation of head; feet and legs remain flexed. Hypotonia, weakness, or cerebral depression may produce a baby who looks like a limp dishrag. Upright suspension with the baby supported by the examiner's hands under the arms (Fig. 27-4) provides good estimation of both tone and strength in the shoulder girdle, since an infant with decreased tone or strength can slip through the examiner's hands. Tone also can be assessed by movement of individual joints.

Strength. Strength and weakness are related to the state of alertness, to gestational age, or to problems in the central or peripheral nervous system, as well as in the muscles. Testing muscle strength is difficult in a newborn infant, and differentiating between muscle weakness and hypotonia may be impossible, since neonates who are weak usually are hypotonic or floppy. However, an adequate screening test of strength in the upper extremities and neck is achieved through a test of the neonate's grasp. The examiner's finger is inserted into the lateral aspect of the neonate's palm, eliciting a reflex palmar grasp. With strong stimulation the strength in the hand in association with this grasp in the normal newborn should be sufficiently strong to partially support the infant's weight as he is lifted from the supine to sitting

A

B

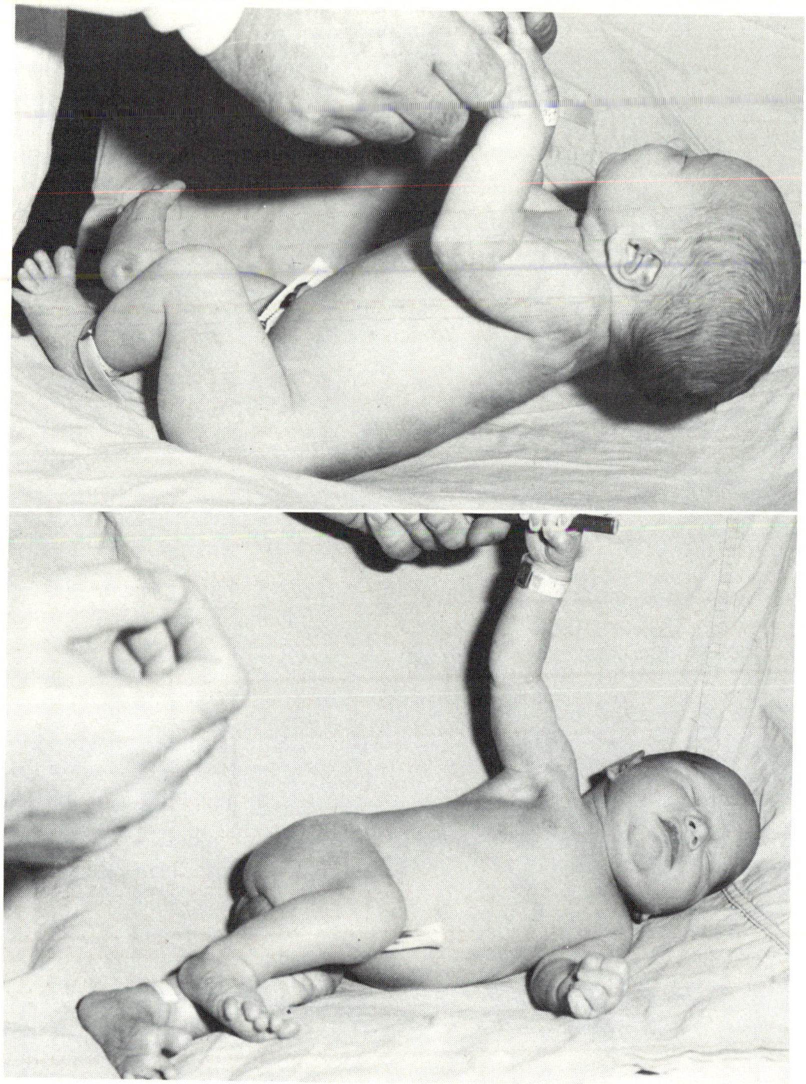

Fig. 27-5. A, Strength may be assessed by lifting the supine infant from the table. The observer's fingers are grasped by the infant; the strength of the grasp, contraction of the biceps, the shoulder girdle, and even the anterior neck muscles are seen and felt. Note this normal newborn's lack of head lag. **B,** An alternative method of testing strength in either arm is shown in this illlustration. The infant is grasping a pencil. Note the tight grip and contraction of biceps as well as of the trapezius and pectorals. The infant can almost be lifted from the sheet.

position. As the neonate is pulled up, the observer should feel contractions in the biceps and the shoulder girdle and some contraction in the sternomastoids, preventing the head from completely falling back (Fig. 27-5). Strength in the lower extremities can be assessed by observing the supporting response, the ability of the newborn to support his weight when the feet are placed on the examining table. Stepping, placing, and the crossed extensor reflexes also may be used to assess strength; asymmetries of strength should be noted.

Observations of the quality of spontaneous movements and movements that can be elicited in response to pinprick stimulation can give considerable information about strength of specific muscle groups. This information is important in localizing the level of a lesion of the spinal cord (Part five).

Movements. Observation of an infant before being touched may reveal a variety of movements. The quantity of spontaneous movement can vary in a range from excessive to decreased. The pattern of movement observed in a normal infant during spontaneous activity can be characterized as random, symmetric, nonstereotyped movements involving all extremities.

In addition to patterned movements, the neonate may have movements that are characterized as either tremors or jitteriness or seizures. Since neonatal seizures are often caused by treatable conditions that, if left untreated, will cause brain damage, it is important to identify and differentiate an infant with this type of activity from an infant who may simply have tremor or jitteriness. Seizures can take various forms, and it should be noted that almost any bizarre alterations of the state of the neonate may represent a seizure. The usual difficulty occurs in distinguishing seizure activity manifested by generalized symmetric tonic-clonic movements from the classic tremulous movements or jitteriness. A few distinguishing clinical features can be helpful. Generalized symmetric tonic-clonic movements are a relatively uncommon manifestation of neonatal seizures. The rhythmic movements of jitteriness or tremors that do not reflect any seizure activity characteristically have equal amplitude without a fast and slow component, as do the tonic-clonic movements of seizures. In a susceptible neonate, jitteriness or tremors are characteristically stimulus sensitive, easily provoked by external stimuli such as a Moro reflex, noise, or simple handling, whereas seizures are not. The movements of tremors or jitteriness usually can be stopped by the examiner passively fixing the affected limb.

The specific causes of seizures are discussed in the section on seizures (Part four). Frequently, abnormalities that cause seizures may also produce jitteriness or tremors. Tremors of high frequency and low amplitude may occur with hypoglycemia or hypocalcemia or in an otherwise normal infant and may disappear within the first week of life. Low-frequency, high-amplitude tremors are often seen in infants who have excessive activity or a low threshold Moro reflex but who are otherwise normal. Coarse tremors occur as a sign of drug withdrawal in infants of addicted mothers (Chapter 37, part four).

Reflexes. The reflexes found to be the most useful in an initial neurologic assessment include the Moro reflex, the tonic neck reflex, the placing and stepping response, sucking, the classic deep tendon reflexes, and palmar or plantar grasp. A multitude of other neonatal reflexes have been described that, although interesting, have limited value in the clinical evaluation of the nervous system. Reflexes are primarily useful when there is a consistent asymmetry identified in association with abnormal findings gained from evaluation of tone, strength, posture, and movement. A reflex also can be useful in indicating CNS dysfunction if it is either obligatory or does not habituate. When either of these two conditions occurs, a sign of CNS dysfunction has been identified. Finally, the absence of these commonly used neonatal reflexes is indicative of abnormal neurologic function.

Sensory system

The primary sensation tested is the neonate's response to superficial pain. To optimally evaluate this sensory modality, the examiner must have the infant in a relatively quiet and preferably alert state. Testing of sensation is most important when one suspects a spinal cord, nerve root, plexus, or peripheral nerve lesion or wants to delineate the sensory level in an infant with a meningomyelocele. Fig. 27-6 is the classic adult dermatome pattern extrapolated to infants and indicates the association of specific motor responses to stimuli. The nerve conduction time in both peripheral nerves and spinal cord is greatly delayed in the newborn; with a pin, a delay as long as 2 or 3 seconds may occur before the infant responds, if he perceives the stimulus. Perception of sensory stimuli by the infant can be manifested by crying, grimacing, alteration in respiratory pattern, or change in level of consciousness or possibly in color. Withdrawal of the extremity is a local reflex phenomenon that does not, by itself, necessarily imply that the sensory stimulus has reached cortical awareness. The truncal incurvation reflex (GALANT) has little value as generally applied; however, it is segmentally innervated. Local stimulation of one area of the trunk may produce local trunk incurvation, indicating that the segmental arc is intact. Therefore this reflex may be helpful in localizing a spinal cord injury.

Cranial nerves

All the cranial nerves of a neonate can be examined easily by modifying the common neurologic examination or by making deductions from neonatal responses involving cranial nerves.

Cranial nerve I. The olfactory nerve can be examined in the neonate but special procedures are required. This examination is not done during the screening examination, since its dysfunction is only rarely associated with neurologic disease in the neonate.

Cranial nerve II. Vision can be tested readily in the neonate (Chapter 26), and its presence indicates that the entire visual system is intact, including the existence of a functional occipital cortex. Blinking in response to a light stimulus indicates only that the visual system is intact to the level of the superior colliculi but is not evidence of visual cortex function. Presence of vision is tested by observing the neonate fix on an object such as the human face, and follow it through an arc of approximately 60 degrees. Since the neonate is myopic, the test object should be placed within 10 to 12 inches of the infant's face. This test should be included in the neurologic screening assessment of all neonates. A more

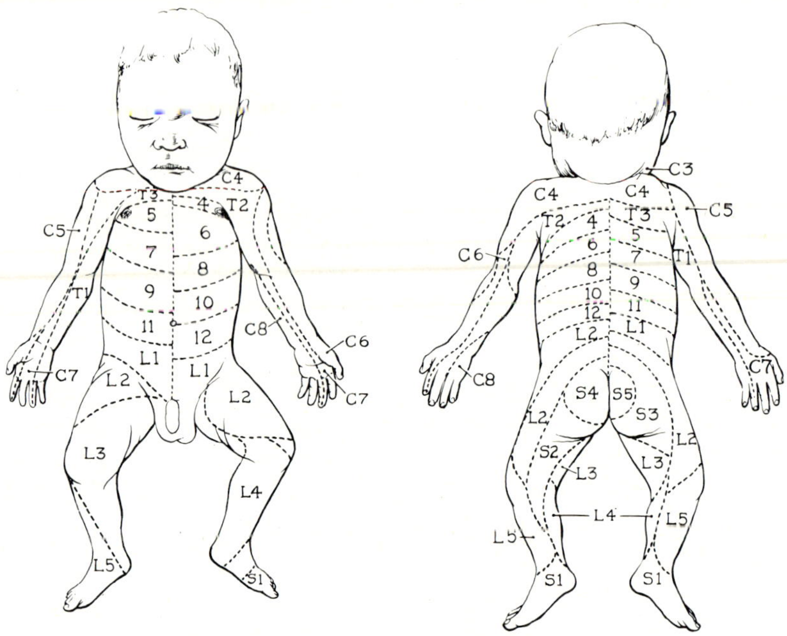

Fig. 27-6. Sensory dermatomes extrapolated from the adult to the infant. As noted on the two sides of the infant, there is considerable overlap of sensory innervation.

refined examination of vision to determine visual acuity consists of producing opticokinetic nystagmus (Chapter 39). A large drum with black and white stripes of varying widths is moved in front of the neonate's eyes. This usually should produce some following movements of the eyes and occasionally nystagmus back in the opposite direction. With gradations of distance and width of stripes on the drum, visual acuity can be estimated.

The remaining part of the evaluation of cranial nerve II involves a thorough evaluation of the external characteristics of the eye and a funduscopic examination. The external eye findings that may be associated with diseases of the nervous system include cataracts, cloudy cornea, irregular shape or asymmetric size of the pupil, vascular hemangioma of the sclera, and microphthalmos. Funduscopic examination is difficult but extremely rewarding, since this is the only chance for the examiner to see actual nerve cells. The ophthalmoscope should be set at −2 to −4 diopters for the best visualization of the optic fundus. Optic disc pallor may be a normal feature, so-called pseudooptic atrophy of the newborn. Retinal hemorrhages, reported to occur in 8% to 50% of neonates, are not always associated with significant neurologic abnormalities; however, subhyaloid hemorrhages usually are associated with subdural hematomas in the infant. Retinal lesions of chorioretinitis secondary to toxoplasmosis, cytomegalovirus, rubella, or syphilis are seen only rarely in the neonatal period, as are fungal balls secondary to *Candida* infection.

Cranial nerves III, IV, and VI. The third cranial nerve must be intact for normal pupil function. The pupils should be equal and respond to light even at 28 to 30 weeks of gestation. The optimum functioning of cranial nerves III, IV, and VI, connected via the medial longitudinal fasciculus, can be assessed by watching the conjugate eye movements while an infant is fixating and following. In addition, conjugate eye movements can be evaluated during the observation of normal doll's eye movement, assessed by holding and rotating the infant at arm's length in an upright posture. This rotation stimulates the semicircular canals, and the impulses travel through the vestibular portion of cranial nerve VIII to the brainstem via the medial longitudinal fasciculus and innervate cranial nerves III and VI. This stimulation causes the eye to tonically deviate away from the direction of the rotation. Rotation should be performed in both directions. When it is impossible to rotate the neonate as mentioned, the semicircular canals may be stimulated by introducing cold water into the ear canal. In this maneuver the eyes deviate to the side of the cold water. When the eyes remain in a fixed position regardless of stimulation or head movement, serious brainstem dysfunction is usually present. A loss of doll's eye movement can be seen when an excessive amount of barbiturates has been administered. A repetitive failure of the eye to move in a single direction should be noted and considered abnormal. Dysconjugate eye movements with some nystagmoid movements may not be uncommon during these maneuvers when they are performed during the first 3 weeks of life. However, when there is a repetitive failure of movement of the eyes in a single direction, persistent dysconjugate eye movements, or continuous nystagmus at rest, significant neurologic dysfunction is present.

Cranial nerves V, VII, IX, X, XI, and XII. The sensory portion of the fifth cranial nerve can be tested by eliciting the corneal reflex or using a pinprick on the face and watching for grimacing movements. In some observers' experience the corneal reflex is not a reliable test of sensation in the newborn. The motor function of cranial nerve V is judged to be intact if the infant can close the mouth through effective masseter strength. The other cranial nerves that must be intact for an effective suck to occur are cranial nerve VII for pursing of the lips and cranial nerve XII for the milking action of the tongue. The observation of effective swallowing indicates adequate function of cranial nerves IX and X. The function of cranial nerve XI can be estimated by visualization of the sternocleidomastoid muscle when the infant is held in the supine position. There should be an ability to maintain the head in an extended position for brief periods of time. Presence of any mass in the sternocleidomastoid muscle, such as a hematoma, can be observed at this time.

Cranial nerve VIII. Examination of the vestibular portion of cranial nerve VIII has been mentioned under the sections on cranial nerves III, IV, and VI. Examination of the auditory portion of this nerve can be tested in the newborn only in a gross fashion. Auditory evoked potential using electroencephalography now can be used for more accurate testing. At the bedside, evidence of the infant's hearing can be assessed by using a graded noise stimulus. This can be in the form of either an electrical noisemaker giving a graded noise or simply a small hand bell. To confirm whether the infant hears the noise, observations of the infant being alerted from sleep or being quieted if awake can be taken as evidence that the neonate hears. Repeated examinations may be necessary, since there may be a lack of response or a variable response of the neonate to the noise stimulus.

Hearing screening. The importance of screening for hearing loss in early infancy is gaining wide recognition, particularly as the incidence of congenital hearing loss becomes more apparent. Screening procedures implemented within the hospital nursery involve the detection of either a behavioral or an electrophysiologic response of the infant to a sound stimulus. Mass experimental auditory screening of neonates has revealed an expected incidence of approximately 1 in 50 deaf infants in the intensive care nursery. The first of these methods to gain wide acceptance, as well as support by the Joint Committee on Infant Hearing Screening, is a seven-item high-risk register. This well-researched and established register identifies infants at risk for hearing loss by means of history and physical examination. However, actual audiologic testing takes place only on a follow-up basis after hospital discharge. Application of a protocol using an arousal response criterion during the infant's light sleep state has also been recommended by the Joint Committee on Infant Hearing Screening, as a supplement to the seven-item high-risk register. However, a recently developed automated screening system, the Crib-O-Gram, is rapidly becoming the behavioral test method of choice. It uses a motion-sensing transducer placed beneath the infant's mattress, which detects changes in neonatal motor activity coincident with the introduction of a calibrated sound stimulus. These changes are entirely integrated, analyzed, and scored by computer algorithms, thus permitting greater objectivity, ease of presentation, and usage than any other method currently available. The Brainstem Evoked Response (BER) technique is the only one of several electrophysiologic test methods (i.e., electrocochleography, respiratory responses, cardiovascular responses) found adequate for screening purposes. Clinical application of BER measurement has been demonstrated in premature infants, wherein consistent responses may be obtained without sedation in quiet infants. Additionally, limited muscle activity, vigilance, and sleep state have shown negligible effects on the response. Many of the abnormalities detected by screening BER are transient. The screening method of choice ultimately should be dictated by the individual facility, available personnel, and number of infants to be served. However, any protocol is effective only when implemented as part of an overall program that also incorporates a longitudinal follow-up approach.

Interpretation of the neurologic assessment

The neurologic assessment is particularly valuable when used to detect treatable diseases, to diagnose specific neurologic disorders, and to assess gestational age. The use of the neurologic assessment for the prognostic identification of neonates at risk for later abnormal development must be interpreted with caution, except in situations where multiple unequivocal signs indicate severe damage. Data suggest that the developing nervous system has the capacity for reorganization of connections following certain kinds of injury. This may account for some of our inability to prognosticate accurately from abnormal neurologic signs found in the neonatal period.

Data and extensive past experience permit some definitive statements regarding the association between some abnormal neonatal neurologic signs and the later appearance of cerebral palsy, mental retardation, and epilepsy. These include:

1. The full-term neonate with a negative family history, a negative prenatal, intrapartum, and neonatal history, a normal neurologic and pediatric examination,

and a negative metabolic screen has a negligible chance of subsequent abnormal neurologic development related to perinatal causes.

2. Signs of neurologic dysfunction occur in a full-term neonate who has acute damage to a previously normal nervous system. A neonate with long-standing absence of a part of the nervous system may not show signs of neurologic dysfunction.
3. Certain neurologic signs, even though infrequent in their occurrence, have considerable predictive power for later abnormal neurologic function and include persistent abnormalities in tone, especially hypotonia; diminished level of activity; weak cry for more than 24 hours; and an inability to suck, requiring gavage feedings. Each of these signs carries a 10-fold to 20-fold increased risk of the subsequent development of cerebral palsy. A neonate with an Apgar score of 3 or less at 10 minutes or neonatal seizures, especially if associated with intrapartum asphyxia or trauma, has a greater than 50-fold increased risk for subsequent development of cerebral palsy.
4. Combinations of signs are more significant than a single abnormality.
5. The total duration of the presence of an abnormal neurologic sign does not necessarily add to or detract from its significance. Clear-cut signs of neurologic dysfunction may be present only a few days and then disappear, with the child later developing signs of frank neurologic dysfunction as development progresses.
6. Unequivocal signs of neurologic dysfunction will appear in the first 7 days of life in a normal full-term neonate who has sustained, during the intrapartum period, a CNS insult severe enough to lead to long-term neurologic sequalae.
7. Assymmetric signs are usually more significant than symmetrical findings, not so much in helping to localize the area of brain involved but simply in indicating that an underlying abnormality exists.
8. Signs of neurologic dysfunction occurring in the presence of identifiable neuropathologic lesions are more predictive of subsequent neurologic abnormality than signs with no association to a demonstrable brain lesion.
9. A neonate with signs of neurologic dysfunction at time of discharge has a 50-fold increased risk of having subsequent abnormal neurologic development.

There is a need for further development of more sophisticated, noninvasive techniques for identifying pathologic changes in the fetal and neonatal brain, thus facilitating more accurate neonatal clinicoNeuropathologic correlation and enhanced predictability of long-term sequelae from the findings of the neonatal neurologic examination.

At discharge an updated complete neurologic assessment should be done, including a neurologic examination, a review of previous signs of neurologic dysfunction, and any specific laboratory or roentgenologic data relative to the nervous system. At that time the neonate should be placed in one of three categories (low risk, high risk, or suspect) regarding risk for subsequent delayed or abnormal development. This designation is for the purpose of planning for the child's optimum health supervision, specifically for detection of developmental delays. As stimulation programs are evaluated and deemed useful, the entry of a child into one of these programs is best done when the child first shows delayed development.

The use of findings from the neonatal neurologic assessment to counsel parents about the risks of subsequent abnormal neurologic development requires considerable discretion. The physician must be honest with the parents but should not destroy all hope, since the ultimate functional state of the child cannot be predicted accurately from the neonatal discharge examination. Moreover, most children with significant neurologic dysfunction are cared for at home during their early years of life. Overt motor dysfunction, secondary to brain insult during the intrapartum or neonatal periods, will appear during the child's first 3 years of life. With optimum health supervision this child can be helped to maximize assets and minimize deficits.

NONINVASIVE DIAGNOSTIC TOOLS

Transillumination

See Part five.

Ultrasonography

The use of ultrasound scans has been a major advance in the definition of normal intracranial anatomy and identification of intracranial pathology. The principles of ultrasonography and its use in the early evaluation of anatomic structures within the brain are discussed in Chapter 12. In the postnatal period, ultrasound has been used most extensively to identify various degrees of subependymal/intraventricular hemorrhage and provides excellent data on the degree and distribution of ventricular dilation. In addition to the fact that the instrument is portable, the major advantages of ultrasonography include the apparent safety of the pulsed ultrasonic waves and the relatively low cost. A real-time sector scanner—handled by highly experienced personnel—applied over the skin of the anterior fontanel can provide excellent coronal and sagittal views of the brain that may be at least as reliable as computed axial tomography (CT) scanning in the identification of both small and large subependymal, intraventricular, and intracerebral hemorrhages. However, CT scans may be preferable for subarachnoid bleeding and indentification of intracranial calcifications.

Computed axial tomography

CT scanning affords an excellent means of identifying the site and extent of neonatal intraventricular hemorrhage. In addition, the size of ventricles and the presence of major parenchymal lesions also may be defined. However, despite the undeniable value of the procedure, it does require moving an infant who is often in a precarious state with regard to maintenance of ventilation, perfusion, temperature, and metabolic status. Moreover, the long-term effects of the radiation exposure from multiple studies remain unknown. Thus, when portable ultrasound is available, the need for a CT scan is diminished considerably (Chapter 13).

Intracranial pressure monitoring

A variety of catheters and pressure transducers have been developed for measuring neonatal intracranial pressure (ICP). These techniques are useful for monitoring an infant's ICP under special circumstances, such as hydrocephalus, brain tumors, and trauma. However, their invasive nature precludes their use in other clinical circumstances where they are needed and may be of similar clinical value.

In neonates the open anterior fontanel provides a unique site for noninvasive ICP assessment. Measurements of anterior fontanel pressure (AFP) can be obtained by applying a small, flat surface-pressure transducer directly on the fontanel; this can be accomplished alternatively by using a fluid-filled system connected to a pressure transducer or using a transducer containing a photoelectric detector and an activated bellows (Chapter 24, part three).

AFP measurements have been compared to the manometric pressure of CSF obtained at the time of lumbar and ventricular punctures in humans and to ventricular pressure in experimental animals. These comparisons have demonstrated positive correlation between ventricular or CSF pressures and AFP. AFP measurement has advantages over the invasive techniques, since penetration of the dural barrier is not required, thus preventing infection and inadvertent CSF loss. The precise diagnostic role of AFP measurements in preterm infants at risk for intracranial hemorrhage or raised intracranial pressure remains to be determined.

Doppler measurement of cerebral blood flow velocity

The study of cerebral blood flow (CBF) velocity by external Doppler technique may offer a new noninvasive tool to gain information related to changes in cerebral hemodynamics. This has been assessed from changes in pulsatile flow in the anterior cerebral arteries using an ultrasonic transducer placed on the anterior fontanel. Proper recording requires exact standards concerning beam angulation and type of transducer. The Doppler technique measures the shift in frequency of an incoming ultrasound beam created in large part by the movement of red blood cells under the instrument. The resultant changes in pulsatile flow calculated from Doppler frequency shifts have been expressed primarily as pulsatility index measurements. Preliminary data with this technique have demonstrated altered cerebral blood flow patterns during asphyxia, at the time of pneumothorax, and in association with left-to-right shunting through a patent ductus arteriosus.

Perlman and associates found an increased incidence of intraventricular hemorrhage in premature infants (<1,500 gm) when an abnormal fluctuating pattern of cerebral blood flow velocity was demonstrated by Doppler ultrasonography. Furthermore, they determined that paralysis with pancuronium (Pavulon) decreased the incidence of intraventricular hemorrhage in this high-risk group of infants. The cause of the fluctuating cerebral blood flow pattern as yet is unknown but may be related to the infants' expiratory efforts against the ventilator. General use of this technique to prevent intraventricular hemorrhage must await confirming studies, as well as more commonly available alternative methods for evaluating cerebral blood flow (Chapter 28, part four).

Alfred W. Brann, Jr.
James F. Schwartz

BIBLIOGRAPHY

Neonatal neurologic assessment

American Speech and Hearing Association, American Academy of Ophthalmology and Otolaryngology, and American Academy of Pediatrics: Supplementary statement of Joint Committee on Infant Hearing Screening, A.S.H.A. **16**:160, 1974.

Clark, D.B.: Abnormal neurologic signs in the neonate: physical diagnosis of the newly born. In Kay, J., editor: Report of the Forty-Sixth Ross Conference on Pediatric Research, 1964.

Dubowitz, L.M.S., Dubowitz, V., and Goldberg, C.: Clinical assessment of gestational age in the newborn, J. Pediatr. **77**:1, 1970.

Hogan, G.R., and Ryan, N.J.: Neurological evaluation of the newborn, Clin. Perinatol. **4**:31, 1977.

Illingworth, R.S.: The development of the infant and young child: normal and abnormal, ed. 4, Baltimore, 1970, The William & Wilkins Co.

McFarland, W.H., Simmons, F.B., and Jones, F.R.: An automated hearing screening technique for newborns, J. Speech Hearing Disorders **45**:495, 1980.

Nelson, K.B., and Ellenberg, J.H.: Neonatal signs as predictors of cerebral palsy, Pediatrics **64**:225, 1979.

Parmalee, A.H., and others: Neurological evaluation of the premature infant, Biol. Neonate **15**:65, 1970.

Prechtl, H.: Prognostic values of neurological signs, Proc. R. Soc. Med. **58**:3, 1965.

Prechtl, H., and Bientema, D.: The neurological examination of the full term newborn infant. In Clinics in developmental medicine, no. 12, London, England, 1964, William Heinemann Ltd.

Schulman-Galambos, C., and Galambos, H.: Brainstem auditory evoked responses in premature infants, J. Speech Hearing Res. **18**:456, 1975.

Thorne, I.: Cerebral symptoms in the newborn, Acta Paediatr. Scand. (Suppl.) **9**:15, 1969.

Noninvasive diagnostic tools

Bada, H.S., and others: Noninvasive diagnosis of neonatal asphyxia and intraventricular hemorrhage by Doppler ultrasound, J. Pediatr. **95**:775, 1979.

Bejar, R., and others: Diagnosis and follow-up of intraventricular and intracerebral hemorrhages by ultrasound studies of infant's brain through the fontanelles and sutures, Pediatrics **66**:661, 1980.

Hill, A., and Volpe, J.J.: Measurement of intracranial pressure using the Ladd intracranial pressure monitor, J. Pediatr. **98**:974, 1981.

Lipman, B., Serwer, G.A., and Brazy, J.E.: Abnormal cerebral hemodynamics in preterm infants with patent ductus arteriosus, Pediatrics **69**:778, 1982.

Pape, K.E., and others: Ultrasound detection of brain damage in preterm infants, Lancet **1**:1261, 1979.

Perlman, J.M., Hill, A., and Volpe, J.J.: The effect of patent ductus arteriosus on flow velocity in the anterior cerebral arteries: ductal steal in the premature newborn infant, J. Pediatr. **99**:767, 1981.

Perlman, J.M., McMenamin, J.B., and Volpe, J.J.: Fluctuating cerebral blood flow velocity in respiratory distress syndrome, N. Engl. J. Med. **309**:204, 1983.

Perlman, J.M., and others: Reduction in intraventricular hemorrhage by elimination of fluctuating cerebral blood flow velocity in preterm infants with respiratory distress syndrome, N. Engl. J. Med. **312**:1353, 1985.

Philip, A.G.S., Long, J.G., and Donn, S.M.: Intracranial pressure: sequential measurements in full-term and preterm infants, Am. J. Dis. Child. **135**:521, 1981.

Volpe, J.J.: Neonatal intraventricular hemorrhage, N. Engl. J. med. **304**:886, 1981.

PART TWO

Birth injury

In 1862, W.J. Little, an orthopedic surgeon, was the first person to propose a causal link between suboptimal perinatal events and subsequent neurologic dysfunction and brain damage. From this article and other classic retrospective clinical-neuropathologic studies using human autopsy material, the term "birth injury" was coined. The designation was intended to be all-inclusive, encompassing most of the then known causes of major childhood developmental disabilities (cerebral palsy, mental retardation, and epilepsy). Subsequently, the phenomenon known as birth injury was correctly classified as either birth asphyxia or birth trauma. However, the use of the word *birth* before either asphyxia or trauma was used to imply that problems during the birthing process were thought to be central both to the cause and pathogenesis of most of these disabilities.

In 1897 Sigmund Freud, while he was a neurologist, developed another concept in a series of three monographs, which he believed explained more completely the various manifestations of cerebral palsy: "the anomaly of the birth process, rather than being the causal etiologic factor, may itself be the consequence of the real prenatal etiology." This concept is quite different from Little's view that all cerebral palsy occurs as a consequence of abnormal parturition.

Since the introduction of the original term, our knowledge has expanded significantly regarding the vulnerable periods of embryonic and fetal development during which insults could occur and the increased numbers of confirmed causes of childhood developmental disabilities. In addition to asphyxia and trauma during the intrapartum period, a variety of known causes, acting at various periods during gestation, now includes chromosomal abnormalities, dysmorphic syndromes, drugs, alcohol, environmental toxins, infections, inherited metabolic diseases, intracranial hemorrhage, and the transient neonatal metabolic disorders of hypoglycemia, hyperbilirubinemia, and hypernatremia. However, even with this expanded knowledge, the causes of most of the cases of cerebral palsy remain unknown.

Even though there is no doubt now that both significant asphyxia and trauma during the intrapartum period can lead to cerebral palsy, current data do not now support Little's original view that intrapartum asphyxia and trauma are the leading causes of cerebral palsy and related developmental disabilities. At the present time the data support the position that only a small percentage of developmental disabilities are related to intrapartum asphyxia or trauma. In children who were full-term infants, the percentage ranges from 3% to no more than 15% at best. From interpretations of both old and new data, Freud's concept that most cases of cerebral palsy have a prenatal origin is gaining increased support.

In the "birth injury" section, birth asphyxia and birth trauma will be discussed separately in an effort to document more clearly the current state of knowledge in each of these areas.

BIRTH ASPHYXIA

Although suggestions appeared in classic retrospective clinical and neuropathologic studies that asphyxia was one of the causal factors in brain damage, most of our information concerning the specific effects of intrauterine asphyxia on the fetus has evolved since the development of techniques for determining blood pH and blood gases. Asphyxia, as used in this discussion, is defined biochemically as having three components: hypoxemia, hypercapnia, and mixed acidosis (metabolic and respiratory). Recent human and animal studies have provided a clearer distinction between the effects of asphyxia and trauma on the fetal nervous system.

Two distinct sites of neuropathologic involvement have been identified in brains of neonates thought to have experienced intrapartum asphyxia. The two principal sites are the cortical and subcortical gray matter and the region of the subependymal germinal matrix. As babies were classified by gestational age, a difference in the locus of lesions in preterm versus full-term neonates became apparent. The pattern of damage in the full-term infant is located principally in the peripheral and dorsal areas of the cerebral cortex, with the lesions involving gyri at the depths of sulci and the neuronal nuclei of the basal ganglia. This pattern of neuropathologic observation is seen in neonates with hypoxic ischemic encephalopathy (HIE). The pattern of damage in the preterm infant is located principally at the center of the hemisphere in the germinal matrix and surrounding periventricular region, with relative sparing of the cortical mantle. Lesions in the preterm infant are principally hemorrhagic and are termed subependymal germinal matrix hemorrhage/intraventricular hemorrhage (SEH/IVH). Lesions in the white matter in the area of the periventricular region were first described by Banker, and they can be seen in both preterm and full-term infants.

The delineation of differences in locus of lesions by gestational age has contributed greatly to our understanding of brain disorders in the perinatal period and their influence on the later appearance of cerebral palsy and related disorders. Each of these entities is discussed in a separate section.

Hypoxic ischemic encephalopathy

During the intrapartum period each normal fetus experiences an episode of hypoxemia, hypercapnia, and a mixed acidosis (i.e., a mild asphyxial episode). This occurs as a consequence of impaired blood flow in the uterus during labor. There are no signs of neurologic dysfunction following this mild asphyxial episode.

Hypoxic ischemic encephalopathy (HIE) is the term used to designate the clinical and neuropathologic findings of an encephalopathy that occurs in the full-term infant who has experienced a *significant* episode of intrapartum asphyxia. In our new and more complete understanding of significant asphyxia during the intrapartum period, it is important to recognize that the child who subsequently will develop cerebral palsy secondary to a presumed intrapartum asphyxial insult will demonstrate unequivocal clinical signs of HIE during the neonatal period, usually during the first 2 to 7 days of life. In an effort to highlight the clinical entity of HIE and its very special significance, the clinical and pathologic features, pathogenesis, and treatment of HIE are described in the following paragraphs.

Clinical features

As the physician attempts to assess the relative risk to a fetus experiencing intrapartum asphyxia, some obstetric conditions, if present, can be considered to put the fetus at increased risk. These include conditions associated with increased risk for fetal asphyxia:

1. Altered placental exchange
   a. Abruption
   b. Placenta previa
   c. Postmaturity
   d. Prolapsed cord
   e. Cord around neck
   f. Intrauterine fetal growth retardation
   g. "Placental insufficiency"
2. Altered maternal blood flow to placenta
   a. Maternal hypotension
   b. Maternal hypertension—pregnancy induced
   c. Maternal hypertension—nonpregnancy induced
   d. Abnormal uterine contractions
3. Reduced maternal arterial oxygen saturation
   a. Maternal hypoventilation
   b. Maternal hypoxia
   c. Maternal cardiopulmonary disease

It is important to note that being at risk for an episode of asphyxia and actually experiencing one are not synonymous. In a prospective study by Nelson and Ellenberg (1983) the relative risk of cerebral palsy in infants weighing 2,500 gm or more following certain obstetric events was described in relation to the Apgar scores. The 18 obstetric complications evaluated in this study were placenta previa, abruptio placentae, breech delivery, face or brow presentation, cord prolapse, placental infarction (2+), toxemia, lowest fetal heart rate (less than 100 beats per minute), oxytocin augmentation, nuchal cord, meconium, uterine dysfunction, use of mid- or high forceps, second stage of labor longer than 59 minutes, chorioamnionitis, prolonged rupture of membranes (longer than 24 hours), short cord (less than 40 cm), and polyhydramnios. Infants whose births were associated with these "anoxigenic" obstetric complications had no greater risk for developing cerebral palsy than did infants whose births were uncomplicated, if their 5-minute Apgar scores were 7 or higher. This group comprised about 62% of the study group and accounted for less than its proportional share of cerebral palsy. An increased risk for cerebral palsy was evidenced when the infant born with an obstetric complication had a 5-minute Apgar score less than or equal to 3. Although these patients represented only 1.5% of the total population, they accounted for 17% of infant deaths and 13% of infants with cerebral palsy in the study population. These data demonstrate that an obstetric complication per se does not increase the infant's risk for cerebral palsy, unless the complication is associated with a significantly low Apgar score.

Data now show that a score of 0 to 3 at 5 minutes is a significantly low Apgar score. Infants who have Apgar scores of 7 to 10 have demonstrated very low risk for an abnormal transition to extrauterine life and for later abnormal neurologic development. The score range of 0 to 3 is significant because of the higher mortality and central nervous system (CNS) morbidity among infants in this range than among infants with scores of 4 to 6 or 7 to 10. The longer the score remains low, the greater is its significance. An infant with a 0 to 3 score at 1 minute has a mortality of 5% to 10%, which rises to approximately 53% if that score is maintained for 20 minutes. In full-term surviving neonates with an Apgar score of 0 to 3 at 5 minutes, the incidence of cerebral palsy is approximately 1%. If this is sustained for 15 minutes, 9% of the survivors will have cerebral palsy, with a dramatic rise to 57% for infants who sustain an Apgar score of 0 to 3 for 20 minutes. It is interesting to note that the remaining 43 percent of neonates in this study with a 0 to 3 Apgar score at 20 minutes were completely normal at 7 years of age, compared to the 57% who had severe cerebral palsy.

The low Apgar score indicates an abnormal condition but does not imply any specific cause. Low scores can be the result of any one of the following six major causes: asphyxia, drugs, trauma, hypovolemia, infection, or anomalies. If a low Apgar score is ascribed to asphyxia, signs known to occur during intrapartum asphyxia should be present and the other causes of low Apgar scores can be eliminated.

The Apgar score can give only an estimate of severity of a process such as asphyxia, not a duration. In the case of asphyxia some estimate of the duration of the episode is very important regarding the potential effect of that insult on the nervous system. This can be estimated from other observations in the newborn. When a low Apgar score occurs, infants tend to lose their color, respirations, tone, reflexes, and heart rate, in the order listed. After effective resuscitation, these functions tend to reappear but in a different order: heart rate, reflexes, color, respirations, and tone. The time required for tone and respirations to return may indicate the severity or duration of the asphyxial insult to the CNS. Delay of greater than 2 hours in return of tone is associated with an increased incidence of HIE, as well as significant neurologic sequelae in surviving neonates. The mean age at onset of spontaneous respirations in an infant asphyxiated during labor and delivery is significantly greater in neonates who developed seizures, a major sign of HIE. Other delivery room observations that may help estimate the length or severity of the intrapartum asphyxial episode are delay in return of the heart rate if resuscitation efforts are considered adequate, meconium present in the trachea, and meconium staining of the umbilical cord, skin, or nails. The last observation indicates previous exposure to meconium for at least 3 to 6 hours.

In the past the clinical course of the full-term infant who experienced intrapartum asphyxia was thought primarily to reflect altered brain function. It is now known, however, that because of the variable involvement of different organ systems, such infants can have quite different clinical courses. The variation in clinical signs is caused in part by the ability of the fetus to redistribute blood flow to protect vital organs, as well as by the difficulty in accurately establishing the length, severity, and acuteness of the onset of the asphyxial episode. In addition, there may be unidentified factors in the mother, fetus, or neonate that can influence the occurrence or severity of asphyxia.

This varied clinical course was documented in a retrospective study by Sexson of 6,045 consecutive deliveries. Fifty-three full-term infants had an Apgar score of 5 or less at 1 and 5 minutes and were thought to have suffered intrapartum asphyxia. Eighteen infants had no apparent disease throughout their hospitalization; however, 35 infants had at least one or as many as five abnormal organ systems. Of these 35 infants, 19 had more than one abnormal system. The 35 affected infants with low Apgar scores had problems (in order of decreasing frequency) with their pulmonary, cardiovascular, CNS, gastrointestinal, and renal systems. None of the infants in this study had clinically significant coagulation problems, although disorders of hemostasis have been described. Nine of these 35 died during the neonatal period. The most common cause of death was persistent pulmonary hypertension, which occurred in four infants. No one system or group of systems appeared to be the primary target of the intrapartum asphyxial episode. Only one third of the infants had clinical signs that suggested CNS involvement. Of the nine infant deaths only two were caused by CNS disturbances. These two infants had massive brain swelling with cortical necrosis. From either the intrapartum course or the status of the neonate in the delivery room, it was not possible to predict whether the CNS or any other organ system was going to be affected.

Data indicate that full-term neonates at risk of developing long-term neurologic sequelae from an intrapartum asphyxial episode will demonstrate signs of neurologic dysfunction at least within the first week of life, most usually within the first 12 hours after birth. Such a neonate does not necessarily need to have a low Apgar score. The major signs of CNS dysfunction in HIE include seizures, abnormalities in state of consciousness, tone, posture, reflexes, respiratory pattern, oculovestibular response, autonomic function, and tenseness of the anterior fontanel. Of these the first three are the most significant and are described in the following discussion.

Neonatal seizures (Part four) frequently are secondary to intrapartum asphyxia. Seizures have been reported in 30% to 69% of infants with abnormal neurologic examinations after an intrauterine asphyxial episode. Typically, seizure onset has been reported to occur at 12 to

24 hours after delivery. If signs other than tonic-clonic movements are used to identify a seizure, however, the onset may be as early as 2 to 6 hours. Seizures per se are not associated exclusively with late neurologic sequelae; however, the seizure occurrence within the first 12 hours, the seizure requiring more than one drug for control, the appearance of status or serial seizures, or a persistently abnormal electroencephalogram (EEG) (electrical silence, burst suppression, or low voltage background) are signs of significant neonatal neurologic dysfunction. Infants with HIE who have seizures as just described have a 30% to 75% likelihood of long-term neurologic sequelae.

Abnormalities in the level of consciousness are helpful in delineating the severity of an asphyxial insult and in predicting which infants may have neurologic sequelae if they survive. In a recent study by Sarnat, full-term asphyxiated infants who were believed to have an encephalopathy were grouped into three clinical states according to the neonate's level of consciousness, neuromuscular control, complex reflexes, autonomic function, seizures, EEG findings, and duration of abnormality. Although all of these factors were important in delineating the three states of encephalopathy, the level of consciousness seemed to be the primary determinant. In state 1, the level of consciousness is hyperalertness; state 2, lethargy; and state 3, stupor. The state of encephalopathy and duration of a given state were the two factors that determined the severity of HIE and were most closely associated with the predictability of long-term outcome. Infants who did not enter state 3, and who had signs of state 2 for fewer than 5 days, appeared normal later in infancy. Infants who entered state 3, who had signs of state 2 for more than 7 days or whose EEG failed to revert to normal, either developed significant neurologic sequelae or died. Infants who showed signs compatible with state 2 had a 5% chance of death and a 20% chance of developing significant neurologic sequelae. These results have been confirmed by Finer in another study using the same scoring system, even without EEG criteria.

When abnormalities of tone were isolated as a predictor of severe handicap in full-term neonates whose history and clinical course were compatible with asphyxia, the risk for cerebral palsy among children surviving the neonatal period was 25%.

A chronologic combination of abnormal signs is more helpful than a single sign in predicting outcome. The most helpful cluster of signs includes an Apgar score below 3 obtained at 5 minutes or longer, together with other factors (e.g., reduced activity levels, tone, reduced consciousness lasting longer than 1 day, need for gavage feeding, hypotonia, or single or multiple episodes of apnea during the first week). The cluster also may include the previously described state 3 or state 2 lasting longer than 7 days, asymmetric neurologic signs, seizures with onset during the first day of life, and an overall impression of abnormal brain function during the time the infant was in the nursery.

More work is needed to define the predictive powers of the neonatal neurologic examination; however, an abnormal neurologic examination (as already defined) of a full-term infant with a history of probable intrapartum asphyxia is an extremely powerful tool in establishing the presence and severity of HIE, in predicting early death, and in identifying neonates who should be observed for later development of neurologic sequelae. As treatment for neonatal HIE is evolving and as potential treatments for children with early developmental delays are appearing, it becomes extremely important to identify the presence and severity of neonatal HIE.

In summary, the full-term neonate at risk for developing cerebral palsy and related disorders from an intrapartum asphyxial episode will demonstrate signs of neurologic dysfunction (HIE) in the first week of life. The reported incidence of moderate to severe cerebral palsy in asphyxiated, surviving full-term neonates varies from 4.7% to 57.1%. The incidence of cerebral palsy and related disorders varies with the severity of the neonatal encephalopathy following the intrapartum asphyxial episode. The typical cluster of neurologic deficits in a severely affected child at follow-up includes spastic quadriplegia, severe mental retardation, seizures, hearing deficits, and microcephaly (Part six).

In the past, intrapartum asphyxia was thought to be the leading cause of cerebral palsy. In its pure form, if that ever is the case, this cause accounts for probably only 3% and no more than 15% of the cases of cerebral palsy. When mental retardation and epilepsy occur with cerebral palsy, they can reasonably be considered components of a nervous system impaired by the perinatal asphyxia. However, when mental retardation and epilepsy occur in the absence of cerebral palsy, the risks attached to perinatal asphyxia are uncertain and may well be insubstantial.

Even though more is known about the etiology and pathogenesis of some cases of cerebral palsy, the most significant aspect of our new knowledge is that the cause of most cases of cerebral palsy is still unknown. If we are to reduce the occurrence of cerebral palsy, increased understanding of the factors that influence the integrity of the developing nervous system during the prenatal period appear to have immense importance.

Pathologic features

The pathologic changes in the brain of a full-term infant who has experienced an episode of asphyxia during the intrapartum period are determined by the length of survival of the patient and the length and severity of the asphyxial episode. There may be no gross or microscopic changes in those patients who die in the first few hours after birth. Animal studies, however, suggest that changes detectable by light and electron microscopy may occur in both neurons and astrocytes shortly after an asphyxial insult. Full-term neonates who die after the first 24 hours of life frequently have brain swelling and cerebral necrosis. Brain swelling was found as an isolated lesion in as many as 39% of cases. The cerebral necrosis involves the cortical gray matter (especially at depths of sulci), underlying white matter, and the gray matter of the basal ganglia. In some patients, cerebral necrosis is most severe in the region of the postcentral gyrus similar to that found in the full-term newborn monkey following experimentally produced intrapartum asphyxia. Areas of petechial periventricular hemorrhage and leukomalacia also can be seen. The pattern of cerebral damage in the full-term infant does not usually include subependymal and/or intraventricular hemorrhage.

Those full-term infants who survive the perinatal asphyxial episode and neonatal period will have two primary neuropathologic conditions—ulegyria and status marmoratus of the basal ganglia. The reader is referred to Gilles for a detailed description and excellent discussion of the variety of changes seen in the nervous system following perinatal insults.

Pathogenesis

Based on human and animal data, a proposed pathogenesis for HIE in the full-term infant and its sequelae in the surviving neonate are outlined in Fig. 27-7. The major components of the diagram have been assembled from data from two rhesus monkey models, acute total asphyxia, and prolonged partial asphyxia (Table 27-1). The two models closely replicate the two different types of perinatal asphyxial events that most frequently occur in the human fetus or neonate—an acute asphyxial episode resulting from cord prolapse and a prolonged partial asphyxial episode resulting from a placental abruption. In most human cases the total perinatal insult probably results from a partial, prolonged asphyxial episode combined with a terminal episode of acute total asphyxia.

Acute total asphyxia of 8 to 10 minutes produces a long-term neurologic dysfunction in the term neonatal monkey similar to that seen in patients with spastic quadriplegia. In the neonatal period neither seizures nor brain swelling is seen. The neuropathologic findings occur primarily in the nuclei located in the brainstem, thalamus, and basal ganglia, while the cerebral cortex is spared.

Prolonged partial asphyxia of 1 to 3 hours in the term fetal monkey produces a clinical course in the neonatal period that is similar to that seen in the depressed human neonate following, for example, a placental abruption.

Table 27-1. Asphyxia in the full-term newborn rhesus monkey

		Partial prolonged asphyxia	Acute total asphyxia
Insult	Length	3-4 hours	12 minutes
	pH	6.9	6.9
	PO_2	15 mm Hg	3 mm Hg
	PCO_2	90 mm Hg	120 mm Hg
	Blood pressure	40 mm Hg	5 mm Hg
Clinical course	Resuscitation	Yes	Yes
	Seizures	Yes	No
	Retinal hemorrhage	Yes	No
	Survival	Variable	Variable
	Sequelae	No dysfunction detected	Spasticity Sensory loss
Pathologic aspects	Brain swelling	Yes	No
	Site of edema	Intracellular	
	Brain necrosis	Yes	Yes
	Locus of necrosis	Cerebral cortex Basal ganglia Thalamus	Brainstem Thalamus Basal ganglia Spinal cord
	Cerebral blood flow	Cortex abnormal at birth	Brainstem abnormal at birth

Seizures occur in approximately 50% of the monkeys within the first 24 hours of life; cytotoxic brain edema occurs in this neonatal monkey after partial prolonged asphyxia. Cerebral blood flow studies in this same animal model show that the brain is abnormal at birth, as demonstrated by the focal areas of ischemia (Fig. 27-8). Brain lesions in the cortex are similar to those in neonates who die following intrapartum asphyxia, as well as in children or adults said to have cerebral palsy secondary to a perinatal insult. The surviving monkey, unlike the human, has no motor deficit despite significant areas of ulegyria in the association areas of cortex.

These animal studies suggest strongly that prolonged partial asphyxia from any cause in the fetus, even in the absence of fetal circulatory collapse or fetal head compression, is the primary event that sets in motion a vicious spiral of cytotoxic edema with impaired cerebral blood flow leading to cerebral necrosis or ulegyria.

The clinical course and the extent of neuropathologic changes in a neonate can vary depending on the acuteness of onset and the length and severity of the asphyxial episode. The entire sequence of events leading to the various types of neuropathologic outcome is not totally clear from current data, although the points represented in each of the squares in the diagram of the proposed pathogenesis (Fig. 27-7) have been demonstrated in either animal or human studies.

The diagram of proposed pathogenesis (Fig. 27-7) is

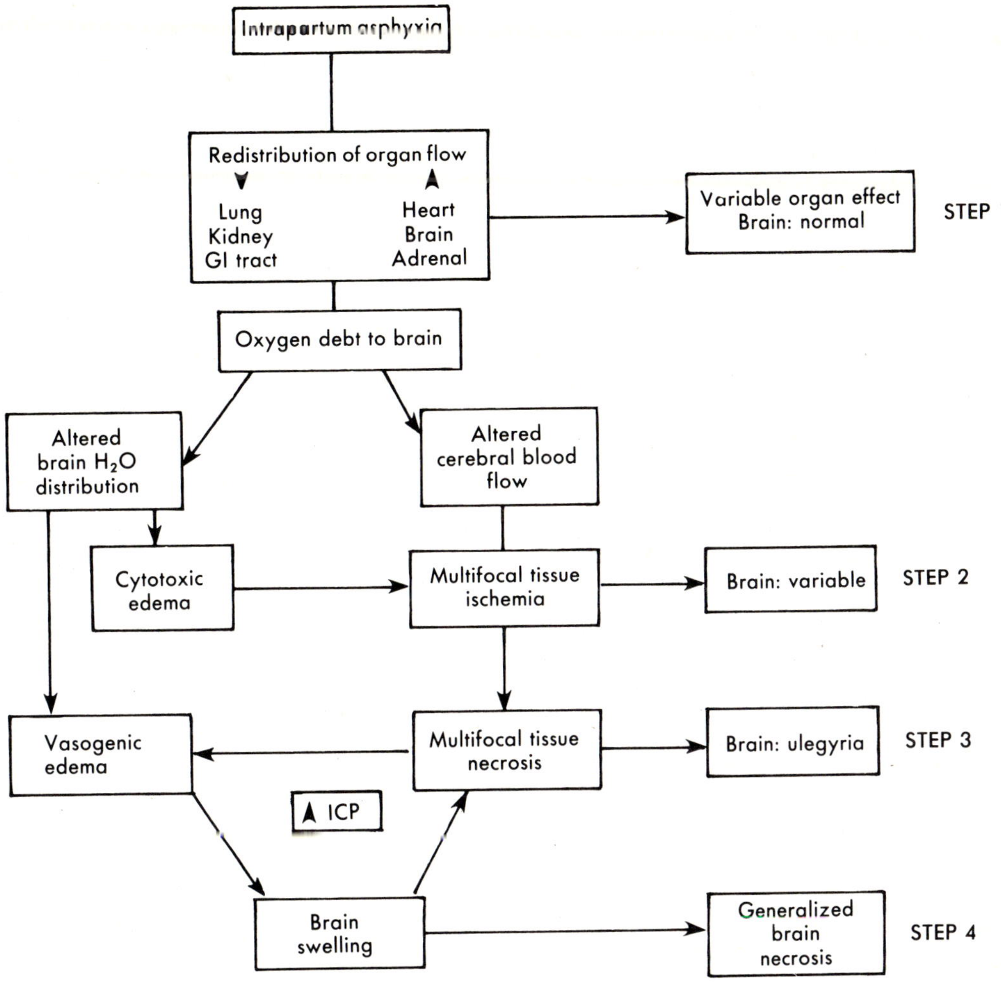

Fig. 27-7. Proposed pathogenesis for the development of hypoxic-ischemic brain damage.

drawn as though there were a continuum of the intrapartum asphyxial episode from top to bottom with the outcomes seen on the right side of the figure. Many newborns with low Apgar scores after intrapartum asphyxial episodes have no evidence of HIE (Fig. 27-7). This has been seen in asphyxiated infants who die because of other organ system failures related to the asphyxia, such as persistent fetal circulation. The lack of findings in the CNS following intrapartum asphyxia could be explained by the known occurrence of the redistribution of cardiac output, resulting in an increased percentage of cardiac output going to the brain. This process of redistribution of flow attempts to maintain adequate tissue oxygenation and prevent tissue ischemia.

If the intrauterine asphyxial episode continues and homeostatic mechanisms that maintain blood oxygenation begin to fail, changes begin to occur in brain-water distribution and continue to take place in cerebral blood flow. These alterations are thought to act synergistically, contributing to the multifocal tissue ischemia described in the fetal monkey, in whom there is a general reduction of blood flow with focal areas of total ischemia. Increasing degrees of ischemia are seen in the brains of fetal monkeys that are subjected to increasing degrees and length of asphyxia. Central to our understanding of the pathogenesis of neonatal HIE and the subsequent development of atrophic cortical sclerosis are the multiple foci of cerebral tissue ischemia. The numerous factors that lead to this multifocal tissue ischemia are poorly understood. The length of time required for tissue ischemia to cause tissue death in the cerebral cortex is uncertain. It is conceivable that, if the asphyxiated fetus is delivered and treated appropriately soon after the development of mild multifocal tissue ischemia, the brain in the surviving infant could escape evidence of tissue necrosis (Fig. 22-7).

When the intrapartum insult is more severe or is not terminated quickly, small areas of multifocal tissue ne-

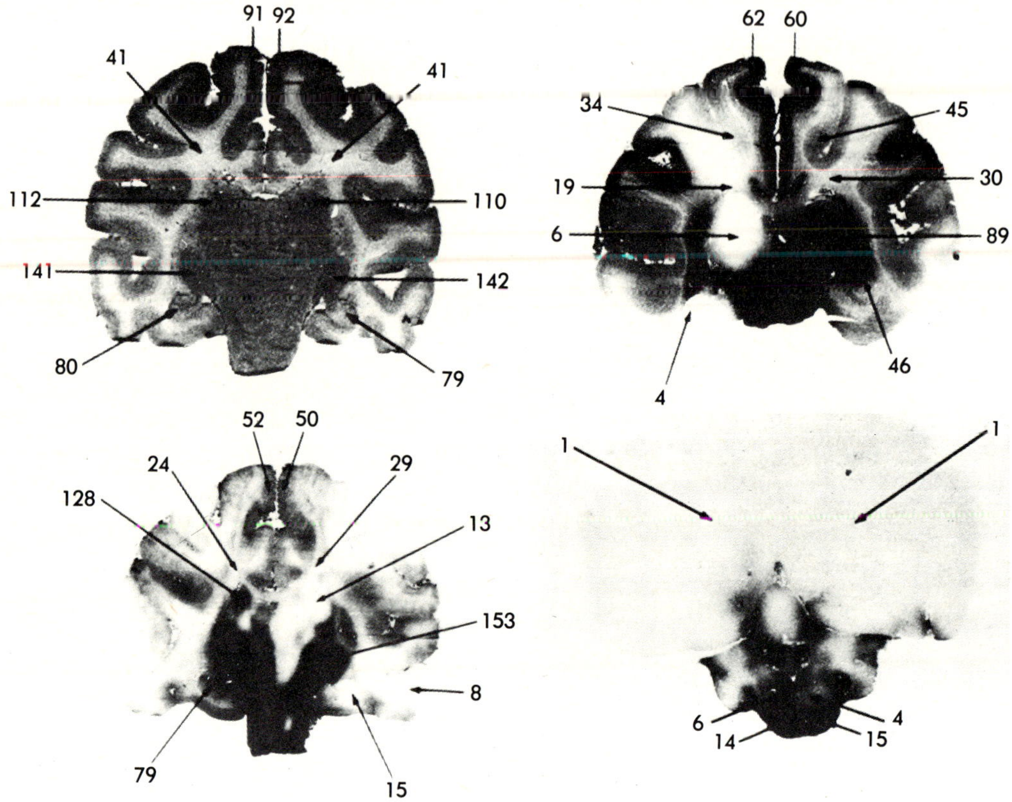

Fig. 27-8. Autoradiograms of coronal sections from full-term monkeys. **A,** Normal; **B,** mild prolonged partial asphyxia (PPA); **C,** moderate PPA; **D,** severe PPA. Numbers represent cerebral blood flow values in ml/gm/minute.

crosis do occur. If these areas are small, they may not lead to significant areas of vasogenic edema with the subsequent development of severely increased intracranial pressure. Brain repair processes convert these areas of multifocal tissue necrosis into areas of ulegyria as described in the monkey brain. The extent and pattern of ulegyria are dependent on the degree and location of cerebral ischemia and necrosis (Fig. 27-7).

If the intrapartum episode is severe and prolonged, multifocal areas of tissue ischemia located at the depths of sulci and within neuronal nuclei are severe and spread to involve the entire cerebral hemisphere. The existing tissue ischemia leads to tissue necrosis. Vasogenic edema develops in and around the areas of multifocal tissue necrosis. This type of edema develops following disruption of the tight junctions of the capillary endothelium with leakage of osmotic materials into the interstitial spaces of the brain, pulling water from the intravascular space. As the multifocal areas coalesce, significant increases in intracranial pressure begin to occur in association with vasogenic edema. From animal data it is known that when intracranial pressure reaches one half to two thirds of the mean arterial pressure, reduced cerebral blood flow can be severe enough to cause tissue ischemia, especially in areas of cortex at depths of sulci. The triad of multifocal tissue necrosis, vasogenic edema, and brain swelling with increasing intracranial pressure leads to a vicious downward spiral with an ever-increasing oxygen debt in the brain, almost total cerebral necrosis, and death (Fig. 27-7).

In some asphyxiated neonates, increased intracranial pressure or brain edema at autopsy are not found. The absence of these findings may be related to redistribution of flow to protect the brain, while supplying inadequate oxygen to the lung, kidney, or gastrointestinal tract. This may lead to dysfunction of these organs and subsequent death. Since brain edema in the monkey that experiences acute total asphyxia is consistently absent, the absence of edema may be related to the type and length of the asphyxial episode. When the asphyxial episode is sudden and complete for 10 to 15 minutes, there can be enough neuronal necrosis confined to the brainstem and basal ganglia to lead to death through impaired respiratory control.

Unknown or poorly quantitated factors leading to thromboembolism and cerebral infarction may play a key

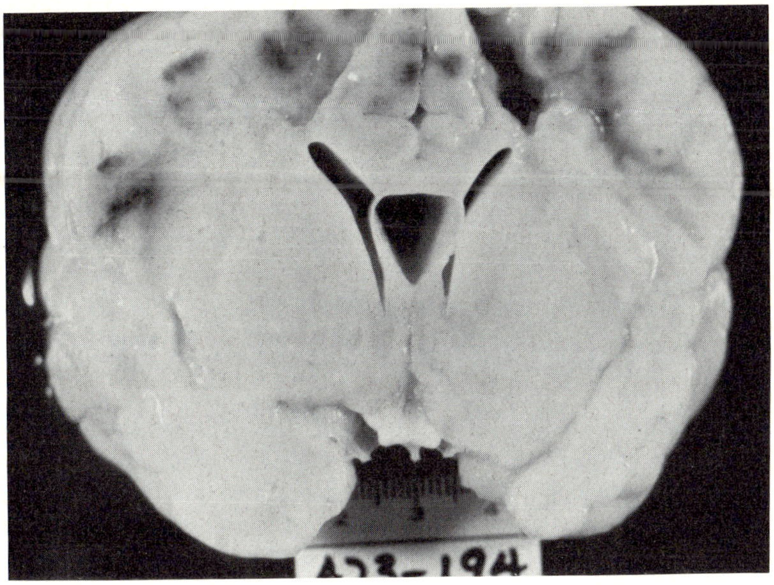

Fig. 27-9. Full-term asphyxiated infant brain with hemorrhagic cortical necrosis.

role in the pathogenesis of ulegyria both with and without a phase of brain swelling during the neonatal period (Fig. 27-9).

Treatment

The general guidelines for treatment of the asphyxiated neonate involve first eliminating the original hypoxia and second alleviating tissue ischemia if present. Specific management, beyond the immediate resuscitation in the delivery room, is still under considerable discussion. When a particular organ is the principal target of the asphyxial episode, such as with the lungs and persistent fetal circulation (Chapter 29), the kidneys and acute tubular necrosis (Chapter 35), or the GI tract and necrotizing enterocolitis (Chapter 33), the management of a specific process assumes central importance. In addition, there are other physiologic and biochemical factors that if left uncorrected can affect brain homeostasis. Most of these factors are altered in the asphyxiated full-term neonate and must be dealt with in the overall therapeutic plan. This discussion is directed toward the management of the neonate with HIE; other deranged organ systems will be discussed only if they directly affect brain homeostasis.

Four questions in regard to the therapeutic management of the neonate with HIE remain unanswered.

1. Can the asphyxiated fetus or neonate whose CNS is altered enough to leave permanent damage be identified?
2. Can this asphyxiated fetus or neonate profit from any therapeutic intervention?
3. If therapeutic intervention is possible, is there a critical time after which treatment is ineffective in eliminating or significantly reducing permanent brain damage?
4. What is the appropriate intervention for this asphyxiated fetus or neonate?

The first question probably is the most important one. Current data increasingly support the position that the full-term neonate who has had a history of fetal distress, a low Apgar score requiring resuscitation, and altered tone or level of consciousness during the first 2 to 6 hours of life is manifesting early findings of HIE. Data from human studies seem to suggest that any infant who develops these signs has a 50% chance of having neonatal seizures and at least a 20% chance of developing cerebral palsy.

Rarely have neonates with an Apgar score of 7 to 10 developed neurologic findings and a clinical course consistent with HIE. It is extremely important in such cases to be sure that the neurologic dysfunction is not secondary to some other cause. It is rare for a neonate to have signs of neurologic dysfunction secondary to intrapartum asphyxia after 24 hours of age with no clinically apparent alteration in the nervous system before that time.

The remaining three questions most specifically concern therapy. The first two questions relate to the stage of the asphyxial process. Certainly, if the neonate is born after a prolonged intrapartum asphyxial episode and has advanced degrees of vasogenic edema and raised intracranial pressure, therapeutic intervention may have minimal benefit.

The therapeutic management of the term fetus at significant risk for developing HIE is first directed toward eliminating the hypoxic environment by immediate delivery of the fetus with institution of adequate oxygenation of the neonate. However, after birth the central role of therapy should be directed at relieving any existing brain ischemia or reducing the brain's metabolic requirements. The first phase of any therapeutic plan for a neonate who either has HIE or is at risk for developing HIE is the institution of a very careful monitoring system. For a patient who may have brain ischemia, the system should include serial neurologic assessment by clinical examination, detection of reduced cerebral perfusion pressure through monitoring of blood pressure and intracranial pressure, structural status of the brain by either CT scan or ultrasound, and evidence of suppressed electrogenesis by electroencephalogram or evoked potentials. All these functions can be measured in the neonate with fairly standard clinical tools. An adequate monitoring system is extremely important not only in initiating therapy in a neonate who becomes abnormal but also in following the progress of any therapeutic intervention once initiated. Other systemic parameters that should be monitored continuously include arterial pH and blood gases, temperature, blood glucose levels, serum and urine electrolytes and osmolality, serum blood urea nitrogen (BUN), serum creatinine, and accurate fluid input and output.

Once the hypoxic environment has been eliminated, efforts should be directed at promoting adequate brain tissue oxygenation by maintaining or restoring cerebral perfusion in an attempt to relieve ischemia. Signs of systemic hypoperfusion should be identified by findings such as an inadequate heart rate, poor capillary refill, abnormal arterial and venous blood pressure, and insufficient urine output. The causes of hypoperfusion in the neonate may be secondary to asphyxia, hypovolemia, or, rarely, septic shock. Hypovolemia should be suspected in situations where the mother has had vaginal bleeding (abruption or placenta previa). Peripheral vasoconstriction may result initially in normal or near normal blood pressure and hematocrit even in the presence of hypovolemia. As the acid-base status normalizes and the peripheral vascular bed opens up, blood pressure may fall. Also the acid base status may deteriorate as sequestered lactic acid is released into the circulation.

The neonate's blood pressure should be maintained at levels that allow adequate perfusion to all body tissues. It is more important to observe the patient's degree of peripheral perfusion and urinary output than to maintain specific levels of blood pressure as outlined in neonatal blood pressure charts (Chapters 21 and 29 and Appendix C). The relationship of low cerebral blood flow to hypotension and adverse neurologic outcome has been documented. Likewise, a loss of autoregulation of cerebral blood flow has been documented, suggesting that hypertension may be equally hazardous to brain tissue as is hypotension. Volume expansion must therefore be undertaken with careful and continual monitoring of the circulatory status. Dopamine at levels of 2 to 5 μg/kg/minute may have a role in normalizing blood pressure and renal blood flow, although the efficacy and safety of this drug are being more fully explored in the newborn.

For adequate oxygen-carrying capacity a normal hematocrit level (45 to 60) should be maintained (Chapter 32). Patients with hematocrits greater than 65 should be considered polycythemic; they are candidates for a partial exchange transfusion to reduce hyperviscosity and enhance tissue oxygenation.

Once adequate oxygenation is established, administration of sodium bicarbonate may be indicated with a severe, persistent metabolic acidosis documented by arterial pH and blood gases (Chapter 22). Rapid infusion of bicarbonate should be avoided to prevent hazardous increases in serum osmolality and the adverse effects of alkalinization on cerebral blood flow.

In the normal state it is important that the brain receive a continuous supply of both oxygen and glucose, the two primary sources of energy for neurons and glia. This is necessary because these cells do not have the capacity to store energy in any chemical form. There is a controversy concerning the appropriate levels of glucose in the brain to be maintained following an asphyxial insult. Data support the view of increasing glucose supply to the brain, which is unable to appropriately use glucose in the postasphyxial state. The opposing view is also supported, however. It suggests a possible deleterious effect of high glucose levels because of the potential hazard of promoting the development of local lactic acidosis, which may be associated with an increase in brain damage seen in the asphyxiated brain. A glucose infusion should be established and monitored with Dextrostix and blood glucose determinations to maintain glucose levels of 45 to 90 mg/dl, not only for cerebral but also for myocardial tissue function. Hypocalcemia may be seen in association with hypoglycemia in the asphyxiated full-term neonate, and calcium in the form of calcium gluconate may be required for calcium levels less than 7.5 mg/dl (Chapter 37, part two).

Fluid overload can be a distinct but avoidable hazard in the treatment of an asphyxiated neonate. The status of the kidney regarding potential acute tubular necrosis or the presence of inappropriate secretion of antidiuretic hormone may materially affect fluid output. Fluid and electrolyte monitoring can detect the presence of either of these conditions. While this monitoring is going on, it is suggested that the asphyxiated neonate initially be started on an electrolyte-free dextrose solution (10%) restricted to a rate of 50 ml/kg/day. Changes in fluid volume and content should be altered as frequently as every 12 hours, depending on data from continuous monitoring of serum electrolytes, serum osmolality, urine output, and body weight.

Seizures, when present, should be recognized and vigorously treated in these patients (Chapter 27, part four). This is particularly important because cerebral oxygen use is increased almost fivefold during a seizure. In the brain with HIE the ability to autoregulate flow in response to energy requirements is altered, making it imperative to eliminate any increases in energy requirements of the brain.

At the present time the treatment of brain edema/ischemia in the asphyxiated neonate remains an area of controversy and speculation. The two phases of cerebral edema in the clinical course of HIE may require different therapeutic approaches. Therapy during the initial stage of cytotoxic edema and focal ischemia without significant increase in intracranial pressure would be directed at reducing local increases in pressure through the use of fluid restriction, osmotic agents such as mannitol, and diuretics such as furosemide. At the same time, while initial tissue ischemia is present, the use of agents that would reduce the energy requirements of the brain, such as barbiturates, may have a specific role.

If the patient is seen for the first time during the second phase of HIE, when there is clinical evidence of a significant increase in intracranial pressure, a more vigorous approach to reducing intracranial pressure by fluid restriction, osmotic agents, and diuretics has been suggested. Barbiturates in large doses have been shown to reduce intracranial pressure in the adult, and their role in HIE is being studied in the neonate.

The use of steroids in cytotoxic edema initially had some appeal on theoretical grounds, but currently there is no proof of their effectiveness. In vasogenic edema characterized by breakdown of the brain capillary with disruption of the blood brain barrier, steroids have been thought to be effective, although this has not been established clearly.

Subependymal germinal matrix hemorrhage/intraventricular hemorrhage

Subependymal germinal matrix hemorrhage/intraventricular hemorrhage (SEH/IVH) is the most common neuropathologic finding in preterm neonates. (See also Part three of this chapter). Although the cause and pathogenesis are not understood fully, they are mentioned in this section because the interpretation of data still strongly links SEH/IVH to hypoxic ischemia. A more recent interpretation seems to support the position that SEH/IVH may not be the significant process. Hypoxic ischemia that affects not only the subependymal germinal matrix but also the white matter throughout the centrum semiovale seems to be the more important global event in understanding the cause, pathogenesis, and ultimately the prevention of developmental disabilities in children who were preterm infants.

BIRTH TRAUMA

The frequency of overt physical traumatic injury because of abnormal position and size of the fetus before delivery, abnormal patterns and length of labor, and abnormal pelvic size and shape has been reduced significantly over the past 40 years through improved obstetric care, especially during labor and delivery. However, the same types of pathologic conditions that were seen in the past are continuing, but at a much lower frequency. These included intracranial hemorrhage of various types (exclusive of SEH/IVH), skull fracture, cephalohematoma, spinal cord trauma, brachial plexus palsy, and facial nerve palsy. The life-threatening or severely handicapping disorders caused by intrapartum trauma per se have been almost completely eliminated. At present, brachial plexus palsy and facial nerve palsy are the only types that occur with any frequency.

Intracranial hemorrhage

All types of intracranial hemorrhage (ICH) that have been described in adults have occurred in newborn infants. However, the various types of ICH occur with different frequencies and different degrees of severity. In the newborn infant more than one type of hemorrhage can and does frequently occur in the same patient. The types of hemorrhage that are thought to be primarily associated with trauma are dealt with in this section.

Subarachnoid hemorrhage, perhaps the most frequent form of neonatal intracranial bleeding, is usually of limited degree and is rarely of clinical significance. A high percentage of newborns will have some erythrocytes (RBCs) in their cerebrospinal fluid (CSF). In one study RBCs in preterm infants ranged from 0 to 39,000/mm^3 with a median of 112/mm^3. Furthermore, small amounts of subarachnoid blood may be detected in postmortem examinations of newborns who were neither clinically symptomatic nor suspected of having suffered intracranial bleeding. Most commonly the RBCs in CSF are an incidental finding, perhaps a result of mild trauma during delivery.

The ease with which one can produce a traumatic lumbar puncture can make interpretation of bloody CSF difficult. In the evaluation of bloody CSF specimens, to distinguish subarachnoid bleeding from a traumatic lumbar puncture, it is necessary to count the number of RBCs in first and third (or fourth) tubes of CSF and also to examine centrifuged CSF supernatant for xanthochromia; the latter finding is indicative of subarachnoid blood and is not the result of a traumatic lumbar puncture.

Significant degrees of subarachnoid hemorrhage can occur with asphyxia, particularly in preterm infants; the bleeding is related to asphyxial injury of capillaries and small veins, with or without the added effect of trauma in the course of delivery. Clinically significant subarachnoid bleeding, especially in the full-term infant, can result from trauma alone. This can occur as an isolated process or in association with hemorrhage in other areas (subdural, epidural) with or without cerebral contusion. When the subarachnoid hemorrhage is associated with other types of bleeding or signs of physical injury, as documented by CT scan or ultrasound examination and caused by difficult delivery, the outcome is frequently poor, with either death in the early neonatal period or profound brain damage in survivors.

The clinical presentation of the full-term infant with isolated subarachnoid hemorrhage can vary considerably. Most commonly there are no clinical signs, and the infant is totally asymptomatic and diagnosed only because of an abnormal lumbar puncture. On occasion an infant appears normal initially and then develops seizures on the second or third day of life as the only clinical manifestation. The infant may look remarkably well between seizures and subsequently have a benign course, with no apparent sequelae. In contrast, the initial clinical manifestations of neonatal subarachnoid hemorrhage may be the early onset of alternating depression and irritability with refractory seizures. It may be impossible in such an infant to establish the primary role of birth trauma or asphyxia as the cause of the subarachnoid hemorrhage and its manifestations. Such infants may develop hydrocephalus as a late complication of subarachnoid bleeding, with obstruction of CSF circulation and reabsorption, as well as other later signs of neurologic impairment and delayed development.

Subdural hemorrhage has become a very rare neonatal neurologic disorder. The two principal locations of subdural hemorrhage are over the cerebral hemispheres and in the posterior fossa. When this type of bleeding has occurred, common historical events include the mother being primiparous with the total labor and delivery occurring in less than 2 or 3 hours, a difficult delivery involving high or midforceps application, or the infant being large for gestational age. In this type of hemorrhage the events of labor simply produce excessive molding of the calvarium with relatively sudden stretching and tearing of the superficial venous channels over the cerebral hemispheres or venous sinuses in the posterior fossa. The clinical presentation depends on the quantity and location of blood.

Subdural hemorrhage over the cerebral hemispheres occurring at the time of birth may be clinically silent, clinically apparent in the first few days after birth, or not apparent until as late as the sixth week of life. When this type of hemorrhage is manifested early, the signs are those of increasing intracranial pressure in the presence of jaundice or anemia. When an infant shows evidence of a convex subdural hematoma as late as the fourth to sixth week, there is usually an increasing head circumference, poor feeding or vomiting, failure to thrive, altered states of consciousness, and occasionally seizures. Even though an increasing head size with signs of increased intracranial pressure usually means hydrocephalus, one must always consider a subdural hematoma in the differential diagnosis, especially with the previously mentioned historical events occurring during labor and delivery. CT scan is a very rapid method of diagnosing this condition and quantifying the amount of blood present. Management of subdural collections of fluid usually involves watching for reabsorption of fluid. Only occasionally does management involve the use of subdural taps or the removal of fluid. The decision depends on the amount of fluid, the rate of evolution of the clinical syndrome, and the presence of signs of increased intracranial pressure.

Subdural hemorrhage, when occurring in the posterior fossa, is secondary to marked molding of the calvarium with tears of the falx or tentorium. This can occur in either full-term or preterm infants. Because of the limited space around the brainstem for collection of blood before function is compromised, this type of hemorrhage is usually lethal in a very short time after the onset of bleeding.

Cerebellar hemorrhage

Massive hemorrhagic destruction of the cerebellum, although infrequent, may occur in low birth weight infants in association with perinatal trauma and asphyxia. At the present time the exact cause and pathogenesis are not fully understood. The clinical course is characterized by severe progressive apnea, a falling hematocrit level, and death.

More mildly affected infants may survive with residual damage. Infants with these sublethal retrocerebellar or intracerebellar hematomas can be suspected from changes in respiration, a high-pitched or hoarse cry, vomiting, hypotonia, and an absent Moro reflex. Rapid enlargement of the head may occur toward the end of the first week of life. Diagnosis is made by CT scan. Surgical drainage of the subdural hemorrhage may be life saving.

Epidural bleeding

This type of bleeding is extremely rare in the newborn, especially since the use of high or midforceps has been almost totally eliminated in obstetric practice. The origin of this type of bleeding is from a laceration of the middle meningeal artery following a skull fracture of the temporal bone, which usually occurs after a slippage of the forceps in a very difficult delivery. The clinical course includes signs of a rapidly appearing anemia, signs of increased intracranial pressure, and asymmetric or focal neurologic signs. When any of these signs are present following a difficult delivery, an aggressive diagnostic approach must be taken to rule out one of the treatable forms of intracranial bleeding. Diagnosis of this condition depends on clinical suspicion, the presence of a fracture in the temporal bone, and blood confirmed by CT scan. Treatment involves evacuation of blood and ligation of the site of arterial bleeding.

Cephalhematomas

See Chapter 20.

Fractures of the skull

See Chapter 20.

Spinal cord trauma

See Chapter 20.

Acute transection of the spinal cord may occur in difficult breech deliveries with hyperflexion or extension of the body in relation to the after-coming head. Much less frequently cord transection may occur with vertex presentation and deliveries in which there has been considerable lateral and direct traction. Mechanisms postulated for injury have included excessive longitudinal stretching of the cervical cord with hyperextension or excessive flexion of the neck, as well as torsional forces. Transection is most common at C5 and C7 levels. Complete lesions at higher cervical cord levels may be incompatible with survival.

The infant initially appears profoundly hypotonic, with no spontaneous movements of the legs and limited movements of the arms and hands, depending on the exact level of the cervical cord injury. Respiratory movements may be entirely abdominal because of intercostal muscle paralysis. In many reports the affected infant resembles an infant with congenital Werdnig-Hoffmann disease (Part five), but in infants with cord injury a level of sensory deficit may be determined if the examiner will carefully observe the infant's facial response, grimace, and cry on pinprick stimulation. The level of motor deficit may be determined by observation of movement of the hands and arms. Urinary and anal sphincter impairment is also evident. Spinal fluid is bloody and xanthochromic. Magnetic resonance imaging (MRI) (Chapter 13) establishes the diagnosis and level of lesion. Direct observation of the cord at operation or after death reveals swelling, maceration, and hemorrhage. Use of steroids soon after injury to reduce spinal cord swelling may provide the only potential beneficial form of therapy. In the child who survives the neonatal period, attention must be directed toward care of the bladder and kidneys, as in children with meningomyeloceles. Physical therapy is useful in preventing contractures. Children with intact arm musculature may eventually be able to ambulate with a swing-through gait.

Complete spinal cord transection is a well-recognized entity, both clinically and pathologically, but is now a very rare event because of improved obstetric care. Attention is being directed to less dramatic forms of cervical cord and brainstem injury, which are rarely recognized clinically.

Brachial plexus palsy

See also Chapter 20.

Brachial plexus palsy in the neonate has an incidence of 0.37 to 1.89 per 1,000 live births. This type of injury usually occurs from traction on the head and neck in the vertex delivery, not from arm traction. The classical descriptions of brachial plexus palsy have identified lesions affecting the upper plexus (Erb's palsy—C5, C6, C7) and lesions affecting the lower plexus (Klumpke's palsy—C8, T1). However, recent statistics on incidence do not reflect such a clear separation. Erb's palsy comprises 58% to 72% of the cases, with the entire plexus being involved up to 25% of the time and isolated Klumpke's palsy being involved only rarely. Bilateral brachial palsy is not common, occurring in 8% to 22% of cases.

In Erb's palsy the most commonly involved neural structures are the fifth and sixth cervical roots or upper trunk of the brachial plexus. Characteristic posture includes an adducted shoulder and an internally rotated arm, with the elbow extended, forearm pronated, and wrist flexed. Because of an associated involvement of higher cervical roots (C4 to C5) from which the phrenic nerve arises, diaphragmatic paralysis on the same side as the brachial plexus may occur in 5% to 9% of the cases. Other causes of diaphragmatic palsy include thoracic surgical procedures involving the thorax.

In lower plexus injury involving roots C7, C8, and T1 the weakness primarily affects the forearm and hand, particularly the flexors of wrists and fingers and intrinsic muscles of the hand. Horner's syndrome may coexist with these lower brachial plexus injuries.

The prognosis for recovery of function varies with the severity of the injury. In studies of infants with brachial plexus injury where all cases were followed, 70% to 92% showed complete recovery, and most of the remaining infants demonstrated some degree of improvement. Collective experience from the literature indicates that, in the infant who does recover completely, some improvement will be seen by 2 weeks, and most infants will achieve full recovery by 1 month and no later than 5 months. With infants who show partial recovery, improvement begins after 2 weeks, but it may be delayed as much as 4 to 6 weeks with decreasing intensity of improvement over the following 12 to 24 months. Improvement after 2 years is not known to occur.

The treatment plan for brachial plexus injury has two phases. The arm or hand or both should be kept in a functional position for the first 7 to 10 days; passive movements should be avoided because of pain during the acute period of traumatic neuritis. Following this phase, an aggressive program of physical therapy should be initiated to include prescribed range of motion exercises directed at reducing contractures during the prolonged healing stage and the return of muscle strength and voluntary movement. Surgical intervention during the healing phase has not been demonstrated to achieve better results than conservative management, including physical therapy. Corrective orthopedic surgery directed at a dysfunctional extremity may have a role in the treatment plan, after 1 to 2 years, when no further recovery is expected.

Facial nerve palsy

See also Chapter 20.

Congenital facial paralysis, present at birth with impaired eye closure and facial movements involving the entire face, as well as flattening of the nasolabial fold on the affected side, is a common birth injury with an incidence of 0.7 to 1.4 of 1,000 live births. The cause is generally considered to be the result of pressure from either obstetric forceps application or pressure on the face, with facial nerve compression in utero against the mother's sacral prominence. Alternative explanations seem necessary, since there are infants with facial nerve paralysis on delivery to whom forceps were never applied. This traumatic facial paralysis at birth has a good prognosis, and usually complete recovery occurs spontaneously within the first month. Taping the eyelid closed and the frequent use of artificial tears is necessary, if the upper eyelid does not cover the cornea during sleep. Surgical exploration is used only when the nerve is severed.

Another disorder of facial muscles, occasionally confused with peripheral facial nerve injury, is the syndrome of asymmetric crying facies in the newborn, which may resemble congenital facial palsy at first glance. However, in this condition, which is considered to be caused by congenital absence or hypoplasia of the angular depressor muscles of the mouth on one side, there is no distortion of the nasolabial fold nor impairment of eye closure. The asymmetry of the face is evident only when the infant cries or at a later age laughs. The corner of the mouth on the affected side is not pulled down. This may confuse the unwary examiner, who may consider the abnormal side to be that on which the corner of the mouth is pulled down when the infant cries. It is not known whether the primary pathology is absence of the depressor muscle or congenital absence of the branch of the facial nerve that innervates the muscle. This condition is occasionally familial and also may be associated with other congenital anomalies, including cardiac malformations in the so-called cardiofacial syndrome.

Weakness of facial muscles, either unilateral or bilateral, when associated with coexistent external rectus muscle palsies with restricted lateral movement of one or both eyes, is referred to as the Möbius syndrome; this condition should be distinguished from isolated facial palsy. The degree of facial paralysis may vary; some limited mobility is noticeable in some infants only when they cry or have difficulty feeding. Careful examination will reveal a rather flat or immobile face with limited expression, and the eyes may remain open when the infant sleeps. In the Möbius syndrome, in addition to impaired abduction of the eyes, lower cranial nerves may be involved with impaired palate and pharyngeal function. This can produce marked dysphagia, severe feeding difficulties, nasal regurgitation and possible aspiration, and speech problems at a later age. Nasogastric tube feedings or gastrostomy may be required. The pathologic basis for these multiple cranial nerve palsies is considered to be absence of their nerve nuclei in the brain stem, although pathologic studies on affected infants have varied considerably.

Congenital ptosis, caused by weakness of the levator palpebrae muscles, may occur as an isolated entity, with the site of the primary disorder being unknown. This tends to persist into later life. If, in addition to the ptosis, the infant has a smaller pupil on the same side, this is most likely congenital Horner's syndrome, which rarely can be an isolated congenital defect but is more commonly associated with a lower brachial plexus palsy and involvement of sympathetic outflow, with traction or avulsion injury affecting the upper thoracic roots.

Alfred W. Brann, Jr.
James F. Schwartz

Bibliography

Anderson, D.C., and Cranford, R.E.: Corticosteroids in ischemic stroke, Stroke, **10:**68, 1979.

Baldy-Mouliner, M., and Frerebeau, P.: Blood flow of the cerebral cortex in intracranial hypertension, Scand. J. Clin. Lab. Invest. **102**(suppl.), VG, 1968.

Banker, B.P.: The neuropathological effects of anoxia and hypoglycemia in the newborn, Dev. Med. Child. Neurol. **9:**544, 1967.

Bondareff, W., Myers, R.D., and Brann, A.W.: Brain extracellular space in monkey fetuses subjected to prolonged partial asphyxia, Exp. Neurol. **28:**167, 1970.

Brann, A.W.: Factors during neonatal life that influence brain disorders. In Freeman, J.M., editor: Prenatal and perinatal factors associated with brain disorders, NIH Pub. No. 85-1149, Bethesda, Md. 1985, National Institutes of Health.

Brann, A.W., and Myers, R.E.: Central nervous system findings in the newborn monkey following severe in utero partial asphyxia, Neurology **25:**327, 1975.

Brann, A.W., Myers, R.E., and DiGiacomo, R.: The effects of halothane-induced maternal hypotension on the fetus. In Med Primator 1970, Proceedings of the Second Conference of Experimental Medical and Surgery in Primates, Basel, Switzerland, S. Karger, 1971.

Brown, J.K., Cockburn, F., and Forfar, J.O.: Clinical and chemical correlates in convulsions of the newborn, Lancet **1**:135, 1972.

Brown, J.K. and others: Neurological aspects of perinatal asphyxia. Develop. Med. Child. Neurol. **16**:567, 1974.

Clark, D.B.: Abnormal neurologic signs in the neonate: physical diagnosis of the newly born. In Kay, J., editor: Report of the Forty-Sixth Ross Conference on Pediatric Research, Columbus, Ohio, 1964.

Clifford, S.H.: The effects of asphyxia on the newborn infant, J. Pediatr. **18**:567, 1941.

Courville, C.B.: Birth and brain damage, Pasadena, Calif., 1971.

DeSouza, S., and Richards, B.: Neurological sequelae in newborn babies after perinatal asphyxia, Arch. Dis. Child. **53**:564, 1978.

Drage, J.S., and Kennedy, C.: The Apgar scores as an index of infant morbidity, Develop. Med. Child. Neurol. **8**:141, 1966.

Dweck, H.S., and Huggins, W.: Developmental sequelae in infants having suffered severe perinatal asphyxia, Am. J. Obstet. Gynecol. **119**:811, 1974.

Ergander, V., and Erikson, M.: Severe neonatal asphyxia, Acta Paediatr. Scand. **72**:321, 1983.

Finer, N.N.: Hypoxic-ischemic encephalopatthy in term infants: perinatal factors and outcome, Pediatrics **98**:112, 1981.

Finer, N.N., and others: Factors affecting outcome in hypoxic-ischemic encephalopathy in term infants, Am. J. Dis. Child. **137**:21, 1983.

Fitzhardinge, P.M., and Flodmark, O.: The prognostic value of computerized tomography as an adjunct to assessment of the term infant with postasphyxial encephalopathy, J. Pediatr. **99**:777, 1981.

Fiyikura, T., and Klionsky, B.: The significance of meconium staining, Am. J. Obstet. Gynecol. **121**:45, 1975.

Freeman, J.M., editor: Prenatal and perinatal factors associated with brain disorders, NIH Pub. No. 85-1149, Bethesda, Md., 1985, National Institutes of Health.

Friedman, S.P., and Courville, C.B.: Atrophic lobar sclerosis of early childhood (Klegyria): report of two verified cases with particular reference to their asphyxial etiology, Bull. Los Angeles Neurol. Soc., **6**:32, 1941.

Gilles, H.: Neuropathologic indicators of abnormal development. In Freeman, J.M., editor: Prenatal and perinatal factors associated with brain disorders, NIH Pub. No. 85-1149, pp. 53-107, Bethesda, Md., 1985, National Institutes of Health.

Goldstein, G.W.: Pathogenesis of brain edema and hemorrhage: role of the brain capillary, Pediatrics **64**:357, 1979.

Hagberg, B.: Epidemiological and preventive aspects of cerebral palsy and severe mental retardation in Sweden, Eur. J. pediatr. Res. **7**:691, 1971.

Katzman, R., and others: Brain edema in stroke, Report of Joint Committee for Stroke Resources, Stroke **8**:512, 1977.

Koops, B.L., and Harmon, R.J.: Studies on long-term outcome in newborns with birth weights under 1500 grams, Adv. Behav. Pediatr. **1**:1, 1980.

Leech, R.W., and Alvord, E.C.: Anoxic ischemia encephalopathy in the human neonatal period: the significance of brain stem involvement, Arch. Neurol. **34**:109, 1977.

Little, W.J.: On the influence of abnormal parturition, difficult labours, premature birth, and asphyxia neonatorum on the mental and physical condition of the child, especially in relation to deformities, Trans. Obstet. Soc. Lond. **3**:293, 1961.

MacDonald, H.M., Neonatal asphyxia. II.: relationship of obstetric and neonatal complications to neonatal mortality in 38,405 consecutive deliveries, J. Pediatr. **96**:898, 1980.

Marchal, C., and others: Traitement des souffrances cérébrales néonatales: action des perfusions répetées de mannitol, Pédiatrie **27**:700, 1972.

Marsh, M.L., Marshall, L.F., and Shapiro, H.M.: Neurosurgical intensive care, Anesthesiology **47**:149, 1977.

Mulligan, J.C., Neonatal asphyxia. II. Neonatal mortality and long-term sequelae, J. Pediatr. **96**:903, 1980.

Myers, R.E.: Experimental models of perinatal brain damage: relevance to human pathology. In Gluck, editor: Intrauterine asphyxia and the developing fetal brain, Chicago, Year Book Medical, 1977.

Nelson, K.B., and Broman, S.H.: Perinatal risk factors in children with serious motor and mental handicaps, Ann. Neurol. **2**:371, 1977.

Nelson, K.B., and Ellenberg, J.H.: Neonatal signs and predictors of cerebral palsy, Pediatrics **64**:225, 1979.

Nelson, K.B., and Ellenberg, J.H.: Apgar scores as predictors of cerebral palsy, Pediatrics **68**:36, 1981.

Nelson, K.B., and Ellenberg, J.H.: Apgar scores as predictors of chronic neurologic disabilities, Pediatrics **68**:36, 1981.

Nelson, K.B., and Ellenberg, J.H.: Obstetric complications as risk factors for cerebral palsy or seizure disorder, JAMA, **251**:1843, 1983.

Nelson, K.B., and Ellenberg, J.N.: Antecedents of cerebral palsy: multivariate analysis of risk, N. Engl. J. Med. **315**:81, 1986.

Nordstrom, C.H., Rehncuoma, S., and Siesjo, B.K.: Effects of phenobarbital on cerebral ischemia. II.: restriction of cerebral energy state as well as glycolytic metabolites, citric acid cycle intermediates, and associated amino acids after pronounced incomplete ischemia, Stroke **9**:335, 1978.

Painter, M.J., and Bergman, I.: Obstetrical trauma to the neonatal central nervous system and peripheral nervous system, Semin. Perinatol. **6**:89, 1982.

Peeters, L.H., and others: Blood flow to fetal organs as a function of arterial oxygen content, Am. J. Obstet. Gynecol. **135**:1071, 1979.

Raichle, M.E.: The pathophysiology of brain ischemia, Ann. Neurol. **13**:1, 1983.

Ranck, J.B., and Windle, W.F.: Brain damage in the monkey, *Maraca mulatta* by asphyxia neonatorum, Exp. Neurol. **1**:130, 1959.

Reivich, M., and others: Regional cerebral blood flow during intrauterine prolonged partial asphyxia. In Myers, S.S., Reivich, M., and Erickhorn, O. editors: Research on the cerebral circulation. Fifth International Salzburg Conference, Springfield, Illinois, 1972, Charles C Thomas.

Robertson, C.M.: Unpublished data.

Sarnat, H.B., Sarnat, M.S.: Neonatal encephalopathy following fetal distress: a clinical and electroencephalographic study, Arch. Neurol. **33**:696, 1976.

Scott, H.: Outcome of very severe birth asphyxia, Arch. Dis. Child. **51**:712, 1976.

Sexson, W.R., and others: The multisystem involvement of the asphyxiated newborn, Pediatr. Res. **10**:432, 1976.

Smith, D.S., and Rehncuoma, B.K.: Barbiturates as protective agents in brain ischemia and as free-radical scavengers in vitro, Acta Physiol. Scand. **492**:129, 1980.

Steen, P.A., and Michenfelder, J.D.: Mechanisms of barbiturate protection, Anesthesiology **53**:183, 1980.

Steiner, H., and Neligan, G.: Perinatal cardiac arrest: quality of survivors, Arch. Dis. Child. **50**:696, 1975.

Storcz, J., and Mestyan, J.: Long-term prognosis of asphyxic neonates from an intensive care unit: intrauterine retarded infants at high risk of cerebral palsy, Acta Paediatr. Acad. Sci. Hungavicae **23**:361, 1982.

Susser, M., and others: Quantitative estimates of prenatal and perinatal risk factors for perinatal mortality, cerebral palsy, mental retardation and epilepsy. In Freeman, J.M., editor: Prenatal and perinatal factors associated with brain disorders, NIH Pub. No. 85-1149, Bethesda, Md. 1985, National Institutes of Health.

Terplan, K.L.: Histopathologic brain changes in 1,152 cases of the perinatal and early infancy period, Biol. Neonate **11**:348, 1967.

Thomson, A.J., and Searle, M.: Quality of survival after severe birth asphyxia, Arch. Dis. Child. 50:620, 1977.

Todd, M.M., and others: The neurologic effects of thiopental therapy following experimental cardiac arrest in cats, Anesthesiology 57:76, 1982.

Towbin, A.: Central nervous system damage in the human fetus and newborn infant: mechanical and hypoxic injury incurred in the fetal-neonatal period, Am. J. Dis. Child. 119:259, 1970.

Volpe, J.J.: Neonatal seizures, Clin. Perinatol. 4:43, 1977.

Wilkenson, H.A., Wepsic, J.J., and Austin, B.S.: Diuretic synergy in the treatment of acute experimental cerebral edema, J. Neurosurg. 34:203, 1971.

Ziegler, A.L., and others: Cerebral distress in full-term newborns and its prognostic value: a follow-up study of 90 infants, Helv. Paediatr. Acta 31:299, 1976.

PART THREE

Periventricular-intraventricular hemorrhage

Periventricular-intraventricular hemorrhage is one of the most common types of acute perinatal brain injury encountered in the neonatal period and is second only to hyaline membrane disease as a major cause of death, in preterm infants. Until a decade ago it was presumed that periventricular-intraventricular hemorrhage was an invariably fatal lesion and that, among the few infants who survived, severe neuromotor handicaps were inevitable. Recent development and subsequent clinical application of noninvasive cranial imaging techniques, particularly CT scanning and cranial ultrasonography, have drastically altered this perception. It is now evident that approximately one third of all very low birth weight infants who are discharged from hospital to home from a level III newborn intensive care unit (NICU) have incurred a periventricular-intraventricular hemorrhage and that the majority are free from major neurologic sequelae. Moreover, with the clinical use of noninvasive cranial imaging techniques, investigators have been able to delineate the incidence, site, and extent of hemorrhage; the presence and degree of ventricular dilation; and the neuropathologic sequelae.

INCIDENCE

Periventricular-intraventricular hemorrhage is essentially a condition of premature infants, although occasionally it is seen in full-term neonates. The incidence of periventricular-intraventricular hemorrhage in preterm infants less than 1,500 gm birth weight or 35 weeks' gestation is reported to vary between 40% and 50%. In fact, the true incidence of periventricular-intraventricular hemorrhage may be lower, since the reported incidence is derived from level III NICU populations and, as such, excludes preterm infants who do not require transport to a level III facility. Most hemorrhages occur within the first 2 postnatal days and virtually all occur within a week of birth. For preterm infants who die within the first few days of life, the frequency of periventricular-intraventricular hemorrhage is approximately 50%, whereas infants who survive the neonatal period have a 30% frequency of hemorrhage. An inverse relationship exists between gestational age and periventricular-intraventricular hemorrhage with the most immature infants having the highest risk. The reported mortality figures for infants with hemorrhage range from 27% to 50%. When deaths are grouped according to the severity of hemorrhage, a positive correlation exists between the extent of hemorrhage and mortality; approximately 50% of premature infants with severe hemorrhage, 15% of those with moderate hemorrhage, and 5% of those with small hemorrhage die. Survival also is influenced by the number and extent of other clinical conditions associated with prematurity.

NEUROPATHOLOGY

Subependymal germinal matrix

The germinal matrix layer is a periventricular structure that is located between the caudate nucleus and the thalamus at the level of, or slightly posterior to, the foramen of Monro. Although it is relatively prominent from 26 to 34 weeks' gestation, it is essentially exhausted by term. Within the matrix are pleuropotential cells that are the precursors for neurons and glia. Although the neuronal elements have migrated out of the germinal matrix layer by 26 weeks' gestation, primitive glial cells can be found within the matrix until near-term gestation.

The germinal matrix is a gelatinous area that contains a rich vascular network and essentially is devoid of supportive stroma. The major blood supply to the area occurs through Heubner's artery, a branch of the anterior cerebral artery. The vessels that traverse the matrix are primitive in appearance and, as such, cannot be categorized as arterioles, venules, or capillaries. At 26 to 34 weeks of gestation the walls of these vessels consist of a single layer of endothelium without smooth muscle, elastin, or collagen. Their morphologic appearance has been characterized as an "immature vascular rete." There are conflicting opinions as to the fate of these vessels on involution of the germinal matrix layer. Whether they will become either veins belonging to the deep venous system or capillaries is unknown.

Subependymal germinal matrix hemorrhage

The bleeding in periventricular-intraventricular hemorrhage usually arises from the "capillary" network of the subependymal germinal matrix layer, although, in term infants and approximately 10% of preterm neonates it may originate from the choroid plexus or the roof of the fourth ventricle. The site of hemorrhage within the germinal matrix layer tends to shift with increasing gesta-

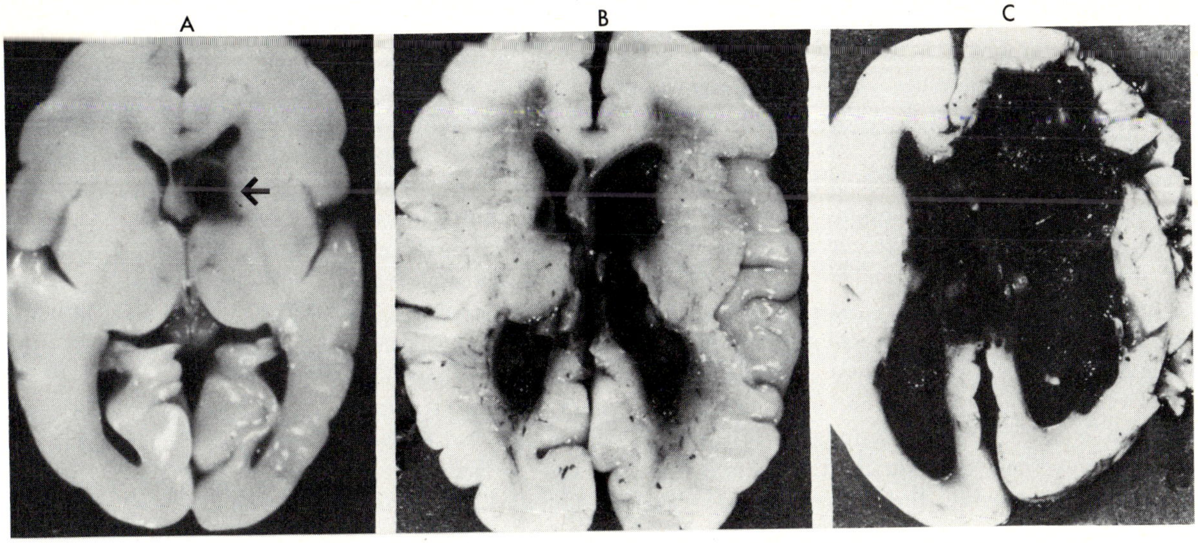

Fig. 27-10. A, Arrow indicates a subependymal cystic lesion that developed at the site of a previous isolated germinal matrix hemorrhage. **B,** Intraventricular hemorrhage with acute dilation of both lateral ventricles. **C,** Extensive parenchymal hemorrhage into the right frontoparietal region producing a mass effect with shift of midline from right to left.

tional age. In infants less than 28 weeks' gestation, hemorrhage occurs mainly in the matrix overlying the body of the caudate nucleus, but in more mature infants the primary site is at the head of the caudate nucleus at the level of the foramen of Monro. Data from animal studies indicate that there is a posteroanterior gradient for both cerebral blood flow and glucose metabolism in the germinal matrix layer and that this regional heterogeneity parallels the direction of involution of the germinal matrix layer. This may, in part, explain the variable location of periventricular-intraventricular hemorrhage at different gestational ages.

The chronic neuropathologic change seen after an isolated germinal matrix hemorrhage is a subependymal cystic lesion at the site of the hemorrhage (Fig. 27-10). Theoretically, destruction of an area of the germinal matrix layer before migration of glial cells may disturb normal cytoarchitectonic relationships among neuron-glial units. To date, no long-term clinical consequences have been attributed to this lesion.

Intraventricular hemorrhage

Intraventricular hemorrhage occurs when hemorrhage in the subependymal germinal matrix ruptures through the ependyma into the lateral ventricles (Fig. 27-10). The extravasated blood spreads throughout the ventricular system and into the posterior fossa, inciting arachnoiditis. If the hemorrhage is extensive, large clots will form within the ventricles.

Acute dilation of the ventricular system is a frequent complication of intraventricular hemorrhage. Approximately 50% of surviving infants with hemorrhage will develop acute ventricular dilation; in the majority of infants it will resolve spontaneously or remain static. The cause of the acute dilation appears to be compromised cerebrospinal fluid absorption secondary to plugging of the arachnoid villi by particulate matter from the intraventricular hemorrhage or blood clot.

Posthemorrhagic hydrocephalus, that is, progressive ventricular dilation, is the major sequela of intraventricular hemorrhage. Data on the incidence of posthemorrhagic hydrocephalus have been obscured by the inclusion of infants with acute ventricular dilation that is transient or static in nature or infants with ventricular dilation associated with cerebral atrophy. In studies in which clinical hydrocephalus was considered the end point of posthemorrhagic hydrocephalus, the incidence is 14%.

The hydrocephalus may be communicating or noncommunicating. In noncommunicating hydrocephalus obstruction of the aqueduct of Sylvius, the foramen of Monro, or the outlet foramina of Luschka and Magendie by a clot impedes the flow of cerebrospinal fluid. Ventricular dilation is usually rapid and clinical hydrocephalus is evident within 2 weeks of hemorrhage. Communicating hydrocephalus may be secondary to an obliterative arachnoiditis at the posterior fossa or obstruction to cerebrospinal fluid absorption anywhere along the path of cerebrospinal fluid flow by debris from an intraventricular blood clot. The clinical course is more indolent, and clinical hydrocephalus may not be evident for several weeks or more following intraventricular hemorrhage (Part five).

Parenchymal hemorrhage

The most extensive periventricular-intraventricular hemorrhage involves hemorrhage into the periventricular white matter (Fig. 27-10). Although this type of hemorrhage occurs in only 15% to 20% of infants with hemorrhage, it is an important cause of subsequent neurodevelopmental handicap. The chronic neuropathologic change that is seen following a parenchymal hemorrhage is the development of a porencephalic cyst at the site of the original hemorrhage.

The exact nature of the intraparenchymal hemorrhage has not been defined; however, there is evidence to support three separate mechanisms. The lesions commonly are described as a "parenchymal extension" of the germinal matrix hemorrhage. This implies that the bleeding into the matrix dissects into the periventricular white matter and forms a hematoma that causes secondary infarction of the adjacent tissue. Other neuropathologic data suggest that occlusion of the veins traversing the germinal matrix by the acute hemorrhage leads to venous engorgement or stasis and subsequent parenchymal hemorrhage. More recently, positron emission tomographic studies of infants who have incurred parenchymal hemorrhages demonstrated that blood flow was decreased to an extensive area of the affected cerebral hemisphere, implying that the intraparenchymal hemorrhage was part of a larger lesion, ischemic in nature. Since the parenchymal hemorrhages in these infants were massive, it is difficult to ascertain whether the bleeding represented a hemorrhagic infarct that was secondary to an ischemic event or whether the massive hemorrhage *per se* led to compromised cerebral perfusion that, in turn, caused widespread ischemia. Necropsy data supporting the positron emission tomography study did not delineate if the ischemia was primary or secondary in the development of intraparenchymal hemorrhage.

Periventricular leukomalacia

Cranial ultrasonographic and neuropathologic data indicate that periventricular-intraventricular hemorrhage may not be an isolated phenomenon but may be a marker for more extensive brain injury. Of note is the association of periventricular leukomalacia, an ischemic lesion, with hemorrhage. Although neuropathologic observations suggest that these two lesions can coexist, they may have separate pathogenic mechanisms.

Periventricular leukomalacia is an ischemic lesion leading to areas of necrosis in the periventricular white matter largely in the regions adjacent to the external angles of the lateral ventricles. The lesion, as originally described, begins as areas of ischemic coagulation necrosis followed by macrophage and astrocytic proliferation eventually, either bands of gliosis or cysts are formed. Ultimately, thinning of the white matter occurs with secondary enlargement of the lateral ventricles. Cavitation of tissue and cystic changes in periventricular regions become apparent. Because the involved area includes white matter through which long descending motor tracts descend from the motor cortex, with the leg fibers being closest to the ventricles and therefore more likely to be damaged, the clinical sequela is most commonly spastic paresis of the legs. With lateral extension of the lesion there also may be involvement of the arms, resulting in spastic quadriplegia. Another possible sequela is visual deficits, presumably related to involvement of optic radiations. Although this lesion occurs predominantly in the preterm infant, it has been described in term infants and is usually associated with evidence of neuronal necrosis.

The precise incidence of this lesion is not known. Although extensive periventricular leukomalacia is uncommon, its recognition is of great importance because of its poor outcome. Unlike periventricular-intraventricular hemorrhage, leukomalacia often occurs beyond the first week of life. Ultrasound may reveal a progression from initial congestion to relative normalization followed by development of cysts and finally to the resolution of cysts but the development of ventricular enlargement. Thus ultrasound evaluation of the neonatal brain in high-risk and very low birth weight infants also should be performed around the time of hospital discharge.

PATHOGENESIS

Although many perinatal and neonatal events have been linked to periventricular-intraventricular hemorrhage, the cause and pathogenesis of periventricular-intraventricular hemorrhage have remained elusive. Prospective clinical studies in which noninvasive cranial imaging techniques were used to identify infants with periventricular-intraventricular hemorrhage have demonstrated clearly that two factors, prematurity and acute respiratory failure requiring assisted ventilation, are strongly associated with periventricular-intraventricular hemorrhage. The connection with prematurity relates to the presence of the subependymal germinal matrix. Indeed, a baseline incidence of periventricular-intraventricular hemorrhage seems to occur in 12% of healthy preterm infants. The role of respiratory failure in the genesis of periventricular-intraventricular hemorrhage is less well delineated. Alterations in cerebral blood flow induced by hypoxia and/or hypercapnia and hypoxic/ischemic injury to the endothelium of the germinal layer capillaries have been offered as possible mechanisms.

Other neonatal events such as pneumothorax, hypotension, acidosis, coagulopathy, transport, volume expansion, and bicarbonate infusion have been correlated with an increased risk for periventricular-intraventricular hemorrhage. However, the associations may reflect the severity of the infant's disease, along with the need for aggressive treatment, rather than a cause and effect relationship with hemorrhage. Additionally, recent clinical obstetric studies demonstrated that perinatal factors including labor, vaginal delivery, and breech presentation do not significantly increase a preterm infant's risk for hemorrhage.

The prevailing hypothesis, based on the neuroanatomic studies of Hambleton and Wigglesworth, is that perturbations in arterial pressure and blood flow to the immature subependymal germinal matrix vascular bed initiate periventricular-intraventricular hemorrhage. Two mechanisms have been proposed (Fig. 27-11). The first suggests that cerebral vasodilation resulting from systemic hypoxia and/or hypercapnia is the initiating event. When cerebral vascular resistance is reduced concurrent with normal or increased arterial pressure, the intravascular pressure in the capillary bed may exceed the interstitial pressure in the germinal matrix. This, in turn, may lead to rupture of the immature capillary plexus and hemorrhage. The alternative theory proposes that alterations in blood flow to the germinal matrix, which are induced by systemic hypotension, lead to disruption of capillary integrity. A subsequent increase in arterial pressure causes rupture of the damaged capillaries. To delineate the impact of alterations in cerebral blood flow on the germinal matrix, laboratory animals have been used to define the physiology of cerebral blood flow during the perinatal period and to serve as models for periventricular-intraventricular hemorrhage.

Autoregulation of cerebral blood flow has been demonstrated in preterm and term experimental animal models. This refers to the maintenance of cerebral blood flow in the face of changes in perfusion pressure. With decreasing maturity the range of autoregulation narrows and resting mean arterial blood pressure shifts left from the middle of the autoregulatory plateau to the lower limit of the plateau. These findings suggest that the immature brain is vulnerable to fluctuations in blood pressure, particularly hypotension. Although the limits of autoregulation have not been defined in the preterm and term infant, preliminary data indicate that autoregulation is intact.

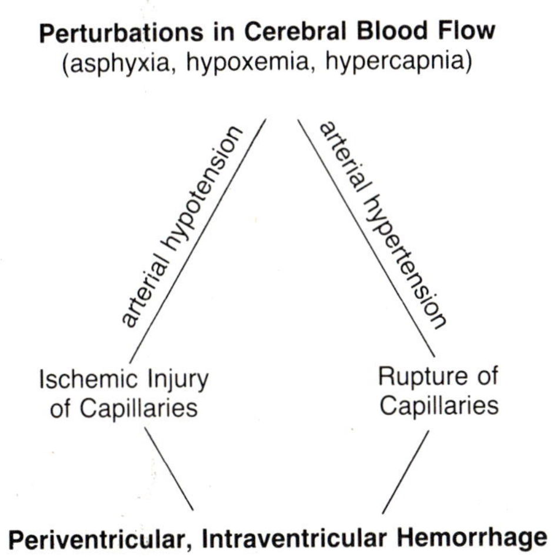

Fig. 27-11. Two proposed mechanisms for the pathogenesis of periventricular-intraventricular hemorrhage.

Data from animal studies indicate that, similar to the adult animal, arterial blood oxygen and carbon dioxide tensions in the perinatal and neonatal animal are potent regulators of cerebral blood flow. Both hypoxia and hypercapnia cause a marked increase in cerebral blood flow. Conversely, hyperoxia and hypocapnia produce a less dramatic reduction in cerebral blood flow. The cerebral blood flow response to hypoxia occurs only after the blood oxygen tension falls to a critically low level, whereas the relationship of carbon dioxide tension ($PaCO_2$) and cerebral blood flow is nearly linear over the physiologic range of $PaCO_2$. Below a $PaCO_2$ of 12 to 15 mm Hg, little or no further decrease in cerebral blood flow is observed. Hypoxia and hypercapnia can reversibly override pressure autoregulation by causing dilation of cerebral blood vessels. When this occurs, vascular resistance-mediated changes in cerebral blood flow in response to alterations in perfusion pressure are minimized and the cerebral circulation is rendered "pressure passive.

In an attempt to clarify the contributions of asphyxia and changes in arterial blood pressure to the pathogenesis of periventricular-intraventricular hemorrhage, studies of two animal models, the newborn beagle and the midterm fetal sheep, have been utilized. Both models have a germinal matrix zone that resembles the subependymal germinal matrix of a human infant at approximately 30 weeks' gestation. Experimental investigations have demonstrated that asphyxia or hypotension alone did not produce periventricular-intraventricular hemorrhage. However, when asphyxia or hypotension was followed by the rapid induction of raised arterial or venous pressure, hemorrhage occurred. Although isolated arterial hypertension, either spontaneous or induced by catecholamines, did cause periventricular-intraventricular hemorrhage, the blood pressures achieved in these studies approached values that exceed the upper limit of the autoregulatory plateau.

The most extensively studied method for producing experimental periventricular-intraventricular hemorrhage is hemorrhagic hypotension followed by rapid volume infusion. Measurements of regional cerebral blood flow in this model indicate that germinal matrix blood flow increased significantly during hypotension and that this increase in flow was sustained up to 1 hour after the restoration of blood pressure. Pretreatment with pharmocologic agents that affect prostaglandin synthesis did not alter the regional blood flow response but did result in a marked reduction in the frequency of hemorrhage.

These experimental investigations indicate that alterations in arterial pressure and blood flow play a major role in the initiation of hemorrhage. Nonetheless, since the impact of perturbations in cerebral circulatory physiology on the germinal matrix layer can be blunted by the inhibition of prostaglandin synthesis, other factors necessary for hemorrhage to occur must be localized within the matrix. Cerebral angiographic studies of the preterm brain have demonstrated a vascular border zone in the germinal matrix, making it an area especially vulnerable to injury when cerebral perfusion pressure falls. Moreover, brain capillary endothelial cells have been shown to contain a large amount of mitochondria, suggesting that these cells are dependent on oxidative metabolism and, as such, may be readily injured by any compromise in oxygen delivery. Most probably, the pathophysiology of periventricular-intraventricular hemorrhage involves a combination of factors whose cumulative effect on the vascular bed of the germinal matrix culminates in hemorrhage.

DIAGNOSIS

The most accurate and reliable method for detecting periventricular-intraventricular hemorrhage is noninvasive cranial imaging. Before the availability of CT scanning and cranial ultrasonography, the diagnosis of periventricular-intraventricular hemorrhage was predicated on the presence of a constellation of clinical signs that were thought to be specific for hemorrhage. Two clinical courses were described, one catastrophic in nature and the other saltatory or stuttering. The catastrophic course included an abrupt deterioration of clinical status including hypotension, apnea and severe metabolic acidosis, and bulging of the anterior fontanel, with rapid progression to death. In the saltatory course, sudden clinical deterioration was followed by recovery. Over the next 48 hours, the cycle usually was repeated several times until death or clinical recovery occurred. Prospective clinical studies employing noninvasive cranial imaging techniques have indicated that these events are not specific for periventricular-intraventricular hemorrhage and, in fact, may be elicited in preterm infants who have no demonstrable neurologic lesion. Moreover, approximately 50% of preterm infants who have a periventricular-intraventricular hemorrhage detected by noninvasive cranial imaging techniques do not have clinical evidence of the hemorrhage. Other infants who incur a hemorrhage may manifest neurologic signs that are so subtle that they may be readily overlooked or attributed to other nonneurologic problems associated with prematurity.

Cranial ultrasonography employing the anterior fontanel as an acoustic window is the most widely used technique for the detection of periventricular-intraventricular hemorrhage and its sequelae. The advantages of ultrasonography when compared to computed tomographic brain scanning include its portability that permits evaluation at the infant's bedside, the use of sound rather than ionizing radiation, and the ability to image in two planes. Several limitations of the technique are the inability to delineate small amounts of blood in the lateral ventricles, especially if they are normal in size, the inaccuracy in distinguishing small subependymal hemorrhage from the germinal matrix, and the overall quality of the scan. Despite these limitations, the specificity and sensitivity of cranial ultrasonography are high enough to warrant its use as the technique of choice for the diagnosis of periventricular-intraventricular hemorrhage.

The optimal timing for detecting periventricular-intraventricular hemorrhage with cranial ultrasonography is the latter part of the first week of life with a follow-up study at 2 weeks of age to determine the extent of the hemorrhage. The presence of ventricular dilation is optimally ascertained at 2 weeks of age; if present, weekly serial scans are helpful in delineating whether the ventricular dilation is transient, static, or progressive. Later follow-up scans may be needed to diagnose periventricular leukomalacia.

Many attempts have been made to develop a descriptive, yet simple method for classifying the spectrum of hemorrhage. Although there is no consensus among diagnosticians, the classification outlined in Fig. 27-12 is the most widely employed.

Small Hemorrhage
- Grade I
  - Isolated germinal matrix hemorrahge
- Grade II
  - Intraventricular hemorrhage with normal ventricular size

Moderate Hemorrhage
- Grade III
  - Intraventricular hemorrhage with acute ventricular dilation

Severe Hemorrhage
- Grado IV
  - Intraventricular hemorrhage with parenchymal hemorrhage

Fig. 27-12. Classification for the spectrum of periventricular-intraventricular hemorrhage.

MANAGEMENT

The clinical management of infants who have sustained a periventricular-intraventricular hemorrhage is identical to that for any sick preterm infant. Two primary goals are the maintenance of adequate perfusion pressure and ventilation. A concerted and continuous effort must be made to monitor and maintain normal PaO_2, $PaCO_2$, pH and osmolality, and adequate perfusion pressure. This includes the judicious use of volume expanders and blood products. Attempts should be made to mitigate wide swings in arterial and venous pressure (e.g., apnea, pneumothorax, crying), to avoid noxious procedures whenever possible, and to limit unnecessary handling and stimulation. If seizure activity is suspected, treatment with the appropriate anticonvulsant medication is indicated.

Acute intraventricular hemorrhage does not require treatment, because the blood within the ventricular system ultimately will dissipate even without intervention. The initiation of serial lumbar punctures shortly after an acute episode of intraventricular hemorrhage has been tried in an attempt to prevent the development of posthemorrhagic hydrocephalus. Although blood and protein were removed and intracranial pressure was lowered, the frequency of posthemorrhagic hydrocephalus remained unchanged.

The treatment of progressive posthemorrhagic hydrocephalus includes serial lumbar punctures, hyperosmolar therapy (e.g., glycerol), drugs that decrease cerebrospinal fluid production (e.g., acetazolamide, furosemide), ventriculostomy, and ventriculoperitoneal shunt placement. Each of these procedures has had varying degrees of reported success and complications. The response to therapy most likely depends on whether the hydrocephalus is obstructive or communicating (Part five).

Noncommunicating or obstructive hydrocephalus usually is characterized by rapid ventricular dilation accompanied by an increase in intracranial pressure. The progressive ventricular dilation is relentless, and attempts to remove large amounts of cerebrospinal fluid by serial lumbar punctures have been unsuccessful. In this situation, surgical ventricular drainage is indicated. Although ventriculoperitoneal shunt placement is the definitive therapy, a ventricular reservoir that can be tapped on a daily basis may be useful as a temporizing measure if the infant is too small or too sick to undergo shunt placement.

Slowly progressive ventricular enlargement associated with normal intracranial pressure is most probably communicating in nature. When evidence of progressive ventricular dilation is present, intervention with daily serial lumbar punctures or drugs that decrease cerebrospinal fluid production is warranted. The optimal duration of therapy is unknown. Serial lumbar punctures are usually done for 3 to 4 weeks or until the amount of cerebrospinal fluid removed is less than 5 ml for several days; drug therapy may continue for months. With both types of intervention, weekly cranial ultrasounds are necessary to monitor the effectiveness of the treatment in arresting or resolving the hydrocephalus. To determine whether or not further intervention will be required, surveillance of ventricular size for several weeks after stopping therapy is appropriate.

A general approach to the management of posthemorrhagic ventricular dilation is as follows. Serial ultrasonographic measurement of ventricular size is obtained at weekly intervals. When rapid, relentless, progressive dilation is documented, surgical ventricular drainage is indicated. Conversely, when ventricular dilation is static, continued observation without specific intervention is appropriate. Finally, when slowly progressive ventricular dilation is observed over at least a 3-week interval, a trial of pharmacologic agents to decrease cerebrospinal fluid production or serial lumbar punctures is warranted. If ventricular dilation progresses in spite of treatment, surgical ventricular drainage may be required.

NEURODEVELOPMENTAL OUTCOME

Although the spectrum and sequelae of periventricular-intraventricular hemorrhage have been well documented with noninvasive cranial imaging techniques, the impact of these lesions on the neurologic and developmental outcome of affected infants remains ill-defined. Clinical studies that compared infants with periventricular-intraventricular hemorrhage to a control group without hemorrhage indicate that infants with small hemorrhages have the same risk for major neurodevelopmental handicaps at 1 to 2 years of age as their counterparts without hemorrhage. The incidence of handicaps in both groups is approximately 11%. Among infants with moderate and severe periventricular-intraventricular hemorrhage, the risk for major handicaps is increased threefold and sevenfold respectively. Although the development of posthemorrhagic hydrocephalus *per se* does not seem to increase an infant's risk for neurodevelopmental handicaps, these children tend to have a more global injury encompassing both neuromotor and cognitive development. Conversely, hydrocephalus ex vacuo, that is, ventricular dilation associated with diffuse cerebral atrophy, has been linked with an adverse outcome.

Data on preschool and early school-age children, although sparse, suggest that children with periventricular-intraventricular hemorrhage who did not have major handicaps at 1 to 2 years of age are at risk for hyperactivity. As more information is forthcoming, awareness of the magnitude and scope of these problems will be enhanced. At present it would appear that extensive periventricular-intraventricular hemorrhage is a marker for severe motor and intellectual deficits. Very likely it is not the hemorrhage per se but concomitant and attendant events associated with the hemorrhage as periventricular leukomalacia that cause the brain injury. Until these events are better understood, it is not possible to predict the neurodevelopmental outcome of an individual child (Part six).

PREVENTION

The most effective means of eliminating periventricular-intraventricular hemorrhage is the prevention of preterm birth. Short of this outcome, efforts to minimize hemorrhage have been directed at modulating wide swings in systemic blood pressure (e.g., with phenobarbital, indomethacin, pancuronium bromide) and/or stabilizing the capillary endothelium of the germinal matrix (e.g., with ethamsylate, vitamin E, indomethacin).

Phenobarbital

See also Chapter 28, part four.

The role of prophylactic phenobarbital therapy in the prevention of periventricular-intraventricular hemorrhage is controversial. An initial prospective, randomized clinical trial demonstrated a dramatic reduction of 70% in the overall incidence of hemorrhage, but no decrease in the frequency of severe hemorrhage was noted when phenobarbital was given during the first 6 days after birth. Several subsequent randomized controlled studies failed to confirm this observation and, in fact, showed that prophylactic postnatal phenobarbital therapy had no impact on the occurrence of hemorrhage.

A preliminary study in which prophylactic phenobarbital was administered antenatally to women in active preterm labor and/or with spontaneous rupture of fetal membranes demonstrated a significant lowering of the incidence and severity of hemorrhage, as well as the mortality rate, for infants in the group given phenobarbital. Until this study is duplicated, no conclusions can be drawn about the efficacy of antenatal phenobarbital for the prevention of hemorrhage.

Indomethacin

In the beagle pup model of periventricular-intraventricular hemorrhage, indomethacin virtually eliminated hemorrhage. The neuroprotective effect was attributed to the inhibition of the cyclooxygenase pathway of prostaglandin synthesis in the cerebral microvasculature, reduction in cerebral blood flow, and the prevention of free radical production. Based on the experimental data, a prospective, randomized clinical study was conducted in which preterm infants were given five doses of indomethacin intravenously, beginning at 6 hours after birth. Infants who were given indomethacin incurred half as many hemorrhages as the control group; however, there was no difference in the distribution of hemorrhages. An incidental finding in several prospective studies of indomethacin prophylaxis for patent ductus arteriosis was a reduced incidence of periventricular-intraventricular hemorrhage for infants in the group given indomethacin.

Pancuronium

See also Chapter 28, part four.

Among infants who require mechanical ventilation, a strong association has been observed between a pattern of fluctuating arterial blood pressure and cerebral blood flow velocity and the subsequent development of periventricular-intraventricular hemorrhage. Paralysis with pancuronium, a competitive nondepolarizing neuromuscular blocking agent, has been shown to stabilize cardiorespiratory variables, including fluctuating patterns of blood pressure. A prospective clinical trial in which pancuronium was administered to preterm infants who required mechanical ventilation and who had abnormal fluctuations in arterial blood pressure and cerebral blood flow velocity demonstrated an immediate abolition of the fluctuating patterns and a significant reduction in the incidence and severity of hemorrhage for infants in the pancuronium group. Although the results of this study are encouraging, the particular subset of infants selected for the study accounted for only 40% of all infants who incurred a hemorrhage. Moreover, the use of pancuronium in extremely immature infants has been associated with serious adverse effects, including edema and renal failure.

Ethamsylate

A preliminary observation on the clinical use of prophylactic ethamsylate for the prevention of periventricular-intraventricular hemorrhage suggested a significant reduction in the frequency of hemorrhage among infants who were treated with the drug within 2 hours of birth. However, the mortality rate for the ethamsylate-treated infants who incurred a hemorrhage was double that for control infants with hemorrhage. No other studies have been reported. Based on experimental data, the proposed mechanisms of action for ethamsylate include reinforcement of the capillary basement membrane by enhancement of hyaluronic acid polymerization, increased platelet adhesiveness, and inhibition of prostacyclin and thromboxane synthesis.

Vitamin E

It has been suggested that vitamin E, an antioxidant and free radical scavenger, might prevent periventricular-intraventricular hemorrhage by stabilizing the endothelial membrane of the capillary network in the germinal matrix. Several clinical investigators have reported a significant decrease in the frequency and severity of hemorrhage in infants who received parenteral vitamin E supplement on the first postnatal day. Conversely, other researchers have observed an alarming increase, especially in the severity of hemorrhage, for infants treated with vitamin E. Thus, at present, it would appear that vitamin E supplementation is not effective in preventing periventricular-intraventricular hemorrhage and may actually increase the risk for hemorrhage.

Summary

Available studies do not support the routine clinical use of any drug to prevent periventricular-intraventricular hemorrhage. The administration of any therapy with the sole intent of preventing hemorrhage still needs to be done within the context of a research protocol, since the safety, efficacy, and risk benefit ratio of most proposed treatments are still unknown.

Lu-Ann Papile

BIBLIOGRAPHY

General

Ahmann, P.A., Lazzara, A., and Dykes, F.D.: Intraventricular hemorrhage in the high-risk preterm infant: incidence and outcome, Ann. Neurol. **7**:118, 1980.

Burstein, J., and others: Intraventricular hemorrhage and hydrocephalus in premature newborns: a prospective study with CT, A.J.R. **102**:631, 1979.

Deonna, T., and others: Neonatal intracranial hemorrhage in premature infants, Pediatrics **56**:1056, 1975.

Donat, J.F., and others: Intraventricular hemorrhages in full-term and premature infants, Mayo Clin. Proc. **53**:437, 1978.

Hawgood, S., Spong, J., and Yu, V.Y.H.: Intraventricular hemorrhage incidence and outcome in a population of very-low-birth-weight infants, Am. J. Dis. Child. **138**:136, 1984.

Hayden, C.H., Shattuck, K.E., and Richardson, C.J.: Subependymal germinal matrix hemorrhage in full-term neonates, Pediatrics **75**:714, 1985.

Holt, P.J., and Allan, W.F.: The natural history of ventricular dilatation in neonatal intraventricular hemorrhage and its therapeutic implications, Ann. Neurol. **10**:293, 1981.

Kosmetatos, N., and others: Intracranial hemorrhage in the premature, Am. J. Dis. Child. **134**:855, 1980.

Lacey, D.J., and Terplan, K.: Intraventricular hemorrhage in full-term neonates, Devel. Med. Child. Neurol. **24**:332, 1982.

Leech, R.W., and Kohnen, P.: Subependymal and intraventricular hemorrhages in the newborn, Am. J. Pathol. **77**:465, 1974.

Palma, P.A., and others: Intraventricular hemorrhage in the neonate born at term, Am. J. Dis. Child. **133**:941, 1979.

Shinnar, S., and others: Intraventricular hemorrhages in the premature infant: a changing outlook, N. Engl. J. Med. **306**:1464, 1982.

Volpe, J.J.: Neurology of the newborn, Philadelphia, 1981, W.B. Saunders Co.

Neuropathology

Armstrong, D., and others: Another look at the pathology of intraventricular hemorrhage. In Lucey, J., editor: Syllabus, Ross Symposium on Perinatal Intracranial Hemorrhage, Columbus, Ohio, 1980, Ross Laboratories.

Barth, P.G., and others: On the relationship between germinal layer hemorrhage and telencephalic leukoencephalopathy in the preterm infant, Neuropadiatrie **11**:17, 1980.

DeReuck, J.: Cerebral angioarchitecture and perinatal brain lesions in premature and full-term infants, Acta Neurol. Scand. **70**:391, 1984.

DeVries, L.S., Regev, R., and Dubositz, L.M.S.: Late onset of cystic leukomalacia, Arch. Dis. Child. **61**:298, 1986.

Grunnet, M.: Periventricular leukomalacia complex, Arch. Pathol. Lab. Med. **103**:6, 1979.

Hambleton, G., and Wigglesworth, J.S.: Origin of intraventricular haemorrhage in the preterm infant, Arch. Dis. Child. **51**:651, 1976.

Hill, A., Schackelford, G., and Volpe, J.J.: A potential mechanism of pathogenesis for early posthemorrhagic hydrocephalus in the premature newborn, Pediatrics **73**:19, 1984.

Larroche, J.C.: Post-haemorrhagic hydrocephalus in infancy, Biol. Neonat **20**:287, 1972.

Ment, L.R., and others: Post hemorrhagic hydrocephalus, J. Neurosurg. **60**:343, 1984.

Pape, K.E., and Wigglesworth, J.S.: Haemorrhage, ischaemia and the perinatal brain, Philadelphia, 1979, J.B. Lippincott, Co.

Pasternak, J.F., and Groothuis, D.R.: Regional variability of blood flow and glucose utilization within the subependymal germinal matrix, Brain Res. **299**:281, 1984.

Pasternak, J.F., Groothuis, D.R., and Fischer, J.M.: Porencephaly from periventricular intracerebral hemorrhage in a premature infant, Am. J. Dis. Child. **134**:673, 1980.

Rorke, L.B.: Pathology of perinatal brain injury, New York, 1982, Raven Press.

Takashima, S., and Tanaka, K.: Microangiography and vascular permeability of the subependymal germinal matrix in the premature infant, Can. J. Neurol. Sci. **5**:45, 1978.

Pathogenesis

Ashwal, S., and others: Patterns of fetal lamb regional cerebral blood flow (CBF) during and after prolonged hypoxia, Pediatr. Res. **14**:1104, 1980.

Betz, A.L., and Goldstein, G.W.: Developmental changes in biochemical properties of isolated brain capillaries, Pediatr. Res. **13**:355, 1979.

deCourten, G.M., and Rabenowicz, T.H.: Analysis of 100 infant deaths with intraventricular hemorrhage: brain weights and risk factors, Dev. Med. Child Neurol. **23**:287, 1981.

Dykes, F.D., and others: Intraventricular hemorrhage: a prospective evaluation of etiopathogenesis, Pediatrics **66**:42, 1980.

Fujimura, M., and others: Clinical events relating to intraventricular haemorrhage in the newborn, Arch. Dis. Child. **54**:409, 1979.

Goddard, J., and others: Moderate, rapidly induced hypertension as a cause of intraventricular hemorrhage in the newborn beagle puppy, J. Pediatr. **96**:1957, 1980.

Goddard-Finegold, J.: Periventricular, intraventricular hemorrhages in the premature newborn, Arch. Neurol. **41**:766, 1984.

Goddard-Finegold, J., Armstrong, D., and Zeller, R.S.: Intraventricular hemorrhage following volume expansion after hypovolemic hypotension in the newborn beagle, J. Pediatr. **100**:796, 1982.

Goddard-Finegold, J., and Michael, L.N.: Cerebral blood flow and experimental intraventricular hemorrhage, Pediatr. Res. **18**:7, 1984.

Goldstein, G.W.: Pathogenesis of brain edema and hemorrhage: role of the brain capillary, Pediatrics **64**:357, 1979.

Haruda, F., and Blanc, W.A.: The structure of intracerebral arteries in premature infants and the autoregulation of cerebral blood flow, Ann. Neurol. **10**:303, 1981.

Hernandez, M.J., Brennan, R.W., and Bowman, G.S.: Autoregulation of cerebral blood flow in the newborn dog, Brain Res. **184**:199, 1980.

Hernandez, M.J., and others: Cerebral blood flow and oxygen consumption in the newborn dog, Am. J. Physiol. **234**:R209, 1978.

Hill, A., Perlman, J.M., and Volpe, J.J.: Relationship of pneumothorax to occurrence of intraventricular hemorrhage in premature infants, Pediatrics **69**:144, 1982.

Levene, M.I., Fawer, C.L., and Lamont, R.F.: Risk factors in the development of intraventricular haemorrhage, Arch. Dis. Child. **57**:410, 1982.

Lou, H.C.: Perinatal hypoxic-ischemic brain damage and intraventricular hemorrhage: a pathogenetic model, Arch. Neurol. **37**:575, 1980.

Lou, H.C., Lassen, N.A., and Friis-Hansen, B.: Low cerebral blood flow in hypotensive neonatal distress, Acta Neurol. Scand. **56**:343, 1977.

Lou, H.C., Lassen, N.A., and Friis-Hansen, B.: Is arterial hypertension crucial for the development of cerebral haemorrhage in premature infants? Lancet **1**:1215, 1979.

Ment, L.R., Stewart, W.B., and Duncan, C.C.: Beagle puppy model of intraventricular hemorrhage: effect of superoxide dismutase on cerebral blood flow and prostaglandins, J. Neurosurg. **62**:563, 1985.

Ment, L.R., and others: Beagle puppy model of intraventricular hemorrhage: effect of indomethacin on cerebral blood flow, J. Neurosurg. **58**:857, 1983.

Murton, L.J., and others: Perinatal factors: periventricular haemorrhage and mortality in very low birthweight infants, Austr. Paediatr. J. **21**:39, 1985.

Oldendorf, W.H., Cornford, E.M., and Brown, W.J.: The large apparent work capability of the blood-brain carrier: a study of the mitochondrial content of capillary endothelial cells in brain and other tissues of the rat, Ann. Neurol. **1**:409, 1977.

Papile, L.A., Rudolph, A.M., and Heymann, M.A.: Autoregulation of cerebral blood flow in the preterm fetal lamb, Pediatr. Res. **19**:159, 1985.

Pasternak, J.F., and others: Regional cerebral blood flow in the newborn beagle pup: the germinal matrix is a "low flow" structure, Pediatr. Res. **16**:499, 1982.

Purves, M.J.: The physiology of the cerebral circulation, New York, 1972, Cambridge University Press.

Purves, M.J., and James, I.M.: Observations on the control of cerebral blood flow in the sheep fetus and newborn lamb, Circ. Res. **25**:651, 1969.

Reynolds, M.L., and others: Intracranial hemorrhage in the preterm sheep fetus, Early Hum. Dev. **3**:163, 1979.

Rosenberg, A.A., and others: Response of cerebral blood flow to changes in P_{CO_2} in the fetal newborn and adult sheep, Am. J. Physiol. **242**:H862, 1982.

Schimmel, M.S. Wund, J.T., and Kairam, R.: Tension pneumothorax and intraventricular haemorrhage, Lancet **1**:413, 1983.

Shapiro, H.M., and others: Heterogeneity of local cerebral blood flow—Pa_{CO_2} sensitivity in neonatal dogs, J. Appl. Physiol. **49**:113, 1980.

Speer, M.E., and others: Intraventricular hemorrhage and vitamin E in the very low-birth weight infant: evidence for efficacy of early intramuscular vitamin E administration, Pediatrics **74**:1107, 1984.

Strauss, A., and others: Perinatal events and intraventricular/subependymal hemorrhage in the very low-birth weight infant, Am. J. Obstet. Gynecol. **151**:1022, 1985.

Szymonowicz, W., Yu, V., and Wilson, F.E.: Antecedents of periventricular haemorrhage in infants weighing 1250 grams or less at birth, Arch. Dis. Child. **59**:13, 1984.

Volpe, J.J., and others: Positron emission tomography in the newborn: extensive impairment of regional cerebral blood flow with intraventricular hemorrhage and hemorrhagic cerebral involvement, Pediatrics **72**:589, 1983.

Wimberley, P.D., and others: Hypertensive peaks in the pathogenesis of intraventricular hemorrhage in the newborn, abolition by phenobarbitone sedation, Acta Paediatr. Scand. **71**:537, 1982.

Diagnosis

Bowerman, R.A., and others: Periventricular leukomalacia in the preterm newborn infant: sonographic and clinical features, Radiology **151**:383, 1984.

Dolfin, T., and others: Diagnosis and evolution of periventricular leukomalacia: a study with real-time ultrasound, Early Hum. Dev. **9**:105, 1984.

Donn, S.M., Roloff, D.W., and Keyes, J.W., Jr.: Lumbar cisternography in evaluation of hydrocephalus in the preterm infant, Pediatrics **72**:670, 1983.

Dubowitz, L.M.S., and others: Neurologic signs in neonatal intraventricular hemorrhage: a correlation with real-time ultrasound, J. Pediatr. **99**;127, 1981.

Fitzhardinge, P.M., Flodmark, O., and Ashby, S.: The prognostic value of computed tomography of the brain in asphyxiated premature infants, J. Pediatr. **100**:476, 1982.

Lazzara, A., and ohters: Clinical predictability of intraventricular hemorrhage in preterm infants, Pediatrics **65**:30, 1980.

Pape, K.E., and others: Diagnostic accuracy of neonatal brain imaging: a postmortem correlation of computed tomography and ultrasound scans, J. Pediatr. **102**:275, 1983.

Papile, L.A., and others: Incidence and evolution of subependymal and intraventricular hemorrhage: a study of infants with birth weights less than 1500 grams, J. Pediatr. **92**:529, 1978.

Partridge, J.C., and others: Optimal timing for diagnostic cranial ultrasound in low-birth-weight infants: detection of intracranial hemorrhage and ventricular dilation, J. Pediatr. **102**:281, 1983.

Rumack, C.M., and Johnson, M.L.: Perinatal and infant brain imaging, Chicago, 1984, Year Book Medical Publishers, Inc.

Prevention

Bedard, M.P., and others: Effect of prophylactic phenobarbital on intraventricular hemorrhage in high-risk infants, Pediatrics **73**:435, 1984.

Donn, S.M., Roloff, D.W., and Goldstein, G.W.: Prevention of intraventricular hemorrhage in preterm infants by phenobarbitone, Lancet **2**:215, 1981.

Hensey, O.J., Morgan, M.E.I., and Cooke, R.W.I.: Tranexamic acid in the prevention of periventricular haemorrhage, Arch. Dis. Child. **59**:719, 1984.

Hittner, H.M., and others: Retrolental fibroplasia: efficacy of vitamin E in a double-blind clinical study of preterm infants, N. Engl. J. Med. **305**:1365, 1981.

Kauffman, R.E.: Therapeutic interventions to prevent intracerebral hemorrhage in preterm infants, J. Pediatr. **108**:323, 1986.

Kuban, K.C.K., and others: Neonatal intracranial hemorrhage and phenobarbital, Pediatrics **77**:443, 1986.

Mahony, L., and others: Indomethacin therapy on the first day of life in infants with very low birth weight, J. Pediatr. **106**:801, 1985.

Ment, L.R., Stewart, W.B., Duncan, C.C.: Beagle puppy model of intraventricular hemorrhage: ethamsylate studies, Prostaglandins **27**:245, 1984.

Ment, L.R., and others: Randomized indomethacin trial for prevention of intraventricular hemorrhage in very low birth weight infants, J. Pediatr. **107**:937, 1985.

Morales, W.J., and Koerten, J.: Prevention of intraventricular hemorrhage in very low birth weight infants by maternally administered phenobarbital, Obstet. Gynecol. **68**:295, 1986.

Morgan, M.E.I., Benson, J.W., and Cooke, R.W.I.: Ethamsylate reduces the incidence of periventricular haemorrhage in very low birth-weight infants, Lancet **2**:830, 1981.

Morgan, M.E.I., Massey, R.F., and Cooke, R.W.I.: Does phenobarbitone prevent periventricular hemorrhage in very low-birth-weight babies?: a controlled trial, Pediatrics **70**:186, 1982.

Perlman, J.M., and others: Reduction in intraventricular hemorrhage by elimination of fluctuating cerebral blood-flow velocity in preterm infants with respiratory distress syndrome, N. Engl. J. Med. **312**:1353, 1985.

Phelps, D.L.: Vitamin E and CNS hemorrhage, Pediatrics **74**:1113, 1984.

Reynolds, E.O.R., Hope, P.L., and Whitehead, M.D.: Muscle relaxation and periventricular hemorrhage, N. Engl. J. Med. **313**:955, 1985.

Setzer, E.S., and others: Prophylactic indomethacin and intraventricular hemorrhage in the premature, Pediatr. Res. **18**:345, 1984.

Shankaran, S., and others: Antenatal phenobarbital for the prevention of neonatal intracerebral hemorrhage, Am. J. Obstet. Gynecol. **154**:53, 1986.

Whitelaw, A., and others: Phenobarbitone for prevention of periventricular haemorrhage in very low birth weight infants, Lancet **2**:1168, 1983.

Neurodevelopmental outcome

Allan, W.C., Dransfield, D.A., and Tito, A.M.: Ventricular dilation following periventricular, intraventricular hemorrhage: outcome at age 1 year, Pediatrics **73**:158, 1984.

Krishnamoorthy, K.S., and others: Neurologic sequelae in survivors of neonatal intraventricular hemorrhage, Pediatrics **64**:233, 1979.

Krishnamoorthy, K.S., and others: Neurodevelopmental outcome of survivors with post-hemorrhagic hydrocephalus following grade II IVH, The Second Special Ross Laboratories Conference on Perinatal Intraventricular Hemorrhage, p. 1302, Columbus, Ohio, 1982, Ross Laboratories.

Liechty, E.A., Bull, M.J., and Bryson, C.Q.: Developmental outcome of very low birth weight infants requiring ventriculoperitoneal shunt, Childs Brain **10**:340, 1983.

McMenamin, J.B., Schackelford, G.D., and Volpe, J.J.: Outcome of neonatal intraventricular hemorrhage with periventricular echo-dense lesions, Ann. Neurol. **15**:285, 1984.

Naulty, C.M., and others: Developmental outcome of infants with grade III intraventricular hemorrhage, South. Med. J. **76**:158, 1983.

Papile, L.A., Munsick-Bruno, G., and Schaefer, A.: The relationship of cerebral intraventricular hemorrhage and early childhood handicaps, J. Pediatr. **103**:273, 1983.

Williamson, W.O., and others: Survival of low-birth-weight infants with intraventricular hemorrhage, Am. J. Dis. Child. **137**:1181, 1983.

PART FOUR

Seizures

Seizures are the most frequent and distinct neurologic sign occurring in the neonatal period and result in the most requests for consultation and evaluation. They may represent primary CNS disease or they may be manifestations of systemic or metabolic insults. The incidence of seizures in the newborn varies, depending on the population—full-term or preterm infants—and the time of onset—first week or first month of life. Estimates of frequency of seizures in the newborn vary from as low as 0.8% of an entire nursery population to 25% in an intensive care unit of sick preterm infants. Of neonatal seizures 85% begin in the first 15 days of life with approximately 65% occurring between the second and fifth days of life.

Seizures at this time represent a relative medical emergency, since they are usually the signal of a life-threatening underlying disease or disorder that can produce irreversible brain damage. Furthermore, experimental evidence suggests that seizure activity in the immediate postnatal period, a time of both active myelination and continuing cell division, may result in reduction in DNA content and brain cell number. It is therefore important to diagnose and treat neonatal seizures and their underlying causes with great dispatch.

CLINICAL MANIFESTATIONS

Seizures in the older child are classified by their clinical manifestation and at times by their site of origin, since both may have etiologic, therapeutic, and prognostic implications. Seizure phenomena in the newborn differ greatly from those observed in older infants and children in that only rarely will newborns have well-organized symmetric generalized tonic-clonic seizures. The explanation for these differences is related to the status of the neuroanatomic and physiologic organization of the neonatal brain referred to later. Various neonatal seizure manifestations follow:

A. Abnormal movements or alterations of tone in trunk and extremities
   1. Fragmentary clonic—multifocal, migratory (non-jacksonian)
   2. Alternating hemiclonic
   3. Tonic
      a. Single extremity
      b. Extension of arms and legs (decerebrate)
      c. Extension of legs, flexion of arms (decorticate)
   4. Myoclonic—isolated or generalized
   5. Bicycling movements of legs
   6. Rowing or drum-beating movements of arms
   7. Loss of tone with generalized flaccidity
   8. Generalized tonic-clonic

B. Facial, oral, lingual movements
   1. Sucking
   2. Grimacing, twitching
   3. Chewing, swallowing, yawning

C. Ocular movements
   1. Tonic horizontal eye deviation
   2. Staring, blinking
   3. Nystagmoid jerks

D. Respiratory manifestations
   1. Apnea, usually preceded or accompanied by one of the other subtle manifestations of seizures
   2. Hyperpneic or stertorous breathing

In addition to these very specific clinical manifestations, any alteration in the state of the infant that is "on-off" in character and is repetitive or paroxysmal in occurrence may be a seizure. Such activity must be differentiated from tremors (Part one), as well as from decerebrate or decorticate posturing indicative of progressive rostrocaudal pressure and herniation. This can be a difficult distinction, even for the experienced clinician.

PATHOPHYSIOLOGY

A seizure requires that the synchronous firing of adjacent neurons reach a critical mass to produce clinical manifestations. Epileptic neurons recruit adjacent neurons to fire synchronously and thereby produce a seizure. Although the neonatal cortex has a relatively complete complement of neurons, there is a relative paucity of dendrites and synaptic connections, with the neuropile having not yet reached its full stage of growth and complexity. The neuronal membranes, which are leaky, allow sodium to enter and potassium to exit from the cell far more easily than from more mature membranes. With the level of sodium-potassium ATP well below mature levels, the cell is less able to pump out sodium efficiently and become repolarized. Thus the newborn's neurons remain relatively hyperpolarized, making it more difficult for the epileptic neuron to have rapid and repetitive firing and to permit recruitment of other neurons for synchronous discharge. These reasons primarily account for the infrequency of cortical seizures in the newborn. The temporal lobe and subcortical structures are more mature and therefore better able to sustain epileptic activity and produce a clinical seizure. This may explain the propensity of the newborn to have such temporal lobe and subcortical manifestations of seizures as grimacing, chewing, repetitive swallowing, staring, or altered respiratory rhythm.

ETIOLOGY

The causes of neonatal seizures are varied, and many seizures respond to specific treatment. Therefore determining the cause is critical. Etiologies are determined on the basis of historical data, physical findings, and clinical observations, plus a variety of laboratory tests and observation of clinical response to various therapeutic measures.

Asphyxia is the most frequent cause of seizures in the full-term infant. Seizures occur not only in those infants whose asphyxia is evident at birth but also in infants whose asphyxia occurred before delivery, which may not have been documented by fetal monitoring. At times seizures caused by asphyxia also may be associated with subarachnoid bleeding, but this is not invariable. The incidence of seizures in asphyxiated infants is reported to vary between 22% and 60%. They most commonly begin early, between 6 and 18 hours of life. Seizures in severely asphyxiated infants are among the most difficult of seizures to control and generally carry the poorest prognosis of all neonatal seizures.

Intracranial hemorrhage historically has been considered the most common cause of neonatal convulsions, with the frequent implication that birth trauma was the primary event. Subarachnoid bleeding may be the result of trauma but is also common with asphyxia. It is difficult to separate the asphyxial insult from the subarachnoid bleeding as the cause of seizures. Furthermore, small amounts of subarachnoid bleeding are frequently noted in infants who have a single seizure on the second or third day of life, who in all other respects appear well and who have a good prognosis. Seizures also have been reported by some to be extremely common in small preterm infants with intraventricular hemorrhage. Intraventricular hemorrhage has been cited as the cause of the vast majority of seizures in infants weighing less than 2,500 gm. In other studies, however, only 11% of infants with intraventricular hemorrhage diagnosed and documented by CT scan have had seizures; these seizures occurred almost entirely in those infants with marked degrees of hemorrhage. Abnormal movements other than seizures also may occur in the infant with intraventricular hemorrhage; decerebrate or opisthotonic posturing due to extensive rostrocaudal pressure and brainstem herniation may occur in such infants, and these movements should be distinguished from seizure activity, particularly by the other associated clinical findings. Seizures occurring in infants with subdural bleeding are not infrequent, although subdural bleeding is a rather rare event in the neonate at the present time. Seizures occurring in the infant with subdural hemorrhage are more likely to be caused by the associated traumatic cerebral contusion producing the bleeding than by the blood in the subdural space.

Infectious causes of neonatal seizures include sepsis, meningitis, TORCH agent infections, and Coxsackie B encephalitis. The mechanism by which sepsis is associated with neonatal seizures is unclear, but the association is real. Seizures occur in approximately 55% of infants with neonatal meningitis, whether caused by group B streptococci, gram-negative organisms, or *Listeria* species. Of the TORCH agents causing neonatal seizures, herpesvirus is particularly important, since it is the only TORCH agent that does not produce subclinical or silent CNS infection. Seizures in congenital herpes infection may occur with generalized disseminated herpetic infection or in association with localized infection primarily involving skin, eye, or oral mucosa, with additional involvement of brain. Infants with generalized systemic disease have evidence of multiple organ involvement in addition to seizures. The viral infection in the CNS may be associated with only a single or few herpetic vesicles on the scalp at the site of a fetal scalp monitor, on an extremity, on the buttocks in association with breech presentation, or in the eye (Chapter 31).

Coxsackie B encephalitis may occur as an isolated infection or in neonatal epidemics resulting in seizures and at times myocarditis.

Hypoglycemia is a cause of neonatal seizures that, if untreated, may lead to acute brain damage. Transient hypoglycemia is particularly likely to occur in association with asphyxia in the stressed low birth weight infant (Chapter 7). In general, hypoglycemia as a direct cause of seizures is no longer a major problem in most neonatal units because of the emphasis that has been given to (1) the frequent use of Dextrostix and blood glucose determinations for detection of infants at risk before seizure occurrence, (2) early provision of supplemental intravenous glucose to infants at risk, and (3) careful monitoring of blood glucose following identification of hypoglycemia and initiation of appropriate treatment. Most important is the necessity of continuing monitoring for possible recurrence of hypoglycemia after it has been detected and treated, because of the possibility of hypoglycemia recurring without resultant further seizures. Increasing numbers of infants have persisting hypoglycemia as a result of identifiable disorders that cause hyperinsulinism, such as nesidioblastosis or islet cell adenoma with inborn metabolic defects. Any infant who is not being weaned from intravenous glucose initiated for hypoglycemia by 7 to 10 days should be considered a candidate for one of these disorders.

Hypocalcemia, with serum calcium levels of less than 7.5 mg/dl and phosphorus levels greater than 8 mg/dl, may occur early, in association with hypoglycemia in the stressed or asphyxiated low birth weight infant (Chapter 37, part two). Despite this association, it is rarely the cause of seizures at that time. More commonly, hypocalcemia is a cause of seizures in the older infant, after the fifth day of life, particularly in the mature formula-fed infant. Maternal hyperparathyroidism caused by parathyroid adenoma should be considered in such instances. The DiGeorge phenotype may on rare occasion be recognized in infants with hypocalcemia and seizures after the first week of life, and hypocalcemia that persists may be due to chronic idiopathic hypoparathyroidism, which can occur in infancy and which requires further laboratory tests for verification. Hypomagnesemia as a cause of neonatal convulsions is extremely uncommon and, when it does occur, is usually associated with hypocalcemia. Fewer than 10% of infants with hypomagnesemia have normal calcium levels. Hypomagnesemia as a cause of seizures should be considered in a patient whose hypocalcemic seizures did not clear after the hypocalcemia was corrected.

Hyponatremia may be a cause of neonatal seizures in infants born of toxemic mothers who were given not only salt-poor diets but also extremely hypotonic intravenous fluids during labor, such as 5% dextrose in water (Chapter 4). Associated symptoms in the symptomatic newborn with hyponatremia include lethargy, irritability, and tremors. The seizures may be refractory to treatment. Increasingly, hyponatremia is being identified in high-risk neonates in whom seizures are secondary to the syndrome of inappropriate secretion of antidiuretic hormone (SIADH). SIADH may occur with CNS diseases such as meningitis or asphyxial encephalopathy, with intraventricular hemorrhage, or in the presence of pulmonary atelectasis and pneumothorax.

Hypernatremia in the sick preterm infant occurs frequently when the infant is being given care under an open radiant warmer. Evaporative fluid losses can be quite high, producing hypernatremia. In addition, hypernatremia may be a result of iatrogenic factors, such as incorrect administration of sodium-containing parenteral fluids, including sodium bicarbonate, the inadvertent substitution of mislabeled intravenous solutions, or the substitution of table salt for sugar in formula preparation.

Neonatal drug withdrawal (Chapter 37, part four) is manifested by tremulousness, irritability, and seizures. It may occur following chronic maternal intake of narcotics, including methadone and pentazocine (Talwin), analgesics such as propoxyphene (Darvon), sedatives, including ethchlorvynol (Placidyl), hydroxyzine hydrochloride (Atarax), and barbiturates. Seizures are less common than tremulousness and constant agitation and generally occur after the first 48 hours of life.

Disorders of amino acid and ketoacid metabolism that may initially manifest as seizures include maple syrup urine disease, nonketotic hyperglycinemia, and methylmalonic acidemia. Other commonly associated findings are hypotonia, feeding difficulties, and severe metabolic acidosis with ketonuria. These disorders are the only inheritable disorders that usually occur in the neonatal period. Hyperbilirubinemia should now be an extremely uncommon cause of neonatal seizures because of the early diagnosis and treatment of this condition. However, seizures will occur in approximately half of infants with kernicterus. Seizures immediately after delivery, which are extremely refractory to anticonvulsant therapy, have resulted from intoxication of infants by maternal anesthetic agents, such as mepivacaine, that were inadvertently injected into the infant by a misplaced catheter and needle at the time of caudal anesthesia; or these seizures have been caused by high local concentrations of mepivacaine at the time of paracervical block anesthesia (Chapter 14).

Pyridoxine dependency is a rare cause of neonatal seizures that may occur in utero or in immediate postnatal life and may be familial. The primary defect may be a deficiency in binding of the coenzyme pyridoxal phosphate to glutamic decarboxylase, the enzyme involved in the formation of gamma-aminobutyric acid (GABA). The absence of GABA, a presumed CNS inhibitor, could produce seizures. Such seizures can be immediately controlled by intravenous injection of 25 to 50 mg of pyridoxine.

Seizures caused by congenital cerebral malformations may begin in the neonatal period but rarely in the first several days. The diagnosis of the malformation may be suspected on the basis of abnormal facies, small or large head size, or multiple congenital anomalies. However, in otherwise normal appearing infants the anomalies may be evident only by special roentgenographic techniques, such as computed tomography, cranial ultrasonography, or rarely with transillumination alone.

DIAGNOSIS

Each infant must be considered to have a potentially treatable disease, regardless of antecedent history. Important historic data should be obtained from the mother's chart and from the mother herself, and one should also be aware of the availability of illicit drugs, any drugs she may have been taking at her physician's direction, and her prior obstetric history. History of previously affected newborn infants also should be obtained. Intrapartum monitoring may provide significant data regarding the possibility of intrauterine asphyxia, although the infant at birth may not have low Apgar scores, since some infants with hypoxic ischemic encephalopathy with seizures suffer their asphyxial insult before birth.

The day on which seizures begin also may be a clue to cause. For example, stressed low birth weight infants with first-day seizures are more likely to have hypoglycemia and hypocalcemia. Neonatal seizures due to intracranial infection are more frequent after the first 48 hours. Seizures caused by hypoxic ischemic encephalopathy most commonly begin within 12 hours of birth and become progressively more frequent and severe during the next 24 to 48 hours. Seizures beginning after the fifth day of life are more likely related to classic hypocalcemia, congenital development defects, or TORCH infections. Such temporal relationships are not invariable but may be helpful in diagnostic evaluation.

Every infant with seizures must be screened for systemic and intracranial infection with immediate blood culture and lumbar puncture. Analysis of spinal fluid should include smear with Gram stain, glucose and protein determinations, and erythrocyte and differential leukocyte counts. Even in the presence of blood in spinal fluid, presumably the result of a traumatic tap, the fluid should be centrifuged and xanthochromia sought, as evidence of prior subarachnoid blood. If adequate spinal fluid is obtained, erythrocyte counts should be compared in the first and third or fourth tubes.

Immediate skull roentgenograms are rarely of value. Although not every infant with seizures requires complex roentgenographic evaluation, CT scans may be helpful in revealing subependymal or intraventricular hemorrhage or subdural blood. Postasphyxial or hypoxic ischemic encephalopathy also may be manifested by striking alterations of cerebral perfusion evident on enhanced CT scans or as areas of diminished attenuation or density on nonenhanced scans obtained 5 to 7 days after the asphyxial event. CT scans also may identify intracranial calcifications caused by congenital TORCH infections, even when these are not evident on skull roentgenograms. Cranial ultrasound appears to have similar diagnostic potential in the neonate, and it is indicated, if available, for all newborns with seizures.

An electroencephalogram (EEG) may confirm the diagnosis of seizures through the correlation of the paroxysmal electrical discharge with the clinical manifestations. However, an EEG is rarely helpful in determination of the cause of seizures, except in the very rare example of pyridoxine-dependent seizures; infants with this problem and profoundly abnormal paroxysmal electrical activity on EEG will show almost immediate normalization of the EEG, as well as seizure cessation, following intravenous injection of pyridoxine. Despite the availability of EEG laboratories in almost all hospitals and published EEG standards in the term and preterm infant, very few EEG laboratories will have knowledgeable pediatric electroencephalographers to interpret their records. The EEG may, however, be more helpful in determination of prognosis.

TREATMENT

While the physician is awaiting results of laboratory tests and reviewing historic data and physical findings, treatment should be administered. There is no reason to withhold treatment for seizures until after EEG, CT scan, or ultrasound examination has been completed. After initial determination of blood glucose level by Dextrostix, if hypoglycemia is present, 10% glucose is given intravenously, 4 to 9 ml/kg (Chapter 37, part one), and this should be continued with constant pump infusion of a 10% to 15% glucose solution, depending on response to therapy and further blood glucose determinations. If hypocalcemia is documented or highly suspected, calcium gluconate is given intravenously as a 5% solution, in a dosage of 200 mg/kg or 4 ml/kg.

The dosage of anticonvulsants in the neonatal period is shown in Table 27-2. Phenobarbital is the initial drug of choice, effective not only in controlling status but also protective against recurrent seizures. The initial loading dosage of phenobarbital is 20 to 30 mg/kg to achieve effective plasma levels in the range of 20 μg/ml. Daily maintenance dosage of phenobarbital of 5 mg/kg/day will not result in excessive accumulation of phenobarbital or sedation, and this should be started within 24 hours after the initial loading dose. If phenobarbital is not effective in terminating seizures, phenytoin (Dilantin) should be administered intravenously, 15 to 20 mg/kg, at a rate of injection not to exceed 50 mg/minute. This will achieve

Table 27-2. Dosages of anticonvulsants for the neonate*

Drug	Dosage for loading	Dosage for maintenance	Route of administration
Phenobarbital	20-30 mg/kg	5 mg/kg/day	IV; maintenance can be given IM or PO
Phenytoin	15-20 mg/kg	3-5 mg/kg/day	IV only; do not administer at rate faster than 50 mg/minute
Paraldehyde	4%-8% solution	Not used for maintenance	IV

*See also Appendix B.

therapeutic levels of between 10 and 20 μg/ml in the neonate. Following this the phenytoin maintenance dosage is 3 to 5 mg/kg/day. These maintenance doses must be administered intravenously, since the newborn infant does not absorb oral phenytoin with a predictable result. Not only do intramuscular phenytoin injections result in unpredictable plasma concentrations because of poor absorption but the drug is irritating and may form crystals following intramuscular injection.

For seizures that persist despite intravenous phenobarbital and phenytoin, paraldehyde may be administered intravenously as a 4% to 8% solution. This is both safe and effective, and the limiting factor for paraldehyde is usually the volume of fluid that the infant can tolerate, rather than total quantity of undiluted paraldehyde.

Diazepam (Valium) is not recommended for neonatal seizures. It is no more effective than intravenous phenobarbital, and it cannot be used for maintaining seizure control, since plasma concentrations of diazepam are not maintained for more than 30 minutes after intravenous injection. It has the disadvantage of producing or enhancing respiratory depression and hypotension, even if given alone, and particularly if administered along with phenobarbital. Because of its sodium benzoate carrier, it may be particularly disadvantageous in the patient with or at risk for indirect hyperbilirubinemia, since the sodium benzoate may take up all available albumin binding sites, increasing the infant's chance for kernicterus.

PROGNOSIS

Neonatal seizures are one of the strongest predictors of later motor or intellectual deficit. Prognosis of neonatal seizures is clearly related to cause and to a lesser extent the degree of infant maturity. Data from the Collaborative Perinatal Cerebral Palsy Project, relating neonatal characteristics of children with later severe neurologic handicaps, compared a number of antecedent variables, including Apgar score, birth weight, and clinical and laboratory evidence of intracranial hemorrhage and seizures. Of the severely handicapped children 30% had seizures in the first month of life, whereas only 0.3% of the neurologically intact survivors had neonatal seizures. Infants of less than 34 weeks' gestational age with neonatal seizures have a fourfold increase in mortality as compared with full-term infants with convulsions. However, cerebral palsy is not as severe in surviving children.

Perinatal asphyxia clearly indicates the poorest prognosis for neonatal seizures both for preterm and full-term infants. Approximately 60% of infants with seizures caused by perinatal asphyxia are likely to have permanent neurologic sequelae. Apgar scores of 0 to 3 at 5 minutes, while associated with a 16-fold increase in death risk and a 17-fold increase in cerebral palsy, were not associated with seizure disorders in children without cerebral palsy. Similarly, obstetric problems such as breech delivery, abruptio placentae, and placenta previa, if associated with low Apgar scores, increased the risk of cerebral palsy and death. However, no significant association occurred with childhood seizure disorders in children without cerebral palsy. The prognosis for infants with seizures related to intraventricular hemorrhage appears to be poor, since seizures in this group are most likely to occur in infants with marked degrees of bleeding; infants with severe intraventricular hemorrhage are at greater risk than those with mild or moderate amount of bleeding. The infant with subarachnoid hemorrhage who has a seizure without pronounced asphyxia has a good prognosis.

Among those infants with seizures related to a primary metabolic disorder, infants with hypoglycemia and late onset hypocalcemia, if treated promptly, have a good prognosis. Preterm infants with significant and/or prolonged hypoglycemia and early onset hypocalcemia, even when treated early, may have a poor prognosis. The associated perinatal stress in the preterm infant may, however, be the more profound determinant of poor outcome. The outcome for infants with other metabolically determined seizures is related more to the primary disorder, for example, maple syrup urine disease, than to the seizures. Infants with seizures related to intracranial infections generally have a poor prognosis, but outcome often depends on rapidity of diagnosis and treatment of the infection.

Prognosis also can be related to time of onset of seizures in the neonate. Early onset of seizures, in the first 24 hours, is more likely to be associated with a poorer prognosis than seizures beginning after that time. Seizure duration is also important, and those infants whose seizures persist and recur for more than 24 hours are at a greater risk of later neurologic sequelae than those with a single brief seizure or multiple seizures that cease or are controlled within 24 hours. The interictal EEG may offer significant help in predicting outcome. The presence of either a flat or periodic EEG or bilateral multifocal electrical discharges in the EEG are predictive of an unsatisfactory outcome. Those infants with a normal interictal EEG and a normal neurologic examination at time of discharge are likely to have a favorable outcome.

Alfred W. Brann, Jr.
James F. Schwartz

BIBLIOGRAPHY

Bejsovee, M., Kulenoa, Z., and Ponca, E.: Familial intrauterine convulsions in pyridoxine dependency, Arch. Dis. Child. **42**:201, 1967.

Brann, A.W.: Factors during neonatal life that influence brain disorders. In Freeman, J.M., editor: Prenatal and perinatal factors associated with brain disorders, Pub. No. 85-1149, Bethesda, Md., April 1985, National Institutes of Health.

Donn, S.M., Grasela, T.H., and Goldstein, G.W.: Safety of a higher loading dose of phenobarbital in the term infant, Pediatrics **75**:1061, 1985.

Freeman, J.M.: Neonatal seizures, diagnosis and management, J. Pediatr. **77**:701, 1970.

Painter, M.J., and others: Phenobarbital and diphenylydantoin levels in neonates with seizures, J. Pediatr. **92**:315, 1978.

Paunier, L., and others: Primary hypomagnesemia with secondary hypocalcemia in an infant, Pediatrics **41**:385, 1968.

Prichard, J.S.: The character and significance of epileptic seizures in infancy. In Kellaway, P., and Petersen, I., editors: Neurologic and encephalographic correlative studies in infancy, New York, 1964, Grune & Stratton, Inc.

Rabe, E.F.: The hypotonic infant, J. Pediatr. **64**:422, 1964.

Rose, A.L., and Lombroso, C.T.: Neonatal seizure states, Pediatrics **45**:404, 1970.

Schulte, F.J., and Schwenzel, W.: Motor control and muscle tone in the newborn period: electromyographic studies, Biol. Neonate **8**:198, 1965.

Schulte, F.J., and others: Maternal toxemia, fetal malnutrition and motor behavior in newborn, Pediatrics **48**:871, 1971.

Smith, B.T., and Masotti, R.E.: Intravenous diazepam in the treatment of prolonged seizure activity in neonates and infants, Dev. Med. Child Neurol. **13**:630, 1971.

Volpe, J.J.: Neonatal seizures, Clin. Perinatol. **4**:43, 1977.

Wasterlain, C.G.: Inhibition of cerebral protein synthesis in status epilepticus, Neurology **22**:427, 1972.

Wasterlain, C.G., and Plum, F.: Vulnerability of developing rat brain to electroconvulsive seizures, Arch. Neurol. **29**:38, 1973.

PART FIVE

Developmental anomalies and neuromuscular disorders

ABNORMALITIES OF HEAD SIZE

The enlarging head

Hydrocephalus is the most common cause of an excessive rate of head growth in the neonatal period, but it must be differentiated from subdural effusions and hematomas, porencephalic cysts, megalencephaly (enlargement of the brain), and the normal rate of growth of premature and full-term infants (Fig. 27-13). Hydrocephalus is not of itself a disease but is the end result of a number of disease processes that produce an accumulation of cerebrospinal fluid (CSF) (see also Part three).

Pathophysiology

CSF is produced by the choroid plexus, as well as from the brain substance, at a relatively constant rate of 0.37 ml/minute (0.26 to 0.65 ml/minute). CSF produced in the lateral ventricles flows through the foramen of Monro, the third ventricle, down the aqueduct to the fourth ventricle, and exits through the foramina of Luschka and Magendie. The fluid then flows along the base, up the sylvian fissures, and over the surface of the hemispheres to be absorbed through valves along the sagittal sinus by bulk flow. The amount of spinal fluid made within the cerebral cortical substance and transported across the ependyma to the ventricles or absorbed by this route is still a matter of investigation. Studies using infusions of artificial CSF have indicated that pressures at which bulk absorption begins to occur are variable. In most individuals the pressure required is around 60 mm of water; in others the pressure may have to reach 180 mm before bulk absorption occurs. The ability of the newborn's head to expand without reaching these higher pressures may account for some forms of hydrocephalus; the arrest of hydrocephalus may occur in some infants when the sutures close firmly enough to achieve that pressure.

In addition to the increased pressures, the undamped pulsations of the choroid plexus are felt to play an important role in the dilation of the ventricles. With progressive ventricular dilation, compression of the cortical mantle occurs before expansion of the cranium and suture separation. Thus considerable reduction in cortical mantle thickness may occur before hydrocephalus becomes evident by measurable increases in the occipitofrontal head circumference. Ventricular enlargement, which is not a uniform process, occurs chiefly at the expense of periventricular white matter. The gray matter, including cortex and basal ganglia, is relatively spared, with little neuronal loss until extreme thinning (less than 0.5 cm) has occurred. Following adequate treatment of moderate hydrocephalus or with spontaneous resolution the cortical mantle may be restored to its former normal thickness, and there may not be any neurologic deficit.

Etiology

Hydrocephalus formerly was classified as obstructive or communicating. However, with the exception of hy-

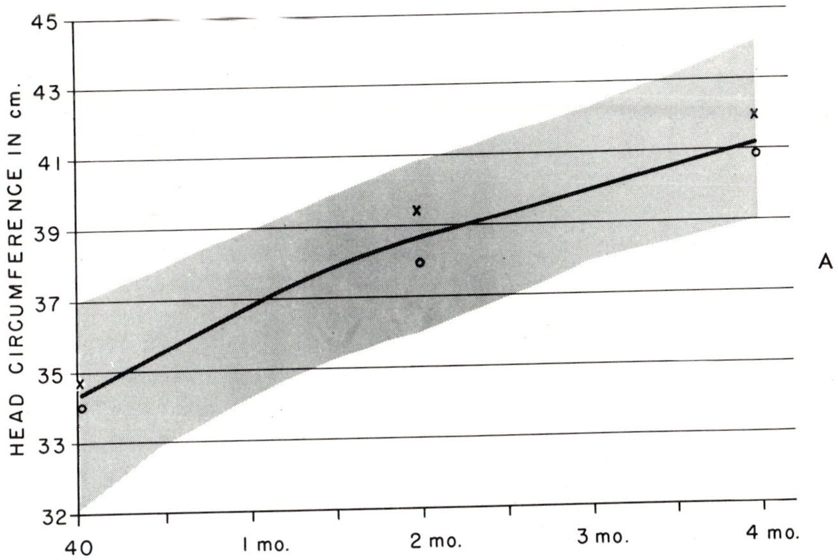

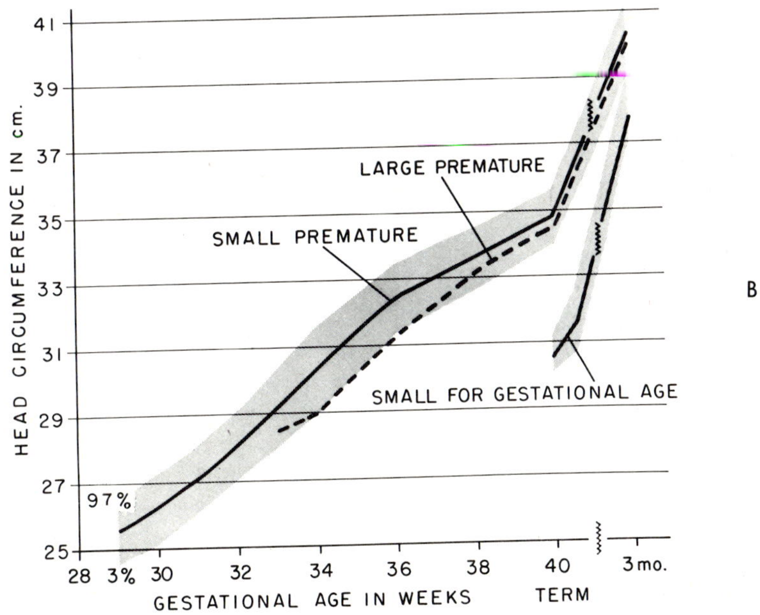

Fig. 27-13. A, Head growth of full-term infants. Birth weight greater than 2,500 gm. The solid line is a combination of males and females. (Redrawn from O'Neill, E.M.: Arch. Dis. Child. **36:**241, 1961.) *X* represents males: *O,* females. **B,** Head growth of low birth weight infants (less than 2,500 gm): the small premature of appropriate size for gestational age (27 to 29 weeks' gestation); the large premature of appropriate size for gestational age (31 to 33 weeks' gestation); and the severely underweight or small for gestational age full-term infant (gestation greater than 38 weeks, weight less than 2.0 kg). (**A** from Nellhaus, G.: Pediatrics **41:**106, 1968. **B** adapted from Babson: J. Pediatr. **77:**11, 1970.) (See also growth charts in Appendix C.)

drocephalus secondary to cortical atrophy (hydrocephalus ex vacuo) and the rare hydrocephalus secondary to overproduction of CSF by a choroid plexus papilloma, all hydrocephalus is caused by an obstruction. The obstruction may lie within the ventricular system, as in aqueductal stenosis, the Dandy-Walker syndrome, or tumors; or it may lie outside the ventricular system, as with arachnoidal adhesions. Obstruction outside the ventricular system was formerly called communicating hydrocephalus because dye placed in the ventricle appeared in the lumbar subarachnoid space.

Overproduction—choroid plexus papillomas. Overproduction of CSF, although rare, is associated with papillomas of the choroid plexus and probably with no other lesion. Infants with choroid plexus papillomas have a communicating hydrocephalus. Elevated CSF protein and xanthochromia are common, and an intraventricular mass can be identified readily by computerized tomography or by air study. These can be surgically removed, with resultant cure of the hydrocephalus.

Obstruction to CSF flow

Congenital malformations

AQUEDUCTAL STENOSIS. The aqueduct is a common location for obstruction producing hydrocephalus in the neonatal period. Normally a single channel, in congenital aqueductal stenosis the aqueduct often is found to be broken into many small channels with varying degrees of occlusion but without evidence of inflammation. Previously, aqueductal stenosis was considered a developmental abnormality, but identical lesions in rodents have been produced by neonatal infection with mumps, influenza, and parainfluenza viruses. No pathologic evidence of the preceding infection could be demonstrated at the time the animals developed hydrocephalus. Thus "congenital" aqueductal stenosis in some cases may be caused by unrecognized viral disease.

THE DANDY-WALKER SYNDROME. The Dandy-Walker syndrome produces a clinically recognizable form of hydrocephalus. The large cystic fourth ventricle causes a prominent occipital shelf, occipital transillumination, and elevation of tentorium and venous sinuses on roentgenographic film.

In addition to the large cystic dilation of the fourth ventricle, there is defective development of the cerebellum with the vermis being smaller than normal and only small amounts of laterally displaced tissue thought to be remnants of cerebellar hemispheres. Despite the marked atrophy of the cerebellar vermis, infants with this syndrome are not ataxic in later life.

THE ARNOLD-CHIARI MALFORMATION. This malformation occurs in varying degrees of severity. In its most severe and classic form it is characterized by downward displacement of the cerebellar tonsils through the foramen magnum, downward displacement, elongation, and folding of the medulla oblongata and fourth ventricle on the cervical cord, and downward displacement of the cervical cord. It is most commonly seen in patients with spinal dysraphia, such as meningomyeloceles. Aqueductal stenosis and micropolygyria often are associated with the Arnold-Chiari malformation. The cause of this malformation is unknown; however, it is not the result of traction on the fixed spinal cord.

The distortion of the medulla, fourth ventricle, and CSF circulation pathways, both at the exit of the fourth ventricle and around the brainstem, may be sufficient to obstruct CSF flow and produce hydrocephalus. Therefore either this anatomic malformation or the associated malformation of aqueductal stenosis may cause hydrocephalus, which may be the only clinical manifestation of this extensive malformation of the lower brainstem, cervical cord, and cerebellum. On rare occasions lower cranial nerve palsies with vocal cord or laryngeal paralysis and respiratory obstruction may be an early manifestation of the Arnold-Chiari malformation.

VEIN OF GALEN MALFORMATIONS. Vein of Galen malformations are another rare cause of hydrocephalus. The markedly dilated vein of Galen compresses the aqueduct, producing the picture of aqueductal stenosis. This large malformation, which may cause heart failure in the early days or weeks of life, produces a loud bruit that may be heard over the vertex of the skull. Arteriography delineates the malformation. With neonatal cardiac failure direct attack on the malformation may be necessary despite the high mortality. If hydrocephalus is the only symptom, treatment usually consists of shunting rather than a direct attack on the malformation.

POSTHEMORRHAGIC HYDROCEPHALUS. The most common form of hydrocephalus in the newborn is posthemorrhagic hydrocephalus, occurring as a sequel to intraventricular hemorrhage. In these infants hydrocephalus is secondary to obliterative arachnoiditis in the posterior fossa, resulting from the blood, with impaired CSF flow out of the fourth ventricle or impaired flow of CSF through the subarachnoid pathways and cisterns at the level of the tentorial notch. Rarely intraventricular blood may cause aqueductal obstruction (Part three).

INFLAMMATORY OR POSTINFLAMMATORY PROCESSES. Fibrosis and adhesions at the exit of the fourth ventricle or along subarachnoid pathways of CSF circulation also may be the result of neonatal bacterial meningitis, with hydrocephalus occurring immediately or at a later time.

Pathology

The pathology of hydrocephalus is the progressive thinning of cortical white matter, with reduction of oligodendroglial cells and astrocytes. The neurons and axons seem quite resistant to the effects of pressure. The hydrocephalus causes greater thinning of the vertex and occipital cortex, since the basal ganglia tend to buttress the lower part of the ventricular wall. Because of the thinning at the vertex (leg area) and because fibers from the leg area undergo the greatest stretch in circumventing the dilated ventricles, patients with hydrocephalus tend to develop a paraparesis with the preservation of the arms. The compressed cerebrum shows a loss of lipids and proteins from white matter with an increase in water content. The lipid and protein loss presumably can be reconstituted with relief of the hydrocephalus. Since the neurons and axons remain intact, there may be no residual deficit.

Clinical manifestations

Few clinical manifestations of hydrocephalus occur in the neonatal period other than enlargement of the head. Since the head can easily enlarge, intracranial pressure is dissipated, and the signs and symptoms of increased intracranial pressure are rare. Vomiting and lethargy are uncommon, and papilledema is rarely if ever seen. Neurologic disability and seizures, if present, are usually the result of the underlying disease process rather than of the hydrocephalus.

As the head enlarges, the fontanel is tense when felt with the infant in the upright position. Suture separation occurs as the fontanel tension increases. Since the sutures of the newborn, especially the small preterm infant, normally may be widely separated, in the absence of increased intracranial pressure or ventricular dilation it may be difficult to use the degree of suture separation, at least in the sagittal suture, as a clinical sign of pressure. However, the squamosal suture, which runs horizontally slightly above the ear in between the temporal and parietal bones, is a sensitive indicator of pressure. Separation of more than a few millimeters of that suture after the first few days of life is a useful sign of increased intracranial pressure, most commonly a result of hydrocephalus.

The frontal bones are prominent in contrast to the parietal bossing classically seen in subdural hematomas; the scalp veins protrude. The setting sun sign, the appearance of sclera above the pupil, is a moderately late sign probably caused by pressure in the region of the superior colliculi. The posterior shelf of the Dandy-Walker malformation has been described. The most significant clinical manifestation of hydrocephalus is enlargement of the head. Plotting serial head measurements on an appropriate head circumference chart is the only clinical method of diagnosing progressive hydrocephalus and is far more accurate than a single measurement.

Diagnosis

The most important element in the diagnosis of hydrocephalus is suspicion. Early detection can come only from plotting serial head circumference measurements with a metal tape. The greatest head circumference obtained should be recorded on a standard head growth chart. Measurements should be made in centimeters; although growth from 13¼ inches to 14¼ inches does not seem great, growth from 34.9 cm to 36.2 cm is more likely to alert the physician. Head circumference measurements should be a recorded part of every baby visit in the first months of life. The diagnosis of hydrocephalus is suggested when the rate of head growth is greater than the norm (i.e., when the rate is crossing percentiles). The absolute head circumference is of less significance than the rate of growth. It is just as significant if the head grows from the third percentile to the fiftieth percentile as if the growth is from the seventy-fifth to greater than the ninety-fifth percentile.

A complete history and physical examination are obviously important in the initial workup of an infant with a large head. However, unless the head circumference exceeds the ninety-seventh percentile or the rate of head growth is currently greater than the norm, more definitive evaluations need not be undertaken; the infant's course should be followed.

Transillumination also should be a part of the initial evaluation of a large head. Transillumination must take place in a totally dark room with a flashlight that has a light-tight seal on the end. Sufficient time must be spent in the room to allow adequate adaptation to the dark. The whole head, including the occiput, should be transilluminated. Transillumination giving a ring greater than 1 cm around the seal (1.5 cm in the frontal area and in premature infants) is abnormal. Abnormal transillumination is seen in chronic subdural hematomas, edema of the scalp, cortical atrophy, porencephaly, hydranencephaly, and hydrocephalus if the cortical mantle is less than 1.0 cm in thickness.

Further definitive diagnostic evaluation may include skull films, cranial ultrasonography, and CT scanning. Intracranial pressure monitoring may be helpful in differentiating hydrocephalus from megalencephaly. Arteriograms rarely are indicated. Pneumoencephalography and ventriculography have been almost entirely replaced by CT scanning and cranial ultrasound examination. All these techniques provide high resolution of ventricular size and identification of intraventricular, intracerebral, subarachnoid, or subdural blood, as well as revealing various malformations, including localized areas of porencephaly, absence of the corpus callosum, and forebrain cleavage anomalies. CT scanning involves transport to the x-ray department and occasional sedation for scanning. It can be repeated serially, as indicated, and provides a noninvasive method of following the progression or resolution of ventricular dilation with or without treatment. Ultrasound examinations, which are totally without any radiation hazard and which can be performed in the special care nursery at the bedside, may provide an even more readily available, nontraumatic, and noninvasive method for obtaining the same information as does CT scanning. This has become the technique of choice.

Differential diagnosis

The differential diagnosis of an enlarging head in the neonate is between hydrocephalus and a number of other, less common causes (Table 27-3).

Subdural hematomas, which may be secondary to perinatal or postnatal trauma, are more common with bleeding disorders. The initial manifestation may be subtle, such as enlargement of the head with no other symptoms, or may include symptoms of increased intracranial pressure or failure to thrive. A boxlike head configuration with biparietal bossing may suggest that the enlargement is caused by subdural hematomas rather than hydrocephalus. Transillumination is usually abnormal in chronic subdural hematomas but may be absent during the acute phase.

The diagnosis of subdural hematoma is made by CT scanning with and without enhancement or by ultrasound examination. Subdural taps rarely are indicated, and the subdural needle should become an object of antiquarian interest in the newborn unit. If subdural blood or effusion is present, treatment by subdural taps should be reserved for those infants with focal neurologic deficits or symptoms and signs of increased intracranial pressure, such as enlarging head size, tense fontanel, or evidence of deterioration in degree of consciousness and awareness. In the absence of such findings, there is little rationale for treatment.

Hydranencephaly is a congenital absence of the brain, but with normal coverings of dura, skull, and scalp, thus differentiating it from anencephaly. It is probably caused either by bilateral carotid occlusion in utero, with resorption of the cerebral hemispheres, or by intrauterine infection. Hydranencephalic infants often appear normal at birth and demonstrate few neurologic abnormalities other than lack of fixing and following an object with the eyes. A large head is a common initial manifestation. Transillumination of marked degree serves to identify these infants on initial screening, but the entity still must be differentiated from large subdural hematomas or severe hydrocephalus.

Table 27-3. Causes of hydrocephalus and differential diagnosis of the enlarging head in the neonatal period

Hydrocephalus	Differentiate from

Overproduction
  Choroid plexus papilloma
Obstruction
  Aqueductal stenosis or occlusion
    Congenital
    Viral
  Vein of Galen
    Familial
  Dandy-Walker syndrome
  Arnold-Chiari syndrome (meningomyelocele)
  Obstruction at base or absorption
	Subdural hematomas
	Hydranencephaly
	Porencephaly
	Megalencephaly
	  Familial
	  Canavan's disease
	  Alexander's disease
	Normal growth of premature and full-term infant
	Growth after feeding malnourished infant
	Subgaleal hematomas
	Achondroplasia
	Normal head/dwarf body

CT scanning or cranial ultrasound examination should make the definitive diagnosis. Shunting may result in collapse of what little tissue is present, with secondary rupture of blood vessels and rapid deterioration of the infant.

Porencephaly is a cavitation of the brain that usually communicates with either the ventricle or the subarachnoid space. The cavitation is commonly the result of prenatal vascular occlusion with resorption of the dead tissue. Developmental arrests at the site of fissures (schizencephaly) produce similar clinical features. Porencephaly may be associated with hydrocephalus or with subdural fluid collections. Infants may have seizures, focal neurologic deficits, or hydrocephalus. Transillumination often is localized. Treatment of the hydrocephalus is indicated; intractable focal seizures secondary to porencephaly may respond to drainage of the cyst.

Arachnoid cysts are uncommon lesions of unknown cause. Many of them appear to be the entrapment of CSF in the pia-arachnoid. They often mimic hydrocephalus but are usually asymmetric. They may produce localized transillumination and local erosion of bone. When occurring in the posterior fossa, they may produce hydrocephalus by aqueductal compression.

Arachnoid cysts may be extremely difficult to differentiate from porencephalic cysts except by injection of air, as with pneumoencephalography or metrizamide cisternography.

With ventriculocardiac shunts the cardiac (atrial) end of the shunt may become infected and produce chronic bacteremia or septicemia. Cardiac shunts may embolize to the lungs, producing pulmonary hypertension, or may occasionally break off in the heart. All shunts may become plugged or obstructed at either end, with resultant signs of increased intracranial pressure. Those shunts inserted in infancy require replacement as the infant grows, unless the hydrocephalus becomes arrested (see later discussion). There are indications that shunts from the ventricle may cause aqueductal stenosis and shunt dependence.

Despite all these complications, an alternative to shunting is unavailable for the infant with progressive hydrocephalus whose ventricles continue to dilate with progressive thinning of cortical mantle.

Enlargement of the head may be caused by enlargement of the brain substance, *megalencephaly*. In such patients, head growth is rarely as rapid as in hydrocephalus. Megalencephaly may be familial, with or without mental retardation, but often is associated with structural abnormalities such as overgrowth of glial cells, astrocytosis, or microgyria. Megalencephaly may be seen with storage of materials within the brain substance, as in Alexander's disease, Tay-Sachs disease in its later stages, or Canavan's disease (spongy degeneration of the white matter). However, enlargement of the brain in these diseases is not noted until after the first 6 months of age. Differentiation from hydrocephalus may be suggested by the rate of head growth and confirmed by CT.

Normal growth of the head of a *premature infant* from 32 to 40 weeks is almost twice as fast as that of a full-term infant up to 2 months of age (see Fig. 27-13). Therefore, unless the rate of head growth is plotted on an age-specific graph, the rate of head growth of small babies will appear to be excessive. This may lead to the erroneous diagnosis of hydrocephalus.

With malnutrition there is a relative sparing of the brain. However, small head size, small brain size, and retardation may result from severe malnutrition. The effect of in utero malnutrition on cerebral development is less well defined. With *feeding of malnourished infants* there may be a *rapid growth* in head circumference, with spreading of the sutures demonstrable on a skull film. This is thought to be catch-up growth secondary to increase in cell size. This catch-up growth also may be seen in the head growth of babies who are small for gestational age (SGA) (Fig. 27-13, *B*).

Achondroplasia is characterized by hypotonia, developmental delay, and an enlarged head. These infants consistently have a large head, greater than the ninety-seventh percentile. However, growth usually parallels the ninety-seventh percentile, and the infants do not exhibit a tense fontanel or dilated scalp veins characteristic of hydrocephalus. Air studies reveal only moderately dilated ventricles, and the infants rarely require shunting. Occasionally, the small foramen magnum does cause cervical cord compression and may interfere with CSF flow at the base. However, unless the rate of head growth continues to exceed the norm, the patient does not require evaluation or shunting. Although the marked hypotonia results in marked delay in the development of motor milestones, these infants are rarely retarded.

Dwarfs and SGA babies may be seen in the neonatal period with what appears to be an enlarged head. It is important in these patients to measure head circumference in relation to gestational age and to follow the rate of head growth rather than rely on a single measurement.

Treatment

At the present time surgery, which is the definitive treatment for hydrocephalus, is less than satisfactory. It consists of shunting the fluid around the obstruction. Currently most shunts are placed from the cerebral ventricles into the peritoneum. The shunts consist of varying types of tubing, with variable types of openings at either end and several types of one-way valves.

The role of medical management of hydrocephalus is not currently clear, especially for posthemorrhagic hydrocephalus, which is an increasingly common problem after intraventricular hemorrhage. The exact role of serial lumbar puncture, a carbonic anhydrase inhibitor such as acetazolamide (Diamox), or osmotic agents such as sorbitol, is not clear. In view of the occurrence of spontaneous arrest and resolution of hydrocephalus in some infants, very careful observation with repeated CT scans or cranial ultrasound, as well as clinical evaluations, is indicated before surgical treatment is undertaken. If the hydrocephalus spontaneously arrests and ventricular dilation subsides, further conservative care is indicated.

The success of shunting depends to a large extent on the experience and interest of the neurosurgeon. However, even in the best of hands, there are complications. The shunts may become infected at either end, although infants with thin cortical mantles may do exceedingly well (see further); infants with thicker cortical mantles do better.

Prognosis and follow-up care

Since shunting in infants with hydrocephalus carries the risks and complications just enumerated and is obviously palliative rather than curative, to estimate the prognosis one must understand the natural history of both treated and untreated hydrocephalus. Infants with uncomplicated hydrocephalus usually require shunting. In one randomized, controlled series, all but two of fifteen unoperated control patients ultimately required surgery. Even those two seemed to have slowly progressive hydrocephalus. Spontaneous arrest of hydrocephalus undoubtedly does occur, but the true frequency is difficult to determine. Arrest of the process should be documented not by head circumference, but by ventricular size and cortical mantle thickness. Serial CT offers a better method of following the course of these infants and determining when true arrest occurs.

In cases of uncomplicated hydrocephalus the infants should be evaluated when the physician documents a progressive and definite increase in head circumference. At this time the ventricles usually are moderately dilated, but even marked thinning of the cortical mantle should not be a deterrent to surgery. It has been shown that even when the cortical mantle is less than 10 mm in thickness, the prognosis may be good (Fig. 27-14). In one series, half the infants whose mantle was less than 10 mm in thickness at the time of surgery had normal IQs.

Hydrocephalus associated with meningomyeloceles has a worse prognosis than hydrocephalus unassociated with spinal dysraphia. The reasons for this difference are

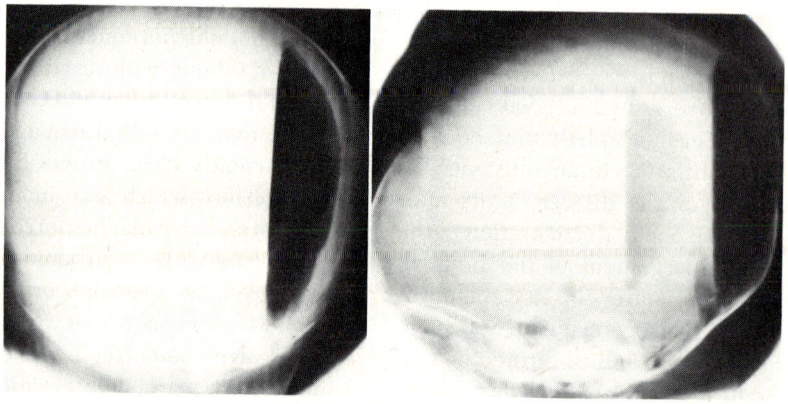

Fig. 27-14. Pneumoencephalogram of a newborn with congenital hydrocephalus. The ventricles are markedly enlarged with virtually no cortical mantle in the left parietooccipital area. The infant had aqueductal stenosis and a possible occlusion of the left posterior cerebral arteries. The infant was shunted at 2 days of age, and at 5 years had no demonstrable neurologic or psychologic deficit.

not entirely clear. In one series, children with hydrocephalus and meningomyeloceles had only a 20% chance of reaching adulthood. The average IQ of the untreated survivors was less than 70. It is Lorber's recommendation that in hydrocephalus associated with meningomyelocele, if the cortical mantle is 26 to 35 mm in thickness, the patient should be watched, and only one third will require surgery; whereas if the mantle thickness is less than 16 mm, surgery is urgently required.

Perhaps one of the differences between those in the meningomyelocele group and those in the uncomplicated hydrocephalus group is that the former are watched more closely. They are in the hospital from birth, and the physician is constantly measuring head size and performing definitive studies. In this sense, perhaps physicians have been too vigorous and aggressive in the early diagnosis and treatment of complicated hydrocephalus. In uncomplicated hydrocephalus, patients are more likely to have large heads and definite ventricular dilation.

Arrested hydrocephalus

Arrest of the hydrocephalic process after shunting has been defined as a cessation of head growth until the head reaches approximately the ninetieth percentile. Growth after that should parallel the normal curve. The fallacy in this definition is that ventricular enlargement with mild increase in pressure may occur without abnormal enlargement of the head. The cortex, therefore, may become markedly thin without evidence of increased intracranial pressure or increasing head size. Children with arrested hydrocephalus often show impaired intellectual performance on reaching school age. These children also may decompensate acutely or die from infections or minor head trauma. Therefore children who have had shunts should be followed carefully with head size measurements and serial charting on appropriate graphs of head circumference; periodic CT scanning or cranial ultrasonography also should be performed to assess the size of the ventricles and thickness of the cortical mantle. Further, the physician should be aware that, following the shunting procedure, collapse of the cortex may lead to subdural hematomas, which also can produce enlargement of the head or increased pressure. In a child whose head continues to grow after shunting, subdural hematomas should be suspected.

The small head

Microcephaly, a small head, is always caused by microencephaly, a small brain, and the two terms have been used interchangeably. A small head circumference, *corrected for gestational age*, suggests the diagnosis. In the normally shaped head the occipital frontal circumference is an index of cranial volume. Where the head shape is abnormal, as in certain forms of craniosynostosis, the head circumference is not a valid index of cranial volume and does not correlate with microcephaly.

Microcephaly has been defined as an occipital frontal circumference greater than 3 SD below the mean, or less than the third percentile. It has generally been equated with mental retardation. The populations used in most studies of microcephaly have had mental retardation or neurologic handicap, and a correlation between the degree of microcephaly and the degree of mental handicap has been established. However, the incidence of microcephaly in the general population and the possibility of an infant with a small head having a normal IQ are not known. Twenty-five percent of hypopituitary dwarfs with normal IQ were microcephalic. Normal intelligence was also measured in 40% of those infants born microcephalic after exposure to the atomic bomb as fetuses. In one group of children examined because of neurologic or cognitive handicaps, 40% were found to be microcephalic, and 14% of those children were found to have normal intelligence. Thus, although mental retardation often is associated with a small head, a small head does not necessarily mean retardation.

Microcephaly may be either congenital or acquired. Congenital microcephaly may follow intrauterine infections with rubella virus, cytomegalovirus, or congenital *Toxoplasma gondii* (Chapter 31, parts two and three). These infections may be apparent from chorioretinitis or the constellation of abnormalities seen with the rubella syndrome, or they may be inapparent and suggested by specific seriologic testing for TORCH infections. Congenital microcephaly is also a part of many chromosomal abnormalities and of other syndromes.

One form of microcephaly is familial and inherited as an autosomal recessive trait. The characteristic appearance of children with this form of microcephaly consists of a normal body and face, with a markedly furrowed brow, a backward sloping of the forehead, and a very small cranial volume. This appearance usually serves to identify the familial form. Genetic counseling is indicated.

Acquired microcephaly may result from perinatal infections such as herpes simplex, from intrapartum or neonatal hypoxic-ischemic insults, and from metabolic causes, including aminoacidurias and hypothyroidism. In these patients the head circumference is normal at birth, but the rate of brain growth is impaired, with resultant microcephaly.

Each infant with microcephaly deserves a complete evaluation and determinations of the cause if at all possible. This should include serologic studies for TORCH agent infections, skull x-ray films, and amino acid screening. The presence of other somatic abnormalities may lead to a chromosomal evaluation. Microcephaly must be differentiated from craniosynostosis (see further). There is no treatment for microcephaly, since it is secondary to microencephaly. In some instances, however, the microencephaly can be prevented.

ABNORMALITIES OF HEAD SHAPE

Abnormalities of head shape may occur in the newborn period and may require surgical intervention. These abnormalities include the large head with frontal bossing and the distended veins seen in hydrocephalus, the large head with parietal bossing seen in chronic subdural hematomas, and the small head with furrowed brow and backward sloping forehead of familial microcephaly. The broad forehead with wide bridge of the nose and hypertelorism may suggest arhinencephaly and other disorders of midline cerebral structures. One of the most common entities causing abnormalities of head shape in the neonatal period is craniosynostosis (Chapter 17).

Craniosynostosis

Craniosynostosis is the premature closure of one or more of the cranial sutures. Since the suture closure and consequent head deformity usually occur prenatally, diagnosis often can be made within the neonatal period. The fontanels as well as the sutures should be evaluated, since their presence or absence has great significance. The anterior fontanel normally closes between the tenth and sixteenth month of life; the posterior fontanel closes between the last 2 months before birth and the first 2 months following birth.

Etiology. The cause of primary (or congenital) craniosynostosis is unclear. It is thought to be a disorder of the membranous bones of the skull and not related to any local underlying growth failure of the brain. Postnatal or secondary craniosynostosis can result from rickets, hypophosphatasia, idiopathic hypercalcemia, or growth failure of the entire brain.

Pathophysiology. In the normal newborn the cranial bones are separate; however, during the first few hours or days of life the cranial bones override one another. This is easily detectable by palpating ridges and feeling the mobility of the bones in relation to one another. This mobility allows the circumference of the head to be molded or reduced in size as the cranial bones slide over one another during passage through the birth canal. Within several hours or days after birth the bones are no longer overriding. Soon after birth the definite sutures are established, and the edges of the flat bones are separated by fibrous tissue. Growth occurs perpendicular to the line of the suture.

The principal sutures of the infant skull are the sagittal, coronal, lamboid, and metopic. Closure of a suture inhibits growth of the skull perpendicular to the fusion. The normal increase in brain volume requires expansion of the skull, which is forced to grow parallel to the fused suture. Deformity results from two factors; restriction of the growth of the vault at right angles to the involved suture and compensatory growth in the areas where the sutures are open. Closure of one of paired sutures results in inhibition of growth and flattening of the skull on that side. Closure of all sutures results in a marked distortion of skull shape as the brain expands through whatever fontanels are opened. Closure of sutures results in distortion of head shape if the underlying brain is normal. The small head with closed sutures whose shape is normal is the result of failure of the brain to grow. In these patients, closure of the sutures is secondary to failure of brain growth; failure of brain growth is not secondary to suture closure.

Sagittal synostosis

Sagittal synostosis is the most common form of craniosynostosis. It occurs predominantly in males and may be familial. It is seen in the neonatal period as a long, narrow head, scaphocephaly, whose circumference is often slightly greater than normal (Fig. 27-15). Sagittal synostosis is rarely associated with other somatic abnormalities and is uncommonly associated with ocular abnormalities, increased intracranial pressure, or mental retardation. Operative correction (see later discussion) is purely for cosmetic purposes. The time of closure of the sutures relative to the amount of cerebral growth remaining determines the degree of cosmetic deformity. Since correction is a cosmetic procedure, it is difficult to establish firm guidelines for operation. An undocumented suspicion also exists that many scaphocephalic heads spontaneously tend to assume a more normal shape with time.

Coronal synostosis

Unilateral and bilateral coronal synostoses are approximately equal in incidence. Coronal synostosis usually is seen as a short broad head with an increase in height. The head circumference tends to be small, although the cranial volume may be normal. The orbits may be shallow and oblique, causing proptosis. Coronal synostosis occurs predominantly in females. A higher incidence of developmental abnormalities and associated mental retardation is seen with this entity than with sagittal synostosis. The stenosis is commonly associated with closure of sutures at the base, giving an appearance similiar to Crouzon's disease. The short anterior fossa may lead to angulation and compression of the optic nerve, with resultant optic atrophy. The cosmetic deformity produced by coronal stenosis is more severe than that with sagittal stenosis, but the surgery is still cosmetic.

Unilateral coronal synostosis produces flattening of the forehead on the affected side and accentuation of the frontal bossing on the opposite side. The orbits may be at different levels, interfering with the development of binocular vision. For this reason, surgery usually is indicated. Synostosis of one coronal suture may result in severe deformity with ipsilateral involvement of the face and orbit. Other complications are exophthalmos, strabismus, nystagmus, papilledema, optic atrophy, and loss of vision. Even more serious malformation and resultant complications are present in patients with bilateral coronal synostoses or in whom multiple sutures are involved.

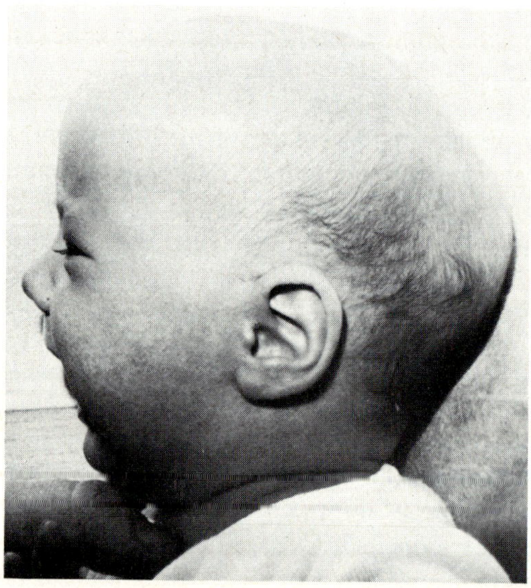

Fig. 27-15. Infant with posterior sagittal synostosis. Note the elongation of the posterior area of the skull, which was also narrow. Ridging of the posterior sagittal suture was present.

Lambdoid stenosis

Premature closure of both lambdoid sutures produces a small, flattened occiput and often broadening and increased height of the skull. Unilateral closure produces flattening on the affected side. The flattening of the occiput in a child with unilateral closure must be differentiated from positional flattening (see further). The absence of a ridge over the lambdoidal suture and skull roentgenograms (Towne's view) should adequately differentiate these entities. Surgery is cosmetic.

Metopic suture

Early closure of the metopic suture during intrauterine life may produce a keel-shaped deformity of the forehead. Surgery for this deformity is purely cosmetic.

Multiple sutures

Closure of multiple sutures produces varied types of severe deformity of the head (Fig. 27-16). Since sufficient room for expansion of the brain is lacking, increased intracranial pressure may occur, and surgery should be carried out as early as possible. Although an increased incidence of mental retardation is evident, many children with multiple suture closures have normal intelligence.

Diagnosis and treatment of craniosynostosis

Diagnosis. Several physical findings should alert the examining physician to suspect a diagnosis of premature craniosynostosis. These findings are an irregular or asymmetric skull, detection of one area where the overriding sutures cannot be felt, the inability of the physician to move the cranial bones in relation to one another in the early days of life, and a bony ridge along the suture line. Hypertelorism, difference in level or position of the eyes, ocular proptosis, strabismus, and optic atrophy also may be present. Signs and symptoms of increased intracranial pressure include funduscopic changes (Chapter 39), a cracked-pot percussion note of the skull too marked for age, bulging of any patent fontanel, and marked irritability.

Radiographic studies are essential to determine the status of the sutures, shape of the skull, skull base, and facial structures. The affected sutures may be totally obliterated or indicated by a thin radiolucent line. Frequently, thickening of bone along the suture, with bone bridging, is present. It is important to recognize that the entire length of a given suture does not need to be involved. In the normal situation the suture closes from posterior to anterior (sagittal suture) and from lateral to medial (coronal sutures). In premature synostosis the closures occur in the same directions. Consequently, prompt diagnosis may be postponed because the portion of the suture best visualized by early radiographic examination may be normal. The *devil's eye configuration*, observed on the posteroanterior radiographic projection, results from the lateral elevation of the lesser wing of the sphenoid. This finding is a clue to unilateral (if it occurs on only one side) or to bilateral coronal synostoses. Radiographic evidence of increased intracranial pressure is manifested by excessive separation of the normal sutures or a beaten silver appearance of the skull.

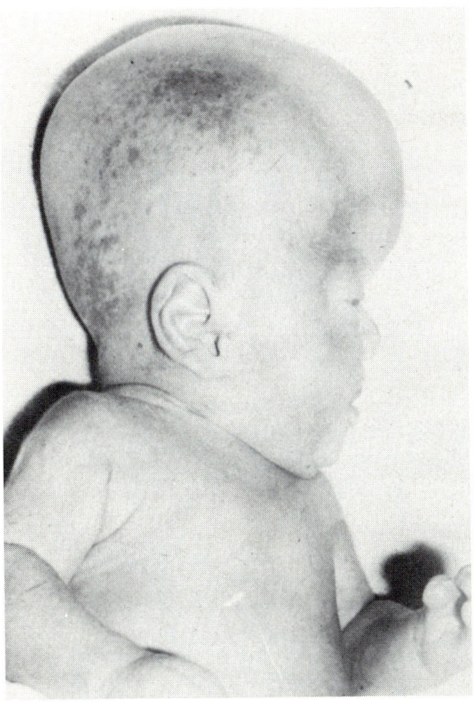

Fig. 27-16. Infant with Apert's syndrome. The shape of the head indicates closure of the lambdoid and coronal sutures. Deformities of the face are caused by closure of sutures at the base of the skull.

The question of synostosis often arises when the anterior fontanel is thought to be too small or closed too soon. Frequently the suspicion proves to be correct. On the other hand, the anterior fontanel may be patent, even though the metopic, sagittal, or one or both coronal sutures are closed. Since the anterior fontanel is open in approximately 50% of patients with each type (sagittal and unilateral or bilateral coronal) of synostosis and with multiple suture closures, it is important not to be lulled into a false sense of security simply because the anterior fontanel remains patent.

Craniosynostosis may be an isolated defect or a component of a syndrome. When craniostenosis is suspected or proved, the pediatrician should be alerted to seek the presence of other malformations. Associated malformations include syndactyly, defects of elbow and knee joints, cardiac anomalies, and choanal atresia. Specific combinations, particularly those involving the limbs, constitute genetically distinct syndromes. The most common syndromes involving premature closure of the sutures are acrocephalosyndactyly (Apert's syndrome) and craniofacial dysostosis (Crouzon's disease). Apert's syndrome consists of acrocephaly, or pointing of the head anteriorly, irregular abnormalities of the sutures, midfacial hypoplasia, and syndactyly of the hands and, occasionally, of the feet. In this syndrome the coronal suture is primarily involved, although other sutures may be involved as well. Crouzon's disease includes shallow orbits and maxillary hypoplasia, as well as premature craniosynostosis, especially of the coronal, lambdoidal, and sagittal sutures. Mental deficiency has been reported more frequently in Apert's syndrome than in Crouzon's disease.

Differential diagnosis. The differential diagnosis of the varied deformities of craniosynostosis rarely should present a problem. A small, normally shaped head with closure of the sutures always represents primary microencephaly and never requires surgery. Confusion of the distorted head shapes comes mainly from the positional flattenings. The long, narrow head of the premature infant is the result of the infant's lying on one side. The roentgenogram shows no ridging of the sagittal suture and no fusion of that suture. Unilateral occipital flattening may be the result of unilateral lambdoidal stenosis. More commonly, it is positional, resulting from an infant's lying on one side of the occiput. Torticollis and bed position relative to light and activity may play a role. Often flattening is seen when lack of interest in the environment is present, and the infant lies on the occiput with little movement. Occipital flattening should alert the physician to the possibility of developmental delay. The absence of ridging of the sutures and x-ray studies should serve to differentiate positional flattening from lambdoidal stenosis.

Treatment. The surgery for craniosynostosis is cosmetic except where multiple sutures are involved. There is little or no indication that these patients develop increased intracranial pressure; there is no evidence that the mental retardation sometimes associated with suture closure can be prevented by surgery; and there is no evidence that surgery prevents the optic atrophy sometimes seen with coronal stenosis. General agreement prevails that the constricting effect of total synostosis on the otherwise normal brain will cause increased intracranial pressure during the period of rapid brain growth and produce brain damage.

Cosmetic indications for surgery are difficult to evaluate, particularly since the procedure should ideally be done before 6 months of age, preferably between the second and third month. Surgery thus is cosmetically prophylactic, and a skilled and experienced neurosurgeon often can restore normal appearance to the infant's head.

The surgical technique involves creating new sutures parallel to the fused suture. It is important that the newly created sutures cross two suture lines (i.e., in coronal stenosis the new suture must cross both the sagittal and squamosal sutures). If two sutures are not crossed, then the newly created suture will not allow sufficient expansion to correct the cosmetic deformity. The new suture line must be treated with phenol or lined with an inert material to prevent refusion. In Shillito's hands the mortality at the operation was only 0.4%; there was a 14% morbidity from wound infections, cardiac arrests, leptomeningeal cysts, and anesthetic complications. It is against these risks that cosmetic indications must be weighed.

DEVELOPMENTAL ABNORMALITIES

Defects in closure of the neuraxis

During the third and fourth weeks of gestation, differentiation of the neural plate occurs, with invagination and dorsal closure to form the neural tube. The neural tube gives rise to the central nervous system, and neural crest cells that form during the process of closure give rise to dorsal root ganglia, sensory ganglia of cranial nerves, and autonomic ganglia. Initially the neural tube closes in the region of the medulla and then proceeds, in a zipperlike fashion, rostrally and caudally. Interruption of the process of closure results in a variety of midline defects, from the cranium down to the lowest level of spinal cord. Because mesodermal differentiation into the dura, vertebrae, and cranium surrounding the differentiating neural tube occurs as an interaction of the neu-

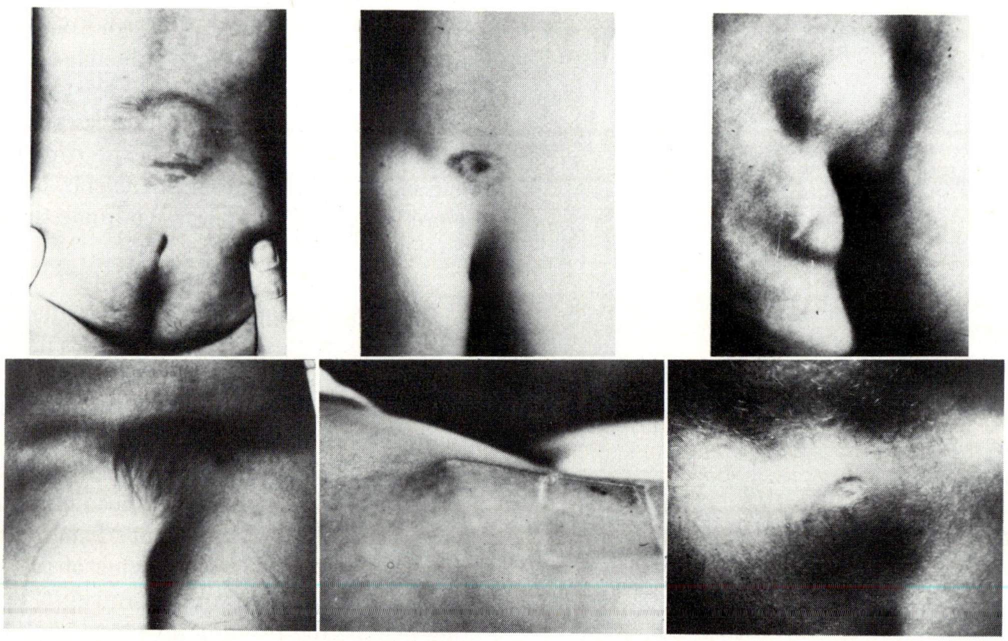

Fig. 27-17. Lesions of the back associated with spina bifida occulta and spinal cord problems. *Top: Left,* Lipoma with hairy patch above hemangioma; *center,* hemangioma; *right,* lipoma. All had tethered cords and intradural lipomas. *Bottom: Left,* Patch of fine hair; *center,* bony spur; *right,* midline scar. Defects shown at bottom left and center were associated with diastematomyelia.

ral tube with surrounding mesoderm, defects in closure of the neural tube involve neural elements and their coverings, including meninges and overlying bony structures. Defects in closure of the neuraxis result in the most common major structural developmental abnormalities of the newborn central and peripheral nervous systems. See Chapter 16 for prenatal diagnosis.

Classification of abnormalities of closure of the spinal cord–spina bifidas

Defects in closure of the spinal canal, termed *spina bifidas*, may be associated with abnormalities of the cord and meninges of varying severity. Their classifications follow.

Meningocele. Meningocele is a cystic dilation of the meninges associated with spina bifida and a defect of the overlying skin. The spinal cord and nerve roots are normal. There is no neurologic deficit.

Meningomyelocele. Meningomyelocele is a lesion identical to the meningocele but with associated abnormalities of the spinal cord and nerve roots. There is neurologic deficit below the level of the lesion. The extent of the deficit depends on the location of the lesion (see further).

Myeloschisis (spina bifida aperta). This is a spina bifida with exposure of the spinal cord and roots and with no cystic covering of meninges. This defect may be small or may extend the whole length of the spinal axis. The clinical significance is identical to that of meningomyelocele.

Spina bifida occulta. This is nonfusion of one or more posterior arches of the spine, usually lumbosacral. A common abnormality found at L5 in 30% of adults, it is of consequence only when associated with underlying abnormalities or when found at other levels. Significant associated abnormalities usually are signaled by a hemangioma, a patch of abnormal hair, a dimple, or a lipoma in the lumbosacral area (Fig. 27-17). The underlying abnormalities include diastematomyelia, spinal lipomas or dermoids, and dermal sinuses (see later discussion).

Embryology

One of the more recent theories suggests that damage to ectoderm produces a bleb of fluid from the neural cleft, which results in embryonic scarring. The degree of damage to ectodermal and mesodermal tissue and the success of the healing and scarring process determine the resultant defect.

Meningomyeloceles and myeloschisis

Clinical manifestations. The degree of neurologic deficit associated with these defects is determined by the level of the lesion. Accurate diagnosis and prognosis for ambulation can be determined to a large degree at birth by careful sensory and motor testing of the infant. The sensory level, in general, gives an approximation of the motor level in these children (Table 27-4) but may be several segments lower. The prognosis can be predicted with a high degree of certainty at birth (Table 27-5), thus helping with the evolution of plans for therapy.

Treatment. A newborn with a meningomyelocele presents the pediatrician with difficult decisions about what to tell parents and whether to recommend surgical closure of the defect. Closure, although usually not technically difficult, carries significant implications. It greatly increases the chances of the infant's survival, but in doing so it initiates an obligation for total care of the child. This places a considerable emotional and financial burden on the family for the numerous surgeries and the rehabilitation that will be required. It also involves appreciable

Table 27-4. Motor examination of lower extremities in children with meningomyeloceles

Movement	Spinal segment: Lumbar	Spinal segment: Sacral	Muscle
Hip			
Flexion	1, 2, 3, 4		Iliopsoas, rectus femoris
Adduction	2, 3, 4		Adductors
Abduction	4, 5	1	Gluteus medius
Extension	4, 5	1, 2	Gluteus maximus, obturator
Knee			
Extension	2, 3, 4		Quadriceps
Flexion	5	1, 2	Hamstrings
Foot			
Dorsiflexion	4, 5	1	Tibialis anterior
Plantar flexion	5	1, 2	Soleus, gastrocnemius

Table 27-5. Deficit and prognosis of meningomyeloceles as related to site of lesion

Motor/sensory level	Maximum motor deficit	Prognosis for ambulation	Risk of hydrocephalus
L5-S1	Dorsiflexion and plantar flexion of feet, weakness of glutei	Will ambulate with or without short leg braces; outlook good	60%
L3-L4	Involvement of quadriceps and hamstrings, plus above	May be able to ambulate with long leg braces and crutches; paralytic hip dislocation	86%
L1 and L2 or above	Complete paraplegia	No functional ambulation	96%

suffering for the infant. Furthermore, the decision to operate must be made promptly, for there is reasonable evidence to suggest that it should take place within the first 24 hours to prevent further deterioration of the spinal cord and roots.

Numerous factors may influence the decision. These should include the size of the lesion and the technical feasibility of closure, the location of the lesion and the prognosis for ambulation of the child, the presence or absence of associated abnormalities (such as hydrocephalus, kyphosis, or other major structural abnormalities), the presence of personnel and facilities to provide adequate care for the infant, and the infant's family structure and the attitudes of the family toward the defect and its consequences. Keeping these factors in mind, the physician must weigh the consequences of the following three possible courses of action.

1. *Immediate closure of the defect*. If the defect is closed immediately, the infant will have approximately a 90% chance of survival. The chance of developing hydrocephalus requiring repetitive shunt procedures will depend on the site of the lesion (Table 27-5). Urologic involvement will occur in about 90%. Fecal soiling can be controlled with rigorous management. Orthopedic care involving braces and transplants of muscles, tendons, and cortex will depend on the site of the lesion, as will the prognosis for ambulation. Psychologic help and social-work assistance will be required for these children. Closure of the defect obligates the physician and society to provide optimum care in each of these areas for the survivors. Despite this care, the function of the child with spinal cord involvement will only approximate normal, the degree of normality depending primarily on the severity of the original lesion.

2. *Passive euthanasia*. See also Chapter 18. Many physicians faced with an infant with a meningomyelocele wish that the problem would go away. However, it has been said that the problem does not go away; only the physician goes away. Even if these infants receive no treatment, 15% to 30% of them will survive. Feeding, antibiotics, and care of the sac will each increase the number of survivors without affecting their quality of life. Figures on the natural history of untreated meningomyeloceles are difficult to find. One series suggests that 40% are stillborn or die within the first week of life. Forty percent of the survivors die by 2 months of age, another 30% die by 2 years of age, and 30% survive. Causes of death are not listed, but many of the late deaths are related to neurologic deterioration secondary to hydrocephalus and to renal deterioration secondary to the neurogenic bladder. Death may occur soon after birth, but for many, death occurs weeks, months, or years later. Thus lack of therapy results not only in more deaths but in the survival of infants who are less functionally able to compete.

3. *Active euthanasia*. This solution to the problem has many moral objections and currently is illegal.

Most children with a meningomyelocele should have active comprehensive therapy. The use of such therapy will not alter the degree of paralysis, but with a vigorous team approach most children will lead happy, useful lives. With normal intelligence these children can be in regular schools despite their paralysis. This course of action is better for the child, the family, and society than providing no therapy and awaiting the child's death.

Management. The quality of survival is paramount, and the preservation of existing function in the lower extremities requires early surgery to close the spinal defect. Where a high lesion has produced complete paraplegia, early surgery does little to improve the quality of survival; the hydrocephalus and the neurogenic bladder will require treatment at the appropriate time. Although closure of the spinal defect takes initial precedence, evaluation of the hydrocephalus and of the renal and bladder status, as well as orthopedic consultation, should take place in the early weeks of life.

An infant born with a meningomyelocele should be transferred immediately to the care of a physician experienced in dealing with the problem. The decision of whether to operate on these infants requires someone who has worked with and followed the course of such infants. The techniques of closure and exploration of the sac may require both neurosurgeons and plastic surgeons, and an orthopedic surgeon may be needed at the initial operation to deal with spinal anomalies. Both survival itself and the quality of that survival may be determined during this neonatal period. After closure of the sac, the infant's course must be followed closely for the progression of existing hydrocephalus. Hydrocephalus may cause bulging of the wound and its breakdown, as well as thinning of the cortex. Evaluation and shunting for hydrocephalus are discussed earlier in the chapter. An intravenous pyelogram and voiding cystoureterogram also should be performed as soon as feasible in the neonatal period. Hydronephrosis may be present at birth, and urinary tract infection may be a continuing problem.

Diastematomyelia

Diastematomyelia is a division of the spinal cord or roots by a bony spicule or fibrous or cartilaginous band that pierces the cord in an anteroposterior direction. This lesion often is associated with a spina bifida occulta at one or more levels and is usually accompanied by a cutaneous lesion such as a hemangioma, a patch of long, fine hair, a lipoma, or a dimple (Fig. 27-17).

At birth there is no neurologic deficit associated with diastematomyelia; but as the infant grows, the spinal cord is not able to ascend because of the bone. Traction on the spinal cord produces neurologic deficit. The deficit may range from persistent enuresis to a neurogenic blad-

A 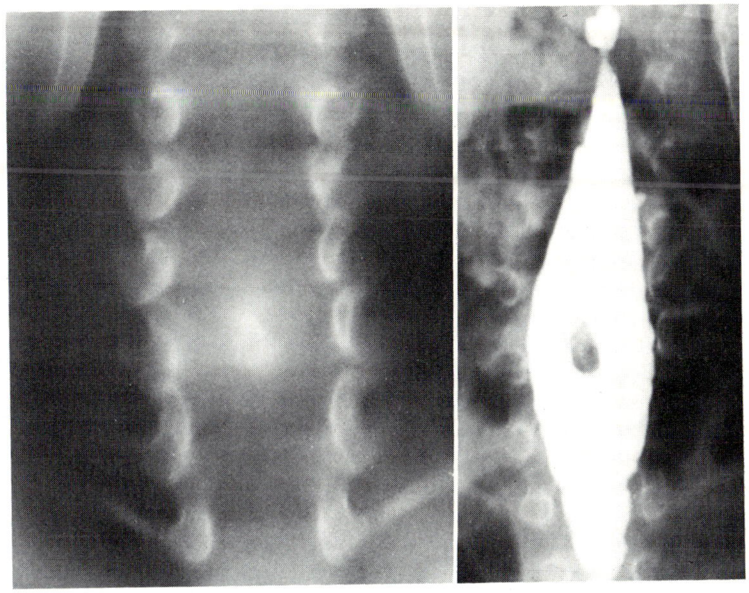 B

Fig. 27-18. A, Tomogram of the spine of an infant with diastematomyelia. The bony spur protruding through the spinal canal and widening of the canal at that area is shown. **B,** Myelogram of the same patient. The spinal cord split around the spur and refused. Same patient as in Fig. 27-18, *bottom center*. The patient was asymptomatic.

der with hydronephrosis. Pain in the legs, weakness, or growth failure of a foot or leg all may be later manifestations. The cutaneous manifestations should suggest the diagnosis. Spine films show a spina bifida and usually a widening of the canal. A midline bony defect confirms the diagnosis (Fig. 27-18). Infants with cutaneous lesions should be followed every 2 to 3 months. A myelogram needs to be done if any neurologic deficit appears. Treatment consists of removal of the bony spicule and release of any tethering of the spinal cord. The surgery is prophylactic rather than curative; an established neurologic deficit may be permanent.

Dermal sinuses and dermoids

Dermal sinuses may occur anywhere along the midline of the back or head but are most common in the occipital area of the skull and in the lumbar region. The sinus is 1 to 2 mm in diameter and may be accompanied by hemangioma or a tuft of hair. These sinuses are to be differentiated from the common superficial dimples seen at the upper end of the gluteal crease. The dermal sinus may extend variable depths into the skin and may continue into the intraspinal space. This lesion should be ruled out on the initial newborn examination. In some cases the sinus has passed unnoticed until it shows redness and swelling associated with infection or is carefully looked for in the patient with meningitis. Roentgenograms of the spine may show a spina bifida, and a widening of the spinal canal may occur if an associated dermoid or lipoma is present. If a sinus is associated with meningitis or with superficial infection or if there is neurologic deficit, the sinus must be removed. Excision should follow the sinus tract to its end. Since intraspinous hematomas may be at the end of a dermal sinus in a significant number of cases, laminectomy may be necessary to remove the tumor.

Lipomas

Lipomeningoceles are large, amorphous accumulations of fatty tissue beneath the skin that may be associated with meningeal defects and may resemble meningomyeloceles. Smaller subcutaneous lipomas may be associated with spina bifida occulta. They may occur at any level of the subcutaneous tissue and may involve the cord itself. It is the intraspinal extensions of these lipomas that become neurologically significant. Widening of the spinal canal shown on a roentgenogram or the development of a neurologic defect suggests the intraspinal process. Surgery should be prophylactic, and, as in diastematomyelia, neurologic deficit may not be reversible. Therefore these infants must be followed frequently and surgery performed at the earliest sign of neurologic involvement.

Encephaloceles

Encephalocele is the name given to cranial anomalies that are similar to the spina bifidas. The term includes craniomeningoceles, encephalomeningoceles, and cranium bifidas. These lesions may occur anywhere along the midline of the head, including the nose, the nasopharynx, and the orbit, but are most common in the occipital area. It usually is not possible to determine the extent of brain involvement before surgery. The size of the lesion should not be a deterrent to surgery, since large lesions may be meningoceles or small lesions may contain cerebral tissue. Roentgenograms of the defect, ultrasound, CT scan, and ventriculograms or pneumoencephalograms are indicated before surgery. Surgery should be undertaken as soon as feasible in the neonatal period to prevent infection and to facilitate care and feeding of the child. Surgery is similar to that undertaken for closure of the back in meningomyeloceles. These children should be evaluated for other structural anomalies of the cervical spine or back and should be followed closely in the postoperative period for the development of hydrocephalus and neurologic signs or symptoms. Prognosis for encephalocele is poor.

THE FLOPPY NEONATE

Hypotonia is one of the most common and often nonspecific signs of illness in the newborn (Fig. 27-19). It may be related to the infant's intrauterine environment, reflecting the effects of maternal disease or drug administration on the fetus. Impaired placental function, circulation and oxygen transport in labor resulting in fetal hypoxia, hypercapnia, and acidosis may be similarly reflected at birth or postnatally in decreased muscle tone, decreased activity, and other evidence of central depression. Sepsis, respiratory distress syndrome, and other systemic diseases also may be associated with hypotonia. The physician therefore must determine whether it is secondary to metabolic abnormalities or to cerebral disease states, including hypoxic ischemic encephalopathy (Part two), intraventricular hemorrhage, and meningitis. Less commonly the hypotonia may be the earliest sign of neuromuscular disease. A key problem in the hypotonic neonate is determination of whether the hypotonia is associated with weakness, since even with repeated careful examination it may be difficult or impossible to make the distinction between weakness and hypotonia in the newborn.

Weakness is the result of anatomic or physiochemical events within the motor system. This motor system or pathway comprises the upper motor neuron, including the motor nerve cells in the cerebral cortex; the descending corticospinal tracts that pass through the brain, brainstem, and the spinal cord; and the motor unit, which includes the anterior horn cells of the spinal cord, the peripheral nerve, the neuromuscular junction, and the muscle. Using clinical observations of tone and movement, muscle bulk, deep tendon reflexes, and response to sensory stimuli, the physician may be able to define the site of anatomic lesions or disease in the motor pathway. Disorders of the upper motor neuron, that is, above the level of the anterior horn cell, are commonly man-

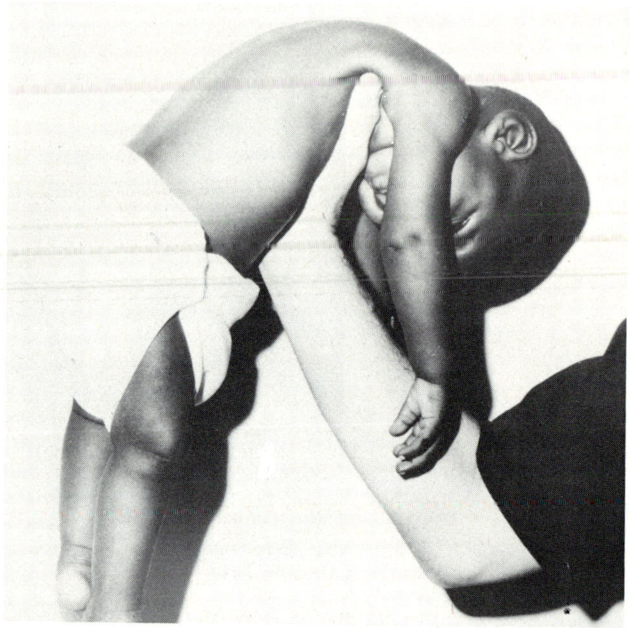

Fig. 27-19. A markedly floppy child in ventral suspension. Contrast this child with the infant shown in Fig. 27-3. This infant showed no flexion of the legs or back and no elevation of the head. The child has Werdnig-Hoffmann disease.

ifested by hypotonia in the newborn rather than by spasticity, as in the older infant or child; however, even with hypotonia, deep tendon reflexes may be increased. In contrast, lesions of anterior horn cell and peripheral nerve are invariably associated with diminished or absent reflexes in the newborn. The deep tendon reflexes in neonates with muscle disease may rarely be present. Disorders of the neuromuscular junction are associated with normally active reflexes. Sensory responses manifested either by limb withdrawal, gross trunk movements, or, in the case of infants with profound weakness with limited trunk or extremity movement, by grimace or crying, indicate in the weak infant that sensory pathways are intact; absence of any response to sensory stimuli in the awake newborn usually is indicative of either spinal cord or peripheral nerve disease. The course of the infant's hypotonia and weakness may also be helpful in establishing a diagnosis, since weakness and hypotonia that are most pronounced at delivery and then improve are more likely the result of intrapartum events, whereas progression of the hypotonia and weakness postpartum over days or weeks may be more indicative of neuromuscular disease.

After determining that the problem is related to neuromuscular and not systemic or central nervous system disease, one attempts to localize the site of the weakness. Important signs of neuromuscular disease in the neonate, in addition to hypotonia, weakness, and altered deep tendon reflexes, are poor sucking and swallowing asso-

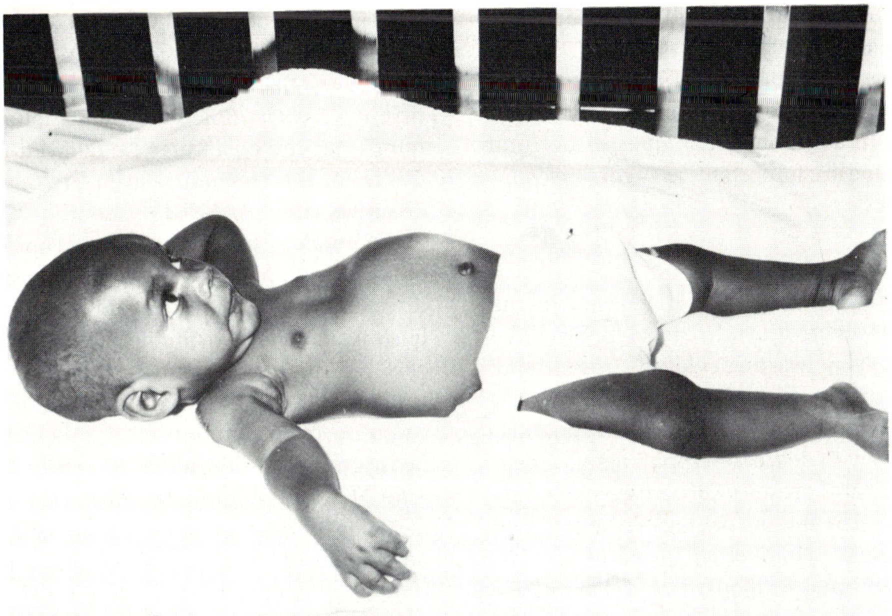

Fig. 27-20. The clinical picture of Werdnig-Hoffmann disease, or marked hypotonia of many causes. The legs are externally rotated and slightly flexed at the knees (the frog-leg position). Note the abdominal breathing and retraction of the chest. There is minimal movement of the arms, as seen by their asymmetry. Note also the alertness of the infant.

ciated at times with aspiration or nasal regurgitation, respiratory distress related to impaired chest movement with diaphragmatic breathing, weakness of facial movements, varying degrees of ophthalmoplegia, fasciculations of the tongue, which must be distinguished from the tremulous tongue movements of the crying infant, and joint contractures.

With careful examination and serial observation of the hypotonic and inactive weak infant, with the additional help of electromyography, and with muscle biopsy with histochemical analysis, specific diagnosis of neuromuscular disorders in the newborn can be determined. Older terms such as *the hypotonic infant, floppy baby syndrome*, or *amyotonia congenita* may be discarded. Recognition of the existence of these disorders and understanding the multiplicity of causes of neonatal hypotonia and weakness may result in the diagnosis of conditions that perhaps are treatable or that may improve with time, provided the infant is given adequate support. Some of the conditions are severe and may be progressive and fatal. Even for these infants, diagnosis is important, not only for prognosis but also for genetic counseling.

Discussion of the differential diagnoses of the floppy or hypotonic newborn, with or without weakness from various causes, follows.

Disorders with neonatal hypotonia and weakness

Spinal cord dysfunction

See discussion in preceding section.

Anterior horn cell disease

Degeneration of the anterior horn cell is the most common definable cause of motor unit dysfunction and is known as Werdnig-Hoffmann disease, an autosomal recessive disorder (Fig. 27-20). It is characterized by extensive widespread muscular atrophy caused by progressive denervation and loss of motor neurons in spinal cord and brainstem, which usually begins in utero. A maternal history of decreased fetal movements may exist, although usually the first manifestations occur after delivery. Clinical manifestations are reported in one third of cases in the neonatal period, with more than half becoming symptomatic by 3 months of age. The disorder is usually lethal by the first year in patients with neonatal onset.

Clinical manifestations. The cardinal manifestations in the symptomatic newborn are inactivity, generalized hypotonia, weakness, and small muscle bulk, and the infant lies in the frog-leg posture. Breathing is abdominal with little or no intercostal or chest movement, and there is marked head lag. Because of weakness of bulbar musculature, impaired sucking and weak cry are noted early, as are fasciculations of the edges of the tongue. Reflexes are absent, but the infant does show response to painful stimuli.

Diagnosis. The diagnosis may be suggested by the classic history and physical findings, especially with the history of a similarly affected sibling. Confirmation requires evidence of denervation on electromyogram

(EMG), and muscle biopsy shows atrophy of motor units. No methods of prenatal detection are available.

Treatment. Therapy is supportive, with attention given to feeding techniques to prevent aspiration and provide sufficient nutrition. In addition, techniques of postural drainage and suctioning are important, as is genetic counseling of the family.

Peripheral neuropathy

Peripheral neuropathies are rarely diagnosed in the neonatal period. However, a syndrome of progressive muscular weakness and wasting closely resembling Werdnig-Hoffmann disease has been described.

Clinical manifestations and diagnosis. Hypotonia, generalized weakness with decreased spontaneous movements, and areflexia are present. Progressive feeding difficulties may occur. The finding of elevated spinal fluid protein, prolonged nerve conduction in motor nerves, and group atrophy on muscle biopsy are the bases for diagnosis.

Treatment. Neuropathies in infants tend to be chronic and may be nonprogressive. Response to steroid therapy may occur.

Neuromuscular junction disease: myasthenia gravis

Two forms of myasthenia are seen in the newborn. Transient neonatal myasthenia gravis is seen in 12% of infants whose mothers have myasthenia gravis. However, maternal myasthenia may not be clinically evident at delivery, and some of these mothers may not have required anticholinesterase medication during pregnancy. No correlation exists between the severity and duration of the mother's illness and the degree of weakness of the newborn, although the birth of one affected infant increases the likelihood of subsequent children being similarly affected. This neonatal disease presumably is caused by a circulating factor transplacentally transmitted to the infant (Chapter 30). These infants almost always show improvement and full recovery within a period of 5 to 47 days. Congenital myasthenia gravis occurs in infants of normal mothers and has a rare familial tendency for occurrence in other siblings. The myasthenia in these infants may be persistent, and involvement of extraocular muscles is common, with little or no generalized weakness.

Clinical manifestations. The initial features of both forms of myasthenia are similar; feeding difficulty is the most common initial manifestation. Despite eagerness to feed, the infant's sucking quickly fatigues so that adequate intake of formula is impossible. Respiratory distress, generalized weakness, hypotonia, and a feeble cry occur and may be the first and most urgent signs of distress shortly after birth in severe cases. Weak facial movements are also common. Ocular muscle weakness is uncommon, as is ptosis in the transitory neonatal form, whereas extraocular muscles are commonly involved in the congenital form, in the absence of generalized weakness. The onset of weakness is noted usually within the first day, with rapid worsening followed by improvement, but the onset may be delayed until the third day of life; in the congenital form the diagnosis often is delayed for several weeks or months.

Diagnosis. The physician must maintain a high level of suspicion, particularly when knowledge of maternal disease, even in complete remission, is available. Infants born to known myasthenic mothers should be followed closely through the first 24 to 36 hours of age for signs just mentioned. The clinical diagnosis is made by the response to intramuscular or subcutaneous injection of neostigmine methylsulfate, 0.125 to 0.5 mg, with atropine, 0.1 mg. Within 10 minutes a measurable increase in strength, facial movements, and sucking ability should be evident. The infant's state before and after administration of neostigmine should be documented. Edrophonium (Tensilon), 0.5 to 1 mg, also may be used, but the brevity of its action makes evaluation of drug response difficult. A negative response with this drug does not rule out the disease.

Treatment. Infants responding to intramuscularly administered neostigmine should be maintained with oral administration of 1 mg neostigmine given 20 minutes before feeding. The dosage must be individually titrated. Periodic attempts to decrease the dosage, with observation of the effect on the infant, should help the physician determine duration of treatment. Supportive measures include gavage feeding and suction.

Muscle diseases

In recent years, increasing use of muscle biopsies and the application of histochemistry to muscle pathology, plus electron microscopic analysis of muscle ultrastructural changes, has resulted in the delineation of a number of congenital, inherited disorders of muscle. Some of these are nonprogressive and appear to have a relatively good prognosis, whereas others have been found to be the cause of profound neonatal weakness and hypotonia with a variable and sometimes fatal outcome.

Myotonic dystrophy

Myotonic dystrophy is probably the most commonly found severe congenital myopathy in the neonatal period. The mother is the affected parent in over 90% of the severely affected infants, although neonatal disease is not related to the severity of maternal disease. Polyhydramnios is a common complication of pregnancy.

Clinical manifestations. The most common clinical manifestations, present at birth, include profound hypotonia and inactivity, feeding and swallowing difficulties, and arthogryposis involving the lower limbs, with talipes equinovarus deformities. Reflexes are either diminished or absent, and in addition to pharyngeal weakness causing feeding problems, there may be bilateral facial weakness and a characteristic tented upper lip. Smooth muscle involvement in the disease may result in abdominal distension and varying degrees of ileus. Severe chest weakness can lead to respiratory distress. With the added problem of diaphragmatic muscle weakness, diagnosis may be difficult, since electromyography rarely reveals myotonic discharge in the affected newborn, and both serum enzymes (CPK, SGOT) and muscle biopsy are normal. The most helpful clues to the diagnosis are the characteristic facial appearance in a hypotonic infant, with a mother who has the classic features of the adult form of myotonic dystrophy—myotonia, distal muscle weakness, characteristic facies, and cataracts. Treatment is limited to supportive care. At times assisted ventilation, as well as parenteral hyperalimentation, may be necessary.

Other muscular dystrophies

Duchenne muscular dystrophy, the most common muscle disease of childhood, is never symptomatic in the neonatal period. Not until 1 year is it possible to recognize the characteristic hypotonia. The other characteristics of this sex-linked recessively inherited disease are not noted until several years of age. However, in the male newborn infant at risk, that is, with affected brothers or maternal uncles, a presumptive chemical diagnosis can be made in the first week of life by determination of the CPK level, which is dramatically elevated.

Congenital muscular dystrophy is a term that has been used as a diagnosis for a poorly defined muscle disease in infancy with symptoms of weakness and flexion contractures. This does not appear to be a distinct disease with specific histologic features, and these cases await further clarification.

Central core disease

Central core disease, one of the first morphologically distinct congenital myopathies, initially was clinically characterized by nonprogressive weakness and hypotonia in children whose motor development was delayed and who also had kyphoscoliosis and other skeletal deformities, including hip dislocation. Since the condition has been more completely delineated, apparently it is a cause of congenital hypotonia at birth or shortly thereafter. Deep tendon reflexes are usually present but may be reduced in proportion to the degree of weakness. No cranial muscles are involved. With the passage of time, delay in motor milestones is evident, as is proximal weakness. Muscle biopsy shows central areas in many but not all muscle fibers in which histochemical reactions for oxidative enzymes are absent. In many patients a marked predominance of type I histochemically determined muscle fibers is present.

Centronuclear (myotubular) myopathy

This was described initially as a disorder of children with congenital, slowly progressive weakness, whose muscle biopsies were characterized by the presence of centrally placed nuclei in muscle fibers. The condition was termed *myotubular myopathy*, with the suggestion that the abnormality in muscle fibers causing the weakness was the result of arrested fiber development at the fetal myotubular stage. In addition to the originally described cases of children with slowly progressive limb weakness, ptosis, and extraocular and facial weakness, a form of this disease is manifested in the immediate neonatal period by profound generalized hypotonia and weakness. The affected infants may have respiratory failure caused by a combination of intercostal and bulbar muscle weakness. These infants also have profound weakness of extraocular and facial muscles, so that eye and facial movements and tendon reflexes are absent. Diagnosis is established by the clinical presentation, histologic and histochemical description of muscle fibers with marked variation in size, and many small fibers with a myotubular structure and centrally placed muscle nuclei. The neonatal weakness may be so profound that a fatal outcome may result. However, some infants who are provided adequate care and support may survive to later infancy and childhood with a nonprogressive course and variable degrees of persisting weakness. The severe congenital disease affects only males.

Congenital muscle fiber type disproportion

Muscle fibers are characterized as either type I or type II on the basis of differing histochemical stains. Muscle biopsy reveals small type I muscle fibers and normal size type II fibers in a rather heterogeneous group of children with variable degrees of muscle weakness. In addition, a homogenous group of infants with small size type I fibers appears to have a congenital myopathy evident at birth. Characteristics are hypotonia, decreased movements, and congenital contractures of joints involving hands or feet. Congenital hip dislocations also are commonly present. Such joint contractures and deformities may be labeled as arthrogryposis. They may be the predominant clinical manifestation of this congenital myopathy, in which presumably restricted limb movements in utero have resulted in the deformed joints. Associated abnormalities in congenital muscle fiber type disproportion myopathy include short stature, high arched palate, long thin face, and kyphoscoliosis, which become evident as the child grows older. The course of the disorder, often familial, is nonprogressive; improvement can be anticipated with survival into childhood and adult life.

Other congenital myopathies

Other congenital muscle conditions occasionally are manifested by hypotonia but no significant weakness in the first weeks or months of life. Nemaline or rod-body myopathy, one of the earliest disorders of muscle weakness with a nonprogressive course, categorized initially on the basis of histochemical and ultrastructural abnormalities, is commonly manifested by hypotonia and variable degree of weakness with delayed motor development. However, most children with this disease have not been symptomatic as neonates. A number of more rare congenital myopathies, characterized strictly on the basis of morphologic changes in muscle fibers, are not well delineated as clinical entities. Multicore myopathy, fingerprint body myopathy, sarcotubular myopathy, reducing body myopathy, and at least five other different types of myopathy with unusual mitochondria have been described. Some patients may show neonatal hypotonia and weakness, but their clinical descriptions remain incomplete at present. Undoubtedly some infants with congenital hypotonia and weakness that is not progressive have these or other as yet undescribed disorders of muscle structure or metabolism. Many such infants are undoubtedly still currently described under the rubric *benign congenital hypotonia*, which appears to be a diagnostic label for children with a clinical syndrome of generalized hypotonia from birth, minimum or mild weakness, a nonprogressive course, and a normal muscle biopsy. The use of this diagnosis is at present a reflection more of our lack of knowledge than of neurologic sophistication.

Muscle biopsy, a feasible procedure in even the weakest infants, until recently has been considered primarily an investigative rather than diagnostic tool in the neonatal period. For muscle biopsy to achieve its potential as a diagnostic test in the evaluation of the hypotonic and weak infant, modern histochemical techniques and electron microscopy must be used in the pathologic examination of tissue. Used in this manner, with biopsies taken from clinically weak muscles, muscle biopsy is a low-risk procedure with great potential for the diagnosis of many neuromuscular and metabolic diseases for which the initial symptoms in the neonate are hypotonia and weakness.

Arthrogryposis multiplex congenita

Arthrogryposis is a condition of multiple causes characterized by fixed deformity of one or more joints at birth. It is not a disease. Clubfoot, either unilateral or bilateral, may be one form of this disorder. The joint fixation is secondary to lack of movement of the joint in utero for periods of time. This could result from fetal malposition or intrauterine paralysis. The weakness or paralysis may be caused by anterior horn cell disease, neuropathies, or congenital myopathies such as congenital fiber type disproportion and neonatal or congenital myotonic dystrophy.

ACUTE METABOLIC DISEASE

Acute metabolic disease in the neonatal period is uncommon, but its prompt recognition may determine the mental outcome of the infant or may even be life saving. The hallmark is the abrupt onset of lethargy, vomiting, and coma in a previously well infant. These findings often are accompanied by seizures. Onset may take place in the first hours or days of life. This constellation of symptoms also suggests the diagnosis of sepsis, meningitis, or intracranial hemorrhage. Immediate evaluation should include blood cultures and lumbar puncture. Urinalysis for acetonuria often will lead to the diagnosis of ketoacidosis found in several of the metabolic diseases. Ketoacidosis otherwise is uncommon in the first month of life, even with starvation, vomiting, or diarrhea. Its presence should therefore suggest the possibility of a metabolic disorder. Specific diagnosis requires the prompt performance of metabolic screening procedures and chromatography of serum and urine for amino acids. For some diseases, such as hyperammonemia, chromatography will be normal, and diagnosis requires specific testing. Acute therapy in most of these diseases consists of removal of protein from the diet and the administration of glucose and intravenous fluids while awaiting the diagnosis. Exchange transfusions occasionally may be life saving. A family history of siblings or relatives with acute neonatal disease should increase suspicion of a metabolic disorder. A discussion of each of the metabolic disorders that may include seizures and other neurologic manifestations is found in Chapter 36.

Alfred W. Brann, Jr.
James F. Schwartz

BIBLIOGRAPHY

Abnormalities of head size

Bergman, E.W., Freeman, J.M., and Epstein, M.H.: Treatment of infantile hydrocephalus with acetazolamide and furosemide: three- to four-year follow-up, Ann. Neurol 8:227, 1980.

Cutler, R.W.P., and others: Formation and absorption of cerebrospinal fluid in man, Brain **91**:707, 1968.

DeLevie, M., and Nogrady, M.B.: Rapid brain growth upon restoration of adequate nutrition causing false radiologic evidence of increased intracranial pressure, J. Pediatr. **76**:523, 1970.

Dobbing, J.: Undernutrition and the developing brain, Am. J. Dis. Child. **20**:411, 1970.

Dodge, R.P., and Porter, P.: Demonstration of intracranial pathology by transillumination, Arch. Neurol. **5**:594, 1961.

Gilles, F.H., and Shillito, J.: Infantile hydrocephalus: retrocerebellar subdural hematoma, J. Pediatr. **76**:529, 1970.

Gold, A.P., Ransohoff, J., and Carter, S.: Vein of Galen malformation, Acta Neurol. Scand. **40**(Suppl. 11):1, 1964.

Johnson, R.T., and Johnson, K.P.: Hydrocephalus as a sequela of experimental mixoviruses, Exp. Mol. Pathol. **10**:68, 1969.

Lorber, J.: Medical and surgical aspects in the treatment of congenital hydrocephalus, Neuropaediatrie **2**:239, 1971.

Lorber, J.: Results of treatment of myelomeningocele, Dev. Med. Child. Neurol. **13**:279, 1971.

Lorber, J., and Zachary, R.B.: Primary congenital hydrocephalus, Arch. Dis. Child. **43**:516, 1968.

Martin, H.P.: Microcephaly and mental retardation, Am. J. Dis. Child. **119**:128, 1970.
Scarf, J.E.: Treatment of hydrocephalus: an historical and critical review of methods and results, J. Neurol. Neurosurg. Psychiatry **26**:1, 1963.
Schick, R.W., and Matson, D.D.: What is arrested hydrocephalus? J. Pediatr. **58**:791, 1961.

Abnormalities of head shape

Freeman, J.M., and Borkowf, S.: Craniostenosis, Pediatrics **30**:57, 1962.
Shillito, J., and Matson, D.D.: Craniosynostosis, Pediatrics **41**:829, 1968.

Developmental abnormalities

Freeman, J.M., editor: A practical approach to the problems of meningomyeloceles, Baltimore, Md., 1974, University Park Press.
Haworth, J.C., and Zachary, R.B.: Congenital dermal sinuses in children: their relationship to pilonidal sinus, Lancet **2**:10, 1955.
Laurence, K.M.: The survival of untreated spinal bifida cystica, Dev. Med. Child Neurol. **1**(suppl.):10, 1966.
Lorber, J.: The prognosis of encephalocele, Dev. Med. Child Neurol. **13**(suppl):75, 1967.
Sieben, R.L., Hamida, M.B., and Shulman, K.: Multiple cranial nerve deficits associated with the Arnold-Chiari malformations, Neurology (Minneap.) **21**:673, 1971.

The floppy neonate

Barwick, D.D., and Walton, J.N.: Polymyositis, Am. J. Med. **35**:646, 1000.
Blattner, R.J.: Arthrogryposis multiplex congenita, J. Pediatr. **71**:367, 1967.
Dodge, P.R., and others: Myotonic dystrophy in infancy and childhood, Pediatrics **35**:3, 1967.
Dubowitz, V.: The floppy infant. In Clinics in developmental medicine, no. 31, London, England, 1969, William Heinemann, Ltd.
Dubowitz, V.: Infantile muscular atrophy, Brain **87**:707, 1976.
Landau, W.M.: Spasticity and rigidity, Recent Adv. Neurol. **6**:1, 1969.
Paine, R.S.: The future of the "floppy infant"; a follow-up study of 133 patients, Dev. Med. Child Neurol. **5**:115, 1963.
Taksuji, N., Brown, B., and Brob, D.: Neonatal myasthenia gravis, Pediatrics **45**:488, 1970.
Taskar, W., and Chutorian, A.M.: Chronic polyneuritis of childhood, J. Pediatr. **74**:699, 1969.
Zellweger, H., and others: Severe congenital muscular dystrophy, Am. J. Dis. Child. **114**:591, 1967.

PART SIX

Follow-up for high-risk neonates

Advances in obstetric and neonatal care have been responsible for the improved survival of high-risk neonates. A major concern persists, however, that neonatal intensive care may result in an increased number of permanently handicapped infants. The earliest follow-up studies of preterm infants following the introduction of modern methods of neonatal intensive care in the 1960s described a decrease in adverse neurodevelopmental sequelae as compared to the preceding era. More recently, despite a continued decrease in mortality, the incidence of neurodevelopmental sequelae has not continued to decrease but has remained fairly constant. Thus the absolute number of both healthy and neurologically impaired survivors has increased. Furthermore, the increased survival of extremely immature low birth weight infants has resulted in a relatively high handicap rate in the subpopulation of infants born weighing less than 750 gm (Fig. 27-21). It is important to realize that conditions of presumed genetic and prenatal origin account for more children with neurodevelopmental dysfunction than disorders arising out of the perinatal period. Infants who are at highest risk for later neurodevelopmental problems include those who had severe asphyxia, severe intraventricular or other intracranial hemorrhage, meningitis, seizures, respiratory failure, or multisystem congenital malformations and those born with very low birth weight (VLBW).

Follow-up clinics should be an integral extension of every neonatal intensive care unit. Specialized care must be made available for problems of growth, development, and chronic disease and is best provided within the setting of a neonatal follow-up program. The follow-up care should initially be provided by the neonatologists together with the family pediatrician and then gradually transferred to a developmental specialist. This initial continuity of care is important to reassure the family that the same persons responsible for the life-saving decisions are continuing to assume responsibility for the child's adaptation into home life. Furthermore, even if the neonatal staff members do not continue the follow-up for a long period, they will benefit greatly by maintaining contact with the infants leaving the nursery and recognizing the sequelae of early neonatal interventions. Growth (weight, height, and head circumference), neurologic development, psychomotor development, vision, and hearing should all be sequentially assessed.

Comparisons will inevitably be made with results of follow-up at other tertiary centers. Weight-selected samples from different units may not be comparable, however, since outcome will be heavily influenced by (1) the socioeconomic profile of the parents, (2) the incidence of extreme prematurity, (3) a selective admission policy, and (4) the percentage of inborn patients at any center. Regional results reflect a more accurate picture of outcome because they include all infants born in an area. This is the ideal situation, but such studies are rarely available.

MEDICAL PROBLEMS

Neonatal intensive care has resulted in an increased morbidity resulting from various medical complications, including chronic pulmonary disease, increased susceptibility to respiratory infection, sequelae of necrotizing enterocolitis, and cholestatic jaundice. These in turn may contribute to multiple rehospitalizations, poor physical growth, and an increase in postneonatal deaths. Up to

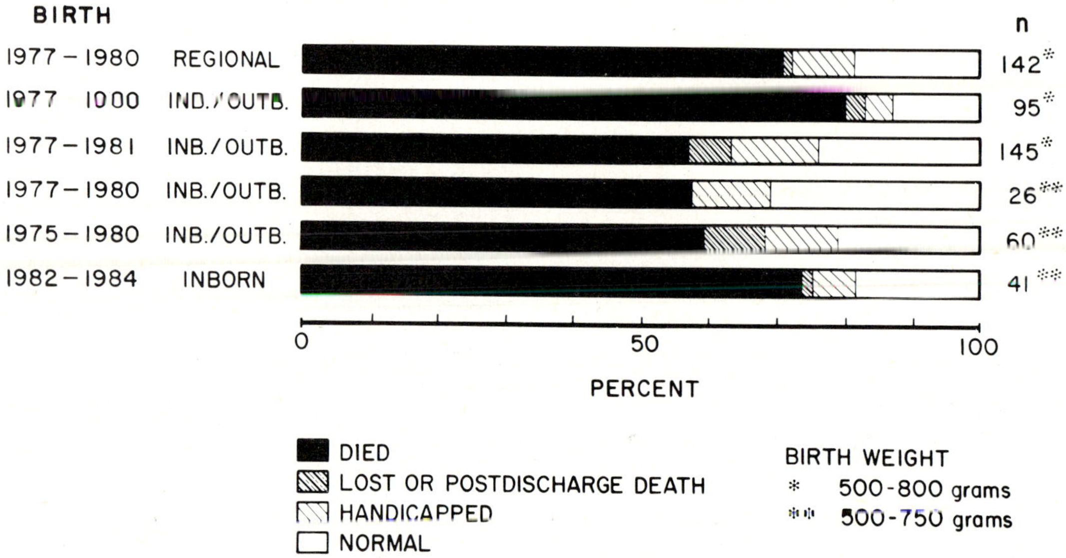

Fig. 27-21. Outcome of extremely small infants. Percentage of infants from selected reports who died during the initial neonatal hospitalization, were lost to follow-up or died after discharge, survived handicapped, or survived normal. Most infants were followed to at least 2 years of age. Handicap was defined as moderate to severe neurosensory impairment and/or developmental or intelligence quotient less than 80. (Modified from Hack, M., and Fanaroff, A.A.: N. Engl. J. Med. **314:**660, 1986. Reprinted by permission of the New England Journal of Medicine.)

33% of (VLBW) infants (less than 1.5 kg) are rehospitalized during the first year of life and up to 10% during the second and third years. Children with neurologic sequelae such as cerebral palsy or hydrocephalus have an even higher rate of rehospitalization for such reasons as shunt complications, orthopedic correction of spasticity, and eye surgery.

Physical growth

Intrauterine and/or neonatal growth retardation occurs in up to 50% of VLBW infants. The poor neonatal growth is related to inadequate nutrition during the acute phase of neonatal disease and to chronic medical sequelae that result in increased caloric requirements. These include chronic lung disease and malabsorption secondary to necrotizing enterocolitis or cholestatic liver disease. Poor feeding in neurologically impaired children and the lack of an optimum nurturing environment in the nursery may also affect neonatal growth. As these conditions gradually resolve and an optimum home environment is provided, catch-up body growth may occur during the first 2 to 3 years of life. Nonetheless, up to 20% of appropriate for gestational age (AGA) and as many as 50% of small for gestational age (SGA) VLBW infants remain subnormal in weight by their third year of life. (See also Chapter 7.)

Intrauterine and neonatal brain growth failure and lack of later catch-up growth may affect cognitive functioning. Fifty percent of SGA VLBW infants are born with subnormal head growth, and brain growth failure may occur during the neonatal period in up to 20% of AGA VLBW infants. Catch-up brain growth may occur during infancy in both AGA and SGA VLBW infants; however, up to 10% of AGA and 25% of SGA VLBW infants will still have a subnormal head size at 2 to 3 years of age.

Growth after discharge is a good measure of physical, neurologic, and environmental well-being. To promote optimum catch-up growth of high-risk infants, neonatal nutrition needs to be maximized and sufficient calories provided during the recovery phase. This is especially important because catch-up of head circumference in both AGA and SGA children only occurs during the first 6 to 12 months after term.

NEURODEVELOPMENTAL OUTCOME

Transient neurologic problems

A very high incidence of transient neurologic abnormalities, ranging from 40% to 80%, occurs in high-risk infants. These include abnormalities of muscle tone such as hypotonia or hypertonia (presenting as poor head control at 40 weeks' postconceptional age), poor back support at 4 to 8 months, or a slight increase in muscle tone of the upper extremities. Since some degree of physiologic hypertonia normally exists during the first 3 months, it may be difficult to diagnose the early developing spasticity related to cerebral palsy. Children who will later develop cerebral palsy initially have hypotonia (poor head control and back support) and only later spasticity of the extremities. Spasticity during the first 3 to 4 months is a poor prognostic sign. Persistence of primitive reflexes might also be a sign of early cerebral palsy. Although mild hypertonia or hypotonia persisting at 8 months usually resolves by the second year, it might indicate later subtle neurologic dysfunction.

Major neurologic sequelae

Major neurologic sequelae can usually be diagnosed during the latter part of the first year of life in up to 10% of high-risk newborns, or even earlier if very severe. Major neurologic handicap is usually classified as cerebral palsy (spastic diplegia, spastic quadriplegia, or spastic hemiplegia or paresis); hydrocephalus (with or without accompanying cerebral palsy or sensory deficits); blindness (usually caused by retrolental fibroplasia); seizures; or deafness (see boxed material and Table 27-6). The intellectual outcome of these children may differ greatly according to the neurologic diagnosis. For example, children with spastic quadriplegia usually have severe mental retardation, whereas children with spastic diplegia or hemiplegia may have intact mental functioning. This is not always measurable until after 2 to 3 years of age.

Most neurologic or physical problems either resolve or become permanent during the first year of life. During the second year the environmental effects of maternal education and social class begin to play a major role on the various cognitive outcome measures. Further problems may emerge, usually subtle motor, visual, and behavioral difficulties. These are best diagnosed and treated in an psychologic and educational rather than a medical follow-up setting.

Timing of follow-up visits

The initial follow-up visit should be 7 to 10 days after discharge. This is important in order to evaluate how the child is adapting to the home environment. This visit usually occurs around the time of the expected date of delivery. A clinic visit at about 4 months of corrected age is important to document problems of inadequate catch-up growth and severe neurologic abnormality that might require intervention or occupational and physical therapy. Eight months of corrected age is a good time to confirm the presence of cerebral palsy or other neurologic abnormality. It is also an excellent time for the first developmental assessment to be performed, usually the Bayley Scales of Infant Development, since the children show very little stranger anxiety at this age and are most cooperative. Alternatively, this first developmental assessment can occur at 12 months.

By 18 to 24 months of age most transient neurologic findings will have resolved, and the neurologically abnormal child will be showing some adaptation with improving functional ability. Most potential catch-up growth will have occurred and some prediction can be made of the child's ultimate growth attainment. At the same time the mental scale of the Bayley scales will provide some assessment of the child's ultimate mental performance.

The Bayley score attained at 8 to 12 months of corrected age tends to drop about 10 points by the second year. This may be a function of the test rather than the child but may also reflect environmental effects. Nonetheless, subnormal scores are predictive of poor later

Various types of neurologic dysfunction in children who have been high-risk neonates

- Motor deficits
  1. Spastic diplegia
  2. Spastic quadriplegia
  3. Spastic hemiplegia
- Mental retardation
- Seizures
- Sensory abnormalities
  1. Hearing deficits
  2. Visual abnormalities
     a. Retrolental fibroplasia
     b. Eye motility dysfunction
- Posthemorrhagic hydrocephalus
- Microcephaly
- Problems of school-age children
  1. Visuomotor deficits
  2. Learning deficits
  3. Subtle neurologic dysfunction

Table 27-6. Very low birth weight (<1.5 kg) infant outcome: Rainbow Babies and Childrens Hospital, Cleveland, Ohio, 1983 (n = 141)

Outcome	%
Postdischarge deaths	3.5
Rehospitalization	
First year	21
Second year	8
Neurodevelopmental outcome	
Normal outcome	78
Major congenital malformation	2
Neurosensory Impairment	13*
Developmental quotient less than 80	7†

*Includes three children with cerebral palsy, four with hypotonia, three with severe visual impairment, one with deafness, and five shunted for hydrocephalus, four of whom had cerebral palsy.
†Excluding children with neurologic abnormality.

functioning. At 3 years of age a Stanford Binet IQ test can be performed, which further validates the child's mental abilities. Language is well measurable at this age. From 4 years of age more subtle neurologic, visuomotor, and behavioral difficulties are measurable. These difficulties may affect school performance, even in those children who have normal intelligence.

Developmental testing

The child's functional ability at each age is more important than the neurologic diagnosis or IQ score. Neurodevelopmental handicap is usually defined in children who have a neurologic abnormality and/or a developmental quotient or IQ less than 80. Some researchers include only infants with an IQ less than 70, whereas others include all children with an IQ less than 1 standard deviation (less than 85). Neurologic abnormality is usually classified by neurologic diagnosis, which can include hypotonia or hypertonia, cerebral palsy (spastic diplegia or quadriplegia hemisyndrome), hydrocephalus, blindness, or deafness, as listed in the boxed material.

The neurologic examination during infancy is largely based on changes in muscle tone that occur during the first year of life. We use the examination developed by Amiel-Tison, which measure the progressive increase in active muscle tone (head control, back support, sitting, standing, walking) together with the concomitant decrease in passive muscle tone. This also documents visual and auditory responses and some primitive reflexes. This method gives a qualitative assessment of neurologic integrity, which is defined as normal, suspect, or abnormal during the first year. Since the Amiel-Tison method of evaluation extends only to the end of the first year, a conventional neurologic examination should be performed thereafter (see also Part one).

Psychomotor developmental tests include the following:

The Bayley Scales of Infant Development are performed before 2 years of age. They include a mental and a motor subscale, which together give a developmental quotient (DQ) and are standardized with a mean of 100. Before 1 year of age these scales are weighed heavily by motor function. It is only during the second year that mental function can be more reliably tested. For example, children with spastic diplegia will have low Bayley scores before 12 months of age but by 2 years might have a normal mental but low motor score.

The Stanford Binet Test of Intelligence is performed between 2 and 6 years of age and gives a measure of mental function or IQ.

The McCarthy Scales of Infant Development may be performed between 3 and 5 years of age. In contrast to the Stanford Binet, this test has 5 subscales that measure different functions: verbal, perceptual, quantitative, memory, and motor. In addition, a general cognitive index is equivalent to the IQ on the Stanford Binet.

The Denver Test of Development is good for clinical use but does not give a quantitative assessment and thus cannot be used to quantitate outcome in specific high-risk populations.

Ophthalmologic testing should be performed on all high-risk children before discharge. If abnormal, repeat examinations should be done at the discretion of the ophthalmologist. All children should have a repeat eye examination between 12 and 24 months of age (Chapter 39).

Hearing should be screened before discharge from the neonatal intensive care nursery. A behavioral response to sound can be used; however, most nurseries now use the Crib-O-Gram or base of brain–evoked responses. Hearing should be reexamined at 12 to 24 months, since the most common cause of hearing loss is related to middle ear infections that occur after the neonatal period and during the first 2 years of life (see hearing screening in part one of this chapter).

Maureen Hack

BIBLIOGRAPHY

Amiel-Tison, C., and Grenier, A.: Neurologic examination of the infant and newborn, New York, 1983, Masson Publishing USA, Inc.

Berger, R.L., and Schaefer, A.R.: The premature infant goes home: guidelines for primary care, Am. J. Dis. Child. **139**:200, 1985.

Georgieff, M.K., and others: Abnormal truncal muscle tone as a useful early method for developmental delay and in low birth weight infants, Pediatrics **77**:659, 1986.

Hack, M., and Breslau, N.: Very low birthweight infants: effects of brain growth during infancy on intelligence at 3 years of age, Pediatrics **77**:196, 1986.

Hack, M., and Fanaroff, A.A.: Changes in the delivery room care of the extremely small infant (<750 gm): effects on morbidity and outcome, N. Engl. J. Med. **314**:660, 1986.

Hack, M., and others: The very low birthweight infant: the broader spectrum of morbidity during infancy and early childhood, Dev. Behav. Pediatr. **4**:243, 1983.

Hagberg, B., Hagberg, G., and Olow, I.: Gains and hazards of intensive neonatal care: an analysis from Swedish cerebral palsy epidemiology, Dev. Med. Child Neurol. **24**:13, 1982.

Horwood, S.P., and others: Mortality and morbidity of 500-1499 gram birthweight infants live-born to residents of a defined geographic region before and after neonatal intensive care, Pediatrics **69**:613, 1982.

Kiely, J., Paneth, N., and Stanley, F.: Monitoring the morbidity outcomes of perinatal health services. In Stanley, F., and Alberman, E., editors: The epidemiology of the cerebral palsies. Clinics in developmental medicine, No. 87, SIMP, Philadelphia, 1984, J.B. Lippincott Co.

Nelson, K.B., and Ellenberg, J.H.: Antecedents of cerebral palsy, N. Engl. J. Med. **315**:81, 1986.

Shapiro, S., and others: Changes in infant morbidity associated with decreases in neonatal mortality, Pediatrics **72**:408, 1983.

Stewart, A.L., Reynolds, E.O.R., and Lipscome, A.P.: Outcome for infants of very low birth weight: survey of world literature, Lancet **2**:1038, 1981.

CHAPTER 28

The respiratory system

PART ONE

The developmental biology of the lung

The lung is clearly a critical organ in early adaptation to extrauterine life. At birth, interruption of the fetal-placental circulation requires the newborn infant to immediately achieve effective gas exchange. Sufficient prenatal maturation of the respiratory system therefore is an essential aspect of intrauterine development. Differentiation of the lung requires carefully regulated coordination of anatomic, physiologic, and biochemical processes. The ultimate product of these maturational events is an organ having adequate surface area, blood supply, and metabolic capability to sustain oxygenation and ventilation during the neonatal period. Particularly important from a biochemical viewpoint is the capacity for rapid synthesis of surface-active phospholipids, which are necessary in establishing normal lung function after birth.

The elucidation of processes leading to lung maturity has depended on multidisciplinary research approaches that have been closely linked to improved clinical understanding of neonatal respiratory disorders. Information on the developmental biology of the respiratory system has provided important insights into pulmonary dysfunction after birth, as well as explanations for developmental anomalies of the lung. Indeed full appreciation of the pathophysiology of disorders such as the respiratory distress syndrome (RDS) requires one to develop a thorough understanding of the process of fetal lung maturation and the biology of pulmonary surfactant. Accordingly the purpose of this section is to review fundamental aspects of fetal lung development, including the physiology and biochemistry of surfactant. Because of the relatively high incidence and major significance of respiratory distress in neonatal-perinatal medicine, and in an effort to provide a frame of reference for the clinician, an attempt is made to relate the basic information to pertinent clinical problems of the newborn.

HISTORICAL PERSPECTIVE

Ever since pulmonary surfactant deficiency was recognized as an underlying problem in neonates with RDS, major efforts have been devoted to investigations concerning the physiology and biosynthesis of this phospholipid-rich substance that lines the respiratory epithelium. In some instances basic research approaches have paid rich dividends in enhancing care of the sick neonate. Advances that have bridged the gap from the laboratory to the bedside are the development of tests of fetal lung maturity, based on amniotic fluid analyses, and the use of corticosteroids for accelerating lung maturation in utero. Table 28-1 presents a chronologic outline of the advances in understanding surfactant and a description of the related discoveries concerning RDS.

The first 50 years were dominated by morphologic studies directed at either pulmonary hyaline membranes (PHM) or structural features of fetal lung development, particularly the glandular and canalicular phases in early gestation. In addition, during this period the effects of surface forces acting at the air-fluid interface of the lung were described by von Neergaard, providing the first experimental observation of the potential significance of pulmonary surfactant.

The next 20 years, from approximately 1950 to 1970, featured clinical studies on the pathophysiology of RDS and basic investigations on the nature and role of pulmonary surfactant. This era of research began with the recognition that PHMs represent a secondary, nonspecific phenomenon occurring because of tissue damage and transudation of protein into the alveoli. Soon thereafter surfactant was "rediscovered" in pulmonary edema foam and lung extracts by Pattle and Clements, respectively. Such parallel advances culminated in the observation by Avery and Mead that lungs of immature fetuses

Table 28-1. Chronology of advances in understanding of pulmonary surfactant and RDS

Date	Observations and research trends
1902	Initial description of pulmonary hyaline membranes (PHM)
1923	First English description of PHM in association with neonatal pneumonia
1929	Discovery of the effects of surface forces at the air-water interface of the lung
1930-1949	Prevailing view that PHM resulted from aspirated amniotic sac contents
1936-1942	Description of structural features of fetal lung development, including three stages *(glandular, canalicular, and alveolar)*
1949	Proposal that an interval of air breathing was prerequisite to development of PHM
1950	Association of PHM with prematurity, fetal anoxia, maternal diabetes, and cesarean section
1950	Description of the clinical respiratory abnormalities associated with PHM
1951	PHM considered to be a secondary phenomenon resulting from tissue damage
1953-1955	Roentgenographic description of the reticulogranular pattern in generalized atelectasis
1954-1959	Elucidation of major pulmonary function abnormalities in RDS
1955-1957	Discovery of surfactant in pulmonary edema foam and lung extracts
1955-1958	Proposal that atelectasis is significant factor in respiratory distress with PHM
1955-1960	Clarification of the clinical pattern of RDS
1959	Demonstration of pulmonary surfactant deficiency in infants succumbing to RDS
1961	Identification of phosphatidylcholine (lecithin) as the major surfactant component
1961-1965	Lowered RDS mortality with intensive respiratory and metabolic care
1962-1967	Description of the timing of lung surfactant appearance during late gestation
1965-1967	Observation that lung phosphatidylcholine concentrations are decreased in RDS
1965-1970	Demonstration that aggressive mechanical ventilation improves survival in severe RDS but causes bronchopulmonary dysplasia
1971	Discovery of the predictability of amniotic fluid lecithin/sphingomyelin ratios, allowing prevention of *iatrogenic RDS*
1971	Improved oxygenation with continuous positive airway pressure
1971-1973	Discovery of the physiologic and biochemical effects of corticosteroids on the fetal lung
1971-1975	Demonstration of enhanced neonatal care via regionalized perinatal programs
1972	Direct demonstration by electron microscopic autoradiography of the role of type II pneumonocytes
1972	Prevention of RDS with antenatal corticosteroid administration
1974	Clarification of pathways for de novo biosynthesis of lung phosphatidylcholine
1975	Discovery of phosphatidylglycerol as a significant component of surfactant
1975-1980	Growing interest in surfactant secretion and turnover
1981-1985	Exogenous surfactant therapy by airway instillation
1983-1985	Emphasis on lung injury and repair (pathogenesis of bronchopulmonary dysplasia, lung antioxidants, new modes of mechanical ventilation)
1985-	Molecular biology of surfactant components being defined, including apoprotein

and infants succumbing to RDS were deficient in surfactant, thus explaining the alveolar collapse and also providing a basis for more rational approaches to both research and treatment of RDS. Subsequently the timing of the appearance of surfactant in the fetal lung has been carefully defined, particularly during late gestation, when the major maturational changes take place. Improved understanding of the basis of pulmonary dysfunction in RDS and the role of surfactant also has facilitated serial improvements in techniques for mechanical ventilatory support of premature infants.

During the past decade there has been somewhat of a shift in emphasis from the anatomic and physiologic approaches to the study of fetal lung development toward biochemical studies and efforts to stimulate intrauterine lung maturation by administration of hormones and other pharmacologic agents. As a result, the metabolic regulation of surfactant production and turnover has become a major focus of research. Elucidation of the phospholipid composition of surfactant has encouraged basic scientists to concentrate their efforts on phosphatidylcholine (lecithin) and phosphatidylglycerol, whereas clinicians have used measurements of these compounds in amniotic fluid for routine prenatal assessment of lung maturation. This has permitted perinatologists to better time the delivery and prevent a substantial number of premature infants from developing RDS.

THE MORPHOLOGY AND HISTOLOGY OF LUNG DEVELOPMENT

Architecture of the respiratory system

Simply stated, the respiratory system may be divided into three components: (1) the upper airways (from the nose and mouth to the trachea), which are mainly extrathoracic and of relatively large diameter, (2) the gas-distributing system of the lungs, or lower conducting airways, which begins with the main stem bronchi and extends to the terminal bronchioli, and (3) the acinar region, which is responsible for carrying out exchange of oxygen and carbon dioxide.

The air-conducting portion of the lung is lined by ciliated epithelium. Bronchi are distinguished as airways that contain cartilage; large bronchi contain cartilage in any cross section, whereas small bronchi show less cartilage, which in fact may not be present in some cross-section histologic examinations. The most peripheral conducting airways (bronchioli) are distal to the last plate of cartilage. Clusters of three to five terminal bronchioli with their associated acini are grouped into lobules. In fully developed lungs the acinar regions feature respiratory bronchioli, alveolar ducts, and alveoli, whereas the immature lung contains saccules that originate from respiratory bronchioli. Saccules and alveoli are distinguished as narrow-walled structures with a characteristic epithelium containing both thin cells (type I) with few subcellular organelles and larger pneumonocytes (type II) with abundant mitochondria, endoplasmic reticulum, Golgi apparatus, and osmiophilic lamellar bodies known to contain surfactant.

The pulmonary vasculature is an essential component of a functional lung that allows gas exchange to take place efficiently. The mature lung has a dual arterial supply and dual venous drainage system. Branches of the pulmonary arteries supply the terminal respiratory units and most of the pleura, and bronchial arteries originating from the aorta supply the airway walls and hilar regions of the lung, including pleural surfaces and the walls of large blood vessels emerging from the mediastinum. The systemic circulation via the bronchial arteries has relatively low flow compared with the pulmonary artery circuit and only accounts for 10% or less of the total pulmonary blood flow. Equally insignificant from a quantitative viewpoint are the bronchial veins that drain from the hila to the azygos or systemic vessels; most of the venous return from the lung occurs via the pulmonary veins.

Development and growth of the airways, pulmonary vasculature, and acinar region

The cardinal features of lung maturation are presented in Fig. 28-1, together with a list of important temporally related events in fetal development. Differentiation of the respiratory system can be conveniently divided into five phases: (1) the embryonic phase, comprising the first 5 weeks after conception and leading to initiation of airways formation; (2) the glandular or pseudoglandular stage from 5 to 16 weeks of gestation, during which time the lower conducting airways are formed; (3) the canalicular phase, which begins at the seventeenth week with the "birth of the acinus" and concludes at 24 to 26 weeks of gestation; (4) the terminal sac period, during which time the first respiratory units are formed; and (5) the alveolar phase, which is initiated in the perinatal period and continues until approximately 8 years of age.

The respiratory system first appears after 3½ to 4 weeks of gestation as an outgrowth of the foregut. The lung bud then divides into two components to form the main stem bronchi, which subsequently branch within the enclosing mesenchyme to form the gas-conducting portion of the lung by the end of the sixteenth week after conception. Although the early stages of intrauterine lung development are defined primarily by changes in appearance of the airways, marked changes also occur in the vascular component of the lung (Fig. 28-1).

The overall pattern of formation of the respiratory system can be summarized by Reid's laws of lung development, a modified version of which follows:

1. The bronchial tree is developed by the sixteenth week of intrauterine life. Differentiation of the airways and the progressively increasing formation of cartilage occur in a centrifugal manner, that is, from hilum to periphery.
2. The preacinar blood vessels follow the development of the airways, whereas the intraacinar arteries and veins develop parallel with the alveoli. Although the main pulmonary veins develop later than do the arteries, the adult pattern of vessels connecting heart with lungs, as well as the ductus arteriosus, is formed by the seventh week of gestation, whereas the preacinar arterial branching takes place alongside the dividing airways, and the developing veins are enveloped by mesenchyme. From 7 to 16 weeks after conception, the main feature of arterial growth is an increase in number of branches. By the sixteenth week virtually all preacinar vessels are present. Thereafter the existing vessels grow in size and length, while new vessels appear in the intraacinar region.

   The canalicular phase of lung development (after the seventeenth week) is characterized by slow invasion of the developing acinus by capillaries. This vascularization process occurs in a centripetal fashion, with the last phase being an extension to the respiratory bronchioles. During fetal life the diameter of blood vessels increases more rapidly at the proximal end than in the distal portions; this is in contrast to the similar rate of growth along an axial pathway following birth. In the fetus the arteries are more muscular than in the adult (wall thickness being higher relative to external diameter). In contrast, the walls of fetal veins have less muscle than those in the adult.
3. Alveoli develop mainly after birth, increasing in number from 20 million in the newborn to approximately 300 million at 8 years of age. There is marked expansion of the acinus after birth. For instance, by 2 months of age the length of the acinus has nearly doubled its neonatal size. A striking observation is that the alveoli develop in a centripetal direction, first on the saccules and their derivatives (the alveolar ducts), then on the respiratory bronchioles. In later childhood alveoli will develop on terminal bronchioles. The size of the alveoli continues to increase until growth of the chest wall ceases with attainment of adult thoracic size.

Cytodifferentiation of the respiratory epithelium

The lung is an extremely complex and heterogeneous organ, containing approximately 40 different cell types. Fortunately the distal respiratory epithelium responsible for gas exchange is more simplified and features mainly two distinct cells in the mature human lung. The ultra-

Gestational Age (weeks)	Pulmonary Morphology	Concurrent Changes	Associated Clinical Disorders
3-4	**Lung Bud** **First Division** 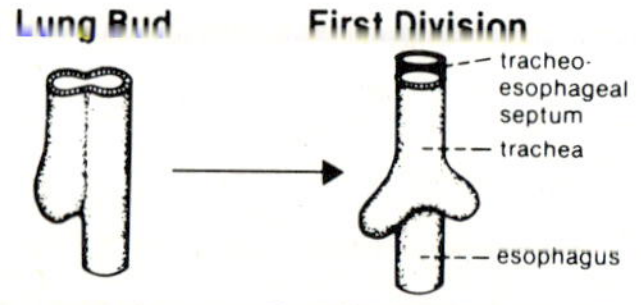 First division airway branching. Lung bud appears from foregut endoderm. Separation of trachea & esophagus.	Beginning of cardiac chamber definition. Sixth aortic arch gives off branches to lung buds and will form the pulmonary arteries. Mesonephric tubules appear signaling early renal formation. Neural tube closes.	Pulmonary agenesis. Bronchial malformations (isomerism syndromes). Tracheoesophageal fistula. VATER complex. Vascular ring. Renal agenesis with lung hypoplasia (Potter's syndrome).
5-6	**Beginning of Pseudoglandular Period** 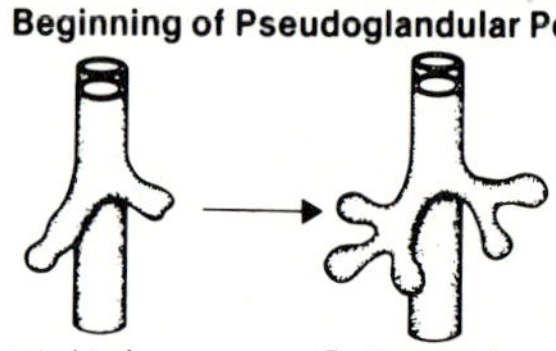 Elongated to form mainstem bronchi. Further division to form lobar bronchi.	Formation of aorta and pulmonary arteries. Pharyngeal pouches yield parathyroid glands and thymus. Mesonephros enlarges and contributes to development of the adrenal cortex, along with coelomic epithelium. Primordium of spleen appears.	
7	**Further Airway Divisions** 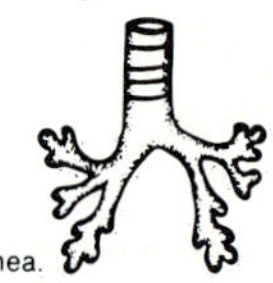 Cartilage present in trachea. Segmental bronchi have formed and subsegmental branches are first appearing.	Branching of pulmonary vasculature parallels the development of the airways. Formation of nasal passage-ways.	Choanal atresia. Tracheomalacia. Bronchial malformations (usually additive). Bronchomalacia. Ectopic lobes. Congenital pulmonary cysts.
8-10	**Closure of Pleuroperitoneal Canals** 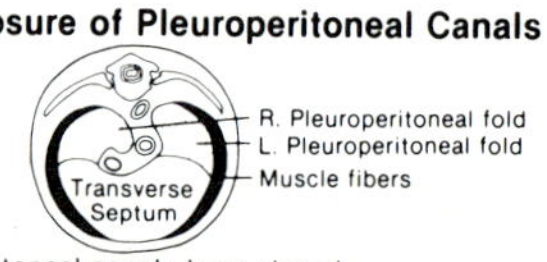 Pleuroperitoneal canals have closed. Branching of airways continues within the enclosing mesenchyme. Distal extension of airway cartilage.	Pulmonary lymphatics appear. Histiogenesis of thyroid is complete. Gut migrates back into abdomen.	Diaphragmatic hernia (with ipsilateral lung hypoplasia). Congenital eventration or accessory diaphragm. Congenital pulmonary lymphangiectasia. Omphalocoele (may restrict the thorax)

Fig. 28-1. Major structural features of lung maturation, concurrent events in morphogenesis, and temporally associated malformations of the respiratory tract. Gestational ages listed refer to weeks of *postconceptional* development, that is, fetal age is dated from the time of ovulation (assumed to be 2 weeks after the beginning of the last menstrual period), as opposed to clinical gestational age, calculated from the first day of the last menstrual period. (From Perelman, R., Engle, M.J., and Farrell, P.: Lung **159:**53, 1981.)

structural features of the cytodifferentiation of the respiratory epithelium have been described for many mammals. In lower animal species, which have been studied in greatest detail, a characteristic sequence of changes has been identified. The same cellular phases of lung development also are present in the human fetus.

In early gestation the epithelial cells are simple and columnar in type and show few signs of organelle differentiation. Specific cell types are not recognizable until the canalicular stage of development. Subsequently, before surfactant is present, large quantities of glycogen accumulate within the respiratory epithelium. Finally during the last 10% to 20% of gestation in most species certain lining cells of the terminal respiratory units undergo alterations, permitting them to be distinguished as type II pneumonocytes. Although type II pneumonocytes have been identified in the human fetus between 22 and 26 weeks of gestation, these cells become more prominent at 34 to 36 weeks of gestation. The major change allowing these cells to be readily identified is the appearance of osmiophilic lamellar bodies in the cytoplasm (Figs. 28-1 and 28-8). There is a very close correlation between the presence of these lamellar inclusions and the appearance of surface-active material in lung extracts.

In addition to the lamellar bodies, other features of the type II pneumonocytes allow them to be distinguished from type I cells of the respiratory epithelium. For instance, type II pneumonocytes have abundant mitochondria, endoplasmic reticulum, polyribosomes, and

Gestational Age (weeks)	Pulmonary Morphology	Concurrent Changes	Associated Clinical Disorders
16	**Beginning of Canalicular Period** **Conducting Airways** **Pulmonary Acinus** 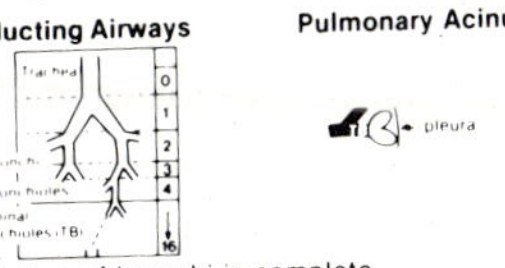 Segmentation of bronchi is complete. Early formation of pulmonary acinus. Ciliated columnar epithelium lines the airways.	Formation of preacinar blood vessels is complete. Kidney is anatomically formed. CNS myelinization begins. Intrauterine movement is present.	Lung hypoplasia.
20	**Pulmonary Vascularization** 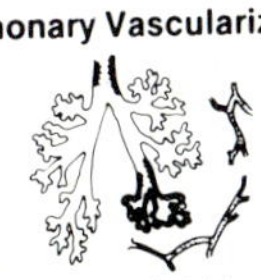 Canalized airways lined by cuboidal epithelium. Decrease in mesenchyme. Capillaries penetrate early saccules.	Fetal "breathing" present. Pancreatic exocrine and endocrine function has been initiated. Thyroxin secretion.	Lung hypoplasia.
26	**Beginning of Terminal Sac Period** 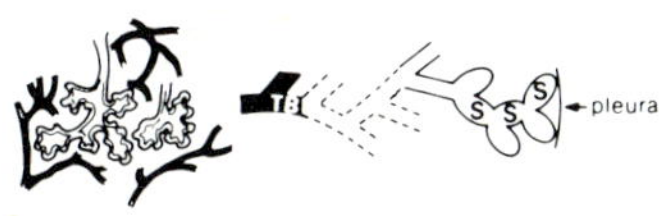 Respiratory saccules (S) appear from transitional ducts. Epithelium attenuates forming septae.	Eyelids unfused. Testes descending.	Respiratory insufficiency.
32-36	**Type II Pneumonocytes** 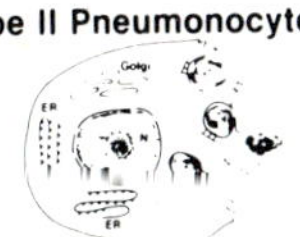 Increased number of type II pneumonocytes with lamellar bodies. Abundant fetal pulmonary fluid present in potential airspaces.	Surfactant may be present but is often deficient. Increased adrenocorticoids. Accumulation of subcutaneous adipose tissue begins. Auricular cartilage present.	Hyaline membrane disease. Transient tachypnea. Apnea of prematurity.
Infancy to 8 Years	**Continuing Alveolar Proliferation** 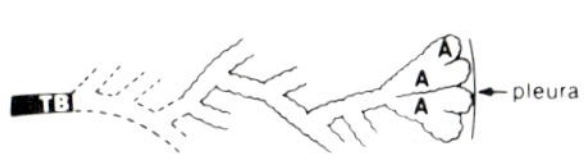 Alveoli (A) form and increase in both size and number (from 20 × 10^6 to 300 × 10^6 alveoli per lung).	Growth of the lungs approximates linear growth. Continued maturation of central ventilatory control mechanisms.	Cystic fibrosis. Lobar emphysema. Pectus excavatum.

Fig. 28-1, cont'd. For legend see p. 560.

Golgi apparatus, suggesting the capability for a high rate of metabolic activity. Indeed histochemical and ultrastructural autoradiographic techniques have confirmed the role of the type II pneumonocyte in the synthesis, storage, and secretion of pulmonary surfactant. These studies also have indicated that the osmiophilic lamellar bodies are the intracellular deposits of surfactant. In essence they may be viewed as secretory granules of unique morphology and composition. The synthesis of surfactant phospholipid has been traced by sequential electron microscopic analysis after administration of a radioisotopic precursor (usually, ^{3}H-choline, which labels phosphatidylcholine almost exclusively). Such studies revealed a sequence typical for exocrine cells: rapid uptake of precursor from capillaries, transfer to endoplasmic reticulum, synthesis of phospholipids, transfer via the Golgi apparatus and perhaps transfer of special proteins to the osmiophilic lamellar bodies for "packaging," and then secretion into the alveolar space.

Although more ultrastructural morphometric analysis of the developing lung is needed, it has been estimated that type II pneumonocytes normally account for no more than 15% of the lung acinar cell population. Despite being similar in number, type I pneumonocytes cover the major part of the alveolus by virtue of their larger size and the long cytoplasmic extensions characteristic of these cells. Because of their thin nature and proximity to capillary endothelial cells, type I pneumonocytes are ideally suited to assist in the transfer of oxygen and carbon dioxide. Therefore gas exchange occurs primarily across that portion of the respiratory epithelium comprised of type I pneumonocytes.

Clinical correlation

The intrauterine timing of pulmonary anomalies can be appreciated from the foregoing review of the sequence of changes taking place during development of the respiratory system. Fig. 28-1 lists several malformations and gives an indication of the approximate time in gestation when the abnormality originates. It is evident, for instance, that *all* malformations of the conducting airways must take place before 16 weeks of gestation. Thus upper airway abnormalities take place between conception and 5 weeks of gestation. Bronchial malformations, which are usually additive and lead to duplicated airways, occur between 5 and 16 weeks, whereas lung hypoplasia, characterized by inadequate development of pulmonary acini, would be evident after 16 weeks.

Knowledge about the process of fetal lung development also provides insights into the age at which the respiratory system is capable of supporting satisfactory gas exchange. Given the present limits of our clinical technology, fetal viability may be first expected at 24 to 26 weeks of gestation. This is when the respiratory saccules have developed, and adequate vascularization by capillary invasion has taken place. Before this time some exchange of oxygen or carbon dioxide may take place, but generally inadequate surface area exists to support continued respiration.

THE PHYSIOLOGY OF PULMONARY SURFACTANT

Role of surfactant in respiratory mechanics

Because of the rapid development of high surface forces along the respiratory epithelium when breathing is first initiated, the availability of adequate quantities of pulmonary surfactant in terminal air spaces is of paramount importance in successful postnatal lung function. Surface forces have interested physiologists since 1929, when von Neergaard noted their effect on the pressure-volume characteristics of liquid- and air-filled lungs. From these early experiments it was theorized that the retractive tendency of air-filled lungs was not only a result of tissue elastic recoil but also of surface forces operating at the gas-liquid interface of the respiratory system. This work and subsequent investigations have defined the contribution of surface factors to the overall collapsing tendency of the lung. Of great interest is the finding that surface tension accounts for approximately two thirds of the total retractive force of the air-inflated lung. The magnitude of surface forces therefore may be viewed as a major obstacle to the neonatal lung. The early research on pressure-volume relationships also established the phenomenon of *hysteresis*, or separation of

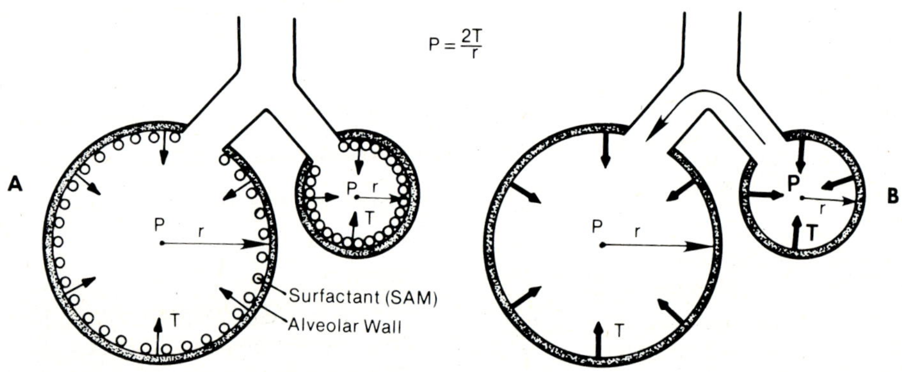

Fig. 28-2. Relationship of Laplace's law to alveolar stability in the normal and surfactant-deficient lung. Although schematically represented as spherical, terminal respiratory units tend to be polygonal in the mature lung. Laplace's law states that the pressure *(P)* within a sphere is directly proportional to surface tension *(T)* and inversely proportional to the radius of curvature *(r)*. **A,** Normal lung. As alveolar size diminishes, surface tension is reduced in the presence of SAM, thereby decreasing the collapsing pressure to be opposed. The pressure within the small and large interconnected alveoli is equal, negating the tendency for transfer of gas. **B,** Surfactant-deficient lung. Without the surface tension–lowering capacity of SAM, alveoli become unstable at low volume and tend to collapse. Some alveoli may empty into large ones to equalize pressure between the two in accordance with Boyle's law. (Modified from an original painting by Frank H. Netter, M.D., from THE CIBA COLLECTION OF MEDICAL ILLUSTRATIONS, copyright by CIBA Pharmaceutical Co., Division of CIBA-GEIGY Corporation.)

inflation and deflation curves on expansion with air but not with liquid. Contrary to expectations based on Laplace's law, experimental observations suggested that the collapsing forces of the lung normally decrease as the alveolar diameter is reduced via deflation or simulated expiration (Fig. 28-2).

Although the studies of von Neergaard led to the prediction of a surface tension–lowering substance in the alveoli, several decades passed (Table 28-1) before other investigators conclusively demonstrated surface-active material, that is, surfactant, in pulmonary fluid (edema foam) and lung extracts. In the key experiments performed with a modified Wilhelmy surface balance it was observed that, when surface films derived from lung extracts were compressed, the surface tension decreased to very low levels and then rose rapidly on expansion. In addition, surface tension tracings during cyclic expansion and compression of the films were widely separated, thus duplicating the hysteresis loop of the intact lung.

Considered collectively, research advances have evolved a biophysical view of pulmonary surfactant as an antiatelectasis factor located in the "alveolar lining layer" that provides a low and variable surface tension and imparts hysteresis to the air-tissue interface. Surface-active material, then, is capable of performing the twofold function of (1) decreasing the pressure required to distend the lung and (2) maintaining alveolar stability over a wide range of local volumes. These functions and the importance of surfactant can be better appreciated by further discussion of relevant experimental techniques and observations.

Laboratory assessment of surfactant

In the laboratory setting pressure-volume and surface balance experiments allow physiologic assessment of surface-active material, lung stability, and distensibility, or compliance, and thus an evaluation of maturity. In its simplest form, a surface balance consists of a Teflon trough, a movable barrier, and a platinum plate (Fig. 28-3). After a surface film is layered over a line in the trough, the barrier is cycled to expand and compress the film. The surface tension is measured from the force exerted on the platinum plate, provided the angle of contact between the plate and liquid approximates zero. As shown in Fig. 28-3, pressure-volume relationships for whole lungs or isolated lung lobes are studied in a closed system by instilling air or saline from a reservoir into the respiratory system under pressure produced by raising a fluid-filled buret. After stabilization at a maximum pressure (usually 30 or 35 cm H_2O), the buret is lowered in a stepwise fashion to empty the lung. At points of no gas flow, relating the change in pressure to change in volume (slope of the P/V curve) yields an estimate of distensibility or static compliance ($\Delta V/\Delta P = C$). As represented in Fig. 28-4, saline-filled lungs establish maximum volume at considerably lower inflation pressures than do air-filled lungs. In the absence of a gas-liquid interface the effects of surface force are eliminated, resulting in a greater tendency to collapse on deflation and much less hysteresis. Retention of volume on deflation to zero pressure in the air-filled, mature lung is an expression of intrinsic alveolar stability. Immature lungs require considerably higher pressures to initiate air filling (opening pressure), have a lower volume at any pressure, and have little or no residual volume on deflation. Therefore maturation of the lung is associated with an increased peak volume as well as an improved capacity to retain air on deflation, that is, deflation stability.

Appearance of surfactant and importance in the perinatal period

Although some evidence suggests surfactant may appear in the human lung as early as 24 weeks of gestation,

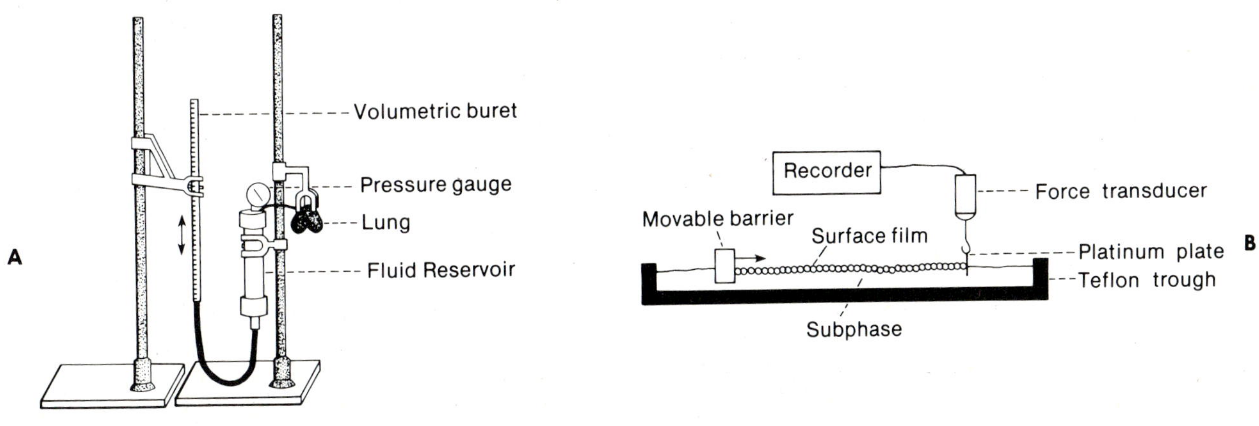

Fig. 28-3. Schematic representation of a pressure-volume apparatus **(A)** and surface balance **(B),** the operation of which is discussed in text.

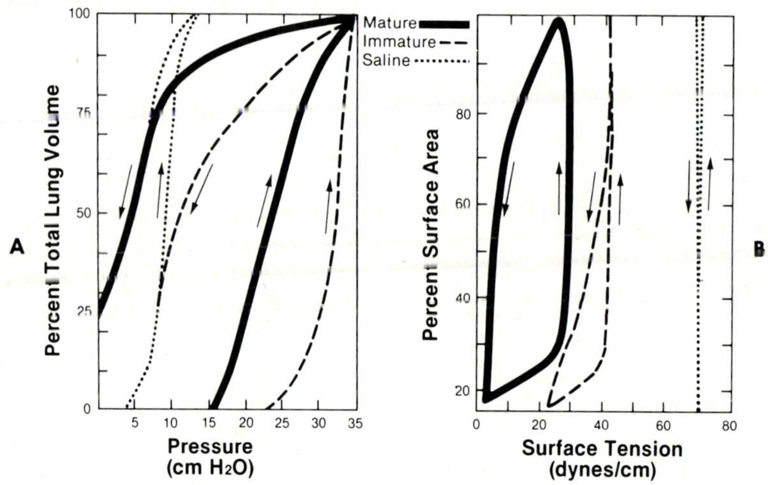

Fig. 28-4. Contrast between mature and surfactant-deficient (immature) fetal lungs as studied with the pressure-volume apparatus **(A)** and surface balance **(B)**. **A,** Representative pressure-volume curves for air-filled mature lungs *(solid line)* and for air-filled surfactant-deficient lungs *(dashed line)*. Note that the mature lung shows lower opening pressure, relative stability of deflation, and maintenance of residual volume. The pressure-volume curve generated by saline filling of the mature lung *(dotted line)* is also shown and emphasizes the lack of surface forces when no air-liquid interface is present. It is further evident that less pressure is required for complete filling with saline than air and that there is less hysteresis between the inflation and deflation portions of the curve. **B,** Representative tracings resulting from cyclical compression and expansion of extracts from a mature lung *(solid line)* and an immature lung *(dashed line)*. The dotted line represents a saline reference tracing. In contrast to the immature lung, mature lung extracts achieve a low surface tension value (<10 dynes/cm) at maximal compression, that is, minimal surface area. (Modified from Kotas, R.V., and others: J. Appl. Physiol. **43:**92, 1977.)

functional surfactant is generally evident in developing mammalian lungs at 80% to 90% of gestation. When surfactant is present, it is noteworthy that deflation stability indicated by $\%V_{10}$ is maximized (Fig. 28-5). These pulmonary maturational events during late gestation portend a successful transition from maternal/placental–dependent gas exchange to extrauterine ventilation.

With the onset of postnatal breathing considerable force is required to overcome the high viscosity and inertia of the fetal pulmonary fluid that fills the potential air spaces at birth. The high pressures generated in the first few breaths not only are required for expansion but are also quite important in moving lung liquid and establishing an air-liquid interface. As air enters the lung and the size of the airways diminishes in the periphery, the surface tension at the junction between lung fluid and air increases. The clearance of fluid from smaller airways may be more efficient in the presence of adequate surfactant. Since the shape of the meniscus at the air-liquid interface depends on the surface tension of liquid molecules at the surface, pulmonary surfactant enhances lung fluid movement by increasing the area of the air-liquid interface over which pressure can be exerted. Therefore, if sufficient surface-active material is present, less effort is required to replace each unit of lung fluid with air.

Once the mature lung has been expanded, the surfactant film lining the alveoli and terminal bronchioles tends to increase surface tension at high lung volumes, promoting emptying, and lower it at diminished lung volume (Fig. 28-2). Lowering surface tension as the size of terminal air spaces decreases prevents collapse at end expiration. The remaining volume of gas, termed *functional residual capacity* (FRC), acts as a reservoir that prevents wide fluctuations in blood oxygen and carbon dioxide levels during respiration. Furthermore a partially expanded air space, that is, the lung at FRC, requires less effort to reexpand than one that is completely collapsed.

Neonatal surfactant deficiency

The physiologic consequences of surfactant deficiency are manifested clinically in the premature neonate as RDS. The classic association of tachypnea, grunting, retractions, hypoxemia, and characteristic chest roentgenogram for the most part can be related to the changes in surface properties of the thin layer of liquid lining the air spaces. As discussed previously, in air spaces devoid

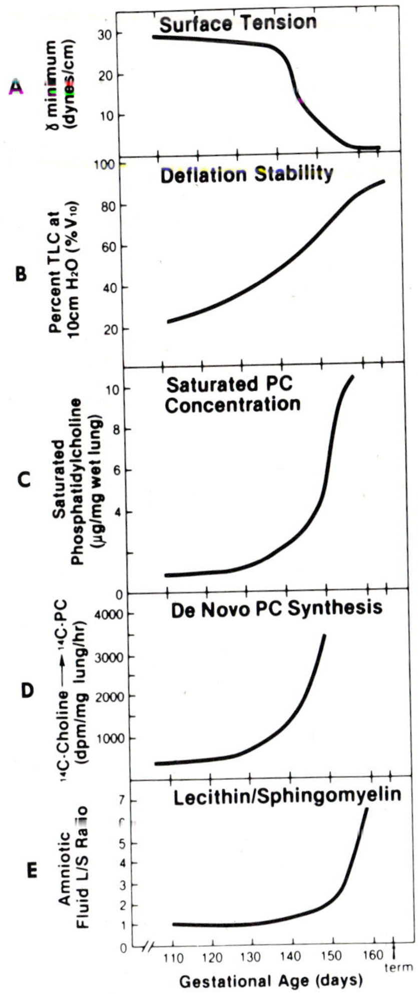

Fig. 28-5. Representative curves depicting the correlation between biochemical and physiologic events during fetal lung maturation in the rhesus monkey. **A,** Surface tension. **B,** Deflation stability. **C,** Saturated PC concentration. **D,** De novo PC synthesis. **E,** Lecithin/sphingomyelin. (Modified from Kotas, R.V., and others: J. Appl. Physiol. **43:**92, 1977.)

of surfactant, surface forces (and therefore pressure) rise rapidly on deflation, leading to instability, further loss of volume, and consequently atelectasis. The reduced volume at end expiration not only negates the buffering capacity afforded by a normal FRC but also requires the generation of high pressures to reexpand the lung with each breath. Large pressure changes coupled with the very compliant thorax of the premature neonate result in retractions. With the stresses of increased oxygen consumption and the work of breathing, metabolic demands are markedly augmented. Because of immaturity and minimum substrate reserves, the prematurely delivered infant with RDS is ill equipped to meet these demands.

Clinical observations have revealed that grunting, a common finding in RDS, improves oxygenation. It has been suggested that the consequences of the grunt are to prolong end expiration, maintain the surfactant-deficient lung at slightly larger volumes, and afford increased time for gas exchange to take place. The clinical application of continuous positive airway pressure (CPAP) was theorized to serve the same physiologic function as the grunt.

The use of positive end-expiratory pressure (PEEP) may have an effect over and above the mechanical one leading to improved gas exchange. This additional role, termed *conservation* of pulmonary surfactant, has stimulated research concerning the influence of current modes of therapy for RDS on surfactant turnover. Investigations have shown that increased ventilation can affect pulmonary surfactant and pressure-volume characteristics. Reduced compliance observed in hyperventilated lungs has been attributed to a decrease in surfactant and corroborated by reduced surface tension–lowering capacity of lung extracts. It has been suggested that ventilation enhances the movement of surfactant from alveoli into the airways, and PEEP hinders this phenomenon. According to this hypothesis the degree and rate of spread of surface-active material would depend on the volume of the alveoli at end expiration. The smaller the alveolus, the greater the flux. Other studies involving injection of various radioactive phospholipid precursors suggest that hyperventilation promotes release—then inactivation of surface-active material—and that end-expiratory pressure, by preventing surface film collapse, negates these adverse effects.

Neurohumoral regulation of surfactant secretion

Evidence accumulated in recent years from multidisciplinary studies supports the concept that the autonomic nervous system or its mediators may influence pulmonary surfactant by regulating the rate of secretion or possibly by controlling in part the turnover of surface-active phospholipids. These studies have used pharmacophysiologic approaches applied primarily to mechanically hyperventilated animals. As mentioned previously, the hyperventilation model is advantageous because this system features increased release of surfactant into the air spaces. Of great interest is the observation that β-adrenergic antagonists (e.g., propranolol) can prevent this respose to increased ventilation. In addition, β_2 agonists terbutaline and isoxsuprine, which are both used clinically for suppression of premature labor, have been shown to stimulate a significant increase in the amount of phospholipid recovered from lung lavages; this effect can be blocked by prior administration of propranolol. These observations suggest that adrenergic mechanisms can control surfactant concentrations in the terminal air spaces. Since other studies have demonstrated that α-adrenergic agents do not affect lung surfactant, it may be concluded that the β-adrenergic receptors are specifically involved in regulating pulmonary phospholipid metabolism.

Cholinergically mediated regulation also has been suspected for many years, ever since studies revealed evidence of decreased surfactant in lungs from vagotomized animals. Subsequent observations in such animals have demonstrated decreased numbers of lamellar bodies ("secretory granules") in type II alveolar pneumonocytes and the presence of generalized atelectasis. Administration of relatively large amounts of acetylcholine and electrical stimulation of the vagus nerve will result in changes implying augmented secretion of pulmonary surfactant. Prior treatment with atropine eliminated increased surfactant secretions and thus confirmed involvement of cholinergic stimulation, but the physiologic significance of this remains uncertain.

Thus β-adrenergic receptors, cholinergic receptors, and (based on other more preliminary data) certain prostaglandins are potential regulators of surfactant turnover. Whether these alter surfactant metabolism during hyperventilation by increasing secretion or by slowing degradation remains unclear. The more precise delineation of the effect of the aforementioned mediators on surfactant kinetics offers an important challenge to the understanding of pulmonary phospholipid metabolism.

THE BIOCHEMISTRY OF PULMONARY SURFACTANT

Chemical composition

Because phospholipids are ideally suited as surface-active agents in interfacial films, the biophysical behavior of pulmonary surfactant provided an early clue to its composition. Studies initiated shortly after the rediscovery of surfactant indicated that the liquid obtained by lung lavage was largely composed of lipid, particularly phospholipid, with smaller amounts of protein. Accordingly, pulmonary surfactant has been defined by Farrell and Avery as "a unique lipoprotein, particularly rich in highly saturated lecithins (saturated phosphatidylcholine molecules) and containing lesser amounts of cholesterol, neutral lipid, and other phospholipids." The predominance of phosphatidylcholine is evident from the data presented in Fig. 28-6, which also illustrates the percentage of contribution from other lipids. The uniqueness of phosphatidylcholine in the respiratory system stems from its fatty acid substructure. Unlike most tissues that exhibit phosphatidylcholine molecules having a saturated fatty acid at the 1-carbon position and an unsaturated fatty acyl constituent at the 2-carbon position, lung parenchyma and bronchoalveolar fluid contain a high proportion of disaturated phosphatidylcholine. In fact, from analysis of extensively purified surfactant fraction, results have been obtained indicating that approximately 60% of the total lipid is 1,2-dipalmitoyl-phosphatidylcholine; the structure of this compound is shown in Fig. 28-6. The highly saturated nature of lung phosphatidylcholine molecules appears to be essential in relation to the surface tension–lowering capability of the alveolar lining layer.

A second phospholipid marker of surfactant, also structurally depicted in Fig. 28-6, is phosphatidylglycerol. After a period of controversy concerning its identity, this special constituent has only recently been identified unequivocally in preparations of lung tissue. In essence this

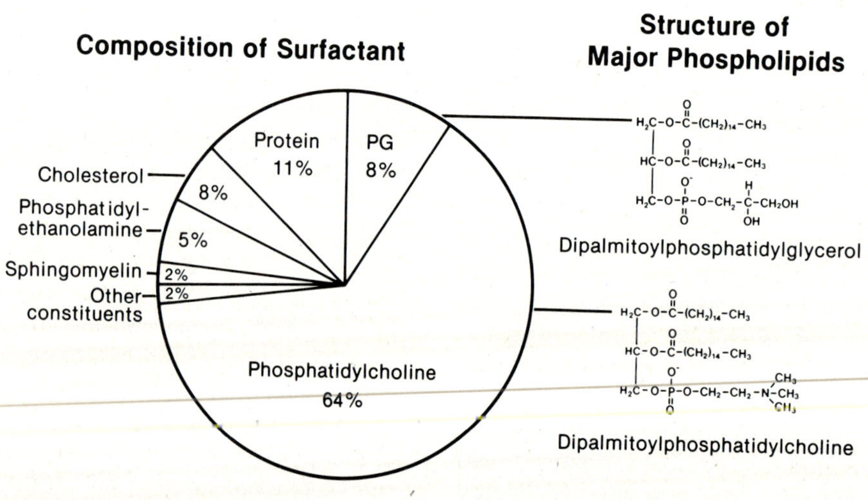

Fig. 28-6. Composition of surface-active material, obtained by lung lavage, and the structure of major phospholipids present in pulmonary surfactant. (From Perelman, R., Engle, M.J., and Farrell, P.: Lung **159:**53, 1981.)

compound was originally misidentified by some investigators as phosphatidyl-*N*,*N*-dimethylethanolamine, or PDME; concurrently, other investigators reported the presence of phosphatidylglycerol and the absence of significant phosphatidyl-*N*,*N*-dimethylethanolamine. The fallacious recognition of phosphatidyl-*N*,*N*-dimethylethanolamine on thin-layer chromatograms promoted an unfortunate misunderstanding of pathways for phosphatidylcholine biosynthesis. Not until recent years has this issue been resolved and the following points established: (1) phosphatidylglycerol is present in whole lung tissue, where it accounts for approximately 3% of the total phospholipid; (2) phosphatidylglycerol is enriched in bronchoalveolar fluid and accounts for approximately 8% of the total phospholipid; (3) phosphatidylglycerol, like saturated phosphatidylcholine, is actively synthesized in the lung and appears to undergo relatively rapid turnover; and (4) the fatty acid composition of phosphatidylglycerol is also similar to that of phosphatidylcholine in that it contains highly saturated constituents.

The proteins present in pulmonary surfactant are also unique. Although there may be as many as 20 different nonserum proteins associated with surfactant material, two proteins in particular seem to be essential components of the surface-active material and function as the matrix for phospholipid molecules. Apoproteins are detectable in human amniotic fluid by 26 weeks gestation with concentrations increasing in parallel with rising surfactant phospholipids by sixfold to tenfold at term.

Mechanisms for production of phosphatidylcholine

Two pathways exist for the de novo synthesis of phosphatidylcholine. The first of these is the choline-incorporation mechanism or cytidine diphosphocholine pathway. As shown in Fig. 28-7, this is a three-reaction metabolic sequence, involving phosphorylation of choline, activation by conversion of choline phosphate to the cytidine diphosphate *(CDP)* derivative, and final transfer of the phosphorylcholine portion of the activated compound to diglyceride, yielding phosphatidylcholine. It is actually the cooperative interaction of these three reactions and the biochemical processes leading to phosphatidic acid formation and hydrolysis that finally produces phosphatidylcholine. In the second de novo mechanism, termed the *methylation pathway*, ethanolamine undergoes similar steps of phosphorylation, activation, and linkage to diglyceride to form phosphatidylethanolamine, which then undergoes three successive methylations to produce phosphatidylcholine. It had been proposed at one time that phosphatidylethanolamine methylation was a major pathway in the fetal primate lung before term gestation. This conclusion was based on misidentification of phosphatidyl-*N*,*N*-dimethylethanolamine, several unwarranted assumptions, and erroneous interpretation of indirect evidence. Subsequently from studies using direct biochemical techniques it has been determined conclusively that the cytidine diphosphocholine pathway is the primary mechanism for biosynthesis of phosphatidylcholine in the developing mammalian lung. The evidence for this conclusion is reviewed in detail by Farrell and Hamosh.

The mechanism by which saturated phosphatidylcholine molecules are specifically formed in the mature lung has stimulated great interest in recent years. The consensus at present, based on a variety of experimental observations, is that the cytidine diphosphocholine pathway despite its predominance does not yield saturated phospholipids, but rather mixed molecules with respect to fatty acid composition. This has led to the current view that the phosphatidylcholine-lysophosphatidylcholine cycle, shown in Fig. 28-7, *F*, is the mechanism operating to control the fatty acid substructure of the final product. Thus there is evidence suggesting that either deacylation-reacylation or deacylation-transacylation reactions are important in the formation of saturated phosphatidylcholine. This question, however, has not been fully resolved. Other possibilities such as a specific transfer protein leading to enrichment of surfactant in saturated phospholipid require further study.

Appearance of increased phosphatidylcholine in the fetal lung

As shown in Fig. 28-5, fetal lung development is characterized by major biochemical changes during late gestation. Most of the studies of phospholipid concentrations and their rates of synthesis have been conducted in either lower animal species or nonhuman primates such as the rhesus monkey. This work has revealed a considerable degree of uniformity in regard to the period of gestation when biochemical changes take place. Irrespective of the total duration of a species' pregnancy, it has been found that augmented lung phosphatidylcholine production is characteristically demonstrable at 85% to 90% of gestation. For instance, in rhesus monkey fetuses increased saturated phosphatidylcholine concentration takes place at approximately 145 to 150 days of the 168-day intrauterine period; this would correspond to 34 weeks of human gestation. At this time or shortly thereafter phosphatidylcholine concentrations in amniotic fluid rise, indicating to the clinician the attainment of fetal lung maturity. As further illustrated in Fig. 28-5, there is a very close correlation between the biochemical changes and their physiologic counterparts. Therefore one can logically assume that the fetal lung is endowed with special regulatory mechanisms operating to control the timing of the biochemical maturation process. This ensures accumulation of a reservoir of phosphatidylcholine before

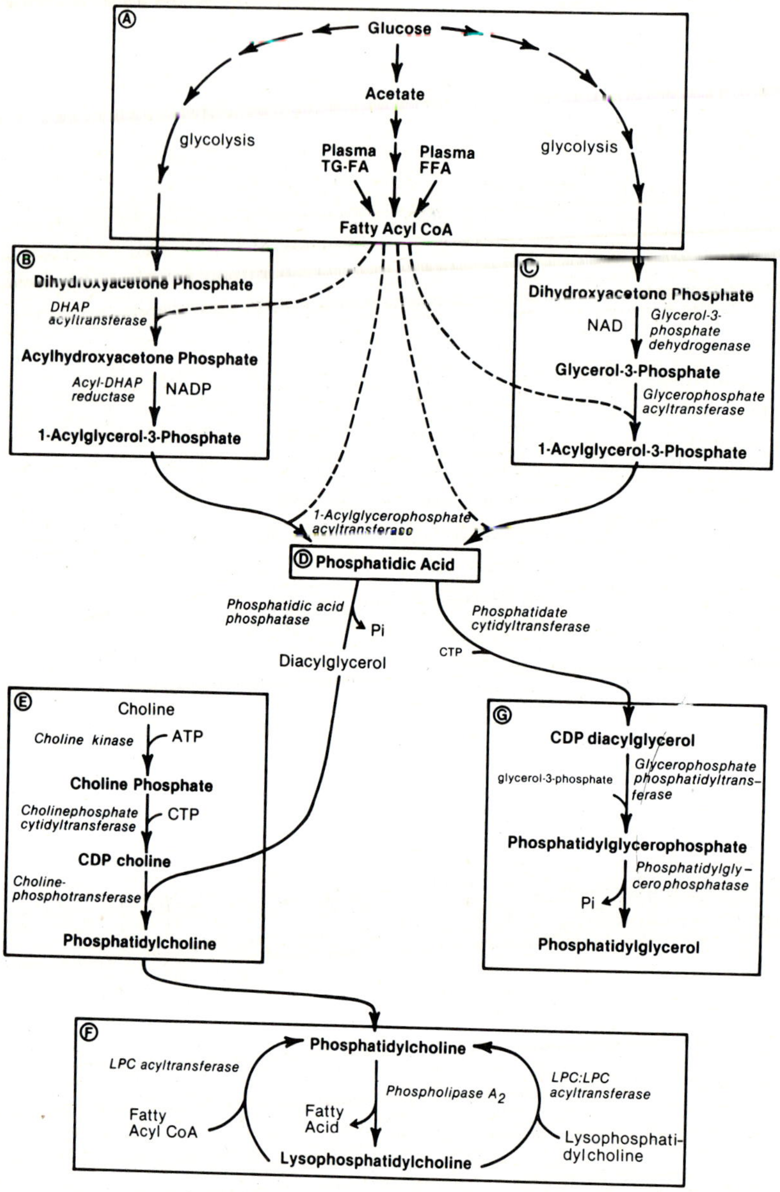

Fig. 28-7. Pathways of phosphatidylcholine and phosphatidylglycerol biosynthesis. *TG-FA,* Triglyceride fatty acids; *FFA,* free fatty acids; *DHAP,* dihydroxyacetone phosphate; *LPC,* lysophosphatidylcholine. (From Perelman, R., Engle, M.J., and Farrell, P.: Lung **159:**53, 1981.)

delivery. Once this increased concentration of phosphatidylcholine is present, increased phosphatidylcholine also is seen in both lung and amniotic fluid, providing further evidence of fetal lung maturity.

Regulation of phosphatidylcholine synthesis

The major emphasis of present research deals with regulatory mechanisms for phosphatidylcholine synthesis and study of pharmacologic agents that accelerate the process of fetal lung development. Fig. 28-8 presents schematically some of the factors of potential importance in controlling the turnover of surfactant phospholipid. These factors include exogenous precursors, key enzymes, and certain hormones.

Substrates

Because an abundance of precursor substrate must be supplied for phosphatidylcholine biosynthesis, the circulatory system is essential in supporting lung metabolism. Furthermore nutrients from the placenta during gestation and from the diet after birth potentially could play an important role in facilitating surfactant produc-

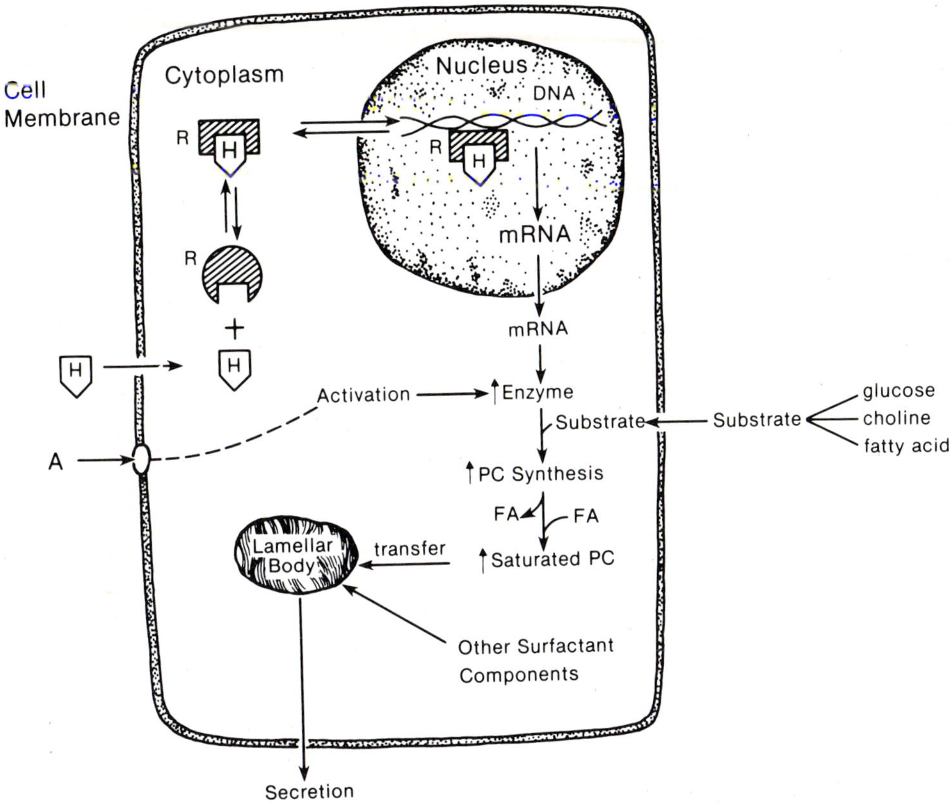

Fig. 28-8. Hypothetic scheme of the production and delivery of surfactant to the "alveolar lining layer" by a type II pneumonocyte. Various potential regulatory steps illustrate hormone-mediated control mechanisms, regulation by substrates, and the key role of enzymes in phospholipid production. *A,* Activator; *H,* hormone, particularly corticosteroid; *R,* receptor; *FA,* fatty acid; *DNA,* deoxyribonucleic acid molecule stimulated by hormone to increased "expression"; *mRNA,* messenger ribonucleic acid molecules coding for increased synthesis of specific enzymes. (Reprinted from Ballard, P.L. In Hodson, W.A., editor: Development of the lung, New York, 1977, Marcel Dekker, Inc. By courtesy of Marcel Dekker, Inc.)

tion. Substances of special interest in this regard are glucose, fatty acids, and choline. Endogenous glucose stored as glycogen in the type II pneumonocyte can contribute to the surge in phosphatidylcholine synthesis during late gestation according to several studies performed with cultured fetal lung. After birth, neither glycogen nor exogenous choline seem to have a regulatory influence on lung lipid synthesis, but glucose continues to be an important precursor. Stored triglycerides and exogenous fatty acids may also contribute fatty acyl substrates.

Enzymes

The rate of product formation in various metabolic pathways often is governed by key enzymes. From biochemical studies of the past two decades there is evidence that phosphatidylcholine biosynthesis might be regulated by some of the enzymes shown in Fig. 28-7. In particular, data have been obtained suggesting that phosphatidic acid phosphatase, choline kinase, cholinephosphate cytidyltransferase, and cholinephosphotransferase all might play a role in elevating fetal lung phosphatidylcholine levels in late gestation. The influence of enzymes on overall pathway rates may be exerted by either adjustments in enzyme concentration or by direct modulation of enzyme activity through altered kinetic properties. Increases in enzyme concentrations often are achieved by augmented protein (enzyme) synthesis through expression of specific genes (Fig. 28-8).

The second general mechanism—direct modulation of enzyme activity via kinetic properties—also seems operative in the developing lung. For instance, the first enzyme of the cytidine diphosphocholine pathway (choline kinase) shows unique kinetic properties in lung tissue that account for the active use of this pathway rather than the methylation mechanism during fetal lung development.

Nonsurfactant proteins

It has recently been hypothesized that two nonsurfactant proteins, epidermal growth factor and fibroblast pneumonocyte factor, may be associated with lung phospholipid biosynthesis.

Fibroblast pneumonocyte factor (FPF) is a heat-stable dialyzable polypeptide produced by fetal lung fibroblasts, which stimulates phospholipid synthesis by the alveolar type II pneumonocyte in vivo or in tissue culture. It has been suggested that FPF may be mechanistically involved with fetal lung responsiveness to antenatal glucocorticoids, modulate target organ response to other growth factors such as thyroid hormone, or both.

Epidermal growth factor (EGF), a powerful mitogen for both epidermal and nonepidermal cells, is a heat-stable nondialyzable single polypeptide chain of 53 amino acid residues. In limited animal studies the principal morphologic effects of EGF on the lung appear to be enhanced growth of cells that were least differentiated (i.e., tracheal and bronchial epithelia develop faster than that of distal airways).

The definitive mechanisms and practical significance of nonsurfactant proteins as potential regulators of fetal lung development remain unclear. However, the relationship of these polypeptides to pulmonary maturation underlines the complexity of the process and the importance of cell-to-cell interactions during development.

Hormones

Various hormones are known to influence the rate of phosphatidylcholine biosynthesis in fetal lung cells. For instance, corticosteroids have a powerful effect on the rate of the cytidine diphosphocholine pathway. Other stimulatory agents include thyroid hormones, estrogens, and theophylline. Evidence also has been obtained suggesting that lung metabolism can be stimulated by cyclic AMP, which probably acts via enzymes as a second messenger. In addition, labor and/or oxytocin have been shown to stimulate the process of fetal lung development; it is possible that the mechanism for this effect involves endogenous corticoids secreted in increased concentrations as a response to stress. Results of recent studies further indicate that some hormones such as insulin may retard surfactant formation. This might explain the clinical observation that hyperinsulinemic fetuses (principally in gestations complicated by maternal diabetes) often show delayed lung maturation.

As shown in Fig. 28-8, hormone receptors are present in the cytoplasm and nucleus of type II pneumonocytes. The developmental pattern for lung receptors is of obvious interest in connection with corticosteroids. In this regard it appears that the presence of the receptor system is not a limiting factor in the stimulation of lung development. The cytoplasmic binding activity for steroid hormones has been detected as early as 9 weeks of gestation, and nuclear transfer of receptor-hormone complexes occurs in lungs of 16-week-old fetuses. Cytoplasmic receptors are present in the fetal lung throughout gestation and have been detected in the lungs of premature and term newborn infants. The concentration of binding sites is constant in lungs studied from 12 to 20 weeks of gestation, whereas lower levels are found between 27 and 40 weeks of gestation. The high concentration of corticosteroid receptors in type II pneumonocytes indicates that the lung is a target tissue for this class of hormones. Although there is considerable evidence that endogenous corticosteroids participate in regulating lung differentiation, this has not been conclusively demonstrated and the potential role of other endogenous substances is presently even less certain.

Biochemical role of corticosteroids

Biochemical studies dealing with the stimulatory influence of corticosteroids on the fetal lung were pursued shortly after Liggins discovered their maturational effect (based on clinical and morphologic observations on lambs) and after Kotas and Avery demonstrated the accelerated appearance of surfactant in hormone-treated rabbit fetuses. Most biochemical studies have used rats and rabbits in which cortisol analogues are directly administered to immature fetuses. Data obtained with these short gestational species support the following conclusions: (1) corticosteroids increase de novo synthesis of phosphatidylcholine, promoting accumulation of this phospholipid in the fetal lung; (2) corticosteroids specifically stimulate the cytidine diphosphocholine pathway, without altering the phosphatidylethanolamine methylation mechanism; (3) corticosteroids cause an increase in the activity of several enzymes essential to synthesis of phosphatidylcholine. Although these changes could be secondary phenomena, they probably represent primary, gene-mediated effects of hormones on type II pneumonocytes. The same effects demonstrated with rabbits and rats also have been observed with cultured human fetal lung explants incubated in the presence of cortisol. Not only have increased phospholipids been repeatedly demonstrated in lung parenchyma, but it also has been determined that fetal pulmonary fluid shows increased saturated phosphatidylcholine after steroid administration. Curiously, however, amniotic fluid phospholipids are not markedly altered after corticosteroid administration; this is probably because of a time delay after metabolic stimulation before newly synthesized phosphatidylcholine molecules can reach the amniotic cavity.

The net biochemical effect of the hormone, through an apparent induction of key enzymes, is to enhance the capacity of the fetal lung to produce the surface-active phospholipids of the respiratory system, as summarized in the following outline on the effects of corticosteroids on fetal lung development:

A. Anatomic*
    1. Increased potential air space
        a. Attenuation of alveolar cells
        b. Narrowing of septa
        c. Greater "alveolarization"
    2. Increased prominence or numbers of type II pneumonocytes
B. Physiologic
    1. Greater distensibility
    2. Greater deflation stability
    3. Earlier appearance of surfactant
C. Biochemical
    1. Increased concentration and/or degree of saturation of phosphatidylcholine in
        a. Lung parenchyma
        b. Lung lavage fluid
    2. Increased conversion of choline to phosphatidylcholine; that is, the apparent rate of the cytidine diphosphocholine pathway is enhanced
    3. Increased activities of lipoprotein lipase, cholinephosphotransferase, lysophosphatidylcholine acyltransferase, and glycerolphosphate phosphatidyltransferase.†

Because of exogenous corticosteroids, the capacity for pulmonary surfactant production is developed at an earlier time in gestation than would normally occur. The hormone therefore acts as a stimulus capable of changing the timing of fetal lung development such that the maturation process is accelerated. Although limited observations suggest that corticosteroids may be the natural inducer for biochemical maturation of the lung in late gestation, this has not been substantiated. Furthermore it has been shown that cortisol alone is not the physiologic stimulus for intrauterine lung maturation.

Further studies on the role of endogenous substances and the triggering of physiologic and biochemical processes leading to lung maturation are required.

SUMMARY

After the embryonic period of development, comprising the first 5 weeks after conception, there are three major stages of fetal lung development: the pseudoglandular, the canalicular, and the terminal sac phases.

The overall pattern of the formation of the respiratory system can be summarized by Reid's laws: (1) the conducting airways are developed by the sixteenth week of gestation; (2) alveoli develop mainly after birth, increasing in number until age 8 years and in size until growth of the thoracic cavity ceases; and (3) the preacinar blood vessels follow development of the airways, whereas the intraacinar vessels develop parallel with the alveoli.

During cytodifferentiation of the respiratory epithelium, type II pneumonocytes containing osmiophilic lamellar bodies become more prominent, implying increased levels of intracellular surfactant.

Pulmonary surface-active material (surfactant) is an antiatelectasis factor located in the "alveolar lining layer" that provides a low and variable surface tension and imparts hysteresis to the air-tissue interface. Functional surfactant decreases the pressure required to inflate the lung postnatally and maintains stability over a wide range of lung volumes.

Although many substances are present in pulmonary surfactant, the predominant and functionally essential constituent is saturated phosphatidylcholine, or lecithin. Lung cells and bronchoalveolar fluid are unique in showing high concentrations of saturated phosphatidylcholine and significant amounts of phosphatidylglycerol.

One benefit to basic research as regards current investigations involving exogenous surfactant therapy in RDS may be a clearer understanding of the importance of various constituents of surfactant compounds to biophysical function.

The major biochemical feature of fetal lung development is an increase in the concentration of saturated phosphatidylcholine, a change that occurs by approximately 90% of term gestation. Shortly after the appearance of increased surfactant phospholipid in lung extracts and in the airways, marked changes take place in lung distensibility and deflation stability, reflecting attainment of functional maturity.

Phosphatidylcholine is synthesized de novo in the lung by the cooperative interaction of the cytidine diphosphocholine pathway and the sequence of metabolic reactions leading to formation of diglyceride through phosphatidic acid.

Regulation of phosphatidylcholine synthesis, secretion, and turnover in the developing lung involves complex mechanisms, including hormonal control of enzyme activities.

Philip M. Farrell
Robert H. Perelman

*The anatomic effects of glucocorticoids in the fetal lung require further definition.

†There is a dispute in the literature regarding specific enzyme changes occurring after fetal or maternal administration of corticosteroids.

BIBLIOGRAPHY
General

Avery, M.E., and Fletcher, B.D.: The lung and its disorders in the newborn infant, ed. 3, Philadelphia, 1974, W.B. Saunders Co.

Farrell, P.M., editor: Lung development: biological and clinical perspectives, New York, 1982, Academic Press, Inc.

Farrell, P.M., editor: Nutrition and infant lung functions: report of a National Heart, Lung, and Blood Institute Symposium, Pediatr. Pulmonol. **2**:44, 1986.

Nelson, G.H., editor: Pulmonary development: transition from intrauterine to extrauterine life, New York, 1985, Marcel Dekker, Inc.

Perelman, R.H., and others: Developmental aspects of lung lipids, Annu. Rev. Physiol. **47**:803, 1985.

Perelman, R.H., and others: Discordance between male and female deaths due to the respiratory distress syndrome, Pediatrics **78**:238, 1986.

Raivio, K.O., Hallman, N., Kouvalainen, K., and Valimaki, I., editors: Respiratory distress syndrome, New York, 1984, Academic Press, Inc.

Shapiro, D.L., and others: Double-blind, randomized trial of a calf lung surfactant extract administered at birth to very premature infants for prevention of respiratory distress syndrome, Pediatrics **76**:4, 1985.

Stern, L., editor: Hyaline membrane disease: pathogenesis and pathophysiology; New York, 1984, Grune & Stratton, Inc.

Developmental anatomy

Boyden, E.A.: Development and growth of the airways. In Hodson, W.A., editor: Development of the lung, New York, 1977, Marcel Dekker, Inc.

Burri, P.H., and Weibel, E.R.: Ultrastructure and morphometry of the developing lung. In Hodson, W.A., editor: Development of the lung, New York, 1977, Marcel Dekker, Inc.

Gilbert, E.F., and Opitz, J.M.: Genetic disorders of the respiratory system. In Jackson, L.G., and Schimke, R.N., editors: Clinical genetics: a sourcebook for physicians, New York, 1979, John Wiley & Sons, Inc.

Hislop, A., and Reid, L.M.: Formation of the pulmonary vasculature. In Hodson, W.A., editor: Development of the lung, New York, 1977, Marcel Dekker, Inc.

Landing, B.H.: Congenital malformation and genetic disorders of the respiratory tract, Am. Rev. Respir. Dis. **120**:151, 1979.

Meyrick, B., and Reid, L.M.: Ultrastructure of alveolar lining and its development. In Hodson, W.A., editor: Development of the lung, New York, 1977, Marcel Dekker, Inc.

Reid, L.: The embryology of the lung. In de Revck, A.V.S., and Porker, R., editors: CIBA Foundation Symposium on Development of the Lung, London, 1967, Churchill Livingstone.

Schumacher, R.E., and Farrell, P.M.: Congenital diaphragmatic hernia, Perinatol. Neonatol. **9**:29, 1985.

Physiology

Avery, M.E., and Mead, J.: Surface properties in relation to atelectasis and hyaline membrane disease, Am. J. Dis. Child. **97**:517, 1959.

Brumley, G.W., and others: Correlations of mechanical stability, morphology, pulmonary surfactant, and phospholipid content in the developing lamb lung, J. Clin. Invest. **46**:863, 1967.

Clements, J.A.: Surface tension of lung extracts, Proc. Soc. Exp. Biol. Med. **95**:170, 1957.

Clements, J.A., Brown, E.S., and Johnson, R.P.: Pulmonary surface tension and the mucous lining of the lungs: some theoretical considerations, J. Appl. Physiol. **12**:262, 1958.

Faridy, E.E., Permutt, S., and Riley, R.L.: Effect of ventilation on surface forces in excised dogs' lungs, J. Appl. Physiol. **21**:1453, 1966.

Jobe, A., Kirkpatrick, E., and Gluck, L.: Lecithin appearance and apparent biologic half-life in term newborn rabbit lung, Pediatr. Res. **12**:669, 1978.

Jobe, A., Mannino, F., and Gluck, L.: Labeling of phosphatidylcholine in the alveolar wash of rabbits in utero, Am. J. Obstet. Gynecol. **132**:53, 1978.

Kotas, R.V., and others: Fetal rhesus monkey lung development: lobar differences and discordances between stability and distensibility, J. Appl. Physiol. **43**:92, 1977.

von Neergaard, K.: Neue Auffassungen uber einen Grundbegriff der Atemmechanik: die Retraktionskraft der Lunge, abhangig von der Oberflachenspannung in den Alveolen, Z Gesame. Exp. Med. **66**:373, 1965.

Young, S.L., and Tierney, D.F.: Dipalmitoyl lecithin secretion and metabolism by the rat lung, Am. J. Physiol. **222**:1539, 1972.

Biochemistry

Bourbon, J.R., and others: Utilization of glycogen for phospholipid synthesis in fetal rat lung, Biochim. Biophys. Acta **712**:382, 1982.

Brown, L.A.S., and Longmore, W.J.: Adrenergic and cholinergic regulation of lung surfactant secretion in the isolated perfused rat lung and in the alveolar type II cell in culture, J. Biol. Chem. **256**:66, 1981.

Epstein, M.F., and Farrell, P.M.: The choline incorporation pathway: primary mechanism for de novo lecithin synthesis in fetal primate lung, Pediatr. Res. **9**:658, 1975.

Farrell, P.M., and Hamosh, M.: The biochemistry of fetal lung development, Clin. Perinatol. **5**:197, 1978.

Farrell, P.M., and Zachman, R.D.: Induction of choline phosphotransferase and lecithin synthesis in the fetal lung by corticosteroids, Science **179**:297, 1973.

Gluck, L., and others: Diagnosis of the respiratory distress syndrome by amniocentesis, Am. J. Obstet. Gynecol. **109**:440, 1971.

Godinez, R.I., Sanders, R.L., and Longmore, W.J.: Phosphatidylglycerol in rat lung. I. Identification as a metabolically active phospholipid in isolated perfused rat lung, Biochemistry **14**:830, 1975.

King, R.J.: Composition and metabolism of the apolipoproteins of pulmonary surfactant, Annu. Rev. Physiol. **47**:775, 1985.

King, R.J., and Clements, J.A.: Surface active materials from the dog lung. II. Composition and physiological correlations, Am. J. Physiol. **223**:715, 1972.

Kotas, R.V., and others: Evidence for independent regulators of organ maturation in fetal rabbits, Pediatrics **47**:57, 1971.

Liggins, G.C.: Premature delivery of foetal lambs infused with glucocorticoids, J. Endocrinol. **45**:515, 1969.

Notter, R.H., Finkelstein, J.N., and Taubold, R.D.: Comparative adsorption of natural lung surfactant, extracted phospholipids, and artificial phospholipid mixtures to the air-water interface, Chem. Phys. Lipids **33**:67, 1983.

Oldenborg, V., and van Golde, L.M.G.: Activity of cholinephosphotransferase, lysolecithin–lysolecithin acyltransferase and lysolecithin acyltransferase in the developing mouse lung, Biochim. Biophys. Acta **441**:433, 1976.

Smith, B.T.: Lung maturation in the fetal rat: acceleration by the injectional fibroblast-pneumonocyte factor, Science **204**:1094, 1979.

Smith, B.T., and Bogues, W.G.: Effects of drugs and hormones on lung in experimental animals and man, Pharmacol. Ther. **9**:51, 1980.

Stern, W., Kovac, C., and Weinhold, P.A.: Activity and properties of CTP: cholinephosphate cytidyltransferase in adult and fetal rat lung, Biochim. Biophys. Acta **441**:280, 1976.

van Golde, L.M.G.: Metabolism of phospholipids in the lung, Am. Rev. Respir. Dis. **114**:977, 1976.

van Golde, L.M.G.: Synthesis of surfactant lipids in adult lung. Annu. Rev. Physiol. **47**:765, 1985.

PART TWO

Assessment of pulmonary function

The majority of neonates requiring intensive care have respiratory problems. In recent years newer methods for evaluating pulmonary function in neonates with suspected abnormalities of the cardiopulmonary system have been developed. Whereas standard techniques for assessing pulmonary function can be applied in a healthy infant, special limitations and problems are encountered in very small or sick babies. A practical clinical approach to disordered cardiopulmonary function is presented in this section, and an attempt is made to facilitate the differentiation between heart and lung disease.

CLINICAL OBSERVATIONS

Five common presenting physical signs relay indirect information regarding pulmonary function. These are respiratory rate, retractions, nasal flaring, grunting, and cyanosis.

Respiratory rate

Precise monitoring of respiratory rate is invaluable, since significant deviation from the normal is observed with mechanical pulmonary dysfunction, acid-base imbalances, or arterial blood gas abnormalities. A detailed discussion of respiratory control and apnea of prematurity appears in Part five.

The range over which respiratory rate can achieve successful gas exchange when the infants are breathing spontaneously is limited. At high rates increased dead space ventilation occurs, whereas at low rates decreased alveolar ventilation results. Infants with lung disease attempt to minimize the work of breathing by controlling the respiratory rate. The total work of breathing consists of elastic and resistive components. The elastic component represents the work required to stretch the lungs during a tidal inspiration, whereas the resistive component is the work required to overcome the movement of air through the airways. In patients with RDS respiratory rate is rapid and shallow, whereas infants with upper airway obstruction, exemplified by subglottic stenosis, may exhibit respiration that is slower and deeper. Fig. 28-9 shows that the work of breathing depends on respiratory rate and the type of pulmonary dysfunction.

Retractions

The diaphragm is the principal mechanical driving force for ventilation, creating a negative intrapleural pressure during inspiration. The pressure generated is ultimately determined by a combination of (1) the force

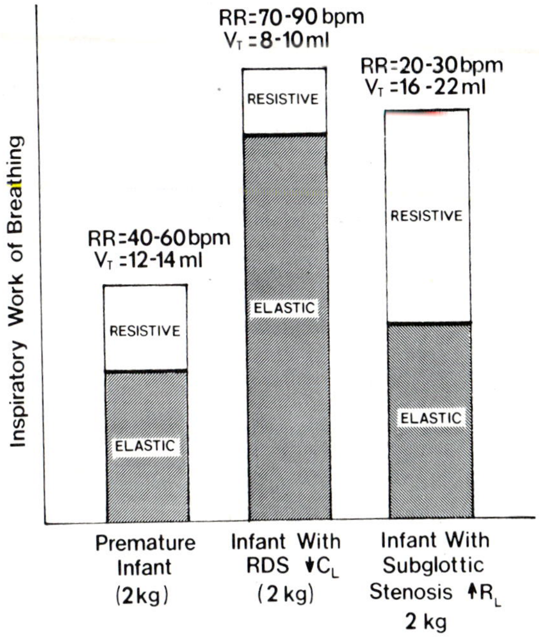

Fig. 28-9. Relative contributions of the elastic and resistive components of work of breathing in infants with normal pulmonary function, decreased compliance *(C_L)*, and increased resistance *(R_L)*.

of the diaphragm; (2) the mechanical properties of the lung; and (3) the stability of the chest wall.

The neonatal chest wall is very compliant, and substernal, subcostal, and intercostal retractions are readily observable with relatively small changes in lung mechanics. In infants with very stiff lungs and marked retractions the chest configuration resembles that seen in pectus excavatum. In neonates with respiratory distress, retractions become more apparent as the lungs become stiffer. Apart from their characteristic appearance in RDS, severe retractions also can signal complications of respiratory disease such as airway obstruction, misplacement of an endotracheal tube, pneumothorax, or atelectasis. Diminishing retractions suggest that lung compliance is improving. The significance of retractions often is overlooked when defining respiratory failure in neonates. In smaller infants (especially those weighing less than 1,500 gm) the progression of retractions should be closely monitored, since many of these infants may exhibit increased retractions even before blood gases demonstrate frank respiratory failure.

Nasal flaring

Nasal flaring is another sign of respiratory distress frequently observed in infants. Nasal flaring is occasionally observed in the absence of other signs of respiratory distress, particularly during feeding and active sleep. The enlargement of the nostrils, produced by activation of the alae nasi results in a marked reduction in nasal resistance. Since newborns are considered obligate nose breathers and nasal resistance contributes up to 50% of the total lung resistance, nasal flaring would be expected to markedly decrease the work of breathing. The early onset of activation (firing) of the alae nasi, when compared with both the diaphragm and inspiratory airflow, may be an important mechanism that prepares the upper airway for peak inspiratory flow. Activation of other respiratory muscles such as the genioglossus (tongue) and the laryngeal muscles is also important for optimum function of the upper airways. The genioglossus muscle protrudes the tongue and, in part, maintains pharyngeal patency while the laryngeal muscles move the vocal cords and regulate airflow, particularly during expiration. The activity of these muscles is modulated by changes in chemical (chemoreceptor) and mechanical (mechanoreceptor) stimulation.

Grunting

With respiratory muscle activity the vocal cords abduct during inspiration and adduct (without any sound) during expiration. When respiratory function is disrupted, however, the work of breathing is greatly increased, and neonates attempt to compensate by closing their vocal cords during expiration. Expiration through partially closed vocal cords produces the grunting sound. Grunting may be either intermittent or continuous, depending on the severity of lung disease. During the initial phase of expiration, the infant closes the glottis, holds air in the lungs, and produces an elevated transpulmonary pressure in the absence of airflow. During the last part of the expiratory phase, gas is expelled from the lungs against partially closed vocal cords, causing an audible grunt. It is not actually the grunt, then, that produces the elevated transpulmonary pressure but the ability of the infant to partially close the vocal cords after end inspiration. During the expiratory phase, when the vocal cords are partially or completely closed, there is an improved ventilation/perfusion ratio because of increased airway pressure and increased lung volume. The end result of this airway closure may be an improvement in gas exchange.

Harrison and others, who demonstrated the significance of grunting in RDS, noted that, when grunting was abolished by endotracheal intubation, arterial oxygen tension (Pa_{O_2}) decreased. They concluded that grunting was responsible for stabilizing lung volume and improving arterial oxygenation. Other studies have suggested that the grunting mechanism can maintain a FRC and a Pa_{O_2} equivalent to those maintained during the application of 2 or 3 cm H_2O of CPAP (see Part four).

Cyanosis

Cyanosis, best observed by examining the lips and tongue, is an insensitive indicator of pulmonary dysfunction. Several types of pulmonary dysfunction, including airway obstruction, ventilation-perfusion inequality, intrapulmonary shunting, and, rarely, diffusion abnormalities, in addition to cardiac disease, may result in cyanosis. The clinical features of cyanosis and their significance are discussed in detail in Chapter 29.

BLOOD GASES

Blood gases are the most widely used clinical method for assessing pulmonary function in neonates and form the basis for diagnosis and management of infants with cardiorespiratory disease. The purpose of this section is to discuss how changes in arterial oxygen (Pa_{O_2}) and carbon dioxide (Pa_{CO_2}) tension reflect disordered pulmonary function in different clinical situations. Techniques of blood gas determination in infants with RDS are discussed in Part three. Normal blood gas and acid base interpretation is discussed in Chapter 25, part three.

Arterial oxygen tension

Oxygen is carried in the blood both in chemical combination with hemoglobin and also in physical solution. The oxygen taken up from the lungs is dependent on the alveolar/capillary pressure gradient. At ambient pressures the amount of dissolved oxygen is only a small fraction of the total quantity carried in whole blood (0.3 ml of oxygen/100 ml of plasma/100 mm Hg at 37° C). Most of the oxygen in whole blood is bound to hemoglobin (1 gm of hemoglobin combines with 1.34 cc of oxygen at 37° C). The quantity of oxygen bound to hemoglobin depends on the partial pressure and is described by the oxygen dissociation curve (Fig. 28-10). The blood is almost completely saturated at a Pa_{O_2} of 90 to 100 mm Hg. The flattening of the upper portion of the S-shaped dissociation curve makes it virtually impossible to monitor oxygen tension above 60 to 80 mm Hg by following arterial oxygen saturation alone. Cyanosis generally is noted only at a Pa_{O_2} of less than 40 mm Hg in neonates. The dissociation curve of fetal (as compared with adult) blood is shifted to the left and at any Pa_{O_2} below 100 mm Hg fetal blood binds more oxygen. The shift appears to be the result of the lower affinity of fetal hemoglobin for diphosphoglycerate. Note that pH, Pa_{CO_2}, temperature, and 2,3-diphosphoglycerate (DPG) content all influence the position of the dissociation curve.

The partial pressure of oxygen in arterial blood not only depends on the ability of the lung to transfer oxygen as determined by alveolar ventilation but also is largely influenced by the *ventilation/perfusion relationships* (*V/Q ratio*) within the lung. For normal gas exchange the

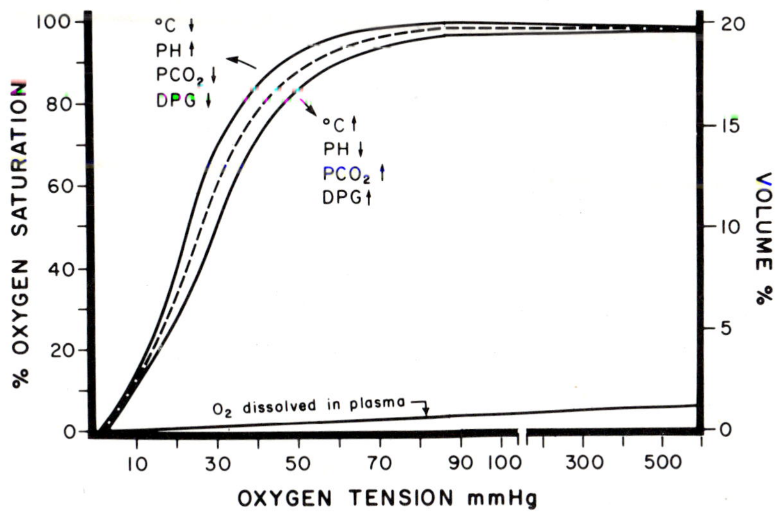

Fig. 28-10. Factors shifting the oxygen dissociation curve of hemoglobin (fetal hemoglobin is shifted to the left). (From Martin, R.J., Klaus, M., and Fanaroff, A. Respiratory problems. In Klaus, M., and Fanaroff, A., editors: Care of the high risk neonate, Philadelphia, 1986, W.B. Saunders Co.)

ventilation and perfusion should be similarly proportioned. The ratio should be very close to 1; that is, for every milliliter of ventilated air there should be a proportionate degree of perfusion. In healthy adults this V/Q ratio is about 0.8 because of variations in the ratio in different parts of the lung. In the presence of cardiopulmonary disease the V/Q ratio may be abnormal, depending on the nature of the pulmonary pathologic condition. In cases of intrinsic pulmonary disease associated with hypoventilation the V/Q ratio will be less than 1. In cardiac anomalies with right-to-left shunt and in pulmonary disease where a large portion of the lung is ventilated but underperfused, a V/Q ratio greater than 1 will be observed.

The most common disturbance in V/Q relationships in neonates is intrapulmonary shunting, which is a consequence of atelectasis. Areas of the lung in which intrapulmonary shunting occurs are perfused but not ventilated and thus have a V/Q of 0. Areas of gas trapping that are virtually nonventilated but perfused also function essentially as a shunt. The result of intrapulmonary shunts is a decrease in PaO_2 similar to that which occurs when there is a right-to-left shunt in the heart or through a patent ductus arteriosus with pulmonary hypertension. Similar arterial unsaturation may occur when the alveoli are well ventilated but not perfused. Right-to-left shunts may occur at three levels: interatrial through the foramen ovale, through the ductus arteriosus, or within the lung itself. In infants with RDS, V/Q abnormalities typically result from a combination of all the above mechanisms (see Part three). Preterm infants both with and without respiratory disease frequently exhibit a fall in PaO_2 during crying, which may be explained on the basis of increased right-to-left shunting resulting from the large intrathoracic pressure changes.

Arterial carbon dioxide tension

$PaCO_2$ is a major determinant of pulmonary function in neonatal respiratory disease, directly reflecting alveolar ventilation and in most situations minute ventilation. As tissue levels of CO_2 increase above those of arterial blood, molecules diffuse into the capillaries and are transported in red blood cells and plasma. Unlike the S-shaped dissociation curve for O_2, the relationship between CO_2 content and tension is almost linear over the physiologic range. $PaCO_2$ is maintained in a range of 35 to 45 mm Hg in healthy infants, although levels below this range are sometimes seen in spontaneously breathing, full-term infants with transient tachypnea or meconium aspiration syndrome. In these conditions hyperventilation is common and results in the decrease in $PaCO_2$. An elevated $PaCO_2$ level is one of the major indicators of respiratory failure.

As a determinant of pulmonary function, an increased $PaCO_2$ is generally a result of one of two major abnormalities in pulmonary physiology. The first condition, atelectasis, is exhibited in RDS and associated with decreased lung compliance, increased respiratory rate, and increased work of breathing. As the infant develops respiratory failure, carbon dioxide retention occurs. The second condition resulting in carbon dioxide retention is alveolar overdistention. The overaeration caused by air trapping is common in meconium aspiration syndrome and may be produced in infants with respiratory disease

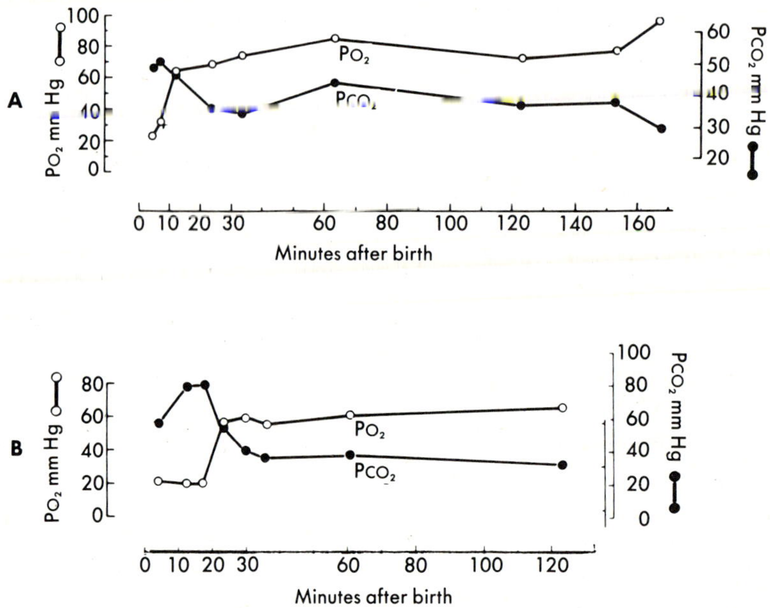

Fig. 28-11. Changes in PO_2 and PCO_2 during the first minutes after birth in a normal infant **(A)** and an asphyxiated infant **(B)** with delayed onset of respiration. (Courtesy R. Tunell, M.D.)

by the use of assisted ventilation. Alveolar overdistention causes lung stiffening, increased work of breathing, and carbon dioxide retention. In addition to measurement of $PaCO_2$, pH must be always determined and HCO_3^- concentration calculated to assess the status of any infant with pulmonary disease.

The initiation of ventilation with the *first breath* after normal delivery results in a rapid fall in $PaCO_2$ within minutes of birth. PaO_2 rises equally rapidly to levels of 60 to 90 mm Hg, although some degree of mismatching of V/Q is evident in the first 1 to 2 hours of life. This is thought to be the result of intracardiac and/or pulmonary right-to-left shunting. The effects of this sudden adaptation on the blood gases are illustrated in Fig. 28-11, which shows the rapid change in PaO_2 and $PaCO_2$ under normal conditions and when there is asphyxia with delayed onset of breathing. The speed with which pulmonary ventilation and perfusion are uniformly distributed is an indication of the remarkable adaptive capacities of the newborn infant for the maintenance of normal homeostasis.

Hyperoxia-hyperventilation test

The hyperoxia test is performed by placing the infant in a 100% oxygen concentration for 5 to 10 minutes and then sampling arterial blood gas or monitoring transcutaneous PO_2 (see Part three). The underlying physiology for this method is that 5 to 10 minutes of oxygen exposure should diffuse oxygen even into the poorly ventilated areas and improve oxygenation. If hypoxia remains after 5 to 10 minutes of 100% oxygen exposure, it suggests the presence of direct right-to-left shunting. Whereas the test was used to evaluate the degree of shunting in RDS to predict outcome, its most useful current application is to differentiate between primary lung and congenital heart disease with right-to-left shunting. A modification of the hyperoxia test combining hyperoxia with hyperventilation is a possible method to distinguish between structural congenital heart disease and persistent fetal circulation (PFC), both of which have right-to-left shunting. During normal ventilation exposure to 100% oxygen in both cyanotic heart disease and PFC will result in virtually no change in PaO_2. However, by hyperventilating the infant for between 5 and 10 minutes and decreasing the $PaCO_2$ to ranges of 18 to 25 mm Hg, infants with PFC may exhibit PO_2 levels greater than 100 mm Hg, if only transiently. In contrast, patients with anatomically fixed right-to-left shunting and particularly those with transposition of the great vessels rarely generate a PO_2 above 40 mm Hg, even with hyperventilation.

Evaluation of ductal shunting

If right-to-left ductal shunting occurs, desaturated blood from the right side of the heart enters the main pulmonary artery and crosses the ductus to the descending aorta. Since the ductus almost always enters the aorta after the origin of the right subclavian and carotid arteries (and therefore temporal arteries), blood arriving at these two sites will be well oxygenated, whereas blood samples from the left subclavian artery and aorta will be (relatively) less oxygenated. Thus preductal gases can be obtained from the right radial artery and postductal gases are drawn through the left radial artery or descending aorta. Alternatively placement of two transcutaneous Po_2 electrodes, one on the right upper chest and the other on the abdomen, accomplishes the same effect in differentiating preductal and postductal Pao_2.

A study of almost 100 patients with RDS demonstrated only a 5 mm Hg difference between preductal and postductal gases. This indicates that right-to-left shunting through the ductus arteriosus is not a major component of the pathophysiology of RDS. In patients with persistent fetal circulation (persistent pulmonary hypertension) there may be right-to-left shunting through both the foramen ovale and ductus arteriosus; this can be demonstrated by either simultaneously obtained preductal and postductal arterial gases, during echocardiography, or by contrast injection at cardiac angiography.

PHYSIOLOGIC MEASUREMENTS

Tests of cardiopulmonary function performed on sick neonates ideally should involve as little additional stress to the infant as is feasible. Roentgenographic evaluation of the chest is an integral part of the diagnostic evaluation of respiratory disorders and is discussed in Chapter 13. Measurements of central venous pressure and pulmonary artery pressure are techniques that may indirectly give useful information regarding pulmonary function and are discussed in Chapter 21. Furthermore the effects of varying levels of CPAP or assisted ventilation on blood gases will provide useful insight into the specific alterations in pulmonary mechanics in infants with respiratory disease (see Part four).

Measurement of airflow

Nasal thermistors can be sensitive enough to detect the small temperature gradients that exist between inspired and expired air. Such a qualitative determination of flow can be very useful in conjunction with standard impedance pneumography and heart rate monitoring (see Chapter 21). In this way the careful characterization of episodes of central apnea, obstructive apnea, and bradycardia (or combinations of all three) can be readily made (see Part five).

Quantitative measurement of airflow can be obtained from an infant pneumotachometer consisting of a fine-mesh screen that provides a known resistance to the flow of air through it. Measurement of the pressure gradient across the screen will be directly proportional to airflow, and the latter then can be directly calculated and integrated into tidal volume. A variety of infant face masks, nosepieces (as for the administration of CPAP), and even endotracheal tube connectors have been fitted with screens to function as neonatal pneumotachometers.

Measurement of lung volumes

The total volume of air in the lungs can be measured and subdivided into lung volumes (Fig. 28-12). Body plethysmography and gas dilution studies are the methods usually employed for making these determinations but are cumbersome and time consuming and thus confined mainly to research.

FRC is the volume of gas that is in direct communication with the airways at the end of expiration. Helium dilution or nitrogen washout techniques have been adapted to measure FRC in infants. The volume of gas in the FRC serves as a buffer to the inspired gas so that large changes in alveolar gas tension are reduced. Thoracic gas volume is the total volume of gas in the thorax at the end of expiration and, in contrast to FRC, includes gas that is not in communication with the airways. Thoracic gas volume is measured by placing an infant inside a body plethysmograph and performing end-expiratory occlusion. Tidal volume (V_T), the volume of gas exchanged during a normal breath, can be measured either with a pneumotachograph as just described or with a plethysmograph. Vital capacity (VC) cannot be measured in infants because of lack of cooperation; but crying VC, the V_T during crying, may be alternatively obtained. Numerous attempts have been made to quantitate V_T from surface measurements of chest wall motion, although these techniques also require complex calibrations and have met with variable success. The size of the lung compartments is related to the height, weight, and surface area of the subjects.

One of the principal functions of the first breath is to transform the fluid-filled fetal lung from an airless organ to one with an appropriate FRC. The ability of the lung to maintain a volume of gas at end expiration depends on two factors. One is the chest wall, which acts as a support for the lungs, and the other is the ability of the lung to produce surfactant to stabilize the expanded alveoli. Both these functions are less well developed in the premature infant.

The factor or factors responsible for the *first breath* are unknown. Multiple stimuli such as exposure to a cold environmental temperature and tactile changes play a role. However, the exact interrelationships of pH, Po_2, and Pco_2 that combine to induce breathing in the human neonate are still to be determined. The pressure change of the first breath must overcome the effects of viscosity of fluid in the airway, the effects of surface tension, and the effects of tissue resistance. Roentgenographic studies of the lung indicate that inflation with air occurs immediately with the first breath. FRC is rapidly established, with little change throughout the first week of life. There is some evidence for gas trapping for 2 or 3 days, which may be related to the gradual disappearance of lung fluid during this period.

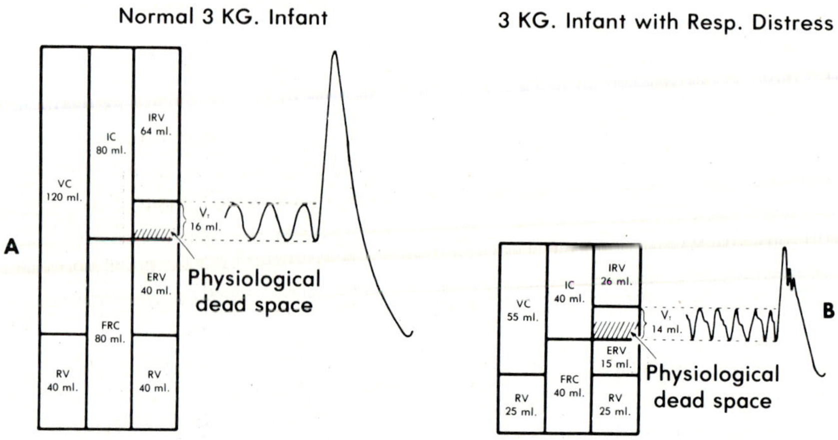

A	Measure	B
36	Respiratory rate/minute	70
0.3	Dead space/tidal volume ratio	0.6
5	Intraesophageal pressure diff. (cm. H_2O)	18
4.4	Compliance (ml./cm. H_2O)	1.0
29	Resistance (cm. H_2O/liter/sec.)	23
40	Total work/breath (gm. cm.)	111
1440	Total work/minute (gm. cm.)	7770

Fig. 28-12. Partitioning of lung volumes and other measures of pulmonary function in a normal infant **(A)** and one with RDS **(B).** (From Avery, M., Fletcher, B., and Williams, R.: The lung and its disorders in the newborn infant, Philadelphia, 1981, W.B. Saunders Co.)

Dead space is that portion of the tidal volume not involved in gas exchange, and thus it will vary with the presence or absence of areas of high V/Q. The dead space is divided into several compartments. Anatomic dead space is the constant airway volume not involved in gas exchange and is made up of the air passages from nares to terminal bronchioles. Alveolar dead space is the volume of gas in alveoli that are well ventilated but underperfused. Physiologic dead space is the sum of anatomic and alveolar dead space. In the normal newborn physiologic dead space is 6 to 8 cc; smaller values are obtained in premature infants. The relationship of dead space to V_T is physiologically significant and normally in the range of 0.3. It is of practical importance to minimize the dead space added by apparatus for assisted ventilation or measurement of lung function to prevent rebreathing and accumulation of carbon dioxide.

Esophageal pressure determinations

Studies have shown that measurements of esophageal pressure in infants closely reflect intrapleural pressure. Pleural pressure can be determined relatively simply by using esophageal balloons or esophageal catheters. Most balloons are made of hand-dipped latex and measure approximately 0.5 cm in diameter and 2 to 3 cm in length. The esophageal catheter is usually placed approximately 12 cm from the gum margin in term infants, and, if cardiac artifact is observed, the catheter is withdrawn until the cardiac artifact diminishes. At first esophageal tone will be increased, so the catheter should remain in place long enough for this tone to diminish before measurements are made. The balloon/catheter is connected to a pressure transducer and may remain in the esophagus for extended periods without producing symptoms in the infant. In conjunction with flow and volume tracings this technique can be used to determine dynamic lung compliance (change in volume per unit change in intrapleural pressure) and pulmonary resistance (change in pressure divided by flow). Esophageal pressure also has been described as a useful technique for evaluation of optimum levels of CPAP in infants with RDS (see "Compliance").

Compliance

Lung compliance depends not only on the intrinsic elasticity of pulmonary tissue but also on the level of FRC. *Compliance* is expressed as change in volume per unit change in pressure. Compliance can be measured during spontaneous breathing using a device to measure airflow and volume (such as a pneumotachograph) and a catheter to measure esophageal pressure. With this method *dynamic compliance* is calculated by dividing the V_T changes by the esophageal pressure changes between points of no airflow at the airway opening (i.e., between end inspiration and end expiration). Alternatively, *static compliance* may be calculated by employing occlusion of the airway as described later.

The degree of elasticity can be estimated from specific

compliance (lung compliance divided by FRC), which corrects for the absolute level of lung volume. Whereas lung compliance in the normal neonate (3 to 6 ml/cm H_2O) is comparable to that of the adult when corrected for unit body weight, compliance of the thorax is relatively much higher in infants.

In normal newborns the lung compliance is low at the initiation of the first breath. With the establishment of respiration and with gradual clearance of lung fluid during the first 3 to 6 hours of life the FRC increases with concomitant improvement in lung compliance. Since the improvement in lung compliance is a result of improvement in FRC, the specific compliance is unchanged. Pathophysiologic factors that may increase the amount of fluid or impede the clearance of lung fluid may delay this improvement in lung compliance. Placental transfusion with subsequent increase in the blood volume and transudation of fluid into the interstitial tissue of the lung is an example of this phenomenon. The variability of compliance values in the first 2 hours of life, in part the result of physiologic variation, also may account for the frequent observations of higher respiratory rates in some infants during this period.

In distressed infants in whom lung compliance is markedly reduced, the compliant immature chest wall poses a disadvantage in that, as the infant attempts to increase negative intrathoracic pressure, the chest wall collapses (retracts). The more compliant airway of the smaller infant may predispose him or her to actual airway collapse during expiration and result in distal gas trapping.

Resistance

Total pulmonary resistance results from airflow through the nasopharynx, trachea, and bronchi and depends on the airway caliber, flow rate, and resistance imposed by lung tissue. In the full-term infant total pulmonary resistance is around 30 cm H_2O/L/sec, approximately six times greater than that in the adult. A major site of airway resistance in the neonate is the nasopharynx. In the normal infant, airway resistance (resistance that is imposed by the breathing tubes) is approximately 18 to 20 cm H_2O/L/sec and viscous resistance (the resistance caused by tissues) is 8 to 10 cm H_2O/L/sec. This latter value is also larger than that in adults. Because of the higher resistances that occur in infants, respiratory apparatus that would materially increase airway resistance further must be avoided where possible.

Time constant of the respiratory system is the duration necessary for a step (e.g., pressure) change to partially equilibrate throughout the lungs. As discussed in Part four, the time constant of the respiratory system can be calculated from the product of lung compliance and the total pulmonary resistance.

The *work of breathing* is a measure of the energy expended in inflating the lungs and moving the chest. In general terms work is the cumulative product of pressure and the volume of air moved at each instant. In the normal infant total pulmonary work has been determined to equal an average value of 1,440 gm·cm/min. In an infant with respiratory distress the total pulmonary work may increase as much as six times. This becomes most important when considered in terms of the oxygen cost of breathing. The neonate requires a greater caloric expenditure to breathe than does the adult, and the distressed infant requires an even greater caloric expenditure for this function. In the full-term infant the work of breathing is minimum when the infant has a respiratory rate of 30 breaths per minute.

Newer techniques to measure pulmonary mechanics

With the sophistication of medical care for critically or chronically ill infants, techniques to assess pulmonary mechanics in adult subjects are being adapted for use in infants. Pulmonary mechanics may be measured by end inspiratory occlusion and the *passive flow and volume* that follow the release of this occlusion. Static lung compliance is calculated by dividing the total exhaled volume by the pressure changes between end inspiration (during the occlusion) and end expiration. The time constant of the respiratory system is obtained from the plot of flow and volume. With this plot, the slope during the relaxed expiration is the time constant. Resistance can then be calculated from the time constant and compliance.

Multiple brief *interruptions of expiratory airflow* may also be used for measurements of pulmonary mechanics. During each brief interruption, there is pressure equilibration throughout the respiratory system, and the static lung compliance can be calculated from the changes in pressure and volume from each interruption to the end of expiration. Resistance of the respiratory system is calculated by dividing the pressure during each brief interruption by the flow that preceded that interruption. The advantages of the multiple-interruption technique over the passive expiration technique is that during a single breath, multiple measurements of pulmonary mechanics can be obtained. Furthermore, the multiple interruption technique will reveal whether pulmonary mechanics vary at different times within a single breath. On the other hand, the single occlusion and passive expiration technique requires minimum equipment.

Many techniques used to measure pulmonary mechanics in older children and adults require patient cooperation. Until recently, techniques such as *forced expiratory maneuvers* were unavailable to study infants. A respiratory jacket surrounding the chest and abdomen may be suddenly inflated to produce a forced expiration. Flow rates at different times during expiration and forced expiratory volumes can be measured. Flow-volume curves can be used to distinguish between restrictive and obstructive pulmonary diseases.

Recent advances in computer technology for analysis of pulmonary function have made such evaluations available to the clinician. By using high-speed microprocessor technology, the clinician can assess the mechanical function of the lungs and energetics of breathing at the bedside and have access to immediate results that may allow ventilator or drug therapy to be optimized.

Information about pulmonary mechanics may be used in the diagnosis and management of infants with acute or chronic pulmonary disorders. In the next few years these new techniques will be added to the armamentarium of providers of neonatal care.

William W. Fox
Thomas H. Shaffer
Waldemar A. Carlo

BIBLIOGRAPHY

Avery, M.E., Fletcher, B.D., and Williams, R.G.: The lung and its disorders in the newborn infant, ed. 4, Philadelphia, 1981, W.B. Saunders Co.

Berman, L.S., and others: Optimum levels of CPAP for tracheal extubation of newborns, J. Pediatr. **89**:109, 1976.

Carlo, W.A., and others: Alae nasi activation (nasal flaring) decreases nasal resistance in preterm infants, Pediatrics **72**:338, 1983.

Chernick, V., and Avery, M.E.: The functional basis of respiratory pathology. In Kendig, E., and Chernick, V., editors: Disorders of the respiratory tract in children, ed. 2, Philadelphia, 1977, W.B. Saunders Co.

Comroe, J.H.: Physiology of respiration, ed. 2, Chicago, 1974, Year Book Medical Publishers, Inc.

Dinwiddie, R., and Russell, G.: Relationship of intraesophageal pressure to intrapleural pressure in the newborn, J. Appl. Physiol. **33**:415, 1972.

Gottfried, S.B., and others: Interrupter technique for measurement of respiratory mechanics in anesthetized humans, J. Appl. Physiol. **59**:647, 1985.

Harrison, V.C., deV., Heese, H., and Klein, M.: The significance of grunting in hyaline membrane disease, Pediatrics **41**:549, 1968.

LeSouef, P.N., England, S.J., and Bryan, A.C.: Total resistance of the respiratory system in preterm infants with and without an endotracheal tube, J. Pediatr. **104**:108, 1984.

Olinsky, A., Bryan, A.C., and Bryan, M.H.: A simple method of measuring total respiratory system compliance in newborn infants, S. Afr. Med. J. **50**:128, 1976.

Peckham, G.J., and Fox, W.W.: Physiological factors affecting pulmonary artery pressure in infants with persistent pulmonary hypertension, J. Pediatr. **93**:1005, 1979.

Scarpelli, E.M.: Concepts in respiratory pathophysiology. In Scarpelli, E.M., Auld, P., and Goldman, H., editors: Pulmonary disease of the fetus, newborn, and child, Philadelphia, 1978, Lea & Febiger.

Schlueter, M.A., and Tooley, W.H.: Right-to-left shunt through the ductus arteriosus in newborn infants, Pediatr. Res. **8**:354, 1974.

Smith, C.A., and Nelson, N.M.: The physiology of the newborn infant, Springfield, Ill., 1976, Charles C Thomas, Publisher.

Thomson, A., and Silverman, M.: Single-birth measurement of lung mechanics in very low-birth-weight infants, Crit. Care Med. **13**:4, 1985.

PART THREE

The respiratory distress syndrome and its management

Despite the enormous strides that have been made in understanding the pathophysiology of RDS and more particularly the role of surfactant in its cause, RDS, or hyaline membrane disease, as it is still commonly known, remains by far the most frequent clinical problem encountered among preterm infants. Furthermore this has persisted despite real progress made in preventing RDS either by pharmacologic inhibition of premature labor, prevention of iatrogenic prematurity (specifically that related to elective cesarean section), or accelerating pulmonary maturity. The improved outcome in RDS, which can be attributed directly to the application of many technologic advances, has raised questions as to whether it is still the major cause of death in low birth weight infants. Because the management of RDS has become more complex, there has been a dramatic increase in the complications of treatment and sequelae of the disease process. Thus autopsy studies show an increase in the incidence of air leak syndromes, bronchopulmonary dysplasia, and intracranial hemorrhage. In this section the clinical features and evaluation of infants with RDS are discussed and current therapeutic approaches short of assisted ventilation outlined.

INCIDENCE

RDS continues to be one of the most important causes of mortality and morbidity in newborn babies, although lack of a precise definition necessitates cautious interpretation of statistics regarding incidence, mortality, and outcome. The diagnosis can be clearly established pathologically or by documentation of surfactant deficiency; nonetheless most series refer only to a combination of clinical, biochemical, and roentgenologic features. Approximately 10% to 15% of babies weighing less than 2.5 kg at birth will manifest RDS, the highest incidence being observed among the lowest birth weight groups. The greatest risk factor appears to be gestational age, whereas other risk factors include maternal diabetes, maternal bleeding, and perinatal asphyxia. The incidence varies inversely with advancing gestational age; thus only exceptional cases are encountered at 37 weeks or beyond, whereas RDS occurs in greater than 70% of newborns at 28 to 30 weeks of gestation. The disease occurs throughout the world with a slight male predominance.

PHARMACOLOGIC ACCELERATION OF PULMONARY MATURATION

See also Chapter 9.

If premature delivery of any infant appears probable

or necessary, the ability to hasten lung maturity is available. Schutte has demonstrated that the incidence and severity of RDS are reduced when labor can be postponed for 12 hours to 3 weeks after admission, either in the presence or absence of therapeutic intervention. In recent years much attention has been focused on hormonal and other pharmacologic agents that achieve this result (see Part one). The effects of various catecholamines as well as aminophylline have been studied; however, the most promising method at this time appears to be prepartum glucocorticoid administration. Although conflicting evidence has appeared in the literature, it appears that these agents, when administered to the mother at least 24 to 48 hours before delivery, decrease both the incidence and severity of RDS. Corticosteroids appear to be only effective before 34 weeks of gestation and when administered at least 24 hours and no longer than 7 days before delivery. Furthermore, very small premature infants do not appear to benefit. Ballard's data indicate that prenatal beta-methasone therapy is less effective in male than in female infants in decreasing the incidence of RDS. Similar sex differences in response to maternal dexamethasone have been reported in the collaborative study and require further study to define the mechanism underlying this apparent male disadvantage. Postpartum administration of corticosteroids to the infant is of no benefit. To date, there are no proven complications of this treatment, but concern has been expressed about the possibility of increased infection in both mother and infant, as well as potential effects on the infant's later growth and development.

PATHOPHYSIOLOGY

The lungs of infants who succumb from RDS have a characteristic uniformly ruddy and airless appearance, macroscopically resembling hepatic tissue. On microscopic examination the striking feature is diffuse atelectasis such that only a few widely dilated alveoli are readily distinguishable (Fig. 28-13). An eosinophilic membrane lines the visible air spaces that usually constitute terminal bronchioles and alveolar ducts. This characteristic membrane (from which the term *hyaline membrane disease* is derived) consists of a fibrinous matrix of materials derived from the blood and contains cellular debris derived from injured epithelium. The recovery phase is characterized by regeneration of alveolar cells, including the type II cells, with a resultant increase in surfactant activity.

The development of RDS is thought to begin with impaired or delayed surfactant synthesis followed by a series of events that may progressively increase the severity of the disease for several days (Fig. 28-14). Surfactant synthesis is a dynamic process that depends on factors such as pH, temperature, and perfusion and may be compromised by cold stress, hypovolemia, hypoxemia, and acidosis. Other unfavorable factors such as exposure to high oxygen concentration and the effects of respirator management may further damage the alveolar epithelial lining, resulting in reduced surfactant synthesis. In fact, as the number of very low birth weight infants with RDS requiring assisted ventilation has dramatically grown, such a prolonged, complicated, clinical course has become the rule rather than the exception. Deficiency of surfactant and the accompanying decrease in

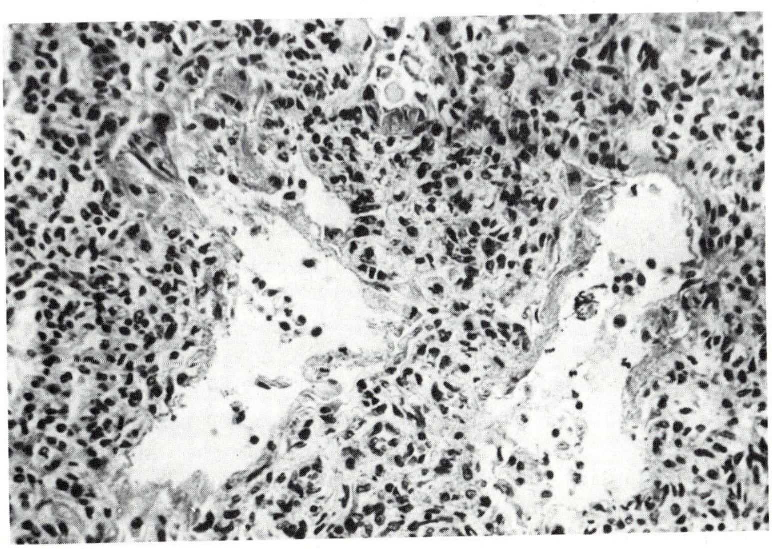

Fig. 28-13. Photomicrograph of lungs of infant with RDS. Note marked atelectasis and hyaline membrane lining the dilated alveolar ducts.

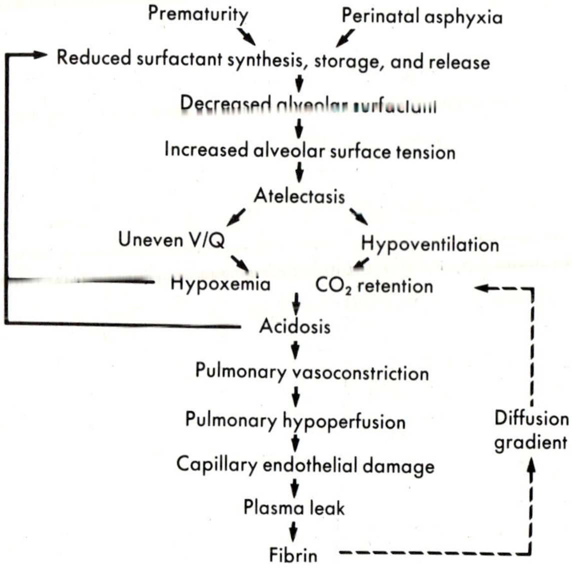

Fig. 28-14. Pathogenesis of RDS.

lung compliance lead to alveolar hypoventilation and V/Q imbalance. The resultant hypoxemia and hypercarbia in turn may reduce surfactant production. Severe hypoxemia will result in lactic acidosis secondary to systemic hypoperfusion and anaerobic metabolism. Hypoxemia and acidosis also result in pulmonary hypoperfusion secondary to pulmonary vasoconstriction, and the result is a further aggravation of hypoxemia as a result of right-to-left shunting at the level of the ductus arteriosus and foramen ovale and within the lung itself. The role of decreased pulmonary blood flow in reducing surfactant production after birth, however, has not been clearly established. It is important to note that the relative roles of surfactant deficiency and pulmonary hypoperfusion in the overall clinical picture of RDS will vary somewhat with each patient.

CLINICAL FEATURES

Infants with RDS characteristically are seen either immediately after delivery or within several hours of birth with the typical signs of neonatal respiratory distress, as outlined below and in Part two. It should be emphasized that continuing close observation and careful physical examination of the infant are as essential as roentgenographic studies in evaluating the clinical status of any infant with respiratory distress. The hazards of hastily concluding that all infants with respiratory distress have RDS are discussed in Part five.

Infants with RDS typically are initially seen with a combination of tachypnea, nasal flaring, subcostal and intercostal retractions, cyanosis, and an expiratory grunt. Respiratory rate is usually regular and increased well above the normal range of 30 to 60 breaths per minute. The presence of apneic episodes at this early stage is an ominous sign that may reflect thermal instability or sepsis but more often is a sign of hypoxemia and respiratory failure. Retractions are prominent and are the result of the very compliant rib cage being drawn in on inspiration as the infant generates high intrathoracic pressures to expand the poorly compliant lungs. The typical expiratory grunt is an early feature of the clinical course and may subsequently disappear. It is thought to result from partial closure of the glottis during expiration and in this way acts as a means of trapping alveolar air and maintaining the FRC (Part two). It should be noted that, although these signs are characteristic for neonatal respiratory distress, they may result from a wide variety of nonpulmonary causes such as hypothermia, hypoglycemia, anemia, or polycythemia (Part five), and furthermore such nonpulmonary conditions may complicate the clinical course of RDS.

Additional clinical features include pallor, resulting from either anemia or peripheral vasoconstriction. The blood pressure must be closely monitored in infants with RDS (see Appendix C). Cyanosis, which may be masked by pallor, is a consequence of right-to-left shunting in RDS and is typically relieved by administering a higher concentration of oxygen. In severe respiratory distress oxygen may not relieve cyanosis (see hyperoxia test, Part two), and ventilatory support or other measures need to be initiated. Acrocyanosis of the hands and feet is a common finding in normal infants and should not be confused with central cyanosis, which always must be investigated and treated. Peripheral edema is frequently present in RDS and of no particular prognostic significance.

Auscultation of the chest is seldom rewarding in infants, since the breath sounds are widely transmitted and cannot always be relied on to reflect pathologic conditions. In moderate to severe RDS breath sounds may be harsh or markedly decreased because of atelectasis. Unilaterally decreased breath sounds (with mediastinal shift to the opposite side) or bilaterally decreased air entry are indicative of pneumothorax, and immediate transillumination is performed (Part five). The detection of a murmur in a cyanotic infant with respiratory distress may indicate underlying cardiac disease or reflect increased pulmonary vascular resistance. The murmur of a patent ductus arteriosus (PDA) is most frequently audible during the recovery phase of RDS when pulmonary vascular resistance has fallen below systemic levels and there is left-to-right shunting (Part four). Distant, muffled heart sounds should alert one to the possibility of pneumopericardium or rarely a pericardial effusion. Percussion of the chest is of no diagnostic value in preterm infants.

A constant feature of RDS is the early onset of clinical

signs of the disease, within the first 6 hours of delivery. Inadequate observation may lead to the impression of a symptom-free period of several hours. The uncomplicated clinical course is characterized by a progressive worsening of symptoms with a peak severity by days 2 to 3 and onset of recovery by 72 hours. When the disease process is severe enough to require assisted ventilation or complicated by the development of air leaks, significant shunting through a PDA, or early signs of bronchopulmonary dysplasia, recovery may be delayed for days, weeks, or months.

ROENTGENOGRAPHIC FINDINGS

See Chapter 13.

The diagnosis of RDS is based on a combination of the previously described clinical features, evidence of prematurity (including biochemical pulmonary immaturity [Chapter 9]), exclusion of other causes of respiratory distress (Part five), and the characteristic roentgenologic appearance. The typical roentgenographic features consist of a diffuse reticulogranular pattern in both lung fields with superimposed air bronchograms (Fig. 28-15). The granular pattern is primarily caused by alveolar atelectasis, although there may be some component of pulmonary edema. The prominent air bronchograms represent aerated bronchioles superimposed on a background of nonaerated alveoli. An area of localized air bronchograms may be normal in the left lower lobe overlying the cardiac silhouette, but in RDS they are widely distributed particularly in the upper lobes. Heart size is typically normal or slightly increased. Cardiomegaly may be prominent as a consequence of birth asphyxia, in infants of diabetic mothers, or because of the development of congestive cardiac failure from a PDA. It is not uncommon for the granularity to be distributed asymmetrically throughout the lung fields in RDS with aeration most diminished on the right. It is important to note that the roentgenologic appearance of RDS, typical or atypical, cannot be reliably differentiated from that of neonatal pneumonia, most commonly caused by group B streptococci. This problem has been the major reason for the widespread use of antibiotics in the initial management of infants with RDS. The increased use of various means of ventilatory support and the enhanced survival of infants with more severe pulmonary disease have resulted in the more frequent roentgenographic recognition of complications such as pulmonary air leaks (Part five) and bronchopulmonary dysplasia (Part six) in the sickest infant. Recent evidence indicates that infants with RDS have a larger thymic silhouette compared with infants of comparable size without RDS. This supports the theory that patients with RDS had inadequate exposure to endogenous corticosteroids during fetal life.

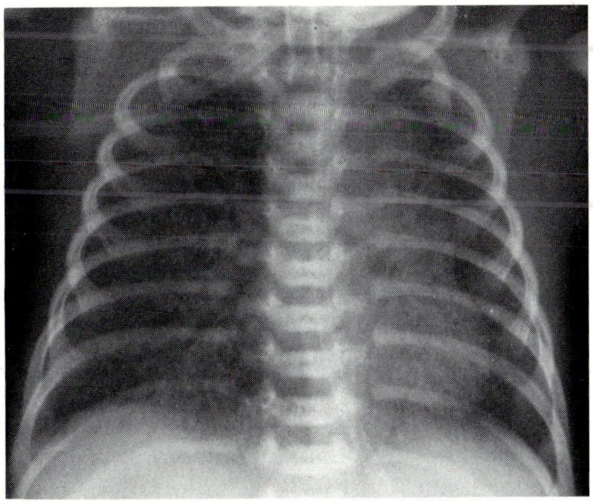

Fig. 28-15. Typical roentgenographic appearance of RDS with reticulogranular infiltrate and an air bronchogram.

Echocardiographic evaluation of infants with RDS may be of value in the diagnosis of a PDA, to quantitate elevations in pulmonary artery pressure (Part five and Chapter 29), and to exclude congenital heart diseases.

ASSESSMENT OF BLOOD GASES

See also Part two.

The ability to accurately monitor and interpret the blood gas status of infants is essential in all cases of neonatal respiratory disease. In its most basic form this involves intermittent arterial sampling usually via an indwelling umbilical arterial catheter or less commonly a radial arterial line. Infants with acute respiratory distress requiring an increased inspired oxygen concentration or assisted ventilation should have blood gases sampled every 4 hours or more often as their clinical condition dictates to minimize morbidity from oxygen toxicity (Parts four and six). Although the various techniques for continuous Po_2 monitoring are widely and very successfully employed, controlled studies that demonstrate decreased morbidity from their use are not available. The practical aspects of oxygen administration are discussed in Chapter 24.

Arterial sampling

The precise measurement of arterial oxygen tension (Pao_2) has been enhanced by incorporating an oxygen electrode into the tip of an umbilical arterial catheter. After appropriate in vivo calibration such an intravascular electrode allows Pao_2 to be continuously monitored while minimizing the need for frequent arterial sampling. A closely related but less popular technique has been to fit a fiberoptic oximeter into the umbilical arterial catheter to continuously measure oxygen saturation instead of the more conventional PaO_2. The latter is customarily maintained between 50 and 90 mm Hg in infants with RDS. Even with these newer techniques intermittent arterial sampling still is required to maintain the arterial carbon dioxide tension ($PaCO_2$) at less than 55 mm Hg and the pH at least 7.25 (see also Chapter 22).

The technique of umbilical catheterization, its complications, and their management are discussed in detail in Chapter 24. It should be noted that, although umbilical arterial catheters still form the basic means of arterial sampling in infants with RDS, the list of catheter-related complications is formidable. The most frequent visible problem from an umbilical or radial line is blanching or cyanosis of part of or all the distal extremity, resulting either from vasospasm or a thrombotic or embolic incident. This complication may be reduced in the case of an umbilical catheter by high placement with the catheter tip at the level of the seventh or eighth thoracic vertebra as opposed to lower placement at the third or fourth lumbar segment just above the aortic bifurcation. Tyson and colleagues have observed thromboatheromatous complications resulting from umbilical arterial catheters in 33 of 56 neonates at autopsy. Hypertension may result if a renal artery is involved, and passage of a catheter past the origin of the superior mesenteric artery has been suggested to increase the risk of necrotizing enterocolitis. Abdominal aortic thrombosis should be diagnosed by careful ultrasound examination. Butt has documented retrograde blood flow into the proximal aorta during flushing of radial and umbilical arterial lines. As this may cause transient blood pressure elevation, routine flushing should be performed with a small volume over a period of seconds. The risk of arterial thrombi appears to be reduced by the addition of small amounts of heparin to the continuous infusion and the use of siliconized rubber catheters with decreased thrombogenicity. All these complications illustrate the importance of applying rigid criteria for the insertion and removal of indwelling arterial catheters and the need for less hazardous methods of monitoring blood gases.

Transcutaneous monitoring

Transcutaneous measurement of PO_2 ($TcPO_2$) has emerged as an important technique for indirectly determining PaO_2 in a noninvasive and continuous manner. Electrodes for $TcPO_2$ monitoring consist of modified Clark electrodes (as used in blood gas analyzers) that are attached to the skin and can be heated to a desired temperature. A good correlation between $TcPO_2$ and PaO_2 can be obtained at a skin electrode temperature of 44° C in both term and preterm infants in the presence or absence of respiratory disease and over a wide range of PaO_2 (Fig. 28-16). The precise reasons for the close relationship between PO_2 in the arterial blood and at the skin surface are quite complex, although it clearly depends on adequate vasodilatation of the capillary bed under the electrode with increasing temperature. It appears that the increase in PO_2 at the skin surface caused by heating to 44° C approximates the decrease in PO_2 caused by O_2 consumption during passage from blood to skin surface, resulting in no net change between the arterial and surface PO_2 values.

For infants with mild respiratory distress $TcPO_2$ monitoring is extremely valuable and may make it unnecessary to insert an umbilical arterial catheter, provided intermittent assessments of pH and PCO_2 are made. Gen-

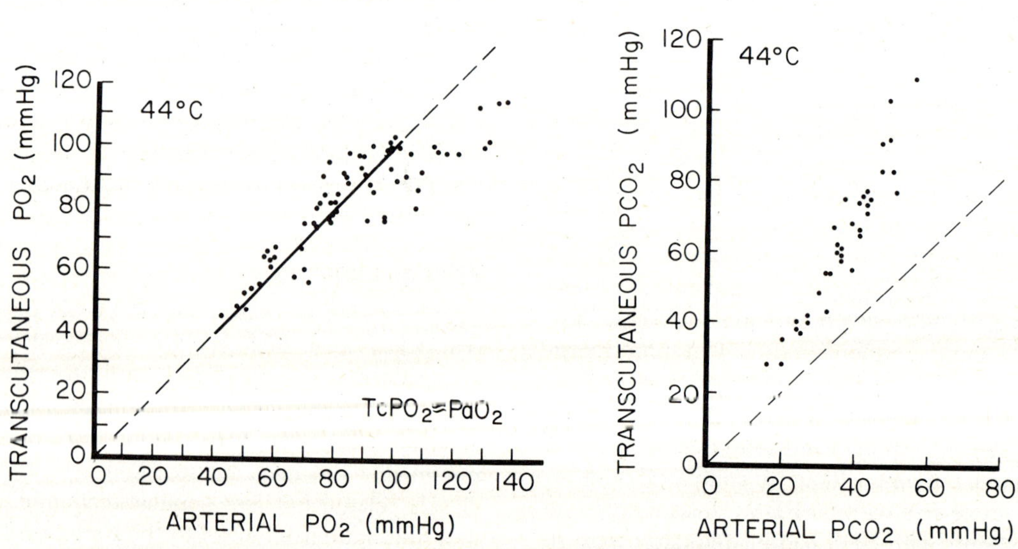

Fig. 28-16. *Left,* Correlation between transcutaneous and arterial PO_2 in preterm infants with RDS. *Right,* Correlation between transcutaneous and arterial PCO_2 in preterm and term infants with cardiopulmonary disease (see text).

erally, this is not the case in infants with moderate or severe respiratory difficulty in whom $TcPo_2$ measurement remains an important adjunct rather than a substitute for arterial blood gas sampling. In profoundly ill neonates with tissue hypoperfusion $TcPo_2$ measurements may somewhat underestimate the infant's level of Pao_2. As levels of Pao_2 exceed 90 mm Hg, $TcPo_2$ will underestimate Pao_2, and the scatter between these two parameters will increase (Fig. 28-16). Thus $TcPo_2$ should be maintained at less than 90 mm Hg to ensure an optimum correlation with Pao_2 and to minimize the risk of hyperoxemia.

The major impact of $TcPo_2$ monitoring in these acutely ill infants has been to rapidly optimize respiratory care and drastically reduce the time required to determine optimum inspired oxygen concentrations, levels of CPAP, and respirator settings. Other benefits include the ability to determine responses to all procedures. Furthermore complications such as pneumothorax, endotracheal tube dislodgment, disconnection from oxygen supply, or respirator malfunction will be rapidly recognized so that immediate corrective treatment can be initiated. A major contribution of $TcPo_2$ monitoring has been the repeated observation that excessive and vigorous handling of sick infants results in hypoxemia. Long and associates noted that the use of continuous oxygen monitoring resulted in a reduced amount of both hypoxia and hyperoxia and furthermore that many episodes of inappropriately low or high oxygen levels would go undetected without continuous monitoring. Nonetheless there are conflicting data as to whether transcutaneous monitoring has reduced the number of arterial blood gas samples in acutely ill neonates.

$TcPo_2$ also has proved invaluable in the longer term care of small premature infants recovering from RDS and requiring oxygen for weeks or even months. Recently we have observed that nursing such infants in the prone rather than the supine position resulted in an increase in $TcPo_2$ especially in those infants who had residual cardiopulmonary disease. It should be noted that in older infants with a postnatal age in excess of 2 months $TcPo_2$ may underestimate Pao_2 (by a mean of approximately 15 mm Hg), although relative changes in oxygenation still can be readily discerned.

The temperature of the skin electrode must be carefully controlled to avoid burns to the skin, and for this reason the electrode is repositioned approximately every 4 hours. Transient areas of erythema are common and usually disappear within hours, although blister formation may occur, particularly in very sick infants with poor perfusion. Quantitation of the heat output of the skin electrode to maintain a temperature at 44° C may be a useful measure of tissue perfusion provided the electrode is properly insulated.

Transcutaneous measurement of Pco_2 offers a useful adjunct to $TcPo_2$ monitoring, increasingly by means of combined electrodes. In contrast to $TcPo_2$ measurements, a surprisingly good correlation between $TcPco_2$ and $Paco_2$ can be obtained using an electrode heated to only 37° C. This may relate to the more ready diffusibility of carbon dioxide compared with oxygen. Nonetheless the correlation can be significantly improved when the electrode is heated to either 42° or 44° C (Fig. 28-16), the latter being the optimum temperature for combined electrodes. The Pco_2 measured at the skin surface in this way is higher than the comparable arterial values. This appears to result from a combination of carbon dioxide production by the skin as a result of local metabolism, the heating effect on Pco_2 as it is warmed beneath the electrode, and other as yet undetermined factors. Transcutaneous Pco_2 electrodes respond to changes in carbon dioxide relatively slowly with an in vivo response time of approximately 60 to 90 seconds, compared with the brisk (5 to 10 seconds) response time for $TcPo_2$. Furthermore, $Paco_2$ does not change nearly as briskly as does Pao_2. Under conditions of profound hypoperfusion and shock the elevation of $TcPco_2$ over the simultaneous value of $Paco_2$ will be further increased, presumably as a result of CO_2 accumulation in tissues. The continuous measurement of tissue pH is being evaluated in infants; however, this requires the insertion of a small needle beneath the skin.

As poor perfusion, hyperoxemia, and advancing postnatal age may make $TcPo_2$ somewhat unreliable as a measure of Pao_2, the technique of continuous noninvasive measurement of arterial hemoglobin O_2 saturation has gained considerable acceptance (see also Chapter 21). This typically employs a microprocessor-based pulse oximeter comprising a light-emitting probe attached to the distal extremity of the infant. Oxygen saturation is computed from the light absorption characteristics of the pulsatile flow (containing both oxygenated and nonoxygenated hemoglobin) as it passes beneath the probe. The resultant monitor readings closely correlate with saturation measurements obtained from arterial samples. Deckardt has demonstrated that maintenance of an O_2 saturation above 80% should ensure a Pao_2 in excess of 40 mm Hg. On the other hand, as hyperoxic levels of Pao_2 are approached, saturation becomes less sensitive with flattening of the hemoglobin dissociation curve, and large changes in Pao_2 will cause only minor alterations in saturation. Thus, in the absence of arterial sampling both O_2 saturation and $TcPo_2$ must be interpreted with caution if hyperoxemia is to be avoided.

TREATMENT

Therapy for RDS comprises the careful application of general supportive measures supplemented by various specific means of controlling and/or assisting ventilation. Close and detailed supervision of small infants requires a dedicated, trained staff experienced and interested in problems specific to the newborn and skillful in the technical procedures involved.

Thermoregulation

Infants with respiratory difficulty require an optimum thermal environment to minimize oxygen consumption and oxygen requirements (Chapter 24). Infants who are hypoxic lose the ability to increase metabolic rate when cold stressed, and a fall in body temperature may be noted. Thus meticulous attention must be paid to the temperature and humidity of the infant's environment and inspired air so that the appropriate neutral thermal environment may be maintained.

Fluid, nutrition, and diuretics

See also Chapter 25.

The ability to supply an adequate caloric intake to the critically ill infant receiving respiratory assistance has been facilitated by the availability of intravenous amino acid–glucose and lipid solutions. The role of nutritional support for these infants cannot be overemphasized. Anderson demonstrated that premature infants receiving as little as 60 calories/kg/day with 10% of the calories provided as protein could remain in positive nitrogen balance (Chapter 25). In many units therefore it has become commonplace to start administration of an amino acid–glucose solution on the second or third day of life, especially for infants weighing less than 1,500 gm and receiving mechanical ventilation. An alternative is to begin small volume gavage feeds of formula or breast milk at this time. Fluid balance must be closely watched, since overenthusiastic attention to calories may result in fluid overload, PDA, and congestive heart failure. Maintenance fluid requirements usually begin at 60 to 80 ml/kg/day as a 10% dextrose solution and increase gradually to 150 ml/kg/day by the fifth day of life. However, these fluid requirements will be greatly modified by many additional factors, particularly the very high insensible water loss experienced by many very low birth weight infants under radiant warmers or phototherapy and the limited concentrating ability of immature kidneys (Chapter 25).

The precise role of diuretics during the acute phase of RDS remains somewhat uncertain, even though pulmonary interstitial edema may significantly influence gas exchange in these infants. Early studies demonstrated a variable improvement in oxygenation associated with diuretic administration. More recent data have revealed that spontaneous diuresis precedes improvement in lung function and recovery from RDS, suggesting a causal relationship. Yeh evaluated the role of early furosemide therapy at 1 mg/kg/day over three intravenous doses in a randomized controlled trial of infants with RDS receiving mechanical ventilation. Although the control group had increased urine output and decreased ventilator mean airway pressure at 48 to 72 hours after initiation of the study, these effects were enhanced in the furosemide group, who also showed improved oxygenation at that time. The facilitated ventilator weaning associated with furosemide may have resulted from the diuretic or systemic vascular effects of the drug. Contrary to a previous report, the incidence of PDA was not increased, nor was there any improvement in longer term morbidity (such as bronchopulmonary dysplasia) or mortality. Furosemide caused an increased renal excretion of sodium, chloride, and calcium, and renal calcification has been reported following longer term drug administration in preterm infants. Thus the short-term improvement in pulmonary status must be weighed against possible long-term side effects, and so routine use of furosemide is not recommended.

In a retrospective study Stevenson found that premature infants with RDS accompanied by a PDA had received larger volumes of fluid during the 2 days before the diagnosis of PDA than did control infants without evidence of a PDA. In a prospective study using sequential analysis, Bell showed that the risk of a PDA with congestive heart failure was greater in infants receiving a high-volume regimen (169 ± 20 ml/kg/day) than those on a low-volume regimen (122 ± 14 ml/kg/day) designed to meet average estimated water requirements (Chapter 25). In the high-volume group 35 out of 85 (41%) developed murmurs consistent with a PDA, and 11 of these were associated with congestive heart failure. In contrast, only 9 of 85 (10%) of the infants in the low-volume group had a PDA murmur, and two developed congestive heart failure. More cases of necrotizing enterocolitis also were observed in the high-volume group. This, together with other recent data, indicates that limitation of fluid intake could possibly reduce the risk of PDA, necrotizing enterocolitis, and bronchopulmonary dysplasia. The fluid therapy in infants with RDS is thus a critical aspect of care.

The renal inability to conserve salt together with a low sodium intake, overzealous use of diuretics, or the osmotic diuresis associated with hyperglycemia all may precipitate hyponatremia, particularly in infants weighing less than 1,500 gm. Maintenance of sodium balance usually is achieved by the administration of 2 to 4 mEq/kg/day of sodium, commencing at 24 to 48 hours, and close monitoring of serum sodium levels. Potassium balance is accomplished by adding 1 to 2 mEq/kg/day to the intravenous infusion from the second day of life.

Intravenous lipid seldom is used in the acute states of respiratory disease because the infants often have hyperbilirubinemia. Orogastric feeding is not often recommended while infants are receiving nasal CPAP. Infants to whom intermittent positive-pressure ventilation (IPPV) is being administered by means of a respirator may be fed with caution. We have reported that, in infants who had recovered from RDS, nasogastric feeding did not change PaO_2.

Acid-base therapy

The need to correct acid-base disturbances should be determined by evaluation of pH, PCO_2, bicarbonate, and changes in buffer base (Chapter 25). Metabolic acidosis is most often encountered when the infant has been depressed at birth and required resuscitation. (See Chapter 22 for emergency treatment in the delivery room of acidosis associated with asphyxia.) A subsequent metabolic acidosis out of proportion to the degree of respiratory distress may signify hypoperfusion, sepsis, or an intraventricular hemorrhage.

Respiratory acidosis may require transient or prolonged ventilation therapy (Part four). Administration of sodium bicarbonate to infants with respiratory acidosis provides only transient correction at best and may further increase the PCO_2. It usually is not necessary to correct a respiratory acidosis if the pH is greater than 7.25 unless an infant's condition is unstable or deteriorating. Severe acidosis, respiratory or metabolic, especially when coupled with hypoxia, may result in pulmonary arterial vasoconstriction and ventilation-perfusion abnormalities or may result in dysrhythmia or decreased cardiac output or both. In severe respiratory acidosis, alkali therapy should be withheld until some form of assisted ventilation has been initiated. If this fails to improve oxygenation and raise the pH, sodium bicarbonate may be administered while continuing with assisted ventilation and always attempting to determine the cause of the acidosis.

Antibiotics in RDS

See also Parts four and five.

Neonatal pneumonia (most commonly caused by group B streptococci) may mimic RDS both clinically and roentgenographically and thus be indistinguishable from it. Such infection usually is acquired around the time of delivery either through ascending infection or passage through a colonized genital tract. The potentially fulminant course of neonatal pneumonia and the difficulty in distinguishing it from RDS have led to the recommendation that all infants with significant respiratory distress receive antibiotics following appropriate cultures. Features suggestive of neonatal infection include maternal fever, prolonged rupture of membranes, persistent hypotension and/or metabolic acidosis, early onset of apnea, organisms in the gastric aspirate, neutropenia, and neutrophilia (Chapter 31). Nonetheless the absence of these features does not exclude the diagnosis of pneumonia. A pencillin combined with an aminoglycoside is the antibiotic regimen of choice, and should be discontinued after 72 hours if cultures are negative.

Transfusion

See also Chapter 32, part two.

It is customary to maintain a venous hematocrit of 40% to 45% during the acute phase of RDS to support an adequate oxygen-carrying capacity. The use of exchange transfusion also has been proposed as a means of increasing the delivery of oxygen to tissues. Delivoria-Papadopoulos demonstrated significantly improved survival after exchange transfusion with fresh adult blood. The presumption was that provision of red blood cells with an increased DPG content would shift the oxygen affinity curve to release more oxygen to tissues. On the other hand, exchange transfusion has a morbidity of its own and there may be an increase in the risk of retrolental fibroplasia following exchange transfusion. Therefore the latter has not been accepted as an established mode of therapy for RDS.

Surfactant therapy

The discovery that surfactant deficiency was key in the pathophysiology of RDS led several investigators to administer artificial aerosolized phospholipids to infants with RDS. In these studies only limited therapeutic success was encountered. In contrast, animal models in which natural surfactant compounds were used yielded more promising results. This stimulated Fujiwara to develop a mixture of both natural and synthetic surface-active lipids for use in humans. The goal was to achieve alveolar stability with less potential risk for a reaction to foreign protein than would be the case with exclusively natural surfactant. When administered to an initial group of 10 preterm infants with severe RDS who were not improving despite artificial ventilation, a single 10 ml of surfactant instilled into the endotracheal tubes resulted in a dramatic decrease in inspired oxygen and ventilator pressures. None of the infants in this uncontrolled series subsequently succumbed from RDS. Recovery, however, was complicated by clinical evidence of a PDA in nine of the infants, possibly the result of a prompt fall in pulmonary vascular resistance with the resultant left-to-right shunting following surfactant therapy. This observation has been confirmed by Clyman in preterm lambs.

Some of the major resolved and unresolved issues related to exogenous surfactant administration are summarized here. Much current enthusiasm is directed toward the use of reconstituted bovine surfactant as described by Fujiwara. This has proved effective in the neonatal baboon model in improving pulmonary compliance and oxygenation, although increased lung blood flow resulting from a PDA was again apparent. Nonetheless, Durand has also demonstrated improved pulmonary function and survival in preterm lambs treated with a purely synthetic protein-free surfactant preparation. Thus the issue of natural versus synthetic surfactant is not entirely resolved, although purely synthetic surfactant has not proved beneficial in human infants.

Surfactant therapy for RDS

KNOWN

Improvement in arterial oxygenation and ventilation
Major ingredient: Dipalmitoyl phosphatidylcholine—Dose of 50 to 100 mg/kg
Administration of fluid suspension by means of endotracheal tube
Natural surfactant more efficacious than synthetics
Instillation before first breath optimal

UNKNOWN

Optimum preparation: natural/synthetic, combination and stability
Duration of effect and need for retreatment
Risk of infection
Pharmacokinetics/metabolism of surfactant preparation
Timing and proper administration for established RDS
Effects on ductus arteriosus
Interaction with endogenous surfactant
Immunologic effects

Modified from Taeusch, H.W., Clements, J., and Benson, B.: Am. Rev. Respir. Dis. **128:**791, 1983. Adaptation by M.S. Kwong.

Various other forms of largely natural surfactant are giving impressive results in preterm infants with RDS. Hallman employed pooled human surfactant obtained from term amniotic fluid in a controlled trial of infants less than 30 weeks of gestation and demonstrated improved oxygenation and mean airway pressure. Meanwhile, randomized controlled clinical trials performed in Buffalo, Rochester, and Toronto have all employed surfactant obtained from calf lungs. In each case a volume of approximately 3 ml of a surfactant preparation that was predominantly phospholipid (80% phosphatidylcholine with only 1% protein) was instilled into the infant's trachea. The data of Enhorning from Toronto clearly demonstrated that surfactant instillation before the first breath improved gas exchange and lowered respiratory support over the first 72 hours in infants of less than 30 weeks gestation (Fig. 28-17). The Rochester trial suggested that one dose of surfactant administered at birth may be insufficient for some infants. Thus both clinical and in vitro data point to the ability of bovine lung extract to exhibit the important surface tension–lowering properties of human surfactant. Optimum timing of administration and duration of effectiveness still need clarification. The unresolved issues of possible complications and recognition of infant populations for whom instillation of surfactant at birth is appropriate await wider clinical trials (see box).

Extracorporeal membrane oxygenation

Extracorporeal membrane oxygenation (ECMO) is an innovative technique that offers promise as a means of supporting life during intractible respiratory failure in

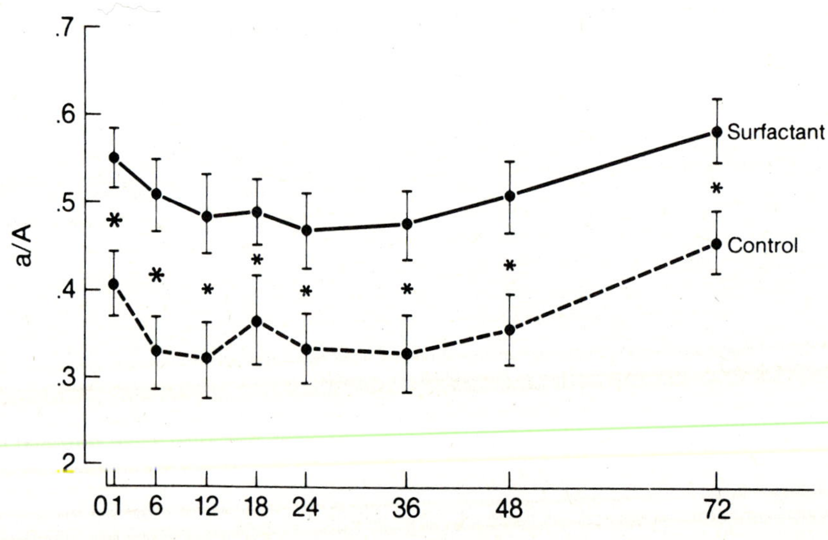

Fig. 28-17. Arterial/alveolar (a/A) Po_2 ratio for surfactant-treated and control infants. Asterisks indicate significant differences. (From Enhorning, G., and others: Pediatrics **76:**145, 1985.)

selected patients. It has also been suggested as an alternative or adjunct to conventional respirator therapy in the hope of decreasing acute and chronic lung damage. Perfusion and gas exchange are performed by means of prolonged venoarterial or venovenous cardiopulmonary bypass through a membrane lung. This allows the infant's heart and lungs to recover at low ventilator settings and inspired oxygen concentrations. This experimental approach has had some encouraging results in the management of neonatal respiratory failure in a limited number of very sick infants with RDS, PFC, meconium aspiration syndrome, and diaphragmatic hernia.

Despite the technical challenge and manpower expenditure involved in its delivery, ECMO is considered a useful therapeutic option for respiratory failure in several major neonatal centers. Although data from a conventional clinical trial have not been collected, Bartlett has reported on 11 ECMO survivors weighing more than 2 kg who were in respiratory failure on standard therapy. Preliminary follow-up data indicate no evidence of neurologic injury that could be specifically attributed to carotid ligation or to the use of ECMO per se. Nonetheless, the technique is invasive, has inherent risks, and should only be employed by teams who are familiar with the procedure.

Richard J. Martin
Avroy A. Fanaroff

BIBLIOGRAPHY

General

Ablow, R.C., and others: A comparison of early onset group B streptococcal neonatal infection and the respiratory distress syndrome of the newborn, N. Engl. J. Med. **294**:65, 1976.

Avery, M.D., Fletcher, B.D., and Williams, R.G.: The lung and its disorders in the newborn infant, ed. 4, Philadelphia, 1974, W.B. Saunders Co.

Ballard, P.L., and others: Fetal sex and prenatal betamethasone therapy, J. Pediatr. **97**:451, 1980.

Boyle, R.J., and Oh, W.: Respiratory distress syndrome, Clin. Perinatol. **5**:283, 1978.

Bryan, M.H., and others: Pulmonary function studies during the first year of life in infants recovering from the respiratory distress syndrome, Pediatrics **52**:169, 1973.

Chu, J., and others: The pulmonary hypoperfusion syndrome, Pediatrics **35**:733, 1965.

Papageorgiou, A.N., and others: The antenatal use of betamethasone in the prevention of RDS: a controlled double-blind study, Pediatrics **63**:73, 1979.

Perelman, R.H., and Farrell, P.M.: Analysis of causes of neonatal death in the U.S. with specific emphasis on fatal hyaline membrane disease, Pediatrics **70**:570, 1982.

Reynolds, E.O.R., and Taghizadeh, A.: Improved prognosis of infants mechanically ventilated for hyaline membrane disease, Arch. Dis. Child. **49**:505, 1974.

Robert, M.F., and others: The association between maternal diabetes and the respiratory distress syndrome in the newborn, N. Engl. J. Med. **294**:357, 1976.

Schutte, M.F., Treffers, P.E., and Koppe, J.G.: Threatened preterm labor: the influence of time factors on the incidence of respiratory distress syndrome, Obstet. Gynecol. **62**:287, 1983.

Strang, L.B.: Hyaline membrane disease. In Neonatal respiration, ed. 1, Oxford, England, 1977, Blackwell Scientific Publications, Ltd.

Tooley, W.H.: Hyaline membrane disease, Am. Rev. Respir. Dis. **115**:19, 1977.

Blood gas assessment

Butt, W.W., and others: Complications resulting from use of arterial catheters: retrograde flow and rapid elevation in blood pressure, Pediatrics **76**:250, 1985.

Cassady, G.: Transcutaneous monitoring in the newborn infant, J. Pediatr. **103**:837, 1983.

Conway, M., and others: Continuous monitoring of arterial oxygen tension using a catheter-tip polarographic electrode in infants, Pediatrics **57**:244, 1976.

Deckardt, R., and Steward, D.J.: Noninvasive arterial hemoglobin oxygen–saturation versus transcutaneous oxygen–tension monitoring in the preterm infant, Crit. Care Med. **12**:935, 1984.

Huch, R., and others: Transcutaneous Po_2 monitoring in routine management of infants and children with cardiorespiratory problems, Pediatrics **57**:681, 1976.

Long, J.G., Philip, A.G.S., and Lucey, J.F.: Excessive handling as a cause of hypoxemia, Pediatrics **65**:203, 1980.

Martin, R.J., Herrell, N., and Pultusker, M.: Transcutaneous measurement of carbon dioxide tension: the effect of sleep state in term infants, Pediatrics **67**:622, 1981.

Martin, R.J., and others: Effect of supine and prone positions on arterial oxygen tension in the preterm infant, Pediatrics **63**:528, 1979.

Mokrohisky, S.T., and others: Low positioning of umbilical artery catheters increases associated complications in newborn infants, N. Engl. J. Med. **299**:561, 1978.

Peabody, J.L., and Emery, J.R.: Noninvasive monitoring of blood gases in the newborn, Clin. Perinatol. **12**:147, 1985.

Tyson, J.E., deSa, D.J., and Moore, S.: Thromboatheromatous complications of umbilical arterial catheterization in the newborn period, Arch. Dis. Child. **51**:744, 1976.

Wilkinson, A.R., Phibbls, R.H., and Gregory, G.A.: Continuous measurement of oxygen saturation in sick newborn infants, J. Pediatr. **93**:1016, 1978.

Fluid, nutrition, and diuretics

Anderson, T.L., and others: A controlled trial of glucose versus glucose and amino acids in premature infants, J. Pediatr. **94**:947, 1979.

Bell, E.F., and others: Effect of fluid administration on the development of symptomatic patent ductus arteriosus and congestive heart failure in premature infants, N. Engl. J. Med. **302**:598, 1980.

Fanaroff, A.A., and Klaus, M.: The gastrointestinal tract—feeding and selected disorders. In Fanaroff, A.A.., and Klaus, M., editors: Care of the high risk neonate, ed. 3, Philadelphia, 1986, W.B. Saunders Co.

Green, T.P., and others: Diuresis and pulmonary function in premature infants with respiratory distress syndrome, J. Pediatr. **103**:618, 1983.

Stevenson, J.G.: Fluid administration in the association of patent ductus arteriosus complicating respiratory distress syndrome, J. Pediatr. **90**:257, 1977.

Yeh, T.F., and others: Early furosemide therapy in premature infants (2000 gm) with respiratory distress syndrome: a randomized controlled trial, J. Pediatr. **105**:603, 1984.

Transfusion

Delivoria-Papadopoulos, M., and others: The role of exchange transfusion in the management of low-birth-weight infants with and without severe RDS, J. Pediatr. **89**:273, 1976.

Surfactant therapy

Avery, M.E.: On replacing the surfactant, Pediatrics **65**:1176, 1980.
Clyman, R.I., and others: Increased shunt through the patent ductus arteriosus after surfactant replacement therapy, J. Pediatr. **100**:101, 1982.
Durand, D.J., and others: Effects of a protein-free, synthetic surfactant on survival and pulmonary function in preterm lambs, J. Pediatr. **107**:775, 1985.
Enhorning, G., and others: Prevention of neonatal respiratory distress syndrome by tracheal instillation of surfactant: a randomized clinical trial, Pediatrics **76**:145, 1985.
Fujiwara, T., and others: Artificial surfactant therapy in hyaline membrane disease, Lancet **1**:55, 1980.
Halliday, H.L., and others: Controlled trial of artificial surfactant to prevent respiratory distress syndrome, Lancet **1**:476, 1984.
Hallman, M., and others: Exogenous human surfactant for treatment of severe respiratory distress syndrome: a randomized prospective clinical trial, J. Pediatr. **106**:963, 1985.
Kwong, M.S., and others: Double-blind, clinical trial of calf lung surfactant extract for the prevention of hyaline membrane disease in extremely premature infants, Pediatrics **76**:585, 1985.
Notter, R.H., and Shapiro, D.L.: Lung surfactant in an era of replacement therapy, Pediatrics **68**:781, 1981.
Shapiro, D.L., and others: Double-blind, randomized trial of a calf lung surfactant extract administered at birth to very premature infants for prevention of respiratory distress syndrome, Pediatrics **76**:593, 1985.
Vidyasagar, D., and others: Bovine surfactant (Surfactant TA) therapy in immature baboons with hyaline membrane disease, Pediatrics **75**:1132, 1985.

ECMO

Bartlett, R.H., and Gazzaniga, A.B.: Extracorporeal circulation for cardiopulmonary failure, Curr. Probl. Surg. **15**:5, 1978.
Bartlett, R.H., and others: Extracorporeal circulation in neonatal respiratory failure: a prospective randomized study, Pediatrics **76**:479, 1985.
Kirkpatrick, B.V., and others: Use of extracorporeal membrane oxygenation for respiratory failure in term infants, Pediatrics **72**:872, 1983.

PART FOUR

Assisted ventilation and the complications of respiratory distress

Respiratory disease and its complications are the most common causes of neonatal mortality and morbidity. Nonetheless, assisted ventilation has contributed to a substantial improvement in outcome of infants with respiratory disorders. The actual practice of assisting ventilation varies widely between centers, and few controlled studies support the various approaches used. Regardless of the techniques employed, a thorough understanding of pulmonary mechanics is essential for assisted ventilation to be successfully administered to ill neonates (see Part two).

PULMONARY MECHANICS DURING ASSISTED VENTILATION

The mechanical properties of the total respiratory system, or parts of it such as the lungs or chest wall, may be described according to their elastic and resistive forces. The elastic forces of the respiratory system may be estimated from simultaneous changes in volume and pressure. *Compliance* is the term used to describe the elastic properties of a system and is calculated as follows.

$$\text{Compliance} = \frac{\Delta\text{Volume}}{\Delta\text{Pressure}}$$

Thus the higher the compliance, the larger the delivered volume per unit of pressure. In neonates the chest wall is very distensible and does not contribute a substantial elastic load when compared with the lungs. Respiratory system compliance in infants with normal lungs ranges from 0.003 to 0.006 L/cm H_2O. The most striking abnormality of pulmonary mechanics in neonates with RDS is decreased lung compliance, which ranges from 0.0005 to 0.001 L/cm H_2O. Therefore, for the same pressure gradient, the delivered tidal volume (V_T) will be reduced in infants with RDS, or, conversely, the pressure gradient would have to be increased to maintain a normal V_T.

Resistance is a property of the inherent capacity of the lungs to resist airflow. Therefore, in addition to the pressure required to overcome the elasticity of the respiratory system, pressure is needed to force gas through the airways (airway resistance) and exceed the viscous resistance of the lung tissue (tissue resistance). Resistance may be expressed as the change in pressure per unit change in flow as follows.

$$\text{Resistance} = \frac{\Delta\text{Pressure}}{\Delta\text{Flow}}$$

The mathematical product of these two mechanical characteristics of the respiratory system, compliance × resistance, may be used to calculate the time necessary for an instantaneous or step change in airway pressure or volume to equilibrate throughout the lungs. Thus the *time constant* (expressed in seconds) of the total respiratory system, or parts of it such as the lungs or chest wall, may be calculated as follows.

$$\text{Time constant} = \text{Resistance} \times \text{Compliance}$$

A duration equal to one time constant will allow a 63% equilibration of pressure or volume. If a longer duration is allowed for the step change to equilibrate, a higher percentage of the pressure (or volume) will be delivered (Fig. 28-18). Nonetheless, as can be seen from the shape of the curve in Fig. 28-18, little further equilibration of the change occurs beyond three to five time constants. The time necessary for the lungs to inflate and deflate will depend on the inspiratory and expiratory time constant, respectively. For example, in a healthy infant with a resistance of 30 cm H_2O/L/sec and a compliance of 0.004 L/cm H_2O, one time constant will be 0.12 second. For a fairly complete equilibration of pressure (five time constants or 5 × 0.12 second) an inspiratory or expiratory phase of 0.6 second will be necessary (assuming equal inspiratory and expiratory time constants). In contrast, since infants with RDS typically have a decreased compliance, their time constant and corresponding time for pressure and volume equilibration will be shorter. Therefore the stiff lungs of an infant with RDS will complete inflation and deflation in a shorter time than normal lungs. The application of the concept of time constant becomes particularly important when high frequencies are employed and inspiratory times, expiratory times, or both are so short that inspiration, expiration, or both are incomplete. If expiratory time is insufficient, expiration may not be complete, leading to an increase in FRC and inadvertent PEEP. Because infants with RDS have a decreased time constant, short inspiratory and expiratory times may be appropriate during the period of peak severity of their disease but insufficient after recovery from RDS when compliance is much higher. It is important to note that the mechanical properties of the ventilator and delivery system have to be considered when determining the times necessary for complete inspiration and expiration. For example, since resistance increases with decreasing radius of a lumen, infants intubated with small endotracheal tubes will have prolonged inspiratory and expiratory time constants.

In summary, it is important to consider the mechanical characteristics of the respiratory system to better understand the physiologic rationale for the blood gas responses that occur after ventilator setting changes. This is especially true in neonates with RDS whose disease is characterized by rapidly changing pulmonary mechanics and in whom high ventilatory frequencies are being increasingly employed.

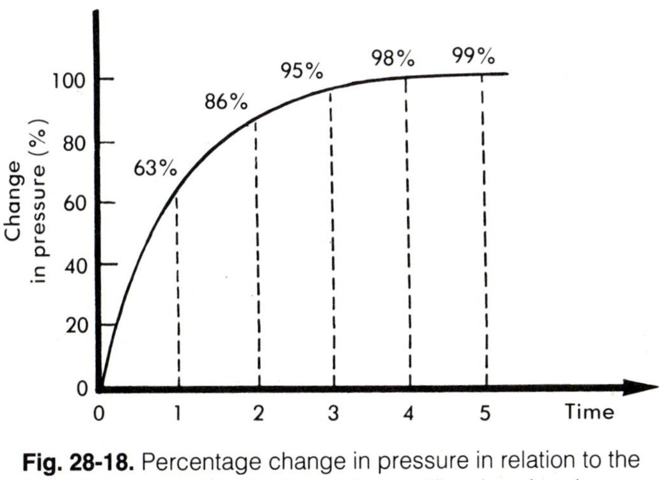

Fig. 28-18. Percentage change in pressure in relation to the time (in time constants) allowed for equilibration. As a longer time is allowed for equilibration, a higher percentage change in pressure will occur. The same rules govern the equilibration for step changes in volume. (Modified from Carlo, W.A., and Martin, R.J.: Pediatr. Clin. North Am. **33**:221, 1986.)

GAS EXCHANGE DURING ASSISTED VENTILATION

Carbon dioxide

Carbon dioxide (CO_2) diffuses readily from the blood into the alveoli and its elimination largely depends on the total amount of air that goes through the alveoli (alveolar ventilation). Since some of the V_T is distributed to parts of the lungs (such as the airways) that are not involved in gas exchange (dead space), alveolar ventilation per minute is calculated as follows:

$$\text{Minute alveolar ventilation} = (\text{Tidal volume} - \text{Dead space}) \times \text{Frequency}$$

In this calculation frequency is the number of breaths per minute. Since dead space stays relatively constant, increases in V_T or frequency increase alveolar ventilation, enhance the elimination of CO_2, and reduce $Pa{CO_2}$.

For a given compliance, V_T is largely determined by the pressure gradient between expiration and inspiration. Under special circumstances (short inspiratory time and long inspiratory time constant), the inspiratory duration may partially determine V_T. For example, a very short inspiratory time may not allow pressure to be equilibrated throughout the respiratory system in an infant with normal lungs (relatively long time constant), resulting in a decreased V_T. Thus, despite an apparent constant pressure gradient and compliance, V_T would be reduced. Frequency is the other major determinant of alveolar ventilation. Fig. 28-19 illustrates the interrelationship between the ventilator settings (on a standard pressure-limited ventilator) and the mechanical properties of the respiratory system as they determine minute ventilation and thus CO_2 elimination.

Oxygen

Oxygen exchange is not only affected by ventilation but also largely depends on the matching of perfusion with ventilation. Several studies in infants, mostly with RDS, have concluded that during assisted ventilation oxygenation is largely determined by the mean airway pressure applied (Fig. 28-20). Mean airway pressure is a measure of the average pressure to which the lungs are exposed during the respiratory cycle and may be calculated by dividing the area under the airway pressure curve by the duration of the cycle or from the following equation.

$$Paw = K(PIP - PEEP)[T_I/(T_I + T_E)] + PEEP$$

where Paw is mean airway pressure, K is a constant that

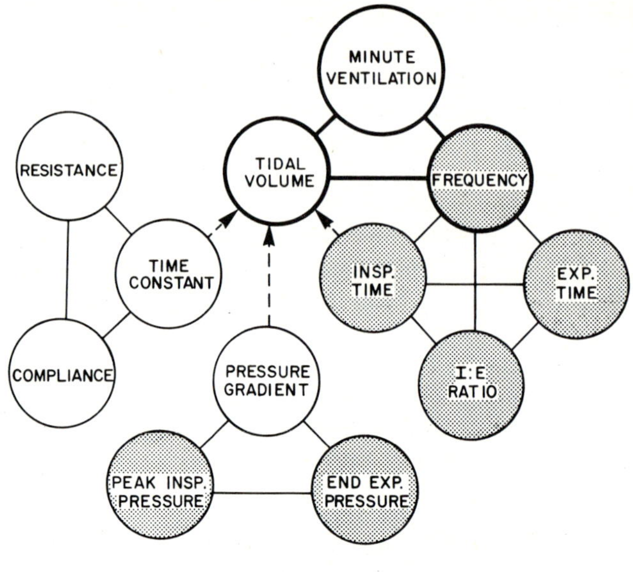

Fig. 28-19. Relationship between ventilator-controlled variables *(shaded circles)* and pulmonary mechanics in determining minute ventilation during pressure-limited, time-cycled ventilation. The relation between the circles that are joined by solid lines is described by simple mathematical equations. Thus simple mathematical equations determine the time constant of the lungs, the pressure gradient, and inspiratory time. These in turn determine the delivered tidal volume, which when multiplied by the respiratory frequency gives the minute ventilation. Alveolar ventilation may be calculated from the product of tidal volume and frequency when dead space is subtracted from the former. (Adapted and reproduced with permission from Chatburn, R.L., and Lough, M.D. In Lough, M.D., Doershuk, D., and Stern, R., editors: Pediatric respiratory therapy, ed. 3, Chicago, 1985, Year Book Medical Publishers.)

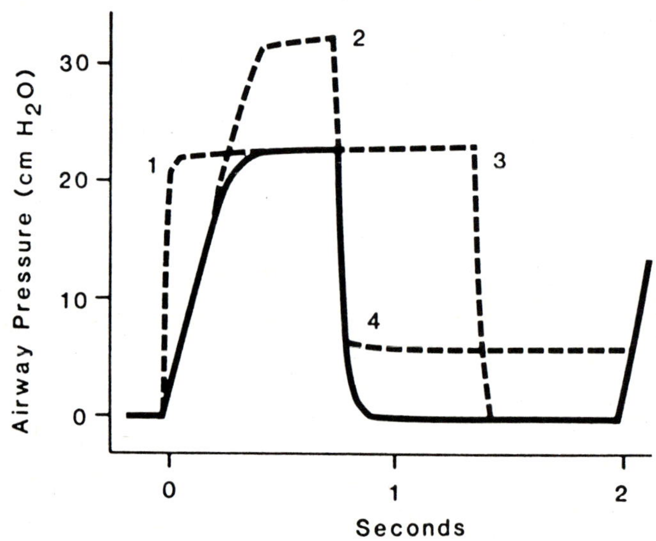

Fig. 28-20. Four different ventilator setting increases that augment mean airway pressure: (1) inspiratory flow, (2) peak inspiratory pressure, (3) I:E ratio, and (4) positive end-expiratory pressure. (From Harris, T.R. In Goldsmith, J.P., and Karotkin, E.H., editors: Assisted ventilation of the neonate, Philadelphia, 1981, W.B. Saunders Co. In Reynolds, E.D.R.: Int. Anesthesiol. Clin. **12:**259, 1974.)

depends on the rate of rise of the airway pressure curve (in clinical situations, K is always less than 1 and usually ranges from 0.8 to 0.9), PIP is peak inspiratory pressure, PEEP is positive end-expiratory pressure, T_I is inspiratory time, and T_E is expiratory time. Therefore Paw will be augmented by increasing any of the following (Fig. 28-20).

1. Inspiratory flow (will increase K)
2. PIP
3. Ratio of inspiratory time to expiratory time (I/E ratio)
4. PEEP

It is unclear precisely why Paw determines oxygenation, but this is probably related to prevention of atelectasis and optimization of lung volume, thus improving V/Q relationships. Although a direct relationship between Paw and oxygenation may exist, there are several limitations: (a) for the same change in Paw, increases in PIP and PEEP enhance oxygenation more than do changes in I/E ratio; (b) very high Paw may cause overdistension of airways and alveoli, leading to an increase in dead space and right-to-left shunting of blood in the lungs; (c) if a very high Paw is transmitted to the intrathoracic structures, cardiac output may decrease; despite adequate oxygenation, oxygen transport (arterial oxygen content × cardiac output) may decrease.

VENTILATORY MANAGEMENT

Continuous positive airway pressure

In 1971 Gregory introduced a new approach for management of RDS with the application of CPAP by means of head box or endotracheal tube to infants who were breathing spontaneously. The initial results were encouraging, since they not only demonstrated significant increase in PaO_2 with a resultant decrease in oxygen requirements, but the outcome data also suggested improved survival. Soon thereafter multiple reports describing different techniques of application appeared. These included a pressurized face chamber, face mask, plastic bags, and nasal prongs. Other investigators chose to indirectly produce positive transpulmonary pressure by exerting continuous negative pressure (CNP) around the chest wall either with a modified negative pressure ventilator or a chamber within the incubator to which a vacuum was applied. The purpose of all these different modes of therapy is to achieve continuous distending pressure (CDP) throughout the respiratory cycle. It should be apparent that this may be accomplished either by exerting a positive pressure on the airway (CPAP) or by exerting negative pressure around the thorax (CNP). Debate continues as to the most efficacious method by which to deliver CDP as well as the optimum time to initiate therapy.

The physiologic basis for the use of continuous distending airway pressure was first suggested by Harrison, who investigated the role of grunting in RDS. He concluded that grunting (exhaling against a partially closed glottis with active contraction of the abdominal muscles) represented an attempt by the infants to overcome atelectasis (Part two). When grunting was eliminated with endotracheal intubation, a fall in PaO_2 ensued. The grunting resumed after extubation, and PaO_2 rose promptly. Although it has been widely accepted that CPAP increases PaO_2, thereby allowing a reduction in fractional inspired O_2 concentrations (FiO_2), it is not entirely clear what physiologic factors account for these effects. It has been postulated that recruitment of previously collapsed alveoli results in better oxygenation by improving ventilation-perfusion relationships within the lungs. After application of CPAP, there is an increase in FRC, which presumably decreases intrapulmonary right-to-left shunting, lending credence to this idea. However, there is a variable effect on lung compliance, which usually decreases. This suggests that, in addition to recruitment of some alveoli, there also may be overdistention of others. With application of CDP the breathing pattern becomes more regular and slower, and grunting generally ceases. Because of the rapidity with which these changes occur, it has been postulated that the changes in frequency are mediated via the Hering-Breuer reflex because of the increase in FRC (Part five).

The optimum level of CDP may be defined as that airway pressure at which PaO_2 is maximum with minimum effect on cardiovascular function. If the pressure is increased above this level, $PaCO_2$ usually rises, probably owing to the decrease in lung compliance. Monitoring of esophageal pressure reveals a sharp rise when optimum CDP is achieved, suggesting recruitment of alveoli and enhanced transmission of airway pressure to the intrapleural space. The optimum level of CDP is not static in any given patient.

The initial report by Gregory described the use of either a pressurized head box or an endotracheal tube. Various modifications were suggested including a face mask that covered only the nose and mouth but required the exertion of great pressure on the head and face to maintain an adequate seal. Devices for CNP administration also were developed; however, an obvious drawback to these is that therapy must be interrupted for any procedure to be performed on the infant.

There are several advantages to the use of nasal prongs for CPAP delivery. This technique is relatively atraumatic, avoids the need for an endotracheal tube, allows constant access to the baby, is simple to set up and care for, and requires lower flow rates than do head or face chambers. An alternative method to the short nasal prongs is the use of nasopharyngeal tubes placed in one or both nares. There is a considerably higher work of breathing with nasal prongs compared with a face mask, which is thought to be a result of the resistance of the tubing. The systems for delivery of continuous distending airway pressure, therefore, continue to be modified.

Increases in the FiO_2 represent the minimum level of respiratory support that an infant with RDS may require. Such support is, however, frequently insufficient, and further assistance is required. Because CPAP almost invariably has a beneficial effect on PaO_2, hypoxemia remains the most universally accepted rationale for institution of this therapy. Specific guidelines, however, are still quite variable. In our nursery the inability of the infant to maintain a PaO_2 of greater than or equal to 60 mm Hg in an FiO_2 of 0.7 constitutes adequate indication for initiating CPAP in RDS. CPAP is applied earlier under certain circumstances, particularly in infants with early onset of severe RDS. The place for routine early administration of CDP to infants with RDS remains to be determined. Because CPAP has a variable effect on $PaCO_2$, one must monitor the blood gases closely, and if respiratory failure ensues (i.e., $PaCO_2$ greater than 55 to 60 mm Hg, pH less than 7.20), endotracheal intubation with mechanical ventilation should be instituted.

In summary, CDP has proved an extremely effective tool for the management of RDS. The level and duration of high oxygen concentration required by these infants are both reduced, and the need for mechanical ventilation appears to be decreased. In addition, CPAP is extremely useful as an intermediate step in weaning infants from mechanical ventilation, and there is evidence that the duration of intubation is decreased. Several studies have additionally shown an improved outcome with decreases in both the mortality and the incidence of bronchopulmonary dysplasia among survivors. If the need for, and duration of, endotracheal intubation are truly decreased, this could lead to a decline in the incidence of the long-term airway problems that sometimes follow this procedure. Despite over a decade of experience, the indications for elective intervention with CDP remain controversial.

Conventional mechanical ventilation

In 1929 Drinker introduced the negative pressure ventilator for adults, and positive pressure ventilators followed thereafter. Although sporadic reports on the use of mechanical ventilation in infants appeared as early as the 1940s, it was many years before ventilators appropriate for use with small infants were available. By the late 1960s the use of ventilators in newborns became more widespread, and in the 1970s mechanical ventilation appears to have contributed significantly to the reduction in perinatal mortality.

Early uncontrolled trials described the use of both intermittent negative pressure ventilation (INPV) and intermittent positive pressure ventilation (IPPV). INPV was delivered initially with a ventilator-incubator combination that enclosed the infant's entire body from the neck down. The smallest babies were tossed about by the relatively large flows and changes in pressure, became bruised, developed skin breakdown beneath the seals at the neck, and also experienced significant thermal stress. Later modifications attempted to stabilize the infant's body by limiting the negative pressure chamber to extend only from the neck to the hips. Stahlman and associates reported a series of 80 patients treated with INPV. Although these patients were severely ill, the derangements of pH, $PaCO_2$, and PaO_2 were corrected in many, and 39% survived.

In simultaneously conducted controlled and uncontrolled studies employing IPPV by means of both pressure and volume ventilators, the efficacy of this mode of therapy in correcting arterial blood gas status was subsequently demonstrated. Proponents of INPV argued that it eliminated the morbidity of endotracheal intubation, still a major problem in neonatal intensive care units, and that this mode of therapy was associated with a reduced incidence of air leaks and chronic lung disease. Access to the infant, however, was considerably more difficult and required interruption of mechanical ventilation, thereby limiting its usefulness, and few neonatal centers employ this mode of therapy today. Because of their greater versatility, positive pressure ventilators are used almost exclusively today.

With the original positive pressure ventilators, gas flow to the patient occurred only during the inspiratory phase of the cycle. Attempts at spontaneous ventilation during the expiratory phase of the ventilator would have entailed markedly increased work of breathing for the patient as well as inhalation of recently exhaled and therefore carbon dioxide–enriched gas. It was thus necessary to abolish spontaneous ventilation either by increasing alveolar ventilation to the point that respiratory drive was overcome or by neuromuscular blockade. This type of ventilation is called controlled because initiation of inspiration is independent of the patient's efforts and strictly controlled by the ventilator. With other ventilators, inspiration is delivered in response to a patient's effort alone (assist ventilation) as well as in combination with a preset number of times per minute (assist-controlled ventilation). Because infants' respiratory efforts are frequently weak and irregular, these ventilators had fallen into disuse. The alternative concept of intermittent mandatory ventilation (IMV), during which a fresh flow of gas is delivered to the patients throughout the respiratory cycle, represented a major step forward in mechanical ventilation of neonates. This mode permits both spontaneous and artificial ventilation to occur concurrently. A further major advantage of IMV is that it has facilitated and simplified weaning from mechanical support. Most ventilators used today have capabilities for IMV.

The application of distending airway pressure throughout the respiratory cycle combined with assisted ventilation and known as PEEP followed naturally. The addition of positive pressure throughout the cycle is thought to prevent collapse of alveoli and improve oxygenation by enhancing V/Q ratios.

Ventilators may also be classified according to the way gas delivery during inspiration is limited. Thus "pressure" ventilators limit the peak inspiratory pressure applied to the airways during inspiration, whereas "volume" ventilators limit the delivered volume. In addition to limiting pressure or volume the inspiratory cycle may be terminated after a certain preset time or volume is reached. These ventilators are thus time-cycled or volume-cycled, respectively. For safety purposes some ventilators may also be made to cycle when a preset PIP is reached independent of their time or volume-cycling mechanisms. Because of ease of use, most neonatal ventilators are pressure-limited time-cycled ventilators commonly called "pressure" ventilators. "Volume" ventilators are less frequently used as attempts are made to ventilate infants with low pressures. Controversial data are presently available regarding differences in outcome of infants treated with "volume" versus "pressure" ventilators.

Using a volume-cycled machine, one presets the V_T (generally 7 to 10 cc/kg) delivered to the patient and adjusts the flow rate to determine the time over which it is delivered, thus determining the I/E ratio. It must be recognized, however, that such ventilators will deliver these volumes irrespective of the pressure generated unless pressure limits are set. This assumes increasing importance in infants with severe RDS in whom compliance is so markedly diminished that delivery of a "normal" V_T requires a tremendous PIP. Furthermore the high flow rates limit the adjustment of the I/E ratio. The alternative is the use of a "pressure" ventilator, wherein flow is delivered to the patient until the predetermined PIP is reached. At this point the pressure may be immediately allowed to return to end-expiratory levels, producing a sawtooth pressure curve, or it may be maintained at peak levels for some time before the expiratory phase begins, producing a pressure curve with plateaus. Thus the "pressure" ventilator used in this way is really time-cycled and pressure-limited.

We recommend initiation of assisted ventilation if any of the following is present.

1. Respiratory acidosis with a pH of less than 7.20 to 7.25
2. Severe hypoxemia ($Pa{O_2}$ less than 50 to 60 torr) despite a high $Fi{O_2}$ (70% to 100%)
3. Apnea complicating the clinical course of RDS

Although a controversial practice, elective intubation has been shown in a prospective randomized trial to increase survival of very low birth weight infants. We prefer to perform endotracheal intubation with tubes of 2.5 or 3 mm internal diameter to minimize damage to the airway. However, as a greater number of smaller babies are being ventilated, 2.5 mm tubes are being used increasingly.

The effect that specific changes in ventilator settings have on blood gases are detailed below.

Peak inspiratory pressure

Changes in PIP (or V_T with volume ventilators) will, in part, determine the pressure gradient between onset and end of inspiration and thus affect alveolar ventilation. An increase in PIP will thus increase tidal volume, increase CO_2 elimination, and decrease $Pa{CO_2}$. Furthermore, increases in PIP will raise Paw and thus improve oxygenation. Use of elevated PIP increases the risk of barotrauma with resultant air leaks, bronchopulmonary dysplasia, and impaired cardiac function; thus caution must be exercised when high levels of PIP are used.

Positive end-expiratory pressure

Adequate PEEP prevents alveolar collapse, maintains lung volume at end expiration, and improves ventilation-perfusion relationships. Because changes in PEEP alter the pressure gradient between inspiration and expiration, elimination of CO_2 may be affected. Thus elevation of PEEP may decrease tidal volume and CO_2 elimination and therefore increase $Pa{CO_2}$. Furthermore, the use of high PEEP (greater than 5 to 6 cm H_2O) may decrease lung compliance, which will be manifested as decreased V_T on a pressure-limited time-cycled ventilator or as increased PIP on a volume ventilator. Thus alveolar hypoventilation could occur with a corresponding increase in $Pa{CO_2}$. Increases in PEEP will raise Paw and improve oxygenation. Nonetheless, use of a very elevated PEEP does not benefit oxygenation substantially. In addition, use of very high PEEP may impair venous return, decrease cardiac output, and decrease oxygen transport. A minimum PEEP of 2 to 3 cm H_2O is recommended because endotracheal intubation eliminates the active maintenance of FRC that infants accomplish by vocal cord adduction.

Frequency (or rate)

Changes in frequency will substantially alter alveolar ventilation and thus $Pa{CO_2}$. Use of moderately high frequencies (60 breaths per minute) has allowed the use of a lower PIP and reduced incidence of pneumothorax. Contrary to earlier observations, recent studies suggest that adequate oxygenation can be maintained at high frequencies. Nonetheless, it appears that the incidence of chronic lung disease or mortality is not altered by ventilation at these moderately high frequencies. When very high frequencies are used, T_I is shortened and tidal volume may decrease. In infants with RDS ventilated with pressure-limited time-cycled ventilators, the delivery of V_T is maintained fairly constant as long as T_I is longer than 0.4 second. Furthermore, if a very short T_E is employed while using high ventilatory frequencies, expiration may be incomplete. The gas trapped in the lung would increase and place the infant on the flat part of the pressure-volume curve, thus decreasing lung compliance. As discussed for PEEP, the gas trapping, also known as inadvertent PEEP, that may accompany the use of a very short T_E would result in reduction of the pressure gradient and elevation of $Pa{CO_2}$.

It is important to note that frequency changes alone (with a constant I/E ratio) usually do not alter Paw and do not substantially affect $Pa{O_2}$. Nonetheless, because it takes a certain time for a pressure plateau to be reached, changes in T_I that accompany frequency adjustments may affect the airway pressure waveform and thus Paw. Therefore the decreased oxygenation observed by some investigators when high frequencies are employed is probably due to an inadvertent reduction in Paw. In addition, a small increase in $Pa{O_2}$ may be expected as frequency is increased owing to a reduction of alveolar $P{CO_2}$ and corresponding increase in alveolar $P{O_2}$. If pulmonary artery hypertension and right-to-left shunting are prominent, the increased pH and reduced $Paco_2$ that accompany the use of high frequencies may reduce shunting and markedly increase Pao_2 in the absence of any increase in Paw.

Ratio of inspiratory to expiratory time

The major effect of changes in I/E ratio is on Paw and thus oxygenation. Reversed I/E ratios (longer T_I than T_E) of as high as 2:1 have been shown to be effective in increasing Pao_2. Although a retrospective study suggested a decreased incidence of bronchopulmonary dysplasia with the use of reversed I/E ratios, a large, well-controlled, randomized clinical trial has revealed only a reduction in the duration of high inspired O_2 concentration and PEEP exposure with reversed I/E ratios but no difference in morbidity or mortality. When corrected for Paw, changes in I/E ratio are not as effective in increasing oxygenation as changes in PIP or PEEP. Furthermore, a prolonged inspiratory time may impede venous return. Changes in I/E ratio do not usually alter V_T unless T_I or T_E becomes too short. Thus CO_2 elimination is usually not altered by changes in I/E ratio.

Inspired oxygen concentration

Changes in Fio_2 alter alveolar oxygen tension and thus oxygenation. Since Fio_2 and Paw both determine oxygenation, they should be balanced. Nonetheless, insufficient data on oxygen versus pressure-related lung injury are available, particularly during increasing ventilatory support. During weaning, maintenance of an appropriate Paw may allow a substantial reduction in Fio_2. However, Paw should be reduced before a very low Fio_2 is reached. A higher incidence of air leaks has been observed if distending pressures are not weaned until a low Fio_2 is reached.

Flow

Changes in flow have not been well studied in infants but probably affect arterial blood gases minimally as long as a sufficient flow is used. High inspiratory flows are needed when inspiratory time is shortened to maintain a square waveform and adequate PIP and V_T.

The use of neuromuscular blockade has been advocated in infants who require mechanical ventilation with high rates or pressures and become increasingly agitated when their attempts at spontaneous respiration are out of phase with the ventilator. This results in decreased effectiveness of mechanical support, and, when oxygenation has become inadequate, paralysis may improve the blood gas status of some of these infants, particularly those with PFC. Neonates with or without lung disease who have persistence of the fetal circulation are particularly susceptible to the effects of agitation, and in these patients neuromuscular blockade may result in a decrease in right-to-left shunting and increased oxygenation. Generalized edema that appears to be the result of absent muscular activity and the roentgenologic appearance of a gasless abdomen are common complications. There remains much controversy surrounding the use of such agents, however, since there are little data available on the indications, efficacy, and complications of their use, especially in very low birth weight infants. Sedation with morphine may stabilize cerebral blood flow in infants at risk for intraventricular hemorrhage. The administration of phenobarbital has led to conflicting results on the incidence of intraventricular hemorrhage in infants with RDS receiving ventilatory support.

Weaning the infant from ventilatory support is frequently a difficult and prolonged process. In milder cases it may be accomplished easily, but with severe disease the superimposition of iatrogenic lung disease may make the process difficult. The approach is usually to decrease PIP as tolerated until 20 to 25 cm H_2O and chest rise is diminished and then to direct one's attention to Fio_2 and IMV. It has been suggested that treatment with aminophylline to stimulate respiratory drive will facilitate the weaning process, but evidence for this is scanty. In most infants, when a low IMV of approximately 10 breaths per minute is tolerated, a short trial of endotracheal CPAP is in order. Prolonged periods of endotracheal CPAP in small infants with resolving lung disease are usually unsuccessful. This is because the infant may be incapable of sustaining the additional work of breathing associated with an increased airway resistance together with the added dead space of the endotracheal tube. Endotracheal CPAP should be maintained at around 4 cm H_2O during the weaning process. The infant is then extubated but may benefit from nasal CPAP. Steroids are not routinely used before extubation, but if stridor caused by laryngeal edema develops, racemic epinephrine aerosols may be administered. Atelectasis after extubation is common in preterm infants recovering from RDS, particularly those of very low birth weight. Application of nasal CPAP after extubation may prevent the development of atelectasis (see discussion later).

There have been some advocates of vigorous chest physiotherapy for infants with severe RDS especially while receiving assisted ventilation. Although some infants undoubtedly benefit from the therapy, many will show deterioration of blood gases. Continuous transcutaneous monitoring of Po_2 is recommended if physical therapy is prescribed, and, unless there is evidence of a beneficial effect, the principle of minimum handling of these fragile infants should be adhered to. During suctioning the catheter should not be inserted beyond the lower end of the endotracheal tube to minimize damage to the airway. During the accompanying bagging periods,

O_2 concentration may be increased 10% over the infant's current requirement, and a pressure manometer must be in place to ensure that comparable pressures are maintained off the ventilator.

High-frequency ventilation

New modes of assisted ventilation, including high-frequency positive-pressure ventilation, high-frequency jet ventilation, high-frequency flow interruption, and high-frequency oscillation (Fig. 28-21), deliver small volumes of gas at high frequencies and limit the development of high airway pressure. Since high ventilatory pressures and the resultant pulmonary barotrauma and cardiovascular compromise are thought to be major contributory factors to complications associated with assisted ventilation, these new modes of ventilation in neonates have aroused considerable interest. Although all these techniques of ventilation have the use of high frequencies and small volumes in common, marked differences exist in both ventilator design and the airway pressure waveforms generated.

High-frequency positive-pressure ventilation is a mode of assisted ventilation that employs standard ventilatory techniques modified with low-compliance tubing and connectors so that an adequate V_T is delivered despite

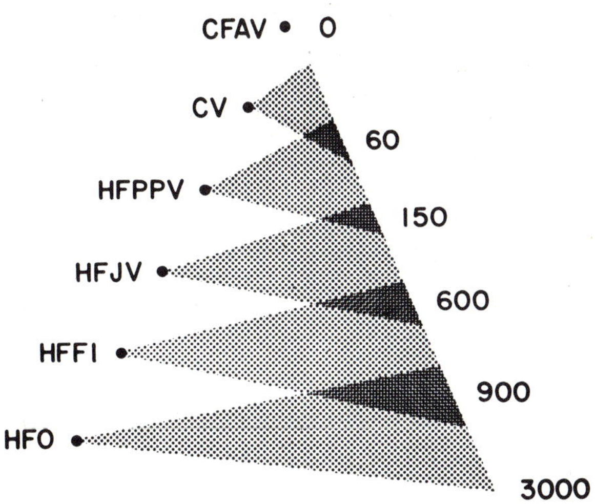

Fig. 28-21. Frequency spectrum for assisted ventilation of neonates. The numbers (on the right) represent approximate ranges of cycles per minute because strict limits of frequency for each mode of ventilation do not exist. Constant flow apneic ventilation *(CFAV)* maintains normal blood gases in animals despite the absence of a cycling frequency but has not been evaluated in human infants. *CV*, Conventional ventilation; *HFPPV*, high-frequency positive pressure ventilation; *HFJV*, high-frequency jet ventilation; *HFFI*, high-frequency flow interruption; *HFO*, high-frequency oscillation. (Modified from Carlo, W.A., and Martin, R.J.: Pediatr. Clin. North Am. **33:**221, 1986.)

short inspiratory times and frequencies between 60 to 150 per minute. Studies with this mode of assisted ventilation revealed a decreased incidence of pneumothorax and high survival rates.

High-frequency jet ventilation uses a completely different system of assisted ventilation that is characterized by the delivery of gases from a high-pressure source through a small-bore cannula. In neonates, frequencies of 150 to 600 per minute have been commonly used. Data from a rabbit model of surfactant deficiency suggest that there may be a relatively narrow range of frequencies, I/E ratios, inspiratory times, and expiratory times at which jet ventilation maximally reduces airway pressures and prevents gas trapping. Although it has been assumed that gas from the surrounding areas is added to that of the ventilator (entrained gas), gas entrainment may occur only at ventilator settings characterized by high flow of gases. During jet ventilation, humidification of gases is particularly difficult, and inadequate humidification may cause tracheal lesions. It cannot, therefore, be assumed that entrainment contributes to the delivered volumes, and humidification should not depend on this phenomenon. We have used jet ventilation at rates of 250 per minute in preterm infants with severe RDS for short periods and observed adequate gas exchange at PIP and Paw levels lower than those required during conventional ventilation. A similar ventilator has been employed in preterm neonates with respiratory failure and intractable air leaks, with observed reductions in alveolar arterial Po_2 gradient and $Paco_2$. The effectiveness of jet ventilation in other respiratory disorders such as meconium aspiration syndrome is still controversial.

Like jet ventilators, *high-frequency flow interruptors* deliver small volumes at high frequencies by interrupting a flow or high-pressure source. In contrast to jet ventilators, there is no injector, no gas entrainment, and probably less turbulence. Humidification of the gas source does not appear to be a problem. Using a high-frequency flow interrupter, Frantz and associates successfully ventilated 10 neonates with RDS and 5 with pulmonary interstitial emphysema and maintained adequate gas exchange at lower airway pressures than those required during conventional ventilation.

Finally, *high-frequency oscillation* is a different technique of high-frequency ventilation that delivers extremely small volumes (even less than dead space) at very high frequencies (up to 3,000 per minute) with the use of a piston pump or acoustic speaker. Furthermore, oscillation is unique because expiration is actively generated by the ventilator in marked contrast to the other modes of high-frequency ventilation in which expiration is passive. Marchak and associates successfully used an oscillator to ventilate a group of infants with severe RDS. Since preliminary animal studies suggest that intermittent sighs may be necessary during oscillation, a combination of this technique with conventional ventilation may be advantageous. Most recently, animal studies have shown the feasibility of applying high-frequency oscillations by chest wall compression.

Although these preliminary data are encouraging, larger controlled trials are required to determine whether high-frequency ventilation is superior to conventional ventilation and whether complications from barotrauma are reduced by this therapy.

COMPLICATIONS OF RDS

Complications related to RDS may occur spontaneously but are more commonly the result of well-intended therapeutic interventions. The major complications are consequent on the placement of arterial catheters (Chapter 24 and elsewhere in this chapter), oxygen administration, mechanical ventilation, and the use of endrotracheal tubes. The complications of assisted ventilation include the following.

1. Pulmonary air leaks: pneumothorax, pneumomediastinum, pulmonary interstitial emphysema (see Part five)
2. Endotracheal tube complications: displacement, dislodgment, occlusion, atelectasis after extubation, palatal grooves
3. Tracheal lesions: erosion, granuloma, subglottic stenosis, necrotizing tracheobronchitis
4. Infection: pneumonia, septicemia
5. Impaired cardiac function
6. Chronic lung disease: bronchopulmonary dysplasia
7. Miscellaneous: intracranial hemorrhage, PDA, retrolental fibroplasia

The liberal use of total parenteral nutrition together with other pharmacologic interventions also has contributed to morbidity. The reader is referred to detailed discussions of these conditions in the relevant sections of this book.

Patent ductus arteriosus

See Chapter 29.

Clinical features of a PDA with left-to-right shunting may be noted in infants recovering from RDS. The incidence of PDA ranges from 15% to 36% in preterm infants and is more prevalent in very low birth weight infants or those with pulmonary disease. A PDA should be suspected when there is a delay in clinical improvement from RDS and the infant still requires the respirator or is oxygen dependent. Aggressive management is indicated if a PDA is confirmed. Evaluation of the left-to-right shunting through the ductus is achieved by echocardiography (measuring left atrial size, left ventricular end-diastolic dimension, or left atrial/aortic ratio) or contrast roentgenographic studies by means of an umbilical arterial catheter. Recognition of a hemodynamically significant PDA is enhanced by using clinical criteria in conjunction with echocardiographic evidence of left atrial/aortic ratio >1.4 and left ventricular systolic time interval ratio <0.27. Therapy includes fluid restriction, medical management of congestive heart failure, and either pharmacologic or surgical closure of the ductus. The PDA has been implicated in the cause of bronchopulmonary dysplasia because it presumably prolongs the duration of ventilatory assistance. Excess fluid intake has been associated with both bronchopulmonary dysplasia and PDA. Pharmacologic or surgical closure of the ductus in these infants is often followed by a dramatic decrease in ventilatory and oxygen requirements. Surgical ligation remains a proved and effective method of treating a PDA in the preterm infant, with a very low operative mortality. Whether this should be the treatment of choice or pharmacologic closure should be initially attempted is not always clear. Ultimately survival following ligation largely depends on the severity of RDS, timing of the surgical procedure, and size of the infant.

A multicenter collaborative trial has studied the efficacy of indomethacin therapy for preterm infants with a hemodynamically significant PDA. A ductal closure rate of approximately 70% was achieved when indomethacin was given either concurrently with, or after failure of, usual medical therapy, without any apparent benefit between these two strategies. This was almost double the spontaneous closure rate. After indomethacin treatment, there was a reopening rate of approximately 25%, although most of these PDAs subsequently closed without need for surgery. Birth weight, gestational age, or age at time of drug administration did not significantly modify drug efficacy. To investigate the optimum timing for indomethacin therapy, Mahony administered the drug at a mean age of 15 hours to a group of preterm infants without any effort made to document presence or absence of ductal shunting before treatment. In this double-blind controlled trial, indomethacin did reduce the frequency of large left-to-right ductal shunts without evidence of drug-related side effects. Despite the decreased incidence of large shunts, longer term morbidity was unaffected by indomethacin administration. Thus its routine use on the first day of life could not be supported before evidence of a PDA became clinically apparent.

Infection

Early in the course of experience with mechanical ventilation infection was extremely prevalent, and mortality was high. This was most commonly associated with gram-negative organisms including *Pseudomonas* and *Klebsiella* organisms and *Escherichia coli*. More recently infection as a complication of mechanical ventilation appears to be less common. *Candida* organisms, *Staphylococcus epidermidis*, *S. aureus*, and gram-negative organisms are the most common offenders, particularly in infants with birth weights less than 1 kg who have required prolonged mechanical ventilation, multiple courses of antibiotic therapy, and indwelling vascular lines. Although cultures of endotracheal aspirates are usually negative, positive cultures do not necessarily indicate clinically significant lower respiratory tract infection.

In the neonate requiring mechanical ventilation careful attention must be given to aseptic technique, particularly at the time of endotracheal intubation and during suctioning. Changing all equipment related to mechanical ventilation every 24 hours is also effective. The prophylactic use of antibiotics under these conditions is of no proved value.

Endotracheal tube complications

Accidental displacement of an endotracheal tube into a main stem bronchus or into the hypopharynx or esophagus is a well-recognized and extremely hazardous complication of mechanical ventilation. The frequency with which such complications occur has been estimated to be from 2% to 40%. Accidental tube displacement usually is associated with ipsilateral hyperinflation and contralateral collapse and clinically characterized by deterioration in the patient's condition, often with cyanosis. Auscultation of the chest may suggest this complication, but roentgenographic studies may be needed to resolve the issue. Similarly, accidental extubation usually is accompanied by sudden deterioration with cyanosis, bradycardia, and respiratory collapse. It is necessary to quickly determine whether there is any mechanical failure in the ventilator and to assume manual ventilation with mask and bag. If any doubt exists, tube position should be inspected visually and the tube replaced if necessary. Note that clinical examination of the chest may be unreliable in determining tube position because of the transmission of breath sounds across the thorax in small infants. Sudden deterioration from tube displacement always must be differentiated from a pneumothorax, and immediate x-ray confirmation of tube position should be undertaken. Although it has been stated that both the quantity and tenacity of secretions increase with assisted ventilation in infants with RDS, tube occlusion because of secretions has become a very infrequent complication, since adequate humidification is available with current ventilators.

The frequency with which serious tracheal lesions complicate endotracheal intubation and IPPV of the newborn infant is difficult to determine. Following extubation edema of the cords may result in transient hoarseness and stridor in many infants. The use of dexamethasone before extubation or epinephrine-isoxsuprine inhalations has not provided universal relief, although there are strong advocates of both these measures. Both gross and histologic evidence of inflammation and epithelial erosions of the trachea have been noted at postmortem examination of infants dying after prolonged endotracheal intubation. Furthermore fiberoptic inspection of the airways of infants who have been intubated for a significant period will reveal some pearly lesions below the cords, although most of these prove to be insignificant. More recently partial or complete occlusion of the trachea and even the main stem bronchi at the site of suction catheter injury has been noted. Recent reports have recommended the use of smaller endotracheal tubes that ensure the presence of an air leak when the tube is in place, securing the tube well so that movement of the tube within the trachea is minimum when infants are moved, careful suctioning techniques using side-hole catheters, and not allowing the catheters to go too far below the distal end of the endotracheal tube to diminish the incidence of severe tracheal lesions.

Prolonged use of orotracheal tubes has been associated with palatal groove formation, although subsequent growth and remodeling of the palate probably repair any early deformation. Esophageal and pharyngeal perforations may rarely occur during endotracheal or nasogastric tube placement and be confined to the mediastinum or extend into the pleural cavity. They require early recognition, intensive medical therapy, and close observation for potential surgical intervention. *Necrotizing tracheobronchitis* is a newly described lesion that has been reported at autopsy (or less frequently on bronchoscopy) in some ventilated infants. Airway obstruction is caused by necrosis and detachment of epithelium, with airway injury extending into the submucosal tissues. The most common mode of clinical presentation appears to be sudden severe hypercarbia with decreased air entry that may require bronchoscopy to remove obstructing necrotic debris from the airway. This entity appears to represent iatrogenic injury, and inadequate humidification during either conventional or high-frequency ventilation has been implicated although not proved as the major etiologic factor.

Subglottic stenosis has been noted in approximately 1% of survivors of mechanical ventilation with birth weights less than 1.5 kg (Fig. 28-22). These infants may be seen initially with airway obstruction during a superimposed respiratory infection. Tracheostomy may be necessary for this small group of infants. Whether the complications of endotracheal tubes can be reduced or eliminated by avoiding prolonged intubation and performing earlier tracheostomy in some infants remains to be proved.

Atelectasis after extubation occurs frequently in infants recovering from RDS. Clinically the infants demonstrate increased respiratory difficulty, retraction, and cyanosis;

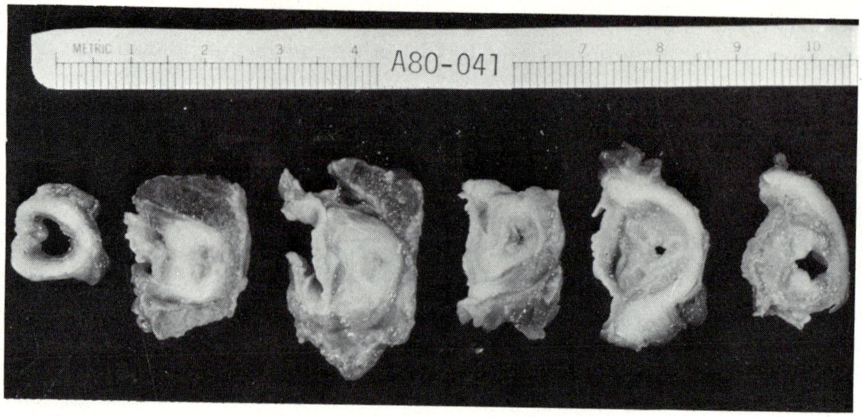

Fig. 28-22. Sequential sections taken through the larynx and upper trachea of an infant who died at 8 months following orotracheal intubation for 4 months. There is complete occlusion of the glottis by granulation tissue. (Courtesy Drs. R.E. Wood and B. Dahms.)

A

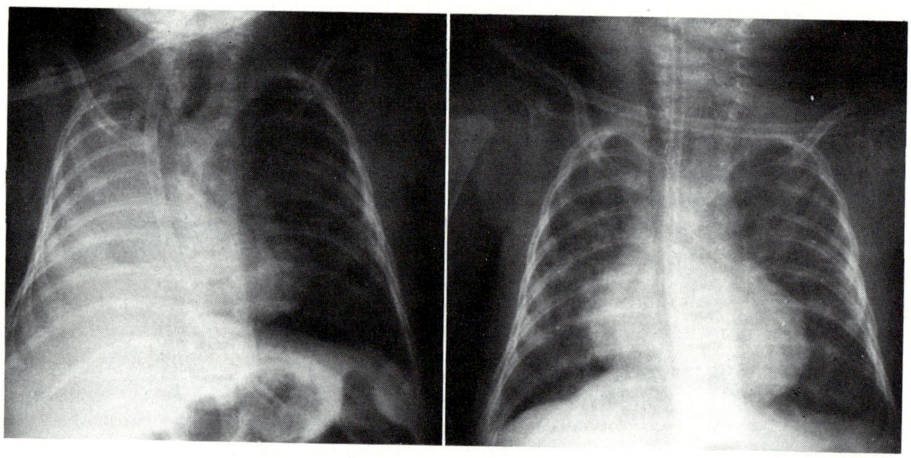

B

Fig. 28-23. Chest roentgenograms of a 1.1 kg infant with **(A)** massive atelectasis of the right lung following extubation and **(B)** reexpansion of the collapsed lung immediately following bronchoscopic removal of a large mucus plug from the right main stem bronchus. (Courtesy Dr. R.E. Wood.)

their blood gases show respiratory failure with hypoxemia and hypercarbia. Roentgenographically the right upper lobe is the most frequent site affected, and shift of the mediastinal structures is common. The approach to treatment comprises physiotherapy with postural drainage and repeated endotracheal suctioning if reintubation is necessary. Availability of the flexible fiberoptic bronchoscope has alleviated the problem, and it is possible to keep the infant well oxygenated while suctioning the bronchial tree. Mucus plugs or even bronchial casts sometimes are removed intact, and prompt clinical and roentgenographic improvement may be noted (Fig. 28-23).

Residual pulmonary disease

See Part six.

Residual pulmonary disease occurs in a significant number of infants surviving mechanical ventilation for severe RDS. The spectrum ranges from infants with minimum roentgenographic changes associated with slight cardiorespiratory distress to crippling cardiorespiratory failure seen after prolonged ventilation with high concentrations of oxygen. The infants may develop restrictive and/or obstructive lung disease, abnormal chest roentgenograms, and cor pulmonale. The pathogenesis and management of these infants are considered in Part six.

Intracranial hemorrhage

See Chapter 27.

Subependymal and/or intraventricular hemorrhage occur frequently, especially in very immature infants with severe pulmonary disease. As discussed elsewhere, numerous causes for intraventricular hemorrhage have been proposed, including neonatal asphyxia with hypotension, rapid volume expansion, changes in serum osmolarity resulting from excessive bicarbonate administration, coagulation abnormalities, hypoxemia, and hypercarbia. It is difficult to clearly establish a relationship between intracranial hemorrhage and bicarbonate administered to infants with RDS. Undoubtedly many preterm infants have received too much bicarbonate, but the proof of a relation to intracranial hemorrhage is not convincing.

Since these factors are all closely interrelated with severe RDS, it is not surprising that intraventricular hemorrhage has been further correlated with mechanical ventilation employing high peak inflation pressures, prolonged inspiratory times, and especially the development of alveolar rupture and air leaks, all of which would be expected to alter cerebral blood flow or volume by impairing venous return. There is considerable interest in the roles of sedation and muscle paralysis on the incidence of intraventricular hemorrhage during assisted ventilation. Despite initial enthusiasm, widespread prophylactic use of phenobarbital does not appear to decrease the incidence of subependymal and/or intraventricular hemorrhage in ventilated preterm infants. Perlman performed a controlled trial of muscle paralysis by randomizing only those infants who demonstrated fluctuating cerebral blood flow velocity patterns on bidirectional Doppler flowmeter. Although the group numbers were small, paralysis of the ventilated infants decreased both cerebral blood flow velocity fluctuations and the incidence of severe intracranial bleeding. Thus, appropriate noninvasive screening techniques to determine risk for intraventricular hemorrhage may allow selection of those infants who will benefit from muscle paralysis, sedation, or both during assisted ventilation.

Even though intracranial hemorrhage is a clearly recognized complication of RDS, it is often unclear at autopsy whether RDS or intraventricular hemorrhage is the cause of death when both are present, and this may be as much a matter of guesswork as of knowledge. The discovery that intracerebellar hemorrhage may result from tight-fitting face masks used for the administration of CPAP was first reported by Pape and associates and noted to be accompanied by extensive molding and displacement of the infant's skull. Martin subsequently reported a series of asphyxiated preterm infants with massive cerebellar hemorrhage in whom mask CPAP had not been employed. These observations further illustrate the importance of continually evaluating the role of iatrogenic factors in the cause of intracranial hemorrhage. This is especially important because recent prospective studies using ultrasound or computed tomography (CT scans) have demonstrated a much higher incidence of subependymal and intraventricular hemorrhage in surviving infants than was previously suspected. This trend will persist as respiratory care for infants with RDS continues to improve and less infants die from pulmonary disease per se.

Oxygen toxicity

See Part six.

Administration of oxygen is an essential component of the care and survival of neonates with respiratory problems. The two major manifestations of oxygen toxicity involve damage to the immature retina (Chapter 39) and lungs (Part six). Pulmonary tissue appears particularly sensitive to the toxic effects of oxygen to which its cells are directly exposed.

There has been ongoing speculation as to the relative roles of prolonged oxygen exposure, endotracheal intubation, immaturity, and technique of assisted ventilation in the genesis of chronic pulmonary disease in infants. Nonetheless there is clearly an association between oxygen therapy and the development of lung injury. The goals of therapy for respiratory distress are to achieve adequate tissue oxygenation while maintaining PaO_2 between 50 and 80 mm Hg, using the lowest environmental oxygen concentration and avoiding excessive barotrauma to limit potentially damaging effects.

Follow-up evaluation

See also Chapter 27 and Part six.

In evaluating the neurodevelopmental outcome of infants with RDS, members of each unit should follow their own infants and closely evaluate growth, intellectual development, vision, and hearing. Major factors influencing the outcome include the fact that the populations comprise mixtures of inborn and transported infants, socioeconomic variables, infants with wide variations in birth weight and gestational age, infants with varying degrees of asphyxia, and differing indications and techniques of ventilation at different centers.

Stahlman, as early as 1973, presented a most encouraging report on the outcome of 85 infants treated for RDS. She found no difference in intelligence or handicap between ventilated and nonventilated infants of the same birth weight. No cases of cerebral palsy or hydrocephalus were identified. It should hastily be pointed out that all but three of her ventilated infants weighed more than 1,500 gm. Today at most centers similar excellent results can be predicted for these relatively large infants if they have not suffered significant perinatal asphyxia.

It is the infants with birth weights below 1,500 gm who are of major concern, as documented by Fitzhardinge in her referral population. Factors associated with poor outcome include a neonatal history of seizures or intracranial hemorrhage and other severe neurologic sequelae. Twenty-nine percent of infants born between 1970 and 1973, requiring mechanical ventilation, had neurologic deficits, and 44% were handicapped on assessment at 2 years. Because of a number of changes in her nursery, including changes in techniques of ventilation and improved nutrition, survivors of mechanical ventilation between 1974 and 1975 showed only an 11% incidence of neurologic deficit, and 28% were handicapped.

The current developmental outcome for infants with mild or moderate RDS is probably comparable to that of infants without RDS. Bennett has shown that birth weight and gestational age have a much stronger influence on mental and motor developmental scores of preterm infants at 2 years than either the presence or severity of RDS. Rothberg has demonstrated a less favorable neurodevelopmental outcome for ventilated versus nonventilated infants weighing <1 kg at birth. Such an association may, however, have little to do with respiratory disease per se because indications for prolonged assisted ventilation in these very low birth weight infants are multifactorial and vary widely between centers. There is some evidence that late abnormalities of pulmonary function are detectable in the premature survivors of RDS. Nonetheless, in the absence of progression to bronchopulmonary dysplasia in infancy, this has not been a clinical problem in childhood. Bertrand has compared pulmonary function and airway reactivity in preterm survivors of RDS at 7 to 12 years of age. The RDS infants did have higher ratios of residual volume to total lung capacity and lower forced expiratory volumes then appropriately matched controls. Airway reactivity was elevated in the children who had been premature (and their mothers) both in the presence or absence of a history of RDS. This area requires further study as more sensitive techniques become available to assess pulmonary function.

Waldemar A. Carlo
Richard J. Martin
Avroy A. Fanaroff

BIBLIOGRAPHY

Pulmonary mechanics

Cartwright, D.W., Willis, M.M., and Gregory, G.A.: Functional residual capacity and lung mechanics at different levels of mechanical ventilation, Crit. Care Med. **12**:422, 1984.

LeSouef, P.N., England, S.J., Bryan, A.C.: Total resistance of the respiratory system in preterm infants with and without an endotracheal tube, J. Pediatr. **104**:108, 1984.

Simbruner, G., and Gregory, G.A.: Performance of neonatal ventilators: the effects of changes in resistance and compliance, Crit. Care Med. **9**:509, 1981.

Gas exchange

Chatburn, R.L., and Lough, M.D.: Mechanical ventilation. In Lough, M.D., Doershuk, C., and Stern, R.: Pediatric respiratory therapy, ed. 3, Chicago, 1985, Year Book Medical Publishers, Inc.

Harris, T.R.: Physiological principles. In Goldsmith, J.P., and Karotkin, E.H.: Assisted ventilation of the neonate, Philadelphia, 1981, W.B. Saunders Co.

Reynolds, E.O.R.: Effect of alterations in mechanical ventilator settings on pulmonary gas exchange in hyaline membrane disease, Arch. Dis. Child. **46**:152, 1971.

CPAP

Ahlstrom, H., Jonson, B., and Svenningsen, N.W.: Continuous positive airways pressure treatment by a face chamber in idiopathic respiratory distress syndrome, Arch. Dis. Child. **51**:13, 1976.

Bancalari, E., Garcia, O.L., and Jesse, M.J.: Effects of continuous negative pressure on lung mechanics in idiopathic respiratory distress syndrome, Pediatrics **51**:485, 1973.

Bonta, B.W., and others: Determination of optimal continuous positive airway pressure for the treatment of RDS by measurement of esophageal pressure, J. Pediatr. **91**:449, 1977.

Boros, S.J., and Reynolds, J.W.: Hyaline membrane disease treated with early end-expiratory pressure: 1 year's experience, Pediatrics **56**:218, 1975.

Fanaroff, A.A., and others: Controlled trial of continuous negative external pressure in the treatment of severe respiratory distress syndrome, J. Pediatr. **82**:921, 1973.

Goldman, S.L., Brady, J.P., and Dumpit, F.M.: Increased work of breathing associated with nasal prongs, Pediatrics **64**:160, 1979.

Gregory, G.A., and others: Treatment of the idiopathic respiratory-distress syndrome with continuous positive airway pressure, N. Engl. J. Med. **284**:1333, 1971.

Kattwinkel, J., and others: A device for administration of continuous positive airway pressure by the nasal route, Pediatrics **52**:131, 1973.

Rhodes, P.G., and Hall, R.T.: Continuous positive airway pressure delivered by face mask in infants with the idiopathic respiratory distress syndrome: a controlled study, Pediatrics **52**:1, 1973.

Tanswell, A.K., and others: Individualized continuous distending pressure applied within 6 hours of delivery in infants with respiratory distress syndrome, Arch. Dis. Child. **55**:33, 1980.

Yu, V.Y.H., and Rolfe, P.: Effect of continuous positive airway pressure breathing on cardiorespiratory function in infants with respiratory distress syndrome, Acta Pediatr. Scand. **66**:59, 1977.

Conventional mechanical ventilation

Boros, S.J.: Variations in inspiratory: expiratory ratio and airway pressure wave form during mechanical ventilation: the significance of mean airway pressure, J. Pediatr. **94**:114, 1979.

Carlo, W.A., and others: Efficacy of computer assisted management of respiratory failure in neonates, Pediatrics **78**:139, 1986.

Chatburn, R.L., Carlo, W.A., and Lough, M.D.: Clinical algorithm for pressure-limited ventilation of neonates with respiratory distress syndrome, Respir. Care. **28**:1579, 1983.

Ciszek, T.A., and others: Mean airway pressure—significance during mechanical ventilation in neonates, J. Pediatr. **99**:121, 1981.

Drew, J.H.: Immediate intubation at birth of the very low-birth-weight infant: effect on survival, Am. J. Dis. Child. **136**:207, 1982.

Finer, N.N., and Tomney, P.M.: Controlled evaluation of muscle relaxation in the ventilated infant, Pediatrics **67**:641, 1981.

Herman, S., and Reynolds, E.O.R.: Methods for improving oxygenation in infants mechanically ventilated for severe hyaline membrane disease, Arch. Dis. Child. **48**:612, 1973.

Manginello, F.P., and others: Evaluation of methods of assisted ventilation in hyaline membrane disease, Arch. Dis. Child. **53**:878, 1978.

Murdock, A.I., and others: Mechanical ventilation in respiratory distress syndrome: a controlled trial, Arch. Dis. Child. **45**:524, 1970.

Pollitzer, M.J., and others: Pancuronium during mechanical ventilation speeds recovery of lungs of infants with hyaline membrane disease, Lancet **1**:346, 1981.

Spahr, R.C., and others: Hyaline membrane disease: a controlled study of inspiratory to expiratory ratio in its management by ventilator, Am. J. Dis. Child. **134**:373, 1980.

Stahlman, M.T., and others: Negative pressure assisted ventilation in infants with hyaline membrane disease, J. Pediatr. **76**:174, 1970.

Stern, L., and others: Negative pressure artificial respiration: use in tretment of respiratory failure in the newborn, Can. Med. Assoc. J. **102**:595, 1970.

Stewart, A.R., Finer, N.N., and Peters, K.L.: Effects of alterations of inspiratory and expiratory pressures and inspiratory/expiratory ratios on mean airway pressure, blood gases, and intracranial pressure, Pediatrics **67**:474, 1981.

High-frequency ventilation

Bland, R.D., and others: High frequency mechanical ventilation in severe hyaline membrane disease: an alternative treatment? Crit. Care Med. **8**:275, 1980.

Boros, S.J., and Campbell, K.: A comparison of the effects of high frequency–low tidal volume and low frequency–high tidal volume mechanical ventilation, J. Pediatr. **97**:108, 1980.

Boros, S.J., and others: Using conventional infant ventilators at unconventional rates, Pediatrics **74**:487, 1984.

Boros, S.J., and others: Neonatal high-frequency jet ventilation: four year's experience, Pediatrics **75**:657, 1985.

Boynton, B.R., and others: Combined high-frequency oscillatory ventilation and intermittent mandatory ventilation in critically ill neonates, J. Pediatr. **105**:297, 1984.

Carlo, W.A., and others: Decrease in airway pressure during high-frequency jet ventilation in infants with respiratory distress syndrome, J. Pediatr. **104**:101, 1984.

Field, D., Milner, A.D., and Hopkin, I.E.: High and conventional rates of positive pressure ventilation, Arch. Dis. Child. **59**:1151, 1984.

Frantz, I.D., III, Werthammer, J., and Stark, A.R.: High-frequency ventilation in premature infants with lung disease: adequate gas exchange at low tracheal pressures, Pediatrics **71**:483, 1983.

Heicher, D.A., Kasting, D.S., and Harrod, J.R.: Prospective clinical comparison of two methods for mechanical ventilation of neonates: rapid rate and short inspiratory time versus slow rate and long inspiratory time, J. Pediatr. **98**:957, 1981.

Heijman, K., and Sjöstrand, U.: Treatment of the respiratory distress syndrome—a preliminary report, Opusc. Med. **19**:235, 1974.

Marchak, B.E., and others: Treatment of RDS by high-frequency oscillatory ventilation: a preliminary report, J. Pediatr. **99**:287, 1981.

Pokora, T., and others: Neonatal high-frequency jet ventilation, Pediatrics **72**:27, 1983.

PDA

Baylen, B.G., and others: The critically ill infant with patent ductus arteriosus and pulmonary disease—an echocardiographic assessment, J. Pediatr. **86**:423, 1975.

Friedman, W.F., and others: The patent ductus arteriosus, Clin. Perinatol. **5**:411, 1978.

Gersony, W.M., and others: Effects of indomethacin in premature infants with patent ductus arteriosus: results of a national collaborative study, J. Pediatr. **102**:895, 1983.

Jacob, J., and others: The contribution of patent ductus arteriosus in the neonate with severe RDS, J. Pediatr. **96**:79, 1980.

Johnson, G.L., and others: Echocardiographic characteristics of premature infants with patent ductus arteriosus, Pediatrics **72**:864, 1983.

Mahony, L., and others: Indomethacin therapy on the first day of life in infants with very low-birth-weight, J. Pediatr. **106**:801, 1985.

Endotracheal tube complications

Erenberg, A., and Nowak, A.J.: Palatal groove formation in neonates and infants with orotracheal tubes, Am. J. Dis. Child. **138**:974, 1984.

Johnson, D.E., and others: Management of esophageal and pharyngeal perforation in the newborn infant, Pediatrics **70**:592, 1982.

Kirpalani, H., and others: Diagnosis and therapy of necrotizing tracheobronchitis in ventilated neonates, Crit. Care Med. **13**:792, 1985.

Ratner, I., and Whitfield, J.: Acquired subglottic stenosis in the very low-birth-weight infant, Am. J. Dis. Child. **137**:40, 1983.

Wood, R.E.: The flexible fiberoptic bronchoscope as a diagnostic and therapeutic tool in infants. In Milner, A.D., and Martin, R.J., editors: Neonatal and pediatric respiratory medicine, London, 1985, Butterworth and Co.

Intracranial hemorrhage

Bedard, M.P., and others: Effect of prophylactic phenobarbital on intraventricular hemorrhage in high-risk neonates, Pediatrics **73**:435, 1984.

deLemos, R.A., and Tomasovic, J.J.: Effects of positive pressure ventilation on cerebral blood flow in the newborn infant, Clin. Perinatol. **5**:395, 1978.

Dykes, F.D., and others: Intraventricular hemorrhage: a prospective evaluation of etiopathogenesis, Pediatrics **66**:42, 1980.

Finberg, L.: The relationship of intravenous infusions and intracranial hemorrhage, J. Pediatr. **91**:777, 1977.

Martin, R., Roessmann, U., and Fanaroff, A.A.: Massive intracerebellar hemorrhage in low-birth-weight infants, J. Pediatr. **89**:290, 1976.

Pape, K.E., and Wigglesworth, J.S.: Haemorrhage, ischaemia, and the perinatal brain, Clinics in Developmental Medicine 69/70, London, 1979, William Heinemann, Ltd.

Perlman, J.M., and others: Reduction in intraventricular hemorrhage by elimination of fluctuating cerebral blood-flow velocity in preterm infants with respiratory distress syndrome, N. Engl. J. Med. **312**:1353, 1985.

Follow-up

Bennett, F.C., Robinson, N.M., and Sells, C.J.: Hyaline membrane disease, birth weight, and gestational age: effects on development in the first 2 years, Am. J. Dis. Child. **136**:888, 1982.

Bertrand, J.M., and others: The long-term pulmonary sequelae of prematurity: the role of familial airway hyperreactivity and the respiratory distress syndrome, N. Engl. J. Med. **312**:742, 1985.

Fitzhardinge, P.M., and others: Mechanical ventilation of infants of less than 1501 grams birth weight: health, growth and neurologic sequelae, J. Pediatr. **88**:531, 1976.

Johnson, J.D., and others: Prognosis of children surviving with the aid of mechanical ventilation in the newborn period, J. Pediatr. **84**:272, 1974.

Lindrough, M., and others: Evaluation of mechanical ventilation in newborn infants, Paediatr. Scand. **69**:151, 1980.

Rhodes, P.G., Hall, R.T., and Leonidas, A.C.: Chronic pulmonary disease in neonates with assisted ventilation, Pediatrics **55**:788, 1975.

Rothberg, A.D., and others: Infants weighing 1000 grams or less at birth: developmental outcome for ventilated and nonventilated infants, Pediatrics **71**:599, 1983.

Stahlman, M., and others: A six-year follow-up of clinical hyaline membrane disease, Pediatr. Clin. North Am. **20**:433, 1973.

Stahlman, M., and others: Role of hyaline membrane disease in production of later childhood lung abnormalities, Pediatrics **69**:572, 1982.

PART FIVE

Other pulmonary problems

MECONIUM ASPIRATION SYNDROME

Meconium staining of the amniotic fluid or fetus is usually considered to be indicative of fetal distress. The passage of meconium in utero accompanies 8% to 20% of all deliveries and is seen predominantly in small for gestational age (SGA) and postmature infants, as well as those with cord complications or other factors compromising the in utero placental circulation. Although knowledge of the pathophysiologic stimuli in the fetus that govern the passage of meconium in response to stress is still incomplete, this phenomenon is almost never observed before a gestational age of 34 weeks. Many infants with meconium-stained amniotic fluid exhibit no signs of depression, although some brief period of asphyxia may well have induced the passage of meconium before delivery. Nonetheless the presence of meconium in the amniotic fluid necessitates careful supervision of labor and close monitoring of fetal well-being (Chapter 8). The accoucheur must be alerted to the possibility of a depressed fetus, and someone skilled in newborn resuscitation must be present in the delivery room. With appropriate management of the airway the meconium aspiration syndrome and complications thereof can be largely prevented.

Pathophysiology

The quantity of meconium will affect the appearance and viscosity of the amniotic fluid, which ranges from a green-tinged, lightly meconium-stained fluid to one with a thick, pea soup consistency. Under normal circumstances fetal respiration is associated with movement of fluid from the airways out into the amniotic fluid. With fetal distress gasping may be initiated in utero. Under these circumstances amniotic fluid and particulate matter contained therein may be inhaled into the large airways. The meconium inhaled by the fetus may be present in the trachea or larger bronchi and be manifested as airway obstruction at delivery. Because of the viscosity of the fetal lung fluid, it is uncommon for inhaled meconium to penetrate into the smaller air spaces before delivery. Nonetheless meconium and squames may be found as far as the alveoli in stillborn infants. After air breathing has commenced, especially if accompanied by gasping respirations, there is a rapid distal migration of meconium within the lung. Roentgenographic studies by Gooding, who instilled tantalum-labeled meconium into the trachea of neonatal puppies before their first breath, confirmed that this can occur within 1 hour.

Pathophysiologically the pulmonary problems relate to airway obstruction and a ball valve phenomenon created by the presence of meconium within the airways. Thus there are areas of atelectasis resulting from total small airway obstruction, adjacent to areas of overexpansion from gas trapping in areas with partial obstruction (Fig. 28-24). In rabbits, after insufflation of the lungs with a meconium-saline mixture, a consistent increase in FRC and expiratory lung resistance occurs. Air leaks, including pneumomediastinum and pneumothorax, often occur after aspiration of meconium and cellular debris.

Whereas PFC can be a major clinical problem in infants with meconium aspiration, the nature of the accompanying pulmonary hypertension is somewhat controversial. Hypoxic pulmonary arterial vasoconstriction is most likely responsible for the PFC. Murphy has applied morphometic techniques to study the pulmonary vascular bed in infants with fatal meconium aspiration. In almost all cases there was abnormal muscularization of the smallest intraacinar arteries that must have developed before birth. Thus both prenatal and perinatal maladaptation of the pulmonary circulation may contribute to the development of PFC in infants with meconium aspiration syndrome.

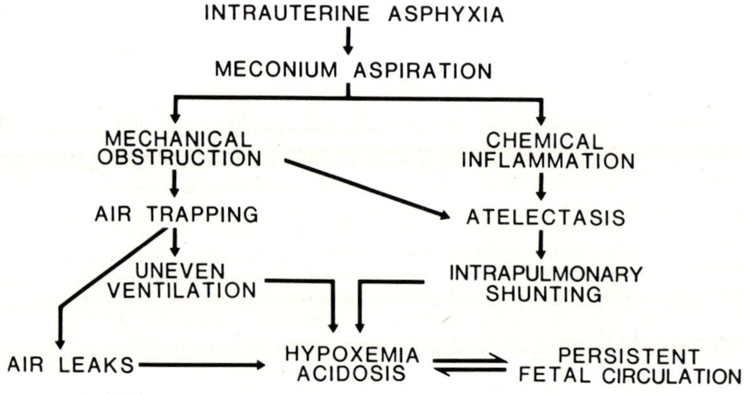

Fig. 28-24. Pathophysiology of meconium aspiration syndrome.

Clinical features

The infant with meconium aspiration syndrome frequently exhibits the classic signs of postmaturity with evidence of weight loss together with nails, skin, and umbilical cord that are heavily stained with a yellowish pigment. The infants often are depressed at birth. In fact the initial clinical picture may be dominated by neurologic and respiratory depression secondary to the hypoxic insult precipitating the passage of meconium. Respiratory distress with cyanosis, grunting, flaring, retractions, and marked tachypnea soon ensues. Characteristically the chest acquires an overinflated appearance, and rales may be audible on auscultation. The chest roentgenogram shows coarse, irregular pulmonary densities with areas of diminished aeration or consolidation (Fig. 28-25). Pneumothorax and pneumomediastinum are noted in up to 50% of infants with meconium aspiration syndrome. Hyperinflation of the chest may be noted roentgenographically with flattening of the diaphragm. Massive aspiration is characterized by a "snowstorm" appearance, and cardiomegaly also may be detected. Arterial blood gases characteristically reveal hypoxemia with evidence of right-to-left shunting. Hyperventilation may result in a respiratory alkalosis, although infants with severe disease usually will have a combined respiratory and metabolic acidosis secondary to the asphyxia and respiratory failure. One should be alerted to the possible development of PFC, which frequently accompanies meconium aspiration syndrome and appears to be the most common cause of a fatal outcome (Chapter 29).

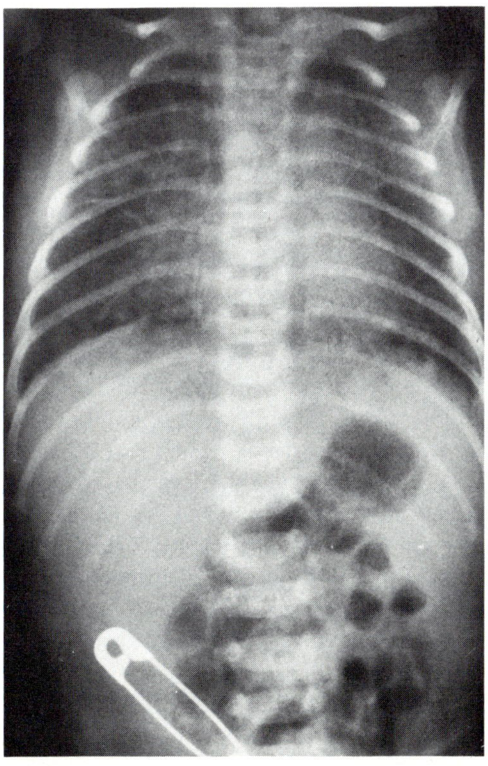

Fig. 28-25. Chest roentgenogram showing multiple linear streaks of meconium aspiration pneumonia.

Management

The key to management of this disorder lies in its prevention. The presence of meconium in the amniotic fluid, however, is not an indication for panic. Although it is clear that meconium staining of the amniotic fluid may signal fetal hypoxia, if other parameters such as fetal heart rate (FHR) and pH remain in the normal range, then the outcome is usually favorable. The combination of meconium-stained amniotic fluid and ominous FHR patterns is associated with significant fetal and neonatal asphyxia with accompanying morbidity, and appropriate interventions should be instituted.

Independent studies from several centers have demonstrated clearly that a combined obstetric and pediatric approach can almost entirely eliminate this major neonatal problem. The cooperative team approach should begin with upper airway suctioning by the obstetrician after delivery of the head. The obstetrician should suction the nose and pharynx with a DeLee suction catheter. Tracheal suctioning under direct vision is ideally performed before the first breath and always must be completed before the initiation of positive pressure ventilation when resuscitating an infant. The controversy is whether all infants with meconium staining of the amniotic fluid should be suctioned. The impressive outcome data when such management is carried out argue strongly for the suctioning of all infants, a position we would advocate. Most significantly, Gregory and associates have found a 56% incidence of meconium in the trachea of meconium-stained infants, in 9% of whom meconium was visualized below the cords despite being absent in the mouth or pharynx. Retrospective data have indicated the benefits of immediate tracheal suctioning of meconium-stained infants in the delivery room, with a marked reduction in morbidity and mortality from meconium aspiration syndrome. Gage documented that catheter suctioning of meconium from the airway of kittens was clearly more effective than bulb suctioning of the upper airway under experimental conditions. He furthermore observed that meconium remained in the trachea for periods exceeding 20 minutes despite spontaneous respirations. These studies underline the importance of tracheal aspiration by the most experienced person in the delivery room before positive pressure resuscitation is begun.

The subsequent management of this disorder consists of supportive respiratory therapy. Little can be done to enhance the mechanisms by which meconium is phagocytosed and removed from distal portions of the respiratory tract. Supportive management includes the use of antibiotics, because bacterial sepsis may have precipitated the passage and subsequent aspiration of meconium, and bacterial pneumonia may be indistinguishable roentgenographically from meconium aspiration syndrome. Furthermore, even though the meconium should be considered sterile, it enhances bacterial growth in vitro. Some authors have advocated the use of steroids; however, in a controlled study hydrocortisone was shown to be of no benefit in the management of this syndrome.

Ventilatory assistance is indicated when adequate levels of PaO_2 cannot be maintained in a high inspired oxygen concentration. Specific details of respiratory management are considered in Part four. Arterial oxygen tension should be maintained at the upper recommended levels, that is, 80 to 90 mm Hg, to minimize hypoxic pulmonary vasoconstriction. Although in initial reports the use of CDP was contraindicated for meconium aspiration, some infants do indeed respond favorably. Truog studied experimental meconium aspiration syndrome in lambs and noted decreased shunting, and improved PaO_2 (without any detrimental effect on pulmonary blood flow) after early application of PEEP. These measures may, however, further increase the risk of air leaks, which is already high because of the many overdistended alveoli. Assisted ventilation is indicated for impending respiratory failure and may be required for a prolonged period. Infants struggling against the ventilator are usually paralyzed, and oxygenation may dramatically improve. A significant mortality can be expected in those infants who require assisted ventilation. Persistence of the fetal circulation is managed with a regimen of minimum disturbance for the infant, hyperventilation (maintaining pH at approximately 7.5), and pulmonary vasodilators such as tolazoline. Transcutaneous monitoring has permitted better control of these potentially unstable infants. The asphyxial complications are treated appropriately and efforts made to prevent hypoglycemia, particularly in SGA infants. The ultimate prognosis may depend not so much on the pulmonary disease as on the accompanying asphyxial insult. No specific long-term deficits in pulmonary function have been described attributed to this disorder, although bronchopulmonary dysplasia may result from prolonged assisted ventilation.

Other aspiration syndromes

At the time of delivery the neonate may aspirate clear amniotic fluid or fluid mixed with pus or blood. It remains unclear whether infants can aspirate a sufficient volume of clear amniotic fluid to interfere with normal ventilation. In deliveries where the amniotic fluid is purulent, the risk of bacterial pneumonia necessitates appropriate antibiotic therapy after evaluation is made for sepsis. Aspiration of either fetal or maternal blood requires no specific therapy and appears to resolve rapidly. Squamous debris associated with amniotic fluid aspiration may persist in the lung for some days. Unless the material is assumed to be infected, therapy should be merely supportive. Aspiration after regurgitation is most likely to be seen in preterm infants, those with disorders of swallowing, and infants with esophageal atresia and tracheoesophageal fistula. Small preterm infants are at greatest risk when fed excessive volumes per gavage. These infants may initially be seen with airway obstruction or apnea and subsequently develop respiratory distress with pulmonary infiltrates visible on roentgenograms. The severity of disease varies, and it may be indistinguishable from an inflammatory pneumonitis. Aspiration syndromes associated with disorders of the swallowing mechanisms may be suspected from the perinatal history (asphyxia), feeding history (color changes, excessive drooling, poor suck), and physical examination. The precise cause, however, may not be readily apparent, and these infants require extensive neurologic evaluation. Neonates with tracheostomies or gastrostomies are at risk for aspiration. Infants with recurrent aspiration, particularly those with disorders of the swallowing mechanism, present complex management problems.

NEONATAL PNEUMONIA

See Chapter 31.

The lungs represent the most common site for the establishment of sepsis in the neonate. Such infection, be it bacterial or viral in origin, may be acquired before or at the time of birth or in the early postnatal period. Since bacterial pneumonia carries a substantial mortality in the neonate, an extremely high index of suspicion must be maintained for all infants, preterm and term alike, in whom signs of respiratory distress are observed.

Etiology

Congenital bacterial pneumonia may be acquired by the fetus via transplacental passage of organisms, although ascending infection from the genital tract before or during labor appears to predominate. It follows that prolonged rupture of membranes in excess of 24 hours is a major predisposing factor, although it is possible that bacteria may gain access to the fetus by ascent through intact membranes. Since bacterial contamination of the infant always occurs during vaginal delivery, neonatal pneumonia may well occur in the absence of prolonged rupture of membranes or any maternal symptoms. Gasping during delivery as a result of fetal asphyxia may predispose the infant to aspirate contaminated amniotic fluid. After the infant is admitted to the neonatal nursery, the risk of acquiring bacterial pneumonia will be largely influenced by the rate of nosocomial infection within the hospital environment.

Over recent years group B streptococci have emerged as the major pathogen producing neonatal pneumonia, with a mortality from 20% to 50%. The organism is characteristically acquired from the maternal genital tract during labor or delivery, and overt group B streptococcal sepsis develops in approximately 1% of infants colonized in this way. This represents an overall infection rate of approximately 1 to 4 per 1,000 live births. Incidence and mortality rate are considerably higher in small preterm infants. Other bacteria to be considered when pneumonia is acquired in utero or in the immediate perinatal period include *Escherichia coli*, *Klebsiella* organisms, group D streptococci, *Listeria* organisms, and pneumococci, acquired via vertical transmission from the mother. When neonatal pneumonia develops several days or even weeks after birth, in addition to these organisms, infections from *Staphylococcus* and *Pseudomonas* organisms and fungi should be considered. Although infection with *Chlamydia trachomatis* does appear to be acquired during parturition, pneumonia caused by this organism typically has a gradual onset of respiratory symptoms beyond 3 weeks of postnatal life. Viral pneumonia can be acquired by the fetus from transplacental passage of organisms, as may be the case in the congenital intrauterine infections (TORCH syndromes) (Chapter 31). Viruses probably also account for a substantial number of postnatally acquired pneumonias. Viral pneumonia is not frequently recognized as such in the neonate, although epidemics resulting from respiratory syncytial virus infection and adenovirus have been described with significant morbidity and mortality.

Clinical course

The nonspecific nature of the clinical signs that are characteristic of neonatal sepsis make a high index of suspicion the key to early diagnosis. In some cases of severe pneumonia the infants may be totally lacking in pulmonary symptoms and present only mild or severe neurologic depression. Other alerting features include thermal instability, apneic spells, abdominal distension, or jaundice. The presence of tachypnea, cyanosis, or other signs of respiratory distress may focus attention on the lungs in these infants. Chest roentgenogram findings range from unilateral or bilateral streaky densities, which may progress to confluent mottled opacified areas, to a diffusely granular appearance with air bronchograms. This may make it impossible to roentgenographically differentiate bacterial pneumonia from RDS, particularly when caused by group B streptococci (Part three). Problems also may be experienced in differentiating severe neonatal pneumonia on roentgenogram from the "snowstorm" appearance of meconium aspiration. The difficulty in making a definitive diagnosis of neonatal pneumonia by roentgenogram has led to the widely accepted practice of administering antibiotics to infants with respiratory distress (particularly RDS) after appropriate cultures have been obtained. White cell count with differential, platelet count, or Gram stain of tracheal aspirate indicates an increased likelihood of respiratory distress being caused by neonatal sepsis but may not differentiate overt pulmonary infection from early colonization.

Latex agglutination assay of body fluids for group B streptococcal polysaccharide antigen allows a specific diagnosis to be made before results of blood and CSF cultures are known. In blood culture–positive infants urine latex assay is almost invariably positive initially or within 12 hours of clinical presentation. It is unclear whether the presence of antigen on assay in infants with negative cultures should be treated as true infection or exposure through colonization with group B streptococcus.

Serologic studies should be performed if congenital intrauterine infection is suspected, and cord blood immunoglobulins should be measured, although not all infants with intrauterine pneumonia will have elevated IgM levels. Chlamydial pneumonitis may be diagnosed by culturing nasopharyngeal or tracheobronchial secretions under appropriate laboratory conditions.

Treatment almost invariably is instituted before the pathogenic organism is identified and its antibiotic sensitivities determined. Broad-spectrum coverage, including a penicillin and aminoglycoside, is the initial line of treatment. For pneumonia of later onset, agents specific for staphylococcal infection should be added. Once the responsible bacterium has been isolated and antibiotic sensitivies identified, the single most effective drug should be continued for 10 days or longer depending on the infant's clinical course. Although antibiotics form the mainstay of treatment, good supportive care is essential. This must include careful fluid management, blood gas monitoring, and ventilatory assistance, as indicated. The duration of chlamydial pneumonia in the neonate appears to be shortened by a 14-day course of oral erythromycin. Early onset bacterial pneumonia, usually caused by group B streptococci, carries a substantial mortality in preterm infants, despite the early administration of appropriate antibiotic therapy.

Persistent fetal circulation may complicate the clinical course of neonatal pneumonia. Animal studies have confirmed that intravenous infusion of group B streptococci rapidly increases pulmonary arterial pressure (with accompanying falls in cardiac output and oxygenation) that may be mediated via thromboxane or prostacyclin metabolites. Pulmonary vascular injury also may be aggravated by granulocytes trapped at sites of injury in the neonatal lung. The efficacy of therapy with granulocyte transfusions or specific anti–group B streptococcal antibody remains undetermined. Administration of prophylactic penicillin at birth to low birth weight infants is not recommended. Bacterial and viral pneumonias of later onset are a cause of considerable morbidity in neonatal intensive care units, but the risk of a subsequent fatal outcome is small.

PULMONARY HEMORRHAGE

Massive pulmonary hemorrhage in the newborn often is associated with RDS and in many instances may be roentgenologically indistinguishable from it. It is usually a preterminal event that has been reported in association with intrauterine asphyxia, neonatal cold injury, aspiration of gastric contents or maternal blood, cerebral edema, severe Rh immunization, kernicterus, congenital heart disease, oxygen administration, widespread viral infection, and bleeding disorders, in addition to RDS. Massive bleeding also may be observed as a complication of procedures to the upper airway, producing erosion or ulceration, and in most instances these will be self-evident. Esterley and Oppenheimer observed massive pulmonary hemorrhage in more than 45% of autopsied neonates with birth weights exceeding 2,500 gm, especially in infants with evidence of intrauterine growth retardation. Frederick and Butler reported massive pulmonary hemorrhage in about 10% of neonatal autopsies, although this incidence probably has decreased because of improved neonatal care. The antecedents of pulmonary hemorrhage are mostly conditions associated with hypoxia, hypervolemia, or congestive heart failure in which an acute rise in lung capillary pressure may be expected. Cole observed that, in infants with massive pulmonary hemorrhage, the hematocrit of the fluid from the endotracheal tube was significantly lower than the venous hematocrit and usually less than 10%. Gel filtration of the proteins from the hemorrhagic fluid and plasma provided clear evidence of molecular sieving, indicating passage of molecules through a porous medium. The most likely interpretation is that massive pulmonary hemorrhage represents the buildup of the capillary filtrate in the interstitial space; when it can no longer be accommodated, it bursts through the pulmonary epithelium into the air spaces. Whereas in most instances pulmonary hemorrhage is thus a reflection of advanced pulmonary edema, in some infants it represents true hemorrhage. Under these circumstances the hematocrit of the pulmonary effluent will be close to the venous hematocrit. The likely reason for the increase in pressure is that severe asphyxia causes acute left-sided heart failure and an acute rise in filtration pressure in the pulmonary capillaries, resulting in generalized lung edema. The factors predisposing to the increased capillary pressure that occurs in neonates with hemorrhagic edema include those favoring filtration of fluid such as hypoproteinemia, overtransfusion, and those causing damage to lung tissue, such as infection, RDS, mechanical ventilation, and excessive oxygen administration. Massive bleeding into the lungs seems relatively uncommon, occurring in association with coagulation disorders, pneumonia, or direct trauma.

Clinically the onset of massive pulmonary hemorrhage is heralded by sudden deterioration of the infant with pallor or shock, cyanosis, bradycardia, and often apnea. Pink or red frothy liquid drains from the mouth and may be seen arising from the trachea between the vocal cords or may be suctioned through an endotracheal tube. In many infants, however, it should be noted that blood will not be observed arising from the endotracheal tube. The diagnosis has been suspected by the finding of diffuse infiltrates or opacification of the lung fields. On autopsy the lungs may appear grossly hemorrhagic and heavy and histologically may reveal intraalveolar hemorrhage.

Hemorrhagic pulmonary edema can be successfully treated by prompt institution of assisted ventilation and transfusion of fresh blood. In some instances exchange transfusion has been successful. Prevention of asphyxia at birth and episodes of asphyxia in infants with predisposing conditions is most important.

TRANSIENT TACHYPNEA

Transient tachypnea often presents a diagnostic dilemma. The disorder is very common and has many overlapping features with respiratory distress caused by surfactant deficiency. Since the infants almost invariably recover fully, it is difficult to define pathologically transient tachypnea of the newborn. The preferred explanation for the clinical features is delayed resorption of fetal lung fluid; thus it is seen more commonly after cesarean section, ostensibly because the infant's thorax is not subjected to the same pressures as when delivery takes place per vaginum in "the big squeeze."

Prolonged labor with a high incidence of failure to progress and greater likelihood of cesarean section has been associated with transient tachypnea. Prolonged maternal administration of hypotonic fluids may occur in this situation and reduce the osmotic gradient that favors resorption of lung fluid in the neonate.

Milner attempted to determine whether vaginal compression has any measurable effect on lung mechanics and lung volume in the hours immediately after birth. Lung function tests were carried out in the first 6 hours of life on 26 babies delivered vaginally and 10 delivered by cesarean section. Striking differences in the thoracic gas volume measurements were observed. The mean thoracic gas volume after vaginal delivery was 32.7 ml/kg; after cesarean section it was only 19.7 ml/kg. Chest circumferences were the same in both groups. He concluded that infants not exposed to vaginal compression have excessively high volumes of interstitial and alveolar fluid for the first few hours, so that thoracic gas volume is reduced, but overall thoracic volume remains within the normal range. In other words, liquid volume is increased, while the gaseous component is decreased.

The syndrome of transient tachypnea typically presents as respiratory distress in nonasphyxiated term infants or preterm infants who are close to term. The clinical features comprise various combinations of cyanosis, grunting, flaring, retracting, and tachypnea in the first few hours after birth. Arterial blood gases reveal varying degrees of hypoxemia, although respiratory failure is uncommon. The chest roentgenogram is the key to the diagnosis. The characteristic finding is prominent perihilar streaking and fluid in the interlobar fissures. The prominent perihilar streaking may represent engorgement of the periarterial lymphatics that appear to participate in the clearance of alveolar fluid. In most instances the roentgenographic appearance can be readily distinguished from the diffuse reticulogranular pattern with air bronchograms that is characteristic of RDS.

The "transient" nature of this disease is quite variable, and it lasts anywhere from 12 to 24 hours in its mildest form to in excess of 72 hours in severe cases. Transient tachypnea must be differentiated from other causes of neonatal respiratory distress. Initially great difficulty may be encountered in distinguishing this disorder from RDS and group B streptococcal pneumonia. Evaluation, monitoring, and basic supportive care must cover all these contingencies. Transient tachypnea of the newborn by definition is self-limiting with no risk of recurrence or residual pulmonary dysfunction. Oral furosemide does not affect the clinical course.

Transient tachypnea also must be distinguished from the clinical syndrome of *cerebral hyperventilation*. This usually is seen in term infants with history of birth asphyxia. The infants are profoundly tachypneic with minimum roentgenographic changes apart from occasional asphyxia-related cardiomegaly. Respiratory alkalosis is typical and is thought to be the result of respiratory center irritation, although there may be a component of postasphyxial pulmonary edema. The prognosis is related primarily to the nature and extent of the accompanying asphyxial insult.

PNEUMOTHORAX AND OTHER AIR LEAK SYNDROMES

Pulmonary air leaks comprise a spectrum of disease that includes pneumothorax, pneumomediastinum, pneumopericardium, and pulmonary interstitial emphysema. If significant morbidity and even mortality are to be minimized with these conditions, particularly tension pneumothorax, a high index of suspicion is essential to initiate early diagnosis and aggressive management.

Incidence

Pneumothorax is far more frequent in the neonatal period than any other time of life. The incidence varies widely depending on selective features such as frequency of neonatal asphyxia, techniques of resuscitation, incidence of respiratory problems, methods of administering assisted ventilation, and even the quality of x-ray examinations and experience of personnel interpreting the films (Chapter 13). Based on numerous roentgenographic surveys, the overall frequency of pneumothorax approximates 1% of all live births.

The likelihood of a pneumothorax being symptomatic in an infant without underlying lung disease is small, and many of these go undetected. Several interventions and disease states markedly increase the risk of pulmonary air leaks. These include vigorous resuscitation at birth, RDS, meconium aspiration syndrome, and pulmonary hypoplasia. In infants treated with assisted ventilation the incidence of pneumothorax and other air leaks is higher in most series, with some variability according to the technique employed. An incidence of 5% to 20% has been documented in RDS both with and without the use of CPAP. At our institution there is a 25% incidence of air leaks in infants weighing less than 2 kg, requiring early onset of assisted ventilation. In term infants with meconium aspiration syndrome the incidence of air leaks is reported to range from 20% to 50%, often occurring early in the course of the disease.

Pathophysiology

Macklin first described, in the overdistended cat lung, the passage of air from a ruptured alveolus, moving up the vascular sheath into the mediastinum and from there into the pleural cavity. Both uneven alveolar ventilation and air trapping would appear to figure prominently in the pathophysiology of the air leak syndromes. On the one hand, inhomogeneity of ventilation is a result of both the atelectatic alveoli in RDS and the small airway plugs of meconium aspiration syndrome. The relatively more distensible areas of the lung receiving most of the ventilation are subjected to exceedingly high transpulmonary pressures, leading to an increased risk of alveolar rupture. On the other hand, during partial airway obstruction full expiration is prevented, and with subsequent inspirations accumulation of air may rupture the alveolar space. The susceptibility to pulmonary rupture is further enhanced in the neonate by a reduction in alveolar connecting channels (pores of Kohn) that would allow air to redistribute between ventilated and nonventilated units. Finally, many cases of pneumothorax and pneumomediastinum may originate at birth as a result of the high initial pressures that may be generated with the first few breaths. If this high pressure is transmitted to units already open, they may rupture as a result of these large pressure changes. High pressures are often necessary in infants with hypoplastic lungs; thus rupture is common.

The high incidence of air leaks during assisted ventilation has been attributed to barotrauma caused by high levels of peak inspiratory pressure (Part four). While optimal ventilator regimens need to be clarified, excessive prolongation of inspiratory time during conventional ventilation may be the major risk factor in the pathogenesis of air leaks. Furthermore, while airway disruption has been thought to occur at the alveolar or saccular level, airway wall disruption may also contribute, as is seen in a baboon model of pulmonary interstitial emphysema.

Clinical features

Extrapulmonary extravasation of air should be suspected in any infant with respiratory disease whose condition suddenly deteriorates. Tachypnea is a uniform finding and may be accompanied by grunting and increasing pallor or cyanosis. If there is a unilateral pneumothorax, the cardiac apex may be shifted away from the affected side and breath sounds decreased, although this is a less reliable sign. Some infants may develop distention of the involved hemithorax or a tensely distended abdomen from downward displacement of the diaphragm. Signs of shock may be present because of compression of the great veins and decreased cardiac output.

Sudden onset of hypertension has also been reported. In pneumothorax, hypoxemia results from both decreased alveolar ventilation and right-to-left shunting of pulmonary blood flow through the atelectatic areas. In preterm infants with RDS a pneumothorax frequently develops beyond the first days of life, when the severity of disease is decreasing and lung compliance increasing. Pneumothorax also may be suspected by a precipitous fall in transcutaneous oxygen tension, diminished excursion of the arterial pressure tracing, or reduced thoracic impedance. Because of a paucity of clinical signs, pneumomediastinum without accompanying pneumothorax frequently escapes clinical detection but is readily identified roentgenographically. Pneumopericardium is a less common complication that may accompany a pneumomediastinum, possibly because of air tracking along pleural reflections around the great vessels. Although it is frequently stated that pneumomediastinum in the neonate precedes pneumopericardium, there is no good evidence to substantiate this. Pneumopericardium may be present as a cardiac tamponade with reduced stroke volume and venous return. Thus there is a fall in systolic blood pressure, and the heart sounds are absent or muffled. Pneumoperitoneum secondary to passage of air from the chest through the diaphragmatic apertures is a rare occurrence that needs to be differentiated from free intraabdominal air secondary to a perforated viscus, and may require contrast bowel studies for confirmation.

Large bilateral pneumothoraces often are observed in infants with the hypoplastic lungs accompanying renal agenesis (Potter's syndrome), other forms of renal dysplasia, or congenital diaphragmatic hernia. The presence of otherwise unexplained extrapulmonary air in the early neonatal period should raise the question of underlying renal malformations, and a thorough physical examination together with the appropriate investigations should be promptly undertaken (Chapter 35; see also later in this chapter).

There appears to be an association between the occurrence of a pneumothorax and intraventricular hemorrhage in preterm infants. Hill has reported a marked increase in anterior cerebral artery blood flow (with a noninvasive Doppler technique) followed by hemorrhage in infants after a pneumothorax has developed. Thus it is proposed that a pneumothorax may increase the risk of intraventricular hemorrhage by impairing venous return to the heart and increasing cerebral arterial blood flow, which results from hypercarbia and raised systemic diastolic pressure.

Extrapolating from newborn dog experiments, Batton suggested that intraventricular hemorrhage is most likely to be precipitated at the time of pneumothorax evacuation, when there may be an instantaneous rise in arterial

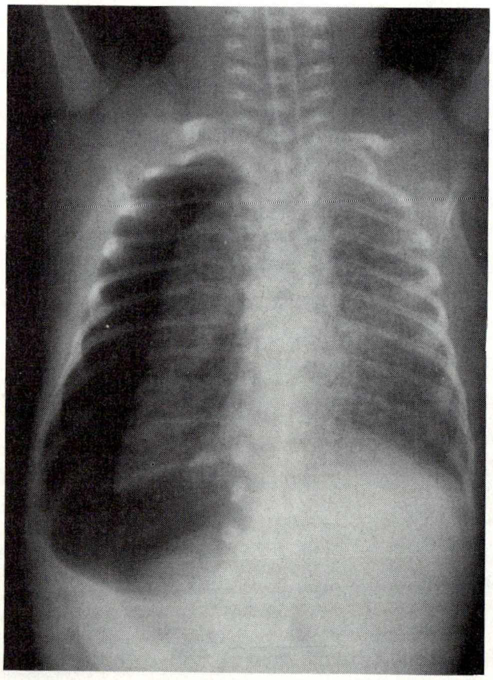

Fig. 28-26. Tension pneumothorax on the right. An endotracheal tube is in place.

blood pressure and cerebral blood flow velocity. (See also Chapter 27.)

Diagnosis

Transillumination of the chest is an extremely useful technique for immediate diagnosis of pneumothorax and is invariably positive if the pneumothorax is large. Its principal benefit is to detect sudden life-threatening air leaks, which require immediate therapy before a definitive roentgenographic diagnosis can be obtained. The technique involves the use of a fiberoptic light probe at the end of a flexible tube that is placed on the infant's chest wall while the nursery is darkened. In the presence of a large pneumothorax the entire hemithorax on the affected side lights up, while the opposite side shows diminished transillumination because of lung compression on that side. Decompression should be accomplished without awaiting roentgenographic confirmation. When there are lesser or questionable areas of abnormal transillumination and the infant's condition is stable, roentgenographic confirmation is indicated before therapeutic intervention is undertaken. This will allow precise localization of the pneumothorax and differentiation from a pneumomediastinum or pneumopericardium.

Good roentgenographic techniques (Chapter 13) are basic to the accurate localization of accumulations of extrapulmonary air in the neonate. A large tension pneumothorax is readily diagnosed by the presence of air in the pleural cavity separating the parietal and visceral pleura, collapse of the ipsilateral lobes, displacement of the mediastinum to the contralateral side, and downward movement of the diaphragm (Fig. 28-26). Because of the decreased compliance of the lung in infants with severe RDS, total collapse is not seen even with a tension pneumothorax, and there may be only minimal shift of the mediastinal structures. A useful roentgenologic sign of pneumothorax is a prominent curvilinear marking above the heart that reflects displacement of the bulging mediastinal pleura across the midline to the contralateral side. The classic roentgenographic appearance can be readily overlooked in an anteroposterior film taken with the patient in the supine position if a large amount of the intrapleural air is situated just behind the sternum. In such instances a horizontal-beam lateral film with the infant supine will identify the retrosternal accumulation of air. If an isolated pneumomediastinum is present on anteroposterior film, there will be a hyperlucent rim of air lateral to the cardiac borders and thymus, elevating the latter away from the pericardium in a characteristic crescent or "spinnaker sail" configuration. This must be roentgenographically differentiated from a pneumopericardium in which air completely surrounds the heart, including its inferior border (Fig. 28-27).

Management

In an infant who does not have any underlying pulmonary disease, no specific management is necessary for an asymptomatic pneumothorax. The presence of an iso-

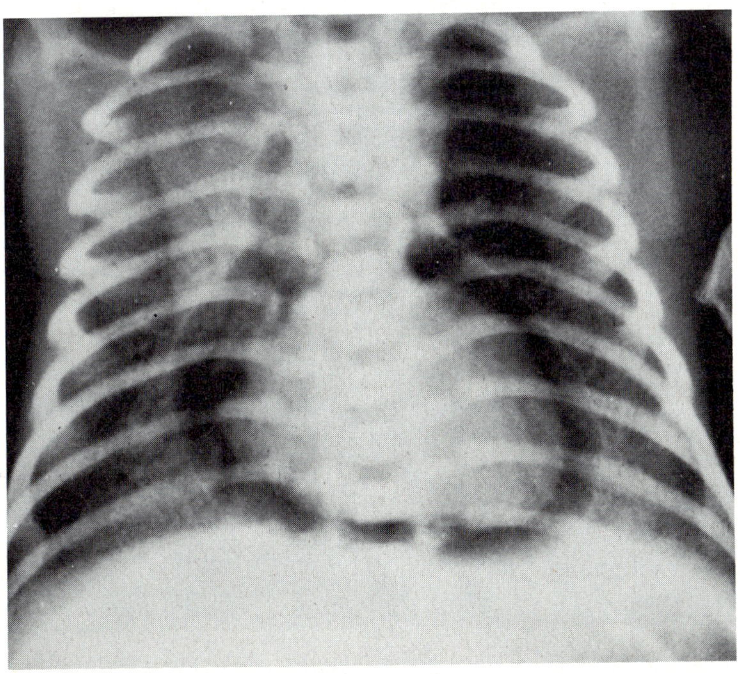

Fig. 28-27. Pneumopericardium in a newborn.

lated pneumomediastinum requires close observation of vital signs and frequent clinical assessment, since this may progress to a pneumothorax at any time. In infants with lung disease the presence of a pneumothorax accentuates the respiratory difficulty and requires prompt if not urgent intervention. This consists of the placement of a large-bore, multiple-holed chest tube into the pleural space, preferably anterior to the lung. Anterior placement in the pleural space is best achieved by insertion of the tube into the chest at or just lateral to the anterior axillary line. This should be connected to an underwater seal at a suction pressure of from 10 to 20 cm H_2O, since reaccumulation of air may occur if suction is not applied.

The chest tube should be introduced under sterile conditions and secured with a pursestring suture. Lung perforation has been described at autopsy in infants who required pleural drainage for pneumothorax. Such iatrogenic lung perforation may well prolong the period of recovery from pulmonary disease or even contribute to death in these infants (Fig. 28-28). Great care therefore must be exercised during chest tube insertion, with curved mosquito clamps used rather than a trocar to guide the catheter into the pleural space. Dramatic improvement in color and circulation follows the relief of a tension pneumothorax, which can be confirmed by repeat transillumination. The ease with which the lung

A

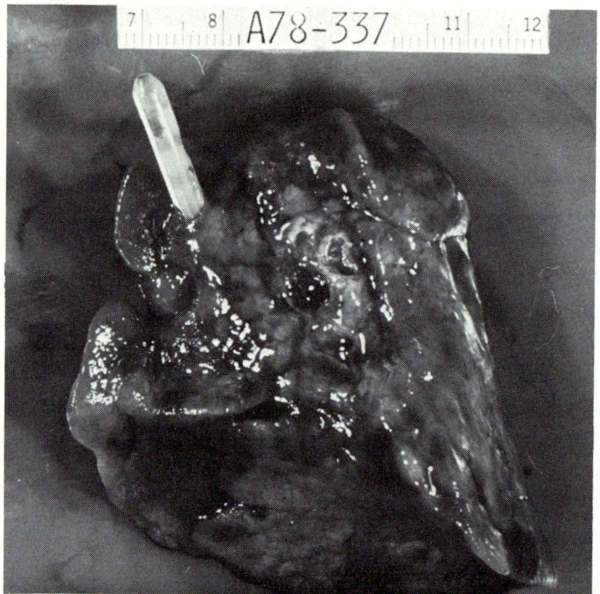

B

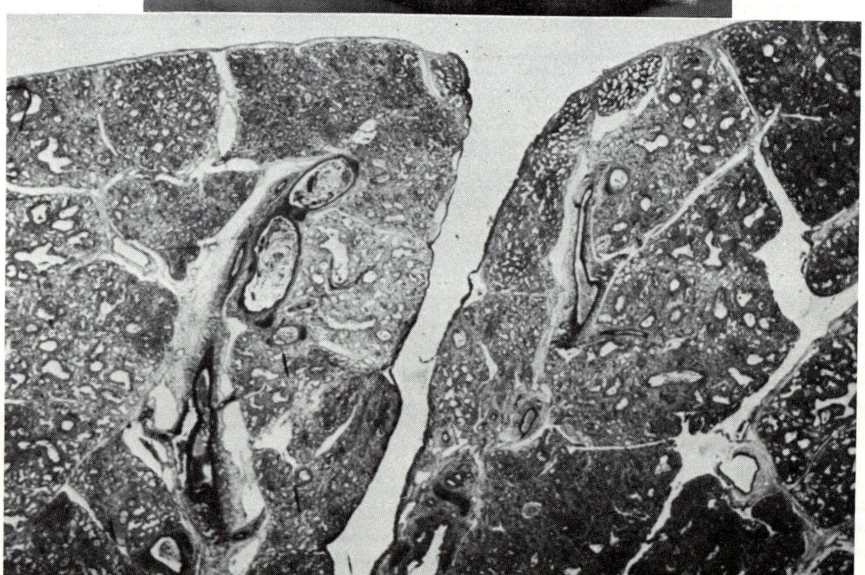

Fig. 28-28. Perforation of the lung associated with insertion of chest tube by means of trocar and cannula. **A,** Gross appearance. **B,** Histologic features demonstrating tract into the lung.

can be reexpanded depends to a large extent on the compliance of the underlying pulmonary tissue. Expansion is particularly slow in infants with hypoplastic lungs associated with a congenital diaphragmatic hernia. Fluid intake may need to be reduced during the acute phase of a pneumothorax, since an increase in vasopressin release has been documented at this time, as assessed by urinary excretion of the hormone. Suction should be maintained until fluctuation of air in the tube and active bubbling have ceased. At this time the tube should be clamped and removed within 24 hours if there has been no reaccumulation of air in the pleural cavity.

Infants who are symptomatic from a large pneumomediastinum rarely benefit from decompression via an anteriorly placed chest tube. Conservative therapy is followed in isolated cases of pneumopericardium, although, if there is an accompanying gas tamponade, pericardiocentesis may be life-saving. Data from experimentally induced pneumopericardium in puppies suggest that a reduction in cardiac size is indicative of drastic hemodynamic compromise, requiring immediate pericardiocentesis.

Pulmonary interstitial emphysema

Pulmonary interstitial emphysema (PIE) is primarily a roentgenographic and pathologic diagnosis made when air ruptures from alveoli or small airways into the perivascular tissues of the lung. Pathologic examination reveals multiple irregular air-filled cysts varying in diameter from 0.1 to 1 cm, localized to interlobular septa, and extending radially from the hilum. PIE is seen predominantly in preterm infants who require the prolonged use of assisted ventilation, and is thought to signal barotrauma. It may result in a vicious cycle by causing compression atelectasis of the adjacent lung, necessitating a further increase in ventilatory pressure and permitting still more escape of air into the interstitial tissues. From this location air may further progress into the mediastinum and pleural space, although it is uncommon for air to track into the neck during the neonatal period.

Two forms of PIE are characteristically described—a diffuse variety and a localized variety—although their causes do not appear to differ. Diffuse PIE usually has been associated with prolonged artificial ventilation and a high incidence of bronchopulmonary dysplasia (Part six). The infants with PIE at highest risk for death are those of lowest birth weight and gestational age, in whom PIE appears within the first 24 hours of life. In this population the subsequent incidence of bronchopulmonary dysplasia may exceed 50%. During management of diffuse PIE every attempt must be made to maintain mechanical ventilatory pressures at a safe minimum. High-frequency ventilation shows real promise as a means of alleviating or even eliminating PIE (Part four).

The localized form is characterized on roentgenogram by discrete involvement of one or more lobes and is usually accompanied by mediastinal shift to the opposite side. The severity of symptoms will depend on the size of the uninvolved area and the ability of the uninvolved lung to adequately meet the infant's ventilatory needs. Both forms of PIE frequently show spontaneous regression over time. Conservative management of localized PIE is recommended as an initial step. Positioning the infant such that the emphysematous lung is always dependent may lead to clinical and roentgenographic improvement within 48 hours. Localized PIE has also been successfully treated by selective intubation of the main stem bronchus on the uninvolved side, and this may hasten resolution in as little as 24 hours. Although technically difficult, this procedure should be attempted before any surgical intervention is attempted. Lobectomy will be indicated in a small number of cases of localized PIE when spontaneous regression is not occurring and medical management has failed. Although clear guidelines for surgical intervention are difficult to establish, it should be reserved for infants in whom the risks of recurring complications outweigh those of surgery.

Massive *air embolism* (or pulmonary venous air embolism) is a dramatic complication of assisted ventilation when high pressures are employed. The air embolism is thought to arise from rupture of alveoli into small pulmonary veins. The diagnosis is made by the roentgenographic appearance of intravascular air, or withdrawal of air from an umbilical arterial catheter, with accompanying clinical signs of shock. The outcome is almost invariably fatal.

DEVELOPMENTAL ANOMALIES

Pulmonary hypoplasia

Pathophysiology

Bilateral pulmonary hypoplasia represents a broad spectrum of anatomic malformations ranging from total bronchial and parenchymal agenesis to mild pulmonary parenchymal hypoplasia. Complete pulmonary agenesis is almost always unilateral (usually involving the left lung) and is frequently accompanied by other congenital anomalies. The lung on the opposite side is typically hypertrophied and often herniates across the midline to occupy part of the affected hemithorax.

Pulmonary hypoplasia, on the other hand, may be either unilateral or bilateral. It may be seen as an isolated entity (so-called primary pulmonary hypoplasia) or be secondary to lesions restricting lung growth. A classification of neonatal pulmonary hypoplasia is as follows:

A. Primary
   1. Pulmonary agenesis (unilateral) with or without other malformations
   2. Idiopathic pulmonary hypoplasia (bilateral)

B. Secondary
   1. Congenital diaphragmatic hernia (unilateral)

2. Oligohydramnios
    a. Chronic amniotic fluid leak (bilateral)
    b. Renal agenesis and dysplasia (bilateral)
3. Skeletal and neuromuscular disease (bilateral)

The result of pulmonary hypoplasia is a decreased number of alveoli, peripheral bronchioles, and arterioles, the latter often leading to medial muscular hypertrophy. A histologic diagnosis involves the demonstration of a low ratio of lung-to-body weight, low lung DNA content, or a decreased radial alveolar count. The diagnosis of primary pulmonary hypoplasia implies a lack of any specific pathophysiologic process that could cause fetal lung compression. Nonetheless it has been proposed that decreased fetal respiratory movement, as might result from hypoxia, neuromuscular disease, or chest wall abnormalities in utero, could result in some degree of functional lung compression and hypoplasia. Another possible explanation of primary pulmonary hypoplasia is that, for as yet unknown reasons, morphologic development of the lungs simply progresses at a slower than normal rate in some infants.

The severity of secondary pulmonary hypoplasia depends on the degree to which thoracic size is reduced. A modest degree of lung restriction results in a histologically normal but undersized lung, whereas severe restriction additionally causes a significant reduction in the extent of bronchiolar branching. The association between unilateral pulmonary hypoplasia and congenital diaphragmatic hernia has been well documented and appears to result from the presence of bowel within the thorax, mechanically restricting lung growth (Chapter 33). In this situation the affected lung may exhibit severe immaturity as well as being small, although the reason for this interruption of pulmonary maturation is unclear. The characteristic increase in pulmonary vascular resistance is the result of a decrease in size of the total pulmonary vascular bed, an increase in pulmonary arterial smooth muscle, and a decrease in the number of vessels per unit of lung. After the hernia is repaired the number of airway branchings and alveoli remains reduced, whereas the pulmonary blood vessels show a persistently increased muscularity for several months. Pulmonary hypoperfusion on the affected side has been demonstrated to persist for years in these infants.

Bilateral pulmonary hypoplasia commonly occurs in association with oligohydramnios caused by either renal disease in the fetus or chronic leakage of amniotic fluid. The presence of pulmonary hypoplasia in infants with bilateral renal agenesis was first recognized by Potter in 1946. It has since become apparent that a similar picture of lethal pulmonary hypoplasia is seen in conjunction with bilaterally dysplastic kidneys with or without cyst formation. Characteristic features include premature birth in the breech position, a typical facial appearance, limb malformations, and severe respiratory insufficiency often complicated by air leaks and invariably resulting in a fatal outcome (Chapter 35). In cases of renal agenesis the reduction in lung volume and number of alveoli is greater than in renal dysplasia, where these changes are more variable in their severity. Infants subjected to oligohydramnios resulting from a chronic leakage of amniotic fluid over many weeks may similarly exhibit a variable degree of pulmonary hypoplasia. Oligohydramnios may act by compressing the fetal thorax or altering the dynamics of lung fluid so that expansion of the lungs cannot be maintained. Pathologic findings by Hislop imply that an interference in normal lung growth has occurred before 16 weeks' gestation in these infants. Since the contribution of fetal urine to amniotic fluid becomes important relatively late in pregnancy, oligohydramnios is unlikely to be the sole cause of the hypoplastic lung. Thus renal agenesis appears to have some direct but as yet unidentified effect on early pulmonary maturation. During fetal development the kidney appears to be an important source of proline, and this has been proposed to contribute to the formation of collagen and mesenchymal tissue in the developing pulmonary parenchyma. Further insight is needed into the interaction between early renal and pulmonary maturation in the fetus.

Thibeault found that in infants with normal kidneys oligohydramnios can be associated with a spectrum of fetal positional and compression abnormalities (Chapter 6). Preterm infants of 34 weeks' gestation or less with premature rupture of membranes for a mean of 19 days (range, 6 to 90 days) and accompanying positional deformities at birth almost invariably had clinical or autopsy evidence of lung hypoplasia. In the absence of positional deformities a small number of comparable infants with prolonged rupture of membranes also showed signs of pulmonary hypoplasia, although this tended to be less severe. It is possible that antenatal evidence of oligohydramnios with decreased fetal mobility may predict relative risk of lung hypoplasia in these infants.

Clinical course

In infants with unilateral pulmonary agenesis the diagnosis may be suspected by unilaterally decreased breath sounds and displacement of the mediastinum to the affected side. Some breath sounds, however, may be audible over the affected side if a portion of normal lung has herniated across the midline. The roentgenographic appearance of a radiopaque hemithorax will help confirm the diagnosis, and accompanying vertebral defects are not uncommon. Treatment is largely of symptoms and prognosis will depend on the presence or absence of other anomalies.

The diagnosis of bilateral primary pulmonary hypoplasia may be readily overlooked. Swischuk reported on eight infants with hypoplastic lungs that did not appear to be accompanied by other organ system disease. These infants were seen with characteristic features of respiratory distress immediately after birth, associated with hypoxemia, hypercarbia, and acidosis. They exhibited clinical evidence of persistent fetal circulation, and all demonstrated small but clear lung fields on chest roentgenogram, accompanied by a pneumothorax in seven out of eight infants. Two infants survived, indicating that a favorable outcome is possible if pulmonary hypoplasia is not pronounced. This entity should be considered in infants with persistent fetal circulation who have the previously stated roentgenographic criteria of bilateral pulmonary hypoplasia.

The clinical course and outcome of infants with pulmonary hypoplasia secondary to congenital diaphragmatic hernia are dependent largely on the degree of herniation and ability to accomplish adequate surgical repair in addition to the extent of the pulmonary hypoplasia and accompanying increase in pulmonary vascular resistance. In classic Potter's syndrome bilateral renal agenesis is easily diagnosed on ultrasound and will always result in the infant's death. A favorable outcome is possible when renal dysplasia is less severe or pulmonary hypoplasia is associated with oligohydramnios of shorter duration.

Congenital lobar emphysema

Congenital lobar emphysema is characterized by overdistention of one or more lobes of an infant's lung caused by trapping of air within the affected area. The relative frequency of involvement of the various pulmonary lobes is illustrated in Fig. 28-29. A variety of conditions, as outlined subsequently, may contribute to this inability of the affected lung to deflate normally, although frequently a specific cause cannot be established. Partial intraluminal bronchial obstruction may result from a deficiency of bronchial cartilage restricted to one lobe or even from inflammatory exudate or aspirated mucus. Similarly bronchial compression may be caused by adjacent vascular structures such as blood vessels or mediastinal and intrapulmonary masses. Finally, partial airway collapse has been proposed to result from the high compliance of the airways of the neonate. It can be seen that congenital lobar emphysema generally cannot be attributed to a single cause but should be considered as a symptom complex rather than a specific disease entity.

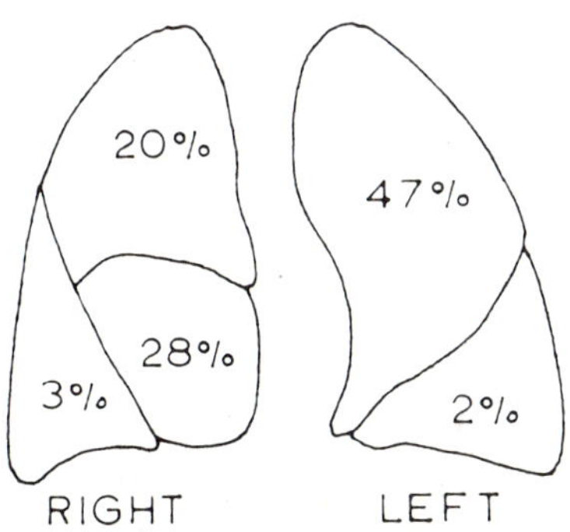

Fig. 28-29. Distribution of congenital emphysema by percentage of lobar involvement. (From DeLuca, F.G.: Clin. Perinatol. **5:**377, 1978.)

The severity of symptoms depends on the size of the overinflated lobe and the resultant compression of surrounding lung tissue and degree of mediastinal shift. These infants may exhibit symptoms soon after birth, but more commonly symptoms begin at 1 or 2 months of age. Respiratory distress frequently is accompanied by wheezing. Physical findings include hyperresonance to percussion, decreased breath sounds over the affected lobe, and shift of the apical heart beat to the contralateral side. Chest roentgenogram clearly demonstrates a hyperinflated lobe that may have herniated across the midline and caused mediastinal shift and compression of the adjacent lung. Roentgenologic differentiation from lung cysts or even a pneumothorax may be difficult but will be aided by the presence of linear bronchovascular and alveolar markings within the emphysematous lobe. Localized PIE will have a preceding history of assisted ventilation at high pressures, resulting in barotrauma. Angiography may be indicated because of the increased incidence of coexisting congenital heart disease and to visualize adjacent pulmonary vascular structures.

Treatment should begin with bronchoscopy in an attempt to identify and remove any cause of airway obstruction. Excision of the affected lobe is generally indicated if the infant remains symptomatic after bronchoscopy and may be life-saving if respiratory failure is severe. If symptoms are minimal or the infant is asymptomatic, conservative management probably should be attempted. After removal of an emphysematous lobe, ventilation rapidly improves with expansion of the previously collapsed lobes. The long-term prognosis is thought to be excellent, although adequate follow-up studies of the effects of lobectomy performed in the neonatal period are not yet available.

Lung cysts

Congenital lung cysts are a rare cause of respiratory distress in neonates that should be readily differentiated from acquired cystic lesions. The latter are typically the result of severe RDS that has required prolonged assisted ventilation or has been complicated by the development of an air leak syndrome (Chapter 28, part five). Acquired cysts or pneumatoceles rarely result from staphylococcal, *Klebsiella*, or other bacterial pneumonia in the neonate and may be large and persist for several months.

There is still considerable controversy concerning the cause of congenital lung cysts. Their presence in stillborn infants, albeit rare, indicates that they truly may be congenital. Nonetheless they are almost never associated with cystic disease in other organs or with any other specific malformation. Congenital lung cysts commonly are located at the periphery of the lung and may represent a disorder of bronchial development occurring in later fetal life. The infants may be seen initially with respiratory distress caused by overdistention of a cyst, recurrent infection, or wheezing caused by partial airway obstruction. The diagnosis is made roentgenologically by recognizing round or oval translucent areas within the pulmonary parenchyma. It should be noted that cysts arising from bronchi may change in size depending on the degree of bronchial obstruction, and on the first day of life they may not even be apparent on roentgenogram because of the presence of fetal lung fluid within the cyst. Multiple cysts must be distinguished roentgenographically from a diaphragmatic hernia (Chapter 33) where air-filled loops of bowel within the thorax may present a similar appearance.

Conservative therapy is appropriate if the infant is asymptomatic. Operative resection of congenital lung cysts, however, will be indicated as a result of complications from pressure effects on adjacent areas of normal lung. Urgent surgical intervention may be needed if pulmonary function is acutely compromised. Surgical resection usually is indicated for the rare case of *cystic adenomatoid malformation*, which is a form of congenital cystic lung disease generally confined to a single lobe. These infants show a roentgenographic density (which probably represents a hematoma) surrounded by scattered radiolucent areas and progressive compression of the surrounding lung.

Chylothorax

Chylothorax is an extremely unusual entity in the neonate that usually is associated with nonspecific respiratory symptoms in the first days of life. The cause is unknown although presumably related to either traumatic injury of the thoracic duct at delivery or some congenital malformation of the duct wall. Other lymphatic vessels in the body tend not to be affected in most cases. Since chylothorax is typically unilateral, there may be decreased breath sounds over the side of the effusion and mediastinal shift to the contralateral side. The characteristic roentgenographic appearance is of a large *pleural effusion* depressing the adjacent diaphragm and displacing the mediastinum.

Pleural effusion at this age may also be a manifestation of infection or heart failure, may accompany hydrops fetalis, or may result from extravasated fluid caused by an improperly placed central venous line. The definitive diagnosis is made by thoracentesis, which will reveal clear fluid rich in lymphocytes during the first day, changing to markedly opalescent fluid with a high protein and fat content after the introduction of milk feeding. The majority of infants recover completely after single or multiple thoracenteses. If continuous drainage of chyle via a chest tube is required, this may result in severe malnutrition, and under these circumstances administration of total parenteral nutrition is indicated. During the administration of intravenous hyperalimentation a marked decrease in the fat content of the pleural fluid has been observed. Although it has been recommended to feed a formula rich in medium-chain triglycerides, this does not appear to significantly reduce the triglyceride and fatty acid content of the fluid accumulating in the pleural space.

Mediastinal masses

Mediastinal masses are rare in the newborn, and, when present, they are usually cystic structures that represent some congenital remnant or malformation. They must be clearly differentiated roentgenographically from a normal thymus, which frequently occupies a prominent place in the anterior mediastinum of neonates. Lesions causing narrowing or significant displacement of the mediastinal trachea will be associated with wheezing, and in addition to the mass noted on roentgenogram, the lung fields may appear hyperinflated.

Miscellaneous intrapulmonary malformations

It has been customary to subdivide congenital lobar malformations within the pulmonary parenchyma into accessory and sequestered lobes. Accessory lobes may reflect an early defect in lung development in which pulmonary tissue has separated from the rest of the lung, although connections with an airway or portion of the gut may persist. These lobes characteristically produce no symptoms but present uncertainty as to their identity when they appear on chest film. Sequestered lobes, on the other hand, are intralobar structures that probably originate from an anomaly in the blood supply to that area of the lung. They do not have any connection to bronchi or the gastrointestinal tract but do have their own independent blood supply arising from the aorta. Respiratory symptoms attributable to a sequestered lobe are unlikely to occur in infancy. They may be confused roentgenographically with an area of atelectasis or pneumonia.

Congenital pulmonary lymphangiectasia is a rare entity in which there is congenital dilation of the lymphatic channels in the lung. The lungs are bulky at autopsy with visible lobulation caused by diffuse dilation of subpleural lymphatics and thickening of interlobular septa. The cause of this disorder appears to be an early cessation of growth of the lymphatic trunks in the septa, leading to the diffuse pattern of cystic lymphatic spaces seen microscopically. These infants typically are seen at term with respiratory distress that progresses to a fatal outcome. There may be coexistent lymphedema in other areas of the body, and congenital cardiac malformations frequently are found at autopsy. Chest roentgenograms reveal a variable pattern of hyperinflation and diffuse granularity with prominent interstitial markings. It follows that diagnosis of this rare condition is not easy, since the roentgenologic and clinical picture simulates those of the common causes of respiratory distress in the neonate.

Pulmonary arteriovenous fistula is an extremely rare cause of respiratory distress in the newborn that may be associated with hemangiomas in other areas such as the skin. This is a potentially curable disorder with single or multiple communications between pulmonary arteries and veins that require surgical intervention.

RESPIRATORY CONTROL AND APNEA OF PREMATURITY

Preterm infants normally exhibit varying patterns of breathing that range from regular respiration to frequent pauses or apneic episodes. Although recent advances have greatly increased our understanding of the pathophysiology of apnea, a disproportionate amount of time in neonatal intensive care units continues to be spent evaluating, monitoring, and treating apneic episodes. The extent of the problem is illustrated by the fact that more than 50% of all surviving infants from our neonatal intensive care unit with birth weights less than 1.5 kg require either respiratory support or pharmacologic intervention for recurrent prolonged apneic episodes. Nonetheless a greater awareness of the influence on the immature respiratory center of various components of respiratory control, such as chemoreceptors and pulmonary stretch receptors, is slowly emerging (Fig. 28-30). A more complete understanding of respiratory control will permit a rational approach to the management of apnea in the neonate.

Maturation of chemical and reflex control of breathing

Spontaneous and sustained breathing movements alternating with episodes of apnea have been well documented in the human fetus. Recent studies have further established that in mature fetal lambs breathing efforts increase in response to elevated levels of arterial PCO_2 ($PaCO_2$). Both full-term and preterm infants also increase minute ventilation in response to small increases in inspired carbon dioxide concentration. Recent evidence indicates that carbon dioxide responsiveness, which reflects predominantly central chemoreceptor activity and is a traditional measure of respiratory drive, is progressively less well developed in the more immature infant. Infants of less than 33 weeks' gestational age exhibit reduced ventilatory responses to inspired carbon dioxide. It is unclear whether this reduced ventilatory response to carbon dioxide in small preterm infants is primarily the result of decreased central chemosensitivity or mechanical factors preventing an appropriate increase in ventilation. It has been proposed that the carbon dioxide response curve has a decreased slope (indicating less respiratory drive) in preterm infants who exhibit apnea (Fig. 28-31), but a cause-and-effect relation between decreased carbon dioxide responsiveness and apnea of prematurity has not been clearly established. In older infants beyond the immediate neonatal period, Shannon observed impaired carbon dioxide responsiveness in those

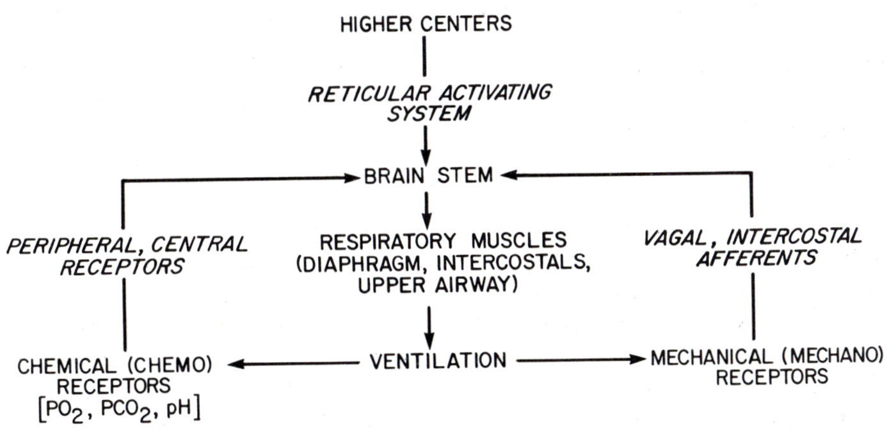

Fig. 28-30. Simplified diagrammatic representation of the various afferent inputs to the neonatal respiratory center. (From Martin, R.J. In Lehrman, R., and Vaughan, V., editors: In Nelson's textbook of pediatrics, ed. 13, Philadelphia, 1987, W.B. Saunders Co., [In press.])

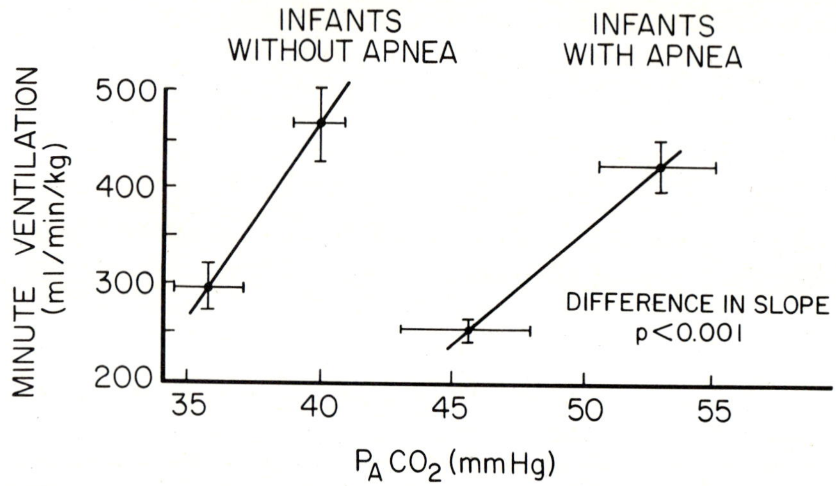

Fig. 28-31. The ventilatory response to carbon dioxide has a decreased slope in infants with apnea. (From Gerhardt, T., and Bancalari, E.: Pediatrics **74:**58, 1984. Reproduced by permission of Pediatrics.)

at risk for sudden infant death, although other investigators have not confirmed these findings.

Rigatto observed that preterm infants respond to a fall in inspired oxygen concentration with a transient increase in ventilation over approximately 1 minute, followed by a sustained depression of ventilation. In term infants a similar response has been observed during the first week of life. This biphasic response to hypoxemia in the neonate is in marked contrast to the ventilatory response in adults, where a low oxygen concentration results in a sustained increase in ventilation. The characteristic response to low oxygen in infants may be due to initial peripheral chemoreceptor stimulation followed by overriding depression of the respiratory center as a result of hypoxemia. Consistent with these findings is the observation that a progressive decrease in inspired oxygen concentration causes a significant flattening of carbon dioxide responsiveness in preterm infants (Fig. 28-32). The magnitude of the fall in Po_2 necessary to depress ventilation remains to be determined. Nonetheless this unstable response to low inspired oxygen may play an important role in the etiology of neonatal apnea.

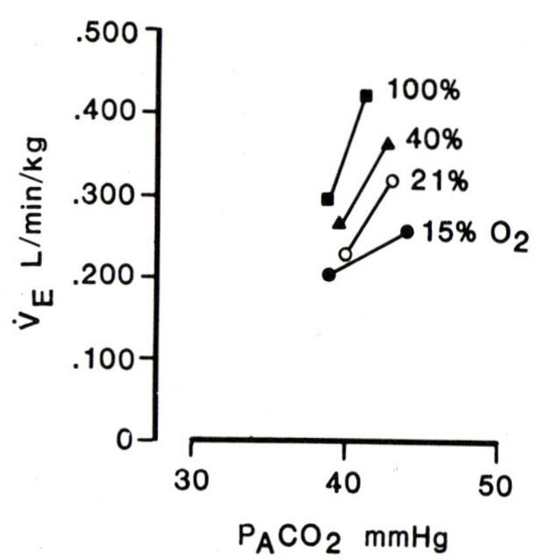

Fig. 28-32. Steady-state carbon dioxide response curves at different inspired oxygen concentrations. The more hypoxic the infant, the flatter the response to carbon dioxide. (From Rigatto, H., de la Torre Verduzco, R., and Cates, D.B.: J. Appl. Physiol. **39:**896, 1975.)

The effects of pulmonary stretch receptors in altering the timing of respiration at varying lung volumes are more readily elicited in the newborn than in the adult. During the first days of life sudden lung inflation results in an initial gasp (Head's reflex) followed by prolonged apnea (the so-called Hering-Breuer inflation reflex). Similarly a small but sustained increase in lung volume (as with the administration of CPAP) causes a significant prolongation of expiratory time and a concomitant decrease in respiratory rate. The ease with which this apparent reflex activity can be elicited in the term neonate suggests that it may play an important role in stabilizing respiration at this age. The Hering-Breuer deflation reflex, consisting of an increase in respiratory rate in response to a diminished lung volume, is probably of significance in preterm infants, who invariably develop areas of atelectasis. The increase in breathing rate is primarily caused by a shortening of expiratory time and may assist in maintaining an adequate FRC in these infants. Pulmonary irritant reflexes also have been elicited in the neonate. Direct stimulation of the tracheal wall with a fine catheter threaded through the endotracheal tube of intubated infants results in augmented respiratory efforts. Such a response is rarely present before 35

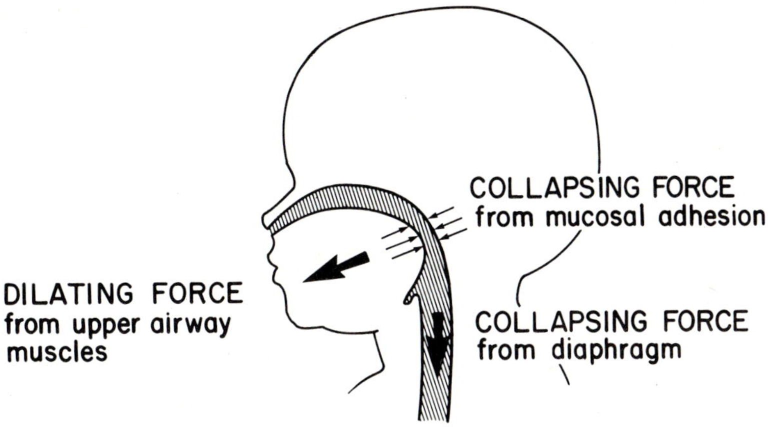

Fig. 28-33. Patency of the upper airway is controlled by the balance of dilating and collapsing forces. (From Martin, R.J., Miller, M.J., and Carlo, W.A.: J. Pediatr. **109:**733, 1986.)

weeks' gestational age. This is suggestive of a functional immaturity of pulmonary irritant receptors at an earlier gestational age, which may be a factor in the increased risk of aspiration in small preterm infants.

Patterns of respiration

Respiration in immature infants is characterized by a wide spectrum of breathing patterns ranging from regular respiration to frequent and even prolonged pauses. Periodic breathing, defined as recurrent sequences of pauses in respiration lasting 5 to 10 seconds and followed by 10 to 15 seconds of rapid respiration, is so common as to be considered normal in preterm infants. It can be abolished by increasing environmental oxygen, but in view of the fact that periodic breathing is considered harmless, this is *not recommended*. The cyclic changes in frequency and tidal volume observed during periodic breathing may be due to instability of the respiratory control center, which is also manifested in apnea or prematurity.

Apneic episodes generally are defined as periods during which there is cessation of respiration for at least 10 to 15 seconds, frequently complicated by cyanosis, pallor, hypotonia, or bradycardia. Small preterm infants exhibit these systemic responses more readily than do more mature infants, even when the apnea is of shorter duration. Since a fall in heart rate frequently occurs very early in the apneic episode, bradycardia may result primarily from vagal influences on central cardiorespiratory control. The problem of recurrent apneic episodes increases both in incidence and severity with decreasing gestational age.

In preterm infants, as well as in adults, apnea may be accompanied by airway obstruction at the level of the pharynx. Negative pharyngeal pressure generated during inspiration may produce pharyngeal collapse, particularly if upper airway muscle activity is decreased (Fig. 28-33). Diaphragmatic activity may then continue, although no airflow results. Indeed the most common type of apnea observed in premature infants is mixed apnea, in which a central respiratory pause is preceded or followed by obstruction. Purely obstructive or purely central apneas are observed less frequently. Prolonged obstructive apneas of 20-second duration may be correlated with abnormal neurologic development in the first year of life. The natural history of apnea in premature infants shows a gradual decrease in frequency of all types of apnea over the first month of postnatal life. In some infants, however, apneas may persist up to 42 weeks' postconceptional age, either as isolated events during sleep or accompanying feeding.

Respiratory control and sleep state

There has been considerable recent interest in the relation between sleep state and respiratory control in the neonate. Although discrepancies exist in criteria for the determination of sleep state, apnea occurs predominantly during active (or REM) and indeterminate (or transitional) sleep in both preterm and term infants. It is uncommon for prolonged apnea to be observed during quiet sleep, when respiration is characteristically regular with little breath-by-breath change in tidal volume or respiratory frequency, although periodic breathing may be seen in quiet sleep.

Several mechanisms have been proposed to explain the high incidence of apnea during active sleep. Chest wall movements are predominantly out of phase (or paradoxical) during active sleep, in contrast to quiet sleep. In other words, abdominal expansion during inspiration is almost always accompanied by inward movement of the rib cage during active sleep, whereas during quiet sleep rib cage and abdomen expand together. These paradoxical chest wall movements during active sleep appear to be the result of decreased intercostal muscle activity and are more common in preterm than term infants. We determined the effect of sleep state on PaO_2 in an attempt to correlate any changes in PaO_2 with altered chest wall movements. In all 10 infants studied, PaO_2 was consistently lower (6 to 10 mm Hg) and more variable during active sleep than during quiet sleep. A fall in FRC also has been observed in infants during active sleep, and this, together with the decrease in PaO_2 during active sleep, would be expected to increase the infant's vulnerability to apneic episodes. Furthermore it has been proposed that electromyographic changes suggestive of diaphragmatic fatigue accompany these paradoxical chest wall movements in normal preterm and term infants without evidence of pulmonary disease. Ventilatory responses to increased carbon dioxide and decreased oxygen concentrations have been compared during active and quiet sleep, and preliminary data would indicate that steady-state carbon dioxide responses are unaffected by sleep state, whereas the depression of ventilation observed in response to hypoxia is accentuated during active sleep. The relative contributions of chest wall movements, neurochemical control, and central respiratory rhythmicity to respiratory control during sleep remain to be unraveled.

Causes of apnea

Recurrent apnea occurs predominantly in preterm infants who weigh less than 1.5 kg and manifest no other overt abnormality. Designated *idiopathic apnea of prematurity* in these infants, this disorder probably involves incomplete organization and interconnections among the respiratory neurons within the brainstem. In many premature infants apnea may represent a final common response of the immature respiratory control system to afferent stimuli of diverse types. Apneic episodes are less frequent over the first few days of life in infants with RDS, and if present at this time should suggest a specific problem that needs to be evaluated (Fig. 28-34). Some of the pathophysiologic disorders associated with apnea of prematurity are tabulated in Fig. 28-35. All these must be considered and appropriate diagnostic tests performed before a label of "idiopathic apnea" is affixed. For example, when apnea is seen shortly after birth, the history may indicate a traumatic delivery or excessive maternal drug administration. Under these circumstances an EEG, CAT scan, or measurement of drug levels may be appropriate. It is not uncommon for a septic infant to develop apnea as the sole or major presenting symptom. A history of prolonged rupture of membranes, foul-smelling amniotic fluid, or maternal fever might suggest such an infectious origin. The thermal environment should be carefully evaluated, since Perlstein has clearly documented that apneic episodes are frequently preceded by rises or falls in the environmental temperature. During the physical examination special note must be taken of clinical evidence for decreased oxygen delivery such as pallor, shock, or left-to-

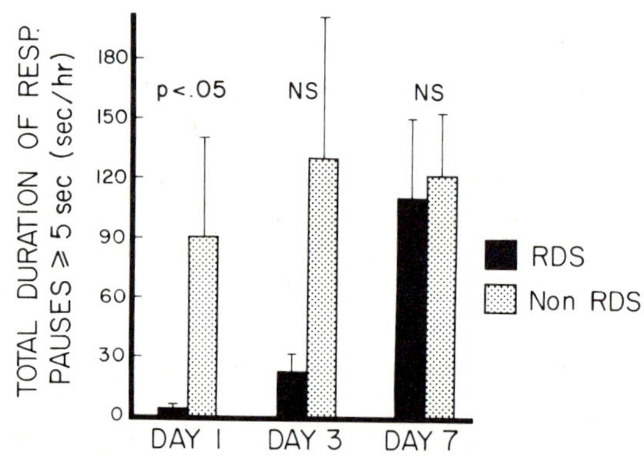

Fig. 28-34. Comparison of the total duration of respiratory pauses (≥5 seconds) in two comparable groups of preterm infants with and without RDS over the first week of life. (From Carlo, W.A., and others: Am. Rev. Respir. Dis. **126:**103, 1982.)

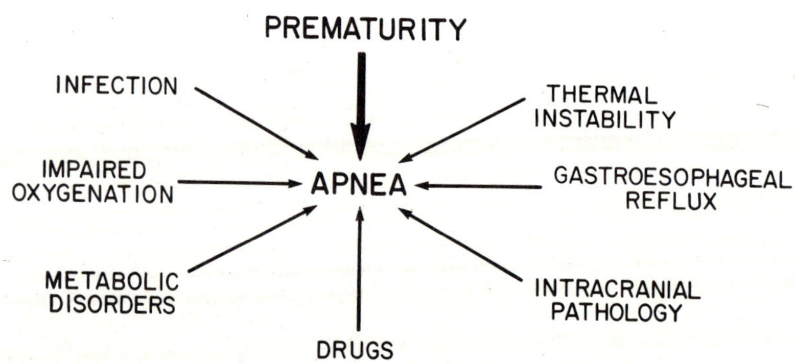

Fig. 28-35. Specific contributory causes of apnea. (From Martin, R.J., Miller, J.J., and Carlo, W.A.: J. Pediatr. **109:**733, 1986.

right shunting through a patent ductus arteriosus. Apnea associated with metabolic disturbances, such as hypoglycemia, may be eliminated by simple measures to correct the metabolic abnormality. The clinical status of the infant, time of onset, and degree of severity of the apneic episodes determine the extent of metabolic evaluation and septic workup. Sound clinical judgment and experience together with continuous surveillance of the infant are necessary.

Management of idiopathic apnea

The principle that should be followed in managing infants with recurrent idiopathic apnea is to commence with that therapy that carries the least potential for short- or long-term side effects. In general, the following steps in management should be followed when apneic episodes do not resolve with gentle tactile stimulation but require vigorous stimulation or intermittent mask-and-bag ventilation to reinitiate respiration.

A variety of modes of sensory stimulation have been shown to decrease apnea in preterm infants, notably irregularly oscillating water beds. The latter can be simulated by connecting a ventilator to an inflatable air mattress. The mechanism whereby apnea is reduced by this means is unclear, although it is tempting to speculate that the neonatal respiratory center responds to a variety of nonspecific sensory inputs such as vestibular or proprioceptive stimulation. Oscillating water beds do not appear to significantly alter the amount of time spent in quiet sleep, active sleep, or wakefulness.

A low CPAP of 3 to 5 cm H_2O, most simply administered via the nasal route, decreases the incidence of apnea in the majority of preterm infants. The main disadvantage of this technique is that it becomes cumbersome over a prolonged period and makes gavage feeding difficult because of the increased risk of aspiration. The precise means by which apnea is decreased on CPAP is unclear. Proposed mechanisms include the stabilization of PaO_2 by increasing FRC, an effect of the stretch receptor influence on respiratory timing, or possible splinting of the upper airway. The latter hypothesis is suggested by the observation that CPAP specifically eliminates those apneas with an obstructive component in preterm infants. It should be noted that with or without the use of CPAP any increase in inspired oxygen concentration beyond 21% must be accompanied by close monitoring of PaO_2 via either intermittent sampling or the transcutaneous route.

The increased use of xanthine drugs (such as theophylline and caffeine) has had a major impact on the management of neonatal apnea. Methylxanthines (theophylline and caffeine) appear to act primarily on brainstem respiratory neurons, producing a central stimulatory effect. Additional contributory effects may include adenosine antagonism, enhanced diaphragmatic contractility, and increased 3′,5′-cyclic AMP. The recommended dose of theophylline (the most widely used drug) is 5 mg/kg loading dose followed by 1 mg/kg every 8 hours to achieve an adequate therapeutic plasma level of approximately 5 to 10 μg/ml. This is substantially lower than the originally described dose because of the slow elimination of xanthines by preterm infants compared with older individuals. More recently it has been proposed that caffeine may be superior to theophylline because of slower excretion, less toxicity, and the fact that theophylline is metabolized to caffeine in substantial amounts in the neonate. At high dosage levels carbon dioxide, responsiveness is increased in the neonate, but at the currently recommended dose, carbon dioxide responses appear to be unaffected by theophylline despite a beneficial therapeutic effect. Care must be taken to avoid short-term toxicity, notably tachycardia or a diuresis. Long-term sequelae of theophylline or caffeine administration have not appeared, and most methylxanthines remain the most accepted pharmaceutical intervention for apnea of prematurity.

EXTRAPULMONARY CAUSES OF RESPIRATORY DISTRESS

In a newborn infant manifesting respiratory embarrassment, there is a tendency to conclude that underlying pulmonary parenchymal disease is present. However, the differential diagnosis of respiratory disease in the newborn is extensive. Disorders of the major airways, chest wall, central nervous system, cardiovascular system, and musculoskeletal system, together with hematologic or metabolic problems, easily may be confused with lung disorders. To avoid serious diagnostic and therapeutic errors, a broad and flexible approach encompassing extrapulmonary causes of respiratory distress in the etiologic considerations is essential. The time-tested approach includes review of historical information related to pregnancy, delivery, and neonatal transition, meticulous observation and careful physical examination of the infant, and analysis of simple laboratory data, including blood gases, hematocrit, and blood sugar, together with appropriate roentgenographic studies. An approach to the classification of extrapulmonary causes of respiratory distress is as follows:

A. Neuromuscular disorders
    1. Brain: asphyxia, drugs, hemorrhage, infection
    2. Spinal cord: trauma, Werdnig-Hoffmann disease
    3. Nerves: injury (phrenic nerve)
    4. Myasthenia gravis
    5. Muscular dystrophies
B. Mechanical-restrictive problems
    1. Airway obstruction
    2. Rib cage abnormalities
        a. Thoracic dystrophies
        b. Generalized bone disease

3. Diaphragmatic disorders
   a. Phrenic nerve injury; congenital eventration of diaphragm
   b. Congenital diaphragmatic hernia
   c. Pleural effusion or chylothorax
   d. Abdominal distension

C. Hematologic disorders
   1. Anemia
   2. Polycythemia

D. Disturbances of acid-base equilibrium: metabolic acidosis

E. Cardiovascular disorders
   1. Congenital heart disease
   2. Congestive heart failure and/or pulmonary edema
   3. PFC

Central nervous system

In the newborn, respiratory distress based on intracranial pathology is most commonly secondary to cerebral edema or intracranial hemorrhage, usually as a consequence of anoxia or birth trauma. These infants present a wide range of respiratory symptoms, including apnea, cyanosis, irregular respiration, and tachypnea, which may be accompanied by grunting, flaring, and retractions. The respiratory symptoms usually resolve, and ultimate prognosis depends on the severity of the hypoxic insult. Medications administered to the mother may have a significant depressant effect on the infant's respiratory center (Chapter 28, part five), and infants of drug-addicted mothers demonstrating withdrawal symptoms also may initially exhibit primarily respiratory symptoms (Chapter 37, part four).

Spinal cord injury

See Chapters 20 and 27.

Injury to the spinal cord occurs predominantly with breech deliveries or with shoulder dystocia. Vigorous traction on the infant's trunk while the head is firmly engaged in the mother's pelvis may result in fractures of the vertebrae with transection of the cord. Initially it may be impossible to distinguish neurologically between hemorrhage and edema of the cord and transection. There is complete paralysis below the level of the injury, which often is the level of the seventh cervical vertebra.

Infants are depressed at birth, often being seen initially with delayed or absent respiratory excursions, shock, respiratory failure, and absence of spontaneous movement. Some withdrawal responses mediated by a spinal reflex distal to the site of injury may be elicited after painful stimuli, and this may confuse the clinical picture. The infants otherwise are flaccid and immobile with absent tendon reflexes. Associated neurologic features are dependent on the level of the lesion. High lesions are associated with phrenic nerve injury and result in diaphragmatic paralysis, producing cyanosis, feeble cry, and irregular respiration. The abdomen does not bulge with inspiration, and roentgenologically the diaphragm will be noted to be markedly elevated. Therapy is largely supportive.

Neuromuscular disease

See Chapter 27.

In the newborn, respiratory failure caused by muscle weakness may be caused by abnormalities of the nervous system or muscles or deformity of the chest wall itself. To recognize these entities, which in and of themselves are all rare, it is necessary to have a high index of suspicion.

The transition to extrauterine life for infants with neuromuscular disorders often is characterized by depression with low Apgar scores and even failure to establish spontaneous respiration. There may be antenatal polyhydramnios as a result of poor fetal swallowing. The subsequent lethargy, hypotonia, diminished spontaneous activity, difficulty with feeding, and weakness then may be attributed to the accompanying perinatal asphyxia. However, telltale signs, including short stature, limb deformities, arthrogryposis, muscle wasting, fasciculation of the tongue, absent tendon reflexes, ptosis, or facial diplegia, may focus attention on a primary neuromuscular disorder. Specific steps then can be taken to establish the primary diagnosis.

Werdnig-Hoffmann disease (infantile spinal muscular atrophy) is a hereditary disease associated with degeneration of anterior horn cells of the cord, resulting in symmetric muscular atrophy (Chapter 27). In its severe forms the bulbar motor nuclei also are involved, and the onset may be early, often in utero, with the mother observing a cessation or pronounced reduction of previously active movements. The infants show generalized hypotonia and paralysis of the limbs and trunk, although the face is spared. Bulbar weakness results in difficulty in sucking and swallowing with noisy respiration caused by an accumulation of mucus in the pharynx, and death from aspiration pneumonia is thus common. Fasciculation of the tongue is diagnostic but may be difficult to ascertain in the newborn.

Respiratory involvement, when seen in infants during the first month, is severe. Diaphragmatic pull results in retraction and abdominal distention, and intercostal muscle function is ineffective. Cunningham and Stocks studied pulmonary function in nine infants with Werdnig-Hoffmann disease. Because of diminished fetal movement and hypotonia at birth, five infants were considered to have had intrauterine onset of the disease. These infants demonstrated significantly reduced thoracic gas volumes, whereas infants with postnatal onset had normal lung volume. The reduction in lung volume correlated only with time of onset of disease, not with duration or degree of muscle weakness. Their findings suggest that fetal breathing is a prerequisite for normal fetal lung development, which is supported by data from Wigglesworth. There is no specific therapy, and respiratory failure is frequently precipitated by infection.

Myasthenia gravis is rare in the newborn infant and appears in two forms (Chapter 27). Neonatal myasthenia gravis is a transient illness that occurs only in children born to mothers with myasthenia gravis. There has been no correlation between the severity of neonatal myasthenia and the severity or duration of the mother's illness. The second form is congenital myasthenia gravis, which is a rare persistent illness occurring in children of normal mothers. Neonatal myasthenia gravis begins shortly after birth and disappears within 6 to 8 weeks. It has been repeatedly suggested that this form may be caused by placental transmission of a neuromuscular blocking substance.

The incidence of symptomatic neonatal myasthenia gravis in babies born to myasthenic mothers is approximately 12%. The dominant clinical manifestations include feeding difficulty, generalized weakness, respiratory difficulty, feeble cry, and facial weakness, including ptosis. Respiratory difficulty occurs in two thirds of the patients and appears to be a result of weakness of their respiratory muscles and inability to handle pharyngeal secretions. Respiratory failure plays a dominant role in those infants who die, and at autopsy examination atelectasis, pulmonary congestion, and evidence of bronchial obstruction or pneumonia may be observed. The diagnosis is based on the observation of weakness in the newborn offspring of a mother with myasthenia gravis and alleviation of the weakness after administration of an anticholinesterase compound. The diagnostic test is best carried out with neostigmine, since edrophonium (Tensilon) has too short a period of action. A positive test is characterized by increase in tone and strength, often detectable as improved suck, stronger respiratory activity, and relief of ptosis.

The neonatal form of *dystrophia myotonica* (Chapter 27) is now recognized as a clinical entity that is quite different from the adult form of the disease. The clinical picture consists of extreme hypotonia and generalized muscle atrophy combined with polyhydramnios, insufficient respiratory activity after birth, joint deformities, and facial diplegia, resulting in a tent-shaped mouth. It should be noted that all infants who are diagnosed in the neonatal period have respiratory problems and that there is a high mortality (50%). The main presenting features in the newborn period are generalized hypotonia together with poor suck and difficulty with swallowing. In addition, the infants exhibit respiratory insufficiency, joint deformities, facial diplegia, and edema most noticeable on the limbs and head with sparing of the trunk. Mental retardation is a common feature of the neonatal form of dystrophia myotonica. Because the baby fails to breathe adequately immediately after birth and usually the mother is not known to have dystrophia myotonica, the diagnosis usually is made when the baby has already been mechanically ventilated. It is a difficult moral and ethical problem to decide whether and to what extent treatment should be continued. Infants who survive the first few weeks of life show gradual improvement in respiration followed by improved swallowing and muscle tone. Subsequent development is slower than normal, and the long-term prognosis is poor. There is little hope of an independent life because of the combination of severe mental retardation and muscle weakness.

Airway obstruction

In the neonate upper airway obstruction occurs infrequently; however, the presentation is often dramatic, and significant respiratory distress may occur. The characteristic clinical presentation depends on the degree and site of obstruction. The following is an anatomic approach to the causes of airway obstruction in the newborn:

A. Nose
   1. Choanal atresia
   2. Drugs: reserpine
   3. Infection: syphilis
   4. Iatrogenic: tubes or tape

B. Mouth and jaw
   1. Pierre Robin syndrome
   2. Hypoplastic mandible
   3. Tongue: enlargement and/or paralysis
   4. Cysts: thyroglossal; gingival

C. Larynx
   1. Floppy epiglottis
   2. Laryngeal web
   3. Cord paralysis
   4. Reflex: laryngospasm

D. Trachea and bronchi
   1. Tracheomalacia
   2. Tracheal stenosis
   3. Tracheal cyst
   4. Bronchostenosis
   5. Bronchomalacia
   6. Lobar emphysema

E. Extrinsic
   1. Goiter
   2. Vascular ring
   3. Aberrant vessels
   4. Hemangiomata
   5. Cystic hygroma
   6. Teratoma
   7. Tracheoesophageal fistula
   8. Mediastinal masses

Developmental anomalies affecting the larynx and trachea have initial symptoms of noisy respiration and often a high-pitched inspiratory stridor, whereas wheezing is more likely with lesions of the mediastinal trachea. Since the newborn infant is a preferential nose breather, infants with nasal obstruction may manifest severe respiratory difficulty, including cyanosis and retractions. The diagnosis is easily established by inability to advance a catheter through the nose into the pharynx. Examination of the size and motion of the tongue also may give a clue as to the cause of upper airway obstruction. Infants with the Pierre Robin syndrome, Möbius syndrome involving cranial nerve palsies, and macroglossia all may be seen to have respiratory difficulty. Stridor, hoarseness, and the character of the cry may alert the examiner to the location of the airway obstruction.

External pressure on the airway, as with goiters, cystic hygromas, hemangiomas, and other masses, all may result in airway obstruction. When upper airway obstruction is suspected clinically, roentgenograms of the chest should include the facial region and neck; specific coned views of the neck and facial soft tissue may be required to establish the diagnosis. One always should carefully inspect the airways on the chest film, looking particularly for displacement or narrowing. Fluoroscopic examination of the airway may be necessary to establish the cause of upper airway obstruction. Development of a fiberoptic bronchoscope suitable for preterm and term infants permits direct visualization of the upper respiratory tract without compromising oxygenation of the infant. This technique is ideal for evaluation of stridor in the newborn as well as identifying vocal cord deformities.

A normal cry generally rules out lesions affecting the vocal cords. If the newborn is aphonic or hoarse, this suggests a congenital laryngeal abnormality or involvement of the recurrent laryngeal nerve. Unilateral vocal cord paralysis is commonly caused by birth trauma, whereas bilateral paralysis is commonly secondary to brain damage; prolonged endotracheal intubation also may damage the vocal cords (Chapter 28, part four). Lesions causing narrowing or significant displacement of the mediastinal trachea usually are characterized by hyperaeration of the lung fields. A vascular ring will be noted to produce an anterior indentation of the trachea. The lesion then can be precisely defined anatomically with angiocardiography.

Congenital choanal atresia

Choanal atresia is a rare malformation; the reported incidence is 0.02% to 0.04% of live births with two thirds of the cases being unilateral. The anomaly is twice as frequent in girls as in boys and involves the right side twice as often as the left. Most cases of choanal atresia occur sporadically. Associated congenital anomalies occur as frequently as 50% of the time and include defects of the heart, eyes, and gastrointestinal tract or syndromes such as Apert's or Treacher Collins.

In view of the fact that newborn infants are preferential nasal breathers, bilateral choanal atresia is first seen as an acute picture with respiratory distress and cyanosis. The diagnosis usually is established by probing both sides of the nose with a firm catheter. These infants are at risk of suffocation until they have learned mouth breathing. They require close observation and monitoring during the first weeks of life, and an oral airway should be established. Early surgical treatment now is recommended with transendonasal perforation of the atretic membrane. In approximately 90% of cases of choanal atresia there is an osseous wall, and only 10% are membranous.

Unilateral choanal atresia, in contrast to the severe life-threatening symptoms of the bilateral variety, may escape detection for many years. Infants may initially have mucous or foul-smelling secretions from the affected side. Many are seen with respiratory distress associated with upper respiratory tract infections. Hall reported a series of 17 patients in whom choanal atresia was associated with multiple anomalies, including mental retardation, hypogonadism (males), small ears, cardiac defects, micrognathia (hypoplastic mandible), postnatal microcephaly, and ocular coloboma. The prognosis for these infants was poor.

Pierre Robin syndrome

The Pierre Robin syndrome comprises micrognathia, cleft of the soft palate, and upper airway obstruction caused by the tongue falling back into the hypopharynx. The infants are seen initially with varying degrees of respiratory difficulty from none to retractions, cyanotic spells, poor feeding, and failure to thrive. Subsequently cyanosis and cor pulmonale may supervene. An airway can be maintained by nursing the infants when they are prone with the head down; this allows the tongue to fall forward and thus prevent obstruction of the airway. Many infants, however, cannot be successfully maintained this way and continue to have frequent bouts of cyanosis and aspiration.

Some investigators have established an airway by positioning an endotracheal tube through a nostril into the hypopharynx. Suturing the tongue forward also has been recommended but is often unsuccessful, with the suture tearing out. Tracheostomy may be necessary, particularly if there is difficulty in maintaining the airway, and gastrostomy also may be indicated. With time the mandible develops, and the muscles of the jaw become strong enough to keep the tongue forward.

Rib cage abnormalities

Thoracic cage and skeletal abnormalities are a rare group of conditions that may cause respiratory distress by restriction of thoracic volume. They include a number of entities incompatible with life. In this group of diseases are those with hypoplasia of the ribs and thorax, including asphyxiating thoracic dystrophy (Jeune's syndrome), thanatophoric dwarfism, achondrogenesis, homozygous achondroplasia, osteogenesis imperfecta (severe form), Ellis-van Creveld syndrome (chondroectodermal dysplasia), hypophosphatasia, spondylothoracic dysplasia, and rib-gap syndrome.

Respiratory distress caused by structural abnormalities of the chest wall should be readily apparent; however, with marked narrowing of the thorax attention may focus on what appears to be a distended abdomen, and the respiratory problem may be erroneously attributed to an intraabdominal pathologic condition. The presence of other associated anomalies, for example, short-limbed dwarfism, together with close observation of respiratory excursions, examination of the bony thorax, and measurement of the circumference of the chest, will establish the diagnosis even before a review is made of the thoracic and skeletal roentgenograms.

With structural abnormalities of the chest wall, asphyxia and respiratory distress are present from birth. The infants are blue and tachypneic and demonstrate severe retractions and characteristically a virtually immobile chest. Diaphragmatic excursions are prominent; thus respiration appears entirely abdominal. Pulmonary hypoplasia accompanies the thoracic dystrophy, and roentgenographically the lungs may appear airless.

Infants with asphyxiating thoracic dystrophy, thanatophoric dwarfism, achondrogenesis, homozygous achondroplasia, or Ellis-van Creveld syndrome have chests with a squared-off appearance, and the posterior rib arcs all appear the same length. The clavicles appear very high, and the diaphragms are low (Fig. 28-36). The transverse diameter of the thorax may appear diminished in comparison with the vertical diameter. On a lateral view the ribs are very short and may appear clubbed anteriorly. The anteroposterior diameter of the thorax is decreased.

The lungs may be poorly aerated, infiltrates are frequently present, and the heart may appear enlarged. Differentiating between the various syndromes of thoracic cage and skeletal abnormalities usually is accomplished by means of skeletal survey. Multiple fractures and bone demineralization are characteristic of osteogenesis imperfecta and hypophosphatasia.

Asphyxiating thoracic dystrophy

The hallmarks of asphyxiating thoracic dystrophy are extreme constriction and narrowing of the thorax, short ribs, and short-limbed dwarfism with abnormalities of the bones of the pelvis and extremities. Associated anomalies include polydactyly and deformed teeth. Renal abnormalities may be present, and renal failure may occur later. The syndrome is inherited as an autosomal recessive trait. As mentioned previously, the chest appears narrow with prominence of the sternum. The thorax is relatively immobile, and the ribs are horizontally directed and short and have bulbous ends. In addition to the thoracic abnormalities, the infants have trident iliac bones with a double-notch appearance of the acetabula.

Thanatophoric dwarfism

Thanatophoric dwarfism was differentiated from achondroplasia in 1967. The disorder has been uniformly fatal in the perinatal period and probably is the most common form of lethal neonatal dwarfism. Appearance at birth is characteristic and includes striking micromelia in association with a normal trunk, a large head, and a narrow thorax. The radiographic findings include se-

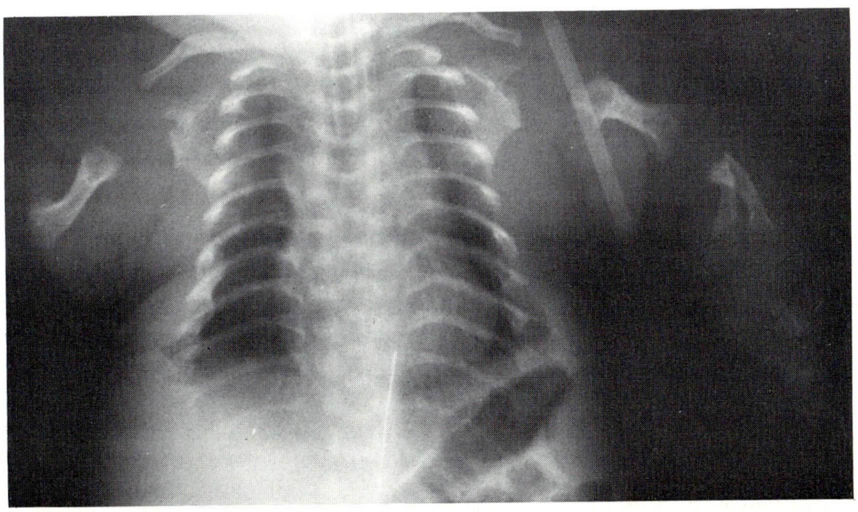

Fig. 28-36. Roentgenographic appearance in thanatophoric dwarfism showing the narrow thorax, low diaphragm, and foreshortened humeri.

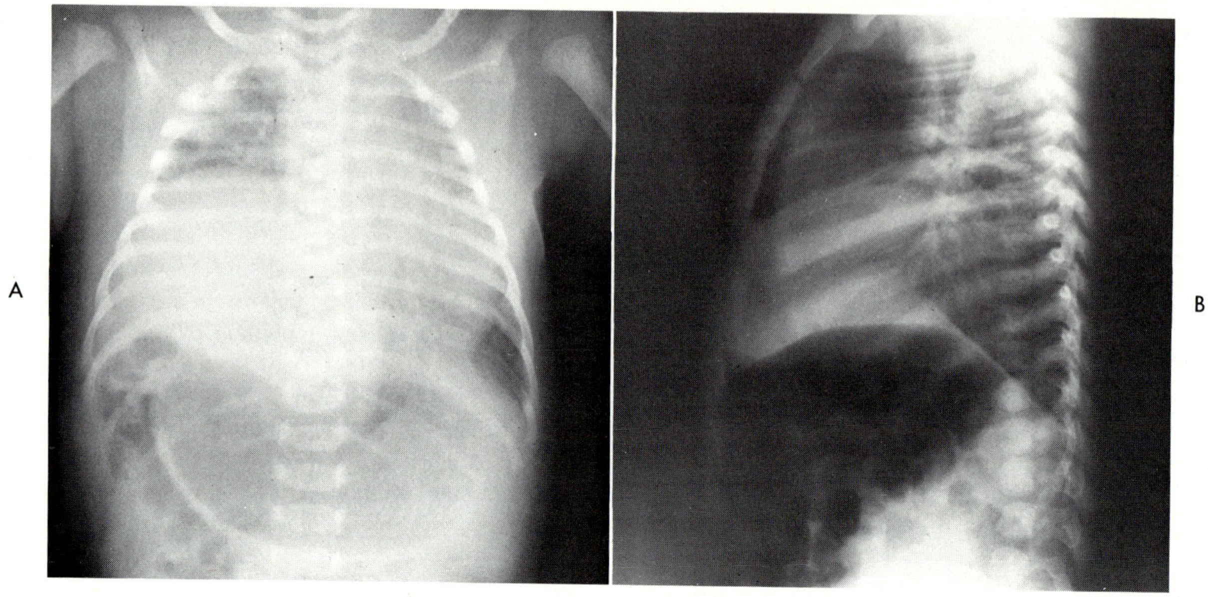

Fig. 28-37. A, Phrenic nerve palsy. Note elevated right dome of diaphragm. **B,** Lateral view.

verely flattened vertebral bodies with markedly widened intervertebral disk spaces, small iliac rings, and flaring of the metaphyses of the long bones. There is a high incidence of polyhydramnios, and the infants often present in the breech position. The condition is inherited as an autosomal recessive trait, occurring more frequently in the black population.

Diaphragmatic disorders

Phrenic nerve paralysis

See Chapter 20.

Phrenic nerve injury with paralysis of the diaphragm is an unusual cause of respiratory distress. It is most commonly present on the right side and follows birth trauma; thus an associated brachial plexus injury or Horner's syndrome may coexist in approximately 75% of the patients. The injuries are observed in large for gestational age infants, particularly those larger than 4 kg, after shoulder dystocia or difficult breech extractions. Fractures of the humerus or clavicle frequently are observed and attest to a violent delivery. The nerve roots of C3 to C5 are stretched, with lateral hyperextension and traction on the neck. Recovery is dependent on the degree of injury; avulsion is obviously permanent, and diaphragmatic eventration secondary to muscle atrophy will ensue.

Lesser injury or edema of the nerve roots results in a spectrum of respiratory symptoms, which may include cyanosis, weak cry, tachypnea, or apnea, and decreased movement is noted on the affected side. On x-ray examination the involved hemidiaphragm is elevated, and atelectasis frequently is observed on that side. The heart and mediastinum are shifted away from the affected side (Fig. 28-37). Fluoroscopically the paralyzed hemidiaphragm is seen to elevate with inspiration and descend on expiration (paradoxical movement), contrasting with the normal diaphragmatic descent on inspiration. Congenital eventration of the diaphragm also results in an elevated hemidiaphragm with paradoxical movement. The major complication to be anticipated is pneumonia superimposed on the atelectasis, which accounts not only for the major morbidity but for the mortality as well. Treatment of phrenic nerve palsy initially is supportive, and in the absence of avulsion spontaneous resolution is to be expected. Surgical plication of the diaphragm may be indicated for selected infants with avulsion. Congenital diaphragmatic hernia is discussed in Chapter 33.

Avroy A. Fanaroff
Richard J. Martin
Martha J. Miller

BIBLIOGRAPHY

Meconium

Fox, W.W., and others: The therapeutic application of end-expiratory pressure in the meconium aspiration syndrome, Pediatrics **56**:214, 1975.

Gage, J.E., and others: Suctioning of upper airway meconium in newborn infants, JAMA **246**:2590, 1981.

Gooding, C.A., and others: An experimental model for the study of meconium aspiration of the newborn, Radiology **100**:137, 1971.

Gregory, G., and others: Meconium aspiration in infants—a prospective study, J. Pediatr. **85**:848, 1974.

Matthews, T.G., and Warshaw, J.B.: Relevance of the gestational age distribution of meconium passage in utero, Pediatrics **64**:30, 1979.

Murphy, J.D., Vawter, G.F., and Reid, L.M.: Pulmonary vascular disease in fatal meconium aspiration, J. Pediatr. **104**:758, 1984.

Ting, P., and Brady, J.: Tracheal suction in meconium aspiration. Am. J. Obstet. Gynecol. **122**:767, 1975.

Tran, N., and others: Sequential effects of acute meconium obstruction on pulmonary function, Pediatr. Res. **14**:34, 1980.

Truog, W.E., and others: Effects of PEEP and tolazoline infusion on respiratory and inert gas exchange in experimental meconium aspiration, J. Pediatr. **100**:284, 1982.

Vidyasagar, D., and others: Assisted ventilation in infants with meconium aspiration syndrome, Pediatrics **56**:208, 1975.

Yeh, T.F., and others: Hydrocortisone therapy in meconium aspiration syndrome: a controlled study, J. Pediatr. **90**:140, 1977.

Pneumonia

Friedman, C.A., Wender, D.F., and Rawson, J.E.: Rapid diagnosis of Group B streptococcal infection utilizing a commercially available latex agglutination assay, Pediatrics **73**:27, 1984.

Pyati, S.P., and others: Penicillin in infants weighing two kilograms or less with early-onset Group B streptococcal disease, N. Engl. J. Med. **308**:1383, 1983.

Rojas, J., and others: Pulmonary hemodynamic and ultrastructural changes associated with Group B streptococcal toxemia in adult sheep and newborn lambs, Pediatr. Res. **17**:1002, 1983.

Runkle, B., and others: Cardiovascular changes in Group B streptococcal sepsis in the piglet: response to indomethacin and relationship to prostacycline and thromboxane A_2, Pediatr. Res. **18**:874, 1984.

Sherman, M.P., Chance, K.H., and Goetzman, B.W.: Gram's stains of tracheal secretions predict neonatal bacteremia, Am. J. Dis. Child. **138**:848, 1984.

Pulmonary hemorrhage

Cole, V., and others: Pathogenesis of hemorrhagic pulmonary edema and massive pulmonary hemorrhage in the newborn, Pediatrics **51**:175, 1973.

Esterley, J., and Oppenheimer, E.: Massive pulmonary hemorrhage in the newborn. I. Pathologic considerations, J. Pediatr. **69**:3, 1966.

Frederick, J., and Butler, N.: Certain causes of neonatal death. IV. Massive pulmonary hemorrhage, Biol. Neonate **18**:243, 1971.

Transient tachypnea

Avery, M.E., Gatewood, O.B., and Brumley, G.: Transient tachypnea of the newborn: possible delayed resorption of fluid at birth, Am. J. Dis. Child. **111**:380, 1966.

Kuhn, M.P., Fletcher, B.C., and deLemos, R.A.: Roentgen findings in transient tachypnea of the newborn, Radiology **92**:751, 1969.

Milner, A.D., Saunders, R.A., and Hopkin, I.E.: Effects of delivery by cesarean section on lung mechanics and lung volume in the human neonate, Arch. Dis. Child. **53**:545, 1978.

Rawlings, J.S., and Smith, F.R.: Transient tachypnea of the newborn, Am. J. Dis. Child **138**:869, 1984.

Wiswell, T.E., and others: Effect of furosemide on the clinical course of transient tachypnea of the newborn, Pediatrics **75**:908, 1985.

Air leaks

Ackerman, N.B., and others: Pulmonary interstitial emphysema in the premature baboon with hyaline membrane disease, Crit. Care Med. **12**:512, 1984.

Allen, R.W., Jung, A.L., and Lester, P.D.: Effectiveness of chest tube evacuation of pneumothorax in neonates, J. Pediatr. **99**:629, 1981.

Batton, D.G., Hellmann, J., and Nardis, E.E.: Effect of pneumothorax-induced systemic blood pressure alterations on the cerebral circulation in newborn dogs, Pediatrics **74**:350, 1984.

Brooks, J.G., and others: Selective bronchial intubation for the treatment of severe localized pulmonary interstitial emphysema in newborn infants, J. Pediatr. **91**:648, 1977.

Gaylord, M.S., and others: Predicting mortality in low-birth-weight infants with pulmonary interstitial emphysema, Pediatrics **76**:219, 1985.

Higgins, C.B., and others: The hemodynamic significance of massive pneumopericardium in preterm infants with respiratory distress syndrome, Radiology **133**:363, 1979.

Hill, A., Perlman, J.M., and Volpe, J.J.: Relationship of pneumothorax to occurrence of intraventricular hemorrhage in the premature newborn, Pediatrics **69**:144, 1982.

Kuhns, L., and others: Diagnosis of pneumothorax or pneumomediastinum in the neonate by transillumination, Pediatrics **56**:355, 1975.

Macklin, C.C.: Transport of air along sheaths of pulmonic blood vessels from alveoli to mediastinum, Arch. Intern. Med. **64**:913, 1939.

Madansky, D.L., and others: Pneumothorax and other forms of pulmonary air leaks in newborns, Am. Rev. Respir. Dis. **120**:729, 1979.

Moessinger, A.C., Driscoll, J.M., and Wigger, H.T.: High incidence of lung perforation by chest tube in neonatal pneumothorax, J. Pediatr. **92**:635, 1978.

Primhak, R.A.: Factors associated with pulmonary air leak in premature infants receiving mechanical ventilation, J. Pediatr **102**:764, 1983.

Stern, P., LaRochelle, F.T., and Little, G.A.: Vasopressin and pneumothorax in the neonate, Pediatrics **68**:499, 1981.

Swingle, H.M., Eggert, L.D., and Bucciarelli, R.L.: New approach to management of unilateral tension pulmonary interstitial emphysema in premature infants, Pediatrics **74**:354, 1984.

Weiner, J.H., and others: Pulmonary venous air embolism in the neonate, Crit. Care Med. **14**:67, 1986.

Developmental anomalies

Askenazi, S.S., and Perlman, M.: Pulmonary hypoplasia: lung weight and radial alveolar count as criteria of diagnosis, Arch. Dis. Child. **54**:614, 1979.

Avery, M.E., Fletcher, B.D., and Williams, R.G.: The lung and its disorders in the newborn infant, ed. 4, Philadelphia, 1981, W.B. Saunders Co.

Deluca, F.G., and Wesselhoeft, C.W.: Surgically treatable causes of neonatal respiratory distress, Clin. Perinatol. **5**:377, 1978.

Hislop, A., Hey, E., and Reid, L.: The lungs in congenital bilateral renal agenesis and dysplasia, Arch. Dis. Child. **54**:32, 1979.

Levin, D.L.: Morphologic analysis of the pulmonary vascular bed in congenital left-sided diaphragmatic hernia, J. Pediatr. **92**:805, 1978.

Potter, E.L.: Bilateral renal agenesis, J. Pediatr. **29**:68, 1946.

Swischuk, L.E., and others: Primary pulmonary hypoplasia in the neonate, J. Pediatr. **95**:573, 1979.

Thibeault, D.W., and others: Neonatal pulmonary hypoplasia with premature rupture of fetal membranes and oligohydramnios, J. Pediatr. **107**:273, 1985.

Wohl, M.E.B., and others: The lung following repair of congenital diaphragmatic hernia, J. Pediatr. **90**:405, 1977.

Respiratory control and apnea of prematurity

Aranda, J., and others: Pharmacokinetic aspects of theophylline in premature newborns, N. Engl. J. Med. **295**:413, 1976.

Bryan, A.C.: Diaphragmatic fatigue in newborns, Am. Rev. Respir. Dis. **119**:143, 1979.

Butcherfuetch, M.C., and others: Relation between apnea duration and type and neurologic status of preterm infants, Arch. Dis. Child. **66**:953, 1985.

Fleming, P.J., Bryan, A.C., and Bryan, M.H.: Functional immaturity of pulmonary irritant receptors and apnea in newborn preterm infants, Pediatrics **61**:515, 1978.

Frantz, I.D., and others: Maturational effects on respiratory responses to carbon dioxide in premature infants, J. Appl. Physiol. **41**:41, 1976.

Gerhardt, T., and Bancalari, E.: Apnea of prematurity. I. Lung function and regulation of breathing, Pediatrics **74**:58, 1984.

Kattwinkel, J.: Neonatal apnea: pathogenesis and therapy, J. Pediatr. **90**:342, 1977.

Martin, R.J., Miller, M.J., and Carlo, W.H.: Pathogenesis of apnea in preterm infants, J. Pediatr. **109**:733, 1986.

Martin, R.J., Okken, A., and Rubin, D.: Arterial oxygen tension during active and quiet sleep in the normal neonate, J. Pediatr. **94**:271, 1979.

Martin, R.J., and others: Effect of lung volume on expiratory time in the newborn infant, J. Appl. Physiol. **45**:18, 1978.

Perlstein, P., Edwards, N., and Sutherland, J.: Apnea in premature infants and incubator air temperature changes, N. Engl. J. Med. **282**:461, 1970.

Rigatto, H., and Brady, J.P.: Periodic breathing and apnea in preterm infants. II. Hypoxia as a primary event, Pediatrics **50**:219, 1972.

Rigatto, H., de la Torre Verduzco, R., and Cates, D.B.: Effects of O_2 on the ventilatory response to CO_2 in preterm infants, J. Appl. Physiol. **30**:896, 1975.

Schulte, F.J., Busse, C., and Eichhorn, W.: Rapid eye movement sleep, motoneuron inhibition, and apneic spells in preterm infants, Pediatr. Res. **11**:703, 1977.

Shannon, D.C., Kelly, D.H., and O'Connell, K.: Abnormal regulation of ventilation in infants at risk for sudden infant death syndrome, N. Engl. J. Med. **297**:747, 1977.

Thach, B.T., and Stark, A.R.: Spontaneous neck flexion and airway obstruction during apneic spells in preterm infants, J. Pediatr. **94**:275, 1979.

Extrapulmonary causes of respiratory distress

Berdon, W.E., and Baker, D.H.: Vascular anomalies and the infant lung: rings, slings and other things, Semin. Roentgenol. **7**:39, 1972.

Carpenter, R.J., and Neil, H.B.: Correction of congenital choanal atresia in children and adults, Laryngoscope **87**:1304, 1977.

Cremin, B.J.: Infantile thoracic dystrophy, Br. J. Radiol. **43**:199, 1970.

Cunningham, M., and Stocks, J.: Werdnig-Hoffmann disease: the effects of intra-uterine onset on lung growth, Arch. Dis. Child. **53**:921, 1978.

Denson, S.E., Taussig, L.M., and Pond, G.D.: Intraluminal tracheal cyst producing airway obstruction in the newborn infant, J. Pediatr. **88**:521, 1976.

Gibson, G.J., and others: Pulmonary mechanics in patients with respiratory muscle weakness, Am. Rev. Respir. Dis. **115**:389, 1977.

Hall, B.D., Choanal atresia and associated multiple anomalies, J. Pediatr. **95**:395, 1979.

Harper, P.S.: Congenital myotonic dystrophy in Britain. I. Clinical aspects, Arch. Dis. Child. **50**:505, 1975.

Jesarty, R.M., Huzar, R.J., and Basu, S.: Pierre Robin syndrome: cause of respiratory obstruction, cor pulmonale and pulmonary edema, Am. J. Dis. Child. **117**:710, 1969.

Kohler, E., and Babbitt, D.P.: Dystrophic thoraces and infantile asphyxia, Radiology **94**:55, 1970.

Langer, L.O., Jr., and others: Thanatophoric dwarfism, Radiology **92**:285, 1969.

Mamba, T., Brown, S.B., annd Grob, D.: Neonatal myasthenia gravis: report of two cases and review of the literature, Pediatrics **45**:488, 1970.

Mellins, R.B., and others: Respiratory distress as the initial manifestation of Werdnig-Hoffmann disease, Pediatrics **53**:33, 1976.

Pagtakhan, R.D., and Chernick, V.: Intensive care of respiratory disorders. In Kendig, E.L., Jr., and Chernick, V., editors: Disorders of the respiratory tract in children, ed. 3, Philadelphia, 1977, W.B. Saunders Co.

Pearse, R.G., and Howeler, C.J.: Neonatal form of dystrophia myotonica, Arch. Dis. Child. **54**:331, 1979.

Simpson, K.: Neonatal respiratory failure due to myotonic dystrophy, Arch. Dis. Child. **50**:569, 1975.

Smith, R.J.H., and Catlin, F.I.: Congenital anomalies of the larynx, Am. J. Dis. Child. **138**:35, 1984.

Stahl, R.S., and Jurkiewicz, M.J.: Congenital posterior choanal atresia, Pediatrics **76**:429, 1985.

Wesenberg, R.L.: The newborn chest, Baltimore, 1973, Harper & Row Publishers, Inc.

Wigglesworth, J.S., Winston, R.M.L., and Bartlett, K.: The influence of the central nervous system on fetal lung development: an experimental study, Arch. Dis. Child. **52**:965, 1977.

Yang, S.S., and others: Lethal short limbed chondrodysplasia in early infancy. In Rosenberg, H.S., and Boland, R.P., editors: Perspectives in pediatric pathology, Chicago, 1976, Year Book Medical Publishers, Inc.

PART SIX

Chronic neonatal lung disease

Prolonged respiratory difficulty in infants is a relatively new and challenging problem in neonatal intensive care. The increased incidence of chronic respiratory disease can be directly related to the more aggressive respiratory management and increased survival of small preterm infants. Fortunately most infants with acute pulmonary disease in the first days of life make a rapid and complete recovery and subsequently have normal lungs. Nonetheless a substantial number of survivors are left with persistent pulmonary sequelae, the precise cause of which remains to be elucidated.

Bronchopulmonary dysplasia is the major form of chronic pulmonary disease in neonates. In 1967 Northway introduced the term *bronchopulmonary dysplasia* to describe chronic pulmonary insufficiency subsequent to severe RDS in infants who had been treated with artificial ventilation and prolonged high oxygen concentrations. Subsequent reports have described a similar disorder after prolonged assisted ventilation for meconium aspiration syndrome, PFC, and various forms of congenital cardiopulmonary disease. Although this section focuses primarily on bronchopulmonary dysplasia, prolonged pulmonary disease is not limited to infants who have received assisted ventilation. Chronic aspiration syndromes caused by functional or structural abnormalities of the gastrointestinal tract are a cause of persistent respiratory distress (Chapter 33). Infants with pulmonary hypoplasia secondary to a diaphragmatic hernia frequently exhibit chronic pulmonary problems postoperatively. Pulmonary infections caused by viruses or *Candida* or *Chlamydia* organisms may result in a prolonged course of respiratory symptoms, whereas cystic fibrosis may be seen rarely in early infancy. The following is the roentgenographic differential diagnosis of bronchopulmonary dysplasia*:

1. Wilson-Mikity syndrome

*From Edwards, D.K.: J. Pediatr. **95**:823, 1979. With permission.

2. Meconium aspiration syndrome
3. Pulmonary interstitial emphysema (PIE)
4. Pulmonary edema
5. Pneumonia (especially viral or fungal)
6. Total anomalous pulmonary venous return (type III)
7. Pulmonary lymphangiectasia
8. Recurrent pneumonitis or aspiration (immune deficiency, gastroesophageal reflux, H-type tracheo-esophageal fistula, etc.)
9. Cystic fibrosis
10. Idiopathic pulmonary fibrosis (Hamman-Rich syndrome)

Krauss first described a clinical syndrome of delayed or prolonged respiratory distress in infants weighing less than 1.25 kg. This came to be known as chronic pulmonary insufficiency of prematurity and was associated with a fall in FRC of unknown cause late in the first week of life. The slowly progressive atelectasis is accompanied by hypoxemia, hypercarbia, apneic episodes, and a requirement for supplemental oxygen. Roentgenograms taken during this period may be normal or show only minimum haziness. Gradual resolution can be expected during the third to fourth week of life.

Of all the differential diagnostic possibilities, Wilson-Mikity syndrome has probably engendered the greatest confusion with bronchopulmonary dysplasia (Fig. 28-38). The roentgenographic similarities have caused some investigators to associate the two conditions, although differences appear to exist in terms of their clinical course. Patients with Wilson-Mikity syndrome generally have an initially benign course, frequently with normal early chest roentgenograms, and an insidious onset of respiratory difficulty and roentgenographic abnormalities. In contrast, patients who develop bronchopulmonary dysplasia initially have severe respiratory disease (usually RDS) and a need for high inspired oxygen concentrations and assisted ventilation. Thus, even though the roentgenographic appearance of the two can be indistinguishable, the characteristic clinical histories usually will permit easy distinction of these conditions. For unknown reasons there has been a dramatic decline in the incidence of the Wilson-Mikity syndrome in recent years, and in its typical form this entity is rarely seen. Most centers have now adopted a more liberal definition of bronchopulmonary dysplasia and include all patients who, after requiring mechanical ventilation during the first week of life, remain oxygen dependent for more than 28 days and have persistent increased densities with or without hyperinflation on chest roentgenograms. This disease is being referred to with increasing frequency as chronic lung disease rather than bronchopulmonary dysplasia.

CLINICAL AND ROENTGENOGRAPHIC FEATURES

Bronchopulmonary dysplasia has been estimated to occur in approximately 5% of all infants admitted for neonatal intensive care and requiring IPPV. Epidemiologic studies, however, do vary widely in defining precise

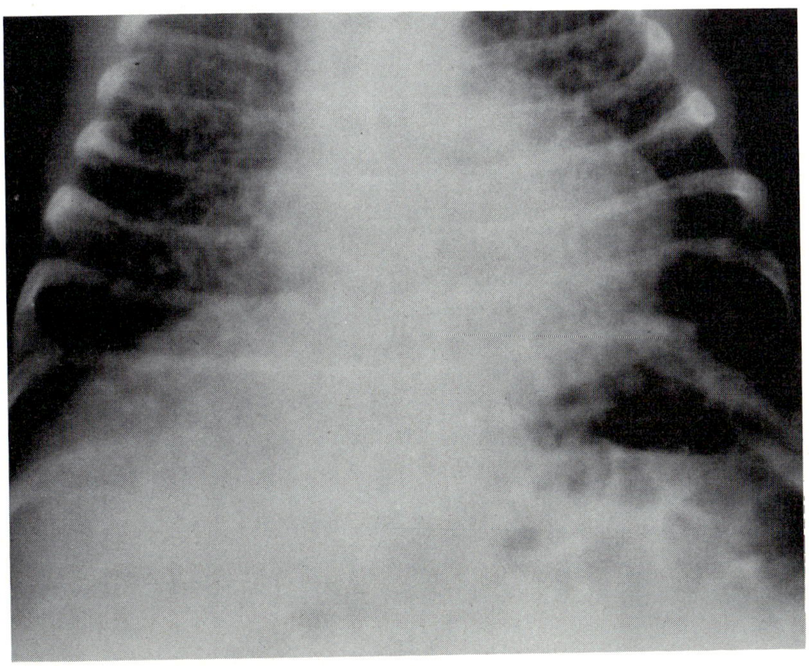

Fig. 28-38. Roentgenogram of an infant with Wilson-Mikity syndrome. Note hyperaeration and bubblelike appearance of the lung.

diagnostic criteria and appropriate neonatal population denominators for comparative studies. Hodson reported an overall incidence of 18% in infants weighing less than 1,500 gm, whereas Tooley observed chronic lung disease in 35% of survivors of RDS who weighed less than 1,500 gm. Most of these infants, however, had only minimal abnormalities when compared with the roentgenographic findings originally described by Northway.

Bronchopulmonary dysplasia is a disease of varying severity that encompasses a relatively broad spectrum of pulmonary complications. At one end are the mildest cases that typically consist of premature infants recovering from RDS who may demonstrate a plateau in both ventilator settings or inspired oxygen requirements during weaning. This plateau phase may be relatively short (24 to 48 hours) and associated with roentgenographic findings of mild pulmonary infiltrates. Some clinicians would still classify these babies as having severe RDS, whereas others would call it early or mild bronchopulmonary dysplasia. At the other end of the spectrum bronchopulmonary dysplasia is characterized by severe cystic emphysema. Bronchopulmonary dysplasia is not specifically confined to preterm neonates but may develop in large term or postterm infants with meconium aspiration syndrome or PFC. These babies usually require higher ventilator settings or more prolonged inspired oxygen exposure to develop the disease than do premature infants. In addition, after surgery some infants such as those recovering from repair of a diaphragmatic hernia, tetralogy of Fallot, and omphalocele may be ventilated for extended periods and develop bronchopulmonary dysplasia.

Nearly all reported cases of bronchopulmonary dysplasia have occurred in infants who required some form of IPPV. The development of bronchopulmonary dysplasia often is suspected when substantial ventilator and oxygen dependence extends beyond 7 days. Nonetheless definitive roentgenographic features do not typically develop until later in the course, usually around the third week of life. The roentgenographic progression of bronchopulmonary dysplasia through the sequence of four stages originally described by Northway is no longer commonly seen. The roentgenographic appearance of stage I is essentially indistinguishable from that of uncomplicated RDS. Dense parenchymal opacification, as seen in stage II bronchopulmonary dysplasia, may commonly simulate another process, such as congestive heart failure from a PDA, fluid overload, or pulmonary hemorrhage. The bubbly pattern of stage III bronchopulmonary dysplasia is not necessarily seen, and when it does appear, it may not follow a period of parenchymal opacity. Finally, the roentgenographic development of chronic lung disease (stage IV) may be more insidious than originally described. The characteristic picture of chronic lung disease ultimately appears at around 20 to 30 days of age. The major features of stage IV disease include hyperinflation and nonhomogeneity of pulmonary tissues, with multiple fine lacy densities extending to the periphery (Fig. 28-39). In conclusion, the radiographic progression through the four classical stages of bronchopulmonary dysplasia is now uncommon, so that absence of stages I to III does not rule out the diagnosis of bronchopulmonary dysplasia. Only a radiographic picture showing chronic pulmonary involvement plus a clinical course that is compatible with bronchopulmonary dysplasia justifies this diagnosis with some degree of consistency.

Complete or partial roentgenographic healing is the usual course of infants who survive the acute phases of their disease. Bronchopulmonary dysplasia typically runs a protracted course punctuated by a variety of complications that lead to acute exacerbations of respiratory symptoms. Cor pulmonale frequently is observed, presumably secondary to pulmonary hypertension resulting from extensive parenchymal disease and chronic hypoxia. Episodes of congestive heart failure will be seen with increasing respiratory distress and hepatomegaly and may be associated with roentgenographic enlargement of the cardiac silhouette. Absolute cardiomegaly, however, is observed infrequently because of pulmonary hyperexpansion, and changes in the pulmonary vasculature may be obscured by the parenchymal disease. Pneumonia commonly complicates the course of bronchopulmonary dysplasia during the first months of life. These pulmonary infections are usually nonspecific in appearance and location and frequently related to the aspiration of feedings. Recurrent atelectasis is a frequent problem in patients with bronchopulmonary dysplasia. Subsegmental or segmental collapse may occur anywhere in the lungs, although the left lower lobe is frequently involved. Atelectasis may be distinguished from consolidation by compensatory emphysema of the remaining lung and a change in the position of fissures. Absence of an air bronchogram in the affected portion of the lung suggests an obstructive cause of the atelectasis. Active intervention, including fiberoptic bronchoscopy, may be indicated.

PATHOPHYSIOLOGY

Several pathogenetic mechanisms are thought to be responsible for the structural changes that characterize bronchopulmonary dysplasia. The term *bronchopulmonary dysplasia* appears to imply a disorder of growth accompanied by abnormal histologic features. A detailed account of the various maturational changes in the developing premature lung is given elsewhere (Chapter 28, part one). In addition to the degree of pulmonary immaturity, Reid has proposed that an understanding of the process of healing after RDS is key to understanding the development of bronchopulmonary dysplasia. After

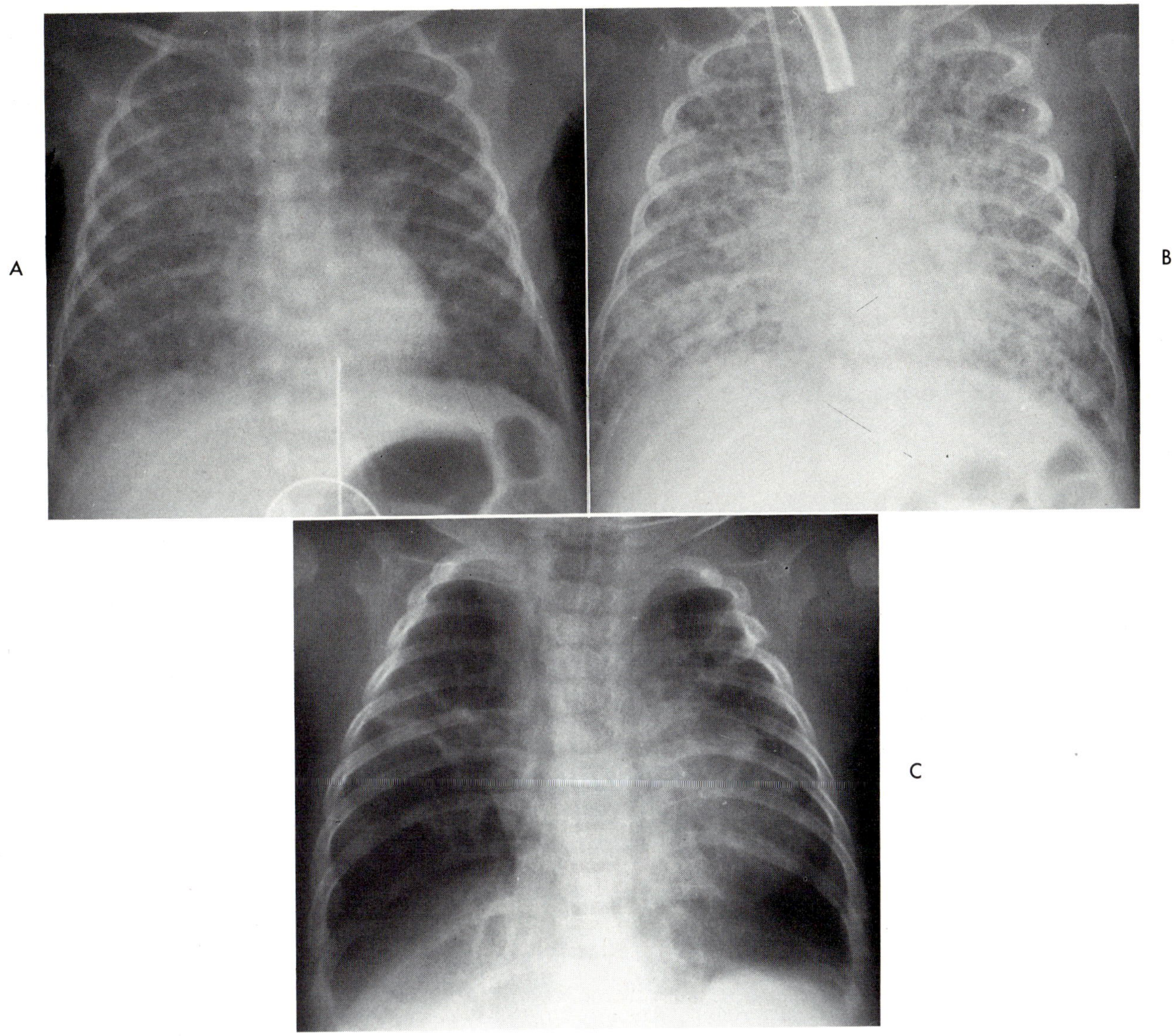

Fig. 28-39. Typical roentgenographic progression of BPD from early BPD **(A),** through stage III **(B),** and later stage IV disease **(C).**

resolution of RDS intraalveolar exudate is cleared to leave a normal lung; the exudate is absorbed into the alveolar wall, resulting in interstitial fibrosis, or organized in situ so that there is an obliteration of the alveolar space. The lung also may become airless and solid because of simple alveolar collapse. In either case the lung is not contributing to gas exchange. Nonaerated regions may reaerate or, if they continue airless, will form scars of condensed lung tissue and fibrose. The bronchiolar mucosa is markedly abnormal with dysplasia and peribronchiolar inflammation. There is bronchiolar muscular hypertrophy and fibrosis of structural portions of the pulmonary lobule. Arterioles are variably hypertrophic, and there is significant involvement of lymphatic and perilymphatic areas. There seems to be a stage when shadows on roentgenographic examination represent transudate/exudate or collapse, but this stage is transient and thus reversible. When the fleeting shadows give way to a static picture, the pattern of scarring may be established (Fig. 28-40).

The typical macroscopic appearance in bronchopulmonary dysplasia is a coarse pattern of scarring mixed with regions of emphysema. The emphysema arises in at least three ways: (1) scarring means that the emphysema of the intervening lung arises in part from overinflation, or can be considered compensatory; (2) there is a failure of multiplication of the alveoli within at least some units, which indicates that there is also a hypoplastic form of emphysema; (3) inflammation and destruction of the alveolar wall or of its capillary bed lead to a

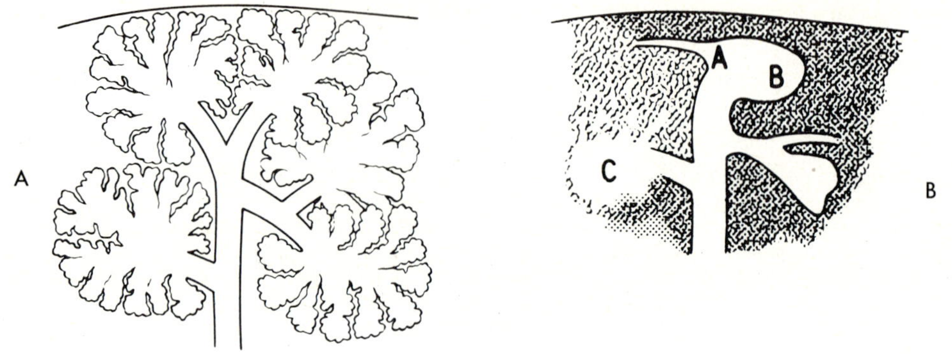

Fig. 28-40. Mechanism whereby inflammatory scarring can lead to alternating regions of scarring and emphysema. *A*, Obliterated bronchiolus; *B*, bronchiolar cyst; *C*, alveolar cyst. **A,** Normal lobule. **B,** After fibrosis. (From Reid, L.: J. Pediatr. **95:**836, 1979.)

destructive form of emphysema; this is particularly relevant to the damage done by high levels of oxygen. Reid notes that the emphysema in bronchopulmonary dysplasia arises from these three processes. Parts of the vascular bed are condensed in the scars, and these arteries develop smaller than normal arterial diameters and thicker muscular walls. Since the latter encroaches on the lumen, the vascular bed is further reduced in volume. In the intervening aerated regions the arteries grow but receive an abnormally large part of the cardiac output. Their growth is also abnormal and will be compensating to some extent for the changed hemodynamic state.

Watts has examined pulmonary function in a group of 10 preterm infants with severe bronchopulmonary dysplasia (stages III and IV of Northway). The most striking finding was a severe maldistribution of ventilation in these infants, as determined by nitrogen washouts. The bronchopulmonary dysplasia group had a pulmonary clearance delay of 223% versus 60% for a comparable group of preterm infants who also had been ventilated but subsequently developed no signs of bronchopulmonary dysplasia. Minute volumes were normal in the infants with bronchopulmonary dysplasia, with increased respiratory frequency, decreased tidal volume, and hypercarbia with a mean Pa_{CO_2} of 55 mm Hg.

Infants with bronchopulmonary dysplasia characteristically have a marked increase in airway resistance. This is associated with a decreased dynamic compliance and a large increase in the work of breathing. Static compliance has been found to be normal or increased, indicating that the decrease in dynamic compliance is due mainly to the increased airway resistance. In the face of airway obstruction, dynamic compliance becomes frequency-dependent and decreases at higher respiratory rates (see Part two of this chapter). FRC may be decreased, normal, or increased, depending on the severity and stage of the pulmonary involvement. Because of the maldistribution of inspired gas in infants with bronchopulmonary dysplasia, measurements of FRC by gas dilution must be interpreted with caution.

Most infants with severe bronchopulmonary dysplasia have marked hypoxemia and hypercapnia and require supplemental oxygen to maintain a Pa_{O_2} above 50 mm Hg. The amount of required oxygen decreases gradually as the disease process improves, but it increases during feeding and physical activity or during episodes of pulmonary infection or edema.

ETIOLOGY

Several clinical factors have been implicated in the etiology of bronchopulmonary dysplasia. Most discussions of etiology have focused on the relative effects of oxygen toxicity and mechanical ventilators on the disease process, whereas the importance of pulmonary immaturity has not received enough attention. The smallest infants have poorly developed surfactant systems, decreased pulmonary stability, and ill-defined structures of both interstitium and alveoli, placing them at highest risk. The lungs of these infants are still developing and require less extrinsic airway pressure or toxic gas exposure to produce significant pulmonary changes. One developmental factor that probably has major significance in the disease is that a neonate of 7 months' gestational age has inadequately developed elastic and connective tissue elements. Stress to these structural elements may be important in the production of emphysema. A clinical comparison can be made to long-time smokers with chronic lung disease and emphysema, in whom elastic tissue is the first pulmonary tissue element to be disrupted.

The role of infection in the origin of bronchopulmonary dysplasia is not clear. Pneumatoceles and cystic lung disease occur in neonatal lungs secondary to infections by *Escherichia coli* or *Pseudomonas*, *Klebsiella*, or *Staphylococcus* organisms. If these infections are chronic, they might result in bronchitis or small airway disease. Recurrent infections appear, on the other hand, to be a common complication of long-term bronchopulmonary dysplasia. Birth asphyxia may be an important factor in predisposing infants to development of bronchopulmonary dysplasia. Asphyxia causes two problems that result in higher oxygen and ventilator requirements. Disruption of surfactant synthesis may result in more severe atelectasis and acidosis, whereas hypoxemia predisposes the infant to increased pulmonary vascular resistance and right-to-left shunting. Interstitial emphysema is a diffuse form of alveolar air leak in which small bubbles of air move along the interstitial spaces of the lung. This condition has been reported to predispose infants to bronchopulmonary dysplasia, but the cause and effect relation between these two conditions is not fully established (Chapter 28, part five).

Oxygen toxicity

Clinical and experimental evidence has suggested that pulmonary oxygen toxicity is a major factor in the cause of bronchopulmonary dysplasia. Although many body tissues can be injured by sufficiently high oxygen concentrations, the lung is exposed directly to the highest partial pressure of inspired oxygen. The precise concentration of oxygen that is toxic to the lung probably depends on a large number of variables, including maturation, nutritional and endocrine status, and duration of exposure to oxygen and other oxidants. Although a safe level of inspired oxygen has not been established, concentrations in excess of 50% carry a substantial risk of lung damage when administered over a period of many days. The pathogenesis of oxygen toxicity, according to studies in both animals and human beings, is nonspecific and consists of atelectasis, edema, alveolar hemorrhage, inflammation, fibrin deposition, and thickening and hyalinization of alveolar membranes. There is early damage to capillary endothelium in animals, and plasma leaks into interstitial and alveolar spaces. Pulmonary surfactant may be altered, adding to the formation of atelectasis. Type I alveolar lining cells also are injured early, and bronchiolar and tracheal ciliated cells can be damaged by 80% to 100% oxygen. Total resolution after oxygen toxicity is possible if the initial exposure is not overwhelming. It is presumed that cellular pathologic processes similar to those in animals also occur in humans.

The contribution of the alveolar macrophage to pathologic effects in the lung is not clear. Continued exposure to high O_2 is accompanied by an influx of polymorphonuclear leukocytes containing proteolytic enzymes. In addition, Bruce has observed that the antiproteinase defense system is significantly impaired in infants exposed to greater than 60% inspired O_2 for 6 or more days. Therefore proteolytic damage of structural elements in alveolar walls may be an important pathogenic factor.

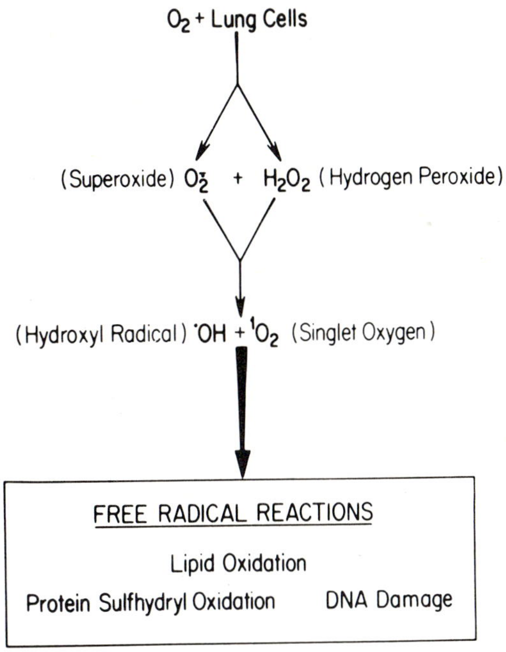

Fig. 28-41. Chemical mechanisms of oxygen toxicity. (From Deneke, S.M., and Fanburg, B.L.: N. Engl. J. Med. **303:**76, 1980. Reprinted by permission of the *New England Journal of Medicine.*)

Although the cellular basis for oxygen toxicity has not been completely elucidated, the principal mechanisms involve the univalent reduction of molecular oxygen and formation of free radical intermediates. The latter can react with intracellular constituents and membrane lipids, thus initiating chain reactions that may result in tissue destruction. An oxygen-radical mechanism of toxicity is consistent with the known chemical reactivity of oxygen, hydrogen peroxide, and superoxide radical. Chemical interactions between oxygen and various radicals can result in singlet excited oxygen formation. Singlet excited oxygen is a highly reactive, electronically excited state of molecular oxygen that is toxic to many biologic systems. At present hydrogen peroxide, superoxide radical, hydroxyl radical, and singlet excited oxygen all are considered possible agents of hyperoxic tissue damage. The term *oxygen radical* sometimes is used very loosely to mean any of these species, since all have been implicated in lipid peroxide formation and subsequent free-radical chain reactions (Fig. 28-41).

To resist the detrimental effects of oxygen toxicity, the body has evolved various antioxidant enzymes such as superoxide dismutase, which eliminates the superoxide radical, whereas other compounds such as vitamin E and selenium also may offer endogenous antioxidant protection. Studies designed to enhance antioxidant protection in the neonate, as by the administration of high doses of vitamin E, however, have failed to demonstrate any sustained beneficial effect.

The natural susceptibility of animals to oxygen varies widely among species. The response also seems to be age dependent, since immature animals survive continuous oxygen exposure longer than do adults of the same species. Loss of mucociliary function may be an additional pathogenic component of bronchopulmonary dysplasia, since exposure to 80% oxygen has resulted in a cessation of ciliary movement after 48 to 96 hours in cultured human neonatal respiratory epithelium. Further understanding of the role of maturation in the response of the lung to high oxygen concentrations should offer greater insight into both the harmful and protective influences on pulmonary oxygen toxicity.

Assisted ventilation

In their initial observations Northway and associates concluded that administration of high concentrations of oxygen was the major agent responsible for the production of bronchopulmonary dysplasia. Nonetheless they indicated that the use of intermittent positive pressure respirators and endotracheal intubation also may contribute to the pathologic state (Fig. 28-42). Clinical experience with newborn infants, however, has not borne out the role of oxygen alone in the pathogenesis of this syndrome. This is supported by the observation that bronchopulmonary dysplasia is virtually unheard of in infants treated with negative-pressure ventilation without the use of endotracheal tubes, despite high concentrations of oxygen being administered. Furthermore bronchopulmonary dysplasia is infrequently observed as a complication of nasal CPAP despite prolonged oxygen requirements.

It has become generally accepted that barotrauma resulting from high pressures used in assisted ventilation is the major culprit in the development of bronchopulmonary dysplasia. The role of the endotracheal tube itself may be difficult to separate from that of either the oxygen or the respirator under these circumstances. Endotracheal tubes would appear to hinder the drainage of tracheal secretions. They further increase both the dead space and the resistance to airflow and may cause a diminution in arterial P_{O_2} by preventing closure of the glottis when the tube is in place.

Although peak inspiratory pressure (PIP) is one of the major factors implicated in the cause of bronchopulmonary dysplasia, it is difficult to determine whether the high pressures have a casual effect on the chronic lung damage or whether these high settings are required after lung damage is already established. No prospective study controlling for other variables that may influence the development of bronchopulmonary dysplasia has shown a relationship between peak or mean airway pressure and bronchopulmonary dysplasia. Bancalari showed no significant differences in the incidence of chronic lung disease between infants ventilated with low pressures and prolonged inspiration and those ventilated with higher pressures and shorter inspiration. Airway resistance appears to be increased after 3 to 5 days in infants mechanically ventilated for RDS who subsequently develop bronchopulmonary dysplasia. Increased airway resistance could result in either partial or complete airway obstruction, predisposing to air trapping, air leak syndromes, and maldistribution of ventilation. The advent of high-frequency ventilation (see Part four) has raised hopes that these techniques (oscillation or jet ventilation) may decrease the incidence of bronchopulmonary dysplasia.

Finally, the duration of both assisted ventilation and oxygen therapy may be a key etiologic factor. This is difficult to substantiate, since it is impossible to separate the time factor from the initial severity of the underlying disease. The more severe the disease, the longer the time required for assisted ventilation.

Fluid therapy

The precise relationship between fluid therapy, PDA, and bronchopulmonary dysplasia has not yet been completely established. Bell has demonstrated that the incidence of both PDA and congestive heart failure in low birth weight infants is increased when high volumes of

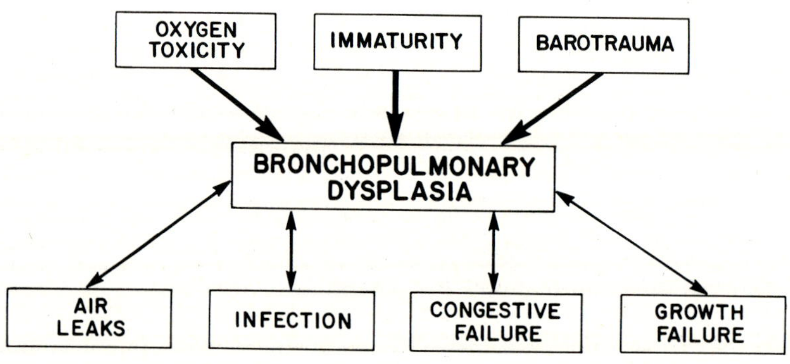

Fig. 28-42. Schematic representation of the pathophysiologic events that contribute to the progressive development of chronic lung injury.

maintenance fluids are used. Evidence by Brown indicates that the presence of a PDA complicating the course of RDS increases the risk of bronchopulmonary dysplasia. Spitzer has proposed that the time taken for maximum urinary output to occur during recovery from RDS is related to the time in an increased O_2 environnment and may predict the development of bronchopulmonary dysplasia. These findings suggest that an increased pulmonary blood flow or interstitial fluid in the lung is another factor that increases the risk of bronchopulmonary dysplasia in preterm infants. Increased pulmonary blood flow caused by PDA and the resulting increase in interstitial fluid cause a decrease in pulmonary compliance and increase in airway resistance. These two changes may prolong the need for mechanical ventilation, with higher ventilatory pressures and oxygen concentrations increasing the risk of bronchopulmonary dysplasia.

MANAGEMENT

Prevention of prematurity and the major causes of neonatal respiratory distress would probably eliminate bronchopulmonary dysplasia as a clinical problem. Since this has not yet been accomplished, all our attention should be directed toward the difficult task of reducing the concentration of supplemental oxygen and minimizing ventilator pressures within the constraints of appropriate management for acute respiratory distress. In spite of our best efforts at prevention, bronchopulmonary dysplasia remains a clinically significant problem. Successful treatment of severe bronchopulmonary dysplasia may require a long-term multidisciplinary commitment, since some infants require care for many years.

Respiratory support

A rational approach to the respiratory care of infants with bronchopulmonary dysplasia requires an understanding of the abnormalities of pulmonary function inherent in the disease. In infants with bronchopulmonary dysplasia the low dynamic lung compliance and high airway resistance result in an increased work of breathing. Hypercarbia will result, since the neonate cannot sustain an appropriately high level of minute ventilation. Intermittent mandatory ventilation (IMV) is a form of assisted ventilation that allows the infant to breathe spontaneously between a set number of mechanical breaths per minute. This technique is of particular value in infants with bronchopulmonary dysplasia who may require prolonged ventilatory support. An IMV rate is selected that allows $PaCO_2$ to be maintained in a high normal range. A PEEP of 2 to 4 cm H_2O is used to stabilize lung volume. An increased inspired oxygen concentration is required to maintain a PaO_2 in the 50 to 70 mm Hg range. Adequacy of gas exchange should be monitored by arterial blood gases at intervals dictated by the child's clinical condition. During times of stability transcutaneous PO_2 measurements are satisfactory although they underestimate PaO_2 by approximately 15 mm Hg beyond 2 to 3 months of age. Oxygen saturation monitors are not influenced by advancing postnatal age. $PaCO_2$ can be approximated from venous samples, which will average 5 mm Hg above arterial values.

Long-term mechanical ventilation requires the presence of a secure airway. If the use of such support is for 1 to 2 months or less, a well-secured endotracheal tube is sufficient, provided that attention is given to fit. An appropriately sized endotracheal tube will leak when 30 cm H_2O positive pressure is applied to the airway. If no leak occurs the endotracheal tube is too large and should be replaced with a smaller tube. If mechanical ventilation is required for more than 1 to 2 months, tracheostomy is a more appropriate form of airway control. Prolonged use of oversized endotracheal tubes may result in a high incidence of subglottic stenosis (Chapter 28, part four).

Inspired gases must be humidified to prevent damage to the respiratory tract mucosa that may be caused by exposure to dry gas. Chest physiotherapy is performed at variable intervals (depending on secretions) in an attempt to prevent atelectasis and the pooling of secretions. This generally includes chest percussion and vibration, followed by airway suctioning. Meanwhile every effort should be made to keep the inspired oxygen concentration and ventilator pressures as low as possible to prevent further pulmonary oxygen toxicity.

Weaning from IMV may be a long, slow process, taking many months in extreme cases. Intercurrent illnesses such as upper or lower respiratory tract infections, bronchospasm, or congestive heart failure may interrupt the weaning process and should be treated aggressively. After IMV has been discontinued the infant may benefit from endotracheal CPAP for 1 to 2 weeks. Weaning from oxygen should progress concurrently and with even greater caution. Reduction in inspired oxygen of as little as 2% may result in a profound change in the infant's clinical condition and requires constant reassessment. Halliday has documented echocardiographic evidence suggesting a mild increase in pulmonary vascular resistance with small decreases in inspired O_2.

Infants with bronchopulmonary dysplasia are being increasingly discharged from the hospital before they are weaned from supplemental inspired oxygen. Whereas the cost-effectiveness and psychologic benefits of home management are clearly enormous, considerable responsibility is placed in the hands of parents or other caretakers and the physician team, who must frequently monitor the infant's well-being. Equipment failure and medication errors must be guarded against. Clinic visits must ensure that congestive failure is well controlled, weight gain and nutritional support are appropriate, and that oxygenation is adequate. Furthermore infants with resolving bronchopulmonary dysplasia do appear to be at increased risk for sudden infant death. Thus parents must be instructed in suctioning techniques and cardiopulmonary resuscitation and must be well prepared, capable, and willing to accept the responsibilities to which they will be exposed.

Nutritional management

Adequate nutrition is a key aspect of care for the infant with bronchopulmonary dysplasia, who may have a 25% increase in resting O_2 consumption over controls. This is partially contributed by the elevated work of breathing. Malnutrition will delay somatic growth and the development of new alveoli, making weaning from mechanical ventilation almost impossible. The malnourished patient is also more prone to infection. For these reasons an aggressive approach should be taken toward supplying a parenteral or oral caloric intake that is adequate for growth. High-calorie formulas and supplements may be used to maximize the intake of calories while restricting fluid intake to prevent congestive heart failure. Dietary management of the infants with bronchopulmonary dysplasia who fail to thrive is complicated by the fact that at glucose intakes exceeding 20 gm/kg/day, CO_2 production exceeds O_2 utilization, further compromising respiratory function. Glucose intake must thus be restricted below this level. If for any reason enteral nutrition is precluded for more than 3 or 4 days, peripheral hyperalimentation with glucose, amino acids, and subsequently fat should be substituted until the gastrointestinal tract again becomes available. Adequacy of nutrition should be closely monitored, and growth charts for height, weight, and head circumference need to be kept. Other means of assessment include arm anthropometry to determine muscle mass and fat deposits and measuring serum levels of albumin. Rib fractures noted on routine chest roentgenograms together with generalized bone demineralization are not infrequently observed in bronchopulmonary dysplasia and are usually a manifestation of rickets. Their cause may relate to dietary or parenteral deficiency of calcium or vitamin D. Another contributing factor might be the calciuria resulting from chronic furosemide therapy, and extra calcium and vitamin D intake are indicated (Chapter 37, part two).

Fluid management

Many infants with severe bronchopulmonary dysplasia have roentgenographic, electrocardiographic, and echocardiographic evidence of cor pulmonale, which appears to resolve as lung function improves. These infants may have fewer problems with congestive heart failure if they are treated by fluid restriction and chronic diuretic administration until cor pulmonale disappears. Infants with bronchopulmonary dysplasia are particularly susceptible to pulmonary edema, perhaps because of abnormal lymphatic drainage or the deleterious effects of right-sided heart failure on left ventricular function. The importance of left ventricular hypertrophy in these infants has additionally been confirmed by both echocardiographic and pathologic studies without accompanying elevation of pulmonary vascular resistance. Fluids are restricted as much as possible, considering the need for a high caloric intake, and chronic diuretic therapy is instituted with a thiazide or a loop diuretic such as furosemide. The use of oral or intravenous diuretics in these infants is associated with a rapid improvement in lung compliance and decrease in resistance, and blood gases may show significant improvement. The reduction in pulmonary capillary pressure observed after furosemide administration is not entirely due to the increased elimination of sodium and water, but seems to be, in part, due to an increase in venous capacitance and reduced venous return. Complications of chronic diuretic therapy include hypokalemia, hyponatremia, metabolic alkalosis, hypercalciuria, and hypochloremia. Parameters that need frequent monitoring include intake and output, electrolytes, urine specific gravity, body weight, rales, peripheral edema, and liver enlargement.

Control of infection

Even though many types of infection can have serious consequences for the child with bronchopulmonary dysplasia, bacterial and fungal sepsis generally result in the most profound setback. As a result, the child needs to be closely watched for early evidence of infection. Tracheal secretions are obtained biweekly for culture and Gram stain, or more often if a change in the quality and quantity of secretions indicates possible infection. A complete blood count, blood culture, and chest roentgenogram are obtained if pneumonia is suspected. Although it is difficult to distinguish between colonization of the airway and true infection, this distinction is important because overtreatment with antibiotics may result in the emergence of more virulent organisms. Selection of antibiotics is based on the sensitivity of the implicated organism, and treatment is continued for a minimum of 1 week or until the infection has been controlled. Clinical measures to prevent pulmonary superinfection are important. These include changing tracheostomy tubes twice weekly and careful hand washing before handling the infant.

Bronchodilator therapy

Infants with both subacute and chronic forms of bronchopulmonary dysplasia may exhibit clinical elements of bronchospasm. Mechanical ventilation and oxygen therapy during the early stages of disease result in hypertrophy of peribronchiolar smooth muscle and increase in airway resistance in addition to the decrease in lung compliance. Rooklin reported that theophylline therapy produced a trend toward decreased pulmonary resistance and increased dynamic compliance at 2 and 24 hours after treatment in infants with bronchopulmonary dysplasia who were less than 30 days of age. Older infants in this study demonstrated no improvement in pulmonary function after bronchodilator therapy, possibly because higher doses were required or because there was a greater degree of fibrosis. Inhalation bronchodilators have also been used in patients with bronchopulmonary dysplasia, and a marked decrease in airway resistance followed their use. Administration of dexamethasone may transiently improve lung function, but the increased risk of major infection and hypertension may not justify its use.

Infant stimulation

The infant with severe bronchopulmonary dysplasia may be ventilator dependent for many months and thus deprived of normal parental stimulation. Developmental delays are the invariable result, which are compounded if any gross neurologic handicap exists. A well-organized program of infant stimulation may help the infant achieve maximum potential. Such a program will instruct the caretakers in helping the infant with various social, language, cognitive, and motor skills. As the child grows, speech therapy is useful in teaching communication skills, especially important for children with a tracheostomy. Beanbag chairs, strollers, and other adaptive tools are employed to mobilize the child and teach gross motor skills. Progress is monitored by periodic developmental evaluations, and emphasis is placed on areas where delay is evident.

Parental support

The parents of an infant with severe bronchopulmonary dysplasia lose considerable control of their child to the hospital staff, particularly in areas related to medical care. Parental participation in other aspects of child care is critical for the child's development and for establishment of normal relationships. Therefore parents are encouraged to visit as frequently as possible and to participate in the day-to-day care of their child. They are educated about relevant medical equipment and procedures. In time many are able to assume complete responsibility for procedures such as chest physiotherapy and tracheal suctioning in addition to holding and playing with their child. During the prolonged hospitalization every effort must be made to assign a consistent physician and nursing team to oversee the child's care and be available for continuing parental support. Parental support groups may also offer a valuable resource for these families.

OUTCOME

During the first year of life the mortality of infants with severe bronchopulmonary dysplasia is high, usually as a result of respiratory failure, sepsis, or intractable cor pulmonale. Eighty percent of these deaths occur during the initial hospitalization. Nonetheless, with adequate nutrition, somatic growth, and control of infection and heart failure, gradual improvement in pulmonary function may be accompanied by resolution of cor pulmonale and roentgenographic healing. Increasing recognition of milder forms of bronchopulmonary dysplasia may also result in improved prognosis. Unfortunately the degree of impaired gas exchange as assessed by need for supplemental O_2 greater than 40% at 1 month has not been able to predict mortality.

Lower respiratory tract infections are common during the first year of life in patients with bronchopulmonary dysplasia, although their exact incidence is difficult to ascertain from the literature. Frequently no specific organisms are isolated, and the disease resolves with broad-spectrum antibiotic therapy. Among survivors of bronchopulmonary dysplasia hospitalization for episodes of wheezing suggestive of bronchiolitis or asthma is common during the first 2 years of life. Acute roentgenographic evidence of hyperinflation may be difficult to appreciate in infants with bronchopulmonary dysplasia, who generally already are hyperinflated. Such episodes of bronchiolitis may be accompanied by focal, transient areas of atelectasis. Pulmonary function studies of infants with a history of bronchopulmonary dysplasia indicate that pulmonary function may be impaired beyond 2 years in many cases, even though the infants may be asymptomatic. Smyth observed a high incidence of obstructive airway disease at 8 years in a small group of survivors of bronchopulmonary dysplasia. Data on longer term follow-up studies of pulmonary function in larger numbers of these infants are currently unavailable, although these clearly will be very important to ascertain in the future.

Myers and colleagues have recently compared the respiratory morbidity in preterm infants surviving RDS, preterm infants who did not have RDS, and appropriately matched term infants. They were unable to demonstrate an increased frequency of respiratory illness for preterm infants with or without RDS when compared with the term infants. Survivors of RDS did, however, experience their first lower respiratory illness earlier and had an increased severity when compared to the term control infants. This latter difference was related to more severe respiratory disease among the infants with residual or chronic lung disease. Thus infants who have roentgenologic evidence of pulmonary abnormalities at discharge are at increased risk for subsequent respiratory illness.

In infants weighing less that 1.5 kg at birth, Vohr demonstrated that infants with bronchopulmonary dysplasia also had more neurodevelopmental sequelae at 2 years when compared to comparable control groups. They also exhibited transiently impaired growth curves, although growth appeared comparable by 2 to 3 years. All these infants had roentgenologic criteria of bronchopulmonary dysplasia as defined by Northway; thus the increased morbidity originally described by Northway in bronchopulmonary dysplasia patients is confirmed. Meisels also observed that infants with bronchopulmonary dysplasia defined by the Northway criteria were at higher risk for growth and developmental delays in the second year of life than infants with RDS. While data from longer term studies are not yet available, it is clearly apparent that neurodevelopmental prognosis will also depend on the diagnostic criteria used to define chronic lung disease in neonates (see also Chapter 27, part six).

William W. Fox
Jeffrey P. Morray
Richard J. Martin

BIBLIOGRAPHY

General

Avery, G.B., and others: Controlled trial of dexamethasone in respiratory dependent infants with bronchopulmonary dysplasia, Pediatrics **75**:106, 1985.

Bancalari, E.: Bronchopulmonary dysplasia. In Milner, A.D., and Martin, R.J., editors: Neonatal and pediatric respiratory medicine, Boston, 1985, Butterworth Publishers.

Bancalari, E., and Gerhardt, T.: Bronchopulmonary dysplasia, Pediatr. Clin. N. Am. **33**:1, 1986.

Bronchopulmonary dysplasia and related chronic respiratory disorders. Report of the Ninetieth Ross Conference on Pediatric Research, Columbus, Ohio. 1986, Ross Laboratories.

Bryan, M.H., and others: Pulmonary function studies during the first year of life in infants recovering from respiratory distress syndrome, Pediatrics **52**:169, 1973.

Donn, S.: Cost effectiveness of home management of bronchopulmonary dysplasia, Pediatrics **70**:330, 1982.

Edwards, D.K., Dyer, W.M., and Northway, W.J., Jr.: Twelve years experience with bronchopulmonary dysplasia, Pediatriccs **59**:839, 1977.

Gersony, W.M.: Patent ductus arteriosus in the neonate, Pediatr. Clin. N. Am. **33**:545, 1986.

Goldman, S.L., and others: Early prediction of chronic lung disease by pulmonary function testing, J. Pediatr. **102**:613, 1983.

Halliday, H.L., Dumpit, F.M., and Brady, J.: Effects of inspired oxygen on echocardiographic assessment of pulmonary vascular resistance and myocardial contractility in bronchopulmonary dysplasia, Pediatrics **65**:536, 1980.

Hodson, W.A., and others: Bronchopulmonary dysplasia: the need for epidemiologic studies, J. Pediatr. **95**:848, 1978.

Kao, L.C., and others: Furosemide acutely decreases airways resistance in chronic bronchopulmonary dysplasia, J. Pediatr. **103**:624, 1983.

Kraus, A.N., Klain, D.B., and Auld, P.A.M.: Chronic pulmonary insufficiency of prematurity (CPIP), Pediatrics **55**:55, 1975.

Markestad, T., and Fitzhardinge, P.M.: Growth and development in children recovering from bronchopulmonary dysplasia, J. Pediatr. **98**:597, 1981.

McCann, E.M., and others: Controlled trial of furosemide therapy in infants with chronic lung disease, J. Pediatr. **106**:957, 1985.

Meisels, S.J., and others: Growth and development of preterm infants with respiratory distress syndrome and bronchopulmonary dysplasia, Pediatrics **77**:345, 1986.

Melnick, G., and others: Normal pulmonary vascular resistance and left ventricular hypertrophy in young infants with bronchopulmonary dysplasia: an echocardiographic and pathologic study, Pediatrics **66**:589, 1980.

Myers, M.G., and others: Respiratory illnesses in survivors of infant respiratory distress syndrome, Am. Rev. Respir. Dis. **133**:1011, 1986.

Northway, W.J., Jr.: Observations on bronchopulmonary dysplasia, J. Pediatr. **95**:815, 1980.

Northway, W.H., Jr., Rosan, R.C., and Porter, D.Y.: Pulmonary disease following respirator therapy of hyaline membrane disease: bronchopulmonary dysplasia, N. Engl. J. Med. **276**:357, 1967.

Reid, L.: Bronchopulmonary dysplasia—pathology, J. Pediatr. **95**:836, 1979.

Rooklin, A.R., and others: Theophylline therapy in bronchopulmonary dysplasia, J. Pediatr. **95**:882, 1979.

Rome, E.S., and others: Limitations of transcutaneous PO_2 and PCO_2 monitoring in infants with bronchopulmonary dysplasia, Pediatrics **74**:217, 1984.

Spitzer, A.R., Fox, W.W., and Delivoria-Papadopoulos, M.: Maximum diuresis—a factor in predicting recovery from respiratory distress syndrome and the development of bronchopulmonary dysplasia, J. Pediatr. **98**:476, 1981.

Smyth, J.A., and others: Pulmonary function and bronchial hyperreactivity in long-term survivors of bronchopulmonary dysplasia, Pediatrics **68**:336, 1981.

Tooley, W.H.: Epidemiology of bronchopulmonary dysplasia, J. Pediatr. **95**:851, 1979.

Truog, W.E., and others: Bronchopulmonary dysplasia and pulmonary insufficiency of prematurity, Am. J. Dis. Child. **139**:351, 1985.

Vohr, B.R., Bell, E.F., and Oh, W.: Infants with bronchopulmonary dysplasia: growth pattern and neurologic and developmental outcome, Am. J. Dis. Child. **136**:443, 1982.

Watts, J.L., Ariagno, R.L., and Brady, J.P.: Chronic pulmonary disease in neonates after artificial ventilation: distribution of ventilation and pulmonary interstitial emphysema, Pediatrics **60**:273, 1977.

Weinstein, M.R., and Oh, W.: Oxygen consumption in infants with bronchopulmonary dysplasia, J. Pediatr. **99**:958, 1981.

Werthammer, J., and others: Sudden infant death syndrome in infants with bronchopulmonary dysplasia, Pediatrics **69**:301, 1982.

Wilson, M.G., and Mikity, V.G.: A new form of respiratory disease in premature infants, Am. J. Dis. Child. **99**;489, 1960.

Workshop on Bronchopulmonary Dysplasia, J. Pediatr. (Suppl.) **85**:815, 1979.

Etiology

Bell, E.F., and others: Effect of fluid administration on the development of symptomatic patent ductus arteriosus and congestive heart failure in premature infants, N. Engl. J. Med. **392**:598, 1980.

Boat, T.F., and others: Toxic effects of oxygen on cultured human neonatal respiratory epithelium, Pediatr. Res. **7**:607, 1973.

Brown, E.R., and others: Bronchopulmonary dysplasia: possible relationship to pulmonary edema, J. Pediatr. **92**:982, 1978.

Bruce, M., and others: Proteinase inhibitors and inhibitor inactivation in neonatal airways secretions, Chest **81**:44S, 1982.

Deneke, S.M., and Fanburg, B.L.: Normobaric oxygen toxicity of the lung, N. Engl. J. Med. **303**:76, 1980.

Merritt, T..A., and others: Newborn tracheal aspirate cytology: classification during respiratory distress syndrome and bronchopulmonary dysplasia, J. Pediatr. **98**:949, 1981.

Stern, L., and others: Negative pressure artificial respiration: use in treatment of respiratory failure of the newborn, Can. Med. Assoc. J. **102**:595, 1970.

Taghizadeh, A., and Reynolds, E.O.R.: Pathogenesis of bronchopulmonary dysplasia following hyaline membrane disease, Am. J. Pathol. **82**:241, 1976.

CHAPTER 29

The cardiovascular system

Congenital cardiovascular disease is a major health problem in the neonatal period. The newborn with a severe cardiac malformation usually will have difficulties in this period or at least in the first 6 months of life. If he survives this critical period without problems, it is likely that he will remain asymptomatic for many years, as in patients with mild pulmonic or aortic stenosis, or decades, as in patients with an atrial septal defect (ASD).

The practice of pediatric cardiology thus tends to be partitioned, on the one hand, into care of the older child with easily identifiable, electively correctable heart disease—such as ASD and ventricular septal defects (VSD), patent ductus arteriosus (PDA), aortic and pulmonic stenosis, postductal coarctation of the aorta, and most cases of tetralogy of Fallot—and, alternatively, into care of the newborn with life-threatening malformations such as transposition of the great arteries, hypoplastic left-heart syndrome, preductal coarctation of the aorta, and a host of complex malformations. In general, the outlook for the older child with one of the seven most common malformations just noted is now excellent, whereas the prognosis for the sick neonate with cardiac disease may vary from excellent (as in infants with transposition of the great arteries with low pulmonary arterial pressure or severe isolated pulmonic stenosis) to bad (as in infants with a hypoplastic left ventricle with diminutive aorta). This chapter discusses those severe lesions which present problems in the first month of life. However, the majority of infants born with heart disease manifest no problem in the neonatal period, and recent advances in diagnosis and corrective surgery allow survival with normal life expectancy in the majority of children with congenital heart disease.

INCIDENCE OF STRUCTURAL CONGENITAL HEART DISEASE

Precise figures of the incidence of structural congenital heart disease probably will never be attainable. Some cardiac defects (such as VSD and PDA) close spontaneously, whereas others (such as ASD) may not become manifest until late in childhood. A recent study of 56,109 infants monitored for an average of 3 years after birth disclosed an incidence of 8.14 infants with congenital heart disease per 1,000 births. Approximately one fifth of all infants born alive with a congenital heart defect die within the first month of life. However, many of these infants have multiple cardiac defects together with congenital defects of other organ systems.

ETIOLOGY OF CONGENITAL HEART DISEASE

Although several causes of congenital heart disease have been firmly identified, in the majority of patients no antecedent factor can be determined. Some cardiac malformations (such as PDA) are more common in girls, whereas others (such as aortic stenosis) are more common in boys; the overall sex ratio is approximately 1:1. Prematurity, calculated by both gestational age and weight, is approximately 2½ times more frequent in infants born with heart disease. However, it has been suggested that infants with transposition of the great arteries tend to be heavier than average, but this finding has been questioned.

Factors known to be associated with congenital heart disease include maternal ingestion of thalidomide and possibly other chemicals, such as dextroamphetamine, phenytoin (Dilantin), phenobarbital, lithium carbonate, ethyl alcohol, and progestogens, maternal infection with rubella virus and possibly with other viruses, season of the year, high altitude (PDA only), major chromosomal disorders such as Down's syndrome and Turner's syndrome, disorders of connective tissue such as Marfan's syndrome and Ehlers-Danlos syndrome, and maternal diabetes. The influence of ionizing radiation is unknown.

McCue and associates have described an association between complete congenital atrioventricular (AV) heart block in the fetus and neonate and maternal connective tissue disease, especially systemic lupus erythematosus. It appears likely that antinuclear antibodies of the IgG class cross the placenta and affect the fetal cardiac conduction tissues.

Common major chromosomal disorders

The incidence of structural congenital heart disease is high in infants with major chromosomal disorders. For trisomy 13 syndrome the incidence is approximately 90%; for trisomy 18 it is greater than 95%. Heart disease is also common in Down's syndrome (40%) and in Turner's syndrome (approximately 20%). In Down's syndrome the heart defect is frequently severe (for example, common AV canal). Occasionally a Turner-like syndrome (Noonan's syndrome) is encountered. In this instance the child has the phenotypic features of Turner's syndrome but no demonstrable chromosomal abnormality; heart disease, especially pulmonic stenosis, is common.

Heart disease caused by maternal rubella

The frequency of fetal infection from mothers having rubella during the first trimester is about 50% (Chapter 31). The heart may be affected in a variety of ways; PDA, peripheral pulmonary artery stenosis, systemic arterial stenosis, and myocarditis are common. Recognition that cardiovascular disease is a part of a general disorder is paramount to the multidisciplinary approach necessary for the adequate management of associated mental retardation, deafness, cataract, and glaucoma, although, in general, the presence of other system malformations does not alter the treatment of the cardiovascular problem.

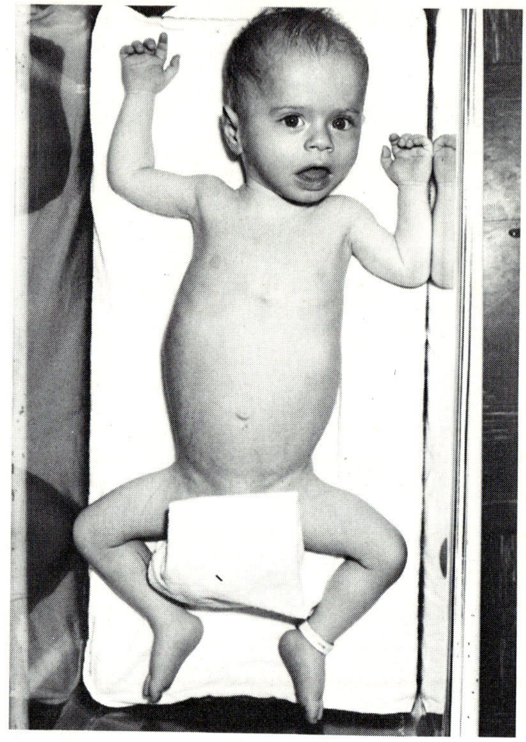

Fig. 29-1. Three-month-old infant with glycogen storage disease (Pompe's disease). Note hypotonic posture and large tongue. There was considerable hepatomegaly.

Infantile hypercalcemia and vascular disease

A broad maxilla, full prominent upper lip, and small anteverted nose characterize the infant with idiopathic infantile hypercalcemia. The hypercalcemia, when detected, is generally present only in infancy, and the association with vascular disease is based on the observation that a number of children with supravalvular aortic stenosis (stenosis of the ascending aorta) or peripheral pulmonary artery stenosis or both have a very similar facial appearance. The disease can occur in siblings, but it remains to be established whether treatment of idiopathic hypercalcemia in infancy will prevent the occurrence of arterial stenoses or the associated mental retardation.

Hereditary disorders of connective tissue

The cardiac defects associated with Marfan's syndrome (aortic regurgitation and aortic aneurysm) do not usually lead to problems in infancy. Similarly neonatal problems are unusual with Ehlers-Danlos syndrome. Spontaneous rupture of a renal artery has been described in a 6-day old infant with osteogenesis imperfecta.

Glycogen storage disease

Pompe's disease is the only type of glycogen storage disease causing cardiac symptoms in the newborn period. The disease is suggested by a positive family history, large tongue, hepatosplenomegaly, and muscular hypotonia. The left ventricle is grossly enlarged. Definitive diagnosis can be made by biochemical and enzymatic examinations of the skeletal muscle (Fig. 29-1).

Other syndromes associated with cardiovascular disease

In addition to the syndromes already referred to, a number of cardiac anomalies are associated with recognizable patterns of human malformation (Table 29-1).

Genetics and congenital heart disease

The question frequently asked of the pediatrician is what the risk is of a malformed heart when a first-degree relative (mother, father, sibling, or child of index case) has congenital heart disease. The question is even more pertinent now that many patients who previously would have died before reproductive age undergo successful surgery. Nora studied the children of 308 adults with ASD or VSD, most of whom had had surgical correction. Parents with ASD had 2.6% of their children affected with ASD, which is 37 times greater than the estimated population frequency. For VSD 3.7% of the children of parents with this heart defect were similarly affected. The data approximate closely with predictions of the mul-

Table 29-1. Less common syndromes sometimes associated with cardiovascular abnormality

Syndrome	Congenital heart defect
VATER	VSD, tetralogy of Fallot
Cerebrohepatorenal	PDA with or without septal defect
Holt-Oram	ASD and other types of congenital heart disease
Hurler's	Cardiomyopathy
Friedreich's ataxia	Cardiomyopathy
XXXXX	PDA
Carpenter's	PDA, VSD, transposition
Cornelia de Lange's	Variable
Cri du chat	Variable
Ellis-van Creveld	Septal defects
Radial aplasia and thrombocytopenia	Variable
XXXXY	PDA
Laurence-Moon-Biedl-Bordet	Tetralogy of Fallot
Charge association	Tetralogy of Fallot, DORV, AV canal, PDA

tifactorial inheritance hypothesis. This states that the incidence in first-degree relatives of an individual with a malformation transmitted by multifactorial inheritance approaches the square root of the population frequency of that lesion (for example, if the population frequency is 0.001 [1 per 1,000], the increase is to $\sqrt{0.001}$, [0.032, or 32 per 1,000]). For ASD the number of offspring affected is very close to the multifactorial prediction; for VSD the 3.7% of children with cardiac malformations approximates the 4.2% prediction. When the mother herself has congenital heart disease, the risk to each child appears to be on the order of 1:7. In the future more marriages will occur between adults who both have corrected or uncorrected congenital heart disease. The risk presumably will be further increased, as has been shown to occur in the case of cleft lip and palate.

Despite the multiple factors known to be associated with congenital heart disease, in approximately 75% of infants afflicted no cause is evident: the family history is negative, pregnancy has been uncomplicated, and no other disease exists in the baby. In the majority therefore the disease is unexpected and is not repeated in siblings. Environmental factors such as ionizing radiation or undiagnosed fleeting infections during embryogenesis also influence the incidence of congenital heart disease. The question frequently asked by the mother who has just given birth to a heart-diseased infant is, naturally, what the risk is for future infants. At the present state of our knowledge a general answer should be that the risk is approximately 1:25. Whittemore and associates have shown that the incidence of heart abnormality in the offspring of a mother who has congenital heart disease is much higher than previously suspected—14%. When there are additional first- or second-degree relatives with congenital heart disease, an assessment cannot be given. There are occasional families in which congenital heart disease occurs at a rate greatly exceeding the multifactorial inheritance hypothesis prediction.

RECOGNITION OF CARDIOVASCULAR ABNORMALITY IN THE FETUS

Structural congenital heart disease

Ultrasonography to detect cardiovascular disease in the fetus may sometimes be desirable because of a strong family history of congenital heart disease, especially if the mother is the survivor of a life-threatening condition such as pulmonary atresia or transposition of the great arteries. The mother-to-child transmission (usually of the same lesion) is believed to be approximately 14%, and delivery in a center equipped for rapid intervention is indicated.

Sometimes severe fetal heart disease—especially single ventricle—is associated with fetal bradycardia, fetal dysrhythmias or fetal death: under these circumstances careful monitoring and sometimes early delivery is indicated. A review by Allan and associates highlighted the finding that the prenatally discovered heart lesions tend to be severe, and in her series of 72 fetuses with a structural heart abnormality there were 34 terminations of pregnancy, 13 interuterine deaths, 20 neonatal deaths, and only 5 survivors.

Fetal dysrhythmias

Equally important is the discovery of fetal dysrhythmia, usually revealed by the obstetrician or ultrasonographer as fetal bradycardia, fetal tachycardia, or fetal heart irregularity. These occurrences are discussed later in this chapter.

Recognition of cardiovascular abnormality in the newborn

The presence of cyanosis or the signs of heart failure are the most frequent reasons for suspecting serious heart disease in the newborn. Less commonly heart disease appears as a shocklike picture, with pallor, flaccidity, and hypoactive arterial pulses; occasionally the presenting abnormality is an arrhythmia, especially supraventricular tachycardia (SVT) or complete heart block.

Uncommon signs of serious neonatal heart disease include isolated tachypnea, isolated liver enlargement, a loud cardiac murmur in a temporarily asymptomatic infant, "failure to thrive," prenatal stethoscopic detection of a loud heart murmur or arrhythmia, hyperdynamic cardiac impulse, abnormal cardiac pulses, systemic hypertension, unsuspected electrocardiogram (ECG) or x-ray film abnormality, and central nervous system symptoms secondary to a cerebral arteriovenous fistula or cerebral hypoxia.

PHYSICAL EXAMINATION OF THE INFANT WITH SUSPECTED CARDIOVASCULAR DISEASE

History

The family history should be reviewed for evidence of congenital heart disease, diabetes, connective tissue disorder, glycogen storage disease, hypercalcemia, or unusual hereditable disease. Questions relating to the present pregnancy should include inquiries about rubella, Coxsackie virus infection, unusual radiation exposure, or threatened abortion.

General appearance

The pedigree, history, and general appearance of the infant may reveal evidence of a major chromosomal defect, hypercalcemia, rubella, connective tissue disorder, glycogen storage disease, or rare syndrome. Early recognition that heart disease is but one manifestation of a complex disorder is essential to proper management.

Behavior of the infant

A general appraisal of the infant's spontaneous activity and response to stimuli often provides insight into the seriousness of the disease. A baby with reduced oxygen delivery to the tissues—whether from cyanotic heart disease or from heart failure—may show little spontaneous movement presumably in an attempt to conserve available oxygen for basal metabolic requirements. In the extreme case a newborn with severe heart failure from prenatal asphyxia, myocarditis, or the hypoplastic left-heart syndrome may be flaccid and apathetic and show almost no response to external stimuli.

Breathing patterns

Tachypnea, altered depth of respiration, intercostal retractions, flaring of the alae nasi, grunting, stridor, and apneic spells all may be observed in infants with cardiovascular disease. It cannot be assumed that the presence of these respiratory symptoms automatically implies that there is primary lung disease. Severe heart failure may mimic pulmonary disease in this regard.

Arterial pulses and measurement of blood pressure (Table 29-2)

See also Chapter 21 and Appendix C.

The radial, posterior tibial, and dorsalis pedis pulses are readily palpable in the normal newborn. Feeling one strong foot pulse that is synchronous with the radial is sufficient to rule out significant adult-type postductal coarctation. In contrast, it *is* necessary to feel both radial pulses, since supravalvular aortic stenosis, aortic isthmus stenosis, and juxtaductal coarctation all may lead to an increased pressure in the right arm when compared with pressure in the left. A reasonable approach therefore is for the physician to feel both radial (or brachial) pulses simultaneously and then to palpate a radial and foot pulse simultaneously, feeling for evidence of pulse delay in the leg (characteristic of mild or moderate coarctation). The more common form of coarctation found in sick neonates is the juxtaductal or preductal form, in which the lower half of the body is perfused with blood originating from the right ventricle. In this situation the femoral and foot pulses are often normal, and one should be able to observe cyanosis of the feet compared with the appearance of the hands. In practice this sign often is missed until after the angiocardiogram has disclosed the true anatomy. If hyperactive pulses are suspected, one may move peripherally and feel the palmar pulses or even the digital pulses (not normally palpable).

If the pulses are judged equal in arm and leg, it is necessary to measure only brachial blood pressure. Arm blood pressure usually can be measured with a 1- to 2-inch cuff and with a stethoscope over the brachial artery; however, the Doppler technique is a significant advance in the accurate measurement of systolic blood pressure in sick neonates, premature babies, and infants in neonatal intensive care units. A major advantage of this technique is that one can easily detect systolic blood pressures with accuracy in the 20 to 40 mm Hg range. Doppler leg blood pressure is most easily assessed by placing the cuff around the calf and interrogating the posterior tibial artery, behind the medial malleolus. The flush technique for measurement of blood pressure remains useful for the detection or confirmation of postductal coarctation. The normal blood pressure (descending aorta) was found by Moss to average 72/47 mm Hg for the resting full-term infant and 64/39 mm Hg for the premature. Crying caused an elevation of approximately 20 mm Hg in both systolic and diastolic measurements. Therefore a baby in whom coarctation is being considered should be quiet while upper and lower limb pressures are measured.

Venous pressure

See also Chapter 21.

Assessment of venous pressure is of very limited diagnostic aid. Burnell compared a group of infants not in heart failure with a group in clinical right-sided heart failure (hepatomegaly) undergoing cardiac catheterization. The group in heart failure had a central venous pressure of approximately 6 mm Hg, whereas the group not in heart failure had a mean pressure of 3 mm Hg. The newborn liver appears to act as a readily distensible sponge, giving rise to gross hepatomegaly rather than allowing much rise in central venous pressure. Occasionally one may observe distended neck veins in the upright infant and rarely a prominent A wave, suggesting obstruction to right atrial emptying (for example, tricuspid atresia or Ebstein's anomaly of the tricuspid valve).

Table 29-2. Peripheral arterial pulse abnormalities (excluding arrhythmias)

Condition	Characteristics
Full-term infants resting	72/47 mm Hg (aortic); brachial, femoral, radial, and dorsalis pedis pulses easily felt when baby is warm and still
Premature infants resting	64/39 mm Hg (aortic); brachial and femoral pulses easily felt; radial and dorsalis pedis pulses felt with difficulty when baby is warm and still
PDA Aortopulmonary window Peripheral arteriovenous fistula Truncus arteriosus Hyperthyroidism Aortic regurgitation	Widened pulse pressure; typical value 90/30 mm Hg; radial and foot pulses bounding; palmar and digital pulses often palpable
Severe aortic stenosis Hypoplastic left-heart syndrome Cardiogenic shock (especially myocarditis) Hemorrhagic or endotoxin shock Advanced heart failure	Narrowed pulse pressure; typical value 55/45 mm Hg; foot and wrist pulses impalpable; brachial and femoral pulses barely palpable; Doppler technique may be only accurate noninvasive method for obtaining blood pressure
Postductal coarctation (adult type)	Arm pulses normal or increased; typical value 90/50 mm Hg; leg pulses absent, diminished, or delayed; flush or Doppler technique usually necessary for lower limb (foot); typical value 60/50 mm Hg; adequacy of collaterals, as well as severity of coarctation, determines gradient
Preductal coarctation Juxtaductal coarctation	Arm and leg pulses may be normal if ductus is open; right ventricular blood perfuses descending aorta; differential cyanosis present but hard to recognize; when ductus is closed, pressure is as with postductal coarctation; absolute values depend on length of coarcted segment, degree of heart failure, and presence of associated lesions (frequent)
Supravalvular aortic stenosis Aortic isthmus stenosis	Right arm pressure may be higher than left arm pressure; typically 80/50 (right) versus 65/50 (left) mm Hg
Juxtaductal coarctation with aberrant right subclavian artery	Left arm pressure may be higher than right arm pressure
Pericardial tamponade Constrictive pericarditis	Pulsus paradoxus; arterial pressure falls by more than 10 mm Hg during inspiration (Doppler technique needed); very rare in infancy; tamponade more likely to be suggested by rapidly increasing venous pressure and liver size
Left ventricular failure	Pulsus alternans; strong pulses alternating with weaker ones; reflects rapidly failing left ventricle; occasionally observed in infants with myocarditis and terminal congenital heart disease

Liver size

Normally the liver may be palpable 2 or sometimes 3 cm below the right costal margin, measured in the nipple-umbilicus line. The size of the liver is a highly reliable index of the severity of right-sided heart failure; in this condition it is frequently 5 or 6 cm below the costal margin. Liver enlargement occurs in a number of other neonatal conditions, including sepsis, congenital rubella, toxoplasmosis, cytomegalic inclusion disease, metastases of neuroblastoma, and hemolytic anemias. However, the observation of an enlarged liver should lead to a strong consideration of heart failure even in the absence of cyanosis or heart murmur. A centrally placed or left-sided liver, if associated with levocardia, frequently is associated with complex congenital heart disease.

Spleen

Splenic enlargement is not a sign of heart failure; however, congenital absence of the spleen, when associated with an abnormally placed liver and evidence of heart disease, frequently portends a complex inoperable abnormality. Congenital absence or hypoplasia of the spleen is suggested by excessive numbers of Heinz bodies within the red cells. Heinz bodies, however, are seen in a variety of situations in the newborn, and their presence especially in the premature infant should be interpreted with caution. (See Chapter 32.)

Peripheral edema

Occasionally the backs of the hands and dorsum of the feet may show pitting edema as a consequence of heart failure. Rarely there is more widespread edema, with sacral pitting and puffy eyelids. In general, however, the lack of a major rise in central venous pressure in infants with congestive heart failure appears also to preclude the development of marked edema, presumably because the high systemic capillary pressures occurring in adult congestive heart failure are not found in infancy. Severe widespread peripheral edema is, accordingly, a more ominous sign in infants than in adults. Etiologic possibilities in "nonimmune" hydrops fetalis include prenatal paroxysmal supraventricular tachycardia (SVT), α-thalassemia, disseminated intravascular coagulation with sepsis, cystic adenomatoid malformation of the lung, and congenital nephrosis. Ultrasonography of the fetus may reveal ascites or pleural effusion. The lymphedema characteristic of Turner's syndrome, especially if associated with organic heart disease, may give the erroneous impression of heart failure.

Ascites and pleural and pericardial effusion

If ascites is observed in the newborn, heart failure is an unlikely cause because of the rarity of high systemic capillary pressures. Before ascribing ascites to heart failure, one should give careful consideration to primary liver disease, primary kidney disease, chylous ascites, and peritonitis. Similarly pleural effusion should prompt consideration of chylothorax or lung disease rather than heart failure. Pericardial effusion or pericarditis in the newborn period is rare and is usually caused by bacterial sepsis.

Precordial impulse and thrills

Considerable information can be gained by laying a warm hand over the left side of the infant's chest. The cardiac impulse of a normal full-term baby is barely palpable, so that if the impulse is readily felt, ventricular volume overloading as from a left-to-right shunt or valvular regurgitation is likely. Right ventricular enlargement and overactivity is indicated by a hyperdynamic quality at the cardiac apex. A hypodynamic or impalpable heart suggests tetralogy of Fallot if the infant is not in heart failure. If heart failure exists, the observation of a hypodynamic impulse may simply reflect low cardiac output.

A number of thrills are diagnostically very useful in the newborn. Fig. 29-2 indicates the site, location, significance, and timing of the four most common systolic thrills. A pulmonic stenosis thrill occurs with tetralogy of Fallot and a VSD thrill with tricuspid atresia. Isolated diastolic thrills are uncommon in the newborn period but occasionally may be felt with congenital valvular regurgitation, especially of the pulmonary valve. A continuous or near-continuous thrill suggests a PDA; the thrill and its accompanying murmur may be maximum in the second, third, or fourth left intercostal space. When the pulmonary artery pressure is sufficiently low to cause a continuous runoff of blood from the aorta through a PDA, the continuous murmur or thrill is nearly always accompanied by bounding arterial pulses.

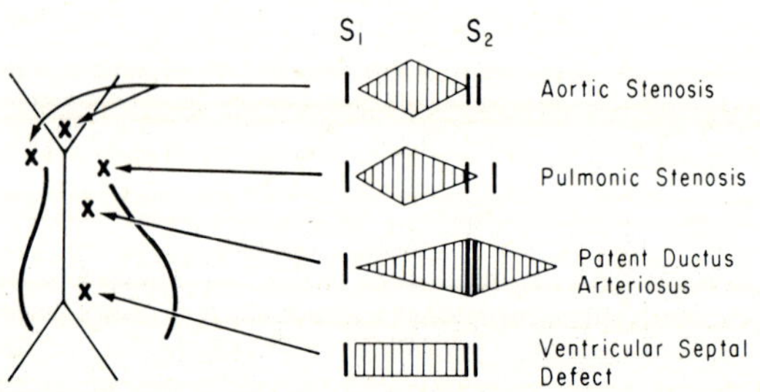

Fig. 29-2. Site, location, significance, and timing of the four most common systolic thrills felt in the newborn.

Heart rate and regularity in normal infants

See also Chapter 21.

The heart rate in quiet full-term infants averages 130 beats per minute, but the range may vary from 70 to 180 beats per minute during the first week of life. A mild sinus arrhythmia occurs in most newborns and is more pronounced in premature infants. The use of long-term ECG recordings in full-term newborns has revealed the existence of clinically unsuspected and presumably benign arrhythmias. A study of 56 full-term infants revealed isolated sinus arrest in one baby, a few premature supraventricular beats in three, and premature ventricular beats in two, one of whom had a premature ventricular beat every fourth beat but a normal ECG by age 14 days. A similar study of 20 premature infants revealed sinus bradycardia in eight and very marked sinus bradycardia (rate below 50 beats per minute) with nodal escapes in an additional five. All infants with birth weights below 1,500 gm had one or more periods of marked sinus bradycardia with or without nodal escape; none of the 50 full-term infants studied by the same group had sinus bradycardia (below 70 beats per minute) or had a nodal rhythm.

Therefore the finding of an occasional premature beat or of a short period of sinus bradycardia or sinus tachycardia is not in itself ominous. However, in the presence of severe heart disease such arrhythmias may portend serious trouble. Long-term ECG tape recording and the use of continuous ECG monitors equipped with a memory loop, whereby the minute preceding and including an arrhythmia can be printed out, have greatly facilitated the unraveling of intermittent arrhythmias in newborns. In instances where an arrhythmia is infrequent and the parents live at a distance from a medical center, use of transtelephonic ECG transmission (Cardiotel program) has been useful.

Heart sounds

The diaphragm side of the stethoscope is usually preferable for auscultation of both heart sounds and murmurs, since it is not necessary for the whole diaphragm (in contrast to the bell) to make contact with the chest wall. There is no advantage to use of the pediatric size stethoscope, but it is of help always to use the same type of stethoscope, preferably one of longer length, to manipulate through incubator portholes.

Infant heart sounds have a ticktock quality because of the more equal duration of systole and diastole (with faster heart rates), the presence of slight pulmonary hypertension (for the first few days), and the proximity of semilunar valves to the chest wall. Compared with that in older children, the infant's apical first sound is particularly well heard, and the small size of the chest allows simultaneous assessment of first and second sounds with the stethoscope at the lower left sternal border. In the normal infant splitting of the first sound should lead one to suspect that one is hearing either a fourth sound (atrial sound) plus a first sound or a first sound plus an ejection click (as in aortic or pulmonic stenosis). A third possibility is that the extra sound is a mitral midsystolic click, suggesting congenital mitral valve prolapse or prolapse associated with Marfan's syndrome. Narrow splitting of the second sound is apparent in most babies; widening and narrowing of the second sound with respiration is usually apparent when the respiration rate is normal. An unusually obvious persistent wide splitting of the second sound may indicate an ASD or total anomalous pulmonary venous return. Singleness of S_2, when combined with a cardiac murmur and cyanosis, raises the possibility of pulmonary atresia or tetralogy of Fallot.

Ejection clicks, although uncommon, are useful physical signs, since when loud and obvious they are characteristic of aortic and pulmonic valvular stenosis. Soft ejection clicks sometimes are heard in normal babies. The ejection click is heard at the onset of an ejection murmur and resembles in timing, although not in character, a widely split first heart sound. The two may be distinguished, if necessary, by the recording of a simultaneous ECG and phonocardiogram; the ejection click is characteristically at least 0.09 seconds after the Q wave of the ECG, whereas the first heart sound (mitral and tricuspid valve closure) finishes earlier.

Cardiac murmurs

Certain murmurs are of major diagnostic help in the newborn period; however, the frequent presence of "innocent" murmurs and of transient ductus arteriosus murmurs renders their interpretation more difficult and more subject to error than in the older child. The situation is complicated by the fact that there are no absolute criteria for loudness, and the fast heart rate of babies sometimes makes it difficult to differentiate ejection from pansystolic murmurs. Characteristic heart murmurs of common heart defects appearing as problems in the neonatal period are discussed later in this chapter when specific lesions are considered. Serious heart disease may exist without any murmur, and conversely a grade 5 or 6 murmur may indicate a benign closing VSD. An organic systolic murmur present at the initial physical examination is more likely to be caused by an obstructive lesion such as aortic stenosis, pulmonic stenosis, or coarctation, whereas a murmur that is first heard at 2 or 3 months of age suggests a septal defect or ductus arteriosus, since the left-to-right shunt "opens up" as pulmonary vascular resistance falls in the first days and weeks of life.

Chest roentgenogram

See also Chapter 13.

Every newborn suspected of having a serious heart disease requires a well-centered anteroposterior chest roentgenogram and preferably a lateral film in addition. The lateral film may disclose left atrial enlargement or an unsuspected pathologic condition in the lung that is not evident on the anteroposterior film. The chest roentgenogram serves two broad purposes: (1) to evaluate the type and severity of heart disease and (2) to detect some of the many simulators of heart disease, including a wide variety of primary lung diseases and mechanical interference with lung function. In the evaluation of heart disease the following features should be considered.

1. **Expansion of the lungs.** Atelectasis or hypoventilation may give the spurious impression of cardiomegaly; correspondingly, overaerated lungs (as in lobar emphysema) may disguise cardiac enlargement.
2. **Heart size.** Unfortunately no firm criteria exist with which to assess cardiomegaly, and except in extreme situations (such as a cardiothoracic ratio greater than 0.75) pronouncements are mostly intuitive. A normal-sized heart is compatible with serious heart disease (such as transposition of the great arteries in the first day of life or anomalously draining pulmonary veins, with obstruction of the common pulmonary vein collecting trunk). A very large heart may be present without heart disease, as is the case in hypoglycemia or high hematocrit syndrome, or the heart may appear spuriously large because of the thymus gland.
3. **Shape of the heart.** The shape is often of considerable help, as in the "egg-on-side" heart of transposition, the boot-shaped heart of tetralogy of Fallot, the globular heart of Ebstein's anomaly, or the "snowman" heart of total anomalous pulmonary venous return into the left superior vena cava. Usually, however, the heart is simply large; useful signs such as prominence of the ascending aorta (aortic stenosis), prominence of the main and left pulmonary artery (pulmonic stenosis), square-shaped heart of tricuspid atresia, and the high origin of the pulmonary arteries (truncus arteriosus) often have not had time to develop or are obscured by the thymus gland.
4. **Pulmonary vascularity.** Three basic abnormalities can be recognized: oligemic lungs, hyperemic lungs, and lungs in which there is obstruction to pulmonary venous return. The pulmonary venous distension of this last category may lead to a "ground-glass," "snowstorm," or reticulated pattern (Fig. 29-3). It is quite different from the pulmonary hyperemic appearance where prominent large vessels appear to emanate from a single source, the hilum, and reflect a different

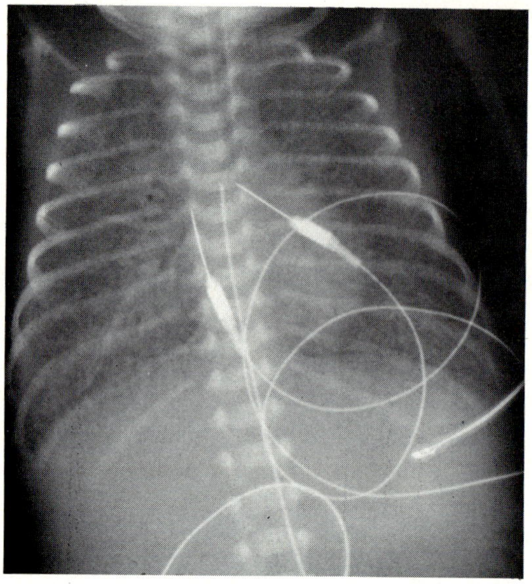

Fig. 29-3. Anteroposterior chest film of neonate with total anomalous pulmonary venous return to portal vein. Note small heart and "reticulated" lung fields, both caused by obstruction to pulmonary venous return.

spectrum of pathologic conditions (mitral valve disease, total anomalous pulmonary venous return with obstruction, or cor triatriatum).

5. **Specific appearances.** In the scimitar syndrome, one lung, usually the right, is supplied by systemic arteries, and a single large pulmonary vein (the "scimitar" on the roentgenogram), joins the inferior vena cava just below the diaphragm. Usually the affected lung is hypoplastic, and the heart is shifted to the right (dextroposition).

The electrocardiogram

The neonatal ECG and especially the ECG taken during the first 24 hours of life show great variability within the range of normal. The changes probably are secondary to the rapidly changing circulation (closing foramen ovale and ductus arteriosus, removal of the placental circulation, and the falling pulmonary artery pressure). Other influences are the infant's gestational age, pH, and levels of sodium, potassium, and calcium. Despite the wide variability of the normal newborn ECG, it is still an extremely useful diagnostic tool; and since it is such a simple noninvasive procedure, it is mandatory in the assessment of any neonate suspected of having cardiovascular disease.

The QRS complex

The newborn's ECG exhibits prominent and prolonged anterior forces resulting in a tall and broad R wave in the right chest leads and often a deep S wave in the left chest leads. The leftward vector in the newborn is small; consequently the R wave in the left precordium has low amplitude initially, but this increases rapidly in the first few months. The posterior vector, although variable, is frequently small in the newborn period and appears late. Thus the S wave in leads V_1 and V_2 is small.

The initial, or septal, vector may be to the left in the newborn period (less so in the premature infant). Rarely this may result in a qR complex in lead V_{4R} or even in V_1 and absent or small Q waves in the left chest leads. With aging, the initial vector extends further to the right, and the Q wave increases in the left precordium. The terminal rightward force is prominent in the newborn and gradually decreases over months to years. This explains the deep S wave in the left chest leads, which decreases with age. The newborn's ECG almost invariably demonstrates clockwise rotation in the frontal plane and usually (but less often) also in the horizontal plane.

The QRS patterns in the chest leads are classified into the following:

1. Adult R/S progression: S wave has higher amplitude than R wave in right chest leads and smaller than R wave in left chest leads.
2. Partial reversal of R/S progression: R wave amplitude is higher than that of S wave in both right and left chest leads
3. Complete reversal of R/S progression: R wave is larger than S wave in the right and smaller than S wave in the left chest leads (Fig. 29-4).

The newborn has either complete (50%) or partial reversal (50%) of R/S progression in the precordial leads, but no adult progression (with rare exceptions) of the R/S ratio is seen. By 1 month of age complete reversal disappears, and adult R/S progression is common. A pure R wave in lead V1 is rare, and a qR is only exceptionally seen in newborns.

T vector

Major changes occur in the T vector following birth. Within the first 5 minutes following birth this vector is oriented to the left anteriorly and minimally inferiorly; by 1 to 6 hours it has shifted much more inferiorly and to the right. Over the next several days the vector rotates markedly to the left and eventually becomes oriented to the left and posteriorly. In the series of Hastreiter and Abella during the first 24 hours the T vector was still oriented to the left anteriorly and inferiorly; at 2 to 7 days it was oriented to the left posteriorly and inferiorly. These changes explain the upright T in lead V_1 and the negative or flat T in lead V_6 that are characteristic of the very early neonatal period.

Electrocardiographic time intervals

Fast paper speeds (100 or 200 mm/second) increase the accuracy of the measurement of the short time in-

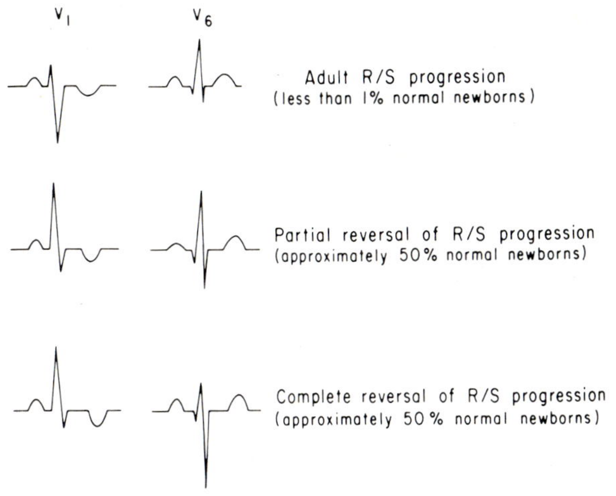

Fig. 29-4. QRS patterns in V_1 and V_6 of normal newborns. Note that adult R/S progression is sufficiently unusual to prompt consideration of left ventricular hypertrophy (or underdevelopment of the right ventricle).

tervals found in the newborn. However, the standard 25 mm/second is usually adequate. At birth the average heart rate is 140 beats per minute, but the rate drops to approximately 120 in the quiet infant during the first several hours. Premature infants have slightly higher heart rates. Although variations in heart rate from 70 to 200 beats per minute are compatible with a normal cardiovascular system, extremes should prompt ECG confirmation that the rhythm is sinus tachycardia or bradycardia. In general, one should be concerned if the *resting* rate is below 90 or above 170 beats per minute. The PR interval should be recorded as the longest observable in a standard or unipolar limb lead (usually the longest is lead II). The normal range is between 0.07 and 0.12 second, influenced slightly by heart rate and the time of cord clamping. The QRS duration averages 0.065 second at birth, falls to about 0.055 second at the end of the first week, and gradually increases to 0.068 second at 12 months. The QT interval is greatly influenced by heart rate and therefore is expressed as QT observed or QT_c (QT corrected to a heart rate of 60). At birth the average observed QT interval is relatively long (0.30 second), decreasing to 0.24 second at 3 weeks and to 0.27 at 1 year. The QT_c is much more constant, averaging 0.40 second.

Electrical axes of the newborn heart

A consideration of the frontal plane QRS axis (assessed from the standard and unipolar limb leads) can be of considerable diagnostic help. The normal newborn has a QRS axis of approximately +35 to +180 degrees. The normal P-wave axis should lie between 0 and +90 degrees (that is, upright in leads I and a V_F). The T-wave axis in the frontal plane is much more labile after birth than is the P or QRS axis. The T axis averages +7 degrees at 1 to 5 minutes after birth, then shifts to +115 degrees at 2 to 4 hours after birth; this is followed by a gradual return to approximately the previous level (+10 degrees) during the following 2 to 7 days. From the first week to the beginning of the third month of life the frontal T-wave axis gradually increases to reach a maximum of +60 degrees. The T wave therefore always should be upright in lead I except for a brief period in the first 24 hours of life, when it may be biphasic or on rare occasion inverted. The T waves are frequently of low amplitude during the first week of life. In the horizontal plane (that is, the precordial leads V_{4R} through V_6) the mean QRS axis has an average value of +130 degrees during the first day of life and decreases gradually to about +110 degrees at the end of the first week; it remains stationary throughout the first month. Thus in all but an occasional infant the QRS axis is a predominantly positive deflection in the right precordial leads. The T wave is usually negative in V_1 immediately after birth but becomes positive in this lead at 2 to 6 hours, after which it usually becomes negative successively in V_1, V_2, V_3 and V_4. On occasion the T wave may be partially negative (biphasic) in V_5 and V_6. This characteristic has been correlated with a left-to-right shunt through the ductus arteriosus in the first 10 hours of life. After the first month of life the T wave always should be upright in V_6. A clearly negative T wave in V_5 or V_6 should suggest an abnormality such as myocarditis, left ventricular hypertrophy, conduction abnormality, or electrolyte disturbance. Whatever the cause of a negative T wave in V_6, follow-up ECGs are indicated.

The ECG of the premature and postmature infant

A number of comprehensive studies have failed to resolve the question of whether the premature infant's ECG has characteristic features different from those of a mature newborn. In part this is because the premature newborn's ECG shows even more variability than that of the full-term infant. Generally, however, there is less right ventricular dominance (also lower right ventricle–to–left ventricle weight ratio) in the ECG of the premature and more right ventricular dominance in the postmature infant.

The ECG in diagnosis during the newborn period

The newborn's ECG is most useful in the unraveling of an arrhythmia, the detection of gross atrial and ventricular hypertrophy, and the occasional almost pathognomonic finding such as myocardial infarction, indicating an anomalous left coronary artery (Fig. 29-74), or left axis deviation and left ventricular hypertrophy typical of tricuspid valve atresia (Fig. 29-57). The ECG plays a supportive role in the detection and assessment of severity of electrolyte disorders and myocardial disorders (Figs. 29-5, 29-69, and 29-70). The major area of uncer-

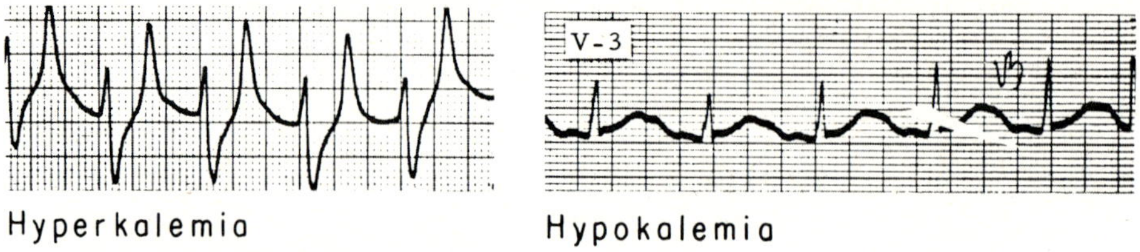

Fig. 29-5. ECG changes of advanced hyperkalemia (lead II). Note tall "tented" T waves, ST depression, and barely visible P waves on downslope of T wave. In the example of hypokalemia (lead V_3) there is a prominent U wave—the second component of what appears to be a double-peaked T wave. In other examples there would be P wave prolongation or prominence, ST depression, or low-voltage T waves. The changes of hypokalemia are much less distinctive than those of hyperkalemia.

tainty is in the diagnosis of right ventricular hypertrophy. This is related to the rapidly changing hemodynamics and individual right/left ventricle weight ratios. Later in infancy and in childhood (when the left ventricle far outweighs the right) the opposite is found: the ECG is a sensitive indicator of right ventricular hypertrophy, but the voltage criteria for left ventricular hypertrophy are unreliable.

Diagnosis of atrial hypertrophy. The diagnosis of atrial hypertrophy is relatively straightforward. A P wave that is peaked and more than 3 mm (0.3 mV) in any standard or unipolar lead indicates probable right atrial hypertrophy (P pulmonale); if the P wave is 4 mm, right atrial hypertrophy is certain. Left atrial hypertrophy is characterized by broadening and notching of the P wave, so that the duration (in a limb lead) is 0.10 second or greater, and the Macruz index (the ratio of P-wave duration to the remainder of the PR interval) is increased (greater than 1.6:1).

Diagnosis of ventricular hypertrophy. The following outline shows the criteria for the diagnosis of ventricular hypertrophy. No single measurement is diagnostic; all values are possible in normal newborns, but many are statistically unlikely.

CRITERIA FOR RIGHT AND LEFT VENTRICULAR HYPERTROPHY IN THE NEWBORN

A. Right ventricular hypertrophy
   1. An R in lead aV_R of greater than 7 mm
   2. A qR pattern in V_1
   3. An RV_1 greater than 28 mm
   4. SV_6 greater than 13 mm
   5. A pure R wave (no q or S) in V_1 of 10 mm or greater
   6. Positive T in V_1 after day 5
B. Left ventricular hypertrophy
   1. R in aV_L greater than 9 mm
   2. R in V_6 greater than 17 mm in first week
   3. R in V_6 greater than 25 mm in first month
   4. Inverted TV_6 or T_1 with voltage changes
   5. Adult R/S progression; that is, SV_1 greater than RV_1 and RV_6 SV_6 (before day 3)

Electrolytes and the ECG in the neonatal period

Although abnormal serum calcium and serum potassium levels sometimes are associated with characteristic ECG abnormalities, undue reliance should not be placed on the ECG to *detect* electrolyte disturbances, since intracellular as well as extracellular electrolyte levels are responsible for the disordered waveform. Magnesium and sodium ion levels and pH disturbances are not generally considered primary determinants of the ECG waveform but are thought to act predominantly by their effects on the intracellular and extracellular levels of potassium.

Hyperkalemia produces a succession of changes in the ECG, with tall, narrow, "tented" T waves progressing to ST segment depression, QRS widening, and a lengthened PR interval (Fig. 29-5). Finally, with severe hyperkalemia the QRS blends with the T wave to produce the "sine-wave" effect. This type of ECG often is observed in the dying neonate, especially following external cardiac massage. *Hypokalemia* leads to ST depression, low-voltage T waves, and development of a prominent U wave (Fig. 29-5). The PR interval may be prolonged with prominent P waves. The changes are much less apparent than those of hyperkalemia.

Serum calcium changes. It is now realized that the levels of intracellular and extracellular calcium ions are basic determinants of the speed of myocardial depolarization and repolarization. Hypocalcemia lengthens the QT interval, whereas hypercalcemia shortens it.

Significance of common electrocardiographic abnormalities in the neonate

Sinus arrhythmia may be obvious in the full-term neonate and very marked in the premature infant. Marked sinus arrhythmia requires ECG confirmation.

Tachycardia (rate over 170 beats per minute) may reflect fever, hyperthyroidism, or excessive activity or may

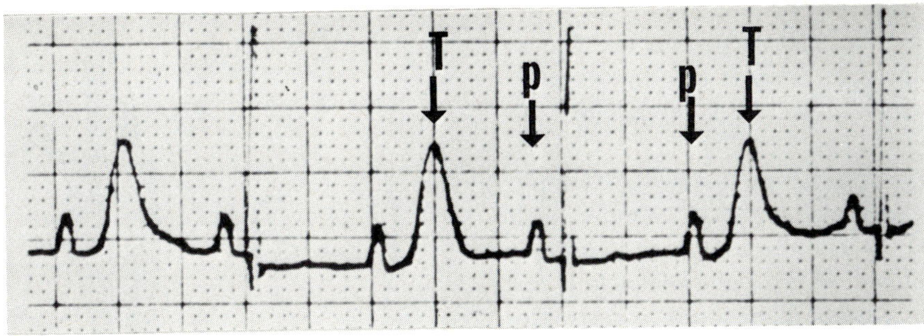

Fig. 29-6. Prolonged QT interval syndrome. Neonatal ECG after observation of fetal bradycardia. QT interval is 0.7 second. QRS rate is 60 per minute with atrial rate 120 per minute. Alternate P waves are blocked, probably by ventricular myocardial refractoriness.

on occasion be physiologic. Sinus tachycardia rates up to 200 beats per minute in the full-term infant and 210 beats per minute in the premature infant have been described. These rates (over 170 beats per minute) necessitate an ECG to distinguish between sinus tachycardia, paroxysmal SVT, atrial flutter with 2:1 AV conduction, and paroxysmal ventricular tachycardia. The major problem that arises is the distinction between paroxysmal SVT and sinus tachycardia.

Bradycardia is when the rate is under 90 beats per minute. Rates down to 90 beats per minute in the full-term infant and 70 beats per minute in the premature infant have been found in the absence of disease. Even lower rates occur during defecation and breath holding with crying. The ECG will distinguish pathologic sinus bradycardia (from apneic spells, pathologic conditions of the central nervous system, gross hypoxia, and so on) from specific bradycardia (such as complete heart blocks, second-degree AV block, and atrial flutter or SVT with a high degree of AV block). Bradycardia and tachycardia may be seen in infants with sinus node dysfunction (sick sinus syndrome) (see Fig. 29-33).

Prolongation of the PR interval indicates first-degree AV block. If the PR interval is constant, no treatment is required; but one should be alerted to the possibility that first-degree AV block may progress to second-degree AV block, especially if digitalis is being administered. Hyperkalemia, hypokalemia, and acidosis also should be considered. In most instances no abnormality exists, and the condition is a benign variant. *Shortening of the PR interval* indicates an ectopic atrial pacemaker (close to the AV node) or the Wolff-Parkinson-White syndrome (short PR, broad QRS).

Variation of the PR interval with equal atrial (P) and ventricular (QRS) rates may indicate premature atrial beats or, if the PR interval has three or more different durations with P waves or varying forms, the benign "wandering pacemaker." *Absence of the P wave* usually indicates an AV nodal pacemaker.

Variation of the PR interval with the atrial rate faster than the ventricular rate (a P wave rate in excess of the QRS rate), when there is no relationship between the two, indicates complete heart block (third-degree AV block), incomplete AV dissociation with ventricular captures, or second-degree heart block.

Variation of the PR interval with the atrial rate slower than the ventricular rate is a rare situation (sometimes called AV dissociation by interference) which implies that a lower pacemaker (usually AV nodal) beats somewhat faster than the sinoatrial (SA) pacemaker. Thus the ventricular rate is rarely as slow as in complete heart block. The most common causes are digitalis intoxication and myocarditis.

A wide QRS indicates right or left bundle branch block, complete AV block, or the Wolff-Parkinson-White syndrome. Random wide QRS complexes indicate ventricular ectopic beats or supraventricular beats with aberrant ventricular conduction. Hyperkalemia, hyponatremia, acidosis, and drugs such as quinidine and phenytoin may broaden the QRS.

A shortened QT_c interval is characteristic of hypercalcemia and of digitalis effect. Hyponatremia also may cause slight QT_c shortening. A *lengthened QT_c interval* is characteristic of hypocalcemia, hypokalemia, drug intoxication (especially from quinidine and phenothiazine derivatives), and patients with cerebrovascular disease. QT_c prolongation also is seen in children with congenital deafness, a heritable form of QT_c prolongation associated with syncopal spells and sudden death (Fig. 29-6).

Right axis deviation +90 to +180 degrees) is a normal finding in the first month of life. An axis between +35 and +90 degrees may be normal in the newborn period, and axes between 0 and +35 degrees occasionally are seen in a newborn. *Left axis deviation (0 to −90 degrees)* is very rare in a normal infant and is highly suggestive of endocardial cushion defects (ostium primum ASD, common AV canal) and tricuspid atresia. A northwest axis (−90 to −180 degrees), if close to −90 degrees, usually represents extreme left axis deviation; if closer to −180 degrees, it is usually extreme right axis deviation. Clockwise inscription of the vector loop in the frontal plane implies the latter, counterclockwise inscription the former.

Right atrial hypertrophy is common with tricuspid atresia and Ebstein's anomaly. It is less common with transposition, tetralogy of Fallot, pulmonary hypertension, and any situation where the right ventricle is operating at systemic pressure. Right atrial hypertrophy also is seen where pulmonary hypertension is secondary to lung disease or when heart failure is present, as in SVT. *Left atrial hypertrophy* is common with mitral insufficiency and may occur with left ventricular failure (especially secondary to isolated aortic stenosis). *Right ventricular hypertrophy* is demonstrated in the ECG in a wide variety of conditions in which the right ventricle operates at systemic pressure. It also is seen in many neonates with pulmonary disease. Extreme right ventricular hypertrophy suggests isolated pulmonic stenosis. *Left ventricular hypertrophy* strongly supports a diagnosis of tricuspid atresia (especially if there is associated left axis deviation) or isolated severe aortic stenosis. Secondary T-wave changes (inverted TV_6 or T_1 or both) may be present with either diagnosis.

The Wolff-Parkinson-White syndrome may be a chance finding and in most cases indicates no underlying heart disease. A wide variety of organic heart diseases may be associated, but especially common are Ebstein's anomaly and corrected levotransposition (*l*-transposition).

A myocardial infarction pattern (abnormal Q waves) is almost diagnostic of anomalous origin of the left coronary artery from the pulmonary artery (see Fig. 29-74). Endocardial fibroelastosis on rare occasions may produce the ECG pattern of infarction, secondary to widespread myocardial fibrosis.

Echocardiography in the neonate

Ultrasound is defined as sound waves that are above the frequency audible by humans (20,000 cycles/second, or 20,000 Hz). For standard cardiac diagnostic purposes frequencies of 2 million to 5 million cycles/second (2 to 5 MHz) are used. Electrical energy is fed into the transducer for very brief periods, or pulses, which are repeated 1 to 2,000 times per second. Ninety-nine percent of the time the transducer acts as the receiver for the second waves, which are reflected from the objects on which they have impinged. The short pulse duration, with a long interval between each, allows for a low energy level. This makes pulsed reflected ultrasound well within all known limits of safety for biologic tissues.

Currently, three types of echocardiographic studies are used in clinical practice. These are M-mode, two-dimensional, and Doppler echocardiography. Each of

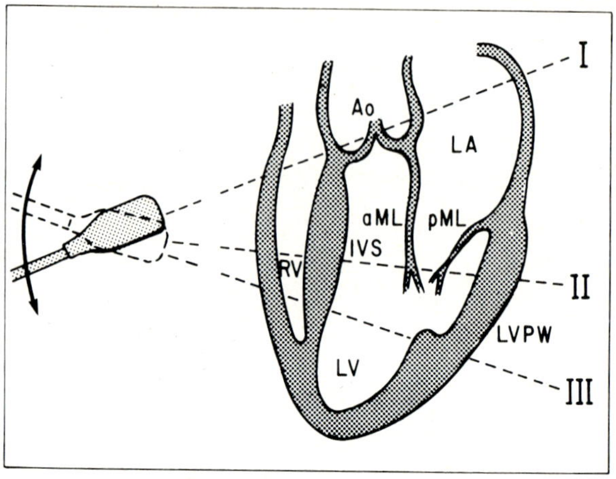

Fig. 29-7. Diagramatic cross section of heart. Echo transducer transects heart at levels *I*, *II*, and *III* for the three standard M-mode echo views. For M-mode sweep (as in Fig. 25-11), transducer is rotated, as shown, through three levels during recording. *Ao*, Aorta; *RV*, right ventricle; *aML*, anterior mitral valve leaflet; *pML*, posterior mitral valve leaflet; *LV*, left ventricle; *LVPW*, left ventricular posterior wall; *LA*, left atrium; *IVS*, interventricular septum. (Modified from Roelandt, J.: Practical echocardiography, Portland, 1977, Research Studies Press. Copyright 1977. Reprinted by permission of John Wiley & Sons, Ltd.)

these studies is reviewed in detail in the following section. Specific application of these studies to isolated congenital heart defects may be found in the sections on common cardiovascular disorders.

M-mode echocardiography

The standard M-mode study is recorded on a moving paper chart recorder so that many cardiac cycles can be recorded for future study. The study is obtained by angling the transducer, transecting the heart at three levels (Fig. 29-7). Area *I* in the figure transects the heart at the level of the aortic valve and left atrium. Here the aortic root and left atrial size may be measured. The aortic valve cusps can be seen in the center of the aorta and form a boxlike configuration when open (Fig. 29-8). The aorta moves anteriorly with systole.

Area *II* transects the heart at the level of the mitral valve (Figs. 29-7 and 29-9). At the onset of ventricular diastole (point *D* in Fig. 29-9) the mitral valve opens, and the anterior and posterior leaflets move in opposite directions. The *E* point represents the maximum anterior excursion of the anterior leaflet during early diastole. Following the rapid filling phase the leaflets tend to close (point F_O in Fig. 29-9) as ventricular filling slows. With atrial systole the leaflets again open (*A* wave in Fig. 29-9) as blood flows from the atrium to the left ventricle. An A wave (atrial systole) should be identified in both

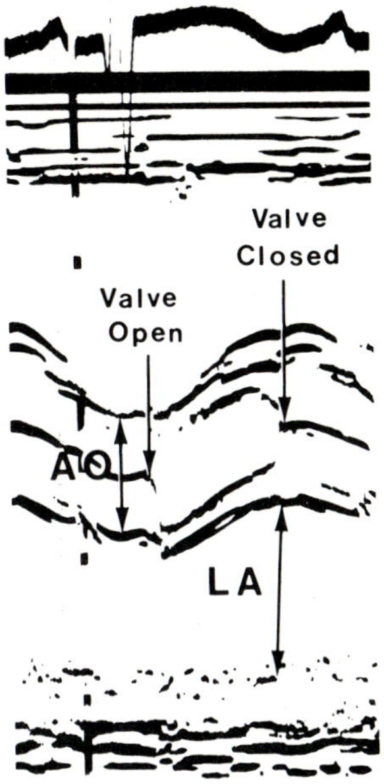

Fig. 29-8. Aorta *(AO)*, left atrium *(LA)* study; corresponds to level I in Fig. 29-7. Aorta is measured at onset of QRS, as shown with double arrow. Left atrium is measured at completion of ventricular systole (when left atrium has been filling), as shown with double arrow.

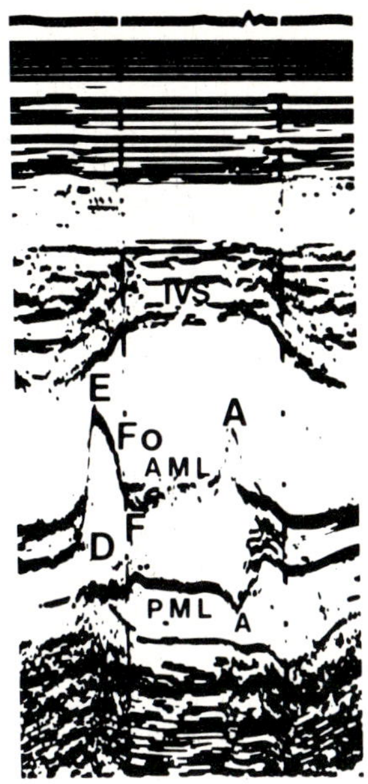

Fig. 29-9. Normal mitral valve study; corresponds to level II in Fig. 29-7. *AML*, anterior mitral leaflet; *PML*, posterior mitral leaflet; *IVS*, interventricular septum; *Fo*, rapid early closure of mitral valve.

the anterior and posterior leaflets. Normally the anterior leaflet motion is the mirror image of that of the posterior leaflet. In mitral valve stenosis the two leaflets have a parallel motion, and the A wave is not identifiable in the posterior leaflet.

The third area is at the left ventricular cavity (Figs. 29-7, area *III*, and 29-10) and transects the anterior heart wall, right ventricular cavity, interventricular septum, left ventricular cavity, some part of the chordae tendineae or papillary muscle apparatus, left ventricular posterior wall, and pericardium. The anterior heart wall echoes are usually diffuse and difficult to define. This makes the right ventricular cavity measurement frequently unreliable. Fig. 29-10 identifies the measurements usually made in this view. The left ventricular cavity internal dimension is measured in systole and diastole. The percentage change in cavity dimension is called the fractional shortening and is obtained by subtracting the left ventricular systolic dimension *(LVS)* from the diastolic dimension *(LVD)* and dividing by the diastolic dimension. Normally this should be at least 25%.

The thickness of the interventricular septum and left ventricular posterior wall *(LVPW)* is measured in systole *(S)* and diastole *(D)* (Fig. 29-10). Normally the interventricular septum moves posteriorly with systole, and the left ventricular posterior wall moves anteriorly. Abnormal septal motion, either flat or paradoxical, occurs

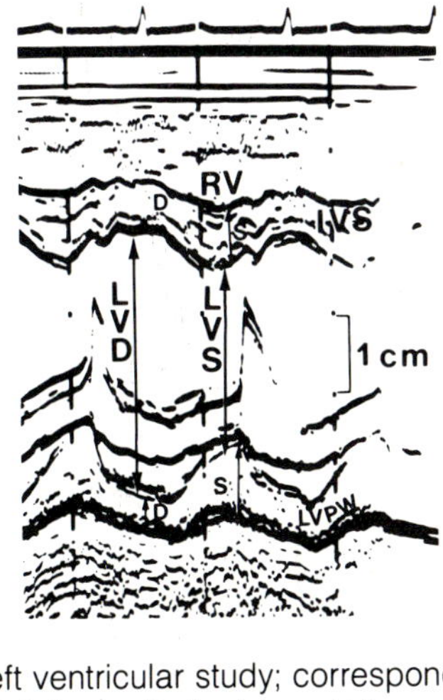

Fig. 29-10. Left ventricular study; corresponds to level III in Fig. 29-7. *LVD*, left ventricular internal dimension in diastole, measured as shown by double arrow; *LVS*, left ventricular internal dimension in systole, measured as shown by double arrow; *LVPW*, left ventricular posterior wall, measured in diastole, *D*, and systole, *S*; *IVS*, interventricular septum, measured in diastole, *D*, and systole, *S*; *RV*, right ventricle.

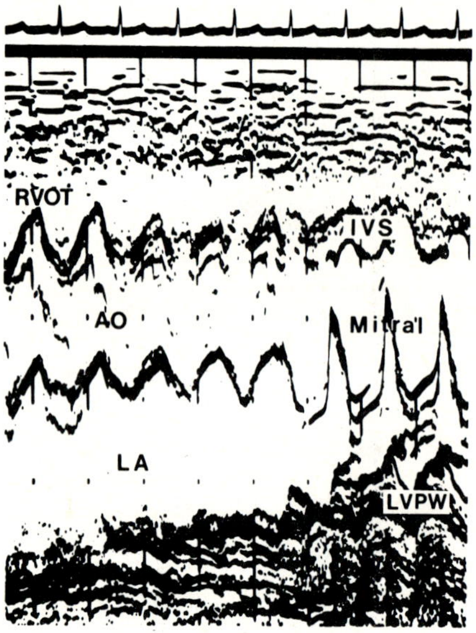

Fig. 29-11. M-mode scan (sweeping from level *I* to *II* to *III* in Fig. 29-7), showing continuity of anterior aortic wall with interventricular septum *(IVS)* and continuity of posterior aortic wall with mitral valve. *LA*, Left atrium; *RVOT*, right ventricular outflow tract; *AO*, aorta, *LVPW*, left ventricular posterior wall.

in some pathologic states such as right ventricular volume overload, myocardial dysfunction, and pulmonary hypertension. When the ventricular muscle function is normal, it thickens with systole.

There is normally minimal space between the epicardium and pericardium so that these structures are seen as a single echo. When a pericardial effusion occurs, there will be a space between these structures, usually more visible posteriorly than anteriorly (Fig. 29-19).

In addition to these three areas being recorded individually, a sweep is made, rotating the transducer through all three levels (Fig. 29-7) and recording this on paper. The transducer will pass through area I, identifying aorta *(AO)* and the left atrium *(LA)*. As the transducer moves into the mitral valve (area *II*) and left ventricle (area *III*), the anterior aortic wall is seen to be continuous with the interventricular septum and the posterior aortic wall with the mitral valve (Fig. 29-11). The normal anterior aorta–interventricular septum relationship is lost in conditions such as tetralogy of Fallot where the aorta overrides the interventricular septum and the interventricular septum *(IVS)* comes in at the level of the aortic valve cusps. The normal posterior aortic continuity with the mitral valve is lost in conditions such as when there is a double-outlet right ventricle and transposition of the great arteries.

The following are the usual measurements made in the three standard views:

A. Aorta—left atrium (Fig. 29-8)
   1. The aortic root dimension *(AO)* is measured at end-diastole (onset of QRS).
   2. The left atrial cavity *(LA)* is represented as the echo-free space behind the posterior wall of the aorta. The echo identifying the left atrial posterior wall at times may be difficult to define. The left atrium is measured at end-systole (at aortic valve closure).

B. Mitral valve (Fig. 29-9)
   1. Amplitude of opening or excursion is measured from point D to E; normally this is greater than 20 mm.
   2. E-F_O slope; or early diastolic closing rate, is normally 70 mm/second or greater.
   3. Mitral valve motion: normally the two leaflets have opposite directions of motion. With mitral stenosis this may become parallel. The A wave should be identifiable in the posterior leaflet; its absence may indicate mitral stenosis.

C. Ventricles (Fig. 29-10)
   1. Right ventricular internal dimension *(RV)* is measured at end-diastole (onset of QRS complex) from anterior heart wall to the right side of the interventricular septum. Because of the difficulty in accurately defining the anterior heart wall, this measurement may be unreliable.
   2. Left ventricular end-diastolic dimension *(LVD)* is the distance between the left side of the interventricular septum and the endocardial surface of the left ventricular posterior wall at end-diastole (onset of QRS).
   3. Left ventricular end-systolic dimension *(LVS)* is the distance between the left side of the interventricular septum and the endocardium of the left ventricular posterior wall at end-systole.
   4. Fractional shortening is normally at least 0.28, or (LVD − LVS) ÷ LVD.
   5. Interventricular septum thickness is measured at end-diastole (D-IVS) and end-systole (S-IVS). Normally systolic thickness is at least 30% greater.
   6. Left ventricular posterior wall thickness is measured at end-systole (S-LVPW) and end-diastole (D-LVPW). Normally systolic thickness is at least 30% greater than end-diastolic.

Table 29-3 lists standard values in normal full-term newborns. Table 29-4 lists standard values in preterm infants without evidence of heart or lung disease.

Systolic time intervals

Systolic time intervals are measurements of the components of electromechanical systole (Fig. 29-12). These consist of the preejection period (PEP) and the ventricular ejection time (VET). Measurement of the systolic time intervals of the left ventricle has been accomplished

Table 29-3. Echocardiographic values in normal newborns based on seven published studies (633 patients, age 1½ hours to 1 month and weighing 1.9 to 4.9 kg)

	Number of studies	Range (mm)
Aortic root diameter	540	7-13.6
Left atrial dimension	540	4-13.5
Interventricular septal thickness (diastole)	440	1.8-4.5
Left ventricular posterior wall (systole)	200	2.5-6
Left ventricular posterior wall (diastole)	440	1.6-4.6
Left ventricular dimension (systole)	211	8-18.6
Left ventricular dimension (diastole)	351	12-24.1
Right ventricular dimension (systole)	200	5.5-11.4
Right ventricular dimension (diastole)	540	6.1-17.7

Modified from Moss, A.J., Gussoni, C.C., and Isabel-Jones, J.: Echocardiography in congenital heart disease, West. J. Med. **124:**102, 1976.

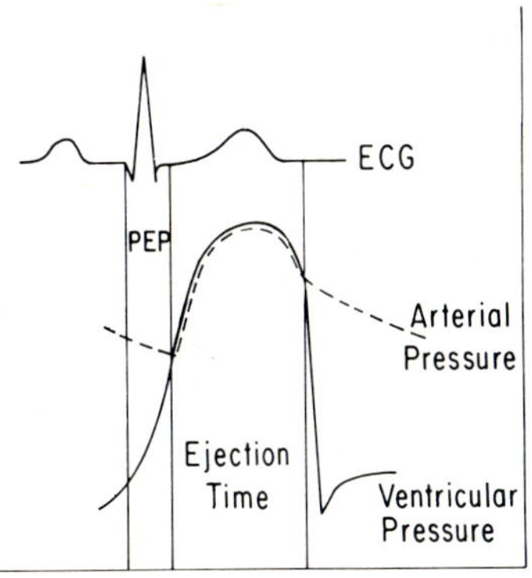

Fig. 29-12. Systolic time intervals. During PEP the ventricle develops sufficient pressure to equal that in great artery (point where ventricular pressure crosses arterial pressure). At this point semilunar valve opens, and ejection phase begins. During ejection time, semilunar valve is open, and flow occurs from ventricle to great artery. When ventricular pressure drops below that in great artery (point where pressures again cross), semilunar valve closes, and ejection phase ends. (See Fig. 29-13.)

Table 29-4. Left atrial dimension (LAD) and left ventricular internal diastolic dimension (LVID) in normal premature infants

	LAD		LVID	
Weight (gm)	Mean (cm)	Normal range (±2 SD)	Mean (cm)	Normal range (±2 SD)
600-900	0.60	0.5-0.7	1.07	0.9-1.2
901-1,200	0.65	0.5-0.8	1.08	0.9-1.3
1,201-1,500	0.69	0.5-0.9	1.18	1.0-1.3
1,501-1,800	0.79	0.6-1.0	1.37	1.2-1.5
1,801-2,200	0.88	0.7-1.1	1.39	1.1-1.6

From Meyer, R.A.: Pediatric echocardiography, Philadelphia, 1977, Lea & Febiger.

noninvasively using the indirect carotid arterial pulse, the ECG, and the phonocardiogram. Abnormal systolic time intervals, measured this way, have been found in left ventricular dysfunction and aortic stenosis.

Echocardiographically it is possible to record both the opening and closing of both the pulmonary and aortic valves. This, combined with the ECG, makes it possible to measure both right- and left-sided heart systolic time intervals. A good correlation exists between the left-sided heart systolic time intervals measured by echo and carotid pulse. Hirschfeld and co-workers have shown a good correlation between echo and pulmonary artery pressure analysis for the right-sided heart systolic time intervals.

The echocardiographic systolic time intervals that are measured include the following (Fig. 29-13):

1. Preejection period (PEP): measured from the onset of the QRS complex to semilunar valve opening
2. Ventricular ejection time (VET): measured from semilunar valve opening to semilunar valve closing
3. PEP/VET: ratio of the preejection period to the ejection time

These intervals are measured for both ventricles. High-quality recordings, where both the opening and the closing of the semilunar valve may be clearly identified, are necessary for the systolic time intervals to be measured by this method. The opening and closing of the aortic valve usually are recorded without difficulty. High-quality echocardiograms, recording both the opening and closing of the pulmonary valve, are less consis-

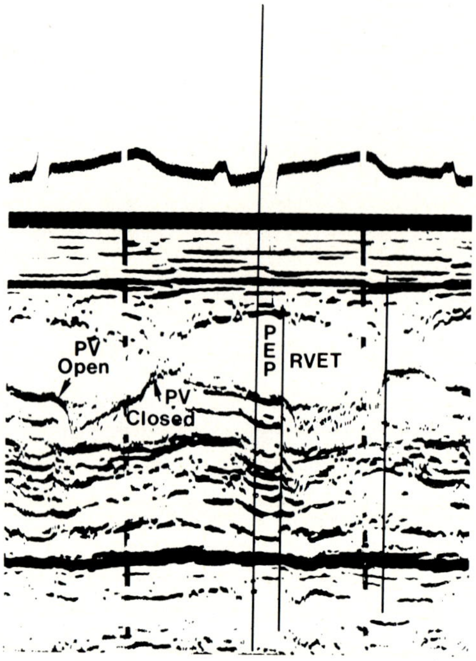

Fig. 29-13. Right-sided heart systolic time intervals. PEP is measured from onset of QRS complex to pulmonary valve opening. Ejection time (RVET) is measured from valve opening to valve closing. This figure is from normal preterm infant. RVPEP = 50 msec, RVET = 220 msec, and RVPEP/RVET = 0.23. (See Fig. 29-12.)

tently recorded. Halliday and co-workers have been able to record both the opening and closing of the posterior pulmonary valve leaflet in 70% to 80% of infants and 50% to 60% of children (Table 29-5).

In normal children the PEP of the right ventricle is shorter than that of the left ventricle, and the ejection time of the right ventricle is longer than that of the left ventricle. In the absence of disorders of contractility the pressure in the great artery determines the systolic time intervals. A rise in the diastolic pressure in the great artery usually results in prolongation of the PEP and thus in an alteration of the ratio between the PEP and VET (PEP/VET).

The relationships have resulted in the application of systolic time–interval measurements to the evaluation of pulmonary artery hypertension and persistent fetal circulation. Increase in the pulmonary vascular resistance has been shown to be associated with alterations in the right ventricular systolic time intervals. Accurate prediction of the level of pulmonary artery pressure using the systolic time intervals has not been possible. However, there has been some correlation between the ratio of the pulmonary to systemic vascular resistance and the ratio of the right-sided heart to left-sided heart systolic time intervals. In some studies a ratio of 0.3 or greater for right ventricle PEP/VET ratio has been associated with a pulmonary artery diastolic pressure of 30 mm Hg or higher.

Table 29-5. Systolic time intervals

Systolic time intervals	All infants	Age <5 days	Age ≥5 days	*p* Value
Preterm infants				
Left ventricle				
Heart rate (beats per minute)	131 ± 14	137 ± 13	143 ± 16	<0.025
PEP (msec)	63 ± 12	66 ± 11	55 ± 9	<0.005
VET (msec)	183 ± 16	187 ± 15	175 ± 15	<0.005
PEP/VET	0.34 ± 0.07	0.36 ± 0.07	0.32 ± 0.06	<0.005
Right ventricle				
PEP (msec)	57 ± 9	60 ± 8	51 ± 7	<0.005
VET (msec)	197 ± 21	201 ± 21	186 ± 18	<0.005
PEP/VET	0.29 ± 0.05	0.30 ± 0.05	0.28 ± 0.04	<0.025
Full-term infants				
Left ventricle				
Heart rate (beats per minute)	132 ± 18	131 ± 19	141 ± 13	<0.01
PEP (msec)	69 ± 10	70 ± 10	65 ± 7	<0.005
VET (msec)	194 ± 17	196 ± 17	185 ± 14	<0.005
PEP/VET	0.36 ± 0.05	0.36 ± 0.05	0.36 ± 0.04	NS
Right ventricle				
PEP (msec)	67 ± 11	69 ± 10	57 ± 8	<0.005
VET (msec)	203 ± 18	203 ± 19	206 ± 19	NS
PEP/VET	0.33 ± 0.06	0.34 ± 0.06	0.28 ± 0.05	≤0.005

From Halliday, H., and others: Pediatrics **62**:317, 1978. Copyright American Academy of Pediatrics 1978.

SPECIFIC APPLICATIONS OF M-MODE ECHOCARDIOGRAPHY IN NEWBORNS

Left-to-right shunts: patent ductus arteriosus

Persistent patency of the ductus arteriosus is common in premature infants (see Chapter 28). Usually clinical problems do not arise as a result of this lesion, and generally the PDA closes at or near term. The large left-to-right shunt that may occur as a result of the low pulmonary vascular resistance in the preterm infant can cause congestive heart failure. RDS thus may be complicated by patency of the ductus arteriosus in the premature infant. Echocardiography has made it possible in most cases to assess noninvasively the magnitude of the left-to-right shunt through the PDA.

The absolute left atrial size determined by echo does not always correlate well with the size of the left-to-right shunt found at cardiac catheterization because of transducer angle and differences in infant size. It has been helpful to relate the left atrial size to that of the aorta, which is positioned in front of the left atrium. Normally these structures have equal dimensions when the aorta is measured at the end of ventricular diastole and the left atrium is measured during ventricular systole (see Fig. 29-8). In normal premature infants the ratio of the left atrial dimension to the aortic dimension has been shown to be 1 or less. In the series, reported by Silverman and co-workers, of premature infants with a clinically significant PDA, requiring surgery, the mean left atrium/aorta ratio was 1.38 ± 0.19. After surgery the ratio returned to normal levels (0.87 ± 0.12).

Figs. 29-14 and 29-15 show an echocardiogram from an infant with RDS with an echocardiogram that showed a left atrium/aorta ratio of 2.4 and increased left ventricular diastolic dimension with normal fractional shortening.

Before treatment (medical or surgical) one must be sure that a ductus-dependent congenital heart lesion such as pulmonary atresia is not present. This is easily accomplished by comprehensive echo studies.

Evaluation of left ventricular function

Ventricular function may be reduced in structural heart disease with congestive heart failure, endocardial fibroelastosis, anomalous origin of the left coronary artery, and cardiomyopathy. In the newborn a cardiomyopathy may occur as part of an infectious process, either intrauterine or postnatally acquired; it may be secondary to generalized hypoxia during the perinatal period and occurs in the infant of a diabetic mother. Echocardiographic demonstration of reduced left ventricular function provides a noninvasive method of diagnosing a cardiomyopathy and may eliminate the need for subjecting an already compromised infant to cardiac catheterization. The echocardiographic finding of reduced left ventricular function before cardiac catheterization contributes important information for directing the study, when the infant's course and clinical findings warrant an invasive procedure.

The following list of echocardiographic abnormalities (Fig. 29-16) indicates reduced left ventricular function.

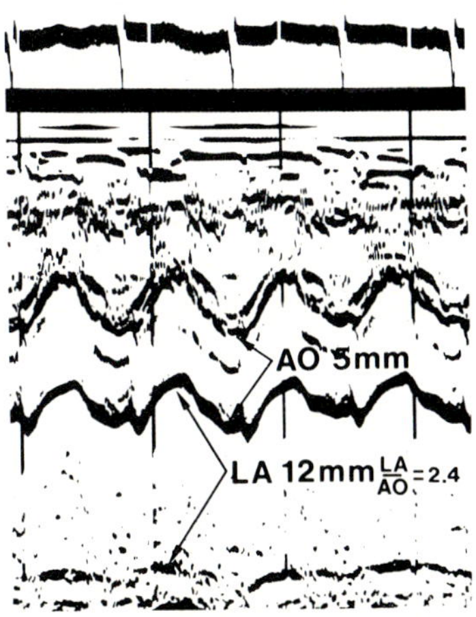

Fig. 29-14. Premature infants weighing 1,200 gm, with RDS and PDA. There is left atrial enlargement (12 mm versus normal of 9 mm). The left atrium/aorta ratio *(LA/AO)* is 2.4 (normal not greater than 1.3).

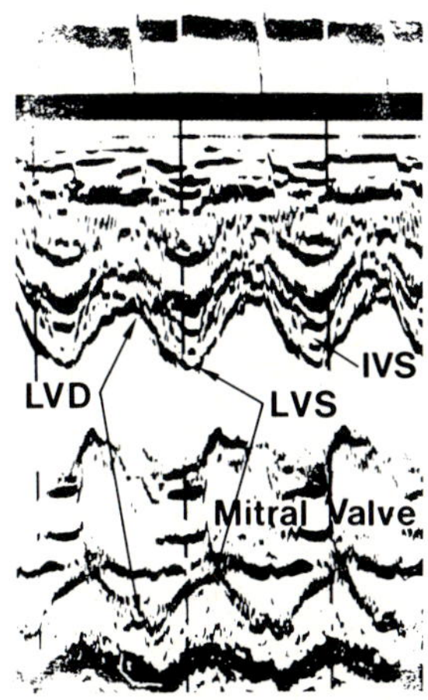

Fig. 29-15. Same infant shown in Fig. 25-13. Left ventricle in diastole *(LVD)* is 19 mm, normal up to 14. Left ventricle in systole *(LVS)* is 12 mm. Fractional shortening is normal (37%) (LVD − LVS) ÷ LVD, or (19 − 12) ÷ 19 = 0.37. Left ventricular enlargement and normal fractional shortening are compatible withh large left-to-right shunt.

1. *Fractional shortening* (below 25%). Fractional shortening is the percentage change of the left ventricular cavity dimension with systole.
2. *Left ventricular enlargement*. The left ventricular diastolic cavity dimension usually will be increased.
3. *Left atrium*. Left atrial enlargement usually will be present.
4. *Mitral valve motion*. The E-F_O slope may be reduced; because of the raised end-diastolic pressure in the left ventricle, there is a reduced rate at which the mitral valve drifts to the closed position following the passive filling phase and prior to atrial systole. This is a nonspecific finding and also is present in mitral stenosis.
5. *Septal motion*. Normally the motion of the interventricular septum is toward the left ventricular posterior wall in systole. Frequently with reduced left ventricular function septal motion is flattened.
6. *Left ventricular wall muscle thickening*. Normally with systole the muscle of the interventricular septum and left ventriclar posterior wall thickens. In a study of 50 normal newborns by St. John Sutton and coworkers the average percentage change in wall thickness was 95% ± 40% for the interventricular septum and about 130% for the left ventricular posterior wall. With left ventricular dysfunction there is reduced muscle thickening with systole.

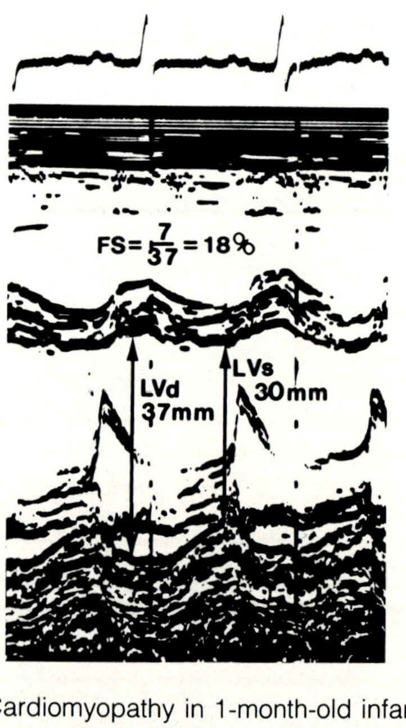

Fig. 29-16. Cardiomyopathy in 1-month-old infant. There is left ventricular enlargement (left ventricle internal dimension, diastole [*LVD*], 37 mm; normal to 25 mm). Fractional shortening *(FS)* is reduced to 18% (normal 25% or greater). *LVS*, left ventricle internal dimension, systole.

TWO-DIMENSIONAL ECHOCARDIOGRAPHY

Two-dimensional cardiac imaging is done primarily with a special type of pulse-echo instrument called a sector scanner. The sector scanners are of two types: (1) mechanical scanners in which the beam is aimed mechanically and (2) electronic scanners (phased array) in which the ultrasonic beam is aimed electronically. In each case the beam of ultrasound is aimed by the instrument in one direction and pulsed. The instrument then waits for and receives all echoes expected to return from the scanning depth chosen. The transducer then is aimed in another direction and the process is repeated. Both types of scanners produce a pie-shaped or sector image.

In pediatric echocardiography most scanning is performed within the first 5 to 6 cm of scanning depth. The original 3.0 MHz sector scanner had very poor near-field resolution, and as a result pediatric imaging was of poor quality. Improved near-field resolution may now be obtained with a higher frequency mechanical sector scanner (i.e., 5.0 or 7.5 MHz) or with phased array instrumentation. Currently, the best images in the premature and newborn infant are obtained with a 7.5 MHz mechanical sector scan. If 7.5 MHz phased array instrumentation becomes available, then near field resolution may be further enhanced.

With two-dimensional echocardiography there are two basic planes used to examine the heart and great vessels: (1) a plane parallel to the major axis of the left ventricle and great vessels and (2) a plane perpendicular to the major axis of the left ventricle and great vessels. To obtain these planes, the transducer is generally applied to four general areas: (1) the parasternal area in the region of the second, third, or fourth left intercostal space, (2) the cardiac apex, (3) the subcostal region, and (4) the susprasternal notch. In each area the transducer can be applied in a long- or short-axis plane, and several different images may be obtained by moving the transducer top-to-bottom or clockwise-to-counterclockwise.

In most systems the video images may be displaced with the apex of the sector either at the top or bottom of the screen, depending on the preference of the echocardiographer. When viewed with the apex at the top, the heart appears "upside down" when viewed from the apical or subcostal region. Although it is still a matter of great debate, most pediatric echocardiographers advocate the display of images with the apex down so that the heart is visualized "right-side up" or in an anatomic position.

The standard two-dimensional echocardiographic examination begins with the parasternal views. These views are best obtained with the patient lying in a left lateral decubitus position with slight cranial elevation. The parasternal long-axis view is obtained by orienting the ultrasound plane along the major axis of the heart from the left hip to right shoulder. In this view the inflow and outflow regions of the left ventricle are well defined (Fig. 29-17). In addition, the superior part of the ventricular septum can be seen contiguous with the anterior aortic root. The outflow portion of the right ventricle is also seen between the chest wall and ventricular septum. From the parasternal long-axis view the transducer can be rotated 90 degrees clockwise to obtain the parasternal short-axis view. The short-axis plane is generally oriented between the right hip and left shoulder. With cranial angulation the right ventricular outflow tract and great vessels are seen. The aortic root appears as a circle with the three aortic valve cusps oriented as an inverted Y. To the left and anterior to the aortic valve, the pulmonary valve and a portion of the main pulmonary artery may be seen. Posterior to the aorta a portion of the left atrium can be visualized. The right ventricle appears sausage shaped as it extends anteriorly from the tricuspid valve and wraps around the aorta to reach the pulmonary artery (Fig. 29-18). With caudal angulation the left ventricular outflow tract is seen bordered anteriorly by the ventricular septum and posteriorly by the anterior mitral leaflet. More caudal angulation reveals the anterolateral and posteromedial papillary muscles.

After examination from the parasternal area the transducer is moved to the cardiac apex and directed cranially to obtain the apical planes. The four-chamber view is obtained with the transducer directed perpendicular to the atrial and ventricular septa and through the plane of the mitral and tricuspid valves (Fig. 29-19). In the four-chamber view the heart is divided into its four chambers by the septa and the mitral and tricuspid valves. The membranous, trabecular, and inlet portions of the ventricular septum are trabecular, and inlet portions of the ventricular septum are well visualized. Although the posterior portion of the atrial septum is well seen, the middle portion is frequently not imaged because the sound beam is parallel to this portion of the atrial septum. Frequently a right and left pulmonary vein can be seen draining into the left atrium. If the transducer is rotated 90 degrees counterclockwise from the apical four-chamber view, the apical long-axis view can be obtained. This view is similar to the parasternal long-axis view; however, more of the cardiac apex and the ascending aorta can be visualized.

The subcostal views are best obtained with the patient supine with the legs flexed at the knees and hips to relax the abdominal muscles. The transducer is oriented initially in the sub-xiphoid region in a sagittal plane. The long axis of the abdominal aorta is visualized in the left paravertebral area. Angling the transducer to the right, the inferior vena cava can be seen. Clockwise and cranial angulation of the transducer reveals the four-chamber view. This view is similar to the apical four-chamber view; however, the atrial and ventricular septa are better visualized. Defects of the atrial septum are especially well seen in this view, as well as the right and left pulmonary veins. Cranial angulation from the four-chamber view reveals the long-axis view of left ventricle, ascending aorta, and portions of the aorta arch and descending aorta (Fig. 29-20). With even more cranial angulation

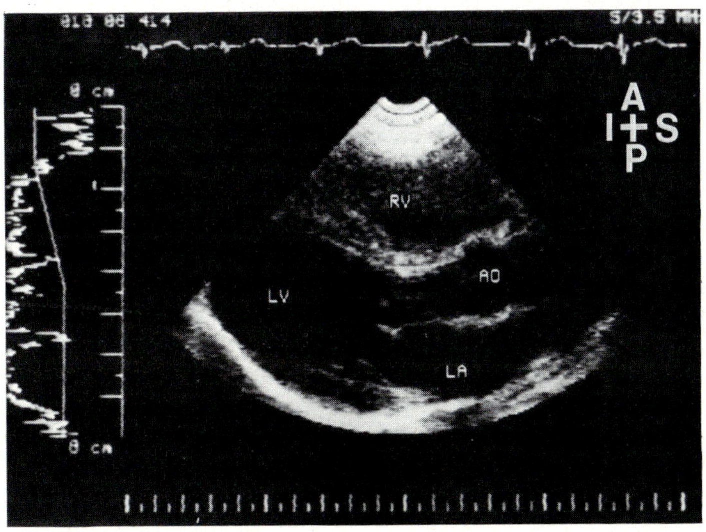

Fig. 29-17. Normal heart. Parasternal long axis view reveals the left atrium *(LA)*, left ventricle *(LV)*, and ascending aorta *(AO)*. The outflow portion of the right ventricle *(RV)* is also well seen with the ventricular septum separating the LV and RV. *A*, Anterior; *I*, inferior; *P*, posterior; *S*, superior.

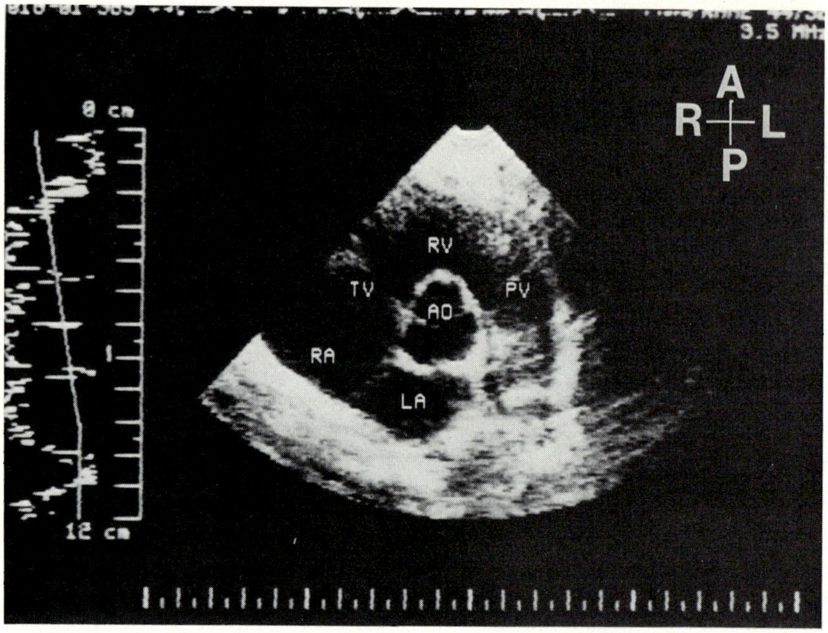

Fig. 29-18. Normal heart, parasternal short axis view. The aortic valve *(AO)* is seen in the center with the pulmonary valve *(PV)* to the left and the tricuspid valve to the right. The right ventricular outflow tract *(RV)* is visualized superior to the *AO* and left atrium *(LA)* inferiorly. The right atrium *(RA)* is also seen rightward and anterior to the left atrium. *A*, Anterior; *L*, left; *P*, posterior; *R*, right.

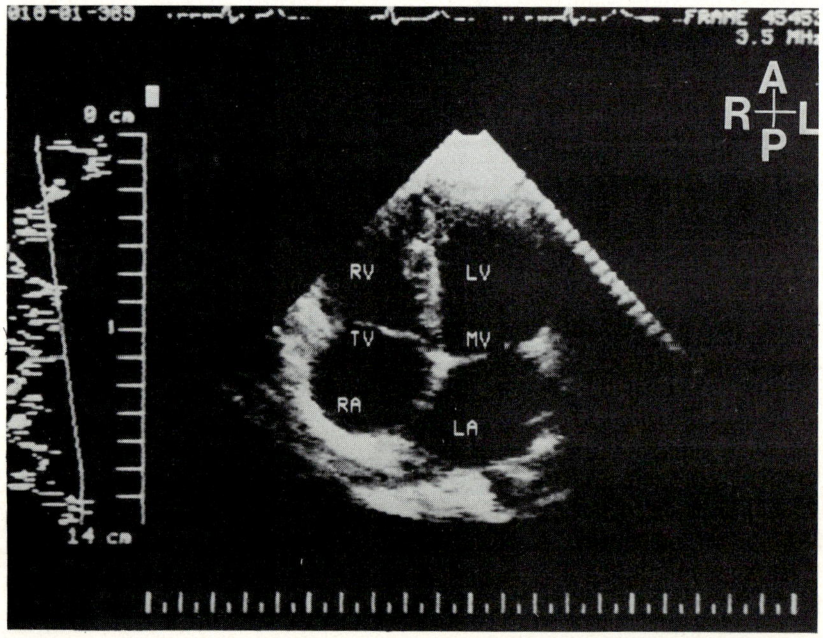

Fig. 29-19. Normal heart. Apical four chamber view: apex is oriented toward the top of the image. The left atrium *(LA)* and left ventricle *(LV)* are divided by the mitral valve *(MV)*. The right atrium *(RA)* and right ventricle *(RV)* are well visualized with tricuspid valve *(TV)* between the RA and RV.

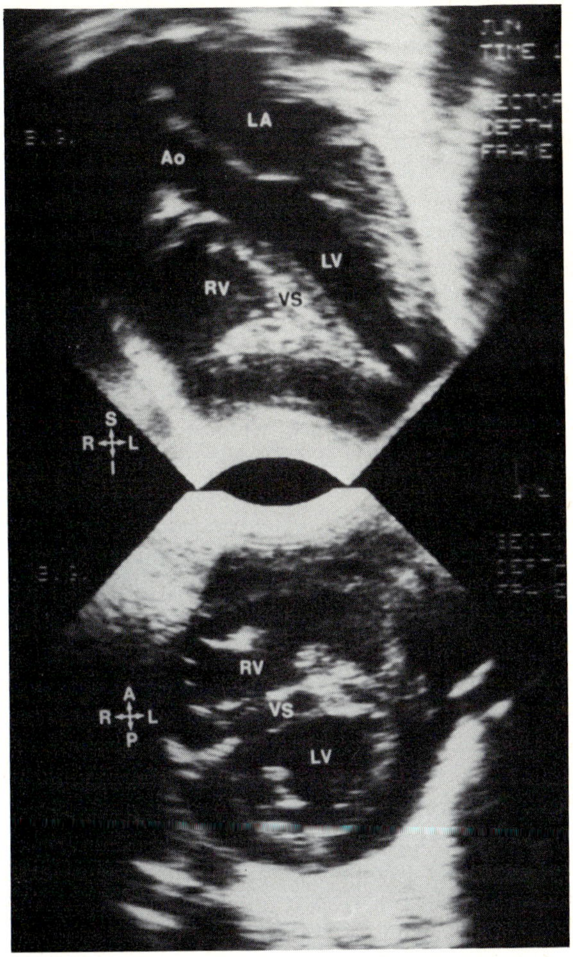

Fig. 29-20. Normal heart. *Top*, Subcostal long axis view of left ventricle *(LV)* reveals the LV outflow tract, ventricular septum *(VS)*, ascending aorta *(AO)*, as well as portions of the right ventricle *(RV)* and left atrium *(LA)*. *Bottom*, Subcostal short axis view shows the left ventricular cavity *(LV)*, muscular ventricular septum *(VS)*, and right ventricle *(RV)*. *A*, Anterior; *I*, inferior; *L*, left; *R*, right; *S*, superior.

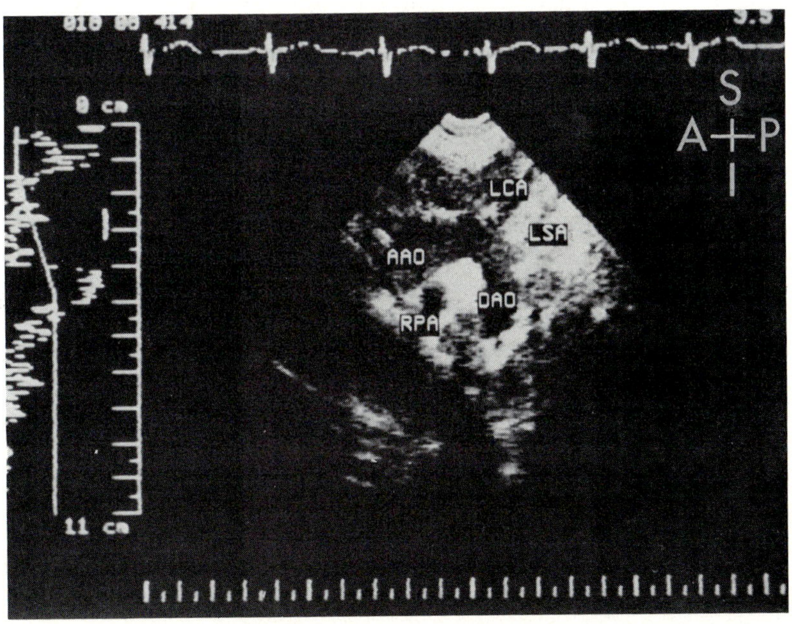

Fig. 29-21. Normal heart: suprasternal long axis view. The ascending aorta *(AAO)* and the branches left carotid artery *(LCA)* and left subclavian artery *(LSA)* are easily identified. Distal to LSA the descending aorta may be identified. The right pulmonary artery *(RPA)* appears in cross-section.

the right ventricular outflow tract and pulmonary arteries can be identified.

To complete the echocardiographic examination, the suprasternal views are obtained. This view is best obtained if the patient's neck is hyperextended with a pillow placed beneath the shoulders. Two basic planes are obtained from the suprasternal notch: the long-axis and short-axis view. To obtain the suprasternal long-axis view, the transducer is positioned with the plane between the right nipple and left scapular tip. In this plane the ascending aorta, aortic arch, and descending aorta are seen in longitudinal section (Fig. 29-21). The right pulmonary artery and innominate vein may also be seen in cross-section. By tilting the transducer to the left, the left pulmonary artery and descending aorta are well visualized, as well as a patent ductus arteriosus if present. The suprasternal short-axis view is obtained by rotating the transducer clockwise into a coronal plane. In this view the ascending aorta appears in cross-section with the right pulmonary artery appearing in transverse section inferior to the aorta. Inferior to the pulmonary artery the left atrium and the pulmonary veins are well delineated (Fig. 29-22).

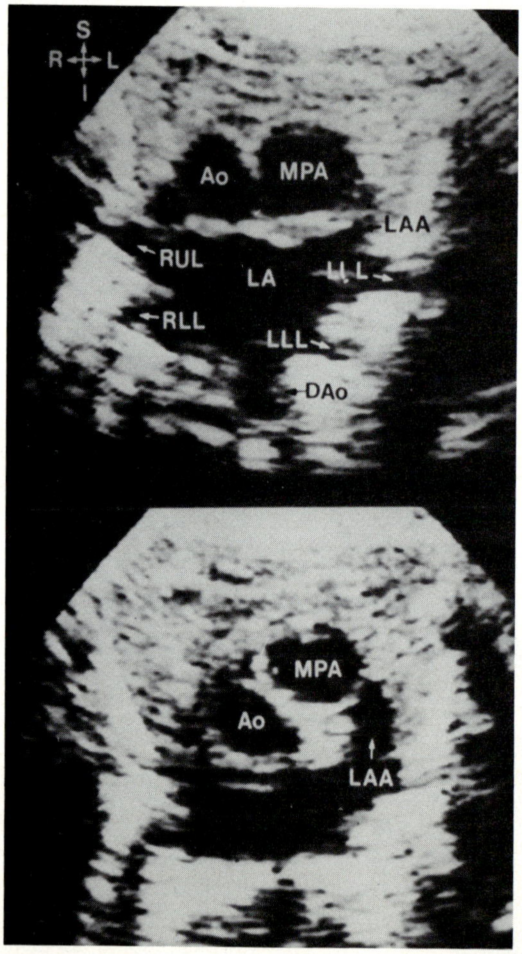

Fig. 29-22. Normal heart. *Top,* Suprasternal short axis view reveals the aortic arch *(AO)* and main pulmonary artery *(MPA)*, in cross-section. Inferiorly the left atrium *(LA)* and the four pulmonary veins are well seen. Inferior to the LA the descending aorta *(DAo)* may be identified. *Bottom,* With slight counterclockwise rotation, the left atrial appendage *(LAA)* may be seen attached to the left superior border of the left atrium. *LUL,* Left upper lobe pulmonary vein, *LLL,* left lower lobe pulmonary vein, *RLL,* right lower lobe pulmonary vein; *RUL,* right upper lobe pulmonary vein.

Doppler echocardiography

A recent addition to two-dimensional echocardiographic systems is the Doppler system. The Doppler system allows the investigator to determine the velocity of red cells within the chambers and across the four valves in the heart. The Doppler principle states that the frequency of a returning ultrasonic signal from a target is proportional to the velocity of that target. The change in frequency, referred to as the *Doppler shift,* is easily converted to velocity. The Doppler freqency shift or velocity then is plotted versus time on a graphic display (Fig. 29-23). By convention, flow toward the transducer is plotted above the baseline and flow away from the transducer appears below the baseline. Blood flow within a vessel or chamber is usually laminar and produces a rather smooth contour on the graphic display. Turbulent or disturbed flow produces a widely dispersed contour referred to as *spectral broadening*. This type of pattern indicates that the red cells at any given point in time during the cardiac cycle have markedly different velocities and are traveling in different directions.

Two types of Doppler systems are used in clinical cardiology: the pulsed and the continuous-wave Doppler. The pulsed Doppler system uses one crystal both for transmitting and for receiving ultrasound waves. Pulsed Doppler is also used in conjunction with a two-dimensional image to localize an area of interrogation. This interrogation in one localized area is referred to as *range-gating*. Range-gating is possible because the speed of ultrasound is constant. Consequently, it is possible to determine when information from a chosen depth will return to the crystal. Analysis of the reflected signal at a given depth is accomplished by analyzing only for that time interval, and information from other depths is disregarded. The continuous-wave Doppler uses two crystals, one that constantly transmits ultrasound waves and another that continuously receives reflected ultrasound waves. As a result, range-gating or flow localization is not possible. The continuous-wave Doppler receives information all along the beam of transmission and does not allow determination of the depth at which a frequency shift occurs.

Color flow mapping by Doppler technique, whereby

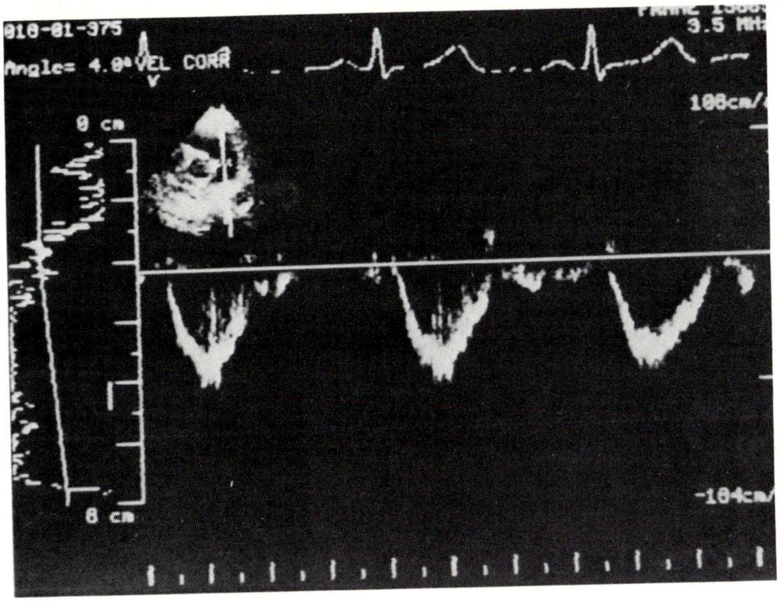

Fig. 29-23. Pulsed Doppler flow tracing obtained from the parasternal short axis with the sample volume in the main pulmonary artery. The flow pattern below the baseline represents normal pulmonary flow in systole. Calibrations for velocity appear on the ordinate and time lines are on the abscissa.

flows moving toward and away from the transducer can be ascribed different colors, represents an important new development. Color Doppler is useful as a qualitative device, by means of which the quantitative Doppler sample volume can be more precisely placed. Color flow mapping also often allows the visualization of septal defects and valvular regurgitations.

In clinical practice pulsed and continuous-wave Dopplers are used in complementary fashion to take advantage of the strength of both systems. The pulsed Doppler has the advantage of permitting Doppler analysis in a precise location guided by the two-dimensional image. However, the pulsed Doppler has velocity measurement limitations that are primarily a function of the transmitting frequency and the depth of sampling. The higher the carrier frequency of the transducer and the greater the depth of sampling, the lower the maximum detectible velocity. In contrast, with the continuous-wave Doppler there is no limitation on the analysis of high velocities. Since it is difficult to differentiate one site of high velocity from another in patients with multiple sites of obstruction, in clinical practice most investigators use the pulsed Doppler to interrogate each valve and the atrial and ventricular septa. If a high velocity is found, the continuous wave instrumentation is used to resolve the velocity.

Current research in Doppler echocardiography revolves around the quantitation of pressure gradients and the determination of pulmonary and systemic blood flow. Hatle and Angelsen first showed that pressure gradients across stenotic valves could be accurately predicted using a modification of the Bernoulli equation. The equation computes the pressure drop across a discrete obstruction, based primarily on an assessment of convective and flow acceleration forces. Although the equation is quite complex, a simplified form appears to be quite accurate in clinical practice:

$$\Delta P = 4V^2$$

where ΔP equals the pressure drop in millimeters of mercury and V equals the peak velocity distal to the valve. Several clinical studies have shown an extremely high correlation between those gradients obtained by cardiac catheterization and those obtained by the Doppler for both pulmonary and aortic stenosis. In many cases the use of the Doppler obviated the need for cardiac catheterization.

The computation of pulmonary and systemic flow is a more recent application of pulsed Doppler technology. The mean velocity across either a semilunar or atrioventricular valve is easily determined by pulsed Doppler. When this valve is multiplied by the cross-sectional area of the valve as determined by two-dimensional echocardiography, the flow across the valve is determined. This technique has been used to estimate pulmonary-to-systemic flow ratios in infants with atrial and ventricular septal defects and has good correlation with cardiac catheterization data obtained by Fick and thermodilution principles. In the next few years this technique should gain widespread clinical acceptance and again eliminate the need for more invasive studies.

Contrast echocardiography

The microbubbles that occur with a small injection of saline into a peripheral vein reflect ultrasound and thus will be recorded by the ultrasound transducer. This technique is used to identify vessels and chambers by the sequential appearance of the saline "contrast" and also to identify intracardiac shunts (Fig. 29-24).

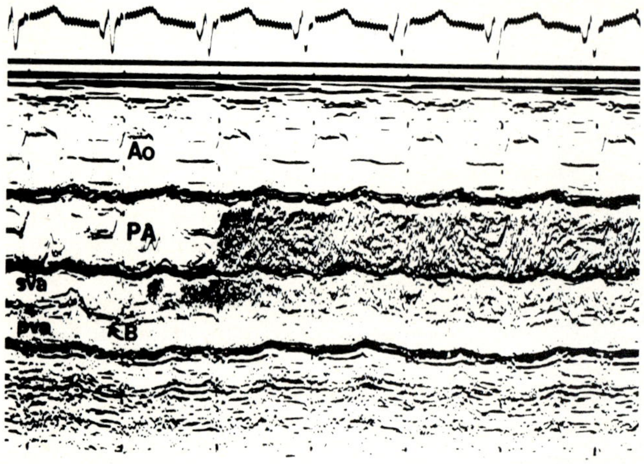

Fig. 29-24. Infant with d-transposition who has undergone interatrial baffle procedure. Five ml saline has been injected into peripheral vein. Saline contrast can be seen appearing in systemic venous atrium *(sva)*, then in pulmonary artery *(PA)*. None appears in pulmonary venous atrium *(pva)* or aorta *(AO)*, indicating there is no leak in baffle *(B)*. (Courtesy Dr. G. Michael Nichols, Boise, Idaho.)

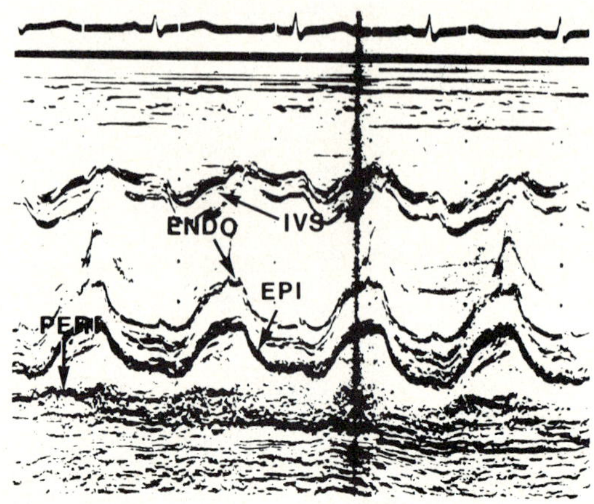

Fig. 29-25. Pericardial effusion in infant. Space between pericardium *(PERI)* and epicardium *(EPI)* contains effusion, *ENDO*, Endocardium; *IVS*, interventricular septum.

Pericardial effusion

Echocardiography has become the most sensitive and reliable method for detecting pericardial effusion. The pericardium produces the brightest echo of the cardiac structures. Normally it is adherent to the epicardium, and no space appears between the two structures. When there is fluid in the pericardial sac, an echo-free space appears between the pericardium and epicardium (Fig. 29-25). Pericardial effusion may occur in the newborn with heart failure and septic pericarditis. Pneumopericardium may occur when there is pneumothorax and also will be seen as an echo-free space between the pericardium and epicardium.

Arterial blood gases and pH

Estimation of arterial P_{CO_2} and pH aids in the quantitative assessment of the seriousness of the condition of infants suspected of having heart disease. If the infant's heel is warm and blood is free flowing, a heel prick provides a worthwhile estimate of arterial P_{CO_2} and pH. Measurement of P_{O_2} from capillary blood is less accurate. In the evaluation of the effect of 100% O_2 breathing on P_{O_2} it is necessary to sample arterial blood (see hyperoxia test, Chapter 28). In the newborn period this usually can be obtained from the umbilical artery, but in older infants the right brachial artery is preferable. Arterial blood collected from anywhere distal to the ductus arteriosus may be "contaminated" by right-to-left ductal shunting and consequently does not accurately reflect pulmonary function. To obtain truly "arterial" blood, it is necessary to sample a pulmonary vein, since in many cyanotic babies the right-to-left shunt is at the atrial level.

Certain deductions may be made from a consideration of the arterial P_{CO_2} and P_{O_2} while the infant is breathing room air and from the P_{O_2} while the infant is breathing 100% O_2 (Table 29-6). Diffusion problems may be ignored, since they do not exist in infants with heart disease. Measurement of transcutaneous P_{O_2} (TcP_{O_2}) has proved a valuable noninvasive alternative to arterial blood sampling in neonates with suspected cyanotic heart disease. Since the infant lies undisturbed with the TcP_{O_2} electrode on the abdominal skin, crying is not a problem; the measurement, although slightly less accurate than Pa_{O_2}, is highly reliable. We have found the combination of TcP_{O_2}, and heelstick pH and P_{CO_2} very useful.

It is commonly stated that, if an infant becomes pink with oxygen administration the hypoxemia is pulmonary in origin, whereas if he or she remains blue, it is cardiac (that is, the problem is a right-to-left shunt). Unfortunately this is an oversimplification. First, there are large intrapulmonary and foramen ovale right-to-left shunts in many neonates with lung disease, who therefore fail to achieve high arterial P_{O_2} with 100% O_2 (especially in RDS). Second, an infant with an isolated PDA may be cyanotic from heart failure, alveolar transudate, and obstructed small air passages. The infant will become pink in 100% O_2 because the mechanism of hypoxemia is alveolar hypoventilation; yet heart disease (PDA) is the problem. Finally, if an infant with transposition is very cyanotic in room air but becomes less cyanotic in 100% O_2, the explanation is not that the cause of the cyanosis is pulmonary but that 100% inspired O_2 has lowered the pulmonary vascular resistance, allowing better mixing through an existing patent ductus. The infant may clinically appear to become pink, but the arterial P_{O_2} will never approach 150 mm Hg. Blood gases and the re-

Table 29-6. Blood gases in the three common mechanisms for arterial unsaturation*

Mechanism	Pa_{O_2} room air (mm Hg)	Pa_{CO_2} room air (mm Hg)	Pa_{O_2} 100% O_2 (mm Hg)
Alveolar hypoventilation	Decreased (<60)	Increased (>50)	Normal (>300)
Right-to-left shunt	Decreased (<60)	Normal† (35 to 45)	Decreased (<300)‡
Ventilation/perfusion unevenness	Decreased (<60)	Normal† (35 to 45)	Normal (>300)

*Pa_{O_2} (room air) provides an estimate of the severity of the problem. An increased Pa_{CO_2} implies alveolar hypoventilation, and failure of the Pa_{O_2} to increase significantly with 100% O_2 implies right-to-left shunting as the problem.
†Rises slowly with prolonged right-to-left shunting or ventilation/perfusion unevenness.
‡With total anomalous pulmonary venous return, neonates with very high pulmonary blood flow may occasionally exceed 300 mm Hg with 100% O_2 breathing.

sponse to 100% O_2 breathing therefore only suggest the disordered pathophysiologic mechanism and the seriousness of the problem rather than identify the problem as pulmonary or cardiac.

Measurement of the arterial or capillary pH is also of value as an estimate of the severity of the problem. Correction of severe acidosis may be partially achieved by the use of sodium bicarbonate. It should be remembered, however, that the use of sodium bicarbonate adds to the total body stores of sodium and of carbon dioxide. Temporary and partial correction of acidosis, however, is often indicated as a prelude to cardiac catheterization and surgery; sodium bicarbonate, 2 to 6 mEq/kg, should be administered over a 2- to 5-minute period into as large a venous pool as possible. Frequently we have used this method of pH adjustment at the beginning of a cardiac catheterization; the usual indication is a sinus bradycardia in a dying infant, and pH is usually 7.1 or lower.

Other laboratory tests

Hypoglycemia

The initial evaluation should include a screening test for hypoglycemia (Dextrostix); when the Dextrostix is low, true blood glucose should be determined. Hypoglycemia may simulate structural congenital heart disease very closely, with cardiomegaly and cyanosis. Hypoglycemia frequently also complicates serious neonatal heart disease, especially the hypoplastic left-heart syndrome. It also is associated with PFC. The hypoglycemia should be treated with intravenous glucose while investigation and treatment of the underlying heart disease are proceeding.

Serum electrolytes

Serum sodium, potassium, and chloride levels should be measured both because electrolyte abnormalities can occur in the infant with serious neonatal cardiovascular disease and because adrenal insufficiency may closely mimic heart disease. Sommerville and colleagues reported on three neonates and one 6-week-old baby (all male) with congenital adrenal *insufficiency* in whom cyanosis and cardiac arrhythmias simulated heart disease.

Methemoglobinemia

Congenital or acquired methemoglobinemia may closely simulate cyanotic congenital heart disease. The infant appears a peculiar lavender or slate blue, and blood from a heel prick appears chocolate colored. Blood from an infant with methemoglobinemia fails to become pink when placed on a glass slide and exposed to room air. The diagnosis can be confirmed by spectroscopy (a characteristic absorption peak at 634 mμ) and by the rapid response to intravenous methylene blue (1 to 2 mg/kg). For long-term medication ascorbic acid (300 to 500 mg/day) administered orally may be preferable but is sometimes less completely effective.

Vectorcardiography

The study of vectorcardiography (VCG) has contributed enormously to our understanding of the scalar ECG (normal 12- or 13-lead ECG). The scalar ECG depicts in two dimensions what is actually a three-dimensional event—the P loop, followed by the QRS and T loops. The small amount of additional information gained from the VCG does not warrant its routine use in the diagnosis of the neonate suspected of having serious heart disease.

CYANOSIS OF THE NEWBORN*

A blue or dusky hue in the newborn frequently is brought to the physician's attention by an experienced nurse. Since the causes may vary from trivial to life threatening, rapid evaluation is essential; those newborns who have persistent central cyanosis usually deteriorate rapidly.

*Modified from Lees, M. H.: Cyanosis of the newborn infant, J. Pediatr. 77:484, 1970.

Recognition of cyanosis

Clinical cyanosis is chiefly dependent on the *absolute* concentration of reduced hemoglobin in the blood rather than on the ratio of reduced hemoglobin to oxygenated hemoglobin. Central cyanosis implies significant arterial unsaturation, whereas "peripheral" cyanosis alone implies normal arterial saturation. In the latter, cyanosis is visible only in the skin of the extremities where a wide arteriovenous oxygen difference leads to a "capillary" reduced hemoglobin content of greater than 4 to 6 gm/dl of blood. It is sometimes stated that it is necessary to have 5 gm of reduced hemoglobin in *arterial* blood before central cyanosis is detectable visibly; clinical experience indicates that this provides a very coarse basis for detection of arterial unsaturation. Were this the case, an infant with a total hemoglobin content of 15 gm/dl of blood would be visibly cyanotic only at an arterial saturation of 67% or less, whereas central cyanosis is detectable by inspection of the tongue and mucous membranes at arterial saturations of 75% to 88% in the presence of about 3 gm of reduced hemoglobin in arterial blood (Fig. 29-26).

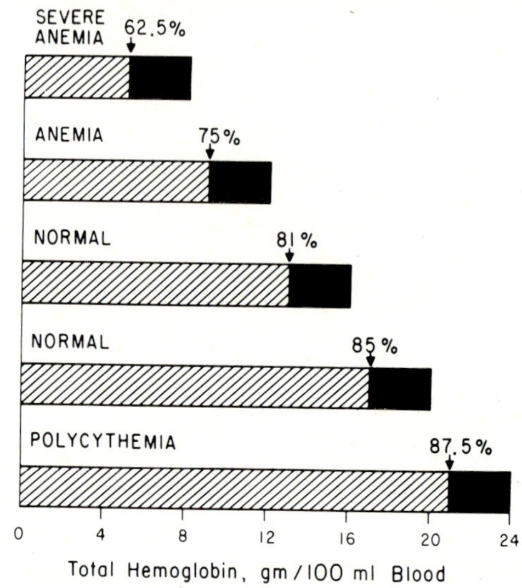

Fig. 29-26. The percentage arterial saturation of blood (diagonally lined portion of each column) when cyanosis will be detected at different total hemoglobin concentrations in the presence of 3 gm/dl of reduced hemoglobin. Central cyanosis is detectable at higher arterial saturations when the total hemoglobin concentration is high. With severe anemia, as for example 8 gm/dl of hemoglobin, central cyanosis may not be apparent until arterial saturation falls to nearly 62%.

Central versus peripheral cyanosis

Infants suspected of being cyanotic are best inspected when they are quiet or sleeping in a thermoneutral environment under a white light, preferably daylight. Central cyanosis is defined as cyanosis of the tongue, mucous membranes, and peripheral skin in the presence of 3 gm or more of reduced hemoglobin in arterial blood. It may be physiologic or pathologic. Peripheral cyanosis is defined as blue discoloration or duskiness confined to the skin of the extremities; it too may be physiologic or pathologic, but the arterial blood will be normally saturated (that is, greater than 94%). There are intermediate conditions in which arterial saturation may be in the range of 90% (for example, 2 gm of reduced hemoglobin out of a total of 20 gm of hemoglobin), and the tongue may appear pink and the extremities cyanotic. Such a baby clinically has peripheral cyanosis as a result of a central disturbance. The clinical distinction of central from peripheral therefore is not always absolute, and elucidation frequently requires the measurement of arterial oxygen saturation or oxygen tension (Pa_{O_2}).

Clinical confirmation that cyanosis of extremities is peripheral in origin often may be obtained by immersing the baby's foot in a pan of 100° F water for 5 minutes; vasodilatation will occur, and the foot will become pink. Reflex vasodilation also may occur in the other foot. Significant arterial unsaturation (central cyanosis) should be considered to be present if the Pa_{O_2} is below 60 mm Hg at 24 hours of age or if the arterial oxygen saturation is below 94%. This does not imply that a Pa_{O_2} of 60 mm Hg or less necessarily represents a pathologic state, but it does mean that the infant either has alveolar hypoventilation or has an alveolar-arterial oxygen difference of about 40 mm Hg.

Peripheral cyanosis

Peripheral cyanosis is common in the neonate and may persist for hours to weeks. It usually is ascribed to "vasomotor instability" and may come and go in an unpredictable fashion. In some instances peripheral cyanosis is clearly caused by cold environment, a high total hemoglobin content, or local venous obstruction (for example, cord around the neck). In other instances the cause is obscure. The most bizarre expression is that of the "harlequin" infant, in whom one quadrant or one side of the body may be cyanotic while the rest is pink; the hands and feet feel warm despite their appearance. Peripheral cyanosis with cold extremities in a relatively warm environment suggests the possibility of peripheral vasoconstriction caused by shock or heart failure. "Differential" cyanosis, that is, pink upper half and blue lower half of the body or vice versa, always in indicative of serious heart disease.

Physiologic central cyanosis

An arterial saturation of less than 94% usually is regarded as abnormal in the awake healthy adult or older child breathing atmospheric air at sea level. However, the critical level of saturation for a newborn depends on the postnatal age, the proportion of adult to fetal hemoglobin, and whether he is crying when the blood sample is taken. Normal newborns have a PaO_2 of around 50 mm Hg by 5 to 10 minutes of postnatal life. The great majority of infants therefore would not be expected to manifest physiologic central cyanosis later than 20 minutes after birth, and many would have a pink tongue and mucous membranes before 10 minutes. Occasionally, a full-term infant who appears normal by standard criteria may require a longer time to achieve a PaO_2 of 60 mm Hg.

The ratio of fetal to adult hemoglobin varies from infant to infant, and the proportions of each hemoglobin affect the oxygen saturation resulting at any given PaO_2 (Chapter 28). Thus, if a baby with a pH of 7.4 and a temperature of 37° C has mostly adult hemoglobin, central cyanosis (arterial saturation 75% to 85%) will be observed at a PaO_2 of 42 to 53 mm Hg, whereas if the baby has mostly fetal hemoglobin, central cyanosis will be observed at a PaO_2 of 32 to 42 mm Hg. *Thus the newborn with a high proportion of fetal hemoglobin may have a serious reduction in oxygen tension before central cyanosis is clinically apparent.* Therefore measurement of oxygen tension is considerably more discriminatory than measurement of oxygen saturation (Fig. 29-27).

The effect of crying on the arterial saturation of the newborn must be considered. Infants age 1½ hours to 3 days have variable responses: 66% have a decrease in oxygen saturation, 27% an increase, and 6.8% no change. Older infants between 4 to 9 days of age respond differently: 21% have a decrease in saturation, 59% an increase, and 22.4% no change. Right-to-left shunting through the ductus arteriosus or foramen ovale is the most likely explanation.

Pathologic mechanisms of central cyanosis

When a resting or sleeping newborn has central cyanosis that persists longer than 20 minutes after birth, an explanation is required. Categories of disease that should be considered are (1) congenital heart disease with right-to-left shunting and diminished pulmonary blood flow, (2) congenital heart disease with right-to-left shunting and increased pulmonary blood flow, (3) congenital heart disease with alveolar hypoventilation secondary to heart failure, (4) primary lung disease, (5) mechanical interference with lung function, (6) PFC syndrome (primary or secondary), (7) central nervous system disease, (8) methemoglobinemia, (9) hypoglycemia, (10) a high hemoglobin level, (11) shock and sepsis, and (12) miscellaneous conditions. There are five mechanisms whereby arterial unsaturation may occur in a patient who is breathing atmospheric air and is not at high altitude: (1) alveolar hypoventilation, (2) diffusion impairment, (3) right-to-left shunting, (4) ventilation/perfusion unevenness, and (5) inadequate transport of oxygen by hemoglobin.

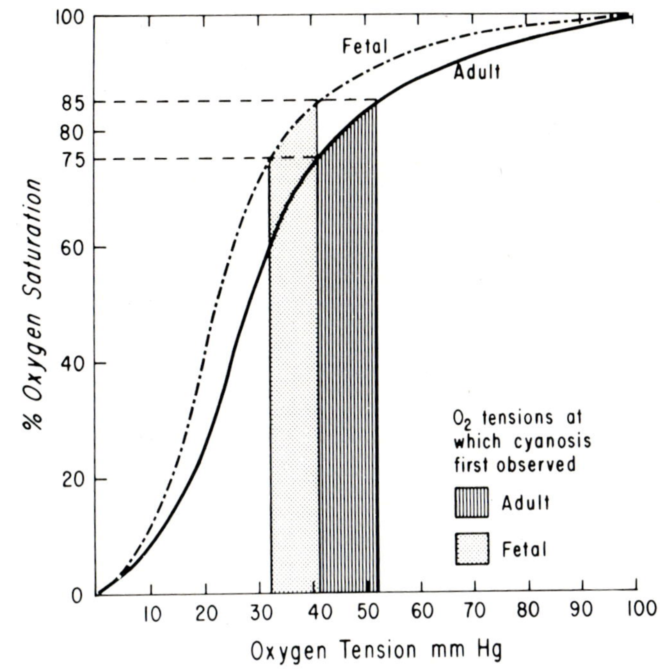

Fig. 29-27. Fetal and adult hemoglobin–O_2 dissociation curves. Note that infant with high proportion of fetal hemoglobin will have a very low PaO_2 (33 to 42 mm Hg) before cyanosis is observed.

A diagnostic approach to central cyanosis

Once it is decided that an infant has central cyanosis (by examination of the tongue, $TcPO_2$, ear oximeter, or direct measurement of arterial PO_2 or O_2 saturation), it is necessary to determine the cause, since the responsible disease process is rarely self-limited. The examination of the cyanotic neonate should proceed along the lines discussed earlier in this chapter, with particular emphasis on the respiratory pattern, spontaneous movement, response to 100% O_2 breathing, arterial pH, PO_2, and PCO_2, chest roentgenogram, and ECG. Use of heel-prick blood to screen for hypoglycemia (Dextrostix) and methemoglobinemia (failure of blood to become pink in air) takes but a moment and rules out two immediately correctable causes of central cyanosis. Measurement of serum electrolytes may reveal hyperkalemia, raising the possibility of adrenal insufficiency or unsuspected sodium or chloride abnormality. If heart disease appears likely, M-mode, two-dimensional, and Doppler echocardiography are very helpful.

Certain clinical patterns may suggest one of the twelve groups of conditions detailed below. However, the clinical signs are capricious, and infants sometimes do not manifest typical findings. The following associations of clinical signs may be helpful (see Table 29-7); however, cardiac catheterization and angiocardiography are sometimes required for the precise anatomic diagnosis of congenital heart disease. An aggressive diagnostic approach

Table 29-7. Elucidation for cause of cyanosis from clinical signs and simple laboratory tests*

Category and pathophysiology	Common underlying disorder	Activity and respiratory pattern	100% O_2 breathing
1. Congenital heart disease Right-to-left shunt; decreased pulmonary blood flow	Tetralogy of Fallot; pulmonary atresia; tricuspid atresia; extreme pulmonary stenosis; Ebstein's anomaly	Respirations 20-50/min; increased tidal volume; total ventilation and alveolar ventilation both increased	No response because pulmonary capillary blood is almost completely saturated
2. Congenital heart disease Right-to-left shunt; increased pulmonary blood flow	Transposition; left-sided heart hypoplasia; preductal coarctation; TAPVR;* truncus arteriosus; very large VSD; AV canal	Respirations 30-60/min; tidal volume normal; total ventilation and alveolar ventilation normal or moderately increased	$Po_2 < 300$ mm Hg. With TAPVR may occasionally exceed 300 mm Hg
3. Congenital heart disease Severe heart failure; shunt or no shunt; alveolar hypoventilation	All in category 2; isolated PDA: isolated VSD; severe aortic stenosis; postductal coarctation; paroxysmal atrial tachycardia	Flaccid with severe heart failure; cyanosis moderate; respirations 40-120/min with rales and rhonchi; decreased tidal volume; total ventilation usually normal with greatly reduced alveolar ventilation, i.e., increased dead space/tidal volume	Usually good response because increasing alveolar oxygen tension to 650 mm Hg overcomes pulmonary capillary unsaturation secondary to alveolar hypoventilation
4. Primary lung disease Alveolar hypoventilation; intrapulmonary right-to-left shunt; $\dot{V}/\dot{Q}$ unevenness; diffusion barrier (RDS)	Atelectasis; atypical RDS; aspiration syndrome; pulmonary hemorrhage; pneumonia; Wilson-Mikity syndrome; lymphangiectasia; pulmonary agenesis; adenomatoid malformation; bronchopulmonary dysplasia	Respirations 30-120/min; typically there is distress, with flaring of alae nasi, grunting, and intercostal and sternal retraction; with severe pathology, tidal volume and alveolar ventilation are greatly decreased; decreased compliance increases work of breathing	Response unpredictable; lack of response indicates intrapulmonary or intracardiac right-to-left shunting as a major factor
5. Mechanical interference with lung function Alveolar hypoventilation	Mucous plugs; lobar emphysema; diaphragmatic hernia; pneumothorax; chylothorax; abnormal thoracic cage; vascular ring; tracheoesophageal fistula; bronchogenic cyst; choanal atresia; Pierre Robin syndrome; mediastinal masses	May closely mimic primary lung disease if lung tissue is compressed; when the airway is partially obstructed, stridor and intercostal retractions are prominent; unreliability of signs underscores need for x-ray film in every infant with cyanosis	Usually good response because alveolar hypoventilation is often the major mechanism of cyanosis
6. Pulmonary hypertension PFC syndrome; gross $\dot{V}/\dot{Q}$ unevenness; intrapulmonary right-to-left shunt; ductal right-to-left shunt	Cause often undetermined; consider asphyxia, meconium aspiration pneumonia	Hyperventilation with increased tidal volume and rate is usual; much of the ventilation is wasted, since it is to underperfused or unperfused alveoli	Variable response depending on the degree of $\dot{V}/\dot{Q}$ unevenness (good response) and intrapulmonary right-to-left shunt (no response); PFC syndrome may respond to oxygen, to intravenous tolazoline, or to induced alkalosis
7. Central nervous system disease Alveolar hypoventilation	Intracerebral hemorrhage; subdural hemorrhage; gross intracranial malformation; meningitis or encephalitis; primary seizure disorder	Apneic spells alternating with periods of normal breathing, or there may be continuous hypoventilation with small tidal volume or bradypnea or both; infant is often apathetic and unresponsive; seizures common	Good response, provided tidal volume is appreciably greater than anatomic dead space and frequency of breathing is not too slow

*Categories 1, 2, 3 and 6 usually require echocardiography and sometimes catheterization and angiography for definitive anatomic diagnosis.
†*TAPVR*, Total anomalous pulmonary venous return; *RVH*, right ventricular hypertrophy; *RVSTI*, right ventricle systolic time interval.
‡Heart may be normal in size in certain varieties of TAPVR.

Heel-prick blood exposed to air	Dextrostix, hematocrit	Arterial pH, arterial P_{CO_2}	Chest x-ray film	ECG and echocardiogram
Dark; becomes pink in air	No abnormality	pH normal unless hypoxemia is extreme; Pa_{CO_2} normal or low	Decreased pulmonary vascular markings; heart may be large or normal	Both usually abnormal; echo usually provides anatomic diagnosis
Dark; becomes pink in air	Hypoglycemia may be present especially with hypoplastic left-heart syndrome	pH normal unless hypoxemia is extreme; Pa_{CO_2} normal	Increased pulmonary vascular markings; heart may be of normal size at first but after a few days is almost always enlarged‡	Both usually abnormal; echo usually provides anatomic diagnosis
Dark; becomes pink in air	Hypoglycemia is frequent, especially with hypoplastic left-heart syndrome	Acidosis and elevated Pa_{CO_2} reflect increasing airway obstruction and alveolar hypoventilation	Enlarged heart; increased vascular markings; often pneumonia	Both usually abnormal; echo usually provides anatomic diagnosis
Dark; becomes pink in air	May be hypoglycemia if glycogen reserves are becoming depleted	Acidosis and elevated Pa_{CO_2} characterize most of the conditions and indicate severity	Each condition has a rather characteristic x-ray appearance, but exceptions occur	ECG normal or RVH*; echo usually normal but may show abnormal RVSTI*
Dark; becomes pink in air	Normal	Elevated Pa_{CO_2} that may or may not be compensated; in severe instances acidosis is present	Characteristic x-ray film in most instances; contrast visualization studies may be needed	ECG normal or RVH; echo usually normal but may show abnormal RVSTI
Dark; becomes pink in air	Normal Polycythemia may be associated with PFC syndrome	May have elevated Pa_{CO_2} due to large arterial-alveolar CO_2 difference caused by the presence of overventilated but underperfused areas; pH depressed	Generally have "snowstorm" or "ground-glass" appearance; heart usually normal in size; x-ray film may be normal with PFC syndrome in absence of meconium aspiration or pneumonia	ECG normal or RVH; echo usually shows abnormal RVSTI and excludes structural congenital heart disease
Dark; becomes pink in air	Normal	Elevated Pa_{CO_2}; combined respiratory and metabolic acidosis is usual	Normal or may show pneumonia	Both usually normal

Continued.

Table 29-7. Elucidation for cause of cyanosis from clinical signs and simple laboratory tests—cont'd

Category and pathophysiology	Common underlying disorder	Activity and respiratory pattern	100% O_2 breathing
8. Methemoglobinemia Reduced oxygen-carrying capacity of blood because of abnormal hemoglobin	Specific enzyme deficiency; abnormal hemoglobin	Infants, although lavender blue. show little distress until over 50% of hemoglobin is methemoglobin; in severe cases tachypnea and hyperventilation closely mimic heart disease	No response
9. Hypoglycemia Probably right-to-left shunting through foramen ovale; hypoventilation	Infant of diabetic mother; small for date baby; idiopathic heart failure, especially from hypoplastic left-heart syndrome	May be apathetic and limp; jitteriness or seizures common; infant may have moderate tachypnea or repetitive apneic spells	Good response to hypoventilation component of cyanosis; variable response to right-to-left shunt
10. High hemoglobin content Increased absolute amount of reduced hemoglobin; arterial blood normally saturated, but increased viscosity and stagnant capillary flow may produce apparent central cyanosis	Maternofetal transfusion; twin-to-twin transfusion; high hematocrit value plus unusually large "placental transfusion"	Usually normal behavior and respirations, but myoclonic jerking, moderate tachypnea, or apneic spells have been reported	Good response because of almost total saturation of hemoglobin when alveolar Po_2 is raised to 650 mm Hg
11. Shock and sepsis Alveolar hypoventilation; $\dot{V}/\dot{Q}$ unevenness	Blood loss; septic shock; septicemia; myocarditis; adrenal insufficiency	Apathetic, hypotonic, and underresponsive to stimuli; respirations rapid and shallow or frequent apneic spells (hypoventilation); low pulmonary artery pressure and blood flow ($\dot{V}/\dot{Q}$ unevenness)	Good response unless hypoventilation or $\dot{V}/\dot{Q}$ disturbance or both are extreme

is justified, since in the majority of instances treatment is available.

Miscellaneous conditions producing generalized cyanosis or differential cyanosis

Cyanosis occasionally may be caused by alveolar hypoventilation secondary to respiratory depression from drugs given to the mother during labor or to the newborn. Transient tachypnea of the newborn occasionally may cause mild cyanosis in addition to extreme tachypnea (see Chapter 28). Neuromuscular disorders, such as Werdnig-Hoffmann disease or incoordination of swallowing with aspiration, may be present with cyanosis. Anomalous systemic venous return to the left atrium produces cyanosis; classically there are no other symptoms. A pulmonary arteriovenous fistula may be responsible for marked arterial unsaturation; such fistulas are frequently multiple and are usually visible on the chest roentgenogram. A bruit is often but not always present.

Preductal coarctation of the aorta with the right ventricle supplying the descending aorta with venous blood via a PDA is the most common cause of cyanosis restricted to the lower half of the body. The less frequent opposite pattern, that is, cyanosis restricted to the upper half of the body, usually occurs in association with d-transposition, a PDA, and pulmonary hypertension.

LUNG DISEASE VERSUS HEART DISEASE

The problem of differentiating lung and heart disease frequently occurs in the neonatal period. Usually the distinction can be made by echocardiography—particularly useful is Doppler interrogation of the heart and blood vessels for directional flow abnormalities and blood-flow velocities. Contrast echocardiography using injections of blood or flush solution containing microbubbles provides a means of seeing PDA, or right-to-left shunts by simultaneous sector scanning. The improvements in echocardiography technology over the past 5 years, including the use of color flow Doppler mapping, have made the need for invasive studies uncommon; however, in occasional instances heart catheterization and angiography are needed.

Persistence of the fetal circulation

The term *persistence of fetal circulation* (PFC syndrome) is applied to the combination of pulmonary hypertension, right-to-left shunting (largely at the foramen ovale but also the ductus arteriosus), and a structurally

Heel-prick blood exposed to air	Dextrostix, hematocrit	Arterial pH, arterial Pco_2	Chest x-ray film	ECG and echocardiogram
Chocolate-colored blood; does not become pink in air or oxygen	Normal	Normal pH; $Paco_2$ may be slightly decreased if infant hyperventilates. Po_2 normal despite cyanosis	Normal	Both usually normal
Dark; becomes pink in air	Dextrostix indicates extreme hypoglycemia; confirm by another method	$Paco_2$ frequently elevated secondary to hypoventilation; pH variable	Mild to massive cardiomegaly	ECG normal; echo shows ventricular enlargement
Dark; becomes pink in air	High hematocrit value (65% to 86%)	Normal	Normal or mild cardiomegaly	ECG normal or mild RVH; echo normal
Dark; becomes pink in air	Normal hematocrit value; hypoglycemia is frequent; hyperglycemia also may occur	Elevated $Paco_2$ and acidosis common	Cardiomegaly frequent	ECG may show ST-T wave abnormalities; echo may show chamber enlargement

normal heart. The PFC syndrome may be idiopathic (primary) or secondary to hyperviscosity of blood, aspiration pneumonia especially meconium aspiration, neonatal sepsis, hypoglycemia, congenital diaphragmatic hernia, or neonatal pulmonary disease (particularly RDS, pulmonary hypoplasia, or diaphragmic hernia). The primary form tends to occur in full-term or postmature infants. The cause is unknown, but it is theorized that the condition results when the normal mechanisms that cause a decline in pulmonary vascular resistance and ductus closure are inadequate. It has been proposed that one cause of PFC syndrome is prenatal transplacental exposure to prostaglandin synthetase inhibitors such as aspirin or indomethacin.

Neonates with PFC syndrome are tachypneic and cyanotic. Right-to-left ductal shunting (when present) may result in a higher $Pa{O_2}$ in the right arm than in the descending aorta or legs. This may produce differential cyanosis and be documented by simultaneous placement of two transcutaneous PO_2 electrodes over the right upper chest and abdomen. The pulmonary closure sound is loud, and there is no diagnostically useful murmur. The ECG characteristically shows mild right ventricular hypertrophy, and the chest x-ray film may be normal or show moderate cardiac enlargement. The infants may have increased total and alveolar ventilation and increased tidal volumes. There is a large arterial-alveolar CO_2 difference, caused by the presence of many overventilated, underperfused alveoli. The cyanosis frequently responds to 100% O_2 breathing initially, with a large increase in pulmonary vein oxygen saturation and a decrease in pulmonary artery pressure.

Echocardiography is invaluable in the evaluation of these infants. M-mode echocardiography reveals a prolongation of right ventricular systolic time intervals in those infants with severe elevation of pulmonary vascular resistance. With two-dimensional echocardiography structural heart disease—particularly total anomalous pulmonary venous return—is easily ruled out. Additionally, the ductus arteriosus and atrial septum are easily visualized, and with pulsed Doppler right-to-left shunting at either the ductal or atrial level, as occurs with PFC syndrome, can be detected.

The infant with PFC syndrome and worsening blood gases despite assisted ventilation may benefit from scalp vein or pulmonary artery tolazoline infusion at a rate of 2 mg/kg/hour, with observations of the effect on transcutaneous or upper and lower limb blood gases. Tolazoline is a systemic vasodilator, as well as a pulmonary vasodilator; it may be necessary to combat systemic hypotension with albumin or blood or pharmacologically (e.g., dopamine). Respirator-induced respiratory alkalosis often proves useful in causing pulmonary vasodilatation. Multiple pulmonary arterial thromboses have been noted in infants dying of PFC syndrome. These infants do not respond to vasodilator therapy.

In the management of the critically sick infant, therapeutic decisions may be aided by observing the effect of interventions on the directly recorded pulmonary artery pressure or by observing changes in the right ventricular systolic time intervals (echocardiogram). The search continues for a therapeutic agent that will cause selective pulmonary arteriolar vasodilatation.*

HEART FAILURE IN THE NEONATAL PERIOD

During the first days of life heart failure may simulate disease of other organs or systems, and conversely other disease entities may have some of the clinical signs of heart failure. Although heart failure is usually the result of structural congenital heart disease or of myocardial disease, it may on occasion be secondary to arrhythmia, respiratory disease, central nervous system disease, anemia, high hematocrit, systemic or pulmonary hypertension intrapartum asphyxia, or septicemia. Thus, when heart failure is diagnosed, it is necessary to determine whether primary structural heart disease is responsible or whether the heart failure is secondary to some other disease.

Recognition of heart failure

Heart failure may be defined as a state in which the heart does not maintain a circulation adequate for the needs of the body despite a satisfactory venous filling pressure. In the newborn, heart failure gives rise to a distinctive clinical syndrome. Common symptoms and signs are feeding difficulties, tachypnea, tachycardia, rales and rhonchi, liver enlargement, and cardiomegaly. Less common manifestations include measurable increase in systemic venous pressure, peripheral edema, ascites, pulsus alternans, gallop rhythm, and inappropriate sweating. Pleural and pericardial effusions resulting from heart failure are exceedingly rare. The distinction between left-sided heart failure (characterized by tachypnea, tachycardia, pulmonary rales, and cardiomegaly) and right-sided heart failure (characterized by liver enlargement, tachycardia, and cardiomegaly) is less obvious in the newborn than it is in the older child or adult. This difference is caused in part by the fact that many of the lesions producing failure give rise first to left ventricular failure, the results of which are elevated left atrial pressure and secondary pulmonary arterial hypertension, which in turn causes right ventricular failure. On occasion one observes "pure" right-sided failure, for example, the newborn with severe isolated pulmonic stenosis, or "pure" left-sided failure, as in the early stages of heart failure associated with aortic stenosis. The signs and symptoms of heart failure in the newborn are considered here in the approximate order of their frequency of occurrence and reliability.

Physical signs of heart failure

Tachypnea. The earliest sign of left-sided heart failure is an increase in respiratory rate to above 50 breaths per minute. It is important that respirations be counted while the baby is sleeping, since the slightest movement or agitation will temporarily elevate the respiratory rate. There is no increase in the depth of respiration (tidal volume), and the baby is not distressed; that is, there is no grunting, flaring of the alae nasi, or intercostal retraction. When a respiratory infection coexists, or when cardiac failure has resulted in the accumulation of pulmonary transudate, the signs of respiratory distress often appear.

Tachycardia. An increase in the resting heart rate to 140 to 180 beats per minute is characteristic of heart failure. The rate tends to be constant, and the RR interval on the ECG varies little. A rate of over 180 beats per minute suggests the possibility of SVT.

Liver enlargement. Liver enlargement is best assessed if one measures the distance between the liver edge and the right costal margin in a line joining the right nipple and umbilicus. When measured in this way, the normal liver may extend as much as 2 cm below the costal margin, but in heart failure it is frequently 3 to 5 cm or more below the costal margin.

Cardiomegaly. The silhouette of the heart as seen on the chest roentgenogram must be carefully interpreted. In the normal newborn the cardiac diameter may seem to be as much as 75% of the thoracic diameter. A large thymus gland interferes with an evaluation of heart size. In addition, cardiomegaly is not present in all neonates with heart failure; for example, the heart is frequently small when the failure is caused by total anomalous pulmonary venous drainage with obstruction to pulmonary venous return (Fig. 29-3).

Pulmonary rales and rhonchi. In the early stages of the formation of a pulmonary transudate fine crepitant rales are present at the lung bases. As left-sided heart

*The use of short-term extracorporeal membrane oxygenation (ECMO), whereby the lung is rested while spontaneous healing and improvement take place, is an exciting growing point. Bartlett and coworkers report that all of 11 infants judged likely to die from respiratory failure survived after ECMO therapy for 1½ to 7 days. Until more specific therapy for PFC syndrome is delineated, the use of ECMO therapy for patients with unrelenting deterioration of pulmonary function is a useful therapeutic modality. (See Chapter 28, part three.)

failure progresses and the transudate reaches the bronchioles, the clinical signs often change to those of obstructive airway disease with rhonchi and sometimes with audible wheezing. If the baby is first seen at this stage, the clinical pattern may simulate that of bronchiolitis.

Feeding difficulties. At birth the infant with severe heart disease usually appears well nourished, since the fetal circulation often minimizes the effect of structural heart disease as long as the infant is in utero. After birth, however, the increasing tachypnea and exhaustion of heart failure make it difficult for the infant to suck, and calorie and fluid intakes are below the daily requirements. Mothers frequently say that the infant tires or goes to sleep after the first 1 to 2 ounces, and experienced nurses quickly recognize the poor feeding performance and exhaustion of the newborn with heart disease.

Peripheral edema. Systemic edema may appear as puffiness on the backs of the hands, on the dorsum of the feet, or around the eyes. Sometimes pitting edema also may occur over the tibia or sacrum, but it is unusual for edema to become widespread.

Elevated systemic venous pressure. Because of the short squat conformation of the infant's neck, elevation of venous pressure is not easily detected by inspection of the jugular veins. When venous pressure is extremely high, the scalp veins occasionally may appear distended with the infant in the sitting position. Measurements of venous pressure made during cardiac catheterization indicate that it is rarely more than 7 or 8 mm Hg even in the presence of gross liver enlargement from congestive heart failure.

Inappropriate sweating. Inappropriate sweating at normal room temperature occasionally is observed in the newborn. It probably is caused by the excessive production of catecholamines associated with heart failure.

Gallop rhythm. A diastolic gallop rhythm (accentuated third or fourth heart sound) is suggestive of primary myocardial disease, especially myocarditis, but it also is observed late in the course of left ventricular failure from a variety of other causes.

Pulsus alternans. Alternate strong and weak peripheral pulses are usually evidence of severe left ventricular failure and are particularly common in primary myocardial disease.

Ascites. Ascites caused by heart failure in the newborn is uncommon, and when it does occur, the amount of fluid in the peritoneal cavity is usually small.

Electrocardiogram. The ECG may be helpful in supplying supportive evidence of heart failure, but no single electrocardiographic sign is pathognomonic. Tall peaked P waves (greater than 0.3 mV in the standard limb leads) are common in right-sided heart failure but also are found in situations such as tricuspid atresia, where the right atrium is hypertrophied but heart failure is not present. Wide notched P waves (in the standard limb leads) often are associated with left-sided heart failure but also are seen with mitral regurgitation (as in the endocardial cushion defect complex) when heart failure, as judged by other criteria, is not present.

Echocardiogram. The echocardiogram is extremely helpful in documenting the presence of an anatomic cause for heart failure. If there is no anatomic cause evidenced by echo, a careful consideration of Doppler flow velocities and various M-mode and sector scan findings provides evidence of ventricular dysfunction.

Advanced, near-terminal heart failure

Heart failure may progress very rapidly in the first hours and days of life. The delay of long-distance transportation, suboptimal environmental temperature, aspiration pneumonia, and other complications may lead to the hospital admission of a near-moribund infant in heart failure. Frequently there is no heart murmur, and the clinical picture is more one of advanced cardiogenic shock, with pallor, apathy, minimal spontaneous movement, greatly diminished peripheral pulses, bradycardia, and diminished heart sounds. The respiratory rate may be very rapid with widespread rales, or the infant may have become exhausted with slow respirations or apneic periods. The liver is usually very large, and the spleen also may be enlarged. Sometimes there is peripheral edema. The clinical picture may closely simulate that of septicemia, meningitis, or pneumonia. However, the presence of a very large liver and gross cardiomegaly usually indicates that heart failure is the major problem.

Heart failure without structural congenital heart disease

The following are situations in which heart failure occurs without structural congenital heart disease:

1. Myocarditis
2. Endocardial fibroelastosis
3. Glycogen storage disease
4. Congenital heart block
5. Paroxysmal supraventricular tachycardia
6. Intrapartum asphyxia

Other arrhythmias. Atrial fibrillation, atrial flutter, and second-degree AV block also may be associated with neonatal heart failure.

Central nervous system disease. Heart failure may be a consequence of pulmonary hypertension secondary to alveolar hypoventilation or apneic periods or both that are caused by cerebral hemorrhage or other major central nervous system disease. An intracranial arteriovenous fistula may cause heart failure with or without clinical evidence of central nervous system disease.

Anemia. Severe anemia (hemoglobin level less than

3.5 gm/dl) occasionally causes heart failure because of the sustained attempt to maintain an increased cardiac output. The most common example is hydrops fetalis caused by Rh incompatibility.

High hematocrit value. Infants with very high hematocrit values may manifest some of the signs of heart failure, with cardiomegaly, slight liver enlargement, and tachypnea; venesection with volume replacement should be performed.

Systemic hypertension. See discussion later in this chapter.

Pulmonary hypertension. Pulmonary hypertension may result from many disease entities. The clinical picture and hemodynamic findings may be secondary to multiple small pulmonary emboli originating from peripheral venous thromboses, to thrombi building up on a Spitz-Holter valve (used in the treatment of hydrocephalus), or to emboli that are septic in origin. Pulmonary hypertension also may be secondary to the acidosis and hypoxia associated with obstructive airway disease (for example, choanal atresia and tracheomalacia), to multiple peripheral pulmonary artery stenoses (common in the rubella syndrome), or to obstructive disease of the left side of the heart (for example, cor triatriatum or mitral stenosis). Occasionally the cause of pulmonary hypertension cannot be determined even at autopsy (primary pulmonary hypertension). In severe cases of pulmonary hypertension not only is the baby in heart failure, but he is also usually deeply cyanotic as the result of right-to-left shunting through the ductus arteriosus or foramen ovale.

Septicemia. Septicemia may be responsible for heart failure in the neonatal period by infection of the myocardium or by the effects of bacterial toxins on the myocardium. The liver and spleen are usually grossly enlarged; the baby is pale and apathetic and may have apneic spells. If the baby is first seen in the near-moribund state, the distinction between heart failure caused by structural heart disease and heart failure caused by septicemia may be especially difficult. Blood culture, white blood cell count, and chest roentgenography may resolve the issue, but usually an echocardiogram is necessary.

MANAGEMENT

General considerations: indications for cardiac catheterization

When clinical evidence indicates that structural heart disease is the cause of heart failure in a newborn, medical treatment should be initiated immediately and a definite anatomic diagnosis made. Although in the past invasive studies were usually necessary, it is now more and more possible to rely on the echocardiogram.

Thus firm information on which to base surgical intervention may be made in a host of neonatal heart lesions, including hypoplastic left heart syndrome, critical aortic stenosis, transposition of the great arteries, and pulmonary atresia. If, following noninvasive assessment the diagnosis is in doubt and the infant is critically ill and not improving, cardiac catheterization and angiography may be indicated.

Routine measures

Chart. A chart for recording the baby's major physical signs and drug dosages at 4-hour intervals is of great assistance in evaluating the response to medical treatment. Respiratory rate (basal or sleeping), heart rate, liver size (centimeters), weight, rales (+ to + + +), dose of digoxin (Lanoxin, either oral or parenteral), doses of other drugs, and other pertinent physical signs such as gallop rhythm, puffy hands or feet, and intercostal retractions should be recorded. The development of apneic periods or apathy and lethargy in a baby with heart failure usually indicates that he or she is becoming exhausted, probably from the additional work of respiration and lack of sufficient oxygen transfer across the lungs to maintain necessary oxidative metabolism. It is also possible that the glycogen reserve in the diaphragm becomes exhausted, as has been described in RDS.

Digitalis. Infants with heart failure may benefit from digitalis. The data of white and Leitman show that in general infants with myocardial failure are more likely to benefit than those with obstructive lesions or left-to-right shunts. The preferred preparation is digoxin. This drug is available in a pediatric elixir and in a parenteral solution. The 24-hour digitalizing dose depends on the age and maturity of the infant (Table 29-8). The newborn and especially the premature infant are more liable to

Table 29-8. Twenty-four-hour digitalizing dose (oral digoxin)*

Age	Digitalizing dose (oral digoxin) first 24 hours (μg/kg)
Premature infants 0-2 weeks or < 1500 gm	10-20
Premature infants 2-4 weeks or < 2500 gm	30
Term newborns 0-1 week	30
Term newborns 1-4 weeks	35

*The parenteral dose should be two thirds of the oral dose. The 24-hour maintenance dose is approximately one fourth of the digitalizing dose. For urgent digitalization give half the digitalizing dose initially, followed by two doses of one fourth each after 8 hours and 16 hours, respectively. The schedule will be safe in at least 95% of infants, but frequent clinical and electrocardiographic examinations are mandatory to detect signs of toxicity such as second-degree AV block, sinus bradycardia of less than 100 beats per minute, and multiple ectopic beats. Digitalis toxicity is potentiated by hypokalemia. Because of individual variations in the amount of digitalis that is required to be effective, increases in the projected digitalizing dose will be needed in many instances.

digitalis toxicity than is the older infant. Any suspicion of digitalis intoxication (arrhythmia, tachycardia, or bradycardia) is an indication for an ECG, for a digoxin blood level determination, and possibly for temporarily withholding the drug and then reducing the dose. Serum digoxin levels in the newborn can be very misleading, since normal undigitalized neonates have been shown to have false positive digoxin levels of 1 to 2 ng/ml due to cross-reactive substances that effect the digoxin assay.

Incubator. An incubator aids in the management of a neonate in heart failure in several ways. The baby can be clothed only in a diaper so that chest movements can be observed from across the room. He or she can be easily positioned to lie on a 10- to 30-degree head-up incline. The oxygen-enriched atmosphere necessary to minimize cyanosis can be provided, and at the same time heat loss and oxygen consumption can be minimized by controlling the environmental temperature in a neutral thermal range. The incubator also allows maintenance of optimal humidity, protects the infant from nursery infections, and facilitates the use of intravenous infusions and cardiac and respiratory monitoring equipment.

Monitoring. Infants who have bradycardia or arrhythmia or who have had apnea or a cardiac arrest require continuous electrocardiographic monitoring.

Feeding. Infants who tire easily often benefit by being fed smaller volumes every 3 or even every 2 hours. Moderately sick infants find even short periods of feeding difficult because of dyspnea, and they may aspirate milk. Gavage feeding is often useful to lessen this danger. A low-salt milk may be used for a few days, but there is a danger of salt depletion from continued use of such formulas. A good compromise between high- and low-salt formulas is a milk moderately low in mineral content, such as Similac PM 60/40 (Ross Labs). Increasing the concentration to 24 calories per ounce (30 ml) may be desirable to increase caloric intake. Frequently even gavage feeding provokes vomiting and aspiration. Under these circumstances it is important for the baby to receive his fluid requirements intravenously even though his caloric intake will fall short of normal daily requirements; the goal is to approach daily basal requirements. Severely ill infants should be given intravenous infusion initially.

Posture. Young infants in heart failure should lie on a 10- to 30-degree incline inside the incubator. This allows venous blood to pool in the legs and probably decreases the work of breathing by lessening the compression of the diaphragm by the abdominal contents. If the slope is steeper, it may be necessary to put tape from the axillae to the mattress to avoid sliding.

Oxygen. The infant with heart failure may benefit considerably from breathing an oxygen-enriched atmosphere, generally 30% to 35%. Even if pulmonary venous and arterial blood is fully saturated, additional dissolved oxygen can be carried in physical solution in plasma, thus decreasing the circulatory needs by a small factor. In the premature infant this additional advantage must be weighed against the risk of retrolental fibroplasia. Arterial blood P_{O_2} should be monitored and maintained between 60 and 70 mm Hg.

Treatment of anemia. The oxygen-carrying capacity of blood will be increased by correcting anemia. The optimal hematocrit value for the acyanotic baby with heart failure is probably between 40% and 50%. A transfusion usually is indicated if the hematocrit reading is below 30% when the infant's state of hydration is normal. Exchange transfusions should be given very slowly as packed cells in increments of 10 ml/kg, while continuously and carefully observing the response (respirations, heart rate, and liver size). Heart failure can be aggravated by hypervolemia from transfusion.

Diuretics (Table 29-9). Furosemide is used in infants and children with congestive heart failure. The suggested dose is 0.5 to 3 mg/kg. Where a rapid response is mandatory, intravenous furosemide is the diuretic of choice. Serum potassium should be monitored and, if necessary, potassium chloride supplied orally.

Long-term diuretic administration is rarely indicated in the management of the newborn; however, hydrochlorothiazide (Hydrodiuril) may be useful occasionally. Infants under 6 months of age require 0.5 to 0.75 mg/kg/day in two doses. Hypokalemia may be a complication. Patients on long-term thiazide therapy also should have determination of hematocrit, white blood cell, and platelet counts repeated at monthly intervals. The principal indication for the use of hydrochlorothiazide is the infant with chronic congestive heart failure for whom nothing surgical can be done or for whom surgery at best would be temporarily palliative. Spironolactone (Aldactone) is an aldosterone antagonist. It causes decreased sodium and water retention, whereas potassium is retained. It sometimes is useful in long-term management at a dosage of 1 to 3 mg/kg/day.

Fluid and electrolytes. Despite heart failure, the newborn has continued need for fluid to replace insensible and urinary water losses and for electrolytes to maintain normal body fluid tonicity. Serum sodium, potassium, and chloride levels should be measured as soon as possible; the amount and type of fluid administered intravenously will depend on serum electrolyte concentrations and the estimated degree of fluid retention. In general, fluid restriction should not be as aggressive as in the older child or adult with heart failure. The problem of prolonged intravenous fluid therapy does not often arise, because the newborn with heart failure who is sick enough to require intravenous fluids generally requires rapid hemodynamic assessment and often surgery. Approximately 80 to 100 ml/kg/24 hours of fluid will be

Table 29-9. Drugs useful in the treatment of heart failure in the neonatal period (for digitalis see Table 29-8) (for vasoactive medications see Tables 29-10 and 29-11)

Drug	Administration	Dosage	Frequency	Indications, response, complications
Spironolactone (Aldactone)	Oral (in divided doses)	1-3 mg/kg/day	Suitable for long-term therapy	For diuresis; 4- to 16-hour response; risk of hyperkalemia and of hyponatremia; contraindicated in renal dysfunction, anuria, or hyperkalemia
Furosemide	IV over 2 minutes	0.5-3 mg/kg	Can be repeated after electrolyte check	For diuresis; 1- to 1½-hour response, risk of deafness if renal failure present; renal calcification
Furosemide	Oral (in 2 divided doses)	1-5 mg/kg	Suitable for long-term therapy	For diuresis: 1- to 6-hour response; risk of hypokalemia
Hydrochlorothiazide (Hydrodiuril)	Oral (in 2 divided doses)	0.5-0.75 mg/kg/day	Suitable for long-term therapy	For diuresis; slow response; risk of hypokalemia
Sodium bicarbonate	IV over 12-hour period	Desired bicarbonate concentration (usually 23 mEq/L) minus existing bicarbonate concentration × 0.6 × body weight (kg) = mEq bicarbonate dosage	Usually given once before planned therapy	For partial correction of metabolic acidosis; risk of hypernatremia, water retention, and alkalosis
Sodium bicarbonate	Large vein (umbilical) or intracardiac; over ½-1 minute	2-5 mEq/kg	Administer one time	Last resort as a resuscitative procedure in cardiac arrest or extreme bradycardia
Tromethamine buffer	IV into large vein, over 5-10 minutes	2-5 ml/kg as a 0.3M solution in 5-10% glucose at pH 8.4	Administer one time usually before planned surgery if hypernatremia contraindicates sodium bicarbonate	For partial correction of metabolic acidosis; an alternative to sodium bicarbonate when hypernatremia is present; risks of hypoglycemia, respiratory depression, and severe local irritation at site of administration
Morphine sulfate	Subcutaneously	0.1-0.2 mg/kg/dose	May be repeated as needed	Useful where signs of left-sided heart failure predominate and the baby is very restless and agitated; risk of respiratory depression

required. The requirement for sodium will vary from 1 to 4 mEq/kg/24 hours and that for potassium from 0 to 3 mEq/kg/24 hours, depending on the serum electrolyte levels. The neonate in heart failure cannot tolerate sudden increases in circulating blood volume. If these daily requirements are distributed evenly throughout the 24 hours and a careful check is made on the presence of pulmonary rales, the liver size, systemic edema, and weight, their administration will not worsen the baby's heart failure by producing hypervolemia and hyponatremia and will prevent him from developing hypernatremia from too severe water restriction. If the baby is first seen when heart failure is in an advanced state with evidence of peripheral edema and widespread pulmonary rales, then intravenous administration of fluid should be reduced to 40 to 80 ml/kg/24 hours pending the baby's improvement from medical measures or following surgery.

With mild heart failure there is commonly no disturbance of pH or $PaCO_2$, but there may be some lowering of PaO_2, owing to intrapulmonary right-to-left shunting or to uneven perfusion of the lung. When a baby is in severe heart failure, a combined metabolic and respiratory disorder may be encountered.

Antibiotics. Some neonates with heart failure have increased pulmonary perfusion, which makes them more susceptible to respiratory tract infections. It is often difficult to be certain whether pulmonary infection is present. Antibiotics may be commenced while awaiting culture results.

Infusion of β-adrenergic drugs. Infants with severe heart failure from left-to-right shunts may improve temporarily following infusion of catecholamines. These agents act by direct inotropic effect. Isoproterenol (Isuprel) is a suitable β-adrenergic stimulator and may be particularly useful when bradycardia is present in advanced cardiogenic shock. The initial dose is approximately 0.1 μg/kg/minute, increasing to 0.4 μg/kg/minute until a heart rate of approximately 140 to 160 beats per minute is achieved. Isoproterenol should be continued throughout anesthesia until the underlying cause of heart failure has been corrected. It is then discontinued slowly during monitoring of the blood pressure and recording of the ECG. Dopamine is also useful in the treatment of cardiogenic shock and refractory heart failure. The drug is diluted in 5% dextrose and infused at a rate of 2 to 5 μg/kg/minute. Dopamine increases cardiac output, blood pressure, and urine flow in patients unresponsive to other catecholamines.

Resuscitative measures. These measures are a last resort when extreme bradycardia or cardiac arrest occurs in an infant who has an operable heart lesion. Usually they will take place on the operating table while the surgeon is preparing for the operation. They are external cardiac massage, pulmonary ventilation via an endotracheal tube, use of rotating tourniquets, intracardiac injection of epinephrine (1 ml of 1:10,000 solution), and intracardiac injection of calcium chloride or calcium gluconate (1 to 2 ml of 10% solution).

Morphine sulfate. Morphine sulfate is indicated in instances where a baby is in heart failure, that is, extremely restless and agitated. Such occasions are more likely to occur in a 3- to 4-week-old infant in whom signs of left-sided heart failure predominate. The dose is 0.1 to 0.2 mg/kg given subcutaneously. A risk of respiratory depression must be considered.

CARDIOGENIC SHOCK

The term *cardiogenic shock* implies acute primary failure of the heart as a pump, although the distinction between cardiogenic shock and severe heart failure is somewhat arbitrary; yet the two do appear as different clinical pictures. In the neonate the clinical picture of cardiogenic shock is encountered infrequently, but it is most common with intrapartum asphyxia, myocarditis, and overwhelming septicemia.

Pathogenesis

The evidence that primary failure of the heart as a pump is the cause of shock is (1) the elevation of systemic venous pressure to 10 to 15 cm H_2O, as compared with the low venous pressure associated with endotoxin and hemorrhagic shock, (2) the presence of a triple or quadruple rhythm, (3) enlarged liver or pulmonary rales, (4) gross cardiomegaly evident on the chest roentgenogram, (5) low-voltage QRS complexes, indicating rapid dilation of the heart, (6) primary T-wave abnormalities on the ECG, and (7) severe acidosis.

Clinical manifestations

Arterial pulses are almost impalpable; the infant is bradycardic and tachypneic, and blood flow through the blanched skin is extremely slow. Often the whole skin has a mottled blue-white appearance. The liver may be enlarged, and there may be rales in the lungs, but these signs of heart failure may be absent if the heart has failed very rapidly and peripheral circulatory failure with deficient tissue blood flow is extreme. The picture then is dominated by evidence of greatly reduced tissue perfusion rather than the signs of traditional heart failure. The resemblance to endotoxic shock and to hemorrhagic shock is close.

Differential diagnosis

The need for urgent treatment of the bradycardic, mottled, dying baby precludes a complete diagnostic evaluation. Cardiogenic shock often is caused by viral myocarditis, but the differential diagnosis also should include the following possibilities: (1) bacterial sepsis with myocarditis and pericarditis, (2) end-stage left ventricular failure from congenital heart disease (usually coarctation), severe aortic stenosis, interrupted aortic arch, or hypoplastic left heart syndrome, (3) anomalous left coronary artery arising from the pulmonary artery, causing myocardial infarction, (4) adrenal insufficiency, especially that caused by congenital adrenal hyperplasia, (5) extreme hypoglycemia with or without heart disease, (6) bacterial or viral myocarditis, (7) primary thoracic conditions such as bilateral pneumothorax, pneumopericardium, or congenital lobar emphysema, (8) hemorrhagic shock with concealed bleeding, as in ruptured spleen, (9) complete heart block with very slow rate, (10) prolonged rapid supraventricular tachycardia, (11) ventricular tachycardia (especially associated with cardiac tumor), and (12) ventricular fibrillation (especially suggestive of the "prolonged QT interval" syndrome).

Intrapartum asphyxia and cardiogenic shock

Cabal and associates have emphasized that cardiogenic shock may occur secondary to severe perinatal asphyxia. There are three major clinical presentations. Some infants show evidence of marked fetal acidemia with abnormal fetal heart rate patterns during labor, depressed fetal scalp pH, and elevated neonatal serum lactic acid values. At birth these infants may have reduced arterial pulses, tachypnea, pulmonary rales, hepatomegaly, and gallop rhythm. There is usually raised central venous pressure, lowered arterial blood pressure, and the radiologic observations of cardiomegaly and pulmonary vascular congestion.

In other infants cardiomegaly and massive tricuspid insufficiency caused by papillary muscle infarction dominate the picture; there is frequently a raised creatine kinase MB fraction.

Still other infants with myocardial dysfunction have had a relatively mild prenatal and immediate postnatal course but have developed cyanosis, tachypnea, and heart failure during the first 24 hours of life. In these infants it has been postulated that the disorder is one of impaired coronary perfusion to portions of the right and left ventricular myocardium through increased work demands created by unusually severe pulmonary vasoconstriction from hypoxia. This postulate was strengthened by electrocardiographic evidence of ischemia and by poor myocardial uptake of thallium 201. In all groups an association with hypoglycemia has been noted.

Treatment

The following plan is suggested for the emergency room management of the moribund infant with the clinical diagnosis of cardiogenic shock.

Record the ECG to rule out complete heart block and to monitor heart rate. Insert a central venous catheter (umbilical vein or femoral vein to right atrium). Measure the central venous pressure (expressed in centimeters of water). Withdraw blood for immediate Dextrostix test, and send sample for blood glucose and serum electrolyte determination. Blood culture (bacterial and viral), hematocrit reading, complete blood count, blood urea nitrogen level, pH, P_{CO_2}, blood type, and crossmatch also should be obtained. If the venous pressure is low (less than 4 cm H_2O), give blood or blood substitute. In endotoxic or hemorrhagic shock very large volumes (up to 40 ml/kg) may be needed to raise the central venous pressure and increase cardiac output. If the venous pressure is high (over 12 cm H_2O in a neonate), cardiogenic shock is probably present, in which case digitalize the baby and start an isoproterenol infusion. (Dose is highly variable.) Mix 1 mg in 100 ml of 5% dextrose to give 10 µg/ml. This solution then can be infused by pump at 0.1 ml/minute or 1 µg/minute (0.4 to 1.0 µg/kg/minute). A satisfactory response is indicated by a falling venous pressure and a rise in heart rate to 100 to 140 beats per minute. Dopamine also may be effective in patients refractory to isoproterenol. Studies by Perkin and co-workers and Schranz and associates involving infants suggests that dobutamine at a dosage of 2.5 to 10 µg/kg/mm may be beneficial in both septic and cardiogenic shock. If the blood glucose level is low, infuse 10% dextrose in addition to maintenance fluid. A high serum potassium or low sodium level is highly suggestive of adrenal insufficiency. These findings may require treatment with rehydration, salt replacement, and the administration of adrenocorticoids (Chapter 37, part five). Take a chest and abdominal film as soon as possible to exclude diagnoses such as pneumothorax and peritonitis with free air in the peritoneal cavity. A lumbar puncture may be indicated, depending on whether there is a strong possibilty of meningitis. Correction of acidosis may require assisted ventilation rather than alkali therapy. Myocarditis, if present, is usually of viral origin. However, once the cultures have been taken, if myocarditis is presumptively diagnosed, antibiotic treatment for sepsis is indicated because of the possibility of a bacterial cause. The death rate from viral myocarditis appearing as a shocklike state in the neonate is approximately 75%. In a dying infant,

Table 29-10. Therapeutic strategies and the use of vasoactive medication in the newborn*

Clinical observations	Likely etiologies	Vasoactive medications
Inadequate cardiac output *with hypoxemia* apparently precipitated by spontaneous closing of the ductus arteriosus	Pulmonary atresia, severe P.S. Tricuspid atresia; TGA	PGE_1
Inadequate cardiac output apparently precipitated by spontaneous closing of the ductus arteriosus	Complex coarctation of aorta; interrupted aortic arch; hypoplastic left heart syndrome; critical aortic valve stenosis	PGE_1 If response inadequate consider intermediate dose dopamine with or without sodium nitroprusside
Myocardial dysfunction without evidence of systemic vasoconstriction	Myocarditis; immediate postoperative period, following cardiac surgery; many forms of severe CHD	Digoxin; low dose dopamine or dobutamine
Myocardial dysfunction with evidence of systemic vasoconstriction and normal BP	Same as above	Moderate dose of dopamine; sodium nitroprusside; if response inadequate, consider dobutamine (instead of dopamine); consider isoproterenol if heart rate slow
Myocardial dysfunction with vasoconstriction and hypotension	Same as above	High dose dopamine; consider epinephrine
Myocardial dysfunction with sinus bradycardia	Same as above	Atropine; isoproterenol
Cardiac arrest		Epinephrine followed by intermediate dose dopamine; isoproterenol if sinus bradycardia

*Treatment of hypovolemia, hypoxemia, hypercarbia or acidosis must accompany drug therapy. Always consider major mechanical interference to cardiac or lung function, such as cardiac tamponade, pneumothorax or diaphragmatic hernia. Chest x-ray film and echocardiogram are of major importance in assessing the problem.

corticosteroids such as hydrocortisone sodium succinate (Solu-Cortef), 50 mg/kg, may be tried; if the heart rate is slow (<80 beats/min), transvenous pacing is an option. If anomalous origin of the left coronary artery is suspected, consider an emergency aortogram.

USE OF VASOACTIVE MEDICATIONS IN THE NEWBORN

Clinical observations of cyanosis, systemic vasoconstriction, arterial hypotension, elevated central venous pressure (liver enlargement), heart rate, and urine output—together with simple laboratory, radiologic, and echocardiographic tests—may define a broad category of circulatory abnormality as suggested in Table 29-10. In this table vasoactive medications most likely to be helpful are suggested, although the use of each of these medications is a "therapeutic trial." Dosages, indications, and effects are described in Table 29-11.

Treatment of hypovolemia, hypoxemia, hypercarbia, or acidosis must accompany drug therapy. One should also consider major mechanical interference to cardiac or lung function such as ventilator dysfunction, cardiac tamponade, pneumothorax, or diaphragmatic hernia.

ARRHYTHMIAS IN THE PERINATAL AND NEONATAL PERIOD

Considerable evidence indicates that after birth there is continued development of the cardiac conduction system and an increase in the sympathetic innervation of the heart. These factors may account for the observed heart rate variability and for the frequency of benign arrhythmias in the newborn. Premature supraventricular and ventricular beats, brief periods of sinus arrest, ectopic atrial rhythms, and wandering atrial pacemaker all have been observed during electrocardiographic monitoring of asymptomatic newborn infants.

Before embarking on the treatment of a tachycardia, bradycardia, or irregular heart beat, one must decide if the arrhythmia is benign and likely to resolve spontaneously or if it is potentially dangerous. Sometimes an arrhythmia indicates underlying extracardiac disease such as central nervous system disease, sepsis, hypoglycemia, drug toxicity (especially digitalis), severe tissue hypoxia, adrenal insufficiency, or electrolyte and acid-base abnormalities. One also must decide if the treatment is likely to be more dangerous than the arrhythmia. In deciding to treat or not to treat, major consideration should be given to whether the ventricular rate and rhythm are compatible with a normal cardiac output.

Mechanisms of arrhythmias

Most arrhythmias are thought to arise either from a disorder of automaticity or impulse formation or from alterations in impulse conduction within the heart. Both mechanisms may be combined.

The SA node, AV node, and His-Purkinje system are pacemaker tissues because they are capable of spontaneous depolarization during electrical diastole (phase 4 of the action potential). The SA node is normally the pacemaker for the heart because it has the fastest rate of spontaneous depolarization. Dysrhythmias caused by altered automaticity may occur when the inherent rate of phase-4 depolarization of the SA node falls below that of other latent pacemaker tissue in the heart. Thus "escape" rhythms will occur when sinus bradycardia is present and the junctional tissue of the AV node depolarizes faster than that of the SA node.

Arrhythmias also result when the automaticity of "ectopic" pacemaker tissue and of pacemakers below the SA node is enhanced, which is promoted by hypoxia, acidosis, digitalis toxicity, sympathetic nerve stimulation, increased wall tension, and altered electrolyte concentrations, particularly sodium, potassium, and calcium.

When local membrane characteristics are altered, as by stretch deformation (increased wall tension), thermal injury, scarring and fibrosis, or a previous premature beat, then disturbances of conduction can occur. Such activity is promoted by (1) cardiac enlargement, (2) nonhomogeneity of recovery from refractoriness in the cell population, (3) shortened refractory periods, and (4) slowed conduction. When a propagating impulse reaches the area of altered conduction (Fig. 29-28), propagation will be through an alternate pathway (area *A*). The impulse having traversed an alternate route now may reach the distal end of the previously blocked pathway, and the original pathway (*B*) is now sufficiently recovered to permit the impulse to be propagated retrogradely through it, setting up a reentrant activation front.

Drug therapy

Drug therapy for arrhythmias is based on the ability of certain drugs to alter or affect electrophysiologic properties of the cardiac tissue.

Many antiarrhythmic drugs act directly to alter the electrophysiologic properties of single fibers, usually resulting in decreased automaticity because the rate of rise of diastolic depolarization is slowed. In addition, because of altered membrane characteristics, the conduction velocity and refractory period will be affected, resulting at times in interruption of reentry pathways. Examples of such drugs are quinidine, procainamide (Pronestyl), lidocaine (Xylocaine), and phenytoin.

Other drugs act on arrhythmias by affecting directly or indirectly autonomic nervous system activity. Thus vagal tone may be directly increased by cholinergic agents such as edrophonium (Tensilon) chloride or neostigmine (Prostigmin) bromide or reflexly increased following the rise in blood pressure induced by sympathomimetic α-agonists such as phenylephrine (Neo-synephrine) hydrochloride. Propranolol hydrochloride (Inderal)

Table 29-11. Vasoactive medications comomonly used in the newborn*

Vasoactive agent	Principle modes of action	Major hemodynamic effects	Administration and dosage	Indications
Digoxin	Increased positive inotropy; enhanced vagal activity; slows conduction through AV node	Increased cardiac output; increased arterial pressure; decreased venous pressure; decreased heart rate	See Table 29-8	Diminished myocardial contractility; treatment of SVT
Epinephrine	Alpha and beta agonist	Increases heart rate and myocardial contractility by activating β_1 receptors	0.1 ml/kg of 1:10,000 solution given IV, IC or ET 0.05 to 1.0 μg/kg/min IV	Cardiac resuscitation Short term use when severe heart failure resistant to other drugs
Dopamine				
Low dose	Stimulates dopamine receptors	Decrease in vascular resistance in splanchnic, renal and cerebral vessels	1 to 5 μg/kg/min IV	Useful in the management of cardiogenic or hypovolemic shock or following cardiac surgery
Intermediate dose	Stimulates β_1 receptors; Myocardial norepinephrine release	Inotrophic response	2 to 20 μg/kg/min IV	
High dose	Stimulates alpha receptors	Increased peripheral and renal vascular resistance	>20 μg/kg/min IV	Septic shock with low SVR
Dobutamine	Synthetic β_1 agonist in low dosages; Alpha and β_2 effects in higher dosages	Increased cardiac output; increased arterial pressure; less increase in HR than dopamine	1 to 10 μg/kg/min IV	Useful alternative to dopamine if increase in heart rate undesirable
Isoproterenol	β_1 and β_2 agonist	Increased cardiac output by positive inotropic and chronotropic action and increase in venous return; SVR generally reduced; PVR generally reduced	0.05 to 0.5 μg/kg/min IV	Useful in low output situations especially when heart rate is slow
Sodium nitroprusside	Direct-acting vasodilator that relaxes arteriolar and venous smooth muscle	Afterload reduction, reduced arterial pressure	1 to 10 μg/kg/min IV (for up to 10 min) 0.5 to 2 μg/kg/min IV	Hypertensive crisis Vasodilator therapy
Hydralazine	Direct-acting vasodilator with major action on arteriolar vascular bed	Afterload reduction; reduced arterial pressure	0.1 to 0.5 mg/kg IV, IM or PO q3 to q6h (PO dose generally twice the IV dose)	Vasodilator therapy Systemic hypertension
Atropine	Competitive inhibitor of the muscarinic effects of acetylcholine	Increases heart rate; cardiac output increased proportionately to tachycardia	0.01 mg/kg IV over 1 min; May be repeated q15 min; up to 4 times.	Sinus bradycardia due to predominant parasympathetic influence (e.g., digoxin or β blocker induced)
Propranolol	β_1 and β_2 blocker	Reduced myocardial contractility; reduces heart rate; reduces arterial pressure; increased refractory period of AV node	0.25 to 4 mg/kg/dose PO q6h 0.01 to 0.15 mg/kg/dose IV q6h	Systemic hypertension; Arrhythmias, especially SVT, Counteracting use of β agonists

*See section on antihypertensive and antiarrhythmic medications for more information. Also see section on use of prostaglandin E_1. For a comprehensive review of cardiovascular drugs in the newborn see Roberts, R.J.: Drug therapy in infants, Philadelphia, 1984, W.B. Saunders Co.

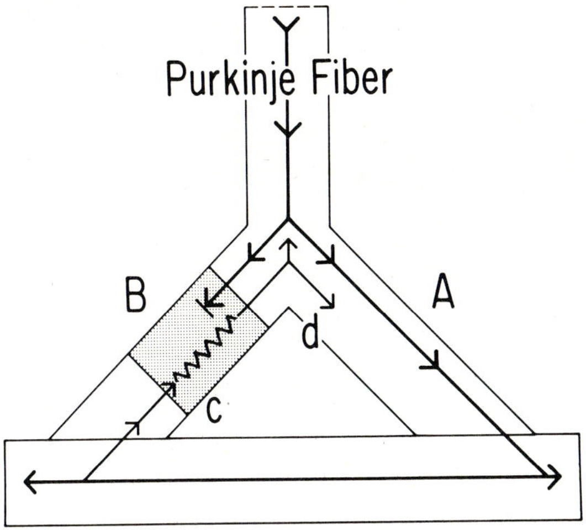

Fig. 29-28. Mechanism of unidirectional block and reentry. Impulse is propagated through Purkinje system and encounters Y-shaped fiber with its two branches terminating on ventricular muscle. Zone of unidirectional block is present in branch *B*. Impulse traverses branch *A* and is propagated through ventricular muscle. The impulse reaches distal end of block in B and is propagated slowly, retrogradely through it *(C)*. Branch A now has become sufficiently repolarized to be depolarized by reentering impulse *(D)*. One such reentrant circulation of impulses may produce premature beat. Repetition of this sequence in circuit produces reentrant tachycardia.

is a β-adrenergic blocker. Digoxin exerts part of its chronotropic action via the sympathetic and parasympathetic nervous system, although its inotropic action is independent of the autonomic nervous system.

FETAL DYSRHYTHMIAS

Fetal tachycardia. Sustained rates greater than 220 per minute are usually due to supraventricular tachycardia, but atrial flutter/atrial fibrillation and ventricular tachycardia have also been described. Fetal tachycardia is an obstetric emergency requiring close cooperation between obstetrician and pediatric cardiologist. Serous effusions and fetal edema may occur rapidly, especially with very fast rates and fetal immaturity. When there is evidence of fetal heart failure, the choice is between early delivery (if the L/S ratio is favorable) and maternal administration of antiarrhythmic drugs. Kleinman and coworkers found that the most commonly administered maternal medications are digoxin, digoxin and Verapamil, and digoxin and propanolol. When maternally administered drugs fail to convert the compromised fetus, immediate delivery is indicated, accepting the consequences of prematurity (Fig. 29-29).

Fetal bradycardia. Sustained fetal bradycardia with normal fetal movements is usually due to complete atrioventricular heart block, and in about 50% of cases there is clinical or serologic evidence of maternal collagen vas-

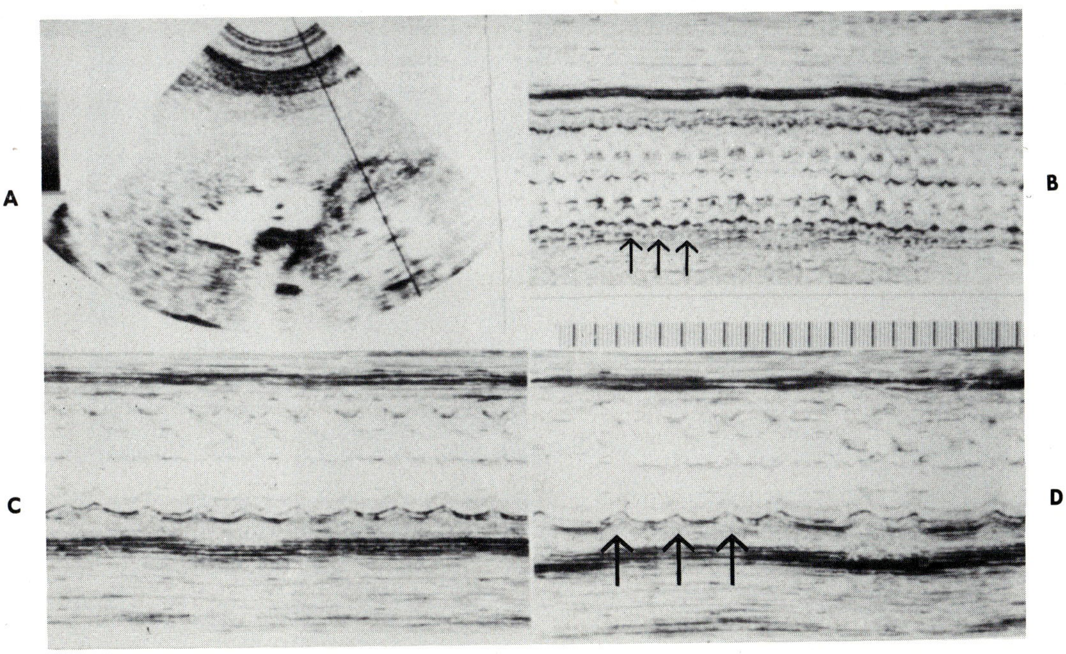

Fig. 29-29. Fetal echocardiograms before (**A** and **B**) and after (**C** and **D**) conversion to sinus rhythm by maternal administration of digoxin. SVT rate is 230 beats per minute *(arrows)*; after digoxin, rate is 120 beats per minute *(lower arrows)*.

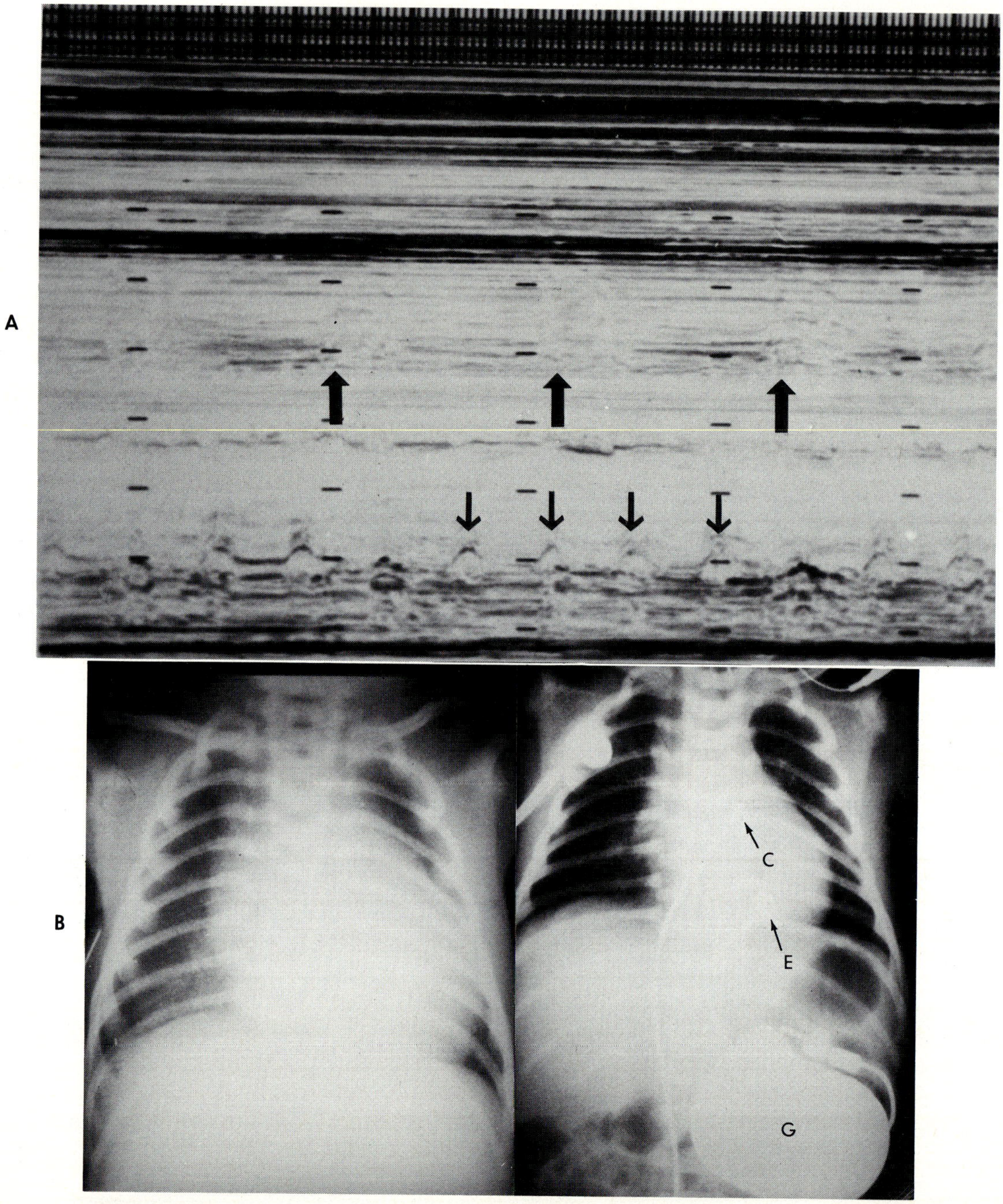

Fig. 29-30. A, Fetal echocardiogram. Complete atrioventricular heart block. Atrial rate is 137 beats per minute *(lower arrows)*; ventricular rate is 50 beats per minute *(upper arrows)*. **B,** Complete atrioventricular block. *A,* At 6 hours after birth (birth weight, 2.7 kg). *B,* At 57 hours of age after placement of a temporary transvenous pacing catheter *(C)*, permanent epicardial lead *(E)*, and 29 g pulse generator *(G)*. The pacing catheter was removed 3 hours later.

cular disease, especially lupus erythmatosus or Sjogren's syndrome.

Other causes of fetal bradycardia are severe structural congenital heart disease (especially single ventricle and truncus arteriosus) and the prolonged QT interval syndrome with a 2:1 atrioventricular "block" due to ventricular refractoriness (see Fig. 29-6).

Complete AV block is fairly easily identified by fetal echocardiography with simultaneous imaging of a ventricle and an atrium (Fig. 29-30). Complete AV block is potentially hazardous to the fetus, and fetal demise has occurred following its discovery. Hard and fast guidelines have yet to be established, but if the ventricular rate is consistently under 60 per minute, the mother should be instructed to keep close account of fetal movements. Any suspicion of diminishing fetal activity calls for preterm delivery, especially if there is echocardiographic evidence of structural heart disease (Fig. 29-30).

Fetal heart irregularity. The nature of the dysrhythmia can usually be determined by studying the motion of the ventricular and atrial walls and the atrioventricular and semilunar valve by M-mode echocardiography.

The more common causes of fetal heart irregularity are premature atrial contractions and premature ventricular contractions. The literature suggests that, when associated with normal fetal movements and unassociated with structural heart disease, these are benign.

Sometimes one encounters a bigeminal or trigeminal rhythm, and under these circumstances it is important to determine the adequacy of cardiac output by interrogating the umbilical artery to see if the premature beats provide a strong systolic flow signal. It is equally important to rule out serious structural disease, of which the dysrhythmia may be a symptom (Fig. 29-31).

Fetal vascular malformation. As obstetric ultrasound becomes more commonly used and ultrasonographers routinely screen the fetal heart for structural abnormalities and dysrhythmia, there will be more frequent and earlier diagnoses of fetal cardiovascular abnormalities. Thus in a series of 6,500 obstetric sonograms, Hegge and associates found seven major cardiac malformations, nine abnormal cardiac positions, and thirteen sustained dysrhythmias. There was also the incidental finding of a centrally placed intracranial sonolucency that was shown by Doppler interrogation to have a continuous flow pattern. The diagnosis of cerebral AV fistula led to elective cesarean section because of the risk of rupture with vaginal delivery (Fig. 29-32).

NEONATAL DYSRHYTHMIAS

Benign arrhythmias

Sinus bradycardia, sinus tachycardia, and sinus arrhythmia

Healthy full-term and premature neonates have heart rates that range from 90 to 195 beats per minute. Rates above and below this range, which are sustained for 15 seconds or more, should have electrocardiographic documentation of the rhythm. In some healthy infants rates during sleep as low as 70 beats per minute are seen. It is important to rule out QT prolongation in this group.

Transient periods of sinus bradycardia may occur during straining, micturition, or crying (Valsalva). Up to 35% of normal premature infants have been noted during monitoring to have brief periods of sinus bradycardia. The bradycardia that occurs with cord clamping or compression of the anterior fontanel may be caused by parasympathetic stimulation. Some maternal medications, such as reserpine or propranolol, may result in bradycardia in the newborn (Chapter 21).

Sinus tachycardia occurs with periods of increased

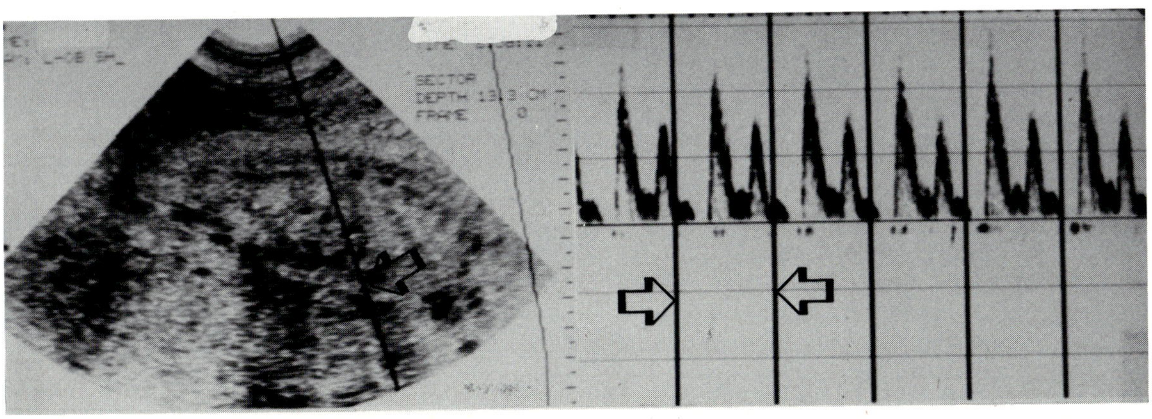

Fig. 29-31. Bigeminal rhythm in a 34-week fetus. Doppler sample volume is in aorta *(arrow)*. Doppler signal indicates alternating normal velocity and lower velocity beats. Although the rate counting all beats is 120/min, the effective rate counting only the higher velocity beats is only 60/min (time between arrows is 1 second). The infant also had truncus arteriosus.

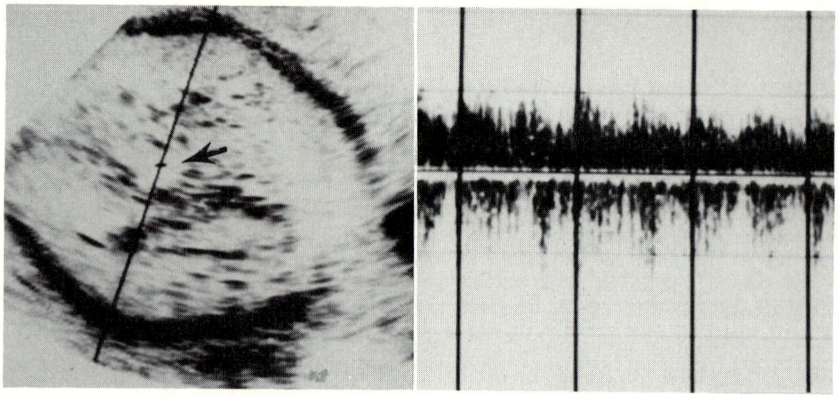

Fig. 29-32. Fetal echocardiogram. **A,** A sonolucent spherical structure was detected at the site of the great vein of Galen *(arrow)*. **B,** Doppler interrogation revealed a high velocity continuous flow pattern. The infant was delivered by cesarean section, and subsequent angiography confirmed the presence of a large cerebral arteriovenous fistula.

activity and crying and also with fever and hyperthyroidism.

Sinus arrhythmia is a phasic variation in the heart rate that may or may not be associated with respiration.

Pathologic arrhythmias

Supraventricular tachycardia

Supraventricular tachycardia (SVT) is the most common tachyarrhythmia in the newborn. It may be caused by dual AV nodal pathways with antegrade conduction down one pathway and the completion of a circle by retrograde conduction up the other (Fig. 29-28). It may be caused by rapid conduction through an accessory bundle (Wolff-Parkinson-White syndrome) or by the existence of an ectopic atrial focus with an automaticity faster than that in the SA node. There is an increased incidence of the Wolff-Parkinson-White syndrome with SVT in Ebstein's anomaly of the tricuspid valve and also with l-transposition of the great arteries. Gillette has investigated the mechanism of this disorder by electrophysiologic studies during cardiac catheterization of 35 children. These studies demonstrated at least seven different mechanisms, most involving some form of reentry. Between 8% and 26% of infants and children with SVT are estimated to have congenital heart disease.

Newborns with SVT are either those in whom the arrhythmia is discovered during the first few days after birth when they are relatively asymptomatic or those who are brought to the hospital in heart failure having had the arrhythmia for several days.

The history usually reveals that the infant has become anxious, restless, tachypneic, or "not well" 1 to 2 days before there is serious concern. Neonates then usually become "wheezy," and at this stage it is easy for both parent and physician to diagnose a lower respiratory tract infection. As the SVT persists, the infant becomes pale, apathetic, and obviously very sick, with signs of congestive heart failure (pulmonary rales, hepatomegaly) and poor skin perfusion. Even at this stage it is possible for one to overlook, because of noisy respiration, the fact that the heart is beating at 280 beats per minute.

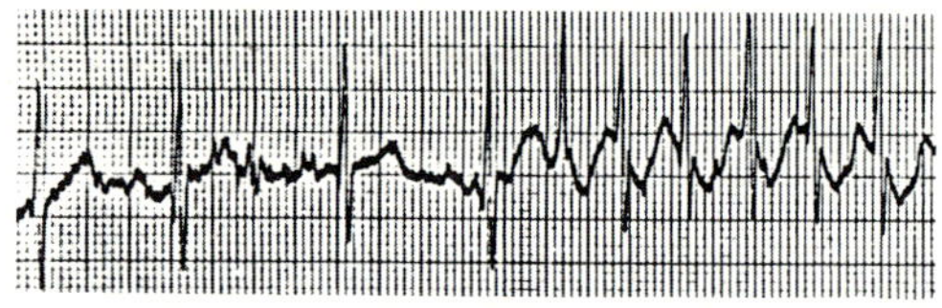

Fig. 29-33. Onset of PAT. Tracing obtained by telemetry. The rate increases from 75 to 200 beats per minute. Note the unchanging RR interval in the last six complexes and that the P waves are masked by the preceding T waves. (Courtesy Dr. Herbert Semler.)

In the absence of AV block the ventricular rate may be very rapid. With AV block the ventricular rate will be variable.

The time taken for an infant to develop heart failure depends mainly on the ventricular rate (180 to 300 beats per minute) and the presence or absence of structural heart disease. An infant with serious cyanotic heart disease who develops SVT during the course of cardiac catheterization may seriously worsen in a few minutes, whereas an infant with a normal heart may tolerate a rate of 220 beats per minute indefinitely.

Recognition of SVT is based on (1) a persistent ventricular rate of over 180 beats per minute, (2) a fixed or almost fixed RR interval on the ECG (Fig. 29-33), (3) abnormal P-wave shape, P-wave axis, or PR interval or total absence of P waves, and (4) little change in heart rate with activity, crying, or breath holding. The surface

ECG may provide clues to the underlying mechanism. Thus, if no P waves are seen, a reentry mechanism is likely. If P waves are seen and there is one-to-one AV conduction, a reentry mechanism is also likely. SVT caused by an ectopic atrial pacemaker often is characterized by unconducted atrial beats, and SVT from an accessory pathway usually will show the typical Wolff-Parkinson-White abnormality on the after-tachycardia ECG. There is rarely any difficulty in diagnosis when the rate is over 210 beats per minute, but frequently the question arises as to whether a tachycardia is sinus or paroxysmal supraventricular when the rate in 180 to 210 beats per minute. Slight variations in the RR interval favor the diagnosis of sinus tachycardia. The QRS complex may at times be wide because of aberrant conduction, and the tracing may resemble that of ventricular tachycardia.

Treatment

Countershock. If the infant's condition is critical, DC countershock provides the most immediate method of terminating the attack. An alternative is the use of IV verapamil with appropriate precautions as detailed in the discussion on drug therapy. In more elective situations drug therapy can be used. Whichever method is chosen, acidosis, electrolyte abnormalities, hypothermia, and hypoxemia should be corrected as far as possible. Vagal stimulation maneuvers are generally unsuccessful and may waste valuable time.

DC countershock (½ to 1 W-second per kg) usually will be successful for cardioversion. It is advisable to start at the lower dose and increase by 2 W-second increments. This may be repeated two or three times. After cardioversion digitalization is begun orally or parenterally, depending on the infant's condition.

Drug therapy

Digoxin. If countershock is unsuccessful, or if the infant is not critically ill, conversion may be accomplished by parenteral digitalization, giving half the digitalizing dose by slow intravenous push. The next two doses, each a fourth the digitalizing dose, may be given 4 to 8 hours after the preceding dose, depending on the response. Administration of digoxin should be continued for maintenance. When renal function is impaired, the digoxin dose should be reduced considerably, since the compound is eliminated almost entirely unchanged by the kidney. Serum digoxin levels and ECG monitoring are the best guides. Use of digoxin in patients with Wolff-Parkinson-White syndrome is controversial.

Propranolol hydrochloride. Propranolol is a β-adrenergic blocking agent that may be administered orally or intravenously. Intravenous administration should be reserved for emergency control of an arrhythmia at a dose of 0.01 to 0.15 mg/kg IV (Table 29-11). The drug is almost completely metabolized in the liver, with less than 2% excreted by the kidneys unchanged; however, reduced doses are still recommended in individuals with impaired renal function. β-Blocking agents should be used with caution in patients with heart failure, since maintenance of adequate cardiac output is dependent on circulating catecholamines in these patients. Atropine sulfate and isoproterenol should be immediately available to treat propranolol-induced bradycardia or hypothermia. Propanalol is especially effective in the treatment of automatic focus tachycardia. It should be used with great caution if Verapamil has been used, since the side effects tend to be additive.

Verapamil. Verapamil is a drug that acts by blocking the slow inward current of calcium, in contrast to most antiarrhythmic drugs, which block the rapid influx of sodium into cells. Verapamil has been reported to be highly effective in slowing the ventricular response of adults with atrial flutter and fibrillation and also in converting SVT to sinus rhythm. The drug must be used with caution in patients with sick sinus syndrome and is contraindicated in patients receiving β-blocking agents.

Verapamil is given as an intravenous dose of 0.1 to 0.2 mg/kg over one minute, carefully observing the ECG and blood pressure response. A second dose may be used within 2 to 3 minutes, however, Epstein and co-workers found that bradycardia and hypotension may occur. For this reason the medication should be used in an intensive care environment, with CPR equipment available. There should be two intravenous lines established, and solutions of dopamine and a calcium preparation should be ready-mixed.

Overdrive pacing. Overdrive pacing, which is pacing the heart at a rate faster than that of the tachyarrhythmia, requires introduction of a pacing wire, usually transvenously, and a pacemaker that is capable of pacing at rates up to 600 beats per minute. This technique has been used successfully in adults for conversion of tachyarrhythmias. Garson and co-workers report the successful use of this technique for cardioversion in four of the five patients in whom it was tried.

Resistant cases. If therapy proves difficult and recurrences are common, it is sometimes necessary to determine the exact mechanism of the SVT by intracardiac electrography. Different mechanisms are more likely to be suppressed by different drugs.

Surgical treatment. The majority of cases of SVT in infants and children are successfully managed medically. Gillette and co-workers report nine pediatric patients ranging in age from 6 months to 14 years with WPW syndrome who underwent surgical division of an accessory connection, or Kent's bundle, for medically unresponsive SVT. There was one death. The survivors have experienced no complications. For refractory SVT, Ott and associates reported excellent results after intraoperative electrophysiologic mapping and surgical division or cryoablation of an abberant conduction pathway or atrial ectopic focus.

Maintenance treatment. A newborn who has had one attack of SVT has an approximately 20% recurrence risk, and continued maintenance of digoxin for 6 months after the last attack is indicated. Recurrences are more likely in those with underlying Wolff-Parkinson-White syndrome, and in these patients continued maintenance of digoxin, sometimes supplemented by quinidine or propranolol, may be indicated.

Prognosis. Nadas and associates have divided infants into prognostically useful clinical groups. The first group consists primarily of boys under 4 months of age without structural heart disease; the second group is composed of older infants of both sexes with or without heart disease. Recurrences after the age of 1 year are unlikely with the first group, but recurrences are frequent with the second group, particularly if the Wolff-Parkinson-White syndrome is present.

Atrial flutter and fibrillation

Atrial flutter is infrequent in the neonate and is likely to be associated with organic heart disease, especially mitral valve disease, endocardial fibroelastosis, Ebstein's malformation of the tricuspid valve, pulmonary atresia, VSD, coarctation, and complex heart defects. Atrial flutter has been diagnosed in utero.

Atrial flutter is diagnosed when (1) the atrial rate is 220 to 400 beats per minute; (2) the atrial mechanism is regular; and (3) there is a characteristic sawtooth pattern of the flutter wave in leads II and III (Fig. 29-34). There is usually some degree of AV block. The ventricular rate will depend on the degree of AV block. If the AV block is fixed, the ventricular rate will be regular; if it is variable, the ventricular rate will be irregular.

Atrial fibrillation is rare in the newborn (Fig. 29-35). It is likely to be associated with serious organic heart disease, especially those conditions associated with left atrial enlargement. The arrhythmia may appear clinically as a tachycardia, but it is more likely to be recognized as a chaotic rhythm. The ECG shows characteristic fibrillation *f* waves and an irregular QRS response.

The clinical picture is similar to that of SVT, and the congestive heart failure may be life threatening, as in SVT.

Treatment is the same as in SVT. DC countershock is usually the most rapid method for cardioversion and should be followed by digoxin maintenance. Occasionally other drugs, such as propranolol hydrochloride, procainamide, or quinidine, may be necessary for cardioversion and/or maintenance. Verapamil has had success in infants with SVT and might be successful in treating atrial flutter or fibrillation. Campbell and associates report atrial overdrive pacing successfully used by both the transvenous and transesophageal routes.

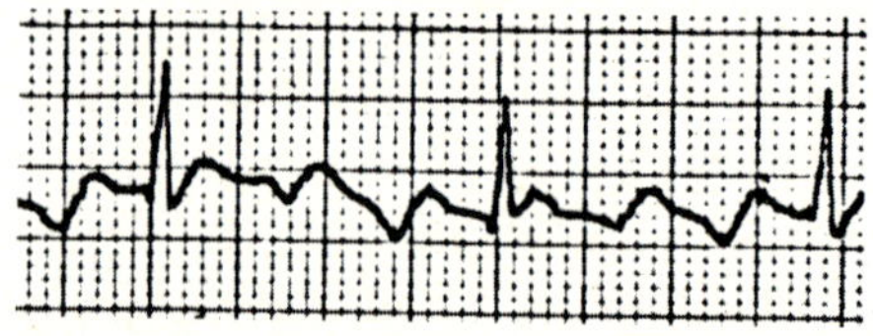

Fig. 29-34. Atrial flutter with 3:1 ventricular response. Ventricular rate is 80, atrial rate 240. The flutter waves have a "sawtooth" appearance.

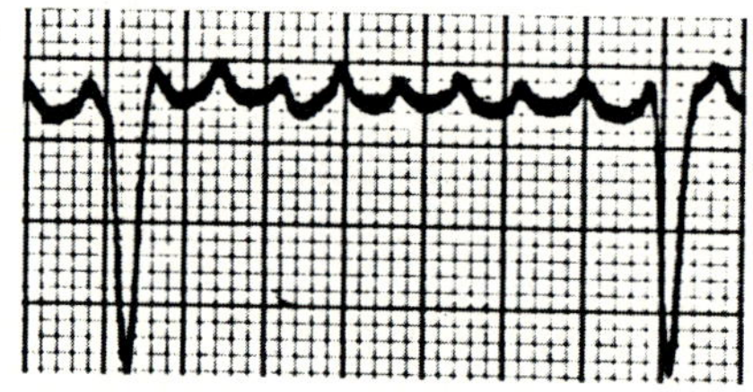

Fig. 29-35. Atrial fibrillation (12-year-old child). Ventricular rate 50 per minute, atrial rate ("f" waves) 400 per minute. On a long tracing it would be seen that the ventricular response is totally irregular.

Preexcitation syndrome (Wolff-Parkinson-White syndrome)

This syndrome (short PR interval and initial slurring and widening of the QRS) is caused by early excitation of the ventricles by an anomalous conducting bundle that conducts faster than the AV node, which it bypasses (hence the short PR interval). Recognition of the syndrome is important because of (1) the high incidence of SVT, and (2) the frequent misinterpretation of the ECG as left bundle branch block, left ventricular hypertrophy, myocardial infarction, or ventricular tachycardia. Wolff-Parkinson-White syndrome may be transient and may alternate with normal conduction (intermittent Wolff-Parkinson-White) (Fig. 29-36). The syndrome may be associated with congenital heart disease, particularly Ebstein's malformation, corrected transposition of the great arteries, dextrocardia, and complex malformations. The treatment for this condition is that of the symptomatic arrhythmias which may occur.

Ventricular tachycardia

Ventricular tachycardia in neonates most commonly occurs in the presence of organic heart disease but is rare, except as a complication of cardiac surgery, anesthesia, or cardiac catheterization. The presence of incessant ventricular tachycardia is highly suggestive of a cardiac tumor.

With the type of tracing shown in Fig. 29-37 there are four possibilities: (1) ventricular tachycardia, (2) SVT with

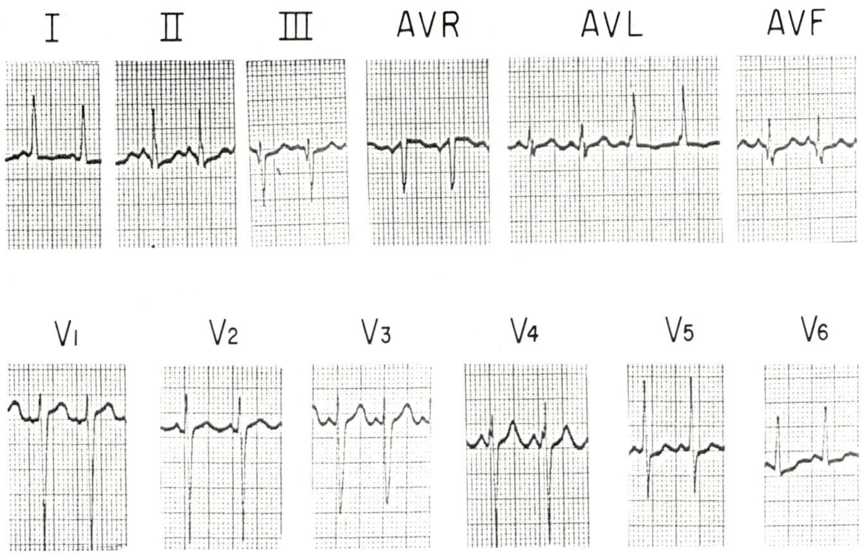

Fig. 29-36. Wolff-Parkinson-White syndrome in the neonate. PR interval is shortened (evident in most leads). QRS is slightly prolonged to 0.08 second (leads II, III, and AV_F), and there is a slurred upstroke in the R wave (lead I). The first two complexes in aV_L show normal ventricular excitation, while the next two show Wolff-Parkinson-White (ventricular preexcitation) syndrome.

aberrant conduction, (3) atrial flutter with aberrant conduction, and (4) WPW with antegrade conduction along an accessory connection. Hyperkalemia may both cause and mimic ventricular tachycardia, and the ECG changes may appear over 1 or 2 minutes. If hyperkalemia is a possibility a trial infusion of 3 ml calcium gluconate, one unit of regular insulin, and 15 ml of 25% glucose should be administered over a 5 minute period. If doubt exists, it is best to proceed directly to DC countershock (unless digitalis toxicity is thought to be present) of 5 to 15 W-seconds in a newborn. Lidocaine may be tried at a dosage of 1 to 2 mg/kg as a single rapid infusion at 20 to 30 μg/minute with continuous cardiac monitoring to warn of premature ventricular contractions or a recurrence of the ventricular tachycardia. Oral phenytoin, propranolol, bretylium tosylate, and Tocainide (a lidocaine analogue) all have been used, but the major experience is in adults.

Stevens and co-workers report four cases of ventricular tachycardia in the neonatal period. One case was detected in utero. All patients survived, two with asymptomatic episodes of ventricular ectopia on long-term follow-up analysis. In their review of the literature, of a total of 45 cases of ventricular arrhythmia in the perinatal period, nine were detected in utero, three persisted beyond the perinatal period, and two resulted in death with associated disorders.

Ectopic beats

Ectopic beats are common in healthy newborn infants, with a reported incidence of between 21% and 31% for healthy premature infants and of up to 23% for full-term newborns. Supraventricular ectopic beats are more common than ventricular ones and may arise in the atrium or AV junctional tissue. They usually are identified by a P wave of abnormal configuration, appearing earlier than the expected PP interval. The QRS that follows may be widened because of aberrancy and because the His-Purkinje system may not be fully repolarized from the preceding normal beat.

Multiple ectopic beats usually pose no threat to life unless they occur within the framework of organic heart disease. Thus the infant with tight valvular pulmonic stenosis may develop heart failure when multiple ectopic beats develop; the relative inefficiency of the ectopic beats leads to a lowered cardiac output. By contrast, normal infants may have alarming runs of ectopic beats and be asymptomatic.

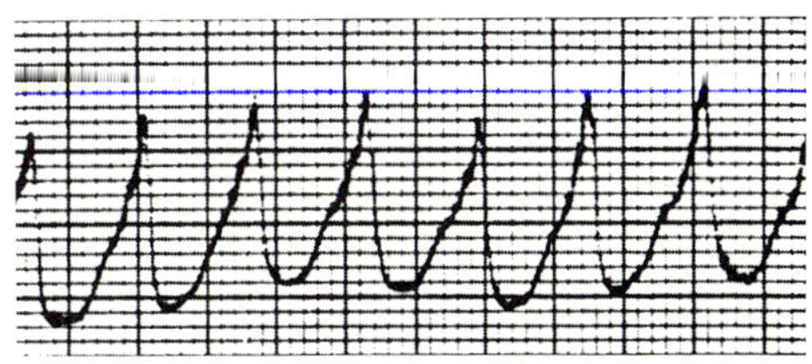

Fig. 29-37. Ventricular tachycardia. Rate is 200 per minute, and there is grossly abnormal ventricular conduction with wide bizarre QRS complexes. (For differential diagnosis, see text).

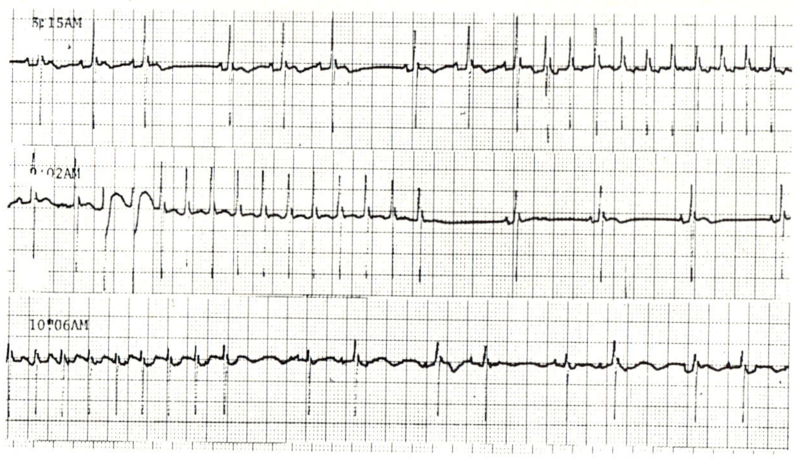

Fig. 29-38. Sinus node dysfunction (sick sinus syndrome) in 2-day-old infant. Note periods of sinus bradycardia and periods of SVT. This child was treated with pacemaker for periods of sinus bradycardia that were frequent and symptomatic. Another child in the family was a victim of SIDS.

Ventricular ectopic beats should be regarded more seriously than atrial ectopic beats, especially if they are multifocal, or if there are short runs of ectopic beats, since these may portend the development of ventricular tachycardia or fibrillation. Treatment of ectopic beats in the asymptomatic infant is usually not indicated because the antiarrhythmic drugs have a negative inotropic action and because ventricular tachycardia is a rare complication.

When heart disease is present and it appears likely that ectopic beats are compromising cardiac output, an attempt should be made to suppress them with drugs. The drugs most likely to be successful are phenytoin, propranolol, and quinidine.

Sinoatrial node disorders

SA node disorders are rare in newborns and children and, when they occur, are usually the result of surgery. When there is failure of impulse formation within the sinus node or of transmission of the sinus node impulse to the rest of the atrium, the heart rhythm will be dependent on the escape rhythm arising in the AV junctional tissue. Symptoms from sinus node disease therefore only result when there is also disease in the conducting tissue beyond the sinus node. Sick sinus syndrome has been divided into type I, characterized by periods of bradycardia and sinus arrest, the type II, with paroxysmal tachycardia.

Yabek and co-workers performed electrophysiologic studies on 18 children with sinus node dysfunction and were able to identify at least three different mechanisms. Lev and co-workers studied the conduction system in two children who had prolonged sinus node dysfunction and found degeneration and fibrosis of the approaches to the SA and AV nodes and atrial preferential pathways in one child and fatty infiltration of these areas in the other.

Management consists of appropriate treatment for the tachyarrhythmias. However, sometimes pacemaker implantation is necessary because the bradycardia becomes life threatening. We have seen one newborn with intermittent symptomatic bradyarrhythmias with sinus arrest and paroxysmal tachyarrhythmias (Fig. 29-38). She was treated with prophylactic pacemaker implantation. A previous child in the family had been the victim of sudden infant death syndrome (SIDS).

Atrioventricular block

AV block in newborns is unusual, but when it occurs, it is usually asymptomatic. It may be secondary to digitalis administration or viral infections. Some types of congenital heart disease have an increased incidence of AV block. These include corrected transposition of the great arteries, ASD, Ebstein's anomaly of the tricuspid valve, and complex cyanotic cardiac defects.

When the PR interval is prolonged, first-degree AV block is said to be present. In normal newborns the PR interval may range from 0.08 to 0.12 seconds. The most common cause of first-degree heart block in the newborn is digitalis effect.

Second-degree AV block is present when not all atrial beats are conducted to the ventricle. The most common form was first described by Wenkebach and is also called Mobitz type I. In Mobitz type I the PR interval progressively lengthens until an atrial beat fails to be conducted to the ventricles and there is a dropped beat. Mobitz type II block also occurs in the newborn (Fig. 29-39). In this form of second-degree AV block, ventric-

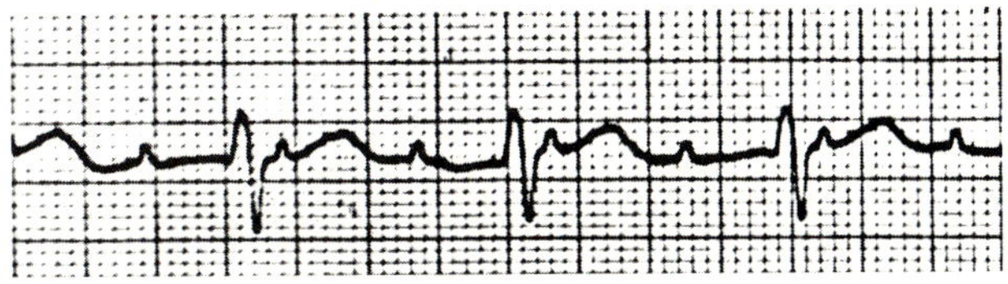

Fig. 29-39. Second-degree AV block (Mobitz type II). Every second P wave gives rise to a QRS complex after a long PR interval.

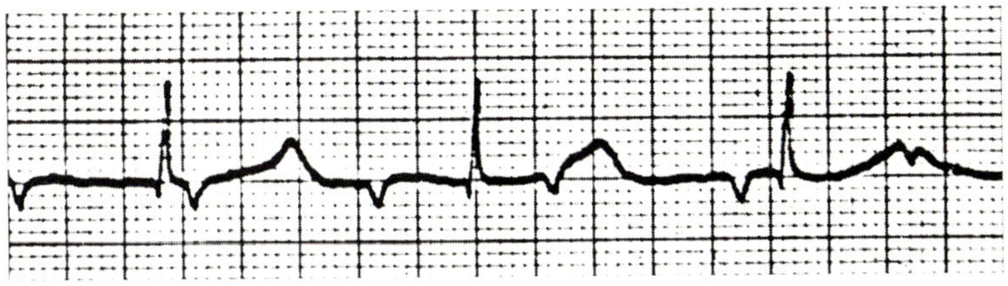

Fig. 29-40. Complete (third-degree) AV block. Note that the P wave rate exceeds the QRS rate and that there is no constant PR interval.

ular beats are dropped without preceding PR-interval prolongation. The PR interval for conducted beats usually is constant.

Third-degree heart block (complete heart block) in the newborn is most often congenital (Fig. 29-40). In an international cooperative study on congenital complete heart block it was estimated that 1 in 20,000 live-born infants has congenital complete heart block.

There is an association with various forms of congenital heart disease, the most common of which is corrected transposition of the great arteries. Familial clusterings have been reported, and in the cooperative study there were 599 patients, among whom were 14 families with two siblings affected. Approximately a third (181 of 599) of the patients in the study had complicating heart disease.

For those without complicating heart disease the risk of death was greatest in early infancy. Approximately three fourths passed their fifth birthday, and a third were older than 10 years. Ninety-two percent of the 418 subjects without complicating heart disease were alive at last examination.

For those patients with associated congenital heart disease the prognosis was not as good, with the risk of dying highest in early infancy. Of 181 patients, 71% were alive at the last examination. Thirty of the 36 deaths were in the first week of life.

In addition to associated heart disease, the risk factor most prevalent for early death was slow ventricular rate and rapid atrial rate. The prognosis was better for infants whose ventricular rate was greater than 55 and whose atrial rate was less than 140 beats per minute.

The occurrence of congenital complete heart block in infants of women with connective tissue disorders has been recognized. McCue and co-workers report 22 children with congenital complete heart block, of whom 14 were born to 11 mothers with clinical or laboratory evidence of connective tissue disorder, primarily lupus erythematosus. This association has been further documented by other groups. Complete AV block is now often discovered prenatally (see section on prenatal arrhythmias) (see Fig. 29-29).

Drug treatment to increase the heart rate, such as with atropine and isoproterenol, has had only limited success. Pacemaker therapy, particularly before congestive heart failure occurs, has been the most successful intervention. The judgment regarding timing of pacemaker implantation remains difficult, particularly since in the absence of associated heart disease the individual who survives infancy with congenital complete heart block probably will do well for many years. Benrey and associates reviewed the indications for and results of pacemaker implantation in children at Baylor. The indications included symptoms of cerebrovascular insufficiency and congestive heart failure and, in a newborn, a ventricular rate below 50 and an atrial rate over 150 beats per minute.

Levy and associates monitored 20 children with congenital complete heart block and found many with bradyarrhythmias, particularly during sleep. These authors recommend that all children with complete heart block have electromagnetic tape recordings at fairly frequent intervals.

CARDIAC ARREST AND EXTREME BRADYCARDIA

Apparent cardiac arrest—that is, lack of audible heartbeat, cardiac impulse, or peripheral pulse—usually is caused by ventricular asystole or extreme bradycardia

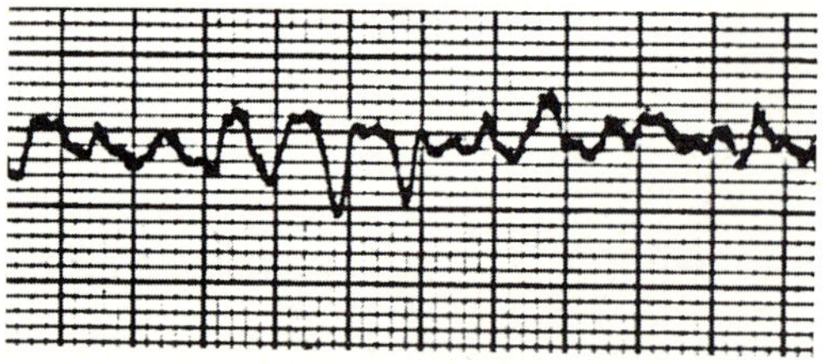

Fig. 29-41. Ventricular fibrillation. Chaotic electrical ventricular activity associated with complete ineffectiveness of ventricular contraction.

rather than by ventricular fibrillation (Fig. 29-41). Either of these two events may be the result of primary respiratory failure. Ventricular asystole and ventricular fibrillation can be distinguished by an ECG. However, it is essential that treatment be started immediately without losing valuable minutes locating an ECG machine and attaching leads. In many neonates there is no doubt as to whether cardiac arrest has occurred. The majority of sick neonates are already having their heart rates monitored, and the alarm is set to sound at a rate of 80 beats per minute. By the time someone reaches the baby, the rate may have fallen to 60 and be continuing to decrease. Treatment should be initiated without waiting for the infant to deteriorate further. It first needs to be determined whether bradycardia or cardiac arrest is primary or is secondary to respiratory failure. In many immature and sick infants bradycardia is secondary to respiratory arrest, and prompt respiratory resuscitation takes first priority and often restores the heart rate to normal. When respirations cease, heart rate and cardiac output fall. In other instances the neonate has become too hypoxemic and acidotic for respiratory resuscitation alone to restore the heartbeat. In this situation cardiac resuscitation is required. Pupillary dilation begins within 45 seconds after circulation stops and is complete by about 1 minute 45 seconds.

Cardiac resuscitation of the neonate

Bradycardia with a heart rate falling to 40 beats per minute or below is the most frequent indication for cardiac resuscitation in the neonate. Ventricular asystole without prior bradycardia is unusual, and ventricular fibrillation is rarely observed except in the terminal stages of advanced heart disease.

The following guidelines assume that pulmonary ventilation is being assisted either by face mask or endotracheal tube and that the heart rate is either inaudible or below 50 beats per minute. Check for audible heart sounds. The hearing of regular heart sounds, however slow, rules out ventricular fibrillation. Flick the precordium over the midsternum, and listen again (equivalent to the chest "thump" in adults). If the heart rate is still inadequate, immediately start external massage. If two people are present, try to alternate cardiac massage and ventilation (40 seconds of cardiac massage to 20 seconds of ventilation). Examine ECG to distinguish ventricular asystole (straight line or occasional bizarre QRS complexes), ventricular fibrillation (irregular chaotic line) (Fig. 29-41) and complete heart block (Fig. 29-40). Precordial compression causes an obvious artifact. If ventricular fibrillation is present, defibrillate with external DC countershock until conversion (usually 5 to 15 W-seconds). If an acceptable rhythm with evidence of adequate cardiac output does not occur, resume cardiac massage. After 4 or 5 minutes of cardiac arrest and reduced cardiac output during external massage, the blood will be acidotic; sodium bicarbonate should be given intravenously (2 to 6 mEq/kg). If there has been no response after 5 to 10 minutes of ventilation, external cardiac massage, and alkali therapy, consider the use of pharmacologic agents and cardiac pacing. The pharmacologic agents that may be tried include:

1. Epinephrine: 0.2 ml/kg of a 1:10,000 solution, intravenous or intracardiac.
2. Isoproterenol: 0.1 to 0.4 μg/kg/minute by intravenous infusion or single doses of 1 μg/kg by intravenous or intracardiac route every 5 minutes.
3. Calcium chloride: 0.5 to 1 ml of 10% solution administered intravenously or by intracardiac route every 5 minutes.
4. Atropine may be indicated if second or third-degree AV block is present; intravenous dose of 0.01 mg/kg.
5. Lidocaine may be indicated in the rare instance where ineffective contraction is caused by ventricular arrhythmias that are resistant to DC countershock alone; in infants 0.5 to 2.0 mg/kg may be given immediately before countershock and repeated every 10 to 15 minutes.

If effective cardiac contraction cannot be restored with one of these agents, it is advisable to pause and determine whether brain damage is irreversible and resuscitation should be stopped or whether an attempt at cardiac pacing is warranted.

Cardiac pacing

Indications for cardiac pacing include bradycardia, cardiac arrest, digitalis intoxication, and complete heart block. The temporary bradycardia associated with the salt-losing crisis of congenital adrenal hyperplasia or any other condition from which it is possible for the infant to recover may warrant pacing. By contrast, a neonate with bradycardia from the terminal stages of RDS or the hypoplastic left-heart syndrome would not be a candidate for a pacemaker.

External pacing is rarely effective. Internal transvenous pacemaker catheters may be placed via the external jugular vein, with the tip lodged in the trabeculations of the right ventricle (see Fig. 29-30) or, if the AV node is functional, in the right atrium. An alternative short-term route is the femoral vein (usually it is not possible to enter the right ventricle from the umbilical vein). The pacing rate should be 100 to 140 beats per minute. Usually a current of 0.5 to 1.0 MA is necessary to obtain a response. Because electrical response is no guarantee of mechanical response, heart sounds and pulses should be checked before it is concluded that the heart is actually propelling blood. The Doppler ultrasound flowmeter is particularly useful for this purpose. If temporary transvenous pacing is successful and the source of the bradycardia is not removed (as in complete AV block), it will be necessary to implant long-term epicardial or myocardial pacemaker wires.

COMMON CARDIOVASCULAR DISORDERS PRODUCING SERIOUS DISEASE IN THE NEONATE

A classification of the structural disorders more commonly encountered in neonatal practice is offered in the outline below.

A. Transposition of the great arteries
   1. D-transposition
   2. L-transposition
B. Left-sided heart obstruction
   1. Hypoplastic left-heart syndrome
   2. Congenital aortic stenosis
   3. Preductal and juxtaductal coarctation of the aorta
   4. Postductal coarctation
C. Right-sided heart obstruction
   1. Pulmonary atresia or extreme pulmonic stenosis with intact ventricular septum
   2. Pulmonary atresia with open ventricular septum, and severe tetralogy of Fallot
   3. Peripheral pulmonary artery stenosis
   4. Tricuspid atresia with and without transposition
   5. Ebstein's anomaly of the tricuspid valve
D. Lesions that produce common mixing of venous and arterial blood
   1. Truncus arteriosus
   2. Single ventricle
   3. Double-outlet right ventricle without pulmonic stenosis
   4. Total anomalous pulmonary venous return
E. Left-to-right shunts
   1. PDA
   2. VSD
   3. Combined PDA and VSD
   4. Common AV canal
   5. Systemic arteriovenous fistula
F. Myocardial disorders
   1. Myocarditis
   2. Endocardial fibroelastosis
   3. Anomalous left coronary artery
   4. Glycogen storage disease
   5. Diabetic cardiomyopathy
G. Miscellaneous
   1. Absent pulmonary valve
   2. Tricuspid insufficiency
   3. Cor triatriatum
   4. Dextrocardia

Transposition of the great arteries

Incidence

The incidence of transposition is between 0.022% and 0.047% of live births (1:2,130 to 1:4,500). Transposition is a common defect, and early recognition is of major importance; hundreds of neonates born with complete transposition of the great arteries have had the defect corrected and are leading normal lives. Males outnumber females 2 to 1, and there is some evidence that they have a higher-than-average birth weight.

Pathology

The aorta arises anteriorly and from the venous ventricle, whereas the pulmonary artery arises posteriorly and from the arterial ventricle. With dextrotransposition (d-transposition) the aortic valve is to the right of the pulmonary valve, whereas with levotransposition (l-transposition) the aortic valve is to the left of the pulmonary valve (Fig. 29-42). There is a well-developed muscular subaortic infundibulum, in contrast to the muscular subpulmonary infundibulum characteristic of the normal heart.

D-transpositions outnumber l-transpositions as a cause for major concern in the newborn period by at least 10 to 1. As a generalization, one can say that d-transposition is a relatively "pure" lesion usually associated only with patent foramen ovale, PDA, and VSD. L-transposition, by contrast, often is associated with dextrocardia, situs inversus, and asplenia when it appears in the newborn period. When it appears in older infants and children, it is usually physiologically "corrected," most commonly by ventricular inversion; unfortunately there are almost always additional lesions present, such as mitral regurgitation, VSD, and subpulmonic stenosis.

Transposition of the great arteries is sometimes associated with a very large VSD or common ventricle, in which case the fact that the great vessels are transposed becomes of secondary importance. The association of tri-

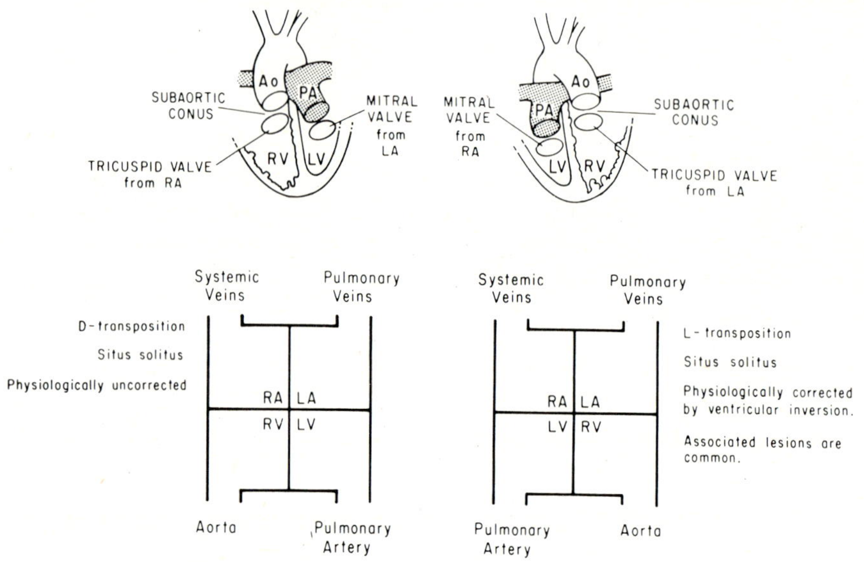

Fig. 29-42. The two most common types of transposition of the great arteries leading to problems in the neonatal period. In both types the aortic valve is high and anterior and arises from the coarsely trabeculated right (venous) ventricle. d-Transposition (left panel) is the common transposition causing problems in the newborn period.

cuspid atresia and transposition is not unusual and leads to common mixing at the left atrial level. The adequacy of systemic (aortic) flow then depends on the size of an associated VSD or PDA.

The major emphasis in this section, then, is on the common d-transposition with situs solitus (normal location of the heart and viscera). Brief mention is made of the most common form of l-transposition—the physiologically corrected (by ventricular inversion) transposition in which the frequently associated VSD and left AV valve regurgitation may give rise to heart failure in the neonate.

D-transposition of the great arteries

D-transposition with intact ventricular septum and small or absent ductus arteriosus. Neonates with transposition and intact ventricular septum are extremely cyanotic and if untreated, usually die in the first few days of life as the ductus arteriosus closes. Conversely, if the ductus arteriosus remains open, there is better mixing of venous and arterial circulations but usually at the expense of pulmonary artery hypertension. If there is only a foramen ovale or ASD, it is necessary for bidirectional shunting to occur at the atrial level; whereas if the duct also is open, a common sequence is for right-to-left shunting to occur at the atrial level and for there to be left-to-right (aorta to pulmonary artery) shunting at the ductal level. The latter situation might seem hemodynamically acceptable; but unfortunately the ductus is frequently very large, and pulmonary artery pressure is at systemic levels.

Clinical manifestations. Cyanosis is present from birth, although the temporary patency of the ductus arteriosus may allow some shunting, and the recognition of cyanosis may be delayed. The breathing rate is characteristically increased to 45 to 80 breaths per minute; there are usually no signs of respiratory distress unless the infant has associated respiratory tract infection. The peripheral pulses are normal. The cardiac impulse is often normal for the first hours or days but thereafter becomes hyperdynamic. The heart sounds are normal, and frequently there is no cardiac murmur. If a heart murmur is audible, it is likely to be nondescript and grade 3 or less in intensity, probably representing the murmur of a closing ductus. As time passes, the neonate becomes progressively more cyanotic; and when arteriovenous mixing is inadequate over a prolonged period, respiratory and metabolic acidosis ensues. Finally if untreated, the infant dies from a combination of hypoxemia and acidosis during the first or second week of life if there is only a patent foramen ovale for exchange of arterial and venous blood.

Diagnosis. Initially the chest roentgenogram may appear normal. However, as time passes, it becomes apparent that the heart is abnormally large and somewhat eggshaped and that the pulmonary vascular markings are increased (Fig. 29-43). The classic roentgenogram of transposition shows, in addition, a narrow mediastinum when viewed anteroposteriorly and a widened mediastinum when viewed laterally. There is usually nothing diagnostically helpful in the ECG tracing. Almost always a mild degree of right ventricular hypertrophy is present, similar to that seen in a wide variety of cardiac and pul-

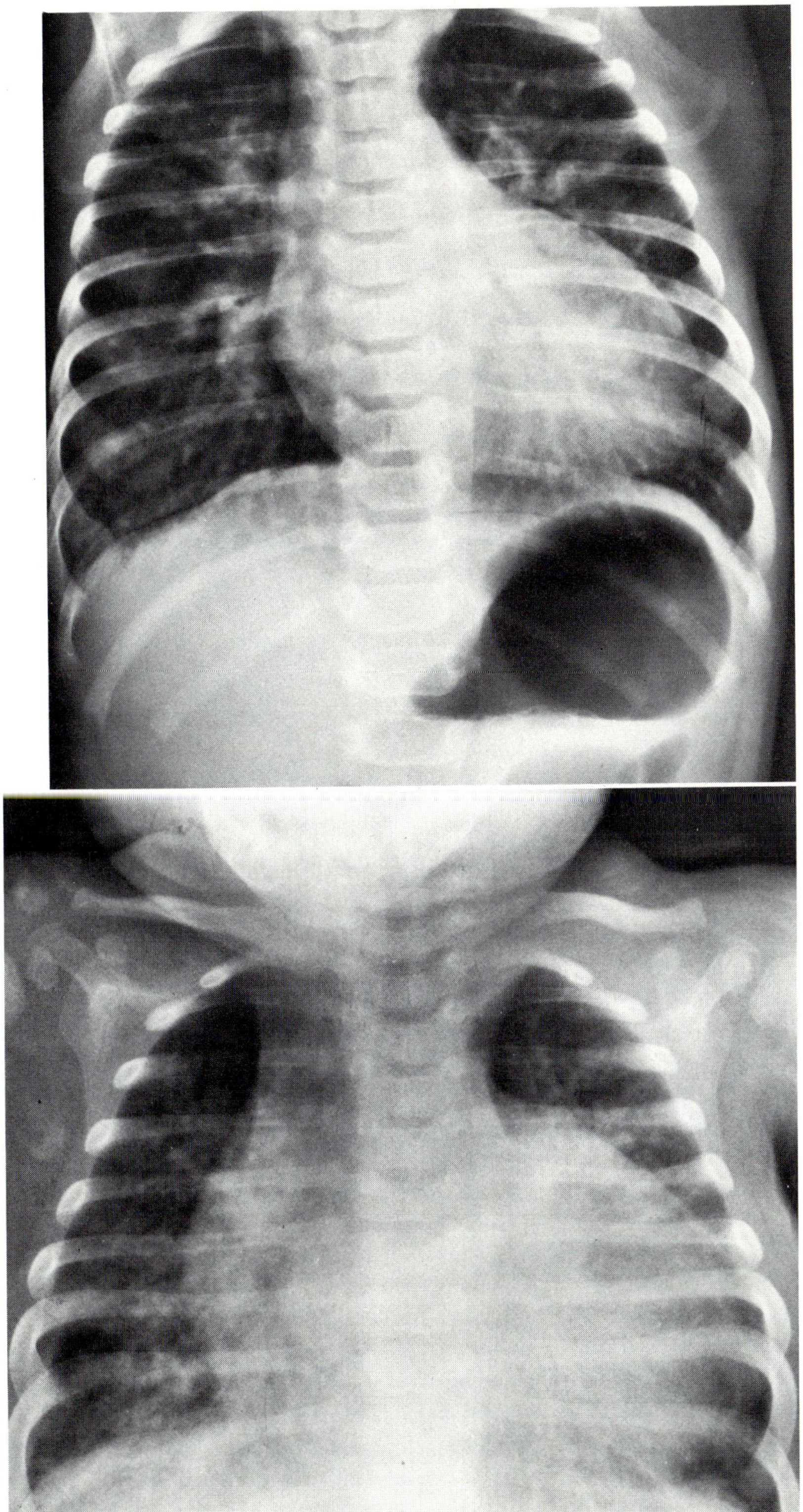

Fig. 29-43. Anteroposterior chest films of two neonates with d-transposition of the great arteries. **A,** Note narrow mediastinum, "egg-on-side" appearance, cardiomegaly, and pulmonary plethora. **B,** Note massive cardiomegaly caused by heart failure.

monary diseases in which the right ventricle is working at systemic pressure.

The arterial oxygen saturation while the infant is breathing room air is usually in the 30% to 70% range, corresponding to a PaO_2 of approximately 15 to 33 mm Hg. The $PaCO_2$ may remain normal or even decreased for surprising periods because of some alveolar hyperventilation. The $PaCO_2$ usually rises on the second or third day of life to 50 or 60 mm Hg, higher in the very severely hypoxemic baby. Similarly the arterial pH may remain normal for a time (because of an increase in plasma bicarbonate level), but it inevitably declines in the severely sick infant because of a combination of the accumulation of the products of anaerobic metabolism and the failure of the lungs to eliminate adequate CO_2. Although the total lung blood flow is increased in infants with transposition, the effective pulmonary blood flow (that fraction derived from the systemic venous return) is decreased.

In most infants 100% O_2 breathing will increase arterial PO_2 by only a few millimeters of mercury (because of the slightly increased O_2 content of pulmonary capillary blood). An occasional infant with transposition, however, shows a much more dramatic response to 100% O_2, with arterial PO_2 increasing from 30 to 70 mm Hg and the infant changing from cyanotic to nearly acyanotic. This change is the result of the effect of oxygen on pulmonary arterioles, causing a fall in pulmonary vascular resistance and allowing an increase in existing atrial, ventricular, and ductus shunts. The net effect is greater crossover between venous and arterial circuits.

Echocardiography. An accurate noninvasive technique, two-dimensional echocardiography, is used for establishing the diagnosis of transposition and revealing associated anomalies. Imaging from the subcostal position allows one to visualize the great arteries and their respective ventricular alignments. Specifically, in the newborn infant the echocardiographer can easily visualize the main pulmonary trunk and its branches originating from the left ventricle confirming the diagnosis (Fig. 29-44). Rare but clinically important atrioventricular valve abnormalities such as a straddling tricuspid valve, anomalous mitral valve attachments, and accessory tricuspid valve tissue aneurysms can be detected with careful imaging.

After cardiac catheterization, two-dimensional echocardiography can also be used to assess the adequacy of a balloon atrial septostomy. Direct visualization of the interatrial septum is easily accomplished, and the tear in the septum primum of the fossa ovalis can be directly measured.

Hemodynamics and angiocardiography. The major problem is lack of communication between pulmonary and systemic circulations after birth. Transposition is of little consequence while the baby is in utero. Infants with

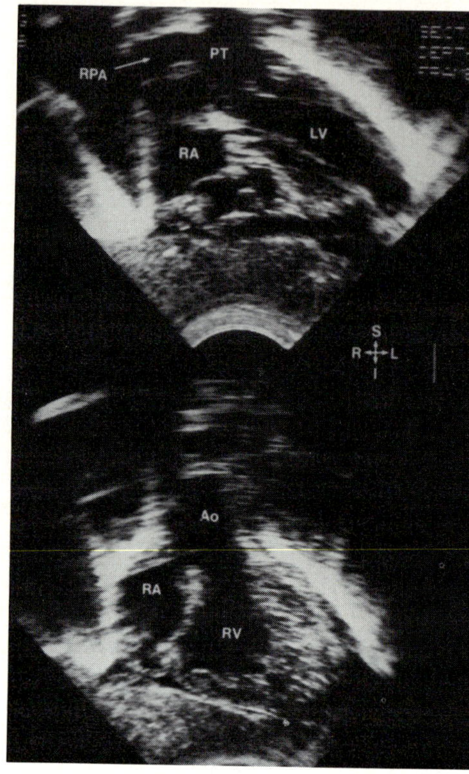

Fig. 29-44. Transposition of the great arteries with intact ventricular septum. *Top,* Subcostal long axis view of the left ventricle *(LV)* revealing the pulmonary trunk *(PT)* originating from the LV. *Bottom,* Anterior angulation from subcostal long-axis view reveals origin of the aorta *(Ao)* from the right ventricle *(RV)*. *I,* inferior; *L,* left; *R,* right; *RA,* right atrium; *RPA,* right pulmonary artery; *S,* superior.

transposition are typically large, well-nourished infants and frequently give no cause for concern during the first minutes and hours of life. The deterioration of the infant thereafter corresponds to gradual constriction of the ductus arteriosus. The low PO_2 perfusing this structure appears to lose its vasodilating effect within hours to a day or two after birth. When the ductus arteriosus closes, the infant is totally reliant on a foramen ovale or ASD for the exchange of venous and arterial blood; unless the ASD is large, death will rapidly ensue from hypoxemia, hypercapnia, and acidosis (Fig. 29-45).

The major abnormal hemodynamic findings are a right ventricular pressure that is at systemic level and a left ventricular pressure (left ventricle supplies the pulmonary artery) that may be high or low, depending on the pulmonary blood flow and pulmonary vascular resistance (assuming there is no pulmonic stenosis). Aortic oxygen saturation is lower than pulmonary artery saturation; arterial oxygen saturations of about 30% to 40% are not uncommon. The catheter passes easily from the inferior vena cava to the right atrium, right ventricle, and out

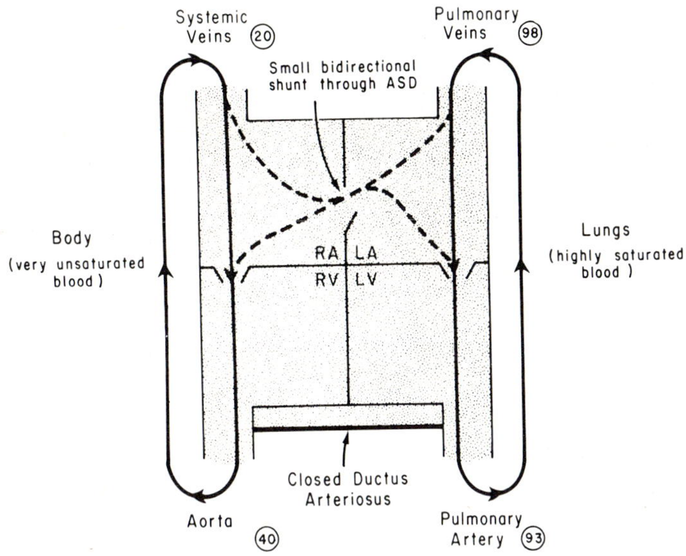

Fig. 29-45. The course of the circulation in d-transposition with intact ventricular septum. Typical oxygen saturations are circled. Small bidirectional shunts of equal magnitude across the atrial septum allow insufficient oxygen to reach the tissues for the maintenance of adequate oxidative metabolism.

into the anteriorly placed aorta. In the majority of cases it also can be passed easily across the foramen ovale into the left atrium and left ventricle.

Right ventricular angiography in the lateral projection reveals the high, anterior location of the aortic valve and the presence or absence of a VSD. Left ventricular angiography discloses the posteriorly located pulmonary artery.

Treatment. Prostaglandin E_1 is indicated as initial therapy whenever acidosis or severe hypoxemia appears to be due to a closing ductus arteriosus. The improvement may be marked and allow subsequent balloon atrial septostomy to be performed on a more metabolically stable infant. Balloon septostomy has allowed definitive treatment frequently to commence during the course of cardiac catheterization. The pressure gradient between the left and right atrium is measured; the larger the gradient, the smaller the foramen ovale or ASD. Patients with a demonstrable gradient will benefit from enlargement of the communication, and even those without a gradient may obtain some beneficial effect from balloon septostomy. Our policy has been to proceed with septostomy from the femoral vein approach whether or not a gradient is demonstrable. Opening of the atrial septum by balloon is achieved by placing the tip of a balloon catheter in the left atrium, inflating it with 2 to 3 ml dilute contrast agent, and rapidly pulling it back across the atrial septum to rupture the thin "membrane" covering the foramen ovale, and in some cases to tear the adjacent interatrial septum. Several results may follow balloon septostomy:

1. Balloon septostomy may be dramatically successful in some babies. Arterial O_2 saturation increases from a moribund 40% to a respectable 80%, and the improvement is maintained. The infant survives and can be operated on with a baffle procedure at the age of 4 to 12 months.
2. The balloon septostomy may be partially successful. The baby's arterial saturation remains satisfactory for days or weeks, but then increasing cyanosis recurs. A second balloon septostomy after the age of 6 weeks is not usually beneficial. The choice is surgical removal of part of the atrial septum versus repair by means of a baffle procedure (switching of the venous return to match the transposed arteries). The choice depends on the weight of the infant (although total repair is now possible at 3 kg) and the experiences and preferences of the surgeon.
3. The balloon septostomy may be totally unsuccessful; early atrial septectomy or baffle procedure is desirable. Our choice is now that of the Senning baffle procedure, which has been successful even in a 2,500 gm infant.

The procedure is not totally corrective in as much as the right ventricle is required to perform systemic work for the rest of the child's life. Early attempts at an arterial switch operation were fraught with high mortality often caused by the unpreparedness of the left ventricle to work against the systemic vascular resistance. There is now a resurgence of interest in the arterial switch operation because of the concept of "preparing" the left ventricle by prior (2 to 3 months) pulmonary artery banding. In some centers the "arterial switch" procedure is being used as the definitive treatment for the neonate with d-transposition of the great arteries. The rationale is that the left ventricle is most prepared to undertake systemic work in the first few days after birth.

D-transposition with open ventricular septum. The presence of a moderate or large VSD might appear to be advantageous to the baby with transposed great arteries because of the better mixing of venous and arterial streams. Any small advantage, however, is more than offset by the greater frequency of pulmonary hypertension and heart failure. In addition, surgical correction is more difficult.

Clinical manifestations. The symptoms tend to be those of right- and left-sided heart failure rather than severe cyanosis. Neonates with transposition and large VSD frequently appear only mildly cyanotic. The cardiac impulse is hyperdynamic; the signs of heart failure are present; and a loud lower left sternal border pansystolic murmur suggests a VSD.

Diagnosis. This condition may simulate a large VSD, common ventricle, or even truncus arteriosus. On the roentgenogram the heart is seen to be large and the pulmonary vascular markings increased. The ECG shows right ventricular hypertrophy and is frequently helpful.

Hemodynamics. The large interventricular communication usually results in both pulmonary hypertension and greatly increased lung blood flow. The latter leads to a raised left atrial pressure and more rapid onset of pulmonary vascular obliterative disease. Right and left ventricular pressures are equal. Pulmonary arterial saturation is higher than aortic saturation.

Echocardiography. Details of the intracardiac anatomy and great arteries are usually well seen on two-dimensional echocardiographic examination.

Cardiac catheterization and angiocardiography. The catheter course may proceed from the inferior vena cava to the right atrium, to the right ventricle, and to the aorta, or it frequently crosses the VSD to enter the posteriorly placed pulmonary artery. The lateral angiocardiogram reveals the VSD.

Treatment. The neonate with transposition, a large VSD, pulmonary hypertension, and increased pulmonary vascular resistance may make good progress during the neonatal period at the expense of progressive pulmonary vascular obliterative disease. Neonates with transposition appear to do fairly well yet almost invariably develop rapidly advancing pulmonary vascular resistance. One approach is pulmonary artery banding (to reduce distal pulmonary artery hypertension) with or without atrial septectomy, followed by baffle procedure at the earliest possible time. An alternative approach is that of early total correction (by arterial switch and closure of VSD) before pulmonary vascular obliterative disease has advanced too far.

D-transposition with other anomalies. PDA is common with transposition, and life expectancy is reduced in infants with these conditions when compared with those having similar transposition but without PDA. Pulmonic stenosis is also common but usually is recognized only in the older infant or child. The site of obstruction is commonly below the pulmonary valve, and it is a progressive lesion. Relief of subpulmonic stenosis is surgically difficult. Recent experience indicates that the atrial baffle correction of venous inflow, leaving the subpulmonic stenosis intact, may be the optimal treatment for infants. If subpulmonic stenosis is severe, an anterior (Waterston) shunt may be indicated.

L-transposition of the great arteries

The presence of a VSD or left AV valve regurgitation complicating l-transposition (the common form of "corrected" transposition) may lead to heart failure in the newborn period. As in "uncorrected" transposition, pulmonary vascular disease appears to advance at a faster rate than is the case with normally placed great arteries. On occasion a newborn is encountered with corrected transposition, a VSD, and pulmonary hypertension leading to heart failure. These infants may require pulmonary artery banding to limit pulmonary artery blood flow in an attempt to prevent the progress of pulmonary vascular disease. An alternative approach to the infant with l-transposition of the great arteries with VSD and evidence of early onset of pulmonary vascular obliterative disease is that of early surgical closure of the VSD; however, the defects tend to be large, and mortality from corrective surgery in infancy is high.

Left-sided heart obstruction

Left-sided heart obstructive disease is a frequent cause of death in the neonatal period. The designation left-sided heart obstruction is misleading, since various lesions frequently coexist. The following fairly distinctive entities are the most commonly encountered: (1) hypoplastic left-heart syndrome, (2) isolated valvular aortic stenosis, (3) preductal and juxtaductal coarctation of the aorta, and (4) postductal coarctation.

Hypoplastic left-heart syndrome

The term hypoplastic left-heart syndrome covers a group of left-sided heart defects commonly associated with each other. The major components are mitral valve atresia, underdevelopment of the left ventricle (small cavity), aortic valve atresia, and hypoplasia of the ascending aorta. A clinical diagnosis of the syndrome is often possible, but exact delineation of the anatomy requires echocardiography and/or angiocardiography. The hypoplastic left-heart syndrome has some overlap with the preductal coarctation syndrome; however, we shall consider the latter diagnosis to apply only to those cases with a normal-sized left ventricular cavity and normal ascending aorta.

Clinical manifestations. The age at diagnosis is usually from 1 to 21 days. The signs and symptoms are most often those of left-sided failure and varying degrees of cyanosis. The typical infant is apathetic and has reduced skin blood flow. Central cyanosis is present, and the arterial pulses are of reduced volume. Doppler measurement of blood pressure commonly is about 60/30 mm Hg in all limbs. The infant breathes rapidly, and frequently there are rales. The precordial impulse is a slightly overactive unless the neonate is in the final cardiogenic shock phase of his disease. Auscultation most frequently reveals normal timing of the heart sounds but a pulmonary closure sound of increased intensity. Gallop rhythms are common.

Diagnosis. The chest roentgenogram shows that the heart is large, but the contour is not usually diagnostically helpful. If mitral atresia is dominant, the characteristic vascular pattern of pulmonary venous engorgement may be present. The ECG frequently shows a right ventricular hypertrophy pattern (accentuated by the small-sized left ventricle). There may be signs of left, right, or biatrial hypertrophy.

Echocardiography. Two-dimensional echocardiography has become a valuable diagnostic tool for the noninvasive visualization of the hypoplastic left ventricle. With subcostal imaging one can readily see a greatly enlarged right ventricle and pulmonary artery (Fig. 29-46). The left ventricle cavity may vary from slitlike to mildly hypoplastic depending on the size of the mitral valve annulus. From the suprasternal notch view the diminutive ascending aorta can be identified, and patent ductus arteriosus can usually be seen connecting the main pulmonary artery and the descending aorta. Pulsed Doppler may be used to help confirm the diagnosis of either aortic or mitral atresia by demonstrating the absence of prograde flow across each valve. Many centers now regard the typical echocardiogram as obviating the need for cardiac catheterization. Our own approach is to supplement the echocardiogram with an aortogram using the umbilical artery catheter for injection. The stringlike hypoplastic ascending aorta is easily recognized (Fig. 29-47). If the diagnosis is in doubt following these studies, a diagnostic cardiac catheterization may be necessary.

The pH is usually normal unless hypoxemia is extreme. The Pa_{CO_2} is normal until left-sided heart failure has produced alveolar transudate and alveolar hypoventilation. Intially there is little response to oxygen breathing because pulmonary capillary blood is almost completely saturated; however, when left-sided heart failure ensues,

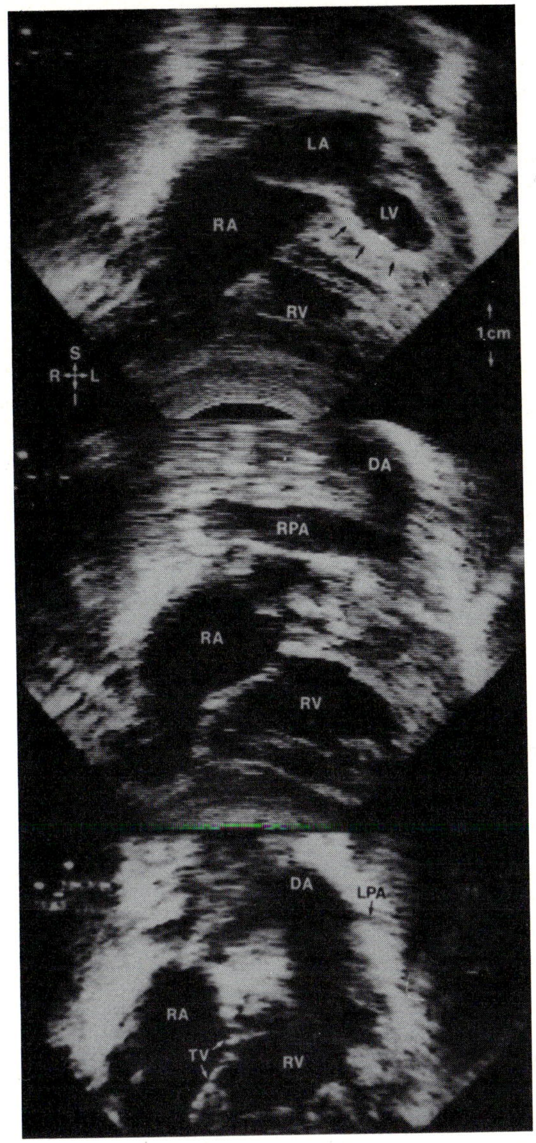

Fig. 29-46. Hypoplastic left heart syndrome. *Top,* Subcostal four chamber view showing a hypoplastic left ventricle *(LV)* and echodensity of the ventricular septum *(black arrows)* suggesting LV fibrosis. *Center,* Cranial angulation reveals a dilated right pulmonary artery *(RPA)* and ductus arteriosus *(DA). Bottom,* Increased cranial angulation reveals a dilated right ventricle *(RV)* in continuity with the main pulmonary and DA. *LA,* left atrium; *LPA,* left pulmonary artery; *RA,* right atrium; *TV,* tricuspid valve. (Courtesy James C. Huhta, Houston, Tex.)

the hypoxemia caused by alveolar hypoventilation is abolished, whereas that caused by right-to-left shunting remains. Hypoglycemia is frequent, and its recognition and correction improve the chances for survival.

Hemodynamics. The hemodynamics are variable. With mitral atresia it is necessary for blood to flow from left

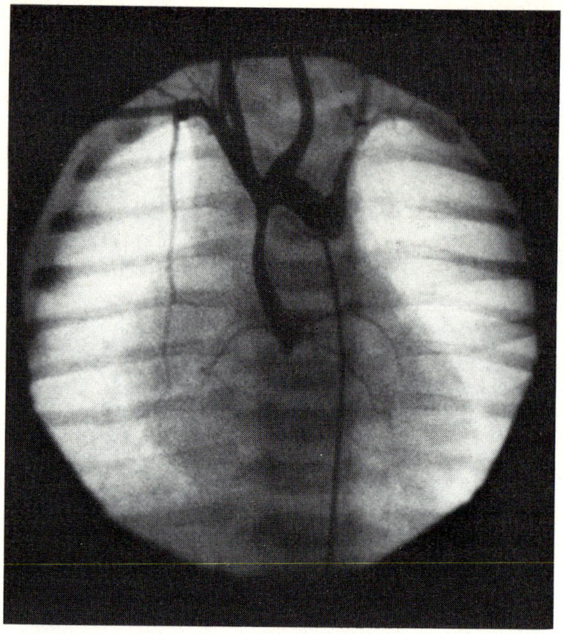

Fig. 29-47. Aortogram in hypoplastic left-heart syndrome. Note diminuitive aortic valve and ascending aorta. There is aortic valve atresia and inadequate coronary flow that is received retrogradely from PDA.

to right across the atrial septum; it then regains the systemic circulation either by way of a VSD or PDA. If aortic atresia is present, a ductal right-to-left shunt is necessary to ensure brachiocephalic artery perfusion and, most important, coronary artery perfusion. In aortic atresia, perfusion of the upper half of the body requires the pulmonary artery pressure to be at systemic levels. The poor prognosis is probably most immediately related to inadequate coronary perfusion.

Treatment. Infants with hypoplastic left-heart syndrome are frequently hypoglycemic as well as acidotic and may benefit from infusion of glucose and sodium bicarbonate in addition to the usual management of heart failure. Prostaglandin E_1 usually produces marked (but temporary) improvement. Reopening of the ductus arteriosus improves coronary blood flow and systemic perfusion via right to left ductus shunting. If mitral atresia or mitral stenosis is a dominant lesion, balloon atrial septostomy during cardiac catheterization may increase left-to-right shunting at the atrial level and allow the left atrial pressure to fall.

The major defect is usually hypoplasia of the left ventricle, and for this there is no direct therapy. The management of hypoplastic left heart syndrome is controversial at this time. Surgical options include the Norwood procedure in which stage I involves anastomosis of the diminutive ascending aorta to the main pulmonary artery, and control of pulmonary blood flow by a Goretex conduit; stage II, usually performed 6 to 24 months later, provides "Fontan" hemodynamics, whereby the right atrium is the pulmonary pumping chamber and the single ventricle is committed to the systemic circulation. Only 10% to 15% survive both procedures, and even survivors have Fontan hemodynamics. There is increasing interest in the use of neonatal cardiac transplantation.

Congenital aortic stenosis

It is unusual for this lesion to produce symptoms in the neonate. However, the clinical picture is distinguishable from that of the hypoplastic left-heart syndrome and must be differentiated because of its operability. Isolated congenital aortic stenosis producing serious illness in the neonatal period is practically always valvular, and usually no other cardiac or systemic abnormality is present.

Clinical manifestations. Failure of the left side of the heart leads to tachypnea, inappropriate sweating, and pulmonary rales. Right-sided heart failure with liver enlargement follows, but characteristically pulmonary symptoms continue to predominate. The infant may have surprisingly normal arterial pulses. A systolic murmur is usually obvious and loudest to the right of the sternum or in the suprasternal notch; an accompanying thrill may or may not be present. A gallop rhythm (presystolic) is common. The second sound is usually single, and an aortic ejection click is frequently heard.

Diagnosis. In contrast to the older child, the infant with critical aortic stenosis almost always has conspicuous left ventricular and left atrial enlargement, as shown on a chest roentgenogram. The lung fields appear passively congested. Severe left ventricular hypertrophy with secondary T-wave changes is apparent in most patients. This characteristic helps distinguish the condition from the hypoplastic left-heart syndrome and also provides an index of severity (secondary T-wave changes indicate critical obstruction).

The combination of an ejection systolic murmur maximal at the upper right sternal border, cardiac enlargement, and an ECG showing left ventricular hypertrophy is very suggestive of critical congenital aortic stenosis. Myocarditis usually gives rise to low ECG potentials, whereas with endocardial fibroelastosis murmurs are not so obvious. Occasionally endocardial fibroelastosis with secondary obstruction to left ventricular outflow may closely simulate congenital aortic stenosis. The presence of pathologic Q waves on the ECG favors a diagnosis of anomalous origin of the left coronary artery from the pulmonary artery rather than aortic stenosis.

Echocardiography. On two-dimensional echocardiography the aortic valve appears extremely dysplastic and thickened. The aortic valve annulus is usually less than 8 mm in size and the ascending aorta is frequently dilated (Fig. 29-48). In patients without additional aortic obstruction the ratio of the ascending aorta to that of the aortic valve annulus is usually greater than 1.7. Addi-

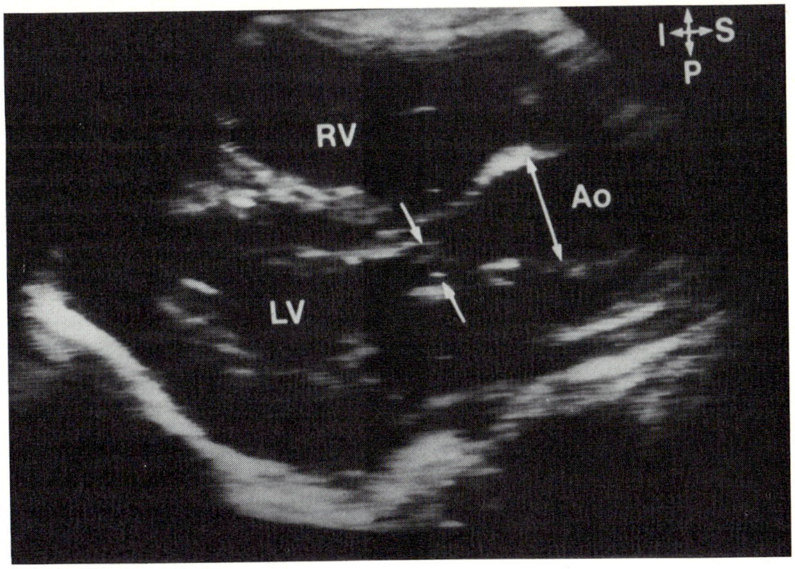

Fig. 29-48. Critical aortic stenosis. Parasternal long axis view of left ventricle *(LV)* showing a thickened aortic valve *(small arrows)* and poststenotic dilation of the aorta *(Ao)* *(large arrow)*. The right ventricle *(RV)* is also mildly dilated. *I*, inferior, *S*, superior, *P*, posterior. (Courtesy James C. Huhta, Houston, Tex.)

tional echocardiographic features include concentric left ventricular hypertrophy and increased echo density of the left ventricular papillary muscles and mitral valve support apparatus. Pulsed Doppler will confirm the diagnosis by revealing turbulence in the ascending aorta, and with continuous wave Doppler the gradient across the aortic valve can be estimated.

The neonate with heart failure from aortic stenosis usually has alveolar hypoventilation from alveolar transudate. The $Pa{CO_2}$ is raised and the $Pa{O_2}$ lowered. The $Pa{O_2}$ while the infant is breathing 100% O_2 should increase to above 150 mm Hg unless right-to-left intrapulmonary shunting is occurring through areas of pneumonia or atelectatic lung.

Hemodynamics. Critical aortic stenosis becomes worse with the passage of time. It is difficult to measure left ventricular pressure, since the foramen ovale is often functionally sealed by the raised left atrial pressure, and entry through the aortic valve, even when technically possible, is hazardous. There is increasing reliance on the echocardiogram to provide a definitive qualitative and quantitative (by Doppler interrogation of the supravalvar area) diagnosis allowing surgical intervention without invasive studies. Occasionally an aortogram is necessary. This angiogram will reveal the caliber of the ascending aorta and an indirect assessment of aortic valve area from the diameter of the stream of unopacified blood coming from the left ventricle.

Treatment. Surgery for aortic stenosis in infancy is difficult when compared with that for severe pulmonic stenosis. Residual obstruction and some aortic insufficiency are frequent. If the infant can be brought through the first critical years, further surgery involving the use of valved conduits and aortic homografts to bypass the obstruction may be possible. The role of balloon angioplasty remains controversial, and long-term follow-up of those infants so treated is necessary before its place is established.

Preductal coarctation of the aorta

The syndrome of preductal coarctation encompasses a wide spectrum of anatomy. The narrow aortic segment may be discrete and located immediately adjacent to or just above the entry of the ductus (juxtaductal or discrete preductal), or, as is often the case, the obstructed segment may be long and involve the aortic arch. If the *ascending* aorta is hypoplastic, the condition is usually classified as hypoplastic left-heart syndrome. Infants with preductal coarctation almost always have an open ductus so that blood flow to the lower half of the body is from the right ventricle by way of the ductus arteriosus. This would not of itself be dangerous were it not for the fact that right-to-left ductal shunting necessitates extreme pulmonary hypertension and consequent damage to the pulmonary vascular bed. The lungs of the baby with preductal coarctation are faced with a double problem; not only are they subjected to a high vascular pressure, but also the flow through them is reduced (the right-to-left ductal shunt acting as a "runoff" from the pulmonary artery).

Clinical manifestations. The syndrome is quite common (approximately 4%) in infants having cardiac catheterizations. There is a high incidence of associated defects; PDA is almost always present, and VSD, transposition of the great arteries, and complex lesions are common. Neonates with preductal coarctation usually develop tachypnea and cyanosis in the first to third weeks of life. It may be possible to recognize differential cyanosis (blue legs and pink arms). The femoral pulses are frequently palpable and may be entirely normal. This characteristic reflects the normal perfusion of the lower limbs via the patent ductus at normal systemic artery pressure. In some neonates the femoral pulses come and go, presumably secondary to variations in the pulmonary artery pressure. Usually there is either normal pulmonary artery pressure and deficient blood flow to the lower half of the body or high pulmonary artery pressure and normal blood flow to the lower half of the body. The latter is more common and preserves adequate kidney perfusion. Eventually the infant with severe preductal coarctation (and usually associated cardiac anomalies) develops right-sided heart failure. One may hear the characteristic murmur of a coarctation, and sometimes, if hypoplasia of the arch involves the left but not the right subclavian artery, the right arm blood pressure may be higher. Often the signs of an associated VSD predominate.

Diagnosis. The clinical diagnosis is suggested by a neonate who has a loud pulmonary closure sound, a murmur suggestive of a VSD, and signs of left-sided, or left- plus right-sided, heart failure. If the baby shows diminished or varying femoral pulses, the diagnosis is strengthened; and if differential cyanosis is observed, it is virtually certain. The heart is usually slightly enlarged, and the pulmonary arteries appear enlarged (secondary to pulmonary hypertension) on the roentgenogram. The ECG almost always indicates right ventricular hypertrophy. Preductal coarctation may closely simulate PFC syndrome.

Typically the $PaCO_2$ (blood sampled from the right arm) is 50 to 60 mm Hg, and the PaO_2 is 30 to 40 mm Hg. When blood is sampled from the femoral or umbilical artery, the PaO_2 is further lowered by right-to-left ductal shunting to 15 to 30 mm Hg, whereas the $PaCO_2$ is increased only by 2 or 3 mm Hg above that of the right arm sample (because of the small arteriovenous PCO_2 difference). This wide difference in PaO_2 between the right arm and leg and the narrow difference in $PaCO_2$ can be used as a test for right-to-left ductal shunting.

Echocardiography. Two-dimensional echocardiography usually reveals a dilated, poorly contractile left ventricle. Using a combination of high parasternal and suprasternal notch views, the coarctation appears as an area of narrowing in the descending thoracic aorta 2 to 3 mm distal to the origin of the left subclavian artery. Many times the discrete coarctation has the appearance of the ledge

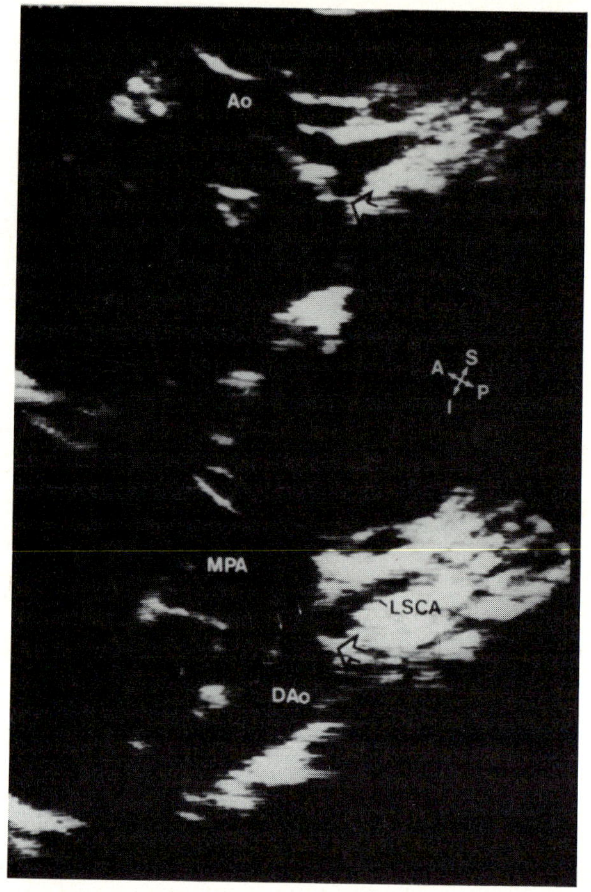

Fig. 29-49. Coarctation of the aorta. *Top,* Suprasternal long axis view of the ascending and descending aorta *(Ao)* showing a discrete coarctation ledge distal to the left subclavian artery *(black arrow). Bottom,* High parasternal view showing the coarctation and patent ductus arteriosus after the administration of prostaglandin E. *A,* anterior; *DAO,* descending aorta; *I,* inferior; *MPA,* main pulmonary artery; *S,* superior.

of tissue emanating from the posterior wall of the descending aorta (Fig. 29-49). Distal to the coarctation ledge there is usually poststenotic dilatation of the descending aorta. In addition, a lack of pulsations in the descending aorta compared to the ascending aorta helps confirm the diagnosis.

Hemodynamics. Cardiac catheterization of the neonate with uncomplicated preductal coarctation reveals severe right ventricular and pulmonary hypertension. The catheter passes from the pulmonary artery to the descending aorta by way of the usually present PDA. Contrast visualization of the right ventricle discloses filling of the pulmonary artery system and of the descending aorta (via the ductus). Increasing degrees of aortic arch atresia are associated with contrast agent also filling the brachiocephalic arteries, and in the extreme case of aortic valve hypoplasia the coronary arteries will fill from the right ventricular injection. However, at this stage the condi-

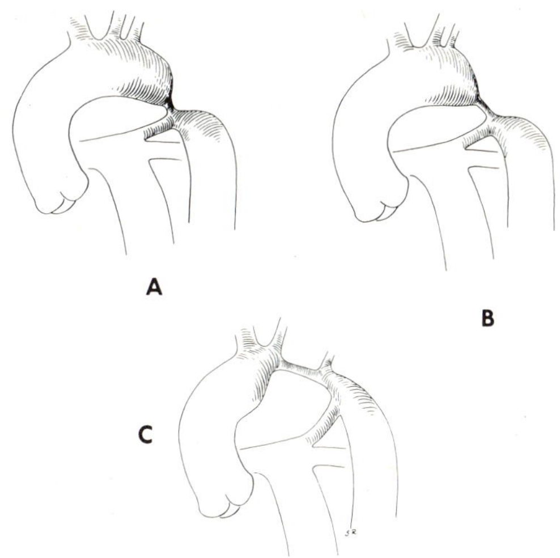

Fig. 29-50. Preductal coarctation of the aorta. Three of the more common variants are *(A)* juxtaductal localized coarctation, *(B)* preductal long-segment coarctation with hypoplasia of the left subclavian artery, and *(C)* aortic isthmus hypoplasia with hypoplasia of the left brachiocephalic arteries. Many other anatomic variations occur, but the physiology is usually that of a "systemic" right ventricle, whereby the descending aorta receives "venous" blood and the pulmonary artery pressure is usually at systemic levels.

tion is best regarded as hypoplastic left-heart syndrome rather than preductal coarctation syndrome.

The left ventricle usually can be entered by the foramen ovale and mitral valve, and opacification of this structure will define the aortic valve, coronary arteries, and aorta up to the point where the contrast agent meets the stream of right ventricle—derived blood. Most characteristically the brachiocephalic arteries fill from the left ventricle, and the descending aorta fills from the right; but the pattern in each patient is dependent on the aortic arch anatomy and the vascular resistance in the various organs of the body (Fig. 29-50).

Treatment. The extreme manifestation of preductal coarctation is complete interruption of the aortic arch. In this condition flow to the descending aorta is governed by patency of the ductus arteriosis. If the ductus begins to close, renal failure, acidemia, and other complications rapidly ensue. The infusion of PGE_1 into the pulmonary artery end of the ductus or intravenously has brought about major improvement in renal and metabolic status, allowing surgical intervention to be much more successful. PGE_1 also is often of value in improving the metabolic and pulmonary status in isolated coarctation, apparently not only by dilating the ductus arteriosus but also—as in one neonate that we have observed—by causing relaxation of the "aberrant ductus tissue" component of the coarctation.

Medical treatment of the neonate with preductal coarctation usually results in only temporary improvement. Surgical repair depends on the extent of aortic arch hypoplasia and the presence of associated anomalies. In most cases it is possible to bring down the left subclavian artery and anastomose it directly to the descending aorta (the ductus tissue is usually too friable for this purpose); in other cases an end-to-end anastomosis or Dacron graft replacement is possible. The ductus is divided. Unfortunately pulmonary hypertension may remain (especially if there is an associated VSD); however, in others it is completely reversible. The surgical mortality for those under 1 month of age requiring surgery is approximately 25%.

Postductal coarctation of the aorta (with closed ductus arteriosus)

Isolated postductal aortic coarctation sometimes causes problems in the neonatal period. Problems are most commonly encountered when other lesions, especially VSD and PDA, coexist. Infants with simple coarctation of the aorta often can be brought out of heart failure by medical means; operation can be deferred until the infants are of an appropriate age. An infant with absent femoral pulses and heart failure and who is deteriorating requires urgent hemodynamic and angiographic assessment; experience indicates that such infants nearly always have complicating lesions, such as aortic arch hypoplasia or VSD.

Clinical manifestations. The neonate with isolated coarctation of the aorta usually has moderately severe, predominantly left-sided heart failure. Occasionally hypertension may be the initial sign. Physical examination reveals the usual signs of heart failure. A diagnosis of coarctation is suggested by a late systolic ejection murmur heard well posteriorly and is made virtually certain by the absence of palpable femoral pulses. In lesser degrees of coarctation or where a good collateral circulation exists, the femoral pulses may be palpable, but there is a time lag between the brachial and the femoral pulse (normally synchronous). The diagnosis can be strengthened by a comparison of arm and leg systolic pressures with the Doppler technique, and in rare instances the coarctation can be visualized by the imprint of prestenotic and poststenotic dilatation on the barium-filled esophagus. Usually there is little doubt about the diagnosis; the only doubt is whether other lesions coexist.

Diagnosis. The heart is enlarged, and the lung fields frequently show the appearance of pulmonary venous engorgement. Right ventricular hypertrophy is usual. It is unusual to find left ventricular hypertrophy from isolated aortic coarctation before the infant is 6 months of age. The echocardiogram is useful in the assessment of coexisting lesions. Left-sided heart failure causes an alveolar transudate and impairment of respiratory gas exchange because of alveolar hypoventilation. The breathing of 100% O_2 increases PaO_2 to above 150 mm Hg, but $PaCO_2$ is unchanged.

Echocardiography. Direct visualization of the coarctation by sector scanning is usually possible. However, sometimes with ventilator-supported infants overinflation of the lungs makes this impossible. The gradient across the coarctation usually can be determined by Doppler interrogation in the prestenotic and poststenotic segments, and often considerable detail of the aortic arch and brachiocephalic vessels is possible. Sometimes, however, the complex anatomy of the aortic arch and the presence of hypoplastic segments makes angiographic examination mandatory so that surgical planning is well informed.

Hemodynamics. Frequently there is systemic hypertension above the coarctation. In the presence of heart failure right-sided heart pressures are slightly elevated. The coarctation may be delineated in several ways: by left ventricular opacification, by right ventricular opacification and subsequent levocardiogram phase, or, if necessary, by aortography. If the infant is less than 10 days old, the umbilical artery may be used; in older neonates the femoral artery can be located by the Doppler technique and entered percutaneously. A third alternative is the right brachial artery. The objective of hemodynamic study is usually not only the delineation of the coarctation but also the search for a PDA, VSD, bicuspid aortic valve, hypoplastic aortic arch, and so on.

Treatment. The infant with uncomplicated coarctation often responds excellently to medical management. Occasionally a neonate will have a systolic arm blood pressure of 150 mm Hg or higher, and the question arises as to whether antihypertensive treatment is indicated. Current practice is to regard systemic hypertension as an indication for operative relief. If antihypertensive medications are used, they must be used with great caution and with careful observation of the effect on urine production, serum creatinine, and blood urea nitrogen. Drugs that may be used are discussed in Table 29-13. Use of the right subclavian artery to swing down and patch the obstructed area has greatly diminished the need for second operations later in childhood. An alternative approach is "patch" angioplasty if the right subclavian artery is small or too distant from the coarctation site.

Right-sided heart obstruction

Classification of obstructive disease of the right side of the heart is somewhat arbitrary. The following are the more common entities that produce life-threatening illness in the neonatal period: pulmonary atresia with intact ventricular septum, pulmonary atresia with open ventricular septum (pseudotruncus arteriosus, extreme tetralogy of Fallot), tetralogy of Fallot, isolated valvular pulmonic stenosis, multiple peripheral pulmonary arterial stenosis, tricuspid atresia, and Ebstein's anomaly of the tricuspid valve.

Pulmonary atresia or extreme pulmonic stenosis with intact ventricular septum

Pulmonary atresia with intact ventricular septum is relatively common and is probably underestimated, since afflicted infants may die rapidly after birth. The only sources of blood to the lungs are the ductus arteriosus and the bronchial arteries. In most instances the ductus closes on the first, second, or third day of life even though it is being perfused by blood of low oxygen tension. In a few instances the ductus remains patent (perhaps predestined to be a PDA); consequently older children occasionally are encountered with complete pulmonary atresia and associated ductus arteriosus. The incidence in a series of sick neonates is 9% to 13%. Since the conditions of severe pulmonic stenosis and pulmonary atresia are closely related clinically, hemodynamically, and therapeutically, they are considered here as a single entity. A baby who angiographically appears to have pulmonary atresia sometimes is found at surgery to have a pinhole pulmonary valve orifice.

Clinical manifestations. Neonates with pulmonary atresia show early evidence of distress, presumably corresponding to closure of the ductus arteriosus. Cyanosis is marked. The respirations are characteristically deep, and alveolar ventilation is greatly increased in an unsuccessful attempt to attain physiologic respiratory gas tensions in arterial blood. The infants usually have a good Apgar score, but their color and breathing are noticed to be abnormal a few hours after birth. The cardiac impulse and peripheral pulses are normal, and frequently there is a loud, blowing, systolic murmur at the lower left sternal border, probably representing massive tricuspid regurgitation. A separate continuous murmur of a PDA is frequently heard. The second heart sound is single.

Diagnosis. The most striking finding on the chest roentgenogram is decreased pulmonary vascularity. The heart may be large and often appears egg shaped because of right atrial enlargement; there may be radiologic absence of the main pulmonary artery (Fig. 29-51). Cardiac enlargement is mainly a function of time; the heart may be normal in size during the first hours and days, whereas it is usually greatly enlarged in the occasional infant who survives beyond the neonatal period. There is a spectrum of right ventricular size so that the ECG may show marked right ventricular hypertrophy in those with a large right ventricular cavity, or it may show left ventricular hypertrophy if the right ventricle is hypoplastic, as is frequently the case. Electrocardiographic evidence of right atrial hypertrophy is usually present.

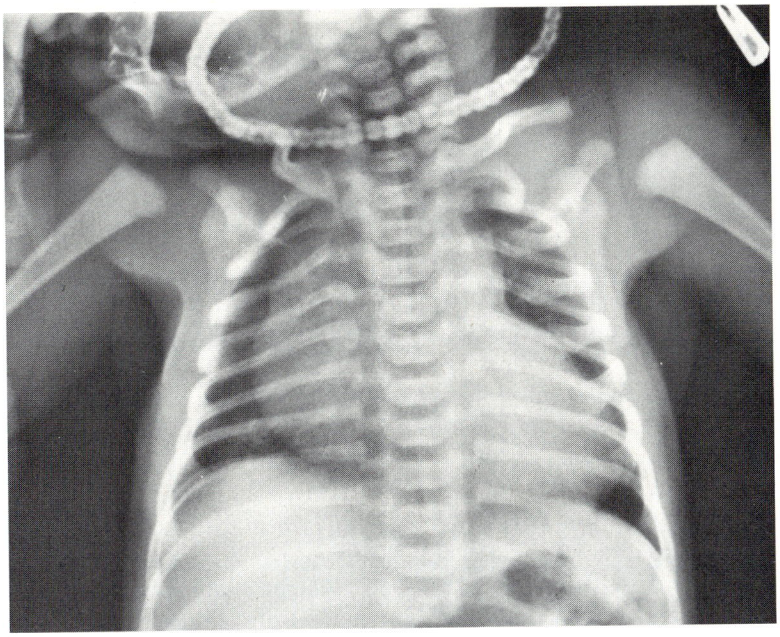

Fig. 29-51. Posteroanterior film of newborn with pulmonary valve atresia and intact ventricular septum. Note large heart and marked decrease in pulmonary vascular markings.

Increased alveolar ventilation results in a pulmonary vein P_{CO_2} of about 25 mm Hg and a pulmonary vein P_{O_2} of about 90 mm Hg. The gross right-to-left atrial shunt results in an arterial P_{CO_2} of about 31 mm Hg and a greatly reduced arterial oxygen saturation. There is no response to oxygen breathing. The arterial pH is often surprisingly normal until the infant is too exhausted to continue the high rates of ventilation necessary to maintain a normal Pa_{CO_2}.

Echocardiography. Parasternal and subcostal imaging show the imperforate pulmonary valve as a thick band of echos. The right atrium is always enlarged, and the atrial septum bulges toward the left atrium. The right ventricle may vary in size from a "cherry pit" with an extremely hypoplastic annulus (Fig. 29-52) to a normal-size chamber frequently with an Ebstein-type deformity of the tricuspid valve. Suprasternal notch views reveal that the pulmonary arteries can vary in size from normal to hypoplastic. The ductus arteriosus also is easily seen from suprasternal and high parasternal views. Pulsed Doppler may be used to assess the patency of both the pulmonary valve and ductus arteriosus and to determine whether tricuspid insufficiency is present.

Hemodynamics. The hemodynamics of pulmonary atresia and extreme pulmonic stenosis are similar. The right atrial pressure is moderately raised, and the right ventricular pressure is usually in the 70 to 100 mm Hg systolic range (only slightly above normal for age). Lack of marked elevation of the right ventricular pressure appears to be caused by the gross tricuspid insufficiency that is often present in infants with pulmonary atresia. Right ventricular angiography is pathognomonic; there is often gross tricuspid regurgitation and either complete absence of pulmonary artery filling or very minor opacification of this structure. The size of the right ventricle can best be assessed angiographically. Many appear hy-

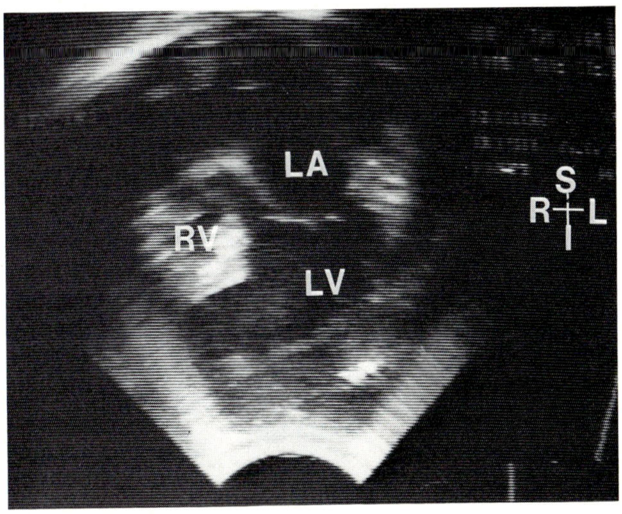

Fig. 29-52. Pulmonary stenosis with intact ventricular septum. Apical four chamber view shows an extremely small right ventricle *(RV)* with a dilated left ventricle *(LV)* and left atrium *(LA)*.

poplastic, but both the ECG echocardiogram and angiogram can be deceptive in the assessment of the adequacy of the right ventricle as a pumping chamber.

Treatment. The treatment has been revolutionized by the use of PGE_1. At the time most infants are referred for diagnosis (6 to 72 hours), the ductus is in the process of closing. PGE_1 infusion at a dose of 0.05 to 0.1 μg/kg/min IV is indicated as soon as the diagnosis is suspected from clinical findings or from echocardiography. After 10 or 15 minutes the ductus dilates, allowing an increase in pulmonary blood flow and an increase in PaO_2 from about 20 mm Hg to 35 to 40 mm Hg; arterial pH increases, and after a period of several hours the infant is in sufficiently good metabolic condition to allow a surgical procedure to be performed with minimal risk.

The outcome of surgery depends to a major extent on the adequacy of the right ventricle. However, in our opinion no neonate should be turned down for surgery because of a hypoplastic right ventricle. In those infants with an adequate right ventricle and isolated critical valvular pulmonic stenosis, a pulmonary valvotomy (transventricular or transpulmonary-arterial) is dramatically successful. Those infants with right ventricular hypoplasia often will require a pulmonary artery-to-aorta shunt instead of, or in addition to, relief of right ventricular outflow obstruction. Although mortality is still significant at the present time, the use of PGE_1 and greater alertness and speed at every stage of referral, combined with surgical advances, are steadily improving the prognosis.

Pulmonary atresia with open ventricular septum and severe tetralogy of Fallot

Pulmonary atresia with open ventricular septum may be thought of as the extreme form of tetralogy of Fallot; there is complete obstruction to right ventricular outflow. It has been referred to at times as pseudotruncus arteriosus, or type IV truncus arteriosus, since the source of lung flow is the aorta (bronchial arteries). The distinction between severely symptomatic tetralogy of Fallot (that is, continuity between right ventricular outflow tract and pulmonary arteries) and complete pulmonary atresia with open ventricular septum usually is not possible to make clinically. It is readily made by echocardiography and, if necessary, angiography.

Clinical manifestations. Infants are cyanotic from birth but usually do not cause concern until a few hours after birth, because temporary patency of the ductus arteriosus allows adequate pulmonary artery blood flow. On the first or second day of life the ductus closes, and the neonate becomes strikingly symptomatic with deep, sighing respirations, increasing central cyanosis, and lethargy. The cardiac impulse is hypodynamic, or one

A

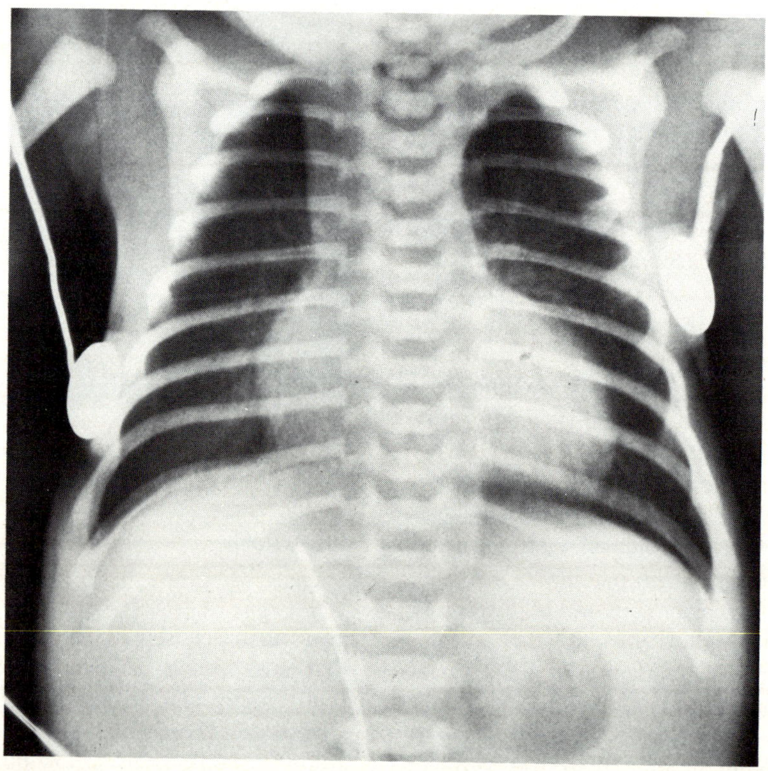

Fig. 29-53. A, Severe tetralogy of Fallot. Note normal-size heart with marked decrease in pulmonary vascular markings.

may feel a right parasternal tapping impulse. The second heart sound is single and maximal at the second right interspace (aortic valve closure), and there is frequently an aortic ejection click. There may be no murmur, or there may be a short ejection murmur of tight infundibular stenosis at the third left interspace.

Diagnosis. The heart is small or normal in size (in contrast to most other cyanotic lesions) and the pulmonary vasculature strikingly diminished. Even on the first day of life the heart may have the characteristic *coeur en sabot* shape of tetralogy (Fig. 29-53, *A*). Moderate right atrial and right ventricular hypertrophy is usual but is not diagnostically helpful. Alveolar hyperventilation produces a high pulmonary venous Po_2 and low pulmonary venous Pco_2, when pulmonary venous blood is admixed with systemic venous blood (at atrial and ventricular levels), hypoxemia and hypercapnia result in acidosis. In the first hours after birth surprisingly normal arterial blood gases can be found; but as the infant tires, ventilation falls, and acidosis results. There is no response to the breathing of 100% O_2, since hypoxemia is secondary to right-to-left shunting.

Echocardiography. Parasternal views reveal a dilated aorta overriding the ventricular septum. Subcostal imaging reveals that the right ventricular outflow tract appears to end blindly and the main pulmonary artery cannot be visualized. The suprasternal notch view reveals the confluence of the right and left pulmonary arteries and a prominent patent ductus arteriosus (Fig. 29-53, *B*). Approximately 25% of patients will have a right aortic arch, with careful attention to the branching pattern of the ascending aorta, this anomaly is easily identified.

Hemodynamics. Diminished pulmonary blood flow leads to diminished left atrial pressure, with consequent right-to-left atrial shunting across the foramen ovale. Blood enters the right ventricle and, in the case of total outflow tract obstruction, leaves to enter the aorta (in systole) and the left ventricle (in diastole). The only source of lung blood flow is via bronchial arteries and in some instances a ductus arteriosus. Clearly the baby's survival is unlikely unless bronchial artery flow is excessive or the ductus remains open. Right ventricular systolic pressure is at systemic level, and the catheter usually enters the aorta readily (across the VSD). Diagnosis is confirmed by angiocardiography.

Treatment. A neonate with pulmonary atresia and open ventricular septum is practically always going to require palliative surgery. In the critical time between diagnosis and surgery the use of PGE_1 to dilate the ductus usually proves lifesaving. Total correction in the neonatal age group has proved difficult, since reconstruction of the outflow tract and atretic pulmonary valve and artery requires the use of a homograft or synthetic conduit. In many centers the Goretex shunt (U-shaped prosthesis between aorta and pulmonary artery) or the modified Blalock (Goretex extension of subclavian artery to pulmonary artery) has supplanted the Blalock and Potts shunt as the first choice for increasing the pulmonary blood flow in the newborn. In selected cases, where an adequate-sized main pulmonary artery exists, a Brock procedure (transventricular "reaming out" of infundibular obstruction) may be preferable. At the time of surgery the presence and size of the main pulmonary artery are noted, since this structure will be hard to visualize later in the child's life and a knowledge of its size is mandatory before plans are made for total correction in early childhood. It is important to note that infants with numerous systemic-pulmonary collateral arteries (SPCAs) will often appear only slightly cyanotic yet re-

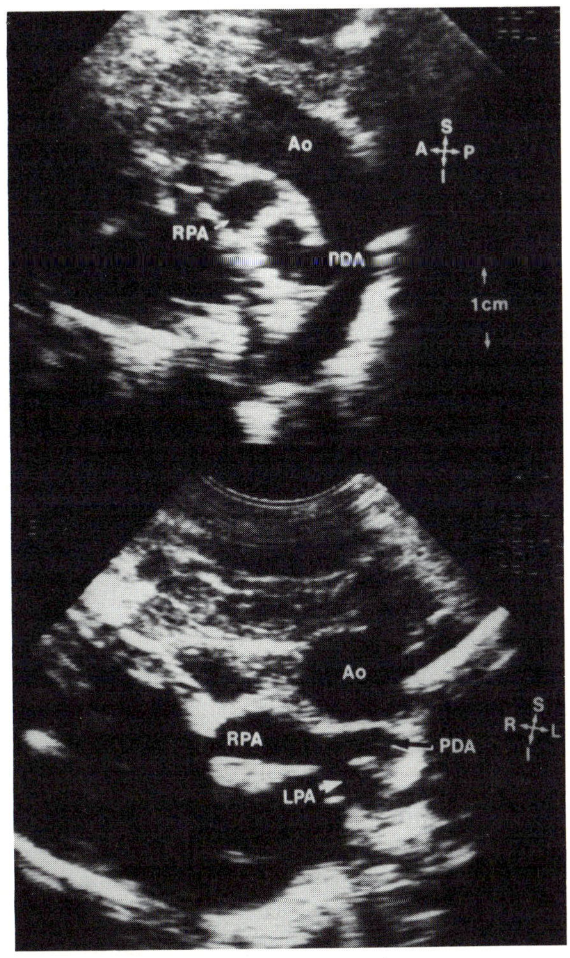

Fig. 29-53, cont'd. B, Pulmonary atresia with open ventricular septum. *Top,* Suprasternal long axis view reveals a curvilinear ductus arteriosus *(PDA)* and a dilated ascending aorta *(Ao)*. *Bottom,* Suprasternal short axis view reveals the pulmonary artery confluence of the right *(RPA)* and left *(LPA)* pulmonary arteries and the PDA.

quire central surgical shunt procedures to cause growth of the central pulmonary arteries and allow ultimate total correction. The results of palliative surgery for pulmonary atresia with open ventricular septum are complicated by the fact that there is frequently coexistent right ventricular hypoplasia and hypoplasia of the pulmonary arterial system. Rudolph and associates have reported the use of formalin infiltration of the walls of the ductus arteriosus in neonates as a palliative technique for maintaining pulmonary blood flow when suitable vessels for a shunt procedure cannot be found.

Pseudopulmonary valve atresia

There exists a rare but important entity where pulmonary atresia can be simulated, although the heart is anatomically normal. This situation can exist within the framework of PFC syndrome when the pulmonary artery pressure is higher than the RV pressure (because of a right-to-left ductus shunt) and the pulmonary valve is closed during the entire cardiac cycle. The RV angiogram may show no RV-to-PA continuity, and the echo shows no moving pulmonary valve. Treatment is that of PFC syndrome with, if possible, placement of a transpulmonary valvar line for the infusion of vasodilator agents.

Multiple peripheral pulmonary arterial stenoses

The most frequent cause of important pulmonary arterial stenoses giving rise to symptoms in the neonate used to be intrauterine rubella infection (Chapter 31). A familial incidence of peripheral pulmonary arterial stenosis also has been recognized, and there is evidence that idiopathic hypercalcemia of infancy is frequently associated with combined pulmonary arterial and supravalvular aortic stenosis. On occasion peripheral pulmonary artery stenosis is associated with various forms of congenital heart disease, especially tetralogy of Fallot. Cases of cutis laxa (generalized elastolysis), Ehlers-Danlos syndrome, arteriohepatic dysplasia, William's syndrome, and Takayasu's disease all have been reported in association with peripheral pulmonary arterial stenosis.

Clinical manifestations. The symptoms are those of predominant right-sided heart failure unless there is a PDA (as is frequently the case), in which case right-to-left ductal shunting leads to cyanosis. In severe cases the lungs are underperfused so that there is an increase in pulmonary ventilation similar to that seen in severe tetralogy or pulmonic stenosis. Classically, continuous murmurs are heard in several areas of the chest; however, in many instances only nondescript systolic murmurs are heard. The pulmonary closure sound may be very loud, since, although there are peripheral areas of obstruction, central pulmonary arterial pressure is greatly increased.

Diagnosis. The areas of stenosis are associated with poststenotic dilatation (Fig. 29-54). These may be visible occasionally on the plain film and may give a spurious impression of adequate or even increased vascular markings. The heart is usually small, unless it has dilated from right-sided heart failure. Right ventricular hypertrophy, often of severe degree, is typical. As the child grows and the obstruction becomes relatively more severe, right ventricular hypertrophy increases and is a useful measurement of progress or deterioration. Signs of right atrial hypertrophy are common. Alveolar hyperventilation is also common. Alveolar hyperventilation without right-to-left shunting produces lowered Pa_{CO_2} and increased or normal O_2 saturation. Ductal right-to-left shunts are frequent, in which case cyanosis, unresponsive to 100% O_2 breathing, is present.

Determination of IgM fraction and rubella antibody titer is indicated. If a generalized disorder, such as cutis laxa or Ehlers-Danlos syndrome, is suspected, a skin biopsy may be worthwhile. Serum calcium and phosphorus levels should be determined because of their association with hypercalcemia.

Echocardiography. From the suprasternal notch view the proximal left and right pulmonary arteries may be imaged and the stenosis characterized. However, the distal pulmonary arteries are better visualized with angiography.

Hemodynamics. Very high (200 mm Hg) right ventricular and central pulmonary arterial pressures may be found. Right atrial pressure rises as a consequence of raised right ventricular end-diastolic pressure, and right-to-left shunting through the foramen ovale is common. Definitive diagnosis can be made by observing pressure gradients within the pulmonary arterial system, but pulmonary angiography is essential if surgery is contemplated. Selective angiography defines the exact location and length of stenotic areas and determines the feasibility of corrective surgery.

Treatment. Total correction is rarely possible, since almost invariably the stenotic areas are very numerous. Occasionally a single stenosis in the main pulmonary artery or a small number of stenoses in primary, secondary, and tertiary divisions can be patch grafted. Such a patient is illustrated in Fig. 29-54. Although the surgery is time consuming, one advantage is that cardiopulmonary bypass usually is not necessary, since one lung may be operated on while the other serves for gas exchange.

Tricuspid atresia

Atresia of the tricuspid valve may occur with normally placed great arteries; tricuspid atresia without transposition is invariably associated with right ventricular hypoplasia and frequently with pulmonary valve hypoplasia. The presence of a VSD or PDA is necessary for blood to gain access to the pulmonary artery. Because the coexistence of transposed great arteries produces a very

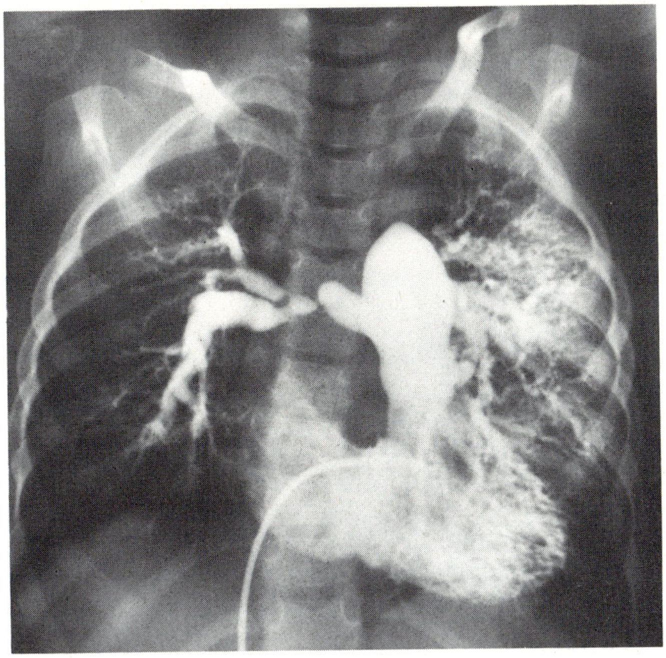

Fig. 29-54. Angiographic appearances in multiple peripheral pulmonary artery stenoses. In this particular case Ehlers-Danlos syndrome was present, and there were associated abnormalities of systemic arteries. The left lung had been operated on, but many areas of stenosis remain in the right lung.

different clinical picture from that in patients with normally positioned great arteries, tricuspid atresia and tricuspid atresia with transposed great arteries are considered separately in the following sections.

Tricuspid atresia with ventricular septal defect and normally positioned great arteries

Clinical manifestations. Cyanosis is present from birth. Infants with a small VSD have greatly diminished pulmonary blood flow, whereas those with a large VSD may have increased pulmonary blood flow. Diminished lung blood flow is more frequent; and it tends to diminish further with time, since there is evidence that the VSD becomes progressively smaller with growth. A further limitation to pulmonary blood flow is the size of the foramen ovale or ASD (Fig. 29-55). Pulmonary underperfusion leads to hyperventilation; and the respirations, although not unduly rapid, are increased in tidal volume. The cardiac impulse is quiet; frequently a thrill caused by a VSD is present at the lower left sternal border. The arterial pulses are normal. The second sound is frequently single, and a loud grade 4 pansystolic VSD murmur is heard maximally at the fourth left interspace. The clinical findings suggest a VSD, except that the infant is cyanotic.

Diagnosis. A few infants have a characteristic square-shaped heart, but the radiologic appearances are very variable and are influenced by the size of the ASD and VSD. In the majority of cases pulmonary vasculature is obviously diminished (Fig. 29-56). The ECG is of major diagnostic significance. In over 80% of the cases both left axis deviation and left ventricular hypertrophy are present. T-wave inversion in leads V_5 and V_6 is frequent. A typical ECG is shown in Fig. 29-57.

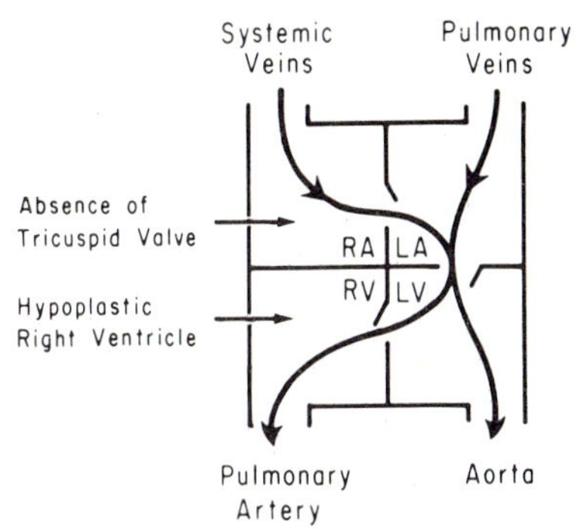

Fig. 29-55. The circulation in tricuspid atresia with patent foramen ovale and VSD.

Pulmonary underperfusion and overventilation produce a low P_{CO_2} and high P_{O_2} in pulmonary vein blood. However, since there is almost complete mixing at the left ventricular level, the final arterial blood gas tensions

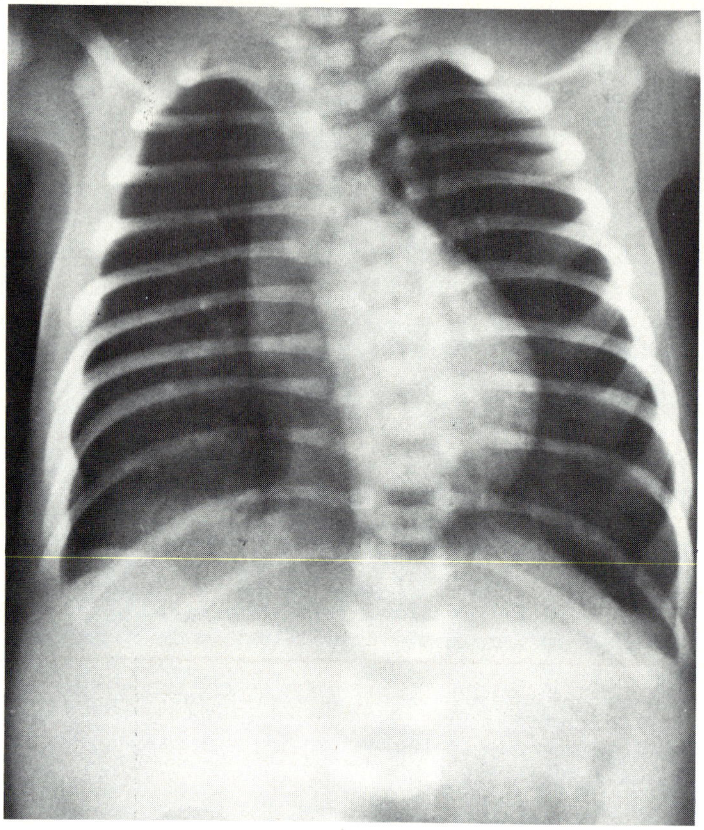

Fig. 29-56. Posteroanterior chest film of a neonate with tricuspid atresia. Note small heart, straight right cardiac border, and decreased pulmonary vascular markings. The plain chest film in tricuspid atresia shows considerable variation in the cardiac contour between patients.

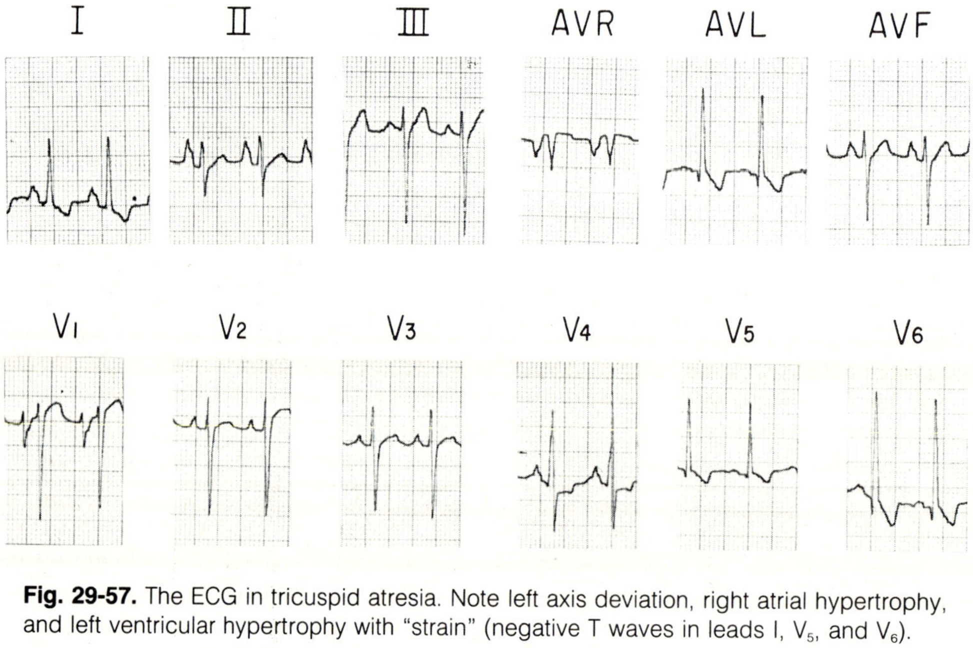

Fig. 29-57. The ECG in tricuspid atresia. Note left axis deviation, right atrial hypertrophy, and left ventricular hypertrophy with "strain" (negative T waves in leads I, V_5, and V_6).

A 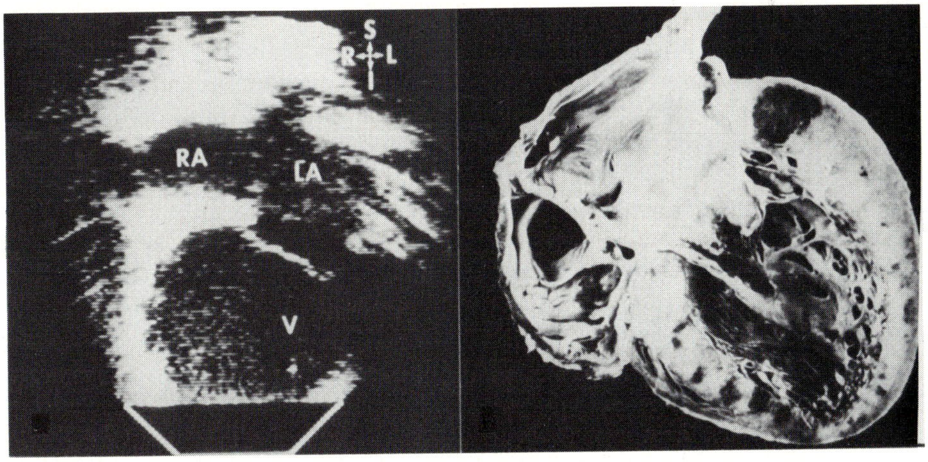 B

Fig. 29-58. Tricuspid atresia. **A,** Apical four-chamber view reveals a dilated left ventricular chamber *(V)*. Mitral valve is seen between left atrium *(LA)* and V. Right atrium *(RA)* is seen however no tricuspid valve is seen. **B,** Pathologic specimen cut in a plane similar to the echocardiographic view. (Courtesy James C. Huhta, Houston, Tex.)

depend largely on the ratio of pulmonary venous to systemic venous return. The pH and $PaCO_2$ are usually normal, although the PaO_2 is greatly reduced because of the very wide arteriovenous PO_2 difference. The breathing of 100% O_2 has almost no effect on arterial PO_2.

Echocardiography. The diagnosis of tricuspid atresia is easily made when the tricuspid valve leaflets cannot be imaged from either the parasternal apical or subcostal planes (Fig. 29-58). The right ventricular size may vary from extremely hypoplastic to slightly smaller than normal depending on the amount of the left-to-right shunting at the ventricular level. The right ventricular size may be estimated from the apical four-chamber view and the parasternal short-axis view. The left ventricle is usually dilated and is best seen in the apical subcostal views. Similarly the right atrium also is enlarged and the atrial septum bulges toward the left atrium.

The ventriculoarterial connection (transposed versus normal) is easily determined from parasternal and short axis views. In patients with normally related great arteries the pulmonary valve is anterior to and to the left of the aortic valve. In patients with transposition the great vessels exit in parallel from the heart and the bifurcation of the posterior pulmonary artery can be readily imaged from the subcostal view.

Frequently pulmonary atresia or stenosis is associated with tricuspid atresia, and this is appreciated from parasternal and subcostal views. In patients with pulmonary stenosis the pulmonary valve annulus is considerably smaller than the aortic valve annulus in the short-axis view.

The pulmonary artery branches visualized from the suprasternal notch view also are smaller than normal. In patients with pulmonary atresia an imperforate membrane is usually present in the pulmonary annulus. Pulsed Doppler can be quite helpful in confirming the diagnosis of pulmonary valve stenosis by revealing systolic turbulence in the main pulmonary artery and its branches. With pulmonary valve atresia the Doppler examination frequently will reveal continuous turbulence confirming the presence of a patent ductus arteriosus.

Hemodynamics. The diagnosis is usually obvious without cardiac catheterization, but the hemodynamics are very characteristic. It is impossible to direct the catheter tip into the right ventricle (ordinarily accomplished without delay). Instead the catheter passes immediately from the right atrium into the left atrium and can be manipulated into the pulmonary veins and left ventricle. Right atrial angiography reveals the sequence of right atrium, left atrium, left ventricle, and then simultaneous filling of the aorta and pulmonary artery. There may be an unopacified corresponding to the hypoplastic right ventricle. On occasion the pulmonary artery can be entered (across a VSD); the pressure is low unless the defect is substantial. The aorta usually can be entered with a flow-guided catheter and is easily visualized by contrast opacification of the left ventricle.

Treatment. Prostaglandin E_1 administration often is beneficial in those with ductus-dependent pulmonary blood flow. There is no definitive correction for tricuspid atresia at the present time. The limiting factor is the hypoplastic right ventricle. There are, however, various palliative maneuvers. If a gradient is found between the right and left atria, a balloon septostomy may aid systemic venous return and lower right atrial pressure. Palliative surgery is designed to increase pulmonary blood flow by means of an ascending aorta-to-right pulmonary artery or modified Blalock shunt. The Fontan procedure, whereby a conduit is placed between the right atrium and pulmonary artery, is the second-stage procedure and is used in the first year of life.

Tricuspid atresia with transposed great arteries. The neonate with this condition has also a large ventricular septal defect. The problem is not so much hypoxemia as pulmonary overcirculation and pulmonary hypertension. The defect may become apparent on the first day of life or after the neonatal period.

Clinical manifestations. Neonates with transposition and tricuspid atresia are cyanotic but usually not as blue as those without transposition. Respirations are rapid but of small or normal volume, typical for the infant with overperfused lungs. The cardiac impulse is hyperdynamic, and the arterial pulses are normal. If pulmonary overcirculation is marked, the signs of left-sided heart failure appear, followed by those of right-sided failure. In severe cases there are pulmonary rales, and the infant dies from hypoxemia, hypercapnia, and acidosis.

Diagnosis. The heart is frequently very large and similar to that of uncomplicated transposition. The pulmonary vascular markings are increased. Some infants show the classic left axis deviation and left ventricular hypertrophy of uncomplicated tricuspid atresia. Others display normal axis or right axis deviation.

$Pa{CO_2}$ is usually normal. $Pa{O_2}$ is decreased and unresponsive to the breathing of 100% O_2. Initially the arterial pH is normal; but when heart failure supervenes and $Pa{CO_2}$ rises, acidosis develops.

The echocardiogram is useful in defining chamber and great vessel localization (see previous section on echocardiography).

Hemodynamics. The catheter course follows the right atrium, left atrium, left ventricle route. Left ventricular angiography, when filmed in the lateral projection, reveals the transposed great arteries. The aorta frequently can be entered by passage of the catheter from the left ventricle across a large VSD. Most patients have severe pulmonary hypertension and greatly increased pulmonary blood flow.

Treatment. Tricuspid atresia with transposed great arteries is one of the more difficult entities to treat. Theoretically pulmonary artery banding should limit pulmonary blood flow and protect the lungs from developing vascular obliterative changes. In practice, however, the small hemodynamic advantage gained from pulmonary artery banding does not offset the hazard of thoracotomy in a small, sick infant, and the immediate mortality is high. Long-term management should be directed toward ensuring that the pulmonary vascular resistance stays low enough for the pulmonary arteries to accept a Fontan (right atrium to pulmonary artery) conduit.

Ebstein's anomaly of the tricuspid valve

The tricuspid valve is malformed and is attached partly to the anulus fibrosus and partly to the right ventricular endocardium. The posterior leaflets—often grossly malformed, sometimes vestigial or absent—are usually displaced downward. The resulting tricuspid valve is typically stenotic and incompetent; it is displaced deeply into the right ventricular cavity, dividing it into two chambers. The area of the right ventricle proximal to the valve is abnormally thin and sometimes aneurysmal.

Incidence. Ebstein's anomaly is uncommon (about 1 in 50,000 to 1 in 100,000), but its clinical recognition is important. The diagnosis is most easily established by echocardiography; one should be cautious in considering cardiac catheterization because of the risk involved in precipitating an arrhythmia. Spontaneous improvement in the first months of life is not unusual. Congenital Ebstein's anomaly often is undetected in the neonatal period, and such infants have no symptoms unless there is a bout of SVT.

Clinical manifestations. The initial symptom in the neonatal period is usually cyanosis. This is caused by right-to-left shunting across a patent foramen ovale or ASD secondary to raised right atrial pressure. Frequently there is a triple or quadruple rhythm caused by third or fourth heart sounds. A systolic murmur of moderate intensity is heard at the middle or lower left sternal border, and a presystolic murmur is often present. The presence of multiple heart sounds and murmurs when combined with the rapid heart rate of the neonate leads to a confusing auscultatory picture. Although the right atrial pressure may be raised slightly, congestive heart failure is uncommon, since right-to-left shunting limits the elevation of right atrial pressure. Where the foramen ovale is small, however, congestive heart failure may ensue.

Diagnosis. The classic findings are those of gross cardiomegaly with pulmonary undercirculation, as shown by a chest roentgenogram. The right atrium accounts for most of the cardiac enlargement. In symptomatic neonates the right atrium is enlarged; however, the roentgenogram may closely simulate that of pulmonic stenosis or pulmonary atresia with intact ventricular septum. Arrhythmias are frequent; ectopic beats, SVT, atrial flutter, and atrial fibrillation are all common; nodal rhythm and AV dissociation are less common. The Wolff-Parkinson-White syndrome occurs in approximately 9% of cases. Many infants have electrocardiographic evidence of right atrial hypertrophy, and some have prolongation of the PR interval. Right bundle branch block is common in older children and, although uncommon in the neonate, is very suggestive of Ebstein's anomaly. The symptomatic newborn with Ebstein's anomaly invariably has right-to-left atrial shunting, and the blood gases reflect the situation. The $Pa{CO_2}$ and pH are normal, but the $Pa{O_2}$ is low and is not significantly increased by the infant's breathing 100% O_2.

Echocardiography. Two-dimensional echocardiography provides an accurate method for diagnosing this anomaly. In the apical four-chamber view the septal leaflet of the tricuspid valve is displaced downward toward the ventricular apex. The tricuspid valve leaflets are thickened and deformed, and the anterior tricuspid valve leaflet is redundant. The portion of the right ventricle between the atrioventricular groove and the displaced tricuspid valve is the atrialized right ventricle and is easily seen in the four-chamber view (Fig. 29-59). In the parasternal long-axis view the dilated right ventricle and the thickened anterior tricuspid valve leaflet can be seen. In the parasternal short-axis views the displacement of the septal leaflet of the tricuspid valve into the right ventricular outflow tract can be seen. Pulsed Doppler interrogation of the right atrial chamber will reveal tricuspid insufficiency when present.

Hemodynamics. It is usually possible to make a firm diagnosis of Ebstein's anomaly in the neonate, based on physical signs with characteristic roentgenographic, echocardiographic, and ECG findings. Hemodynamic study is usually not indicated, since spontaneous improvement is common and catheterization may precipitate an arrhythmia. Cardiac catheterization, if performed, will show a high right atrial pressure, evidence of right-to-left atrial shunting, and difficulty or inability to cross the tricuspid valve. If the tricuspid valve can be crossed, there is a characteristic short ejection phase on the right ventricular pressure tracing; the intracardiac ECG may demonstrate that, although the catheter tip is in the right atrium, a right ventricular intracavity ECG is being recorded (because of the prolapse of the atrium into the ventricle). Angiocardiography is very helpful in disclosing the anatomy of tricuspid valve.

Treatment. Treatment is rarely required in the neonatal period and can be deferred until the child is large enough to undergo replacement of the anomaly with a prosthetic valve or to undergo tricuspid valvuloplasty. If treatment in the neonatal period is essential for survival, consideration should be given to the use of tolazoline (Priscoline) to lower pulmonary vascular resistance.

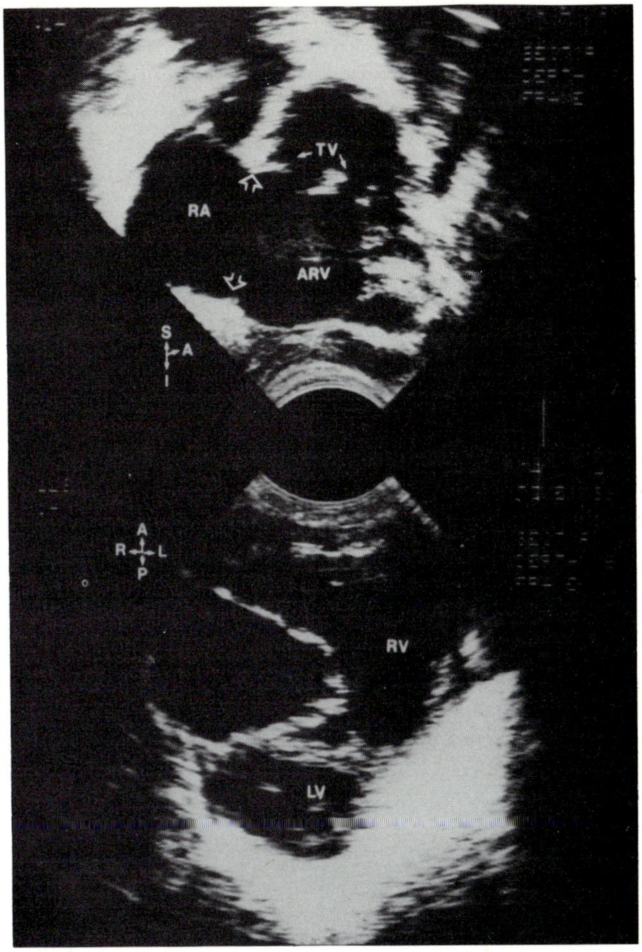

Fig. 29-59. Ebstein's anomaly of the tricuspid valve. *Top,* Subcostal four-chamber view shows a dilated right atrium *(RA)* and an atrialized portion of the right ventricle. The tricuspid valve *(TV)* can be seen extending into the right ventricular outflow tract. *Bottom,* Parasternal short axis through the right ventricle *(RV)* and left ventricle *(LV)*. The tricuspid valve leaflets extend well into the right ventricle. Open white arrows demarcate the tricuspid valve annulus.

Lesions that produce common mixing of venous and arterial blood

The four most important lesions that produce common mixing of venous and arterial blood are truncus arteriosus, very large VSD or common ventricle, double-outlet right ventricle without pulmonic stenosis, and total anomalous pulmonary venous return. A single atrium produces common mixing but rarely gives rise to serious illness in the neonate. Patients with these lesions tend to have certain features in common: mild cyanosis, a hyperactive cardiac impulse, cardiomegaly with increased pulmonary blood flow, and pulmonary hypertension. The cyanosis may go undetected, since the volume of well-oxygenated pulmonary vein blood exceeds that of the systemic vein blood. The resulting admixed arterial saturation is closer to pulmonary vein levels than it is to systemic vein levels. Frequently the saturation is 88% to 90%, and cyanosis will be obvious only when the hematocrit value is high.

Persistent truncus arteriosus

Two percent to 4% of severely sick neonates with heart disease have this lesion. The recognition of truncus arteriosus, although a relatively uncommon lesion, has become important since the advent of palliative and corrective surgery.

Pathology. The designation *truncus arteriosus* implies that only one artery arises from the heart and that this artery (the truncus arteriosus) gives rise to coronary arteries, pulmonary arteries, and the aorta. The truncus arteriosus almost always overrides a large VSD. The fact that the pulmonary arteries are of normal size necessitates the existence of severe pulmonary hypertension or greatly increased pulmonary blood flow; usually both are present. Various anatomic subtypes exist, depending on the exact point of origin of the pulmonary arteries from the truncus arteriosus. The so-called pseudotruncus, or type IV truncus, in the Collet-Edwards classification is now classified as tetralogy of Fallot with pulmonary atresia, the blood supply to the lung being bronchial-arterial rather than pulmonary-arterial.

Clinical manifestations. The major problem facing neonates born with a persistent truncus arteriosus is gross pulmonary overperfusion and pulmonary hypertension (usually at systemic artery pressure). In rare instances the pulmonary arteries are somewhat hypoplastic, allowing near-normal pulmonary blood flow and pulmonary artery pressure. Neonates with truncus arteriosus appear only *mildly cyanotic;* respirations are rapid but not deep. When left-sided heart failure supervenes, the signs of respiratory distress appear. The cardiac impulse is hyperactive, and the peripheral arterial pulses are bounding. The second heart sound is single and loud; there is commonly a loud, pansystolic murmur of a VSD at the lower left sternal border and on occasion a loud, continuous murmur at the upper left sternal border or an early diastolic murmur of truncal insufficiency. The general picture resembles that of a neonate with a large PDA (a neonate with a large PDA is frequently cyanotic from alveolar hypoventilation secondary to left-sided heart failure).

Diagnosis. The heart size is frequently massive, and the pulmonary vascular markings are very prominent. The sign of "high" origin of the pulmonary artery is not useful in the newborn period. Right ventricular hypertrophy is almost always present, and sometimes there is biventricular hypertrophy. Arterial pH and PCO_2 are normal unless the neonate is in heart failure. PaO_2 is low and unresponsive to the infant's breathing of 100% O_2. If heart failure supervenes, that part of the PaO_2 depression caused by hypoventilation is improved by 100% O_2 breathing.

Echocardiography. In the parasternal long-axis view most patients are indistinguishable from those with tetralogy of Fallot or pulmonary atresia with a ventricular septal defect. However, with high parasternal and suprasternal imaging the pulmonary arteries can be seen arising directly from the ascending aorta confirming the diagnosis (Fig. 29-60). With subcostal imaging, anterior angulation from the standard four-chamber view reveals the ascending aorta and the pulmonary arteries can be seen to arise from the left lateral aspect of the aorta.

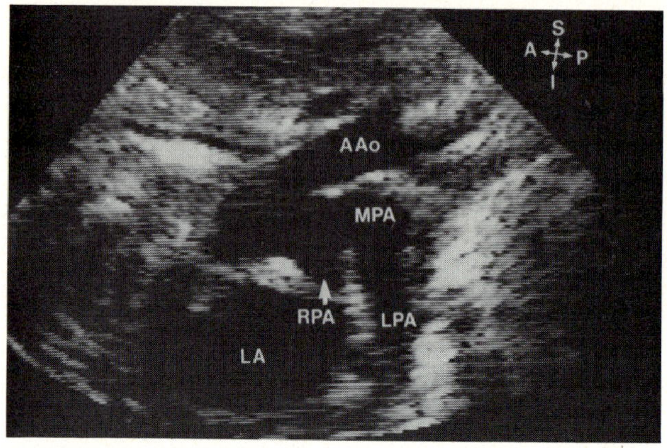

Fig. 29-60. Persistent truncus arteriosus. Suprasternal long axis view reveals origin of the main pulmonary artery *(MPA)* from the ascending aorta *(AAo)*. The branches of left *(LPA)* and right *(RPA)* pulmonary arteries are also well seen. *LA,* Left atrium.

Pulsed Doppler interrogation of the left ventricular outflow tract is extremely useful to rule out truncal valve insufficiency.

Hemodynamics. There is right ventricular hypertension, and the catheter passes from the right ventricle into the truncus arteriosus. That the pulmonary arteries can usually be entered from the common trunk suggests the diagnosis, which is confirmed by contrast visualization of the truncus arteriosus. The lateral view is useful in defining the exact site of origin of the pulmonary artery (Fig. 29-61).

Treatment. Although truncus arteriosus is a difficult lesion to manage, some neonates respond well to medical measures. However, the response is at the expense of increasing pulmonary vascular resistance. Our policy has been to treat the neonate medically and then, in consultation with the thoracic team, to make a decision as to whether the baby will grow rapidly enough to allow a total correction in the first year of life. Banding of the pulmonary artery is usually not helpful because it tends to increase truncal valve insufficiency. Definitive surgical repair consists essentially of closing the VSD, disconnecting the pulmonary artery from its truncal origin, and joining the pulmonary artery to the edges of the right ventriculotomy by means of a valved woven Dacron graft or valved aortic homograft. Our experience has been that, when faced with a neonate in chronic heart failure, surgery is indicated early because of rapidly decreasing ventricular function.

Single ventricle

A single ventricle is very commonly associated with other anomalies: pulmonic stenosis, common atrium, ASD, and endocardial cushion defects. Among neonates

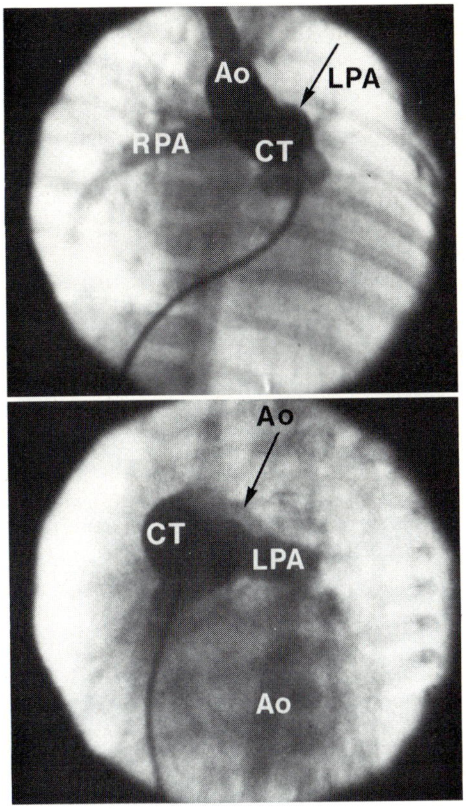

Fig. 29-61. Truncus arteriosus. Single frames taken from cineangiogram. **A,** Anteroposterior projection. Note right *(RPA)* and left *(LPA)* pulmonary arteries arising from the common trunk *(CT)*. Some truncal valve regurgitation is evident. **B,** Lateral projection showing the left pulmonary artery arising from the posterior aspect of the trunk. The trunk continues as the aorta *(Ao)*.

with this anomaly 15% to 20% die in the first week of life.

Clinical manifestations. Mild to moderate cyanosis is present depending on the ratio of pulmonary to systemic blood flow. There is usually no murmur, or there is a nondescript left parasternal systolic murmur. Most infants without pulmonic stenosis have greatly increased pulmonary blood flow so that respirations tend to be rapid. If heart failure ensues, other signs of respiratory distress appear.

Diagnosis. The heart is large, and pulmonary vascularity is increased. Usually the ECG signs of biventricular hypertrophy are present. In the majority of cases normal Q waves are seen. The echocardiogram confirms absence of the septum.

Echocardiography. Echocardiography is an extremely helpful tool in assessing the many different varieties and additional malformations associated with the single ventricle. There are several excellent texts on pediatric echocardiography available.

Hemodynamics. Common mixing occurs at the ventricular level so that arterial saturation is in the 88% to 92% range. If no other lesions are present, there is increased pulmonary blood flow and pulmonary hypertension. The large number of associated lesions makes selective angiography mandatory for detailed diagnosis.

Treatment. Surgical treatment is possible by converting the single ventricle to a systemic ventricle and providing pulmonary blood flow with a Fontan conduit. In the neonatal period banding of the pulmonary artery may be required to allow survival to the age for definitive repair.

Double-outlet right ventricle without pulmonic stenosis

Double-outlet right ventricle occurs in 2% to 3% of neonates with congenital heart disease. The lesion almost always is associated with anomalies of the aortic arch and with VSD. There may be associated transposition of the great arteries. Extracardiac defects are common, and there is an association with trisomy 18 syndrome.

Clinical manifestations. Mild cyanosis is present. The obligatory increase in pulmonary artery pressure and pulmonary blood flow rapidly produces tachypnea followed by right-sided heart failure. The outcome often is determined by the degree of hypoplasia of the aortic arch and by the location of the VSD. The murmur of a VSD is usually present.

Diagnosis. Gross cardiomegaly and increased pulmonary vascular markings are characteristic. There is usually combined ventricular hypertrophy. The diagnosis rests on angiographic evidence of the great artery origins. The aortic and pulmonary valves both arise from the right ventricle (anterior ventricle) and at the same level (normally the pulmonary valve is higher). Frequently there is hypoplasia of the aortic arch.

Treatment. Infants may benefit from pulmonary artery banding to allow survival, however, primary repair is often indicated in early infancy when there is chronic heart failure or pulmonary hypertension. The VSD patch is positioned in such a way as to incorporate the aortic origin into the left ventricle. Double-outlet right ventricle *with* pulmonic stenosis is rarely observed in the neonatal period; the obstruction is often subvalvular in location.

Total anomalous pulmonary venous return

Total anomalous pulmonary venous return (TAPVR) implies the return of all pulmonary venous blood directly or indirectly to the right atrium and requires the presence of an ASD in order that blood may reach the left atrium, left ventricle, and systemic circulation. The lesion is important, since it is frequently surgically correctable. The incidence is 2% to 4%.

Clinical manifestations. The lesion appears at all ages in childhood. The most important determinant of the

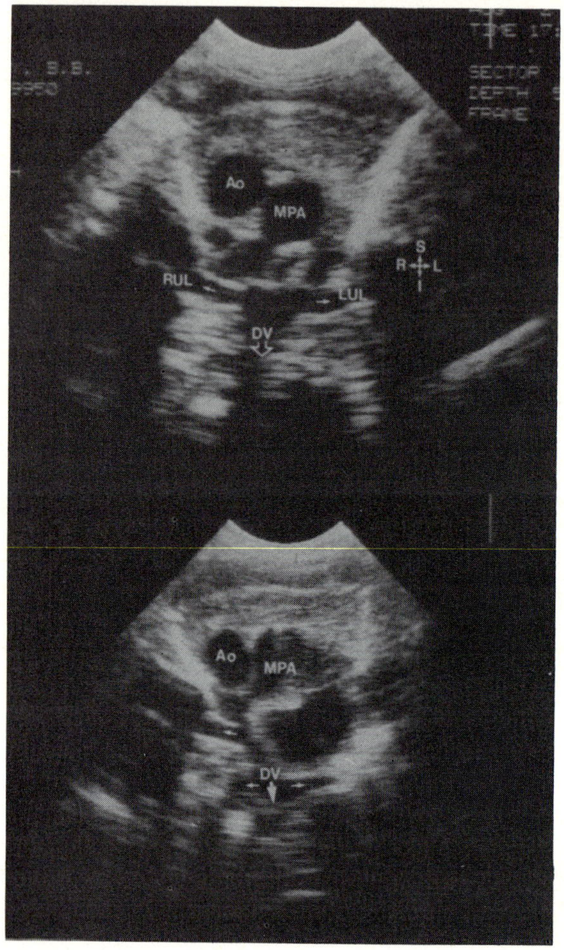

Fig. 29-62. Total anomalous pulmonary venous return, infradiaphragmatic type. *Top,* Suprasternal short axis view reveals the left *(LUL)* and right *(RUL)* upper lobe pulmonary veins entering a pulmonary vein confluence, which then drains through a descending vein *(DV)*. The aorta *(Ao)* and main pulmonary artery *(MPA)* are seen in cross-section. *Bottom,* With scanning from the suprasternal notch more inferiorly the two lower lobe pulmonary veins *(small horizontal arows)* can be seen entering the descending vein. (Courtesy James C. Huhta, Houston, Tex.)

time of presentation appears to be the degree of obstruction to pulmonary venous return. Infants with total anomalous pulmonary venous return, who become seriously sick in the newborn period, almost always have a degree of obstruction to the return of pulmonary venous blood. There is increased pulmonary vein pressure, increased pulmonary capillary pressure, and increased pulmonary artery pressure. When the pulmonary veins drain directly into the right atrium and there is a large ASD, the hemodynamics are very similar to those of an ASD. The mild arterial unsaturation that is present may go unnoticed for many years.

Clinically there is marked tachypnea, and pulmonary rales are heard if pulmonary venous pressure is elevated. Less commonly the signs of right-sided heart failure develop secondary to raised right atrial pressure. The infants are mildly or moderately cyanotic. A gallop rhythm is frequently present, and there is marked right ventricular overactivity. Commonly there is no murmur. If present, the murmur often resembles that of an ASD with a midsystolic ejection component at the upper left sternal border and a flow murmur of relative tricuspid stenosis at the lower left sternal border. Frequently the second heart sound is widely split and fixed with regard to respiration.

Pathology. There are four main types, according to the mode of entry of the pulmonary veins into the right side of the heart: (1) drainage of pulmonary veins into the right atrium, directly or via the coronary sinus, (2) drainage into the right superior vena cava or azygos vein, (3) drainage into a persistent left superior vena cava, which then empties into the left innominate vein, and (4) drainage of a common pulmonary venous collecting trunk below the diaphragm into the portal vein or ductus venosus. There are a large number of variations of these four basic types.

Diagnosis. The radiographic contours considered characteristic of the condition (figure-of-eight and so on) are not often seen in the newborn, presumably because insufficient time has elapsed for superior vena caval distension to occur. In the newborn the observation of a small heart with the pattern of pulmonary *venous* congestion is very suggestive of total anomalous pulmonary venous return with obstruction (see Fig. 29-3). In those without obstruction but with overwhelming pulmonary blood flow there is cardiomegaly and an increase in pulmonary *arterial* markings. The ECG shows moderate right ventricular hypertrophy. There is usually complete reversal of R/S progression in the precordial leads. Signs of right atrial hypertrophy are frequent. The arterial pH and P_{CO_2} are usually normal unless heart failure is present. The Pa_{O_2} is inevitably lowered, although cyanosis may not be clinically apparent (arterial saturation 88% to 92%). The Pa_{O_2} usually will not exceed 300 mm Hg during 100% O_2 breathing but occasionally may go higher because of torrential pulmonary blood flow compared to the volume of systemic flow.

Echocardiography. Two-dimensional cardiography in TAPVR reveals an enlarged right atrium and left ventricle. Of more importance is the fact that the pulmonary veins do not appear to enter the left atrium as visualized in the subcostal and apical four-chamber views. In these cases evaluation of the extracardiac vascular structures will usually reveal the site of drainage of the pulmonary venous confluence. In TAPVR to the coronary sinus an enlarged coronary sinus may be visualized in several echocardiographic planes. In most cases the connection

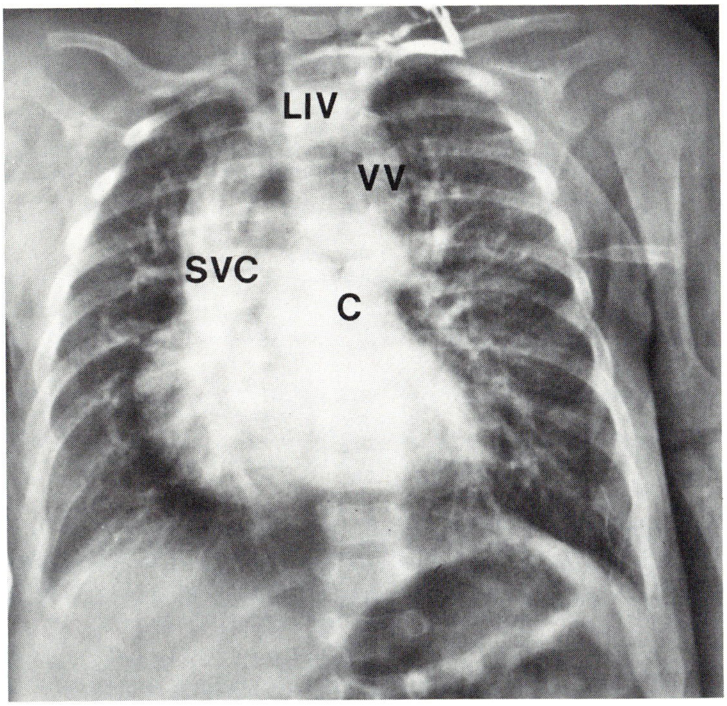

Fig. 29-63. Total anomalous pulmonary venous return. Contrast agent has been injected into a peripheral vein. The levocardiogram phase shows the confluence of pulmonary veins *(C)* ascending via a vertical vein *(VV)* into the left innominate vein *(LIV)* to enter the superior vena cava *(SVC)*.

of the common pulmonary venous chamber to the coronary sinus and right atrium usually can be visualized. In TAPVR to the superior vena cava both the innominate vein and superior vena cava are dilated as seen from suprasternal notch views. In addition, a left vertical vein is easily identified.

TAPVR of the infradiaphragmatic type may be more difficult to identify by two-dimensional echocardiography. However, an important clue to the diagnosis is the appearance of a large vascular structure in the abdomen seen in the subcostal view, which is distinct from the IVC and aorta. Careful imaging from the suprasternal notch view will often reveal the connection of the pulmonary venous confluence to the descending vein, which confirms the diagnosis of infradiaphragmatic TAPVR (Fig. 29-62).

Hemodynamics. The hemodynamics are extremely variable and are dependent on the presence of obstruction to pulmonary vein return, the adequacy of the ASD, and the presence of additional defects. Typically right atrial pressure is slightly elevated; and if the anomalous pulmonary collecting trunk can be entered with the catheter (which it frequently can), a rise in pressure can be demonstrated as the catheter advances retrogradely toward the pulmonary capillary bed. The point of entry of pulmonary venous blood into the right side of the heart frequently can be identified by a sudden rise in oxygen saturation. Pulmonary arterial saturation is generally about 2% higher than systemic arterial saturation (because of streaming effects within the right atrium); the degree of pulmonary hypertension is variable, depending on the pulmonary blood flow and pulmonary vein pressure.

Angiography is occasionally needed for detailed diagnosis. Ideally the anomalous pulmonary vein trunk can be carefully opacified; a second choice is opacification of the main pulmonary artery or right ventricle, with filming of the levocardiogram phase (Fig. 29-63). It is important to determine the exact relationship between the collecting trunk and the left atrium if surgery is contemplated. If the infant has not received excessive contrast agent, opacification of the left atrium and left ventricle is desirable, since these structures frequently are undersized and may determine the surgical outcome.

Treatment. The presence of a significant gradient across the atrial septum is an indication for a balloon septostomy, and this alone sometimes will decompress the right atrium sufficiently to allow the infant to achieve a better respiratory and metabolic status in preparation for open-heart surgery.

Vigorous treatment of heart failure is indicated; but, if the infant is deteriorating, thoracic surgical consultation should be sought and plans made for immediate correction. In the majority of instances the anomalous pulmonary venous collecting trunk runs immediately behind the left atrium so that surgery consists of performing an anastomosis between these two structures.

Prognosis. The mortality is high because the infants are small and frequently very sick, and open-heart surgery may have to be performed under emergency conditions. The mortality in infants is approximately 10%. The mortality is similar regardless of the anatomy. A major determinant appears to be the adequacy of the left ventricle to handle the additional volume load and avoid pulmonary edema following surgical repair.

Left-to-right shunts

Four types of left-to-right shunts are considered in the following sections: PDA, VSD, combined PDA and VSD, endocardial cushion defect (common AV canal), and systemic arteriovenous fistulas. ASDs are present in the newborn period but rarely cause symptoms. Total anomalous pulmonary venous return is considered as a "common mixing" lesion rather than a left-to-right shunt. Infants with left-to-right shunts have certain clinical characteristics in common. The neonates are acyanotic, the cardiac impulse is hyperactive, and the chest roentgenogram shows cardiac enlargement with an increase in pulmonary vascular markings.

Patent ductus arteriosus

See also Chapter 28, part four.

Indirect evidence indicates that the normal human ductus arteriosus undergoes fairly rapid initial constriction during the first few hours after delivery of the baby, followed by a more gradual final functional closure over 1 to 8 days. In premature infants closure of the ductus may be delayed up until the time of full gestational age and beyond. Thus surgical closure of a PDA is not indicated in the asymptomatic premature infant, since spontaneous closure can be anticipated in most instances. PDA ligation sometimes is indicated in the premature infant who has recovered from RDS but in whom a large left-to-right shunt is causing heart failure unresponsive to medical management, including a trial of indomethacin.

Clinical manifestations. In the neonate it is common to hear a soft inconstant systolic murmur at the upper left sternal border in the first 10 hours of life. The closure of the ductus arteriosus is strongly influenced by the Po_2 of the blood perfusing it. However, there are paradoxes; thus the ductus arteriosus remains widely patent in infants with severe RDS but unfortunately does not always remain open in infants with pulmonary atresia and hypoxemia, even though arterial and ductus Po_2 may be at fetal levels.

A widely patent ductus arteriosus is an important and fairly frequent cause of serious illness in the neonate. Such neonates may be in serious heart failure and frequently have associated pneumonia. Neonates with symptomatic ductus arteriosus are tachypneic and later exhibit pulmonary rales and the signs of right-sided heart failure. In advanced left-sided heart failure they are cyanotic from alveolar hypoventilation. The peripheral pulses are bounding, and the cardiac impulse is hyperdynamic. There is usually no thrill, but a harsh multifrequency systolic murmur is evident at the left sternal border. The murmur resembles that of a VSD but is slightly higher in location and more "grating" in character. The "swishing" continuous murmur heard in some neonates with PDA requires a low pulmonary artery pressure; such infants are rarely in serious trouble in the neonatal period.

Diagnosis. The heart is enlarged, and the pulmonary vascular markings are increased. The classic roentgenographic contour is that of left ventricular and left atrial enlargement; however, in most cases the cardiomegaly is nonspecific. The ECG is almost always abnormal in seriously sick neonates. Both right ventricular hypertrophy and biventricular hypertrophy are seen. Flow reversal in the descending aorta, respresenting diastolic runoff down the PDA, can be detected and quantitated by the directional Doppler. The infant in heart failure from a PDA is frequently hypoxemic from alveolar hypoventilation and mistakenly may be thought to have a right-to-left shunt. The pH is usually normal (compensated respiratory acidosis), the $Paco_2$ elevated, and the Pao_2 depressed. Since the depressed Pao_2 is caused by hypoventilation, the breathing of 100% O_2 should result in a level of 150 mm Hg or greater.

Echocardiography. With high resolution two-dimensional echocardiography it is possible to image a patent ductus arteriosus in greater than 90% of premature and newborn infants. The PDA is best visualized using a combination of high parasternal and suprasternal notch views (Fig. 29-64). The addition of pulsed Doppler increases the sensitivity of detection of ductal patency to near 100%.

When evaluating a PDA it is extremely important to rule out the presence of a "ductus-dependent" congenital heart lesion such as pulmonary or tricuspid valve atresia. As mentioned in previous sections, a complete echocardiographic study can easily document associated defects.

Although two-dimensional and pulsed Doppler echocardiography are highly sensitive and specific in the diagnosis of a PDA, quantitating the amount of left-to-right shunt is much more difficult. Studies are currently under way to validate the clinical utility of estimating pulmonary-to-systemic flow ratios by Doppler techniques. Presently most echocardiographers determine the he-

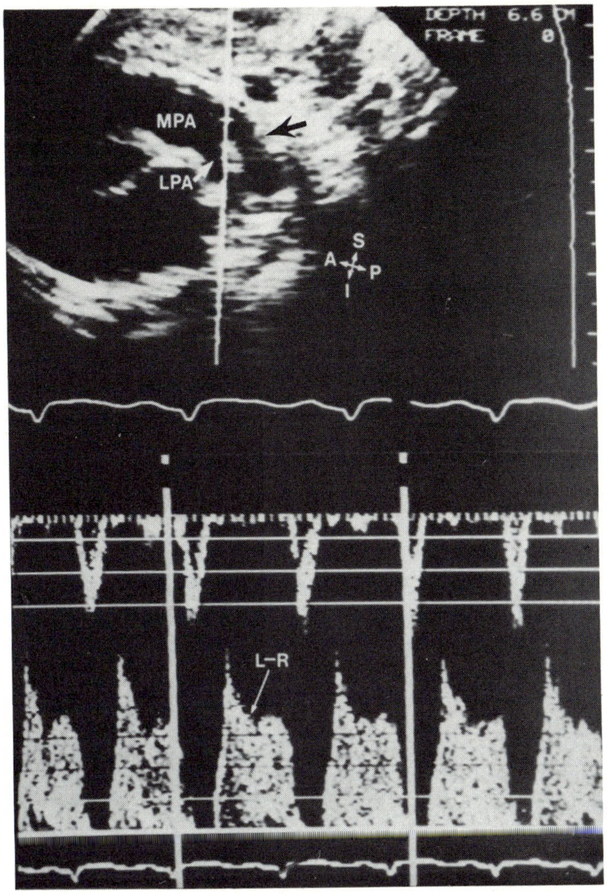

Fig. 29-64. Patent ductus arteriosus. *Top,* High parasternal view shows the main pulmonary artery *(MPA),* left pulmonary artery *(LPA),* and patent ductus arteriosus *(large arrow).* Sample volume for pulsed Doppler is in the pulmonary end of the ductus arteriosus. *Bottom,* Pulsed Doppler recording with the sample volume as indicated above. Velocity display extending above the baseline represents the left-to-right shunt through the ductus during both systole and diastole.

modynamic significance of a PDA by documenting left atrial and left ventricular enlargement in conjunction with clinical evidence of respiratory distress.

Hemodynamics. The diagnosis is easily and rapidly confirmed by right-sided heart catheterization; however, this is now rarely necessary since the introduction of two-dimensional and Doppler echocardiography. There is usually right ventricular and pulmonary arterial hypertension, and the catheter readily traverses the patent ductus to enter the descending aorta. There is a step-up in O_2 saturation at the pulmonary artery level and left-to-right shunting. Often the catheter enters the left atrium across a foramen ovale; the left atrial pressure and left ventricular end-diastolic pressures are raised. When necessary (chiefly to rule out other lesions, such as VSD or aortic arch hypoplasia), left ventricular angiography filmed in the left anterior oblique projection visualizes the ductus and excludes the aforementioned complicating lesions. If doubt exists as to the status of the left ventricle and proximal aorta, occasionally it may be necessary to perform retrograde arterial catheterization using the transfemoral approach or the umbilical artery (if the infant is less than about 7 days of age).

Treatment of full-term infants. Full-term infants may have an isolated pathologic (permanent) patency of the ductus arteriosus. Symptomatic medical treatment of heart failure and pneumonia should be pursued vigorously, since the majority of full-term infants with isolated PDA survive the neonatal period, and surgery can be performed electively when the infant reaches age 1 or 2 years. In a minority, symptoms progress; and in the event that indomethacin administration fails to produce improvement, ligation of the ductus is indicated. The cause of the heart failure and pneumonia is totally removed by surgery. A neonate may appear to be in irreversible pulmonary edema, yet with careful medical management before surgery and with the operation performed by an experienced surgeon, the infant's recovery is rapid.

Premature infants. Most premature infants with a ductus arteriosus have a temporary (physiologic) patency. The ductus arteriosus will eventually close, however, serious prolonged respiratory distress and even death may result especially under 34 weeks' gestational age. In these infants indomethacin (a prostaglandin synthetase inhibitor) has proved extremely effective, and surgical ligation is now rarely required.

Oral doses have been 0.2 mg/kg given by nasogastric tube, repeated if necessary for up to three doses at 8-hour intervals. In general, infants who have shown the highest incidence of successful indomethacin ductus closure have been less than 30 weeks of gestational age and less than 10 days chronologic age, although older or later responders are not unusual. Lyophilized intravenous indomethacin is a useful alternative to the oral preparation. Its advantages are that a therapeutic blood level is more reliably achieved without gastric irritation. With oral indomethacin gastric perforation and necrotizing enterocolitis have been reported.

Contraindications to the use of indomethacin are the following: (1) total serum bilirubin >10 mg/dl, (2) blood urea nitrogen >25 mg/dl, (3) serum creatinine >1.2 mg/dl, (4) platelet count <50,000/mm^3, and (5) signs of necrotizing enterocolitis, or (6) any evidence of internal or external bleeding.

Ventricular septal defect

Isolated VSD is not a common cause of serious illness in the neonate. This is because of the relatively high pulmonary vascular resistance at birth and the probability that the normal postnatal fall in pulmonary vascular resistance in those infants with large VSDs may be delayed or slow. The infant destined to develop heart failure from a large isolated VSD typically develops heart failure at 6 weeks to 4 months of age.

Incidence. VSD is an extremely common lesion in asymptomic newborns and frequently is associated with other congenital heart lesions. The natural history of isolated VSD has been greatly clarified over recent years, and it is now clear that spontaneous closure can be anticipated in approximately one third to one half, a few closures occurring as late as the fifth decade of life. This realization has greatly influenced management and has resulted in the application of stricter criteria before advising surgical closure in asymptomatic children.

Clinical manifestations. The neonate who becomes severely symptomatic from an isolated VSD usually has a very large defect and typically develops heart failure in the third or fourth week of life. There is usually common mixing of venous and arterial blood at the ventricular level, resulting in a mildly cyanotic infant. The physical signs of mild cyanosis, an overactive precordium, and a loud pulmonary closure sound sometimes are accompanied by a typical VSD murmur at the lower left sternal border. However, in other neonates the systemic and pulmonary vascular resistances are almost balanced, and there is little or no murmur. Thus the condition may mimic transposition with VSD, truncus arteriosus, and other "common mixing" situations.

Diagnosis. The heart is large, but the contour usually is not diagnostically helpful. The barium swallow may reveal left atrial enlargement. The pulmonary vasculature is increased. Broad notched P waves indicative of left atrial enlargement are frequent. There may be right or combined ventricular hypertrophy. The neonate with a large VSD who has severe symptoms usually is cyanotic from a combination of alveolar hypoventilation (alveolar transudate) and right-to-left shunting (at the ventricular level). Typically there is a mild compensated respiratory acidosis: the PaO_2 is depressed, and only that fraction of the depression caused by alveolar hyperventilation is responsive to the breathing of 100% O_2.

Echocardiography. Ventricular septal defects greater than 3 mm in size are easily visualized by two-dimensional echocardiography. However, because of the curvature of the septum a variety of echocardiographic planes is necessary for complete examination of each portion of the ventricular septum. Defects in the membranous portion of the ventricular septum are located in a subaortic position beneath the septal leaflet of the tricuspid valve.

Most membranous defects are best imaged in the parasternal long- and short-axis views and in a cranially angulated subcostal four-chamber view (Fig. 29-65). Muscular ventricular septal defects are located in the inferior portion of the ventricular septum between the membranous septum and cardiac apex. These defects are best visualized in the parasternal and subcostal short-axis view. Defects in the inlet septum are located in the posterior part of the septum adjacent to the atrioventricular valves. These defects are best seen in the apical and subcostal four-chamber views scanning at the level of the atrioventricular valves.

In patients with moderate to large ventricular septal defects (i.e., greater than 5 mm in size), the left ventricle and left atrium are usually enlarged secondary to increased pulmonary venous return. The left ventricular enlargement is best seen in the parasternal long-axis view and the apical and subcostal four-chamber views.

With the advent of Doppler technology an accurate estimation of right ventricular and pulmonary artery pressure can be obtained. By using continuous wave Doppler the peak velocity across a VSD can be measured and then converted into a millimeters of mercury pressure drop with a modification of the Bernoulli equation. Subtracting the pressure drop across the VSD from the systolic blood pressure accurately predicts both right ventricular pressure and (in the absence of pulmonary valve stenosis) the peak pulmonary artery pressure. Hemodynamic information such as this helps the clinician to optimize the timing of invasive studies and surgical intervention.

Hemodynamics. The neonate with heart failure from a large VSD has rather different hemodynamics from his older-infant counterpart. The VSD is large, sometimes approaching "single ventricle." In addition, there may be multiple defects, and frequently the muscular part of the septum is involved. At cardiac catheterization the venous approach reveals right ventricular and pulmonary

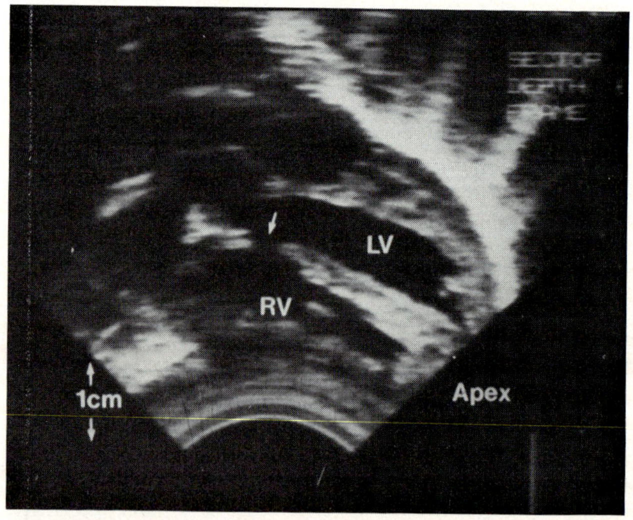

Fig. 29-65. Ventricular septal defect. Subcostal four-chamber view shows a perimembranous VSD *(arrow)* with extension into the trabecular inlet septum. *LV,* Left ventricle; *RV,* right ventricle.

arterial hypertension. The increase in O_2 saturation in the right ventricle may be quite small because of near-equalization of pulmonary and systemic vascular resistances and ventricular pressures. When the left atrium can be entered, the pressure is usually increased, the degree being proportional to the pulmonary blood flow.

Definitive diagnosis rests on echocardiography and angiocardiography; it is important to know not only the size and location of the VSD but also the existence of other cardiac anomalies. Left ventricular opacification in the lateral or left anterior oblique projection is most useful (Fig. 29-66); but if the left ventricle cannot be entered via the foramen ovale (as is frequently the case), right ventricular angiography can outline the ventricular septum. If there is a right-to-left shunt, the left ventricle and aorta also are visualized. Occasionally transarterial catheterization may be necessary to visualize the left ventricle.

Treatment. Medical treatment of heart failure is indicated; but if there is not obvious and sustained improvement within 2 or 3 days, serious consideration should be given to early surgical intervention. There is some evidence that neonates who develop heart failure with isolated VSD are likely to have an accelerated onset of pulmonary vascular obliterative disease. This is especially true of those with left atrial and pulmonary vein hypertension (who are likely to have pulmonary rales). Since this group of neonates is likely to have large or multiple VSDs banding and later total repair sometimes appears to offer less risk compared with attempts at early one-stage total correction or prolonged medical management with the risks of progressive pulmonary vascular obliterative disease. When the VSD is well visualized angiographically, and particularly when the defect is single, the use of hypothermia with limited bypass for one-stage early correction is preferred.

Combined patent ductus arteriosus and ventricular septal defect

The lesions of PDA and VSD frequently are combined and cause symptomatic disease in the neonate. Either lesion may predominate, although frequently the cal-

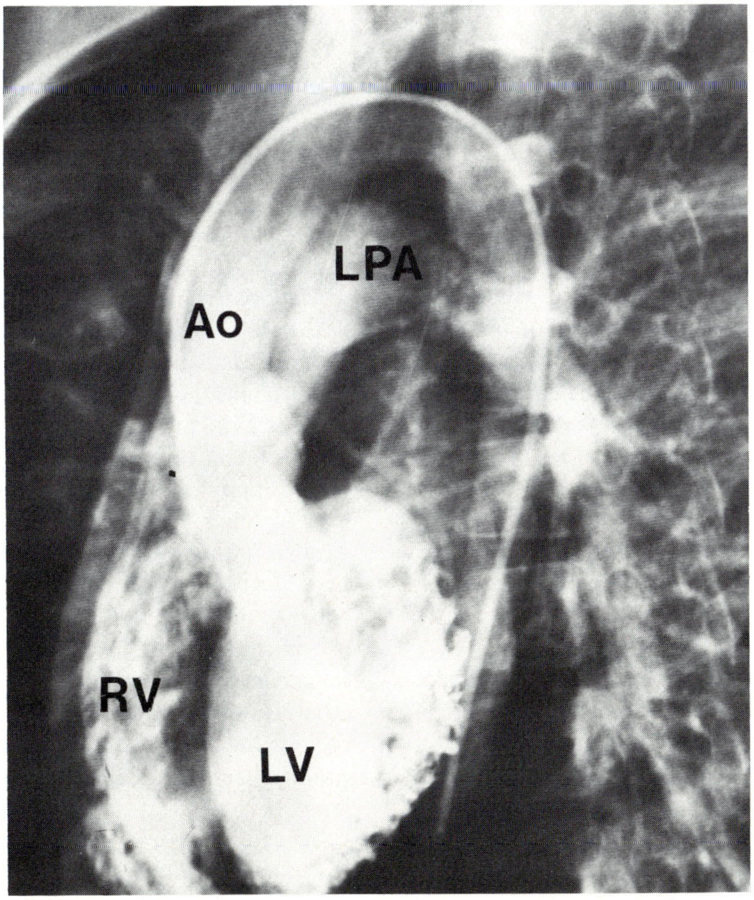

Fig. 29-66. Angiographic appearances of VSD. The catheter is in the left ventricle *(LV)*. Contrast passes through a high VSD into the right ventricle *(RV)* and fills the aorta *(Ao)* and pulmonary artery *(LPA)*.

culated left-to-right shunts through each are approximately equal.

The physical signs are those of a left ventricular hyperdynamic cardiac impulse, bounding pulses (if the PDA component is substantial), and a systolic thrill and murmur at the third or fourth left interspace. The signs vary somewhat according to which lesion is dominant; it is unusual, however, to hear the typical continuous murmur of a PDA. The chest roentgenogram discloses a large heart with increased pulmonary vascularity. The ECG reveals left or combined ventricular hypertrophy except if significant pulmonary hypertension is present, in which case isolated right ventricular hypertrophy may be seen. Echocardiography is valuable in visualizing both VSD and PDA and determining shunt direction at peak flow velocity.

At cardiac catheterization the ventricular defect is detected by the step-up in oxygen saturation at the right ventricular level, and commonly the catheter crosses the ventricular septum to enter the aorta. When necessary, left ventricular angiography secures the diagnosis. The presence of a PDA usually is demonstrated by catheter passage through it into the descending aorta, and the quantitation of left-to-right shunting is assessed by further increase in oxygen saturation at the pulmonary arterial level. If doubt exists, aortography or left ventriculography is indicated to settle the issue.

It is important to try to determine (by oximetry and angiography) which of the lesions is causing the greater left-to-right shunt. The calculations can be misleading because, if a large VSD is present, pulmonary artery pressure may be raised and the ductus shunting reduced (because of a lesser pressure gradient than would exist without the VSD). When both lesions are equally present, division of the ductus usually does not improve the situation. In the case of the neonate in heart failure it seems that the best surgical treatment is division of the ductus, accompanied by banding of the main pulmonary artery, followed by closure of the VSD and unbanding of the pulmonary artery at the appropriate age (usually 1 to 4 years.) If the VSD is single and easily accessible, early primary closure is often now preferred.

Common atrioventricular canal

Common AV canal is virtually the only type of endocardial cushion defect that causes serious problems in the newborn period. There is a large AV septal defect of an elliptic configuration, and the aortic leaflet of the mitral valve and the septal leaflet of the tricuspid valve are both cleft. The result is that all four cardiac chambers are in communication with one another, and additionally there is regurgitation of varying degrees through the cleft mitral and tricuspid valves. The association with Down's syndrome is well known; however, neonates without chromosomal anomaly also may have endocardial cushion defects.

Clinical manifestations. The severity of the hemodynamic abnormality usually results in symptoms appearing in the first or second week of life. The major variable is the degree of valvular regurgitation present, especially mitral regurgitation. A few children remain asymptomatic for many years; such children often turn out to have a major atrial component to their lesion, with a small VSD and minimal valvular regurgitation. Neonates with a common AV canal tend to rapidly develop tachypnea and liver enlargement. They may be mildly cyanotic from right-to-left shunting. The precordial impulse is hyperdynamic; the pulmonary closure sound is loud. Murmurs are variable. The most frequent finding is a loud pansystolic murmur at the lower left sternal border and a more blowing apical decrescendo pansystolic murmur; the former arises from the VSD, the latter from mitral insufficiency. Frequently there is a middiastolic apical murmur caused by increased mitral valve diastolic flow.

It is important to note that some infants with a common atrioventricular canal will have normal auscultatory findings during the first few days of life. This is because of the equalization of the two atrial pressures and the two ventricular pressures associated with elevated neonatal pulmonary vascular resistance. Because the infant with Down's syndrome has a 40% incidence of congenital cardiac disease, it is important for a comprehensive cardiologic examination to be performed in the neonatal period regardless of physical findings. In many instances a chest film and ECG will confirm normality, but in other instances it is necessary to obtain an echocardiogram.

Diagnosis. The heart is enlarged, and the pulmonary vasculature is increased, but the contour is nonspecific. Left axis deviation is present in the majority of patients and is a most helpful diagnostic finding. Biatrial enlargement and right or combined ventricular hypertrophy are also frequent and depend mainly on whether valvular regurgitation or shunting is dominant. Most infants are in mild heart failure so that a compensated respiratory acidosis with elevated $Pa{CO_2}$ and normal pH is present. The $Pa{O_2}$ is depressed from right-to-left shunting and is not responsive to 100% O_2 breathing.

Echocardiography. Two-dimensional echocardiography is especially useful in the evaluation of atrioventricular canal defects. In these defects a large central defect involving the lower portion of the ventricular septum is easily seen in the apical and subcostal four-chamber views (Fig. 29-67).

Instead of separate mitral and tricuspid valves, there is a common atrioventricular valve composed of five leaflets. The morphology of one of these leaflets, the anterior bridging leaflet, forms the basis for the anatomic classification of these defects.

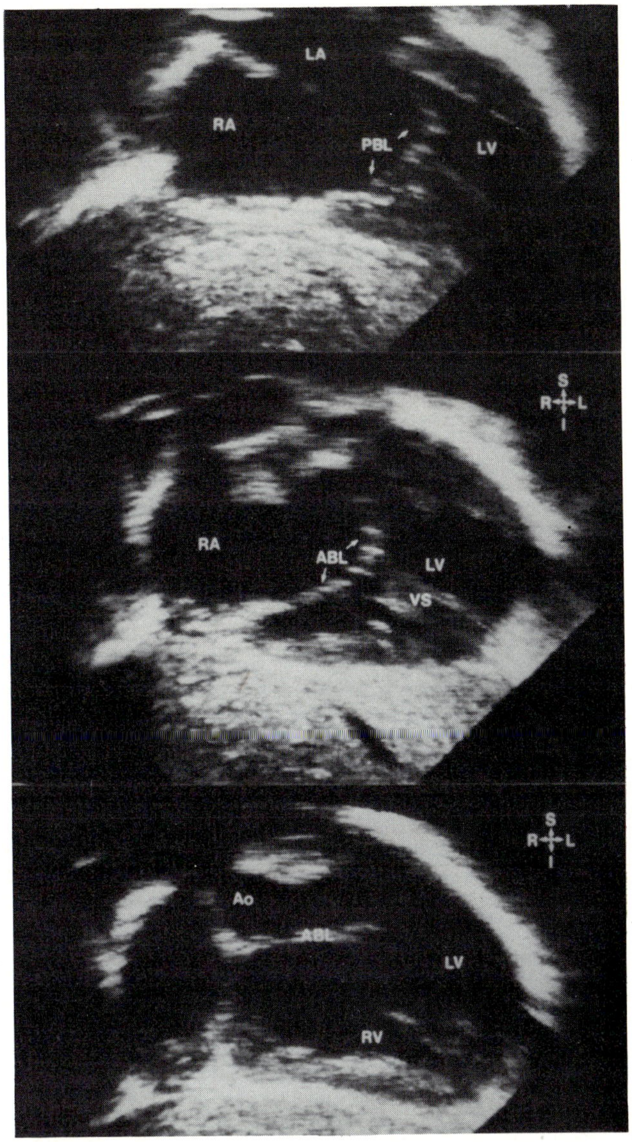

Fig. 29-67. Complete atrioventricular canal. *Top,* Subcostal four chamber view with inferior angulation reveals a large atrial septal defect located between the left atrium *(LA)* and right atrium *(RA)*. The posterior bridging leaflet *(PBL)* of the common AV valve can also been seen with chordal attachments to the ventricular septum *(VS) Center,* More superior angulation reveals the anterior bridging leaflet of the common AV valve. *Bottom,* With increasing superior angulation a large VSD in the inlet septum can be seen between the LV and RV. In addition, the ABL can be seen encroaching on the left ventricular outflow tract, which results in the typical "goose-neck" deformity seen on LV angiogram. *AO,* aorta. (Courtesy James C. Huhta, Houston, Tex.)

The atrioventricular valve anatomy is best visualized with the subcostal short-axis view and is far superior to angiography for valve anatomy. The chordal attachments of the valve leaflet are also well visualized and best seen in the apical four-chamber view.

Hemodynamics. Studies of severely symptomatic neonates usually demonstrate raised atrial and right ventricular pressures. The catheter characteristically can be advanced from the right atrium to the left atrium to the left ventricle and then on withdrawal enters the right ventricle, demonstrating continuity between all four chambers. There is pulmonary artery hypertension and evidence of left-to-right shunting, usually at both the atrial and the ventricular levels. It is important to determine whether the major shunt is at the atrial level or at the ventricular level. Mitral and tricuspid valve regurgitation can best be assessed by Doppler echocardiography.

Treatment. Medical treatment allows the infant to gain sufficient weight for total correction. The results of total correction of the common AV canal have improved markedly in the last years. In most centers the trend is toward total correction at the age of 2 to 4 months, an age at which pulmonary vascular disease should not have progressed far.

Prognosis. The child with common AV canal who fares best following corrective surgery appears to be the one in whom the major shunt is at the atrial level (ostium primum ASD) and in whom the ventricular component is small. Such children are likely to have a near-normal pulmonary artery pressure. Many infants have residual mitral valve insufficiency, and in perhaps 10% a further operation on the mitral valve is required. A further surgical hazard is that of complete heart block, requiring permanent pacing. This occurs in 5% to 10% of cases. The overall surgical mortality is now approximately 5% to 10%.

Systemic arteriovenous fistula

Systemic arteriovenous fistulas are relatively uncommon as a cause of severe illness in the neonate; but their recognition is important because some are treatable and, if they go untreated, they may cause death early in the neonatal period. They may be seen on fetal echocardiography (see Fig. 29-32). The most common sites associated with severe heart failure appear to be the brain and the liver. Serious consideration should be given to the possibility of a systemic arteriovenous fistula whenever heart failure of obscure cause occurs in a neonate.

Intracranial arteriovenous fistula. Cerebral malformations involving the great vein of Galen are the most frequent intracranial arteriovenous fistulas. The clinical presentation includes tachypnea, pallor, dyspnea, and cyanosis. Signs of respiratory distress and congestive heart failure may be prominent. A cranial bruit usually but not invariably is heard. Skull measurements and transillumination may be normal. The cardiac impulse is often hyperdynamic and maximal at the lower left sternal border. There may be a systolic regurgitant murmur. The liver edge usually is enlarged below the right costal margin when congestive heart failure occurs.

The chest roentgenogram may show massive cardiac enlargement as well as active and passive pulmonary vascular engorgement. The ECG may suggest right ventricular hypertrophy. CT scan and ultrasonography of the head usually reveal the lesion. Hemodynamic studies may reveal systemic pressures in the pulmonary artery and right ventricle and oxygen saturation as high as 94% in the superior vena cava. Cineangiography with injection of contrast material into the left ventricle shows an intact ventricular septum and normal aortic root. Following opacification of the aortic arch and brachiocephalic vessels there can be extremely rapid recirculation of the contrast agent so that the jugular veins, superior vena cava, and right atrium become rapidly and densely opacified. The mean left atrial and left ventricular end-diastolic pressures may be elevated, confirming the impression of left ventricular failure. Cerebral angiography confirms the diagnosis (Fig. 29-68).

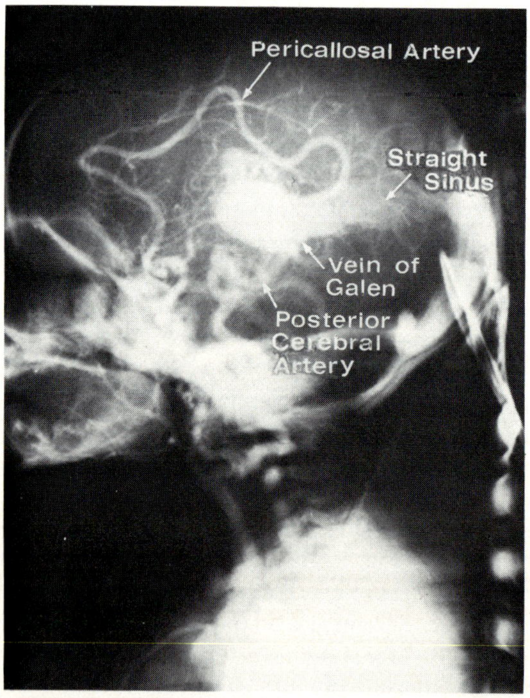

Fig. 29-68. Arteriovenous fistulas; intracranial communication. Right innominate artery injection demonstrates aneurysmal vein of Galen, which is fed directly by the right posterior cerebral artery and an enlarged, tortuous pericallosal artery. A markedly dilated straight sinus in seen draining from the vein of Galen into the transverse sinus.

These infants may respond satisfactorily to medical management. However, most infants with intracranial arteriovenous fistulas deteriorate rapidly. Some have medically irreversible heart failure, whereas in others central nervous system symptoms predominate. Occasionally surgical clipping of feeding arteries has been successful.

Giant hemangioma of the liver. Giant hemangioma of the liver may cause heart failure in the newborn period. There is a hyperactive cardiac impulse, gross hepatomegaly, and cardiac failure of obscure origin. Cardiac catheterization reveals highly saturated blood in the inferior vena cava. The blood supply (portal vein or hepatic artery) can be determined by selective angiography, and the lesion can be successfully removed, with resolution of heart failure.

Other systemic arteriovenous fistulas. Many variants occur and give rise to "high output" heart failure. They often can be surgically corrected. Occasionally a cutaneous hemangioma is large enough to cause death from congestive heart failure in the neonatal period.

Myocardial disorders

The more common conditions giving rise to neonatal heart failure through primary myocardial dysfunction are myocarditis, endocardial fibroelastosis, diabetic cardiomyopathy, glycogen storage disease (type II, or Pompe's disease), and anomalous origin of the left coronary artery from the pulmonary artery. The latter condition is actually a form of structural cardiovascular disease, but the clinical presentation is frequently that of a myocardiopathy. A large number of rare conditions may produce myocardial dysfunction both as primary disorders (such as tumors of the heart) and as disorders secondary to systemic disease such as muscular dystrophy, myotonic dystrophy, or pyruvate dehydrogenese enzyme deficiency. Anomalous left coronary artery, endocardial fibroelastosis, and glycogen storage disease usually appear in infants in the second to sixth month of life. The neonatal series underrepresents the true incidence.

Myocarditis

Neonatal myocarditis may be viral, bacterial, or protozoal *(Toxoplasma gondii)*. Viral myocarditis is the most common, although frequently it is not possible to grow any organism from body tissues. The most common responsible viruses are the Coxsackie virus B group, the rubella virus, and cytomegalovirus. The newborn may have active rubella myocarditis with or without other stigmata of intrauterine rubella infection. Coxsackie virus myocarditis can occur in epidemics during the neonatal period. Septic (bacterial) myocarditis has been rarely encountered since the widespread use of antibiotics. In the past bacterial myocarditis has been especially associated with pneumonia and diphtheria. *Toxoplasma* organisms may cause myocarditis by direct invasion of the heart by the parasite.

Clinical manifestations of viral myocarditis. The neonate may appear in a critical state of peripheral circulatory collapse, although in some the onset is more insidious. Frequently there is a history of a viral infection in the mother during the last 2 weeks of pregnancy. Characteristically the infant is normal at birth but rapidly develops the signs and symptoms of heart failure at 3 to 20 days of age. Auscultation usually reveals a gallop rhythm but no murmur. Sometimes the heart sounds are pathologically quiet.

Diagnosis. In the majority the heart is enlarged, and the lungs show the pattern of pulmonary venous congestion. Characteristically the QRS voltages on the standard leads are reduced (Fig. 29-69), and the T waves are frequently inverted or flattened in the left precordial leads. Although the diagnosis may seem obvious, it is important to rule out septic myocarditis (by blood culture). Any suggestion of anomalous coronary artery (infarct pattern on the ECG or appearance of a mitral regurgitation murmur) may warrant sector scan echo visualization of the coronary arteries or aortography. *Toxoplasmosis* or cytomegalovirus is suggested by abnormal head size, microphthalmia, and chorioretinitis.

Treatment. The mortality from viral myocarditis is very high. Heart failure should be treated and the infant given antibiotics to cover the possibility of septic myocarditis, at least until negative blood cultures are certain. Digitalis should not be given if the infant's heart rate falls below 100 beats per minute. Great attention should be paid to achieving a neutral thermal environment to minimize metabolic needs. The critically sick infant should receive his total nutritional support intravenously. Occasionally one is confronted with a moribund bradycardic infant as a result of myocarditis. In this situation the use of isoproterenol (0.05 to 0.2 μg/kg/minute or sufficient to raise the heart rate to 120 beats per minute) administered intravenously seems justified. Dopamine, 1 to 10 μg/kg/minute in 5% dextrose may provide useful inotropic support.

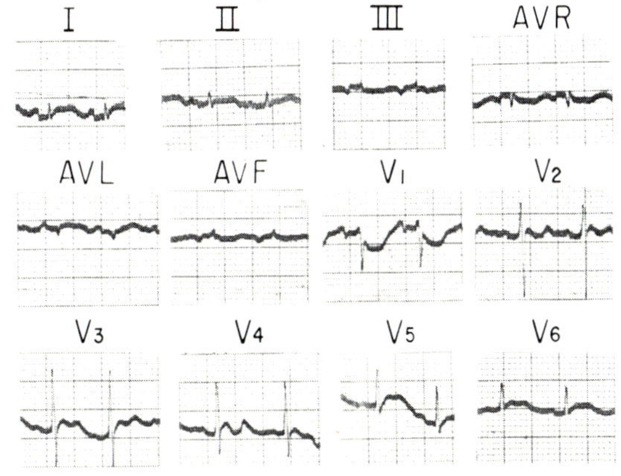

Fig. 29-69. ECG of a baby with proved Coxsackie virus myocarditis. At 1 month of age there is low QRS amplitude and ST depression (V_1). By 2 years of age the cardiogram had returned to normal.

Endocardial fibroelastosis

Endocardial fibroelastosis occurs both as a primary condition, where the cause is unknown, and as a secondary phenomenon, particularly in association with left-sided heart obstruction. The primary form is now unaccountably rare. A smooth, glistening, yellowish membrane lines the left ventricle, with varying degrees of encroachment into the mitral and aortic orifices. The left atrium and very rarely the right atrium occasionally are involved. Usually the left ventricle is greatly dilated, but a contracted type of ventricle does occur, especially in the newborn. Theories of causation include genetic determination by an autosomal recessive gene, a form of end-stage myocarditis caused by Coxsackie virus or mumps virus, and a theory that the condition may be caused by a primary metabolic defect of cardiac muscle such as carnitine deficiency. Primary endocardial fibroelastosis has been seen much less frequently in recent years, for unknown reasons.

Clinical manifestations. Most infants with endocardial fibroelastosis are referred to diagnostic centers at 2 to 4 months of age with an admission diagnosis of "failure to thrive," heart failure, or cardiomegaly of unknown origin. The history usually reveals that the infant was abnormal during the neonatal period, but the absence of cardiac murmur commonly delays recognition of heart disease. The symptoms and signs of the primary form of endocardial fibroelastosis are characteristic. Infants are undernourished and show evidence of predominantly left-sided heart failure with tachycardia, tachypnea, and inappropriate sweating. The peripheral pulses are normal, and the heart is not hyperdynamic (although it may be large). The heart sounds are normal; some have no murmur, whereas others have the murmurs of mitral or aortic valve disease.

Diagnosis. There is often gross cardiac dilatation (except the contracted form), and evidence of pulmonary venous congestion is usually present. Marked left ventricular hypertrophy is almost always present. This is manifested not only by the voltage changes but also by secondary T-wave changes. On occasion pathologic Q waves are present. The echocardiogram will show a dilated left ventricle and poor left ventricular function; serial studies will help evaluate the response to therapy.

Differential diagnosis. Endocardial fibroelastosis is usually distinguishable from acute viral myocarditis by the shorter history and by the ECG. Neonates with glycogen storage disease (type II) are hypotonic, have large tongues, and frequently have a positive family history.

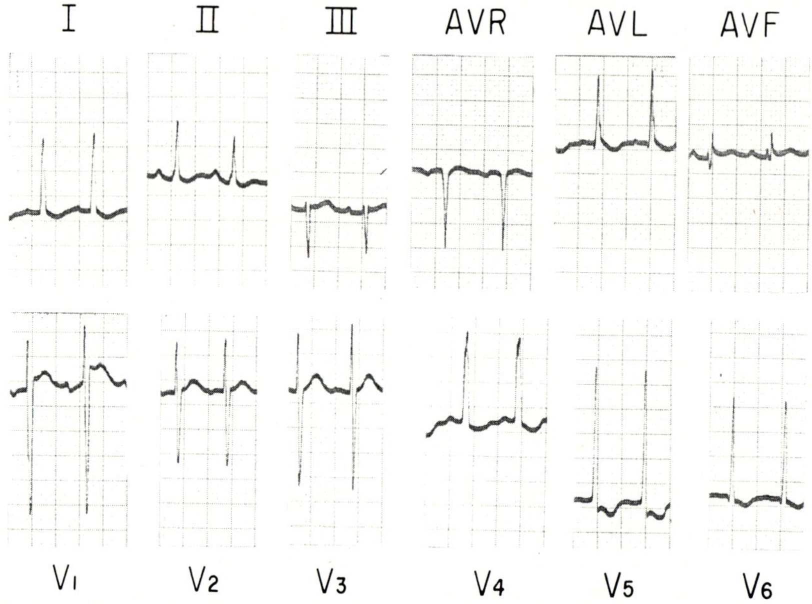

Fig. 29-70. ECG of an infant with endocardial fibroelastosis. All leads are recorded at half standard. There is marked left ventricular hypertrophy with secondary T wave changes (leads I, V_5, and V_6).

Skeletal muscle biosy shows a greatly raised glycogen content in type II glycogen storage disease. Carnitine deficiency can be diagnosed by determination of serum carnitine level and if necessary by skeletal muscle biopsy (Fig. 29-70). The most important differential diagnosis is that of an anomalous left coronary artery arising from the pulmonary artery. This produces a clinical picture and a chest roentgenogram almost identical to those of endocardial fibroelastosis. The diagnosis of anomalous left coronary is strongly suggested by an infarct pattern on the ECG and by the murmur of mitral regurgitation (caused by papillary muscle infarction). Since the anomalous left coronary artery can be surgically treated and mimics endocardial fibroelastosis very closely, it has become our policy to perform an aortogram on every infant with a clinical diagnosis of endocardial fibroelastosis.

Hemodynamics. The left ventricle is large and fails to empty adequately. Left ventricular end-diastolic pressure is raised, and, if there is mitral valve involvement, there is frequently a diastolic gradient across the mitral valve, with greatly raised left atrial pressure. Right-sided heart pressures are elevated secondary to left-sided heart pressure elevation. If the patient is undergoing diagnostic studies, it is important to confirm the presence of two normally placed coronary arteries either by left ventricular or aortic root angiography. The cardiac output is frequently low and is reflected by a widened arteriovenous oxygen content difference.

Prognosis. Manning and associates reported 31 of 56 infants surviving over 2 years, although many survivors had large hearts and abnormal ECGs. The rapid reversion of the abnormal T waves was a favorable prognostic sign. Since the diagnosis of endocardial fibroelastosis (primary form) is essentially a pathologic one and it is likely that it is a disease of multifactorial causes, it is extremely difficult to provide parents with a reliable prognosis.

Treatment. There is no specific therapy except where carnitine or other metabolic deficiency can be shown. Heart failure should be treated and the metabolic needs of the critically sick infant minimized by intravenous feeding and the careful maintenance of thermoneutrality. Digitalis is particularly important, and some infants demonstrate an unusual degree of dependency on digitalis.

"Diabetic cardiomyopathy"

The infant of a diabetic mother has been known to be at increased risk for cardiac defects and other heart disease (see Chapter 3). The recent literature documents in these infants the occurrence of a cardiomyopathy which may be associated with respiratory symptoms and congestive heart failure. The cardiomyopathy occurs in infants whose mothers have gestational or overt diabetes. Echocardiographic studies by Gutgesell and co-workers, Way and co-workers, and Mace and co-workers document abnormal thickness of the right ventricular wall and interventricular septum in infants of diabetic mothers when compared with normal babies of comparable gestational age. This was not explainable by the increased size of the infants, since the same measurements in large

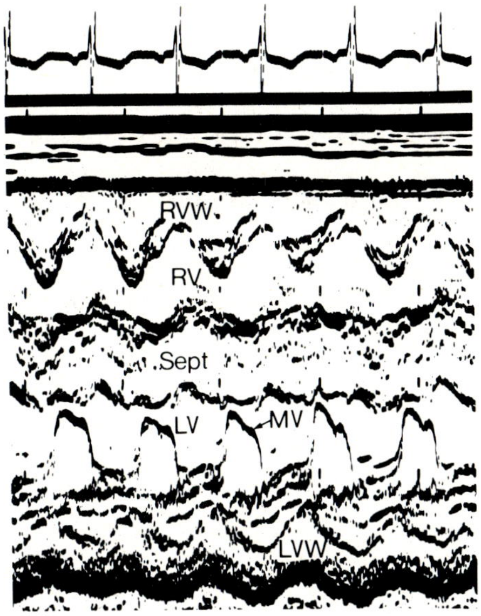

Fig. 29-71. M-mode echocardiogram from 3-day-old infant of diabetic mother. There is generalized thickening of cardiac walls; however, septum *(SEPT)* is thickened to much greater degree than left ventricular wall *(LVW)*. *LV*, left ventricle; *MV*, mitral valve; *RV*, right ventricle; *RVW*, right ventricular wall. (Courtesy Drs. R. Snider and N. Silverman.)

for gestational age normal infants were significantly smaller. In the study by Way and co-workers of 11 infants of diabetic mothers with congestive heart failure and/or respiratory symptoms, all had disproportionate thickening of the interventricular septum, although not all had evidence of left ventricular outflow obstruction. This is comparable to the autosomal dominant disease of idiopathic hypertrophic subaortic stenosis in which the interventricular septum is asymmetrically hypertrophied with respect to the left ventricular posterior wall. (Normally the interventricular septum/left ventricular posterior wall does not exceed 1.3.) In the hypertrophic cardiomyopathy of infants of diabetic mothers the interventricular septum/left ventricular posterior wall may range from 1.3 to greater than 2 and has been called disproportionate septal hypertrophy (Fig. 29-71). Obstruction, demonstrated by cardiac catheterization or by echo, may or may not be present.

Symptoms may be worsened by treatment with digitalis, and improvement may occur with propranolol administration. For this reason an echocardiogram probably is indicated in all infants of diabetic mothers. The natural history appears to be benign and the abnormality usually resolves in 3 to 12 months.

Glycogen storage disease

See also Chapter 36.

The only type of glycogenosis in which the heart is involved to a major extent is type II (Pompe's disease). In this condition there is a defect in the enzyme α-1,4-glucosidase, resulting in the accumulation of glycogen in heart, liver, and skeletal muscle. The disease is usually lethal within the first year.

Clinical manifestations. Infants affected with Pompe's disease display a very characteristic clinical picture with failure to thrive, muscular hypotonia, hepatomegaly, and large tongue (see Fig. 29-1). Usually there is no cardiac murmur or a nondescript systolic murmur that may reflect outflow tract obstruction. Affected infants lie quietly, usually supine and in the hypotonic frog-leg position. The respirations are rapid.

Diagnosis. The heart is large, and the lung fields may show passive pulmonary venous engorgement. A characteristic but not pathognomonic ECG has been described (Fig. 29-72). The PR interval is short, the QRS voltages are greatly increased, and deep Q waves over the left precordium are frequently seen. In some cases there is T-wave inversion in leads V_5 and V_6.

The echocardiogram shows LVH, usually with the picture of a dilated cardiomyopathy. The diagnosis may be confirmed by the finding of greater than 1.5% glycogen by wet weight in skeletal muscle biopsy; levels of 8% to 10% are not unusual.

Treatment. No definitive treatment is available; the major contribution the pediatrician can make is in counseling and alerting the parents to the possibility of diagnosis early in the gestation of future offspring by means of examination of the amniotic fluid for α-1,4-glucosidase activity.

Anomalous origin of the left coronary artery from the pulmonary artery

Early recognition of the anomalous left coronary artery is important; if the condition is untreated, the mortality in infancy is high, and both palliative surgery and corrective surgery are available. The incidence is 0.4 to 0.5% of patients with congenital heart disease. The condition often is not recognized in the neonatal period, but symptoms tend to become obvious at age 2 to 4 months. Occasionally the lesion escapes recognition until later childhood or even adult life.

Clinical manifestations. The major symptoms are failure to thrive and the manifestations of left ventricular failure. Occasionally parents will observe episodes that could be interpreted as angina pectoris or coronary occlusion, but in the majority of infants the symptoms differ little from those of endocardial fibroelastosis. There may be no murmur, or the apical systolic murmur of mitral insufficiency may be present. Mitral insufficiency is probably secondary to infarction of the papillary muscles of the mitral valve.

Diagnosis. The heart is characteristically large and

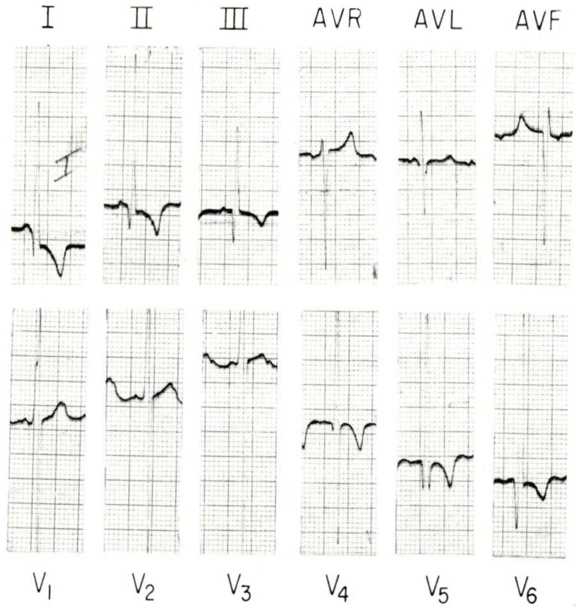

Fig. 29-72. ECG of an infant with type II glycogen storage disease. The PR interval is short. There is left axis deviation, right ventricular hypertrophy, and left ventricular hypertrophy with "strain" (inverted T waves in leads V_5, V_6, and I).

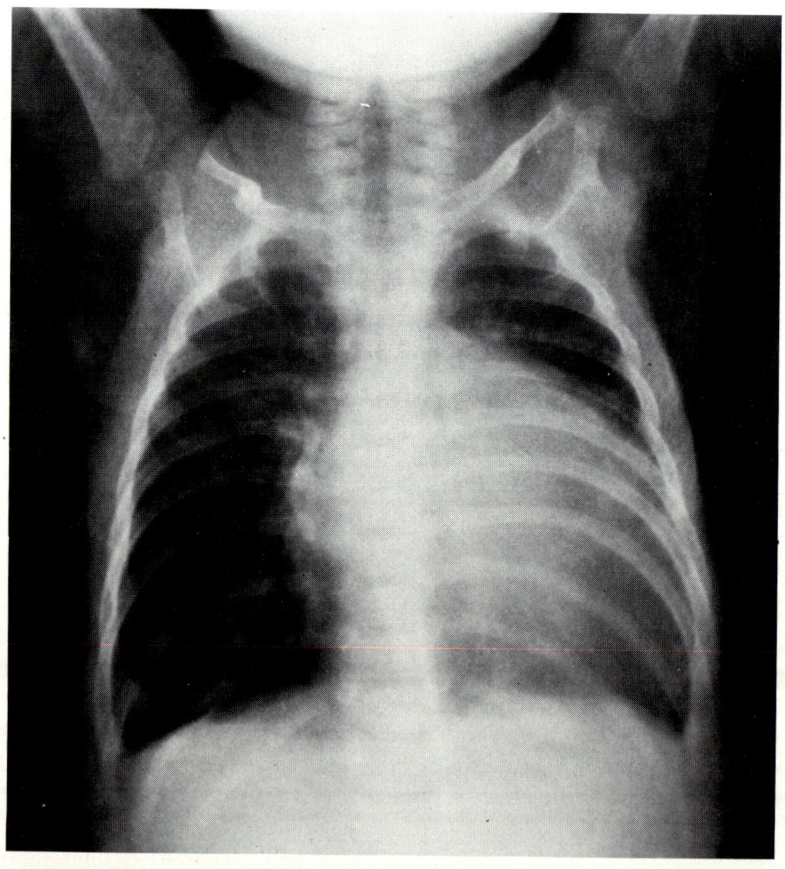

Fig. 29-73. Chest film of an infant with anomalous origin of the left coronary artery from the pulmonary artery. Note extreme cardiomegaly. Fluoroscopically the heart changed very little in volume between systole and diastole.

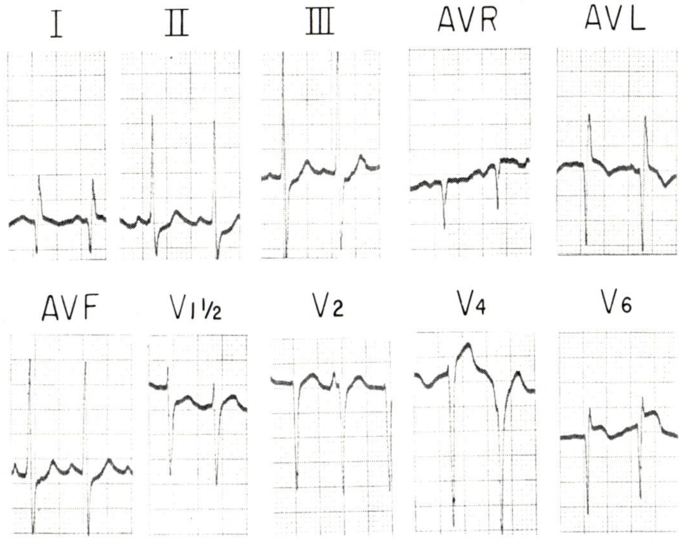

Fig. 29-74. Anomalous origin of the left coronary artery from the pulmonary artery, producing myocardial infarction. Note pathologic Q waves in leads I, aV_L, and V_6. At surgery (ligation of anomalous coronary) the apex and posterior wall of the left ventricle showed widespread infarction.

empties poorly with each systolic contraction (Fig. 29-73). The most characteristic ECG is that of myocardial infarction (Fig. 29-74). However, in some the appearance is that of ischemia; in a small number only the voltage changes of left ventricular hypertrophy are present.

The echocardiogram shows a greatly dilated LV and LA, often without mitral valve insufficiency. Since the anomalous left coronary artery arises from the posterior aspect of the main pulmonary artery, it is hard to image; however, failure to see the left coronary artery leaving the aorta is suggestive evidence.

Hemodynamics. The hemodynamics are greatly influenced by the size and number of anastomoses between the right and left coronary arterial systems and by the pulmonary arterial pressure. Thus infants with many anastomoses and low pulmonary artery pressure have a left-to-right shunt from the aorta to the pulmonary artery by means of the anomalous left coronary artery. This "runoff" into the pulmonary artery compromises coronary capillary–filling pressure and myocardial blood flow to all areas of the heart. Temporary elevation of the pulmonary artery pressure may account for the rarity of diagnosis during the neonatal period. It is important therefore to measure pulmonary artery pressure, assess the degree of the left-to-right shunt, and visualize the coronary arterial system. The typical infant shows rapid opacification of the normal right coronary artery, followed by opacification of the anomalous left coronary artery and pulmonary artery.

Treatment. Management is controversial at the present time. Some cardiologists favor medical treatment of the infant with high pulmonary artery pressure, little or no left-to-right shunt, and a stable clinical course. Prolonged survival of these infants is possible, and the anomalous left coronary artery can be anastomosed to the ascending aorta by means of a saphenous vein graft when the child is larger. The sick infant with low pulmonary artery pressure and left-to-right shunting presents a dilemma. Simple ligation of the anomalous coronary artery improves myocardial perfusion but leaves a single coronary system. Recently, direct attachment of the anomalous coronary artery to the aorta by a variety of techniques in both types during infancy has been gaining popularity. We have recently treated an infant by an anastomosis to the aorta, with restoration of almost normal LV function over the period of a year.

Miscellaneous congenital heart conditions

A large number of rare heart lesions may produce symptomatic disease in the neonate. Four of these conditions are mentioned briefly in the following sections: absence of the pulmonary valve, isolated tricuspid insufficiency, cor triatriatum, and dextrocardia.

Isolated congenital absence of the pulmonary valve

Absence of the pulmonary valve is rare as an isolated anomaly and occasionally is associated with tetralogy of Fallot. Diagnosis of the isolated lesion is suggested by a diastolic murmur, heard maximally at the second left interspace, that is slightly delayed in onset after the pulmonic closure sound. There is an associated systolic murmur because of increased systolic pulmonary valve flow. Pulmonary insufficiency characteristically produces very marked dilatation of the main pulmonary arteries. The diagnosis can be made by echocardiography and is confirmed by the absence of a diastolic gradient across the pulmonary valve and by pulmonary artery angiography. The disease either has a rather benign course, or the patient dies soon after birth. The poor outcome in some newborns may be because of associated physiologic pulmonary hypertension, causing a significant backward driving force from pulmonary artery to right ventricle and an impairment of adequate right ventricular emptying.

Isolated congenital tricuspid insufficiency

This is rare and appears to be caused by congenital short chordae tendineae or by papillary muscle infarction secondary to coronary and myocardial hypoxemia. The closure of apparently adequate valve cusps is prevented. Occasionally tricuspid insufficiency has been reported in association with the PFC syndrome or secondary to papillary infarction from profound fetal asphyxia and hypoxemia. The diagnosis is suggested by cyanosis (from right-to-left atrial shunting), a loud pansystolic murmur at the lower left sternal border, evidence of grossly raised venous pressure, hepatomegaly, and a large heart with an especially large right atrium. The diagnosis can be made by echocardiography by interrogation of the tricuspid valve. Catheterized neonates have had greatly raised right atrial pressures, and right ventricular angiography has disclosed massive tricuspid regurgitation. When the condition is secondary to fetal asphyxia, there is often spontaneous improvement or complete resolution, but when the condition appears life threatening, the lowering of pulmonary vascular resistance (by increasing inspired oxygen tension or administering vasoactive drugs such as tolazoline into the pulmonary artery) might allow improved right ventricular emptying.

Cor triatriatum

The division of the left atrium into an inner chamber receiving the pulmonary veins and an outer chamber leading to the mitral valve constitutes cor triatriatum. The communication between the two left atrial chambers is inadequate for the free efflux of pulmonary vein blood, so that pulmonary venous pressure rises, and the infant dies with the signs of left ventricular failure; failure of the accessory left atrial chamber would be a more accurate description of the hemodynamics.

The condition is rare but important because it is surgically correctable. The first sign is tachypnea, followed by pulmonary rales. Pulmonary hypertension ensues, with a loud pulmonic closure sound. The ECG shows right ventricular hypertrophy. The chest roentgenogram discloses a somewhat enlarged heart with the vascular pattern typical of pulmonary venous engorgement, a lacy pattern throughout the lung fields, often with the Kerley B lines of engorged lymphatics. The echocardiogram may be pathognomonic with visualization of the accessory chamber. There is usually no murmur so that the condition mimics PFC and a variety of primary respiratory conditions, including pulmonary lymphangiectasia and atypical RDS. The condition also mimics other causes of left-sided heart obstruction, especially total anomalous pulmonary venous return with obstruction to pulmonary venous return, pulmonary vein stenosis, and mitral atresia.

Diagnosis is confirmed if necessary by cardiac catheterization. There is a discrepancy between pulmonary artery wedge pressure (reflecting the inner chamber) and left atrial pressure. Occasionally the catheter can be passed across the diaphragm connecting the two left atrial chambers, and the gradient can be demonstrated. The anomalous left atrial septum also can be demonstrated angiographically following pulmonary artery contrast agent injection. Surgical relief is possible early in life by excision of the anomalous septum.

Dextrocardia and levocardia with situs inversus

Dextroposition of the heart is to be distinguished from true dextrocardia. With dextroposition other noncardiac conditions are responsible for rightward displacement of the heart. In these situations careful appraisal of the lungs and gastrointestinal tract reveals the true nature of the problem. If there is true dextrocardia or true levocardia with situs inversus (that is, no pathologic condition present to cause mediastinal shift), then it is likely that the child will have associated structural congenital heart disease.

Neonates who have either dextrocardia or levocardia with situs inversus account for less than 3% of congenital heart malformations discovered in the newborn period. Dextrocardia with abdominal situs inversus is not infrequently associated with cyanotic cardiac lesions. Neonates with dextrocardia and normally placed viscera or partial situs inversus have a very high incidence of complex cyanotic congenital heart disease, particularly if there is splenic agenesis or polysplenia. Similarly those with splenic agenesis and levocardia frequently have complex heart disease, whether or not there is abdominal situs inversus.

In management of the neonate with apparent dextrocardia one should consider the following:

1. The possibility of dextroposition being caused by movement of the mediastinum secondary to lung agenesis, lobar emphysema, diaphragmatic hernia, and so on should be ruled out. Pulmonary arteriography may be required.
2. An increase in the number of Howell-Jolly and Heinz bodies and an elevated reticulocyte count suggest splenic agenesis. Splenic agenesis may be confirmed by aortography or by an abnormal spleen scan.
3. An abnormal P axis (such as negative P wave in lead

I) may indicate atrial inversion. It also may be caused by an ectopic atrial pacemaker (sometimes in the left atrium).

4. Echocardiography usually provides the definitive diagnosis by not only defining the intracardiac anatomy but also the extracardiac venous and arterial connections as well.
5. Cardiac catheterization and angiocardiography are occasionally necessary for precise chamber localization. The venous atrium and sometimes other chambers are easily reached. There is a high incidence of systemic venous anomalies that may complicate cardiac catheterization.
6. Other congenital defects, especially gastrointestinal and genitourinary tract anomalies, should be looked for.

Treatment. Infants with dextrocardia and levocardia with situs inversus tend to have complex heart disease. This is particularly true if the spleen is absent or rudimentary. If surgical treatment is required, it usually can be only palliative and most often consists of decreasing or increasing pulmonary blood flow by pulmonary artery banding or aortopulmonary shunt.

OTHER CARDIOVASCULAR CONDITIONS

Vascular rings

The incidence of symptomatic vascular rings is not known. Out of 6,647 children recorded in the Toronto Heart Registry, 0.95% had vascular rings or allied aortic arch anomalies. The overwhelming majority of the estimated 900,000 persons in the United States with an anomalous origin of the right subclavian artery arising from a left descending aorta are asymptomatic and have no positive physical signs. The more important lesions to be considered in the symptomatic newborn are double aortic arch, right aortic arch with left ligamentum arteriosum, anomalous innominate artery, anomalous origin of the right subclavian artery, and anomalous origin of the left pulmonary artery. Most clinically significant vascular rings (for example, double aortic arch and right aortic arch with left ligamentum arteriosum) encircle both the trachea and the esophagus. Some (for example, anomalous origin of the right subclavian artery) give rise to only partial encirclement. The anomalous left pulmonary artery runs between the trachea and esophagus, partially compressing both structures.

Clinical manifestations

See also Chapter 28.

Neonates with significant constriction usually have respiratory difficulty, often in the first few days of life. Stridor, wheezing, and intercostal retractions all indicate airway obstruction and give rise to hypoventilation, with arterial hypoxemia and hypercapnia when the obstruction is critical. Symptoms related to esophageal compression are usually present and cause aspiration pneumonia. However, it is not usually obvious that the baby has a swallowing difficulty until he or she takes solid foods. Vascular rings may mimic many other causes of respiratory distress.

Diagnosis

Contrast esophagograms should be performed by an experienced radiologist because of the risk of aspiration. Radiologists frequently choose a thin barium mixture, and many prefer to record the swallow on videotape for later repeated viewing. Each lesion has rather characteristic features. The double aortic arch produces a constant compression deformity at the level of the aortic arch, with marked posterior indentation and lesser left and right indentations (Fig. 29-75). The features of the right aortic arch with left ligamentum arteriosum are similar, but the indentation on the left side is nonpulsating and sharper (ligamentum arteriosum). The anomalous right subclavian artery produces an oblique or spiral indentation on the posterior esophageal wall, pointing upward and to the right. The anomalous innominate artery arises to the left of the midline and passes in front of the trachea to compress the trachea; the barium swallow is normal. The anomalous left pulmonary artery arises from the main pulmonary trunk just to the right of the midline. It then proceeds anterior to the esophagus and behind the trachea to compress both structures. An anterior indentation on the esophagus is therefore highly suggestive of an anomalous left pulmonary artery (Fig. 29-76). If the trachea shows signs of posterior compression or narrowing, the diagnosis is virtually certain. Frequently the esophagogram is pathognomonic, and no further studies are necessary. Echocardiography is of considerable help. Because the structures to be imaged are nearly stationary, CT scanning and nuclear magnetic resonance imaging can be very helpful. In cases of doubt aortography resolves the issue, although several projections may be necessary. A pulmonary arteriogram usually discloses the anomalous left pulmonary artery. However, a 40-degree angle anteroposterior projection may be necessary to spatially separate the main and branch pulmonary arteries.

Treatment

Neonates with symptomatic double aortic arch, those with right aortic arch with left ligamentum arteriosum, and those with anomalous left pulmonary artery almost always require surgical correction. Occasionally a neonate with a large retroesophageal right subclavian artery has respiratory symptoms (usually caused by repeated aspiration pneumonia) sufficiently severe to warrant surgical division of the aberrant vessel. The treatment of the anomalous innominate artery is controversial; it has been suggested that occasionally it may be associated

A

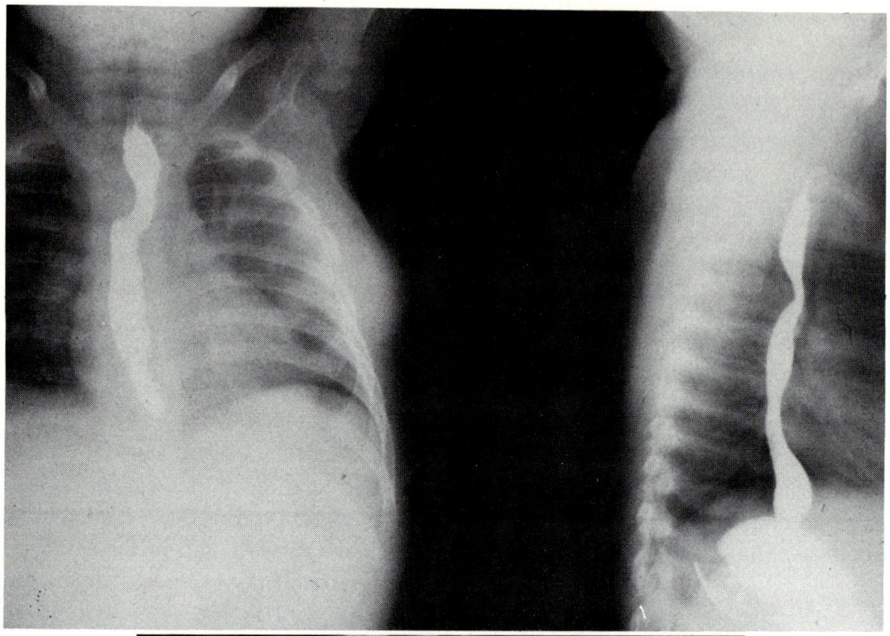

B

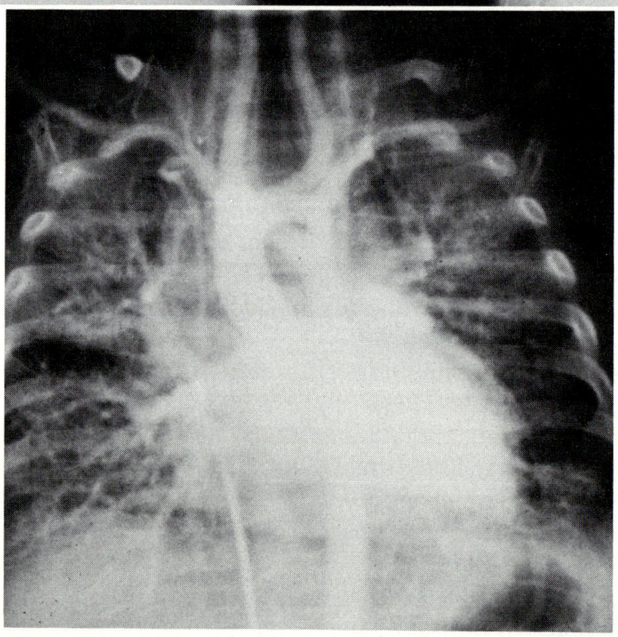

Fig. 29-75. Double aortic arch. **A,** Note imprint of posterior aortic arch on posterior and right aspect of esophagus. **B,** Angiogram discloses double arch. Anterior arch gives rise to left subclavian artery, whereas the other three brachiocephalic arteries arise from the posterior arch. (Courtesy Dr. John R. Campbell.)

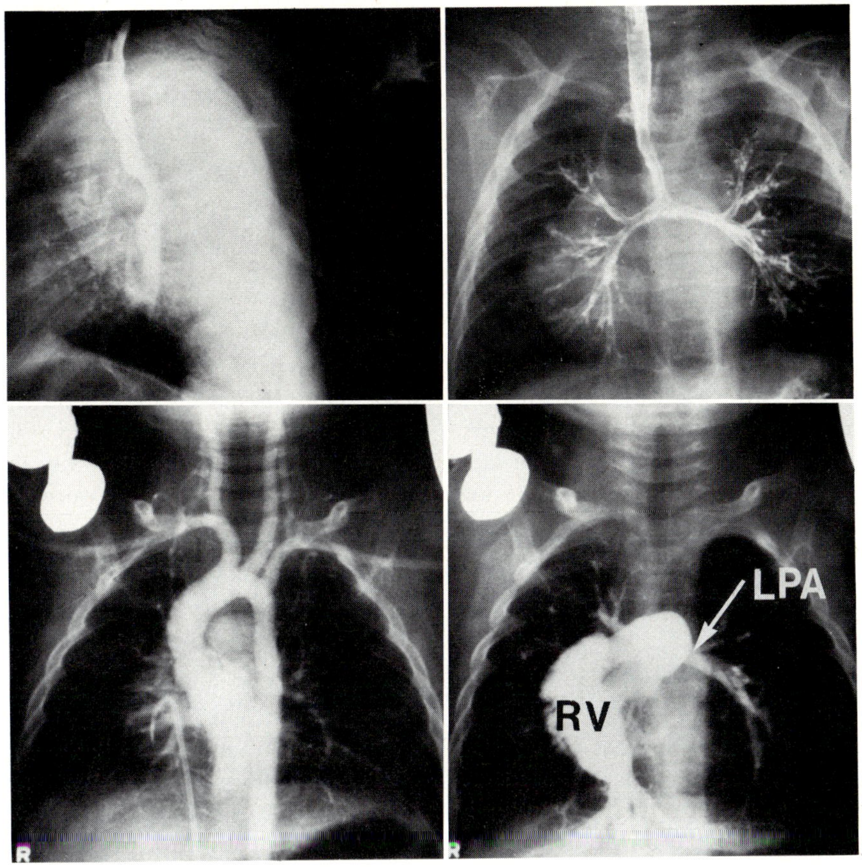

Fig. 29-76. Anomalous left pulmonary artery. The left pulmonary artery proceeds rightward as it leaves the heart. To regain the left lung, it loops leftward between the esophagus and trachea. **A,** Anterior indentation on esophagogram. **B,** Diffuse tracheal narrowing secondary to posterior compression. **C,** Normal levocardiogram. **D,** Right atrial injection. The heart is dextroposed; the right ventricle *(RV)* is in end-systole and has filled an abnormal pulmonary artery (the right ventricle and right atrium are overlapped in this projection). The left pulmonary artery *(LPA)* appears to arise from behind the main pulmonary artery rather than as the usual direct continuation. A more caudally angled and anteroposterior projection is necessary to spatially separate the main and branch pulmonary arteries. (Courtesy Dr. John R. Campbell.)

with reflex bouts of apnea. Gross has achieved surgical correction of this anomaly by pulling the vessel forward and attaching it to the sternum. It is, however, a common anomaly and, like the aberrant right subclavian artery, produces no symptoms in the vast majority of patients.

Systemic hypertension

Although rarely an emergency, systemic hypertension in a neonate always requires an explanation and usually requires treatment. Even though antihypertensive treatment may be needed urgently to combat heart failure or minimize the risk of cerebrovascular accident, the cause must be established even if the hypertension can be successfully controlled with drugs. (See also Chapter 21 and Appendix C.)

Etiology

Hypertension in the neonate is now being more frequently recorded, and it seems likely that the increased incidence is a result of increased use of umbilical artery catheterization. Thus catheters with the tip located between T4 and T12 are above the level of origin of the renal arteries, and unilateral or bilateral renal artery thrombi are more common than previously realized. Nephrogenic hypertension also may be caused by congenital renal artery stenosis, renal vein thrombosis, polycystic kidneys, and a wide variety of congenital and acquired renal diseases. Coarctation of the aorta remains an important treatable cause. Less likely possibilities include pheochromocytoma, Cushing's syndrome, congenital adrenal hyperplasia, primary hyperaldosteronism, and neuroblastoma (secretion of catecholamines or partial obstruction to the renal artery).

Diagnosis

The accurate estimation of systemic blood pressure has been much improved by the Doppler reflected ultrasound technique. In many neonates the indwelling umbilical artery or radial artery line can supply direct measurements. For both Doppler and direct auscultation methods the cuff width should be approximately 50% of the extremity circumference; for most full-term newborns this will mean a bladder 2.5 to 4 cm wide and 5 to 10 cm in length. It is very easy to gain a spurious impression of hypertension from using too small a cuff. The leg pressure should be within 20 mm Hg of arm pressure; if it is significantly higher, it suggests that too small a cuff is being used on the leg. We have found blood pressure measurements in the leg, made with the cuff placed around the calf and Doppler interrogation at the posterior tibial artery (behind the medial malleolus) to be accurate. Fundal examination may reveal features of a hypertensive retinopathy similar to that found in adults. Brachial and femoral pulses should be felt simultaneously to be sure they are synchronous.

Examination of the urinary sediment may reveal evidence of underlying acute or chronic renal disease, either of which may be associated with hypertension. Blood urea nitrogen, creatinine, sodium, potassium, and bicarbonate levels should be obtained. A coagulation profile should be obtained if there is reason to suspect a hypercoagulable state. A 24-hour urine sample can be collected for vanillylmandelic acid (VMA), metanephrines, urinary steroid excretion, and, if appropriate, pregnanetriol. A clinical diagnosis of renal disease should be followed by intravenous urography and if necessary, by renal angiography. If an umbilical artery catheter is present, it may be both suspected as causative (possible renal artery thrombosis) and used for aortography. Many nephrologists consider persistent hypertension of unknown cause to necessitate the estimation of plasma renin activity (to rule out primary hyperaldosteronism) and renal biopsy (to rule out the possibility of occult underlying renal disease). Renal scans are sometimes useful for comparing the function of the two kidneys and are useful for comparative follow-up studies.

Normal blood pressure

Systolic blood pressure in the arm was measured in infants at the ages of 4 to 6 days and 5 to 7 weeks by deSwiet and co-workers using the Doppler ultrasound technique (Table 29-12).

In 391 infants in whom measurements were made on both occasions, blood pressure at 4 to 6 days was significantly related to blood pressure at 5 to 7 weeks. Fig. 29-77 was constructed by Dr. Stephen Alexander from the data of Bucci and associates relating to preterm infants. Note that a factor is added for postnatal age, that is, a 2,000 gm infant 30 hours of age would be expected to have a systolic blood pressure of 60 mm Hg. (See also Chapter 21.)

Table 29-12. Systolic blood pressure in newborns

Age	Number	State	Blood pressure (mm Hg) (SEM)
4-6 days	469	Sleeping	70.7 ± 0.3
5-7 weeks	144	Sleeping	89.7 ± 0.9
5-7 weeks	252	Awake	96.8 ± 0.6

Modified from deSwiet, M., Fayers, P., and Shinebourne, E.A.: Br. Med. J. **2**:9, 1976.

Management

An initial decision needs to be made as to whether the hypertension is imminently life threatening. If immediate control is necessary, a sodium nitroprusside drip at a dose of 2.5 to 5 μg/kg/minute is recommended. Mild hypertension frequently responds to diuretics (chlorothiazide or furosemide) whereas with severe hypertension therapy usually should begin with hydralazine.

In resistant situations multiple-drug therapy involving various combinations of furosemide, hydralazine, and methyldopa has been successful.

The question of nephrectomy for unilateral renal involvement is controversial. Plumer and co-workers reported that their hypertensive neonates generally responded poorly to medical management and suggested nephrectomy for unilateral renal involvement if blood pressure was not controlled within 24 hours. Adelman and associates successfully managed all of 17 hypertensive neonates with diuretics and anti-hypertensive agents, often with rather high drug dosages (Table 29-13).

Use of the specific angiotensin 1 converting enzyme (ACE) inhibitor—captopril—has greatly facilitated control of hypertension in the premature and neonatal infant. The necessary prolonged use of umbilical arterial lines has led to recognition of systemic hypertension of a mild degree as a fairly frequent occurrence after several weeks of umbilical arterial line use. Frequently there is left ventricular hypertrophy by echocardiography, and the thickened, less compliant left ventricle appears to impede filling, leading to tachypnea or respirator dependency. Under these circumstances captopril at a dose of 0.1 mg to 1.0 mg/kg PO q6h to q12h has proved rapidly effective. It is important to give a test dose of 0.2 mg/kg PO and to have dopamine (5 μg/kg/min) and normal saline on hand if the blood pressure should fall precip-

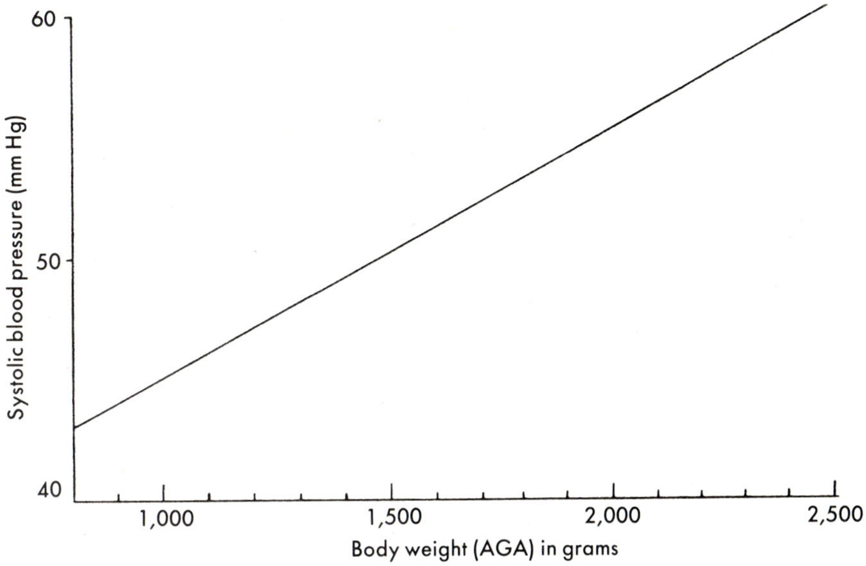

Add for postnatal age:

Hours	3-7	8-12	13-18	19-24	25-32	33-40	41-54
mm Hg.	1	2	3	4	5	6	7

Fig. 29-77. Systolic blood pressure in AGA underweight newborns. (Courtesy Dr. Stephen Alexander; data from Bucci, G., and others: Acta Paediatr. Scand. [Suppl.] **299:**5, 1972.)

Table 29-13. Drugs useful in the management of neonatal hypertension

Drug	Dose range	Comments
Chlorothiazide	10 to 20 mg/kg PO q12h	Diuretic; suitable for mild hypertension
Furosemide	1-4 mg/kg IV, PO q6 to q24h	Diuretic; suitable for mild and moderate hypertension
Hydralazine	0.1 to 0.5 mg/kg IV, PO q3 to q6h	Vasodilator; moderate and severe hypertension
Methyldopa	2 to 12 mg/kg IV, PO q6 to q8h	Central acting; used in combination with other drugs
Diazoxide	2 to 5 mg/kg/dose IV q2 to q6h	Vasodilator; rapid action; for severe hypertension
Propranolol	0.5-2.0 mg/kg PO q6 to q8h or 0.05-0.15 mg/kg IV q6 to q8h	β-adrenergic blocker; seldom indicated in neonates
Sodium nitroprusside	0.5 to 8.0 μg/kg/minute IV	Vasodilator; rapid action; for severe hypertension
Captopril	0.2 mg/kg PO as test 0.1 mg to 1.0 mg/kg P0 q6 to q12h	Specific competitive inhibitor of ACE; useful for renal hypertension; have IV dopamine (5 μg/kg/min) and normal saline available if blood pressure drops precipitously

Modified from Adelman, R.D., and others: Pediatrics **62:**71, 1978.

itously. First reports of captopril usage were in hyperreninemic infants, but it is now clear that the drug is often effective when the plasma renin is normal. Although the medication appears remarkably free of side effects, neutropenia, proteinemia, and azotemia have been reported.

Cyanotic spells and central nervous system problems

Neonates with cyanotic heart disease, especially those with tetralogy of Fallot or pulmonary atresia with open ventricular septum, may develop cyanotic spells that, if severe, can lead to death. Usually these spells follow crying or bowel movement or occur soon after awakening. They are quite different from the apneic spells of immaturity. Typically the child becomes progressively more cyanotic and develops deep, sighing respirations. If the condition is unrelieved, acidosis and hypoxemia lead to circulatory and respiratory depression with pallor, flaccidity, bradycardia, and on occasion convulsions, cardiac arrest, and death. The underlying heart disease is often surgically treatable, and the occurrence of even minor spells always should lead to hospital admission.

Treatment

If the spell is mild, the baby should be comforted to stop the crying. Oxygen should be given by face mask if this can be done without further upsetting the infant. If the spell is more severe, with bradycardia or impairment of consciousness, morphine sulfate (0.1 to 0.2 mg/kg body weight) should be administered subcutaneously. If the infant is profoundly depressed and has a very slow heart rate, sodium bicarbonate (2 to 3 mEq/kg over a 2-minute period) should be administered intravenously and external cardiac massage initiated to try to improve the coronary circulation. Ventilation with oxygen (face mask or endotracheal tube) is indicated if respiration is depressed. Most neonates will recover from this latter situation. However, spells of the severe type are always multiple and progressive, unless appropriate surgery to improve pulmonary blood flow is performed. An exception is the infant who is anemic relative to his degree of unsaturation. Thus an infant with an arterial saturation of 70% is anemic if he has a hematocrit value of 40%. Sometimes the spells can be completely abolished by treating the anemia, but most often surgery is required. Phenylephrine has been used to increase bronchial collateral blood flow and propranolol to decrease β-adrenergic activity. A useful medication to consider in the event of severe unremitting spells is Ketamine hydrochloride. Ketamine can be administered intramuscularly; it both raises the blood pressure and has a dissociative anesthetic effect. A suitable dose is 0.5 to 2.0 mg/kg; the duration of action ranges from 1 to 10 minutes. It should be emphasized that the occurrence of spells always indicates the need for action, usually in the form of total repair or an aortopulmonary anastomosis.

Other central nervous system emergencies associated with cyanotic heart disease

Brain abscess is very uncommon in infants under 2 years of age but should be considered, especially if the baby has the potential for paradoxical embolism, for example, passage of septic material right to left across the VSD in tetralogy of Fallot. Cerebral thrombosis is also rare but occasionally may occur with a very high hematocrit value. Immediate treatment consists of venesection, 10 to 15 ml/kg, with replacement of blood by plasmanate or 5% dextrose. Anticoagulation with heparin (0.5 mg/kg given intravenously) may be considered but should not be used if brain abscess or mycotic aneurysm is a possibility. Anoxic brain damage is far more common in the neonate than is brain abscess or cerebral thrombosis.

Digitalis toxicity

Cardiac glycosides are excreted in an exponential fashion. Digoxin is the most commonly prescribed agent, but ouabain and digitoxin also are used in pediatrics. Toxicity caused by digitoxin is particularly dangerous because of its long biologic half-life (9 days) as compared with that of digoxin (38 hours) and ouabain (22 hours). Ouabain has very little advantage over digoxin. It starts to act slightly faster (3 to 10 minutes as opposed to 5 to 30 minutes for digoxin). However, digoxin is recommended for neonates in need of a cardiac glycoside.

Digitalis toxicity in infants and children is mainly manifested by arrhythmias, but vomiting, lethargy, or anorexia sometimes will call attention to digitalis overdose, and with massive digitalis poisoning there may be convulsions, apnea, or sudden death. A digitalis-induced arrhythmia usually is characterized by bradycardia associated with SA node or AV node inhibition. A variety of arrhythmias occur: (1) marked sinus arrhythmia with a rate variation greater than 50 beats per minute, (2) sinus arrest with escape beats, (3) AV nodal rhythm, (4) second-degree AV block, (5) complete AV block or AV dissociation, (6) atrial or ventricular premature beats, bigeminal rhythm, (7) PAT with or without AV block, and (8) ventricular tachycardia or ventricular fibrillation. Probably the most common arrhythmias warning of digitalis intoxication are SA block, second-degree AV block, or multiple ectopic beats.

Digitalis toxicity is especially likely if there is renal disease or hypothyroidism. Certain pathologic states (myocardial disease, hypokalemia, hypomagnesemia, hypercalcemia, anoxia, and alkalosis) sometimes potentiate the action of digitalis and can result in toxicity with "normal" circulating levels of digoxin.

Digitalis toxicity should be differentiated from digitalis effect. *Digitalis effect* consists of slight slowing of the heart rate, prolongation of the PR interval, shortening of the QT interval, a shift of the ST segment, or a change in the direction of the U wave. These signs merely indicate that digitalis is fixed in the myocardium and do *not* indicate that dosage should be reduced.

Treatment

Treatment of digitalis toxicity involves the following steps.

1. Gastric lavage or emesis is indicated if oral ingestion is recent.
2. Digitalis administration should be stopped and an attempt made to increase the rate of digitalis excretion by fluids given orally or intravenously.
3. The child should be placed in an intensive care unit; the ECG should be monitored and serum electrolyte and serum digoxin levels determined frequently.
4. Correction of any acid-base or electrolyte disturbance should be attempted. If the serum potassium level is low (as after thiazide diuretic administration), potassium chloride (1 gm/10 kg/day) may be given orally.

If the situation is urgent, potassium chloride (0.5 mEq/kg) may be given intravenously in not less than 1 hour, as a solution of 40 mEq (3 gm) potassium chloride in 500 ml 5% dextrose. Potassium should be given intravenously only with a physician present and with constant ECG monitoring and frequent serum potassium determinations. McNamara and associates have suggested that potassium should not be administered routinely to patients with digitalis intoxication, because toxic doses of digitalis inhibit the transfer of extracellular potassium into the cell, and the resulting high concentration of serum potassium produces myocardial depression.

5. There is a possible source of danger in the misplacement of a decimal point when giving intramuscular doses. If the mistake is realized within a few minutes, it may be possible to drain the site of injection or excise the tissue.
6. Specific arrhythmias require specific treatment. The ease of transvenous pacing even in the newborn has revolutionized the treatment of digitalis poisoning. Slow rates associated with digitalis-induced bradycardia or heart block are common and respond very effectively to temporary insertion of a transvenous endocardial catheter pacemaker and to control of the heart rate by electrical stimulation. Propranolol (0.05 to 0.2 mg/kg) may suppress ventricular arrhythmias.
7. Murphy and co-workers found treatment with "Fab" fragments of digoxin-specific antibodies to be highly successful with massive digoxin poisoning. The material is obtainable from many poison control centers.
8. "Overdrive" pacing to break an arrhythmia, followed by transvenous ventricular pacing at a rate of 140 to 160 beats per minute, should be considered even when the problem is a tachyarrhythmia rather than a bradyarrhythmia.

Pericardial effusion and cardiac tamponade

The term *cardiac tamponade* or *acute cardiac compression* denotes an interference with the diastolic filling of the heart and with cardiac contraction because of an increase in intrapericardial pressure. Both pericardial effusion and cardiac tamponade are rare in the newborn period but are most likely to occur as a complication of septic pericarditis. Pericardial tamponade also may be caused by gas in the pericardial space. This is likely to occur with high-pressure respirator settings. Stroke output is diminished because the elevated pericardial pressure compresses the right atrium and interferes with the venous inflow from the great veins. A normal cardiac output is temporarily maintained by a compensatory tachycardia, and the blood pressure at first is sustained by peripheral vasoconstriction. At a critical level of intrapericardial pressure (10 to 15 cm H_2O) there is a sudden reduction in stroke volume and cardiac output, and there is a fall in blood pressure.

Diagnosis

Physical signs include (1) rising venous pressure to 20 cm H_2O or above (considerably higher than the pressure found in heart failure), leading to liver enlargement and neck vein engorgement, (2) falling arterial pressure with narrowed pulse pressure, (3) usually tachycardia and peripheral vasoconstriction, (4) pulsus paradoxus, a distinct diminution in pulse amplitude by 10 to 20 mm Hg during inspiration, (5) quiet heart, and (6) a reduced urine output.

The important step is to suspect the diagnosis. Echocardiography has become the major noninvasive method for detecting and quantitating pericardial effusions (see Fig. 29-25). Angiocardiography is rarely necessary.

Treatment

Pericardiocentesis may be indicated to confirm the diagnosis, determine the causative agent, or relieve the symptoms. The central venous pressure should continue to be monitored as an index of successful treatment. The line may be used for rapid blood replacement, as well as for drug therapy. Pericardiocentesis should be performed under strict sterile conditions with a 3-inch short-bevel 18- or 20-gauge needle to which is attached the V electrocardiographic lead. If the ventricle is touched by the exploring electrode, there is great amplification of existing recorded QRS complexes, or ventricular ectopic beats are provoked. A preferred alternative is to use two-dimensional echocardiography to guide the needle into the pericardial space. If needle pericardiocentesis is unsuccessful, it is usually because the fluid is too thick for aspiration. In that case surgical therapy involving pleuropericardial drainage of chronic pericardial effusions or pericardiectomy is indicated.

Bacterial endocarditis

Bacterial endocarditis is rare in the neonatal period. When it does occur, it is likely to be part of an acute generalized overwhelming septicemia. Septicemia may be the result of indwelling venous or arterial catheters. Candida endocarditis has been described following umbilical artery catheterization; the classic signs of subacute endocarditis do not occur. Echocardiography can help greatly in the visualization of vegetations.

Syndrome complexes

Despite careful attention to the history, physical examination, ECG, and roentgenogram, it is often not possible to make a precise anatomic diagnosis. This is not a reflection of diagnostic inadequacy but a result of the

Table 29-14. Syndrome complexes and diagnostic possibilities

Syndrome complex	Possible diagnoses
1. Marked cyanosis during first days of life Increased pulmonary blood flow	Transposition of great arteries Hypoplastic left-heart syndrome Preductal coarctation of aorta
2. Cyanosis during first days of life Reduced pulmonary blood flow	Pulmonary atresia with open ventricular septum Pulmonary atresia or extreme pulmonic stenosis with intact ventricular septum Tricuspid atresia Ebstein's anomaly of tricuspid valve Transposition with pulmonic stenosis
3. Mild cyanosis; increased pulmonary blood flow	Truncus arteriosus Large VSD or common ventricle Total anomalous pulmonary venous return Double-outlet right ventricle and variants Transposition of great arteries with large VSD Common AV canal
4. Early heart failure with or without cyanosis secondary to hypoventilation	Arteriovenous fistula (especially cerebral) Severe aortic stenosis, aortic arch hypoplasia, or long-segment aortic coarctation Large PDA Absent pulmonary valve SVT
5. Heart failure at 1 to 4 weeks Insidious onset Murmur present	Large VSD PDA Common AV canal Postductal coarctation Double-outlet right ventricle Truncus arteriosus
6. Heart failure Large heart Acyanotic No murmur	Primary myocardial disorder Myocarditis Endocardial fibroelastosis Anomalous left coronary artery Glycogen storage disease
7. Heart failure with small or normal-sized heart Roentgenogram of pulmonary venous engorgement	Total anomalous pulmonary venous return with obstruction (for example, drains below diaphragm into liver) Cor triatriatum

changing fetal-to-newborn circulation, the presence of heart failure or pulmonary hypertension, and the nonspecificity of some signs. The usual result is that, although one may make an intelligent guess at the structural abnormality, one is left with three or four conditions with which the signs are compatible. Certain syndrome complexes emerge, based on the presence or absence of major physical signs.

Echocardiography and often cardiac catheterization combined with selective angiocardiography are essential for accurate diagnosis except in very rare instances where signs are pathognomonic and the correct treatment is obvious. The syndrome complexes shown in Table 29-14 are intended only to indicate the more likely possibilities.

TALKING WITH PARENTS

Explanation of the baby's specific condition

Many parents do not understand the spoken anatomic description, and statements such as "hole in the heart" often are misinterpreted. A box diagram of the four heart chambers and two great arteries is readily understood by all and can be kept by the parents when they are called on to explain the situation to other relatives. An excellent booklet entitled *If Your Child Has a Congenital Heart Defect* is available from local heart associations and from the American Heart Association, 73 Greenville Ave., Dallas, TX 75231.

The natural history of the lesion should be indicated so that a strong case can be made for or against surgery. Surgery is still hazardous in the neonate, not only because of intraoperative problems but also because of recovery room death on the first days after surgery. Such postoperative deaths usually are caused by low-output states and respiratory complications (atelectasis, airway obstruction, and intrapulmonary right-to-left shunting).

Genetic counseling

The overall incidence of structural heart disease can be stated as being approximately 1%. For parents who already have one affected child, the risk increases to 3% or 4%. These odds are more easily understood if one states that 24 out of 25 times the next child will have a normal heart. If two first-degree relatives are affected, or if multiple second-degree relatives are affected, one would be unwise to quote odds, since an unusual heritable tendency already has been demonstrated. The risk to a child born to a mother who herself has congenital heart disease is 10% to 15%. If the father has congenital heart disease, the risk to the child is probably 5% to 8%.

CARE OF THE NEONATE AFTER CARDIOVASCULAR SURGERY

Recent advances in medical management (such as balloon septostomy for d-transposition of the great arteries and PGE_1 for maintaining patency of the ductus arteriosus) combined with recent advances in surgical techniques (such as subclavian flap operation for severe coarctation) have resulted in the majority of neonates with serious heart disease undergoing successful palliative or reparative heart surgery.

In many of the infants severe hypoxemia and myocardial catecholamine depletion have led to myocardial dysfunction; lack of fluid intake has led to electrolyte imbalance; and hypoglycemia and hypocalcemia may have further added to the precarious state of the infant. The surgical procedure may proceed satisfactorily from a technical point of view, but careful postoperative management is critically important.

The decision as to whether the infant should be cared for in a neonatal or cardiac intensive care unit will depend on local expertise, particularly the experience of nurses and staff. For an in-depth review of the subject the reader is referred to the monograph by Sade and associates.

Postoperative monitoring

Cardiac function

See also Chapter 21.

The standard surface ECG is displayed on an oscilloscope with simultaneous display of heart rate. The occurrence of bradycardia, tachycardia, or irregularity triggers an alarm and also activates a printout from a "memory loop" (a magnetic tape of the ECG of the preceding minute continuously updated). After open-heart surgery temporary atrial and ventricular pacing wires are left in place so that immediate control of a rate or rhythm problem is possible. Temporary pacing wires also facilitate the diagnosis of complex arrhythmias, as well as allow electronic control of the heart rate. The wires are usually pulled out on the fourth postoperative day. One should obtain a follow-up chest film to help rule out bleeding.

After closed heart surgery it is usually sufficient to leave pacing wires in only if a conduction disturbance or rhythm problem is anticipated, since the atrial and ventricular epicardium often is not visualized (for example, coarctation repair and PDA ligation).

Blood pressure in the postoperative period usually is monitored by means of an indwelling radial artery line, an umbilical artery catheter, or, in the more stable infant, by transcutaneous Doppler technique. We regard the lower limits of normal for systolic pressure as 45 mm Hg for the 1,500 gm infant, 60 for the 2,500 gm infant, and 65 for the 3 kg infant (Fig. 29-77).

Right atrial pressure (central venous pressure). It is necessary at times to raise right and left atrial pressures to high levels to ensure adequate ventricular filling and cardiac output. Thus, in the neonate who has undergone total repair of tetralogy of Fallot, a right atrial pressure of 12 to 15 mm Hg is sometimes necessary, and after aortic commissurotomy a left atrial pressure of 15 to 16 mm Hg may be required. When maintenance of adequate filling pressures is critical, it is common practice to leave indwelling lines through the right and left atrial appendages, through widely placed mattress sutures. These lines are pulled out through the chest wound on the second to fifth postoperative day. Central venous pressure also may be monitored from a line inserted into the umbilical vein and advanced through the ductus venosus to the inferior vena cava.

Pulmonary artery pressure. At times it may be desirable to monitor pulmonary artery pressure and have access to a source from which mixed venous blood can be withdrawn. A pulmonary artery line can be inserted through the free wall of the right ventricle at the time of open-heart surgery.

Cardiac output. Most postoperative deaths are caused by low output. The ability to accurately monitor systemic blood flow is advantageous, yet a simple technique is hard to achieve. Current methods include measurement of arteriovenous oxygen difference with assumed oxygen consumption (Fick principle); thermodilution measurements (Swan-Ganz catheter); temporary electromagnetic flow probe placed around the aorta or main pulmonary artery at the time of surgery; and the use of echocardiography. The echocardiographic measurement of cardiac output is made by determining the volume of blood flow through the ascending aorta. This is achieved by a formula that combines the aortic cross-sectional area (by M-mode echocardiography) and the blood flow velocity profile (by Doppler echocardiography).

Pulmonary function

See also Chapter 28, part two.

Almost every neonate who has undergone palliative or corrective cardiac surgery requires temporary ventilator support. Even if the infant was previously free breathing, the effect of anesthesia and of surgery is to depress chemoreceptor function, impair the production of pulmonary surfactant protein, allow the overproduction of bronchial secretions, disturb the ventilation/perfusion ratios, and decrease lung compliance secondary to increased lung water. The use of appropriate respirator settings is guided principally by pH and arterial blood gases.

Blood gases should be maintained close to the physiologic range by adjustments of the respirator settings, the intention being to produce favorable gases with minimal positive pressure because of the risk of pneumothorax and extrapulmonary air.

Temperature requirements

Maintenance of a neutral environmental temperature (at which oxygen consumption is minimum) greatly aids the infant postoperatively by allowing every milliliter of oxygen transferred to be used in maintaining vital body functions rather than being wasted in keeping the infant warm or in satisfying a febrile infant's hypermetabolic state. Usually this environment is achieved by skin servocontrol in an overhead radiant heat warmer; typically an abdominal skin temperature of 97° F is optimal.

Fluid and electrolyte requirements

In general, greater fluid restriction is necessary after cardiopulmonary bypass (60 ml/kg) than after nonpump procedures (100 ml/kg). This is because of the tendency to retain sodium and water from the pump prime. Hyponatremia is common and is usually caused by disproportionate retention of water and usually will respond to fluid restriction or diuretics. If serum sodium declines below 125 mEq/L, there is a risk of seizures. Hypernatremia may be seen in neonates who have received large amounts of sodium bicarbonate. Treatment is by sodium restriction and liberalization of fluids.

Hypokalemia is frequent after cardiac surgery and potentiates the action of digitalis. It can be treated by administration of potassium at 1 mEq/hour for a 3 kg neonate until serum levels reach 4 to 4.5 mEq/L. Hyperkalemia occurs as a result of renal failure. Careful watch also needs to be kept for the development of hypoglycemia and of hypocalcemia.

Chest x-ray examinations

A portable chest film should be obtained as soon as possible after the surgical procedure to check position of the endotracheal tube and to recognize intrathoracic complications such as bleeding, pneumonia, pneumothorax, and pericardial effusion.

Use of cardioactive drugs in the postoperative period

Most infants who have undergone cardiovascular surgery require temporary sympathomimetic drug support. Despite increased biosynthesis of catecholamines by the adrenal glands, the myocardium of the patient in serious heart failure is depleted of catecholamines. An increase in cardiac output sometimes can be obtained by the use of sodium nitroprusside to reduce systemic vascular resistance. The combination of isoproterenol or dopamine to augment ventricular contractility and sodium nitroprusside to diminish afterload is especially effective. The following recommended doses are given in Table 29-15, although there is wide variation in response.

Table 29-15. Recommended doses of cardioactive drugs in postoperative period (See also Tables 29-10 and 29-11)

Drug	Intravenous dose (μg/kg/minute)	Effect
Isoproterenol	0.05-0.5	Predominantly β-adrenergic agonist
Dopamine	2.0-20	May act at special dopamine receptors
Dobutamine	2.5-10	β_1-Receptor agonist
Sodium nitroprusside	0.5-8	Arteriolar vasodilator
Prostaglandin E_1	0.05-0.1	Opens ductus arteriosus

The postoperative use of PGE_1 deserves special mention. This drug acts to maintain patency of the ductus arteriosus and sustains pulmonary blood flow in lesions such as pulmonary atresia. Postoperatively it is often useful to continue infusion of the drug into the aortic end of the ductus or intravenously until it is definitely clear that the surgical aorto-pulmonary shunt is widely and usefully patent. Typically the infant may be weaned from PGE_1, 1 to 2 days after surgical shunting.

TREATMENT OF SPECIFIC POSTOPERATIVE COMPLICATIONS

Blood loss and blood replacement

The guides to blood replacement are the blood pressure, left and right atrial pressures, cardiac output, hematocrit, loss from chest tubes, and skin circulation. Blood volume should be maintained at equal to or 5% over normal values and hematocrit at at least 35% in acyanotic patients and 45% in those who have residual cyanotic heart disease. It is important to use the right blood product: whole fresh blood for bleeding, platelet transfusions for low platelet counts, and packed cells when the hematocrit is to be raised.

Renal failure

Renal failure after neonatal heart surgery is usually the result of a low-output state. The diagnosis is first suggested by a urine output falling to less than 1 ml/kg/hour and is further suspected by a rising urine sodium (greater than 60 mEq/L) and low urine/plasma osmolarity ratio (less than 1.2). A test dose of furosemide, 1 to 5 mg/kg, confirms the diagnosis if urine output does not rise significantly. Occasionally polyuric renal failure is seen with low specific gravity (less than 1.010) and rising serum creatinine and blood urea nitrogen. Treatment of renal failure in the neonate is discussed in Chapter 35.

Cardiac tamponade

Tamponade is suspected when there is hypotension, especially when accompanied by a rising central venous pressure. The suspicion is heightened by the x-ray finding of a widening mediastinum, pulsus paradoxus, or gallop rhythm. Since tamponade is usually caused by an intrapericardial bleed, immediate treatment is imperative with pericardiocentesis or thoracotomy in the cardiac recovery room, if necessary, but usually in the operating room.

Increased chest drainage

The maximum allowable upper limit for drainage in the immediate postoperative period is 5% of blood volume per hour. Blood should be replaced hourly with the appropriate blood product. Greater volumes of blood loss usually require reexploration unless a coagulation defect, such as thrombocytopenia, can be identified.

Continued deterioration with no obvious cause

Most deaths in the postoperative period are caused by low cardiac output. In the problem patient with a seemingly adequately operated lesion and without severe hypoxemia or arrhythmia, the following should be considered: pericardial tamponade, concealed bleeding, hypoglycemia, hypocalcemia, heart failure from hypervolemia, and overwhelming infection.

Failure to establish a positive diagnosis for low-output failure is an indication for echocardiographic and sometimes for hemodynamic and angiocardiographic study. Sometimes this can be accomplished in the recovery room, using the indwelling lines and contrast echocardiography to detect shunts and obstructions. When there is reason to believe that an undiagnosed major hemodynamic lesion is present, the patient should be transferred to the cardiac catheterization laboratory for formal study; a prosthetic patch may have torn loose, a valve inadvertently been rendered incompetent, or other unsuspected complications developed.

PEDIATRIC CARDIOLOGY: THE FUTURE

Exciting and important advances have occurred over the past 5 years in both diagnosis and treatment.

Diagnosis

The use of two-dimensional and Doppler echocardiography has dramatically reduced the need for invasive hemodynamic and angiographic studies in the neonate. Thus PDA and PFC syndrome can be accurately assessed, and appropriate treatment can be instituted based on echocardiographic assessment.

Emerging diagnostic tools include further development of ultrasound; nuclear magnetic resonance (NMR) imaging, especially useful for visualizing extracardiac vascular structures that are relatively stationary (e.g., vascular rings, coarctations); and cine CT scanning whereby moving structures can be imaged by repetitive "slices" gated to the ECG signal.

Treatment

Balloon angiography has found its place in the dilation of stenotic pulmonary valves and recoarctations of the aorta; other applications are controversial. Emerging technologies include laser commissurotomy of stenotic valves, the greater use of conduit surgery, and heart or heart-lung transplantation when all other medical and surgical treatments fail.

Prevention

Whereas advances in fetal echocardiography have certainly allowed early identification of structural heart disease, advances in prevention have been slight. The importance of mother-to-child transmission (about 14%) when the mother has congenital heart disease has strengthened the genetic theory, but the nature of the environmental "trigger" remains elusive. The seminal work of Clark and associates in using the chick embryo to define the effect of physical and chemical interventions on cardiac morphogenesis is of great importance.

DRUGS USEFUL IN THE TREATMENT OF CARDIOVASCULAR DISEASE IN NEONATES

See also Appendix B.

Antiarrhythmic drugs

A. *Atropine*
   1. Dosage: minimum 0.15 mg regardless of weight; 0.01 mg/kg/dose SC may be given IV; may repeat every 4 to 6 hours
   2. Preparation: check bottle, since there are many concentrations available; usual concentration is 0.5 mg/ml.

B. *Digoxin* (Lanoxin)
   1. Therapeutic range: 0.8 to 2.0 ng/ml
   2. PO digitalizing dosage
      a. Premature: <1,500 gm, 0.01 to 0.02 mg/kg
         Premature: <2,500 gm, 0.03 mg/kg
      b. Full-term newborn: 0.03 mg/kg to 0.05 mg/kg
   3. Parenteral digitalization: two thirds of oral dosage
   4. Maintenance: a fourth to a third of digitalizing dosage, in two divided doses (q12h)
   5. Digitalization
      b. Half the calculated digitalizing dosage initially, a fourth in 8 hours and a fourth in another 8 hours; start maintenance 12 hours after last digitalizing dose
      b. Digitalis toxicity may not be manifested by vomiting; arrhythmias on ECG best way to assess possible toxicity
   6. Reduce dose with renal failure
   7. Preparations
      a. Elixir: 0.05 mg/ml
      b. Ampules: 0.25 and 0.10 mg/ml
      c. Tablets, scored: 0.125, 0.25, 0.375, and 0.50 mg (older child and adult use)

C. *Lidocaine*
   1. IV initial dosage: 0.5 to 1.0 mg/kg q 20 to 60 minutes prn
   2. IV maintenance dosage: 10 to 50 μg/kg/minute

3. Half-life: 15 to 30 minutes
4. Preparations: 1% or 2% solution

D. *Phenytoin* (Dilantin)
1. Oral dosage: 2 to 5 mg/kg/day
2. IV initial dosage: 1 to 5 mg/kg slow push
3. Slow gastrointestinal absorption
4. Half-life: 24 hours
5. Metabolism: liver

E. *Procainamide* (Pronestyl) hydrochloride
1. IV dosage: 3 to 8 mg/kg over 5 minutes, to 500 mg
2. IV maintenance dosage: 20 to 80 μg/kg/minute
3. Oral dosage: 15 to 50 mg/kg/24 hours, divided into 4 to 6 doses
4. Oral absorption: 75% to 95%
5. Metabolism: liver
6. Renal excretion unchanged: 50% to 60%

F. *Propranolol* (Inderal)
1. IV initial dosage: 0.05 to 0.15 mg/kg, slowly over 10 minutes
2. Oral dosage: 0.2 to 4 mg/kg/day
3. Half-life: 2 to 3 hours
4. Metabolism: liver

G. *Quinidine*
1. Oral dosage: 15 to 60 mg/kg/day in 4 or 5 doses
2. Gastrointestinal absorption: greater than 95%
3. Metabolism: liver
4. Renal excretion unchanged: 20% to 50%

H. *Verapamil*
1. IV dosage, over 30 seconds 0.1 to 0.2 mg/kg
2. Reflex conversion of SVTs requires agents that increase blood pressure, because of reflex bradycardia, which may be very prominent. Atropine, dopamine, and calcium chloride should be available and a second IV line established.

I. *Methoxamine hydrochloride* (Vasoxyl)
1. Causes increase in peripheral vascular resistance with elevation of systolic and diastolic blood pressure that persists for 60 to 90 minutes
2. Cardiac output unchanged or decreased
3. Renal blood flow decreased
4. Reflex bradycardia prominent
5. Blood pressure should not be raised over 160 mm Hg systolic (125 mm Hg in the neonate)
6. Preparation: ampules, 10 or 20 mg/ml
7. Dosage: 0.25 mg/kg IM or 0.1 mg/kg IV

J. *Phenylephrine* (Neo-Synephrine) *hydrochloride*
1. Vasoconstrictor and pressor chemically related to epinephrine
2. For conversion of SVT, rapid IV infusion is recommended
3. Dosage: 1 ml of the drug contains 10 mg; for use in infants the drug should be appropriately diluted
   a. Infants: 0.005 to 0.02 mg/kg IV, slowly
   b. Adults: 0.15 to 0.8 mg IV push

K. *Edrophonium chloride* (Tensilon)
1. Short-acting anticholinergic agent that results in reflex bracycardia, which responds to atropine
2. Advantages
   a. Rapid acting (within 30 to 60 seconds)
   b. Brief duration of action (lasts average of 10 minutes)
3. Dosage for difficult diagnosis of myasthenia gravis or conversion of SVT: IV, may be repeated
   a. Children up to 75 pounds: 0.1 ml (1 mg)
   b. Children more than 75 pounds: 0.2 ml (2 mg)
   c. Infants: 0.1 to 0.2 mg/kg (single dose)
4. Cardioversion—range of doses
   a. First correct acidosis
   b. SVT
      (1) Premature, newborn, infant: ½ to 1 W-second/kg
      (2) Child: ½ to 2 W-seconds/kg
      (3) Start at lower dose
   c. Ventricular tachycardia or fibrillation: higher energy levels may be required

Antihypertensive drugs

A. *Methyldopa* (Aldomet)
1. Oral dosage: 10 mg/kg/24 hours, divided into 2 or 3 doses
   a. Increase or decrease to effect
   b. Increase at 2-day or more intervals to not more than 65 mg/kg/24 hours
2. IV dosage (crises): 20 to 40 mg/kg/24 hours, divided into four doses IV, then same dosage continued orally when controlled
3. Preparation
   a. Tablet: 250 mg
   b. Solution (injection): 50 mg/ml

B. *Diazoxide* (Hyperstat)—Dosage: 2.5 to 5 mg/kg/dose
1. Initiate therapy at the low dose and give as bolus in peripheral IV (not intracardiac) over a 30-second period
2. May repeat in half hour: then q 2 to 5 hours

C. *Hydralazine* (Apresoline)
1. Oral dosage: 0.4 to 2.0 mg/kg/day, divided into four doses
2. Parenteral dosage alone: 0.1 to 0.5 mg/kg q3h to q6h

D. *Magnesium sulfate*
1. IM dosage: 0.1 gm/kg of 20% to 50% solution, repeated q4h if necessary
2. IV dosage: 2 mg/kg of 3% solution; no more than 75 to 100 mg/hour

E. *Sodium nitroprusside*
1. Fast onset, potent hypotensive agent, quickly reversible
2. Mechanism: peripheral vasodilatation by direct

effect on peripheral vessels, independent of autonomic control

3. Administration: IV drip only in D5W
4. Dosage: 0.5 to 8 μg/kg/minute IV drip
5. Preparation: 50 mg vial of desiccated nitroprusside: dissolve in 2 to 3 ml D5W, then dilute in 250, 500, or 1,000 ml D5W for infusion
   a. 50 mg in 250 ml = 1 mg/5 ml = 200 μg/ml
   b. 50 mg to 500 ml = 1 mg/10 ml = 100 μg/ml
   c. 50 mg in 1,000 ml = 1 mg/20 ml = 50 μg/ml
6. Monitor blood pressure and heart rate closely; if severe hypotension develops, stop IV drip, and blood pressure will increase in 1 to 10 minutes

F. *Captopril*
   1. Angiotensin 1 converting enzyme (ACE) inhibitor, especially useful in hyperreninemic hypertension but has proved effective also when serum renin is normal
   2. Oral administration only, dose 0.1 mg to 1.0 mg/kg q6h to q12h after test dose
   3. Test dose 0.2 mg/kg PO with dopamine (5 μg/kg/min) and normal saline available if BP drops precipitously
   4. Low incidence of side effects, but neutropenia, proteinemia, and azotemia may occur

Diuretics

A. *Chlorothiazide* (Diuril)
   1. Dosage: 10 mg/kg/24 hours, divided into two doses, oral
   2. Preparations
      a. Tablets: 250 to 500 mg
      b. Syrup: 250 mg/5 ml
   3. Risk of hypokalemia

B. *Furosemide* (Lasix)
   1. IV dosage: 0.5 to 1.5 mg/kg
   2. Oral dosage: 1 to 4 mg/kg/day
   3. Preparations:
      a. Tablets, scored: 20, 40, 80 mg
      b. Ampules: 20 mg/2 ml
      c. Oral solution: 10 mg/ml

C. *Hydrochlorothiazide* (Hydrodiuril)
   1. Dosage: tenth of chlorothiazide dosage
   2. Preparation: Tablets, scored, 25 and 50 mg

D. *Mannitol*
   1. For treatment of oliguria and anuria
   2. Test dosage: 0.2 gm/kg; 6 gm/m^2; single IV dose given within 3 to 5 minutes
   3. Dosage for edema, ascites: 2 gm/kg; 60 gm/m^2 of 15% to 20% solution given over 2 to 6 hours IV
   4. Preparation: injection of 50, 100, 150, 200, and 250 mg/ml (5%, 10%, 15%, 20%, and 25%)
   5. CAUTION: circulatory overload, electrolyte imbalance, tremors and convulsions (hyponatremia), headache, nausea, chills, dizziness, tachycardia, intraocular hemorrhage, death in organic central nervous system disease, and pulmonary hypertension; don't mix with infused blood

E. *Spironolactone* (Aldactone)—1.5 to 3.0 mg/kg/day in two to three doses; 4- to 16-hour response; risk of hyperkalemia and hyponatremia, contraindicated in renal dysfunction, anemia or hypokalemia
   Preparation: tablets—25, 50, 100 mg

Miscellaneous

A. *Morphine sulfate*—IM or IV dosage: 0.1 to 0.2 mg/kg

B. *Nalorphine* (Nalline)—dosage: 0.01 mg/kg

C. *Pancuronium bromide* (Pavulon)
   1. Neuromuscular blocking agent
   2. Dosage: 0.04 to 0.1 mg/kg

D. *Prostaglandin E_1*
   1. For maintaining ductal patency
   2. Dosage: 0.1 μg/kg/minute; 500 μg (0.5 mg) (1 vial) in 50 ml; 10 μg/ml

E. *Sodium bicarbonate*—IV dosage: 3 to 5 mEq/kg/dose

F. *Succinylcholine*
   1. Dosage for intubation: 1 to 2 mg/kg IM
   2. Takes two mintues for patient to become paralyzed

G. *Tolazoline* (Priscoline)
   1. Action: vasodilator
   2. Indications: pulmonary vasoconstriction
   3. Dosage:
      a. At cardiac catheterization, to evaluate pulmonary hypertension: 1 mg/kg bolus to pulmonary artery
      b. For PFC: 1 to 2 mg/kg push initially, 1 to 4 mg/kg/hour, drip

H. *Diazepam* (Valium)
   1. Oral dosage: 0.12 to 0.8 mg/kg/24 hours, divided into 3 or 4 doses
   2. IM or IV dosage: 0.2 to 0.5 mg/kg single dose; given slowly

I. *Indomethacin*
   1. IV dosage, 0.2 mg/kg, IV, repeat if necessary at 0.1 mg/kg 12 hours and 24 hours later
   2. PO dosage is same (by nasogastric tube)
   3. Caution with renal failure, jaundice, thrombocytopenia: IV preparation should be used if infant is at risk for necrotizing enterocolitis

J. *Ketamine hydrochloride*
   1. IM dosage, 0.5 to 2.0 mg/kg

K. *Calcium chloride* (27% calcium)
   1. Intracardiac dosage: 10 mg/kg diluted 1:1 with saline; use cautiously if patient is digitalized
   2. IV dosage 10 mg/kg
   3. Preparation: ampules 100 mg/ml (10% solution)

L *Calcium gluconate* (9% calcium)
   1. Dosage 200 mg/kg/dose IV

M. *"Polarizing" solution* for acute hyperkalemia with or without tachycardia; Administer 3 ml calcium gluconate, one unit of regular insulin, and 15 ml of 25% glucose over a 5 minute period to a 2 to 3 kg infant
N. *Kayexalate*—calculate dose required PO or PR every 6 hours as needed; average is 0.5 to 1.0 gm/kg/dose; 1 mEq potassium per 1 gram of resin

Sympathomimetics

A. *Dobutamine* (Dobutrex)
   1. Synthetic catecholamine
   2. β-Receptor stimulator that is more selective for the heart
   3. Has mild chronotropic effects
   4. Helpful in treatment of cardiac decompensation
   5. Administration: IV only
   6. Rate of infusion: 2.5 to 10 μg/kg/minute
B. *Dopamine* (Intropin)
   1. Pharmacologic properties: increased cardiac output, increased blood pressure, increased renal blood flow, useful for shock
   2. Preparation: ampules, 5 ml (40 mg/ml) (total: 200 mg)
   3. Dosage: 5 to 15 μg/kg/minute IV drip
   4. Dilution
      a. 2.5 cc/1,000 ml = 100 μg/ml
      b. 5.0 cc/500 ml = 400 μg/ml
   5. Monitor heart rate, blood pressure, central venous pressure, and urine output
C. *Epinephrine*
   1. Alpha + +, beta + +
   2. Intracardiac dosage: 0.3 to 2.0 cc diluted 1:10,000 (0.1 ml/kg)
D. *Isoproterenol* (Isuprel) (beta only)
   1. Range of recommended dosages includes 0.05 to 0.5 μg/kg/minute IV drip
   2. Should be given by infusion pump
   3. Dosage: 1 ml (200 μg) in 200 ml = 1 μg/ml
   4. Monitor heart rate, blood pressure, central venous pressure, and urine output

Martin H. Lees
Douglas H. King

BIBLIOGRAPHY
General

Ainger, L.E., Lawyer, N.G., and Fitch, C.W.: Neonatal rubella myocarditis, Br. Heart J. **28**:691, 1966.

Beuren, A.J., and others: The syndrome of supravalvular aortic stenosis, peripheral pulmonary stenosis, mental retardation, and similar facial appearance, Am. J. Cardiol. **13**:471, 1964.

Clark, E.B., Hu, N., and Rosenquist, G.C.: Effect of conotruncal constriction on aortic-mitral valve continuity in the stage 18, 21, and 24 chick embryo, Am. J. Cardiol. **53**:324, 1984.

Graham, T.P., Atwood, G.F., and Boucek, R.J.: Use of prostaglandin E_1 for emergency palliation of symptomatic coarctation of the aorta, Cathet. Cardiovasc. Diagn. **4**:97, 1978.

Lees, M.H., Burnell, R.H., Morgan, C.L., and Ross, B.B.: Ventilation/perfusion relationships in children with heart disease and diminished pulmonary blood flow, Pediatrics **40**:259, 1967.

Mitchell, S.C., Korones, S.B., and Berendes, H.W.: Congenital heart disease in 56,109 births; incidence and natural history, Circulation **43**:323, 1971.

Nora, J.J., and others: Medical and surgical management of anomalous origin of left coronary artery from pulmonary artery, Pediatrics **42**:405, 1968.

Nora, J.J.: Multifactorial inheritance hypothesis for the etiology of congenital heart diseases: the genetic-environmental interaction, Circulation **38**:604, 1968.

Olley, P.M., Coceani, F., and Bodach, E.: E-type prostaglandins; a new emergency therapy for certain cyanotic congenital heart malformations, Circulation **53**:728, 1976.

Roberts, R.J., editor: Drug therapy in infants, pharmacologic principles and clinical experience, Philadelphia, 1984, W.B. Saunders Co.

Rowe, R.D., and Uchida, I.A.: Cardiac malformation in mongolism; a prospective study of 184 mongoloid children, Am. J. Med. **31**:726, 1961.

Rudolph, A.M.: Complications occurring in infants and children. In Braunwald, E., and Swan, H.J.C., editors: Cooperative study in cardiac catheterization, Monograph no. 20, 1968, American Heart Association; Circulation, vols. 37 and 38, (Suppl. 3), 1968.

Tripp, M.E., and others: Systemic carnitine deficiency presenting as familial endocardial fibroelastosis: a treatable cardiomyopathy, N. Engl. J. Med. **305**:385, 1981.

Valdes-Dapena, M., and Miller, W.H.: Pericarditis in the newborn, Pediatrics **16**:673, 1955.

Waber, L.J., and others: Carnitine deficiency presenting as familial cardiomyopathy: a treatable defect, J. Pediatr. **101**:700, 1982.

Whittemore, R., Hobbins, J.C., and Engle, M.A.: Pregnancy and its outcome in women with and without surgical treatment of congenital heart disease, Am. J. Cardiol. **50**:64, 1982.

Woolf, P.K., and others: The treatment of cardiomyopathy in pyruvate dehydrogenase deficiency (PDED) (abstract). II. Pediatr. Res. **20**:4, 1986.

Cardiovascular disease (prenatal diagnosis)

Allan, L.D., and others: Spectrum of congenital heart disease detected echocardiographically in prenatal life, Br. Heart J. **54**:523, 1985.

DeVore, G.R.: The prenatal diagnosis of congenital heart disease, a practical approach for the fetal sonographer, J. Clin. Ultrasound **13**:229, 1985.

Hegge, F.N., Lees, M.H., and Watson, P.T.: Fetal cardiac abnormalities identified during obstetrical sonography, J. Reprod. Med. (In press.)

Electrocardiogram

Hastreiter, A.R., and Abella, J.B.: The electrocardiogram in the newborn period. I. The normal infant, J. Pediatr. **78**:146, 1971.

Hastreiter, A.R., and Abella, J.B.: The electrocardiogram in the newborn period. II. The infant with disease, J. Pediatr. **78**:346, 1971.

Michaelsson, M.: Electrocardiographic studies in the healthy newborn, Acta Paediatr. Scand. **48**:108, 1959.

Echocardiography

Allen, H.D., and others: Echocardiographic demonstration of a right ventricular tumor in a neonate, J. Pediatr. **84**:854, 1974.

Bass, J.L., Ben-Schachar, G., and Edwards, J.E.: Comparison of M-mode echocardiography and pathologic findings in the hypoplastic left heart syndrome, Am. J. Cardiol. **45**:79, 1980.

Baylen, B.G., and others: The critically ill premature infant with patent ductus arteriosus and pulmonary disease—an echocardiographic assessment, J. Pediatr. **86**:423, 1975.

Bierman, F.Z., and Williams, R.G.: Prospective diagnosis of d-transposition of the great arteries in neonates by subxiphoid two-dimensional echocardiography, Circulation **60**:1496, 1979.

Bierman, F.Z., and Williams, R.G.: Subxiphoid two-dimensional imaging of the interatrial septum in infants and neonates with congenital heart disease, Circulation **60**:80, 1979.

Cohn, H.E., and others: Cardiovascular responses to hypoxemia and acidemia in fetal lambs, Am. J. Obstet. Gynecol. **120**:817, 1974.

Cotton, R.B., and others: Medical management of small preterm infants with symptomatic patent ductus arteriosus, J. Pediatr. **92**:467, 1978.

Donnelly, W.H., Bucciarelli, R.L., and Nelson, R.M.: Ischemic papillary muscle necrosis in stressed newborn infants, J. Pediatr. **96**:295, 1980.

Gersony, W.M., Morishima, H.O., and Daniel, S.S.: The hemodynamic effects of intrauterine hypoxia: an experimental model in newborn lambs, J. Pediatr. **89**:631, 1976.

Gittenberger-de Groot, A.C., and others: The ductus arteriosus in the preterm infant, histologic and clinical observations, J. Pediatr. **96**:88, 1980.

Goldberg, S.J., and others: Doppler echocardiography, Philadelphia, 1985, Lea & Febiger.

Gutgesell, H.P., Speer, M.E., and Rosenberg, H.S.: Characterization of the cardiomyopathy in infants of diabetic mothers, Circulation **61**:441, 1980.

Gutgesell, H.P., and others: Left and right ventricular systolic time intervals in the newborn, Br. Heart J. **42**:27, 1979.

Gutgesell, H.P., and others: Transient hypertrophic subaortic stenosis in infants of diabetic mothers, J. Pediatr. **89**:120, 1976.

Halliday, H., and others: Respiratory distress syndrome; echocardiographic assessment of cardiovascular function and pulmonary vascular resistance, Pediatrics **60**:444, 1977.

Halliday, H., and others: Echocardiographic ventricular systolic time intervals in normal term and preterm neonates, Pediatrics **62**:317, 1978.

Hernandez, A., and others: Diagnosis of pulmonary arteriovenous fistula by contrast echocardiography, J. Pediatr. **93**:258, 1978.

Hirschfeld, S., and others: Measurement of right and left ventricular systolic time intervals by echocardiography, Circulation **51**:304, 1975.

Hirschfeld, S., and others: The echocardiographic assessment of pulmonary artery pressure and pulmonary vascular resistance, Circulation **52**:642, 1975.

Hirschklau, M.J., and others: Echocardiographic diagnosis: pitfalls in the premature infant with a large patent ductus arteriosus, J. Pediatr. **92**:474, 1978.

Jacob, J., and others: The contribution of PDA in the neonate with severe RDS, J. Pediatr. **96**:79, 1980.

Lendrum, B., and others: Echocardiographic (echo) studies in infants of diabetic mothers, Pediatr. Res. **12**:385, 1975.

Mace, S., and others: Echocardiographic abnormalities in infants of diabetic mothers, J. Pediatr. **95**:1013, 1979.

Meyer, R.A.: Pediatric echocardiography, Philadelphia, 1977, Lea & Febiger.

Sahn, D.J., and Anderson, F.: Two-dimensional anatomy of the heart, New York, 1982, John Wiley & Sons, Inc.

Silverman, N.H., and Snider, A.R.: Two-dimensional echocardiography in congenital heart disease, East Norwalk, Conn., 1982, Appleton-Century-Crofts.

Snider, A.R., Ports, T.A., and Silverman, N.H.: Venous anomalies of the coronary sinus: detection by M-mode, two-dimensional and contrast echocardiography, Circulation **60**:721, 1979.

Tajik, A.J., and others: Two dimensional real-time ultrasonic imaging of the heart and great vessels, Mayo Clin. Proc. **53**:271, 1978.

Way, G.L., and others: Echocardiographic assessment of ventricular dimensions and myocardial function in infants of diabetic mothers, Pediatr. Res. **9**:273, 1975.

Way, G.L., and others: The natural history of hypertrophic cardiomyopathy in infants of diabetic mothers, J. Pediatr. **95**:1020, 1979.

Weinberg, A.G., and Laird, W.P.: Group B streptococcal endocarditis detected by echocardiography, J. Pediatr. **92**:335, 1978.

Cyanosis

Gatti, R.A., and others: Neonatal polycythemia with transient cyanosis and cardiorespiratory abnormalities, J. Pediatr. **69**:1063, 1966.

Goetzman, B.W., and others: Neonatal hypoxia and pulmonary vasospasm; response to tolazoline, J. Pediatr. **89**:617, 1976.

Gootman, N.L., Scarpelli, E.M., and Rudolph, A.M.: Metabolic acidosis in children with severe cyanotic congenital heart disease, Pediatrics **31**:251, 1963.

Lees, M.H., and Jolly, J.: Severe congenital methaemoglobinaemia in an infant, Lancet **2**:1147, 1957.

Oliver, T.K., Jr., Demis, J.A., and Bates, G.D.: Serial blood-gas tensions and acid-base balance during the first hour of life in human infants, Acta Paediatr. Scand. **50**:346, 1961.

Roberton, N.R.C., Hallidie-Smith, K.A., and Davis, J.A.: Severe respiratory distress syndrome mimicking cyanotic heart disease in term babies, Lancet **2**:1108, 1967.

Sommerville, R.J., and others: Adrenal insufficiency mimicking heart disease in infancy, Pediatrics **42**:691, 1968.

Wood, J.L.: Plethora in the newborn infant associated with cyanosis and convulsions, J. Pediatr. **54**:143, 1959.

Lung disease versus heart disease

Persistence of the fetal circulation

Arcilla, R.A., Thinelius, D.G., and Ranniger, K.: Congestive heart failure from suspected ductal closure in utero, J. Pediatr. **75**:74, 1969.

Bartlett, R.H., and others: Extracorporeal circulation in neonatal respiratory failure: a prospective randomized study, Pediatrics **76**:479, 1985.

Corby, D.G.: Aspirin in pregnancy; maternal and fetal effects, Pediatrics **62**:930, 1978.

Csaba, I.P., Sulyok, E., and Ertle, T.: Relationship of maternal treatment with indomethacin to persistent fetal circulation syndrome, J. Pediatr. **92**:484, 1978.

Gersony, W.B.: Persistent fetal circulation; a commentary, J. Pediatr. **82**:1103, 1973.

Haworth, S.G., and Reid, L.: Persistent fetal circulation; newly recognized structural features, J. Pediatr. **88**:614, 1976.

Levin, D.R., Perkin, R.M., and Weinberg, A.G.: Pulmonary microthrombi in newborn infants with unresponsive persistent pulmonary hypertension (abstract), Pediatr. Res. **16**:102A, 1982.

Manchester, D., Margolis, H.S., and Sheldon, R.E.: Possible association between maternal indomethacin and primary pulmonary hypertension of the newborn, Am. J. Obstet. Gynecol. **126**:467, 1976.

Heart failure

Benzing, G., and others: Simultaneous hypoglycemia and acute congestive heart failure, Circulation **40**:209, 1969.

Berdon, W.E., and Baker, D.H.: Giant hepatic hemangioma with cardiac failure in the newborn infant; value of high-dosage intravenous urography and umbilical angiography, Radiology **92**:1523, 1969.

Burnell, R.J.: Venous pressure in congestive heart failure in infancy, Arch. Dis. Child. **45**:360, 1970.

Goldberg, L.I.: Dopamine; clinical uses of an endogenous catecholamine, N. Engl. J. Med. **291**:707, 1974.

Graves, S.W., and others: Endogenous digoxin, immunoreactive substance in human pregnancies, J. Clin. Endocrinol. Metabol. **58**:748, 1984.

Kliegman, R., and Fanaroff, A.A.: Caution in the use of dopamine in the neonate, J. Pediatr. **93**:540, 1978.

Murphy, D.J., and others: Massive digoxin poisoning treated with fab fragments of digoxin specific antibodies, Pediatrics **70**:472, 1982.

Perkin, R.M., and Levin, D.L.: Shock in the pediatric patient. II. Therapy, J. Pediatr. **101**:319, 1982.

Schranz, D., and others: Hemodynamic effects of dobutamine in children with cardiovascular failure, Eur. J. Pediatr. **139**:4, 1982.

White, R.D., and Leitman, P.S.: Commentary: a reappraisal of digitalis for infants with left-to-right shunts and "heart failure," J. Pediatr. **92**:867, 1978.

Cardiogenic shock and perinatal asphyxia

Bucciarelli, R., and others: Serum creatine phosphokinase MB fraction in newborns with transient tricuspid insufficiency, N. Engl. J. Med. **298**:146, 1978.

Cabal, L.A., and others: Cardiogenic shock associated with perinatal asphyxia in preterm infants, J. Pediatr. **96**:705, 1980.

Driscoll, D.J., and others: Hemodynamic effects of dobutamine in children, Am. J. Cardiol. **43**:581, 1979.

Finley, J.P., and others: Transient myocardial ischemia of the newborn infant demonstrated by thallium myocardial imaging, J. Pediatr. **94**:263, 1979.

Lees, M.H.: Perinatal asphyxia and the myocardium, J. Pediatr. **96**:674, 1980.

Nelson, R.M., and others: Serum creatine phosphokinase MB fraction in newborns with transient tricuspid insufficiency, N. Engl. J. Med. **298**:146, 1978.

Riemenschneider, T.A., and others: Disturbances of the transitional circulation: spectrum of pulmonary hypertension and myocardial dysfunction, J. Pediatr. **89**:622, 1976.

Rowe, R.D., and Hoffmann, T.: Transient myocardial ischemia of the newborn infant; a form of severe cardiorespiratory distress in full-term infants, J. Pediatr. **81**:243, 1972.

Dysrhythmias (neonatal)

Berube, S., and others: Congenital heart block and maternal systemic lupus erythematosus, Am. J. Obstet. Gynecol. **130**:595, 1978.

Campbell, R.M., and others: Atrial overdrive pacing for conversion of atrial flutter in children, Pediatrics **75**:730, 1985.

Chameides, L., and others: Association of maternal systemic lupus erythematosus with congenital complete heart block, N. Engl. J. Med. **297**:1204, 1977.

Epstein, M.L., Kiel, E.A., and Victorica, B.E.: Cardiac decompensation following verapamil therapy in infants with supraventricular tachycardia, Pediatrics **75**:737, 1985.

Garson, A., Jr., Gillette, P.C., and McNamara, D.G.: Supraventricular tachycardia in children: clinical features, response to treatment and long term follow-up in 217 patients, Am. J. Cardiol. **45**:430, 1980.

Gelband, H., Myerburg, R.J., and Bassett, A.L.: Management of cardiac arrhythmias. In Roberts, N., and Gelband, H., editors: Cardiac arrhythmias in the neonate, infant and child, New York, 1977, Appleton-Century-Crofts.

Gillette, P.C.: The mechanisms of supraventricular tachycardia in children, Circulation **54**:133, 1976.

Gillette, P.C., and others: Surgical treatment of supraventricular tachycardia in infants and children, Circulation **60**:111, 1979.

Levy, A.M., Camm, A.J., and Keane, J.F.: Multiple arrhythmias detected during nocturnal monitoring in patients with congenital complete heart block, Circulation **55**:247, 1977.

McCue, C.M., and others: Congenital heart block in newborns of mothers with connective tissue disease, Circulation **56**:82, 1977.

Michaelsson, M., and Engle, M.A.: Congenital complete heart block: an international study of the natural history. In Engle, M.A., and Brest, A.N., editors; Cardiovascular clinics, vol. 4, no. 3, Philadelphia, 1972, F.A. Davis Co.

Nadas, A.S., and others: Paroxysmal tachycardia in infants and children, Pediatrics **9**:167, 1952.

Newburger, J., and Keane, J.F.: Intrauterine supraventricular tachycardia, J. Pediatr. **95**:780, 1979.

Ott, D.A., and others: Surgical management of refractory supraventricular tachycardia in infants and children, J. Am. Coll. Cardiol. **5**:124, 1985.

Pearl, W.: Cardiac malformations presenting as congenital atrial flutter, South. Med. J. **70**:622, 1977.

Podrid, P.J., and Lown, G.: Long term therapy with tocainide, Am. J. Cardiol. **45**:452, 1980.

Rosen, M.R., and Hordoff, A.J.: Mechanism of arrhythmias. In Roberts, N., and Gelband, H., editors: Cardiac arrhythmias in the neonate, infant and child, New York, 1977, Appleton-Century-Crofts.

Soler-Soler, J., and others: Effect of verapamil in infants with paroxysmal supraventricular tachycardia, Circulation **59**:876, 1978.

Stevens, D.C., and others: Fetal and neonatal ventricular arrhythmia, Pediatrics **63**:771, 1979.

Williams, D.O., Tatelbaum, R., and Most, A.S.: Effective treatment of supraventricular arrhythmias with acebutolol, Am. J. Cardiol. **44**:521, 1979.

Yabek, S.M., Swensson, R.E., and Jarmakani, J.M.: Electrocardiographic recognition of sinus node dysfunction in children and young adults, Circulation **56**:235, 1977.

Dysrhythmias (fetal)

Huhta, J.C., and others: Pulsed Doppler fetal echocardiography, J. Clin. Ultrasound **13**:247, 1985.

Kleinman, C.S., and other: Fetal echocardiography: a tool for evaluation of in utero cardiac arrhythmias and monitoring of in utero therapy; analysis of 71 patients, Am. J. Cardiol. **51**:237, 1983.

Kleinman, C.S., and others: Treatment of supraventricular tachyarrhythmias, J. Clin. Ultrasound **13**:265, 1985.

Silverman, N.H., and others: Recognition of fetal arrhythmias by echocardiography, J. Clin. Ultrasound **13**:255, 1985.

Transposition of great arteries

Liebman, J., Cullum, L., and Belloc, N.B.: Natural history of transposition of the great arteries; anatomy and birth and death characteristics. Circulation **50**:237, 1969.

Rashkind, W.J., and Miller, W.W.: Creation of an atrial septal defect without thoracotomy; a palliative approach to complete transposition of the great arteries, JAMA **196**:991, 1966.

Aortic stenosis

Huhta, J.C., and others: Echocardiography in the diagnosis and management of symptomatic aortic valve stenosis in infants, Circulation **70**:438, 1984.

Tricuspid atresia

Edwards, J.E., and Burchell, H.B.: Congenital tricuspid atresia; a classification, Med. Clin. North Am. **33**:1177, 1949.

Truncus arteriosus

Collett, R.W., and Edwards, J.E.: Persistent truncus arteriosus; classification according to anatomic types, Surg. Clin. North Am. **29**:1245, 1949.

PDA

Friedman, W.F., and others: Pharmacologic closure of patent ductus arteriosus in the premature infant, N. Engl. J. Med. **295**:526, 1976.

Halliday, H.L., Hirata, T., and Brady, J.P.: Indomethacin therapy for large patent ductus arteriosus in the very low birth weight infant; results and complications, Pediatrics **64**:154, 1979.

Heymann, M.A., Rudolph, A.M., and Silverman, N.H.: Closure of the ductus arteriosus by prostaglandin inhibition, N. Engl. J. Med. **295**:530, 1976.

Huhta, J.C., Cohen, M., and Gutgesell, H.P.: Patency of the ductus arteriosus in normal neonate. Two dimensional echocardiography versus Doppler assessment, J. Am. Coll. Cardiol. **4**:561, 1984.

Neal, W.A., and others: Patent ductus arteriosus complicating respiratory distress syndrome, J. Pediatr. **86**:127, 1975.

Rudolph, A.M., and Heymann, M.A.: Medical treatment of the ductus arteriosus, Hosp. Pract. **12**:57, 1977.

Rudolph, A.M., and others: Formalin infiltration of the ductus arteriosus; a method for palliation of infants with selective congenital cardiac lesions, N. Engl. J. Med. **292**:1263, 1975.

Serwer, J.A., Armstrong, B.E., and Anderson, P.A.W.: Continuous wave Doppler ultrasonograph IC quantitation of patent ductus arteriosus flow, J. Pediatr. **100**:297, 1982.

Thibeault, D.W., and others: Patent ductus arteriosus complicating the respiratory distress syndrome in preterm infants, J. Pediatr. **86**:120, 1975.

Ventricular septal defect

Campbell, M.: Natural history of ventricular septal defect, Br. Heart J. **33**:246, 1971.

Hoffman, J.I.E., and Rudolph, A.M.: The natural history of ventricular septal defects in infancy, Am. J. Cardiol. **16**:634, 1965.

Common ventricle

Van Praagh, R., and others: Diagnosis of the anatomic types of single or common ventricle, Am. J. Cardiol. **15**:345, 1965.

Arteriovenous fistula

Hall, R.J., Nelson, W.P., and Blake, H.A.: Massive pulmonary arteriovenous fistula in the newborn; a correctable form of "cyanotic heart disease," an additional cause of cyanosis with left axis deviation, Circulation **31**:762, 1965.

Myocarditis

Hosier, D.M., and Newton, W.A., Jr.: Serious Coxsackie infection in infants and children, Am. J. Dis. Child. **96**:251, 1958.

Macauley, D.: Acute endocarditis in infancy and early childhood, Am. J. Dis. Child. **88**:715, 1954.

Rosenberg, H.S., and McNamara, D.G.: Acute myocarditis in infancy and childhood, Prog. Cardiovasc. Dis. **7**:179, 1964.

Cor triatriatum

Jegier, W., Gibbons, J.E., and Wigglesworth, E.W.: Cor triatriatum—clinical, hemodynamic and pathological studies; surgical correction in early life, Pediatrics **31**:255, 1963.

Vascular ring

Fearon, B., and Shortreed, R.: Tracheobronchial compression by congenital cardiovascular anomalies in children, Ann. Otol. Rhinol. Laryngol. **72**:949, 1963.

Stewart, J.R., Kincaid, O.W., and Edwards, J.E.: An atlas of vascular rings and related malformations of the aortic arch system, Springfield, Ill., 1964, Charles C Thomas, Publisher.

Hypertension

Adelman, R.D.: Neonatal hypertension, Pediatr. Clin. North. Am. **25**:99, 1978.

Adelman, R.D., and others: Nonsurgical management of renovascular hypertension in the neonate, Pediatrics **62**:71, 1978.

Blaufox, M.D.: Systemic arterial hypertension in pediatric practice, Pediatr. Clin. North Am. **18**:577, 1971.

Bucci, G., and others: The systemic systolic blood pressure of newborns with low weight, Acta Paediatr. Scand. (Suppl.) **229**:5, 1972.

de Swiet, M., Fayers, P., and Shinebourne, E.A.: Blood pressure survey in a population of newborn infants, Br. Med. J. **2**:9, 1976.

Lum, L.G., and Jones, M.D., Jr.: The effect of cuff width on systolic blood pressure measurements in neonates, J. Pediatr. **91**:963, 1977.

Plumer, L.B., Kaplan, G.W., and Mendoza, S.A.: Hypertension in infants—a complication of umbilical arterial catheterization, J. Pediatr. **89**:802, 1976.

Vidt, D.G., Bravo, E.L., and Fouad, F.M.: Captopril, N. Engl. J. Med. **306**:214, 1982.

Postoperative care

Sade, R.M., Cosgrove, D.M., and Castenada, A.R.: Infant and child care in cardiac surgery, Chicago, 1977, Year Book Medical Publishers, Inc.

CHAPTER 30

Immunology

For the human newborn, extrauterine existence is contingent on a delicate balance between hostile microorganisms in the environment and the infant's host defense mechanisms. During the 9 months of gestation the fetus develops in a highly protective environment, whereas during the birth process and thereafter the infant is exposed to a wide variety of microorganisms. Although the antimicrobial defense mechanisms have begun to develop early in gestation, at the time of delivery many of these mechanisms do not function as efficiently as in older children or adults. The relatively high incidence of infectious disease in the prenatal period bears testimony to the fact that the host-parasite balance is precarious in many neonates. Thus there is an increased incidence of neonatal infectious diseases often caused by microorganisms generally considered to be of low pathogenicity.

Host defense mechanisms may be divided into nonspecific and specific categories. Nonspecific mechanisms function effectively without requiring prior exposure to a microorganism or its antigens. These include physical barriers (e.g., intact skin and mucous membranes) and chemical barriers (e.g., gastric acid, digestive enzymes, bacteriostatic fatty acids of the skin) as well as phagocytic cells and the complement system. In contrast, specific host defense mechanisms such as cell-mediated and antibody-mediated immune responses function most effectively if there has been prior exposure to the infecting agent or its antigens (i.e., immunization).

NONSPECIFIC HOST DEFENSE MECHANISMS

Phagocytic mechanisms

The most primitive of the host defense mechanisms involves the ingestion and killing of bacteria and other microorganisms by phagocytic cells. Although polymorphonuclear leukocytes (PMNs) are the most important phagocytic cells, monocytes and the nonmobile phagocytic cells of the reticuloendothelial (RE) system contribute substantially to the function of this system. Protection provided by the nonmobile phagocytes of the RE system is strikingly demonstrated by intravascular microbial invasion in patients with congenital asplenia.

Effective elimination of invading microorganisms by mobile phagocytic cells such as PMNs requires (1) movement of the PMN to the site of infection, (2) adherence of the microorganism to the phagocyte's membrane, (3) ingestion, and (4) killing. Specific defects in some of the phases of phagocytic function have been identified in the normal neonate, as well as in disorders such as chronic granulomatous disease. (See Chapter 32.)

In the neonate, movement of PMNs toward a site of infection (chemotaxis) is defective. The neonatal PMN has a decreased chemotactic response to chemoattractant factors generated from normal adult serum. Moreover, neonatal serum does not generate chemoattractant factors as readily as adult serum. Membrane deformability is closely related to phagocyte movement. The membranes of neonatal PMNs are less deformable (i.e., more rigid) than adult PMN membranes, and this also appears to contribute to the movement disorder of the neonatal PMN. In contrast, neonatal monocytes have no chemotactic defect, and membrane deformability is normal.

Adherence of bacteria to the phagocyte's cell membrane is a prerequisite for ingestion and killing of the invading microorganism. This is an inefficient process in the absence of specific antibody and complement, since many bacteria have polysaccharide capsules that impede their adherence to PMN membranes and impair ingestion. In adult serum diluted to less than 10% ingestion of bacteria by neonatal PMNs is significantly less efficient than by adult PMNs. However, at high serum concentrations ingestion of bacteria by neonatal and adult PMNs is comparable.

Ingestion results in the formation of a phagocytic vacuole within the PMN. Occurring simultaneously with this event is an oxygen-requiring metabolic burst. Normally the enzyme nicotinamide adenosine dinucleotide phosphate oxidase (NADPH oxidase) catalyzes the production of superoxide anion ($.O_2^-$) from NADPH and O_2. Additionally, highly reactive products are generated by related enzymatic reactions. These include singlet oxygen, hydrogen peroxide, and hydrogen radicals. Hydrogen peroxide is thought to play a major bactericidal role by interacting with halide (iodide or chloride) ions in the presence of myeloperoxidase (MPO), resulting in the halidation of the ingested microorganism. The reaction of hydrogen peroxide with halide in the presence of MPO causes the release of light (i.e., chemiluminescence), which is closely correlated with the microbial killing activity of PMNs. Fusion of lysosomes and other intracytoplasmic granules with the phagocytic vacuole occurs, adding lysozyme, lactoferrin, cationic proteins, and other bactericidal and bacteriostatic materials to the contents of the phagocytic vacuoles.

In chronic granulomatous disease there is defective microbial killing, which appears to be due to a defect in the triggering of NADPH oxidase activity. PMNs from neonates show a decreased chemiluminescence response on ingestion of bacteria or other particles, suggesting a diminished bactericidal capacity. Neonatal PMNs kill bacteria as well as adult PMNs do when the bacterium to phagocyte ratio is 1:1; however, when the bacterium to phagocyte ratio is increased to 100:1, neonatal neutrophils demonstrate a markedly depressed bactericidal capacity. Thus, when stressed, the neonatal phagocytic cells perform less well than adult cells under the same conditions.

The complement system

The complement system plays an important role as one of the principal humoral effector pathways of immunity. Its major function is to facilitate the neutralization of foreign substances either in the circulation or on mucous membranes. This is accomplished by a series of plasma proteins that are involved in both specific and nonspecific host defense mechanisms.

The "classic pathway" of complement activation requires the presence of specific antibodies against a particular antigen and the formation of immune complexes. Two antibody molecules of the immune complex are bridged by the first component of complement, C1, which initiates a chain reaction in which one activated component serves as the enzyme that cleaves the next component in line. The order of component activation in the classical pathway is C1, C4, C2, and C3. Fragments with different biologic activities are created, which either remain attached to the site of activation or diffuse into the milieu (Table 30-1). As an example, the third component of complement, C3, is cleaved into the membrane bound C3b and the fluid phase C3a. With the generation of C3b the classical pathway merges with the other mode of complement activation, the "alternative pathway" (Fig. 30-1).

Table 30-1. Biologically active complement fragments

Fragment	Biologic activity
C3a	Anaphylatoxin
C3b	Opsonization, immune adherence
C5a	Leukocyte chemotaxis, increased vascular permeability
C5b6789	Lysis

In contrast to the classic pathway the alternative pathway may be activated by bacterial or mammalian cell surfaces in the absence of specific antibodies. This is possible because small amounts of circulating C3 are constantly being converted to C3b, which can bind to cell surfaces and interact with the next components in line, factors B and D, and in a positive feedback mechanism form a potent enzyme for further C3 activation (C3bBb). C3b, which was originally generated by the classical pathway, may involve this "amplification loop" of the alternative pathway to significantly enhance local C3 activation.

The central location of C3 within the complement pathway is highlighted not only by the fact that classic and alternative pathways converge at this point, but more important, further biologic effects are determined by the interaction of this important molecule with a variety of regulatory systems. The direction in which the complement pathway will proceed depends on the surface to which the C3b molecule is bound. Certain bacteria and other membranes offer a "protective surface" that favors the binding of C3b to factors B and D and the assembly of the enzyme that will convert the next component in line, C5, into C5a and C5b. This remains attached to the membrane and assembles the components of the membrane attack complex C5b, C6, C7, C8, and C9. The insertion of this complex into the cell membrane results in the loss of membrane functions and cellular integrity.

In the absence of a protected site C3b is exposed to factors I and H, which facilitate cleavage of C3b into iC3b and C3dg. All these fragments of C3 can function as ligands for cellular receptors, which are located on erythrocytes and almost all immune-competent cells. The C3b receptor (CR1) is known to mediate adherence of complement-coated complexes to erythrocytes, PMNs, and monocytic phagocytes; it also plays an important role in the clearance of immune complexes, bacteria, and cellular debris from the circulation. Other receptors also have been identified, such as the C3d binding protein, CR2, which is found on B lymphocytes and eosinophils. Its function still awaits clarification, but there is evidence that adherence of the Epstein-Barr virus is mediated by this receptor. Finally, the iC3b receptor, CR3, seems to be important for the ability to overcome bacterial invasion, and patients with a genetic deficiency of CR3 suffer severe recurrent bacterial infections.

The components of the classic complement system, as well as their functional activity, measured by total hemolytic complement (CH_{50}) assay, in full-term neonates is comparable to those of normal adults. In earlier studies in which neonates were compared to their mothers, significant deficiencies in complement components were reported. These studies did not take into account that a number of complement components are acute phase proteins and therefore their concentration in maternal serum is significantly elevated when compared with that of other normal adults. However, preterm neonates have significantly decreased concentrations of C1q, C4, C3, and CH_{50} activity compared with term neonates. Moreover, there was a statistically significant correlation between increasing birth weight or gestational age and serum concentrations of these components. Studies by Johnson and co-workers have shown that the functional activity of the classic pathway (CH_{50}) and the C3 concentration were below the normal adult range in 51% and 63%, respectively, of term newborns. Thus, within the population of term newborns, there are infants with normal and abnormal concentrations and function of the classic pathway components.

Concentrations of factor B of the alternative pathway in newborn serum vary from 35% to 60% of normal adult values and are abnormal in 15% to 30% of infants. There is no correlation between factor B concentration and gestational age. In contrast, properdin concentrations are significantly lower in preterm infants compared with term neonates. Stossel reported defective alternative pathway function in 15% of term neonates using an endotoxin particle opsonization assay. Other studies of alternative pathway function have shown defective function in 75% of term newborns and a significant correlation between increased function and gestational age. Johnston studied function of both the alternative and classic pathways in 27 term newborns. Of these infants 81% had defective alternative pathway function, 51% had abnormal classic pathway activity, 37% had defects in both pathways, and in only 11% were both pathways functionally normal.

Whether deficiencies in the complement system predispose the neonates to infection has not as yet been established. It is likely that defects in the complement system and the alternative pathway, in particular, will ultimately be found to play a role in susceptibility to infection, especially in preterm infants. Newborns have a limited spectrum of circulating antibody transmitted across the placenta; they receive IgG, no IgM, and very little antibody to the entire range of gram-negative bacteria. Thus the classic pathway has relatively little value at and shortly after birth. It follows that, in the absence of specific antibody, nonspecific activation of the biologically active fragments and complexes of the complement system via the alternative pathway becomes an extremely important defense mechanism for neonates during their first encounter with many bacteria. In a majority of neo-

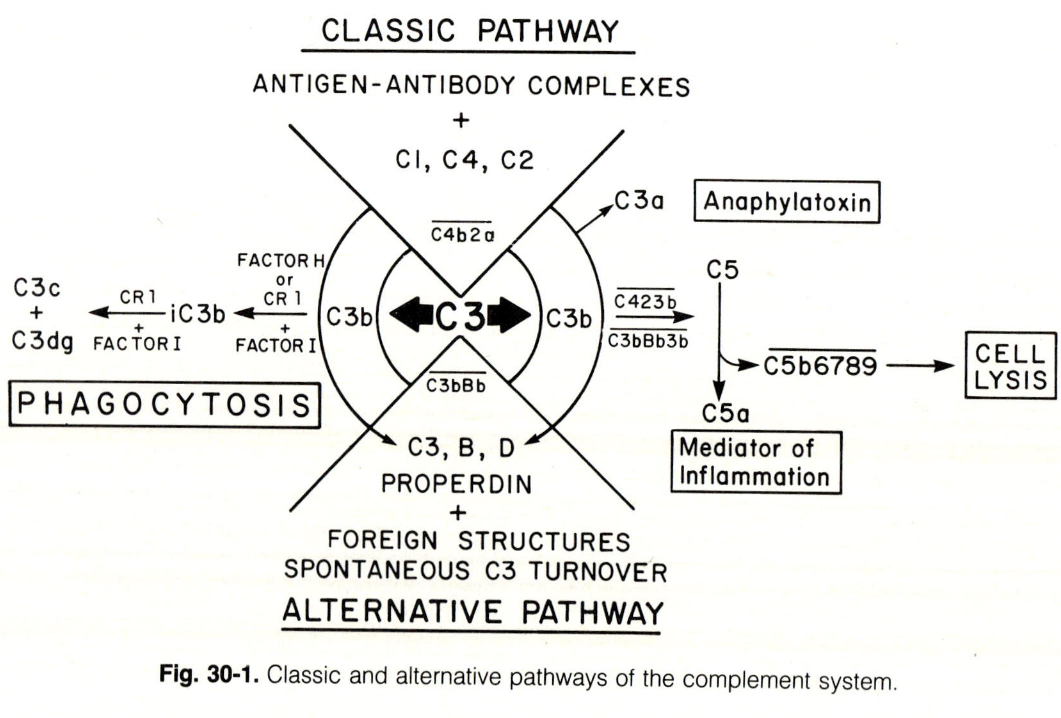

Fig. 30-1. Classic and alternative pathways of the complement system.

nates the functional deficiency of the alternative pathway, in conjunction with impaired function of neutrophils, is likely to be clinically relevant.

SPECIFIC HOST DEFENSE MECHANISMS

The two major specific host defense mechanisms are the antibody-mediated and cell-mediated immune systems. Antibody-mediated immunity is related to B lymphocytes, plasma cells and their products, immunoglobulins, and antibodies. Cell-mediated immunity involves the function of T lymphocytes of various types, their soluble products, and their interaction with macrophages, which are mononuclear phagocytes.

Antibody-mediated immunity

Specific antibody may be produced in response to direct exposure to infection or immunization by an almost infinite spectrum of antigens (e.g., proteins, carbohydrates, bacteria, viruses, fungi, drugs). Antibodies are synthesized and secreted by plasma cells residing in the lymph nodes, spleen, mucosal linings of the gastrointestinal and respiratory tracts, and the bone marrow. The plasma cells arise from B lymphocytes after antigenic stimulation.

Antibodies comprise a unique family of proteins termed *immunoglobulins* (Ig), which consist of five major classes of human immunoglobulins: IgG, IgA, IgM, IgD, and IgE. The basic structure of the immunoglobulin molecule, as illustrated by IgG, is shown in Fig. 30-2. The IgG molecule is composed of four polypeptide chains, two heavy chains and two light chains, held together by covalent disulfide bonds as well as by noncovalent forces. In a given IgG molecule the two heavy chains and two light chains have identical amino acid sequences. The different immunoglobulin classes are distinguished by antigenic and amino acid sequence differences in their heavy chains (Table 30-2). Some of the immunoglobulin classes are composed of subclasses, for example, IgG has four subclasses—IgG_1, IgG_2, IgG_3, and IgG_4—which result from antigenic differences in the heavy chains. In addition to these differences between the immunoglobulin classes and subclasses, there are antigenic and amino acid sequence differences among molecules from the same class and subclass. This molecular heterogeneity is due to amino acid sequence variation in the amino terminal portions of the heavy chains and light chains in the so-called variable regions. The variable regions make up portions of the antibody combining sites of immunoglobulin molecules, and it is the structural variability in this region that permits different antibody molecules to react specifically with different antigens. In contrast, the amino acid sequences of the carboxy terminal portions of the heavy and light chains do not vary between molecules of the same immunoglobulin class or subclass and are termed the *constant regions*. Whereas the variable regions of immunoglobulin molecules confer the antigen-binding specificity, the constant regions are responsible for the biologic functions of the immunoglobulin molecules. Since the structure of the constant regions of the various immunoglobulin classes differs, their biologic properties and functions vary as well. For example, only IgM and IgG activate the complement system via the classic pathway, and only IgG can be actively transported across the placenta.

The chemical characteristics and biologic properties of the immunoglobulin classes are summarized in Table 30-2. IgG is the major immunoglobulin in the serum and interstitial fluid and has a relatively long half-life (20 to 30 days). It is responsible for immunity to bacteria (par-

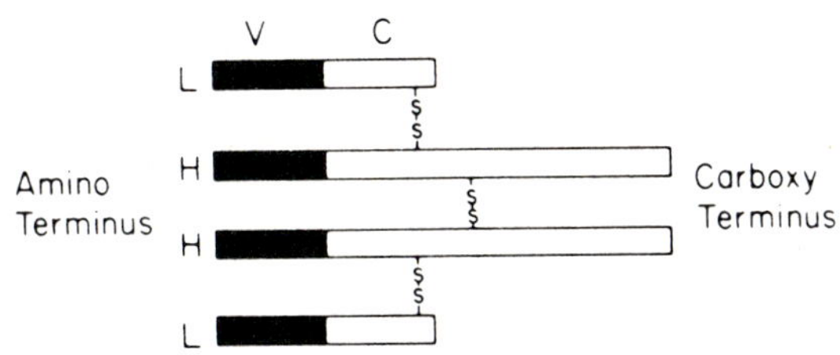

Fig. 30-2. Structure of the immunoglobulin G (IgG) molecule.

Table 30-2. Chemical and biologic properties of human immunoglobulin classes

	IgG	IgA	IgM	IgD	IgE
Heavy chains	γ	α	μ	δ	ϵ
Molecular weight (daltons)	150,000	160,000 400,000*	900,000	180,000	190,000
Biologic half-life (days)	21	5	5	2	2
Adult serum concentration (mg/dl)	1,000	250	100	2.3	0.01
Placental transfer	+	0	0	0	0
Binds complement (classic pathway)	+	0	+	0	0
Reaginic activity	0	0	0	0	+
Mucosal immunity	+	+++	+	0	++

*Secretory IgA.

ticularly gram-positive bacteria), bacterial toxins, and viral agents. IgG antibodies can neutralize viruses and toxins, as well as facilitate the phagocytosis and destruction of bacteria and other particles to which they are bound. This property is termed *opsonization*. Bacteria to which IgG is bound adhere to the surface membranes of neutrophils and monocytes (macrophages) by means of membrane receptors for a portion of the IgG heavy chain. IgG can activate the complement pathway, increase the inflammatory response, and increase neutrophil chemotaxis and complement-mediated opsonization.

IgA is the second most abundant immunoglobulin in serum, but it is the predominant immunoglobulin in the gastrointestinal and respiratory tracts, as well as in human colostrum and breast milk. In secretions, IgA occurs as a dimer joined by a J-chain and bears an additional polypeptide chain termed the *secretory component*. This moiety endows the molecule with resistance against degradation by proteolytic enzymes. Secretory IgA is thus uniquely suited for functioning in the secretions of the respiratory and gastrointestinal tracts. IgA provides local mucosal immunity against viruses and limits bacterial overgrowth on mucosal surfaces. It also may limit absorption of antigenic dietary proteins. IgA does not activate the classic complement pathway but can activate an alternative pathway.

IgM antibodies exist in serum primarily as pentamers joined together by a J-chain. IgM provides protection against blood-borne infection. It occurs in only small quantities in interstitial fluids and secretions. IgM antibodies are potent bacterial agglutinins and activate the classic complement sequence. Through activation of the complement system, IgM antibodies cause deposition of C3b on bacterial cell surfaces and thus facilitate phagocytosis, since neutrophils have receptors for C3b. However, there are no phagocytosis-promoting receptors for IgM. Most serum antibodies to gram-negative bacteria are of the IgM type. Intrauterine and neonatal infections elicit the formation of predominantly IgM antibodies. Since IgM does not cross the placenta, the presence of specific IgM antibody in cord blood to spirochetes, rubella, cytomegalovirus, or other microorganisms can be taken as reliable evidence for intrauterine infection with these agents. The absence of IgM does not, however, exclude the possibility of congenital intrauterine infection.

IgE antibodies are present in very small quantities in serum and secretions. These antibodies play a major role in allergic reactions of the immediate hypersensitivity type. IgE antibodies bind to the cell membranes of basophils (mast cells) via a receptor for the carboxy terminal portion of the heavy chain. Binding of antigen (allergen) to the IgE fixed to the basophil results in the liberation of histamine, slow-reacting substance of anaphylaxis (SRS-A), and other pharmacologic mediators of immediate allergic reactions. IgD, which occurs in low concentration in serum, is present on the surface of B lymphocytes. The role of surface membrane IgD is discussed later.

Table 30-3. Normal values for immunoglobulins at various ages*

Age	IgG (mg/dl)	IgA (mg/dl)	IgM (mg/dl)
Newborn	600-1,670	0-5	5-15
1-3 months	218-610	20-53	11-51
4-6 months	228-636	27-72	25-60
7-9 months	292-816	27-73	12-124
10-18 months	383-1,070	27-169	28-113
2 years	423-1,184	35-222	32-131
3 years	477-1,334	40-251	28-113
4-5 years	540-1,500	48-336	20-106
6-8 years	571-1,700	52-535	28-112
14 years	570-1,570	86-544	33-135
Adult	635-1,775	106-668	37-154

From Buckley, R.H., and others: Pediatrics **41**:600, 1968. Copyright American Academy of Pediatrics, 1968.
*See also Appendix C, Tables 11 and 12.

Levels of immunoglobulins in the serum of newborns change dramatically during the first 2 years of life. Interpretation of normal serum immunoglobulin values requires comparison with age-matched controls. Table 30-3 shows normal immunoglobulin levels for infants and children. (See Appendix C, Tables 11 and 12.)

Cell-mediated immunity

Cell-mediated immunity refers to a group of immunologic responses in which T lymphocytes play a central role; serum immunoglobulins and antibodies cannot produce these reactions or transfer them to another individual. The cutaneous delayed hypersensitivity reaction is a classic example of a cell-mediated immune reaction. An individual who has been exposed to tubercle bacilli or immunized with BCG has T lymphocytes that are sensitized to tuberculin. When such an individual is injected intradermally with turberculin (PPD), sensitized T lymphocytes are activated to divide as well as to secrete a variety of soluble factors known as lymphokines. Some of these lymphokines have chemoattractant properties and cause monocytes (macrophages) and neutrophils to accumulate at the site where sensitized T cells are interacting with antigen. Migration inhibitory factor (MIF) causes macrophages to remain at that site and macrophage activating factor (MAF) *incites* these cells to extreme phagocytic and metabolic activity; these cells are termed *activated*, or "angry," *macrophages*. Antigen-stimulated T cells also secrete lymphokines, which cause

Table 30-4. Lymphokines

Target cell or tissue	Factor	Effect
Macrophages	Migration inhibitory factor (MIF)	Inhibits macrophage migration in vitro; may lead to accumulation of macrophages
	Macrophage activating factor (MAF)	Increases phagocytosis, glycolysis, oxygen consumption
Neutrophils	Leukocyte inhibiting factor (LIF)	Inhibits migration of neutrophils
	Chemotactic factor	Attracts neutrophils
Lymphocytes	Interleukin-2	Promotes proliferation of activated T lymphocytes
	B cell growth factors	Promotes B cell proliferation
	Helper and suppressor factors	Modulate T and B cell responses
Mammalian cells of the same species	Interferon	Inhibits viral replication; may act as immunosuppressive or enhancing agents
Mammalian cells: tumor cells, some bacteria and yeasts	Lymphotoxin (LT)	Inhibition of cell proliferation or frank cell cytotoxicity
Skin	Skin reactive factor (SRF)	Augments capillary permeability in vivo; contributes to infiltration with mononuclear cells

nonsensitized T cells to divide (mitogen factors), and in this way these cells are nonspecifically recruited into the reaction. The accumulation of macrophages, lymphocytes, and neutrophils and the attendant inflammatory reaction at the site of tuberculin injection are what we perceive clinically as a positive delayed hypersensitivity reaction. Granuloma formation is essentially a delayed hypersensitivity reaction initiated by a particle (e.g., tubercle bacillus or fungus) rather than a soluble protein. The extensive tissue damage in the middle of a granuloma is caused by indiscriminate destruction of normal tissue by "angry" macrophages. The basic scheme of cell-mediated immune reactions is that T cells are activated by antigens to which they have been sensitized (i.e., exposed), and these cells liberate lymphokines that modify the behavior of other cells such as macrophages, neutrophils, and other lymphocytes. A list of important lymphokines and their properties is found in Table 30-4.

Other cell-mediated reactions include the killing of tumor cells or virus-infected cells by direct contact of a cytolytic T cell with the target cells, by the liberation of a lymphocytotoxin by the T cell, which kills the target cells, or by the recruitment of lymphokine activated killer (LAK) cells. These nonspecific killer cells are activated by interleukin-2 (IL-2) and are capable of lysing virtually all tumor cells. Another nonspecific cytolytic system, the natural killer (NK) cells, appears to be particularly important in eliminating virus-infected cells.

T lymphocytes also regulate antibody formation to many antigens. A subpopulation of T lymphocytes induces B lymphocytes to differentiate into plasma cells after exposure to antigen. These cells are termed *inducer* or *helper* T cells. B-cells differentiation can be inhibited by other subpopulations of T cells, termed *suppressor* T cells. The actions of both helper T cells and suppressor T cells are often mediated by lymphokines.

Development of T and B lymphocyte populations

Both the T and B lymphocyte populations are derived from pluripotent hematopoietic stem cells arising from the intraembryonic mesenchyme. These cells migrate to the blood islands of the yolk sac, thence to the fetal liver, and later in embryonic life to the bone marrow, where they reside throughout extrauterine life.

Cells destined to become T lymphocytes, the prothymocytes, migrate from the fetal liver or bone marrow to the thymus, entering at the cortex. As these thymocytes migrate toward the thymic medulla, they undergo numerous cycles of cell division, as well as differentiation into functionally different classes of T lymphocytes (e.g., helper-inducer cells, suppressor cells, cytotoxic cells). The thymic microenvironment plays a key role in this differentiation process, and thymic hormones continue to influence T cells even after they have left the thymic microenvironment.

The thymus comprises both epithelial and lymphoid elements. The epithelial components of the thymus are derived from the third and fourth pharyngeal pouches and migrate into the anterior superior mediastinum. The parathyroid glands arise from the same region. The thymic lymphoid cells come from the stem cells just mentioned and first appear in the embryonic thymus at approximately 8 weeks of gestation. T lymphocytes can be detected in the thymus after 11 weeks of gestation and begin to appear in the peripheral blood, spleen, and lymph nodes by 16 to 18 weeks of gestation. By 30 to 32 weeks of gestation the fetus has a near normal (adult) number of circulating T lymphocytes. Thus at birth nor-

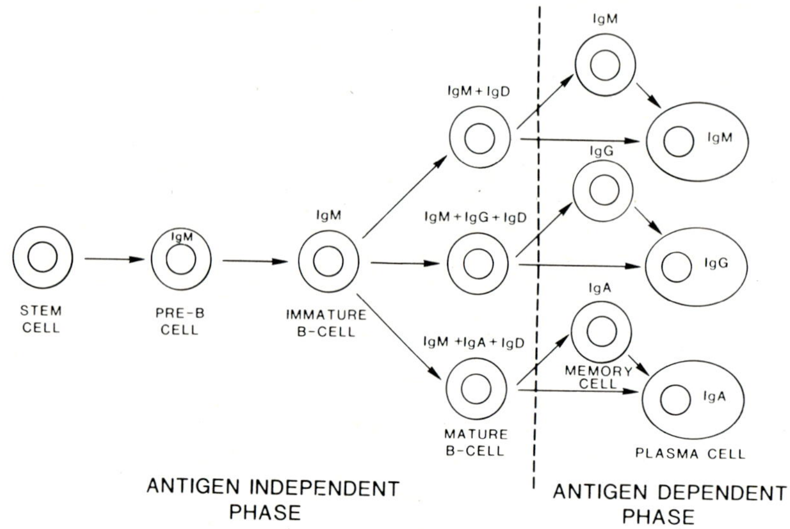

Fig. 30-3. Sequence of B lymphocyte differentiation.

mal newborns and many infants born prematurely will have normal numbers of T lymphocytes detectable in their peripheral blood.

B lymphocytes are the precursors of immunoglobulin secreting (antibody-secreting) plasma cells. B lymphocytes are derived from the same stem cells that give rise to T cells, but B cell differentiation occurs in a different inductive microenvironment. In birds, B cell differentiation occurs in the bursa of Fabricius, an anatomically distinct lymphoepithelial organ in the wall of the hindgut. In humans and other mammals there is no bursa of Fabricius, and the development of B cells occurs first in the fetal liver and subsequently in the bone marrow. B-cell differentiation is represented schematically in Fig. 30-3. The first identifiable cells of the B cell line arise from stem cells in the fetal liver at 8 weeks of gestation. These cells, termed *pre-B cells,* contain small amounts of low molecular weight (8S) IgM in their cytoplasm. At this stage of differentiation the development of clones of cells with different antibody specificities has already begun, that is, different pre-B cells are producing IgM with different variable regions. At approximately 10 weeks of gestation the first "true" B cells can be identified in the liver. These cells synthesize surface membrane IgM (sIgM) only. These B cells, which have been called immature B cells, are exquisitely sensitive to inactivation following contact with antigens. The ease with which these cells may be inactivated is thought to be closely related to the well-established phenomenon of immunologic tolerance in neonatal animals. The immature sIgM + B cells proliferate, and some of their progeny begin to produce other immunoglobulin classes and display them on their membranes. B cell clones of the following types emerge: IgM + IgG + IgD, IgM + IgA + IgD, and IgM + IgD. By the fifteenth week of gestation the normal fetus has levels of circulating B lymphocytes that are as high or higher than those of normal adults. Unlike the immature B cells, B cells bearing surface IgD cannot be readily inactivated by antigen but can be triggered to differentiate into immunoglobulin-secreting plasma cells when exposed to antigen in the presence of helper or inducer T cells. The development of the different B cell clones and antibody diversity occurs in the absence of antigen and is termed the *antigen-independent phase of B cell differentiation.* Differentiation of B cells to plasma cells depends on the presence of antigen and is regulated by inducer and suppressor T lymphocytes; this is the *antigen-dependent phase of B cell differentiation.*

Specific immunity in the neonate

The appearance of specific antibodies or a population of sensitized T cells directed against a specific antigen requires exposure (i.e., immunization or infection) and immunocompetence. For example, in utero the fetus is normally exposed to very few foreign antigens and makes little or no antibody. At birth the only antibodies present are the IgG antibodies transferred from the mother via the placenta, unless there has been a congenital infection, in which case IgM antibodies against the infecting agent are usually detectable. Thus an active immune response requires exposure to antigen.

Second, an infant or fetus must be developmentally capable of responding to an antigen at the time the antigen is presented. The ability to mount antibody or cell-mediated immune responses to specific antigens is acquired sequentially during the course of embryonic development. Early in gestation, fetuses can respond to

Table 30-5. Appearance of immunologic responses in the fetal lamb

Antigen	Days after conception
Bacteriophage	<40
Ferritin	56
Allogenic skin grafts	75
Simian virus 40	90
Ovalbumin	120
Lymphocytic choriomeningitis virus	140
Birth	150
Diphtheria toxoid	>190

Modified from Silverstein, A.M.: Ontogeny of the immune response: a perspective. In Cooper, M.D., and Dayton, D.H., editors: Development of host defenses, New York, 1977, Raven Press.

certain antigens, whereas other antigens will elicit antibody production or cell-mediated immune reactions only after birth. This sequential development of antigen-specific immunocompetence was first described by Silverstein in the fetal lamb (Table 30-5) and has been observed in other mammalian species. The well-known inability to induce antibodies to the polysaccharides from *Pneumococcus* and *Haemophilus* organisms in children under 18 months of age is a clinically important example of the sequential acquisition of antigen-specific immunocompetence in humans.

Antibody responses of the fetus and premature and full-term newborn differ from those of older children and adults. They do not respond to some antigens (e.g., pneumococcal polysaccharide), and the antibody responses to other antigens (rubella, cytomegalovirus, toxoplasma) are predominately of the IgM type. The T lymphocyte population of newborns contains a relatively large number of suppressor cells for B cell differentiation. In addition, the B cells of newborns differentiate predominately into IgM-secreting plasma cells, whereas adult B cells will produce IgG- and IgA-secreting plasma cells as well. The adult pattern of B cell differentiation develops during the first year of life.

There are also deficiencies in cell-mediated immunity in premature and full-term neonates. T cells have reached normal levels by 30 to 32 weeks of gestation and are capable of proliferating at adult levels in response to phytohemagglutinin (PHA), concanavalin A (Con A), and allogeneic cells (mixed lymphocyte reaction). However, T lymphocytes from premature and full-term neonates show markedly reduced ability to secrete migration inhibitory factor or immune interferon and to kill tumor or virus-infected cells when compared with those of normal adults. Cutaneous delayed hypersensitivity reactions are decreased even when there is evidence of adequate exposure. Infants with oral or cutaneous candidiasis may show only weakly reactive *Candida* skin tests, whereas their in vitro lymphocyte proliferation responses to *Candida* may be comparable to those seen in adults. This discrepancy is caused by the decreased inflammatory reactions seen in infants. In general, the recognition, or afferent, phase of cellular immune responses in the neonate is comparable to that seen in the adult, whereas the efferent, or effector, limb of these responses is diminished.

IMMUNOLOGIC ASPECTS OF THE MOTHER-CHILD RELATIONSHIP

Passive immunity is the acquisition of specific antibody or sensitized lymphocytes from another individual and represents a means by which specific immunity may be acquired without prior exposure to antigen or the mounting of a specific immune response. Such immunity is transient but nonetheless may provide sufficient antimicrobial protection during a vulnerable period of life. The development of an antibody response to an antigen seen for the first time requires 7 to 14 days. Thus active antibody-mediated immunity is of little value during the crucial first few days of an infection with a new microorganism. The presence of circulating specific antibody to that organism (i.e., passive immunity) permits the mobilization of multiple host defense mechanisms (i.e., complement system, neutrophils) to eliminate the invading microorganism as well as limit its colonization. In humans the major avenues for the acquisition of passive immunity are the transfer of IgG across the placenta and the transfer of secretory IgA via colostrum and breast milk.

Placental transport of IgG antibodies

Although B lymphocytes are present in the fetus by the end of the first trimester, there is very little active fetal immunoglobulin production, since this process depends on exposure to antigens. Serum immunoglobulin levels in the fetus are extremely low until 20 to 22 weeks of gestation, at which time an accelerated active transport of IgG across the placenta begins. Only maternal IgG is transported; IgA, IgM, IgD, and IgE are not. The specificity of this transport process is caused by the presence of specific receptors on the heavy chain of the IgG molecule. The transport of IgG is an active placental process, and the neonate's serum IgG concentration at birth is 5% to 10% higher than that of the mother. Prematurely delivered infants have lower IgG levels than those delivered at term. Moreover, small for gestational age (SGA) infants have lower IgG levels than their appropriately grown (AGA) peers at any gestational age. Fetal weight loss in utero is often due to placental dysfunction, which reduces the nutrient supply and limits transfer of IgG as well. This phenomenon is further manifested by the progressive decrease in IgG transport after 44 weeks

Table 30-6. Relationship of antibody type with transplacental transfer

Good passive transfer (IgG)	Poor passive transfer (IgA)	No passive transfer (IgM)
Diphtheria antitoxin	*Haemophilus influenzae*	Enteric somatic (O) antibodies *(Salmonella, Shigella, E. Coli)*
Tetanus antitoxin	*Bordetella Pertussis*	Skin-sensitizing antibody
Antierythrogenic toxin	*Shigella flexneri*	Heterophile antibody
Antistaphylococcal antibody	Streptococcus MG	Wassermann antibody
Salmonella flagella (H) antibody		
Antistreptolysin		
All antiviral antibodies present in maternal circulation (rubeola, rubella, mumps, poliovirus)		
VDRL antibodies		

of gestation, a period when the placenta is known to become increasingly dysfunctional.

Elevated levels of IgM or IgA in cord blood usually indicate that the infant has been exposed to antigen in utero and has synthesized antibody itself. Congenital infections with syphilis and rubella characteristically produce elevation of the cord blood IgM concentration, and specific fetal antibody of the IgM type directed against the infecting agent can be detected. Elevated levels of both IgM and IgA also may be found if maternal-to-fetal transplacental bleeding has occurred.

The transfer of IgG antibodies from mother to child across the placenta provides the newborn with a portion of the mother's immunologic experience. Antibodies to viral agents, diphtheria, and tetanus antitoxins, which are usually of the IgG class, are efficiently transported across the placenta and attain protective levels in the fetus. In contrast, antibodies to agents that evoke primarily IgA or IgM antibody responses are transported poorly or not at all, leaving the neonate unprotected against those organisms (Table 30-6). Moreover, an infant cannot be protected against agents to which the mother has not made significant amounts of antibody.

Placental transfer of IgG antibody may have deleterious as well as beneficial effects. Hemolytic disease of the newborn is produced by placental transfer of IgG antierythrocyte antibodies usually directed against Rh or ABO blood group antigens. Transient neutropenia, thrombocytopenia, myasthenia, or hyperthyroidism are also produced in approximately 20% of infants born to mothers with systemic lupus erythematosus, idiopathic thrombocytopenic purpura, myasthenia gravis, or hyperthyroidism by IgG transported across the placenta. These disorders, as well as the protective effects of maternal IgG, are transient, since IgG has a half-life of 20 to 30 days.

Immunologic properties of human breast milk

Specific and nonspecific protective factors transferred to the neonate via the breast milk are listed in Table 30-7. Even though all immunoglobulin classes can be detected in colostrum, secretory IgA comprises the vast majority of the immunoglobulins in human breast milk. Secretory IgA consists of two "serum" IgA subunits, a J-chain and a secretory component, rendering it resistant to digestion by trypsin and pepsin as well as hydrolysis by gastric acid. There is no evidence that immunoglobulins present in breast milk enter the systemic circulation of the human neonate in significant quantities.

Table 30-7. Human milk protective elements

Component	Comment
Cellular factors	
Macrophage	Phagocytosis
	Produces lysozyme, lactoferrin, and complement
	May regulate B lymphocyte immunoglobulin production
Lymphocyte	
B cells	Humoral immunity; IgA synthesis
T cells	Cellular immunity
	Partially regulate humoral immunity
Growth-promoting factors	
DNA synthesis and cell division in vitro	Functional in both animal and human fibroblasts
DNA synthesis and growth by mucosal cells	Described in laboratory animals
Bifidus factor	Nitrogen-containing polysaccharides that specifically enhance the growth of *Lactobacillus bifidus*
Lactoperoxidase	Functions in conjunction with hydrogen peroxide and cyanide to form an in vitro antibacterial system

The levels of IgA, IgM, and IgG have been studied serially in milk. The IgG concentration is relatively constant during the first 180 days of lactation, whereas the IgM and IgA are highest in colostrum, decrease during the first 5 days of lactation, and then remain relatively constant during the next 175 days. Breast milk contains antibodies to a broad spectrum of enteric bacteria and

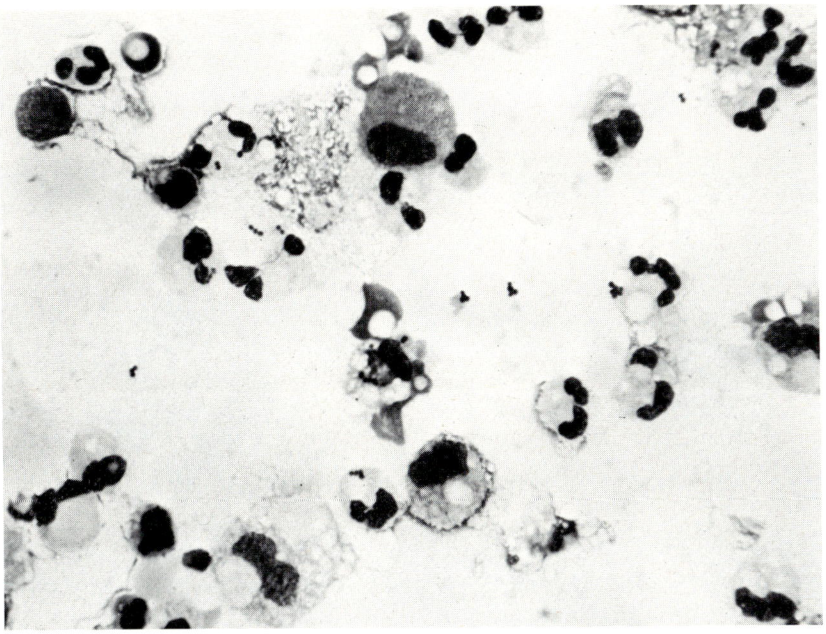

Fig. 30-4. Leukocytes in human breast milk.

viruses (e.g., polio, ECHO, Coxsackie), and the antibody titers to these agents decrease in parallel to the fall in concentration of IgA in the milk.

The majority of immunoglobulins present in human breast milk are thought to be produced by plasma cells located within the breast itself, and very little milk immunoglobulin is derived from maternal serum immunoglobulins. Moreover, milk antibodies are directed predominately against enteric bacterial and viral antigens; the concentration of such antibodies is much higher in colostrum than in maternal serum. Thus the antibody composition of breast milk in part compensates for the deficiency of antibodies directed against enteric antigens in placentally transferred IgG. This unique spectrum of antibody specificity is achieved by the "homing" of B lymphocytes sensitized in the mother's gastrointestinal tract to her mammary glands. B cells stimulated by enteric bacterial or viral antigens in Peyer's patches of the small intestine migrate to the mucosal linings of the lactating mammary gland where they differentiate into plasma cells and secrete their antibodies. Antigens introduced into the gastrointestinal tract will stimulate the development of antibodies in the breast milk, whereas antibodies to these antigens do not develop in the serum. Thus a mother will transfer to her baby via breast milk antibodies specific for microbial agents present in her own gastrointestinal tract. As the neonate is being freshly colonized, these antibodies limit bacterial growth in the gastrointestinal tract and protect against overgrowth.

The cellular components of human breast milk consist of macrophages, T and B lymphocytes, neutrophils, and epithelial cells. The cellular content of colostrum or early milk is higher than that of later milk and varies greatly between women. Neutrophils are present in significant numbers early in lactation, and their presence may be related to breast engorgement during the initial days of lactation. Although the function of the breast milk neutrophil is unclear, its presence does not necessarily imply infection. Epithelial cells occasionally present in milk may originate from the skin of the nipple.

The breast milk macrophage is a mononuclear phagocytic cell that comprises approximately 80% of the leukocytes in milk (Fig. 30-4). This is an active phagocytic cell that contains large amounts of intracytoplasmic lipid and IgA, bears cell surface receptors for IgG and C3b, and synthesizes several important host resistance factors including lysozyme, C3 and C4 complement components, and lactoferrin (Fig. 30-5). Milk macrophages are capable of phagocytizing and killing both gram-positive and gram-negative bacteria and appear to interact with the lymphocytes present in breast milk.

The host defense factors that the breast milk macrophage synthesizes provide important nonspecific antimicrobial protection for the neonate. Lysozyme is capable of lysing the cell walls of many bacteria. This enzyme is synthesized by the milk macrophage, and its concentration in human milk is 300 times that found in cow's milk. It is stable in an acid environment comparable to that of the gastric contents. Lactoferrin is an iron-binding protein that is present in many external secretions. It is synthesized by the milk macrophage, and its concentration in breast milk is higher than in any

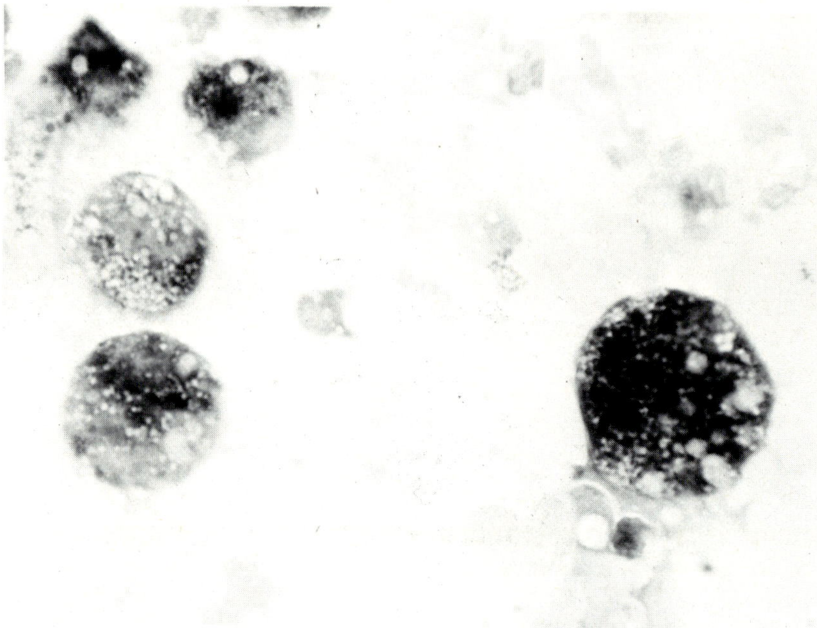

Fig. 30-5. Breast milk macrophages.

other body fluid. Lactoferrin's antimicrobial activity derives from its ability to chelate iron, thus depriving bacteria of a cofactor important for their growth. The growth of both *Staphylococcus* organisms and *E. coli* is limited by lactoferrin. The C3 and C4 complement components are also actively synthesized by breast macrophages. The function of these proteins in milk is unclear, since there is relatively little IgG and IgM or the early complement components, C1 and C2, which are necessary for activation of C3 to its biologically active forms. IgA may activate C3 via the alternative pathway; however, it is not known whether this occurs in milk. IgA is present in highest concentrations within the breast macrophage itself. However, this macrophage-associated IgA is not synthesized by the macrophage. Viable macrophages have been shown to release this IgA slowly, and this has led to the hypothesis that the breast macrophage may represent a vehicle for immunoglobulin transport down the neonate's gastrointestinal tract.

Viable T and B lymphocytes are present in human breast milk. T lymphocytes represent as much as 50% of the milk lymphocytes early in lactation and fall to less than 20% as lactation progresses. Breast T cells can be stimulated by Con A and PHA to undergo blast transformation and DNA synthesis. The spectrum of responses of the breast T cells differ from that of the peripheral blood T cells from the same donor. For example, milk T cells are often unresponsive to *Candida albicans* antigen, whereas the peripheral blood T cells from the same donor are highly reactive. In contrast, milk T cells respond well to the K_1 capsular antigen of *E coli*, whereas peripheral blood lymphocytes responses to K_1 are minimal or absent. This phenomenon may be related to the previously described homing of lymphocytes sensitized in the gastrointestinal tract to mammary glands. The transfer of cell-mediated immunity from tuberculin-sensitive mothers to their breast-fed infants has recently been reported. If these reports are substantiated, this form of passive transfer of cellular immunity could be of major clinical significance. It is unlikely that intact T lymphocytes are passing from the mother's milk across the mucous membranes of the infant's gastrointestinal tract. It is more likely that a soluble T cell factor, for example, transfer factor, might be involved. The B lymphocytes present in milk have IgG, IgA, IgM, and IgD on their surfaces. However, these cells synthesize IgA almost exclusively. The role of B cells in milk is as yet unclear.

Breast milk constituents may interact with the neonate's immune system in ways other than those already mentioned. A significant increase in the secretory IgA content of nasal and salivary secretions has been observed in breast-fed versus formula-fed newborns during the first few days of life. It is postulated that this may reflect the influence of a soluble factor in milk acting to stimulate the mucosal immune system of the breast-fed infant. Factors enhancing IgA synthesis by B cells and epithelial cell growth have also been reported to be produced by milk macrophages.

Many nurseries have tried to take advantage of the antibody content and other antimicrobial properties of human milk by using a variety of breast milk banking systems. All too often these programs either freeze the milk, which destroys the viable cells, or pasteurize the milk, which destroys both the cellular and immunoglobulin content. Other banking systems refrigerate whole "fresh" breast milk for variable periods of time with no milk "treatment." This will preserve intact the antibody content, but cellular viability falls significantly by 24 hours, and the numbers of both macrophages and neutrophils significantly decrease secondary to either cytolysis or adherence to the walls of the storage container. Thus, although human milk banking may make a significant contribution to infant nutrition, its immunologic contribution following storage is uncertain at best.

EVALUATION OF HOST DEFENSE MECHANISM FUNCTION IN THE INFANT

Some disorders of immunologic function may become clinically apparent in the neonatal period or first year of life. Because of differences in the developmental status of the newborn's host defense mechanisms and the lack of exposure to antigens, the evaluation of the function of host defense mechanisms in the infant is somewhat different from that performed for older children and adults. Infants who have experienced two or more significant bacterial or fungal infections should be suspected of having a defect in their host defense mechanisms. Patients with unusual infections (e.g., from *Pneumocystis carinii*) or infections that respond incompletely to therapy and recur are also suspect. Growth failure, chronic diarrhea, chronic dermatitis, hepatosplenomegaly, and recurrent abscesses commonly occur in immunologically deficient infants. Infants having a sibling (and in the case of X-linked disorders a maternal uncle) with a known immunologic defect should receive an appropriate laboratory evaluation even if there has not as yet been any episode of infection.

In evaluating a patient for a possible host defense mechanism defect, all host defense systems, that is, phagocytic, complement, antibody, and cell-mediated immunity, should be considered. The evaluation should be divided into initial screening tests and definitive tests that allow one to establish a specific diagnosis. Whereas screening tests should be obtainable by physicians at all hospitals, definitive tests may be available only at major medical centers. The laboratory tests appropriate for evaluation of host defense mechanisms of the infant are listed in the following material. Those tests considered to be initial screening tests are indicated by an asterisk (*).

A. Phagocytosis
   *1. White blood cell count and differential
   *2. Nitroblue tetrazolium (NBT) dye reduction test (qualitative)
   3. Ingestion of endotoxin-coated Oil Red O particles; quantitative NBT reduction; NBT reduction : ingestion ratio
   4. Quantitative bacterial killing
   5. Chemotaxis analysis using a Boyden chamber
B. Complement
   *1. Total hemolytic complement assay (CH_{50})
   *2. Measurement of C3 by radial diffusion
   3. Measurement of individual components of the classic and alternative complement pathways by radial diffusion
   4. Functional measurement of the alternative pathway
   5. Functional assay for C5 (yeast phagocytosis)
C. Antibody-mediated immunity
   *1. Quantitation of serum IgG, IgA, and IgM by radial diffusion; serum immunoelectrophoresis
   *2. Measurement of specific antibodies after immunization
   *3. Isoagglutinin titer (anti-A and anti-B)
   4. IgE radioimmunoassay
   5. Quantitation of B cells in blood by immunofluorescent techniques with specific antiimmunoglobulin antibodies
   6. B cell differentiation to plasma cells in vitro using pokeweed mitogen stimulation
D. Cell-mediated immunity
   *1. Total lymphocyte count
   *2. Delayed hypersensitivity skin tests to common antigens
   *3. Lymphocyte responses to mitogens (PHA, Con A)
   4. Lymphocyte responses to antigens *(Candida)* and allogeneic cells (mixed lymphocyte reaction)
   5. Quantitation of circulating T lymphocytes by sheep erythrocyte (E) rosette technique and immunofluorescence analysis with monoclonal antibodies specific for T lymphocytes and T cell subpopulations

Phagocytic function

Neutropenia is the most common abnormality related to phagocytic function and may be readily detected by white blood cell count and differential (Chapter 32). Neutropenia may be caused by bacterial or viral infection, antigranulocyte antibodies, as in systemic lupus erythematosus (SLE), or be part of a primary congenital disorder. Persistent neutropenia should prompt bone marrow examination. Disorders revealing morphologic abnormalities, such as Chediak-Higashi syndrome, in which there are giant cytoplasmic granules, may be readily detected by examining the blood smear.

Chronic granulomatous disease (CGD) may appear during the first few months of life. This disorder can be detected by the NBT dye reduction tests. Neutrophils from patients with CGD do not undergo the normal increase in oxidative metabolism that occurs during phagocytosis of particles. NBT reduction occurs concomitantly with particle ingestion in normal individuals but does not occur in patients with CGD. If the NBT test shows reduced or absent dye reduction, suggesting a neutrophil metabolic defect like CGD, a more accurate determination quantitating the amount of NBT reduction for the number of particles ingested (NBT reduction: ingestion ratio) should be performed. This quantitative test is helpful in detecting variants of CGD.

A variety of defects in neutrophil chemotaxis have been described, particularly in patients with recurrent abscesses. Chemotaxis can be evaluated by measuring the movement of neutrophils using a chamber divided by a micropore filter (Boyden chamber). Normally neutrophils will move through a micropore filter toward a chemoattractant produced by incubating endotoxin with fresh serum. Through this method intrinsic defects in neutrophil chemotaxis, as well as defects in the ability of patients serum to produce appropriate chemoattractant factors, may be identified. The hyper-IgE syndrome (Job's syndrome) is an example of a neutrophil chemotactic defect that can become clinically apparent during the first year of life.

Complement system

Both transient and persistent deficiencies of serum complement components have been reported. The total hemolytic complement test (CH_{50}) measures the ability of the patient's serum to serve as a complement source to permit lysis of sheep red blood cells (SRBC) by rabbit antibody to SRBC. This method will detect defects in the classic complement pathway and particularly in the earlier components of that pathway (C1, C4, C2, C3, C5). The CH_{50} test is the best single screening test for complement deficiencies; however, this does not detect deficiencies in the alternative pathway. Individual components of the classic and alternative pathways can be measured by radial diffusion techniques in many laboratories. Functional analyses of the alternative pathway and of the C5 component, important in Leiner's syndrome, are available in relatively few laboratories.

Antibody-mediated immunity

Analysis of antibody-mediated immunity begins with quantitation of serum immunoglobulins (IgG, IgA, and IgM) by radial diffusion. Results must be compared with matched normal values, as shown in Table 30-3. Immunoelectrophoresis is helpful in determining whether the immunoglobulins present are normal; homogenous proteins similar to those seen in multiple myeloma are sometimes seen in patients with congenital infections and certain immunodeficiency diseases. In general, analysis of immunoglobulins has limited value in the first 3 to 4 months of life, since most of the infant's serum immunoglobulin is maternal IgG. However, elevation of IgM in the cord blood may indicate intrauterine infection; elevation of both IgM and IgA suggests maternofetal bleeding. At all ages (except very low birth weight infants) serum IgG values should be greater than 200 mg/dl, and the presence of IgG values below this level requires more extensive investigation. In patients who have received routine immunizations, antibody titers to diphtheria and tetanus toxoids and polio may be studied. To assess antibody responses before and after immunization, serum samples should be tested. Immunization with DPT and Salk killed polio vaccine is useful for this purpose. In children suspected of being immunodeficient, live virus vaccines should be avoided. Cases of paralytic polio from vaccine strains have been reported in immunodeficient children, as have fatal vaccinia and disseminated infections from BCG immunization.

In infants with immunoglobulin deficiency, studies of circulating B lymphocytes should be performed. B lymphocytes are identified using immunofluorescent techniques for the presence of immunoglobulins (mostly IgM and IgD) on their cell membranes. Even in newborns, 5% to 15% of circulating lymphocytes are B cells. B cells are characteristically *lacking* in male infants with X-linked agammaglobulinemia and in some patients with severe combined immunodeficiency disease. Some patients who cannot make immunoglobulins have circulating B cells, but those cells cannot differentiate into plasma cells and secrete immunoglobulins or antibodies. This is characteristic of patients with common variable immunodeficiency (formerly called acquired agammaglobulinemia). Such patients may be evaluated using in vitro B cell differentiation studies. However, normal children show little B cell differentiation in vitro until approximately 6 months of age. Moreover, common variable immunodeficiency is very rare during the first year of life.

Cell-mediated immunity

T lymphocytes comprise 60% to 80% of the peripheral blood lymphocyte population; thus lymphopenia (less than 1,200/mm^3) is characteristic of disorders in which the number of T cells is reduced. In contrast, in B cell deficiency disorders lymphopenia is usually not detectable, since B cells normally comprise only 5% to 15% of the peripheral blood lymphocyte population. Delayed hypersensitivity skin reactions cannot be elicited in patients with cell-mediated immunodeficiencies. Positive delayed hypersensitivity skin tests require both an intact T cell system and exposure to specific antigens. Since neonates have been exposed to very few antigens capable of inducing specific cell-mediated immunity, even delayed hypersensitivity tests to common antigens are normally negative during the first 6 months of life. For this reason screening of infants for delayed hypersensitivity to detect defects in cell-mediated immunity has only limited value. However, normal infants who have had oral candidiasis for more than 1 week or have had a repeated episode will usually have a positive skin test to *Candida* antigen (1:10 dilution). A child with persistent or recurrent candidiasis and a negative delayed hypersensitivity skin test should have additional evaluation of cell-mediated immune functions.

Because of the limited value of delayed hypersensitivity skin testing for detection of cell-mediated immune deficiencies, in vitro lymphocyte responses play an important role in the evaluation of cellular immunity in this age group. Mature T lymphocytes will proliferate and synthesize DNA when incubated with plant lectins such as PHA or Con A. These responses are quantitated by measurement of DNA synthesis in PHA- or Con A-stimulated cultures using tritiated thymidine incorporation into cellular DNA. These studies may be performed on as little as 0.25 ml of whole blood obtained from a finger or heel puncture, making such studies feasible for even very small infants. Thymidine incorporation is absent or reduced in patients who are deficient in T cells (e.g., DiGeorge syndrome and severe combined immunodeficiency disease). Ability to respond to specific antigens such as *Candida* and the ability to recognize foreign (allogeneic) cells are also T cell functions and can be measured using similar methods. In patients with lymphopenia or reduced in vitro lymphocyte responses to PHA or Con A, the number of circulating T cells should be determined. T lymphocytes form rosettes with sheep red blood cells and can be easily identified under a light microscope. Analysis with T lymphocyte–specific monoclonal antibodies should be performed to confirm the diagnosis.

HOST DEFENSE MECHANISM DISORDERS IN EARLY INFANCY

Neutropenia

See also Chapter 32.

Neutropenia is present when fewer than 1,500 neutrophils/mm^3 are present in the peripheral blood. Some of the causes of neutropenia in the neonate are listed in Table 30-8. The patient's prognosis is related to the underlying cause for the neutropenia; however, most neutropenias in the neonatal period are transient and have a good prognosis, unless there is overwhelming neonatal sepsis.

Table 30-8. Causes of neutropenia in the newborn

	Example
Infection (sepsis)	
Maternal autoimmune disease	Systemic lupus erythematosus
Isoimmunization	Antibody to neutrophil antigen
Genetic agranulocytosis	
Neutropenia and malabsorption	Schwachman syndrome
Drug induced (often associated with thrombocytopenia)	Thiazides Phenytoin sodium (Dilantin) Amidopyrine Propylthiouracil Phenothiazines Trimethadione Sulfa drugs
Cyclic neutropenia	
Inborn errors of metabolism	Ketotic hyperglycinemia Methylmalonic acidemia Isovaleric acidemia Propionic acidemia Chronic tyrosinosis Maple syrup urine disease

Chronic granulomatous disease

Chronic granulomatous disease (CGD) is a disorder of white blood cell bactericidal activity. Neutrophils from patients with CGD do not increase their oxidative metabolic activity on ingestion and phagocytosis of bacteria or other particles. Hydrogen peroxide, superoxide, and other reactive radicals necessary for neutrophil bactericidal activity are not produced. In patients with CGD, bacteria may remain viable within the neutrophils for many hours, whereas bacteria ingested by normal neutrophils are quickly killed.

CGD is a hereditary disease with an X-linked recessive pattern of inheritance. However, an autosomal recessive pattern of inheritance and affected females have been reported. The autosomal recessive form of the disease is often less severe than the X-linked form. Children with X-linked CGD generally have recurrent infections during the first few months of life. Infections are predominantly caused by catalase-positive bacteria (*Staphylococcus, E. coli, Serratia marcescens*) and fungi (*Candida, Aspergillus*). These children frequently have adenopathy, draining lymph nodes, or pneumonias that respond slowly to therapy. Hepatosplenomegaly is a common finding and may be associated with liver abscesses. Persistent dermatitis, diarrhea, perianal abscesses, osteomyelitis, and ulcerative stomatitis occur frequently in this disorder.

The neutrophils of patients with CGD are unable to reduce NBT dye on phagocytosing particles. Killing of catalase-positive bacteria is also abnormal. Neutrophil counts are normal or elevated, cell-mediated immunity and antibody-mediated immunity are normal, and serum immunoglobulins become elevated as the children become older. The mothers of CGD patients have intermediate defects in NBT reduction and bacterial killing so that carriers of X-linked CGD may be detected. There is no specific therapy to correct the neutrophil defect in CGD. Individual infections require appropriate antibiotic therapy and frequent prolonged courses of therapy. The prophylactic use of antibiotics in CGD patients is controversial.

X-linked infantile agammaglobulinemia

Children unable to synthesize immunoglobulin or antibodies usually do not suffer from infection before 5 or 6 months of age. During the first 6 months of life maternal IgG antibodies are sufficient to protect the infant from infection provided that the phagocytic, complement, and cell-mediated immune systems are intact. After the first 6 months of life these children suffer repeated infection, particularly with gram-positive encapsulated bacteria *(Pneumococcus, Streptococcus, Staphylococcus)* and some gram-negative encapsulated bacteria (*Haemophilus* and *Meningococcus*); *Pneumocystis carinii* pneumonitis may also occur. Patients with X-linked agammaglobulinemia usually have repeated episodes of pneumonia and otitis media. Sepsis, meningitis, cellulitis, and septic arthritis also are common in this disorder. A fatal meningoencephalitis caused by ECHO virus has been reported in older children with X-linked agammaglobulinemia.

The serum of patients with X-linked agammaglobulinemia lacks all immunoglobulin classes; IgG is less than 100 mg/dl, and IgA, IgM, IgD, and IgE are usually undetectable. They are unable to synthesize antibodies, and B cells are absent from their peripheral blood. Pre-B cells are present in their bone marrow, suggesting that this disorder is the result of a defect in differentiation of pre-B cells to B cells. Normal numbers of T cells are present, and delayed hypersensitivity and other cell-mediated immune functions are intact. Treatment consists of immunoglobulin replacement by infusion of intravenous gammaglobulin at a dose of 400 mg/kg every 3 to 4 weeks.

Transient hypogammaglobulinemia of infancy

Transient hypogammaglobulinemia of infancy (THI) is a self-limited immunoglobulin deficiency that may or may not be associated with an increased susceptibility to infection. The disorder appears to be caused by a maturational delay in the ability of T helper cells to facilitate immunoglobulin production by B cells. Levels of IgG are most significantly depressed in these patients, IgA may be reduced, but IgM levels are usually normal. Patients have normal numbers of B cells, as well as T cells and T cell subpopulations. Antibody synthesis to blood group antigens and to tetanus and diphtheria toxoids is normal; T cell function is also normal. In full-term infants with THI, depressed IgG levels are usually detected between 3 and 6 months of age; these infants rarely suffer life-threatening infections as a consequence of this mild to moderate hypogammaglobulinemia. Immunoglobulin deficiency usually resolves spontaneously before 2 years of age, and immunoglobulin replacement therapy is not recommended. However, in some premature infants hypogammaglobulinemia may be profound (i.e., IgG levels of 50 mg/dl or less) and may result in greater susceptibility to life-threatening bacterial infections. Since the major portion of transplacental passage of IgG occurs after 20 weeks' gestation, infants born before 28 weeks' gestation may have serum IgG levels of only 50% or less of the maternal IgG concentration. After 1 month of postnatal life, their IgG levels may be sufficiently low to make them susceptible to infection, particularly late group B streptococcal infections. We recommend that serum IgG levels be monitored in all premature infants of less than 28 weeks' gestation. Although studies are under way, no data are yet available to indicate that prophylactic immunoglobulin replacement therapy is efficacious in these patients. Immunoglobulin replacement (500 mg/kg of intravenous gammaglobulin) should be considered on a case-by-case basis at the present time.

Although transient hypogammaglobulinemia of infancy in full-term infants is a benign self-limited disorder, it must be distinguished from two more serious disorders that may appear at the same age, namely X-linked infantile agammaglobulinemia (XLA) and severe combined immunodeficiency disease (SCID). T cells are present and functional in THI but absent or nonfunctional in SCID. B cells are present and antibody synthesis to tetanus and diphtheria toxoids can be detected in THI, whereas both are absent in XLA patients. Assuming that a child has THI without adequately ruling out SCID and XLA may put the child at risk for a life-threatening infection and delay appropriate therapy.

Wiskott-Aldrich syndrome

The Wiskott-Aldrich syndrome is an X-linked recessive disorder consisting of the clinical triad of eczema, thrombocytopenia, and increased susceptibility to infection. Gastrointestinal bleeding caused by thrombocytopenia occurs during early infancy in patients with Wiskott-Aldrich syndrome. These patients characteristically have reduced or absent isoagglutinins and do not produce antibodies after immunization with polysaccharides. Infections by bacteria with polysaccharide capsules (e.g., *Pneumococcus* and *Haemophilus*) are a persistent problem. Serum IgM levels are often depressed while serum IgA levels become elevated. These immunoglobulin abnormalities are difficult to detect in early infancy. Antibody-mediated and cell-mediated immunity are relatively normal early in life, but patients with Wiskott-

Aldrich syndrome characteristically lose immunologic function as they grow older. Defects in membrane glycoproteins of both T lymphocytes and platelets have been demonstrated in patients with Wiskott-Aldrich syndrome. These defects result in increased cell destruction, which accounts for the thrombocytopenia, as well as the loss of long-lived memory T lymphocytes and the progressive immunodeficiency seen in these patients. Histocompatible bone marrow transplantation has resulted in immunologic reconstitution and is the treatment of choice for this otherwise fatal disease.

Thymic hypoplasia with hypocalcemia (DiGeorge syndrome)

DiGeorge described the association of thymic hypoplasia with hypoparathyroidism. Patients with this syndrome, DiGeorge syndrome, have congenital hypocalcemic tetany, cardiac anomalies, abnormal facies, and increased susceptibility to infection because of defects in T cell function. Both the thymus and the parathyroid glands are derived from epithelial evaginations from the third and fourth pharyngeal pouches. The aortic arch has its origin in the same area. It is likely that a developmental abnormality involving the third and fourth pharyngeal pouch region during the sixth and eighth week of gestation results in this syndrome. This disorder is usually not familial and is variable in the severity of its clinical expression.

Patients with DiGeorge syndrome most frequently have severe hypocalcemic tetany within a few days of birth. This results from congenital hypoparathyroidism. In addition, over 90% of infants with this syndrome have cardiac anomalies, usually involving the aortic arch. These include interrupted aortic arch, truncus arteriosus, tetralogy of Fallot, and right-sided aortic arch. Facial anomalies include micrognathia, a "fish mouth" appearance, notched pinnae accompanied by the appearance of backward-rotated ears, and hypertelorism. If patients survive the newborn period, recurrent infections with bacteria, viruses, and fungi, particularly *Candida*, occur, as do chronic diarrhea and failure to thrive. Nephrolithiasis also has been reported in these patients.

Immunologic defects in DiGeorge syndrome are related to defective T cell development and function. At autopsy the thymus is either absent or markedly reduced in size (less than 5% normal for age); however, if any thymus tissue is present, it is histologically normal. Patients with DiGeorge syndrome usually have reduced numbers of lymphocytes capable of forming rosettes with sheep red blood cells (T cells), and in vitro lymphocyte responses to PHA, Con A, allogeneic cells, and antigens (e.g., *Candida*) are reduced. Delayed hypersensitivity reactions to antigens to which the patients have been exposed are also absent. The severity of the defects in cell-mediated immunity is variable and is inversely proportional to the amount of residual thymus tissue present. Serum immunoglobulins are present in normal amounts, and serum IgE may be elevated. Antibody responses in DiGeorge syndrome patients are usually poor, since many antigens require T cell help for optimum antibody synthesis.

Fetal thymus transplantation is the treatment of choice for patients with DiGeorge syndrome. This procedure results in extremely rapid restoration of T cell function, suggesting that thymic hormonal factors may play an important role in this process. However, treatment with thymosin, a thymic hormone, has not been successful in reconstituting cell-mediated immunity in DiGeorge syndrome patients with more severe T cell defects. Some patients with this disorder may have sufficient residual thymic tissue to increase their cell-mediated immunity as they become older. These patients usually have less severe cellular immune defects at diagnosis and may not require fetal thymus transplants.

Patients with this syndrome are at risk for development of graft-versus-host reaction (see further) if they are transfused with viable nonhistocompatible lymphocytes. If blood transfusion is necessary, blood should be irradiated with 3,000 rad before administration.

Severe combined immunodeficiency disease

The term *severe combined immunodeficiency disease* (SCID) refers to a group of disorders characterized by the absence of both antibody-mediated and cell-mediated immunity. Some forms of SCID have an autosomal recessive pattern of inheritance, whereas other forms show X-linked recessive inheritance. Deficiency of the enzyme adenosine deaminase (ADA) is responsible for SCID in approximately 50% of patients with autosomal recessive SCID.

The absence of both antibody-mediated and cell-mediated immunity results in profound susceptibility to a broad spectrum of bacterial, viral, and fungal infections. Onset of infections is usually within the first 3 months of life, and, if immunologic reconstitution is not possible, these infants will usually succumb to infection within the first year of life. Because the infants lack cell-mediated immunity, maternal antibodies are insufficient to completely protect SCID infants from infection. Cytomegalovirus pneumonia is common, progressive, and often fatal. Progressive fatal poliomyelitis may result from routine immunization with live polio vaccine as can disseminated fatal vaccinia infections from contact with smallpox vaccine or other vaccinated individuals. Measles and chickenpox infections are usually fatal. Administration of BCG often produces a disseminated and fatal infection with this "attenuated" mycobacterium.

Infections with gram-negative bacteria, especially *E.*

coli and *Pseudomonas* species, predominate in early infancy, although there is some protection from *Pneumococcus* and *Streptococcus* species because of maternal IgG. *Pneumocystis carinii* pneumonitis occurs very frequently in SCID patients, and SCID must be suspected in any infant with pneumocystis infection. Most SCID patients will develop oral candidiasis, which usually progresses to involve the gastrointestinal tract and perineal area. These candidal infections usually do not respond well to conventional therapy. *Aspergillus* infections also occur in these infants. Failure to thrive, chronic diarrhea, and a variety of skin rashes often accompany or precede the onset of infections.

The clinical and immunologic picture of SCID may result from (1) absence of lymphoid stem cells, (2) enzyme deficiencies impairing stem cell or T cell development (e.g., ADA deficiency), or (3) thymic abnormalities (e.g., thymic dysplasia) interfering with T cell development; impairment of B cell function is secondary to the primary T cell defect. As just mentioned, SCID is a group of disorders, and it is likely that these pathogenetic mechanisms occur in different forms of the disease.

The diagnosis of SCID may be made at birth or even prenatally in patients with ADA deficiency by measurement of ADA activity in amniotic fluid cell cultures. SCID patients have markedly reduced lymphocyte counts (less than $1,200/mm^3$), and usually less than 10% are T cells as measured by sheep red blood cell rosetting or by monoclonal antibody immunofluorescence analysis. In some patients T cells of maternal origin may be present, but these cells are usually nonfunctional. Lymphocytes from SCID patients will not respond to PHA, Con A, allogeneic cells, or antigens. Delayed hypersensitivity to *Candida* is absent, even in the face of prolonged *Candida* infection. Defects in antibody-mediated immunity are often difficult to diagnose during the first 3 months of life because of the relatively low level of immunoglobulin synthesis that normally occurs at this age. Most SCID patients will make no immunoglobulins or antibodies of their own and will lack circulating B cells. Sometimes abnormal monoclonal immunoglobulins can be found in these infants. Some patients with SCID may have serum immunoglobulin as well as B cells. This immunologic picture has been termed the *Nezelof syndrome* and is a variant of SCID. Some patients with Nezelof syndrome lose their immunoglobulins and B cells and become indistinguishable from classic SCID patients. This type of progressive immunologic involution occurs commonly in ADA-deficient patients.

The treatment of choice for severe combined immunodeficiency is bone marrow transplantation from a related histocompatible donor matched with the patient by HLA typing and mixed leukocyte reaction testing. Unmatched bone marrow transplants are not successful and produce fatal graft-versus-host (GVH) reactions. GVH reactions occur when histoincompatible immunocompetent lymphocytes (the graft) are infused into an immunoincompetent host such as an SCID patient. Donor cells attack the patient's skin, gastrointestinal tract, liver, lungs, kidneys, bone marrow, and even central nervous system. Symptoms appear in approximately 7 to 14 days after transplantation and may include fever, maculopapular rash, hepatosplenomegaly, diarrhea, and tachypnea. The skin rash may progress to exfoliation, and diarrhea often becomes bloody. Neutropenia, thrombocytopenia, anemia, and increased infections are also common. In their severe form GVH reactions are usually fatal. GVH reactions may also be initiated by transfusing an SCID patient (or DiGeorge syndrome patient) with blood products. This may be avoided by irradiating the blood products with 3,000 rad. Transplantation of T cell–depleted bone marrow from parent to child (haploidentical transplantation) has been found to result in complete or partial reconstitution of immunologic competence in 50% to 70% of patients undergoing this procedure. Return of immunologic function is much slower than in histocompatible bone marrow transplants.

See also Chapter 32, part two.

Histocompatible bone marrow transplantation has been successful in most patients with the ADA-deficient form of SCID; however, these patients do not respond to haploidentical T cell–depleted parental bone marrow transplants as well as non-ADA–deficient patients. This may be due to the metabolic toxicity resulting from the accumulation of deoxyadenosine nucleotides in ADA deficiency. Some patients with ADA-SCID have shown both clinical and immunologic improvement after enzyme replacement therapy using monthly infusions of glycerolized (frozen) irradiated normal red blood cells as an enzyme source. Enzyme replacement therapy is considered a temporary measure or adjunctive therapy until more definitive therapy can be implemented.

Acquired immunodeficiency syndrome (human immunodeficiency virus)

Acquired immunodeficiency syndrome (AIDS) is caused by infection with the human T lymphotropic virus type III, human immunodeficiency virus (HIV). Mother-to-child transmission of HIV infection may occur in utero or postnatally by transfusion with HIV-infected blood products. HIV has been isolated from human breast milk, and it has been determined by serologic tests that infants breast-fed by virus-infected mothers have become exposed to the virus. Infants infected in utero by HIV may show symptoms of infection as early as 6 weeks of age, but the average onset of symptoms is at 6 months of life. HIV-induced immunodeficiency affects both antibody-

and cell-mediated immunity in infants, and patients show increased susceptibility to a broad spectrum of infectious agents. Most commonly patients have (1) recurrent bacterial infections, including sepsis, meningitis and pneumonia, (2) persistent and recurrent oral candidiasis, and (3) failure to thrive.

Lymphadenopathy, hepatosplenomegaly, chronic and recurrent diarrhea, and salivary gland enlargement usually occur somewhat later. *Pneumocystis carinii* pneumonitis and pulmonary lymphoid hyperplasia occur commonly in these patients. Susceptibility to opportunistic infection is the hallmark of the acquired immunodeficiency syndrome; some of the opportunists seen in AIDS include *Pneumocystis carinii*, cryptosporidium, *Mycobacterium avium, Strongyloides,* and *Candida* organisms.

Acquired immunodeficiency syndrome should be suspected in infants whose mothers come from a high-risk category (i.e., intravenous drug abusers, sexual partners of bisexual males) and who display the previously described clinical signs and symptoms. Antibody to HIV is transported across the placenta and may be detected in uninfected infants for 3 to 6 months. Although most HIV-infected patients will be seropositive by both enzyme-linked immunosorbent assay (ELISA) and Western Blot analysis, some infants from whom HIV has been grown have no detectable antibody to the virus. Unlike adults with AIDS, infants with AIDS are generally not lymphopenic, and the characteristic reversal of the normal 2:1 ratio of helper cells (T4+) to suppressor cells (T8+) may not be seen until later in the disease. While infants with AIDS are hypergammaglobulinemic, they are also antibody deficient. Proliferative responses of AIDS patients' B cells to stimuli such as pokeweed mitogen and staphylococcus Cowan I strain are abnormally low early in the disease; in contrast, T lymphocyte responses to concanavalin A and allogeneic cells remain normal until late in the disease.

At present there is no specific antiviral therapy for HIV infection, and mortality is greater than 50%. Immunoglobulin replacement therapy with intravenous gammaglobulin at a dose of 400 mg/kg of body weight every 3 to 4 weeks appears to markedly reduce the incidence of bacterial infections but not of opportunistic infections, and the effect of this therapy on long-term survival remains to be determined. Attempts to improve cell-mediated immunity, including interferon and interleukin-2 infusions, have not been successful.

Developmental immunodeficiency of the neonate

In summary, the host defense mechanisms in the neonate function less efficiently than those of the older child or adult. For example, neutrophil chemotaxis and intracellular bactericidal activity are diminished compared with those of adults. The function of the alternative pathway of the complement system is decreased in the majority of both premature and full-term neonates. The neonate cannot make antibody to as many antigens as adults can, and immunoglobulin synthesis appears to be blunted by the presence of suppressor T cells and immature neonatal B cells. Neonatal T cells are also deficient in their effector functions, such as secretion of migration-inhibitory factor and immune interferon. The conclusion that the human neonate is immunodeficient and that multiple host defense mechanisms are operating suboptimally is inescapable. If the infant is sufficiently stressed or the natural barriers are breached, one or more of these mechanisms will fail and infection may result. To prevent this, provision of a protected environment is necessary for the newborn, particularly in the presence of perinatal complications.

Stephen H. Polmar
Uwe Manthei

BIBLIOGRAPHY

General

Fudenberg, H.H., and others: Basic and clinical immunology, Los Altos, Calif. 1984, Lange Medical Publications.

Goldstein, R.A.: Symposium—Childhood immunodeficiency disorders: diagnosis, prevention and management, Clin. Immunol. Immunopath. 10(1):1, 1986.

Rosen, F.S.: Developmental immunology, Clin. Allergy Immunol. 5(2):191, 1985.

Development of specific and nonspecific host defense mechanisms

Ballow, M., and others: Development of immune system in very low birthweight (less than 1500 g) premature infants: concentrations of plasma immunoglobulins and patterns of infections, Pediatr. Res. **20**:899, 1986.

Cooper, M.D., Lawton, A.R., and Kincade, P.W.: A two-stage model for development of antibody-producing cells, Clin. Exp. Immunol. **11**:143, 1972.

Hayward, A.R., and Lydyard, P.M.: B-Cell function in the newborn, Pediatrics **64**:758, 1979.

Hayward, A.R., and Lydyard, P.M.: Suppression of B-lymphocyte differentiation by newborn T-lymphocytes with an Fc Receptor for IgM, Clin. Exp. Immunol. **34**:374, 1979.

Johnston, R.B., Jr., and others: Complement in the newborn infant, Pediatrics **64**:781, 1979.

Owen, J.J.T., Cooper, M.D., and Raff, M.C.: *In vitro* generation of B-lymphocytes in mouse foetal liver: a mammalian "bursa equivalent," Nature **249**:361, 1974.

Pyke, K.W., and Gelfand, E.W.: Detection of T-precursor cells in human bone marrow and foetal liver, Differentiation **5**:189, 1976.

Raff, M.D., and others: Differences in susceptibility of mature and immature mouse B-lymphocytes to anti-immunoglobulin in induced immunoglobulin suppression in vitro: possible implications for B-cell tolerance to self, J. Exp. Med. **142**:1052, 1975.

Reinherz, E.L., and others: Discrete stages of intrathymic differentiation: analysis of normal thymocytes and leukemia lymphoblasts of T-cell lineage, Proc. Natl. Acad. Sci. **77**:1588, 1980.

Silverstein, A.M.: Ontogeny of the immune response: a perspective. In Cooper, M.D., and Dayton, D.H., editors: Development of host defenses, New York, 1977, Raven Press.

Stiehm, E.R., Winter, H.S., and Bryson, Y.J.: Cellular (T-cell) immunity in the human newborn, Pediatrics **64**:814, 1979.

Stossel, T.P., Alper, C.A., and Rosen, F.S.: Opsonic activity in the newborn: role of properdin, Pediatrics **52**:134, 1973.

Wilson, C.B.: Immunologic basis for increased susceptibility of the neonate to infection, J. Pediatr. **108**:1, 1986.

Immunologic aspects of the mother-child relationship

Ahlstedt, S., and others: Antibody production by human colostral cells, I. Immunoglobulin class, specificity, and quantity, Scand. J. Immunol. **4**:535, 1975.

Alford, C.A., Jr.: Immunoglobulin determinations in the diagnosis of fetal infections, Pediatr. Clin. North Am. **18**:99, 1974.

Goldblum, R.M., and others: Antibody forming cells in human colostrum after oral immunization, Nature **257**:797, 1975.

Heird, W.D., and Hansen, I.H.: Effects of colostrum on growth of intestinal mucosa, Pediatr. Res. **11**:406, 1972.

Klagsbrun, M.: Human milk stimulates DNA synthesis and cellular proliferation in cultured fibroblasts, Proc. Natl. Acad. Sci. **75**:5057, 1978.

Parmely, M.J., Beer, A., and Billingham, K.: *In vitro* studies on the T-lymphocyte population of human milk, J. Exp. Med. **144**:358, 1976.

Pittard, W.B.: Breast milk immunology: a frontier in infant nutrition, Am. J. Dis. Child. **133**:83, 1979.

Pittard, W.B., Polmar, S.H., and Fanaroff, A.A.: The breast milk macrophage: a potential vehicle for immunoglobulin transport, J. Reticuloendothel. Soc. **22**:597, 1977.

Udall, J.N., and others: The effect of early nutrition on intestinal maturation, Pediatr. Res. **13**:409, 1979.

Host defense mechanism disorders in early infancy

Buckley, R.H., and others: Development of immunity in human severe primary T-cell deficiency following haploidentical bone marrow stem cell transplantation, J. Immunol. **136**:2398, 1986.

Cleveland, W.W., and others: Foetal thymic transplant in a case of DiGeorge syndrome, Lancet **2**:1211, 1968.

Cooper, M.D., and others: Primary antibody deficiencies, Springer Semin. Immunopathol. **1**:265, 1978.

DiGeorge, A.M.: Congenital absence of the thymus and its immunologic consequences: concurrence with congenital hypoparathyroidism. In Bergsma, D., and Good, R.A., editors: Immunologic deficiency disease in man, New York, 1968, The National Foundation.

Ferguson, A.C.: Prolonged impairment of cellular immunity in children with intrauterine growth retardation, J. Pediatr. **9**:52, 1978.

Hitzig, W.H., Dooren, L.J., and Vossen, J.M.: Severe combined immunodeficiency diseases, Springer Semin. Immunopathol. **1**:283, 1978.

Polmar, S.H.: Metabolic aspects of immunodeficiency. In Meisher, P.A., and Jaffee, E.R., editors: Seminars in hematology, vol. 17, New York, 1980, Grune & Stratton, Inc.

Polmar, S.H., and others: Enzyme replacement therapy for adenosine deaminase deficiency and severe combined immunodeficiency, N. Engl. J. Med. **295**:1337, 1976.

Tiller, T.L., Jr., and Buckley, R.H.: Transient hypogammaglobulinemia of infancy: review of the literature; clinical and immunologic features of 11 new cases and long-term follow-up, J. Pediatr. **92**:347, 1978.

CHAPTER 31

Infections in the fetus and neonate

PART ONE

Postnatal bacterial infections

Infectious diseases continue to be one of the most significant causes of fetal wastage and neonatal morbidity and mortality. Although the first section of this chapter focuses primarily on bacterial infections, viral, parasitic, and fungal infections always must be considered in the differential diagnosis of sepsis during the perinatal period.

NEONATAL SEPTICEMIA

Incidence and mortality

Neonatal septicemia refers to a generalized bacterial infection that has been documented by positive blood culture during the first month of life. Septicemia may be a prelude to infection of specific organ systems (such as meningitis or osteomyelitis) or occasionally may follow unrecognized or inadequately treated localized infection. It has been estimated that neonatal septicemia affects between 1 in 500 and 1 in 1,600 newborns. The incidence of septicemia will be influenced markedly by the quality of intrauterine life, host factors, and environmental factors. In the preantibiotic era mortality from neonatal septicemia exceeded 90%, but with the availability of antibiotics it has fallen to a range of 13% to 50%. The incidence of neonatal septicemia and the mortality have not decreased during the past decade and may even have increased because of the development of life support techniques that have permitted the survival of the extremely premature or otherwise high-risk neonate.

Etiology

A significant proportion of neonatal infections are opportunistic in that the host is infected by organisms that can be cultured readily from the cervix or vaginal canal of normal pregnant women, from the external environment, or from the skin or gastrointestinal (GI) tract of normal individuals. In this setting, a tabulation of microbial agents that may be responsible for neonatal sepsis is inappropriate, since any microorganism can produce disease in an appropriate host. Saprophytic microorganisms recovered from the blood of a neonate should not be assumed to be contaminants. In the following sections, emphasis will be placed on the recognition of specific situations that should permit the clinician to anticipate the possibility of neonatal infection in general and to predict the possibility of disease as a result of specific infectious agents, thereby permitting the rapid initiation of appropriate diagnostic, therapeutic, and supportive procedures.

Sources of infection

Transplacental acquisition of bacteria during the course of maternal bacteremia is difficult to establish, but it has been documented in patients infected with *Listeria monocytogenes* and *Treponema pallidum*. Transplacental acquisition of fungal infection also has been proved in neonates with cryptococcal disease and has been suggested by finding elements resembling *Candida* organisms in calcified brain lesions of neonates with hydrocephalus. Late in pregnancy, transplacental transmission of coxsackieviruses and poliomyelitis viruses has been demonstrated.

Neonatal infection may follow aspiration of infected amniotic fluid, an occurrence that is favored by prolonged rupture of the fetal membranes or contamination of amniotic fluid during the course of a difficult delivery. In some patients, amniotic infection may be found in the presence of intact membranes. Occasionally, septicemia may occur after direct invasion of the chorionic vessels on the placental surface. With ruptured fetal membranes, infection with gram-negative enteric microorganisms, *Staphylococcus aureus*, group B β-hemolytic streptococci (*S. agalactiae*), *Streptococcus faecalis*, and infection by anaerobic microorganisms should be anticipated. Systemic infection occurs in 1% to 4% of infants born to mothers whose amniotic fluid is infected.

Infection also may be acquired during delivery. In these patients, organisms that are inhabitants of the vaginal canal, including *S. agalactiae*, *Escherichia coli*, *L. monocytogenes*, *Acinetobacter* species, α-hemolytic streptococci, *Haemophilus influenzae*, and *Neisseria meningitidis*, should be considered as possible causative agents.

Following birth, bacterial or viral infection may be acquired in the delivery room or newborn nursery via the respiratory and/or GI tract or by invasion of bacteria through the umbilical stump. Occasionally, bacterial invasion may be secondary to an infected circumcision or may result from a cutaneous wound. Infection also may follow the route of an umbilical or peripheral intravenous catheter. The neonate who is exposed to resuscitation or inhalation therapy equipment or who lives in an environment of nebulizers and water-filled incubators has an increased risk of infection due to *Flavobacterium meningosepticum*, *Serratia marcescens*, *Proteus* species, and *Pseudomonas aeruginosa*. The newborn whose skin is bypassed by the use of indwelling umbilical catheters and infants requiring total parenteral nutrition may develop septicemia with *Staphylococcus epidermidis*, *S. aureus*, *Pseudomonas*, *Bacteroides*, *Serratia*, *Citrobacter*, *Candida*, and *Torulopsis*. Bacteremia may be induced in 10% of children during exchange transfusions but only rarely leads to septic complications.

Direct contamination of the newborn by the hands of nursery personnel or by other adults generally occurs when hand-washing techniques are inadequate. Epidemic neonatal infection due to *S. aureus* almost always is transmitted in this manner. Discontinuation of routine hexachlorophene bathing of neonates has been followed by recurrences of epidemic neonatal staphylococcal disease in many nurseries. The role of hand contamination of personnel in the epidemiology of gram-negative neonatal infections due to *Escherichia coli*, *Klebsiella pneumoniae*, *Enterobacter* species, *Serratia marcescens*, *Proteus mirabilis*, and *Pseudomonas* species also has been emphasized. *Salmonella* and *Shigella* infections also have been initiated in neonates by acquisition of these organisms from a maternal carrier followed by infant-to-infant spread as a result of inadequate hand-washing by medical personnel. In addition, direct contamination of the newborn has been associated with neonatal infection caused by *Bacillus subtilis*, *Pasteurella multocida*, *Citrobacter* species, and *Campylobacter fetus*.

Infection may be introduced into an intensive care nursery by the admission of newborns whose infection was acquired in the community. Although this represents a potential threat in referral centers, these infants infrequently serve as a source of infection to others if appropriate precautions are observed.

Maternal factors influencing the development of sepsis

The socioeconomic status, race, and vaginal flora of the mother may influence the likelihood of septicemia in the newborn. In New York City the incidence of neonatal infection in poor families is approximately twice that in the most prosperous families, and the rate in blacks exceeds that in white or Puerto Rican populations. Some studies suggest that these differences reflect differing standards of prenatal care. Others have shown that different economic and racial groups receiving care in the same prenatal clinic had different rates of antenatal and neonatal infection.

Symptomatic bacteriuria during pregnancy is associated with premature births, and treatment of bacteriuria during pregnancy has been followed by a significant decrease in the number of low birth weight babies. Asymptomatic bacteriuria during pregnancy may be associated with prematurity, but this association has not been confirmed by all investigators. Since both prematurity and low birth weight are associated with an increased risk of neonatal infection, symptomatic bacteriuria during pregnancy may be a factor that indirectly influences the development of sepsis in the neonate. Smoking during pregnancy also has been associated with low birth weight and thus also may indirectly influence the development of neonatal sepsis. (See also Chapter 9.)

Mycoplasma hominis, *Ureaplasma urealyticum*, and *M. fermentans* have been isolated from the genitourinary system, and colonization by genital mycoplasmas has been associated with low birth weight. The association of low birth weight with *U. urealyticum* colonization of the maternal birth canal is highly significant but not necessarily related to premature delivery. Colonization of the birth canal with *U. urealyticum* or with *M. hominis* has not been related to a history of previous premature births, stillbirths, abortions, or to the development of toxemia or bleeding in the third trimester of pregnancy. However, it is more prevalent among black women than white women and more common among poor patients in both groups. Mycoplasmas have been isolated more frequently from infertile than fertile couples. They also have been recovered from the fetal membranes of spontaneous abortuses and from the viscera of aborted fetuses and stillborn infants. Colonization of neonates with mycoplasmas may be associated with neonatal *Mycoplasma* infection. *Mycoplasma hominis* has been associated with cervical lymphadenitis, as well as with meningitis and brain abscess in the newborn infant. Maternal colonization by mycoplasmas may influence the development of neonatal sepsis, however, to the extent that low birth weight plays a role in increasing the risk of septicemia. Genital mycoplasmas have been isolated from the blood of patients with fever following abortion and delivery, but bloodstream infection of the fetus or newborn appears to be infrequent.

Factors operative at or near the time of delivery

Infants born to mothers with septicemia or viremia or with infections of the urinary tract, vagina, or cervix have an increased incidence of infection. An increase in neonatal infections also has been observed in infants born to febrile mothers, even when the specific focus of maternal infection cannot be identified. An increased risk of neonatal infection accompanies rupture of the fetal membranes for more than 24 hours before delivery. Excessive bleeding from placenta previa or abruptio placentae, excessive manipulation, and a prolonged second stage of labor and fetal distress during delivery also are factors that have been associated with an increased incidence of neonatal infection. Cephalhematomas (Chapter 20) have been followed by the development of osteomyelitis of the underlying skull or by sepsis and meningitis. Fetal monitoring in utero has been associated with the formation of scalp abscesses in up to 7% of deliveries in which monitoring has been used.

Host factors

Male infants are infected more frequently and have a greater risk of neonatal death than female infants, even allowing for the greater number of male births. A possible exception may be in the risk of infection with group B β-hemolytic streptococci. An increasing number of differences between newborns and older children in their capacity to resist infection have been delineated (Chapter 30). Defects in the response of neonatal leukocytes to chemotactic factors, impaired phagocytosis, and impaired bactericidal capacity have been reported. Deficiencies of several serum complement components including Clq, C3, and C5, deficient opsonic activity of neonatal sera, and low levels of serum properdin also have been observed. IgA and IgM immunoglobulins are not acquired transplacentally; thus most neonates have very low levels of IgA and IgM globulins at birth. Despite transplacental acquisition of IgG globulin, specific antibodies to certain antigens, such as pertussis or varicella, may be lacking because they are absent from maternal blood. The frequency of neonatal infection in general and the incidence of disease caused by organisms indigenous to the host or environment suggest that these infections reflect the deficits in host immunity that have been observed. This fact is highlighted by recent observations that type III, group B streptococcal disease affects newborns with a very low concentration in serum of transplacentally derived antibody to the capsular polysaccharide antigen of type III, group B *Streptococcus*. Susceptibility may be enhanced in premature infants with immature phagocytic capacity and low levels of complement proteins.

Other factors

Bottle feeding may increase the risk of neonatal infection in comparison with infants who are breast-fed, although no in vivo protective effect has been demonstrated. Human colostrum contains agglutinins against gram-negative bacteria; they may be passed along the intestinal tract and provide some local protective effect in the GI tract. Human milk also contains large quantities of iron-binding proteins that are known to exert a powerful bacteriostatic effect on *E. coli*. It also contains macrophages and lymphocytes that may play a role in local immunologic defense (Chapter 30).

Nosocomial infections are common among very low birth weight infants requiring multiple supportive measures. Coagulase-negative staphylococci have emerged as a frequent cause of bacteremia in neonates undergoing prolonged mechanical ventilation and protracted use of vascular access catheters for alimentation, as well as in those with clinical evidence of necrotizing enterocolitis. Contaminated parenteral fluids also may serve as a source of sepsis. An outbreak of polymicrobial bacteremia due to *Klebsiella pneumoniae* and *Enterobacter cloacae* in a neonatal intensive care unit has been associated with the intravenous administration of a contaminated lipid emulsion. Elevated serum levels of vitamin E have been associated with an increased incidence of sepsis in infants with birth weight of 1,500 gm or less. Decreased resistance to infection was thought to have resulted from a vitamin E–related decrease in oxygen-dependent intracellular killing. Nosocomial infection caused by *Candida* organisms is discussed in Part three of this chapter.

Clinical manifestations

Septicemia may occur at any time during the first month of life. Onset within the first 2 days of life is associated more frequently with prenatal or perinatal predisposing factors, whereas onset after 48 to 72 hours of age more frequently reflects disease acquired at or subsequent to delivery.

The evolution of signs and symptoms differs from patient to patient; the course may be fulminant, leading to death in several hours, or it may be more protracted. The earliest clinical signs of neonatal septicemia are characterized by lack of specificity, and they include lethargy, irritability, poor feeding, or only the suggestion by the nursing staff or the mother that the newborn is not doing as well as previously. Since these signs also may accompany noninfectious neonatal problems, such as anemia, cardiac decompensation, central nervous system (CNS) disorders, or metabolic problems, including hypoglycemia, the physician must supplement these clinical findings with additional clinical and laboratory information that may support the possibility of neonatal septicemia. If a diagnosis of septicemia cannot be excluded or an alternative explanation for the findings is not established, appropriate cultures must be obtained and therapy initiated.

Additional clinical manifestations of neonatal septicemia may reflect primary or secondary involvement of any organ system. Fever may be present but is often absent; hypothermia is as common as hyperthermia, particularly in premature infants who frequently experience irregular fluctuations of body temperature. Tachypnea, cyanosis, apnea, tachycardia or bradycardia, and hypotension may be noted. Although these findings may suggest that the patient is in the terminal stages of septicemia, one should not necessarily infer that septicemia has been of long duration, since the infection may become fulminant in a short period of time. The presence of focal neurologic signs, tremors, seizures, or a full fontanel may be noted even in septic neonates without neonatal meningitis. Vomiting, abdominal distension, diarrhea, hepatomegaly, splenomegaly, jaundice, pallor, petechial or purpuric lesions, or bleeding may occur. The onset of jaundice in the first 24 hours of life in the absence of a primary hemolytic disorder always should suggest the possibility of septicemia. Studies of icteric infants with septicemia have revealed that a preponderance of cases are associated with gram-negative bacilli, particularly *E. coli*. The hypothesis for this includes both hemolysis of red blood cells sensitized by bacterial polysaccharides and liver cell destruction or impairment of the bilirubin excretory functions of the liver. Rapidly developing diffuse erythema of the skin in the absence of a discrete eruption, accompanied by sudden development of anemia and leukocytosis in an infant born to a mother with premature rupture of the membranes, should suggest the possibility of *Clostridium perfringens* septicemia. The skin discoloration in these patients has been attributed to deposition of hemoglobin released from erythrocytes by lecithinase, a potent hemolysin elaborated by this organism.

Infections that may precede or accompany septicemia include omphalitis, conjunctivitis, soft tissue or skin abscesses, impetigo, otitis media, meningitis, or osteomyelitis. When cellulitis is found, infection with streptococci should be considered. The presence of impetigo or abscesses should suggest staphylococcal disease. If necrotic skin lesions with a purple hue are noted, infection with *Pseudomonas aeruginosa* or *Aeromonas hydrophila* may exist.

Differential diagnosis

The nonspecificity and wide range of signs and symptoms that may be observed in neonates with septicemia frequently suggest a number of alternative diagnoses. These may include hemolytic anemia, hypovolemic shock, intracranial hemorrhage, respiratory distress syndrome, pneumonia, primary disease of the GI tract, thrombocytopenic purpura, leukemia, hypocalcemia, hypoglycemia, or other metabolic disorders.

Laboratory evaluation

A specific diagnosis can be confirmed only by the presence of a positive blood culture. When septicemia is suspected, two or more blood cultures should be obtained. If the patient is critically ill, one culture is adequate.

Since focal infections may precede or follow septicemia, cultures of other body fluids or orifices may help to establish an etiologic diagnosis. When septicemia is suspected, both urine and cerebrospinal fluid (CSF) should be examined and cultures obtained. Specific morphologic and chemical CSF findings that may suggest the presence of bacterial meningitis are discussed subsequently (neonatal meningitis). If skin lesions or soft tissue abscesses are present, these should be aspirated for smear and culture. When infection is localized in a joint, fluid should be aspirated, examined, and cultured. Stool cultures may be helpful in establishing a diagnosis of septicemia due to *Shigella*, *Salmonella*, *Campylobacter*, and infrequently *S. aureus*. Cultures of gastric aspirate or of cord blood from infants who are clinically well but who were born 24 hours or more after rupture of the membranes are not likely to be of diagnostic value and may be misleading. However, we recommend that two or more blood cultures be obtained from different peripheral venous sites in these infants as a means of screening for the possibility of significant bacteremia.

Neonatal sepsis has been associated with chorioamnionitis. The incidence of umbilical cord neutrophilic infiltrates, however, far exceeds the number of proven cases of fetal or neonatal infection. Their presence, therefore, does not serve to separate definitively the infected from the uninfected neonate but may help to identify a high-risk group of infants. Routine prophylactic antibiotic treatment of all infants with umbilical cord vasculitis is not warranted. The presence of three or more polymorphonuclear leukocytes per high-power field demonstrable on a smear of amniotic fluid or debris in the external auditory canal also correlates significantly with the ultimate demonstration of septicemia. The presence of organisms on Gram stain or recovered by culture of the same material is less specific, but in some patients the organisms that are obtained are identical to those recovered from the blood of the same patient. A smear of the buffy coat should be examined for bacteria by Gram stain.

The white blood cell count should be obtained in newborns with possible septicemia. Leukopenia (less than 3,500 white cells/mm^3) or leukocytosis (greater than 25,000 white blood cells/mm^3) supports a diagnosis of infection. A differential white blood cell count may be of even greater assistance, particularly in septic full-term neonates whose total white blood cell counts are within the normal range. A comparison between the absolute number of band neutrophils found in normal and infected neonates reveals that in infants with bacterial infection (including those with normal neutrophil counts) the band counts are increased significantly beyond the normal range (Table 31-1). A depression in platelet count (less than 150,000 platelets/mm^3) may be noted during septicemia; however, a normal platelet count does not exclude the diagnosis. Similarly, a peripheral smear that suggests a hemolytic process may be found in neonates with septicemia but is also seen in many neonates who are not infected. An erythrocyte sedimentation rate greater than 5 mm/hour within the first 24 hours of life may suggest septicemia. An elevated serum concentration (greater than 0.8 mg/dl) of the C-reactive protein is a useful adjunctive parameter for the early diagnosis of bacterial infection.

Serologic studies, described subsequently, may help to establish a diagnosis of syphilis or infection with various viral, fungal, or parasitic agents. An elevated serum IgM concentration (greater than 17 to 20 mg/dl) during the first week of life suggests that infection has occurred in utero or perhaps at birth. However, infants dying of bacterial infection during the first several days of life may do so with normal serum IgM levels. Conversely, elevated serum IgM concentrations may occur in newborns who have never been infected, because of contamination caused by maternal bleeding into the fetal circulation. If elevated serum IgM has been caused by admixture of fetal with maternal blood, a rapid fall in serum IgM concentration will ensue during the first week of life.

Countercurrent immunoelectrophoresis (CIE) may be effective in establishing the etiologic diagnosis of septicemia or meningitis caused by *Haemophilus influenzae* (type b), *Streptococcus pneumoniae*, and *Neisseria meningitidis* within 30 minutes of the time that blood or CSF samples have been received in the laboratory. It also has been possible to establish a diagnosis of septicemia or meningitis due to K1 strains of *E. coli* by the use of CIE, but appropriate antisera for these diagnostic studies are available at present only in selected research laboratories. Group B streptococcal infections may be diagnosed presumptively, employing latex agglutination test kits that are available commercially. Serogroup-specific antisera are employed for detection of antigen in body fluid specimens. When specimens are processed according to the manufacturer's instructions, the tests are extremely sensitive and reasonably specific for diagnosing group B streptococcal infection.

Hypoglycemia and hyponatremia may accompany septicemia in the newborn. Hypoglycemia has been noted during septicemia with gram-negative bacilli with much greater frequency than during infection with gram-positive organisms. Infection in normal children and adults is accompanied by an increased elaboration of corticosteroids, growth hormone, glucagon, and epinephrine, and by increased glycogenolysis and gluconeogenesis. All these factors tend to promote hyperglycemia rather than hypoglycemia during active infection. Increased peripheral utilization of glucose, perhaps as a result of enhanced insulin sensitivity and lack of glycogen stores, has been suggested as a possible contributing factor for hypoglycemia during neonatal sepsis. Decreased corticosteroid activity has not been documented even when adrenal hemorrhage is found postmortem. Hyponatremia during septicemia probably reflects inappropriate retention of fluid in excess of solute, resulting in dilutional hyponatremia. It also may reflect changes in total body sodium concentration as a result of diarrhea, vomiting, excessive sweating, or insufficient intake. Symptoms of hyponatremia include irritability, lethargy, and seizures, signs that are indistinguishable from those noted in patients with septicemia. Measurement of serum electrolytes should be made in infants with possible or proven septicemia, since the results obtained may support the diagnostic impression, have differential diagnostic value, and are essential in designing specific regimens of sup-

Table 31-1. Absolute number of bands/mm^3 of blood of 169 normal full-term infants

Time of sampling	Mean	Standard deviation	Skewness	Median	Range for 95%	
					Low	High
Birth	358	419	1,371	155	0	1,410
Day 1	531	664	1,771	306	0	2,220
Day 5	282	345	1,948	189	0	1,240

From Akenzua, G.I., and others: Pediatrics **54:**38, 1974.

portive care for each infant. (See Chapter 25, part three; Chapter 37, part one.)

Complications

The complications of septicemia in the neonate are similar to those which accompany this disease in older children and adults. These include congestive heart failure, shock, and disseminated intravascular coagulation. The incidence of mild disseminated intravascular coagulation in neonates with septicemia may be as high as 66%. Focal infection in one or more organ systems also may occur. (See Chapter 32.)

Treatment

The neonate with suspected sepsis must be treated immediately after appropriate diagnostic studies have been initiated and before the etiologic agent is identified or its susceptibility to antimicrobial agents established. The course of neonatal septicemia may be so rapid that the threat to life is greater than the possibility that undesirable side effects may accompany the use of antibiotics in some patients who subsequently prove to be uninfected. The choice of antibiotics must be based on (1) consideration of the type of microorganisms that may be encountered, (2) the sensitivity of those organisms to the antibiotic employed, (3) the likelihood of achieving bactericidal concentrations of antibiotics at the site of infection, and (4) consideration of possible adverse effects of therapy with specific antibiotic agents. Since the sensitivity of various microorganisms to antimicrobial agents may change with time and differs from institution to institution, it is imperative that physicians be aware of the sensitivity pattern of bacteria isolated in their own hospital and community. In addition, immaturity of renal and hepatic function precludes the use of certain drugs entirely and requires that dosage schedules for preferred drugs be adjusted depending on the gestational age, birth weight, and postnatal age of the infant. The dosage recommendations in Table 31-2 are based on consideration of pharmacokinetic information presently available concerning the use of antimicrobial agents in the newborn period. Although general recommendations can be given, specific dosages required by infants may change from day to day. Ideally, serum concentrations of antibiotics should be monitored to ensure therapeutic efficacy while minimizing toxicity.

When septicemia is suspected in the first 72 hours of life and etiologic agent is unknown, the combination of ampicillin and an aminoglycoside should be used. Ampicillin provides effective coverage for all gram-positive organisms except penicillinase-producing staphylococci and is also of value in treating infection with most strains of *H. influenzae*, some strains of *E. coli*, *Salmonella*, *Shigella*, *Proteus mirabilis*, and many strains of *L. monocytogenes*. A synergistic inhibitory effect has been demonstrated in vitro when ampicillin and kanamycin or gentamicin have been tested for activity against various strains of *E. coli*, *Listeria*, and enterococci. Kanamycin and gentamicin are the aminoglycoside drugs used most frequently; choice of one or the other should be dictated by the sensitivity of the enteric organisms found in each community. Gentamicin, however, offers effective coverage for most strains of *Pseudomonas*, whereas kanamycin does not. Tobramycin sulfate offers broad coverage of gram-negative organisms, including *Pseudomonas*, and may be the only aminoglycoside that inhibits the growth of some multiply resistant, nosocomially acquired gram-negative microorganisms. Amikacin is another useful alternative.

When septicemia is suspected after 3 days of age, specific consideration must be given to providing coverage of organisms that may have been acquired from the environment. Consideration should be given to the addition of a penicillinase-resistant penicillin to the regimen until an organism has been identified or, perhaps, to the substitution of methicillin for ampicillin. Methicillin is preferred on our service for coverage of penicillin-resistant staphylococci because it is bound to protein to a much lesser extent than is nafcillin or oxacillin; thus the risk of displacing bilirubin from albumin-binding sites is reduced.

Following identification of the causative agent, a single antibiotic can be employed in most cases. Although specific therapy should be based on the results of antibiotic sensitivity testing, an appropriate choice usually can be made before such results are available. In Table 31-2 are listed the more commonly used antibiotics. Suggested specific indications for their use in neonatal sepsis or meningitis are listed in Table 31-3. The toxicity of these drugs and additional comments, including important pharmacologic considerations, are included.

Antibiotic treatment of neonatal septicemia generally is continued for 7 to 10 days; a longer period of treatment may be required, depending on the clinical response of the patient. Meticulous observation and other supportive measures are indicated. Electronic monitoring is important but cannot be substituted for frequent assessment by skilled nurses and physicians. Oral feeding should be discontinued to decrease the likelihood of aspiration and to permit more precise monitoring of fluid intake. Gastric suction may be required intermittently to prevent or treat gastric dilation. Appropriate quantities of fluids, electrolytes, and glucose should be provided intravenously. Antibiotics may be given by the intravenous route but when added to intravenous solutions should be administered within 1 hour. Two or more antibiotics should not be placed in solutions containing other drugs or vitamins (the latter may inactivate the antibiotic before infusion). The infant's environment should be adjusted to maintain a rectal temperature of 37° to 38° C and a skin temperature of 36° to 37° C. Sponge baths with tepid water, and rarely, antipyretics may be required if temperature exceeds 39.5° C. Oxygen should be provided to relieve hypoxemia if it is present. Hyponatremia should be treated by fluid restriction if there is evidence of inappropriate secretion of antidiuretic hormone. If sodium losses are excessive, sufficient sodium should be given to relieve symptoms of hyponatremia and to raise the serum sodium concentration to 130 mEq/L. Sodium bicarbonate (2 to 3 mEq/kg) or glucose (as required) should be given to counteract profound acidosis and hypoglycemia.

Septic shock should be treated by volume expansion. Optimally, whole blood (10 to 20 ml/kg stat.) should be provided. Hydrocortisone sodium succinate (10 to 20 mg/kg) has been used as an immediate dose in critically ill infants with persistent hypotension and may be continued at 5 mg/kg every 6 hours in some patients. There is little evidence that steroid administration is beneficial, but individual patients may improve after administration of steroids. Disseminated intravascular coagulation often occurs. Although specific treatment of the disease pro-

Table 31-2. Antibiotics that may be employed for treatment of neonatal sepsis or meningitis*

	First week of life or premature			Full-term infant over 1 week of age			
Agent	**Dosage**	**Route**	**Schedule**	**Dosage**	**Route**	**Schedule**	**Comment**
Amikacin	15 mg/kg/day	IM, IV	q12h	22.5 mg/kg/day	IM, IV	q8h	When using IV, infuse over 30 minutes
Ampicillin	100-150 mg/kg/day	IM, IV	q8h or q12h	150-300 mg/kg/day	IM, IV	q6h or q8h	Use highest dosage in meningitis Use 100 mg/kg/day in premature infants between 1 and 4 weeks of age with sepsis
Carbenicillin	225 mg/kg/day	IM, IV	q8h	300 mg/kg/day	IM, IV	q6h	Give loading dose of 100 mg/kg to all patients Full-term infants may be given 300 mg/kg/day even during first week of life
Cefotaxime	100-150 mg/kg/day	IV	q12h	150-200 mg/kg/day	IV	q6h or q8h	Use highest dosage in meningitis
Ceftazidime†	60 mg/kg/day	IV	q12h	60 mg/kg/day	IV	q12h	Experience limited in premature infants
Ceftriaxone	Not established			50-100 mg/kg/day	IV	q12h	Dosage not established for first week of life; use highest dosage in meningitis
Cephalothin	50 mg/kg/day	IM, IV	q8h	50-100 mg/kg/day	IM, IV	q6h	
Chloramphenicol	25 mg/kg/day	IV	q8h	50mg/kg/day	IV	q6h	If used, serum concentrations should be monitored
Clindamycin	20 mg/kg/day	IV	q8h	30 mg/kg/day	IV	q6h	Do not use in patients with meningitis
Colistimethate	5 mg/kg/day	IM	q12h	8 mg/kg/day	IM	q8h	
Erythromycin	Not established			40 mg/kg/day	PO	q6h	Use only for treatment of *Chlamydia trachomatis* pneumonia
Gentamicin	5 mg/kg/day	IM, IV	q12h	7.5 mg/kg/day	IM, IV	q8h	When used IV, infuse over 30 minutes Intraventricular therapy also may be required in patients with meningitis

Continued.

*See also Appendix B: Therapeutic Agents.
†Optimal dosage requires further study.

Table 31-2. Antibiotics that may be employed for treatment of neonatal sepsis or meningitis—cont'd

	First week of life or premature			Full-term infant over 1 week of age			
Agent	**Dosage**	**Route**	**Schedule**	**Dosage**	**Route**	**Schedule**	**Comment**
Kanamycin	15 mg/kg/day	IM, IV	q12h	25 mg/kg/day	IM, IV	q8h or q12h	When used IV, infuse over 30 minutes Recent pharmacologic studies suggest that these dosage recommendations may require revision upward, but clinical studies to support lack of toxicity at increased dosages not available
Methicillin	100 mg/kg/day	IM, IV	q8h	200 mg/kg/day	IM, IV	q6h	Give q12h on first day of life
Mezlocillin	150 mg/kg/day	IM, IV	q12h	300 mg/kg/day	IM, IV	q6h	Premature infants older than 1 week may be given 225 mg/kg/day on a q8h schedule
Moxalactam	100 mg/kg/day	IV	q12h	150-200 mg/kg/day	IV	q8h	Do not use as the only drug for unknown sepsis or meningitis
Nafcillin	100 mg/kg/day	IM, IV	q12h	200 mg/kg/day	IM, IV	q6h	
Neomycin	50-100 mg/kg/day	PO	q6h	50-100 mg/kg/day	PO	q6h	Use only if lack of systemic absorption can be ensured
Nystatin	200,000-400,000 units	PO	q6h	200,000-400,000 units	PO	q6h	Do not use for systemic infections
Oxacillin	100 mg/kg/day	IM, IV	q12h	200 mg/kg/day	IM, IV	q6h	
Penicillin	100,000-150,000 units/kg/day	IM, IV	q8h or q12h	100,000-300,000 units/kg/day	IM, IV	q6h or q8h	Use highest dosage in meningitis
Polymyxin B	3 mg/kg/day	IM, IV	q12h	4 mg/kg/day	IM, IV	q8h	If used IV, infuse over 30 minutes Intrathecal administration also required if used in treatment of meningitis
Ticarcillin	150-225 mg/kg/day	IM, IV	q8-12h	225-300 mg/kg/day	IM, IV	q6h or q8h	Use lower dosage and longer interval for premature infants
Tobramycin	4-5 mg/kg/day	IM, IV	q12h	5-7.5 mg/kg/day	IM, IV	q6h or q8h	If used IV, infuse over 30 minutes; use higher dosage for meningitis
Vancomycin	20-40 mg/kg/day	IV	q12h	30-60 mg/kg/day	IV	q6h or q8h	Use highest dosage in meningitis; infuse over 60 minutes to avoid histamine-like reactions; serum concentrations should be monitored

cess is important, administration of fresh whole blood or packed red blood cells, fresh frozen plasma, and platelets is an important ancillary supportive measure. There has been limited experience recently with the use of white cell transfusions for septic newborns with neutropenia. This technique appears promising, particularly when neutropenia reflects severe bone marrow depletion of neutrophils. The use of exchange transfusion to improve tissue oxygenation and to enhance opsonic activity in septic neonates also has been associated with clinical improvement. There is enthusiasm for the potential of immunoglobulin preparations for intravenous use to prevent or ameliorate bacteremia in premature infants. However, the efficacy of administering exogenously each of these component forms of therapy to alter the outcome of neonatal sepsis will require a large prospective, controlled clinical trial.

See also Chapter 32, part two.

INFECTION OF ORGAN SYSTEMS

Neonatal bacterial meningitis

Incidence

Bacterial meningitis is responsible for 1% to 4% of neonatal deaths and develops in approximately 1 of every 2,500 live births. Meningitis is probably more common during the first month of life than in any succeeding month.

Etiology

The same organisms that are responsible for neonatal septicemia cause neonatal meningitis. *E. coli* and group B streptococci remain the organisms recovered most frequently. Group B β-hemolytic streptococci, *L. monocytogenes,* and *F. meningosepticum* have a predilection for the meninges of newborns, and *F. meningosepticum* tends to produce epidemic disease. Mixed bacterial meningitis and mixed viral and bacterial meningitis also have been reported in the neonatal period.

Pathology

A subarachnoid inflammatory exudate generally is present and is more common at the base of the brain than over the convexity. During the acute stages of the disease the brain may be swollen and hyperemic, and the ventricles may be small. Herniation of cerebral or cerebellar tissue is uncommon. Hydrocephalus occurs frequently, and the degree of ventricular enlargement tends to increase with the duration of the disease. Ventriculitis has been mentioned with increasing frequency in necropsy reports of patients dying of neonatal meningitis; it may be noted in some patients with acellular and sterile CSF. In the first week of disease, polymorphonuclear leukocytes are the predominant cells within both the subarachnoid space and the ventricular system. During the second and third weeks macrophages, histiocytes, and lymphocytes are the predominant cells found in the exudates. Vasculitis is common, and both thrombosis and infarction may occur. A glial reaction is noted in areas directly subjacent to the inflammatory exudate, and diffuse encephalopathy characterized by karyorrhexis and loss of nerve cells may be noted. Hemorrhagic cerebral necrosis occurs commonly in newborns who die of enterobacterial meningitis; this type of reaction is particularly characteristic following *Proteus* infection.

Pathogenesis

The complications of pregnancy and delivery that predispose the newborn to septicemia also increase the risk of meningitis, since in most patients the meninges are seeded hematogenously. Neonatal skin infections, pneumonia, otitis media, and urinary tract infections are also frequently accompanied by bacteremia with the subsequent development of meningitis. Meningitis may be associated with one third of the cases of septicemia and is more common in premature than in full-term infants. The risk of meningitis also is increased in infants with meningomyelocele.

Factors referable to the microorganism itself may be associated with an increased risk of meningitis. Whereas early-onset group B streptococcal septicemia often is related to infection by organisms of serotypes I or II, meningitis (early or late onset) usually is associated with infection by organisms of serotype III. Similarly, meningitis due to *L. monocytogenes* is usually caused by type IV organisms. Most neonatal meningitis caused by *E. coli* is the result of infection by strains containing K1 capsular polysaccharide, an antigen that is immunochemically identical or very similar to meningococcal group B capsular polysaccharide. Thus certain microorganisms appear to possess certain antigens that confer on the organisms specific invasive potential.

Clinical manifestations

Any of the clinical manifestations of neonatal septicemia may herald the presence of neonatal meningitis. Thus in most patients an appropriate diagnostic evaluation for the newborn with possible septicemia includes lumbar puncture. Poor feeding, vomiting, respiratory distress, irritability, and temperature instability are common, and convulsions, paralysis of various cranial nerves, abnormal Moro reflex, abnormal cry, or focal neurologic signs may be seen. A bulging fontanel and stiff neck are late signs; when they appear before initial diagnosis and therapy, the outlook is dismal. Subdural effusions, coma, and hydrocephalus may occur.

Laboratory manifestations

Specific diagnosis is dependent on a careful evaluation of the CSF and ultimately depends on demonstration of organisms on a Gram-stained smear of the CSF and their growth on culture. The number and type of cells and the protein concentration in normal newborns differ from accepted norms in older children. A study of CSF obtained from 117 high-risk newborns who had no evidence of bacterial or viral infection of the CNS revealed an average CSF cell count of 8.4 cells/mm^3 with a range of 0 to 32 cells/mm^3. Approximately 60% of the CSF white blood cells were polymorphonuclear leukocytes. Protein concentration within CSF of normal full-term infants varies from 20 to 170 mg/dl with a mean value of 90 mg/dl. CSF protein concentrations in premature infants vary between 65 and 150 mg/dl during the first 2 weeks of life. The values of premature infants are related inversely to birth weight.

The CSF cell count in newborns with bacterial meningitis may reach 10,000 or more cells/mm^3, but meningitis may be found in the presence of cell counts that are normal. Protein concentration may be elevated or normal. In the presence of meningitis, CSF glucose concentration may be less than half of the blood glucose concentration obtained at the time of lumbar puncture. Occasionally, CSF glucose concentrations of 10 mg/100 ml or less may occur; however, they also occur in newborns who have hypoglycemia or intracranial hemorrhage but no meningitis. A Gram-stained smear of the CSF should be examined by an experienced observer. The CSF always should be cultured even if it appears to be crystal clear or if a bloody tap has been obtained. CSF, serum, and urine also can be evaluated by countercurrent immunoelectrophoresis or latex agglutination tests that may permit an etiologic diagnosis within minutes. Blood cultures should be obtained and are positive in 50% to 60% of cases.

Treatment

Until a definitive diagnosis has been made, antibiotic treatment should be initiated with ampicillin and an aminoglycoside, using dosage schedules shown in Table 31-2. The choice of aminoglycoside should be based on the infant's age and on knowledge of the resistance patterns of nosocomial pathogens in individual intensive care units. Once a specific pathogen has been identified and its susceptibilities are known, the best drug or combination of drugs should be employed (Table 31-3). Penicillin G would be preferred for group B streptococcal disease, and ampicillin is favored for infection with enterococci, *Listeria monocytogenes*, or *P. mirabilis*. Aminoglycoside therapy may add synergy. Methicillin is preferred for staphylococcal infection and an antipseudomonal penicillin plus an aminoglycoside for *Pseudomonas* infection. Treatment of coliforms with both ampicillin and an aminoglycoside antibiotic may be preferred, since the combination may be synergistic against some strains of *E. coli*. In patients with unknown or ampicillin-resistant gram-negative bacterial meningitis, the use of a third-generation cephalosporin also should be considered.

Regimens for the treatment of gram-negative neonatal meningitis have not been particularly effective in sterilizing promptly the CSF. Ventriculitis with sequestration of microorganisms within the ventricular system in infants with gram-negative meningitis is a relatively common occurrence. Aminoglycosides administered intrathecally do not diffuse over the surface of the brain or into the ventricles in a uniform manner.

A collaborative study of neonatal meningitis has shown no decrease in mortality when therapy with intrathecal or intraventricular aminoglycosides was coupled with their parenteral administration, compared with parenteral therapy alone. For this reason, neither intrathecal nor intraventricular aminoglycosides can be recommended.

Recent advances in antimicrobial therapy have resulted in the availability of moxalactam, a drug that is effective for the treatment of gram-negative organisms other than *Pseudomonas*. It is not recommended for the treatment of infection that results from gram-positive organisms. Transport of this drug across the blood-brain barrier is excellent.

In a collaborative study comparing ampicillin plus moxalactam therapy with ampicillin plus amikacin therapy for gram-negative neonatal meningitis, similar case fatality rates, duration of positive CSF cultures, and outcome were found for the two treatment regimens. Despite its superior CSF penetration and bactericidal activity, the use of moxalactam did not significantly improve the outcome of this devastating infection. Moxalactam subsequently has been associated with abnormalities of blood clotting in adults. As a result of the similarity of its gram-negative spectrum with moxalactam and its broader gram-positive spectrum, cefotaxime has been substituted in most centers for situations in which moxalactam formerly would have been chosen for use. Cefotaxime is preferred to other third-generation cephalosporins for neonates both because it has been used more extensively and because it is not excreted in the bile. (Excretion could have an inhibitory effect on the bacterial flora of the intestinal tract.) Thus either cefotaxime or the conventional regimen of ampicillin and an aminoglycoside is satisfactory for treatment of enteric gram-negative meningitis caused by ampicillin-sensitive organisms. If facilities are not available for determining aminoglycoside concentrations, or if the patient has abnormal renal function, cefotaxime is preferred. The effective dosage of cefotaxime is shown in Table 31-2. Other newer third-generation cephalosporins also are being

Table 31-3. Indications, pharmacology, and toxicity of antibiotics

Antibiotic	Indications	Pharmacology	Toxicity	Comments
Amikacin	May be used for gram-negative organisms; preference is to limit its use to kanamycin- and gentamicin-resistant species	Renal excretion; crosses blood-CSF barrier poorly; not absorbed from GI tract in normal host	Possible ototoxicity, nephrotoxicity, and neuromuscular blockade	Toxic-reaction in neonate rare if appropriate dosage used and renal function and/or blood levels of antibiotic monitored
Ampicillin	Initial treatment of neonatal sepsis and meningitis; gram-positive organisms except penicillin-resistant staphylococci; may be used for sensitive strains of *H. influenzae, Salmonella, Shigella;* use for gram-negative infection only on basis of sensitivity test results or for synergistic effect with an aminoglycoside	Renal excretion primarily	Rash, elevated transaminase, eosinophilia; may produce seizures or neuromuscular irritability when administered in high dosages; nephritis may occur rarely	
Carbenicillin Ticarcillin	Treatment of *Providencia;* may be used with an aminoglycoside for *Pseudomonas* infections or susceptible strains of *Proteus*	Renal excretion	Rash, elevated transaminases, nausea, vomiting, diarrhea	May cause platelet dysfunction; theoretic sodium content is 4.7 and 5.2 mEq per gram in carbenicillin and ticarcillin, respectively; sodium load should be considered
Cephalosporins (first generation)	Not the drug of choice for any known infection; alternative drug for treatment of penicillinase-producing staphylococci	Renal excretion; clearance of cephaloridine affected more markedly than cephalothin by renal insufficiency; crosses blood-CSF barrier poorly if at all	Rashes, urticaria, neutropenia (rare); Coombs' test may become positive during therapy; renal tubular damage may occur (more common with cephaloridine)	Phlebitis common during IV administration; use with caution if sensitivity to penicillin has been documented; produce brownish black color of urine when tested with Clinitest tablets
Cefotaxime (third generation)	Septicemia, meningitis, ventriculitis caused by *E. coli, Klebsiella, Serratia, H. influenzae*	Crosses blood-brain barrier; 85% to 90% excreted by kidneys	Possible nephrotoxicity, neutropenia, eosinophilia, elevated transaminases (transient)	Not the drug of choice for any infection due to gram-positive cocci
Ceftazidime (third generation)	May be used in combination with an aminoglycoside for *Pseudomonas* infections	Renal excretion	Possible nephrotoxicity; bone marrow suppression (transient); mild elevation of transaminases	Greater activity against *Pseudomonas* than other cephalosporins; should always be employed in combination with an aminoglycoside for treatment of serious *Pseudomonas* infections
Ceftriaxone (third generation)	Septicemia, meningitis, soft tissue and bone and joint infections due to susceptible organisms; broad spectrum of activity against gram-positive and gram-negative bacteria; most strains of *Listeria,* enterococci, methicillin-resistant staphylococci, *C. difficile,* and many *Pseudomonas* strains are resistant	Penetrates inflamed meninges efficiently; 30% to 65% excreted by kidneys; the rest is excreted in bile	Possible nephrotoxicity, hepatotoxicity; eosinophilia, leukopenia, alterations in prothrombin time have occurred rarely	Approved for use recently; experience to date in neonatal infections is limited

Continued.

Table 31-3. Indications, pharmacology, and toxicity of antibiotics—cont'd

Antibiotic	Indications	Pharmacology	Toxicity	Comments
Clindamycin	May be used in selected neonates with *B. fragilis* septicemia or peritonitis		Pseudomembranous enterocolitis in adolescents and adults—rare in children; little experience in neonates	
Chloramphenicol	*Salmonella* sepsis with ampicillin-resistant strain; *H. influenzae* sepsis or meningitis with ampicillin-resistant strains; may be required in certain cases of anaerobic sepsis (e.g. with *B. fragilis*) or in certain cases of sepsis due to *Serratia*	Blocks protein synthesis acting on ribosomal site; metabolized by liver and conjugated with glucuronide for excretion	Gray baby syndrome characterized by anorexia, vomiting, abdominal distension, followed by hypothermia, shallow irregular respirations, development of ashen gray cyanosis, and death; syndrome related to immature hepatic function and characterized by high blood levels of unconjugated chloramphenicol	Dose-related reversible anemia generally develops when administered for more than 7-10 days
Erythromycin	Penicillin-resistant staphylococcus, *Chlamydia*, pertussis	Crosses blood-brain barrier poorly; excreted in urine, stool, and biliary system	No significant toxicity	
Gentamicin	May be used in initial treatment of neonatal sepsis or meningitis; use for *Pseudomonas*, hospital-acquired *K. pneumoniae*, *Enterobacter*, *Serratia*, and kanamycin-resistant coliform or meningitis; treatment of gram-negative organisms except *Pseudomonas* and kanamycin-resistant coliforms	Inhibits glucuronyl transferase in higher than therapeutic dosages; crosses placental barrier; crosses blood-CSF barrier poorly; not absorbed from GI tract in normal host	Possible ototoxicity, nephrotoxicity, and neuromuscular blockade	Toxic reaction in neonate rare if appropriate dosage used and renal function and/or blood levels of antibiotic monitored
Methicillin Oxacillin Nafcillin	Penicillin-resistant *Staphylococcus aureus* infections	Renal excretion; methicillin protein bound only 20%; oxacillin 88% and nafcillin 92% protein bound	Nephrotoxicity; eosinophilia may precede renal damage	Monitor BUN, creatinine, and observe for hematuria and proteinuria; low protein binding suggests potential advantage for methicillin in neonates with hyperbilirubinemia with regard to minimizing risk of kernicterus; usefulness for treating sepsis and meningitis may be limited by potential toxicity
Moxalactam	Septicemia, meningitis, ventriculitis caused by *E. coli*, *Klebsiella*, *Serratia*, *H. influenzae*	Crosses blood-brain barrier; 60% to 90% excreted by kidneys	Eosinophilia, neutropenia (reversible), disturbances in vitamin K–dependent clotting function	

Table 31-3. Indications, pharmacology, and toxicity of antibiotics—cont'd

Antibiotic	Indications	Pharmacology	Toxicity	Comments
Neomycin	Bacterial diarrhea, enteropathogenic *E. coli*	Not absorbed from normal GI tract	Ototoxic, nephrotoxic, neuromuscular blockade	Do not use parenterally
Penicillin G	*Streptococcus pyogenes,* gram-positive anaerobes, including gram-positive bacilli; *S. pneumoniae,* nonpenicillinase *S. aureus, S. agalactiae, Neisseria gonorrhoeae, N. meningitidis, Bacteroides* except *B. fragilis, Pasteurella multocida, Fusobacterium, Treponema pallidum* (syphilis), *Actinomyces israeli,* and leptospires	Renal excretion	Rare nephrotoxicity, rare neuromuscular toxicity	May be used in initial treatment of neonatal septicemia or meningitis in conjunction with an aminoglycoside; however, this combination may not provide effective coverage for infection with *H. influenzae, Salmonella,* or enterococci
Polymyxin B and colistin (polymyxin E)	Effective against *Pseudomonas* and kanamycin-resistant *E. coli*	Renal excretion; dose not cross blood-CSF barrier; not absorbed from GI tract in normal host	Painful injection, ataxia, drowsiness, peripheral neuropathy; neuromuscular blockade may occur; nephritis and azotemia	Polymyxin B may be given intrathecally
Streptomycin	*Mycobacterium, Francisella tularensis,* and *Pasteurella pestis*	Renal excretion	Cardiovascular collapse, vestibular and auditory damage	Employed infrequently in neonates; if used, provide as 30 mg/kg/day IM q12h; toxic reaction in neonate rare if appropriate dosage used and renal function and blood levels of antibiotic monitored
Tobramycin	Broad coverage of gram-negative organisms including *Pseudomonas*	Renal excretion	Possible nephrotoxicity and ototoxicity	
Vancomycin	Effective against *S. epidermidis* and methicillin-resistant *S. aureus;* most gram-positive aerobes and anaerobes are susceptible; may be employed in combination with gentamicin for enterococcal infections	Renal excretion	Nephrotoxicity, ototoxicity, neutropenia, eosinophilia, combination therapy with aminoglycoside may be synergistically nephrotoxic	Flushing and/or hypotension may result from rapid infusion
Nitrofurantoin	Contraindicated in newborn; may cause hemolytic anemias in patients with glucose-6-phosphate dehydrogenase deficiency			
Sulfonamides	Contraindicated in newborn; predisposes to kernicterus by displacing bilirubin from albumin-binding sites; maternal ingestion of sulfamethoxypyridazene (Kynex) may be followed by hemolysis and jaundice in newborns with glucose-6-phosphate dehydrogenase deficiency			
Tetracyclines	Contraindicated in newborn; administration to pregnant women or newborns may produce permanent brown-yellow or gray-black dental discoloration of deciduous or permanent teeth; may cause enamel hypoplasia; may inhibit bone growth in normal premature infants; may cause increased intracranial pressure (pseudotumor cerebri)			

tested to determine their efficacy in the treatment of neonatal sepsis and meningitis. Data are inadequate at present to determine the specific efficacy of these compounds in the treatment of neonatal infection. The broad spectrum, ease of administration, and low toxicity of the third-generation cephalosporins suggest that this class of antimicrobial agents will play an important role in the treatment of gram-negative meningitis in the future.

Meningitis caused by gram-positive organisms should be treated for 14 days after CSF sterility is documented, but treatment may be indicated for a more extended period of time if the clinical situation dictates. When disease is caused by gram-negative organisms, therapy is continued for 2 weeks after the CSF has been proved sterile or for a minimum of 3 weeks, whichever is longer. Examination and culture of CSF should be repeated before discontinuation of antibiotic therapy.

Supportive care of the newborn with meningitis is similar to that described for the septic neonate. In particular, the possibility of inappropriate secretion of antidiuretic hormone with development of dilutional hyponatremia is best treated by fluid restriction. Seizures may be controlled with phenobarbital (10 to 20 mg/kg loading dose) administered intramuscularly or intravenously or with phenytoin (10 to 20 mg/kg as a loading dose). Intravenous diazepam (0.1 to 1.0 mg) can be administered slowly until seizures are controlled; this drug may displace bilirubin from albumin-binding sites. (See Chapter 27.)

Prognosis

Mortality for newborns with meningitis remains between 20% and 30%, a rate that, in part, is dependent on the gestational age of the infant, the type of microorganisms producing the disease, the duration of disease before initiation of antibiotic therapy, and the sensitivity of the microorganisms to various antimicrobial drugs. A significant risk of death or severe impairment was found among infants with group B streptococcal meningitis who, at hospital admission, were comatose or semicomatose and who had decreased perfusion, leukopenia, low neutrophil counts, or CSF protein exceeding 300 mg/dl. The quantity of *E. coli* capsular polysaccharide material to which the host is exposed also is correlated with outcome. The greater the concentration of K1 antigen and the longer it can be detected in the CSF, the worse the prognosis. Sonographic findings of parenchymal echogenicity and/or moderate to marked ventriculomegaly also are predictive of significant neurologic sequelae. Approximately one half of the survivors of both gram-positive and gram-negative neonatal meningitis experience permanent sequelae resulting in significant neurologic damage.

Pneumonia

Incidence

See also Chapter 28, part five.

Pneumonia is the most common form of neonatal infection and one of the most important causes of perinatal death. In the 1920s and 1930s pneumonia was found at autopsy in 20% to 30% of stillborn and newborn infants; more recently, intrauterine pneumonia has been reported in 5% to 35% of autopsies.

Etiology

Pneumonia may follow infection with the same organisms responsible for neonatal sepsis. When the disease is acquired in utero or at the time of delivery, infection with *E. coli, Klebsiella, Listeria, H. influenzae, Treponema pallidum, Enterobacter, Staphylococcus, Streptococcus pneumoniae, S. agalactiae,* or *Proteus* may be suspected. When disease is acquired shortly after birth, the same organisms may be responsible, but infection with *S. aureus, Pseudomonas, Serratia,* and *Candida* should be considered. Viral pneumonia may be noted at or shortly after birth, and epidemic disease has been reported to follow introduction of respiratory syncytial, ECHO, and adenovirus into the newborn unit. Pneumonia may occur as a manifestation of neonatal herpes simplex infection. *Pneumocystis carinii* pneumonia has been reported in debilitated premature and full-term infants; it also has been observed in a small number of healthy full-term babies. Epidemic pneumonitis due to *Pneumocystis* appears to be more prevalent in Europe than in the United States. *P. carinii* pneumonia has been observed as an incidental finding at necropsy of infants who had been healthy but died unexpectedly.

Pathogenesis and pathology

Pneumonia may be acquired (1) transplacentally in utero, (2) by inhalation of contaminated amniotic fluid before or at the time of delivery, (3) by aspiration of infected materials during or after delivery, (4) by inhalation of aerosols that contain infectious microorganisms in the newborn nursery, or (5) hematogenously from another focus of infection or during the course of septicemia. Intrauterine pneumonia frequently follows prolonged rupture of the membranes. All fetuses swallow amniotic fluid; thus the oropharynx or GI tract may serve as portals of entry for microorganisms. Gasping may be induced as a result of asphyxia, prompting aspiration of infected amniotic fluid. Intrauterine pneumonia acquired transplacentally has been associated with maternal pneumococcal septicemia and with viremia. When intrauterine pneumonia occurs, the process is diffuse, and the alveoli are filled with polymorphonuclear leukocytes and microorganisms. Amniotic debris may be found; this suggests that disease has followed aspiration rather than hematogenous dissemination of microorganisms.

Aspiration during or following delivery may lead to bronchopneumonia, which may be associated with hemorrhage and with evidence of pleural inflammation. Abscesses, empyema, and pyopneumothorax may be found when infection is due to *S. aureus*, although these findings are not restricted to infection with this organism. Pneumatocele formation, found so commonly in association with infection due to *S. aureus*, also has been noted in the newborn with pneumonia due to *E. coli*, *Klebsiella*, *Enterobacter*, or anaerobic organisms. *Pseudomonas* pneumonia may follow septicemia or use of contaminated resuscitation or inhalation therapy equipment. The inflammatory response in these individuals may be perivascular and characterized by necrosis of vessel walls and of alveoli.

Clinical manifestations

Intrauterine pneumonia should be suspected when respiratory distress develops in any infant, but suspicions should be heightened if antecedent problems referable to pregnancy and delivery have been noted. The infant who has acquired pneumonia in utero or during delivery may be ill at birth, and the initial cry may be delayed. Spontaneous respirations may not occur or may be established with difficulty. If respirations are established, tachypnea, moderate retractions, and an expiratory grunt may be observed. Fever may or may not be noted. In most cases there is no cough. Cyanosis may be constant or intermittent, and respirations may be irregular and punctuated by periods of apnea. Dullness to percussion, decreased breath sounds, and rales may be present, but at times these findings are absent throughout the entire course of the disease. Congestive heart failure manifested by cardiac enlargement, hepatomegaly, and tachycardia may complicate the pneumonic process. Neurologic abnormalities also may appear; they include hypotonia, flaccidity, hypertonia, tremors, and convulsions. When neurologic findings are present, the prognosis generally is poor. At necropsy of some newborns with pneumonia who have had neurologic findings, no gross intracranial lesions are found.

Postnatally acquired pneumonia may develop at any time. Symptoms are similar to those occurring in children with pneumonia immediately after birth; the onset may be abrupt or gradual. Chlamydial pneumonia patients classically exhibit a staccato cough; they are afebrile, and frequently they gain weight slowly.

Diagnosis

Roentgenograms are required to support the diagnosis of pneumonia and to distinguish it from other causes of respiratory distress. In some patients no abnormality will be found if roentgenographic studies have been performed early, following the onset of symptoms, but by 24 to 72 hours a diagnosis should be possible. In other patients an area of radiopacification is present, but it may be attributed to atelectasis. Roentgenograms may reveal either bilateral homogeneous consolidation when pneumonia is acquired in utero or diffuse bronchopneumonia when disease has been acquired postnatally. Pneumatoceles may be observed, and occasionally hemothorax or pleural effusions are present. The radiograph of segmental or lobar atelectasis is unlike that of congenital or postnatal pneumonia. Where lobar atelectasis occurs, consolidation of an entire lobe or segment may be noted, but rarely is an entire lung involved. The involved hemithorax is smaller than the opposite side, the diaphragm may be elevated, and the heart is shifted toward the area of presumed atelectasis. In contrast, it may be extremely difficult to distinguish the roentgenogram of pneumonia from that of massive meconium aspiration. In meconium aspiration, opacities may be distributed in the same manner as in bronchopneumonia, but the roentgenographic changes tend to be maximal early and disappear rapidly during the ensuing period of several days. In contrast, the patchy opacifications noted in bronchopneumonia tend to be minimal early and become more impressive during the subsequent period of several days.

Pneumonia caused by the group B streptococci or other bacteria may be indistinguishable roentgenographically from respiratory distress syndrome or transient tachypnea. Pneumonia due to *Chlamydia trachomatis* may produce roentgenographic findings of hyperinflation of the lung associated with diffuse bilateral pulmonary infiltrates.

Tracheal aspirate cultures may not be particularly helpful in establishing an etiologic diagnosis, since they often reveal the same kind of flora as found in the vaginal canal. The presence of polymorphonuclear leukocytes on a tracheal aspirate smear suggests an infectious process, and recovery of *S. aureus* or *Pseudomonas* organisms from the tracheal aspirate may affect the choice of antibiotic therapy. Before 12 hours of age, the presence of bacteria and neutrophils in tracheal secretions may provide helpful adjunctive information for identifying neonates with pneumonia and bacteremia. Tracheal secretions should be processed for viral isolates when nonbacterial pneumonia is suspected. A recently licensed enzyme-linked immunosorbent assay for respiratory syncytial virus is a sensitive, specific, and rapid diagnostic method for testing tracheal secretions or nasal washings.

Blood cultures should be obtained in infants with pneumonia; positive cultures establish an etiologic diagnosis. A definitive diagnosis of *Chlamydia* pneumonia requires isolation of the organism from the lung or lower respiratory tract. Detection serologically of high levels of IgM antibody (greater than 1:32) appears to reflect systemic rather than localized chlamydial infection, but rapid diagnostic tests are not yet available commercially. The white blood cell count and differential appear to be of little value generally, but in individual patients they may reveal a striking leukocytosis (25,000 white blood cells/mm^3) or leukopenia (less than 3,500 white blood cells/mm^3).

Treatment

When a diagnosis is established, treatment should be prompt. If the diagnosis is supported by historical and clinical findings but initial roentgenograms fail to confirm the clinical impression, treatment should not be delayed and should be continued until a chest roentgenogram at 72 hours fails to confirm the diagnosis. Treatment with antibiotics should be directed toward coverage of the same organisms as those that produce neonatal septicemia. Thus ampicillin and kanamycin or gentamicin in dosages similar to those used for septicemia are indicated for early-onset infections (Table 31-2). When infections with *S. aureus* or *P. aeruginosa* are suspected, treatment must be altered. Staphylococcal infection is treated best with methicillin, whereas *Pseudomonas* infections can be treated with ticarcillin together with an aminoglycoside, such as gentamicin or amikacin, which will cover other gram-negative organisms as well. Pneumonia due to *Chlamydia* or *Pertussis* organisms responds best to treatment with erythromycin. Erythromycin can be given in a dosage of 40 mg/kg/24 hours divided into four oral doses. Treatment should be continued for 10 to 14 days or longer as dictated by the clinical course of the patient. Adequate fluids and oxygen, as required to treat hypoxemia, should be administered. Ribavirin small-particle aerosol recently has been licensed for use in the treatment of lower respiratory tract infections associated with respiratory syncytial virus. If sudden deterioration with tachypnea and cyanosis is noted during the course of the disease, pneumothorax should be suspected and relieved promptly.

Prognosis

Intrauterine pneumonia is not necessarily fatal; however, the more critically ill infants are prone to die in utero or within the first 2 days of life despite meticulous care and administration of appropriate antibiotics. The prognosis is worse for premature than for full-term infants. In the absence of other problems, the prognosis for full-term infants who acquire pneumonia postnatally is good.

Gastroenteritis

Incidence

Gastrointestinal tract infections can occur sporadically or as a result of an epidemic outbreak of disease. The incidence varies even within the same nursery from year to year.

Etiology

The agents that have been associated with both epidemic and sporadic diarrheal disease include enteropathogenic strains of *E. coli* (EPEC), *Salmonella*, *Shigella*, *Yersinia*, *Campylobacter*, and on rare occasions *Pseudomonas*, *Klebsiella*, *Enterobacter*, and *C. albicans*. An epidemic of enterocolitis recently was attributed to infection by group A β-hemolytic streptococci. Enteric types of adenovirus, rotavirus, and calicivirus have been identified as causative agents for gastroenteritis in neonates. In many cases the etiologic agent is not identified, and viruses are assumed to be responsible despite negative viral and serologic studies.

E. coli may be subdivided into a number of serogroups depending on their antigenic composition. The somatic O antigen is associated with the cell body, whereas the H antigen is associated with the flagellae. Serogroup A strains, particularly serotypes 055:B5 and 0111:B4, have been associated with epidemic disease more frequently than serotypes of group B. EPEC organisms have been recovered from infants with severe diarrheal disease but also may be found in the stools of certain infants who are asymptomatic or who have mild disease. More recently, diarrhea has been reported in association with colonization by *E. coli* that are not considered enteropathogenic. The frequency with which these enterotoxigenic strains produce neonatal gastroenteritis is unknown. Strains of *E. coli* considered to be enterotoxigenic may elaborate a heat-labile or heat-stable toxin that activates adenylate cyclase and produces a secretory diarrhea. Some strains of *E. coli* produce diarrhea by invasion of the gut wall; these strains may be toxin producers as well. Recently, strains of *E. coli* that adhere to the gastrointestinal mucosa but that neither invade it nor produce toxin have been associated with diarrhea.

Pathology

When diarrhea is associated with EPEC, there may be no lesion in the GI tract. In some patients small ulcerations of the bowel with a scant inflammatory reaction have been noted. *Salmonella* gastroenteritis may be accompanied by superficial mucosal ulceration and occasionally by deeper ulcers, which may be associated with gross bleeding and perforation. Mesenteric lymphadenitis also may be found. *Shigella* gastroenteritis tends to be a superficial mucosal disease with shallow ulcers occasionally associated with fibrinous superficial exudates that coalesce to form pseudomembranes. *Salmonella* gastroenteritis is associated with bacteremia and the development of distant foci of infection more frequently than is infection by *Shigella* or EPEC. *Campylobacter* diarrhea also is accompanied frequently by bacteremia; the course may be rapidly fatal. Meningitis is a frequent complication of this type of infection in the premature infant.

Pathogenesis

The GI tract is colonized initially by organisms that enter the oropharynx at delivery. Maternal carriers of *Salmonella, Shigella, Campylobacter,* and EPEC serve as the initial source of these pathogens in the nursery. Subsequently, infection may spread from patient to patient as a result of inadequate hand-washing by personnel. Asymptomatic personnel who are carriers of these organisms have proved to be the source of several major epidemics. Fomite transmission has been observed, and in rare instances infection has followed ingestion of contaminated milk, water, or materials used for roentgenographic evaluation of the GI tract.

Clinical manifestations

GI tract colonization by microorganisms associated with gastroenteritis may be followed by no symptoms or by severe diarrhea with fever, vomiting, and abdominal distention. Bloody diarrhea containing mucus should suggest *Shigella, Yersinia,* or *Campylobacter* gastroenteritis, but melena and hematochezia have been observed in neonates with gastroenteritis due to *Salmonella* or EPEC. A blue discoloration of the stools or diaper may be found in some patients where *Pseudomonas* species predominate in the stool. Vomiting and respiratory symptoms occur frequently with enteric adenoviral gastroenteritis. Dehydration, acidosis, electrolyte disturbances, and hypotension may occur during the course of disease.

Diagnosis

Stool cultures should be obtained from all infants with gastroenteritis. Recovery of EPEC, *Shigella, Yersinia, Campylobacter,* or *Salmonella* organisms from the stool of an infant with diarrhea is presumptive evidence that disease is due to one of these pathogens. EPEC organisms are identified on the basis of serologic studies in which specific antisera are employed to agglutinate *E. coli* in the laboratory. From 10 to 20 colonies of *E. coli* should be typed before a negative report for EPEC leaves the laboratory. Fluorescent antibody studies also have been employed in screening stool samples for EPEC. Serotyping *E. coli* can be helpful in tracing the course of epidemic disease due to this organism but may be of no value in discerning the etiology of diarrhea in an individual patient. Techniques to ascertain elaboration of *E. coli* toxins are available; they are expensive, time consuming, and generally not used in community hospitals.

When feasible, a stool specimen should be evaluated by direct or immune electron microscopy for the presence of adenoviral particles. In the majority of infants acutely ill with diarrhea, the presence of viral particles is associated causally with the diarrhea. A recently developed enzyme immunoassay* may detect rotavirus in stool specimens although false positive tests may occur in neonates. A stool smear for polymorphonuclear leukocytes also may be of value. Diarrhea due to EPEC, *Yersinia, Campylobacter, Salmonella,* or *Shigella* may be associated with fecal leukocytes; fecal leukocytes generally are not found in patients with nonspecific or viral gastroenteritis. Blood cultures may be helpful in establishing a diagnosis of salmonellosis or *Yersinia* or *Campylobacter* infection and may be positive in rare cases of EPEC and shigellosis.

Treatment

Diarrhea due to EPEC should be treated by oral administration of neomycin in a dosage of 50 to 100 mg/kg/day divided into four doses for 5 days. Polymyxin B or colistimethate sulfate may be given orally if the organisms are resistant to neomycin. *Salmonella* infections that are mild and are not associated with positive blood culture require no antibiotic treatment. If septicemia occurs, ampicillin (as for sepsis) should be provided. Neonates are susceptible to complications of *Salmonella* infection such as osteomyelitis. Parenteral therapy should be initiated if distant foci of infection are suspected. Chloramphenicol can be used if *Salmonella* strains prove to be resistant to ampicillin. *Shigella* infections should be treated with ampicillin orally or with a nonabsorbable oral antibiotic. Kanamycin, colistin, or neomycin may be employed as determined by the sensitivity of the *Shigella* isolate. In many centers *Shigella* species have become resistant to ampicillin; chloramphenicol or kanamycin may be required if systemic therapy is necessary. Amoxicillin should not be substituted for ampicillin even if the *Shigella* isolate proves to be sensitive to ampicillin. *Campylobacter* and *Yersinia* infections can be treated with kanamycin; chloramphenicol can be provided if meningitis follows localized disease. Fluids should be administered intravenously as necessary for treatment of dehydration or maintenance of adequate hydration.

Prevention and prognosis

Infants born to mothers with diarrhea should be isolated until the results of maternal and infant stool cultures are available. Personnel with diarrhea should be excluded from the nursery. Overcrowding must be avoided and proper hand-washing techniques employed. If formulas are prepared in the hospital, use of appropriate procedures to ensure sterility is essential. If epidemic disease as a result of EPEC occurs, the nursery should be closed to new admissions and all infants treated with

*The enzyme immunoassay is available commercially as Rotazyme, produced by the Abbott Laboratories, North Chicago, Ill.

neomycin. The nursery may be reopened 48 hours after neomycin has been initiated and no new cases have appeared. Mortality has varied from 0% to 37% during the course of epidemics due to EPEC.

Necrotizing enterocolitis (NEC)

Although not primarily a diarrheal disease, enterocolitis associated with necrosis and ulceration of the GI tract has been noted in some children with diarrhea due to *E. coli*, *Klebsiella*, *Enterobacter*, *Shigella*, *Clostridia*, *Salmonella*, and rotavirus organisms. Pathologic similarity of pneumatosis intestinalis to gas gangrene of the bowel has suggested the possibility that toxin production plays a significant role in the pathogenesis of necrotizing enterocolitis. Epithelial surfaces of the mucosa are sloughed, and submucosal hemorrhaging may be present. Vomiting, abdominal distension, GI bleeding, peritonitis, and shock may be found. Intramural air or free air within the peritoneal cavity may be noted on abdominal roentgenograms. Blood cultures frequently are positive in affected infants; however, it is likely that septicemia is a secondary event. An infectious etiology for NEC has been postulated because the disease occurs in clusters.

Increased risk of illness among nursery staff caring for neonates with NEC has been cited as additional evidence that a transmissible agent may be responsible for some cases of NEC. Several studies have documented a predilection for NEC when colonization of the GI tract with *Klebsiella* and *Enterobacter* species is observed. These results prompted the use of oral aminoglycosides in attempts to treat or prevent NEC. Many investigators have proposed the prophylactic administration of aminoglycosides for all infants at high risk for NEC. Others, however, have been concerned about the possibility that widespread use of these antibiotics would lead to the emergence of organisms resistant to these drugs. Recent reports have suggested that toxins from *C. difficile* or *C. perfringens* may play a role in some of these cases. Some investigators advocate the initiation of therapy with oral vancomycin for affected infants and their contacts when an outbreak of NEC occurs in a unit where *C. difficile* is endemic (Chapter 33).

Otitis media

Incidence

Retrospective postmortem studies have demonstrated a high (about 70%) incidence of otitis media in premature infants; this suggests that otitis media may play a major role in neonatal mortality, particularly in premature infants. Prospective clinical studies indicate that otitis media develops in a minimum of 0.6% of all live births during the first month of life and that the rate may reach 2% to 3% in premature infants.

Etiology

The organisms producing otitis media in the newborn infant are similar to organisms that cause otitis media in older children. Studies of infants under 6 weeks of age have shown that *S. pneumoniae* was the causative organism in 19% to 30% of cases. *Haemophilus influenzae* was recovered in 14% to 25% of cases and β-hemolytic streptococci (groups A and B) were recovered in 5% of cases. Gram-negative organisms (*E. coli*, *Enterobacter*, *Klebsiella*, and *Pseudomonas*) were found in 7% to 18% of neonates with otitis media. In all studies, between 40% and 50% of cultures obtained by needle tympanocentesis have been sterile or judged nonpathogenic. But included among the "nonpathogenic" are organisms such as *S. aureus*, *S. epidermidis*, and *Neisseria (Branhamella) catarrhalis*, which organisms have been shown to be pathogenic in a selected group of older children. Thus it is likely that these have been responsible for purulent otitis media in some newborns. Since strict anaerobic culture techniques were not employed in most studies, a number of "sterile isolates" may have contained anaerobic microorganisms. Viral infection also has been associated with neonatal middle ear disease.

Pathogenesis and pathology

Otitis media is more common in premature than in full-term infants. This increased risk of infection may be related to the small size of the eustachian tube, with resultant obstruction and secondary infection. Aspiration of infected amniotic fluid is probably the leading cause of otitis media in newborns. The disease increases in frequency in bottle-fed babies, a finding that may be related to the supine position of such infants during feeding or to the possibility that local immunity may be conferred from the IgA in breast milk. Secretory IgA antibodies in breast milk may exert protection by preventing the attachment of otitis media–causing bacterial strains to retropharyngeal cells.

Clinical manifestations

Rhinorrhea is the most common manifestation of otitis media in the newborn period. Irritability, lethargy, vomiting, poor feeding, cough, diarrhea, or fever also may be present. Young infants with otitis media often are asymptomatic. Erythema, dullness, and bulging of the pars flaccida of the tympanic membranes may be noted, and pneumatic otoscopy may reveal a decreased mobility of the tympanic membrane. Infants with typical facial or submandibular group B streptococcal cellulitis generally have ipsilateral otitis media at the time of admission.

Diagnosis

The nonspecificity of clinical signs and symptoms coupled with difficulties in visualizing the tympanic membrane early in life probably accounts, in part, for the discrepancy between incidence figures derived from prospective clinical studies and figures from retrospective postmortem studies. Specific diagnosis should be made by culture and smear of purulent middle ear fluid obtained after perforation or by myringotomy or needle tympanocentesis. Cultures of the nasopharynx may yield the same organism in some cases but cannot be relied on in any individual patient to provide the type of information that may be used to select a specific antibiotic. Blood cultures may be helpful in patients with concomitant septicemia. Lumbar puncture should be performed to exclude meningitis. Meningitis that was not suspected before examination of CSF has been noted in a number of newborns with otitis media, but the specific frequency with which these two problems occur concurrently is unknown.

Treatment

A combination of ampicillin and kanamycin or gentamicin will provide effective treatment for most newborns with otitis media. When culture results are known, antibiotic therapy can be altered appropriately. Treatment should be continued for 14 to 21 days, using the dosages employed for septicemia (Table 31-2).

Prognosis

Recurrent or persistent disease is not uncommon. The results of a recent prospectively performed study indicate that infants with onset of otitis media before 2 months of age are at high risk for developing chronic otitis media with effusion. Careful follow-up evaluation for infection and hearing loss is important. The insertion of plastic tubes may be indicated to ensure adequate drainage of the middle ear.

Omphalitis

Incidence

Omphalitis occurs in many neonates who develop purulent or serosanguineous drainage about the umbilical stump. Umbilical phlebitis and even arteritis may develop spontaneously or follow catheterization of umbilical vessels. Tetanus may follow contamination of the umbilical stump but is rarely encountered in societies that practice routine immunization for tetanus and asepsis at the time of delivery. Necrotizing fasciitis is a life-threatening complication resulting from rapidly spreading destruction of the fascia and subcutaneous tissue.

Etiology

Any organisms that are found on the skin or that may be introduced into the umbilical vessel by catheterization can produce omphalitis.

Pathogenesis

Direct bacterial invasion of the umbilical cord and surrounding skin is common. Bacteria may invade the umbilical artery and spread along its lumen, necrosing the loose connective tissue of the arterial wall. If both the umbilical and iliac ends are occluded, a septic loculated focus of infection may be found. When the umbilical end remains patent, purulent material may drain through the umbilicus. If the connective tissue of the artery is extensively involved, peritonitis may develop, or the infection may extend along its course and appear as a scrotal or deep thigh abscess. If the iliac end of the artery is patent but the umbilical end is sealed, septicemia may ensue.

Clinical manifestations

Purulent drainage may be noted from the umbilical stump at its base of attachment to the abdominal wall or from the navel after the cord has separated. The discharge may be foul smelling. Periumbilical erythema and induration may be noted. If extensive periumbilical edema or involvement of the abdominal wall is noted, the complication of necrotizing fasciitis should be considered.

Diagnosis

When the umbilical stump discharges purulent material, it should be smeared and cultured. When a loculated periarterial abscess is present, material obtained at the time of drainage also should be cultured. Whenever septic umbilical arteritis is suspected, blood cultures should be obtained.

Treatment

In most patients omphalitis without purulent discharge responds to local application of antibiotic ointments containing neomycin, polymyxin, and bacitracin. Parenteral administration of antibiotics may be indicated if a purulent discharge is noted or periumbilical inflammation is present. In such cases, methicillin and gentamicin are logical choices until a specific organism has been identified. Extensive surgical resection is required to achieve cure of necrotizing fasciitis.

Conjunctivitis

See Chapter 39.

Incidence

Conjunctivitis most commonly is due to chemical irritation that follows the prophylactic institution of silver nitrate into the conjunctival sac. Chemical conjunctivitis may be found in almost 100% of infants so treated. Chemical conjunctivitis due to erythromycin or penicillin occurs much less frequently but does occur in some newborns. The incidence of other forms of conjunctivitis is difficult to assess. However, the incidence of gonococcal ophthalmitis has increased in recent years despite presumably effective and mandatory regimens of prophylactic eye care.

Etiology

Neisseria gonorrhoeae and *Chlamydia trachomatis* are the most important causes of conjunctivitis in the newborn period. Other bacteria, including *S. aureus*, group B hemolytic streptococci, *Pseudomonas*, *Streptococcus pneumoniae*, and Koch-Weeks bacillus, also are common causes of this disease. Conjunctivitis is the most common ocular manifestation of neonatal herpes simplex infections.

Pathogenesis

Conjunctivitis due to *N. gonorrhoeae*, *C. trachomatis*, *S. agalactiae*, or herpes simplex generally is initiated by infection with microorganisms acquired during passage through the birth canal. Infection with *S. aureus*, *Pseudomonas*, or other organisms more commonly reflects infection acquired during the neonatal period.

Clinical manifestations

Chemical conjunctivitis usually is noted soon after birth and becomes less prominent after 2 days of age. Bacterial conjunctivitis is most prominent during the first week of life but may occur at any time during the neonatal period. Inclusion conjunctivitis has been noted as early as 24 hours but generally develops during the second week of life. The signs of bacterial conjunctivitis in the newborn are similar to those observed in older individuals. A purulent ocular discharge, erythema and edema of the lids, and injection or suffusion of the conjunctiva or sclera may be found. If the infection is untreated, corneal involvement may occur and will be characterized by punctate corneal epithelial erosions. In the case of disease with *N. gonorrhoeae*, large punctate superficial lesions may be seen, which coalesce and progress to corneal perforation. When staphylococcal conjunctivitis is complicated by corneal involvement, the lower portion of the cornea is infected more frequently than the upper half, and marginal corneal infiltrates with peripheral vascularization may be seen. When a chlamydial agent is involved, inflammatory changes may be barely detectable, or there may be intense inflammation, swelling, and a yellow discharge in association with pseudomembrane formation. The cornea is affected rarely. Necrosis of the cornea has been observed followed by fibrosis and scarring of the lid margin. Chlamydial infections generally are bilateral, whereas unilateral disease is common when staphylococcal disease is present. When chlamydial conjunctivitis is not treated, inflammation persists for 1 or 2 weeks. A subacute phase follows with slight injection of the conjunctiva and an accumulation of purulent material along the lid margins. Occasionally, chronic disease develops.

Diagnosis

The clinical appearance of the patient, coupled with Gram stain and culture of the purulent discharge, establishes a diagnosis. Gram-negative diplococci within leukocytes suggest a diagnosis of gonococcal disease. When gonococcal disease is suspected, purulent material should be plated at the bedside on Thayer-Martin media or placed in special transport media and immediately sent to the bacteriology laboratory. Other organisms are less fastidious, and a swab of purulent material, cultured promptly, is sufficient to establish a diagnosis.

Chlamydial infections can be documented by performing Giemsa stains on material obtained by gently but firmly scraping the lower portion of the palpebral conjunctiva with a blunt spatula or wire loop. Cotton and Calgonite swabs have not proved adequate. Care must be taken not to injure the conjunctiva during the process of obtaining a smear. The smears obtained in this manner may reveal a predominance of neutrophils with smaller numbers of lymphocytes and monocytes. Leber cells (macrophages containing cellular debris) and inclusion-bearing epithelial cells are characteristic. The inclusions are composed of elementary bodies that appear adjacent to the nucleus. Larger inclusions may appear in the form of a cap indented by the nucleus. In many patients inclusion-bearing cells are difficult to find. For this reason it has been suggested that purulent conjunctivitis that develops after day 5, from which no pathogenic bacteria are recovered and that fails to respond to topical application of neomycin/polymyxin ophthalmic ointment, be treated as chlamydial conjunctivitis whether or not inclusions have been demonstrated.

Treatment

Gonococcal ophthalmitis should be treated parenterally with aqueous penicillin G in a dosage of 50,000 units/kg daily in two divided doses for 7 days. The conjunctival sac should be irrigated with sterile isotonic saline. Parenteral treatment with an aminoglycoside and an antipseudomonal penicillin in addition to topical treatment is indicated for conjunctivitis due to *Pseudomonas* organisms. Antibiotics containing various combinations of bacitracin, neomycin, and polymyxin, administered topically as an ophthalmic ointment or solution several times a day for a period of 7 to 10 days, have been recommended for other forms of bacterial conjunctivitis. Inclusion conjunctivitis should be treated with 10% sulfacetamide ophthalmic suspension or ointment or 1% tetracycline ointment applied six to eight times per day.

Erythromycin ophthalmic ointment also may be used. Reduction in erythema and discharge usually follows within 24 hours. The proper duration of treatment is not known, but 14 days is sufficient in most cases. Recurrences and reinfection have been noted, and if this occurs, treatment must be repeated. Since chlamydial pneumonia may accompany or follow chlamydial conjunctivitis, use of erythromycin (40 mg/kg/day in four divided oral doses) should be considered in addition to the topical therapy.

Prevention and prognosis

In most patients prompt recognition and treatment eradicate conjunctival disease. If bacterial conjunctivitis is not treated, corneal involvement with eventual opacification, keratectasia or staphyloma formation, and perforation may ensue. A 1% solution of silver nitrate properly instilled into the conjunctival sac at birth generally will prevent gonococcal ophthalmitis. Topical application of erythromycin or tetracycline ointments also provides effective prophylaxis. Significantly higher rates of infection with ointment rather than liquid preparations have been related to difficulty in application and in the mechanical introduction of bacteria.

Osteomyelitis and septic arthritis

Incidence

Osteomyelitis is a relatively rare but potentially lethal neonatal infection. A referral center may be called on to evaluate and treat two or three newborns per year. Septic arthritis is frequently concomitant, probably reflecting spread of infection via blood vessels that penetrate the epiphyseal plate.

Etiology

S. aureus is the leading cause of hospital-acquired osteomyelitis and septic arthritis in the newborn. *Candida* species and gram-negative enteric bacilli have assumed major roles for nosocomially acquired bone and joint infections. These infections are most commonly isolated in nursery outbreak situations. The most frequent causative agents for community-acquired osteomyelitis and septic arthritis are group B streptococci and *S. aureus*. Some uncommon or rare species that have been isolated include *N. gonorrhoeae*, *H. influenzae*, group A streptococci, and *T. pallidum*.

Pathology

Osteomyelitis usually affects the metaphyseal regions of long bones. However, involvement of the small bones of the hands and feet, the vertebrae, and the ribs has been noted. Multiple foci of osteomyelitis may be seen more frequently in the newborn period than in older individuals; between 10% and 40% of newborns have more than a single locus of infection. The cortical bone is thin, permitting infection to extend readily into soft tissues. Involucrum formation is common, but sequestration is rare if the process is recognized and treated promptly. Infection may extend through the metaphyseal plexus of veins into the joint. The position of the metaphyses of the hip and elbow with relation to the joint capsule permits direct spread into the joint. Destruction of cartilage, dislocations, and pathologic fractures may occur and permanently affect bone growth.

Pathogenesis

Osteomyelitis almost invariably follows hematogenous dissemination of microorganisms. Infection of the skin, omphalitis, umbilical catheterization, and occasionally improperly performed femoral venipunctures are predisposing factors in some cases. Complications of pregnancy have been reported in up to 41% and complications of delivery in 48% of newborns with osteomyelitis. In the majority of cases, some antecedent illness can be identified. Occasionally, osteomyelitis may follow direct extension of a soft tissue infection to bone; this has been noted in neonates with osteomyelitis of the maxilla.

Clinical manifestations

Destructive changes in bone due to osteomyelitis may be quite advanced by the time a definitive diagnosis is made, because of the failure to recognize the subtlety of the initial signs and symptoms. In many patients the disease is not accompanied by systemic signs or symptoms. Fever is absent or is a very late and intermittent finding. Most frequently, swelling, tenderness, and decreased motion of an extremity are the findings that prompt initial appraisal by a physician. In one patient with osteomyelitis of the clavicle, an incomplete Moro reflex was the only finding on physical examination. Localized tenderness, local erythema, and regional lymphadenopathy also may be noted. Heat and fluctuance are rare early in the disease. In some patients, an acute onset of illness with fever, icterus, hemorrhagic manifestations, and hypotension occurs.

Diagnosis

When the history and physical examination suggest the possibility of osteomyelitis, roentgenograms should be obtained. Roentgenographic changes develop 7 to 10 days after the onset of infection; those obtained early may reveal only soft tissue swelling. High resolution bone scintigraphy is more sensitive than radiography in the early stages of infection. Evaluation of small bones is essential to reveal increased radionuclide activity or, occasionally, a "cold" lesion. Later in the course of infection, periosteal thickening, cortical destruction, irregularities of the epiphysis, and periosteal new bone formation may be found. Additional findings may include localized areas of rarefaction, periosteal elevation, a widened joint space, and subluxation or dislocation of the bone from the joint. Since multiple sites of osteomyelitis are not infrequently found, roentgenographic skeletal survey or high resolution bone scintigraphy is warranted in newborns after a single site of osteomyelitis has been confirmed, although other sites are not suggested by the clinical findings. Roentgenographic survey should be delayed for 7 to 10 days after initiation of treatment to maximize the likelihood of defining all possible sites of infection. Fig. 31-1 depicts the roentgenographic findings in a newborn with multiple sites of disease due to *S. aureus*.

Aspiration of soft tissues and of bone is indicated; Gram-stained smears and cultures of this material should be obtained. Blood cultures are essential and in my experience yield the causative agent in 60% of cases. Joint fluid obtained from patients with joint involvement should be smeared and cultured as well. Syphilis, tuberculosis, scurvy, and deep cellulitis are disorders that must be considered in the differential diagnosis.

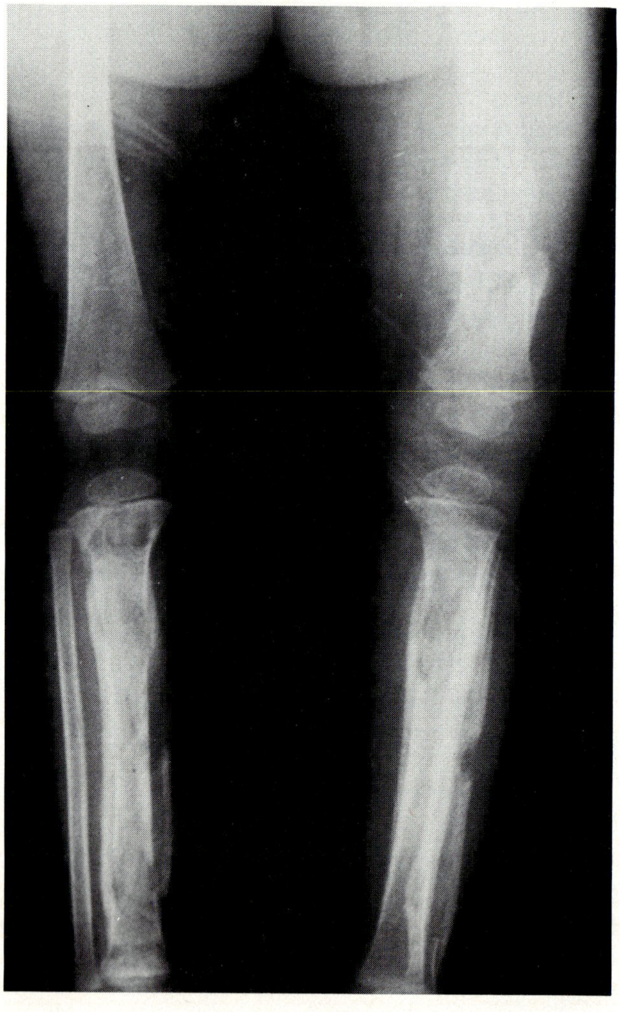

Fig. 31-1. Multiple sites of osteomyelitis in an infant as a result of *S. aureus* infection are demonstrated. Clinical evidence of infection became apparent at 2 weeks of age. Osteolytic lesions can be seen in the right femur, right tibia and fibula, and left tibia. Periosteal new bone formation is visible in many areas.

Treatment

Until the specific etiology has been clarified by culture, treatment should be initiated with methicillin and gentamicin parenterally. When the specific organism and its sensitivity have been identified, treatment should be continued with an appropriate antibiotic (Table 31-3). The dosages employed should be those used for treatment of septicemia or meningitis (Table 31-2). Parenteral therapy should be continued for 3 to 6 weeks, or longer, until clinical and radiographic findings indicate healing and the erythocyte sedimentation rate is normal. Intraarticular administration of antibiotics is not indicated; there is no evidence that such administration is necessary or hastens recovery. There is little or no role for oral antimicrobial therapy in treatment. Surgical decompression may be required if pus is aspirated from the site of involvement. Generally, drilling of bone or windowing to drain medullary collections of pus is not necessary. When the hip joint is involved, prompt surgical decompression and drainage are required.

Prognosis

The degree of residual damage depends on the extent of disease before effective treatment. Permanent disability is more common when joint involvement has occurred. Growth disturbances may result from destruction of the epiphyseal plate. The number of foci of osteomyelitis in a patient who is treated effectively does not appear to correlate specifically with the extent or likelihood of permanent disability. Chronic osteomyelitis is relatively infrequent. Overall, residual effects may be anticipated in 25% of neonates with infection of the bones or joints.

Urinary tract infections

Infection of the urinary tract is discussed in detail in Chapter 35. Most infections of the urinary tract in the newborn occur in association with neonatal septicemia or serve as a focus of infection for the development of septicemia and meningitis. The organisms causing this disease are virtually identical to those that cause neonatal septicemia. Infection with *E. coli* is most common, and epidemics of septicemia and urinary tract infections have been traced to this organism. Infection with other gram-negative organisms, as well as with *S. aureus* and *S. epidermidis*, is not infrequent. Infection is more common in males than females and in association with obstructive abnormalities of the genitourinary system. Symptoms referable to the genitourinary system are rare, and in most patients the symptomatology is nonspecific, similar to that found in neonates with septicemia. In some patients, only poor feeding, weight loss, or diarrhea may be noted. Initial treatment should include parenteral administration of ampicillin and an aminoglycoside.

Infections of the skin and mucous membranes

Incidence

Infection of the skin and mucous membranes is common and may result from infection with bacteria, viruses, or fungi. (See Chapter 38.)

Etiology

Colonization of the skin begins at birth, and the organisms that are acquired reflect those in the environment. During the period of time that hexachlorophene bathing of newborns was a common practice, colonization with gram-negative flora was prevalent. Cessation of hexachlorophene bathing has been accompanied by increases in both the rate of colonization and infection due to *S. aureus*. Cutaneous or mucocutaneous lesions also may result from infection due to group A β-hemolytic streptococci, *P. aeruginosa*, *T. pallidum*, herpes simplex virus, vaccinia virus, variola virus, rubeola virus, and *C. albicans*.

Pathology

Abscesses, pustules, or bullous lesions are caused by *S. aureus* and occasionally by streptococci. Histologic examination of the skin of patients with bullous impetigo may show intraepidermal bullae filled with polymorphonuclear leukocytes. Ritter's disease (Chapter 38), a disorder associated with toxin-elaborating staphylococci, is characterized by a severe bullous eruption and by shedding of the epidermis. Histologic examination of the skin reveals an intraepidermal blister, cellular death and acantholysis, and a striking absence of inflammation. *Pseudomonas* or *Aeromonas hydrophila* infections cause ecthyma gangrenosum, which is characterized by the development of yellow-green pustules that progress rapidly to form hemorrhagic and necrotic ulcers. Skin abscesses with minimal inflammation may be caused by *Candida* species. Their occurrence should be considered diagnostic of invasive infection. (See Part three of this chapter.)

Pathogenesis

Infection generally develops as the result of infection through a small break in the skin and is caused by organisms with which the patient has been colonized. Scalp abscesses may follow intrauterine monitoring of the delivery with scalp electrodes. Nursery personnel or other infants can serve as a source of infection of the neonate with *T. pallidum* or by various viruses. *C. albicans* infection generally follows colonization of the buccal mucosa or GI tract by *Candida* or contamination of the diaper area by *Candida* within stools.

Clinical manifestations

Skin and soft tissue infections should be discovered promptly, since clinical findings generally are apparent to even the casual observer. Bullous lesions that appear after the second day of life generally suggest staphylococcal disease, in contrast to noninfectious blistering diseases that may be manifest at birth (Chapter 38). The blisters range in size from small vesicles to larger bullae filled with straw colored material. When these lesions rupture, an erythematous denuded area is found. In Ritter's disease the epidermis may be shed in sheets, and intact bullae are frequently sterile. A diagnosis of *Pseudomonas* or *Aeromonas* infection should be suspected in patients with ecthyma gangrenosum. Congenital syphilis may be suggested by the presence of maculopapular lesions, and in some cases bullae have been noted at birth, particularly on the palms and soles. The blisters develop on an erythematous base and may contain cloudy or hemorrhagic fluid that contains spirochetes. When the blisters rupture, a macerated area remains on which crusts form. *Candida* infection may be localized to the oral cavity or the diaper area. Paronychia may be seen in infants who suck their thumbs. The early cutaneous lesions are vesicular with a surrounding area of erythema. Pustules may develop, and a confluent erythematous moist erosion is soon noted. Facial or submandibular cellulitis occurs as an unusual manifestation of group B streptococcal infection. Oral moniliasis or thrush is characterized by the appearance of white cheesy material that clings to the oral, buccal, and even pharyngeal mucosa. Variola, vaccinia, herpes simplex, and herpes zoster viruses produce vesicular lesions that initially may be similar in appearance to each other, both clinically and histologically.

Diagnosis

A specific diagnosis should be based on smear and culture of the lesion. In patients with Ritter's disease, however, microorganisms may not be present within the intact bullous lesions. Blood cultures should be obtained and may be positive in neonates with cutaneous staphylococcal or streptococcal disease. *Candida* can be demonstrated by use of a potassium hydroxide preparation that shows pseudomycelia and may be cultured on Sabouraud's medium. Dark-field examination of bullous lesions may reveal *T. pallidum* in patients with congenital syphilis; when this diagnosis is suspected, appropriate serologic studies should be performed. Fluid obtained by aspiration of vesicles may permit identification of disease caused by various viral agents.

Treatment

Bacterial infections of the skin should be treated by systemic administration of antibiotics. Methicillin is appropriate for susceptible strains of staphylococci; penicillin G is used for streptococci or *T. pallidum*, as well as for ecthyma gangrenosum caused by *Pseudomonas* organisms. Intravenous fluid therapy may be required to maintain hydration in patients with Ritter's disease. Specific attention also should be paid to maintenance of adequate hemoglobin and serum albumin concentrations and to maintenance of body temperature. Incision and drainage will be required if abscesses are found. Oral *Candida* infections (thrush) respond well to administration of nystatin (Table 31-2), and *Candida* dermatitis can be treated with saline soaks or with 1:5,000 benzalkonium chloride washes and with nystatin cream. An old but effective treatment is 0.5% aqueous gentian violet applied directly to lesions.

Full evaluation for disseminated disease (Part two) should be carried out and treatment initiated promptly with vidarabine for vesicular lesions presumed to be caused by herpes simplex. Early initiation of treatment will prevent dissemination of localized infection and optimize outcome of generalized herpes infection heralded by cutaneous lesions.

Mastitis

Neonatal mastitis or breast abscess is attributed generally to infection with gram-positive organisms, usually staphylococci. Other organisms, however, may be responsible for mastitis, and cases caused by *E. coli*, *Pseudomonas*, *Proteus*, *Salmonella*, and group B streptococci have been described. The incidence is low; in one large center only 22 cases of neonatal mastitis were seen in a 9-year period.

Mastitis rarely develops during the first week of life but is seen more frequently during the second and third weeks after birth. Infection probably results from invasion of the duct system of the breast by skin flora. The breast may be erythematous, enlarged, and tender but is more likely to be firm than fluctuant. The disorder must be distinguished from enlargement that is physiologic and hormonally induced; the latter more likely will produce swelling bilaterally. Aspiration of the infected area for smear and culture and blood cultures are indicated. Infectious mastitis may be distinguished from milk stasis or noninfectious inflammation by the findings in milk samples of leukocyte counts exceeding 10^6/ml and bacterial counts greater than 10^3/ml. Methicillin should be used to treat staphylococcal disease and kanamycin or gentamicin for infection due to gram-negative microorganisms.

Parotitis

Suppurative parotitis is a rare disease in the newborn period; approximately 100 cases have been reported since 1878. Infection is caused by the ascent of microorganisms through Stensen's duct or may occur hematogenously. Typically, pregnancy and delivery are normal. From 7 to 14 days after birth, parotid gland swelling and fever may be noted. Facial paralysis may be present. The swollen parotid gland is accompanied by an area of erythema in the overlying skin; the gland may be tender, warm, firm, or fluctuant. Purulent material may drain spontaneously from Stensen's duct or may be expressed. Septicemia may accompany localized infection, and dehydration occurs preceding the onset of disease in some patients. Staphylococci are implicated most frequently, but *Pseudomonas* and *E. coli* may be offending agents.

Diagnosis should be made by smear and culture of purulent material obtained from Stensen's duct. Blood cultures should be obtained. Incision and drainage should be performed if the lesions are fluctuant. Systemic antibiotic treatment should be provided, and initial therapy should include coverage for *S. aureus* and *Pseudomonas* species. The disease must be differentiated from infections of the maxilla and from lymphangiomas, hemangiomas, lipomas, and adenomas.

Adrenal abscess

Adrenal abscesses have been reported on several occasions, following localization of microorganisms during an episode of septicemia or as a complication of adrenal hemorrhage. *E. coli*, *Bacteroides*, and group B streptococci have been isolated. This rare lesion must be distinguished from adrenal hemorrhage, suprarenal hematoma, neuroblastoma, and nephroblastoma. Abdominal ultrasonography may be helpful in suggesting the diagnosis.

Meningoencephalitis

Infection of the brain and meninges due to viruses and fungi or protozoal parasites also may be noted during the neonatal period. Transplacental infection with cytomegalovirus, rubella virus, and *Toxoplasma gondii* and perinatal infection with herpes simplex viruses are discussed in Parts two and three of this chapter. Poliovirus, Coxsackie virus, ECHO virus, varicella-zoster virus, and Epstein-Barr virus (EBV) may be acquired before, at, or following the time of delivery. Disorders caused by these agents, as well as tuberculosis and syphilis, are discussed in greater detail later. When conventional bacterial cultures of CSF are sterile in neonates with meningoencephalitis, infection with *Mycoplasma hominis* also should be considered.

Aseptic CNS infections vary in severity; some infants may have devastating disease and die of their infections, whereas in others no symptoms are apparent. In symptomatic infants, signs and symptoms identical to those found in newborns with septicemia or bacterial meningitis occur. Examination of CSF may reveal a pleocytosis that (after the first several days) will be predominantly lymphocytic. The CSF protein concentration may be elevated, but the glucose concentration generally is not depressed when compared with the blood glucose concentration. Etiologic diagnosis depends on isolation of virus from the throat, urine, stool, or CSF and demonstration of a significant rise in antibody titer to the virus that has been isolated. With the exception of vidarabine for herpes simplex meningoencephalitis, there is no antiviral compound for effective specific treatment of viral meningitis.

INFECTION BY SPECIFIC MICROORGANISMS

Anaerobic infection

Incidence

Chow and associates noted an incidence of anaerobic bacteremia of 1.8 cases per 1,000 live births; anaerobic microorganisms accounted for 26% of all cases of neonatal bacteremia. The relative frequency with which anaerobes were recovered from these newborns reflects, in part, their recovery from cord blood cultures; clinically significant anaerobic bacteremia in the neonatal period may be less frequent.

Pathogenesis

Prolonged rupture of the membranes, maternal amnionitis, prematurity, fetal distress, foul odor at birth, and respiratory distress are commonly associated with anaerobic infection. That these conditions might predispose to anaerobic septicemia is consistent with observations that *Bacteroides* and anaerobic streptococci are prevalent inhabitants of the genital tract at or near term and that a variety of anaerobic microorganisms are recovered toward the end of the first week of life from the oropharynx of the normal neonate. Anaerobic septicemia and meningitis also may follow or accompany anaerobic peritonitis in newborns with GI tract obstruction of necrotizing enterocolitis. Anaerobic microorganisms frequently may be recovered from gastric aspirates of newborns of mothers who have had ruptured membranes for more than 24 hours, but their recovery is associated infrequently with clinical disease. Bacteroidaceae, *Clostridium, Peptococcus, Peptostreptococcus,* and *Veillonella* are isolated most frequently from peritoneal fluid. Isolation of more than one anaerobe or of aerobes and anaerobes from the same specimen is common.

Clinical manifestations

The signs and symptoms of anaerobic septicemia or peritonitis are indistinguishable from those described for other forms of neonatal septicemia or in patients with peritonitis. Necrotizing enterocolitis (NEC) is a common finding in neonates with anaerobic peritonitis. Thrombocytopenia is observed commonly in patients with NEC and has been associated with endotoxemia.

Diagnosis

Anaerobic infection may be overlooked unless cultures employing special media and appropriate fermentative and gas-liquid chromatographic procedures are used. The cost of such techniques is high and warranted only in selected tertiary care centers. Where such techniques are available, blood cultures should be inoculated at the bedside into evacuated tubes containing media appropriate for isolation of anaerobic microorganisms.

Treatment

The choice of antibiotic treatment for anaerobic infection ideally should be based on accurate sensitivity data. Sensitivity determinations are difficult to perform with anaerobic organisms and are frequently unreliable indicators of therapeutic response in vivo. In general, penicillin is effective against virtually all gram-positive anaerobic microorganisms and against most gram-negative organisms. A prominent exception is *B. fragilis,* which is resistant to penicillin in most cases. Since this organism is commonly isolated from peritoneal fluid in newborns with intestinal perforation or NEC, consideration must be given to adding chloramphenicol or clindamycin to the therapeutic regimen. Clindamycin should not be used in patients with meningitis. The dosages administered should be those given for septicemia (Table 31-2). Metronidazole may be considered as an alternate therapy.

Prognosis

Mortality secondary to neonatal anaerobic septicemia varies from 4% to 37%.

Infant botulism

Incidence

In 1976, a syndrome suggesting infant botulism was described. Approximately half of all the reported cases have been located in California; however, cases have been confirmed in 25 other states, Great Britain, and Australia.

Etiology

Although extensive epidemiologic studies have been performed, no single source of the organism has been determined. Preformed toxin has not been noted in any food substances, but *C. botulinum* spores have been isolated from honey, vacuum cleaner dust, and soil around the home of one sick infant where excavation had taken place. Ingested spores of *C. botulinum* germinate, and the bacteria colonize the large intestine and elaborate toxin. Approximately 60% of infants studied have had type A organisms and 40% have had type B organisms.

Pathogenesis

C. botulinum toxin blocks the peripheral cholinergic synapses, producing a flaccid paralysis. The colon, where toxin formation and bacterial growth occur, is possibly less permeable to the toxin than is the small intestine. Thus there are low or nondetectable concentrations of toxin in the serum of most affected infants and, correspondingly, a less severe illness occurs than in older children or adults. The incubation period usually is 18 to 36 hours, but it may be as short as several hours or as long as 8 days.

Clinical manifestations

Constipation often is the first sign of illness. Muscle weakness is manifested by a less vigorous sucking ability, weak cry, loss of neck and limb strength, or generalized hypotonia and hyporeflexia. Progressive paralysis may ensue. Difficulty swallowing and absent cough reflex may be noted. Paralysis of the muscles of respiration may be characterized by aspiration pneumonia.

Diagnosis

Both organism and toxin can be found in the feces of the affected infant. Electromyography also may be helpful; brief, small-amplitude motor reaction potentials have been described.

Treatment

Supportive care is necessary for management of neurologic manifestations. Patients should not be fed by mouth until adequate gag reflex and swallowing are observed. Gavage feeding can supply the necessary nutritional intake and may stimulate the elimination of *C. botulinum* toxin and the organism via peristalsis. However, normal bowel motility may not return for several weeks. Respiratory and cardiovascular status should be monitored closely. Antibiotic therapy may eradicate the organism, but it has no effect on toxin that already has been elaborated and that is bound to tissues. Some drugs may eradicate anaerobic microorganisms in the gastrointestinal tract without eradicating *C. botulinum*. Close contact of the infected infant with other infants should be avoided, since the bacteria may be excreted in the stool for a period up to several months.

Prognosis

Complete recovery is generally observed, but it may require several months.

Listeria monocytogenes

Incidence

Although infection with *L. monocytogenes* may produce disease in normal healthy individuals, infection is more prevalent in the neonatal period or in adults with underlying disease.

Etiology

Listeriosis is caused by *L. monocytogenes*, a nonspore-forming, short gram-positive rod. It can be confused with diphtheroids on the basis of colonial morphology, and for this reason it is likely that the frequency with which it is isolated is underestimated. These bacteria may appear to be gram-negative because they decolorize readily during the Gram-staining procedure.

Pathogenesis

Listeriosis may develop at birth or may begin late in the neonatal period. Disease with early onset is acquired transplacentally from a mother with subclinical or clinical infection. Infection acquired early in pregnancy may lead to abortion and, if acquired later, to stillbirth or premature delivery. *L. monocytogenes* may be recovered from the vaginal canal or cervix of pregnant women; thus infection may be acquired at the time of delivery by aspiration or ingestion. *Listeria* organisms are isolated with great frequency from mothers of infants who develop *Listeria* infection during the first 5 days of life (early onset disease). Early onset disease is likely to be associated with maternal fever or other signs of maternal infection and with premature delivery. The development of late onset neonatal disease generally is not associated with maternal illness or maternal carriage of the organism. The distribution of *Listeria* serotypes from neonates with early and late onset disease also differs. Early onset disease is predominantly associated with recovery of serotypes Ia and Ib and occasionally with IVb from the blood of infected infants. Late onset disease is associated primarily with recovery of serotype IVb from the blood and CSF; it is predominantly a meningitic rather than septicemic infection. Several outbreaks of listeriosis, chiefly with serotype IVb, have been reported in newborns after ingestion of contaminated milk.

Clinical manifestation

The initial symptoms of listeriosis in both early and late onset disease are quite variable. Anorexia, lethargy and vomiting, jaundice, respiratory distress, cyanosis, petechial rashes, and evidence of myocarditis all have been noted. A high proportion of newborn infants with early onset listeriosis are meconium-stained at birth, even if they are preterm. Signs referable to the CNS are commonly associated with late onset disease. In some instances initial symptoms are absent, and in a few patients cultures of the meconium have grown *Listeria* without the development of overt infection. Hepatosplenomegaly and granulomas of the skin or posterior pharynx have been noted in some affected infants.

Diagnosis

Blood, CSF, and urine cultures should be obtained in all patients. Cultures of the vagina or cervix may support the diagnosis if *Listeria* organisms are recovered from the mothers of infants with early onset disease. A higher index of suspicion of infection caused by *L. monocytogenes* should exist if the maternal history includes prior stillbirth or repeated spontaneous abortions. CSF findings in cases of *Listeria* meningitis are identical to those observed in patients with other bacterial meningitides, with a predominance of polymorphonuclear leukocytes, an elevated protein concentration, and a depressed CSF glucose concentration. The organism may be seen on smear. Organisms also may be recovered from amniotic fluid or meconium. Enzyme-linked immunosorbent assay (ELISA) also has been used to aid in the diagnosis of listeriosis; this test has only fair sensitivity but good specificity (greater than 90%).

Treatment

Ampicillin is effective in most cases; however, therapy should be guided by sensitivity studies. Aminoglycoside may add synergy.

Prognosis

Mortality may be close to 100% in early onset infection but varies between 20% and 50% if disease develops between the fifth and thirteenth days of age. CNS sequelae are often observed. However, in the absence of meningitis or other CNS complications, the prognosis for normal development, even in premature babies, is good.

Group B β-hemolytic streptococci (*Streptococcus agalactiae*)

Incidence

An increasing number of reports of neonatal sepsis and meningitis due to *S. agalactiae* have appeared. Franciosi and associates reported an incidence of 2 cases per 1,000 live births.

Etiology

Group B streptococcal infection is caused by organisms that are gram-positive cocci that grow on solid media and in broth aerobically. Identification as a group B organism can be suggested by CAMP test and confirmed by specific precipitin or immunofluorescent methods.

Pathogenesis

S. agalactiae may be responsible for disease at or shortly after birth (early onset) or may be associated with infection that develops after 7 days of age. Hood and associates reported that of 151 mothers who had group B streptococci in their genital tracts, 56 (37%) experienced abortion, perinatal infant death, premature births, or serious illness in their infants. Other investigations have not confirmed these findings. Although colonization by group B streptococci was noted in 254 per 1,000 women during the third trimester and 262 per 1,000 newborns, Baker and associates found that the attack rate for neonatal infection was only 2.9 per 1,000 newborns.

Early onset group B streptococcal disease is acquired during passage through the birth canal of colonized women. The subtypes of group B streptococcal organisms isolated from infants with early onset disease are similar to those of the maternal vagina; group BI is the principal offender. In contrast, group BIII was the only subtype isolated by Franciosi and associates from infants with delayed onset disease; this subtype usually is not found in the mother but has been isolated from nursery personnel. Thus early onset disease is acquired intrapartum, whereas delayed onset infection generally is acquired from environmental sources.

The group B streptococcal serotype and its interaction with the host also determine the clinical expression of disease. Klesius and associates reported the presence of nonspecific opsonins for serotypes BIb, BIc, BII, and BIII in 95% of human sera, but only 10% of the population tested had specific BIa opsonizing antibody. These findings suggest a basis for the pathogenic potential of serotype BIa in the early neonatal period; this serotype is a frequent cause of early onset fatal septicemic disease. Type III isolates are the predominant cause of both early and late onset meningitis; this suggests that type III strains possess properties that permit meningeal invasion. The capsule of type III, group B streptococci contains a high content of sialic acid. This moiety apparently is capable of preventing activation of the alternate pathway for complement metabolism. In the absence of type-specific circulating antibody, failure of activation of the alternate pathway for complement metabolism results in inefficient opsonization of the type III, group B streptococcus. Poor opsonization leads to persistence of bacteremia and predisposes to a higher frequency of meningitis.

Clinical manifestations

Two distinct clinical syndromes are seen: an early septicemic form of disease or an illness whose onset is delayed and that is primarily meningitic in type. Early onset disease frequently is associated with obstetric complications. This form of the disease commonly includes acute respiratory distress and is characterized by other signs and symptoms of septicemia. Death occurs within hours to days in most patients and usually is related to pulmonary involvement. In most instances group B streptococci can be seen within and cultured from the lung. Late onset disease generally develops after 7 days of age, and meningitis is frequently noted. In these cases, clinical findings are those of bacterial meningitis. In some patients, usually with late onset disease, otitis media, septic arthritis, osteomyelitis, ethmoiditis, facial cellulitis, necrotizing fasciitis, and conjunctivitis have occurred. Asymptomatic bacteremia with group B streptococci has been documented. Pneumonia without septicemia also has been observed.

Diagnosis

Blood and CSF should be cultured and examined. Where appropriate antisera are available, a rapid diagnosis may be made by examination of blood, CSF, or urine by countercurrent immunoelectrophoresis or latex particle agglutination. Tracheal aspirate also may be acceptable for diagnostic purposes. Gastric washings, however, have not been adequate.

Treatment

Penicillin G or ampicillin should be given as described for septicemia or meningitis. Prophylactic treatment of maternal carriers is not indicated. Use of intravenous ampicillin during delivery of women with positive vaginal, cervical, or rectal cultures for group B streptococci at term has been associated with a significant decrease in colonization of their newborn infants with this organism. This approach may play a role in reducing the incidence of early-onset disease. At least one well-controlled large study suggests that administration of aqueous penicillin G at birth was associated with a decreased incidence of group B streptococcal disease as well as a decrease in disease caused by all penicillin-susceptible organisms. Since a concomitant increase in infection with gram-negative organisms may accompany this approach, it cannot be recommended for general implementation at this time.

Prognosis

Mortality from early onset disease varies from 70% to 100%. Mortality from delayed onset meningeal disease varies from 18% to 45%; survivors may experience hydrocephalus or other neurologic sequelae.

Neisseria gonorrhoeae (gonococcal disease)

Incidence

Gonorrhea is the most commonly reported communicable disease in the world; 100 million new cases are identified each year. In the United States it has been estimated that 2 million unreported cases and 1 million reported cases occur yearly. The incidence of gonococcal infection in pregnant women has ranged from 2.5% to 7.3% in recent studies. In this setting it is not surprising that infection of the neonate by *N. gonorrhoeae* occurs frequently.

Etiology

N. gonorrhoeae is an aerobic gram-negative diplococcus that is fastidious but that grows well on selected media.

Pathogenesis

Gonococcal infection may be acquired in utero as a result of orogastric contamination of an infant with *N. gonorrhoeae* following premature rupture of the membranes in an infected mother. The gonococcus also may invade mucosal surfaces, including the conjunctiva, rectal mucosa, and pharynx. Thus when maternal gonococcal infection is present, the neonate may acquire infection during delivery. Gonococcal infections also may be acquired postnatally from an infected adult or carrier.

Clinical manifestations

The most common neonatal form of disease is ophthalmitis (Chapter 39). Neonatal gonococcal arthritis and septicemia or meningitis also occur. Disseminated infection is more likely to occur when maternal gonococcal disease is symptomatic and associated with premature rupture of the membranes. Gonococcal vaginitis and scalp abscess have been reported in the newborn infant.

Diagnosis

Evaluation and treatment of neonates with possible gonococcal ophthalmitis have been discussed. Diagnosis of other forms of localized or disseminated gonococcal disease is dependent on identification of the organism on smear or culture of blood, pharynx, or localized lesions. Blood should be cultured at the bedside. Cotton swabs free from fatty acids should be used for collection of other specimens. When cultures are obtained, they should be plated on Thayer-Martin media and incubated in a 2% to 10% carbon dioxide atmosphere.

Treatment

Arthritis and septicemia should be treated by administration of aqueous penicillin G in a dosage of 75,000 to 100,000 units/kg/day in three divided doses for 7 days. Meningitis should be treated with aqueous penicillin G (100,000 units/kg/day in three divided intravenous doses for at least 10 days). Gonococci with increased resistance or complete resistance to penicillin have been recovered; in these cases, treatment must be guided by the specific sensitivity of the organism involved.

Management of a neonate born to a mother with gonococcal infection

All pregnant women should have endocervical cultures examined for gonococci near term as a routine part of prenatal care. Specific measures to prevent gonococcal ophthalmitis are indicated (see earlier discussion in this chapter). Orogastric and rectal cultures should be obtained from all patients of infected mothers, and blood also should be cultured if septicemia is suspected. Any positive gonococcal culture should be considered as presumptive evidence of disseminated gonococcal infection, and penicillin treatment as described for gonococcal septicemia should be initiated. Asymptomatic culture-negative infants should be treated with single doses of aqueous penicillin (50,000 units for fullterm infants and 25,000 units for preterm infants). An isolation period for 24 hours in the hospital is recommended. Mothers of these infants should observe them carefully following discharge from the nursery for signs and symptoms of arthritis or generalized infection.

Syphilis

Incidence

In recent years, congenital and neonatal syphilis has resurfaced as a significant problem. The incidence in the United States is currently higher than in other Western countries.

Etiology

Syphilis is caused by *T. pallidum,* a thin spirochetal organism that varies from 5 to 20 μm in length. It is killed by heat (40° to 42° C), by drying, by soap, and by water. It has not been cultured in vitro.

Pathogenesis and pathology

Syphilis in the newborn is a transplacental infection. Spirochetes rarely are found in fetal tissue before 18 weeks of intrauterine life, probably because the well-developed Langhans layer of the chorion presents a barrier to infection. After the sixteenth week of pregnancy, this layer atrophies, and fetal infection may follow. It has been suggested more recently that infections of the fetus may take place much earlier but that pathologic changes in the tissues do not occur until after the fifth month as the fetus becomes increasingly immunocompetent and inflammatory cells are found.

Spirochetemia may cause fetal wastage or death; stillbirths occur in about one fourth of pregnancies in untreated mothers. Normal children are born to only 30% of women who have had an untreated late syphilitic infection and to practically no untreated women who are infected during the first 7 months of pregnancy. The extent of disease in the newborn will depend on the time during gestation that a diagnosis of syphilis was made, the extent of disease in the mother, and the effectiveness of maternal treatment. Treatment of the mother before the eighteenth week of gestation almost always prevents signs of infection in the fetus, whereas treatment after the eighteenth week may cure fetal spirochetemia but will not always prevent the development of late stigmata of congenital syphilis. Since significant infection occurs after the first trimester of pregnancy, organ development is not affected, but all organ systems may be involved. Inflammatory and destructive changes may involve the liver, spleen, lung, bone, bone marrow, kidneys, and adrenal glands. Involvement of the CNS, teeth, and cornea may occur early but may not become apparent until late in infancy. Examination of the placenta in cases of congenital syphilis will reveal focal villitis and endovascular and perivascular proliferation in villous vessels (Chapter 11). Spirochetes may be visible.

Clinical manifestations

Infants who are severely affected may be born *hydropic,* (Chapter 6) a finding reported in up to 40% of cases in some recent series. Severe consolidated pneumonia may be present at birth. Profound anemia and hepatosplenomegaly, which may be related to extramedullary hematopoiesis, are relatively constant findings in these patients. In other patients there are no clinical findings for 1 to 3 weeks. Poor feeding initially and fever may be noted, and snuffles (syphilitic rhinitis) may appear. The nose becomes obstructed and discharges a clear, serosanguineous material. Purulent drainage may reflect secondary infection with streptococci or staphylococci. Cutaneous lesions have been reported at birth but usually are noted after 7 days of age. They are copper-colored maculopapular lesions that characteristically are distributed on the palms and soles and about the perioral, perinasal, and diaper areas. The rash may become vesicular and confluent in areas and may progress to involve the trunk and extremities. Perianal condylomata may form, and mucocutaneous lesions may develop. The lips may be roughened and cracked, and these lesions may evolve into radiating scars known as rhagades. Moist mucous membrane patches, exfoliation of nails, loss of hair, iritis, and choroiditis may occur. Syphilitic hepatitis with jaundice, generalized lymphadenopathy, pancreatitis, orchitis, colitis, and renal involvement characterized by the development of nephrotic syndrome may benoted. CNS involvement probably occurs early but is asymptomatic in most cases. Pleocytosis and increased CSF protein concentration may be found. Pseudoparalysis of the limbs may be observed but is relatively uncommon in comparison with the frequency with which involvement of bone can be noted roentgenographically.

Roentgenograms of the bones may show osteochondritis at the metaphyses and periostitis in over 90% of infants by 3 months of age. A radiolucent area may appear at the medial aspect of the proximal tibial metaphysis; this is called Wimberger's sign (Fig. 31-2). Subepiphyseal fractures or epiphyseal dislocations may occur. Roentgenograms may reveal a dense band at the epiphyseal ends, below which is a band of translucency. The line may be smooth or serrated; a serrated appearance is known as Wegener's sign and represents points of calcified cartilage aimed at the nutrient cartilage canal. Bone lesions may be present despite prenatal treatment

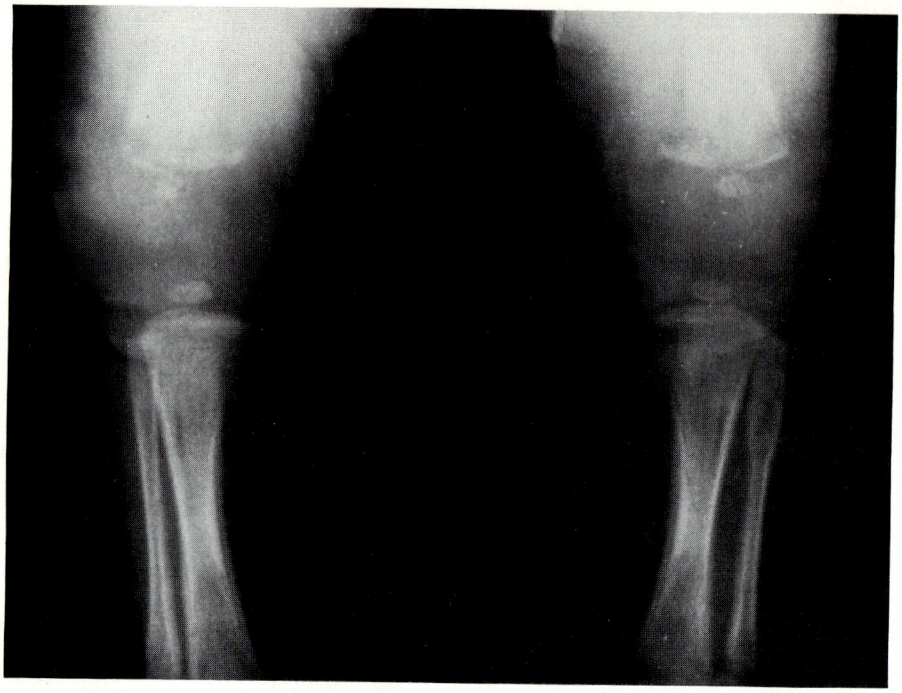

Fig. 31-2. Osteochondritis and periostitis of the bones in both lower extremities in a patient with congenital syphilis. Radiolucent area at the medial aspect of the proximal tibial metaphyses (Wimberger's sign) is present. Zone of translucency is visible proximal to the epiphyseal ends of both tibias (Wegner's sign).

but generally disappear with or without postnatal therapy by 10 months of age.

Diagnosis

It is possible to make a diagnosis of congenital syphilis by dark-field examination and/or direct fluorescent antibody staining of organisms obtained by scraping the skin or mucous membrane lesions or the umbilical cord. More commonly, diagnosis is suggested by the clinical and roentgenographic findings and confirmed by serologic testing. Invasion by *T. pallidum* results in the development of antibodies known as reagins that are not specific for the *Treponema* organism as well as antibodies to the *Treponema* organism itself. Nontreponemal antigens produce two types of antibodies: univalent antibodies that may be detected by complement fixation tests (Kolmer and Wassermann) and bivalent antibodies detectable by flocculation tests (Kahn, RPR, and VDRL). If transplacentally acquired antibody is responsible for a positive test in an uninfected infant, a reduction in infant titer of at least 50% occurs during the first month of life, and the titer returns to normal by 3 months.

Specific treponemal antigen tests include the *T. pallidum* immobilization (TPI) test, the fluorescent treponema antibody absorption test (FTA-ABS), and the FTA-ABS IgM test. Antibodies that react in the TPI and FTA-ABS tests cross the placenta; these tests are specific for infection with *T. pallidum* in the mother, but a single positive test does not document neonatal infection. The FTA-ABS IgM test initially appeared to be a promising diagnostic tool that suggested specific neonatal infection by *T. pallidum*. More recently, evidence has shown that the fetal IgM is directed against maternal IgG rather than against *T. pallidum*. For this reason, false positive results are not uncommon. A positive FTA-ABS or TPI test at or near the time of birth must be repeated at 1 and 2 months of age to determine whether the antibody titer is falling (reflecting maternal but not neonatal infection) or is increasing (suggesting active congenital syphilis). When clinical or serologic tests suggest congenital syphilis, CSF should be examined and a CSF FTA-ABS test performed. Treatment is indicated if any specific antibody test is positive and the physician is uncertain about cooperation with regard to follow-up serologic examinations.

Treatment

Asymptomatic congenital syphilis without CNS involvement (normal CSF) can be treated with an injection of benzathine penicillin G in a single dose of 50,000 units/

kg intramuscularly. Symptomatic congenital syphilis or neurosyphilis should be treated with aqueous crystalline penicillin G, 50,000 units/kg/day in two doses intramuscularly or intravenously for 10 days, or aqueous procaine penicillin G, 50,000 units/kg/day intramuscularly for 10 days.

Febrile reactions (Herxheimer's reactions) have been reported following initiation of treatment. Effective treatment is followed by disappearance of clinical signs, but roentgenographic findings may persist for 3 to 6 months. Blood and CSF serologic tests will become negative in several months.

Complications

When prenatal syphilis is not prevented or is unrecognized, late congenital syphilis may develop. Furthermore, the treatment of congenital syphilis after birth will not always prevent the late complications of the disease; only 60% of infants will have a positive serologic test for syphilis. Complications include interstitial keratitis, which may appear at any time but which generally appears during the second decade of life, deafness, neurosyphilis, Hutchinson's teeth (notched central incisors), mulberry molars, bone and joint involvement (saber shins, Clutton's joints), depressed nasal bridge, fissures about the nose and mouth, and gummas of the skin and other organs.

Prevention

A serologic test for syphilis should be performed early (first trimester) and late (third trimester) to ensure maximum possible protection of the fetus. If an FTA-ABS test performed on maternal serum is positive, maternal treatment should be instituted. Following therapy, the pregnant patient with syphilis should be followed with monthly titers to ensure that they fall as anticipated.

Chlamydia trachomatis

Incidence

Inclusion conjunctivitis and chlamydial pneumonia have been reported with increasing frequency. The number of pregnant women who are vaginally colonized with Chlamydia varies from 2% to 13%. In one study, conjunctivitis was reported in 35% and pneumonia in 20% of infants born to colonized mothers.

Etiology

C. trachomatis is an unusual organism with an intracellular and an extracellular phase; only the latter is infectious. The intracellular phase is necessary for survival of the organism, since chlamydiae cannot synthesize ATP. The organism can be grown in cell culture using McCoy cells, although this technique is available only in selected centers. Presumptive diagnosis can be made by finding inclusion bodies within epithelial cells obtained from conjunctival scrapings and processed using a Giemsa stain.

Pathogenesis

Chlamydial infections are acquired by passage through an infected birth canal. Inclusion conjunctivitis has been noted on the first day of life, suggesting that ascent of the organism may cause infection in utero. Chlamydiae also may be recovered from pharyngeal and rectal cultures.

Clinical manifestations

The most common neonatal form of disease is inclusion conjunctivitis. An afebrile pneumonia syndrome occurring between 2 and 12 weeks of age has been reported with increasing frequency. Chlamydiae also have been incriminated as a cause of otitis media in the newborn infant.

Diagnosis

Chlamydial conjunctivitis is suggested if purulent bilateral conjunctivitis is present from which no organisms are recovered using routine cultures. Identification of inclusion bodies on a Giemsa-stained smear of conjunctival scrapings strongly suggests this diagnosis. If the child has pneumonia, hyperinflation noted on a chest roentgenogram, a staccato cough, eosinophilia, and elevated serum immunoglobulins support the diagnosis of chlamydial infection.

Treatment

Pneumonia should be treated with oral erythromycin in a dosage of 40 mg/kg/day in 4 divided doses for 3 weeks. Conjunctivitis alone may be treated with the same dose of erythromycin for a 2-week period, along with irrigation of the eye with saline or buffered ophthalmic solution daily. Topical antibiotic is not necessary.

Tetanus

Incidence

Neonatal tetanus is usually seen where hygiene is poor; 20 to 30 cases occur in the United States yearly.

Etiology

Clostridium tetani is a slender, gram-positive, anaerobic spore-forming bacillus that is not invasive. It produces disease by elaboration of a soluble exotoxin. Two toxins are produced: tetanospasmin and tetanolysin. Tetanospasmin produces muscular spasms and convulsions; tetanolysin causes hemolysis of red blood cells in vitro but does not have this effect in humans.

Pathology

No specific pathologic lesions are attributed to this infectious agent, although changes in the brain and spinal cord have been described in patients dying of tetanus. Death generally is due to asphyxia, either because of laryngeal spasm, prolonged seizures, direct effect on the medullary center and the brainstem, or as a result of a secondary pulmonary infection.

Pathogenesis

The umbilical stump that is contaminated by soil or by feces or skin lesions may serve as a portal of entry for the organism. When toxin elaboration occurs, it probably reaches the CNS by progressing up the trunks of motor nerves. Muscular contractions are produced by its effect on the neuromuscular end-plates and on the anterior horn cells of the CNS. When toxin becomes fixed to nervous tissue, it cannot be neutralized by antitoxin. Antitoxin crosses the placenta; thus infants born to mothers whose tetanus immunizations are current will have adequate antitoxin levels.

Clinical manifestations

The incubation period ranges from 2 to 10 days. Initial symptoms include difficulty in feeding and excessive crying, and within a brief time trismus is observed, followed shortly by generalized muscle spasms, rigidity, and seizures. Deep tendon reflexes may be absent during spasms or may be increased. Opisthotonos may be extreme but may also be absent. Fever and cardiorespiratory difficulties, including tachycardia, tachypnea, cyanosis, or apnea, may be observed.

Differential diagnosis

When all of the characteristic clinical findings are present, a diagnosis is apparent. Trismus generally is not observed in neonates with meningitis, intracranial hemorrhage, or kernicterus. Hypocalcemia and hypomagnesemia may be associated with seizures, tremors, and laryngospasm, but generalized rigidity and trismus are absent. Phenothiazine derivatives can produce spasms of the muscles of the neck and back, trismus, and dysphagia, but phenothiazine toxicity should be excluded by history or by metabolic studies of blood and urine. The rapid tonic seizures of tetanus are not found in individuals suffering from phenothiazine intoxication.

Treatment

The maintenance of a clear airway and provision of adequate ventilation are most important. Meticulous care must be exercised to decrease the likelihood of secondary bacterial pulmonary infections; this includes frequent suctioning under sterile conditions. Diazepam as required (0.1 to 2.0 mg) is the most effective agent in controlling seizures and rigidity in patients with tetanus. Barbiturates may be indicated as an adjunct to therapy and may help to sedate the patient. Penicillin G should be given intravenously to eradicate *Clostridium* organisms that may continue to elaborate toxin. The bladder may need to be catheterized if it does not empty spontaneously. Although there is little evidence that tetanus antitoxin is efficacious if administered after clinical symptoms are apparent, it is recommended. Human tetanus–immune globulin (1,500 units) should be given intramuscularly. Active immunization against tetanus is still required, since recovery from tetanus does not confer permanent immunity.

Prevention

A well-immunized mother offers the best protection against tetanus neonatorum. Aseptic obstetric and neonatal care minimizes the likelihood of introduction of *Clostridium* organisms.

Tuberculosis

Incidence

Clinical tuberculosis is rare during the first month of life; however, management of the infant born to a mother who has tuberculosis is not an uncommon problem. Tuberculosis that becomes apparent during the first month of life may be congenital in etiology or acquired at or after the time of delivery by aspiration or inhalation.

Etiology

Mycobacterium tuberculosis var. *hominis* is the usual cause of congenital or neonatal disease. Infection with bovine strains of *M. tuberculosis* or with atypical *Mycobacterium* species is rare but has been reported.

Pathology

When disease is acquired via the umbilical vein, a primary complex forms in the porta hepatis of the liver, and miliary tubercles may be found in the spleen, bone marrow, lung, kidney, adrenal glands, and brain and on serosal surfaces. Gross or microscopic placental lesions may be detected. If the primary complex is located in the lungs, it is assumed that infection followed aspiration of amniotic fluid or vaginal secretions contaminated with tubercle bacilli or by inhalation.

Pathogenesis

Most cases of congenital tuberculosis are acquired hematogenously. Although the mother generally has miliary tuberculosis, congenital tuberculosis has been diagnosed in infants born to mothers with endometrial or cervical disease who have no pulmonary involvement and who also have negative tuberculin tests. Uninfected infants have been born to mothers who have miliary disease. Placental tuberculosis may be present without neonatal disease. Proof of congenital tuberculosis requires demonstration of active disease in the mother and child with no postpartum contact between the two and demonstration of a primary complex in the liver. Rupture of a caseating placental or endometrial granuloma may contaminate amniotic fluid, and the neonate may acquire disease by aspiration. Tuberculosis also can be contracted after delivery from other individuals with active pulmonary infection. In these cases, symptoms in the infants generally are delayed beyond 1 month of age. There often is a maternal history of spotty vaginal bleeding during the pregnancy.

Clinical manifestations

Symptoms of tuberculosis in the neonatal period may be nonspecific and include poor feeding, vomiting, weight loss, and fever. Respiratory symptoms may be absent, or cough and severe respiratory distress may develop. Hepatosplenomegaly, generalized lymphadenopathy, and pneumonia may be found. Obstructive jaundice, meningitis, and osteomyelitis are more common in neonates who acquire disease at or after birth than in patients with congenital tuberculosis. Infants with congenital tuberculosis frequently are born prematurely, and signs of disease may not appear for several days or even weeks. Otitis media may be seen, particularly in infants who aspirate infected amniotic fluid. Tuberculous otitis media frequently results in perforation of the tympanic membrane and commonly is associated with deafness and facial nerve paralysis.

Diagnosis

Examination of the placenta should be performed in every mother with possible tuberculosis. If tuberculous granulomas are noted, tuberculosis in the child should be suspected; however, they have been noted in some cases in which no disease developed in the newborn. Demonstration of acid-fast organisms on tracheal or gastric aspirate smears also aids in making a presumptive diagnosis. Gastric washings, urine specimens, and material obtained by aspiration of bone marrow or lymph nodes should be cultured for *Mycobacterium* organisms. Chest roentgenographs may suggest pulmonary tuberculosis. Generally, the tuberculin test is not positive for 4 to 6 weeks, even in neonates who are infected in utero. The tuberculin test may remain negative in the face of active disease. Lumbar puncture should be performed and CSF examined and cultured to exclude CNS involvement.

Treatment

Active neonatal tuberculosis should be treated initially with isoniazid (INH) in an oral dosage of 30 mg/kg/day in two divided doses and streptomycin at 20 to 30 mg/kg/day in two divided doses administered intramuscularly. Streptomycin therapy should be continued for 3 or 4 months. Therapy with isoniazid is continued for 18 to 24 months, and para-aminosalicylic acid (PAS) may be substituted for streptomycin when it is discontinued. Ethambutol and rifampin have not been evaluated in the neonatal period. When necessary because of infection with mycobacteria that are resistant to isoniazid, rifampin may be given in a dosage of 20/mg/kg/day. Ethambutol can be administered in a dosage of 25 mg/kg/day for 2 months followed by reduction in dosage to 15 mg/kg/day. Retrobulbar neuritis with loss of visual acuity is a prominent side effect of ethambutol; hence its use in the neonate whose visual acuity cannot be tested is not recommended unless no alternatives are available. Kanamycin in appropriate dosage may be substituted for streptomycin. Corticosteroids have been used in critically ill infants, particularly in those with CNS infection who have an actual or impending blockage to the flow of CSF or in patients with respiratory distress as a result of endobronchial disease.

Management of the newborn whose mother has tuberculosis

Infants born to mothers known to have active tuberculosis should be separated immediately from their mothers. Appropriate diagnostic studies should be performed to determine the possibility of active tuberculosis in the infant. Treatment with isoniazid also should be initiated in therapeutic dosage. If neonatal tuberculosis is confirmed, streptomycin should be added and treatment carried out as indicated in the previous section. If neonatal tuberculosis is excluded, the isoniazid dosage should be decreased to 10 mg/kg/day and treatment continued with this single drug for a period of 1 year. Alternatively, isoniazid therapy may be provided for only 3 months. At the end of this period, if a chest roentgenogram and tuberculin test are still negative, isoniazid may be discontinued, and BCG vaccine may be administered. If this mode of therapy is chosen and if active disease in the mother is still present, the infant must be isolated from the mother until the tuberculin test in the infant becomes positive (about 6 weeks) or until the mother is no longer considered to have active disease.

When maternal pulmonary tuberculosis has been treated for at least 1 week, and if compliance with regard to maternal therapy is ensured, infant and maternal contact can be permitted provided that isoniazid prophylaxis of the infant also is ensured. In cases of maternal pulmonary tuberculosis that become apparent during pregnancy but for which treatment has been provided and in which the sputum no longer contains *Mycobacterium* organisms, isoniazid at 10 mg/kg/day should be prescribed for the infant for a period of 1 year; a period of separation from the mother is not necessary.

When maternal tuberculosis is active and/or when other cases of tuberculosis are known to be present in the household but compliance with regard to treatment of the adults cannot be ensured, the following are recommended:

1. The baby should be separated from the mother and other household contacts with active disease.
2. Active tuberculosis of the neonate must be excluded by chest roentgenogram and tuberculin testing before BCG administration, unless administration of BCG is carried out before 2 weeks of age.
3. Immunization with BCG should be provided.
4. When the tuberculin test becomes positive as a result of BCG immunization, the infant may be returned to the family setting if, in the interim, efforts have been made to ensure treatment of adults with active disease.

It is also important to observe infants who have received BCG, since BCG failures have been reported, and the infant might have acquired tuberculosis before immunization. One study has shown that preterm infants who are appropriate for gestational age (up to 32 weeks) could be immunized effectively with BCG.

Most commonly, the physician is faced with the delivery of an infant born to a mother with a history of treated tuberculosis who has not received therapy for a number of years before pregnancy and delivery. The possibility of relapse is greatest just after delivery, and the relapse rate is greatest in individuals whose disease has been arrested for less than 5 years. The risk to such an infant is dependent on the likelihood of reactivation of maternal disease; thus frequent examinations of the mother are imperative. Postpartum chest roentgenograms obtained at 1, 3, and 6 months after delivery are indicated. The infant should be tuberculin-tested at 6 weeks of age and at intervals of 3 months during the first year of life. If there is any question with regard to reactivation, treatment of the mother and infant with isoniazid is indicated.

PREVENTION OF INFECTION IN THE NEONATAL UNIT

Barrier nursing technique

Several controlled trials have demonstrated that the use of masks and gowns by nursery personnel affected neither staphylococcal carriage rates nor infectious illness in infants but tended to keep personnel away from their patients. Virtually all controlled clinical trials have demonstrated that effective hand-washing is responsible for the absence of nosocomial infection in nursery units. Conversely, ineffective hand-washing techniques frequently have been associated with epidemic disease. Hexachlorophene (3% as a liquid soap or cream) has proved to be extremely effective in preventing infection by gram-positive bacteria, and various iodinated preparations, including chlorhexidine (0.5%), are effective against gram-negative organisms. These agents have a cumulative effect when used repeatedly for hand-washing. *P. aeruginosa* has been recovered from both types of germicidal solution; thus attention must be paid to sterilization of the containers from which these materials are dispensed. Even a quick dip and rinse followed by the mechanical process of drying the hands with a paper towel is extremely effective in reducing the transmission of organisms from the hands of personnel to patients.

Routine hexachlorophene bathing of infants

Intensive or extensive exposure to hexachlorophene produces vacuolation in myelinated regions of the animal brainstem and cerebellum. Toxic encephalopathy was reported among infants in France, attributable to the accidental incorporation of excessive amounts of hexachlorophene in baby talcum powder. Possible neuropathologic effects have been attributed to the use of three or more daily baths in 3% hexachlorophene, primarily in infants who weighed 1,400 gm or less at birth and who lived in the nursery environment for more than 3 days. Infants receiving fewer than three baths with 3% hexachlorophene or infants bathed in a 100-fold dilution of 3% hexachlorophene were at a much lower risk of disease. None of the infants in the studies reported who weighed more than 1,400 gm and who were bathed fewer than three times in 3% hexachlorophene or who were bathed in a 100-fold dilution of 3% hexachlorophene demonstrated neuropathologic lesions. Clinical correlates of these pathologic findings have not been established in most cases. It is possible that the neuropathology may even be self-limiting or reversible following withdrawal of hexachlorophene.

These findings, however, prompted the recommendation that routine hexachlorophene bathing of neonates be discontinued. Subsequently, some hospital nurseries have experienced an increased incidence of staphylococcal infection. In view of these events, the following recommendations can be made. In the absence of infection, prophylactic bathing with hexachlorophene should not be performed. Rather, emphasis must be placed on reliable surveillance of neonatal disease, prompt isolation and treatment of infected infants, and adequate hand-washing. Hexachlorophene should still be used as an antibacterial agent by personnel working in the neonatal unit. Crowding should be avoided, and cohort nursing techniques should be employed wherever possible. When these practices are inadequate for infection control, antibacterial bathing regimens employing hexachlorophene should be initiated temporarily. If infants are bathed with hexachlorophene, they should be rinsed carefully to ensure that no residual hexachlorophene remains on the surface of the skin. Hibiclens, which is absorbed, has been used for this purpose by some centers.

Antibiotic prophylaxis

There is no evidence that infection is prevented by giving antibiotics to high-risk infants who are not infected. There is also no evidence that antibiotic prophylaxis is required for patients with respiratory distress syndrome or for neonates during and subsequent to exchange transfusion. Prophylaxis, however, is indicated for the prevention of gonococcal ophthalmitis.

Artificial bacterial colonization

The deliberate introduction of a nonvirulent strain of a microorganism to prevent colonization with virulent strains has been recommended and in some nurseries has proved effective in aborting epidemic bacterial infection in the newborn. Deliberate introduction of nonvirulent strains of coagulase-positive staphylococci in the nose and colonization of the umbilicus shortly after birth have been used. Infections have been reported that were related to the nonvirulent staphylococci introduced in this manner, suggesting that application of this technique may be hazardous and should be limited to selected and carefully controlled situations.

Care of the umbilicus

The umbilicus is a direct portal of entry to the bloodstream and also serves as a site from which other areas of the skin may become contaminated or colonized. In instances where the cord will not be used for arterial or venous catheterization, the application of triple dye to reduce bacterial colonization is recommended.

Resuscitation and ventilation equipment

Gram-negative microorganisms, particularly *Pseudomonas*, *Aeromonas*, and *Serratia*, have produced both sporadic and epidemic infection in the neonatal unit. Culturing of medications, nebulizers, and inhalation therapy equipment should be performed routinely, and equipment should be changed frequently to prevent such infections. Use of umbilical, arterial, and venous catheters as well as intravenous catheters for parenteral alimentation also has been accompanied by an increased risk of opportunistic infection. Meticulous care is required in the preparation of solutions for use in total parenteral alimentation and in the insertion and care of catheters. Administration of fluids should be discontinued if signs of inflammation, thrombosis, or purulence are observed. When bacteremia related to intravenous therapy is noted, discontinuation of therapy is imperative; continued infusion of the suspect infusate under coverage of antimicrobials has not altered the course of infection. All apparatus used for intravenous administration should be replaced, both daily and when infusion devices are changed, to decrease the hazard of extrinsic contamination.

Ralph D. Feigin
Stuart L. Abramson
Morven S. Edwards

BIBLIOGRAPHY

Neonatal septicemia

Baker, C.J., and others: Suppurative meningitis due to streptococci of Lancefield group B: a study of 33 infants, J. Pediatr. **82**:724, 1973.

Blanc, W.A.: Pathways of fetal and early neonatal infection, J. Pediatr. **59**:473, 1961.

Bobo, R.A., and others: Nursery outbreak of *Pseudomonas aeruginosa:* epidemiological conclusions from five different typing methods, Appl. Microbiol. **25**:414, 1973.

Edwards, M.S., and others: Long-term sequelae of group B streptococcal meningitis in infants, J. Pediatr. **106**:717, 1985.

Fetter, B.F., Klintworth, G.H., and Hendry, W.S.: Mycoses of the central nervous system, Baltimore, 1967, The Williams & Wilkins Co.

Geil, C.C., Castle, W.K., and Mortomer, E.A., Jr.: Group A streptococcal infections in newborn nurseries, Pediatrics **46**:849, 1970.

Gotoff, S.P., and Behrman, R.E.: Neonatal septicemia, J. Pediatr. **76**:142, 1970.

Hable, K.A., and others: *Klebsiella* type 33 septicemia in an infant intensive care unit, J. Pediatr. **80**:920, 1972.

Kaplan, J.M., and others: Pharmacologic studies in neonates given large doses of ampicillin, J. Pediatr. **84**:571, 1974.

Klein, J.O.: Recent advances in management of bacterial meningitis in neonates, Infection **12**(suppl.):44, 1984.

Knittle, M.A., Etizman, D.V., and Baer, H.: Role of hand contamination of personnel in the epidemiology of gram-negative nosocomial infections, J. Pediatr. **86**:433, 1975.

Laurenti, F., and others: Polymorphonuclear leukocyte transfusion for the treatment of sepsis in the newborn infant, J. Pediatr. **98**:118, 1981.

Lee, Y., and others: The genital mycoplasmas: their role in disorders of reproduction and in pediatric infections, Pediatr. Clin. North Am. **21**:457, 1974.

McCracken, G.H., and Mize, S.G.: A controlled study of intrathecal antibiotic therapy in gram-negative enteric meningitis of infancy. I. Pediatr. **89**:66, 1976.

McCracken, G.H., Jr., and Nelson, J.D., editors: Antimicrobial therapy for newborns, New York, 1983, Grune & Stratton, Inc.

McCracken, G.H., and others: Moxalactam therapy for neonatal meningitis due to gram-negative enteric bacilli: a prospective controlled evaluation, JAMA **252**:1427, 1984.

Okada, D.M., Chow, A.W., and Bruce, V.T.: Neonatal scalp abscess and fetal monitoring: factors associated with infection, Am. J. Obstet. Gynecol. **129**:185, 1977.

Overbach, A.M., Daniel, S.J., and Cassady, G.: The value of umbilical cord histology in the management of potential perinatal infection, J. Pediatr. **76**:22, 1970.

Pryles, C.V., and others: A controlled study of the influence on the newborn of prolonged premature rupture of the amniotic membranes and/or infection in the mother, Pediatrics **31**:608, 1963.

Yeung, C.Y., Lee, V.W.Y., and Yeung, M.B.: Glucose disappearance rate in neonatal infection, J. Pediatr. **82**:486, 1973.

Specific infectious diseases

Atkinson, G.O., Jr. and others: Adrenal abscess in the neonate, Radiology **155**:101, 1985.

Bazay, G.R., and others: *Pneumocystis carinii* pneumonia in three fullterm siblings, J. Pediatr. **5**:767, 1970.

Bland, R.D.: Otitis media in the first six weeks of life: diagnosis, bacteriology, and management, Pediatrics **49**:187, 1972.

Dan, M.: Neonatal septic arthritis, Isr. J. Med. Sci. **19**:967, 1983.

Edwards, M.S., and others: An etilogic shift in infantile osteomyelitis: the emergence of the group B streptococcus, J. Pediatr. **93**:578, 1978.

Esterly, N.B., and Solomon, L.M.: Neonatal dermatology. II. The blistering and scaling dermatoses, J. Pediatr. **77**:1075, 1970.

Forshall, I.: Septic umbilical arteritis, Arch. Dis. Child. **32**:25, 1957.

Goscienski, P.J.: Inclusion conjunctivitis in the newborn infant, J. Pediatr. **77**:19, 1970.

Haltalin, K.C.: Neonatal shigellosis: report of 16 cases and review of the literature, Am. J. Dis. Child. **114**:603, 1967.

Haney, P.J., Bohlman, M., and Sun, C.C.J.: Radiographic findings in neonatal pneumonia, A.J.R. **143**:23, 1984.

Kaslow, R.A., and others: Enteropathogenic *Escherichia coli* infection in a newborn nursery, Am. J. Dis. Child. **128**:797, 1974.

Kohl, S.: *Yersinia enterocolitica:* a significant "new" pathogen, Hosp. Pract. **13**:81, 1978.

Leake, D., and Leake, R.: Neonatal suppurative parotitis, Pediatrics **46**:203, 1970.

McCracken, G.H., Jr., and Sarff, L.D.: Current status and therapy of neonatal *E. coli* meningitis, Hosp. Pract. **10**:57, 1974.

Naeye, R.L., Dellinger, W.S., and Blanc, W.A.: Fetal and maternal features of antenatal bacterial infections, J. Pediatr. **9**:733, 1971.

Nelson, J.D.: Antibiotic concentrations in septic joint effusions, N. Engl. J. Med. **284**:349, 1971.

Pederson, P.V., and others: Necrotising enterocolitis of the newborn—is it gas gangrene of the bowel? Lancet **2**:715, 1976.

Pittard, W.B., Thullen, J.D., and Fanaroff, A.A.: Neonatal septic arthritis, J. Pediatr. **88**:621, 1976.

Prophylaxis of gonococcal ophthalmitis, The Medical Letter **12**:37, 1970.

Robbins, J.B., and others: *Escherichia coli* K1 capsular polysaccharide associated with neonatal meningitis, N. Engl. J. Med. **290**:1215, 1974.

Sarff, L.D., Platt, L.H., and McCracken, G.H., Jr.: Cerebrospinal fluid evaluation in neonates: comparison of high risk infants with and without meningitis, J. Pediatr. **88**:473, 1976.

Shurin, P.A., and others: Bacterial etiology of otitis media during the first six weeks of life, J. Pediatr. **92**:893, 1978.

Tetzlaff, T.R., Ashworth, C., and Nelson, J.D.: Otitis media in children less than 12 weeks of age, Pediatrics **59**:827, 1977.

Torphy, D.E., and Bond, W.W.: *Campylobacter fetus* infections in children, Pediatrics **64**:898, 1979.

Ulshen, M.H., and Rollo, J.L.: Pathogenesis of *E. coli* gastroenteritis in man—another mechanism, N. Engl. J. Med. **302**:99, 1980.

Weissberg, E.D., Smith, A.L., and Smith, D.H.: Clinical features of neonatal osteomyelitis, Pediatrics **53**:505, 1974.

Specific bacterial infections

Albritton, W.L., Wiggins, G.L., and Feeley, J.C.: Neonatal listeriosis: distribution of serotypes, J. Pediatr. **88**:481, 1976.

Alexander, R.R.: Chlamydia: the organism and neonatal infection, Hosp. Pract. **14**:63, 1979.

Baker, C.J.: Group B streptococcal infections in neonates, Pediatr. **64**:P1R5, 1979.

Baker, C.J., and others: Suppurative meningitis due to streptococci of Lancefield group B: a study of 33 infants, J. Pediatr. **82**:724, 1973.

Boyer, K.M., and Gotoff, S.P.: Prevention of early-onset neonatal group B streptococcal disease with selective intrapartum chemoprophylaxis, N. Engl. J. Med. **314**:1665, 1986.

Chow, A.W., and others: The significance of anaerobes in neonatal bacteremia: analysis of 23 cases and review of the literature, Pediatrics **54**:736, 1974.

Franciosi, R.A., Knostman, J.D., and Zimmerman, R.M.: Group B streptococcal neonatal and infant infections, J. Pediatr. **82**:707, 1973.

Handsfield, H.H., Hodson, W.A., and Holmes, K.K.: Neonatal gonococcal infection, JAMA **225**:697, 1973.

Holder, W.R., and Knox, J.M.: Syphilis in pregnancy, Med. Clin. North Am. **56**:1151, 1972.

Hood, M., Janney, A., and Dameron, G.: Beta-hemolytic streptococcus Group B associated with problems of the perinatal period, Am. J. Obstet. Gynecol. **82**:809, 1961.

Horn, K.A., and others: Group B streptococcal neonatal infection, JAMA **230**:1165, 1974.

Howard, J.B., and McCracken, G.H., Jr.: The spectrum of group B streptococcal infections in infancy, Am. J. Dis. Child. **128**:815, 1974.

Kendig, E.L., Jr.: The place of BCG vaccine in the management of infants born to tuberculous mothers, N. Engl. J. Med. **281**:520, 1969.

Klesius, P.H., and others: Cellular and humoral immune response to group B streptococci, J. Pediatr. **83**:926, 1973.

Koutsoulieris, E., and Koslaris, E.: Congenital tuberculosis, Arch. Dis. Child. **45**:584, 1970.

Litt, I.F., Edberg, S.C., and Finberg, L.: Gonorrhea in children and adolescents: a current review, J. Pediatr. **85**:595, 1974.

Mardh, P.A.: *Mycoplasma hominis* infection of the central nervous system in newborn infants, Sex. Transm. Dis. **10**(suppl. 4):331, 1983.

McCracken, G.H., Jr., Dowell, D.L., and Marshall, F.N.: Double blind trial of equine antitoxin and human immune globulin in tetanus neonatorum, Lancet **1**:1146, 1971.

McCracken, G.H., Jr., and Kaplan, J.M.: Penicillin treatment for congenital syphilis, JAMA **228**:855, 1974.

Pinheiro, D.: Tetanus of the newborn infant, Pediatrics **34**:32, 1964.

Ray, C.G., and Wedgwood, R.J.: Neonatal listeriosis, Pediatrics **34**:378, 1964.

Rosen, E.V., and Richardson, J.N.: A reappraisal of the value of the IgM fluorescent treponemal antibody absorption test in the diagnosis of congenital syphilis, J. Pediatr. **87**:38, 1975.

Russell, P., and Altshuler, G.: Placental abnormalities of congenital syphilis, Am. J. Dis. Child. **128**:160, 1974.

Siegel, J.D., and others: Single-dose penicillin prophylaxis against neonatal group B streptococcal infections, N. Engl. J. Med. **303**:769, 1980.

Yow, M.D., and others: Ampicillin prevents intrapartum transmission of group B streptococcus, JAMA **241**:1245, 1979.

Prevention of infection

Drutz, D.J., and others: Bacterial interference in the therapy of recurrent staphylococcal infections: multiple abscesses due to the implantation of the 502A strain of *Staphylococcus,* N. Engl. J. Med. **275**:1161, 1966.

Ehrenkranz, N.J.: Bacterial colonization of newborn infants and subsequent acquisition of hospital bacteria, J. Pediatr. **76**:839, 1970.

Geil, G.C., Castle, W.K., and Mortimer, E.A.: Group A streptococcal infections in newborn nurseries, Pediatrics **46**:849, 1970.

Gezon, H.M., and others: Hexachlorophene bathing in early infancy: effect on staphylococcal disease and infection, N. Engl. J. Med. **270**:379, 1964.

Gluck, L., and Wood, H.F.: Effect of an antiseptic skin-care regimen in reducing staphylococcal colonization in newborn infants, N. Engl. J. Med. **265**:1177, 1961.

Hurst, V., and Grossman, M.: The hospital nursery as a source of staphylococcal disease among families of newborn infants, N. Engl. J. Med. **262**:951, 1960.
Light, I.J., and others: Ecologic relation between *Staphylococcus aureus* and *Pseudomonas* in a nursery population: another example of bacterial interference, N. Engl. J. Med. **278**:1243, 1968.
Lockhart, J.D.: How toxic is hexachlorophene? Pediatrics **50**:229, 1972.
Mortimer, E.A., Wolinsky, E., and Hines, D.: The effect of rooming-in on the acquisition of hospital staphylococci by newborn infants, Pediatrics **37**:605, 1966.
Shuman, R.M., Leech, R.W., and Alvord, E.C.: Neuropathology in newborn infants bathed with hexachlorophene. Morbid. Mortal. **22**:93, March 17, 1973.
Williams, C.P.S., and Oliver, T.K.: Nursery routines and staphylococcal colonization of the newborn, Pediatrics **44**:640, 1969.

PART TWO

Viral infections

It is increasingly apparent that certain viruses and protozoa have a predilection for the fetus and may cause abortion, stillbirth, intrauterine infection, congenital malformations, acute disease during the neonatal period, or chronic infection, with subtle manifestations that may be recognized only after a prolonged period. It is important to recognize the manifestations of viral and protozoal infections in the neonatal period not only to diagnose the acute infection but also to anticipate the potential implication for the subsequent growth and development of the infant.

HERPESVIRUS ORGANISMS

Herpes simplex virus

Recent media coverage of genital herpes infections has resulted in considerable public anxiety. Certainly herpes simplex virus (HSV) infections among neonates are being diagnosed more frequently. Although HSV previously was estimated to occur once in every 8,000 to 10,000 deliveries, more recent data indicate the rate may be twice as high.

Pathogenesis

The herpes viruses belong to a group of DNA viruses that cause latent infection, lasting for the lifetime of the individual and resulting in periodic recurrences. There are no seasonal variations or regional epidemics of HSV infections, and direct contact is necessary for the transmission of the virus. Virus has been shown to survive on fomites for as long as 88 hours, particularly if the surface is moist, but transmission of disease from these fomites has not been proved and must be exceedingly uncommon. The attack rate for HSV-1 infections either in the oral cavity or above the waist is highest among 1- to 3-year-old children. These primary HSV infections in early childhood usually result from contact with a family member and are most often asymptomatic. Most individuals in the lower socioeconomic classes are infected during childhood, but two thirds of those in the middle or upper groups are still uninfected as young adults. Recurrent disease will occur in 20% to 45% of oral infections.

In contrast, genital infections usually are caused by HSV-2 and are transmitted predominantly by sexual contact. They occur most commonly after the age of 15 years. HSV-1, however, now is being isolated from 10% to 40% of teenagers with primary genital infections. The majority of genital infections are asymptomatic, probably because most of the infections involve the cervix, which has few sensory nerve endings.

Maternal clinical manifestations

Primary infection already has occurred in 10% to 35% of women of childbearing age. Genital infection usually begins with local tenderness and burning, involving the labia and vaginal mucosa, 2 to 7 days following sexual contact. Although both symptomatic and asymptomatic individuals may transmit infection, the risk of infection after intercourse is not known. Following a period of paresthesia, vesicles full of seropurulent fluid develop. These vesicles break down easily forming shallow ulcers and releasing fluid containing large numbers of infectious virus particles. There is often copious watery, vaginal discharge, edema, dysuria, and bilateral pelvic and inguinal lymphadenopathy, accompanied by systemic symptoms of fever, malaise, and headache. The pain may last 10 to 14 days with healing occurring 2 to 5 weeks later. Viral shedding is heaviest during the first 3 to 4 days and generally absent from lesions after 2 weeks, but cervical shedding of the virus, which occurs in 80% to 90% of primary infections, may continue for weeks. Asymptomatic primary infections occur in at least 50% of women.

Recurrence is four times greater with HSV-2 genital infection than with HSV-1. The HSV-2 is shed in smaller amounts than in primary infections, and not generally after 7 days. Cervical virus shedding may occur, but it is less frequent. If cervical lesions are not visible, the shedding involves 1,000-fold less virus than in primary infections. However, HSV was isolated from the cervix in 10% of asymptomatic women who had a history of a genital infection within the previous 6 months. Pregnancy increases both the frequency of infection and the persistence of the virus. Whitley and colleagues studied infected neonates and found that 70% of the mothers had no signs or symptoms of infection, although 13% had sexual partners with penile lesions.

Fetal and neonatal transmission

Transplacental transmission of HSV infection to the neonate may occur during maternal viremia. However, an ascending transcervical infection, first involving the intact fetal membranes, then resulting in chorioamnionitis, probably is more common. It is likely that ascending infection is responsible for the premature rupture of membranes, rather than the rupture of membranes leading to infection. The use of fetal monitoring electrodes accelerates the transcervical infection and breaches the infant's skin barrier, increasing the risk of infection. The occurrence of an ascending infection despite intact membranes may be reflected by the tripled rate of spontaneous abortions in the first 20 weeks of gestation with genital HSV infections, the occasional occurrence of fetal malformations of a similar pattern, the development of neonatal herpes infections in infants delivered by cesarean section with intact membranes, and the high rate of prematurity among infected infants. Nonetheless, the majority of infants show no evidence of infection in utero.

Congenital infections

Congenital herpes simplex is rare and probably results from destruction of normally formed organs, rather than defects in organogenesis, since the lesions are similar to those of neonatal herpes. The infants are usually growth-retarded and have severe psychomotor retardation with intracranial calcifications, microcephaly, hypertonicity, and seizures. All of the children have eye involvement, including microphthalmia, cataracts, chorioretinitis, blindness, and retinal dysplasia. Others have patent ductus arteriosus, limb anomalies, and recurrent skin vesicles, with a short life expectancy.

Neonatal infection

The majority of infants are infected directly during passage through the birth canal. The risk of vaginal delivery in the presence of genital herpes has not been clearly delineated. It may be as high as 40% to 60% with active infection at term, and certainly primary infections after 32 weeks' gestation have a higher risk (50%) than recurrent infections (4%). In one prospective study of 16 mothers shedding HSV asymptomatically at delivery, Jenista reported no cases of detectable infection in the infants. The decreased likelihood of cervical involvement and the lower titers of shed virus during recurrent infection probably are responsible.

A few infants (probably less than 10%) are infected postnatally, most frequently via either airborne infection or direct contact with virus from labial lesions (cold sores) on the mother, father, or other nursery personnel. Cold sores are estimated to occur in 16% to 46% of adults. In surveys of nursery personnel, it was found that 15% to 34% had a history of recurrent labial lesions; one in 100 individuals had a cold sore every week, and twice as many were shedding virus asymptomatically in saliva than had cold sores. Transmission from other infants in the nursery has been proved and maternal breast lesions have been suspected as another source of infection. Strain typing may be useful in delineating the source of infection, although infections resulting from the postnatal acquisition of virus are as severe as infections acquired during birth.

Although asymptomatic HSV infections are common in adults, they are exceedingly rare in neonates. No cases of asymptomatic HSV infections were found in over 1,600 infants surveyed from four centers. Of all the neonatal infections, 15% to 20% are caused by HSV-1, rather than HSV-2. Half of the infants are born prematurely, usually between 30 and 37 weeks of gestation, and many have complications of prematurity, particularly respiratory distress syndrome. Two thirds of the term newborns have normal neonatal courses and are discharged before the onset of disease. There appears to be no difference in outcome whether the infant is infected with HSV-1 or HSV-2 or is premature or term at birth.

Clinically, neonatal infections have been classified as disseminated, with or without central nervous system (CNS) involvement, or localized. The latter infections may involve the CNS, the eyes, the skin, or the oral cavity and occur in nearly one third of the infants.

Disseminated infections

Disseminated infections may involve virtually every organ system but predominantly the liver, adrenal glands, and lungs. The infants present usually in the first week of life, but sometimes in the second week, with signs of bacterial sepsis or shock. Only a small percent of infants initially show stigmata identifying the disease (skin vesicles, oral cavity ulcers, or keratitis), but these will occur eventually in half the infants. A bleeding diathesis occurs in one fourth of the infants, often manifested as disseminated intravascular coagulation (DIC) with decreased platelets, petechiae, and purpura. Clinically, bleeding occurs most often in the gastrointestinal tract. Although infants may have jaundice, one fourth of them will have hepatomegaly and abnormal liver function tests without clinical jaundice. Cyanosis and respiratory distress are common, and nearly one fifth of the infants will have pneumonitis or pleural effusion on chest films. Although CNS involvement occurs in half of these infants, many of them will die before manifesting symptoms that include irritability, apnea, a bulging fontanel, focal or generalized seizures, opisthotonous, posturing, or coma. Virus can be isolated from only one third of the infants demonstrating CNS symptoms. In other infants, the cerebrospinal fluid (CSF) may be entirely normal, despite culture-proved infection.

Overall, the mortality rate without antiviral therapy is 82%. With CNS involvement, there is a 91% mortality rate, and only 7% of survivors lack sequelae (usually visual defects and psychomotor retardation). Without CNS involvement, the mortality rate is 73%, and 12% of survivors are free of sequelae. The median duration from onset of symptoms to death is 7 days, with death occurring at a median age of 2 weeks. Death results from CNS progression, respiratory distress and pneumonitis, shock, DIC, and bleeding. In a few infants, bacterial sepsis, necrotizing enterocolitis, or respiratory distress syndrome are the major factors.

Localized infections

In contrast to disseminated infections, infants with localized CNS infections usually have the infection in the second week of life or as late as the fourth week. Although the CSF occasionally is normal, it usually shows a mild pleocytosis (<200 WBC/mm^3) with a predominance of mononuclear cells, an increased protein concentration, and a normal glucose concentration. Red blood cells are often present, reflecting hemorrhage. Lethargy, poor feeding, irritability, and focal or generalized seizures may be the presenting manifestations. Half of the infants have skin vesicles, but some infants will never have mucocutaneous lesions. Nearly all the electroencephalograms are abnormal with a characteristically diffuse, periodic slow and sharp wave pattern. In 41% of the infants, progressive neurologic deterioration results in death as late as 6 months after onset, and another 42% survive with severe neurologic sequelae (microcephalus, hydrocephalus, psychomotor retardation, and blindness or cataracts).

Ocular involvement may occur alone or in conjunction with localized CNS or disseminated disease and may be secondary to either HSV-1 or HSV-2. In addition, ocular disease may not be discovered until months after the disease has started. Microphthalmia, cataracts, optic atrophy, and corneal scarring may result from chorioretinitis, keratitis, and retinal hemorrhage. HSV infections present most commonly with skin findings or, rarely, with isolated oral cavity lesions. Vesicular eruptions are most characteristic, and lesions occur in crops at the same body locations for as long as 5 years; however, erythematous macules, bullae, and purpura also are found. A few infants will have subclinical disease of the eye or CNS and later will have psychomotor retardation or visual impairment, and 70% of the infants having skin vesicles will progress to CNS or disseminated disease.

Antepartum management

The prevention of genital infections is important, and the use of spermicidal foams to kill virus and condoms to prevent direct contact are recommended whenever a sexual partner has genital herpes. Pregnant women particularly should be counseled to avoid sexual contact with men who have either active oral or genital herpes. Although maternal oral or intravenous acyclovir is successful in shortening the duration of virus shedding, the safety of this agent for the fetus, the development of drug resistance, and the efficacy of preventing neonatal infection have not been established. The agent is not currently recommended for use in pregnancy. Genital HSV infections in the first half of pregnancy are associated with an increased rate of spontaneous abortions and an extremely small number of cases of malformations, although the association with malformations remains unproved. Amniocentesis to diagnose congenital infection is unreliable.

A careful history for HSV infections should be elicited from all women during pregnancy. Those who are identified as high-risk individuals for an active genital HSV infection during the third trimester should be monitored weekly from 32 weeks gestation, since these women are more likely to deliver prematurely. High-risk groups include women with a history of prior genital herpes, women with genital herpes detected at any time during pregnancy, women with herpetic lesions on the hands or below the waist, women with a sexual partner who has a history of genital herpes, and women who have had orogenital contact with a partner who has a history of orolabial herpes. Weekly monitoring for genital herpes is based on the premise that most infants are infected during passage through the birth canal. Monitoring should include an examination, cultures of the vagina and cervix, cultures and cytology of any suspicious lesions, and cervical and vaginal Papanicolaou smears. Immunofluorescent, enzyme-linked immunosorbent assay (ELISA), RAI, or immunoenzyme assays for HSV antigen may also be helpful, if available, but antibody screening has no benefit. Most cultures are positive within 3 or 4 days of incubation.

There is consensus that infants should be delivered by cesarean section when an active herpes infection is present at the onset of labor and the amniotic membranes have been ruptured less than 4 to 6 hours, whether or not the infection is primary or recurrent. The pregnant woman should be counseled carefully to come into the hospital as soon as her membranes rupture or labor begins. Nevertheless, the mother must be informed that even a cesarean section gives no guarantee that the baby will be free from infection. The Academy of Pediatrics recommended that a cesarean section be performed only if the membranes have been ruptured less than 12 hours. More recently, Nahmias and colleagues have recommended that infants be delivered by cesarean section if the membranes have been ruptured less than 24 hours. According to their rationale, there may not be an ascending infection with vulvar or lower vaginal infections, and even with cervical involvement and an ascending infection, the quantity of virus reaching the baby may not be sufficient to infect the infant or cause severe disease. The infant also might be delivered by cesarean section in the presence of genital lesions at the time of delivery, since cultures cannot be obtained quickly enough to be of benefit and smears are not sensitive enough to rule out infection. Finally, the use of fetal scalp monitors should be avoided in high-risk women.

Postpartum and neonatal management

All women with either active genital herpes or a history of herpes should be counseled during the postpartum period regarding the recognition of herpetic lesions and the precautions to be taken when touching the infant. Gloves should be worn when handling vaginal secretions, and hand-washing should be emphasized. All infants should be isolated initially and both gown and gloves worn by persons in contact with infants, until the results of the maternal cultures are determined negative. Nursery personnel with cold sores should practice strict hand-washing and wear a mask, but there is no evidence to require their actual removal from the nursery.

An infant has intermediate risk if delivered by cesarean section with intact membranes in the presence of either clinical genital herpes at delivery or a positive culture or cytology within a week of delivery. These infants should be isolated, with care taken to wear gown and gloves, and the eyes, oral cavity, and skin should be inspected carefully for the presence of any lesions, with cultures obtained from the mouth, the eyes, and any possible lesions. Circumcision should be delayed until the infant is discharged, but the infant may be discharged with the mother if the infant's cultures are negative; weekly pediatric appointments should be scheduled for the first month. Breast-feeding is allowable, as long as there are no suspicious lesions on the breast.

The greatest risk is for those infants delivered either vaginally or by cesarean section, after rupture of membranes in the presence of either positive cultures or cytology within a week of delivery. Evidence of clinical genital herpes or a positive Papanicolaou smear at delivery also indicates great risk. These infants need immediate isolation; inspection of the eyes, mouth, and skin; and cultures of eyes, mouth, and any possible lesions. A complete blood count, liver function tests, and herpes serology also should be drawn. Repeat cultures and blood work should be sent for analysis in 3 to 4 days and discharge held until 10 days. Prophylactic topical eye ointment (vidarabine) should be administered for 5 days for prevention of keratoconjunctivitis. There is, however, no evidence to support the need for prophylactic systemic therapy. Blood, urine, and CSF should be cultured when indicated clinically. An opthalmologic consultation should be obtained if there are any suspicious eye lesions, and similarly, neurologic evaluation, EEG, or CT scan should be obtained when clinically indicated. As stated earlier, breast-feeding may be allowed in the absence of breast lesions; circumcision should be delayed until discharge; weekly appointments should be made for the following month; and the parents should be educated regarding signs of infection. If herpetic lesions first occur after 6 weeks of life, no particular therapy needs to be given, since the infants respond similarly to older children.

Apart from general supportive measures, the only therapy shown to have a significant effect on outcome is vidarabine, although a trial of acyclovir currently is being evaluated. There is no hyperimmune globulin available for use and there is little evidence to support the use of gammaglobulin. Any infant who has lesions, is shedding virus, or has suspicious symptoms with a history of exposure to the virus should be treated immediately. Vidarabine is given at 15 mg/kg/day intravenously over 12 hours for 10 days. During clinical trials of vidarabine therapy compared to placebo, Whitley found a reduced mortality rate for disseminated herpes from 85% to 57% and for localized herpes from 50% to 10%. The higher dosage of 30 mg/kg/day was not found to have any greater efficacy and thus is no longer used.

Cytomegalovirus

Cytomegalovirus (CMV) is a double-stranded DNA virus of the herpes family. It is also the most common cause of congenital viral infections in humans, occurring in 1% of all newborns.

Epidemiology and transmission

See also Chapter 32, part two.

Humans are the only known hosts for CMV, and intimate contact is required for transmission of the virus between individuals. The majority of CMV transmissions that occurs between 20 and 40 years of age are by sexual contact. After 40 years of age, transmission may occur with less intimate contact, as it also does in young children in nursery schools. However, the virus can cross the placenta, resulting in intrauterine infection, or it can be transmitted via the cervix (during delivery) or breast milk, resulting in neonatal infection. Indeed, virus shedding in breast milk resulted in neonatal infection in 63% of infants; shedding from the cervix either during the third trimester or the third trimester and postpartum period infected 26% and 57% of infants, respectively. Blood transfusion, renal transplants, and semen serve as other sources.

Race, age, and socioeconomic class of pregnant women are all important factors determining susceptibility to primary infection. By 20 to 25 years of age, most women from poorer socioeconomic classes are infected, but the virus is found in only 20% to 30% of women from middle

Table 31-4. Congenital CMV infection in infants screened by urine culture

Location	Number tested	Percent positive
Bethesda, Md.	545	0.55
Cleveland, Ohio	2,147	1.21
Rochester, N.Y.	1,963	1.01
Birmingham, Ala.	939	2.45
Aarhus and Viborg, Denmark	3,060	0.36
Malmo, Sweden	2,200	0.31
Hamilton, Ontario, Canada	15,212	0.42

From Hanshaw, J.B.: Cytomegalovirus. In Remington, J.S., and Klein, J.O., editors: Infectious diseases of the fetus and newborn infant, Philadelphia, 1983, W.B. Saunders Co.

to upper socioeconomic classes. Blacks appear to become infected at an earlier age and with greater frequency than do whites, although by 60 to 70 years of age, most individuals from all classes and races are infected. However, CMV is a concern for all pregnant women, regardless of the preconceptual humoral immunity of the woman, in contrast to congenital rubella, which endangers only the fetus of a woman lacking prior immunity. Therefore the prevalence of congenital CMV directly correlates with the socioeconomic class of the population, ranging from 0.2% (Manchester, England) to 2.4% (Birmingham, Alabama) (Table 31-4).

Women who work in high-risk settings should have their antibody titers checked before pregnancy. Seronegative pregnant women should not care for infants with known or suspected CMV infection, but they should be allowed to work in the nursery. Isolation of CMV-infected infants and the use of gowns and good hand-washing should be enforced; it should be remembered that CMV can be isolated from a nonabrasive surface up to 8 hours after inoculation with urine. Since aerosal spread of virus has not been documented, respiratory isolation is unnecessary.

Asymptomatic congenital infections

Nearly all congenital infections occur in infants whose mothers had antibody to the virus before pregnancy and represent reactivation of latent infection. Under these circumstances 2.5% of babies will have viruria at birth. Fortunately, the majority of infants born to women with prior immunity are asymptomatic. A clinically apparent infection at birth in the infant of a woman with prior immunity is very rare; however, 10% to 20% of these infants are at risk for late sequelae. Sensorineural hearing loss, which is the most important late development, may be bilateral and significant in magnitude. Reynolds found hearing loss in 25% of infants identified by an elevated cord blood IgM level, whereas Stagno demonstrated it in only 7% to 14% of infants identified by urine screening in the first week of life. Most importantly, in one fourth of the infants the loss only developed or became severe after the first year of life. Likewise, chorioretinitis, which occurs in 1% of asymptomatic infants, may be a late sequela, and microcephaly, mental retardation, and neuromuscular deficits may occur in as many as 2% of these "asymptomatic" infants by 2 years of age. Another 5% of infants are at risk for a defect in tooth enamel, resulting in severe caries.

Cytomegalic inclusion disease

Symptomatic congenital infection, also known as cytomegalic inclusion disease (CID), occurs in only 5% to 10% of infected infants and nearly always represents primary maternal infection around the time of conception. A primary infection during pregnancy carries a 25% risk of congenital infection, although infections occurring late in pregnancy may be less damaging. Asymptomatic congenital infection has been reported in the subsequent pregnancies of three women who had infants who were severely affected or died from congenital CMV. Evidence supports the conclusion that these subsequent infections resulted from reactivation of maternal infection.

Death from symptomatic congenital infection may occur after birth or months later, resulting in an overall mortality as high as 30%; few survivors are normal. In a follow-up study by Pass, half of the infants developed bilateral, severe to profound sensorineural hearing loss progressive in nature; 70% of the infants had microcephaly; 61% had intellectual impairment (the majority had an IQ less than 50); 35% had neuromuscular disorders; and 22% had chorioretinitis or optic atrophy. Periventricular calcifications occur in only 1% of infants with congenital CMV, but they are associated with moderate to profound mental retardation and, occasionally, hydrocephalus. Dental defects and caries in 40% of the infants and inguinal hernias in males are the only definite teratogenic effects.

Most commonly an SGA or a premature infant has hepatosplenomegaly and abnormal liver function tests, especially alkaline phosphatase and serum glutamic-oxaloacetic transaminase (SGOT). Hyperbilirubinemia, which occurs in over half the infants, may be transient, but it is more likely to be persistent with a gradual rise in the direct bilirubin. Petechiae, purpura, and thrombocytopenia (direct suppression of the megakaryocytes in the bone marrow) usually develop after birth and may persist for weeks. A Coomb's negative hemolytic anemia and pneumonitis with peribronchial and diffuse interstitial infiltrates may occur.

Perinatal infections

Perinatal infections acquired from cervical secretions or breast milk are more likely to be asymptomatic, although 4 of 45 infants (8%) in a prospective study developed a prolonged interstitial pneumonitis. A recent study followed 55 infants with acquired CMV infections, prospectively matched with controls, and there was no increase in the risk of sensorineural hearing loss among these perinatally infected infants. However, the acquisition of CMV by premature infants with birth weights less than 2,000 gm, in association with the excretion of CMV at less than 8 weeks of age and with severe neonatal cardiopulmonary disease, was associated with severe handicaps. Transfusion-acquired CMV infections also can be a significant problem and result in a syndrome of rapid deterioration, septic appearance, pneumonia, hemolytic anemia, thrombocytopenia, hepatosplenomegaly, and atypical lymphocytosis, with a mortality rate of 40%.

Symptomatic infections have been reported in 13% of infants of seronegative mothers who received at least one transfusion from a seropositive donor and in 24% of the infants who received more than 50 ml of packed red blood cells. No infections occurred in infants of seronegative mothers who received only seronegative transfusions. The use of blood from seropositive donors did not affect the risk of infection in infants of seropositive mothers and did not result in any morbidity or mortality. Thus three risk factors for a symptomatic infection appear to be a seronegative mother, transfusion of more than 50 ml of packed red blood cells, and low birth weight. More recently, it also has been shown that the use of frozen, deglycerolized blood products may protect the infant from infection (Chapter 32, part two).

Health field personnel

Much concern often exists among women who work in day care centers, institutions for the mentally retarded, or high-risk health fields (nursery, dialysis, laboratories, oncology), concerning their risk of CMV infection during pregnancy. Although some epidemiologic studies indicate increased risk, others fail to document this. Ahlfors showed an increase in seropositivity among women less than 25 years of age who spent more than 6 months caring for infants, but no difference was noted in women over 25 years of age. Yeager showed a seroconversion rate of 4.1% among neonatal nurses and 7.7% among pediatric nurses, but none among personnel with little patient contact, while Haneberg found twice as many seropositive individuals who worked directly with patients compared to those with little patient contact. However, Dvorsky found similar annual attack rates in medical students (0.6%), house staff (2.7%), nurses (3.3%), and young women in the community (2.5% during pregnancy and 5.5% between pregnancies).

Neonatal diagnosis

A diagnosis rarely can be made on the basis of clinical findings alone. Periventricular calcifications are highly suggestive; however, intracranial calcifications also may be found in congenital toxoplasmosis, rubella, or syphilis. Skull films may be adequate to identify the calcifications, but CT scan may be more sensitive and also may demonstrate other abnormalities.

A number of laboratory diagnostic methods are available. The isolation of virus from a fresh urine specimen, liver biopsy, or other organs at autopsy may identify infection, but it does not necessarily indicate that the infant's disease is caused by the infection. Urine refrigerated at 4° C remains 93% infective for 7 days and 50% infective for 1 month. Therefore, if the urine cannot be immediately inoculated into tissue culture, it should be refrigerated or held in wet ice. It is estimated that more than 90% of infants with a systemic infection will have viruria. Viruria at birth is an indication of intrauterine infection, since perinatal infections require at least 30 days before the development of virus shedding in the urine. The shedding of virus from the pharynx is also present at birth with congenital infection, but the virus excretion is not as prolonged as in the urine. Only 20% of infants with viruria and 50% of severely affected infants will show cytopathic effects (inclusion-bearing cells) with Papanicolaou, Giemsa, or hematoxylin and eosin stains; therefore this method should be used only when virologic culture is unavailable. Early CMV nuclear antigens can be detected by anticomplement immunofluorescence within 24 hours of inoculation of urine into tissue culture in 91% of infants with viruria.

Since IgG crosses the placenta, an antibody titer in the infant reflects only maternal antibody titers. The measurement of IgM antibody to CMV is specific for neonatal infection, since IgM does not cross the placenta. Of those infants with viruria, only 76% will have IgM anti-CMV antibody detected, and 21% of infants lacking viruria will also be positive. An elevation of cord blood IgM (>20 mg/dl) has been used as a screening test for congenital infections, since it indicates antigenic stimulation of the fetus in utero. However, an elevation only takes place in one third of asymptomatic congenital infections and also occurs in 1% of uninfected infants. Rheumatoid factor may be elevated in 35% to 45% of CMV-infected infants, but it is nonspecific. The detection of CMV antigens in the urine with an ELISA also has been used more recently. Although this may detect 60% to 80% of infected infants, there is a 20% false positive rate.

Therapy

There is no specific therapy for congenital CMV infection. To date, the antiviral agents have not been shown to alter the progression of the disease. Both cytosine arabinoside (Ara-C) and idoxuridine (IDU) transiently may decrease viral shedding; however, they are quite toxic and do not affect the clinical outcome. Adenine arabinoside (Ara-A) has less effect on the CMV DNA-induced DNA polymerase than with other herpesviruses. Acyclovir is mostly inactive, since it requires the conversion of thymidine kinase to an active form and CMV does not induce this enzyme. The use of interferon, transfer factor, and hyperimmune serum has not been studied for congenital infections. The follow-up of a child with congenital CMV, whether symptomatic or not, is critical and needs to include periodic speech, hearing, visual, and developmental examinations. These children appear to have normal seroconversion rates in response to live virus vaccines during immunization.

Varicella-zoster virus infection

Maternal varicella is rare, occurring in only 5 cases per 10,000 pregnancies, because only 4.5% of pregnant women who were born in the United States lack antibody to varicella-zoster virus. The risks of varicella in pregnant women, however, may be greater than those in nonpregnant, infected adults. Maternal death (3%) may occur, usually from pulmonary disease, but there is no appreciable increase in fetal loss.

Maternal varicella leads to fetal transmission in approximately 26% of the cases. In addition, maternal infection rarely may result in a congenital syndrome of intrauterine growth retardation, aplasia of a single limb with cicatricial lesions of the overlying skin, neurologic damage, and ocular disease. This occurs most frequently after a first trimester infection. An intrauterine infection may be assumed whenever a child under 2 years of age develops a zoster infection.

The incubation period for varicella is 10 to 21 days from exposure to onset of rash. Patients may be infectious 3 days before developing the rash. The use of varicella zoster immune globulin (VZIG) prolongs the incubation period. One fourth of the infants born to mothers with varicella in the 3 weeks before delivery will develop congenital varicella (within 10 days of birth). However, only those infants who develop the rash from 5 to 10 days after delivery (maternal rash up to 4 days before delivery) will lack the transplacental transfer of maternal antibody. These infants have a 30% mortality. Any infant who develops the rash up to 4 days after delivery can be expected to have maternal antibody and survive.

Antepartum management

It has been recommended occasionally that passive immunization with VZIG be given to pregnant women who are exposed to varicella-zoster infection but lack a history of disease. However, only 8% of these women actually develop varicella after exposure. Also, it is unknown whether VZIG can really prevent fetal infection. More important, however, there is insufficient VZIG to allow such use. If assays become available in the future to test for varicella-zoster antibodies, pregnant women lacking a history of infection might be tested for antibodies, and the use of VZIG considered. Severe maternal varicella infections should be treated with supportive measures and antibiotics used only if bacterial superinfection occurs. Efficacy has not been shown for steroids. If supportive measures against life-threatening complications fail, the use of acyclovir may be considered, but this drug has not been demonstrated to be safe or beneficial to the pregnant woman and her infant.

Isolation procedures

Recommendations for isolation are outlined in Table 31-5. Only hospital personnel with a history of varicella or zoster should care for either an infectious mother or her infant. Exposed personnel without a history of disease should be removed from patient care from days 7 to 21 after exposure.

In the event of a first-trimester varicella infection, the infant's postnatal growth and development should be followed carefully, even when there are no congenital deformities. Since ocular damage occasionally has not been reported until several months postnatally, serial eye examinations might be beneficial.

Prophylaxis

Only those infants who lack the transplacental transfer of maternal antibody should receive passive immunization. This includes infants whose mothers develop the rash up to 4 days postpartum, since maternal viremia may precede the onset of rash and these infants may be infected in utero, without receiving maternal antibody. Therefore, if the mother develops the rash from 4 days antepartum to 4 days after delivery, the infant should be treated with 125 units (1.25 ml) VZIG intramuscularly. Since the benefit of passive immunization is decreased significantly whenever immunization occurs more than 72 hours following exposure, VZIG should be given immediately. There are no data supporting administration to infected pregnant women.

The live, attenuated varicella vaccine currently being investigated is not licensed for use in the United States. It has been tested in both children and nurses lacking immunity and appears to be safe. Long-term follow-up of immunity after vaccination is needed.

Therapy

There are no clinical trials of acyclovir for congenital varicella, since the use of VZIG has been so successful. Acyclovir has been shown to be of some benefit, however, for immunocompromised patients with varicella zoster infections. Its use may be considered for an infant who develops varicella from 5 to 10 days after delivery. The dosage is 15 mg/kg/day intravenously for 7 to 10 days. A toxic reaction in adults includes rash, vomiting, and tremors.

Table 31-5. Isolation for varicella-zoster

Type of exposure or disease	Isolation
Mother with a history of varicella-zoster	No isolation necessary for either mother or infant
Mother lacking a history of varicella-zoster	
Exposure more than 21 days before delivery and no lesions present	No isolation necessary for either mother or infant
Exposure from 4 to 21 days before delivery and no lesions present	Both mother and infant require isolation, assuming a 3-day hospital stay The infant should be isolated from the mother to prevent postnatal infection
Exposure less than 4 days before delivery	No isolation necessary for either mother or infant Isolation must begin if still hospitalized 7 days after exposure
Mother develops antepartum varicella	
Lesions present during labor and delivery	Both mother and infant require separate isolation The infant may be isolated with the mother if the infant has lesions
No new maternal lesions developing for 72 hr and all old lesions crusted over	Although the mother is not infectious, the infant is, and should be isolated with the mother
Mother has active herpes zoster lesions	The mother must be isolated separately from the infant
Siblings at home develop varicella at time of discharge	The infant may be sent home after boarding all infected siblings and exposed noninfected siblings with relatives or friends The infant may be given VZIG before discharge

Modified from Young, N.A., and Gershon, A.A.: Chickenpox, measles and mumps. In Remington, J.S., and Klein, J.O., editors: Infectious diseases of the fetus and newborn infant, Philadelphia, 1983, W.B. Saunders Co.

Epstein-Barr virus

The Epstein-Barr virus is also a herpesvirus that most frequently infects young adults. However, it has not been isolated from cervical secretions and, despite the high incidence of infection among young adults, has not been associated with congenital malformations or neonatal disease. An earlier association with poor outcome of pregnancy has not been confirmed.

ACQUIRED IMMUNODEFICIENCY SYNDROME—HUMAN IMMUNODEFICIENCY VIRUS

See also Chapter 30.

Acquired immunodeficiency syndrome (AIDS), first reported in 1981, has now reached epidemic proportions, with over 15,000 cases reported to the Centers for Disease Control (CDC) as of December 1985. Children and adolescents represent 1.1% of the total AIDS population, and 49% of adult and 69% of pediatric patients with AIDS have died.

The definition for AIDS, established by the CDC, is that of a patient diagnosed with an opportunistic infection or malignancy indicating an underlying cellular immunodeficiency for which other etiologies have been ruled out. However, AIDS-associated symptoms (weight loss or failure to thrive, interstitial pneumonitis, hepatosplenomegaly, lymphodenopathy, chronic diarrhea, recurrent infections, persistent oral candidiasis or herpetic lesions, and malaise) can be found in patients of high risk groups who do not have either an opportunistic infection or malignancy. In pediatrics, lymphoid interstitial pneumonitis is now considered a criterion for diagnosis.

Pathogenesis

Although the etiology of AIDS has never been proved, a retrovirus, ribonucleic acid (RNA) virus of the Togavirus group clearly has been implicated. It predominantly affects the T lymphocytes, particularly the helper T cells. Now known as human immunodeficiency virus (HIV), this virus has been called human T lymphotrophic virus, type III (HTLV-III), lymphadenopathy-associated virus (LAV), or AIDS-associated retrovirus (ARV). HTLV-III has been isolated from blood, semen and saliva, breast milk, tears and urine. It also has been isolated from at least 95% of blood donors who have been implicated in transfusion-acquired AIDS. Antibody to HTLV-III has been found in 68% to 100% of AIDS patients and 84% to 100% of patients with AIDS-related symptoms but in less than 1% of individuals with no risk factors for AIDS. Not all individuals exposed to the virus become infected and possibly only 5% to 10% of infected individuals per year show symptoms. Hospital personnel with documented exposure to infected blood or mucous membrane material have rarely ever developed antibody to the virus.

Pediatric high-risk groups

There are two major risk factors in children, 58% of whom are less than 1 year at diagnosis. These include receipt of blood or blood products (16% of pediatric cases) and birth to a mother who has AIDS, is at high risk for AIDS, or is the sexual partner of an infected individual (71% of pediatric cases). The median time interval between birth and onset of symptoms is 4 months; this is shorter than the median interval of 8 months after transfusion-associated disease and is compatible with in utero transmission. The shorter incubation period also might imply increased risk in neonates who have an immature cellular immune system.

Maternal-infant transmission

At least six infants have had signs and symptoms at birth and died within a month. The disease progression has been slower and the mortality lower in infants with a later onset. Infected mothers may be asymptomatic both before and during the pregnancy; indeed, infected individuals may transmit the virus for years before they develop symptoms. The risk of AIDS in infants of infected mothers is unknown; however, in Church's study, eleven mothers who had delivered infected infants had another twelve pregnancies, resulting in four infected infants. In addition, Scott and colleagues followed thirteen mothers identified by the birth of an infant who had AIDS or AIDS-related complex through a subsequent pregnancy. Not only were the mothers themselves at high risk of developing disease during those pregnancies, but six of seventeen infants developed AIDS. Five infants had AIDS-related complex and only six remained clinically normal, which is a 65% risk of an affected child. This does not mean that a mother who is antibody positive but has not delivered an infant with AIDS necessarily has the same risk. Moreover, postnatal transmission has been documented, which might indicate transmission through infected breast milk or close maternal contact.

Neonatal infection

Infected infants are usually symptomatic before 1 year of age with the adult symptoms of lymphadenopathy, hepatosplenomegaly, chronic diarrhea, interstitial pneumonitis, and persistent thrush. In addition, infants have failure to thrive, recurrent severe bacterial infections, and occasionally recurrent enlargement of the parotid glands. *Pneumocystis carinii* has occurred in 70% and Kaposi's sarcoma in 5% of pediatric patients. Viral infection due to cytomegalovirus and Epstein-Barr virus are frequently observed in patients with AIDS. Bacterial sepsis also may be a presenting manifestation.

Laboratory evaluation

A complete blood cell count may show atypical lymphocytes and lymphopenia, although this is not invariably present in infants. In most healthy individuals, helper T cells are twice as frequent as suppressor T cells, but in patients with AIDS, the helper to suppressor ratio of T4:T8 is less than 1.0. Lymphocyte responses to mitogens and antigens are abnormal, and skin test reactions are poor. Serum immunoglobulins are usually very high or normal, but specific immunoglobulin production in response to antigens is abnormal. A determination of antibody to the AIDS retrovirus may be helpful in a child, as well as in an adult.

Antenatal management

There is no effective therapy for AIDS. Bone marrow transplantation has not resulted in relief of symptoms, but gamma globulin may be of some benefit for preventing recurrent sepsis. Clearly, prevention of disease is important. All blood and blood products should be tested for HTLV-III with the ELISA kit. Positive results should be confirmed by Western blot or immunofluorescence assay. This should be used in addition to screening potential donors for high-risk factors, and it is expected to eliminate 95% of potentially infected blood. Since 95% of AIDS patients also have CMV, the use of CMV-negative blood to prevent CMV infection in premature infants may have the added benefit of eliminating some AIDS-infected blood products from transfusion by infected blood. All materials contaminated with blood or mucous membrane secretion should be handled with gloves and disposed of sterilely. Infected individuals should refrain from sexual intimacy. Congenital cases may be prevented with the use of birth control by infected or high-risk mothers. However, the infective risk to the fetus is unknown, even if the mother is antibody positive; thus abortion cannot be recommended. Infants also have developed AIDS after being delivered by cesarean section. The cord blood and placenta should be saved and sent to the CDC for analysis.

Postpartum management

The approach to a child born to an infected or high-risk mother is difficult. These infants are at increased risk of developing perinatal CMV, toxoplasmosis, or hepatitis B from the mother. The mother should be counseled carefully regarding the potential risk of transmitting virus via breast milk. The laboratory analysis should include at least a complete blood count and a lymphocyte ratio of T4:T8. However, it should be emphasized that the prognostic value of a positive test, the length of time before seroconversion in an infected infant, and the false positive rate are unknown. Day-care is usually not recommended because of problems with incontinence, biting, and other infant oral habits. The risk of horizontal transmission from an infected child to household contacts has not been delineated clearly. However, of 251 household contacts studied, only 8% were antibody seropositive and all were in high-risk groups. None of the foster mothers or grandmothers caring for the children with AIDS had antibody against HTLV-III, suggesting that transmission within households, by means other than sexual contact, is infrequent.

Differential diagnosis

In a symptomatic infant, ELISA testing of serum from the parents, siblings, and donors of any blood or blood products may be helpful. The immunodeficiency must be differentiated from congenital causes of immunodeficiencies, such as severe combined immunodeficiency, DiGeorge syndrome, Wiskott-Aldrich syndrome, neutrophil disorders, ataxia telangiectasia, and hypoagammaglobulinemia or agammaglobulinemia. Congenital rubella, cytomegalovirus, toxoplasmosis, and herpes simplex infections in the first 6 months also must be eliminated.

Therapy

Once the diagnosis is made, aggressive therapy is required. All blood must be irradiated to prevent graft versus host disease, and it should be negative for cytomegalovirus. Since infants are particularly susceptible to bacterial sepsis and meningitis, some physicians advocate the use of prophylactic gamma globulin (300 mg/kg biweekly), but this is unproved. Results from a follow-up of 46 children with AIDS indicate that 26 of them had at least one serious bacterial infection. *Streptococcus pneumoniae, Haemophilus influenzae* type B, and *Salmonella species* were most frequently responsible for outpatient bacteremias, and staphylococcal infections were found in conjunction with cellulitis, abscesses or impetigo, and *Esherichia coli* with urinary tract infections. Others advocate *P. carinii* prophylaxis with trimethoprim-sulfamethoxazole, unless rash, fever, or cytopenia occur, in which case pentamidine isethionate should be used. Efficacy has not been demonstrated for any of these. Early in treatment, corticosteroids also should be instituted for lymphoid interstitial pneumonitis, before irreversible pulmonary fibrosis occurs, despite the increased risk of infection. Finally, optimal nutrition may be difficult to achieve because of the chronic diarrhea. Parenteral nutrition has additional risk in these severely immunodeficient children, and high caloric oral feedings should be the goal.

VIRAL HEPATITIS

Hepatitis may result from a variety of viral infections, including cytomegalovirus, herpesvirus, rubella virus, Epstein-Barr virus, and coxsackievirus. Hepatitis B virus (HBV) is, however, the most common etiologic agent and may be responsible for as many as half of the 50,000 to 60,000 new cases of hepatitis reported each year to the CDC. In contrast, the incidence of hepatitis A virus (HAV) infection is decreasing in North America and Europe. Recently hepatitis non-A, non-B (HNANB) and delta agent-associated hepatitis also have been implicated in human disease.

Hepatitis A

HAV is an RNA virus, and infected individuals excrete 27 nm particles in the feces for 2 to 3 weeks before the onset of the disease and lasting for 4 to 6 weeks. Transmission is fecal-oral with an incubation period of 15 to 40 days. Viremia may occur transiently, but chronic, carrier states do not result, and infected children frequently are anicteric. Antibodies are already rising to high titers in the serum at the onset of clinical symptoms. Therefore anti-HAV IgM (RIA or ELISA) that develops at the onset of jaundice and persists for months to a year usually is measured to detect acute infection, rather than anti-HAV IgG. Immunity is long-term but affords no protection against hepatitis B.

Hepatitis A appears to present no risk to either the pregnant woman or her fetus with respect to increased severity of disease during pregnancy, congenital malformations, stillbirths, or intrauterine growth retardation. There may be a risk of prematurity and also infection if the disease occurs in the mother in the third trimester. A single intramuscular dose of immune serum globulin (0.5 ml) shortly after birth may be beneficial to the newborn. Although a few investigators have associated outbreaks of infectious hepatitis at the time of conception with Down's syndrome, this was not confirmed in the more recent studies.

Hepatitis non-A, non-B

The diagnosis of HNANB is made by exclusion in a patient whose anti-HAV titer does not change and who is also negative for hepatitis B surface antigen (HBsAg). The agent has not been identified, but there appears to be more than one, based on differing incubation periods of 28 days versus 59 days. Transmission is usually via blood or blood products, but the fecal-oral route is also possible. During an epidemic it was found that the incidence of infection was higher in women in any trimester of pregnancy (17%), as compared to non-pregnant women (2%), and fulminant hepatitis was more frequent (22% versus 0%). Maternal infection during the third trimester also is associated with the highest risk of transmission to the neonate, as indicated by the elevation of serum alanine aminotransferase (ALT) levels at 4 to 8 weeks of life. Persistent elevation continued through 6 months of age in two of seven infants. Infants born to mothers infected during the third trimester should receive immune serum globulin (0.5 ml) intramuscularly in the first 24 hours of life and again at 28 days. Follow-up of serum ALT levels also may be helpful.

The delta agent, or hepatitis D virus, requires HBV for replication and transmission. Maternal transmission to the neonate has been found, but the importance of this agent in perinatal infections is unknown.

Hepatitis B

HBV is a DNA virus and the viral particle (Dane particle) is 42 nm in diameter. HBsAg, also known as the Australia antigen, and hepatitis-associated antigen (HAA) consist of spherical, 22 nm particles produced from the protein coat. A common surface antigen (a) and subdeterminants (d, w, y, and r) have epidemiologic value but no apparent clinical importance. Removal of the surface antigen yields a 27 nm core, the core antigen (HBcAg). The e antigen (HBeAg) and a DNA polymerase also are associated with the virus, and HBeAg is only found as a soluble antigen in the serum of HBsAg-positive individuals.

Pathogenesis and natural history

HBV is primarily transmitted via blood and blood products. Other body fluids and fomites also may be contaminated, although it is unclear whether or not this results only from traces of blood that may be present. The incubation period varies from 50 to 160 days.

Most infected individuals have a self-limited disease, whether or not clinical hepatitis is present. They become noninfective and develop anti-HBc and anti-HBs antibodies, whereas other individuals become chronic carriers, characterized by the persistence of HBsAg. The latter may by asymptomatic or they may develop chronic active hepatitis.

Perinatal transmission

The pregnancy itself does not affect the severity of the maternal disease. There is also no increase in malformations, stillbirths, or growth retardation, but there is an increased risk of prematurity, as high as 32% in one study. Acute HBV infections occurring in the first and second trimesters of pregnancy rarely are transmitted to the neonate, unless the mother becomes a chronic carrier. However, the risk of transmission increases to 60% to 70%, if the infection occurs in the third trimester or in the first 2 postnatal months. Transmission to the infant is most likely to occur at the time of delivery via contamination by blood and cervical secretions. HBsAg has been detected in the gastric aspirates of 90% of infants delivered to women who are HBsAg and HBeAg positive. Transplacental transmission via maternal-fetal transfusion theoretically is possible and delivery by careful cesarean section does not decrease the risk. It has been shown that 50% of cord blood, 33% of amniotic fluid, and 71% of breast milk from HBsAg and HBeAg-positive women also contain HBsAg, although contamination with trace amounts of maternal blood could account for this. The presence of maternal HBeAg greatly increases the risk, and neonatal transmission occurs in 80% to 90% of HBeAg-positive, anti-HBe-negative women with 85% of the infants becoming chronic carriers. HBeAg-positive women with anti-HBe have a 25% transmission rate, and women with neither HBeAg nor anti-HBe have a 12% rate. The higher transmission rate in infants of Chinese mothers (64%) and black mothers (31%), compared to white mothers (4.4%), probably reflects the carrier rate for HBeAg and HBsAg. Postnatal infection also may occur from the mother or another family member, particularly in low socioeconomic areas. Spread of the virus via breast milk has been argued, but bottle-fed infants also become antigen positive at the same or higher rate.

Laboratory diagnosis

There is considerable variation in the appearance and disappearance of the antigens and antibodies associated with HBV infection. After an incubation period, which varies from 50 to 160 days, there is a prodrome associated with a rise in serum glutamic pyruvic transaminase (SGPT) and SGOT. In adults, this appears 1 to 2 weeks before the rise in serum bilirubin. Also in adults, HBsAg may appear in the serum 4 to 6 weeks after exposure and may last from 1 to 6 weeks and continue up to 20 weeks. In individuals with self-limited disease, there is a window between the disappearance of HBsAg and the development of anti-HBsAg. Thus, when disease is suspected, serial blood samples must be tested. Anti-HBsAg, which confers immunity against future reinfection, usually appears with the onset of clinical symptoms, but it may remain undetectable in 10% of adult patients. After the development of HBsAg, there is a lag of approximately 4 to 10 weeks before anti-HBcAg appears. DNA polymerase can be detected shortly after HBsAg appears. Similarly, HBeAg is measureable shortly after HBsAg is found, but it disappears before the HBsAg does and is found only in association with HBsAg.

In adults with persistent infection, HBsAg may last up to 20 weeks with a large variability in the titers. Thus, when a patient becomes HBsAg-negative, this should be followed by repeat measurements. Anti-HBcAg, however, is always present in chronic infection. The persistence of HBsAg and HBeAg, DNA polymerase, and abnormal liver function tests, along with the absence of anti-HBsAg, is consistent with chronic active hepatitis and implies a poor prognosis. In these individuals a liver biopsy may become advisable.

Neonatal infection

Infected neonates often remain HBsAg positive for prolonged periods, although they appear clinically well; however, fulminant, fatal cases of hepatitis do occur and may be recurrent in successive pregnancies. Also, more recent studies have indicated that significant disease may occur even in asymptomatic infants. In a follow-up of 56 mother-infant pairs over 4 to 39 months, Schweitzer demonstrated that all of the infants remained antigen positive. Twenty other infants were studied more closely, and only two of them developed clinical hepatitis along with anti-HBsAg. Of the other 18 infants, ten remained antigen positive without developing antibody or clinical hepatitis; however, they did have elevations of liver enzymes and chronic hepatitis on liver biopsy. Subsequently, two of the eight remaining infants also developed elevated liver enzymes, fibrosis, and portal infiltration on biopsy.

HBV also is implicated as an infrequent cause of the congenital hepatitis syndrome (see Chapter 34, part two). Compared to other causes, the prognosis is worse with more severe disease. Another association with HBsAg-positive neonatal hepatitis is congenital α_1-antitrypsin deficiency, and it is speculated that HBV infection may act as a trigger for those individuals genetically predisposed to the disease. The prognosis may be poor, but some patients have remained asymptomatic for up to 21 years. Finally, there is considerable evidence linking HBV infection to hepatocellular carcinoma, which is more common in areas with a high prevalence of surface and e antigen.

Prevention

Hepatitis B immune globulin (0.5 ml) should be given intramuscularly within 12 hours of birth, followed by 10 μg of intramuscular hepatitis B vaccine (0.5 ml) within the same 12 hours, to all infants whose mothers are either chronic carriers or who have developed hepatitis during the pregnancy or postpartum period. The vaccine should be readministered at 1 and 6 months of life and should not interfere with other immunizations. Initially it was found that the administration of hepatitis B immune globulin (0.5 ml) at birth and at 3 and 6 months of age to infants in Taiwan reduced both the infection rate (from 94% to 75%) and the carrier rate (from 91% to 22%). After it was demonstrated that HBIG did not interfere with the response to vaccination, combinations of HBIG and the vaccine were shown to reduce further the carrier rate from 25% to a range between 2% to 8%. Similar results have been found in infants whose mothers are HBsAg and HBeAg positive.

RUBELLA INFECTIONS

Rubella is a very mild, but extremely contagious, disease transmitted by droplet contact. Primarily, it manifests as both a maculopapular rash lasting 3 days or less, beginning on the face and spreading to the trunk and extremities, and as postauricular, suboccipital, and posterior cervical lymph node enlargement. Although arthralgias as well as the rare complications of myocarditis, encephalitis, Guillain-Barré syndrome, and thrombocytopenic purpura may occur, recovery is nearly always rapid and complete.

Congenital infection

Congenital rubella infection is the major concern. In the prevaccine period, congenital rubella was the leading cause of deafness in children attending schools for the deaf in the United States. Rubella epidemics used to occur every 6 to 9 years, and the last epidemic in the United States took place in 1964 and 1965. This epidemic is believed to have affected 30,000 pregnancies, resulting in 20,000 infants with congenital rubella syndrome and 11,000 fetal deaths or therapeutic abortions. Although there have been no major epidemics since vaccination was begun in 1969 and congenital rubella cases have been drastically reduced, rubella remains epidemic, and 10% to 30% of young adults continue to be susceptible.

Rubella results in chronic infection of the fetal tissues, causing an inhibition of fetal cell multiplication; thus congenital rubella is not a static disease. As many as 68% of infected infants show no apparent involvement at birth, but they develop consequences years later. Central and peripheral hearing defects are the most common result, appearing to be progressive after birth. The major teratogenic effects of rubella involve the cardiovascular system (pulmonary artery hypoplasia, patent ductus arteriosus, and coarctation of the aortic isthmus) and cataract formation. Multiple other abnormalities commonly occur, including intrauterine and postnatal growth retardation, thrombocytopenic purpura, dermal erythropoiesis, interstitial pneumonia, bony radiolucencies, retinopathy, and hepatosplenomegaly. The more severe infections may result in fetal death. Delayed manifestations also may result in thyroid dysfunction, diabetes, growth hormone deficiency, and progressive rubella panencephalopathy.

The risk of a congenitally infected infant varies with the gestational age of the fetus when maternal infection occurs. A subclinical maternal infection may also infect the infant. In the United States from 1964 to 1965, 50% of infants were infected if they were exposed in the first month of gestation, 22% in the second month, 6% in the third, and 1% in the fourth, with minimal risk after 28 weeks of gestation. In contrast, in Great Britain, more than 80% of infants were infected if exposed in the first 12 weeks of pregnancy, 54% at 13 and 14 weeks, and 25% at the end of the second trimester.

Antepartum management

Rubella immunity should be confirmed in all women before pregnancy, either by verification of rubella immunization or by serologic determination, since history of rubella infection is unreliable. Acceptable tests for immune screening include hemagglutination inhibition (HI), ELISA, radioimmunoassay (RIA), passive hemagglutination (PHA), immunofluorescence assays, and latex agglutination (LA), but HI and single radial hemolysis are most commonly used. Nonimmune women should be immunized, unless there is a current pregnancy or a pregnancy has occurred within 3 months. Nonetheless, fears of the risks to the fetus from rubella vaccine virus have not been substantiated.

The diagnosis of a rubella infection may have critical importance during pregnancy. A serum specimen should be drawn within 10 days of the exposure to a rubella or rubella-like illness. Antibodies begin to appear with the rash (12 to 21 days after exposure) and peak 7 to 10 days after the rash. A high antibody titer within 10 days of exposure is indicative of prior immunity, and no further steps need to be taken. A fourfold or greater rise in titer is evidence of acute rubella infection, and a constant titer is reassuring that rubella infection has not occurred. However, that individual remains at risk for rubella throughout the pregnancy.

Unfortunately, many women wait to seek medical care for 1 to 5 weeks after exposure, and at this time, a serum antibody titer should be obtained and repeated in 2 weeks to determine if there is a subsequent rise in titer. A titer of 1:32 is evidence of a rubella infection at some undetermined time, and a rubella specific IgM should be obtained. The IgM antibody is only detectable for 1 month following infection, and its presence is evidence of an acute rubella infection, although its absence does not exclude rubella infection. A rise in titer after 2 weeks is evidence of acute infection. In the event of a well-documented rubella exposure in a nonimmune woman, counseling must be offered. The use of immune globulin is not recommended, since previous studies of immune globulin have shown no protection. If a woman will not consider a therapeutic abortion under any circumstances, large doses (15 to 20 ml) of immune globulin might be considered. Finally, a new diagnostic approach has been described in which fetal blood sampling of the umbilical cord is performed under ultrasound to measure rubella-specific IgM levels. This procedure may allow a better determination of the risks to the fetus; however, it is not without risk, and it delays the timing of the abortion to very late in the second trimester.

Postpartum management

Any suspect infant, whether or not there are clinical findings, should be isolated, since virus excretion may occur for months after birth. Virus isolation should be attempted by swabbing the nasopharynx soon after birth. The determination of rubella-specific IgM in cord serum is reliable in diagnosing congenital infection. Similarly, the persistence of rubella antibodies at 6 to 12 months is evidence of antibody production against rubella, since maternal antibody should have waned by this time. Ophthalmologic and spinal fluid examinations, radiologic bone surveys, and cardiac evaluation should occur after birth in all infants of infected pregnancies. The physician should be aware of the progressive nature of the disease, in particular with regard to hearing, the central nervous system, and the eye.

In the postpartum period, the use of immunization becomes very important. Hospital personnel and family contacts of infected infants should be immunized, unless they can document immunity or there are contraindications (current pregnancy or one that will occur within 3 months). The infants should be isolated from pregnant women, both in the hospital and at home. Finally, all nonimmune pregnant women detected with the virus during their pregnancies should be immunized after delivery to protect future pregnancies, as long as they will not become pregnant again in the next 3 months. The use of Rh immune globulin does not interfere with effective immunization.

ENTEROVIRUSES

These RNA viruses are a subgroup of the picornaviruses and consist of three main groups, the polioviruses, the coxsackieviruses, and the enteric cytopathogenic human orphan (ECHO) viruses. More recently identified enteroviruses have been designated only by a number. Their distribution is widespread with the human as the only natural host. Transmission occurs via either the fecal-oral or the oral-oral route and is more likely to occur in poor socioeconomic conditions, especially with inadequate sanitation. Infection occurs throughout the year in tropical areas, but it is more common in summer and fall in temperate climates. Asymptomatic reinfection commonly occurs. In critical infection, the virus replicates in the oropharyngeal and intestinal lymphoid tissue, but after 3 to 5 days of incubation, there is a "minor viremia," during which the virus spreads to the reticuloendothelial system. This signals the end of the infection in most individuals, but, in others, widespread dissemination occurs as the "major viremia."

Poliovirus

Maternal poliomyelitis is associated with an increased incidence of spontaneous abortions, stillbirths, and prematurity, but there is little evidence of risk of congenital malformations. The severity of the maternal illness correlates with the fetal loss. Although vaccination of pregnant women is not recommended, follow-up of pregnant women vaccinated inadvertently has not demonstrated any risk of fetal loss, prematurity, or malformations. Congenital poliomyelitis (transplacental transmission) has always been rare, but since the use of the inactivated and live, attenuated vaccines, it is virtually nonexistent. These infants have weakness and paralysis before the fifth day of life. In infants who do develop infection, fever, diarrhea, and, occasionally, meningeal symptoms are present; muscle weakness occurs in more than half of them.

ECHO viruses

The ECHO viruses have not been associated with fetal losses or malformation, although it appears that these viruses do cross the placenta. The passive aquisition of maternal antibody may ameliorate neonatal infections. Infection of the newborn may be either asymptomatic or associated with a nonspecific febrile illness, but it may also occur with disseminated disease and the appearance of sepsis, which has a high mortality rate. These latter infants may exhibit poor feeding, irritability, hypotonia, lethargy, and fever, which proceed to shock, hepatomegaly, disseminated intravascular coagulation, and seizures. Meningoencephalitis is common in infants exhibiting a sepsislike illness. The cerebral spinal fluid findings are quite variable and may resemble bacterial disease. Follow-up of infants with meningitis has suggested that intellectual defects may occur. Respiratory infections, including pneumonia, vomiting and diarrhea, severe hepatitis and fatal hepatic necrosis, and a maculopapular rash have all been noted in association with ECHO viruses.

Coxsackie viruses

Evidence for an association of maternal coxsackie infections with congenital malformations has been accumulated in several large studies. Coxsackie B3 and B4 have been associated with cardiovascular anomalies, Coxsackie B2 and B4 with urogenital anomalies, and Coxsackie A9 with gastrointestinal problems. However, other investigations have failed to associate Coxsackie B infections with congenital heart defects. Although stillbirths and congenital infections have been observed, postnatal transmission is more common within the first 2 days of life. A diphasic course may be noted in which the initial illness appears mild, but more severe disease may occur after recovery begins. Coxsackie B infections, more than any of the other enteroviruses, have been associated with severe and often fatal infections, although asymptomatic infants are still the general rule. Coxsackie B infections are responsible for most cases of neonatal myocarditis; frequently they occur in epidemics and often result in meningoencephalitis. The cerebrospinal fluid findings, again, resemble those of bacterial infections. Coxsackie B infections also have been associated with hepatitis, pancreatitis, necrotizing enterocolitis, pneumonia, and vomiting and diarrhea. Coxsackie A viruses have been cultured from children with the sudden infant death syndrome.

THE MYXOVIRUSES

Mumps

A mumps infection during the first trimester of pregnancy increases the risk of spontaneous abortion (27% compared to 13% in a control group) but not in the second or third trimesters. Although the mumps virus has been isolated from fetal and placental tissue, large studies have not demonstrated any increased risk of congenital malformations. There also are no reports of mumps infections occurring after neonatal exposure; thus the mother with mumps does not need to be isolated from her infant. Neither vaccinations nor the use of immune globulin is recommended for use in the pregnant, exposed woman.

A controversial association of mumps during pregnancy exists with endocardial fibroelastosis in the newborn. The risk is estimated at 2%, although this remains to be proved, since the data are based on the potentially inaccurate mumps skin test reactivity in individuals with endocardial fibroelastosis as compared to members of the control group.

Rubeola

Gestational rubeola (measles) follows the same clinical course as infection in nonpregnant adults, but maternal mortality, usually from pneumonia, may be as high as 14% to 15%. There also may be an increased incidence of abortions, prematurity, low birth weight, neonatal death, and congenital malformations, but the risk appears to be low; thus the varied and nonspecific pattern of malformations is questionable.

All women should be vaccinated against rubeola before reaching childbearing age. If the mother's immunity is not certain, she should be vaccinated and avoid pregnancy for at least 3 months following vaccination. The use of immune globulin in exposed, pregnant women has no demonstrated benefit to either the mother or her fetus. Most women do have immunity before pregnancy. Rubeola is considered congenital when the rash occurs in the first 2 weeks of life. When the mother has the rash at birth, congenital infection may occur in as many as 30% of the newborns. Mortality, which may be higher among premature infants, is estimated at 30%. Postnatal infection (after 14 days of life) usually, but not always, results in a mild disease.

Influenza

A 50% increase in maternal mortality, which was reported in the earliest influenza epidemics, has not occurred since. Thus it is no longer considered necessary to immunize a pregnant women against influenza, unless she is otherwise at high risk. The vaccine is, however, safe for use during pregnancy.

Most of the data demonstrating an association of fetal loss and malformations, particularly of the central nervous system, were collected by maternal history during epidemics rather than by serology. Subsequently it was shown that 39% of individuals denying any illness during an epidemic had titers suggestive of infection during pregnancy, while 24% of history-positive patients lacked serologic evidence of recent infection. Moreover, the anticipated risk of anencephaly was present only in areas where the incidence of influenza was already high. Finally, the use of drugs during pregnancy increased during the epidemics. There has been no documented association of influenza infection with fetal loss or malformations since 1958. Likewise, the data linking influenza virus to childhood leukemia are also unconvincing.

RESPIRATORY SYNCYTIAL VIRUS

Large outbreaks of respiratory syncytial virus (RSV) occur yearly in winter and early spring. Since immunity has short duration, repeated infections are common, and the recurrence may be as severe as the first infection. Disease is transmitted to the eyes or nose via infected secretions, rather than by mouth or aerosol droplets. The virus is highly contagious and may survive for 20 minutes on skin, 30 to 60 minutes on paper gowns, and more than 6 hours on cribs and countertops. Hospital personnel act as significant vehicles for transfer of infection and are probably responsible for nursery epidemics. During an outbreak, 20% to 40% of hospitalized infants exposed to an infected infant will develop infection, and half of them will develop lower respiratory tract disease.

High-risk groups

Young infants, especially from 2 to 5 months of age, are more likely to develop severe disease, even though they have high levels of antibody. Immunodeficiency, prematurity, congenital heart disease, and pulmonary disease (e.g., bronchopulmonary dysplasia) increase the mortality. Pulmonary hypertension, in particular, is a high-risk factor. Poor socioeconomic conditions and passive smoking increase the risk of infection. A normal birth can be expected of a pregnancy complicated by infection with RSV, especially since there is no viremia.

Clinical manifestations

Asymptomatic infections are rare in infants. Among hospitalized babies, 20% initially develop apnea. Lower respiratory tract disease occurs in 40% of infants, and 1% will require hospitalization. Most infants develop bronchiolitis or pneumonia with subsequent coughing, wheezing, cyanosis, and progressive respiratory failure. The chest roentgenogram most commonly shows hyperexpansion, and also infiltrates. Hypoxemia may be marked, but it does not correlate necessarily with the clinical severity of the disease, although more hypoxic infants shed virus longer. Clear nasal discharge, fever, and otitis media may occur also. A shift to the left on white cell differential may confuse the RSV infection with bacterial disease.

Outcome

In one outbreak, intensive care was required for 14% of all infected infants and for 63% of those with congenital heart disease, and mechanical ventilation was needed for 5% and 22%, respectively. Mortality among all infants was 1.5%, but it increased to 37% among those with congenital heart disease. Most of the infants who died had pulmonary hypertension, and others may have increased risk for episodes of wheezing later in their development.

Diagnosis and therapy

Rapid diagnosis is made most conveniently by immunofluorescent staining of RSV antigen on anterior nasal swabs. Diagnosis may be made from a viral culture of respiratory secretions (anterior nasal swab, nasal wash, sputum) or lung biopsy. The cytopathic effects (development of a syncytium) require 4 to 7 days in culture; serology is not helpful.

Therapy primarily has been supportive, and it includes the use of supplemental oxygen and mechanical ventilation. Arterial blood gases must be monitored, since cyanosis is not invariably present in hypoxemic infants. Ribavirin, a synthetic nucleoside that inhibits RNA and DNA viruses, is now available and may have the benefit of promoting a faster recovery, increased arterial oxygen saturation, and decreased viral shedding. This small particle aerosol can be administered through an oxygen hood, tent, or ventilator, and no toxicity has been demonstrated.

ROTAVIRUS

Rotavirus is a widespread pathogen that usually results in asymptomatic or subclinical infections in neonates, but it may be responsible for diarrheal disease in one half to three fourths of infected infants. After an incubation period of 1 to 2 days, the infant may develop irritability and poor feeding, followed by watery stools that are often associated with mucus and increased reducing substances in the stool. Recovery usually begins on the third or fourth day. A few infants develop severe diarrhea and dehydration, which may even be fatal. Therapy consists mainly of rehydration and maintenance of fluids and electrolytes.

Prematurity and low birth weight do not increase the risk of infection. In temperate climates, disease is usually prevalent during cool, dry months, whereas in tropical areas, infection is relatively constant. In nurseries, endemic infection rates may vary from 10% to 50% or may be absent altogether. The frequency of handling and the closeness of infants are probably the most important factors controlling spread of infection. It has been postulated that transmission of the virus may occur at birth, from personnel or family members, from contaminated formula or fomites, or from airborne contamination. Diagnosis most commonly is made by the detection of viral antigens in stool specimens, such as by rotavirus antigen (Rotazyme) assays, and serologic responses also can be measured. Preliminary results of vaccination trials are encouraging.

Jill E. Baley

BIBLIOGRAPHY

Herpes simplex

Blackett, P.R., and others: Intrauterine infection with herpes simplex virus: resultant congenital manifestations, JAMA **225**:129, 1973.

Committee on fetus and newborn. Committee on infectious diseases, American Academy of Pediatrics: Perinatal herpes simplex virus infections, Pediatrics **66**:147, 1980.

Hain, and others: Ascending transcervical herpes simplex infection with intact fetal membranes, Obstet. Gynecol. **56**:106, 1980.

Harger, J.H., and others: Characteristics and management of pregnancy in women with genital herpes simplex virus infection, Am. J. Obstet. Gynecol. **145**:784, 1983.

Hatherly, L.I., Hayes, K., and Jack, I.: Herpes virus in an obstetric hospital. II. Asymptomatic virus excretion in staff members, Med. J. Aust. **2**:273, 1980.

Hatherly, L.I., Hayes, K., and Jack, I.: Herpes virus in an obstetric hospital. III. Prevalence of antibodies in patients and staff, Med. J. Aust. **2**:325, 1980.

Hatherly, L.I., and others: Herpes virus in an obstetric hospital: herpetic eruptions, Med. J. Aust. **2**:205, 1980.

Jenista, J.A.: Perinatal herpesvirus infections. In Amstey, M.S., editor: Virus infection in pregnancy, Orlando, Fla. 1984, Grune & Stratton, Inc.

Linneman, C.C., and others: Transmission of herpes simplex virus type I in a nursery for the newborn: identification of viral isolates by DNA "fingerprinting," Lancet **1**:964, 1978.

Montgomery, J.R., Flanders, R.W., and Yow, M.D.: Congenital anomalies and herpes virus infection, Am. J. Dis. Child **126**:364, 1973.

Nahmias, A.J., Keyserling, H.L., and Kerrick, G.M.: Herpes simplex. In Remington, J.S., and Klein, J.P.: Infectious diseases of the fetus and newborn infant, Philadelphia, 1983, W.B. Saunders, Co.

Nahmias, A.J., and others: Perinatal risk associated with maternal genital herpes simplex virus infection, Am. J. Obstet. Gynecol. **110**:825, 1971.

Parvey, L.S., and Chien, L.T.: Neonatal herpes simplex virus infection introduced by fetal monitor scalp electrodes, Pediatrics **65**:1150, 1980.

Sullivan-Bolijai, J.Z., and others: Disseminated neonatal herpes simplex virus type I from a maternal breast lesion, Pediatrics **71**:455, 1983.

Whitley, R.J., and others: The natural history of herpes simplex virus infection of mother and newborn, Pediatrics **66**:489, 1980.

Whitley, R.J., and others: Vidarabine therapy of neonatal herpes simplex virus infection, Pediatrics **66**:495, 1980.

Whitley, R.J., and others: Neonatal herpes simplex virus infection: follow-up evaluation of vidarabine therapy, Pediatrics **72**:778, 1983.

Witzleben, C.L., and Driscoll, S.G.: Possible transplacental transmission of herpes simplex infection, Pediatrics **36**:192, 1985.

Zervoudakis, I.A., and others: Herpes simplex in the amniotic fluid of an unaffected fetus, Obstet. Gynecol. **55**:165, 1980.

Cytomegalovirus

Adler, S.P., and others: Cytomegalovirus infections in neonates acquired by blood transfusions, Pediatr. Infect. Dis. **2**:114, 1983.

Ahlfors, and others: Risk of cytomegalovirus infection in nurses and congenital infection in their offspring, Acta Paediatr. Scand. **70**:819, 1981.

Anders, B.J., Lauer, B.A., and Foley, L.C.: Computerized tomography to define CNS involvement in congenital cytomegalovirus infection, Am. J. Dis. Child **134**:795, 1980.

Dvorsky, M., and others: Cytomegalovirus infection of breast milk and transmission in infancy, Pediatrics **72**:295, 1983.

Dvorsky, M.E., and others: Occupational risk for primary cytomegalovirus infection among pediatric health-care workers, N. Engl. J. Med. **309**:950, 1983.

Haneberg, B., Bertnes, E., and Haukens, G.: Antibodies to cytomegalovirus among personnel at a children's hospital, Acta Paediatr. Scand. **69**:407, 1980.

Hanshaw, J.B., and others: School failure and deafness after "silent" congenital cytomegalovirus infection, N. Engl. J. Med. **295**:468, 1976.

Huang, E.S., and others: Molecular epidemiology of maternal cytomegalovirus infections and their infants, N. Engl. J. Med. **303**:958, 1980.

Kumar, M.L., and others: Congenital and postnatally acquired cytomegalovirus infections: long-term follow-up, J. Pediatr. **104**:674, 1984.

Paryani, S.G., and others: Sequelae of acquired cytomegalovirus infection in premature and sick infants, J. Pediatr. **107**:451, 1985.

Pass, R.F., and others: Outcome of symptomatic congenital cytomegalovirus: results of long-term longitudinal follow-up, Pediatrics **66**:758, 1980.

Reynolds, D.W., and others: Inapparent congenital cytomegalovirus infection with elevated cord IgM levels: causal relationship with auditory and mental deficiency, N. Engl. J. Med. **290**:291, 1974.

Saigal, S., and others: The outcome in children with congenital cytomegalovirus infection: a longitudinal follow-up study, Am. J. Dis. Child **136**:896, 1982.

Stagno, S., and others: Auditory and visual defects resulting from symptomatic and subclinical congenital cytomegaloviral and toxoplasma infections, Pediatrics **59**:669, 1977.

Stagno, S., and others: Comparative study of diagnostic procedures for congenital cytomegalovirus infection, Pediatrics **65**:251, 1980.

Stagno, S., and others: Congenital cytomegalovirus infection: the relative important of primary and recurrent maternal infection, N. Engl. J. Med. **306**:945, 1982.

Stagno, S., and others: Defects of tooth structure in congenital cytomegalovirus infection, Pediatrics **69**:646, 1982.

Yeager, A.S.: Longitudinal serological study of cytomegalovirus infections in nurses and in personnel without patient contact, J. Clin, Microbiol. **2**:448, 1975.

Yeager, A.S., and others: Prevention of transfusion-acquired cytomegalovirus infections in newborn infants, J. Pediatr. **98**:281, 1981.

Yeager, A.S., and others: Sequelae of maternally derived cytomegalovirus infections in premature infants, J. Pediatr. **102**:918, 1983.

Varicella-Zoster

Balfour, H.H.: Intravenous acyclovir therapy for varicella in immunocompromised children, J. Pediatr. **104**:134, 1984.

DeNicola, L.K., and Hanshaw, J.B.: Congenital and neonatal varicella, J. Pediatr. **94**:175, 1979.

Dodion-Fransen, S., Dekegel, D., and Thirty, L.: Congenital varicella-zoster infection related to maternal disease in early pregnancy, Scand. J. Infect. Dis. **5**:149, 1973.

McIntosh, K.: Varicella vaccine: decisions a little nearer, N. Engl. J. Med. **310**:1456, 1984.

Meyers, J.D.: Congenital varicella in term infants: risks reconsidered, J. Infect. Dis. **129**:215, 1974.

Ndumbe, P.M., and others: Immunization of nurses with a live varicella vaccine, Lancet **1**:1144, 1985.

Preblud, S.R., and others: Management of pregnant patient exposed to varicella, J. Pediatr. **95**:334, 1979.

Stagno, S., and Whitley, R.J.: Herpesvirus infections of pregnancy. II. Herpes simplex virus and varicella-zoster virus infections, N. Engl. J. Med. **313**:1327, 1985.

Weibel, R.E., and others: Live attenuated varicella virus vaccine: efficacy trial in healthy children, N. Engl. J. Med. **310**:1409, 1984.

Epstein-Barr virus

Chang, R.S., and Seto, D.Y.: Perinatal infection by Epstein-Barr virus, Lancet **2**:201, 1979.

Icart, J., and Didier, J.: Infection due to Epstein-Barr virus during pregnancy, J. Infect. Dis. **143**:499, 1981.

Acquired Immunodeficiency Syndrome

Ammann, A.J., and others: Acquired immunodeficiency in an infant: possible transmission by means of blood products, Lancet **2**:956, 1983.

Bernstein, L.J., and others: Bacterial infection in the acquired immunodeficiency syndrome of children, Pediatr. Inf. Dis. **4**:427, 1985.

Centers for Disease Control: Provisional Public Health Service interagency recommendations for screening donated blood and plasma and antibody to the virus causing acquired immunodeficiency syndrome, Morb. Mort. Week. Rep. **34**:5, 1985.

Church, J.A., Allen, J.R., and Stiehm, E.R.: New scarlet letter(s): pediatric AIDS, Pediatrics **77**:423, 1986.

Church, J.A., and Isaacs, H.: Transfusion-associated acquired immune deficiency syndrome in infants, J. Pediatr. **105**:731, 1984.

Hirsch, M.S., and others: Risk of nosocomial infection with human T-cell lymphotrophic virus III (HTLV-III), N. Engl. J. Med. **312**:1, 1985.

Joncas, J.H., and others: Acquired (or congenital) immunodeficiency syndrome in infants born of Haitian mothers, N. Engl. J. Med. **308**:842, 1983.

Kaplan, J.E., and others: Evidence against transmission of human T-lymphotropic virus/lymphadenopathy-associated virus (HTLV-III/LAV) in families of children with the acquired immunodeficiency syndrome, Pediatr. Inf. Dis. **4**:468, 1985.

Mead, P.B., and others: AIDS in mothers and babies, Contemp. Obstet. Gynecol. (special issue), p. 126, 1985.

Progress on AIDS, FDA Drug Bull., **15**:26, 1985.

Rogers, M.F.: AIDS in children: a review of the clinical epidemiologic and public health aspects, Pediatr. Inf. Dis. **4**:230, 1985.

Rubinstein, A., and others: Acquired immunodeficiency with reversed T4/T8 ratios in infants born to promiscuous and drug-addicted mothers, JAMA **249**:2350, 1983.

Scott, G.B., and others: Acquired immunodeficiency syndrome in infants, N. Engl. J. Med. **310**:76, 1984.

Scott, G.B., and others: Mothers of infants with acquired immunodeficiency syndrome (AIDS): evidence for both symptomatic and asymptomatic carriers, JAMA **253**:363, 1985.

Shannon, K.M., and Ammann, A.J.: Acquired immune deficiency syndome in an infant, J. Pediatr. **106**:332, 1985.

Update: acquired immunodeficiency syndrome—United States, JAMA **253**:3398, 1985.

Ziegler, J.B., and others: Postnatal transmission of AIDS-associated retrovirus from mother to infant, Lancet **1**:896, 1985.

Hepatitis

Barin, F., and others: Immune response in neonates to hepatitis B vaccine, Lancet **1**:251, 1982.

Beasley, R.P., and others: Evidence against breast feeding as a mechanism for vertical transmission of hepatitis B surface antigen, Am. J. Epidemiol. **105**:94, 1975.

Beasley, R.P., and others: Hepatitis B immune globulin (HBIG) efficacy in the interruption of perinatal transmission of hepatitis B virus carrier state: initial report of a randomized double-blind placebo-controlled trial, Lancet **2**:388, 1981.

Beasley, R.P., and others: Prevention of perinatally transmitted hepatitis B virus infections with hepatitis B immune globulin and hepatitis B vaccine, Lancet **2**:1099, 1983.

Delaplane, D., and others: Fatal hepatitis B in early infancy: the importance of identifying HBsAg-positive pregnant women and providing immunoprophylaxis to their newborns, Pediatrics **72**:176, 1983.

Derso, A., and others: Transmission of HBsAg from mother to infant in four ethnic groups, Br. Med. J. **1**:949, 1978.

Khuroo, M.S., and others: Incidence and severity of viral hepatitis in pregnancy, Am. J. Med. **70**:252, 1981.

Lee, A.K., Ip, H.M., and Wong, V.C.: Mechanisms of maternal-fetal transmission of hepatitis B virus, J. Infect. Dis. **138**:668, 1978.

Okada, K., and others: e Antigen and anti-e in the serum of asymptomatic carrier mothers as indicators of positive and negative transmission of hepatitis B virus to their infants, N. Engl. J. Med. **294**:746, 1976.

Porter, C.A., and others: Alpha-1 antitrypsin deficiency and neonatal hepatitis, Br. Med. J. **3**:435, 1972.

Recommendations for protection against viral hepatitis, Morb. Mort. Week. Rep. **4**:313, 1985.

Rizzetto, M., and others: Evidence for a variant of hepatitis B virus or a non-A, non-B hepatitis agent, Perspect. Virol. **11**:193, 1981.

Schweitzer, I.L., Edwards, V.M., and Brezina, M.: e Antigen in HBsAg-carrier mothers, (letter to the editor), N. Engl. J. Med. **293**:940, 1975.

Schweitzer, I.L., and others: Hepatitis and hepatitis-associated antigen in 56 mother-infant pairs, JAMA **220**:1092, 1972.

Snydman, D.R.: Current concepts: hepatitis in pregnancy, N. Engl. J. Med. **313**:1398, 1985.

Stevens, C.E., and others: HBeAg and anti-HBe detection by radioimmunoassay: correlation with vertical transmission of hepatitis B virus in Taiwan, J. Med. Virol. **3**:237, 1979.

Tong, M.J., and others: Studies on the maternal-infant transmission of the viruses which cause acute hepatitis, Gastroenterology **80**:999, 1981.

Wong, V.C.W., and others: Prevention of the HBsAg carrier state in newborn infants of mothers who are chronic carriers of HBsAg and HBeAg by administration of hepatitis-B vaccine and hepatitis-B immunoglobulin: double-blind randomized placebo-controlled study, Lancet **1**:921, 1984.

Zanetti, A.R., and others: Perinatal transmission of the hepatitis B virus and of the HBV-associated delta agent from mothers to offspring in northern Italy, J. Med. Virol. **9**:139, 1982.

Rubella

Alford, C.A., Jr.: Congenital rubella: a review of the virologic and serologic phenomena occurring after maternal rubella in the first trimester, South Med. J. **59**:745, 1966.

Bernstein, D.I., and Ogra, P.L.: Fetomaternal aspects of immunization with RA27/3 live attenuated rubella virus vaccine during pregnancy, J. Pediatr. **97**:467, 1980.

Centers for Disease Control: Rubella prevention: recommendations of the Immunization Practices Advisory Committee, Morb. Mort. Week. Rep. **33**:301, 1984.

Daffos, F., and others: Prenatal diagnosis of congenital rubella, Lancet **2**:1, 1984.

Desmond, M.M., and others: The longitudinal course of congenital rubella encephalitis in nonretarded children, J. Pediatr. **93**:584, 1978.

Dudgeon, J.A.: Congenital rubella, J. Pediatr. **87**:1078, 1975.

Fulginiti, V.A., and Alexander, E.R.: Rubella in pregnancy: a guide to rational counseling, JAMA **245**:1666, 1981.

Hinman, A.R.: Prevention of congenital rubella infection: symposium summary, Pediatrics **75**:1162, 1985.

Mann, J.M., and others: Assessing risks of rubella infection during pregnancy, JAMA **245**:1647, 1981.

Miller, E., Cradock-Watson, J.E., and Pollock, T.M.: Consequences of confirmed maternal rubella at successive stages of pregnancy, Lancet **2**:781, 1982.

Modlin, J.F., and others: Risk of congenital abnormality after inadvertent rubella vaccination of pregnant women, N. Engl. J. Med. **294**:972, 1976.

Preblud, S.R., and others: Fetal risk associated with rubella vaccine, JAMA **246**:1413, 1981.

Public Health Laboratory Service Working Party on Rubella: Studies on rubella in pregnancy, Br. Med. J. **3**:203, 1968.

Robinson, R.G., and others: Rubella immunity in older children, teenagers, and young adults: a comparison of immunity in those previously immunized with those unimmunized, J. Pediatr. **101**:188, 1982.

Townsend, J.J., and others: Progressive rubella panencephalitis: late onset after congenital rubella, N. Engl. J. Med. **292**:990, 1975.

Enteroviruses

Bacen, C.J., and Sims, D.G.: Echovirus 19 infection in infants under six months, Arch. Dis. Child **51**:631, 1976.

Bowers, V.M., Jr., and Danforth, D.N.: The significance of poliomyelitis during pregnancy—an analysis of the literature and presentation of twenty-four new cases, Am. J. Obstet. Gynecol. **65**:34, 1953.

Brown, G.C., and Evans, T.N.: Serologic evidence of coxsackie etiology of congenital heart disease, JAMA **199**:151, 1967.

Cramblett, H.G., and others: Nosocomial infection with echovirus type II in handicapped and premature infants, Pediatrics **51**:603, 1973.

Davies, D.P., and others: Echovirus-II infection in a special-care baby unit, Lancet **1**:96, 1979.

Farmer, K., MacArthur, B.A., and Clay, M.M.: A follow-up study of 15 cases of neonatal meningoencephalitis due to coxsackie virus B5, J. Pediatr. **87**:568, 1975.

Hart, E.W., and others: Infection of newborn babies with ECHO virus type 5, Lancet **2**:402, 1962.

Horn, P.: Poliomyelitis in pregnancy: a twenty-year report from Los Angeles County, California, Obstet. Gynecol. **6**:121, 1955.

Kinney, J.S., and others: Risk factors associated with echovirus 11-infection in a hospital nursery, Pediatr. Inf. Dis. **5**:192, 1986.

Krous, H.F., Dietzman, D., and Ray, C.G.: Fatal infections with Echovirus types 6 and 11 in early infancy, Am. J. Dis. Child. **126**:842, 1973.

Marier, R., and others: Coxsackie B5 infection and aseptic meningitis in neonates and children, Am. J. Dis. Child. **129**:231, 1975.

McDonald, L.L., St. Geme, J.W., and Arnold, B.H.: Nosocomial infection with ECHO virus type 31 in a neonatal intensive care unit, Pediatrics **47**:995, 1971.

Miller, D.G., and others: An epidemic of aseptic meningitis, primarily among infants, caused by echovirus 11-prime, Pediatrics **41**:77, 1968.

Modlin, J.F., and others: Perinatal echovirus infection: risk of transmission during a community outbreak, N. Engl. J. Med. **305**:368, 1981.

Nagingten, J., and others: Fatal echovirus II infections in outbreak in special-care baby unit, Lancet **2**:725, 1978.

Philip, A.G.S., and Laroon, E.J.: Overwhelming neonatal infection with ECHO 19 virus, J. Pediatr. **82**:391, 1973.

Sells, C.J., Carpenter, R.L., and Ray, C.G.: Sequelae of central-nervous system enterovirus infections, N. Engl. J. Med. **293**:1, 1975.

Siegel, M., and Greenberg, M.: Poliomyelitis in pregnancy: effect in fetus and newborn infant, J. Pediatr. **49**:280, 1956.

Wilfert, C.M., and others: Longitudinal assessment of children with enteroviral meningitis during the first three months of life, Pediatrics **67**:811, 1981.

Myxoviruses

Canelli, A.F.: Sur le comportement normal et pathologique de l'immunité antimorbilleuse chez le nourrisson jeune, Rev. Franç. de Pediat. **5**:668, 1929.

Centers for Disease Control, Immunization Practices Advisory Committee: Mumps Vaccine, Morb. Mort. Week. Rep. **31**:617, 625, 1982.

Doll, R., Hill, A.B., and Sakula, J.: Asian influenza in pregnancy and congenital defects, Br. J. Prev. Soc. Med. **14**:167, 1960.

Dyer, I.: Measles complicating pregnancy: report of 24 cases with three instances of congenital measles, South. Med. J. **33**:601, 1940.

Gersony, W.M., Katz, S.L., and Nadas, A.S.: Endocardial fibroelastosis and the mumps virus, Pediatrics **37**:430, 1966.

Greenberg, M., and others: Maternal mortality in epidemic Asian influenza, Am. J. Obstet. Gynecol. **76**:897, 1957.

Hakosalo, J., and Saxen, L.: Influenza epidemic and congenital defects, Lancet **2**:1346, 1971.

Hardy, J.M.B., and others: The effect of Asian influenza on the outcome of pregnancy: Baltimore 1957-1958, Am. J. Public Health **51**:1182, 1961.

Karkinen-Jaaskelainen, M., and Saxen, L.: Maternal influenza, drug consumption, and congenital defects of the central nervous system, Am. J. Obstet. Gynecol. **118**:815, 1974.

Kurtz, J.B., Tomlinson, A.H., and Pearson, J.: Mumps virus isolated from a fetus, Br. Med. J. **284**:421, 1982.

Nouvat, J.R.: Rougeole et grossesse, Thesis 113, Bordeaux, 1904.

Overall, J.C., Jr.: Intrauterine virus infections and congenital heart disease, Am. Heart J. **84**:823, 1972.

Packer, A.D.: The influence of maternal measles (morbilli) on the newborn child, Med. J. Aust. **1**:835, 1950.

Ronaldson, G.W.: Measles at confinement, with subsequent modified attack in the child, Br. J. Child. Dis. **23**:192, 1926.

St. Geme, J.W., Jr., and others: Experimental gestational mumps virus infection and endocardial fibroelastosis, Pediatrics **48**:821, 1971.

Shone, J.C., and others: The mumps antigen skin test in endocardial fibroelastosis, Pediatrics **37**:423, 1966.

Siegel, M., Fuerst, H.T., and Press, N.S.: Comparative fetal mortality in maternal virus diseases: a prospective study in rubella, measles, mumps, chickenpox, and hepatitis, N. Engl. J. Med. **274**:768, 1966.

Respiratory syncytial viral infections

Berkovich, S., and Taranko, L.: Acute respiratory illness in the premature nursery associated with respiratory syncytial virus infection, Pediatrics **34**:753, 1964.

Bruhn, W.F., Mokrohisky, S.T., and McIntosh, K.: Apnea associated with respiratory syncytial virus infection in young infants, J. Pediatr. **90**:381, 1977.

Church, N.R., and others: Respiratory syncytial virus-related apnea in infants—demographics and outcome, Am. J. Dis. Child. **138**:247, 1984.

Glezen, W.P., and others: Risk of respiratory syncytial virus infection for infants from low-income families in relationship to age, sex, ethnic group, and maternal antibody level, J. Pediatr. **98**:708, 1981.

Goldson, E.J., and others: A respiratory syncytial virus outbreak in a transitional care nursery, Am. J. Dis. Child. **133**:1280, 1979.

Hall, C.B., Douglas, R.G., and Geiman, J.M.: Respiratory syncytial virus infections in infants: quantitation and duration of shedding, J. Pediatr. **89**:11, 1976.

Hall, C.B., and others: Aerosolized ribavirin treatment of infants with respiratory syncytial viral infection: a randomized double-blind study, N. Engl. J. Med. **308**:1443, 1983.

Hall, C.B., and others: Ribavirin treatment of respiratory syncytial viral infection in infants with underlying cardiopulmonary disease, JAMA **254**:3047, 1985.

Lemprecht, C.L., Krause, H.E., and Mufson, M.A.: Role of maternal antibody in pneumonia and bronchiolitis due to respiratory syncytial virus, J. Infect. Dis. **134**:211, 1976.

MacDonald, N.E., and others: Respiratory syncytial viral infection in infants with congenital heart disease, N. Engl. J. Med. **307**:397, 1982.

MacDonald, N.E.: RSV update: time to alter your clinical approach? J. Resp. Dis. **6**:11, 1985.

Minnich, L., and Ray, C.G.: Comparison of direct immunofluorescent staining of clinical specimens for respiratory virus antigens with conventional isolation techniques, J. Clin. Microbiol. **12**:391, 1980.

Mintz, L., and others: Nosocomial respiratory syncytial virus infections in an intensive care nursery: rapid diagnosis by direct immunofluorescence, Pediatrics **64**:149, 1979.

Neligan, G.A., and others: Respiratory syncytial virus infection of the newborn, Br. Med. J. **3**:146, 1970.

Taber, L.H., and others: Ribavirin aerosol treatment of bronchiolitis associated with respiratory syncytial virus infection in infants, Pediatrics **72**:613, 1983.

Rotavirus

Albrey, M.B., and Murphy, A.M.: Rotaviruses and acute gastroenteritis of infants and children, Med. J. Aust. **1**:82, 1976.

Appleton, H., and others: A search for faecal viruses in newborn and other infants, J. Hyg. **81**:279, 1978.

Bishop, R.F., and others: Diarrhea and rotavirus infection associated with differing regimens for postnatal care of newborn babies, J. Clin. Microbiol. **9**:525, 1979.

Cameron, D.J.S., and others: Pattern of shedding of two noncultivable viruses in stools of newborn babies, J. Med. Virol. **2**:7, 1978.

Chrystie, I.L., Totterdell, B.M., and Banatvala, J.E.: Asymptomatic endemic rotavirus infections in the newborn, Lancet **1**:1176, 1978.

Losonsky, G.A., and others: Safety, infectivity, transmissibility and immunogenicity of rhesus rotavirus vaccine (MMV 18006) in infants, Ped. Infect. Dis. **5**:25, 1986.

Murphy, A.M., Albrey, M.B., and Crewe, E.B.: Rotavirus infections of neonates, Lancet **2**:1149, 1977.

Steinhoff, M.C., and Gerber, M.A.: Rotavirus infection of neonates, Lancet **1**:775, 1978.

van Renterghem, L., Borre, P., and Tilleman, J.: Rotavirus and other viruses in the stool of premature babies, J. Med. Virol. **5**:137, 1980.

Vesikari, T., and others: Increased "take" rate of oral rotavirus vaccine in infants after milk feeding, Lancet **2**:700, 1984.

PART THREE

Fungal and protozoal infections

FUNGAL INFECTIONS

Disseminated candidiasis is occurring with increasing frequency in the very low birth weight infant. Risk factors include very low birth weight, congenital anomalies, abdominal surgery, central lines, and maternal drug abuse, as well as the use of broad spectrum antibiotics, hypertonic glucose solutions, and intralipid. Early recognition is important, since as many as one third of the cases may be diagnosed at autopsy, and 60% to 80% of the remainder may be diagnosed too late to begin effective therapy.

Candida

Incidence

Mucocutaneous, cutaneous, and disseminated candidiasis all have been reported in the newborn. Oral candidiasis (thrush) is common.

Etiology

Candida organisms are yeastlike fungi that produce pseudomycelia and spores. *C. albicans*, *C. tropicalis*, *C. pseudotropicalis*, and *C. stellatoidea* are but a few of the species that have been proved pathogenic for man.

Pathology and pathogenesis

Systemic candidiasis may cause disease in any organ system. *Candida* abscesses have been described in the liver, spleen, lung, brain, kidney, and heart. Superficial infection of the skin and GI tract is even more common and is characterized by invasion of epithelium by hyphae, with penetration of the basement membrane. In some patients, pseudomembranes form. If the infection penetrates the walls of veins, thrombosis and hematogenous infection will develop. Thrush frequently is complicated by esophagitis and GI tract colonization; the latter may develop in the absence of thrush. In general, *C. albicans* has a predilection for stratified epithelium, whereas columnar epithelium resists infection. The umbilical cord and fetal membranes may be involved in patients with congenital candidiasis.

C. albicans may be acquired from the vaginal flora of the mother at delivery, and person-to-person transmission may occur. The increasing use of intravenous and intraarterial catheters has been accompanied by an increased incidence of systemic candidiasis. Prolonged antibiotic therapy has been associated with an increased risk of candidal infection. Superficial and systemic candidiasis also has followed *congenital infection*, which has been reported both in the presence and absence of intact membranes. The infant may have a generalized maculopapular rash, respiratory disease, and white-beaded abscesses on the umbilical cord that are diagnostic.

Clinical manifestations

Oral thrush begins as a small papular lesion that may be associated with or evolve into vesicles. These coalesce to form cheesy white patches that may cover the buccal mucosa, gingiva, and tongue. These membranes may be quite adherent to underlying tissue. No systemic symptoms are apparent. *Candida* esophagitis may be associated with poor feeding, regurgitation, vomiting, and hematemesis. Diarrhea may suggest the presence of candidiasis, but it is necessary to demonstrate mycelial forms in the stool before attributing this symptom to the presence of *Candida* infection. Cutaneous lesions usually are restricted to the diaper area but may be noted in any moist warm area, including the neck, axilla, and the antecubital and popliteal fossae. Generalized cutaneous lesions have been noted at birth in congenital cutaneous candidiasis, which is characterized by maculopapular lesions that become vesicular and rupture, leaving denuded skin with well-defined, raised, scaling borders.

The presentation of systemic candidiasis in the very low birth weight infant is similar to that of bacterial sepsis, and includes apnea and bradycardia, temperature instability, shock, hyperglycemia, glycosuria, and diffuse erythema. The onset of infection occurs late, at a mean of 5 weeks after birth. Infection may involve the pulmonary system, causing aspiration pneumonia at birth or a later-onset pneumonia of hematogenous origin. Gradual respiratory deterioration may result, with generalized haziness or infiltrates visible on chest film. Involvement of the central nervous system (meningitis and brain abscesses) is very common and may leave severe sequelae (aqueductal stenosis, hydrocephalus, and psychomotor retardation) in survivors. Renal disease may be associated with candiduria, acute renal failure with multiple parenchymal abscesses, papillary necrosis, hypertension secondary to renal artery obstruction with fungal masses, or renal enlargement from fungal pelvic bezoars. Joint effusions, arthritis, osteomyelitis, and lytic bone lesions from fungal dissemination are particularly common in the lower extremities, probably because of seeding from an umbilical catheter. Other infants may present a necrotizing enterocolitis-like picture, with feeding intolerance, abdominal distension and occult blood, without pneumatosis cystoides intestinalis. As many as 50% of the infants may have endophthalmitis, demonstrated by the appearance of fluffy or hard, white balls on the retina or in the vitreous on indirect ophthalmoscopy. Finally some infants develop endocarditis or abscesses of subcutaneous or deep tissues.

Diagnosis

Little progress has been made in facilitating the diagnosis of systemic fungal infections. The detection of *Candida* antigens or antibodies has no benefit, as yet. Since cultures are only intermittently positive, multiple cultures should be obtained in a high-risk infant. Cultures should be plated on blood agar and Sabouraud's medium. The presence of fungus in the blood, joint aspirate, spinal fluid, or suprapubic or catheterized urine culture is indicative of infection and should never be disregarded as a contaminant, even if a subsequent culture is negative. Suspicion should be maintained in the presence of a urinalysis showing budding yeasts or hyphae, since only 6% of colonized infants have positive urinalyses, and half of the 6% also will have positive urine cultures. Gram stains of buffy coat smears drawn through umbilical venous catheters may demonstrate the presence of organisms. Potassium hydroxide (KOH) preparations of skin scrapings may show fungal involvement. Invasive disease may be documented by the identification of endophthalmitis on indirect ophthalmoscopy or by lung biopsy, when a progressive pneumonia of unexplained etiology is present. Echocardiography may show valvular fungal endocarditis. In addition, renal ultrasound may show pelvic bezoars or parenchymal abscesses. Although the cerebrospinal fluid (CSF) findings are usually abnormal, the presence of normal CSF indices does not preclude the diagnosis of meningitis. A CT scan also has been used to diagnose brain abscess.

Treatment

Oral moniliasis responds to nystatin (Mycostatin) suspension (1 to 2 ml) provided four times each day for 5 to 10 days. Cutaneous candidiasis will respond to nystatin ointment three times a day for 7 to 10 days; in some cases, secondary bacterial infection requires treatment with another topical or systemic antibiotic. Nystatin with a corticosteroid (Mycolog cream or ointment) may be used in severe cases of *Candida* dermatitis.

Systemic candidiasis should be treated with amphotericin B intravenously. Treatment should be initiated at 0.1 mg/kg in a single daily dose infused over a 4- to 6-hour period. In some patients, responses to relatively low-dosage therapy (0.1 to 0.3 mg/kg/day) is dramatic, whereas in others a dosage of 1 mg/kg/day will be required. Dosages should be adjusted on the basis of the sensitivity of the organism and the blood level of amphotericin B that is achieved. Treatment is continued for 4 weeks. It is important to carefully monitor patients receiving amphotericin B for cardiac arrhythmias and to provide potassium supplementation as needed to replace the increased urinary potassium losses that will occur. Serum electrolyte, blood urea nitrogen, and creatinine levels should be monitored and treatment temporarily discontinued if the blood urea nitrogen reaches abnormally high levels. In conjunction with amphotericin B, 5-fluorocytosine has been used to treat systemic candidiasis effectively. The dosage range is 50 to 150 mg/kg daily, given orally in divided doses every 6 hours. The toxicity of this regimen for neonates has not been well established; complete blood counts and liver enzymes should be monitored. In addition, intravenous miconazole 20 to 40 mg/kg/day in three divided doses has been used, but it should be considered a second-line therapy. Intrathecal amphotericin B may be required in *Candida* meningitis if it does not respond to intravenous therapy.

The development of *Malassezia furfur* pneumonia and sepsis, which occurs only in infants receiving intralipid infusions through central catheters, has become a problem recently. This organism may be present on the skin of one third of very low birth weight infants; it requires high concentrations of medium-chain triglycerides to grow. Infants may respond simply to catheter removal and discontinuation of intralipid infusion.

Coccidioidomycosis

Incidence

Coccidioidomycosis occurs only rarely in the newborn period.

Etiology

Coccidioides immitis is the fungal agent that produces this disease and may be found in tissues as a spherule that has a doubly refractile capsule that contains endospores. On culture media the sporangia develop septate hyphae that are disseminated readily by the aerosol route.

Pathology and pathogenesis

Coccidioidomycosis may be a disseminated granulomatous disease. Multiple small abscesses may develop following hematogenous spread to the lungs, liver, spleen, meninges, and brain. Infection can be acquired by inhalation of spores or by their entry through lacerations or abrasions of the skin. Transplacental passage of the fungus has been reported. Placental lesions have been described in pregnant women who have disseminated coccidioidomycosis, and infection following aspiration of contaminated amniotic fluid also has been documented. Coccidioidomycosis is endemic in the southwestern portion of the United States as well as in Mexico, Argentina, Venezuela, and Paraguay. Disease, however, may occur in any geographic location, since individuals who have been exposed to the disease in an endemic area may develop reactivation of their infection at any time after the initial exposure.

Clinical manifestations

The incubation period ranges from 1 to 3 weeks. Specific signs and symptoms depend on the initial route of infection. When infection is acquired by the aerosol route, pneumonia is common. If the disease becomes disseminated, lesions will appear in the skin, bone, lymph nodes, liver, spleen, and meninges. Fever, respiratory distress, and jaundice frequently accompany neonatal coccidioidomycosis.

Diagnosis

When this disorder is suspected, tracheal and gastric aspirates, urine, CSF, blood, and bone marrow should be examined and cultured for *C. immitis*. Chest radiographs may show focal consolidation or diffuse nodular infiltrates. Materials should be plated on blood agar and on Sabouraud's medium and Mycocel slants and should be cultured both at room temperature and at 37° C. Skin and serologic tests are available but may not be helpful in the initial neonatal period. Complement-fixing antibody may cross the placenta; thus a rise in the infant's titer must be demonstrated to document neonatal infection. A complement-fixing antibody titer of 1:8 or greater generally indicates disseminated disease. Thus if the maternal titer reaches this level, systemic coccidioidomycosis should be considered in the mother and anticipated as a possibility in the infant.

Treatment

Disseminated coccidioidomycosis is a fatal disease that must be treated with amphotericin B intravenously for 4 weeks or longer. Intrathecal administration is necessary if meningitis is present and fails to respond to intravenous medication. Generally, a dosage of 1 mg/kg/day administered as a single daily dose over a period of 4 to 6 hours intravenously is efficacious.

Cryptococcosis

Incidence

Cryptococcal infection is rare in the newborn period. The CNS is involved primarily, but any organ system may be affected. Neonatal infection has been shown to result from transplacental passage of *Cryptococcus* organisms.

Etiology

C. neoformans is a ubiquitous saprophytic fungus that may produce disease. Both in tissues and in culture it appears as a nonsporulating, yeastlike, nonmycelial fungus with a broad capsule. It can be found on the skin as well as in the pharynx, GI tract, and vaginal tract of healthy individuals.

Pathology and pathogenesis

In the presence of underlying or debilitating illness, hematogenous dissemination may occur, and any organ system may be infected. Pathologic findings vary from minor inflammatory responses to abscess formation. Granulomas have been noted, and hepatitis and cirrhosis of the liver are common findings. Meningitis frequently leads to obstructive hydrocephalus. Granulomas of the brain have been reported; they may calcify. Calcifications may be visible on roentgenograms obtained at birth in neonates who have developed intrauterine cryptococcal disease. The fetus can be infected transplacentally, or the organisms may be acquired at or following delivery.

Clinical manifestations

Congenital cryptococcosis frequently is associated with premature birth. Newborns fail to thrive, feed poorly, and may show signs of CNS infection. Lethargy, irritability, and vomiting may be noted initially; this may be followed by seizures, opisthotonic posturing, or hydrocephalus. Chorioretinitis, cataracts, and endophthalmitis all have been reported. Interstitial pneumonia may be present and produce symptoms referable to the respiratory system. Hepatosplenomegaly, jaundice, ulcerative skin lesions, thrombocytopenia, and petechial or purpuric hemorrhages also have been noted. Thus the initial presentation may be identical to that of infants with infection due to cytomegalovirus or rubella virus. In addition, calcific densities may appear along the margins of dilated ventricles, suggesting cytomegalic inclusion disease or, less commonly, toxoplasmosis.

Laboratory manifestations

The CSF may contain between 100 and 1,000 cells/mm^3, but lymphocytes will predominate after the first week of infection. The protein concentration is elevated and the CSF glucose level is depressed compared with the blood glucose level. Organisms may be demonstrable on India ink preparation; however, caution must be exercised in suggesting a diagnosis of cryptococcosis solely on this basis, despite the competence of the observer.

Cultures of CSF, blood, and other body tissue should be obtained. A latex agglutination test for the detection of cryptococcal antigen in CSF has proved to be a rapid and, when properly controlled, effective test for establishing a diagnosis of cryptococcosis. The organism can be grown on blood agar and on Sabouraud's medium. Blood, sputum, abscess cavities, and bone marrow also serve as materials that frequently yield a positive culture.

Treatment

Amphotericin B should be administered as for *Candida;* however, if the patient is critically ill, treatment may be initiated with a dosage of 0.25 mg/kg/day. The drug 5-fluorocytosine may be used in conjunction with amphotericin B, as described previously.

Histoplasmosis

Incidence

Histoplasmosis is a disorder that is rare in the neonatal period. When it occurs, disseminated disease is common and is generally fatal unless treated.

Etiology

Histoplasma capsulatum is the fungus that produces histoplasmosis; it grows in tissues in a yeast phase and is encapsulated.

Pathogenesis

Fungus enters the body through the skin, mucous membranes, and respiratory or GI tract. Focal infections tend to seed the bloodstream, leading to formation of abscesses and granulomas in many organs. Transplacental infection has been suspected in infants born to mothers who have disseminated histoplasmosis during pregnancy. There is little evidence of human-to-human or animal-to-human transmission. Histoplasmosis is endemic in the Mississippi River Basin but has been reported in individuals throughout the United States.

Clinical manifestations

Signs and symptoms of respiratory distress may be noted early. Irritability, poor feeding, failure to thrive, and fever are common. Hepatosplenomegaly and generalized lymphadenopathy may be present. Osteomyelitis and meningitis have been reported.

Laboratory manifestations

CSF will reveal 1 to 1,000 white blood cells/mm^3 that are predominantly lymphocytes after the first several days of illness. The protein concentration will be increased and the glucose concentration depressed. Patients are frequently anemic and may be leukopenic and thrombocytopenic as well.

Diagnosis

Smears and cultures of sputum, blood, bone marrow, and CSF or biopsies of the affected organ may reveal the fungal organisms. Giemsa or Wright's stain is satisfactory, but the use of special silver stains or fluorescent microscopy may facilitate the diagnosis. Complement fixation tests may be employed but can be confused by the presence of maternal antibodies. Both yeast and mycelial phase antibodies should be measured; an elevated yeast phase antigen generally is associated with acute infection.

Treatment

Disseminated histoplasmosis should be treated with amphotericin B as indicated for the treatment of candidiasis. Intrathecal administration will be required in patients with meningitis who fail to respond to intravenous treatment. The drug 5-fluorocytosine may be used in conjunction with amphotericin B.

PROTOZOAL INFECTIONS

Malaria

Incidence

Malaria remains an important cause of abortion, stillbirth, and neonatal death in many parts of the world. Sporadic cases occur each year in inhabitants of North America. Congenital malaria is well documented.

Etiology

Malaria is caused by a protozoal parasite of the genus *Plasmodium*. Neonatal infection has been recorded with all species, including *P. vivax*, *P. malariae*, *P. ovale*, and *P. falciparum*.

Pathology and pathogenesis

Malarial parasites invade erythrocytes, which subsequently adhere to and occlude blood vessels. Red blood cells that are disintegrating accumulate and may blockade the reticuloendothelial system. Anemia is the result of hemolysis. Parasites may be found in other organs of the body, including the intestinal tract, liver, spleen, lung, and brain. The placenta is involved in most women who suffer from malaria during pregnancy. Transplacental transmission of parasites is documented and may take place during the course of symptomatic maternal malaria or may occur many years after women have left an endemic area. In the latter situation, parasitemia may be subclinical; thus congenital malaria may occur without a history of a malarial attack during pregnancy. Mosquito-borne disease may occur in newborns just as in older children or in adults. When malaria occurs in pregnant women, intrauterine infection does not always ensue. In the face of parasitemia the infant may acquire malarial parasites during labor and delivery as a result of contamination of the infant's blood with that of the mother. Blood donated by individuals with malaria may serve as a source of malarial parasites. Neonatal malaria is rare, since IgG antibody to the malarial parasite crosses the placenta, providing some protection for the newborn. This antibody specifically aids in the phagocytosis of merozoites and infected erythrocytes, but it does not alter the hepatic phase of malaria.

Clinical manifestations

If congenital malaria has occurred, disease may become manifest in the early days of life. Malaria acquired postnatally may appear at any time between 8 and 30 days after delivery. The incubation period is dependent on the specific species involved, the size of the inoculum, and the immune status of the host. Congenital malaria may appear relatively late. Specific signs and symptoms can vary from irritability, weight loss, and low-grade fever to devastating disease. Fever, diarrhea, vomiting, tachypnea, cyanosis, and meningeal findings may be present. Anemia and jaundice, which may occur acutely, suggest hemolysis. Hepatosplenomegaly is common, and renal function may be impaired.

Diagnosis

The diagnosis is dependent on demonstration of parasites in the bloodstream. Thick smears should be prepared and examined on several different occasions to maximize the possibility of parasite detection.

Treatment

Chloroquine is indicated for the treatment of acute malaria in a dose of 5 mg/kg diluted in a multiple electrolyte solution containing glucose. This dose may be repeated once in 12 to 24 hours. Chloroquine also can be provided orally in an immediate initial dose of 10 mg/kg followed by a dose of 5 mg/kg at 6, 24, and 48 hours. For strains of *P. falciparum* that are resistant to chloroquine, quinine can be provided orally in a dosage of 20 to 30 mg/kg/day in three divided doses for 7 to 10 days or may be given intravenously in a dose of 10 mg/kg diluted in a multiple electrolyte solution containing glucose and repeated once after 24 hours. Because of the extreme toxicity of this drug, the oral route is preferred.

Pneumocystis carinii

Incidence

Pneumonia may be caused by *Pneumocystis carinii* in newborns whose host resistance is impaired. Rarely, it is associated with pneumonia in healthy normal neonates.

Etiology

P. carinii is a protozoan that only recently has been cultivated in vitro. Morphologic appearance of the cysts in pathologic specimens is so characteristic that diagnosis can be made morphologically.

Pathology and pathogenesis

Pathologic changes are limited to the lungs. Infection begins in pulmonary alveolar spaces, and the exudate that develops contains lymphocytes, plasma cells, polymorphonuclear leukocytes, and histiocytes. An eosinophilic lacelike appearance may be found on stains with periodic acid–Schiff reagent. Cysts can be demonstrated readily by use of methenamine silver stains. Specific modes of transmission are unclear, but nursery epidemics of *Pneumocystis* infection have occurred and suggest an airborne route. In a few patients, intrauterine infection has been described, suggesting the possibility of transplacental transmission. The specific association of *P. carinii* infection with the debilitated host suggests that disease results from some impairment in host-parasite relationships. Nutritional deprivation may be accompanied by *Pneumocystis* infection that clears with nutritional repletion.

Clinical manifestations

The incubation period is approximately 3 weeks. The onset is insidious, and over a short period of time tachypnea, cough, and cyanosis are noted. Rales are unusual, and fever is relatively infrequent. Roentgenograms demonstrate bilateral diffuse infiltrates that tend to extend from the hilus of the lung to the periphery. Frequently, the degree of pulmonary involvement detected clinically and by pulmonary function studies is in excess of that which can be accounted for by the roentgenographic appearance of the lungs.

Diagnosis

Roentgenographic studies may suggest this disease but are not diagnostic. Diagnosis depends on demonstration of *Pneumocytosis* cysts. Although *P. carinii* organisms have been observed in material obtained from tracheal aspirate, gastric aspirates, or by needle biopsy of the lung, the likelihood of establishing a definitive diagnosis is greatest if open lung biopsy is performed. The risk of pneumothorax also is minimized in comparison with needle biopsy.

Treatment

Pentamidine isethionate is effective when given as a single dose of 4 mg/kg intramuscularly for 10 to 14 days. It can be obtained from the Centers for Disease Control in Atlanta, Georgia when a diagnosis of *Pneumocystis* infection is highly suspected or confirmed. This infection is best treated in children over 2 months of age and in adults with trimethoprim-sulfamethoxazole (Bactrim, Septra). There is no reason to believe that this drug combination would be any less effective in the newborn infant. It is well known, however, that sulfa drugs displace bilirubin from albumin-binding sites, predisposing infants to kernicterus at relatively low levels of serum bilirubin. Moreover, the potential for toxicity of trimethoprim in the newborn infant is unknown. For these reasons, although this drug combination is the preferred treatment for *Pneumocystis* infections beyond the newborn period, it cannot be recommended for neonates until additional pharmacologic studies have been performed.

Toxoplasmosis

Incidence

Maternal infection with the parasite *Toxoplasma gondii* is usually asymptomatic. Only 15% of French women with serologic evidence of toxoplasmosis during pregnancy manifested clinical disease, usually a mild febrile illness with cervical adenopathy. Among 23,617 pregnant women analyzed by the Collaborative Perinatal Research Study in the United States, 6.4 per 1,000 developed an infection with *Toxoplasma* organisms, as evidenced by a rise in their antibody titer against this organism. Cats are still believed to be a major source of infection. The susceptibility of patients with AIDS to this organism is high.

Not all infants born to a mother with evidence of toxoplasmosis during pregnancy become infected. One to three infants per 1,000 live births have IgM antibody directed against this organism, indicating intrauterine infection. The incidence of fetal infection increases throughout pregnancy, but the most severe involvement results from maternal infection that occurs during the first and second trimesters. Successful isolation of this parasitic organism cannot be accomplished in most laboratories.

Clinical manifestations

Over 70% of infants born with congenital toxoplasmosis do not manifest signs of clinical illness in the neonatal period. The most common findings during the first few months of life in comparison to congenital rubella and cytomegalovirus (CMV) infection are illustrated in Fig. 31-3. These infants fall into two major groups: (1) infants with generalized disease in whom the primary manifestations of low birth weight, hepatosplenomegaly, icterus, and anemia are observed in the first several weeks of life, and (2) infants with primarily neurologic disease in whom the major findings are abnormal spinal fluid, convulsions, intracranial calcifications, and hydrocephalus or microcephaly. These latter findings, with the exception of the abnormal spinal fluid, are not seen until after 1 month of age in the majority of infants. Chorioretinitis, the most common lesion in congenital toxoplasmosis, occurs in both groups of infants but usually is not apparent in the neonatal period. Postmortem examination of infants who died in the neonatal period reveals multiple foci of necrosis with encysted forms of the *Toxoplasma* parasite in myocardium, renal glomeruli and tubules, the adrenal gland, and the brain. The enlarged liver and spleen are the result of marked extramedullary hematopoiesis; parasites are rarely seen. The overall mortality in Eichenwald's series was 12%; 90% of the survivors developed serious neurologic sequelae, such as mental retardation, convulsions, spasticity, palsies, severely impaired vision, hydrocephalus or microcephaly, and deafness.

The infants with asymptomatic, or silent, congenital toxoplasmosis are diagnosed by the demonstration of a seroconversion or a significant rise in antitoxoplasmic antibodies in the mother during pregnancy or the presence of specific antitoxoplasmic IgM antibodies in the cord blood serum or in serum obtained from the neonate

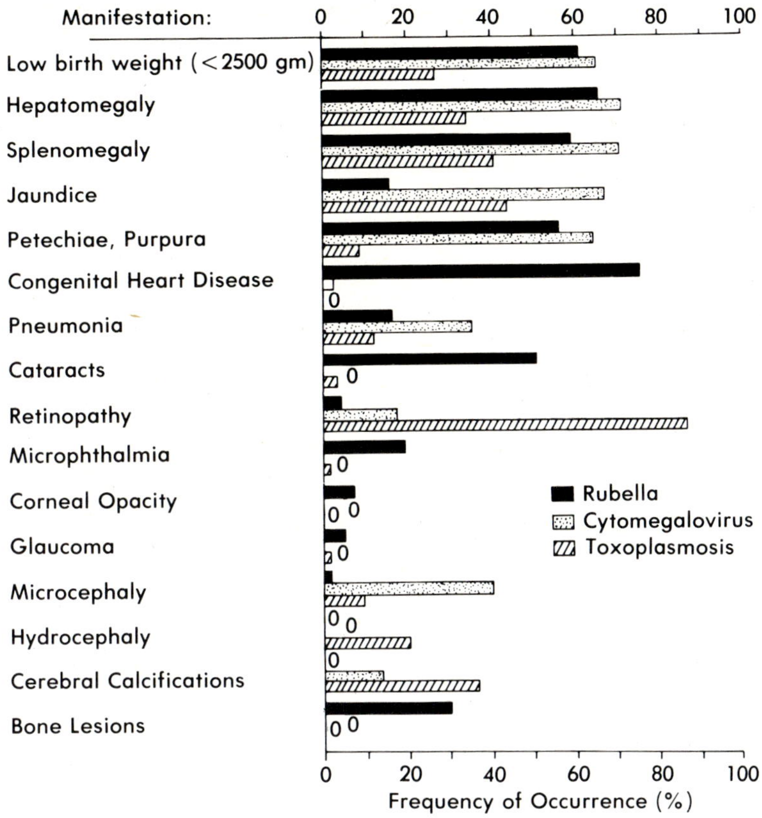

Fig. 31-3. Manifestations of symptomatic congenital rubella and CMV infections and toxoplasmosis in the neonate. (From Overall, J.C., Jr.: Viral infections of the fetus and neonate. In Feigin, R.D., and Cherry, J.D., editors: Textbook of pediatric infectious diseases, Philadelphia, 1981, W.B. Saunders Co.)

soon after birth. These infants usually have abnormal spinal fluid with lymphocytosis and elevated protein levels in the neonatal period. In one study of 13 newborns diagnosed because of routine screening tests or during the evaluation of nonspecific findings, 11 (85%) developed chorioretinitis and 5 (39%) neurologic sequelae. The onset of eye disease occurred as early as 1 month to as late as 9.3 years. Neurologic defects included microcephaly, seizures, severe psychomotor retardation, mild cerebellar dysfunction, and delay in development. In another group of 11 children who were asymptomatic as neonates but who were diagnosed because of the onset of symptoms later in life, 10 of 11 (91%) had chorioretinitis, and 8 of 11 (73%) had neurologic sequelae. Sixteen of the children in these two groups had skull films, and 5 (31%) had intracranial calcifications. All had neurologic sequelae.

These data indicate that a majority of infants with subclinical congenital toxoplasmosis in the neonatal period develop clinical manifestations of their disease later in life.

Diagnosis and treatment

Since the organism cannot be isolated readily, neonatal diagnosis requires testing for specific IgM antibody. A less specific but readily available screen for TORCH infection on serial serum samples is available at state health laboratories. In contrast to active neonatal infection, a serum sample obtained from the infant at 3 to 4 months of age should show a significant drop if the antibody present in the newborn period was passively transferred from the mother.

Present evidence suggests that treatment may decrease the incidence of adverse sequelae. Therapy would appear to be appropriate for a symptomatic newborn and for an asymptomatic infant with proved infection, i.e., a rising titer of antibody or a positive IgM *Toxoplasma* organism fluorescent antibody test on the infant's blood. Therapy consists of oral pyrimethamine, 1 mg/kg/day, and then 0.5 mg/kg/day for 21 to 30 days, along with oral sulfadiazine, 25 mg/kg/day for 21 to 30 days. Folinic acid, 2 to 6 mg, also should be given three times per week to prevent anemia. The treatment may be repeated when evidence of ongoing disease exists after a course of therapy. Close neurodevelopment follow-up should be an integral part of the infant's subsequent pediatric care.

Ralph D. Feigin
Stuart L. Abramson
Morven S. Edwards
Jill E. Baley

BIBLIOGRAPHY

Specific fungal infections

Baley, J.E., Kliegman, R.M., and Fanaroff, A.A.: Disseminated fungal infections in very low birth-weight infants: clinical manifestations and epidemiology, Pediatrics **73:**144, 1984.

Buchs, S.: Candida meningitis: a growing threat to premature and full-term infants, Pediatr. Infect. Dis. **4:**122, 1985.

Child, D.D., and others: Radiographic findings of pulmonary coccidioidomycosis in neonates and infants, A.J.R. **145:**261, 1985.

Dvorak, A.M., and Gavaller, B.: Congenital systemic candidiasis: report of a case, N. Engl. J. Med. **274:**540, 1966.

Emanuel, B., and others: *Cryptococcus* meningitis in a child successfully treated with amphotericin B, with a review of the pediatric literature, J. Pediatr. **59:**577, 1961.

Holland, P., and Holland, N.H.: Histoplasmosis in early infancy, Am. J. Dis. Child. **112:**412, 1966.

Hyatt, H.W.: Coccidioidomycosis in a 3-week-old infant, Am. J. Dis. Child. **105:**93, 1963.

Kozinn, P.J., and Taschdjian, C.L.: Enteric candidiasis: diagnosis and clinical considerations, Pediatrics **30:**71, 1962.

Kozinn, P.J., and others: Neonatal candidiasis, Pediatr. Clin. North Am. **5:**803, 1958.

Schirar, A., and others: Congenital mycosis *(Candida albicans)*, Biol. Neonate **24:**273, 1974.

Smale, L.E., and Waechter, K.G.: Dissemination of coccidioidomycosis in pregnancy, Am. J. Obstet. Gynecol. **107:**356, 1970.

Smith, H., and Congdon, P.: Neonatal systemic candidiasis, Arch. Dis. Child. **60:**365, 1985.

Tudehope, D.I., and Bigby, B.: Neonatal systemic candidiasis treated with miconazole and ketoconazole, Med. J. Aust., May 14, 1983, p. 480.

Specific parasitic infections

Covell, G.: Congenital malaria, Trop. Dis. Bull. **47:**1147, 1950.

Harvey, B., Remington, J.S., and Sulzer, A.J.: IgM malaria antibodies in a case of congenital malaria in the United States, Lancet **1:**333, 1969.

Robbins, J.B.: Immunological and clinicopathological aspects of *Pneumocystis carinii* pneumonitis. In Bergsma, D., and Good, R.A., editors: Immunologic deficiency diseases in man, New York, 1968, The National Foundation, p. 219.

Williams, A.I.O., and McFarlane, H.: Distribution of malarial antibody in maternal and cord sera, Arch. Dis. Child. **44:**511, 1969.

Toxoplasmosis

Alford, C.A., Jr., Stagno, S., and Reynolds, D.W.: Toxoplasmosis; silent congenital infection. In Krugman, S., and Gershon, A.A., editors: Infections of the fetus and the newborn infant, New York, 1975, Alan R. Liss, Inc.

Desmonts, G., and Couvreur, J.: Congenital toxoplasmosis; a prospective study of 378 pregnancies, N. Engl. J. Med. **290:**110, 1974.

Desmonts, G., and Couvreur, J.: Toxoplasmosis; epidemiologic and serologic aspects of perinatal infection. In Krugman, S., and Gershon, A.A., editors: Infections of the fetus and the newborn infant, New York, 1975, Alan R. Liss, Inc.

Eichenwald, H.F.: A study of congenital toxoplasmosis. In Siim, J.C., editor: Proceedings of the Conference on Clinical Aspects and Diagnostic Problems of Toxoplasmosis in Pediatrics, Baltimore, 1956, Williams & Wilkins Co.

Feldman, H.A.: Toxoplasmosis, Pediatrics **22:**559, 1958.

Miller, M.J., Seaman, E., and Remington, J.S.: The clinical spectrum of congenital toxoplasmosis; problems in recognition, J. Pediatr. **70:**714, 1967.

Remington, J.: Toxoplasmosis. In Charles, D., and Finland, M., editors: Obstetric and perinatal infections, Philadelphia, 1973, Lea & Febiger.

Sever, J.L.: Perinatal infections affecting the developing fetus and newborn. In The prevention of mental retardation through control of infectious disease, Washington, D.C., 1966, U.S. Department of Health, Education, and Welfare.

Wilson, C.B., and others: Development of Adverse Sequelae in children born with subclinical congenital *Toxoplasma* infection, Pediatrics **66:**767, 1980.

CHAPTER 32

The blood and hemopoietic system

PART ONE

Hematologic problems in the fetus and neonate

HEMOPOIESIS IN THE EMBRYO AND FETUS

As early as day 14 of gestation, mesenchyme in the blood islands of the yolk sac begins to differentiate into primitive megaloblastic erythroblasts. Intravascular erythropoiesis in the yolk sac persists for about 2 months. Toward the end of the first trimester the liver becomes the major site of hemopoiesis. Granulopoiesis and thrombocytopoiesis begin during the hepatic phase. Blood cell precursors are found in the spleen and thymus as well as in the liver, although these may not be significant hemopoietic organs in the human fetus. Production of monocytes and lymphocytes is evident by the fifth month, when lymph nodes and the thymus have formed. The bone marrow is the major site of hemopoiesis by the last trimester, although the liver continues to make some blood cells as late as the first postnatal week. By 30 weeks all bony cavities contain very cellular hemopoietic marrow tissue. In postnatal life hemopoietic activity recedes from long bones to the skeleton of the trunk, and marrow cellularity diminishes. A newborn must expand the volume of active marrow to increase production of blood cells because the marrow space is already fully active.

Blood cells in utero

The primitive nucleated erythroblasts in the blood are replaced by definitive mature erythrocytes by 16 weeks' gestation. At this stage erythrocytes are considerably larger than those present at birth, and the hemoglobin concentration and red blood cell (RBC) count are lower (Fig. 32-1). The RBC count gradually increases and the size of the cells decreases during the remainder of fetal life. Reticulocytosis decreases from up to 80% at 10 weeks to approximately 4% by 30 weeks. Erythrocyte production is under the control of erythropoietin, produced by the fetal liver and kidney beginning in the hepatic phase, and increases in response to fetal hypoxia.

Leukocytes are present only in small numbers during the first half of gestation. Granulocyte counts increase to adult values after about 26 weeks' gestation (Fig. 32-1). Lymphocyte counts reach approximately two thirds of the values at term by 20 weeks' gestation and then increase gradually.

Small numbers of megakaryocytes have been observed as early as the yolk sac stage of hemopoiesis, and platelets are occasionally seen by 11 weeks' gestation. By 30 weeks the platelet count approaches normal adult values.

NORMAL HEMATOLOGIC VALUES IN THE NEWBORN

Cord blood hemoglobin concentration at birth ranges from 14 to 20 gm/dl, with a mean of 17 gm/dl. The hematocrit ranges from 43% to 63% (mean 55%), and the RBC count is correspondingly elevated, with a mean of $5.5 \times 10^6/mm^3$. These values may be modified by several factors, which must be taken into consideration in interpretation of hematologic data in the newborn.

An important determinant is the duration of gestation. During the final weeks of intrauterine life the hemoglobin concentration of blood undergoes a rapid increase (Fig. 32-1), with average increments of 1 to 3 gm/dl occurring between the thirty-eighth and fortieth weeks. This magnitude of change will be reflected in a correspondingly reduced hemoglobin concentration at birth in prematurely born as compared with full-term infants. In a study of premature infants having birth weights of less than 1,200 gm, a mean hemoglobin concentration of 15.6 gm/dl was found, as compared with 17.1 gm/dl in full-term infants.

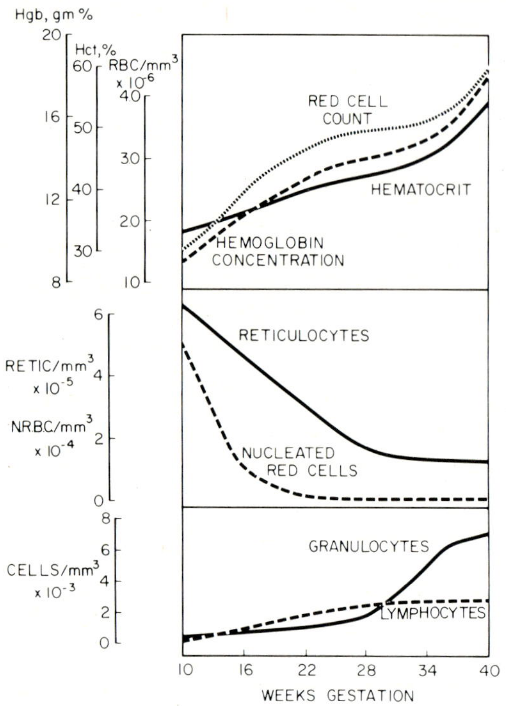

Fig. 32-1. Hematologic changes during prenatal development.

The time allowed to elapse before the cord is clamped at delivery can have a considerable effect on the blood volume and total circulating RBC mass of the newborn. The placental vessels contain approximately 100 ml of blood at term, and transfusion of a major fraction of the blood contained in the placenta can occur under conditions that promote emptying of the placental vessels at delivery. Placing the infant below the level of the placenta and delaying clamping the cord for several minutes after birth can increase the blood volume of the infant by as much as 40% to 60%. One study found that newborns with delayed clamping of the cord had mean blood volumes of 126 ml/kg, as compared with 78 ml/kg in infants whose cords were clamped immediately at birth. In both groups of infants the average hematocrit value was the same at birth, but after 48 hours mean hematocrit values of 65% were obtained in the group with delayed clamping of the cord and 48% in the infants in whom placental transfusion was prevented. Increased hemoglobin and hematocrit values can be demonstrated for at least 3 or 4 days in infants with delayed cord clamping.

The effect of transfusion of placental blood into the infant at birth may result in even greater increases in the blood volume in the premature infant. The quantity of blood in the placenta undergoes little change in the last 2 to 3 months of gestation, during which time the blood volume of the infant increases considerably. The preterm infant can thus receive a proportionately larger fraction of blood volume by the addition of placental blood.

It remains unclear whether the addition of the placental blood to the circulation is advantageous to the infant. Although the rapid increase in blood volume that occurs might impose significant stress on the heart and pulmonary vasculature, it has been reported that a decreased incidence of neonatal respiratory distress may occur in infants in whom clamping the cord is delayed. Furthermore, infants having a larger circulating RBC mass at birth will gain an increased storage supply of iron resulting from breakdown of the additional hemoglobin; however, this may contribute to hyperbilirubinemia in the first week of life. This supplementary iron can be used at a later time for hemoglobin production and will help to prevent iron deficiency if dietary intake is inadequate to supply the iron requirements for rapid growth during later infancy.

During the first week of life, hematocrit and hemoglobin values obtained from capillary blood may be markedly higher than venous samples because of peripheral venous stasis. This may allow significant anemia to be undiagnosed. Warming the infant's heel may decrease the difference between capillary and venous values. Sick infants should always have venipuncture hematocrits, since acidosis and hypotension increase peripheral stasis.

An additional modifying factor that occurs within the first few hours following delivery is a shift in the distribution of fluid to produce a decrease in the circulating plasma volume and a corresponding increase in the RBC concentration in the blood. An elevation in the hemoglobin value of approximately 2 gm/dl above cord blood values persists until the end of the first week of life (Fig. 32-2).

Reticulocyte counts in cord blood of normal infants average 4% to 5%, and in most cord blood samples nucleated RBC precursors are also present. These findings reflect high levels of erythropoietin production, with consequent erythroid hyperplasia in the bone marrow and high levels of RBC production. This results from the relatively low oxygen saturation of fetal blood—65% in the umbilical vein and as low as 30% in the umbilical artery—and the relatively poor oxygen release to the tissues by fetal hemoglobin, which has a high oxygen affinity. Infants with placental insufficiency and intrauterine growth retardation have higher than normal erythropoietin production and a correspondingly greater degree of erythrocytosis (Chapter 7).

The erythrocytes of the newborn are considerably larger than those of adults, reflected in an increase in the mean cellular diameter and mean corpuscular volume (MCV) indices (Table 32-1). The RBCs have in-

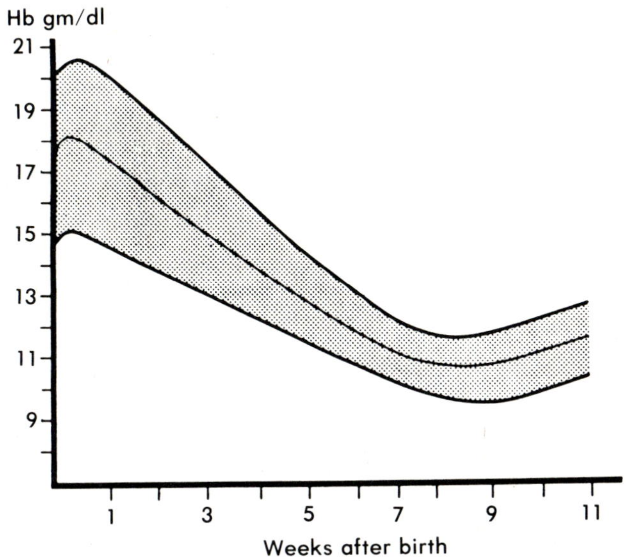

Fig. 32-2. Normal hemoglobin values in full-term infants (mean ± 2 SD).

Table 32-1. Normal hematologic values in cord blood of the full-term newborn

Hemoglobin concentration	14.0-20.0 gm/dl
Red blood cell (RBC) count	4,200,000-5,800,000/mm^3
Hematocrit	43%-63%
Mean cell diameter	8.0-8.3 μm
Mean corpuscular volume (MCV)	100-120 μm^3
Mean corpuscular hemoglobin (MCH)	32-40 pg
Mean corpuscular hemoglobin concentration (MCHC)	30%-34%
Reticulocyte count	3%-7%
Nucleated red blood cell count	200-600/mm^3
White blood cell count	10,000-30,000/mm^3
Granulocytes	40%-80%
Lymphocytes	20%-40%
Monocytes	3%-10%
Platelet count	150,000-350,000/mm^3
Serum iron concentration	125-225 μg/dl
Total iron-binding capacity	150-350 μg/dl

creased hemoglobin content, but the mean corpuscular hemoglobin concentration (MCHC) is within the normal range established for erythrocytes of adults.

Several physiologic and metabolic characteristics of erythrocytes of newborns also differ from those of RBCs of older children and adults. Permeability of the fetal RBC membrane to sodium and potassium is increased, and glucose utilization and adenosine triphosphate (ATP) production by the erythrocytes are correspondingly elevated. The latter changes appear in part to represent compensatory activities that serve to maintain normal concentrations of intracellular cations by means of an augmented rate of energy-dependent ion transport.

RBC survival is shortened to a mild or moderate degree in the full-term infant, as compared with the normal adult erythrocyte survival time of 100 to 120 days. In the premature infant shortening of the RBC life span is even greater, although considerable variability has been reported. The reduced life span of the erythrocytes of the infant may be related to the relatively larger size of the fetal erythrocyte, which, together with greater cell rigidity, renders the erythrocytes less compliant and deformable within the small blood vessels and may cause them to be more susceptible to intravascular damage. In addition, the increased permeability of the RBC membrane to sodium and potassium predisposes the RBCs to the development of adverse osmotic changes within the cells, adding further risk of premature cell destruction, particularly within the spleen and other reticuloendothelial organs.

An increase in the activity of several glycolytic RBC enzymes also has been demonstrated in the blood of newborns. However, these changes may reflect the presence of a larger percentage of young RBCs rather than a specific characteristic of the cells. Other enzymes, including carbonic anhydrase and methemoglobin reductase, dependent on reduced nicotinamide adenine dinucleotide (NADH-dependent reductase), exhibit reduced activity in the RBCs of the newborn. The decrease in the latter enzyme is a major factor in accounting for the elevated levels of methemoglobin in the blood of newborns, particularly in premature infants, as well as the predisposition of young infants to form methemoglobin more readily in the presence of precipitating factors.

From 70% to 90% of the hemoglobin in the blood of the fetus and newborn is fetal hemoglobin. This hemoglobin type continues to predominate through the first weeks of postnatal life, after which it gradually becomes replaced by adult hemoglobin. A functional difference between fetal and adult hemoglobin results from the ability of the latter to interact with low molecular weight phosphorylated compounds in the cell to produce altered oxygen-binding properties of the hemoglobin. When adult hemoglobin combines with these substances, which include 2,3-diphosphoglycerate (2,3-DPG), ATP, and related compounds, a marked decrease in oxygen affinity occurs. Fetal hemoglobin, on the other hand, undergoes virtually no participation in this type of interaction. The result of this difference in the behavior of adult and fetal hemoglobins is a leftward shift of the oxygen dissociation curve of fetal blood as compared with the blood of adults, representing a relatively greater oxygen affinity of the fetal blood. This property may be of considerable benefit to the fetus in utero by facilitating placental oxygen exchange from maternal blood to the fetal erythrocytes. However, because of the high oxygen affinity of the fetal hemoglobin, release of oxygen to the tissues is impeded, which may be disadvantageous to the newborn, particularly if anemia is present. (See Part two.)

The leukocyte count at birth averages approximately 20,000/mm^3, with a wide normal range from 9,000 to 30,000. Approximately 70% of the white blood cells consist of neutrophils, which often include band forms, and occasionally a small number of metamyelocytes and myelocytes. The white count usually drops with bacterial infection, and rare blast forms may appear in the blood smear. After the first week of life the differential count shifts to a predominance of lymphocytes, which persists until 4 or 5 years of age.

Platelet counts of full-term infants range from 150,000 to 300,000/mm^3, which are usually considered to be normal values for adults. Some reports have indicated slightly lower values in some premature infants. In any infant, however, a platelet count of less than 100,000/mm^3 should be considered abnormal.

The bone marrow findings of the newborn reflect the extremely active production of blood cells, particularly erythrocytes, which is characteristic of this period of life. The bone marrow at birth is highly cellular and occupies almost the entire medullary cavity of all the bones. Consequently, diagnostic bone marrow aspiration in young infants can be performed in long bone areas, such as the tibia, whereas in the older child and adult these bones contain primarily fatty tissue. Erythroid precursors comprise approximately 40% of the cellular elements present in aspirated bone marrow specimens.

HEMATOLOGIC CHANGES IN THE NEONATE AND INFANT

Within hours after birth of a normal infant the low oxygen saturation of the blood increases to reach approximately 95% saturation. The striking changes in erythropoiesis that occur in the first weeks of life are largely attributable to the improved oxygenation of the blood and tissues of the infant. Erythropoietin levels, which are elevated at birth, rapidly fall to undetectable levels. In the bone marrow, erythropoietic activity becomes suppressed, with RBC precursors comprising less than 10% of the nucleated elements by the end of the first week of postnatal life. The reticulocytosis, which is characteristic at birth, also decreases rapidly to reach less than 1% by 5 to 7 days. Nucleated RBC precursors disappear even more rapidly and after 2 to 4 days are usually no longer demonstrable in the blood of normal infants.

The postnatal suppression of erythropoiesis, combined with the expansion of the blood volume of the infant caused by rapid growth, produces a progressive decline in the hemoglobin concentration of the infant, beginning near the end of the first week of life and reaching its low point after 2 to 3 months. This physiologic anemia of infancy may result in a hemoglobin concentration of as low as 9.0 gm/dl (11.0 $\pm$ 2.0) in a normal full-term infant. These changes do not represent any abnormality or nutritional deficiency in the infant, and the hematologic events at this stage are not affected by the administration of iron or other hematinic agents. With the resumption of active erythropoiesis following the second to third months, if iron supplies are adequate, the hemoglobin concentration of the infant gradually increases to reach a mean level of 12.5 gm/dl, which persists throughout early childhood.

In premature infants, particularly those with birth weights of less than 1,500 gm, the physiologic decrease in hemoglobin concentration develops earlier than in full-term infants and reaches a lower ultimate level. Minimum values are achieved by 4 to 7 weeks, and hemoglobin concentrations of 7 to 8 mg/dl may occur in apparently healthy infants. Resumption of active erythropoiesis in the premature infant is also initiated earlier in postnatal life than in the full-term infant.

The supply of available iron stores in the full-term infant is usually sufficient to sustain normal RBC production for approximately the first 6 months of life, even without additional exogenous iron. Thereafter the iron needs related to growth require an intake of approximately 1 mg/kg daily if anemia is to be prevented. In the infant whose iron reserve at birth is diminished, the need for additional iron intake develops earlier. Included in this group are premature infants and infants with blood loss during the fetal or neonatal periods.

Although the iron needs of the normal full-term infant during the first year of life can usually be met by adequate dietary intake, some of these infants develop iron deficiency. It has therefore been recommended that iron supplementation be included in the diet of all infants throughout the first year of life. Iron-enriched cereals and milk formulas generally provide the most convenient and reliable means for providing this supplementary iron. In the premature infant dietary iron is almost never adequate, and iron supplementation is mandatory to prevent the development of anemia. In these infants it is desirable to introduce iron-enriched milk formula or other iron-containing preparations into the diet during the early weeks of life. Although exogenous iron is not incorporated into hemoglobin to a significant extent in young infants, orally administered iron is nevertheless absorbed and stored by the infant and can be used for hemoglobin synthesis later when the need for additional iron develops.

All hemoglobin molecules are constructed of four heme groups and four globin chains. The different varieties of hemoglobins vary in their globin chain components. Embryonic hemoglobins produced in the first trimester include Gower 1, composed of four ϵ-chains (ϵ_4), Gower 2 ($\alpha_2\epsilon_2$), and Portland ($\zeta_2\gamma_2$). Beyond early embryonic life all hemoglobins contain two α-chains and vary only in their non-α-globin chains. Hemoglobin F, the major fetal hemoglobin, contains two α- and two γ-chains ($\alpha_2\gamma_2$). The major adult hemoglobin, Hb A, contains two α- and two β-chains ($\alpha_2\beta_2$). A minor constituent of adult hemoglobin is Hb A_2 ($\alpha_2\delta_2$). Newer techniques of molecular biology have yielded much information about the genetics of the hemoglobinopathies and of normal hemoglobin synthesis (Fig. 32-3).

The α-globin chains are carried on chromosome 16 and are duplicated in most populations. Thus most persons have two haploid sets of α-genes, or a total of four gene copies. The non-α-genes are carried on chromosome 11 (Fig. 32-4). The δ- and β-genes are closely linked. There are two γ-genes on the same chromosome that are similar in structure, but one gene produces a protein higher in glutamine ($^G\gamma$) and the other a protein higher in alanine ($^A\gamma$). The ratio of $^G\gamma$ and $^A\gamma$ chain production remains constant at 3:1 throughout fetal life. β-Chain production is detectable by the tenth week of gestation and continues at that rate until late in gestation. Between 32 and 36 weeks' gestation the relative rate of β-chain synthesis increases and γ-chain synthesis decreases. At birth approximately 50% of non-α-chain syn-

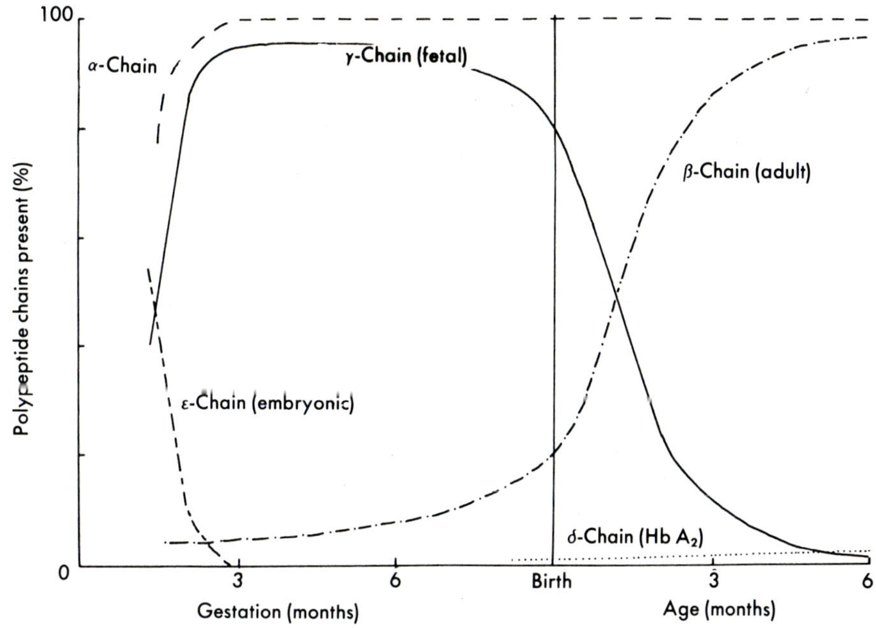

Fig. 32-3. Development of human hemoglobin chains. (From Huens, E.R., and others: Cold Spring Harbor Symp. Quant. Biol. **29:**327, 1964. Copyright 1964.)

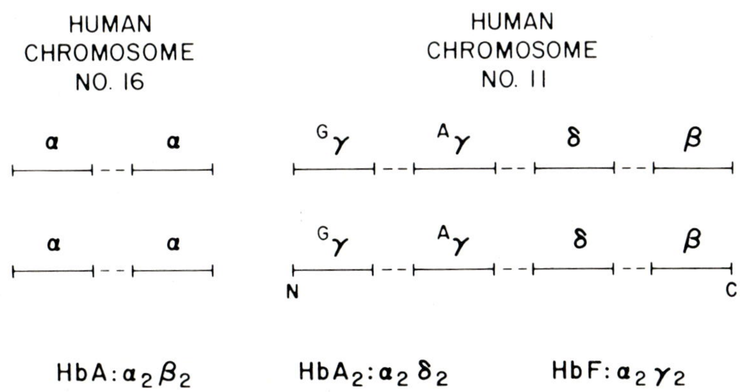

Fig. 32-4. Number and chromosomal arrangement of nonembryonic human globin genes. (From Forget, B.G., and others: Structure of the human globin genes. In Maniatis, T., Axel, R., and Fox, C.F., editors: Eukaryotic gene regulation: ICN-UCLA Symposia on Molecular and Cellular Biology, vol. 14, New York, 1979, Academic Press, Inc.)

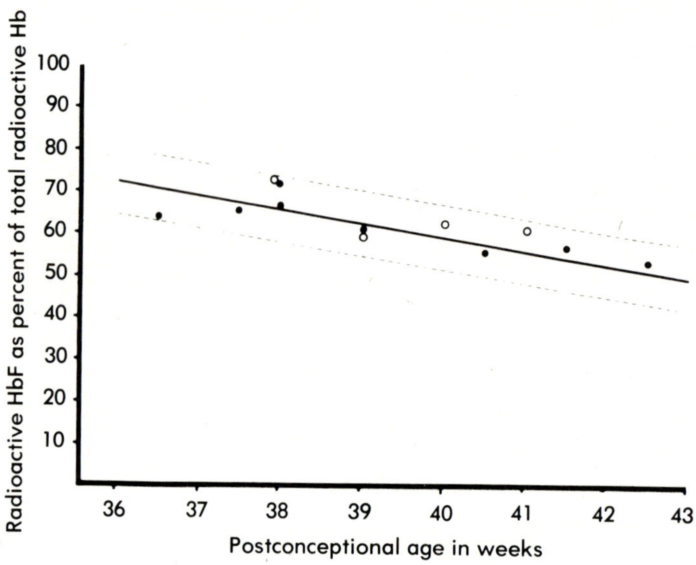

Fig. 32-5. Fetal hemoglobin synthesis as a percentage of total hemoglobin synthesis in relation to postconceptional age. ●, Infants less than 1,000 gm; ○, control term newborn infants. (From Bard, H., and Prosmanne, J.: J. Clin. Invest. **70:**50, 1982.)

thesis consists of β-chains. Over the first few months of postnatal life the $^{G}\gamma$-to-$^{A}\gamma$ ratio changes from 3:1 to 2:3. During the normal period of neonatal depression of erythropoiesis, there is a steady, linear decline in total γ-chain production. The cells that appear in the bloodstream when erythropoiesis resumes after 6 weeks of age contain predominantly HbA. The postnatal period of depressed erythropoiesis makes the "switch" from fetal to adult hemoglobin production appear to be very abrupt, but in fact it is a gradual process that begins prenatally and occurs on schedule even in very premature infants (Fig. 32-5). Infants of diabetic mothers have a delayed γ-to-β switch. Both the switch from embryonic to fetal and from fetal to adult hemoglobin production occur within the same population of erythroblasts. The globin chains that are synthesized do not appear to be affected by the site of erythropoiesis (yolk sac, hepatic, or myeloid) and are controlled by factors determined by the gestational age of the fetus.

ANEMIA IN THE NEWBORN PERIOD

Anemia caused by hemorrhage

Fetal-maternal transfusion

Transplacental transfusion of fetal blood into the circulation of the mother has been known for many years to be the basis for maternal antibody formation against fetal erythrocytes in the pathogenesis of isoimmune hemolytic disease. In a survey of more than 600 pregnancies, fetal erythrocytes were detected in maternal blood in approximately 50% of the cases. In about 1% of the pregnancies the transplacental hemorrhage appeared to be of sufficient magnitude to produce anemia in the infant.

Clinical manifestations. In most patients the bleeding appears to occur at a slow rate over a prolonged period before delivery. The degree of anemia in the newborn can vary widely, ranging from mild to very severe. Jaundice is characteristically absent, the direct antiglobulin test is negative, and the liver and spleen are not enlarged; these findings allow this condition to be readily distinguished from the anemia of isoimmune hemolytic disease. Pallor and tachycardia are present to a degree related to the severity of the anemia. The infant otherwise is usually active and in no apparent distress. The anemia is accompanied by polychromatophilia of the erythrocytes, by elevated reticulocyte counts, and often by increased numbers of nucleated RBCs. If the anemia is severe and is the result of chronic long-term hemorrhage, the hematologic findings characteristic of severe iron-deficiency anemia will be present, including hypochromia and microcytosis of the erythrocytes, decreased serum iron levels, and an absence of stainable iron in aspirated bone marrow. (See Chapter 22.)

If the fetal-maternal transfusion occurs acutely at the time of labor or delivery, the findings in the infant will reflect the rapid reduction in the blood volume (Chapter 24, part one). Loss of more than 40 ml of blood can be sufficient to produce findings of hypovolemic shock. The infant may appear weak and pale, with tachycardia and labored respirations. Anemia can usually be demonstrated, but if insufficient time has elapsed for compensatory hemodilution to occur, the hemoglobin concentration may not be significantly depressed. Acute blood loss usually can be confirmed, however, by decreased arterial or venous pressure. The presumptive diagnosis of severe acute blood loss should be considered in any

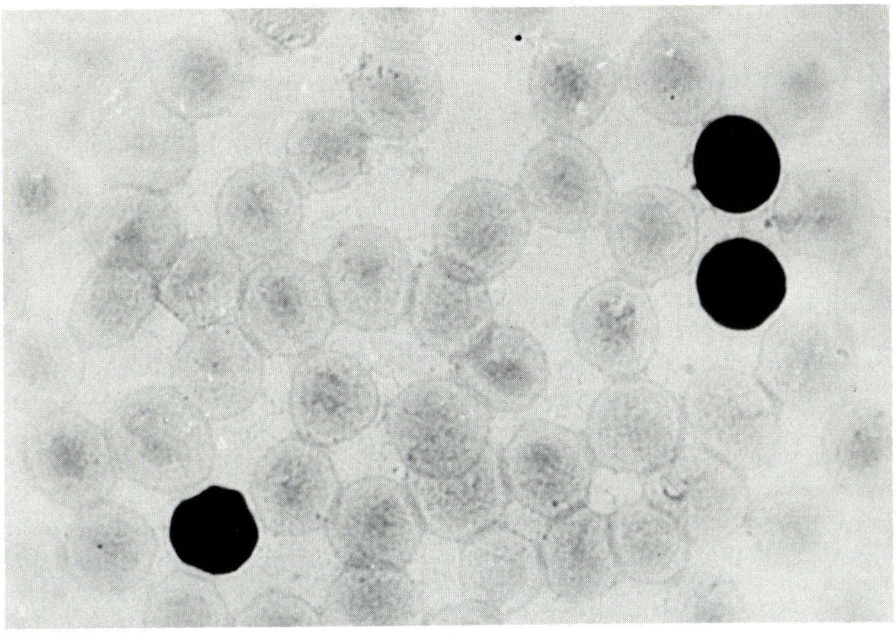

Fig. 32-6. Fetal erythrocytes in maternal blood following a transplacental hemorrhage. The slide was stained following elution of adult hemoglobin by the Kleihauer-Betke procedure. The fetal cells containing HbF are darkly stained, whereas those of the HbA mother are barely visible.

pale neonate in distress when the liver or spleen is not enlarged, and appropriate measures should be undertaken immediately to confirm or disprove this possibility.

Laboratory manifestations. Loss of fetal blood into the maternal circulation can be established by demonstrating the presence of fetal erythrocytes in the mother's blood. The most widely applicable technique is the slide elution procedure of Kleihauer and Betke. In this procedure, which is performed rapidly and easily, unstained blood smears are fixed and then incubated in an acidic buffer that causes adult hemoglobin to be eluted from the erythrocytes. Fetal hemoglobin resists elution under these conditions and remains within the intact RBCs. After staining, the fetal hemoglobin-containing erythrocytes become visible as darkly stained cells, while the erythrocytes of maternal origin, which contain principally adult hemoglobin, appear as clear, ghostlike cells (Fig. 32-6). The presence of even small numbers of fetal cells in maternal blood is readily ascertained by this procedure, and by determination of the percentage of fetal cells present an estimate of the quantity of blood transfused can be made. If major blood group incompatibility exists between the mother and infant, transfused fetal erythrocytes may be rapidly removed from the maternal circulation and may not be detectable in blood smears from the mother. Under these conditions the mother may develop fever or a shaking chill, representing a transfusion reaction to the infusion of incompatible blood. Buffy coat smears of the maternal blood may demonstrate erythrophagocytosis when blood group incompatibility exists and may be helpful in establishing a diagnosis when the slide elution test for fetal cells is negative because of rapid hemolysis.

Treatment. Treatment of the infant depends on both the severity of the anemia and whether the blood loss occurred acutely or chronically. In the infant with a mild degree of anemia, particularly when there is evidence that the blood loss was not acute, no immediate therapy is usually necessary if the infant is vigorous and in no distress. If tachycardia or marked pallor is present, a transfusion of packed RBCs is indicated. In the severely affected infant with findings of iron deficiency caused by prolonged hemorrhage, incipient heart failure may be present, and transfusion may impose a risk of vascular overload. Under these conditions a partial exchange transfusion using packed RBCs is preferable. When transfusions are done in these infants, it is rarely necessary to increase the hemoglobin concentration to more than 11 to 12 gm/dl to achieve complete relief of symptoms of anemia. Iron therapy is essential in subsequent care because of depletion of the iron stores by chronic blood loss. Adequate iron supplementation in these infants can be achieved by the regular use of an iron-enriched milk formula or by oral administration of an iron preparation sufficient to provide 2 to 3 mg of elemental iron per kilogram daily. The iron supplementation should be started in early infancy and continued throughout the first year of life to ensure that the iron needs for growth of the infant are fully met.

In the neonate with findings of hypovolemic shock at birth because of acute bleeding into the maternal circulation shortly before delivery, rapid diagnosis and prompt institution of therapy are essential to prevent irreversible changes. Therapy is directed toward rapid restoration of the infant's blood volume and should be started immediately after the condition is recognized. Fresh type O, Rh-negative blood, 10 to 20 ml/kg, should be injected through an umbilical catheter. When blood is not readily available, albumin solutions, plasma, or dextran may be given in the initial infusion, to be followed by whole blood as soon as it becomes available. The response to blood replacement in these infants is usually dramatic. Tachycardia and tachypnea rapidly subside, and tone and activity improve promptly. Subsequent additional transfusions with packed RBCs are indicated if signs of distress persist or if the hemoglobin concentration falls to less than 8 to 9 gm/dl after fluid equilibration in the plasma has taken place. Orally administered iron should be given to these infants and continued throughout the first year.

Blood loss in utero from one twin to another

See also Chapters 10 and 11.

Incidence and etiology. Newborn monovular twins frequently exhibit large differences in their hemoglobin concentrations at birth, with anemia being present in one twin and polycythemia in the other. In approximately 70% of monovular twin pregnancies the placentas are monochorial and almost invariably contain vascular communications between the fetal circulations (Chapter 11). When a significant degree of arteriovenous anastomosis exists between the placental circulations of one twin and the other, the opportunity exists for the twin on the arterial limb of the communication to infuse blood into the circulation of the other. A study of 130 monochorial twin pregnancies indicated an incidence of at least 15% significant blood loss from one twin to the other. A high mortality of the affected twins occurred, often with death in utero early in the pregnancy. Of 38 of these infants born alive, only 13 survived, suggesting that this complication may be a major factor to account for the higher mortality of monochorial as compared with dichorial twin pregnancies.

Clinical manifestations. In the donor twin, anemia may vary from mild to severe. RBC hypochromia and microcytosis are often present as a reflection of iron deficiency caused by the prolonged blood loss. Elevated reticulocyte counts and large numbers of nucleated RBCs represent a compensatory increase of erythrocyte production. The anemia is often accompanied by oligohydramnios and hypotension. If blood loss has been extensive, the infant may exhibit pallor, weakness, and tachycardia.

The polycythemic infant presents a ruddy appearance and often is larger than the anemic twin. The infant may show evidence of hypertension, which can be associated with heart failure and pulmonary edema. Hyperviscosity of the blood results from the increased RBC mass and can predispose these infants to venous thrombosis or hemorrhage. Hyperbilirubinemia may accompany breakdown of the increased numbers of RBCs.

Treatment. The donor twin may require supportive transfusions if symptomatic anemia is present. With severe anemia a partial exchange transfusion with packed RBCs minimizes the risk of circulatory overload. If the infant is asymptomatic and the anemia is not severe, orally administered iron will usually be sufficient.

In the polycythemic twin, phlebotomy is indicated if complications arise as a result of hyperviscosity of the blood or from circulatory overload. The hemoglobin concentration can be reduced most effectively by performing a partial exchange transfusion using albumin to replace the blood that is removed. Partial exchange transfusion should probably be performed on asymptomatic patients with central venous hematocrits greater than 70% to prevent the complications of hyperviscosity.

Obstetric hemorrhage

Incidence. Anemia in newborns caused by acute obstetric hemorrhage occurs at a rate of approximately 1 per 1,000 live births. This complication to which the infant is predisposed may result from obstetric accidents in otherwise normal pregnancies or to abnormalities of the umbilical cord, umbilical vessels, or placenta.

Etiology. Rupture of the normal umbilical cord has been documented as a cause of neonatal hemorrhage primarily following precipitous, often unattended deliveries. Although this now occurs infrequently, it should be considered when an anemic infant with a history of an uncontrolled delivery is encountered. When the cord is abnormally short or is entangled with the infant, it may become torn in the course of even a normal delivery. Varices or aneurysms of the umbilical vessels may produce areas of focal weakness that predispose the infant to rupture of the cord. When the placental insertion of the umbilical cord is abnormal (Chapter 11), giving rise to anomalous aberrant vessels lying free on the placental surface or to a diffuse velamentous insertion, the unprotected vessels become easily subjected to laceration during the delivery with the risk of considerable blood loss by the infant. A possible anomaly is multilobularity of the placenta, in which one or more accessory lobules exist apart from the main body of the placenta. The lobules are joined by fragile communicating vessels that become easily disrupted during labor and delivery, accompanied by hemorrhage.

In placenta previa and abruptio placentae, hemorrhage

from the placental surface can result in blood loss from the infant as well as from the mother. In these disorders the incidence of stillbirths is high, and surviving infants frequently are severely anemic at birth. Acute blood loss following accidental incision of the placenta at cesarean delivery is also possible, particularly in placenta previa. Tearing or separation of the placenta during delivery of the infant through the uterine incision may also lead to significant blood loss.

Clinical manifestations. In anemia developing as a result of obstetric hemorrhage, the findings in the infant at birth are attributable to acute blood loss; following severe hemorrhage, these may include pallor, tachycardia, irregular respirations, decreased tone, and a weak cry. The central venous pressure will often be reduced. The hemoglobin concentration immediately after delivery may not reflect the true magnitude of blood loss; however, usually 6 to 12 hours later, after hemodilution has occurred, the anemia will be fully apparent.

Treatment. Therapy is directed toward rapid expansion of the blood volume with transfusions of fresh whole blood whenever possible, as described in the preceding sections. Dietary supplementation with orally administered iron should be started early and in adequate amounts to prevent later development of iron deficiency.

Postnatal hemorrhage

Hemorrhage in the first days of life as a cause of anemia most often results from birth trauma. When a congenital or acquired disorder of hemostasis is present in the infant, postpartum hemorrhage may occur, even in the absence of unusual trauma at delivery. Postnatal bleeding may be apparent or occult and in either case may result in gradual or rapidly progressive anemia. The sudden onset of shock in a previously well infant sometimes may be the first indication of occult hemorrhage. In any infant who develops anemia beyond the first day of life, without jaundice or other evidence of hemolysis, every attempt should be made to ascertain or exclude the presence of internal bleeding. In premature infants, in cases of multiple births, and following breech or traumatic deliveries the risk of postnatal hemorrhage is increased.

Hemorrhage into the scalp associated with a caput succedaneum often occurs (Chapter 20) but usually subsides within a few days, producing no untoward effect. Occasionally a substantial quantity of blood may be lost into the scalp, resulting in anemia of sufficient severity to require supportive transfusions of packed RBCs. Subperiosteal hemorrhages (cephalhematomas) occur with or without fracture of the skull (Chapter 20). The hemorrhage is often gradual and may continue for 1 to 3 days, after which it usually subsides spontaneously. Massive blood loss requiring transfusion occurs in rare instances. A more frequent complication in these infants is the development of jaundice following degradation of the extravasated blood. The bilirubin level may become sufficiently elevated to require exchange transfusion if the hemorrhage has been extensive.

Intracranial hemorrhage may result as a complication of birth trauma, and intraventricular hemorrhage is particularly prevalent in premature infants (Chapter 27, part three). Subarachnoid or subdural hemorrhage is rarely of sufficient severity to produce anemia.

Hemorrhage into the liver, spleen, adrenals, or kidneys, following rupture or laceration of these organs, may also produce anemia in the perinatal period. Predisposing factors include traumatic or breech delivery, prematurity, disorders of hemostasis, and conditions that produce swelling or distension of the abdominal organs. The liver is most often affected. Hemorrhage may be mild and limited to subcapsular bleeding or may result from rupture of the parenchyma and capsule of the liver, with massive blood loss into the peritoneal cavity. With progressive subcapsular hepatic hemorrhage the infant may appear well until rupture of the capsule ensues, followed by rapid development of hemoperitoneum and hypovolemic shock. Splenic rupture in the newborn period occurs infrequently but may follow a traumatic delivery (Chapter 20). In most reported examples of this complication, splenic distension associated with splenomegaly caused by isoimmune hemolytic disease was present. Retroperitoneal hemorrhage involving the adrenals, or less often the kidneys, usually follows a traumatic delivery and may produce anemia (Chapter 20). Findings attributable to blood loss often develop soon after birth and are accompanied by an enlarging flank mass. In some infants the adrenal hemorrhage may be manifested as unexplained jaundice together with a mass in the flank in an otherwise healthy-appearing infant. The diagnosis can often be established by the finding of a radiolucent suprarenal mass and downward and lateral displacement of the kidney on an excretory urogram. These findings may be similar to those of congenital neuroblastoma. Arteriography through the umbilical artery will usually show increased vascularity in neuroblastoma, whereas an avascular lesion is seen in adrenal hemorrhage. Ultrasound and CT scans may distinguish those entities without the need for arteriography.

Congenital anemias caused by erythrocyte underproduction

Congenital hypoplastic anemia

Congenital hypoplastic anemia (CHA) has been described under a variety of names, including chronic aregenerative anemia, erythrogenesis imperfecta, pure red cell aplasia, and Diamond-Blackfan anemia. It was initially described as a distinct entity in 1938. There is an equal sex distribution and no clear-cut genetic pattern of inheritance in most cases, although both full- and half-siblings have been affected. Gradual onset of severe anemia occurs in the first months of life, with 72% of patients presenting by the age of 4 months. Reticulocytopenia in the peripheral blood reflects the marked diminution of erythrocyte precursors in the bone marrow (erythroblastopenia). Total white count, absolute neutrophil count, and platelet count are all normal.

Several features characteristic of fetal erythrocytes persist throughout life in these patients, including macrocytosis (MCV usually greater than 100 μm^3), elevated levels of hemoglobin F, heterogeneously distributed among the red cell population, and expression of the "i" antigen on the surface of erythrocytes. These features are often helpful in distinguishing CHA from transient erythroblastopenia of childhood (TEC), in which the MCV is usually less than 90 μm^3 at presentation and hemoglobin F levels and "i" antigen expression are low. This disorder may also appear in the first months of life but requires no specific therapy and has no long-term consequences.

Levels of erythropoietin are elevated in CHA. The mechanism of suppression of erythropoiesis is not known. Immunologic factors are suspected, since both serum and lymphocytes have been found to inhibit bone marrow erythroid colony growth in vitro. Multiple mechanisms probably are active, and CHA does not have a single pathogenesis underlying all cases of the disorder. Neither a nutritional factor nor lack of stimulating hormones, however, appears to contribute to lack of erythrocyte production.

Several constitutional anomalies, including triphalangeal thumbs, have been reported in association with CHA. Peripheral blood lymphocyte and bone marrow chromosomes are normal, in contrast to Fanconi's anemia, which usually appears beyond the neonatal period and involves multiple cell lines. Several patients with CHA have developed acute leukemia in adolescence or young adulthood. Short stature is a consistent finding but is not usually evident at birth, with only about 20% of patients small for gestational age. Short stature may be aggravated by corticosteroid therapy.

Infants have gradually increasing pallor, poor feeding, and listlessness. Physical examination is usually unremarkable except for pallor unless the child is experiencing congestive heart failure, in which case hepatomegaly with or without splenomegaly and flow murmurs suggestive of cardiovascular decompensation may be present. These findings reverse with transfusion. Evaluation includes complete blood count with reticulocyte count, red cell indices, and bone marrow examination.

Most patients respond to corticosteroid therapy with improvement or normalization of the hemoglobin and independence of transfusion therapy. The response to steroids appears to be greatest when treatment is instituted early. Patients started on steroids 6 months or more into their illness have a lower response rate. Some patients fail to respond to steroids and remain transfusion dependent. After initial daily prednisone, erythroid activity may be preserved by every-other-day or other intermittent schedules for steroid therapy to minimize the complications of long-term daily steroid use. Some patients remit with the onset of puberty and become independent of transfusion or steroid therapy, but this is an erratic occurrence. Therapy is begun with the equivalent of 2 mg prednisone/kg body weight, but occasionally higher doses are needed to obtain a response. If the disease is steroid responsive, reticulocytosis is typically seen within 1 to 2 weeks, but occasionally a longer period is required, and 6 to 8 weeks should be completed before concluding that the process is not responsive. Androgens have no place in the management of CHA. The mechanism of action of corticosteroid therapy is unclear, but the observation of its efficacy serves to underscore the possible immune etiology of CHA.

Most patients survive at least into young adulthood. Causes of death include transfusional hemosiderosis and septicemia following splenectomy performed for hypersplenism in chronically transfused patients. Steroid-responsive patients have a far better survival rate but experience the consequences of long term steroid therapy and have markedly short stature.

Anemias of endocrine insufficiency

The normochromic, normocytic anemias of adrenal insufficiency, hypothyroidism, and pituitary insufficiency are usually mild, that is, hemoglobin levels rarely fall below 8 gm/dl. However, in hypoadrenalism the severity of the anemia may be obscured by a contracted plasma volume. Therapy is directed at correction of the underlying deficiency. Although macrocytosis is occasionally noted in this group of disorders, it probably reflects the large red cell size characteristic of the newborn. True megaloblastic changes occur only in the presence of associated folate or vitamin B_{12} deficiency. A modest increase in icterus may also be present as a result of early (intramarrow) red cell senescence.

Osteopetrosis

Osteopetrosis (Albers-Schönberg disease) is an autosomal recessive disease characterized by defective osteoclast and monocyte function that leads to thickened and brittle cortical bone formation, frequent fractures, growth retardation, and diminution in marrow space. The net effect is a compromise of erythroid as well as granulocyte and megakaryocyte development. Hemopoietic adjustment usually occurs via extramedullary hemopoiesis. The resultant normochromic, normocytic anemia is frequently accompanied by immature or nucleated RBCs in the peripheral circulation. The combination of repeated transfusions and extramedullary blood formation ultimately leads to hypersplenism. Although variations in severity are typical, the early-onset form is usually fatal. Until recently, therapy was essentially supportive. For patients with HLA identical, mixed leukocyte culture (MLC) nonreactive donors, it is possible to restore hemopoietic and bone remodeling functions with allogeneic bone marrow transplantation.

Constitutional pancytopenia

The Fanconi variant of constitutional aplastic anemia is characterized by moderate to severe pancytopenia in association with one or more congenital defects. These defects include hyperpigmentation, absent or hypoplastic thumbs, combination of absent radii and thumbs (in contrast to absent radii with thumbs in the radial-platelet hypoplasia syndrome), decreased numbers of carpal bones, microphthalmia, hyperreflexia, microcephaly, short stature, decreased bone age, strabismus, developmental abnormalities of the ears, double ureters, and ectopic and/or horseshoe kidneys.

The phenotypic expression of this disorder may precede the hematologic manifestation by a few months to as many as 15 years. Approximately 10% of these patients never develop hematologic disease.

Chromosomal abnormalities, uniformly seen in this disorder, include increased frequency of breakage, endoreduplications, and defective chromatid exchanges. The precise relationship between the chromosomal abnormalities and the hematologic manifestations is unclear, although the defective DNA repair mechanism (abnormal chromatid exchanges) suggests that the hematologic manifestations, that is, both the aplasia and subsequent leukemia, are secondarily induced. Elevated fetal hemoglobin levels, not uniformly distributed throughout the RBC mass, and the presence of the i antigen are typically seen in this disorder. The leukemic transformation occurs in about 7% of these patients and is almost exclusively of the acute monocytic or monomyelocytic variety.

In most cases androgen therapy effectively increases erythroid production and to a lesser extent granulocyte and platelet production. One such example is oxymetholone, administered orally in a dosage of 1 to 3 mg/kg/day. Once a response is identified, the dosage should be reduced to the minimum amount capable of maintaining a sustained response. Corticosteroids, other than having the ability to diminish testosterone-induced skeletal maturation, offer no additional therapeutic advantage. For the androgen-nonresponsive patient, RBC transfusion support accompanied by iron chelation therapy is the only major alternative. However, marrow transplantation from a genotypically normal HLA identical, MLC nonreactive sibling is an appropriate consideration. Androgen therapy must be carefully monitored because of potential hepatotoxicity and the risk of late-occurring hepatic carcinoma. The familial variant of constitutional aplastic anemia, so-called because of the lack of skeletal and chromosomal abnormalities, is otherwise identical in hematologic expression and therapeutic responsiveness.

Acquired anemias caused by erythrocyte underproduction

Transient erythroblastopenia of childhood

Transient erythroblastopenia of childhood (TEC) is frequently confused with congenital erythroid hypoplasia (CEH). Unlike CEH, however, most cases occur between 6 months and 4 years of age and usually follow viral infections. It rarely lasts longer than 4 months and usually disappears without any sequelae.

Children with TEC experience gradual onset of severe anemia without reticulocytosis. Platelets and leukocytes are normal, and the bone marrow shows erythroid hypoplasia without other abnormalities. The MCV is characteristically normal, in contrast to the macrocytosis seen in CEH. Remission is usually spontaneous and complete, although the anemia may be severe enough to require transfusion. The distinguishing characteristics of CEH and TEC are noted in Table 32-2. TEC has also been noted in infants with inborn errors in carnitine metabolism.

Aplastic crises of hemolytic disease

Transient erythroid hypoplasia may complicate hemolytic disorders. Even brief periods of erythroid aplasia may result in severe anemia if the red cell life span is very short, as in sickle cell disease or enzyme defects such as pyruvate kinase deficiency. Viral infections have been implicated in these aplastic crises, especially human *Parvovirus*, also associated with fifth disease (infectious erythema), which directly infects human erythroid progenitors in tissue culture. Exacerbation of anemia with reticulocytopenia characterizes aplastic crises, which are self-limited. Supportive transfusion may be required.

Acquired aplastic anemia

Acquired aplastic anemia is rare in infancy but has been reported, particularly in association with maternal drug ingestion (e.g., azathioprine) or drugs given to the infant (e.g., chloramphenicol), or as the initial presenting symptom of acute leukemia. Neutropenia, thrombocytopenia, and reticulocytopenia with a hypocellular bone marrow biopsy characterize aplastic anemia. The treatment of choice in older patients is bone marrow transplantation, but little experience with transplantation in neonates with aplastic anemia is available.

Table 32-2. Comparison of congenital erythroid hypoplasia and transient erythroblastopenia

	Congenital	Transient
Onset	Essentially all under 6 months of age	Most between 6 months and 4 years of age
Etiology	Variable inheritance	Viral, idiopathic
Skeletal defects	Present in approximately one third of patients	None
Chromosomal defects	Rare, unrelated	None
Male : female ratio	1 : 1	1 : 1
Hematologic findings		
MCV	Greater than 95 μm^3	Less than 90 μm^3
Pure red cell aplasia	Present	Present
Hemoglobin F	Usually increased	Consistent with age
i Antigen	Usually present	Absent
Therapy	Corticosteroid response in more than 85% of cases	None necessary
Prognosis	Spontaneous remission in 10%-15% of cases; hemosiderosis in long-term RBC-transfused patients	Complete recovery in 6-8 weeks

Folic acid and vitamin B_{12} deficiency

See also Appendix C.

Both folic acid and vitamin B_{12} are required for DNA synthesis and thus for growth. The manifestations of deficiencies of both are protean and include growth failure and neurologic abnormalities in young infants. The hematologic manifestations are usually easily recognized, since erythroid macrocytosis, hypersegmentation of the neutrophils, and hyperplastic bone marrow with megaloblastic changes in all cell lines are characteristic.

Serum folate levels in the newborn are two to three times higher than those in normal adults and fall within the first month of life. In premature infants the serum folate is often below normal levels, although the consequences of this deficiency are unclear. Because of rapid growth the folate requirements for small premature infants are high and may not be met by the amounts present in some modified cow's milk formulas. Recognition of the importance of folate supplementation has reduced the problem of folate deficiency in infants receiving parenteral nutrition. Because folate is heat labile, terminal sterilization of milk may result in significant folate deficiency in infancy. Goat's milk has almost no folate, and infants receiving goat's milk should receive supplemental folate, 1 to 2 mg/week orally. There are rare disorders of folate-binding proteins and folate metabolism that result in clinical and biochemical folate deficiency.

Serum vitamin B_{12} levels are also high at birth and fall in the first month. Milk is usually a good source of vitamin B_{12}, which can be stored for months in infants. The major exception is infants of mothers who are strict vegans and who eat no animal products for several years. The clinical disorders in these infants, especially the neurologic manifestations, are usually much worse than in the mothers who are also deficient in vitamin B_{12} but whose needs are lower. Malabsorption, gastric resection, and resection of the terminal ileum (e.g., in necrotizing enterocolitis) are more common causes of vitamin B_{12} deficiency than is dietary deficiency. Juvenile pernicious anemia may also appear in infancy. All these conditions will respond to parenterally administered vitamin B_{12}, which may be a lifelong requirement for many survivors of perinatal bowel resections and for patients with juvenile pernicious anemia. Other rare disorders of vitamin B_{12} transport and metabolism manifest clinically as megaloblastic anemia. The potential devastation of the neurologic complications of vitamin B_{12} deficiency, particularly during a period of rapid brain growth, demands attention to this possibility in patients at risk. As in adults, vitamin B_{12} should be administered before folate in infants when the nature of the deficiency is not clear.

Anemias caused by cell destruction

Accelerated RBC destruction resulting from intrinsic or acquired abnormalities of erythrocytes is common in the perinatal period. Isoimmune hemolytic disease is unique to this age group. Certain clinical features are prominent in hemolytic disease of the newborn and are affected by physiologic factors characteristic of the neonatal period.

Catabolism of hemoglobin is increased in all hemolytic states. The newborn liver is significantly less able to conjugate bilirubin than the mature liver, and hyperbilirubinemia is predominantly unconjugated, or indirect reacting. One gram of hemoglobin yields approximately 35 mg bilirubin.

Hemopoiesis occurring during the third trimester may be pronounced in hemolytic states. Extramedullary hemopoiesis occurs more readily in this period, and hepatosplenomegaly caused by myeloid metaplasia is often a prominent feature of hemolytic states.

Immature erythroid and myeloid precursors are released more readily from the bone marrow and other sites of hemopoiesis in the newborn period than later in life. Thus circulating marrow elements are frequently found in peripheral blood, a finding termed *erythro-*

blastosis. Young myeloid cells may also circulate when hemopoiesis is particularly brisk.

The blood-brain barrier of newborn infants is unusually permeable to bilirubin in the plasma that is not bound to plasma proteins, particularly albumin. This makes infants susceptible to the development of kernicterus, or bilirubin staining of the brain, which does not occur with higher levels of bilirubin in older children and adults. The damage to nervous system tissue is irreversible. It is seen at relatively low concentrations of bilirubin in premature infants because of low serum albumin, proportionately greater unbound bilirubin, and greater blood-brain permeability (Chapter 34). Drugs and hydrogen ions may displace bilirubin and predispose to development of kernicterus in certain circumstances. Prevention of kernicterus is the major concern in treatment of hyperbilirubinemia caused by hemolytic disease of the newborn.

The major causes of hemolytic disease in the newborn period include immune destruction of RBCs resulting from passively transferred maternal antibody, intrinsic defects in the red cell, and infection.

Isoimmune hemolytic disease

Maternal immunoglobulin G (IgG), or 7S antibody, passes across the placenta. If the antibodies are directed against antigens present on fetal erythrocytes, they bind to the red cell membrane and may cause the target cells to be removed by tissue macrophages. IgM, or 19S antibody, does not cross the placenta and does not cause hemolysis in the fetus. Hemolysis is extravascular. Free hemoglobin is not found in the serum except in rare cases of severe hemolysis. This reflects the fact that the antibodies act by altering the RBC membrane to enhance clearance of the cells and not primarily by fixing complement. Complement components are low even in term infants, and most IgG antibodies fix complement less efficiently than IgM antibodies. The major sites of destruction are the liver and spleen. The efficiency of clearance relates to the amount of antigen on the membrane, the amount of antibody bound to the antigens, the biologic activity of the antibody, and the maturity of macrophage function, particularly splenic function.

Red cell antigens are glycoproteins whose expression is genetically determined. Persons who are type O produce antibodies to blood group antigens A and B, termed *naturally occurring antibodies*. Their production appears to be incited by bacterial glycoproteins that are antigenically similar to the A and B substances. Type A persons produce anti-B, and type B persons produce anti-A. Most of these naturally occurring antibodies are IgM and do not cross the placenta. If a fraction of the antibodies is IgG, they may be passively transferred and may cause hemolysis if the infant carries the RBC antigen. Thus ABO hemolysis is frequently not caused by maternal sensitization but by passive transfer of antibody directed at cross-reacting antigens. In contrast, Rh and minor blood groups do not react with such antibodies, and hemolysis induced by antibodies results from maternal sensitization to fetal antigens.

ABO incompatibility

See also Part two of this chapter.

Individuals who lack the A and B blood group substances normally demonstrate antibodies against the factors that are absent. Type O persons produce anti-A and anti-B antibodies, primarily 19S globulins. Frequently some of the anti-A activity in type O and type B individuals can be demonstrated in the 7S fraction of serum. If this antibody crosses the placenta of an infant whose RBCs bear the A substance, the infant may develop hemolysis. Thus hemolytic disease caused by anti-A may occur following a first pregnancy in an unsensitized mother. Subsequent pregnancies are not likely to produce more severely affected infants. ABO hemolytic disease may also occur because of antibody production in a sensitized mother. Blood group substance A_1 appears to be the most strongly antigenic of the major blood group antigens and is associated with the largest number of cases of clinically apparent hemolysis. Expression of the A and B substances is relatively poorly developed in the fetus and newborn. The antigen density is lower than later in life and probably accounts for the relatively mild hemolysis accompanying many cases of ABO incompatibility. Approximately 40% of infants of type O mothers are either type A (31%) or type B (9%). The cord blood Coombs' test is positive in approximately 33% of these pregnancies, but a relatively small percentage require intervention for control of hyperbilirubinemia or anemia. The spectrum of disease is extremely broad. The incidence and severity may be greater in black than in white infants.

The naturally occurring anti-A IgG is a univalent or "incomplete" antibody that agglutinates type A cells well in 20% albumin but poorly in saline. Thus it may be difficult to demonstrate direct antiglobulin positivity unless appropriate steps are taken. Hemolysis resulting from anti-A and anti-B antibodies is characterized by the presence of spherocytes on the baby's blood smear. Spherocyte formation is thought to result from removal of a portion of the RBC membrane in the spleen, with release of cells containing reduced surface area and somewhat reduced cell volume.

Rh incompatibility

(See also Part two of this chapter.)

The antigens in the Rh system are determined by three closely linked genes that segregate as alleles. The antigens are termed C, c, D, d, E, and e. The d antigen is inferred but has not been demonstrated. Several rare variants have also been identified and have been associated with isoimmune hemolytic disease, including C^w, C^x, and D^u. Individuals are defined as Rh positive if their red cells express the D antigen and may be either homozygous (D/D) or heterozygous (D/d) for the D antigen. Rh-negative individuals are homozygous d/d. The D antigen is highly antigenic and is expressed on the RBC membrane as early as the eleventh week of fetal life. These facts are probably responsible for the severity of Rh hemolytic anemia, which is associated with hemolysis early in fetal life and high titers of antibodies. The incidence of hemolytic disease of the newborn due to Rh antibodies varies with racial groups. Approximately 85% of whites are Rh positive, as are 93% of blacks and 99% of Orientals. Rh incompatibility occurs only if the mother is Rh negative. Hemolytic disease is approximately three times as common in whites as in blacks and is rare in Chinese.

Fetal cells may enter the maternal circulation at any time during a pregnancy, but fetal-maternal transfusion is most common with trauma related to delivery or amniocentesis. Fetal cells can be demonstrated in the maternal circulation of up to 50% of patients following delivery, but the volume of bleeding is rarely more than about 0.2 ml. Approximately 1.0 ml of blood appears to be necessary to sensitize the mother to the antigens of the fetal cells. If the mother has naturally occurring antibodies to one of the major blood group antigens (A or B) present on fetal cells, the fetal cells may be destroyed before the mother has a chance to become sensitized to other antigens (such as D) present on the same cell. This is thought to account for the fact that Rh sensitization is less frequent in pregnancies in which ABO incompatibility also exists. Because most transplacental bleeding occurs around the time of delivery, Rh-negative mothers rarely become sensitized to Rh-positive fetal cells before term in the first pregnancy unless they have had previous transfusion with Rh-positive blood. The probability of sensitization increases with each Rh-positive infant; subsequent pregnancies are more likely to be affected, but fewer than 10% of Rh-negative women who bear Rh-positive infants are eventually sensitized (Chapter 5).

Immunization to the D antigen incites production of both 19S and 7S globulins. The 7S globulins are capable of transplacental transfer and coat fetal cells bearing the D antigen. These cells are then destroyed in the fetal liver and spleen, with resulting anemia and compensatory increase in erythropoiesis. The severity of the disorder varies from minimal hemolysis without clinical manifestations to uncompensated anemia with erythroblastosis and hydrops fetalis. Successive Rh-positive pregnancies in sensitized women incite increasing titers of antibodies, and the clinical severity tends to increase with each affected pregnancy. This is not the case in ABO incompatibility, even when the mother is sensitized to major blood group antigens. The titer of maternal antibody cannot be used as a reliable guide to the severity of disease in the infant, but a high or rising anti-D titer in a sensitized Rh-negative woman suggests significant hemolytic disease in the infant and may be used as an indication for amniocentesis to confirm the diagnosis and assess severity of hemolysis.

Jaundice is usually minimal or absent at birth because bilirubin is rapidly transported across the placenta and metabolized and excreted by the mother. With active hemolysis, however, jaundice is apparent within the first 12 to 24 hours of postnatal life and increases rapidly. The most severely affected infants have hydrops fetalis (Chapter 6), marked pallor, edema, ascites, pleural effusion, and congestive heart failure. The placentas are often also edematous and pale. In the most severe forms, disseminated intravascular coagulation may accompany brisk hemolysis, similar to severe hemolytic transfusion reactions. Anemia at birth is most often associated with Rh incompatibility but may be seen in isoimmune hemolytic disease caused by other blood group incompatibilities.

The incidence of Rh hemolytic disease has been greatly diminished by the prophylactic use of anti-D immune globulin following delivery, abortion, or amniocentesis in unsensitized Rh-negative women. High-titer anti-D serum is obtained from sensitized Rh-negative women or men deliberately immunized with Rh-positive cells. Administration of the γ-globulin at 28 weeks' gestation and within 72 hours of delivery results in clearance of circulating Rh-positive cells and prevents immune recognition of the foreign antigen by the mother. This procedure is not completely effective because transplacental bleeding may occur before delivery, and sensitization may antedate administration of the immune globulin (Chapter 5). Extensive fetal-maternal transfusion results in more circulating Rh-positive cells than can be cleared with the standard dosage of immune globulin, and sensitization may occur unless the dosage is substantially increased in this situation. However, most instances of sensitization of Rh-negative women occur because of failure to administer anti-D globulin following abortion or delivery of an Rh-positive infant.

Because the severity of Rh hemolytic disease tends to become progressively greater with each affected pregnancy, management extends into the prenatal period. Early delivery of severely affected children may facilitate hematologic management if the lung function has matured sufficiently to permit extrauterine survival. Intrauterine transfusion may be given to support the infant until delivery is feasible (Chapter 5).

Spectrophotometric assessment of bilirubin in amniotic fluid is used to determine the need for intervention (intrauterine transfusion or early delivery) in affected infants. If the maternal anti-D titer is greater than 1:16 and rising in a woman who has delivered a previous stillborn infant or an infant requiring exchange transfusion for Rh incompatibility, amniocentesis is performed and the optical density rise at 450 μm is determined. The result is interpreted according to the zone into which the measurement falls related to gestational age of the fetus. More than 95% of severely affected infants can be identified by serial examination of amniotic fluid spectrophotometry, which facilitates selection of infants for intrauterine transfusion and early delivery. Amniocentesis should be performed at about 21 weeks' gestation and repeated every 7 to 21 days, depending on the initial reading, in pregnancies at risk (Chapter 5).

Intrauterine transfusion is feasible because RBCs are absorbed intact from the peritoneal cavity. The cells enter the subdiaphragmatic lymphatics and are transported into the right lymphatic duct and into the circulation over 7 or 8 days. Infusion of excessive volumes of RBCs results in increased intraperitoneal pressure with occlusion of the umbilical vein, so it is important that the volume be limited. Inadvertent trauma to the heart and major arteries is associated with mortality, but many fetal organs have been punctured without apparent adverse effects. Washed, packed O negative RBCs should be used for intrauterine transfusion. Fatal and nonfatal lymphocyte engraftment has been reported, mandating the use of red cells that are at least white-cell poor, and preferably irradiated, to prevent lymphocyte engraftment and graft-versus-host disease.

Recently techniques for intravascular in utero exchange transfusion via percutaneous umbilical blood sampling have been developed. Although available only in specialized centers, these procedures should further improve fetal survival in Rh-affected pregnancies.

Other minor blood group incompatibilities

Sensitization to any of the minor blood group antigens can be associated with isoimmune hemolytic disease. These include Kell, Duffy, Lewis, Kidd, M, S, and others. The less antigenic components of the Rh system—C, c, E, and e—can also be associated with hemolytic disease of the newborn. The spectrum varies from subclinical evidence of sensitization to active hemolysis with hyperbilirubinemia requiring exchange transfusion. Hydrops fetalis with intrauterine or perinatal death has been reported with anti-Kell hemolytic disease.

The following sections discuss the diagnosis, management, delayed manifestations, and prognosis of hemolytic disease of the newborn.

Diagnosis. Jaundice in the first few days of life is the most frequent feature leading to diagnosis of isoimmune hemolysis. The bilirubin in cord blood rarely exceeds 5 mg/dl even in the most severe cases but begins to accumulate within the first 24 hours in most patients. The bilirubin is predominantly unconjugated because of the immaturity of the liver enzymes responsible for glucuronidation (Chapter 34).

Anemia is rarely present at birth except in hemolytic disease caused by Rh incompatibility but develops as hemolysis increases. Hepatomegaly and splenomegaly may be present due to extramedullary hemopoiesis, reticuloendothelial hyperplasia associated with extravascular hemolysis, and occasionally to congestive heart failure with severe anemia.

The blood smear shows evidence of active erythropoiesis, with polychromasia, reticulocytosis, and nucleated RBCs. In severe cases less mature erythroid precursors and sometimes myeloid precursors are found in the peripheral blood. Macrocytosis reflects the increase in young cells as well as the normally elevated RBC volume in the newborn period. Densely stained microspherocytes are often prominent in ABO incompatibility and are associated with increased osmotic fragility of the RBCs (Fig. 32-7). Spherocytes are also seen in minor blood group incompatibilities but not in Rh hemolytic disease. If the rate of RBC production equals the rate of destruction, anemia may be absent despite active hemolysis. When active hemolytic disease is present at birth, the suppression of erythropoiesis, which normally occurs within the first 24 hours of birth because of decreased erythropoietin production, is not seen.

Blood group incompatibility between mother and infant and the presence of antibody bound to the infant's erythrocytes must be demonstrated to establish a definitive diagnosis of isoimmune hemolytic disease. The direct antiglobulin test for detection of bound antibody is the most useful test but may be negative in mild cases of hemolysis if small amounts of antibody are present on the cell. In ABO disease the albumin antiglobulin test is more sensitive than the test performed in saline because the antibodies are often univalent ("incomplete"). An indirect antiglobulin test on the mother's serum may detect free antibodies when these cannot be identified on the infant's cells. Occasionally in Rh hemolytic disease the antibody may mask the D antigen, and the cells may falsely type as Rh negative. This occurs in a setting of severe hemolytic disease in an infant whose Rh-negative mother has a positive indirect antiglobulin test and has previously borne affected infants, but its occurrence should not obscure the diagnosis.

Management. See also Chapter 34.

Management is directed at prevention of the complications of hyperbilirubinemia and anemia. Hyperbilirubinemia is associated with neurologic damage caused by binding of unconjugated bilirubin that is not bound to serum albumin to the brain stem and basal ganglia. Unconjugated bilirubin complexes with phospholipids in

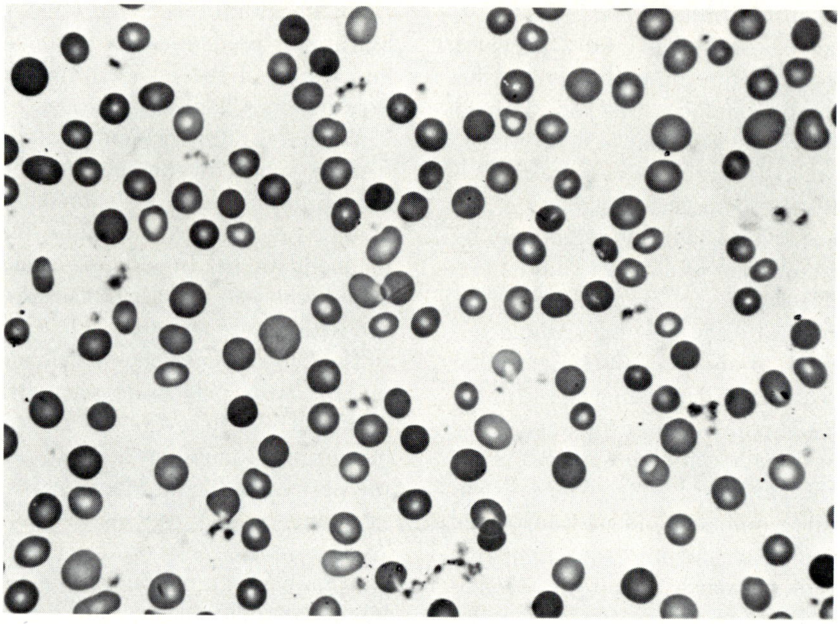

Fig. 32-7. Microspherocytes in ABO incompatibility. (Wright's stain; ×800.)

membranes and binds at lipid-water interphases. Binding to albumin is rapid and reversible, and an equilibrium is rapidly established in plasma and extracellular fluid. Beyond the neonatal period the blood-brain barrier is less permeable to penetration of unconjugated bilirubin, and most pathologic conditions associated with jaundice are accompanied by an increase in direct-reacting bilirubin. Thus the neurologic sequelae of hyperbilirubinemia are rarely seen except in this age group.

The first clinical sign of kernicterus is lethargy. Hypotonia and poor feeding are other early signs associated with loss of the sucking reflex. The hypotonia is replaced by hypertonia within the first few weeks, and most infants become opisthotonic and spastic. Long-term consequences are high-frequency nerve deafness, athetoid movements, mental retardation, and dysplasia of dental enamel. Frequently there is a transient period of clinical improvement that may lead to the impression that damage has not occurred. Kernicterus is never present at birth because of transplacental passage of bilirubin and should be regarded as a preventable disorder. Clinical manifestations in infants with hemolytic disease usually appear between the second and sixth day of life. Kernicterus rarely occurs at bilirubin levels below 20 mg/dl in full-term, otherwise healthy infants. Prematurity and low serum albumin levels also predispose to the development of kernicterus at lower bilirubin levels, as do acidosis and certain drugs by displacing bilirubin from albumin-binding sites. Clinical judgment must be used to facilitate decision making in jaundiced infants by taking into account infant age, birth weight, and the level of bilirubin at which observation, phototherapy, and exchange transfusion are indicated.

Phototherapy. See also Chapter 34.

Exposure of free or bound bilirubin to blue light (wavelengths 400 to 500 nm) causes a change in configuration from the normal Z form to a photobilirubin, termed the E form. Photobilirubin does not form an insoluble acid, is nontoxic to nervous system tissue, and is excreted in the bile without conjugation. The Z configuration is more stable, however, and the E form is readily transformed back to the Z form. These changes occur both in vivo and in vitro. Light exposure of the skin lowers plasma bilirubin through this conversion, and increased excretion of the photobilirubin may prevent the development of high, toxic levels. No serious short-term consequences of phototherapy are known, although deposition of pigments may darken the skin, and biochemical evidence of riboflavin deficiency has been demonstrated. There is concern about possible long-term side effects of phototherapy based largely on the possible carcinogenic hazard of radiation exposure. In vitro tests of mutagenicity have confirmed the theoretic hazards, but the clinical significance is as yet unknown. Continuous exposure to light is less mutagenic than intermittent exposure and is preferred. The infant's eyes must be protected from direct light exposure, and shielding the Isolette may decrease the exposure of nursery personnel.

Exchange transfusion. See also part two of this chapter.

Exchange transfusion has two goals in hemolytic disease of the newborn: (1) removal of sensitized, damaged erythrocytes, which contribute to the rate of hemolysis, and (2) removal of unconjugated bilirubin, which may cause neurologic damage. Exchange of twice the total blood volume (calculated as 80 ml/kg body weight) will replace 85% of the infant's RBCs and a substantial portion of plasma containing both antibody and bilirubin. Both antibody and bilirubin are distributed throughout the extracellular fluid, however, and reenter the plasma following exchange transfusion. In addition, tissue-bound bilirubin may also reenter the circulation, and rebound elevations in bilirubin following exchange transfusion are common. The first exchange transfusion serves to remove sensitized erythrocytes and correct anemia. Subsequent exchange transfusions are directed primarily at removal of bilirubin, much of which is released from tissue-binding sites.

The hazards of exchange transfusion include introduction of infectious agents, either from umbilical vein catheterization or contamination of blood or intravenous infusion solutions; arrhythmias caused by hypocalcemia when blood anticoagulated with acid-citrate-dextrose is used; congestive heart failure or shock, if careful attention is not paid to maintenance of intravascular volume; and thrombosis of the inferior vena cava related to the placement of the catheter. The procedure should be performed under rigidly aseptic conditions, with continuous cardiac and respiratory monitoring, and the infant must be kept warm. The bilirubin and hematocrit levels should be determined immediately after transfusion and again within 2 hours after equilibration has occurred. (See also Chapter 22.)

Delayed manifestations. Anemia occurring late following isoimmune hemolytic disease is not necessarily related to the severity of the acute process. Infants with mild hemolytic disease may experience an abrupt increase in the rate of red cell destruction after 1 week of age. This may be a result of improved splenic function and more effective clearance of sensitized cells. If the liver enzymes responsible for bilirubin metabolism have also matured, jaundice may not accompany the drop in hemoglobin. Infants who have had exchange transfusions continue to have detectable, passively transferred maternal antibody. As their production of erythrocytes bearing the offending antigen increases, hemolysis may accelerate. Infants who are not anemic in the first 48 hours of life normally cease producing erythropoietin and RBCs. Anemia developing in the next few weeks may not incite erythropoiesis, since the bone marrow is relatively less sensitive to stimulation during this period. Thus ongoing hemolysis may lead to anemia after the first week of life, which is not compensated by increased RBC production. Infants with mild hemolysis must be followed closely to detect the occasional infant who develops severe and even life-threatening anemia.

Since the hemolysis is extravascular, iron is stored in the reticuloendothelial cells of the liver and spleen and is available for reuse. Even infants who have had exchange transfusion should not be depleted of iron stores. Infants who have particularly active bone marrow with ongoing hemolysis or early anemia should receive folic acid supplementation to prevent the development of megaloblastic anemia.

A small number of infants with isoimmune hemolytic disease develop persistent jaundice with an elevation in the conjugated, direct-reacting component. This may be associated with abnormalities of liver enzymes and was formerly termed the *inspissated bile syndrome*. Its pathogenesis is uncertain, and in most instances the laboratory abnormalities disappear by 3 to 6 months of age (Chapter 34, part two).

Prognosis. The prognosis for infants with isoimmune hemolytic disease is related to the degree of hyperbilirubinemia. The levels of bilirubin associated with major anatomic abnormalities and gross functional defects are not well known, and it is even less clear whether lower levels of bilirubin elevations are associated with more subtle intellectual or neurologic impairment. These possibilities are under active investigation, and the criteria for therapeutic intervention may be revised as more information becomes available.

Hemoglobinopathies

Abnormalities of globin chain production, both quantitative and qualitative, can be detected prenatally and may have major clinical manifestations in the perinatal period. The quantitative disorders of globin chain production are the thalassemias, which are named according to the globin chain that is underproduced (α or β). Qualitative disorders include the sickle syndromes, hemoglobin E, hemoglobin C, and the M hemoglobins.

Thalassemias. The *thalassemia syndromes* are the result of various mutations that affect the transcription or translation of the globin genes. The α-thalassemias are largely caused by gene deletion and result in an excess of γ- and β-chain production compared to α-chain production. Because α-chain synthesis begins during the first trimester (Fig. 32-3), major abnormalities in which there is no synthesis of α-chains cause severe anemia in the fetus. Four α-genes normally are present in each cell, two on each chromosome 16 (Fig. 32-4). Deletion of one α-gene results in no clinical abnormality and is termed the *silent carrier* state. This is usually suspected from family studies and can be confirmed by measuring the ratio of α-/non-α-chain (γ- plus β-chain) synthesis using radioactive amino acids to label reticulocytes. Deletion of two α-genes leads to microcytosis without anemia. In black populations the two gene deletions are on different chromosomes ("trans"), whereas in Asian populations the two gene deletions are on the same chromosome ("cis"). The result of the different arrangements of the gene deletions is that Asian patients can inherit two chromosomes 16 without α-genes, whereas black patients can inherit at least one α-gene with each chromosome 16. Loss of three α-genes results in microcytosis with mild anemia, and hemoglobin H (β-4-tetramers) on hemoglobin electrophoresis. In the perinatal period the abnormal hemoglobin is Bart's, which is made up of γ-4-tetramers and is evident on cord blood electrophoresis. Globin chain synthesis studies show the α-/non-α-chain ratios that reflect the number of α-genes present: 3:4 with a single gene deletion (silent carrier, three genes present); 1:2 with two gene deletions, either cis or trans; and 1:4 with a single gene present (Bart's in the newborn period, hemoglobin H later in life). When all four globin genes are absent, severe anemia with hydrops fetalis and intrauterine death ensue. (See also Chapter 6.)

Two infants have been successfully delivered with homozygous α-thalassemia and have survived the newborn period with continuing transfusions of packed RBCs. In the Asian populations at risk for homozygous α-thalassemia, only about 1% of the population is Rh negative, and α-thalassemia is the most common cause of hydrops fetalis. Cord blood electrophoresis in these infants demonstrates primarily hemoglobin Bart's, which has a very high oxygen affinity and delivers oxygen poorly, and smaller amounts of hemoglobins H (β_4) and Portland ($\zeta_2\gamma_2$), which are more effective carriers of oxygen. The presence of these latter two hemoglobins is probably responsible for the survival of some infants into the third trimester. The erythrocytes are hypochromic and have inclusions (precipitated globin chains) demonstrable on supravital staining, with reticulocytosis and erythroblastosis on smear. Because the α-thalassemias are caused by gene deletions, carrier detection and prenatal diagnosis using amniotic fluid fibroblasts or chorionic villus biopsy cn be performed using complementary strands of DNA to detect the presence of the genetic material.

β-Thalassemia (Cooley's anemia) consists of a group of related disorders in which β-chain production is diminished (β^+) or absent (β^0). More than 40 different molecular mechanisms have been described that produce the β-thalassemia phenotype and include mutations producing termination codons, errors in splicing of messenger ribonucleic acid (RNA), frameshift mutations, and polyadenylation mutations. Most are not deletions, with the exception of some forms of δ-β-thalassemias, in which both the β-chain and parts or all the δ-chain are deleted. The region that controls β-chain production and the switch from γ- to β-chain synthesis is toward the 5′ end of chromosome 11, close to the δ-gene. If this area is deleted, γ-chain synthesis continues, with hereditary persistence of fetal hemoglobin and mild microcytosis in postnatal life. Because δ- and β-chain production are minimal in fetal life, infants with homozygous β-thalassemia are normal at birth and for the first 6 months of life. During the second half of the first year progressive anemia develops, resulting both from decreased production of hemoglobin and from hemolysis of cells containing precipitated α-chain because of the unbalanced chain synthesis. The deleterious effect of excess α-chains results in destruction of erythrocytes within the bone marrow and ineffective erythropoiesis, which is not a feature of α-thalassemia, since excess β-chains are not as harmful to the cells.

Patients with one normal and one thalassemia gene have microcytosis, mild or no anemia, and basophilic strippling on smear caused by precipitated α-chains. Hemoglobin electrophoresis shows an increase in hemoglobin A_2 and/or hemoglobin F. The only clinical consequence of this condition, called *thalassemia minor*, is the mild anemia and iatrogenic excessive treatment with iron because of the microcytosis. Patients with homozygous thalassemia, or doubly heterozygous for two thalassemia genes, usually depend on transfusions and have severe anemia *(thalassemia major)*. Some patients have moderately severe anemia but are not transfusion dependent, a condition termed *thalassemia intermedia*. These patients show hepatosplenomegaly, osteoporosis from expanded marrow cavities, jaundice from premature destruction of erythrocytes, and extremely bizarre peripheral blood smears with hypochromia, nucleated RBCs, reticulocytosis, and various RBC sizes and shapes. The hemoglobin electrophoresis shows a predominance of hemoglobin F, with either no hemoglobin A (β^0) or up to 30% A (β^+).

Although β-thalassemia is not apparent until late in infancy, it can be detected prenatally or on cord blood. The major method of prenatal diagnosis of β-thalassemia is globin chain synthesis performed on fetal cells obtained by fetoscopy, in which fetal or umbilical vessels are sampled. The widespread application of this technique has permitted prenatal diagnosis on more than 5,000 pregnancies at risk and has greatly reduced the birth rate of new patients with Cooley's anemia in the areas where the disease is endemic, especially Greece, Italy, and Sardinia. As the molecular lesions are better characterized, it is now often possible to use specific probes for the normal or abnormal genes or restriction enzyme polymorphisms to identify genetic sites linked to the abnormal gene. These methods permit analysis of amniotic fluid fibroblasts or chorionic villus biopsies, which are simpler and often easier to interpret.

Several instances of heterozygous γ-thalassemia have been reported. An extensive deletion of the γ-, δ-, and β-genes from chromosome 11 results in hemolytic disease of the newborn with hypochromic, microcytic RBCs. The disease is self-limited and evolves into heterozygous thalassemia minor after the newborn period. Infants with heterozygous isolated γ-thalassemia have also been described, and several instances of homozygous ${}^{G}\gamma$-thalassemia have been reported. These infants, who have a fused ${}^{G}\gamma{}^{A}\gamma$-gene because of an unequal crossover, have higher than normal levels of ${}^{A}\gamma$-chain production and are not anemic. Homozygosity for a form of γ-thalassemia in which both the ${}^{G}\gamma$- and ${}^{A}\gamma$-genes are affected has not been described. Such a condition should be fatal in utero with death in the first trimester.

Abnormalities of globin chain structure. Several abnormalities of γ-chain structure have been detected in the course of cord blood screening for other disorders. None has been associated with anemia or clinical disease and is not detectable past early infancy.

β-Chain abnormalities account for the majority of the known variant hemoglobins. Many are hemoglobins of abnormal (usually increased) oxygen affinity, known as M hemoglobins. The major disorders of clinical significance in the United States are sickle cell disease and hemoglobin C disease. Because of the low levels of β-chain production, these rarely cause any clinical problems in the newborn period. Prenatal diagnosis is possible at about 14 weeks' gestation.

Hemoglobin C disease alone is not associated with significant morbidity or mortality in childhood. Sickle cell disease and hemoglobin SC disease are accompanied by sickling phenomena that may be life threatening, and early diagnosis is advisable to permit management decisions that should prevent much of the early mortality of sickle cell disease. Without early diagnosis, about 12% of infants born with sickle cell disease die by age 2 years. Of these, the majority die of infection, most between 6 months and 2 years. Several infants have been reported who have died of generalized intravascular sickling in the neonatal period and have not had abnormally high levels of sickle hemoglobin. At least two infants have died from exchange transfusion performed with blood containing sickle hemoglobin (sickle cell trait, and SC disease).

Cord blood screening is done in many institutions to identify affected infants. Because of the high levels of hemoglobin F at birth, it may be difficult to accurately quantitate the hemoglobins. However, identification of hemoglobin S with or without hemoglobins A and C permits identification of infants at risk for significant hemoglobinopathies and defines a group of infants who should have a quantitative electrophoresis repeated at 3 to 6 months. Because of the low levels of the S, the hemoglobin solubility tests (Sickledex) are not usually suitable for screening in the newborn period. The metabisulfite tests for sickling may or may not demonstrate abnormalities on cord blood. Prenatal diagnosis of S and C hemoglobinopathies is feasible using globin chain synthesis by fetal reticulocytes or more recently by restriction enzyme analysis of amniotic fluid fibroblasts. These techniques have not been as extensively applied as they have in the thalassemias but have the potential of ensuring that parents who are carriers of the abnormal genes have only healthy children.

Hemoglobin E is a β-chain variant that is unstable and associated with microcytosis. Hemoglobin E occurs often in Southeast Asia, with a gene frequency of 50% in some areas of Thailand. The occurrence of E overlaps with both α- and β-thalassemias, and many interesting combinations of abnormal globin chains are possible. Homozygous E is usually associated with mild to moderate anemia and microcytosis but is not a clinically severe disorder. Hemoglobin E–β-thalassemia is usually more severe and may appear clinically as homozygous β-thalassemia, although the spectrum of disease is wide. With the large influx of immigrants from areas in which hemoglobin E is common, this disorder is being seen more often throughout the United States.

Methemoglobinemia

Methemoglobin is an otherwise normal hemoglobin in which the iron is oxidized and unable to carry oxygen. Normally iron is present in the reduced ferrous state. Oxidation to the ferric state occurs at a slow rate under normal conditions, but methemoglobin is reduced by an enzyme designated NADH-dependent diaphorase. Several other pathways exist but are not responsible for significant regeneration of ferrous iron. Activity of this enzyme is substantially reduced in normal full-term infants and is very low in premature infants; it rises to adult levels in erythrocytes by 4 months of age. In some populations, including Navajo Indians, congenital deficiency of this enzyme persists past early infancy. In newborns, methemoglobinemia is usually associated with oxidant stresses that increase the levels of methemoglobin. In congenital diaphorase deficiency, methemoglobinemia may be present continually without unusual oxidant or drug exposure.

When greater than 10% of hemoglobin is present as methemoglobin, the skin becomes dusky and the blood develops a brown color. The duskiness of the skin does not improve when the patient breathes high concentrations of oxygen. Direct exposure of the blood to oxygen does not affect the brown color, as should occur if the hemoglobin is simply deoxygenated.

A variety of drugs and chemicals precipitate acute episodes of methemoglobinemia in newborns, including phenacetin, certain sulfonamides, aniline and its derivatives, and nitrites, which may contaminate well water and are present in some folk medications ("sweet spirits of nitre"). Infant food prepared from soil-grown vegetables, such as carrots, containing high levels of nitrites from fertilizer have caused clinically significant methemoglobinemia. In many cases the source of the oxidant causing methemoglobinemia is never identified and may include municipal water sources. Most of these infants have been bottle-fed on formulas prepared with tap water. In addition to the reduced level of diaphorase, the γ-chain of hemoglobin F interacts with oxidants in such a way as to make hemoglobin F more susceptible to methemoglobin formation than hemoglobin A. In congenital diaphorase deficiency, significant neonatal methemoglobinemia may be present in heterozygotes as well as homozygotes for this autosomal recessive disorder.

The usual symptoms related to methemoglobinemia are tachypnea and tachycardia, and the major clinical finding is cyanosis at rest. The severity of illness is related to the levels of methemoglobinemia. Since methemoglobin cannot carry oxygen, these patients are functionally anemic. If the condition develops rapidly and methemoglobin levels are 30% or greater, infants may be dyspneic and irritable. Clinically apparent cyanosis implies methemoglobin levels of 10% or greater, but levels as high as 60% to 70% have been described in severely affected infants and may be fatal. A simple screening test for the presence of methemoglobin is performed by placing a drop of the infant's blood and that of a normal control on filter paper, which is waved gently in air for 30 seconds to oxygenate the hemoglobin. Control venous blood should turn red, whereas blood containing elevated levels of methemoglobin remains brown. A spectrophotometric procedure will confirm the diagnosis and quantitate the abnormal hemoglobin.

Once the diagnosis is established, a cause must be sought. Environmental sources of toxins should be reviewed and should include drugs, source of food and water, and topical agents, such as diaper marking dyes, which may be absorbed. If no source is sought, assay of the infant's erythrocytes for NADH-reductase levels and electrophoresis for detection of one of the abnormal M hemoglobins is indicated. The M hemoglobins are caused by single amino acid substitutions that enable the globin chains to form stable complexes with ferric rather than ferrous ions. These hemoglobins are resistant to reduction by the usual intraerythrocyte enzymes. Most M hemoglobins result from β-chain mutations and are not evident in the newborn period. A few result from α-chain substitutions and may manifest neonatal methemoglobinemia. The major problems in differential diagnosis are congenital cardiac conditions such as tetralogy of Fallot and severe respiratory disease, but diagnostic clinical features are usually apparent.

Treatment of methemoglobinemia caused by NADH-reductase deficiency or by oxidant exposure is administration of methylene blue at a dosage of 1 to 2 mg/kg intravenously. Methemoglobin levels fall within 1 or 2 hours. Failure of response suggests an abnormal hemoglobin. Recurrence with reexposure to toxins suggests deficiency of erythrocyte enzymes, especially glucose-6-phosphate dehydrogenase (G6PD), and of glutathione peroxidase and reductase. Ascorbic acid in doses of 300 to 400 mg orally/day may also be effective and sufficient in mild cases. Excessive administration of methylene blue may cause methemoglobinemia and hemolysis and should be avoided.

Unstable hemoglobins

Congenital Heinz body hemolytic anemias are a group of disorders associated with structurally abnormal hemoglobins that precipitate within the cell. Both α- and β-chain mutants have been described. Some are electrophoretically identical to hemoglobin A, and other techniques must be used to establish the existence of an abnormal hemoglobin. All patients are heterozygotes, and almost one third appear to represent spontaneous mutations. These are uncommon genes, and the probability of homozygosity is very low. The spleen selectively removes the precipitated Heinz bodies, so the abnormal hemoglobin comprises 10% to 30% of the total hemoglobin, with the remainder consisting primarily of hemoglobin A. Following splenectomy, the number of Heinz bodies and the proportion of abnormal hemoglobin increase. The peripheral smear may demonstrate slight hypochromia, microcytosis, and basophilic stippling but may be entirely normal. To establish the diagnosis, demonstration of Heinz bodies on a supravital preparation is particularly useful. Incubation of the blood for 24 to 48 hours increases the yield, especially in patients whose spleens are intact. Heating red cell hemolysates to 50° C (122° F) for 1 hour produces a visible precipitate.

Since only about 25% of patients with unstable hemoglobins have α-chain mutations, most are not apparent in the immediate neonatal period. Those who do demonstrate the disorder early may have mild hyperbilirubinemia or significant hemolysis, depending on the variant. Anemia is rarely severe enough to require transfusion. Patients should receive folic acid supplementation, avoid oxidant drugs (which may aggravate Heinz body formation), and may require splenectomy if hemolysis is severe.

Congenital deficiencies of red cell enzymes

Normal fetal erythrocytes differ metabolically from adult erythrocytes in several ways. Some of these differences reflect the fact that the life span of fetal RBCs is approximately half that of adult erythrocytes. Many appear to be instrinsic differences between fetal and adult RBCs. For instance, neonatal eythrocytes have elevated levels of glucose phosphate isomerase, phosphoglycerate kinase, enolase, and glyceraldehyde-3-phosphate, but lower levels of phosphofructokinase. They are deficient in several enzymes that protect against oxidant damage, including NADH-dependent methemoglobin reductase (diaphorase), catalase, and glutathione peroxidase. These may predispose the infant's RBCs to Heinz body formation, methemoglobinemia, and hemolysis with relatively mild oxidant stresses. When hereditary enzyme deficiency is superimposed on the ordinary metabolic alterations of fetal RBCs, significant hemolysis is often more of a problem than it is later in life.

Glucose-6-phosphate dehydrogenase. The gene for G6PD is carried on the X chromosome. More than 100 variants have been identified. Most are distinguishable electrophoretically from the "normal" B enzyme, but relatively few are associated with disease. The enzyme is unstable; intracellular levels of G6PD do not decline to the point that would make the red cell susceptible to oxidant damage before 120 days and thus do not limit the RBC life span. Unstable variants decline in activity at a greater rate. Mature erythrocytes are anucleate and cannot replenish the supply of enzyme by new synthesis. The rate of decay of enzyme activity determines the severity of the disease. Older cells are more susceptible to hemolysis with oxidant damage than young cells, which have higher levels of G6PD.

Because this is an X-linked disorder, males are most often affected. Studies of this enzyme resulted in promulgation of the *Lyon hypothesis*, which holds that one X chromosome is randomly inactivated in individual cells in females. Thus, rather than having a uniform population of cells with enzyme levels and electrophoretic patterns reflecting both the normal and abnormal enzyme, heterozygous females have two populations of cells. In one population the normal enzyme is expressed and no abnormal enzyme is identifiable, and in another population only the abnormal enzyme can be found. Some heterozygous females may have significant G6PD deficiency if a large proportion of their cells express only the abnormal enzyme. Populations with a high frequency of abnormal G6PD enzymes include blacks, Southern Europeans, Sephardic Jews, Chinese, Southeast Asians, and Arabs.

Drug-induced hemolysis is the most characteristic manifestation of relatively mild G6PD deficiency. This is the form most often seen in blacks, with a gene frequency of 11% in American blacks. The RBC survival is normal under ordinary conditions, but acute hemolysis develops with infection or exposure to certain drugs. The concomitant events of infection and drug exposure may result in markedly more severe hemolysis than occurs with either alone. This is particularly relevant for administration of aspirin, which does not appear to cause hemolysis without infection but does so with active infection. The role of infection may relate in part to generation of hydrogen peroxide by phagocytic cells ingesting microorganisms.

Congenital nonspherocytic hemolytic anemia occurs with more severe enzyme deficiencies, such as the Mediterranean variant. Affected individuals have a population of older RBCs that are unable to metabolize the oxidants generated by normal events and thus develop Heinz bodies and are destroyed prematurely. These persons have an additional population of younger RBCs susceptible to hemolysis with oxidant stresses such as infection or drugs and may hemolyze much of their RBC volume with fatal consequences. *Favism* is the term applied to acute hemolysis with ingestion of fava beans in persons with severe G6PD deficiency. Infants with G6PD deficiency may develop acute, severe hemolysis with maternal ingestion of fava beans or oxidant drugs either while the infant is in utero or via breast milk.

The clinical severity of the disorder is determined by the nature of the abnormal enzyme, the maturity of the infant, and the degree and extent of oxygen and/or drug therapy. Many instances of hyperbilirubinemia with hemolysis (fall in hemoglobin and reticulocytosis) associated with neonatal G6PD deficiency may occur without obvious precipitating factors. This may be sufficient to cause kernicterus and require exchange transfusion.

The smear demonstrates some fragmentation and poikilocytosis resulting from removal of cytoplasm and membrane in the spleen. Heinz bodies can be demonstrated by supravital staining with cresyl violet. Several screening tests for G6PD deficiency are easily performed, but the degee of reticulocytosis affects the result. Since young RBCs have higher levels of G6PD, the test should be performed again after recovery when the reticulocyte count is low if a normal result is obtained during an acute hemolytic reaction. An alternative approach is to test only the denser cells by differential centrifugation, since these are the older fraction of RBCs and more likely to be deficient in G6PD.

Drug-induced hemolysis occurs with glutathione synthetase deficiency, glutathione reductase deficiency, and glutathione peroxidase deficiency. The inability to detoxify oxidants is the same as in G6PD deficiency. These are uncommon disorders and are associated with reduced levels of glutathione and formation of Heinz bodies with exposure to acetylphenylhydrazine. G6PD levels are normal. Specific enzymatic assays are required to establish the diagnosis. These disorders may be associated with neonatal hyperbilirubinemia.

Pyruvate kinase. Pyruvate kinase (PK) is carried on an autosomal chromosome, and its deficiency is the most frequently encountered enzymopathy of the glycolytic pathway associated with anemia. It catalyzes the conversion of phosphoenolpyruvate to pyruvate, with gen-

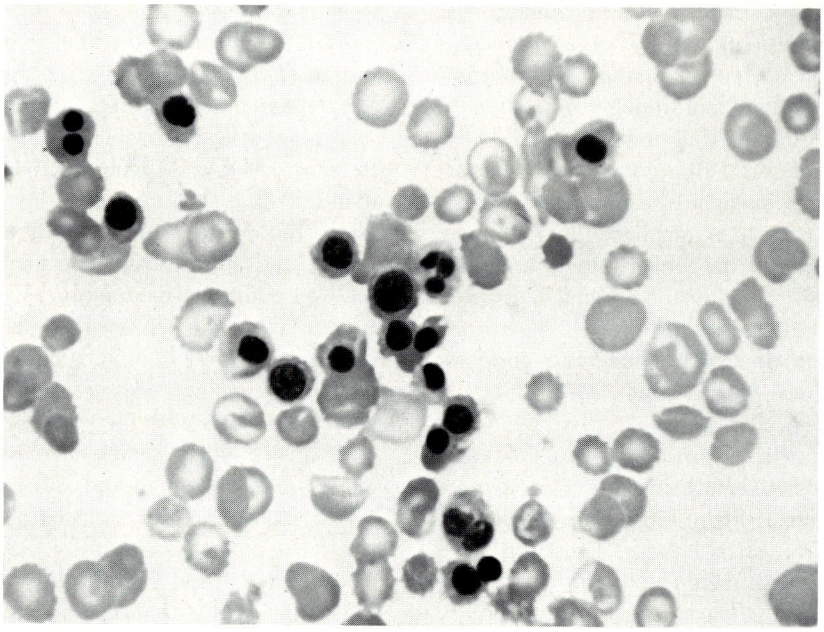

Fig. 32-8. Cord blood smear from an infant with severe pyruvate kinase deficiency and erythroblastosis fetalis. (Wright's stain; ×800.)

eration of ATP. Intracellular levels of ATP are diminished, and the sodium-potassium pump in the RBC membrane does not function well, particularly with incubation. Potassium loss exceeds sodium gain initially, and the cells lose water and become crenated (desiccytes). These cells are poorly deformable and are removed on passage through liver and spleen. There is some evidence that reticulocytes may be selectively destroyed in the bone marrow, liver, and spleen. The reason for this is not clear but may relate to the higher rate of glycolysis seen in reticulocytes. The spleens of these patients are full of reticulocytes, and tagged mature PK-deficient RBCs may have a normal survival time.

Several abnormalities have been described. In some families the level of enzyme activity is diminished. In others the enzyme is kinetically abnormal, and in still others the enzyme is unstable and decreases with RBC age. Since it is autosomally determined, two abnormal enzymes may coexist in the same cell. Carriers for mutant enzymes do not demonstrate hemolysis. The disorder may be difficult to diagnose even with quantitative assays of PK activity, especially if the enzyme has abnormal kinetics and the assay is performed with a high concentration of phosphoenolpyruvate. The buildup of products before this reaction, especially 2,3-DPG, may aid in making the diagnosis.

Certain population groups have a relatively high incidence of PK deficiency, notably Northern Europeans and Amish groups. Persistent jaundice and the presence of a nonspherocytic hemolytic anemia should suggest the diagnosis of PK deficiency. Although morphologic abnormalities of the cells are observed in wet preparations with a phase contrast microscope, the Wright-stained smear is unremarkable except for polychromasia consistent with the degree of reticulocytosis (Fig. 32-8). Despite significant anemia, patients are rarely symptomatic, which probably results in part from the elevated levels of 2,3-DPG, which lower oxygen affinity and improve tissue oxygen delivery.

The clinical course is highly variable. Hyperbilirubinemia in the newborn period is common, and persistent jaundice and transfusion requirement are not unusual. Patients have been described as having a fully compensated hemolytic anemia with persistent hyperbilirubinemia but no anemia. More often the hemolytic rate is significant, and patients are splenectomized early in life with variable response. Most patients derive some benefit from splenectomy, with a rise in hemoglobin and reduction or elimination of transfusion requirement. Occasionally patients do not benefit at all from splenectomy. Bilirubin gallstones frequently occur, and aplastic crises with infection may result in rapid development of severe anemia. Folic acid supplementation is required, but iron is reused, and dietary supplementation should not be given. This is especially true if significant numbers of transfusions have been required.

Disorders of the red cell membrane

The erythrocyte is the model system for the study of all mammalian cell membranes. It is easily available in large quantity, and the membrane can be separated from other cell components simply by lysing and washing the cell, which contains no contaminating organelles. The membrane consists of a lipid bilayer with intrinsic, transmembrane proteins and extrinsic proteins that form a lattice on the cytoplasmic side of the bilayer. Abnormalities of either the lipid or the protein component will alter RBC shape. The lipids of the plasma are in equilibrium with those in the RBC membrane, which can incorporate lipid from the plasma. Most lipid abnormalities (1) are associated with an increase in RBC membrane area without an increase in volume, (2) are acquired disorders, and (3) are manifested by acanthocytes on smear. The intrinsic RBC shape is determined by the protein lattice beneath the lipid bilayer; when the lipid is extracted from erythrocyte ghosts, the shell of protein that remains has the shape of the original, intact cell. The proteins of the RBC membrane and their interactions are known in some detail. The proteins are named according to their migration on polyacrylamide gel electrophoresis. Bands 1 and 2 are the α- and β-chains, respectively, of the protein *spectrin*. Heterodimers of the spectrin chains interact with actin, which attaches to an anchoring protein termed *ankyrin* (band 2.1), which links the spectrin-actin lattice to the major transmembrane protein, band 3, which is the anion channel. Other proteins affect the interaction of these structural units. Abnormalities of these proteins or their associations cause hereditary abnormalities of RBC shape, which are intrinsic to the RBC and cause ongoing hemolysis.

Erythrocytes in the perinatal period are less deformable than are adult RBCs. Deformability is determined by characteristics of the spectrin lattice and by the volume of the cell; larger cells are less deformable. Deformability is important for the cell to be able to transverse capillaries whose internal diameters are smaller than the diameter of the cell. In addition, the erythrocytes of the fetus and newborn have large numbers of "pocks," or autophagic vacuoles, on their surfaces. These pocks are seen when the cells are examined unstained under phase contrast microscopy and are normally present on fewer than 3% of adult RBCs. They increase dramatically in the absence of splenic function and are present on 47% of premature and 24% of full term infants' erythrocytes. They disappear by 2 months of age and are thought to indicate immaturity of splenic function, low rates of blood flow through the spleen, or both. This splenic hypofunction may explain why the neonatal erythrocyte is larger and less deformable than that of older children and adults.

Several defects of cytoskeletal protein function result in congenital hemolytic anemias, all of which may appear in the newborn period. Several of these conditions may be more severe in the neonatal period than later in life, reflecting the combined effects of the inherited disorder and the normal decreased deformability of the neonatal erythrocyte. Hyperbilirubinemia is often a significant problem because of the immaturity of the liver during this period. All these disorders are at least somewhat heterogeneous, and although various abnormalities in erythrocyte membrane proteins have been found, it is not clear how these cause the morphologic abnormalities that are seen.

Hereditary spherocytosis

Loss of surface area is the major effect of the variety of defects seen in hereditary spherocytosis (HS). The autosomal dominant form of the disease appears to result from defects in the binding of spectrin to actin as a result of abnormal binding of another membrane protein, band 4.1. The autosomal recessive form is caused by spectrin deficiency in some family members. The severity of hemolysis varies, from mild and asymptomatic to severe with chronic anemia.

Red cells from patients with HS tend to lose membrane fragments more readily than normal when they are metabolically exhausted but not when they are metabolically replete. These cells have lost 15% to 20% of their membrane lipid and somewhat more of their surface area. The cells have increased permeability to sodium and an increased turnover of ATP, probably because of increased activity of the sodium pump. These metabolic alterations may account for the special hazards posed by passage of HS cells through the spleen.

HS affects about 1 in 5,000 infants and is most common in people of Northern European ancestry. Presentation with jaundice in the neonatal period is typical. Jaundice may be sufficiently severe to require exchange transfusion. The major differential diagnosis is between HS and ABO incompatibility, although a negative direct antiglobulin (Coombs') test strongly suggests HS. Family studies are often useful. About 25% of cases are sporadic. Sometimes an asymptomatic parent will be recognized when an infant has been diagnosed as having HS. All spherocytes are osmotically fragile, so the osmotic fragility test is not a helpful differential feature.

Beyond the newborn period most patients develop a chronic hemolytic anemia whose severity varies from mild (reticulocytosis without anemia) to severe (requiring periodic transfusions). Gallstones eventually develop in many patients with chronic hemolytic anemias but are often asymptomatic and not associated with gallbladder disease. Splenectomy has been accepted treatment to prevent the development of gallstones and usually cures the hemolysis completely, although the morphologic abnormalities persist. Routine splenectomy is being used less as the hazards of postsplenectomy septicemia are better recognized. In general the decision about splenectomy should attempt to balance the risks of leaving the spleen—anemia, the metabolic costs of increased erythropoiesis, severe anemia with aplastic crises, and gallstones in adult life—against the risk of postsplenectomy septicemia, which is rare but may be fatal. These decisions need to be individualized for each patient and family. Since the severity of hemolysis in the newborn period is often greater than it is later in life, the neonatal course should not be used to predict the long-term severity of disease. Unless frequent transfusions are required, splenectomy should be delayed until at least age 2 and preferably 5 years, when humoral immunity is better developed and the risks of postsplenectomy septicemia may be lower.

Hereditary elliptocytosis

The elliptic shape characteristic of RBCs in hereditary elliptocytosis (HE) is acquired by the cells after they enter the circulation (Fig. 32-9). A variety of molecular lesions have been found in HE, which is a heterogeneous disorder. The major abnormality appears to be a defect in association of spectrin dimers, which results in decreased mechanical stability of the membrane. Normal RBCs undergo elliptic deformation under high shear stress, and this may become a permanent condition for HE cells because of this instability. HE is a more common disorder than HS, is an autosomal dominant in inheritance, and in most cases is not associated with disease. Because up to 15% of normal RBCs may be elliptic on smear, greater than 25% elliptocytes is required to make this diagnosis. Hemolysis may be severe in the 10% of patients in whom this condition is more than a morphologic curiosity, most of whom are homozygous for the abnormality. Osmotic fragility and monovalent cation leak are similar to those of HS in HE homozygotes, and splenectomy lessens the hemolysis.

Some patients with HE develop severe poikilocytosis in the newborn period. These patients have moderate to severe hemolytic anemia and thermal instability of the RBCs in the first year of life. All these patients appear to have a defective spectrin dimer association in the RBC membrane. Neonatal jaundice and hemolysis may be severe but abate over the first year of life. The thermal stability improves, and the clinical expression is that of mild heterozygous HE. The improvement coincides with the decrease in fetal hemoglobin in the first year. The reason for this is not clear, but it is thought that high intracellular free 2,3-DPG levels in cells with hemoglobin F may weaken the binding of spectrin to actin.

A disorder related to HE, and perhaps the homozygous form of HE, is hereditary pyropoikilocytosis (HPP). This is a rare disorder described only in black patients in which the mechanical stability of the intact cells and their membrane skeletons are greatly decreased. Extreme RBC fragmentation and poilikocytosis are seen on smear and are accompanied by severe thermal instability in vitro. The cells contain less spectrin than normal cells, but this is thought to reflect loss of unstable spectrin rather than deficient synthesis. These cells are high in calcium. Diminished spectrin self-association is believed

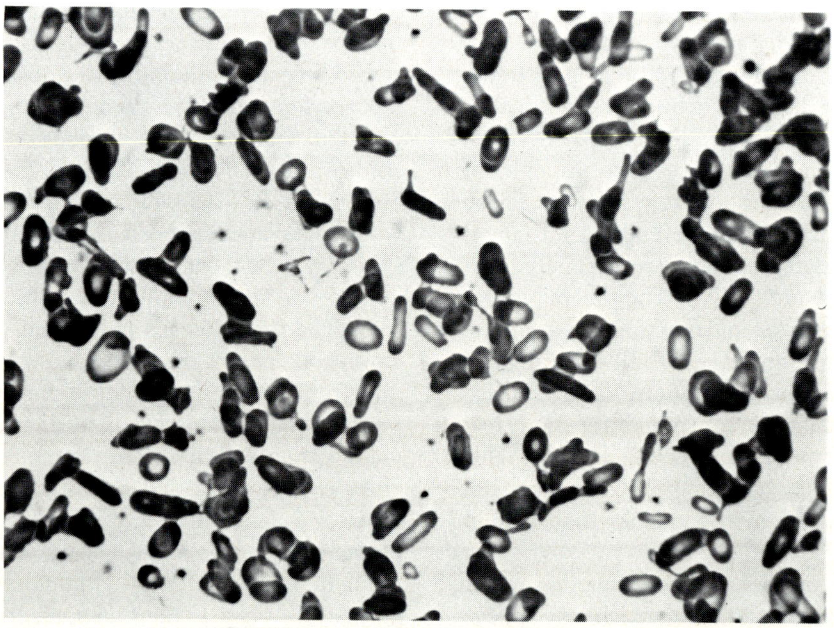

Fig. 32-9. Peripheral blood smear at age 1 week from an infant with hereditary elliptocytosis. (Wright's stain; ×800.)

to cause cell fragmentation and reduce the ratio of surface to volume, which results in cell rigidity. Neonatal jaundice and hemolysis may be severe, but unlike the typical form of HE or HE with neonatal poikilocytosis, jaundice is associated with chronic hemolysis after the first year of life. As with other RBC membrane disorders, splenectomy improves red cell survival. The parents of these patients may be hematologically normal or have mild HE, but all have been found to have the abnormalities of spectrin peptide mapping and dimer association, regardless of their hematologic status.

Hereditary stomatocytosis

In hereditary stomatocytosis the RBCs are swollen and cup shaped and there is an extreme defect in cation permeability. The cells tend to accumulate sodium in excess of potassium loss and gain volume. There is a marked increase in the activity of the sodium-potassium pump in response to the increase in intracellular sodium, with consequent increase in requirement for energy in the form of ATP. In the hypoglycemic, stagnant environment of the spleen, these cells are unable to fulfill their energy needs and are destroyed. Splenectomy reduces the rate of hemolysis but may not eliminate it. These cells are also abnormally rigid and poorly deformable, which contributes to their rapid rate of destruction. In one instance, biochemical correction of the permeability defect, with reduction of the energy requirement and intracellular water, also corrected the abnormality in deformability, which suggests that this is a secondary defect.

As with other defects in the membrane, hereditary stomatocytosis may be accompanied by hyperbilirubinemia in the newborn period and may be severe enough to require exchange transfusion.

Vitamin E deficiency

See also Appendix C.

Vitamin E (α-tocopherol) is one of several free-radical scavengers that serve as antioxidants to protect cellular components against peroxidative damage. Other significant antioxidants include vitamin C; intracellular thiols, particularly reduced glutathione (GSH) and the enzymes that regenerate GSH (GSH peroxidase, GSH reductase, GSH synthetase, G6PD); selenium, which is a cofactor required for enzymatic activity of GSH peroxidase; catalase; and superoxide dismutase. The important function of vitamin E is to protect the double bonds of lipids in biologic membranes in all tissues, including blood cells. It is a fat-soluble vitamin, and conditions that impair fat absorption are associated with vitamin E deficiency. The requirement for vitamin E increases with the dietary content of polyunsaturated fatty acids (PUFA) and with exposure to oxidant stress. Infant formulas are supplemented in proportion to their PUFA content at a ratio of 0.8 IU:1 gm PUFA (13 IU/quart in most cow's-milk formulas). Although dietary deficiency of vitamin E can be produced in animals, relatively few conditions in human beings are associated with vitamin E deficiency. These include premature infants and patients with cystic fibrosis, severe cholestasis, biliary atresia, or severe hemosiderosis, such as thalassemia major. The lipoproteins that transport and bind vitamin E are low in neonates, which contributes to the low serum levels normally seen. Documentation of tissue deficiency of vitamin E can be done with the peroxide hemolysis test, in which the patient's RBCs are incubated with small amounts of hydrogen peroxide and the amount of hemolysis (release of hemoglobin) is measured. For unknown reasons erythrocyte vitamin E in neonatal cells is oxidized at a lower peroxide concentration than it is in adult cells. The hematologic findings in vitamin E deficiency are reticulocytosis, thrombocytosis, and acanthocytosis. Infants often have peripheral edema. The major other findings are neurologic and include spinocerebellar degeneration, ataxia, and peripheral neuropathy.

Infants with low tocopheral levels do not usually develop hemolysis unless their diets high in PUFA are supplemented with iron, which is a powerful oxidant. This complication is virtually limited to premature infants and is now extremely rare following the recognition of the importance of administering vitamin E in formulas and parenteral hyperalimentation mixtures. Other oxidants may also increase the need for vitamin E, especially oxygen itself. The observation that oxygen increases the need for vitamin E has lead to the suggestion that supplementary vitamin E may minimize some of the toxic effects of oxygen on tissues other than blood, particularly the lung and retina. Several studies are now investigating the use of vitamin E for prevention of bronchopulmonary dysplasia and retrolental fibroplasia, but the benefits remain unclear. Since other antioxidants such as selenium and vitamin C are also important in protection against oxidant damage, these factors may need to be considered and controlled in future studies of tocopherol therapy.

A major reason for concern about the efficacy of vitamin E for prevention of oxidant damage is increasing evidence that administration of relatively high doses of tocopheral (25 to 50 mg/day) may be associated with serious morbidity and mortality. An unusually high incidence of sepsis and necrotizing enterocolitis was found in a study of retrolental fibroplasia. A preparation of vitamin E for intravenous use was associated with unexplained pulmonary deterioration, liver and renal failure, and thrombocytopenia in premature infants. This preparation has been removed from clinical use. High doses of vitamin E impair platelet function and may interfere with bacterial killing by phagocytes, which requires generation of reactive oxygen species that are scavenged by tocopherol. Normal adult serum levels of tocopherol range from 0.8 to 1.5 mg/dl, but levels may be lower in persons with low serum lipids despite adequate tissue levels of tocopherol. Clinical problems have been seen with serum levels of 5.1 ± 1.5 mg/dl, achieved with 25 to 50 mg tocopheral/day given orally or parenterally to premature infants. Oral absorption is unpredictable, especially in very small premature infants, who may have serum levels of less than 0.5 mg/dl with normal peroxide hemolysis tests. There is currently insufficient data to guide supplementary therapy in infants exposed to oxidant stresses, but it appears that serum levels of 1.5 mg/dl are adequate for at least some retinal protection, and levels greater than 3.0 mg/dl should be avoided.

POLYCYTHEMIA

Polycythemia, or erythrocytosis, refers to an increase in the number of circulating erythrocytes. Since newborn infants are polycythemic compared to older infants and adults because of intrauterine hypoxia and the presence of a high-affinity hemoglobin, the definition requires that the packed cell volume be even higher than the normal level. An hematocrit over 65% or hemoglobin concentration greater than 20 gm/dl constitutes polycythemia in the newborn.

The causes of polycythemia in the neonatal period include intrauterine hypoxia and transfusion and are only rarely associated with intrinsic bone marrow dysfunction. Twin-twin transfusions, maternal-fetal transfusion, and delayed clamping of the umbilical cord can result in neonatal polycythemia. Maternal toxemia, placenta previa, intrauterine growth retardation caused by placental insufficiency, and postmaturity all may cause fetal hypoxia with a physiologic increase in erythropoietin production and resulting polycythemia in the infant. Several endocrine disorders of the fetus and mother have also been implicated, including congenital adrenal hyperplasia, thyrotoxicosis, and maternal diabetes. Maternal diabetes is also associated with a delay in the switch of γ- to β-chain production, for unknown reasons. Infants with Down's syndrome and hyperplastic visceromegaly (Beckwith-Wiedemann syndrome) may also have polycythemia on the basis of increased erythropoietin production. With rare exceptions, high-affinity hemoglobins are β-chain anomalies and thus are not manifest in utero or at birth by polycythemia. Cardiac shunts do not cause systemic desaturation until after birth, so cyanotic congenital heart disease is also not associated with polycythemia at birth.

The effects of polycythemia relate to (1) blood viscosity increasing at an exponential rate as the volume of packed red cells rises above 65% and (2) the flow of blood through smaller capillaries being greatly impeded at high viscosity. In addition, the high volume of RBCs often results in hyperbilirubinemia as the cells break down. The RBCs of the newborn are less deformable than those of older children and adults, at least in part because of their greater volume. Erythrocytes must assume a cylindric shape in passing through the smallest capillaries, and the smallest cylinder formed by fetal RBCs is 8% greater than than of adult cells. Although this difference is small, it is likely to be important for passage through 3 μm pores in the smallest capillaries and in the spleen. The other major contributor to blood viscosity is the content of plasma proteins, especially fibrinogen. Many of these proteins are present at reduced levels in the neonate, with a concomitant reduction in plasma viscosity.

The poorer RBC deformability and the decreased plasma protein level appear to cancel each other out, and the viscosity of whole fetal blood is equivalent to that of whole adult blood over a wide range of shear rates. As the central venous hematocrit rises above 65%, the viscosity of whole blood increases greatly (Fig. 32-10), and blood flow through the capillaries becomes sluggish. Poor perfusion of tissues further increases the production of erythropoietin, which compounds the problems. Sluggish flow or infarction of tissues may occur in the brain, lungs, bowel, or any other organ, and diffuse thrombotic disease may develop. Infants are usually plethoric, listless, and icteric. Symptoms attributable to polycythemia include respiratory distress, lethargy, jitteriness, edema, and priapism. The infants are also more

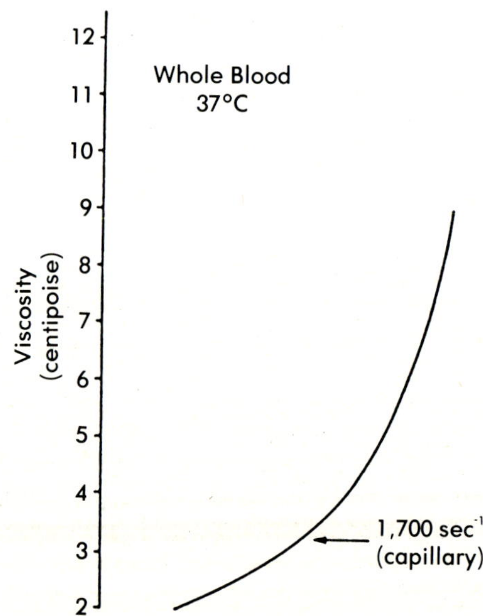

Fig. 32-10. Viscosity versus hematocrit at low shear rate. (From Wells, R.: N. Engl. J. Med. **283:**183, 1970. Reprinted by permission of The New England Journal of Medicine.)

prone to hypoglycemia and hyperbilirubinemia.

Management of patients is designed to reduce RBC mass without loss of blood volume. Infants who are obviously symptomatic and all those with a central hematocrit of greater than 70% even without symptoms should undergo partial exchange transfusion with albumin solutions to reduce the hematocrit to between 45% and 55% (see Part two of this chapter). The goal of treatment of asymptomatic patients is the prevention of the sometimes serious effects of thrombosis. Hyperbilirubinemia may be severe, and early partial exchange with albumin solutions is safer than later double-volume exchange transfusion.

The procedure can be performed using 10% aliquots of the estimated blood volume, with repeat hematocrit determinations at the conclusion of the procedure and 6 to 12 hours later. Mild to moderate thrombocytopenia may accompany severe polycythemia but rarely causes problems and resolves without additional intervention.

Black and associates have extensively studied the effects of partial plasma exchange transfusion on long-term outcome. Ninety-three infants with polycythemia and hyperviscosity were randomly assigned to receive either a partial exchange transfusion or symptomatic treatment. Polycythemic infants demonstrated more neurologic problems than the nonpolycythemic controls. Furthermore, at 2 years the polycythemic infants who had undergone partial exchange transfusions had fewer neurologic problems and fine motor abnormalities than those receiving symptomatic treatment only. However, gastrointestinal injury was prevalent among those receiving partial exchange transfusions. Thus polycythemia with hyperviscosity may result in a major incidence of short- and long-term morbidity, although partial exchange transfusion can cause confounding problems.

In twin-twin transfusions clinical problems are often more severe in the recipient than in the donor infant. The donor infant must be evaluated and managed appropriately, however, and consideration must be given to supplemental iron therapy if the donor twin shows signs of blood loss, even if transfusion is not required. Blood from the polycythemic twin should never be used for transfusion into the anemic twin because of admixture and lack of sterility.

HEMOSTASIS

Overview of coagulation

Development of normal hemostasis

The processes that arrest bleeding following injury are termed hemostasis. These processes involve the vascular wall; the endothelial cells that line the vessels; blood platelets; the coagulation system, including a series of control anticoagulant proteins; and the fibrinolytic enzyme system (Fig. 32-11). The normal values and the functions of the various components change with fetal and neonatal development, and imbalances in the com-

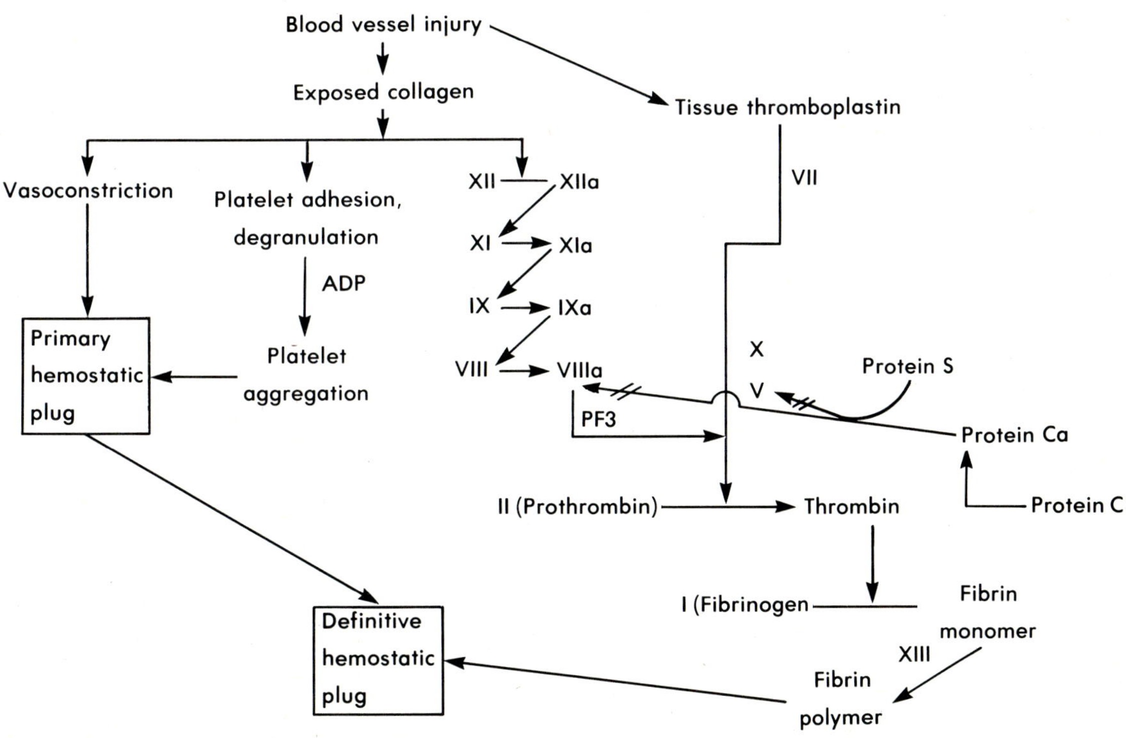

Fig. 32-11. Clotting cascade. Components of normal hemostasis.

plex system may result in excessive bleeding, inappropriate thrombosis, or both.

Vascular wall and endothelium

The smooth muscles of the walls of arterioles and venules contract with injury and reduce the distal pressure and blood loss. Capillaries do not have muscular walls; the blood flow through capillaries is controlled by precapillary sphincters. Control of vascular contraction is accomplished largely via the sympathetic nervous system.

The endothelial cells lining blood vessels, including capillaries, play a major role in both activating and inhibiting coagulation. The endothelial cells themselves are involved in production of factor VIII, antithrombin III, plasminogen activator, and prostacyclin (a vasodilator and inhibitor of platelet aggregation). An intact endothelial lining inhibits platelet adhesion and aggregation.

Platelets

Platelets are produced as early as 11 weeks of gestation, and the count in both preterm and term infants is equivalent to that in adults. Platelet aggregation in response to collagen and epinephrine is reduced in the newborn; data on the response to ADP are conflicting, but it appears that the release reaction is not fully developed. Platelet prostaglandin synthesis is essentially normal. Expression of platelet-specific antigens and of HLA antigens is fully developed in the fetus.

Coagulation factors

Both the prothrombin time (PT) and the activated partial thromboplastin time (aPTT) are significantly prolonged in neonates compared to adults and to infants over 1 month of age. Factors V and VIII and fibrinogen are present at adult levels by birth (Table 32-3), but many other clotting factors are present in reduced amounts. The PT is prolonged because of decreased levels of vitamin K–dependent clotting factors. Adult levels are reached by a few days after birth when vitamin K is administered to the newborn. The aPTT is prolonged because of low levels of the contact factors in the plasma, including factors XI and XII.

Anticoagulants

Several proteins and proteinases function as physiologic anticoagulants and are responsible for maintaining normal balance between hemostasis and thrombosis. These include antithrombin III, α-2-macroglobulin, α-1-antitrypsin, and two vitamin K–dependent proteins that inactivate activated factors V and VIII, protein C and protein S. α-2-Macroglobulin and α-1-antitrypsin levels are higher in the term neonate than in adults. Antithrombin III levels are lower in the newborn and do not reach adult levels until about 1 year of age. Protein C and protein S levels are low, as are all vitamin K–dependent clotting factors, but these deficiencies predispose to thrombosis rather than hemorrhage. Fibrin degradation products act as anticoagulants but are normally removed from circulation by the liver as rapidly as they are formed; they are rarely detectable in normal neonates.

Fibrinolytic system

Plasminogen activator levels are high at birth and may exceed those of adults but fall rapidly in the first few days of life. Plasma plasminogen levels are approximately 50% of adult levels in the newborn and rise to adult norms by 2 weeks of age. Antiplasmin activity (α-2-antiplasmin) is higher in the newborn period than in adult life.

Vitamin K

Vitamin K is a fat-soluble vitamin that carboxylates glutamic acid residues on several proteins important for coagulation. This posttranslational modification of proteins is required to enable factors II, VII, IX, and X and proteins S and C to bind calcium and is essential for their functional activity. Vitamin K deficiency is manifested by a prolongation of the PT; prolongation of the aPTT; decreased coagulant activities of factors II, VII, IX, and X; a decreased ratio of factor II coagulant activity to antigen; the presence of noncarboxylated prothrombin; and the presence of prothrombin that has abnormal calcium-binding patterns.

Vitamin K is not transported across the placenta well, and some infants are vitamin K deficient at birth. The diet is an important source of vitamin K immediately after birth because of the absence of stores. Vitamin K is absorbed in the small intestine and requires the presence of bile acids. Even in infants who are not vitamin K deficient at birth, the levels of vitamin K–dependent factors are approximately 30% of adult levels and rise to adult normals by 6 weeks of age. Dietary vitamin K is phylloquinone, or vitamin K_1. The other major form is vitamin K_2, or menaquinone, which is synthesized by intestinal bacteria that differ widely in their production of vitamin K_2. Human milk contains variable but often low amounts of vitamin K_1, usually less than 20 μg/L, and occasionally less than 5 μg/L. Commercial formulas contain over 50 μg/L. Also, the intestinal flora of breast-fed infants may produce less vitamin K than the flora of the formula-fed infant. Breast-fed infants are at higher risk of vitamin K deficiency than formula-fed infants. Antibiotic administration may increase the risk of vitamin K deficiency after the first month of life by decreasing endogenous production of vitamin K_2.

Classic *hemorrhagic disease of the newborn* occurs

Table 32-3. Hemostatic function

Hemostatic factor or component	Premature infant	Full-term infant	Age adult level is attained
VASCULAR AND PLATELET FUNCTION			
Vasoconstriction	Present	Present	At birth
Capillary fragility	Increased	Normal	At birth
Bleeding time	Normal	Normal	At birth
Platelet count	Normal	Normal	At birth
Platelet function	↓↓ Aggregative ability	↓ Aggregative ability ↓ Clot retraction ↓ Platelet factor 3 availability	Not established
COAGULATION			
Whole blood clotting time	Decreased	↓ Or normal	At birth
Activated partial thromboplastin time (aPTT) (adult normal, 35-45 seconds)	70-145 seconds	45-70 seconds	2-9 months
Prothrombin time (PT) (adult normal, 12-14 seconds)	12-21 seconds	13-20 seconds	3-4 days
Thrombin time (TT) (adult normal, 8-10 seconds)	11-17 seconds	10-16 seconds	Few days
Thrombotest (II, VII, IX, X)	30%-50%	40%-68%	2-12 months
XII (Hageman factor)	10%-50%	25%-60%	9-14 days
IX (PTA)	5%-20%	15%-70%	1-2 months
IX (PTC)	10%-25%	20%-60%	3-9 months
VIII (AHF)	20%-80%	70%-150%	At birth
VII (proconvertin)	20%-45%	20%-70%	2-12 months
X (Stuart-Prower factor)	10%-45%	20%-55%	2-12 months
V (proaccelerin)	50%-85%	80%-200%	At birth
II (prothrombin)	20%-80%	26%-65%	2-12 months
I (fibrinogen) (gm/dl)	150%-300%	150%-300%	2-4 days
XIII (fibrin-stabilizing factor)	100%	100%	At birth
Fibrin split products (μg/ml)	0-10	0-7	
Antithrombin III	48%	55%	

Modified from Bleyer, W.A., Hakami, N., and Shepard, T.H.: J. Pediatr. **79:**838, 1971.

from 1 to 7 days of life. Infants are normal at birth but develop cutaneous or gastrointestinal bleeding. Other common sites include nasal bleeding, bleeding following circumcision, and hematuria. Estimates of the incidence of this complication in the absence of routine vitamin K prophylaxis vary from 0.25% to 1.7% in healthy term infants. Intracranial hemorrhage is not a common complication at this age.

Early hemorrhagic disease of the newborn occurs with maternal exposure to drugs that may affect coagulation, including warfarin, anticonvulsants, and antituberculous chemotherapy. Severe and often life-threatening hemorrhage may occur during delivery or in the first day of life. Rare cases occur without known predisposing factors. Intracranial hemorrhage is a frequent complication, and infants may be rendered severely damaged neurologically.

Late hemorrhagic disease may occur between 1 and 3 months of age. Secondary causes may occur at any age, usually as a complication of gastrointestinal disease (diarrhea, cystic fibrosis, biliary atresia, hepatitis), a β-lipoprotein deficiency, or exposure to warfarin. The idiopathic cases in 1- to 3-month old infants are most common in breast-fed infants and may be aggravated by antibiotic use. Acute intracranial hemorrhage is the most common initial presenting feature of late hemorrhagic disease and is often fatal or neurologically devastating. Cutaneous bleeding is the second most frequent feature, followed by gastrointestinal or mucous membrane bleeding or bleeding following surgery or an intramuscular injection. The breast milk of mothers of these infants contains approximately half the levels of vitamin K in breast milk of control mothers.

The only form of hemorrhagic disease of the newborn that cannot be prevented by prophylactic administration of vitamin K (0.5 to 1 mg given intramuscularly) is the early form, in which bleeding disorders may be incited by the trauma of delivery. The classic and late forms of hemorrhagic disease of the newborn can be prevented by such prophylaxis. Recently when routine prophylaxis was discontinued in England, a resurgence of bleeding caused by vitamin K deficiency in the newborn occurred. Although the incidence of significant bleeding complications is not high in normal term infants, especially those who are not exclusively breast fed, the morbidity and mortality appear to justify prophylaxis of all infants. Several other questions, however, remain unanswered. One is the suggestion that oral vitamin K may be as effective as intramuscular administration, which requires further study before practices are changed. Another question is whether infants who are exclusively breast fed should receive additional prophylaxis after 1 month of age. Again, too little data are available to support routine use of additional vitamin K. A third issue concerns prophylaxis of infants at risk of early hemorrhagic disease whose mothers are receiving anticonvulsants or antituberculous agents. (Warfarin is a teratogen and is containdicated in pregnancy for this reason, but exposed infants would also be at risk.) Oral administration of large doses (20 mg/day) of vitamin K to the mother may improve the coagulation status of the infant, and these infants should be given vitamin K immediately on delivery.

Although proteins C and S, which are anticoagulant proteins, are also vitamin K dependent, thrombotic problems related to their deficient functioning have not been described. This may be a reflection of the more recent identification of these proteins and less detailed study of their role in vitamin K deficiency, but it appears that the clinical significance of vitamin K deficiency is balanced in favor of hemorrhage rather than thrombosis.

Congenital coagulation disorders

Hemophilia

Both classic hemophilia (hemophilia A, factor VIII deficiency) and Christmas disease (hemophilia B, factor IX deficiency) are X-linked and thus occur almost exclusively in males. The severity of factor deficiency determines the severity of bleeding, which rarely occurs spontaneously in patients who have levels greater than 5% of normal. Birth trauma and circumcision may cause severe, life-threatening bleeding. Subgaleal hemorrhage may be massive and may be complicated by secondary consumptive coagulopathy and anemia. Bleeding after circumcision, or less often after heel stick blood sampling, is a frequent sign of hemophilia. A positive family history in two thirds of the cases raises the index of suspicion and helps confirm the clinical diagnosis. Many of the remaining cases are apparently new mutations.

Prolongation of the aPTT with a normal PT is characteristic of hemophilia A and B, but this may be difficult to interpret because the aPTT is normally longer in the neonate than in older children. A specific assay of factor VIII and IX must be run. A very low level of factor VIII activity combined with a normal level of factor VIII antigen confirms the diagnosis of classic hemophilia. The assay must also be performed on the mother. Careful studies permit identification of carriers with a high degree of probability, and prenatal diagnosis is now available for some but not all families at risk for factor VIII deficiency. The risk that a male infant of a carrier mother will be affected with hemophilia is 50%.

Therapy of bleeding episodes consists primarily of factor replacement. In moderate hemophilia A and in von Willebrand's disease, some treatments have now used the vasopressin analog DDAVP (1-deamino-8-*d*-arginine vasopressin), which raises all components of the factor VIII system two- to three-fold after intranasal or intravenous administration, but this experience does not yet extend to the newborn period. For factor VIII deficiency, cryoprecipitate is the treatment of choice and usually permits administration of hemostatic doses of factor VIII without excessive volume. For factor IX deficiency, 10 ml/kg of fresh frozen plasma usually suffices. Every effort should be made to use products that limit the risk of hepatitis B, which has a high fatality rate in the newborn period (see part two of this chapter). All patients with severe hemophilia should receive the hepatitis B vaccine because of the high probability of infection with multiple plasma transfusions. Lyophilized preparations of factor VIII and of factor IX (also containing factors II, VII and X) are the most convenient way of giving high doses of factor replacement without volume overload and permit early treatment of bleeding episodes at home to minimize joint damage. However, these preparations carry a high risk of transmitting the virus of acquired immunodeficiency syndrome (AIDS), as well as other infectious agents. AIDS has become the second most frequent cause of death in patients with hemophilia in the United States. Heat-treated preparations should lessen this risk for future patients. Most infants with hemophilia do not have clinically significant bleeding after the immediate perinatal period until they become mobile and thus rarely require factor replacement between ages 1 week and 6 months.

Von Willebrand's disease

Von Willebrand's disease is usually a relatively mild bleeding diathesis and is transmitted as an autosomal dominant disorder. A less common form involves autosomal recessive transmission, in which the carriers are asymptomatic and homozygous patients are severely affected. The von Willebrand factor is a large, multimeric glycoprotein that circulates in a form that is complexed to the factor VIII procoagulant protein. It plays an important role in platelet function by promoting platelet-vessel wall interactions. The gene for von Willebrand factor has been cloned, and many unanswered questions about the function of this protein should be resolved in the near future. Laboratory tests that confirm the diagnosis of von Willebrand's disease are the bleeding time, factor VIII coagulant activity, factor VIII–related antigen, and ristocetin cofactor, all of which are abnormal. The bleeding time is not useful in young children. Prolonged mucous membrane bleeding is frequent. Neonatal manifestations are extremely rare except in the most severe form, which may behave as hemophilia. Treatment consists of administration of cryoprecipitate or DDAVP.

Other factor deficiencies

Congenital deficiency of factor XIII, fibrin-stabilizing factor, may cause bleeding at several days of age. This is an autosomal recessive disorder in which the factor that stabilizes the fibrin polymer is absent, and the fibrin clot dissolves before wound healing is complete. Bleeding from the umbilical stump or 2 to 3 days after circumcision are the most common manifestations. Routine clotting studies are normal, and diagnosis requires special factor assays. Replacement therapy with fresh frozen plasma can be given but is rarely required except following surgery or major trauma.

Congenital afibrinogenemia is a rare disorder of fibrinogen synthesis in which both the PT and PTT are extremely abnormal. Heterozygous patients are asymptomatic, and homozygous ones may have problems such as easy bruising, hemarthrosis, menorrhagia, bleeding after surgery, and cerebral hemorrhage. Bleeding in the immediate neonatal period is frequent. Dysfibrinogenemias also occur and are usually milder than afibrinogenemia. Therapy consists of infusion of cryoprecipitate.

Congenital deficiencies or abnormalities of prothrombin, factor V, factor VII, and factor X have all been described. All are extremely rare, and all have appeared in the newborn period with excessive bleeding, including intracranial hemorrhage.

Platelet disorders

Platelets are essential for primary hemostasis. Disorders of platelet number or function are usually manifested by cutaneous and mucous membrane bleeding, which may be spontaneous or traumatic. Platelets, anucleate, granule-containing formed elements that normally circulate for about 10 days, are produced by budding from the membrane of the megakaryocyte in the bone marrow. They must be capable of adhering to vessel walls, aggregating with each other, releasing their granule contents and prostaglandins, and interacting with fibrin; they must also refrain from performing these functions within an intact vasculature. Normal numbers in premature and term neonates are 150,000 to 450,000 platelets/mm^3, the same as adult norms. Increased numbers of platelets are rarely a problem in the neonate; thrombocytosis with thrombotic complications is a problem of adults with myelodysplasia. Thrombocytopenia and disorders of platelet function are common in the neonate and may be complicated by significant bleeding problems.

Thrombocytopenia caused by underproduction

Thrombocytopenia may result from deceased production or increased destruction of platelets. Decreased production is less common than increased destruction. Congenital disorders that may be associated with decreased rates of platelet production include the thrombocytopenia–absent radii (TAR) syndrome and isolated megakaryocytic hypoplasia without associated orthopedic abnormalities (Fig. 32-12). These infants may have

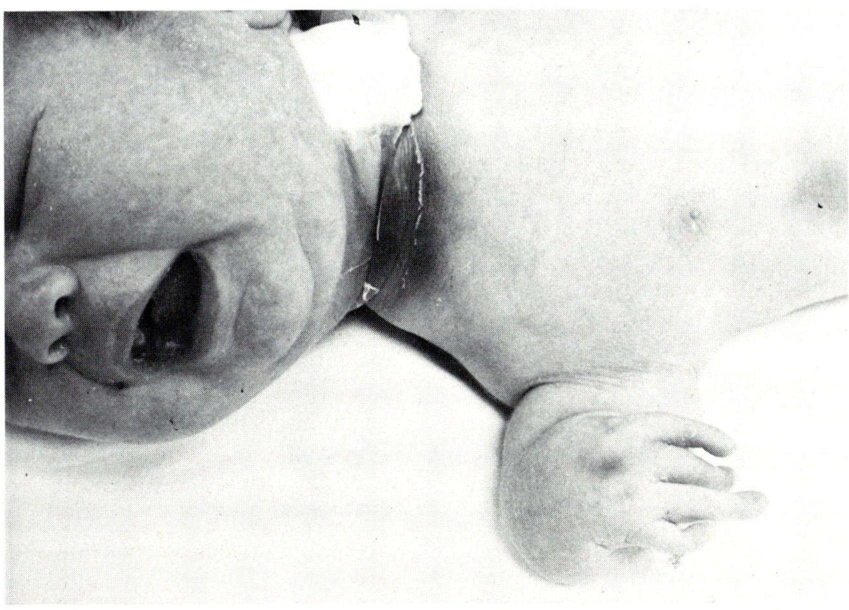

Fig. 32-12. Hand anomalies and skin hemorrhage in a newborn with thrombocytopenia–absent radius syndrome.

intracranial hemorrhage at birth, but the bleeding manifestations tend to lessen as they get older and the platelet count often rises. Affected infants appear to be unduly susceptible to milk allergy and may fail to thrive. Infants with TAR frequently have a transient leukemoid reaction in the newborn period, and about one third have cardiac defects. This may be inherited as an autosomal recessive disorder, but the form of inheritance is not yet proved. Isolated amegakaryocytic thrombocytopenia may be the initial sign of progressive bone marrow failure. Trisomy 13 and trisomy 18 frequently have associated thrombocytopenia, which is usually not severe. Isovaleric acidemia, methylmalonic aciduria, and ketotic hyperglycinemia all have associated decreased platelet production. Congenital infection with cytomegalovirus and rubella is often complicated by thrombocytopenia; both decreased production and increased destruction appear to be involved to varying degrees in different patients. Bone marrow infiltration with leukemia; metastatic tumors, especially neuroblastoma; histiocytosis; and osteopetrosis are manifested by thrombocytopenia, with other cell lines also involved.

Megaloblastic anemias caused by severe folate or vitamin B_{12} deficiency may also be associated with neutropenia and thrombocytopenia. In the newborn period the impairment of DNA synthesis that results from folate or B_{12} deficiency is manifested by growth failure and neurologic difficulties as well.

Wiscott-Aldrich syndrome

Wiscott-Aldrich syndrome is an X-linked congenital immunodeficiency syndrome associated with eczema and thrombocytopenia resulting from decreased platelet production. Both bleeding from thrombocytopenia and immunodeficiency with associated infections and lymphoproliferative malignancies are potentially life-threatening complications for these infants. Only the thrombocytopenia is easily recognizable at birth, and bleeding manifestations in the nursery may be the presenting symptoms. The eczema usually develops in the first few months of life; and the humoral immunodeficiency is masked by passively transferred maternal antibody at birth. Early bone marrow transplantation has greatly improved the outlook for those children who have a compatible donor.

Immune thrombocytopenia

Thrombocytopenia resulting from increased destruction of platelets may be immune or nonimmune. Immune thrombocytopenia is caused by transfer of maternal antibody, either *autoimmune* or *isoimmune*.

Autoimmune neonatal thrombocytopenia is a possible complication when the mother has circulating platelet antibodies due to an autoimmune disease such as lupus erythematosus or idiopathic thrombocytopenic purpura (ITP). This disorder is best diagnosed by maternal history and platelet count. When the maternal platelet count is normal, the infant is rarely affected unless the mother has been splenectomized. However, when the maternal count is low, 50% to 90% of infants are affected. (See Chapter 30.)

Isoimmune thrombocytopenia is analogous to erythroblastosis and can occur alone or in conjunction with RBC sensitization. The incidence of this disorder is about 3 per 10,000 live births. The mother produces an antiplatelet antibody on stimulation by fetal platelets, which cross the placenta. The antibody is most often directed against the Pl^{A1} antigen, since only 3% of the population is negative for this antigen, and therefore a Pl^{A1}-negative mother has a high probability of sensitization.

The major therapeutic dilemma in immune thrombocytopenia is deciding which mothers are at risk of having a thrombocytopenic infant. In autoimmune thrombocytopenia, bleeding is likely if maternal platelets are low. Isoimmune disorders are rarely detected until after an affected child has been born. Since the disorder may occur with subsequent pregnancies, later babies should all be considered to have a high risk for thrombocytopenia. When an infant has a low platelet count, the most risky period is delivery itself. For this reason, cesarean section is recommended for all infants judged at high risk. If the mother's platelet count is less than $60,000/mm^3$ to $100,000/mm^3$, platelet transfusions should be available before surgery.

Once infants are born without problems, they have a very low risk of significant bleeding and rarely need treatment. The parents can be reassured that the disorder is self-limited and will clear when the maternal IgG is metabolized, usually in 4 to 8 weeks. If an infant has more than minor skin bleeding after delivery, the most effective treatment is platelet transfusions. The mother is the ideal platelet donor, since she is Pl^{A1} negative, but she has circulating antibodies that are difficult to remove, even by washing the platelets. If bleeding persists despite platelet transfusions, exchange transfusion with fresh whole blood will eliminate much of the antibody while also raising the infant's platelet count. Babies with significant bleeding into an enclosed space, such as intracranially, may develop delayed jaundice as the blood is resorbed. Fig. 32-13 shows the typical response to transfused platelets in an infant with isoimmune thrombocytopenia. (See also part two of this chapter.)

Nonimmune platelet destruction

Nonimmunologic destruction of platelets may occur in hypersplenism, with mechanical destruction in giant hemangiomata (Kasabach-Merritt syndrome), after cardiac surgery ("Waring blender" syndrome), and with in-

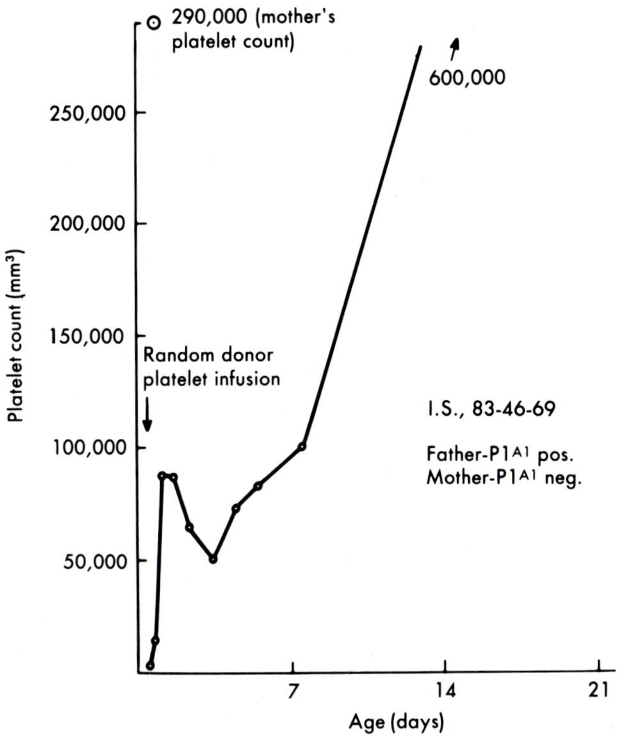

Fig. 32-13. Neonatal response to random donor platelet transfusions in isoimmune disease with low titers of circulating antibody. Survival curves probably represent combined effects of antibody dilution and increasing endogenous platelet survival.

dwelling catheters. A wide variety of drugs may induce thrombocytopenia, possibly because of direct toxic effects or antibody-mediated destruction by hapten binding to platelets. Many common drugs are included in this category, such as antibiotics and anticonvulsants, and these drugs may cross the placenta from the mother into the infant. Heparin may induce thrombocytopenia and is often used to ensure patency of indwelling catheters in sick neonates. Certain fatty acids may cause platelet aggregation and accelerated clearance; most widely used soybean lipid preparations for hyperalimentation are free of this complication. Double-volume exchange transfusion for hyperbilirubinemia may deplete the platelet supply, and infants who receive multiple exchange transfusions with stored components often develop moderate degrees of thrombocytopenia lasting several days. Toxic effects of bacteria and viruses may cause thrombocytopenia without inducing generalized disseminated intravascular coagulation (DIC). Thrombocytopenia associated with infection is one of the most often observed phenomena in neonatal intensive care units. Recurrent episodes of thrombocytopenia with microangiopathic hemolytic anemia have been described with congenital deficiency of a plasma factor, as yet unknown, or recurrent thrombotic thrombocytopenic purpura. Thrombotic complications are usually more significant than bleeding, although both may occur, and all body systems may be involved. Hemolytic uremic syndrome, a closely related disorder, rarely appears before 4 months of age and is more common in older children. Several patients with lifelong recurrent thrombotic thrombocytopenic purpura responding to plasma infusions have thrombocytopenia and hemolysis in the newborn period.

Disorders of platelet function

Disorders of platelet function may also cause hemorrhage in the newborn period. Some of these disorders are associated with thrombocytopenia. The *gray platelet syndrome,* in which the platelets are large and agranular and appear bluish gray on Wright's stained smear, is a familial disorder with absent α-granules. Patients are thrombocytopenic, and the platelet count may rise with splenectomy, although the morphologic and functional abnormalities persist. In *Bernard-Soulier syndrome,* an autosomal recessive disorder in which platelet membrane glycoproteins Ia and Ib are missing, the platelets are large, have markedly abnormal adhesion, and are usually decreased in number. The hemorrhagic complications and prolongation of the bleeding time are out of proportion to the degree of thrombocytopenia. *Glanzmann's thrombasthenia,* also autosomal recessive, is associated with diminished or absent glycoproteins IIb and IIIa, abnormal aggregation, and normal adhesion. This is the most common of the inherited disorders of platelet function and is not associated with thrombocytopenia. *Hermansky-Pudlak syndrome,* a rare autosomal recessive disorder with oculocutaneous albinism, accumulation of ceroidlike pigment in bone marrow macrophages, and platelet storage pool disease, is associated with an abnormal platelet release reaction and mucous membrane bleeding. Platelet function is also abnormal in *Chédiak-Higashi syndrome,* with giant granules and storage pool disease, but bleeding is rarely a clinical problem until the patient develops pancytopenia with an aggressive lymphoproliferative disorder. In the *May-Hegglin anomaly* giant platelets and Döhle bodies in the neutrophils are noted on smear. Platelet function is generally normal, but approximately one third of patients have thrombocytopenia and may have significant bleeding. In each of these disorders platelet transfusions may be indicated when aggressive local measures fail to control bleeding. All these diseases are present at birth and may cause significant bleeding in the newborn.

Acquired disorders of platelet function may be caused by drugs such as aspirin and some of the semisynthetic penicillins (ticarcillin, piperacillin), high-dose vitamin E administration, and uremia. Mucous membrane and cutaneous bleeding are the usual clinical manifestations.

Indomethacin induces platelet dysfunction in a way similar to aspirin. Infants who are receiving indomethacin to induce closure of a patent ductus arteriosus have a prolonged bleeding time. Clinically significant hemorrhage has not been attributed to effects of drugs on platelet function, but these are usually given to infants who are already at risk for intraventricular hemorrhage, and the relative contributions of various risk factors may be difficult to determine.

Disseminated intravascular coagulation

See also Part two of this chapter.

Despite numerous publications on DIC, treatment of this disorder remains difficult and controversial. DIC occurs when the balance between circulating procoagulants, proteases, endothelial lining, and blood flow is upset, either locally or systemically, producing apparent consumption of intrinsic clotting factors. The primary defect also can be an alteration in the fibrinogen molecule itself. It is important to remember, however, that DIC is a *syndrome* that occurs secondary to a variety of primary events, which include*:

A. Hypoxia-acidosis
   1. Hyaline membrane disease (respiratory distress syndrome)
   2. Asphyxia
B. Infectious diseases
   1. Disseminated viral diseases
   2. Bacterial septicemia
   3. Protozoal infections—toxoplasmosis
C. Obstetric conditions
   1. Abruptio placentae
   2. Dead twin fetus
   3. Chorioangioma
   4. Eclampsia and preeclampsia
   5. Infants who are small for gestational age or postmature
D. Miscellaneous diseases and conditions
   1. Severe erythroblastosis fetalis (Rh isoimmunization)
   2. Necrotizing enterocolitis
   3. Shock

This complication typically is recognized in a very sick neonate who suddenly develops generalized bleeding with oozing from puncture sites, catheter insertions, and endoctracheal tubes. Because diagnosis may be difficult in newborns who normally have prolonged clotting studies, all sick neonates should have clotting studies performed on admission as a baseline of comparison should bleeding develop later.

The diagnosis of DIC is based on laboratory findings of thrombocytopenia, increased aPTT and PT, and decreased fibrinogen levels.

A. Minimal criteria for DIC
   1. Thrombocytopenia
   2. ↑ aPTT
   3. ↑ PT
   4. Hypofibrinogenemia
B. Helpful confirmative tests
   1. ↑ Thrombin time (not corrected by protamine)
   2. ↑ Fibrin split products
   3. ↓ Levels of factors V and VIII

If additional tests are available, prolonged thrombin time, fibrin split products, and decreased levels of factors V and VIII will confirm the diagnosis. Once successful therapy is initiated, the intrinsic clotting factors usually increase first, and it may take 5 to 10 days for platelets to revert to normal levels.

The most important issue in therapy of DIC is whether the triggering event (e.g., septicemia, asphyxia) is treatable and reversible. If it is not, the infant may do poorly regardless of how vigorously the blood abnormalities are treated.

Most centers now believe that supportive care with blood components is the best treatment of DIC, having the least chance of causing further stress to an already sick infant. Fresh frozen plasma, 20 ml/kg, provides all intrinsic clotting factors and can be repeated every 12 to 24 hours if bleeding persists. If platelets are less that 20,000 to 40,000/mm^3, one or two platelet packs should also be given. Since one unit of platelets also contains fibrinogen and factor VII, platelets alone frequently are adequate treatment of a bleeding episode and are particularly useful when one does not want to push large intravascular volumes into a small infant. For the rare infant whose bleeding persists despite these measures, exchange transfusion with fresh, heparinized blood will provide clotting factors and platelets while also eliminating some of the circulating fibrin split production.

Heparinization has been effective in reversing DIC in some situations in adults and has occasionally been recommended for children. There has never been any objective evidence that heparin reverses DIC in children, however, and heparinization of small infants frequently triggers even more bleeding in an infant who is already critically ill. In addition, heparin has a prolonged half-life in neonates, and it is very difficult to monitor heparinization accurately, since all clotting tests are prolonged in normal newborns.

Evaluation of a bleeding newborn

In the evaluation of a neonate with bleeding, one should first determine whether the bleeding is localized or generalized. Localized bleeding, such as subperiosteal or intraventricular or intrapulmonary hemorrhage, is al-

*From Corrigan, J.J., Jr.: Am. J. Pediatr. Hematol./Oncol. 1:245, 1979. (Published by Raven Press Ltd., New York.)

Table 32-4. Laboratory evaluation of the bleeding infant

	Platelet count	PT	aPTT	Fibrinogen	Factor VIII
Well infant					
Thrombocytopenia	↓	N	N	N	N
Vitamin K deficiency	N	↑	↑	N	N
Classic hemophilia	N	N	↑	N	↓↓
Sick infant					
DIC	↓	↑	↑	↓↓	↓
Liver disease	N– ↓	↑	↑	Sl ↓	N– ↑
Infection	N– ↓	N	N– ↑	↑	↑

N, Normal; Sl, slightly.

most always a local phenomenon and not a result of a generalized coagulopathy, but the latter two are frequently triggered by asphyxia and may ultimately progress to DIC.

Table 32-4 illustrates the laboratory evaluation of a bleeding infant. Because infection, either viral or bacterial, is the most common cause of neonatal bleeding, all such infants should have a thorough search for infection, including TORCH titers and careful viral and bacterial cultures. A good screening series of clotting tests includes a platelet count, PT, aPTT, and fibrinogen level. If thrombocytopenia is the only abnormality in an otherwise vigorous infant, specific causes such as platelet antibodies, congenital megakaryocytic hypoplasia with absent radius or Wiskott-Aldrich syndrome must be suspected. If platelets are normal, but aPTT and PT are prolonged, the child may have had inadequate vitamin K; an intravenous dose of 1 mg can be given as a diagnostic trial. Healthy males with a prolonged aPTT may have hemophilia; a specific assay for antihemophilic factor or Christmas factor will confirm the diagnosis.

An infant who suddenly becomes ill with generalized bleeding usually has bleeding either from thrombocytopenia plus vasculitis or from thrombocytopenia associated with a full-blown DIC syndrome. Occasionally, liver disease can be confused with DIC, but this is uncommon in neonates. Liver disease must be severe to decrease production of factors II, VII, IX, and X enough to prolong the PTT. Fibrinogen levels never get below 60 to 80 mg/dl without consumption, since a small amount of fibrinogen is made by extrahepatic sources such as vascular endothelium. Therefore a fibrinogen level of less than 50 mg/dl is caused either by DIC or, rarely, by congenital hypofibrinogenemia.

Deficiencies of anticoagulant proteins

Deficiencies of proteins S and C, which are vitamin K–dependent anticoagulant proteins, and of antithrombin III (heparin cofactor) have all been associated with a predisposition to develop thrombosis. Deficiency of protein S has been associated with recurrent venous thrombosis on a familial basis, but all affected patients have been adults. In contrast, homozygous protein C deficiency is associated with severe, often fatal thrombosis in the newborn period. Several patients have developed recurrent purpura fulminans in the immediate newborn period. Alternate-day infusion of a factor IX concentrate containing protein C has permitted survival of one patient for over a year. Chronic anticoagulation with warfarin is an alternate therapeutic option, as yet unproved in this condition. Acquired protein C deficiency as a result of chronic warfarin administration has been implicated in the syndrome of warfarin-induced necrosis, which underscores the delicate balance between the coagulant and anticoagulant proteins in normal physiology.

Recurrent thrombosis has also been described in congenital antithrombin III deficiency. This is a rare disorder. Levels of antithrombin III are low in premature and full-term neonates and may account for newborns appearing to require higher doses of heparin than older children and adults. However, newborns are not unduly resistant to heparin therapy and can usually be effectively anticoagulated with heparin despite low levels of antithrombin III.

DISORDERS OF PHAGOCYTIC CELLS

Polymorphonuclear leukocytes, monocytes, and tissue macrophages are all derived from the bone marrow. A stem cell common to other marrow elements is the ultimate precursor. Myelopoiesis, or production of neutrophils and monocytes, takes place in the liver and bone marrow but apparently does not occur in the yolk sac, which is the site of erythropoiesis in the first trimester. Monocytes leave the marrow and mature into fixed tissue macrophages in other organs, including the liver, spleen, and lungs. Under normal conditions in neonates and adults a reserve of mature neutrophils is present in the marrow that exceeds the circulating pool by a factor of 10. These mature cells are released under conditions of stress or infection. In addition, intravascular neutrophils are free in the circulation and adhere to vessel walls in "circulating" and "marginal" pools that exist in equilibrium. Neutrophils form the first line of defense against bacterial infection and are able to migrate into areas of infection, ingest organisms, and kill them rapidly. Monocytes form the second line of defense, arriving in the inflammatory infiltrate much less rapidly then neutrophils. Monocytes are important for defense against fungal infections as well as against bacteria. Phagocytes are also major factors in wound healing, being needed for removal of necrotic material as well as for prevention of infection. In addition, tissue macrophages are the major site of destruction of sensitized or damaged erythrocytes in hemolytic disease, regardless of the nature of the RBC abnormality.

Phagocytic cells interact in complex fashion with humoral factors, which regulate the recognition of foreign material and the formation of inflammatory exudates. The major humoral factors are immunoglobulins and components of the complement and coagulation systems. IgG, 7S globulin, crosses the placenta and provides the neonate with passive protection against some organisms. The amount of protection varies with the gestational age of the infant (since much of the IgG is acquired in the last month of pregnancy) and with the immune status of the mother. Complement components are synthesized by the infant, with much of the contribution coming from the liver, including its macrophages. Low levels of some components, particularly in the alternative or properdin pathway, even in healthy full-term infants, may contribute to increased susceptibility to infection. Activated complement factors and some coagulation factors are potent "chemoattractants," or stimulators of migration toward a gradient. The factors, although beyond the scope of this section, contribute heavily to normal function of phagocytic cells. (See Chapter 30.)

Neutrophil kinetics

The absolute neutrophil count tends to be markedly elevated at birth and in the first few days of life. Since lymphocytosis is a normal finding at this age, the total white count may be quite high. The high neutrophil count is related to several factors. The rate of marrow *production* is high because of an elevated level of a hormone, termed *colony-stimulating factor*, which increases the rates of division and maturation of marrow precursors. The rate of *release* from the marrow is increased at delivery, perhaps because of the stress of delivery, with release of epinephrine and endogenous cortisol. In addition, the rate of *demargination* of the intravascular pool is increased by the same factors that accelerate release. By 1 week of age the absolute neutrophil count has reached the levels normally seen later in childhood. Because of the lymphocytosis that is normal at this age, the percentage of neutrophils may be lower than in older children, but the absolute numbers should be the same (Fig. 32-14).

Neutropenia

Although normal values vary somewhat with time in the first few days of life, an absolute neutrophil count

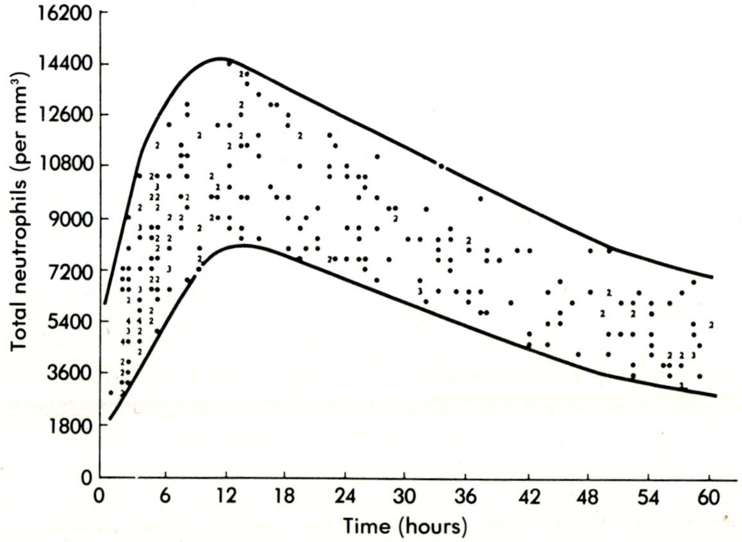

Fig. 32-14. The total neutrophil count reference range in the first 60 hours of life. Dots represent single values; numbers represent the number of values at the same point. Heavy lines represent the envelope bounding these data. (From Manroe, B.L., and others: J. Pediatr. **95:**89, 1979.)

below 1,500 constitutes neutropenia at any age. Genetic or racial factors may affect normal neutrophil counts, but these remain rather poorly defined. As in older patients, significantly increased risk of infection varies inversely with the neutrophil count, and does not become a major risk factor until the neutrophil count is below 500.

Congenital, persistent neutropenia may be severe and life-threatening or mild and relatively benign. *Benign congenital neutropenia* is a relatively common condition and is often picked up as an incidental finding on a routine complete blood count (CBC) or as part of a CBC done for evaluation of infection. The neutrophil count usually ranges from 200 to 800 and may increase somewhat with bacterial infection. Most of these patients do not have severe infections of deep tissues but are bothered by cutaneous infections and mouth sores. Wounds often heal slowly. This may be an inherited problem but often appears to be an isolated finding in the index patient. Because of the relatively mild clinical course, many patients may go undiagnosed for many years, but affected ones may appear in the nursery.

Infantile genetic agranulocytosis, or *Kostmann's syndrome*, is a severe form of hereditary neutropenia with autosomal recessive inheritance. Most reported cases are from Scandinavia, but the disease has occurred in all racial groups. Children are agranulocytic at birth, and there is an associated marked monocytosis, usually greater than 30% of the circulating white cells. Children may develop deep tissue infections, most often in the skin and respiratory tract, that are difficult to control. The bone marrow precursors of neutrophils grow normally in vitro, and no inhibitors of proliferation have been identified. Most children die within the first few years of life from infection, but several patients have survived into adolescence and developed myeloid leukemia. Subtle chromosomal abnormalities have been described. Lymphoid function is normal.

Reticular dysgenesis is the ultimate immunologic deficiency state. Patients have severe combined immune deficiency, without T or B lymphocyte function, and agranulocytosis. Patients are affected early in infancy and die quickly from overwhelming infection unless bone marrow transplantation can be performed. As with other patients with severe combined immunodeficiency, florid graft-versus-host disease from RBC or platelet transfusion is a risk if blood products are not irradiated to prevent lymphocyte proliferation.

Cyclic neutropenia is a disorder of the entire bone marrow with cyclic hematopoiesis, but because of the longer life spans of RBCs and platelets, only neutropenia is clinically significant. This may be inherited as an autosomal dominant condition, or may be sporadic with unclear inheritance. Most patients have cycles of 21 to 28 days in duration and periods of 4 to 5 days of agranulocytosis at the nadir. The neutropenia is associated with severe monocytosis, often with eosinophilia, so the total leukocyte count remains within the normal range despite agranulocytosis. Patients have repeated episodes of fever, mouth sores, and ulceration of all mucosal surfaces and may develop lymphadenitis with cutaneous or oral infections. Bone pain at the time of severe neutropenia is a debilitating problem for some patients. The bone marrow findings vary with the time of the cycle, and reflect the 10- to 14-day gestation of the neutrophil. Humoral immunity and macrophages are normal. The cycle appears to begin in utero, since patients have appeared with agranulocytosis and monocytosis at birth. Frequent blood counts are required to make the diagnosis unless a family history exists. Aggressive therapy of infections usually prevents life-threatening complications in these patients, and late development of leukemia has not been described.

Bone marrow dysfunction with pancreatic insufficiency, or *Schwachman-Diamond syndrome*, includes patients with a variable constellation of clinical problems. Some are affected most by malnutrition and dwarfism, and others have recurrent infections but minimal gastrointestinal difficulties. The sweat test is normal in these patients, but the combination of pancreatic insufficiency with recurrent pulmonary infections may closely mimic cystic fibrosis. Hypoplastic anemia and thrombocytopenia are also present, but neutropenia is usually the most significant component of the marrow dysfunction. Treatment includes pancreatic enzyme replacement and aggressive therapy of infections. This disorder is usually not evident in the newborn period.

There are a wide variety of other persistent neutropenias with variable degrees of monocytosis, eosinophilia, and bone marrow morphologies. At present, no good system exists for classification or for understanding the underlying pathogenesis. Therapy remains preventive with episodic treatment of infections. Chronic prophylactic antibiotics should be reserved for patients who are repeatedly plagued with significant infections, since selection of resistant organisms and development of opportunistic infections and antibiotic-associated colitis and allergy remain real problems for these patients.

Acquired neutropenia is a common problem in the newborn. The major etiologies are immune, drug induced (including maternal drugs), and infection. Several perinatal complications are associated with significant neutropenia, including maternal hypertension, birth asphyxia, periventricular hemorrhage, and reticulocytosis related to hemolysis occurring after 14 days of age. A measure that may be helpful in predicting which infants are infected is the ratio of immature (band forms and younger) to total neutrophils, or I/T ratio. Usually this is less than 0.13, and it may rise to 0.80 or greater in association with documented sepsis. Some evidence suggests that the high I/T ratio may predict which infants have depleted their bone marrow stores of neutrophils, but this is not confirmed.

Isoimmune neutropenia may occur in the same manner as isoimmune hemolytic anemia and isoimmune thrombocytopenia, with transfer of maternal antibodies across the placenta to interact with paternal antigens expressed on the infant's cells. Because autoimmune neutropenia in adults is an uncommon phenomenon, the passive transfer of antineutrophil antibodies associated with maternal disease is rare but may occur as a complication of systemic lupus erythematosus. Isoimmune neutropenia, as with its relatives, is caused by an IgG antibody and is a transient phenomenon. Most infants do not have clinical problems with infections, but if they are sick for other reasons, they may develop significant complications. The neutrophil count usually begins to rise between 2 and 4 weeks and remains normal. Subsequent children will also be at risk of being affected. Specific antibodies can usually be identified in maternal serum, and cytotoxic activity of maternal serum for paternal leukocytes is a good indication that an isoimmune process is responsible for the infant's neutropenia.

Maternal drugs that have caused neutropenia in an infant include sulfonamides, semisynthetic penicillins, propylthioracil, methimazole, and gold salts. These are also self-limited processes, and unless a significant infection intervenes, infants usually do well.

Infection is probably the most frequent cause of neutropenia in the nursery. Congenital viral infections, including cytomegalovirus, herpes, and rubella, may cause neutropenia. Severe neutropenia may be a complication of necrotizing enterocolitis and of group B streptococcal sepsis, as well as other bacterial infections in the newborn period. The neutropenia that complicates these processes often results from depletion of bone marrow stores. The bone marrow is the major site of storage of neutrophils; in the adult approximately seven times as many mature neutrophils are present in the bone marrow as are present intravascularly (circulating and marginal pools combined). Whether as large a reservoir is available in the newborn is unclear, but the infant is already using most of the available marrow cavity for hemopoiesis and clearly does not have the reserve capacity available to the adult. Studies in adult and infant rats have demonstrated rapid depletion of stores and development of neutropenia in neonates, whereas adult animals were able to maintain an elevated neutrophil count. In addition, in necrotizing enterocolitis the release of endotoxin and other bacterial products may cause a shift in the distribution of circulating neutrophils into the marginal pool. A rise in the I/T ratio appears to be an excellent predictor of bacterial infection in the neonate, especially in the presence of respiratory distress. Increases in the total numbers of immature cells are less reliable.

Because of the morbidity and mortality associated with bacterial infections in the neonate and the serious concerns about the consequences of neutropenia in an infected infant, neutrophil transfusions have been advocated. Some encouraging data suggest that neutrophil transfusions may improve the survival of these infants. All the studies performed to date have been small, and none has been initiated comparing plasma infusions to neutrophil transfusion. Because neonates are deficient in many factors important in host defense besides neutrophils, this information will be needed to evaluate neutrophil transfusion. Obtaining adequate numbers of functional neutrophils, which must be freshly prepared in expensive and complex laboratories, remains a difficult undertaking. Neutrophil transfusions have been shown to benefit adult patients with gram-negative infection or infection resistant to antibiotics and are less widely used at present than when first introduced. Whether all or some neutropenic, infected neonates will benefit from plasma or neutrophil transfusion is an important question requiring further study before clinical practices are changed. The hazards of transmission of infectious agents, possible graft-versus-host disease, and leukoagglutination will also need to be considered.

Phagocyte function in the newborn

Detailed studies of phagocyte function are not routinely available in most clinical laboratories. They require special techniques, skilled technicians, freshly prepared living cells, and relatively large volumes of blood. Thus studies of neonatal phagocyte function are frequently performed on cord blood or on blood from infants about to be transfused. These difficulties may account for some of the disparities in reported results. In general, phagocytosis (the ability of cells to ingest particles), killing of bacteria, and the ability of cells to generate the reactive oxygen species needed for bacterial killing are close to normal adult values in premature and full-term neonates. The only function that appears to be reproducibly impaired is chemotaxis, the ability of phagocytes to sense and move in response to a chemical gradient into an area of inflammation. These cells have considerable reserve power, and defects that are statistically significantly different from adult norms may or may not be biologically significant for the patient. Low levels of complement proteins synthesized by the liver, low levels of immunoglobulins passively transferred across the placenta, and the lack of active immunity affect neutrophil function in vivo, since recognition of foreign pathogens depends heavily on humoral immunity. All these defects are more severe in premature than full-term infants. Monocyte production of interleukin 1, or leukocyte pyrogen, which mediates fever, is normal except in infants born by elective cesarean delivery, in whom it is diminished.

Infants with congenital defects in neutrophil function frequently have bacterial infections during the newborn period. The defects that cause ongoing, life-threatening susceptibility to infection include deficiency of membrane-adhesive glycoprotein, Mo1, chronic granulomatous disease, and Chédiak-Higashi syndrome. Some patients with severe chemotactic defects with or without hyperimmunoglobulin E present as newborns.

Disorders of neutrophil function

Mo1 deficiency

Several patients have been described with recurrent invasive bacterial and fungal infections, delayed wound healing, delayed separation of the umbilical cord, granulocytosis, and juvenile periodontitis beginning soon after primary dental eruption. The neutrophils from these patients do not adhere or spread normally, fail to orient in a chemotactic gradient, and do not ingest particles opsonized with C3bi. The neutrophils and monocytes lack the C3bi receptor and are missing a surface glycoprotein, Mo1, whose molecular weight is variably estimated at 110,000 to 229,000 daltons and which reacts with a monoclonal antibody to Mo1. Lymphocytes normally have a surface glycoprotein, LFA-1, which shares a common β-subunit of 94,000 daltons with Mo1. In Mo1 deficiency, the β-subunit is missing from both neutrophils and lymphocytes; the α-subunit of Mo1 is absent from the neutrophil, and the α-subunit of LFA-1 is missing from lymphocytes. The primary defect is thought to be in their common β-chain.

Mo1 deficiency is inherited as an autosomal recessive disorder. Its frequency is not known, but it may be one of the more common major defects in neutrophil function. Infants often have delayed separation of the umbilical cord 4 to 6 weeks after birth, which never heals in some infants, and bacterial infections of the umbilicus, breasts, and other soft tissues beginning within the first few weeks of life. Despite an impressive granulocytosis, pus formation and wound healing are very poor. Death in the first few months of life from relentlessly progressive infection with *Staphylococcus aureus, Pseudomonas,* and many other bacterial and fungal pathogens is common, but a few patients have lived for years. Prenatal diagnosis has not been attempted but should be feasible with fetal neutrophils.

Chronic granulomatous disease and disorders of oxidative killing

See also Chapter 30.

Chronic granulomatous disease (CGD) is a congenital disorder of the membrane-associated oxidase found in all phagocytic cells. The oxidase is inactive in resting cells and is activated by particulate and soluble stimuli that interact with the membrane. In vivo most activation occurs via the receptors that mediate chemotaxis or phagocytosis. When activated, the oxidase catalyzes the first step of a four-electron reduction of molecular oxygen, with production of the superoxide anion (O_2^-). O_2^- forms hydrogen peroxide (H_2O_2) and several other reactive species such as hydroxyl radical that are important in bacterial killing and also cause damage to host tissues. Patients with CGD are susceptible to infection with organisms that contain the enzyme catalase, which detoxifies hydrogen peroxide produced by the bacteria themselves. Neutrophils from patients with CGD can kill many catalase-negative organisms using bacterial H_2O_2 and myeloperoxidase from the neutrophil primary granule within the phagolysosome.

The most common form of this uncommon disease is X-linked, and the overall male-to-female ratio is 7:1. In the usual male variant the cells are lacking a cytochrome b, which is thought to be part of the electron transfer chain of the oxidase system. The mothers of boys with X-linked CGD have two populations of neutrophils: one normal and one deficient in oxidase activity, as determined by reduction of nitroblue tetrazolium (NBT) by stimulated cells. Carriers also have an unexplained susceptibility to develop discoid lupus erythematosus. Patients with CGD may also express the MacLeod phenotype on their RBCs, which lack the Kell precursor substance Kx, which is also inherited as an X-linked chromosome. This can be a cause of erythrocyte and granulocyte sensitization, since absence of Kx is extremely rare in the general population.

In the autosomal recessive form, which includes all females and a minority of males, the parents' neutrophils are normal. Some of the patients with the autosomal recessive form of the disease have small amounts of superoxide production and a kinetically abnormal oxidase. In general these patients have had less severe problems with infection than patients with no oxidase activity at all.

Patients may acquire CGD in the neonatal period, but most do not develop problems with infection until they are several months of age. Lymphadenitis, skin infections, respiratory infections, diarrhea, and failure to thrive are common initial problems. Neutrophils from these patients have normal chemotactic adherence, phagocytosis, and nonoxidative killing. Delayed cord separation is not a feature of CGD, and although infected areas may develop granulomata, uninfected wounds heal well. Pus formation is normal, and granulocytosis is usually associated with acute infections only. Chronic lymphadenopathy, hepatosplenomegaly, the anemia of chronic disease, and hyperimmunoglobulinemia are common.

Chronic prophylactic antibiotics have greatly diminished the frequency of bacterial infections in patients with CGD. Trimethoprim-sulfamethoxazole, 5 mg/kg/day given twice a day, is usually used because it is well tolerated and effective and prevents the development of *Pneumocystis carinii* pneumonia as well as bacterial infections. Identifying and obtaining antibiotic sensitivities of organisms is crucial to the management of patients with immunodeficiency because they may have unusual pathogens; for example, *Chromobacterium violaceum* is a significant pathogen in CGD. Prolonged courses of antibiotics are often needed because the organisms survive within the phagolysosomes of neutrophils, monocytes, and macrophages, where they may proliferate protected from systemically administered antibiotics. Surgical drainage and debridement of infected tissues are important for the management of soft tissue infections. In overwhelming infections, leukocyte transfusion may be beneficial. Deep tissue granulomata may cause problems because of mass effects, such as gastric outlet obstruction and bladder malfunction. Organisms are often difficult to culture from these granulomata because they are intracellular, and surgical management is often required.

With better understanding of the pathogenesis of infection in CGD, better antibiotic therapy, improved and more aggressive surgical management, and use of prophylactic antibiotics, the prognosis for these children is much better than it was when the disorder was first described more than 30 years ago. However, it is still fatal at an early age for many patients and entails prolonged hospitalization and invasive procedures for most patients. Prenatal diagnosis is available using fetal blood obtained by fetoscopy. When the disorder is X-linked, fetoscopy can be performed selectively on male infants, lessening the risk for pregnancies carrying female infants.

Myeloperoxidase deficiency is usually an incidental finding and in most patients does not seem to be associated with increased susceptibility to infection. Myeloperoxidase is an enzyme located in the primary granule of the neutrophil and is different from eosinophil peroxidase, which is present in patients with neutrophil peroxidase deficiency. Myeloperoxidase-deficient neutrophils have a prolonged respiratory burst. Bacterial killing is delayed but effective. Neonatal problems have not been identified, but patients are affected at birth.

Severe G6PD deficiency may be associated with defective oxidative killing and a very abbreviated respiratory burst. The metabolic consequences of G6PD deficiency are depletion of the reduced form of nicotinamide adenine dinucleotide phosphate (NADPH), which is required as an electron donor for the membrane oxidase, and extensive oxidative damage to cellular constituents because of exhaustion of reduced glutathione, which is the major scavenger of oxidants in mammalian systems. Since severe G6PD deficiency also produces a severe chronic hemolytic anemia, the hyperbilirubinemia and hemolysis are usually the initial findings. Few patients have clinical problems with infection, but when enzyme activity is very low, the defect in oxidative metabolism can be as severe as in CGD. C6PD deficiency is X-linked. The combination of chronic nonspherocytic hemolytic anemia and recurrent infection in a male child of Mediterranean or Oriental background should raise the suspicion of G6PD deficiency.

Chédiak-Higashi syndrome

The Chédiak-Higashi syndrome (CHS) is an autosomal recessive disorder characterized by partial oculocutaneous albinism, photophobia, nystagmus, frequent pyogenic infections, intermittent febrile episodes, and abnormally large granules in all granule-containing cells (neutrophils, platelets, melanocytes, neurons, large granular lymphocytes, gastric mucosa, pancreas, thyroid, renal tubular epithelium). Neutrophil chemotaxis and bacterial killing are abnormal, but phagocytosis and oxidative metabolism are normal. Platelet function is also impaired, but clinical problems with bleeding have not been described in patients who are not thrombocytopenic. The large inclusions in the neutrophils consist of fused primary and secondary granules, and degranulation is extremely abnormal, probably accounting for impaired bacterial killing. Microtubular assembly is abnormal, and levels of cyclic adenosine monophosphate (cAMP) are increased. Attempts to normalize microtubular assembly by raising intracellular levels of cyclic guanosine monophosphate (cGMP) improve neutrophil function in vitro (chemotaxis and degranulation). Natural killer cell function and antibody-dependent cellular cytotoxicity are also normal. The deficiency in lymphocyte function may be the most significant clinical problem for these patients. Although intermittent fevers and soft tissue infections, particularly of the skin, are common manifestations of CHS, the major life-threatening complication is the development of the "accelerated," or lymphoma-like, phase, in which patients develop lymphadenopathy, hepatosplenomegaly with pancytopenia, and infiltration of all organs with lymphocytes and histiocytes. Evidence suggests that this may represent a specific immune deficiency in which patients are unable to eliminate the Epstein-Barr virus, analogous to the X-linked lymphoproliferative syndrome. Although various therapies may control the hypersplenism temporarily, the development of the accelerated phase has been uniformly fatal for these patients.

It is common for patients to be infected in the first few months of life, but neonatal presentation of CHS is uncommon. However, the diagnosis can be made at birth or prenatally by recognition of the huge inclusions in nucleated blood cells, particularly neutrophils, on the peripheral blood smear. This is a rare disorder, with only about 100 cases reported worldwide, but considerable research has been done because of the existence of natural animal models in mink, cattle, and mice.

Chemotactic defects

In addition to Mo1 deficiency, CGD, and CHS, two other disorders of neutrophil chemotaxis may be seen in the newborn period. A disorder with severe neutropenia in which the bone marrow has many mature neutrophils that do not appear to be capable of migrating out of the marrow has been termed the *lazy leukocyte syndrome*. These patients are susceptible to multiple bacterial pathogens, especially cutaneous and respiratory infections, and do not make pus or heal wounds well. They are peripherally neutropenic, and a bone marrow examination with chemotactic studies on the marrow neutrophils is required to make the diagnosis. Various chemotactic defects, usually associated with hyperimmunoglobulin E, tend to appear with skin infections, usually from *Staphylococcus aureus*. The hyper IgE is rarely evident in the immediate newborn period but may occur within the first few months of life, and the cutaneous infections and chemotactic defect are often evident within the first month. The IgE itself does not impair chemotaxis, and no serum inhibitors of chemotaxis are identified in most patients. The pathogenesis of this disorder is not clear; it may represent an immunoregulatory defect in which blocking antibodies or hypersensitivity phenomena interfere with neutrophil function. This is more often an acquired than a congenital disorder and usually affects older children and adults.

Eosinophilia

Elevated numbers of eosinophils (greater than 850/μL) are frequently seen in infants in neonatal intensive care units. The etiology of the eosinophilia is usually unclear but may entail allergy to proteins administered as foods. Occasional observation of Charcot-Leyden crystals in the stools of infants with marked peripheral blood eosinophilia enhances the credibility of this impression. Since many proteins that are not absorbed intact in older children and adults are absorbed from the gastrointestinal tract of neonates, transient reactions to these foreign substances could be expected. No adverse effect of eosinophilia in the neonate has been described, and in the overwhelming majority of infants this resolves spontaneously as the child grows.

Congenital asplenia

Congenital asplenia or polysplenia is found as an isolated anomaly or in association with other congenital defects. Asplenia with dextrocardia and cyanotic congenital heart disease is termed *Ivemark's syndrome*. Polysplenia is associated with splenic dysfunction and should be treated as functional asplenia, although it is not as major an immunologic impairment. Diagnosis is suspected in the presence of anomalies known to be associated with asplenia and may be confirmed by splenic scan. Howell-Jolly bodies are sometimes present in normal newborns but are seen in greater numbers in asplenia. It is important to identify these patients early because they are susceptible to development of overwhelming infection with a variety of organisms, including gram-negative organisms and pneumococcus. Administration of prophylactic antibiotics should be seriously considered, and children should be managed similarly to other young children who are splenectomized early in life.

MALIGNANT DISORDERS

Congenital and neonatal leukemia

Leukemia, as defined by the proliferation of hemopoietic blasts with infiltration of nonhemopoietic organs and bone marrow failure, has been described at birth and in neonates. Definition of these entities is difficult because other causes of leukemoid reactions must be excluded (e.g., erythroblastosis, congenital infections) and because transient myelodysplastic syndromes that resolve spontaneously may be seen in the neonatal period and do not constitute leukemia. A disproportionate number of these infants have trisomy 21, including one infant with mosaic trisomy 21 who was phenotypically normal. Disordered regulation of myelopoiesis is thought to play a role in these disorders. In most instances the blasts are in the myeloid cell line or cannot be characterized (acute undifferentiated leukemia). Acute lymphoblastic leukemia in neonates is extremely rare. Acute monocytic leukemia has been described in several infants. Cutaneous involvement is common and may be the initial symptom and antedate identifiable bone marrow involvement. The cutaneous nodules are palpable and are usually pigmented either maroon or bluish gray. The white count is elevated, with aleukemic leukemia being uncommon. Hepatosplenomegaly is typical, and lymphadenopathy occurs infrequently.

Congenital leukemia is usually rapidly fatal. Neonatal leukemia carries a poor prognosis, but survival of several years with chemotherapy-induced remissions has been described. Some encouraging data exist for the treatment of acute monocytic leukemia in the neontal period with epipodophyllotoxins, VP-16 and VM-26, with five of six patients ceasing therapy and free of disease 5 years after diagnosis. A major difficulty in the treatment of these patients arises from the high toxicity of most standard chemotherapeutic regimens in young infants, and the substantial morbidity to growth and nutrition at this crucial period of development. Because these patients usually have extremely high white counts, they fall into the worst prognostic groups. Older children with more responsive forms of leukemia have better ability to tolerate cytotoxic therapy. Neonates are usually excluded from standard protocols for the treatment of childhood leukemia; substantial dosage modifications must be made for chemotherapeutic agents; and the toxicity of therapy directed at the central nervous system in young infants is very high. Because of the significant incidence of spontaneous regression of entities indistinguishable from leukemia and the extremely high toxicity of relatively ineffective therapy, patients are often observed for several weeks with supportive therapy to determine the natural progression of the disorder. Exceptions may be made for infants with monoblastic leukemia, who may respond to the well-tolerated, relatively nontoxic epipodophyllotoxins, and for those with acute undifferentiated or lymphoblastic leukemia, who often attain remission with vincristine and prednisone, which are also usually well tolerated.

Better characterization of the leukemic cells in these infants using cytogenetics, enzyme markers (terminal deoxynucleotidyl transferase, TdT), and a wide variety of monoclonal antibodies may help to define these disorders better, and suggest improved, less toxic methods of therapy.

Solid tumors in the newborn

Although uncommon, several different solid tumors occur in infancy. Because most arise as abdominal masses, a thorough abdominal examination should be a part of all newborn evaluations. Included among the more common abdominal tumors are neuroblastoma, nephroblastoma (Wilms' tumor), rhabdomyosarcoma, hepatoblastoma, and teratoma. Rarely, cases of transplacental passage of tumor from mother to infant have been reported. Most of these incidents have dealt with malignant melanoma in which the placenta was extensively replaced by tumor. Transplacental passage of Hodgkin's disease, lymphosarcoma, and bronchogenic carcinoma also have been reported. In addition, several cases of choriocarcinoma of the placenta with transfer to the mother of the malignant trophoblast have been identified. Retinoblastoma, another relatively common tumor in the neonate, is covered in Chapter 39, part two.

Congenital mesoblastic nephroma and Wilms' tumor

For many years congenital mesoblastic nephroma was thought to be a variant of Wilms' tumor. In 1967 Bolande and associates emphasized the benign nature of this tumor, which may grow to be very large but will not metastasize. Pathologically the tumor consists of mesenchymal elements without the tubular differentiation usually seen in Wilms' tumor. Ultrasonography or computed tomography (CT) performed at birth or shortly thereafter will reveal a large, hard abdominal mass that is part of the kidney. Excisional surgery is curative, since the tumor is benign, and radiotherapy and/or chemotherapy should not be given, especially since these treatments are relatively toxic in small infants unless both kidneys are involved.

Wilms' tumor also occurs in the neonate and should be treated in accordance with the degree of involvement, as outlined in the National Wilms' Tumor Study Programs. Vincristine, actinomycin D, and doxorubicin (Adriamycin) have been used with impressive success in these patients, but the dosage must be modified to account for excessive toxicity in the small neonate. Radiotherapy is also a highly effective modality. The sarcomatous variant of Wilms' tumor, although exceedingly rare, is highly resistant to both radiotherapy and chemotherapy.

Neuroblastoma

The incidence of clinical neuroblastoma is less than 1 per 10,000 live births. However, autopsy series of newborns dying from a variety of causes have shown that 1 in 40 have neuroblastoma in situ on serial sectioning of adrenal glands. Whether this phenomenon is caused by maturation of the tumor or by specific immunologically mediated suppression is a moot point. The tumor arises from neural crest tissue and therefore can occur anywhere along the sympathetic chain. In the neonate the adrenal is a primary site in approximately 70% of the cases, and the tumor is evident as an abdominal mass. Ten percent of the tumors arise from the posterior mediastinum. The liver is the most commonly occurring metastatic site, although almost any area may be involved. On occasion the liver may be so huge as to mimic hydrops fetalis, an impression further intensified by the occurrence of anemia secondary to marrow replacement. Skin metastases appear as bluish subcutaneous nodules and are frequently referred to as "blueberry muffin spots." Orbital metastases, although rare, may produce a disfiguring proptosis. With progression of the disease, severe cachexia is common.

Once neuroblastoma is suspected, 24-hour urine samples should be obtained for quantitative catecholamine assays. If all metabolites are assayed, the test will confirm the diagnosis in more than 95% of patients. Evaluation should also include abdominal films in search of calcific-like densities, intravenous pyelogram, skeletal roentgenograms and bone scans, bone marrow aspiration and biopsy, liver-spleen scan, CT, and ultrasonography. As a single test, ultrasonography is probably the most reliable imaging procedure.

If the tumor is completely resectable, surgery is the most effective therapeutic endeavor. In stage IVS disease (localized abdominal primary tumor with metastases limited to liver, bone marrow, and/or skin), cure is possible with removal of the primary tumor only. Most centers elect merely to observe young infants with localized disease, since urinary catecholamines offer a reliable way to monitor tumor activity. A short course of radiation therapy (up to 500 rad) or a single dose of cyclophosphamide (up to 300 mg/kg) may be sufficient to diminish massive liver involvement in stage IVS patients. For unresectable tumors, increased urinary catecholamine levels will confirm the diagnosis and eliminate the need to obtain biopsy tissue.

Neither chemotherapy nor radiation therapy alters the survival rate in neuroblastoma, although survival time may be prolonged by therapy. Whereas young infants do better than children over 1 year of age, infants affected before 1 month and infants with disease evident at birth may do worse than children affected at 1 to 12 months of age. The high rate of spontaneous regression and tumor maturation have stimulated considerable research and discussion of tumor biology in the neonate.

Rhabdomyosarcoma

Rhabdomyosarcoma, a tumor of striated muscle cells, has a peak incidence at the toddler and teenage ranges but is also seen in newborns. Although head and neck sites are the most common overall, neonates tend to develop abdominal or pelvic tumors, which are usually evident as a mass in the abdomen or pelvis. Symptoms may develop because of ureteral or urethral compression or bowel obstruction. The botryoid sarcoma variant may cause a large nodular mass to protrude from the bladder or vagina.

The four pathologic types of rhabdomyosarcoma are embryonal, alveolar, botryoid, and pleomorphic. The prognosis is best for the embryonal and worst for the pleomorphic type. The botryoid type is a variant of the embryonal type in which the tumor grows in cystic formations beneath a mucosal surface such as the bladder lining.

Because this tumor is highly infiltrative, complete excisional surgery is often difficult. It is important to coordinate therapy between surgeons, radiotherapists, and oncologists, since early radiotherapy and chemotherapy may eliminate the need for radical ablative surgery. Results of the first Intergroup Rhabdomyosarcoma Study showed that pelvic and extremity primary tumors have a high incidence of lymph node spread at diagnosis, but the prognosis is excellent if all gross tumor can be removed at surgery. The most effective drugs for this tumor are vincristine, cyclophosphamide, actinomycin D, and doxorubicin.

Hepatoblastoma

Hepatic tumors are rare in children. When they occur, they are usually seen in small infants. There is a high incidence of associated anomalies, including hemihypertrophy, renal abnormalities, Meckel's diverticulum, and absent adrenal gland. Hemihypertrophy also occurs with increased frequency in patients with Wilms' tumor. Rarely does hepatoblastoma cause jaundice or other abnormalities of liver function. The initial signs include an enlarging abdominal mass, weight loss, and cachexia. Thrombocytosis is often striking, perhaps because of thrombopoietin production by the tumor, and is unusual as a feature of any other tumor. Painful pressure on the celiac nerve axis is frequent. Alpha-fetoprotein levels are usually elevated and serve as a reliable tumor marker if serially obtained. It is important to note, however, that alpha-fetoprotein values tend to be elevated in the normal neonate and thus cannot be relied on as a single determination. Complete resection offers the best chance for cure. If the tumor has not metastasized to lungs or bone and is localized to one lobe of the liver, the long-term survival after surgery is about 60%. Combination chemotherapy is an effective adjunct, whereas radiation therapy has essentially no role.

Teratoma

Sacrococcygeal teratomas (Fig. 32-15) are the most common solid tumors of the neontal period and must be differentiated from myelomeningoceles, pilonidal cysts, hemangiomas, and chordomas. It is important that these

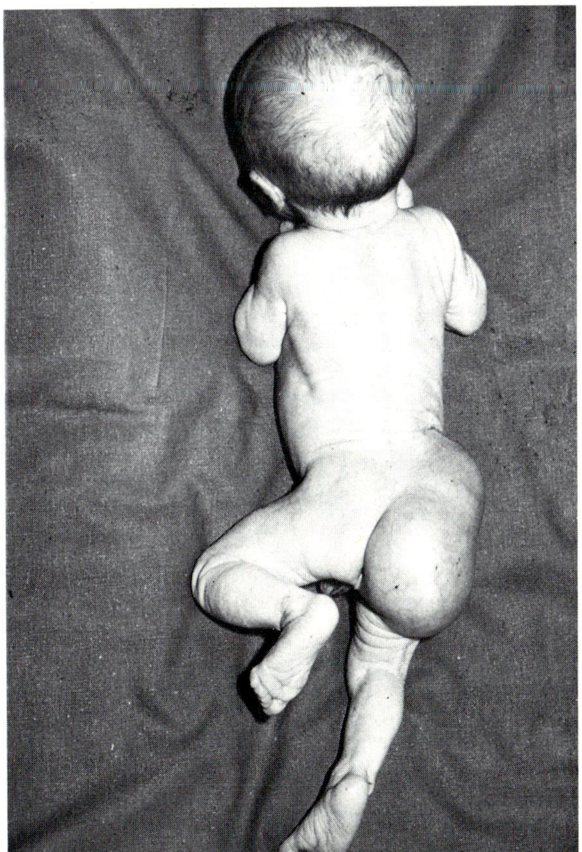

Fig. 32-15. Three-month-old infant with a slowly enlarging, right buttock mass. Excision of the tumor showed sacrococcygeal teratoma.

tumors be diagnosed early, since they may undergo malignant degeneration rapidly, within a few weeks up to 6 months. Often these seemingly benign tumors have associated areas of malignant change. Accordingly, the pathologist must search carefully during histopathologic processing. In the neonate 5% to 10% of these tumors have associated malignant areas, and in older infants the incidence increases to 50% to 60%.

There is extraordinary variation in the size of buttocks or perianal area in such patients. A careful rectal examination, however, invariably reveals a mass because the tumor originates from an area near the anterior surface of the sacrum and within reach of digital examination. On lateral radiographic evaluation the rectum is displaced forward, and calcific-like densities may be visualized occasionally. Complete excision is the major therapeutic modality, since malignant teratomas do not respond well to either radiotherapy or multiagent chemotherapy.

Susan B. Shurin

BIBLIOGRAPHY

Hematopoiesis in the embryo and fetus

Hebert, A.A., and others: Dermal erythropoiesis in Rh hemolytic disease of the newborn, J. Pediatr. **107**:799, 1985.

Oski, F.A., and Naiman, J.L.: Hematologic problems in the newborn, Philadelphia, 1972, W.B. Saunders Co.

Wolf, B.C., and others: Evidence to suggest that the human fetal spleen is not a hematopoietic organ, Am. J. Clin. Pathol. **80**:140, 1983.

Hematologic changes in the neonate and infant

Bard, H.: Postnatal fetal and adult hemoglobin synthesis in early preterm newborn infants, J. Clin. Invest. **52**:1789, 1973.

Bard, H.: Postnatal fetal and adult hemoglobin synthesis in D_1 trisomy syndrome, Blood **40**:523, 1972.

Bard, H., and Prosmanne, J.: Postnatal fetal and adult hemoglobin synthesis in preterm infants whose birth weight was less than 1,000 grams, Clin. Invest. **70**:50, 1982.

Bard, H., and others: The relative rates of synthesis of hemoglobin A and F in immature red cells of newborn infants, Pediatrics **45**:766, 1970.

Bromberg, Y.M., Abrahamov, A., and Salzberger, M.: The effect of maternal anoxaemia on the foetal haemoglobin of the newborn, J. Obstet. Gynaecol. Br. Commonw. **63**:875, 1956.

Gairdner, D., Marks, J., and Roscoe, J.D.: Blood formation in infancy: normal erythropoiesis, Arch. Dis. Child. **27**:214, 1952.

Huehns, E.R., and others: Developmental hemoglobin anomalies in chromosomal triplication: D_1 trisomy syndrome, Proc. Natl. Acad. Sci. USA **51**:89, 1964.

Linderkamp, O., and others: Geometry of neonatal and adult red blood cells, Pediatr. Res. **17**:250, 1983.

Linderkamp, O., and others: Erythrocyte deformability in the fetus, preterm, and term neonate, Pediatr. Res. **20**:93, 1986.

Manroe, B.L., and others: The neonatal blood count in health and disease. I. Reference values for neutrophilic cells, J. Pediatr. **95**:89, 1979.

Perrine, S.P., Greene, M.F., and Faller, D.V.: Delay in the fetal globin switch in infants of diabetic mothers, N. Engl. J. Med. **312**:334, 1985.

Wilson, M.G., Schroeder, W.A., and Graves, D.A.: Postnatal change of hemoglobins F and A_2 in infants with Down's syndrome (G trisomy), Pediatrics **42**:349, 1968.

Wilson, M.G., and others: Hemoglobin variations in D_1 trisomy syndrome, N. Engl. J. Med. **277**:953, 1967.

Wood, W.G., and others: Control of haemoglobin switching by a developmental clock? Nature **313**:320, 1985.

Anemia in the newborn period

Beck, M., and others: Neuraminidase deficiency presenting as nonimmune hydrops fetalis, Eur. J. Pediatr. **143**:135, 1984.

Collins, J.E., and others: Vitamin B12 absorption after necrotizing enterocolitis, Arch. Dis. Child. **59**:731, 1984.

DeWitte, D.B., and others: Neonatal pancytopenia and severe combined immunodeficiency associated with antenatal administration of azathioprine and prednisone, J. Pediatr. **105**:625, 1984.

Frigoletto, F.D., and others: Ultrasonographic fetal surveillance in the management of the isoimmunized pregnancy, N. Engl. J. Med. **315**:430, 1986.

Gorman, J.G., and others: Prevention of Rhesus immunization, Clin. Immunol. Allergy **4**:473, 1984.

Grannum, P.A., and others: In utero exchange transfusion by direct intravascular injection in severe erythroblastosis fetalis, N. Engl. J. Med. **314**:1431, 1986.

Guggenheim, M.A., and others: Progressive neuuromuscular disease in children with chronic cholestasis and vitamin E deficiency: diagnosis and treatment with alpha tocopherol, J. Pediatr. **100**:51, 1982.

Heisel, M.A., and others: Congenital pernicious anemia: report of seven patients, with studies of the extended family, J. Pediatr. **105**:564, 1984.

Hittner, H.M., and others: Retrolental fibroplasia and vitamin E in the preterm infant—comparison of oral versus intramuscular:oral administration, Pediatrics **73**:238, 1984.

Johnson, L., and others: Relationship of prolonged pharmacologic serum levels of Vitamin E to incidence of sepsis and necrotizing enterocolitis in infants with birth weight 1,500 grams or less, Pediatrics **75**:619, 1985.

Lorch, V., and others: Unusual syndrome among premature infants: association with a new intravenous vitamin E product, Pediatrics **75**:598, 1985.

Vanderpas, J., and Vertongen, F.: Erythrocyte vitamin E is oxidized at a lower peroxide concentration in neonates than in adults, Blood **66**:1272, 1985.

Wang, W.C., and others: Differentiation of transient erythroblastopenia of childhood from congenital hypoplastic anemia, J. Pediatr. **88**:784, 1976.

Polycythemia

Black, V.D., and others: Neonatal hyperviscosity: randomized study of effect of partial plasma exchange transfusion on long-term outcome, Pediatrics **75**:1048, 1985.

Black, V.D., and others: Gastrointestinal injury in polycythemic term infants, Pediatrics **76**:225, 1985.

Reinhart, W.H., and others: Rheology of fetal and maternal blood, Pediatr. Res. **19**:147, 1985.

Coagulation

Chaou, W.T., and others: Intracranial hemorrhage and vitamin K deficiency in early infancy, J. Pediatr. **105**:880, 1984.

Clouse, L.H., and Comp, P.C.: The regulation of hemostasis: the protein C system, N. Engl. J. Med. **314**:1298, 1986.

Corazza, M.S., and others: Prolonged bleeding time in preterm infants receiving indomethacin for patent ductus arteriosus, J. Pediatr. **105**:292, 1984.

Corrigan, J.J.: Activation of coagulation and disseminated intravascular coagulation in the newborn, Am. J. Pediatr. Hematol. Oncol. **1**:245, 1979.

Corrigan, J.J., Sell, E.J., and Page, C.: Hageman factor and disseminated intravascular coagulation (DIC) in newborns and rabbits, Pediatr. Res. **11**:916, 1977.

Glader, B.E., and Buchanan, G.R.: The bleeding neonate, Pediatrics **58**:548, 1976.

Hall, J.G., and others: Thrombocytopenia with absent radius, Medicine **48**:411, 1969.

Hathaway, W.E.: The bleeding newborn, Semin. Hematol. **12**:175, 1975.

Lane, P.A., and Hathaway, W.E.: Vitamin K in infancy, J. Pediatr. **106**:351, 1985.

McDonald, M.M., and Hathaway, W.E.: Anticoagulant therapy by continuous heparinization in newborn and older infants, J. Pediatr. **101**:451, 1982.

McDonald, M.M., and others: Role of coagulopathy in newborn intracranial hemorrhage, Pediatrics **74**:26, 1984.

Motohara, K., and others: Severe vitamin K deficiency in breast-fed infants, J. Pediatr. **105**:943, 1984.

Peters, M., and others: Persistent antithrombin III deficiency: risk factor for thromboembolic complications in neonates small for gestational age, J. Pediatr. **105**:310, 1984.

Peters, M., and others: Coagulation and fibrinolytic factors in the first week of life in healthy infants, J. Pediatr. **106**:292, 1985.

Rohyans, J., Miser, A.W., and Miser, J.S.: Subgaleal hemorrhage in infants with hemophilia: report of two cases and review of the literature, Pediatrics **70**:306, 1982.

Seligsohn, U., and others: Homozygous Protein C deficiency manifested by massive venous thrombosis in the newborn, N. Engl. J. Med. **310**:559, 1984.

Sills, R.H., and others: Severe homozygous Protein C deficiency, J. Pediatr. **105**:409, 1984.

Stuart, M.J.: Platelet function in the neonate, Am. J. Pediatr. Hematol. Oncol. **1**:227, 1979.

Warrier, A.I., and Lusher, J.M.: DDAVP: a useful alternative to blood component in moderate hemophilia A and von Willebrand disease, J. Pediatr. **102**:228, 1983.

Zipursky, A., and others: Clinical and laboratory diagnosis of hemostatic disorders in newborn infants, Am. J. Pediatr. Hematol. Oncol. **1**:217, 1979.

Phagocytes

Anderson, D.C., and others: Abnormalities of polymorphonuclear luekocyte function associated with a heritable deficiency of high molecular weight surface glucoproteins (GP 138): common relationship to diminished cell adherence, J. Clin. Invest. **74**:536, 1984.

Bhat, A.M., and Scanlon, J.W.: The pattern of eosinophilia in premature infants: a prospective study in premature infants using the absolute eosinophil count, J. Pediatr. **98**:612, 1981.

Brodeur, G.M., and others: Transient leukemoid reaction and trisomy 21 mosaicism in a phenotypically normal newborn, Blood **55**:691, 1980.

Engle, W.A., Schreiner, R.L., and Baehner, R.L.: Neonatal white blood cell disorders, Semin. Perinatol. **7**:184, 1983.

Frazier, J.P., and others: Leukocyte function in healthy neonates following vaginal and cesarean section deliveries, J. Pediatr. **101**:269, 1982.

Gallin, J.I., and others: Recent advances in chronic granulomatous disease, Ann. Int. Med. **99**:657, 1983.

Gibson, E.L., Vaucher, Y., and Corrigan, J.J.: Eosinophilia in premature infants: relationship to weight gain, J. Pediatr. **95**:99, 1979.

Krause, P.J., Maderazo, E.G., and Scroggs, M.: Abnormalities of neutrophil adherence in newborns, Pediatrics **69**:184, 1982.

Lawrence, R., and others: Eosinophilia in the hospitalized neonate, Ann. Allergy **44**:349, 1980.

Miller, M., and Cosgriff, J.M.: Hematologic abnormalities in newborn infants with Down Syndrome, Am. J. Med. Genet. **16**:173, 1983.

Mills, E.L., and Quie, P.G.: Congenital disorders of the functions of polymorphonuclear neutrophils, Rev. Infect. Dis. **2**:505, 1980.

Newberger, P.E., and others: Prenatal diagnosis of chronic granulomatous disease, N. Engl. J. Med. **300**:178, 1979.

Raghunathan, R., and others: Phagocyte chemotaxis in the perinatal period, J. Clin. Immunol. **2**:242, 1982.

Stoerner, J.W., and others: Polymorphonuclear leukocyte function in newborn infants, J. Pediatr. **93**:862, 1978.

Weston, W.L., and others: Monocyte-macrophage function in the newborn, Am. J. Dis. Child. **131**:1241, 1977.

Splenic function

Freedman, R.M., and others: Development of splenic reticuloendothelial function in neonates, J. Pediatr. **96**:466, 1980.

Majeski, J.A., and Upshur, J.K.: Asplenia syndrome: a study of congenital anomalies in 16 cases, JAMA **240**:1508, 1978.

Ozsoylu, S., Hosain, F., and McIntyre, P.A.: Functional development of phagocytic activity of the spleen, J. Pediatr. **90**:560, 1977.

Waldman, J., and others: Sepsis and congenital asplenia, J. Pediatr. **90**:555, 1977.

Nonhematologic malignancies

Beckwith, J.B., and Perrin, E.V.: *In situ* neuroblastoma: a contribution to the natural history of neural crest tumors, Am. J. Pathol. **43**:1089, 1963.

Blank, E., Neerhout, R.C., and Burry, K.A.: Congenital mesoblastin nephroma and polyhydramnios, JAMA **240**:1504, 1978.

Bolande, R.P., Brough, A.J., and Izant, I.J.: Congenital mesoblastic nephroma of infancy: a report of eight cases and the relationship to Wilms' tumor, Pediatrics **40**:272, 1967.

Dehner, L.P.: Neoplasms of the fetus and neonate. In Naeye, R.L., Kissane, J.M., and Kaufman, N., editors: Perinatal diseases, Baltimore, 1981, Williams & Wilkins.

Isaacs, H.: Perinatal (congenital and neonatal) neoplasms: a report of 110 cases, Pediatr. Pathol. **3**:165, 1985.

Knudson, A.G., and Meadows, A.T.: Regression of neuroblastoma IV-S: a genetic hypothesis, N. Engl. J. Med. **302**: 1254, 1980.

PART TWO

Blood component therapy for the neonate

Transfusion therapy is an essential part of the modern intensive care required to achieve a successful outcome for extremely premature and ill neonates. Many blood components are available for transfusion to the neonatal recipient. The appropriate use of these components requires not only an understanding of normal perinatal hemopoiesis and an accurate clinical and hematologic assessment of the infant, but also a knowledge of the composition and characteristics of each blood component, the changes that occur in the product during storage, the proper transfusion techniques for each component, and the relative risks and benefits of transfusion.

Newborns have some unique needs related to transfusion; however, similarities also exist in acceptable transfusion practice between the neonate and the older recipient. For example, blood should be collected by standard sterile techniques from healthy donors whose medical histories have been appropriately obtained, evaluated, and recorded. Prospective donors at risk for transmission of infectious diseases, especially hepatitis and acquired immunodeficiency syndrome (AIDS), should be deferred. Pretransfusion testing, including at least screening for hepatitis B surface antigen, antibody to human immunodeficiency virus (HIV), syphilis, unexpected red blood cell (RBC) antibodies, and ABO and Rh typing should be completed; appropriate compatibility testing should be performed as well. Records should be kept to document the identity of specific donors and recipients. This information is invaluable in tracking adverse reactions to transfusion, in identifying donors implicated in transfusion-transmitted diseases, and in improving the safety of the blood supply. Blood components, rather than whole blood, should be chosen for transfusion according to the specific needs of the recipient (1) to eliminate the risks associated with unneeded portions, (2) to decrease the risk of circulatory overload, and (3) to make available the other components from each blood donation for transfusion to other patients.

SPECIAL NEEDS OF THE NEONATAL RECIPIENT

Cytomegalovirus

See also Chapter 31, part two.

Human cytomegalovirus (CMV) is a member of the herpes family of viruses with an extremely high prevalence in the population. It has been recognized as a transfusion-transmitted infection since 1966, despite the usual inability of investigators to culture the virus from the blood of seropositive, otherwise healthy blood donors. Restriction endonuclease analysis of CMV deoxyribonucleic acid (DNA) has confirmed transfusion transmission of the virus. Viral isolates from two multiply transfused premature infants infected with CMV within 11 days of each other demonstrated a CMV strain indistinguishable from the virus isolated from their common blood donor. The persistent lifelong nature of the CMV infection is presumed to be responsible for the association between CMV seropositivity and infectivity via transfusion. The incidence of CMV seropositivity among healthy blood donors varies with age and geographic location; however, it averages approximately 50%. Although it has been estimated that only 3% to 15% of blood donations from CMV-antibody-positive donors are actually infectious, at present a more specific method than antibody testing is not available to identify potentially infectious units.

Three types of posttransfusion CMV infection occur: primary infection, reactivation of previous infection, and reinfection with a different CMV strain. Primary CMV infection occurs in previously unexposed (seronegative) patients transfused with blood from a seropositive donor (i.e., one with active or latent CMV infection); is characterized by viremia, viruria, and eventual seroconversion to CMV–immunoglobulin G positivity; and produces little if any significant disease among immunocompetent individuals. Reactivation infection occurs in CMV-seropositive individuals following transfusion of seropositive or seronegative blood, presumably because of endogenous viral reactivation facilitated by transfused leukocytes.

Blood transfusion is a significant source of acquired CMV disease in premature, low birth weight (LBW) infants, and primary CMV disease in these infants is a cause of significant morbidity and mortality. A statistically significant difference has been found between the incidence of postnatal acquired CMV infection in a group of 74 untransfused neonates (11%) and in 77 perinatally transfused infants (25%, $p < 0.05$). Neonatal exchange transfusions have been associated with an increased incidence of acquired CMV infection, with the risk increasing in infants exposed to many blood donors. Three risk factors for the development of significant transfusion-associated CMV disease have been identified: (1) CMV-seronegative mother, (2) perinatal transfusion of more than 50 ml of blood, and (3) low birth weight. Ten of 74 infants (13.5%) of seronegative mothers exposed to CMV-seropositive whole blood or RBC transfusions developed serious CMV infection, with four deaths. In contrast, none of 90 infants of seronegative mothers transfused exclusively with CMV-antibody negative blood components developed CMV infection. No CMV infections were attributable to the transfusion of fresh frozen plasma from CMV-antibody-positive donors. The antibody status of blood donors had no effect on the incidence of CMV infection among infants of CMV-seropositive mothers. None of the infected infants of seropositive mothers developed serious or fatal symptoms attributable to CMV. This suggests that maternally derived CMV antibody is capable of modifying the severity of CMV infections and may protect the infant from a small viral inoculum in transfused blood. Subsequent data suggest that loss of passively acquired maternal CMV antibody, through catabolism and iatrogenic blood loss, may predispose premature infants of seropositive mothers to a higher incidence of symptomatic CMV infection derived from maternal sources. Thus transfusion of only CMV-seronegative blood components to infants of seropositive mothers may actually be detrimental because of lack of antibody in prenatally exposed infants. Passive administration of high-titer anti-CMV plasma has been used successfully to treat at least one case of neonatal CMV infection in a preterm infant. Most large blood centers or transfusion services can now screen blood components for CMV antibody using any of the commercially available test kits.

Because of concern that the high prevalence of CMV seropositivity among blood donors, especially in certain regions of the United States, might severely limit availability of seronegative components, alternative methods of minimizing the risk of posttransfusion CMV infection in these high-risk infants have been investigated. As an intracellular virus, cytomegalovirus is transmitted via transfusion with intact leukocytes. Frozen deglycerolized red blood cells (FDCs) can be prepared in which an average of 93.5% of the original leukocytes has been removed during the freeze-thaw process; in vitro studies show the remainder appear to be nonviable. Exclusive use of such FDCs, whether obtained from CMV-seropositive or -seronegative donors, effectively eliminates transfusion-associated CMV infection in neonates. Saline washing of RBCs without freezing and thawing results in somewhat less effective leukocyte removal (89%) and is not effective in preventing transfusion-acquired neonatal CMV infection. Potential disadvantages of a transfusion program that uses only FDCs rather than screening for CMV-seronegative blood components include:

1. Freezing and deglycerolization is a method applicable only for RBCs. Thus no provision is made for the infant who may require transfusion of platelets and/or white cells, products that carry a high risk of CMV transmission.
2. Approximately 1½ to 2 hours of preparation time are required for FDCs, and the product must be used within 24 hours of thawing. FDCs are thus an inefficient inventory item, particularly for smaller nurseries, and may not be rapidly available in an emergency.
3. Cost may be a factor depending on regional practices. In general, FDCs are more expensive than are liquid-stored RBCs.

Based on this information, the following are recommendations for the use of CMV-seronegative blood components in neonates:

1. CMV-seronegative blood components are very important for LBW infants of CMV-seronegative mothers and may also be appropriate for seronegative neonates of any birth weight requiring transfusion.
2. Blood components requiring CMV screening include only those that contain cellular elements—whole blood, RBCs, platelet concentrates, and leukocyte concentrates. There is no need to provide CMV-seronegative fresh frozen plasma or cryoprecipitate.
3. There is no documentable advantage to the use of CMV-seronegative blood components in infants with CMV-seropositive mothers. Some data suggest this practice may be deleterious by hastening the decline in titer of protective maternal antibody.
4. In practice it is reasonable to transfuse CMV-negative blood components to all neonates until the result of the maternal CMV antibody testing can be obtained.
5. Since infant-to-infant spread of CMV in the neonatal intensive care setting has been shown and the virus can survive on environmental surfaces, the use of CMV-seronegative blood components should be integrated into a comprehensive program for control of neonatally acquired CMV infection.

Graft-versus-host disease

See also Chapter 30.

Graft-versus-host disease (GVHD), resulting from the proliferation of viable donor-derived T lymphocytes in response to major and minor histocompatibility antigens in the severely immunocompromised host, has been reported following blood transfusion. The clinical symptoms and signs of fever, generalized erythematous rash progressing to erythroderma and desquamation, liver dysfunction, jaundice, profuse watery diarrhea, pulmonary insufficiency, and pancytopenia may develop 4 to 30 days following a transfusion, most often within 10 days. A short and fatal course is usual. Posttransfusion GVHD has been reported in infants with impaired cellular immunity such as severe combined immunodeficiency and Wiskott-Aldrich syndrome, in those receiving intrauterine transfusion followed by postnatal exchange transfusion, and rarely in presumably normal preterm or full-term infants following exchange or other transfusion.

In infants receiving transfusion, karyotypic analysis has shown that GVHD results from the postnatal exchange transfusion rather than the intrauterine transfusion. An intrauterine transfusion may induce a state of tolerance to certain histocompatibility antigens in the fetus, which allows subsequently transfused lymphocytes to proliferate rather than be rejected if they share any histocompatibility antigens with the intrauterine transfusion. Interestingly, donor lymphocytes have been demonstrated in 35% of live-born infants following intrauterine transfusion, probably because of variable immunologic immaturity. Occasionally, donor cells persist in surviving infants beyond 1 year. Donor-derived lymphocytes have also been detected following postnatal exchange transfusion in infants who had not received intrauterine transfusion; however, none of these donor cells persisted to a year's duration, and most had disappeared within 4 months. Some donor lymphocytes are detectable in adults after transfusion for about 1 week. It has been suggested that, although fetal lymphocytes theoretically respond to allogeneic cells as early as 12 weeks' gestation, the immune system of the extremely premature infant may not be mature enough to reject foreign lymphoid cells, rendering them susceptible to posttransfusion GVHD. Determining which neonates are at risk for posttransfusion GVHD is complicated. Three factors have been identified that increase the risk of transfusion-associated GVHD: "profound immunoincompetence," low (<500/mm³) absolute lymphocyte count, and the transfusion of more than 10^7 lymphocytes/kg body weight.

Viable lymphocytes capable of initiating acute GVHD in a susceptible host are present in almost all blood components, including fresh or stored whole blood or packed RBCs, leukocyte-depleted or saline-washed RBCs, platelet concentrates, granulocyte concentrates, and fresh plasma. Viable leukocytes (4% of the original number) that retain normal in vitro blast transformation and mitotic activity persist in FDCs, although GVHD has not been reported following transfusion of this product. There is no evidence for the occurrence of GVHD following transfusion of noncellular frozen blood components, fresh frozen plasma and cryoprecipitate, which theoretically do not contain viable lymphocytes. Blood components obtained from family members and from unrelated volunteer donors have been implicated in posttransfusion GVHD. Most implicated transfusions have been from normal unrelated donors; the antigenic disparity between donor and recipient is at least partly responsible for the usually fatal outcome. In any infant with suspected posttransfusion GVHD, attempts to document lymphoid chimerism are recommended. Not all rashes occurring in jaundiced newborns with diarrhea represent GVHD. Recently a nonfatal posttransfusion syndrome of maculopapular rash, thrombocytopenia, and lymphopenia has been described in transfused neonates. Although the skin biopsy histologically resembled that seen in GVHD, the symptoms were transient and all infants recovered without treatment. Eight of the 27 infants described had received only irradiated blood components. The authors speculate that this syndrome may represent an immunologic reaction of the host against the transfused leukocytes.

No effective therapy is available for transfusion-associated GVHD; however, the complication can be prevented by pretransfusion irradiation of the blood component with 1,500 to 6,000 rad. These doses are well above the 500 rad required to abolish lymphocyte proliferation in response to allogeneic cells, as measured in the mixed lymphocyte culture, but they do not functionally damage any other blood cells. No case of transfusion-associated GVHD has been reported resulting from a blood component irradiated with at least 1,500 rad. To date no studies have found adverse reactions to blood components specifically related to the pretransfusion irradiation.

When an infant has been identified as requiring irradiated blood products, all blood components for that infant should be irradiated, since the precise number of viable cells necessary to initiate GVHD is not known, and the degree of immunoincompetence is often difficult to estimate. The known and presumed indications for irradiation of blood components for neonates are listed in the boxed material.

Indications for irradiated blood components in neonates

DEFINITE INDICATIONS

1. Neonate suspected of having a congenital cellular immunodeficiency syndrome, based on family history, clinical appearance, radiologic findings, or laboratory data
2. Intrauterine transfusion at any gestational age
3. All exchange transfusions in infants treated with intrauterine transfusion
4. Infant with malignancy, such as, congenital leukemia or neuroblastoma, receiving intensive therapy

RELATIVE INDICATIONS

1. Extremely premature or very low birth weight infant
2. Infant with acquired immunodeficiency syndrome (AIDS)
3. Blood components containing large numbers of leukocytes, such as platelet concentrate and granulocyte concentrate, to be given to newborns of any birth weight and at any gestational age
4. Absolute lymphopenia (lymphocyte count <500/mm³), as an isolated finding

Modified from Leitman, S.F. and Holland, P.V.: Transfusion **25:**293, 1985.

CONSEQUENCES OF BLOOD STORAGE

The purposes of the anticoagulant/preservative solution in which blood is stored are to prevent clotting and to preserve viable, functional blood elements. Because RBC glycolysis continues, although at a reduced rate, during liquid storage at 1° to 6° C (34° to 43° F), significant biochemical changes occur throughout the storage period that may affect the clinical response to transfusion. The clinical relevance of these biochemical changes depends partly on the volume and rate of transfusion relative to the blood volume of the recipient. Storage-induced changes in whole blood and RBCs that are important in transfusion include the following: (1) a fall in 2,3-diphosphoglycerate (2,3-DPG), (2) a decrease in adenosine triphosphate (ATP) level, (3) an increase in the supernatant plasma potassium concentration, and (4) a decrease in pH.

2,3-Diphosphoglycerate

2,3-DPG is an intracellular RBC organic phosphate that is the most important regulator of hemoglobin's affinity for oxygen. An increase in the 2,3-DPG level leads to a decrease in hemoglobin oxygen affinity and therefore an increase in the delivery of oxygen to the tissues. 2,3-DPG is well maintained for the first 5 to 7 days of RBC storage but falls rather dramatically thereafter. The average transfusion recipient is unaffected by low levels of 2,3-DPG in transfused cells because of rapid in vivo regeneration and the ability to compensate temporarily by an increase in cardiac output. Neonates, however, do not tolerate the transfusion of 2,3-DPG–depleted RBCs well. At birth, infants have mostly fetal hemoglobin, a high oxygen-affinity hemoglobin that interacts poorly with 2,3-DPG. In addition, premature infants have lower endogenous 2,3-DPG levels and regenerate the deficiency less well. Because of the neonate's small size and blood volume, transfused RBCs frequently account for most circulating RBCs. Also, premature infants with pulmonary diseases may already have inadequate tissue oxygenation. Therefore transfusion of 2,3-DPG–sufficient RBCs is indicated for neonates because efficient oxygen delivery is always required, including the period during and immediately following a transfusion. This can be accomplished by choosing the freshest conveniently available, compatible RBC unit that is less than 5 to 7 days from collection, since 2,3-DPG levels are well maintained for this period of storage in all commonly used RBC anticoagulant/preservative solutions.

Adenosine triphosphate

The concentration of ATP, which falls progressively during RBC storage, is an imporant determinant of the RBC viability. ATP depletion during storage is responsible for transformation of RBC shape from disk to sphere, for the loss of RBC deformability, and for most of the potassium leakage from cells into plasma that occurs independently of RBC hemolysis. The addition of adenine to standard RBC preservative solutions has significantly improved ATP maintenance during storage. Normal ATP levels can be expected in RBCs stored up to 7 days in citrate-phosphate-dextrose-adenine (CPDA-1) or in AS-1 (Adsol*). Further, adenine-containing anticoagulant/preservative solutions, acid-citrate-dextrose-adenine (ACD-adenine) and CPDA-1, have been demonstrated to be safe in children and in neonates. Very little clinical experience has been reported with the use in neonates of the new additive solutions for RBC preservation, Adsol, and Nutricel,† which contain 56% and 73% more adenine per unit of RBCs, respectively. No adverse effects have been reported.

Potassium

Despite the improved ATP maintenance during RBC storage, potassium leakage into surrounding plasma does occur, and the high concentrations of potassium found even after only 7 days of storage are of concern to some neonatologists. Rarely hyperkalemia following exchange transfusion has been reported. The etiology of the increased potassium concentration is important. In CPDA-1 red cells stored less than 7 days, the elevated plasma potassium is the result of leakage out of the RBC, not the result of cell lysis. The result is that potassium-deficient RBCs are actually transfused. After transfusion the rejuvenated RBCs will absorb potassium from plasma. Movement of potassium into transfused RBCs is also facilitated by the metabolic alkalosis that results from the metabolism of the citrate to bicarbonate. Posttransfusion hypokalemia is a well-recognized sequelae of massive transfusion in adults. Several investigators, using 7-day-old citrated blood for neonatal transfusion, noted no significant change in the serum potassium following exchange transfusion or transfusion of 10 ml of RBCs/kg. It has been estimated that the net potassium load from a double-volume exchange transfusion using 7-day-old citrated blood is about 3 mEq, considering the potassium withdrawn during the exchange procedure. In unusually sensitive neonates the citrated RBCs can be washed to remove supernatant potassium; however, the washing delays availability of the product, diminishes its shelf life to 24 hours, and is usually unnecessary.

Hydrogen ion concentration

The pH of blood at any time after collection into any of the available anticoagulant/preservative solutions is lower than normal body pH. The metabolic alkalosis accompanying the metabolism of citrate to bicarbonate helps to offset the acid load. Both citrate-phosphate-dextrose (CPD) and CPDA-1 have a higher pH than the previously used ACD. It is recommended that the pH of the neonate be monitored if acidosis is a concern and that the infant be treated with bicarbonate, as indicated by laboratory results, rather than attempting to buffer the blood with THAM or bicarbonate.

COMPATIBILITY TESTING REQUIREMENTS IN THE NEONATAL PERIOD

The Standards of the American Association of Blood Banks define the minimal pretransfusion and compatibility testing requirements for neonatal (infant less than 4 months of age) transfusion as the following:

1. An initial neonatal specimen must be tested for ABO group and Rh type. These tests need not be repeated for the remainder of the neonatal period provided all transfusions are ABO and Rh compatible (Table 32-5).
2. An initial serum sample from either the infant or the mother must be tested for antibodies reactive against RBC antigens. If this initial test reveals no antibodies, it need not be repeated throughout the neonatal period during one hospitalization.
3. If the initial test for unexpected antibodies is negative,

*Fenwal Laboratories, Deerfield, Ill.
†Cutter Laboratories, Emeryville, Calif.

Table 32-5. Criteria for ABO and Rh compatibility of blood components

ABO group: infant	ABO group: red blood cells and granulocytes	ABO group: plasma (FFP) or platelets	
GUIDELINES FOR ABO-COMPATIBLE BLOOD COMPONENTS			
O	O	O, A, B, or AB	
A	A or O	A or AB	
B	B or O	B or AB	
AB	AB, A, B, or O	AB	
Rh type: infant	**Rh type: red blood cells and granulocytes**	**Rh type: plasma**	**Rh type: platelets**
GUIDELINES FOR Rh-COMPATIBLE BLOOD COMPONENTS			
Positive	Positive or negative	Positive or negative	Positive or negative
Negative	Negative	Positive or negative	Negative

and all RBC transfusions given to the infant are either group O or are of an ABO group compatible with both the newborn and the mother, a crossmatch of donor RBCs with the intended recipient's serum is not necessary for any transfusions in the neonatal period during a single hospitalization.

These minimal compatibility testing requirements are suitable because the immunologic system of the newborn is apparently immature and relatively unresponsive to antigenic stimulation during the first 4 months of life. Among 65 neonates who received a mean of 13.1 (range, 2 to 27) transfusions from an average of 8.8 different blood donors during the first 3 months of life, none formed a RBC alloantibody. This study supports the concept that neonates rarely, if ever, form RBC alloantibodies. In addition, nearly all the neonate's immunoglobulins at birth are of maternal origin. Thus antibody screening and crossmatching may be done using maternal serum that has relevant antibodies present in high concentration, and it is relatively easy to obtain a large sample.

These minimal testing requirements of the American Association of Blood Banks describe policies that are permitted, not mandated. Any hospital blood bank or transfusion service may raise the standard to require more testing of neonates, equivalent to that required for all other transfusion recipients, if desired.

Other unique aspects

ABO group

The ABO group of a newborn is based solely on the testing of neonatal RBCs for the A and B antigens, since the isohemagglutinins (anti-A and/or anti-B) appropriate to the neonate's blood group are not present in serum at birth.

Rh type

The Rh type can be difficult to determine if the infant's RBCs are coated with IgG antibody of any specificity, producing a positive direct antiglobulin test. Prenatal Rh immune globulin passively administered to the mother may be present on the infant's cells at birth. Neonatal RBCs that are heavily coated with immunoglobulin G (IgG) antibody may result in a false-positive or false-negative Rh typing results. Antibody-coated Rh-negative RBCs may appear to be Rh positive because the sensitized cells agglutinate with antiimmunoglobulin reagent. False-negative results may occur if the Rh-positive RBCs of the neonate are so fully saturated with maternal anti-D that no D sites remain to react with the reagent anti-D (the phenomenon of "blocking antibodies"). Both these situations should be resolvable by the laboratory, but the techniques required are tedious and time consuming. False-positive results may also be caused by attempting to use a sample of cord blood that has been contaminated with Wharton's jelly. If saline washing does not remove the contamination, a new sample from the baby will be required.

Selection of blood in hemolytic disease of the newborn

Red cells transfused to neonates with immune-mediated hemolysis must lack the antigen corresponding to the antibody responsible for the RBC destruction. If anti-D is responsible, transfused cells must be Rh negative. ABO-hemolytic disease of the newborn occurs most often in group A or group B babies of group O mothers. These infants require group O RBCs for transfusion until the maternally derived antibody has completely disappeared from the serum and the RBCs of the infant. Antibodies of any specificity that occur in maternal serum as IgG have the potential to cause neonatal hemolysis. In most cases, the mother's serum is used for compatibility testing; and the RBCs for transfusion are selected to lack appropriate antigens. Maternal serum may contain antibodies directed against antigens other than those on the baby's cells or may contain IgM antibodies that have not crossed the placenta and are therefore not present in the infant's serum. In these situations the infant's blood is needed for compatibility testing.

Antibodies to low-incidence antigens

It may be difficult to detect a maternal antibody responsible for the destruction of neonatal RBCs if that antibody is directed against a very-low-incidence RBC antigen. In this case a crossmatch between the maternal serum and the paternal RBCs should identify the immune-mediated nature of the hemolysis and often the specificity of the RBC antibody as well.

Antibodies to high-incidence antigens

If the maternal antibody is directed against a very common RBC antigen, it may be difficult to find compatible blood for the infant. Although it is preferable to attempt to locate compatible blood either from family members or through a rare donor registry, exchange transfusion with incompatible cells may be necessary in an emergency. Since the exchange transfusion will also remove some of the offending antibody, the use of incompatible RBCs is preferable to no transfusion.

Red cell typing after intrauterine transfusion

Misleading results of routine blood grouping and direct antiglobulin testing may be obtained in infants who have received intrauterine transfusions. Neonatal RBCs are diluted with donor blood cells. Reactions with anti-A and/or anti-B, which are normally weak in newborns because of the incomplete development of these antigens on neonatal RBCs, may appear falsely negative in the presence of transfused group O cells. The initial direct antiglobulin test may likewise fail to detect a pathogenic antibody if most of the neonate's circulating RBCs are transfused cells lacking the corresponding antigen.

TRANSFUSION THERAPY FOR THE NEONATAL PATIENT

Blood components appropriate for neonates include RBCs, fresh frozen plasma, cryoprecipitate, platelet concentrates, and leukocyte concentrates. These components are transfused either as (1) part of an exchange transfusion, (2) a partial exchange, or (3) a small-volume replacement transfusion. These are considered separately in this section because of differences in indications, techniques, and product requirements.

Exchange transfusion

An exchange transfusion is the replacement of most or all of the recipient's RBCs and plasma with appropriately compatible RBCs and plasma from one or more donors. The amount of blood exchanged is generally expressed in relationship to the recipient's blood volume, for example, double-volume exchange or partial exchange. The technique was first reported by Wallerstein in 1946 as a useful method to treat severely affected erythroblastotic newborns in whom repeated transfusion of appropriately compatible Rh-negative blood was ineffective. He used a 60-minute simultaneous withdrawal and transfusion method requiring two sites of vascular access. The technical improvements described by Diamond and associates in 1951 contributed significantly to the safety and ease of the procedure and included the alternate withdrawal and infusion of blood through a single polyethylene tube in the umbilical vein. The exchange transfusion subsequently has become a common therapeutic modality in the neonatal intensive care nursery, although the indications for its use have changed dramatically with the decline in severe hemolytic disease caused by Rh sensitization.

Indications

Hemolytic disease of the newborn. The clinical syndrome of hemolytic disease is the result of the destruction of fetal RBCs coated with passively acquired maternal antibody. ABO–hemolytic disease is currently the most common cause of neonatal immune-mediated hemolysis. ABO incompatibility between mother and fetus exists in approximately 15% of all pregnancies. The majority of these group A and/or group B infants of group O mothers have demonstrable anti-A and/or anti-B coating their RBCs at birth; however, most have clinically mild disease, and few require exchange transfusion. Almost any blood group antibody that occurs as IgG could potentially cause hemolytic disease, including maternal autoantibodies. The objectives of exchange transfusion in hemolytic disease are:

1. To remove antibody-coated RBCs that will have a shortened intravascular survival
2. To restore oxygen-carrying capacity by providing antigen-negative RBCs that should have a normal intravascular survival
3. To remove free, maternally derived antibody from the plasma
4. To remove potentially toxic bilirubin resulting from RBC destruction
5. To provide additional free albumin to which bilirubin can bind
6. To restore plasma volume with normal human plasma

Hyperbilirubinemia.
See also Chapter 34.

The most common indication for neonatal exchange transfusion is the presence of excessive unconjugated bilirubin, which is potentially dangerous whenever the serum concentration exceeds the level at which damage to the central nervous system occurs. The objectives of exchange transfusion in hyperbilirubinemia are the same as those listed for hemolytic disease. An exchange transfusion is the most effective treatment for immediate reduction of serum bilirubin; and it should be accomplished before the onset of central nervous system damage. Some hyperbilirubinemia-related alterations in the neonatal central nervous system have been shown to be rapidly reversible with exchange transfusion. The usual bilirubin levels at which therapy is required have been defined and are discussed in Chapter 34.

Disseminated intravascular coagulation. See also part one of this chapter.

Disseminated intravascular coagulation (DIC) is an acquired activation of the clotting system characterized by systemic thrombus formation and the consumption of platelets and plasma coagulation factors. DIC in the neonate may be initiated by a variety of conditions, including hypoxia, acidosis, hypothermia, hypotension, respiratory distress syndrome, sepsis, viremia, necrotizing enterocolitis, and intravascular hemolysis. The standard coagulation screening tests (PT, PTT, TT) are usually prolonged in the premature neonate because of developmental factor deficiency. The diagnosis of DIC can be established, however, by a decreasing platelet count, increased fibrin degradation products, and depletion of at least one of the plasma coagulation factors consumed in clotting, which is expected to be normal in the newborn period (i.e., fibrinogen, factor V, factor VIII). These assays may detect only the most severely affected infants. Increased rates of fibrinogen and platelet consumption that were not apparent from standard screening tests have been reported in sick neonates.

There is general consensus that the most important therapy in DIC is directed toward the underlying disease process. Treatment of the coagulopathy per se is controversial. Although at least one study demonstrated that transfusion therapy for the coagulopathy did not improve survival, exchange transfusion is usually recommended, particularly for those infants with hemorrhagic manifestations. Many authors have suggested that the value of exchange transfusion in DIC goes beyond supplying depleted coagulation factors. The objectives of exchange transfusion in DIC are:

1. To replenish depleted plasma coagulation factors and platelets necessary for hemostasis
2. To provide antithrombin III and protein C, naturally occurring anticoagulants deficient in neonates
3. To remove fibrin degradation products that may be poorly metabolized by the immature neonatal liver
4. To remove toxic products that initiated the process
5. To remove damaged erythrocytes
6. To correct anemia and improve tissue oxygenation by replacing fetal RBCs with adult ones
7. To supply deficient host defense proteins

Neonatal sepsis. Overwhelming infection continues to be a major cause of morbidity and mortality in the neonatal period. Multiple defects in the neonatal cellular and humoral immune response have been identified as potential contributors to the compromised host defense system of newborns (Chapter 31 and part one of this chapter).

Several reports have suggested improved survival of septic infants whose therapy included exchange transfusions. Although some of these infants were actually treated with exchange transfusions because of the difficulty in obtaining granulocyte concentrates in a timely manner, the benefits of the exchange transfusion extend beyond the provision of normal neutrophils. Theoretic and documented benefits of exchange transfusion in neonatal sepsis include:

1. Increase in the circulating level of immunoglobulins, particularly IgM and IgA, which may enhance defense mechanisms
2. Removal of bacteria and bacterial toxins
3. Improvement in the opsonic activity against the offending organism
4. Increase in the pool of normal neutrophils
5. Improvement in perfusion and tissue oxygenation
6. Decrease in hemorrhagic complications by correcting the platelet count and plasma coagulation system and removing fibrin degradation products

Although these exchange transfusions for neonatal sepsis were generally performed using fresh whole blood, the demonstration of preserved opsonic activity in bank blood and of viable neutrophils, functional in vitro, in whole blood stored at 4° C (39° F) up to 9 hours suggests that blood products other than fresh whole blood, although unproved, should be investigated. Exchange transfusion for this indication remains controversial and investigational.

Toxin removal. Exchange transfusion of the newborn is a readily available technique for the removal of other toxins, such as drugs or chemicals given to the mother near the time of delivery, potentially toxic doses of antibiotics, and substances such as ammonia or potassium that may accumulate because of enzyme deficiency, prematurity, or renal failure. When exchange transfusion is used to treat hyperkalemia, rapid improvement is expected by physical removal of excessive potassium; however, further lowering of the serum potassium in the subsequent hours is most likely caused by the movement of potassium into the transfused hypokalemic RBCs, facilitated by the metabolic alkalosis that results from metabolism of citrate to bicarbonate, as previously described.

Kinetics

The efficiency of an exchange transfusion is maximal initially and diminishes exponentially as the procedure continues. The kinetics of exchange are very similar, regardless of whether a continuous (simultaneous withdrawal and replacement) or discontinuous (alternating withdrawal and replacement) technique is used. The effect of exchange transfusion varies with the component being removed. Efficiency is the highest for RBC exchange. A one-volume exchange transfusion results in removal of 70% to 75% of the neonate's RBCs; a two-volume exchange replaces 90%. Despite the correction of anemia, neonates continue to produce RBCs and release them into the circulation for up to 6 days. Conversely, the amount of bilirubin and/or maternal alloantibody removed by exchange transfusion is significantly less than seen with RBCs because of the equilibrium that exists for the bilirubin, antibody, and similar substances between the intravascular pool and the extravascular tissue stores.

The amount of bilirubin removed by an exchange transfusion varies with the serum concentration and the rate of the exchange. A double-volume exchange transfusion should eliminate more than 50% of the intravascular bilirubin; however, postexchange equilibration with tissue stores invariably causes a rebound increment in the serum concentration, which may be significant enough to require a second exchange procedure. The efficiency of removal of bilirubin and/or plasma antibody can be increased by 50% by performing the exchange transfusion slowly. This allows the extravascular component to equilibrate more extensively with the intravascular space during the slower and therefore longer procedure. The bilirubin level immediately following a slow exchange may be higher than the dramatic drop seen after a rapid exchange; however, the rebound will be significantly less because more bilirubin has actually been removed. The effect of a double-volume exchange on other cellular components depends in part on the composition of the replacement fluids used. Platelets should be expected to decrease by 50% to 70% or more unless replaced at the end of the procedure. Leukocytes may fall during the procedure; however, most infants have a demonstrable increase in circulating neutrophils following an exchange transfusion.

The optimum volume for an exchange transfusion is twice the infant's blood volume. The kinetics just described demonstrate that a double-volume exchange is more effective than a single-volume exchange; however, little is gained by exceeding two blood volumes. Likewise, little is lost if the exchange transfusion volume is slightly less than two times the neonate's blood volume. In practice the actual volume used should be approximated to the nearest full unit to minimize the number of donor exposures. In very low birth weight (VLBW) infants part of a unit of RBCs is sufficient for a double-volume exchange. The remainder of the same donor unit should be stored unentered in the blood bank and reserved in the event the same neonate requires a second exchange transfusion.

Choice of blood components

Safe, effective exchange transfusions have been performed using many different combinations of blood components. No single product or combination is unequivocally the best, and controlled trials contrasting fresh whole blood with alternate blood preparations are unavailable. Because of the relatively large volumes of anticoagulant/preservative solution administered to a neonate during a double-volume exchange, it is important to be cognizant of the composition of the various preparations and the potential complications of each. The relative advantages and disadvantages of several available blood components are listed in Table 32-6.

The most frequently used products for neonatal exchange are CPDA-1 red cells stored no longer than 5 to 7 days, saline-washed RBCs stored a maximum of 5 to 7 days before washing, or FDCs. There is a theoretic concern about using RBCs for neonatal exchange that have been preserved in Adsol because of the mannitol it contains. No complications have been reported related to this anticoagulant/preservative solution, although the experience with neonates is limited. At the very least these RBCs can be used for neonates as saline-washed cells since the wash procedure removes almost all the preservative solution. For a two-volume exchange transfusion, fresh frozen plasma (FFP) must be added to any of these RBC products to provide plasma coagulation factors, albumin, and other normal plasma proteins. Both stored whole blood and "reconstituted" blood (i.e., RBCs plus FFP) are deficient in platelets. Infants who are significantly thrombocytopenic (platelet count $\leq$50,000/mm^3) following an exchange transfusion, who are bleeding, or who continue to consume platelets should receive additional transfusion with 1 to 2 units of platelet concentrates. A single unit of platelets should be sufficient to increase the platelet count to over 50,000/mm^3 in a stabilized infant with dilutional thrombocytopenia; however, additional units are likely to be required if there is ongoing hemorrhage, sepsis, or consumptive coagulopathy. Platelets may be administered as a separate transfusion at the end of the exchange, or they may be used as the final aliquots of the replacement fluid to complete the procedure. It is recommended that platelets not be added to reconstituted blood during an exchange because this may lead to increased microaggregate formation, a situation associated with pulmonary dysfunction in adults.

Table 32-6. Advantages and disadvantages of various blood components for neonatal exchange transfusion

Component(s)	Advantages	Disadvantages
Red blood cells (CPDA-1) (<5-7 days) plus fresh frozen plasma (FFP)	Readily available 2,3-DPG well preserved Provides coagulation factors Can be pooled in small aliquots in an in-line graduated burette, allowing the hematocrit to be adjusted during exchange No risk of overheparinization	Risk of hypocalcemia from citrate Risk of rebound hypoglycemia No platelets At least two donor exposures
Frozen deglycerolized red cells (FDCs) plus FFP	2,3-DPG levels at least as high as in fresh blood Reduced risk of hypocalcemia Normal electrolytes Minimal number of leukocytes Low risk of CMV transmission Can be pooled as for RBCs plus FFP Allows access to rare blood types for neonates with antibodies Provides coagulation factors	High cost Extra preparation time required; less readily available Short shelf life once thawed Potential risk of hypoglycemia during exchange No platelets At least two donor exposures
Heparinized fresh whole blood	High levels of 2,3-DPG Provides coagulation factors Supplies platelets Reduced number of donor exposures No risk of hypocalcemia	Not readily available Short storage period Risk of hemorrhage from heparin Potential risk of hypoglycemia during exchange Hematocrit cannot be altered during procedure Risk of increase in nonesterified free fatty acids (secondary to heparin), causing uncoupling of bilirubin-albumin binding

In infants who are hypoxic or acidotic, RBCs known to lack hemoglobin S should be chosen for exchange transfusion. Massive fatal intravascular sickling and multiple renal and splenic infarctions have been reported following neonatal exchange transfusion with sickle trait blood. Testing of the unit by the blood bank must be specifically requested.

Supplemental calcium. Neonatal exchange with citrated blood may be associated with a decreased level of ionized serum calcium because of calcium chelation with citrate. Traditionally, intermittent infusions of calcium gluconate have been administered in an attempt to offset this potential complication; however, it is unclear whether this practice is routinely necessary or beneficial. One study found no significant difference in the post-transfusion ionized calcium between a group of full-term infants given 100 mg of calcium gluconate after each 100 ml of a two-volume exchange transfusion and a similar group receiving exchange transfusion without the supplemental calcium. This information from relatively healthy, full-term infants may not directly apply to the VLBW premature infant. If used, prophylactic calcium is usually administered intravenously after each 100 to 200 ml of blood exchanged. The calcium must be infused into a vein not being used for the exchange procedure to avoid clotting of the blood component before its transfusion. Whether or not calcium is given, the infant should be observed carefully for signs of irritability, tetany, or electrocardiographic changes.

Additional albumin. Because albumin binds to unconjugated bilirubin, it is postulated that increased levels of serum albumin allow increased intravascular binding of bilirubin, which in turn promotes bilirubin diffusion from the extravascular tissue stores into the vascular space, thereby increasing the total quantity of bilirubin that can be removed during an exchange transfusion. This is the rationale for the recommendation to administer 25% albumin either 1 hour before an exchange (1 gm/kg) or at intervals during the procedure after each 100 ml of blood is transfused. No evidence shows that this practice is of practical value in neonates with normal albumin levels; it is most likely to benefit those infants with reduced reserve albumin-binding capacity. Also, such albumin infusions should be used cautiously, if at all, in infants who are severely anemic, in congestive heart failure, with elevated central venous pressures, or with other conditions which increase the risk of intravascular fluid overload.

Volume and hematocrit of replacement fluids

An exchange transfusion equal to twice the infant's estimated blood volume is the goal for the most efficient procedure with optimum predicted clinical benefit. Calculations are based on a blood volume of 85 ml/kg for a newborn; a VLBW premature may have a blood volume closer to 100 ml/kg, and this figure can be substituted in the formula as appropriate. If whole blood is used for the exchange transfusion, the volume of blood required in milliliters is equal to the weight in kilograms times 2 times 85. The hematocrit of that whole blood will depend upon the hematocrit of the individual blood donor, but it is usually less than 50%. If "reconstituted" blood (RBCs plus plasma) is used, the following formula will achieve a replacement fluid with a final hematocrit of approximately 50%:

1. Total volume (ml) = weight (kg) × 85 × 2
2. Absolute volume of RBCs needed = result of step 1 divided by 2
3. Actual volume (ml) of RBCs needed = result of step 2 divided by 0.7
4. Actual volume (ml) of FFP needed = step 1 − step 3

If measured, the actual hematocrit of the unit of packed RBCs being transfused can be substituted for the approximate hematocrit (0.7) in step 3 to achieve more precision.

RBCs and FFP may be pooled by the blood bank or at the bedside. If a Y-tubing connection and a graduated burette are used to pool aliquots of 50 to 100 ml, the hematocrit of the replacement fluid may be altered throughout the procedure, enabling very anemic newborns to receive initial transfusions of fluid with a hematocrit of 70% and subsequent infusions gradually lowered to the desired level. This procedure rapidly corrects anemia and achieves initial improvement in tissue oxygenation while avoiding exposure of the infant to a second unit of blood.

Donor blood needs to be kept well mixed throughout the exchange to ensure that the final aliquots will have the desired hematocrit. The last aliquot removed can be used for determination of postexchange hematocrit, bilirubin, and possibly compatibility testing in anticipation of additional transfusions.

Vascular access

Exchange transfusions in the newborn period are usually accomplished via umbilical venous and arterial catheters. These catheters should be radiopaque to allow radiologic documentation of correct location before the infusion of hypertonic solutions and should have end holes only, since side holes promote thrombus formation because of the dead space at the end of the catheter. The umbilical vessels are easiest to catheterize within hours of birth; however, it may be possible to achieve vascular access by this route for several days if necessary. Catheters should be secured with suture, filled with solution at all times, never left open to air, and never completely covered from sight. If umbilical catheters are not available for exchange transfusion or are deemed too risky for use, peripheral arteries and veins may be used. Considerable success has been achieved using the radial artery for withdrawal even in VLBW infants. Occasionally the ulnar or posterior tibial artery has been used without associated morbidity.

Methodology

Two primary methods of exchange transfusion are typically used. The first is the *isovolumetric method*, in which blood is continuously and simultaneously withdrawn and replaced. This technique requires vascular access through two catheters; if automated infusion pumps are used, these catheters must be the same size. A single peristaltic pump regulates the blood withdrawn, usually from the umbilical artery, and the blood infused, usually through the umbilical vein. Two persons simultaneously withdrawing and infusing aliquots of blood may also approximate an isovolumetric exchange. Theoretically the isovolumetric method is more efficient because it eliminates the dead space in the syringe hub and catheter, which is filled with blood that is never exchanged in the discontinuous, push-pull method described next.

The second method of exchange is the *discontinuous technique* described by Diamond and associates, which can be accomplished through a single vascular access. A three-way or four-way stopcock joins a single syringe, the unit of blood, the infant, and the extension tubing leading to the graduated discard container. Disposable kits are now commercially available that allow this entire procedure to be completed in a relatively closed system. A maximum of 5 ml/kg (or 5% of the estimated blood volume) is used for each alternating withdrawal and infusion. A discontinuous exchange transfusion should be performed slowly rather than rapidly to minimize hemodynamic changes associated with each step. In preterm infants the aortic systolic and mean arterial pressures fall during each withdrawal phase and rise during the infusion phase. During slow exchange (5 ml/kg/3 minutes), the arterial pressure returns to baseline during the infusion phase. However, during rapid exchange (5 ml/kg/45 to 60 seconds) arterial pressure rises during the infusion phase but does not reach baseline. Instead, the peak arterial pressure falls progressively below the baseline with each withdrawal/infusion cycle, accompanied by changes in intracranial pressure. These hemodynamic changes and alterations in intracranial pressure are avoided by the use of an isovolumetric technique. In the small, ill neonate, already at risk of intracranial hemorrhage, the slower rate of exchange transfusion is indicated when the discontinuous exchange methodology is used.

Throughout the exchange the neonate should be maintained in a neutral thermal environment because a higher morbidity and mortality is associated with hypothermic neonates. Similarly, blood for exchange transfusion should be carefully warmed to a maximum of 37° C (98.6° F). Infants treated with exchange transfusion using blood at room temperature have been reported to experience a drop in rectal temperature of 0.7° to 2.5° C (mean, 1.3° C) during the procedure, in contrast to those transfused with prewarmed blood, whose rectal temperature decrease averaged 0.3° C (range, 0.1° to 0.6° C). In addition, cold blood transfused through the umbilical vein passes directly to the heart and, in the presence of a patent foramen ovale, may easily reach the left side of the heart and the coronary arteries, precipitating cardiac arrhythmias.

The ideal method of controlled warming of blood is via an in-line blood warmer placed close to the umbilical catheter. Various models of in-line warmers are commercially available. Blood warmers should be regulated precisely and their temperature meter checked with each use. Quality control monitoring of blood warmers should be routine, including periodic verification of the temperature with a mercury thermometer. RBCs readily hemolyze if warmed to 50° C (122° F); some hemolysis is apparent at lower temperatures. Severe hemolytic transfusion reactions have been reported as a result of blood warmer malfunction or careless blood warming by covering the blood tubing with a wet, hot towel. If in-line blood warmers are unavailable, a closed unit of RBCs or whole blood may be gently warmed in a 37° C water bath, which is monitored with a thermometer.

Additional considerations

1. Neonatal exchange transfusion is best performed by experienced personnel with at least one nurse and one physician present throughout the procedure. Because morbidity and mortality of the procedure may be significant, referral to a regional neonatal intensive care unit is advisable. Potential complications of exchange are listed in the boxed material.
2. Hypoglycemia may occur in the neonate (1) during a transfusion, particularly if the anticoagulant/preservative solution used has a low glucose concentration, or (2) following the exchange transfusion if the high glucose load of the blood induces hyperinsulinemia, which persists after the glucose infusion has been discontinued. Blood glucose monitoring during and following an exchange transfusion is recommended.
3. The infant's oxygenation, ventilation, and acid-base balance should be monitored frequently, since the inspired oxygen concentration must often be increased during an exchange transfusion.
4. Postexchange platelet counts should be monitored to ensure that an adequate peripheral blood platelet count is maintained by transfusion, if necessary, especially in the infant requiring more than one exchange.
5. Because exchange transfusion is not a selective procedure, certain drug doses require alteration, whereas others do not.

Potential complications of neonatal exchange transfusion

BLOOD COMPONENT–RELATED COMPLICATIONS

- Transfusion-associated infection: hepatitis, CMV, AIDS, bacterial sepsis
- Hypocalcemia, arrhythmia
- Hyperkalemia, arrhythmia
- Hypoglycemia
- Metabolic acidosis
- Metabolic alkalosis
- Excessive heparinization
- Thrombocytopenia
- Graft-versus-host disease
- Hemolysis caused by incompatible RBCs
- Sickling of cells containing hemoglobin S

CATHETER–RELATED COMPLICATIONS

- Cardiac arrhythmias
- Infection: sepsis, omphalitis, thrombophlebitis, hepatic abcess
- Thrombosis: arterial, hepatic vein, portal vein
- Vessel perforation
- Necrotizing enterocolitis
- Peripheral ischemia and necrosis
- Intravascular catheter loss
- Emboli
- Renovascular hypertension

PROCEDURE–RELATED COMPLICATIONS

- Hypothermia
- Systemic blood pressure fluctuations: hypovolemia, hypervolemia
- Intracranial pressure fluctuations
- Intracranial hemorrhage
- Air embolus
- Accidental hemorrhage
- Thrombocytopenia
- Hemolysis caused by mechanical, thermal, or osmotic damage to RBCs

Partial exchange transfusion

See also Chapters 22 and 32, part one.

Partial exchange transfusion is an effective method of rapidly decreasing the hematocrit and whole blood viscosity in polycythemic neonates with hyperviscosity or correcting severe anemia without the risk of intravascular fluid overload and subsequent heart failure.

The long-term benefit of early partial exchange transfusion in polycythemic, hyperviscous neonates is controversial, at least partly because the prognosis for such infants depends greatly on the etiology. There is general agreement, however, that all newborns with a venous hematocrit exceeding 70%, even without symptoms, should be treated to reduce the hematocrit to at least less than 60%. FFP, plasma protein fraction USP (Plasmanate), 5% albumin, and saline have been used as replacement fluids for the whole blood withdrawn. Albumin solutions are preferred to plasma because the risks of transfusion-transmitted infections associated with plasma, especially hepatitis and AIDS, are eliminated. The volume of exchange required can be calculated using the following formula:

$$\text{Volume of exchange (ml)} = \frac{\text{Blood volume} \times (\text{Observed hematocrit} - \text{Desired hematocrit})}{\text{Observed hematocrit}}$$

To correct severe anemia, packed RBCs are used as the replacement fluid for the whole blood withdrawn. The formula used to calculate the volume required for exchange is similar to the one just given; however, the hematocrit of the unit of RBCs used must be taken into account. RBCs usually have a hematocrit that approximates 70%; thus the formula:

$$\text{Volume of exchange} = \frac{\text{Blood volume} \times (\text{Desired hematocrit} - \text{Observed hematocrit})}{70\% - \text{Observed hematocrit}}$$

This formula is based on the assumption that the rise in hematocrit is a linear function of the volume of blood exchanged. The incremental change in hematocrit progressively diminishes throughout the exchange. This formula therefore may slightly underestimate the actual volume of exchange required to achieve the desired hematocrit.

The technique of partial exchange transfusion is similar to that used to accomplish a larger volume exchange. A discontinuous methodology is most often used, and aliquots of 5 ml/kg or less should be used for each withdrawal and infusion.

Replacement transfusions

Red blood cell transfusions

Indications. Despite observations that (1) ill neonates as a group are more likely to be transfused than any other hospitalized patients and (2) RBCs are the most frequently transfused blood component in neonates, no uniformly accepted criteria exist for the transfusion of premature or term infants. This is partly because of the difficulty in measuring all the parameters that determine oxygen availability, oxygen delivery, and oxygen need in these patients.

Most RBC transfusions in newborns are administered under one of two circumstances. The first and most common indication is the replacement of acute blood loss resulting from hemorrhage or more often from iatrogenic measures required for laboratory testing and monitoring. The amount of blood drawn for testing has been variously estimated between 2% and 8% of the infant's blood volume per 24 hours spent in neonatal intensive care, despite the use of microanalytic techniques. A portion of this blood loss is "hidden loss," that volume of blood lost on cotton swabs or in the dead spaces of tubing or butterfly sets used to draw blood samples. Although neonates are capable of RBC production, their marrow response to anemia is slow compared to a normal adult. Thus the usual approach is to replace iatrogenic blood losses prophylactically rather than to attempt to determine whether an infant can physiologically tolerate the added insult of a falling hematocrit and some hypovolemia. The removal of 5% to 10% of an infant's blood volume over a short period necessitates blood replacement, particularly in an already compromised, sick neonate in whom symptoms of anemia may be difficult to recognize.

The second typical indication for neonatal RBC transfusion is correction of anemia, a determination that must be made by careful clinical assessment of the infant, the laboratory values (hematocrit and reticulocyte count), and other potential compensatory mechanisms such as the increase in intracellular 2,3-DPG, which normally occurs during the "physiologic" anemia of infancy. Signs and symptoms traditionally associated with anemia in a neonate include tachypnea, tachycardia, pallor, lethargy, apnea, and poor weight gain. However, no linear correlation exists between the hemoglobin concentration alone and the presence or absence of the clinical signs of anemia (tachypnea, tachycardia). The correlation that does exist is between the signs and symptoms of anemia and the *available oxygen*, a function of the hemoglobin concentration and the position of the oxygen-hemoglobin dissociation curve. Thus some neonates appear clinically anemic despite measured hemoglobin concentrations in the normal range for age. In contrast, infants undergoing exchange transfusion in the immediate newborn period are more likely to tolerate lower levels of hemoglobin well than are similarly aged infants with no exchange transfusion. Replacement of RBCs containing adult hemoglobin for those containing fetal hemoglobin in these infants results in more available oxygen and less stimulus for reticulocyte production at any given hemoglobin level.

Representative criteria for RBC transfusion of infants with and without respiratory distress are listed in the boxed material. Infants with continued respiratory distress are transfused more aggressively. Preterm infants

Criteria for replacement transfusion in the high-risk infant

WITH RESPIRATORY DISTRESS, TRANSFUSION SHOULD BE GIVEN WHEN:

The hematocrit is less than 40%.
Hypovolemia is present, as judged by (1) pallor, (2) pulse rate greater than 160/minute, or (3) systolic blood pressure less than 50 mm Hg (birth weight greater than 1,000 g).
Greater than 10% of the blood volume has been removed within 48 hours and the hematocrit is less than 45%.

IN THE ABSENCE OF RESPIRATORY DISTRESS, TRANSFUSIONS SHOULD BE GIVEN WHEN:

The hematocrit is less than 30% in the first week of life.
The pulse rate is greater than 160/minute, the respiratory rate is greater than 60/minute, or roentgenograms reveal cardiomegaly.

Modified from Lubin, B.: Clin. Haematol. **7:**19, 1978.

have been shown to have improvements in weight gain associated with a decrease in oxygen consumption and metabolic rate during the week following a RBC transfusion (10 ml/kg), as compared to these same parameters measured before the transfusion. In the treatment of symptomatic anemia, at least 10 ml of RBCs/kg is a typically used dosage.

Red cell preparations. The optimal RBC product for neonatal transfusion is a small sterile aliquot of readily available compatible RBCs with a hematocrit of approximately 65%; well-preserved 2,3-DPG; minimal biochemical changes, particularly a relatively high pH and low supernatant potassium concentration; minimal risk of transmitting infection; and the option to obtain several such aliquots from the same blood donor. Several methods have been developed that address these particular needs.

Quadruple packs. Whole blood collected into CPDA-1 anticoagulant/preservative solution and stored less than 5 to 7 days meets the biochemical criteria for transfusion to neonates. In a quadruple pack, a primary blood collection bag with three integrally connected satellite bags, plasma can be removed into one satellite bag, and the remaining RBCs with a usual hematocrit approximating 70% can be divided into the other three bags. Each bag will contain one third of a unit of RBCs, about 85 ml. Since all these manipulations are performed without entering the quad pack system, each of the one-third units retains it normal shelf life.

Each of the 85 ml aliquots may be further apportioned into two, three, or four pediatric transfer bags, depending on the volume requested for each infant's transfusion. Each of the original one-third units should be entered and appropriately apportioned at the time of use, since they must be transfused within 24 hours of entering. Using this system, several infants can be transfused from a single blood donation. In addition, an infant requiring daily replacement transfusions can receive RBCs, with a maximum pretransfusion storage period of 5 days, from the same blood donor unit on 3 successive days. Minimizing donor exposure is an important way to decrease the risk of transfusion-transmitted infections. Good communication between the nursery and the transfusion service is essential to optimize this blood utilization protocol.

Unit-dose system. Distribution of the precise volume of prefiltered RBCs in syringes is a useful technique in nurseries where several infants receive one or more small volume transfusions per day with a syringe mechanical infusion pump. Whole blood can be collected into a multiple-pack system as just noted and RBCs prepared. A resealable injection site coupler inserted into an access port of the blood bag permits repeated entry into that unit or partial unit over 24 hours. Whenever RBCs are needed, the volume requested is aspirated into a syringe through a needle inserted into the injection site and an appropriate blood filter, usually a neonatal microaggregate filter. A sterile cap is used to cover the filled syringe, and appropriate identifying labels are applied to the syringe. Using this system minimizes wastage of blood through the flexibility in the volume of the component that can be prepared. These small syringe aliquots are sterile and show no deterioration in the quality of the component, as measured by hematocrit, pH, supernatant potassium concentration, lactate dehydrogenase (LDH) level, plasma free hemoglobin, or glucose during the six hours following dispensing. Alternatively, if a blood bank–monitored refrigerator is maintained in the neonatal intensive care unit, partial RBC units may be released daily to the nursery, labeled with identification of the infant or infants for whom each unit is intended. When a transfusion is ordered, nursing personnel who will administer the transfusion follow the same procedure as just described to obtain the precise amount of blood required. This also ensures that many small transfusions to a single neonate within 24 hours will be from the same donor unit.

Half-unit donations. Approximately 225 ml of blood can be collected into a triple-pack system after adjusting the volume of anticoagulant. Removal of the plasma into one of the satellite bags results in two aliquots of RBCs, each with a volume about 60 ml, appropriate for neonatal transfusion. This practice provides an opportunity to use healthy blood donors who do not meet the 50 kg minimum weight requirement for donation of a whole unit of blood. This methodology may be important in expanding the blood donor pool, thereby ensuring the availability of relatively fresh RBCs for neonates.

Individual small units. A full unit of whole blood is composed of the premeasured anticoagulant/preservative solution plus 450 ml ± 10% of donor blood. If the maximum 495 ml is collected into a bag with one satellite bag, 30 to 60 ml can be removed into the satellite bag for neonatal use, and the remainder is enough to serve as an ordinary whole unit. Although this technique could produce many small aliquots of relatively fresh blood without the need to recruit new blood donors, the inability to provide multiple transfusions for a patient from the same blood donor unit is a distinct disadvantage.

Saline-washed red blood cells. Saline-washed RBCs are an alternative product for neonatal use. Two pediatric-sized units of approximately 135 ml each can be produced from a single unit of whole blood using an automated blood cell processor. Both pediatric units have only a 24-hour shelf life after washing. Aliquots can be obtained for neonatal transfusion using either multiple pediatric transfer bags or syringes, as already described. Saline-washed RBC units have a significantly reduced supernatant potassium concentration, essentially no citrate, few leukocytes, and less than 0.2% of the original plasma proteins. Whole blood units less than 1 week from collection are still required to ensure adequate levels of 2,3-DPG.

Frozen deglycerolized red blood cell systems. Small volumes of deglycerolized RBCs can be prepared from a unit of RBCs that are glycerolized in a standard fashion, separated into three equal aliquots, and frozen. When thawed and deglycerolized for transfusion, each aliquot contains 60 to 70 ml of RBCs, with an average hematocrit of 75%. Each aliquot may be thawed as needed but must be transfused within 24 hours of thawing and deglycerolization. A single donor unit may thus be used for a single infant on 3 separate days. Each aliquot could also be further divided into smaller-volume portions for transfusion to several infants within a 24-hour period. FDCs have 2,3-DPG levels equivalent to those in freshly drawn blood, a markedly lower supernatant potassium concentration, very few leukocytes and platelets, and only minute amounts of plasma proteins and anticoagulant. FDCs carry a low risk of CMV transmission. They are, however, generally more expensive and require more preparation time than liquid-stored RBCs.

RBCs nearing their expiration date can be biochemically modified before being glycerolized and frozen as just described. These "rejuvenated" RBC units have improved oxygen transport function at the time of transfusion; 2,3-DPG levels are 150% of normal. The ability to rejuvenate RBCs could decrease the wastage of blood while providing RBCs especially suited for neonates.

Walking donor programs. On-call blood donors, usually hospital personnel, have sometimes been used to provide small volumes of heparinized whole blood, drawn into syringes as needed for neonatal transfusion before the development of alternative methods such as those already described. This methodology is listed here to discourage its use by highlighting its disadvantages:

1. No pretransfusion compatibility testing
2. No pretransfusion screening for hepatitis, AIDS, or CMV
3. Suboptimal donor health history screening
4. No pretransfusion donor and patient samples available to evaluate adverse reactions
5. Generally poor transfusion records
6. Risk of overheparinization of the blood, causing coagulopathy or hemorrhage in the neonate
7. Potential bacterial contamination of the blood through faulty phlebotomy technique
8. Potentially increased risk of hepatitis transmission by using untested blood donors who work in a high-risk hospital environment
9. An increased burden on the nursery staff, who must assume the responsibility for donor recruitment, phlebotomy, and any storage of the blood

Technical aspects. Careful attention to the technical aspects of RBC transfusion is more important to achieving a successful transfusion than is usually appreciated. This is particularly true in neonates, for whom small volumes of RBCs blood cells are variously manipulated in an attempt to meet the perceived needs of the neonatal transfusion recipient more adequately. Because of the small size and relative immaturity of the newborn, seemingly insignificant changes in the RBC component may become major problems in the infant.

Filters. All blood components must be filtered before transfusion. The use of a standard 170 μm blood filter is sufficient for most RBC-containing components in newborns. Microaggregate filters (pore size 10 to 20 μm) with a small internal volume specifically for neonatal use are commercially available, but their value in routine usage is controversial. Microaggregates are the 20 to 120 μm particles of nonviable granulocytes, platelets, and fibrin strands that progressively develop in RBC and whole blood units throughout the storage period. When neonates routinely receive blood stored less than 5 to 7 days, there should be little danger from microaggregates because very few of these particles exist in such fresh blood. If neonatal microaggregate filters are used, care must be taken to follow the manufacturer's instructions exactly. Most neonatal microaggregate filters are made to accommodate only a single, small-volume transfusion; these should not be used for larger transfusions, including exchange transfusion. If unusual resistance is encountered in aspiration of blood through a filter and no visible clots are seen within the RBC unit, the filter should be changed. Two severe hemolytic reactions, one fatal, have been reported resulting from pretransfusion mechanical trauma to RBCs in a microaggregate filter. Measurable hemolysis, which increased as the rate of filtration decreased, has been observed with blood stored for as little as 1 day.

Needle size. For replacement transfusions of RBCs, the optimum needle or catheter size and the rate of infusion that minimize the risk of mechanical hemolysis are not clear. A substantial increment in hemolysis accompanies an increase in flow rate and a decrease in needle size (23- and 25-gauge needles) when 9-day-old RBCs are used. No significant hemolysis of fresh RBCs is noted with different needle gauges (21, 23, 25, 27) and various rates, suggesting that the small-caliber needles required in tiny preterm infants may be adequate for RBC transfusion when all other technical aspects of the transfusion have been optimized.

Infusion pumps. Small-volume RBC transfusions are usually administered slowly using a mechanical infusion pump. Several varieties of pumps are commercially available. Some have been studied and found to be suitable for RBC transfusion, whereas others may not be suitable. Infusion pumps should be tested to determine that hemolysis does not occur before their use in RBC transfusion.

Warming of blood. No published studies address the safety or the consequences of slowly transfusing relatively cold, small-volume RBC aliquots to neonatal patients. Although traditionally considered to be unnecessary, small-volume RBC aliquots in syringes are often warmed before transfusion, presumably based on anecdotal experiences. Various warming techniques are in use. A syringe aliquot cannot be warmed in a conventional water bath because it is an open system and susceptible to spillage and contamination. The large dead space in conventional blood warmers precludes their use for these small volumes. A labeled syringe aliquot of RBCs placed inside the temperature-controlled Isolette of the intended neonatal recipient for 30 minutes before transfusion warms more rapidly than similar aliquots left at room temperature. However, the temperature of the blood inside the Isolette syringes does not reach the temperature set for the Isolette, even after 90 minutes. No evidence of RBC destruction is seen when syringes of RBCs are held for the maximum allowable duration of a transfusion (6 hours) in a 37° C warm air incubator. However, when syringes of RBCs are placed adjacent to a neonate under a radiant warmer, significant erythrocyte damage occurs, as evidenced by increased plasma-free hemoglobin, increased supernatant potassium concentration, and decreased pH. This erythrocyte damage is observed both when the radiant heater is operated at full power and when the infrared energy output is regulated via skin temperature servocontrol. Excessive heating can be avoided and the RBC damage minimized by placing the syringes of blood on a stand beside the radiant warmer rather than directly under it or by shielding the syringe with aluminum foil. RBCs in syringes may be safely and effectively warmed before neonatal transfusion by placing the labeled syringe inside the infant's warm air Isolette. In contrast, when an infant who is being managed under a radiant warmer requires a transfusion, extreme caution must be used to place the syringe aliquot of RBCs beside, rather than under, the radiant warmer. If the syringe and infusion pump must be placed under the radiant warmer beside the infant for the transfusion, the RBCs should be shielded with aluminum foil to minimize hemolysis.

Fresh frozen plasma transfusions

Product definition. FFP is the anticoagulated fluid portion of one unit of blood that has been centrifuged, separated, and frozen solid within 6 hours of collection. FFP contains all the clotting factors including fibrinogen, fibronectin, γ-globulins, albumin, and other plasma proteins in the same concentration as they are present in the normal blood donor. None of the proteins is concentrated during preparation.

Other single-donor frozen plasma products are available in some regions of the United States. These differ only in that they were processed and frozen between 6 and 24 hours of the whole blood collection and therefore contain slightly lower concentrations of the labile plasma coagulation factors, factor V and factor VIII. The maximum expected loss of activity of these coagulation factors is 20% to 25%. Thus the indications for the various frozen plasma products are interchangeable, except for the treatment of severe factor V deficiency, in which FFP is the treatment of choice. The term FFP is used throughout the remainder of this section to refer to all single-donor frozen plasma products.

Indications. Few specific indications exist for the use of FFP in neonates; most indications are associated with correction of acquired or congenital coagulation factor deficiencies.

1. FFP is indicated as part of the replacement fluid in a two-volume exchange transfusion because of the anticipated coagulation factor deficiency that accompanies this procedure.
2. Hemorrhage secondary to vitamin K deficiency and the resultant decreased activity of the vitamin K–dependent coagulation factors—II (prothrombin), VII, IX, and X—is rare except in infants not given prophylaxis. An infant with severe vitamin K deficiency and bleeding should be treated with a single transfusion of FFP, 15 to 20 ml/kg, to supply the deficient factors quickly and to control the bleeding.

Parenteral vitamin K should also be given. If the vitamin K is given, only those infants with severe liver disease resulting in severely impaired coagulation factor synthesis should require a second transfusion of FFP.

3. Transfusion of FFP, either as part of an exchange or as repeated simple replacement transfusions, is indicated for the repletion of coagulation factors that are consumed during DIC. A double-volume exchange transfusion is usually the preferred therapy, particularly in severely affected infants, in very tiny infants unlikely to tolerate the volume of colloid associated with repeated FFP infusions, and in those infants likely to require surgical intervention. Exchange transfusion will result in much higher levels of clotting factor activity than those achievable by simple transfusion. If the hemorrhagic symptoms of DIC are less severe, repletion of clotting factors to hemostatic levels may be achieved by transfusion of 15 ml/kg FFP, followed by careful observation and possibly additional doses of FFP. Replacement transfusion with platelets may also be required because platelets are consumed during the course of DIC. The volume of plasma infused with the platelet transfusion may be subtracted from the volume of FFP required, since platelets are routinely stored in relatively fresh plasma with reasonable clotting factor activity levels. Gross and colleagues have compared exchange transfusion and replacement transfusion in the treatment of the coagulopathy of DIC in neonates. They found no apparent difference between the two treatment groups: (1) those treated with double-volume exchange transfusion every 12 hours and (2) those treated with infusions of 15 ml/kg FFP plus one unit of platelets every 12 hours. Both treatments were continued as long as laboratory criteria for DIC persisted. The outcome depended on the success of the treatment of the primary pathologic process.
4. Congenital factor IX deficiency (hemophilia B, Christmas disease) can be diagnosed in the newborn period; however, serious bleeding as a result of the disorder is unusual. Acute bleeding episodes should be treated with FFP infusion. The minimum hemostatic level of factor IX activity is 20%, but the desired plasma level depends on the site and seriousness of the hemorrhage. One ml of FFP is equivalent to 1 International Unit (IU) of factor IX, and the transfusion of 1 ml/kg will raise the plasma factor IX activity by 1%. The following formula may be used to calculate FFP dose:

$$\text{Volume FFP} = (\text{Desired factor IX activity} - \text{Initial factor IX activity}) \times \text{Weight (kg)}$$

5. Except for congenital afibrinogenemia, hemophilia A (factor VIII deficiency), and von Willebrand's disease, bleeding resulting from other congenital coagulation factor deficiencies should be treated with 15 ml/kg FFP.
6. Infants of mothers who have received certain anticonvulsant or oral anticoagulant medication during pregnancy are at an increased risk of hemorrhage despite aggressive administration of parenteral vitamin K. FFP, 20 ml/kg, is recommended in these infants if the cord blood studies indicate severe deficiency of vitamin K–dependent factors or if any bleeding occurs in the early neonatal period.
7. FFP may be appropriate for infants with protein-losing enteropathies in whom parenteral nutrition has been ineffective.
8. FFP is contraindicated as a colloid for volume expansion or as a nutritional supplement, since safer therapies exist.

Available preparations. FFP is usually frozen in aliquots of approximately 225 ml. Some regions of the United States have available pediatric FFP units, each approximately 100 ml in volume. These large-volume products are appropriate for use in neonatal exchange transfusion but invariably result in significant wastage when used for replacement transfusion. Methods have been described for the preparation of 20 ml aliquots of FFP in sterile, pyrogen-free pharmaceutic vials. Plasma is separated from whole blood as soon as possible after collection and dispensed into the small vials using a laminar airflow hood to minimize the risk of contamination. The FFP is then quickly frozen in the small-vial aliquots. When requested for neonatal transfusion, one or more vials can be quickly thawed and dispensed. Such vials have injectable caps through which precise volumes of plasma can be aspirated. Using this technique, plasma from a single blood donor provides approximately 12 neonatal transfusions.

Technical aspects. Plasma transfusions should be ABO compatible with the neonate's RBCs (see Table 32-5); pretransfusion compatibility testing is not required. FFP may be stored frozen for 1 year. There is no clinical advantage to the transfusion of "fresher" versus "older" frozen units. FFP should be transfused as soon as possible after it has been thawed, but certainly within 6 hours if it is being used for coagulation factor replacement. A thawed unit of FFP may be divided into small aliquots for transfusion; and, if stored in a properly monitored refrigerator between 1° C and 6° C (34° and 43° F), these aliquots may be transfused over the 24 hours following initial entry into the primary unit.

Theoretically, small-volume FFP transfusions should not require prewarming; however, if FFP is prewarmed, care should be taken (as described for RBCs) to avoid overheating because this will denature the coagulation proteins.

FFP should always be administered through a blood filter. Microaggregate filters are superfluous but are probably not harmful to the product.

FFP does not need to be screened for antibody to CMV because of the lack of viable leukocytes in the product. Although FFP has not been shown to transmit CMV, the passive administration of antibody to CMV with this product may cause the CMV antibody test to become positive in the neonate. This does not represent CMV infection, and the antibody will disappear on a time course consistent with the 21-day half-life of γ-globulin.

FFP produced from whole blood units destined for Adsol or Nutricel RBC preservation is satisfactory for transfusion to neonates, since during component production the platelet-rich plasma is separated from the RBCs before the preservative solution is added to the cells. Thus the anticoagulant/preservative solution in these FFP units consists only of a citrate, phosphate, and dextrose solution.

Cryoprecipitate transfusion

Product definition. Cryoprecipitate is the cold-insoluble precipitate remaining when FFP has been thawed slowly. Each unit (bag) of cryoprecipitate is derived from a single blood donation. One unit of cryoprecipitate is 10 to 15 ml in volume and contains factor VIII, both the portion with procoagulant activity, factor VIII:C (at least 80 IU/concentrate), and the von Willebrand's factor, factor VIII:vWF (40% to 70% of the original amount present in the FFP unit); fibrinogen (150 to 250 mg/concentrate); factor XIII (20% to 40% of the original FFP); and fibronectin (20 to 40 mg/cryoprecipitate unit).

Indications. Cryoprecipitate is indicated in the treatment of bleeding episodes associated with severe factor VIII deficiency (classical hemophilia A) or severe von Willebrand's disease. Significant bleeding from either of these disorders is rare in the newborn period. Infusion of 1 IU of factor VIII:C activity/kg should raise the plasma factor VIII:C activity by 2%. It can be assumed that each unit (bag) of cryoprecipitate contains at least 80 IU of factor VIII:C activity. The actual factor VIII:C activity varies among blood donors; the factor concentration is not measured in every unit. For the treatment of hemophilia A–related hemorrhage, the desired factor VIII:C activity depends on the severity of the bleeding. The following formula can be used to calculate the amount of cryoprecipitate required:

$$\text{Factor VIII required (IU)} = \frac{(\text{Desired factor VIII} - \text{Observed factor VIII})}{2} \times \text{Weight (kg)}$$

$$\text{Units (bags) of cryoprecipitate} = \frac{\text{Factor VIII required (IU)}}{80}$$

The number of units of cryoprecipitate administered should be rounded up to the next whole number.

Hemostasis in von Willebrand's disease can be achieved with the transfusion of one to two units of cryoprecipitate, repeated daily.

Cryoprecipitate is the treatment of choice for congenital afibrinogenemia, a rare disorder that manifests in the neonatal period. A plasma fibrinogen level of 100 mg/dl is hemostatic. Since one unit of cryoprecipitate can be assumed to contain an average 200 mg of fibrinogen, one unit (bag) of cryoprecipitate will raise the plasma fibrinogen level of the recipient by 200 mg/dl of recipient blood volume.

Technical aspects. The technical guidelines for the administration of FFP apply also for the transfusion of cryoprecipitate, except that small aliquots of cryoprecipitate should not be withdrawn from a bag being stored at refrigerator temperatures after thawing. Only the amount to be transfused immediately should be requested and thawed.

Platelet transfusion

A normal platelet count for a premature or full-term newborn is between 150,000/mm^3 and 450,000/mm^3. Any platelet count below 100,000/mm^3 is definitely abnormal and should be investigated. Numerous in vitro abnormalities of neonatal platelet function have been identified; however, the clinical significance of the findings is unclear because the bleeding time, considered to be the best in vivo test of platelet function, is normal in the newborn.

The etiology of neonatal thrombocytopenia may be decreased platelet production, increased peripheral platelet destruction, or a combination of both mechanisms. Platelet transfusion may provide information about the mechanism of the thrombocytopenia if posttransfusion platelet counts are obtained at 1, 4, and 24 hours. In disorders of decreased platelet production a predicted posttransfusion platelet count increment is observed, followed by a progressive decline in circulating platelets consistent with a normal platelet survival half-life of 3 to 5 days. A shortened half-life of transfused platelets is characteristic of increased platelet destruction. If very rapid platelet destruction is present, there may be no demonstrable platelet count increment, even 1 hour after transfusion. Immune-mediated destruction, active bleeding, and fever may contribute to reduced platelet survival. If the infant's own platelets do not survive normally because of an intrinsic platelet defect such as that seen in Wiskott-Aldrich syndrome, the normal transfused donor platelets should survive. Finally, in immune-mediated platelet destruction transfused platelets will survive normally if they are compatible with the responsible antibody or antibodies, but they will be rapidly destroyed if they are incompatible (part one of this chapter).

Immune-mediated thrombocytopenia in neonates is caused by maternal IgG that has crossed the placenta during fetal life. Two categories of immune thrombocytopenia are recognized in neonates and the distinction between them is therapeutically important. The first category is maternal autoimmune thrombocytopenia, alone or associated with other collagen-vascular disorders, in which the maternal IgG antiplatelet antibody has broad reactivity against all platelets, thereby causing thrombocytopenia of both the mother and the infant. Transfused random donor platelets, maternal platelets, or platelets from any family member have uniformly very short survival in the neonate. Usually no platelet count increment is detectable 1 hour after the transfusion. Random donor platelet transfusions should be used only to treat acute bleeding episodes in the infant and not prophylactically in an attempt to maintain the infant's platelet count above a certain arbitrary value. Because random donor platelets may survive long enough to contribute to hemostasis, if not to the platelet count, they are superior to no platelet transfusion in the event of bleeding. For severe hemorrhage, a double-volume exchange transfusion is needed to remove circulating antiplatelet antibody so that transfused platelets will survive.

The second category of neonatal immune-mediated thrombocytopenia is alloimmune, or isoimmune, neonatal thrombocytopenia, in which the maternal IgG platelet alloantibody is specifically directed against an antigen present on the fetal platelets that is absent from the maternal platelets. The mother's platelet count remains normal, whereas the infant's platelet count is usually very low. Several dominantly inherited platelet-specific antigens have been implicated in isoimmune neonatal thrombocytopenia. The most common is Pl^{A1}, an antigen present in homozygous or heterozygous form in 98% of unselected individuals. Minimal response should be expected from transfusion of random donor platelets in an infant with this disorder, since 98% of the random donor platelets will be positive for the Pl^{A1} antigen and will be rapidly destroyed by the circulating maternal alloantibody in the neonate. Maternal platelets, which by definition lack the responsible antigen, will be compatible with the alloantibody and survive normally in the neonate. Maternal platelet transfusion is the treatment of choice to support the newborn's platelet count and prevent potentially serious complications. The disorder is self-limited and usually disappears by 3 to 4 weeks of age in surviving infants. Maternal platelets for transfusion should be obtained by a plateletpheresis procedure, during which the mother's platelets are removed but her RBCs and plasma are returned to her. This technique allows the mother to donate platelets again in a few days if they are needed by the infant, and it is safe even in the postpartum period. In the laboratory, alloantibody-containing plasma should be removed before transfusion, and the maternal platelets resuspended in ABO-compatible FFP or in ACD solution. (See Part one.)

Product definition. A standard platelet concentrate prepared from a single donation of whole blood contains a minimum of 5.5×10^{10} platelets in 50 to 60 ml of relatively fresh plasma. Platelets are optimally stored at 20° to 24° C (68° to 75° F) with gentle agitation and have a shelf life of 5 days from collection. One donor unit is usually the only source of a single platelet transfusion for a neonate. Transfusion of one unit of platelets per kilogram body weight should result in a platelet count increment of approximately 250,00/mm³. This is equivalent to an expected increment of 75,000 to 100,000/mm³ in an average term infant from one unit of platelets. This magnitude of increment is often not observed, in part because of the high incidence of destructive thrombocytopenias in the neonatal population. To transfuse a therapeutic dose of platelets without intravascular volume overload, the product may be concentrated to a minimum volume of 15 to 20 ml without functional damage to the platelets. These platelets should be transfused immediately after concentration and resuspension, since their shelf life is only 4 hours after processing.

Plateletpheresis concentrates are available in all areas of the United States but not necessarily in all individual hospitals. These platelet concentrates are produced from a single blood donor, whose plasma and RBCs are returned throughout the procedure. In this way a much larger volume of donor blood can be processed, yielding more platelets per product. The expected yield from plateletpheresis is a minimum of 3.0×10^{11} platelets per product; however, the actual platelet content of an individual product varies according to the donor's predonation platelet count and the volume of donor blood actually processed during a given procedure. It is possible to split a plateletpheresis unit for neonatal use, but this is rarely indicated. The major indication for plateletpheresis products is for those infants with isoimmune neonatal thrombocytopenia for whom the mother is the platelet donor. In this situation the actual platelet donation procedure is frequently abbreviated, resulting in a platelet concentrate of a size more suitable for a newborn. This minimizes the chance of wasting a specially donated component.

Indications. As in older children and adults, platelet transfusions are administered primarily to treat or to prevent the hemorrhagic manifestations of thrombocytopenia in the neonate. The platelet count that indicates significant risk of bleeding is controversial, and in all probability varies with clinical situations, such as coexisting illnesses, required medications that may interfere with platelet function, anatomic lesions, DIC, and many others. Among older patients an inverse relationship has been demonstrated between the platelet count and the bleeding time and also between the platelet count and the frequency and severity of hemorrhage. Significantly more thrombocytopenic neonates (platelet count $\leq$100,000/mm^3) develop skin, renal, pulmonary, or central nervous system hemorrhage than nonthrombocytopenic infants, and the thrombocytopenic infants also have a higher mortality rate.

In practice, platelet transfusions are given to neonates with platelet counts below 30,000/mm^3 to 50,000/mm^3 from any etiology except immune thrombocytopenia, to prevent hemorrhage. Even higher platelet counts may constitute an indication for prophylactic transfusion if surgical intervention is anticipated, if medications that potentially interfere with platelet function are necessary, or if rapid peripheral platelet destruction is present.

Therapeutic platelet transfusions, those given to actively bleeding infants, should be considered for infants with less than 100,000 platelets/mm^3. Data demonstrate that the bleeding time begins to become abnormally prolonged when the platelet count drops below 100,000/mm^3. Platelet transfusions may also be indicated to treat hemorrhage in the presence of qualitative platelet dysfunction. The response to platelet transfusion in these infants is measured by the cessation of bleeding.

Technical aspects

1. Platelets should be ABO and Rh compatible with the recipient whenever possible (Table 32-5). If incompatible platelets must be used, consideration should be given to removal of the incompatible plasma and resuspension of the platelets in compatible plasma. Although Rh matching does not affect posttransfusion platelet survival, RBCs contaminating the platelet concentrate theoretically may cause Rh sensitization in the recipient. This does occur in older patients but has never been well documented in the neonate. Platelet concentrates that are not visibly pink contain less than 0.5 ml of RBCs; whether Rh sensitization actually is a risk from this tiny volume of RBCs in infants who rarely if ever make RBC alloantibodies is unknown. The use of Rh immune globulin in neonates within 72 hours of exposure to Rh-positive RBCs through a platelet transfusion is controversial.
2. No pretransfusion compatibility testing for platelet transfusion is required.
3. The needle gauge used for platelet transfusion is apparently not too critical; however, when this issue has been studied, the conditions did not precisely mimic those in the neonatal intensive care setting. It is probably safe to use the guidelines for needle size for RBCs when transfusing platelets.
4. Platelets must be transfused through a standard 170 μm blood filter. Microaggregate filters should not be used because large platelet losses have been observed during passage through these filters. Moderate impairment of platelet function and fall in pH occur when platelets held in syringes are exposed to radiant heaters or to warm air incubators.
5. Platelets should not be warmed before transfusion.
6. Platelets should not be put into a refrigerator, even for a short period. If a product cannot be used immediately, it may be left at room temperature for a short time or returned to the standard controlled-environment conditions in the blood bank.
7. Various infusion pumps may be used for platelet infusion when precise control over the infusion rate is important or when an extremely slow infusion rate is required.

Granulocyte transfusion

See also Chapter 31, part one.

An alternative therapy to double-volume exchange transfusion for overwhelming neonatal sepsis is the administration of granulocyte concentrates. Unlike other blood components, most granulocyte concentrates are obtained from leukapheresis procedures rather than from the centrifugation and physical separation of this component from single units of whole blood. Some methods of obtaining granulocytes from whole blood have been described; typically the product is called a "buffy coat." There is limited clinical experience using this component.

Several reports have been published suggesting improved survival among neonates treated with granulocyte transfusion. Laurenti and colleagues transfused septic neonates with repeated leukocyte transfusions obtained by filtration leukapheresis, a technique of granulocyte procurement infrequently used because of the high incidence of donor reactions and recipient reactions and the substantial evidence that cells obtained by this method are functionally inferior to almost all other granulocytes. Laurenti reported that when those infants with fulminant disease, negative blood cultures, or an inadequate number of granulocyte transfusions were excluded, an improved survival rate was seen among transfused neonates compared to untransfused neonates (72% survival versus 10%). Christensen and associates showed that granulocytes collected from normal donors by centrifugation using hydroxyethyl starch as an RBC sedimenting agent improved survival among septic neonates with documented depletion of their storage neutrophils. Data of Cairo and co-workers suggest a decreased mortality among infants with clinically suspected sepsis, with or without marrow neutrophil depletion, who were transfused with granulocytes obtained from family members or unrelated donors. Donors were premedicated with steroids to increase the granulocyte yield from the donation. Stork and colleagues used buffy coat concentrates prepared from fresh whole blood (less than 6 hours from collection) for transfusion to neutropenic neonates with presumed sepsis or necrotizing enterocolitis. In this randomized, controlled trial no survival advantage could be demonstrated in the transfused group. In contrast to other reports in which no adverse effects of granulocyte transfusion were observed, these investigators reported respiratory compromise in two infants after repeated granulocyte transfusions. Alternate methods of neonatal granulocyte concentrate production have been described, although clinical experience with these products is limited.

Additional well-controlled prospective studies of neonatal granulocyte transfusion are needed before this therapy is accepted as routine. At least the following issues related to this therapy need to be addressed:

1. The population of infants likely to benefit from this therapy needs to be clearly defined and methods devised by which these infants could be rapidly and reliably identified. The validity of transfusing normal adult granulocytes for neonatal neutrophil dysfunction should be addressed.
2. The optimum granulocyte product needs to be described, considering at least the following: ready availability of a product that cannot be stored as an inventory item, the optimum granulocyte dose, the tolerable limits of volume and hematocrit of the product, the functional characteristics of granulocytes for transfusion, the risk to the neonate, and the risk to the donor.
3. The optimum method of administering the product and the duration of therapy should be addressed.

When granulocyte concentrates are transfused, the following guidelines apply:

1. Because of the large number of RBCs contaminating most granulocyte concentrates, the product must be ABO and Rh compatible with the intended neonatal recipient.
2. Pretransfusion compatibility testing is required.
3. The product must be irradiated.
4. The granulocyte concentrate should be given by partial exchange transfusion if the infant is unable to tolerate the volume or the additional transfusion of RBCs. Hypervolemia and polycythemia with hyperviscosity are potential risks with serious consequences.
5. Granulocyte concentrates should be transfused as soon as available. If any storage is necessary, the product should be stored at room temperature (20° to 24° C) without agitation. It should not be placed in the refrigerator.
6. Granulocyte concentrates should not be warmed above room temperature before transfusion.
7. Standard 170 μm blood filters must be used to administer the transfusion. Microaggregate filters should be avoided because of the probability of large cell losses in these filters.
8. The minimal needle caliber for vascular access is unknown; however, 23-gauge needles were used in published therapeutic trials.
9. At least some of the commercially available electromechanical infusion pumps are satisfactory for granulocyte transfusion.

POTENTIAL INFECTIOUS COMPLICATIONS OF TRANSFUSION

Inherent infectious risks are associated with transfusion, although the incidence, compared to the total number of transfusions administered annually, is very small.

All blood collection agencies take precautions to reduce the risk of transfusion-transmitted diseases, including:

1. Donor health history, which includes specific questions about jaundice, fever, night sweats, lymphadenopathy, exposure to persons with hepatitis or AIDS, and travel outside the United States
2. Specific screening tests on each unit of donated blood for syphilis serology, hepatitis B surface antigen, and antibody to human immunodeficiency virus (HIV)
3. Maintenance of a permanent record of donors who have ever tested positive for any of these

Additional specific measures have been taken to eliminate those persons in high-risk groups for AIDS from the donor pool. The details of these measures vary by geographic location. The list of transfusion-transmitted infections is extensive, as shown in the boxed material. The following sections cover those most relevant to the neonate.

Hepatitis

See also Chapter 31, part two.

Any blood component that has been prepared from whole blood by simple centrifugation and physical separation can potentially transmit hepatitis. Three distinct types of posttransfusion hepatitis are recognized.

Hepatitis A

Hepatitis A (HAV) is an infrequent posttransfusion complication, partly because of the very short period of viremia and the lack of an asymptomatic carrier state associated with HAV. Since the availability of test kits for IgM anti-HAV, the antibody that signifies recent HAV infection, several reports have documented the transfusion transmission of this viral disease in neonates. HAV

Transfusion-transmitted infections

VIRAL
Hepatitis A
Hepatitis B
Hepatitis non-A, non-B
Human immunodeficiency virus (AIDS virus)
Cytomegalovirus
Human parvovirus
Epstein-Barr virus

TREPONEMAL
Syphilis

PARASITIC
Malaria
Filariasis
Trypanosoniasis
Toxoplasmosis
Babesiosis

BACTERIAL
Brucellosis
Multiple other organisms

Modified from Bove, J.R.: Transfusion-transmitted diseases: current problems and challenges. In Brown, E., editor: Progress in hematology, vol. XIV, Orlando, Fla., 1986, Grune & Stratton, Inc.

has been reported in 11 neonates all exposed to the same single blood unit, an epidemic which illustrates one of the potential hazards of using a single unit of blood for transfusion to many infants. Other reports document nursery outbreaks that involve many infants and staff members. In one case two infants exposed to one blood donor became infected, and one of these infants subsequently was responsible for the spread to 15 nurses and one parent. The index case developed asymptomatic HAV from parenteral exposure to a single blood donor who was IgM-anti-HAV positive, despite the fact that, of all the transfusions she received, 39% were from HAV-immune donors. This lack of protection suggests inadequate quantities of specific γ-globulin were passively transferred with transfusion of RBCs.

Hepatitis B

Exposure to blood is the most common source of hepatitis B (HBV) infection. The elimination of paid blood donors and the uniform screening of each blood donation for HBV surface antigen has drastically reduced the incidence of posttransfusion HBV to less than 10% of the total number of reported cases of posttransfusion hepatitis. Posttransfusion HBV is often acutely asymptomatic but may also be rapidly fatal or evolve into a chronic asymptomatic carrier state.

Non-A, non-B hepatitis

Approximately 90% of posttransfusion hepatitis is non-A, non-B (NANB) hepatitis, so called because its etiologic agent, which is most likely viral, remains unidentified but is not HAV or HBV. The incidence of posttransfusion NANB hepatitis is estimated to be between 7% and 17% of blood recipients. Although the acute illnesses are usually asymptomatic, the chronic sequelae may be much more serious, with chronic active hepatitis identified in as many as 60% of patients and cirrhosis in 20%. Since the etiologic agent is unidentified, no specific test exists for NANB hepatitis. Some studies have suggested an association between posttransfusion NANB hepatitis and the receipt of blood from asymptomatic, apparently healthy donors with high levels of serum alanine-aminotransferase (ALT). Many blood centers routinely defer potential donors found to have elevated ALT levels. It is probable that, in the absence of a major breakthrough in the search for the agent responsible for NANB hepatitis, ALT screening of all blood donors will be required. Blood donor ALT screening may decrease posttransfusion NANB hepatitis by 30% to 40%.

HIV infections

Human immunodeficiency virus (acquired immunodeficiency syndrome)

See also Chapters 30 and 31, part two.

Transfusion-associated AIDS (TAA) is defined by the Centers for Disease Control as a condition characterized by the signs and symptoms of AIDS occurring in a person who is not a member of a known high-AIDS-risk group and who has been transfused within the previous 5 years. Fewer than 3% of all known AIDS cases are suspected of having been transmitted via transfusion of a blood component or a blood derivative. Most of these cases are linked to blood donations that occurred before the identification of HIV as the causative agent of AIDS and the availability, in early 1985, of an assay to screen all blood donations for antibody to HIV.

The risk of TAA varies from one region to another. There is a direct relationship between the risk of TAA and the overall incidence of AIDS in the community. TAA is known to have a very long incubation period from exposure to clinical illness (15 to more than 50 months); however, the time from parenteral exposure to the virus via blood transfusion to seroconversion is remarkably short, nearly always less than 6 to 9 months. Any blood component produced by simple centrifugation and separation from an infectious unit of whole blood could potentially be responsible for AIDS transmission. Exposure to large numbers of different blood donors is related to an increased risk of TAA.

TAA is an important and very emotional issue in neonatal intensive care facilities, where many transfusions are administered and severely ill infants are repeatedly transfused. Despite efforts to minimize the number of different blood donors to whom a neonate is exposed, multiple transfusions invariably lead to multiple donor exposures. The first reported case of AIDS suspected to have been transmitted via blood transfusion occurred in a 20-month-old infant who had been transfused shortly after birth with blood components from 19 different blood donors. One of these blood donors, healthy at the time of blood donation, subsequently died of AIDS.

Clearly the elimination of high-risk-group members from the blood donor pool plus the routine laboratory testing of each blood donation for HIV antibody has reduced and should continue to reduce the already small risk of TAA.

Cytomegalovirus

See the previous section on special needs of the neonatal recipient.

Malaria

Transfusion-associated malaria is a rare complication; usually fewer than 10 cases per year are reported in the United States. The disease has been reported, however, in premature infants after the transfusion of very small volumes of RBCs (9, 15, 35 ml). Careful blood donor history is relied on for the elimination of potentially infectious units from the blood supply, since no routine screening test for malaria is used.

Syphilis

Posttransfusion syphilis is so extraordinarily rare that individual cases are generally worth reporting. One recent report documented posttransfusion syphilis after an exchange transfusion with fresh whole blood in an infant of 32 weeks' gestation. Only fresh blood components or those stored at room temperature (i.e., platelet and leukocyte concentrates) have the potential to transmit syphilis, since the causative organism does not survive at 4° C for longer than 120 hours. In addition, few blood donors are potentially infectious because only those in the early stage of disease, where spirochetemia is present before seroconversion occurs, pose any threat. Federal regulations require, however, that every blood component must be negative to a serologic test for syphilis.

Bacterial contamination

Bacteremia resulting from a bacterially contaminated blood component is also an infrequent complication. When it does occur, it is more likely to be related to the transfusion of a blood component that has been stored at room temperature, since most of the bacterial contaminants are skin organisms which do not grow well in the cold. *Yersinia enterocolitica*, a gram-negative enteric organism which grows well at 4° C, is an exception to this generalization; it has been reported recently as the cause of a fatal septic episode that resulted from a RBC transfusion. Blood components pooled before transfusion, such as cryoprecipitate and platelet concentrates, are potentially at higher risk of contamination because of the many manipulations and entries into the component bags required during processing. Repeated entries into a unit of RBCs or plasma for small-volume neonatal transfusions also pose a slightly increased risk of contamination, particularly if diligent attention is not paid to a well-designed protocol to ensure sterile technique during aspiration of a blood component into a syringe and its subsequent transfusion.

Significance of transfusion-associated risks

Neonatal blood transfusion is clearly associated with various known and unknown risks: infectious, immunologic, biochemical, hematologic, cardiovascular, and others. Many of these potential transfusion risks exist for any transfusion recipient; however, at least several pose a greater threat to the neonatal transfusion recipient. None of these potential risks is a contraindication to necessary transfusion. The possibility of a transfusion-associated complication, however, underscores the importance of the appropriate use of blood component therapy for specific indications.

Phyllis I. Warkentin

BIBLIOGRAPHY

Neonatal transfusion therapy

General references

Gray, J.M.: The use of blood components in fetal and neonatal medicine. In Umlas, J., and Silvergleid, A.J., editors: Transfusion for the patient with selected clinical problems, Arlington, Va., 1982, American Association of Blood Banks, pp. 117-179.

Lubin, B.: Neonatal anaemia secondary to blood loss, Clin. Haematol. **7**:19, 1978.

MacMahon, P., Jones, S.T., and Kovar, I.Z.: Hypoglycaemia and blood transfusions in the newborn, Lancet **2**:388, 1985.

Montgomery, R.R., Marlar, R.A., and Gill, J.C.: Newborn haemostasis, Clin. Haematol. **14**:443, 1985.

Murphy, R.J.C., Malhotra, C., and Sweet, A.Y.: Death following an exchange transfusion with hemoglobin SC blood, J. Pediatr. **96**:110, 1980.

Irradiation of blood components

Button, L.N., and others: The effects of irradiation on blood components, Transfusion **21**:419, 1981.

Leitman, S.F., and Holland, P.V.: Irradiation of blood products: indications and guidelines, Transfusion **25**:293, 1985.

Park, B.H., and others: Fatal graft-vs.-host reaction following transfusion of allogeneic blood and plasma in infants with combined immunodeficiency disease, Transplant. Proc. **6**:385, 1974.

Parkman, R., and others: Graft-versus-host disease after intrauterine and exchange transfusions for hemolytic disease of the newborn, N. Engl. J. Med. **290**:359, 1974.

Schechter, G.P., Whang-Peng, J., and McFarland, W.: Circulation of donor lymphocytes after blood transfusion in man, Blood **49**:651, 1977.

Stites, D.P., and Pavia, C.S.: Ontogeny of human T cells, Pediatrics **64**(suppl.):795, 1979.

Thompson, J.E., and others: Development of apparent graft vs host (GVH) reaction following a maternal platelet transfusion in an immunocompetent infant, Pediatr. Res. **15**(4):604, 1981.

Consequences of stored blood

Batton, D.G., Maisels, M.J., and Shulman, G.: Serum potassium changes following packed red blood transfusions in newborn infants, Transfusion **23**:163, 1983.

Heaton, A., and others: Use of Adsol preservation solution for prolonged storage of low viscosity AS-1 red blood cells, Br. J. Haematol. **57**:467, 1984.

Kahn, R.C., and others: Hemodynamic oxygen transport and 2,3-diphosphoglycerate changes after transfusion of patients in acute respiratory failure, Intensive Care Med. **12**:22, 1986.

Latham, J.T., Bove, J.R., and Weirich, F.L.: Chemical and hematologic changes in stored CPDA-1 blood, Transfusion **22**:158, 1982.

Sohmer, P.R., and Dawson, R.B.: The clinical implications of stored blood. In Sherwood, W.C., and Cohen, A., editors: Transfusion therapy: the fetus, infant, and child, New York, 1980, Masson Publishing USA, Inc.

Compatibility testing in the neonatal period

Ludvigsen, C., and others: Failure of neonates to form red blood cell alloantibodies following transfusion, Transfusion **22**:405, 1982.

Mollison, P.L.: Blood transfusion in clinical medicine, ed. 7, Oxford, 1983, Blackwell Scientific Publications, Ltd.

Schmidt, P.J., editor: Standards for blood banks and transfusion services, ed. 11, Arlington, Va., 1984, American Association of Blood Banks.

Technical aspects of neonatal transfusion

Butch, S.H.: Technical aspects of transfusion. In Luban, N.L.C., and Keating, L.J., editors: Hemotherapy of the infant and premature, Arlington, Va., 1983, American Association of Blood Banks.

Herrera, A.J., and Corless, J.: Blood transfusions: effect of speed of infusion and of needle gauge on hemolysis, J. Pediatr. **99**:757, 1981.

Luban, N.L.C., Mikesell, G., and Sacher, R.A.: Techniques for warming red blood cells packaged in different containers for neonatal use, Clin. Pediatr. **24**:642, 1985.

Sagi, E., and others: Exchange transfusion in newborns via a peripheral artery and vein, Eur. J. Pediatr. **137**:283, 1981.

Schmidt, W.F., III, and others: RBC destruction caused by a micropore blood filter, JAMA **248**:1629, 1982.

Strauss, R.G., and others: Effects of environmental warming on blood components dispensed in syringes for neonatal transfusions, J. Pediatr. **109**:109, 1986.

Strauss, R.G., and others: Sterility and quality of blood dispensed in syringes for infants, Transfusion **26**:163, 1986.

Thompson, H.W., Lasky, L.C., and Polesky, H.F.: Evaluation of a volumetric intravenous fluid infusion pump for transfusion of blood components containing red cells, Transfusion **26**:290, 1986.

Exchange transfusion

Aranda, J.V., and Sweet, A.Y.: Alterations in blood pressure during exchange transfusion, Arch. Dis. Child. **52**:545, 1977.

Chopek, M., and McCullough, J.: Protein and biochemical changes during plasma exchange. In Berkman, E.M., and Umlas, J., editors: Therapeutic hemapheresis, Washington, D.C., 1980, American Association of Blood Banks.

Christensen, R.D., and others: Exchange transfusion as an alternative to granulocyte concentrate administration in neonates with bacterial sepsis and profound neutropenia, J. Clin. Apher. **2**:177, 1984.

Delivoria-Papadopoulos, M., and others: Neonatal oxygen transport: the role of exchange transfusion. In Sherwood, W.C., and Cohen, A., editors: Transfusion therapy: the fetus, infant, and child, New York, 1980, Masson Publishing USA, Inc.

Delivoria-Papadopoulos, M., and others: The role of exchange transfusion in the management of low-birth-weight infants with and without severe respiratory distress syndrome. I. Initial observations, J. Pediatr. **89**:273, 1976.

Diamond, L.K., Allen, F.H., Jr., and Thomas, W.O., Jr.: Erythroblastosis fetalis. VII. Treatment with exchange transfusion, N. Engl. J. Med. **244**:39, 1951.

Goldman, S.L., and Tu, H.C.: Automated method for exchange transfusion: a new modification, J. Pediatr. **102**:119, 1983.

Greenberg, J., and Sacher, R.A.: Exchange transfusion in the newborn. In Luban, N.L.C., Keating, L.J., editors: Hemotherapy of the infant and premature, Arlington, Va., 1983, American Association of Blood Banks.

Gross, S.J., Filston, H.C., and Anderson, J.C.: Controlled study of treatment for disseminated intravascular coagulation in the neonate, J. Pediatr. **100**:445, 1982.

Hovi, L., and Siimes, M.A.: Exchange transfusion with fresh heparinized blood is a safe procedure: experiences from 1069 newborns, Acta Paediatr. Scand. **74**:360, 1985.

Nieburg, P.I., Stockman, J.A., III: Rapid correction of anemia with partial exchange transfusion, Am. J. Dis. Child. **131**:60, 1977.

Setzer, E.S., and others: Exchange transfusion using washed red blood cells reconstituted with fresh-frozen plasma for treatment of severe hyperkalemia in the neonate, J. Pediatr. **104**:443, 1984.

Sotelo-Avila, C., Brouillette, R.T., and Gould, S.D.: The hematocrit of reconstituted blood for exchange transfusion in newborn infants, J. Pediatr. **100**:971, 1982.

Vain, N.E., and others: Role of exchange transfusion in the treatment of severe septicemia, Pediatrics **66**:693, 1980.

Vaughan, R.L.: Morbidity due to exchange transfusion with heat-hemolyzed blood, Am. J. Dis. Child. **136**:646, 1982.

Wallerstein, H.: Treatment of severe erythroblastosis by simultaneous removal and replacement of the blood of the newborn infant, Science **103**:583, 1946.

Red blood cell transfusion

Kakaiya, R.M., and others: Pedi-pack transfusion in a newborn intensive care unit, Transfusion **19**:19, 1979.

Kim, H.C.: Red blood cell transfusion in the neonate, Semin. Perinatol. **7**:159, 1983.

Sanner, H.E., and Wooten, M.J.: Analysis of saline-washed red cells for transfusion to neonatal patients, Transfusion **25**:437, 1985.

Staples, J.W., and Fritz, G.E.: Development and use of pediatric frozen red cell packs, Transfusion **16**:566, 1976.

Stockman, J.A., III: Anemia of prematurity. Current concepts in the issue of when to transfuse, Pediatr. Clin. North Am. **33**:111, 1986.

Stockman, J.A., III: Red cell transfusion in the newborn. Indications and unique blood banking needs, Am. J. Pediatr. Hematol. Oncol. **3**:205, 1981.

Stockman, J.A., III, and Clark, D.A.: Weight gain: a response to transfusion in selected preterm infants, Am. J. Dis. Child. **138**:828, 1984.

Transfusion of platelets and plasma

Gill, F.M.: Transfusion therapy for coagulation disorders in the newborn infant. In Sherwood, W.C., and Cohen, A., editors: Transfusion therapy: the fetus, infant and child, New York, 1980, Masson Publishing USA, Inc.

Johnson, C.A., Snyder, M.S., and Weaver, R.L.: Effects of fresh frozen plasma infusions on coagulation screening tests in neonates, Arch. Dis. Child. **57**:950, 1982.

Kevy, S.V., Fosburg, M., and Wolfe, L.: The use of platelets, plasma and plasma derivatives in the newborn. In Luban, N.L.C., and Keating, L.J., editors: Hemotherapy of the infant and premature, Arlington, Va., 1983, American Association of Blood Banks.

Moroff, G., and others: Reduction of the volume of stored platelet concentrates for use in neonatal patients, Transfusion **24**:144, 1984.

Sills, R.H., and Stuart, M.J.: Platelet transfusion in the newborn. In Sherwood, W.C., and Cohen, A., editors: Transfusion therapy: the fetus, infant, and child, New York, 1980, Masson Publishing USA, Inc.

Granulocyte transfusion

Cairo, M.S., and others: Improved survival of newborns receiving leukocyte transfusions for sepsis, Pediatrics **74**:887, 1984.

Christensen, R.D., Anstall, H.B., and Rothstein, G.: Depletion of neutrophils during neonatal septicemia: mechanisms involved and experimental treatments. In Luban, N.L.C., and Keating, L.J., editors: Hemotherapy of the infant and premature, Arlington, Va., 1983, American Association of Blood Banks.

Chistensen, R.D., and others: Granulocyte transfusions in neonates with bacterial infection, neutropenia, and depletion of mature marrow neutrophils, Pediatrics **70**:1, 1982.

Laurenti, F., and others: Polymorphonuclear leukocyte transfusion for the treatment of sepsis in the newborn infant, J. Pediatr. **98**:118, 1981.

Shigeoka, A.O., Hall, R.T., and Hill, H.R.: Blood-transfusion in group-B streptococcal sepsis, Lancet **1**:636, 1978.

Stork, E., Baley, J., and Shurin, S.: A controlled trial of granulocyte transfusions in neutropenic neonates, Pediatr. Res. **19**:336A, 1985.

Potential infectious complications of transfusion

Adler, S.P.: Transfusion-associated cytomegalovirus infections, Rev. Infect. Dis. **5**:977, 1983.

Arnow, P.M., and others: *Escherichia coli* sepsis from contaminated platelet transfusion, Arch. Intern. Med. **146**:321, 1986.

Azimi, P.H., and others: Transfusion-acquired hepatitis A in a premature infant with secondary nosocomial spread in an intensive care nursery, Am. J. Dis. Child. **140**:23, 1986.

Bove, J.R.: Transfusion-transmitted diseases: current problems and challenges. In Brown, E., editor: Progress in hematology, vol. XIV, Orlando, Fla., 1986, Grune & Stratton, Inc.

Curran, J.W., and others: Acquired immunodeficiency syndrome (AIDS) associated with transfusions, N. Engl. J. Med. **310**:69, 1984.

Demmler, G.J., and others: Posttransfusion cytomegalovirus infection in neonates: role of saline-washed red blood cells, J. Pediatr. **108**:762, 1986.

Taylor, B.J., and others: Frozen deglycerolyzed blood prevents transfusion-acquired cytomegalovirus infections in neonates, Pediatr. Infect. Dis. **5**:188, 1986.

Tolpin, M.D., and others: Transfusion transmission of cytomegalovirus confirmed by restriction endonuclease analysis, J. Pediatr. **107**:953, 1985.

Yeager, A.S., and others: Prevention of transfusion-acquired cytomegalovirus infections in newborn infants, J. Pediatr. **98**:281, 1981.

CHAPTER 33

The neonatal gastrointestinal tract

PART ONE

Development

The ability to supply a consistent input of qualitatively and quantitatively normal nutrients to a low birth weight infant is limited by immaturity of gastrointestinal tract (hepatic and intestinal) function. Teleologic principles would suggest there may be certain advantages to this normal developmental phase; survival of the species might not otherwise be possible. This is an important area for further study. In addition, more efficient means of delivery of calories to the low birth weight infant must be devised. Intraluminal nutrients and hormones released from the gastrointestinal tract in response to *consistent* enteral nutrient input play major roles in the interrelated series of events allowing adaptation to extrauterine life.

EMBRYOLOGY

Organogenesis

The developing organism undergoes a series of sequential, coordinated changes in morphology and metabolism that result in the formation of organized arrangements of specialized cells. Table 33-1 summarizes the major events that occur during development of the gastrointestinal tract. By 4 weeks' gestation the hepatobiliary system and pancreatic buds have begun to form. Over the next 1 to 2 weeks the intestine elongates more rapidly than does the embryo itself and forms a loop that protrudes along the yolk stalk into the umbilical cord. Between the sixth and eighth week of fetal development, while the greatest portion of the intestine is still in the umbilical cord, the nascent small intestine rotates around the axis of the superior mesenteric vessels in a counterclockwise fashion. The duodenum and the splenic flexure of the colon do not enter into the cord but are held in position by mesenteric bands. Over the next 2 weeks the small intestine continues to grow and coil inside the cord; at 10 weeks' gestation the intestine reenters the abdominal cavity, with the jejunum leading the way and filling the left portion of the abdominal cavity. The ileum follows and fills the right half of the abdominal cavity; the colon then reenters. The cecum becomes fixed close to the iliac crest, and the ascending and transverse colon come to lie in their respective positions. Abnormalities of exit or return of the intestine lead to various types of nonrotation or malrotation.

Characteristically, during intestinal ontogenesis, differentiation and maturation progress from the proximal to the distal portions of the digestive system. Villi are present in the jejunum by 9 weeks and in the entire small intestine by 14 weeks' gestation, at which time they are lined by a single layer of cells with centrally placed nuclei. Primitive crypts of Lieberkuhn begin to appear by 10 to 12 weeks, and by 19 weeks' gestation well-developed villi and crypts are found even in the ileum. The enterocytes develop microvilli by 3 to 10 weeks of intrauterine life. These are initially short and irregularly spaced, demonstrate different stages of maturity, and have a partially developed glycocalyx. By the tenth week of intrauterine life the microvilli are regular, and many mitochondria are present beneath the microvilli.

Pancreatic parenchymal tissue is derived from the primitive gut. A dorsal and ventral outpouching of the primitive midgut unite to form the pancreas. The dorsal (nascent body and tail) and ventral (gives rise to head of pancreas) anlagen may be evident by the fourth week of gestation as evaginations of the foregut. The anlagen fuse in appropriate position by the sixth week; fusion of the ductular system follows. Anomalies arise from faulty rotation around the duodenum and during fusion of the dorsal and ventral pancreas (e.g., heterotopic or annular, pancreas divisum).

A sparse number of secretory granules are detected

Table 33-1. Development of the human gastrointestinal tract from the entoderm (epithelial lining and glandular epithelium) and a mesoblastic mesenchymal layer (muscular, vascular, serosal elements)

Age (weeks)	Crown-rump length (mm)	Stage of development
2.5	1.5	Gut not distinct from yolk sac
3.5	2.5	Foregut and hindgut present
		Yolk sac broadly attached at midgut
		Liver bud present
		Mesenteries forming
4	5.0	Intestine present as a single tube
		Esophagus and stomach distinct
		Liver cords, ducts, and gallbladder forming
		Omental bursa forming
		Pancreatic buds appear as outpouching of gut
5-6	8.0-12.0	Intestine elongates into a loop and rotates
		Stomach rotates
		Parotid and submandibular buds appear
7	17.0	Circular muscle layer present
		Duodenum temporarily occluded
		Intestinal loops herniate into cord
		Villi begin to develop
8	23	Villi lined by single layer of cells
		Small intestine coiling within cord
		Taste buds appear
		Microvilli short, thick, and irregularly spaced
		Lysosomal enzymes detected
9-10	30-40	Auerbach's plexus appears
		Intestine reenters abdominal cavity
		Crypts of Lieberkühn develop
		Active transport of glucose appears
		Dipeptidases present
		Microvilli of enterocytes more regular and glycocalyx present
		Mitochondria numerous below microvilli
12	56	Parietal cells present in stomach
		Muscular layers of intestine present
		Alkaline phosphatase and disaccharidases detectable
		Active transport of amino acid present
		Mature taste buds present
		Enterochromaffin cells appear
		Pancreatic islet cells appear
		Bile secretions begin
		Colonic haustra appear
		Coelomic extension into umbilical cord obliterated
13-14	78-90	Meissner's plexus appears
		Circular folds appear
		Peristalsis detected
		Lysosomes detected ultrastructurally
16	112	Pancreatic lipase and tryptic activity detected
		Meconium present
		Lymphopoiesis present
		Peptic activity present
20	160	Peyer's patches present
		Muscularis mucosa present
		Mesenteric attachments complete
		Zymogen granules present and well developed in pancreas
24	200	Paneth's cells appear
		Maltase and sucrase and alkaline phosphatase very active
		Ganglion cells detected in rectum
		Amylase activity present
28	240	Lactase activity increasing
		Esophageal glands present
32	270	Circular folds present
		Hydrochloric acid found in stomach
34	290-300	Sucking and swallowing become coordinated
		Esophageal peristalsis rapid, nonsegmental contraction occurs
36-38	320-350	Maturity of GI tract achieved

Modified from Arey, L.B.: Developmental anatomy: a textbook and laboratory manual of embryology, ed. 7, Philadelphia, 1965, W.B. Saunders Co.

by the twelfth week, and detectable levels of pancreatic lipase and trypsin activity are detectable at about the sixteenth week. Well-developed zymogen granules are noted at the twentieth week of fetal life. The activities of the digestive enzymes progressively increase, however, and remain markedly low in the neonate as compared with the older infant.

The esophagus, which develops from the foregut during the fourth week of gestation, has attained its normal position by the seventh week as the stomach has descended into the abdomen. By 13 weeks of intrauterine life the longitudinal muscle layers and muscularis are well formed. The ganglion cell element, although well differentiated, is not evenly distributed until after the eighteenth week of gestation. The epithelial lining is initially columnar and then becomes ciliated by the fifth to sixth month of intrauterine life. Stratified squamous epithelium is present. The esophagus is the only part of the digestive system that apparently has neither digestive nor absorptive function. It serves as a conduit for food from the mouth to the stomach and as a barrier against reflux of gastric contents.

Cellular proliferation, differentiation, and maturation

The functions of the gastrointestinal tract are diversified and include absorption and digestion of nutrients, maintenance of fluid and electrolyte balance and protection of the host from toxins and pathogens. The energy requirements for the rapid growth observed in healthy premature and full-term infants must be met by effective digestion and absorption of protein, fat, and carbohydrate. The gastrointestinal tract undergoes substantial changes during the perinatal period; in the premature infant the gastrointestinal tract may not have reached full functional capacity. After birth the intestine is exposed to a variety of toxins and bacteria at a time when immature immune function increases the susceptibility of the neonate to infection. The capacity of the gastrointestinal tract to meet the digestive and immunologic needs of the infant during the perinatal period will be reviewed.

DEVELOPMENT OF MOTILITY

There is a cranial-to-caudal migration of neuroblasts during the fifth to twelfth weeks of gestation. By 24 weeks the normal distribution of ganglion cells is present so that it is possible to histologically make the diagnosis of Hirschsprung's disease in a premature infant. There is a gradual and steadily progressive maturation of ganglia from early embryonic life throughout childhood. Early immaturity of the cells is physiologic, and maturation takes place gradually over the first several years of life.

Swallowing occurs in the human fetus such that by 16 to 17 weeks of intrauterine life the fetus ingests 2 to 7 ml of amniotic fluid every 24 hours. By 20 to 21 weeks this volume has increased to 16 ml per day, and at term the infant swallows approximately 450 ml of amniotic fluid per day. Although there is marked variation, the coordination of sucking and swallowing is not well developed before 34 weeks' gestation.

Esophageal motility also is poorly developed in the preterm infant. There is poor coordination in response to deglutition, rapid peristaltic waves, and simultaneous nonperistaltic contractions along the entire length of the esophagus. The lower esophageal sphincter pressures are also decreased, and gastric emptying time is delayed—increasing the risk of developing gastroesophageal reflux. As the fetus matures, there is an increased rate of motility through the intestinal tract. For example, administered contrast material would reach the cecum of a 32-week premature infant in 9 hours, and of the full-term infant in 4 to 7 hours. Immaturity of the muscular layers of the intestinal tract, incoordination of peristaltic waves, an increase in the number of antiperistaltic waves, and possibly decreased hormonal secretions all contribute to the prolonged transit time commonly encountered in the preterm infant. Preterm infants rarely pass meconium in utero even when subjected to severe asphyxia, whereas full-term and postterm infants pass meconium readily, even if the asphyxial episode is brief (Chapter 28, part five). Preterm infants, especially those with respiratory distress, have an absent or impaired rectosphincteric reflex and behave similarly to patients with Hirschsprung's disease. Many of these infants temporarily display a pattern that suggests a functional obstruction.

ABSORPTIVE FUNCTION

The postnatal development of essential gastrointestinal functions is governed by interacting determinants: (1) genetic endowment, (2) the "biologic clock" or intrinsic timing mechanisms, (3) environmental influences such as changes in diet composition, and (4) regulatory or "triggering" mechanisms, namely hormonal input. Although exact role of each of these factors in modulating perinatal adaptation needs to be more fully defined, it is important to keep the latter two concepts in mind while planning to feed the low birth weight infant. The major trophic influence on the intestinal tract is the presence of intraluminal nutrients, which is closely related to hormonal release. The sequence of emergence of various digestive enzymes is shown in Table 33-1.

Carbohydrate absorption

Salivary and pancreatic amylase activity are detectable by 22 weeks' gestation, but the amylase content of pancreatic tissue or duodenal juice remains low even after birth. In contrast, glucoamylase, an intestinal brush border enzyme that removes glucose from the nonreducing end of starch, demonstrates activity at 1 month similar to that found in adults. With the exception of lactase, dissacharidase activity reaches adult levels by the twenty-eighth week of gestation. Lactase activity does not reach full-term levels until 36 weeks. In studies using breath hydrogen analysis as a measure of carbohydrate malabsorption most preterm infants demonstrate lactose malabsorption for several weeks. Despite lactose malabsorption, growth rates and stool patterns remain normal in healthy premature infants on lactose-containing formula or breast milk. Fermentation of malabsorbed lactose by the colonic bacterial flora may result in production of volatile organic acids, which are then absorbed by the colon. Absorption of these fermentation products minimizes energy loss by small intestinal malabsorption of lactose. Changes in the colonic flora associated with broad spectrum antibiotics or diversion of the intestinal stream following surgery could place the premature infant at increased risk for significant carbohydrate malabsorption.

Except in the case of lactose, the rate-limiting step in carbohydrate absorption is the ability of the developing intestine to transport glucose. Glucose absorption seemingly is less efficient in developing intestine compared to the mature intestine. Despite the decreased amylase and lactase activity and the diminished capacity of the intestine to transport glucose, carbohydrate malabsorption is not a clinical problem in healthy preterm infants, perhaps because of the colonic salvage mechanism.

Protein absorption

The pH of gastric contents is increased in newborn infants compared to older children and adults because of decreased basal and stimulated HCl secretion and prolonged buffering by stomach contents. As a result, pepsin is inactivated and there is no intragastric digestion of protein in infants 5 to 8 days old. Both chymotrypsin and trypsin activities are decreased at birth in preterm and full-term infants. Mucosal dipeptidase activity and amino acid transport capacity are well developed in early life. Despite decreased activity of enzymes involved in protein digestion, 85% of the dietary nitrogen intake is absorbed by infants regardless of age, diet, or maturity. Newborn infants completely digest cow's milk protein at concentrations similar to the protein concentration in breast milk.

Increased intestinal uptake of intact protein has been demonstrated in newborn compared to adult animals and has been attributed to decreased secretory IgA, decreased proteolysis, or increased mucosal permeability to protein in the developing gut. Enhanced uptake of proteins could sensitize the developing organism to food antigens or permit potentially damaging proteases to enter the portal circulation.

Lipid digestion

The processes mediating the intraluminal phases of fat digestion and the enterohepatic circulation of bile acids mature sequentially to ensure acclimation after the termination of gestation; a considerable degree of coordination exists. Perinatal delay in establishing efficient mechanisms for the absorption of fat (and for the establishment of bile flow) will create a significant nutritional disadvantage for the newborn. The severity of the inefficiency may be inversely related to the length of gestation.

The overall efficiency of intestinal intraluminal and hepatic excretory function for fat digestion depends on effective bile formation. Bile flow is directly dependent on the adequate synthesis, conjugation, secretion, and recirculation of bile acids (i.e., the enterohepatic circulation). Efficient biliary elimination of bile acids, the main determinant of bile flow in the mature animal, allows for the delivery of bile acids, which are critical for lipid digestion, to the intestinal lumen. In utero, the fetus is dependent on the placenta for delivery of nutrients. Progressive maturation occurs in the liver and gastrointestinal tract to permit successful transition from the fetal environment to the extrauterine environment. Failure to adequately adapt to premature exposure to these new demands will be associated with inefficiency of intestinal digestive and absorptive function. Lipids can be absorbed by pinocytosis from the gut of a 12-week-old human fetus; however, efficient postnatal fat digestion and absorption is more complex. The transfer of insoluble dietary lipid, which is the major caloric source in early life, from the gut lumen to the aqueous environment of the body is initiated by key intraluminal events: (1) emulsification of fat globules, (2) enzymatic (lipase) hydrolysis of triglycerides, (3) solubilization of the lipolytic products, and (4) transfer across the intestinal mucosa. The mucosal phase of fat absorption is well developed at birth; therefore luminal events, which require bile acids to function efficiently, are overall rate-limiting in fat absorption. There are sufficient animal data to document an immaturity of many of the processes involved in the enterohepatic circulation of bile acids in early life. (See box.)

Physiologic steatorrhea is primarily due to intraluminal detergent (bile acid) deficiency. Infants will not achieve adult levels of efficiency of fat absorption until approximately age 4 to 5 months. Inefficient use of dietary fats may be exacerbated by predominant long-chain fat inges-

Summation of data from various species that indicates bile acid metabolism and transport function at reduced rates in early life

HUMAN STUDIES

1. ↓ Hepatic bile acid clearance (reflected by ↑ serum bile acid levels and exaggerated postprandial rise)
2. ↓ Bile acid pool size
3. ↓ Bile acid synthetic rate
4. Altered bile acid synthetic pathways (i.e., production of atypical bile acids)
5. Low intraluminal bile acid concentrations
6. ↓ Ileal active transport of bile acids

ANIMAL STUDIES

1. ↓ Hepatic clearance of bile acids reflected by:
   a. ↑ Serum bile acids levels
   b. ↓ Uptake by liver cells/vesicles
2. ↓ Bile acid pool size (? ↓ synthetic rate)
3. ↓ Rate of intracellular metabolism of bile acids
   a. ↓ Conjugation rate
   b. ↓ Sulfation rate
4. ↓ Bile acid secretion rate
   a. ↑ Intrahepatic retention
   b. ↓ Basal levels of bile acid secretion
5. ↓ Ileal active transport of bile acids

From Balistreri, W.F., Heubi, J.E., and Suchy, F.J.: Immaturity of the enterohepatic circulation in early life: factors predisposing to "physiologic" maldigestion and cholestasis, J. Pediatr. Gastrenterol. Nutr. **2:**346, 1983.

tion. The limiting factor appears to be inadequate micelle formation resulting from the low concentration of intraluminal bile acids; therefore there is inadequate solubilization of dietary triglycerides.

Preterm infants who receive only intravenous dextrose for the first few days of life have no postnatal rise in various gastrointestinal hormones. Preterm infants who are fed orally have a dramatic surge in hormonal output. These data have led Lucas to suggest that enteral feeding is a "triggering" mechanism and that, if at all possible, early consistent enteral nutrition, "minimal enteral feeding," is extremely beneficial.

Inherent, specific, compensatory processes may ameliorate the impact of impaired fat absorption. Because of low activity of pancreatic lipase, the newborn must depend on extrapancreatic lipases for adequate fat digestion. For example, lingual lipase, which mediates intragastric lipolysis, partially compensates for the relative pancreatic lipolytic defect. Breast milk, in addition to trophic factors such as epidermal growth factor and hormones, contains a bile salt–stimulated lipase, which can complement the activity of lingual lipase and result in near-complete hydrolysis of dietary triglyceride. Nonnutritive sucking (NNS), via use of a pacifier during gavage feeding of premature infants, may be associated with an accelerated maturation of the sucking reflex, facilitate transition to oral feeding, decrease intestinal transit time, and shorten hospital stay; this needs further study. The physiologic mechanisms of NNS are not defined, although decreased energy expenditure during pacification and improved nutrient absorption are possible. Sucking is an important stimulus for the secretion of lingual lipase.

During the phase of inefficient use of orally administered lipids it may be possible to reduce the critical need for bile acids through the administration of formulas that include medium-chain triglycerides (MCT) as a major caloric source. MCT is well absorbed, even in the face of impaired lipolysis and impaired micellar solubilization.

ROLE OF COLON DURING DEVELOPMENT

In developing and mature animals the colon absorbs Na^+ and H_2O from the intestinal lumen. Active Na^+ absorption can be increased 300% to 400% by the presence of aldosterone, suggesting that the colon plays a critical role in maintenance of salt and water homeostasis. Diversion of the fecal stream after intestinal surgery will increase Na^+ and H_2O requirements in preterm and full-term infants. In contrast to the adult colon, the developing colon may be involved in nutrient absorption. Colonic mucosa from developing rats and second trimester fetuses has well-developed villi. Active transport of glucose and amino acids has been demonstrated by colonic mucosa from developing animals. In addition to involvement with salt and water homeostasis, the developing colon may absorb essential nutrients, partially compensating for decreased absorption of nutrients by the small intestine during development.

GUT IMMUNOLOGY AND PROTECTIVE PROPERTIES OF HUMAN MILK

See also Chapter 30.

The gastrointestinal tract protects the host from a variety of toxins, pathogens, and foreign antigens. Decreased gastric acidity, decreased protease activity, increased permeability of intestinal mucosa to foreign proteins, decreased intraluminal bile acids and dysmotility may compromise local defense mechanisms of the intestine in preterm of full-term infants. Mucosal protection is further compromised by decreased levels of secretory IgA demonstrated in the intestinal secretions of newborn animals.

Numerous studies suggest that breast-feeding protects infants against infections and allergic disorders because of the presence of numerous "protective agents" found in human milk. Growth of lactobacilli is stimulated in the colon of infants fed human milk. Organic acids produced by the bacteria inhibit the growth of enteric pathogens. Bacteriocidal enzymes and high concentrations of secretory IgA are present throughout lactation. Proteins present in human milk bind nutrients essential for bacterial metabolism. These observations suggest that human milk provides mucosal immunity against toxins, antigens, and pathogens until the infant's defense mechanisms mature.

SUMMARY

The gastrointestinal tract is capable of readily adapting to extrauterine life by 36 weeks' gestation; there is sufficient activity of various enzymes, the transport of nutrients is relatively efficient, and the ability to respond to antigenic stimuli is present. However, the *preterm* infant, in whom the intestinal tract has not reached full functional capacity, is vulnerable to the development of necrotizing enterocolitis, enteric infections, and to delayed growth or development. Various physiologic factors interfere with normal gastrointestinal function in preterm infants. These include:

1. Poor coordination of sucking and swallowing
2. Incompetent lower esophageal sphincter
3. Delayed gastric emptying time
    a. Decreased gastric acidity
    b. Decreased pepsinogen production
4. Decreased absorption of fat
    a. Decreased bile acid production and bile flow
    b. Decreased micelle formation
    c. Decreased lipolytic activity
5. Incomplete digestion of protein
6. Decreased activity of lactase
7. Decreased or poorly coordinated GI motility
8. Decreased secretions of immunoglobulins and decreased immunologic response
9. Decreased rate of cellular proliferation and migration

John C. Bucuvalas
William F. Balistreri

BIBLIOGRAPHY

Balistreri, W.F., Heubi, J.E., and Suchy, F.J.: Immaturity of the enterohepatic circulation in early life: factors predisposing to "physiologic" maldigestion and cholestasis, J. Pediatr. Gastroenterol. Nutr. **2**:346, 1983.

Balistreri, W.F., and others: Physiologic immaturity of the enterohepatic circulation of bile acids. In Barbara, L., and others, editors: Bile acids in gastroenterology, Lancaster, Penn., 1983, MTP Press Ltd.

Bernbaum, J.C., and others: Nonnutritive sucking during gavage feeding enhances growth and maturation in premature infants, Pediatrics **71**:41, 1983.

Boyer, J.L.: New concepts of the mechanisms of hepatocyte bile formation, Physiol. Rev. **60**:303, 1980.

Corring, T., Durand, G., and Henry, Y.: Some aspects of development and nutrition in the monogastric animal during postnatal life, World Rev. Nutr. Diet. **39**:124, 1982.

Cotton, P.B.: Congenital anomaly of pancreas divisum as cause of obstructive pain and pancreatitis, Gut **21**:105, 1980.

Ferguson, D.R., and others: Aldosterone induced changes in colonic sodium transport occurring naturally during development in neonatal pig, J. Physiol. **292**:495, 1979.

Ghishan, F.K., and Wilson, F.A.: Developmental maturation of D-glucose transport by rat jejunal brush border membrane vesicles, Am. J. Phys. **248**:G87, 1984.

Goldman, A.S., and Goldblum, R.M.: Protective properties of human milk. In Walker, W.A., and Watkins, J.B., editors: Nutrition in pediatrics: basic science and clinical application, Boston, 1985, Little, Brown & Co.

Grand, R.J., Watkins, J.B., and Torti, F.M.: Development of the human gastrointestinal tract: a review, Gastroenterology **70**:79, 1976.

Hamosh, M.: Lingual and breast milk lipases. In Barness, L.A., editor: Advances in pediatrics, vol. 29, Chicago, 1982, Year Book Medical Publishers.

Hamosh, M., and others: Fat digestion in the newborn: characterization of lipase in gastric aspirates of premature and term infants, J. Clin. Invest. **67**:838, 1981.

Henning, S.J.: Postnatal development: coordination of feeding, digestion and metabolism, Am. J. Physiol. **241**:G199, 1981.

Heubi, J.E., Balistreri, W.F., and Suchy, F.J.: Bile salt metabolism in the first year of life, J. Lab. Clin. Med. **100**:127, 1982.

Hirata, Y., and Matsuo, T.K.: Digestion and absorption of milk protein in infants' intestine, Kobe J. Med. Sci. **11**:103, 1965.

Hofmann, A.F.: The enterohepatic circulation of bile acids, Clin. Gastroenterol. **6**:3, 1977.

Jones, R.S., and Meyers, W.C.: Regulation of hepatic biliary secretion, Ann. Rev. Physiol. **41**:64, 1979.

Kien, C.L., and others: A method for assessing carbohydrate energy absorption and its application to premature infants, Am. J. Clin. Nutr. **36**:910, 1982.

Koldovsky, O.: Digestion and absorption. In Stave, U., editor: Perinatal physiology, New York, 1978, Plenum Publishing.

Koldovsky, O.: Digestion and absorption of carbohydrates, protein, and fat in infants and children. In Walker, W.A., Watkins, J.B., editors: Nutrition in pediatrics: basic science and clinical application, Boston, 1985, Little, Brown & Co.

Lebenthal, E.: Infant nutrition: metabolism and the digestive system, J. Pediatr. Gastroenterol. Nutr. (suppl. 1) **2**:S57, 1983.

Liao, T.H., Hamosh, P., and Hamosh, M.: Gastric lipolysis in the developing rat: ontogeny of the lipases active in the stomach, Biochem. Biophys. Acta **754**:1, 1983.

Lucas, A.: Endocrine aspects of enteral nutrition. In New aspects of clinical nutrition, Basel, Switzerland, 1983, Karger.

MacClean, W.C., Jr., and Fink, B.B.: Lactose malabsorption by premature infants: magnitude and clinical significance, J. Pediatr. **97**:383, 1980.

MacLaurin, J.C., and others: Fat calcium and nitrogen balance in full-term infants, Post Grad. Med. **51**:45, 1975.

Mares, A.J., and Hirsch, M.: Congenital cysts of the head of the pancreas, J. Pediatr. Surg. **12**:547, 1977.

Phillip, J., Koch, H., and Classen, M.: Variations and anomalies of the papilla of vater, the pancreas, and the biliary duct system, Endoscopy **6**:70, 1974.

Signer, E., and others: Role of bile salts in fat malabsorption of premature infants, Arch. Dis. Child. **49**:174, 1974.

Udall, J.N., and Pang, K.: Development of gastrointestinal mucosal barrier. I. The effect of age on intestinal permeability to macromolecules, Pediatr. Res. **15**:241, 1981.

Watkins, J.B.: Mechanisms of fat absorption and the development of gastrointestinal function, Pediatr. Clin. North. Am. **22**:721, 1975.

Weijers, H.A., Drion, E.F., and Van De Kamer, J.H.: Analysis and interpretation of the fat-absorption coefficient, Acta Paediatr. Scand. **49**:615, 1960.

Westergaard, H., and Dietschy, J.M.: Delineation of dimensions and permeability characteristics of the two major diffusion barriers to passive mucosal uptake in rabbit intestine, J. Clin. Invest. **54**:718, 1974.

PART TWO

Selected anomalies and intestinal obstruction

ABDOMINAL WALL DEFECTS

Abdominal wall defects in infants include two subtypes: (1) omphalocele and (2) gastroschisis. Omphaloceles are formed by incomplete closure of the anterior abdominal wall after the return of the midgut during the tenth to twelfth week of gestation. Complete abdominal wall integrity is dependent on appropriate closure of the embryonic cephalic, caudal, and lateral folds of the abdominal wall. Failure of migration and fusion of the lateral abdominal folds is associated with the formation of a central abdominal omphalocele with insertion of the umbilical cord onto the central omphalocele sac with a surrounding fascial defect (Fig. 33-1). Although the size of the fascial defect can vary, with large defects the entire midgut, as well as the stomach, liver, and spleen, may be herniated. The abdominal cavity remains diminutive in the absence of the visceral contents. Smaller defects include only herniated intestine and minimal abnormalities in peritoneal size. Defects of less than 4 cm are classified as hernias of the umbilical cord but require treatment as if they were central omphaloceles. Failure of growth and fusion of the lateral and cephalic folds results in the pentalogy of Cantrell, consisting of a cleft sternum, anterior midline diaphragmatic defects, a pericardial defect, congenital cardiac abnormalities including ectopia cordis, and an upper abdominal omphalocele. Incomplete closure of the caudal and lateral abdominal folds results in cloacal or bladder exstrophy and hypogastric omphalocele.

Rupture of an omphalocele before or at the time of delivery can occur and is associated with evisceration of the abdominal contents through the normal covering membranous sac, exposing the herniated viscera to the amniotic fluid.

Gastroschisis is distinguished from omphalocele by having a defect on the abdominal wall that is of smaller size and lateral to the umbilicus, the umbilical cord being normally attached to the abdominal wall immediately to the left of the defect (see Fig. 33-1). No covering sac is found, and the herniated viscera is usually limited to the small intestine and occasionally a small portion of the liver. In addition, the intestine that has been exposed to amniotic fluid for a prolonged period of time appears foreshortened because of mesenteric thickening and interloop adhesions. Ischemic compromise of the herniated intestine can occur because of mesenteric compression when the abdominal wall defect is extremely small.

The embryologic etiology of gastroschisis is unclear. Rupture of a hernia of the umbilical cord through the site of the obliterated left umbilical vein after completion of the enfolding of the somatic components of the anterior abdominal wall but before closure of the umbilical ring has been postulated by Sharf.

The diagnostic distinction between omphalocele and gastroschisis is of importance because of the difference in the spectrum of associated anomalies seen with each syndrome. Omphaloceles have associated cardiac, neurologic, genitourinary, skeletal, or chromosomal abnormalities in 67% of infants. Cardiovascular malformations occur in 15% to 25% of children with central omphaloceles and are invariably present in infants with Cantrell's pentalogy. Anomalies associated with the lower midline omphaloceles include vesicointestinal fistula, imperforate anus, colonic agenesis, and the exstrophy complex. In addition, in the Beckwith-Wiedemann syndrome (omphalocele, macroglossia, macrosomia, and hypoglycemia), the associated pancreatic hyperplasia or nesidioblastosis can be associated with severe episodes of hypoglycemia within the first hours of life, which can cause permanent neurologic damage if not anticipated and prevented (Chapter 37). In addition, trisomy 13 or trisomy 18 has been associated with the omphalocele complex. Infants with omphaloceles also have a high incidence of gastrointestinal anomalies including malrotation, midgut volvulus, Meckel's diverticula, intestinal atresias or duplication, and diaphragmatic hernias.

Gastroschisis, however, has very few nongastrointestinal anomalies. Gastrointestinal anomalies include malrotation, jejunoileal atresia secondary to ischemic occlusion from constricting abdominal wall defects, and Meckel's diverticula. In addition, prematurity has been seen in up to 60% of patients with gastroschisis.

The preoperative management of all patients with abdominal wall defects is the same regardless of their subtype. A nasogastric tube should be placed for intestinal decompression, and the eviscerated intestine or sac should be covered with warm, moist dressings. An intravenous line should be placed and vigorous fluid resuscitation undertaken. Infants with suspected Beckwith-Wiedemann syndrome should have frequent serum glucose determinations; they require mandatory intravenous glucose support. All infants with exposed eviscerated intestine require immediate surgical intervention after resuscitation, whereas those with a covering sac can receive a more extensive evaluation before surgical intervention. A careful preoperative search should be made for associated anomalies, and congenital cardiac disease should be excluded.

The surgical correction of abdominal wall defects must be individualized in accordance with several factors: the presence of an intact sac, the size of the eviscerated contents relative to the abdominal cavity, the nature of the herniated viscera, and the possibility of associated

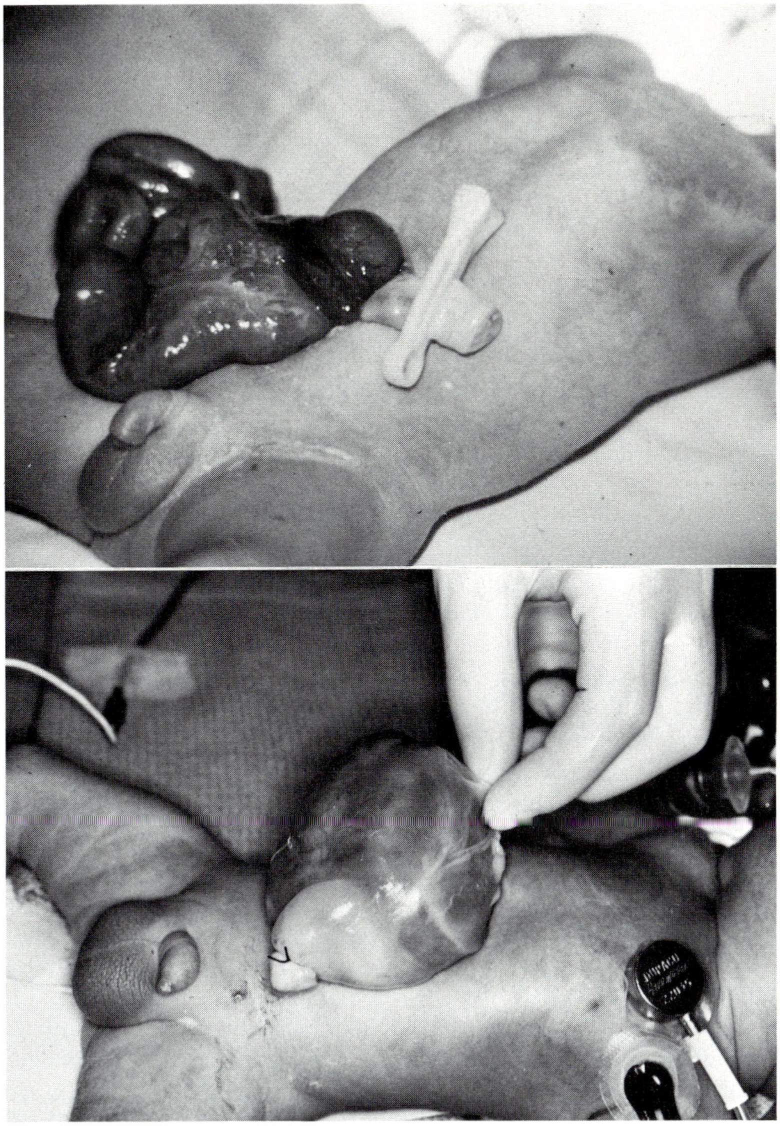

Fig. 33-1. A, Gastroschisis. Herniated midgut with thickened, foreshortened mesentery to the right of the normal umbilical cord insertion site. **B,** Omphalocele. Newborn with intact omphalocele sac containing intestine and liver. The umbilical cord inserts onto the sac. (Photograph courtesy R.J. Stevenson, M.D.)

anomalies. These factors are more important than the primary defect (i.e., gastroschisis or omphalocele). Selective management must be employed to achieve the objectives of prompt visceral coverage and treatment of the associated anomalies. Closure of the abdominal wall defect is ideal but not essential at the first surgical procedure. Four methods are currently used.

1. *Primary repair* of the ventral wall defect with complete reduction of the herniated viscera is preferred but not possible in all cases. Infants with isolated intestinal evisceration are optimal candidates. However, the intestinal contents must not be reduced under conditions that create high intraabdominal pressure while attempting primary closure. Compromise of inferior vena caval (IVC) blood return and diaphragmatic elevation will produce postoperative hemodynamic and respiratory complications. Cardiovascular collapse can also result from kinking of the IVC during reduction of the herniated liver. Attempts to monitor the intraabdominal pressure through gastrostomy tube pressures and distal venous pressures are cumbersome and not as reliable as close vigilance of the infant's vital signs. Even when caution is exercised, infants undergoing primary closure often require prolonged periods of respiratory support and

muscular paralysis. The decreasing morbidity from intubation and ventilation in modern intensive care settings has caused some authors to advocate this method for almost all infants. However, attempts to remove all of the inflammatory peel overlying intestine that has been exposed to amniotic fluid in gastroschisis and ruptured omphalocele are not warranted to facilitate primary closure and can damage the underlying intestine.

2. *Staged reduction* of the herniated viscera is best suited for infants with large defects containing the liver and intestine, and those that cannot tolerate primary repair. Staged reduction requires the placement of a prosthetic silo of mesh-reinforced silastic material to allow progressive daily reduction of the abdominal contents. These daily reductions can be done in the nursery without anesthesia, which allows assessment of the degree of respiratory and vascular compromise. It has been our policy to *construct* the silos using local anesthesia when staged reduction appears prudent, reserving general anesthesia for the final abdominal closure. Reduction can take up to 10 days. At its completion the silo is removed and the ventral abdominal wall defect is closed. Mesenteric vascular compromise can occur within the silo, and frequent inspection of the herniated contents should be carried out through the opaque sac. Local infection is controlled by the application of antibacterial ointment (e.g., Betadine) to the silo and the suture lines. Staged reduction using sequential ligation of the omphalocele sac itself has been reported, but it has not been widely adapted.

3. *Skin flap closure* over the herniated viscera without ventral wall repair is used primarily in infants with multiple complex congenital anomalies. The presence of a sac overlying the viscera facilitates this closure method. The skin flaps are mobilized laterally and inferiorly, but not superiorly, so as not to impede thoracic growth. Skin closure prevents local infection while more immediate associated anomalies and problems are addressed. The ventral hernia is then repaired at 6 to 12 months of age. During this interval the progressive growth of the peritoneal cavity can be encouraged by allowing the infant to sleep in a prone position.

4. *Nonsurgical methods* employing desiccation of the sac are indicated only in children with uncorrectable congenital anomalies or in those that cannot tolerate surgical interventions. It can also be employed when staged reduction fails because of infectious complications. The sac is painted with 0.5% Mercurochrome in 65% alcohol on 3 successive days and then is allowed to air dry. Epithelialization will proceed over several weeks. The ventral hernia can be repaired at a later date.

The definitive care of abdominal wall defects requires a thoughtful use of all these treatment options. Overzealous use of primary repair or rapid silo reduction will precipitate mesenteric ischemia and intestinal damage. Even under optimal closure conditions prolonged intestinal dysfunction can result; early institution of hyperalimentation will allow maintenance of normal nutrition and healing.

INTESTINAL DUPLICATIONS

Duplications of the intestinal tract are recognized because of a palpable mass, intestinal obstruction, pain, or bleeding. Only rarely do they perforate. Their individual surgical care is directed by the location of the duplication and its relationship to the neighboring intestine.

The vast majority of duplications involve the small intestine. These are primarily spherical or cylindric. Isolated spherical cystic duplications are best treated by segmental resection of the involved intestine. When long cylindric duplications involve a significant portion of the intestine, resection of the mucosa within the duplication—leaving the muscular wall of the duplication within the mesentery—allows preservation of the native intestine. The high incidence of peptic hemorrhage from ectopic gastric mucosa within these long tubular duplications makes complete mucosal excision mandatory. Intramural cystic duplications at the ileocecal valve region have been responsible for both obstruction and intussusception and are best treated by ileocecal resection.

Colonic duplications frequently occur with the long segment involvement having proximal continuity with the colon, while the distal duplicated intestine forms a second anus. Associated duplication of the genitourinary tract is common. Division of the entire septum between the duplicated rectum and the colon above the anus allows the formation of a single lumen within the intestine. Isolated division of the rectosigmoid septum establishes only distal continuity and has also been successful. When isolated cystic duplications occur in the proximal colon, only segmental resection is necessary. Cystic duplications may also occur posterior to the anorectum, causing rectal obstruction or prolapse of the posterior rectal wall. Transsacral resection is curative, but these masses must be distinguished from sacrococcygeal teratomas and anterior meningoceles. In rare cases these cystic pelvic duplications can occur as masses in the buttock or perineum from herniation through the sciatic notch or obturator foramen.

Stomach and duodenal duplications are much less common than those of the small and large intestine. Gastric duplications should be resected when possible or marsupialized into the normal stomach. Duodenal duplications can only occasionally be resected completely because of involvement of the pancreatic and biliary ducts. Cyst duodenostomy with excision of the duplication mucosa is an acceptable alternative.

INTESTINAL OBSTRUCTION

The differential diagnosis of intestinal obstruction occurring in the newborn period spans a wide spectrum of diagnostic possibilities. Obstruction can arise secondary to a lesion located anywhere from the high esophagus to the anus and can be caused by intrinsic blockade, extrinsic compression, or nonocclusive functional obstruction. Division of these lesions into preampullary, postampullary small intestinal, and colonic obstructions allows their symptoms and presentations to be clearly characterized. The antepartum use of ultrasonography has allowed early recognition of polyhydramnios, distended intestinal loops, and conditions such as abdominal wall defects and congenital diaphragmatic hernia often associated with intestinal developmental abnormalities (Chapter 12). When these complications are suspected after antepartum examination, plans for transport of the mother allowing for delivery of the infant in a medical center capable of neonatal resuscitation and surgical treatment is appropriate.

Preampullary obstructions include tracheoesophageal fistula, pyloroantral mucosal webs, pyloric atresia, and hypertrophic pyloric stenosis. Rarely, duodenal atresia can also occur with preampullary obstruction. Polyhydramnios often occurs because the infant cannot ingest and absorb the appropriate amount of amniotic fluid. Toxemia, diabetes mellitus, multiple gestation, and anencephaly have all been associated with polyhydramnios; any infant with these findings should be suspected of having a high intestinal obstruction. Excessive salivation and frequent nonbilious vomiting are common, but abdominal distension is infrequent and confined to the high epigastric areas. Generalized distension can indicate perforation at the site of obstruction.

Obstruction beyond the ampulla of Vater is characterized by bilious vomiting. All infants seen with bilious vomiting or high volumes (more than 15 ml) of bilious gastric fluid after passage of a nasogastric tube require immediate investigation. As the level of obstruction proceeds distally in the intestinal tract, intestinal and abdominal distension become more prominent features. Delayed or absent passage of meconium is also seen with increasing frequency as the level of the intestinal obstruction proceeds toward the anus. Conditions within this group include duodenal atresia, duodenal webs, annular pancreas, malrotation, jejunoileal atresia, and meconium ileus.

Colonic obstructions are associated with delayed or absent passage of meconium. Once the spectrum of imperforate anus lesions is excluded, most colonic obstructions represent meconium plug syndromes or Hirschsprung's disease. Acquired lesions secondary to necrotizing enterocolitis are also seen in older infants. Delayed passage of meconium is also associated with some metabolic disorders (i.e., hypothyroidism, hypomagnesemia, prematurity, sepsis, and narcotic administration); these all must be excluded.

Physical examination can help define the cause of the obstruction in selected cases, but in the majority of infants, physical examination early following delivery is deceptively normal. The classic auscultatory findings of intestinal obstruction are absent in most infants who may instead have a silent abdomen. Palpable masses are commonly appreciated with meconium ileus and intestinal duplications and are occasionally seen with malrotation and volvulus. Abdominal wall tenderness, erythema, edema, and induration all suggest perforation and peritonitis. Signs of progressive fluid depletion from third space losses are common in late presentations.

Abdominal radiographs are the single most helpful test for defining the cause and level of the intestinal obstruction. Plain supine, upright, and decubitus views give adequate diagnostic information to define the level of obstruction with high gastroduodenal or jejunal lesions. High complete lesions rarely require additional contrast radiographs unless surgical intervention is going to be delayed, in which case malrotation with volvulus must be excluded. Duodenal obstructions caused by atresia, annular pancreas, preduodenal portal vein, and malrotation can all occur with a "double bubble" sign caused by the dilated duodenum and stomach. High jejunal obstructions show dilated loops of proximal bowel with air-fluid levels and no distal air passage. Distal jejunal-ileal and colonic obstructions show numerous loops of dilated intestine with air-fluid levels. A water soluble contrast enema is helpful to define the level of the lesions and will demonstrate an unused "microcolon" in low jejunoileal lesions. Normally, air should reach the large intestine within 8 to 12 hours; failure of distal progression suggests complete obstruction. Calcification within the peritoneal cavity occurs secondary to in utero intestinal perforation and meconium peritonitis. The characteristic changes of meconium ileus, Hirschsprung's disease, and the meconium plug syndromes are also best defined with a contrast enema. The position of the cecum is also noted; however, a right lower quadrant cecum does not unequivocally exclude malrotation. In cases of low colonic obstruction a suction mucosal biopsy to exclude Hirschsprung's disease and a diagnostic sweat chloride for cystic fibrosis will be necessary to confirm the suspected radiographic diagnosis.

In all infants with bilious vomiting and signs of probable intestinal obstruction an orderly but rapid diagnosis should be reached. Plain abdominal radiographs should be taken as fluid resuscitation is begun. Appropriate contrast studies are immediately undertaken when necessary to define the level of obstruction and to exclude malrotation with volvulus. Although central nervous system disease, sepsis, and metabolic disturbances can all lead to bilious vomiting, intestinal obstruction must primarily be excluded. Special care must be given to avoid any delay in the diagnosis and treatment of malrotation with volvulus in all infants with bilious vomiting.

Preampullary obstruction of the intestine

Preampullary obstructions in the intestinal tract primarily involve the stomach and its pyloric outlet. The high level of the obstruction within the gastrointestinal tract precludes abdominal distension, although vomiting, abdominal pain, and occasional gastric bleeding are encountered in these infants. The absence of bile staining of the vomitus is characteristic of the preampullary location. These obstructions include gastric antral mucosal webs, pyloroantral atresia, hypertrophic pyloric stenosis, and the antral dysmotility syndrome.

Gastric antral mucosal webs and pyloroantral atresia

Obstruction of the distal stomach and pylorus can be classified into two types, pyloric and antral (1 cm or more proximal to the pylorus). In each case the obstruction can be complete or partial and occur with a spectrum from a thin membrane to complete atresia. Infants with complete obstruction will have maternal hydramnios and nonbilious vomiting, whereas those with only partially obstructing webs may not show symptoms until several weeks of age with failure to thrive. Failure of coalescence of the vacuoles within the developing stomach epithelium, which establish intestinal patency during the first trimester, is believed to be the embryologic mechanism of these abnormalities. Variability of this failure of coalescence explains the broad spectrum from partially obstructing webs to complete atresia.

The diagnosis is suggested by nonbilious vomiting, dysphagia, dyspnea, excessive salivation, and no palpable "tumor" characteristic of hypertrophic pyloric stenosis. Radiographic confirmation by upper gastrointestinal examination is diagnostic. Thick webs or atresias are easily recognized, although air contrast techniques are often necessary to visualize thin webs. Upper gastrointestinal endoscopy can help confirm the diagnosis in difficult cases.

Surgical therapy for infants with a complete or incomplete pyloroantral web includes a longitudinal gastrotomy overlying the defect, allowing visualization of the web and the associated pyloric outlet. Excision of the web with closure of the stomach mucosa and a Heineke-Mikulicz pyloroplasty is curative. Pyloroantral atresia requires resection of the atretic margin of the stomach and duodenum with reconstruction as a gastroduodenostomy. Gastric decompression is necessary during the healing phase after both surgical procedures, requiring gastrostomy tube drainage or a suitable nasogastric tube.

Nonsurgical therapy has been recommended by some authors for patients with incomplete antral webs and moderate symptoms. Small curd formula and antispasmodics were successful in four patients reported by Tunnell. Although no web was seen on follow-up radiographs at 1½ to 3 years, long-term follow-up is not available and the significance of this observation is unclear. The occurrence of obstructing gastric webs in adults, many of whom had persistent vomiting as infants, suggests that these do not regress, making surgical excision the wisest recourse.

Hypertrophic pyloric stenosis

Hypertrophic pyloric stenosis is an enlargement of the pyloric musculature, causing gastric outlet obstruction in infancy. The cause is unclear, but immature ganglion cells, abnormal ganglion cell distribution, or ganglion cell degeneration have all been proposed by some authors and refuted by others. Hereditary factors are also involved, with male babies affected more often that female babies at a ratio of 4:1. The first-born male seems most often affected. Associations with blood groups O and B, as well as maternal stress in the last trimester of pregnancy, have also been noted. The absence of pathologic changes of pyloric stenosis at birth suggests postnatal "work" hypertrophy or congenital delay of pyloric sphincter development as associated factors.

Nonbilious vomiting is the most common initial symptom associated with later dehydration and hypochloremic hypokalemic metabolic alkalosis. Symptoms can occur as early as the first week of life and as late as 5 months, although the average infant is 3 to 6 weeks of age at presentation. Progressive and protracted vomiting develops, with symptoms evolving over a 1-week period. The diagnosis of pyloric stenosis is confirmed by the presence of visible peristaltic waves in the epigastrium and a palpable pyloric "olive." Radiographic confirmation is unnecessary when the characteristic physical findings are present. In questionable cases ultrasonography can visualize the hypertrophic pyloric musculature, and upper gastrointestinal radiographs will demonstrate pyloric obstruction, with the characteristic "string sign" and enlarged "shoulders" bordering an elongated obstructed pyloric channel (Fig. 33-2).

Preoperative evaluation should include treatment of the hypochloremic hypokalemic alkalosis and vigorous rehydration. Approximately 2% of infants with pyloric stenosis develop indirect hyperbilirubinemia, which is postulated to be secondary to defective hepatic glucuronyl transferase activity, starvation, and increased absorption of unconjugated bilirubin. Spontaneous resolution after pyloromyotomy can be expected.

Hypertrophic pyloric stenosis should be treated by surgical pyloromyotomy after adequate fluid and electrolyte resuscitation. Myotomy throughout the length of the hypertrophic muscle on the anterior gastric wall re-

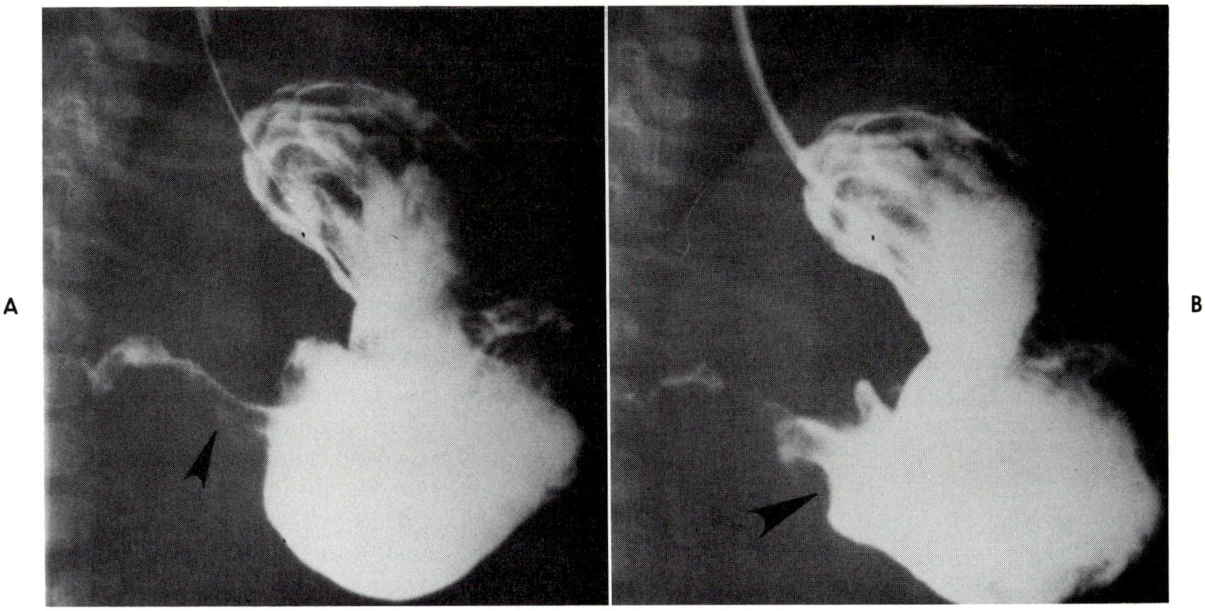

Fig. 33-2. A 5-week-old infant with hypertrophic pyloric stenosis. **A,** Elongated pyloric outlet with "double-tract" sign. **B,** Hypertrophic pyloric muscular "shoulders."

lieves the gastric outlet obstruction. Feedings can be commenced after 6 to 8 hours. In the unlikely event of mucosal perforation, closure of the perforation with placement of an omental patch, or mucosal and muscular closure with repeat myotomy on the posterior gastric wall are acceptable treatment. After perforation the patient should remain NPO with nasogastric decompression until mucosal sealing occurs. Persistent vomiting is uncommon after the first several feedings and is suggestive of an inadequate myotomy. Repeat surgical intervention is indicated after radiographic confirmation.

In infants with nonbilious vomiting and no palpable tumor additional diagnostic considerations include severe pylorospasm secondary to sepsis, salt-losing adrenogenital syndrome and increased intracranial pressure. Cystic pyloric duplications and ectopic pancreatic tissue can both cause nonbilious vomiting and a palpable mass and are distinguishable from hypertrophic pyloric stenosis at laparotomy or by radiographic examination.

Gastric volvulus

Volvulus of the stomach occurs in one of two forms. Volvulus may occur along the long axis of the stomach from the gastric cardia to the pylorus, referred to as *organoaxial volvulus,* or it may rotate in mesenterioaxial fashion twisting anteriorly on an axis crossing from the greater to the lesser curvature. Mesenterioaxial volvulus is more common in infants and produces the characteristic "upside-down" stomach. Acute volvulus produces dramatic symptoms of occlusion of the cardia and pylorus with acute gastric distension and epigastric fullness, whereas partial or recurrent volvulus can cause intermittent and variable symptomatology. Volvulus may occur in conjunction with other associated anomalies such as eventration of the diaphragm, diaphragmatic hernias, and abnormalities of foregut rotation. A lack of peritoneal fixation with ligamentous laxity or abnormal enteromesenteric bands or adhesions have been implicated as an associated cause.

The diagnosis in acute cases is suspected in infants with upper gastric tympany and severe distress associated with retching, abdominal pain, and occasional vomiting. Difficulty passing a nasogastric tube is characteristic. Abdominal radiographs reveal a distended left upper quadrant stomach and occasionally a beaklike narrowing at the obstructed pylorus, twisted gastric mucosal folds, and variable obstruction at the cardia.

Prompt surgical therapy is indicated in all cases of recurrent volvulus or acute gastric volvulus. Reduction of the volvulus and resection of any nonviable regions of the stomach are undertaken, followed by gastric fixation. This can be accomplished using anterior gastropexy associated with a temporary Stamm gastrostomy for decompression. Recurrence after anterior gastropexy and gastrostomy fixation is uncommon but has been reported.

Pyloroantral dysmotility syndrome

Pyloroantral dysmotility syndromes are functional gastric outlet obstructions associated with nonbilious emesis, distinguishable from the anatomic obstructive syndromes only by radiographic investigation. Upper gastrointestinal radiographs disclose delayed gastric emptying with absent antral peristalsis and mild associated gastroesophageal reflux. A characteristic elongated and conical antrum is often seen. These functional obstructions most often respond to positional therapy and small-curd, low-volume feedings, as well as medication (metoclopromide). In those infants who are unresponsive to medical therapy with associated failure to thrive, Heineke-Mikulicz pyloroplasty with extension at least 3 cm onto the antrum and 1 cm onto the pylorus has been successful in improving gastric emptying. Catch-up growth and diminished vomiting have followed surgical intervention in most cases. Gastrostomy tube placement should be undertaken to allow postoperative gastric decompression and later gradual controlled feedings.

Lactobezoars

Lactobezoars are a not uncommon complicaton of feeding high caloric density formulas to small preterm infants. Susceptible patients include those with birth weights of 1,500 gm or less who receive a formula containing 24 calories/ounce, wherein 40% to 50% of the fat content is medium-chain triglycerides (MCT). MCT is absorbed from the stomach, theoretically creating the possibility of a residual nidus for bezoar formation; however, this remains to be proven. Affected infants become symptomatic 3 to 12 days after the onset of feeding. Symptoms usually include abdominal distension, increased gastric residuals, vomiting, diarrhea, and heme-test positive stools. Several infants have been asymptomatic, and the bezoar was found serendipitously. The diagnosis is often made by palpating a mass in the left upper quadrant or by routine radiologic evaluation of the abdomen. A well-formed intraluminal cast surrounded by air may be seen. The injection of 2 to 3 ml/kg of air into the stomach will often outline the bezoar; contrast studies with barium or other imaging agents are not usually needed. The cause of lactobezoars is unknown. Several factors have been cited, such as the delayed gastric emptying time of a sick, premature infant, decreased gastric acidity, the higher caloric density of formulas developed for administration to premature infants, the calcium content of the formula, or the quality and quantity of the fat or the protein. Treatment is initially conservative—nasogastric decompression and lavage have not been necessary in the management of the majority of infants. However, gastric perforation associated with lactobezoars has been reported. Prevention of lactobezoar formation may be possible by delaying the introduction of high caloric density formulas until the infant reaches 2 to 3 weeks of age. The disorder has been encountered, however, in premature infants receiving lower density formulas as well. Bezoars have also been identified in patients who have received antacids as therapy for acute gastritis or for upper gastrointestinal hemorrhage.

Gastric perforation

Gastric perforation in the newborn occurs most often during the first 5 days of life. Spontaneous gastric perforation necessarily excludes perforations secondary to trauma from gastric intubation, distal intestinal obstruction, or accidental insufflation of the stomach during assisted ventilation. Perinatal stress seems to be a causative factor in over 80% of cases with an ischemic mechanism proposed. Infants with perinatal ischemia from placental abruption or placenta previa, those delivered by emergency cesarean section, and those with postnatal asphyxia or shock, and infants requiring exchange transfusion are particularly prone to develop this syndrome. Experimental evidence by many authors has demonstrated prolonged arterial spasm, intravascular capillary stagnation with coagulation, and disruption of capillary vessel walls after ischemic damage. It would appear that this mechanism is common to both gastric perforations and necrotizing enterocolitis. However, in 20% of cases of acute gastric perforation no ischemic stress can be identified. These infants usually have a reluctance to feed after an initial satisfactory feeding period.

Perforation characteristically occurs on the third to fourth day with the abrupt onset of abdominal distension and marked respiratory distress. Vomiting is an inconsistent feature. Radiographic confirmation of massive pneumoperitoneum is suggestive, and contrast studies to confirm the diagnosis are not indicated. Signs of hyvolemic shock and sepsis complete the clinical picture.

Gastric perforation in a newborn represents an immediate surgical emergency. Because of the large size and proximal nature of the perforation, these infants may develop rapidly progressive pneumoperitoneum with associated cardiorespiratory compromise (Fig. 33-3). Emergency bedside paracentesis, using a large intravenous catheter to decompress the abdomen, is often necessary while surgical preparations are being made. A nasogastric tube should be placed while prompt resuscitation is undertaken. Surgical intervention should not be delayed.

The surgical correction of gastric perforation involves debridement of the perforation margins and two-layer closure of the stomach. Gastrostomy tube decompression should be used. The tear often involves the posterior wall of the stomach along the greater curvature, making division of the gastrocolic omentum and exploration of the posterior gastric wall necessary even if a disruption is also found on the anterior wall. Multiple areas of injury must be excluded. The entire intestinal tract should also be examined to exclude other ischemic injuries. The use of near-total gastrectomy for the unfortunate but rare infants with complete gastric necrosis has occasionally lead to survival.

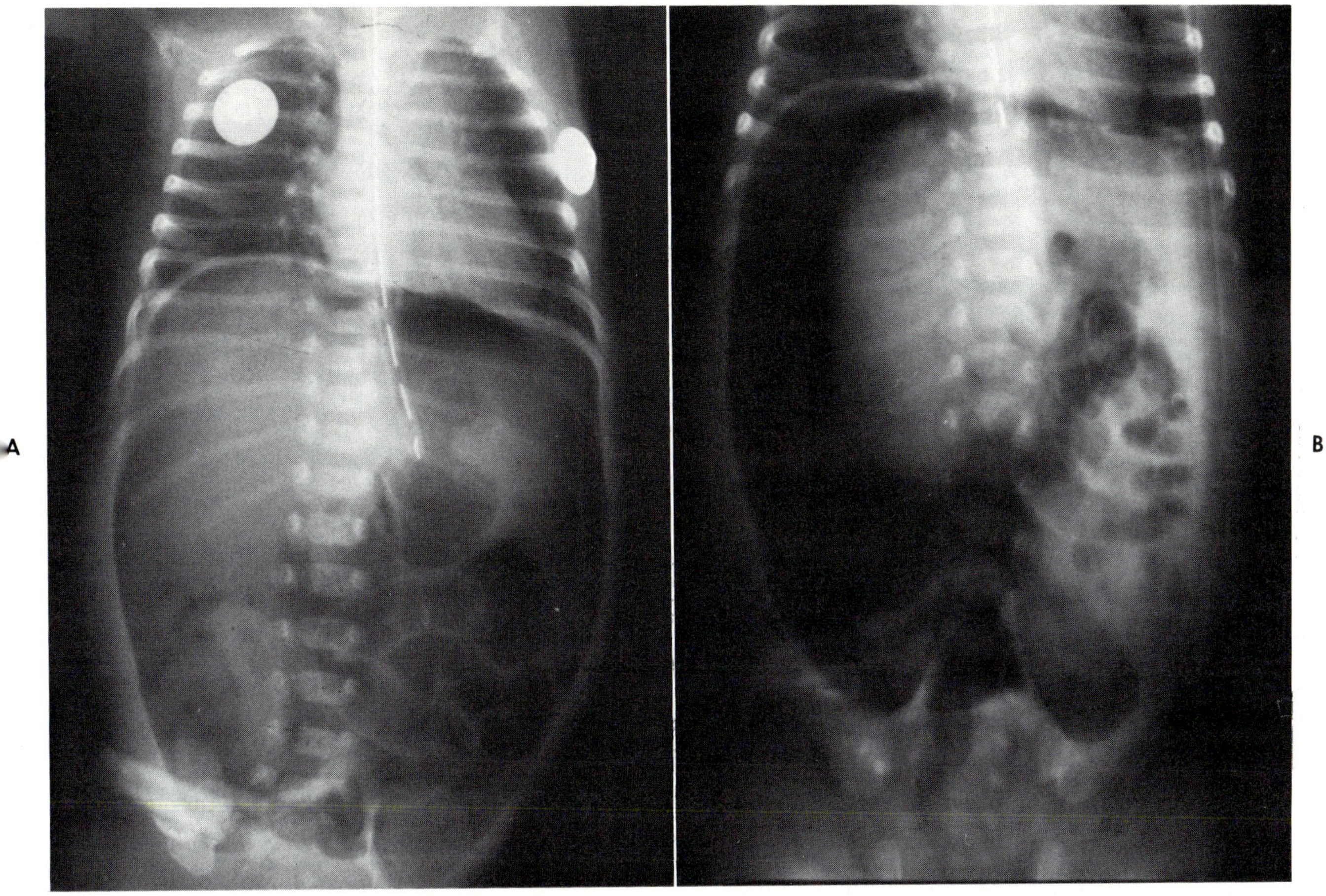

Fig. 33-3. A 3-day-old infant with severe birth asphyxia and acute gastric perforation. Radiographs show massive pneumoperitoneum, **A,** which is confirmed by a left lateral decubitus view. **B,** A large disruption of the greater curvature of the stomach was found at laparotomy.

Postoperative vigorous supportive therapy coupled with broad spectrum intravenous antibiotics is necessary. In spite of optimal intensive care management, mortality continues to be in excess of 50% in many series. The most important factors affecting survival appear to be the interval between the onset of symptoms and definitive therapy, the extent of peritoneal contamination, the degree of prematurity, and the severity of other associated consequences of asphyxia.

Postampullary obstructions

Intrinsic duodenal obstruction

Duodenal atresia is responsible for over 50% of all instances of intrinsic duodenal obstruction. The pathogenesis of this malformation is unknown; however, it appears to result from failure of recanalization of the gastrointestinal tract during the second month of fetal life. This is often found in association with other anomalies, including Down's syndrome, intestinal malrotation, congenital heart disease, tracheoesophageal anomalies, and renal anomalies.

Approximately 20% of patients with congenital intrinsic duodenal obstruction will be found to have an annular pancreas, secondary to persistence of the left bud of the ventral pancreas (Figs. 33-4 and 33-5). There is an association with intrinsic stenosis or atresia of the duodenum. In infants with duodenal obstruction failure to thrive and hyperbilirubinemia may also be present. However, the earliest clue to the possible existence of duodenal obstruction is polyhydramnios. The great majority of lesions are located in the postampullary region of the duodenum; therefore most affected infants will have the onset of bilious vomiting during the first 24 hours of life. Abdominal distension will be localized in the upper abdomen. Respiratory distress secondary to abdominal distension may occur, and meconium is normally passed in the majority of cases. Radiologic evaluation may reveal the classic "double bubble" appearance of duodenal atresia. Bar-

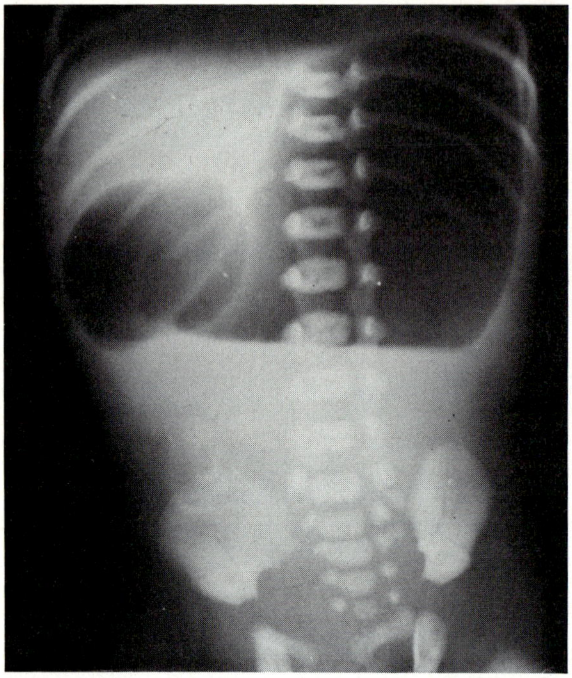

Fig. 33-4. Newborn infant with duodenal atresia. Classical "double bubble" sign with air-fluid levels and no distal intestinal air.

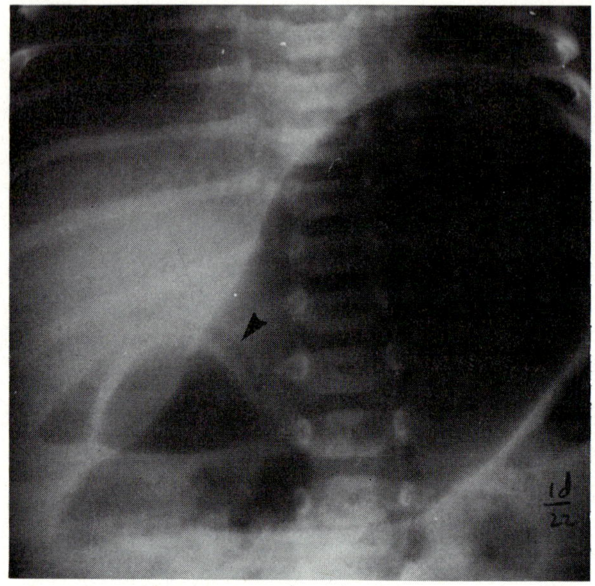

Fig. 33-5. Annular pancreas in a 1-day-old infant. "Double bubble" pattern is seen with distal intestinal air indicating high grade partial obstruction. Air within the common bile duct *(arrow)* and gallbladder is visualized.

ium enema may be helpful to differentiate malrotation and partial duodenal obstruction secondary to fibrous band formation. Contrast studies of the upper gastrointestinal area may be necessary to document the presence of an incomplete duodenal obstruction.

The surgical correction of duodenal obstruction is dictated by the pathologic lesion. Intrinsic lesions must be distinguished from extrinsic compression to allow appropriate therapy.

Duodenal atresia or high grade duodenal stenosis requires reconstruction using a side-to-side duodenostomy. A similar reconstruction is used in cases of annular pancreas to avoid division of the encircling pancreatic ducts within the annular segment. Duodenal webs may occur as an isolated septum or elongate as a "wind sock" within the lumen. Duodenotomy with resection of the web and transverse closure of the duodenum is necessary. Special care must be exercised in all duodenal lesions to identify and protect the biliary and pancratic ducts. These ducts often enter the duodenum along the medial aspect of a duodenal web and are easily traumatized during web resection. Subtotal resection of the web leaving the medial portion in place will avoid injury to these ducts. Similarly, they can occur along the margin of the atretic duodenum and must be identified before a reconstructive anastomosis is undertaken. As in all cases of intestinal atresia, the distal bowel should be carefully inspected for other areas of discontinuity.

The surgical repair of this spectrum of anomalies is often characterized by a long period of delayed gastric emptying after reconstruction. Placement of a gastrostomy tube at the time of correction allows decompression, as well as gradual feeding advancement, to be undertaken. Intravenous hyperalimentation or jejunal feedings distal to the reconstruction allows maintenance of adequate nutrition during this often prolonged period.

Extrinsic duodenal obstruction

Extrinsic compression of the duodenum is most often caused by malrotation and associated volvulus or annular pancreas. Uncommon causes include duplications and retroperitoneal tumors.

Malrotation. Failure of normal rotation and subsequent fixation of gastrointestinal tract result in variable clinical symptoms. This is a potentially lethal disorder. The complications of malrotations are due to intestinal obstruction or vascular compromise (Figs. 33-6 and 33-7). The pathophysiology is due to arrest of the cecum in the upper abdomen, which results in fibrous band formation between the cecum and the posterior peritoneum, causing partial duodenal obstruction (Ladd's bands). Failure of the normal posterior fixation of the small intestine mes-

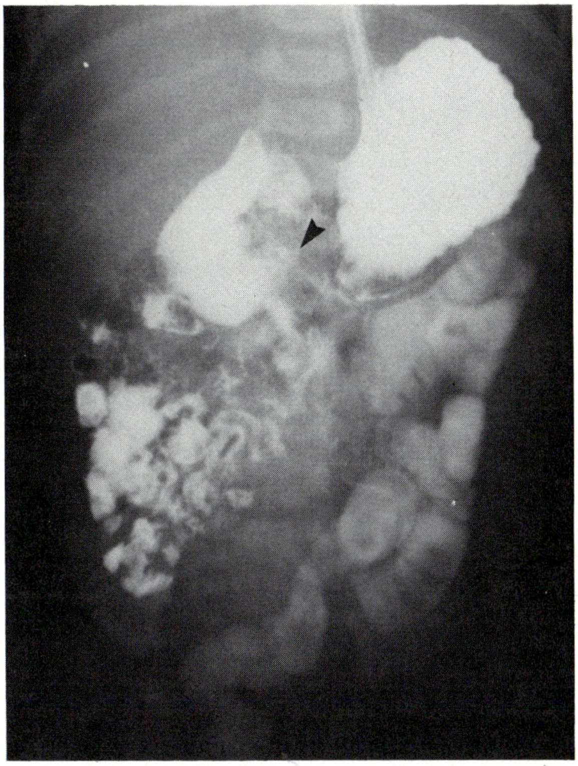

Fig. 33-6. Newborn with bilious vomiting and malrotation. Contrast enema shows the colon within the left abdomen, whereas barium upper gastrointestinal series defines the right abdominal position of the small intestine. Duodenal dilation from partially obstructing Ladd's bands and a low medial displacement of the duodenojejunal junction *(arrow)* can be appreciated.

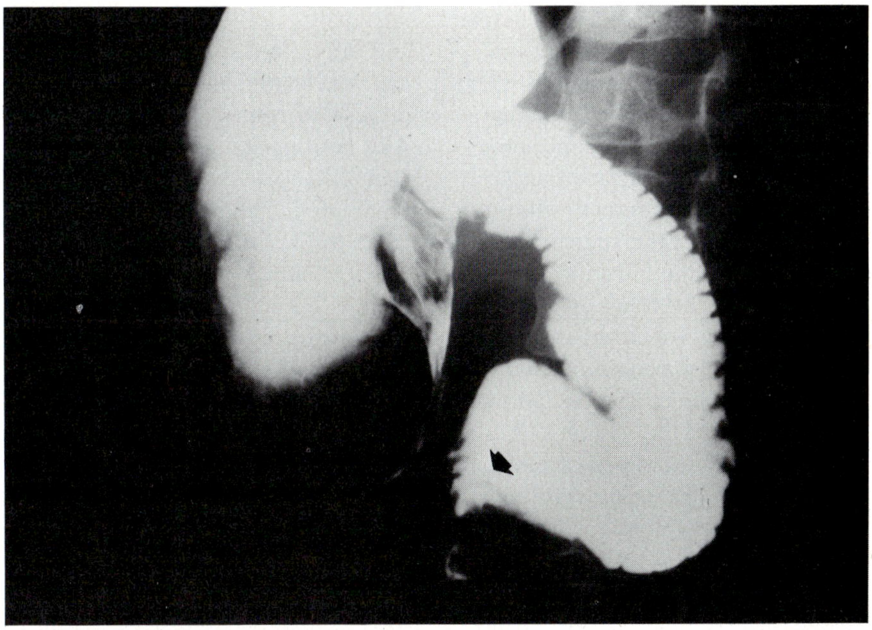

Fig. 33-7. Newborn with malrotation and midgut volvulus. Duodenal obstruction with duodenal distension and an absent ligament of Treitz associated with the corkscrew contrast pattern at the point of volvulus are characteristic of the volvulus about the superior mesentery vascular pedicle *(arrow)*.

entery allows the midgut to be suspended on the pedicle of the superior mesenteric vessels, creating an abnormally narrow and horizontal base around which midgut volvulus can occur. Malrotation may occur as an isolated anomaly or in association with other malformations of the gastrointestinal tract such as omphalocele, gastroschisis, diaphragmatic hernia, or duodenal atresia. Approximately 80% of patients with malrotation who develop symptoms will do so within the first month of life. The signs of intestinal obstruction may develop at any time. The sudden onset of bilious vomiting in a previously well neonate is suggestive of malrotation with volvulus formation, which needs immediate confirmation. The formation of a volvulus will result in severe midintestinal ischemia and bilious vomiting, occasional rectal bleeding, and shock. A contrast enema will reveal obstruction to retrograde flow at the level of the midtransverse colon. This is an acute surgical emergency that requires immediate surgical intervention. Similar to other instances of partial duodenal obstruction, malrotation without volvulus formation may be a difficult diagnostic problem. Infants may have protracted vomiting, manifestations of abdominal pain, or failure to thrive. Barium enema or upper gastrointestinal radiography may help identify these patients by demonstrating a dilated duodeum, abnormal positioning of the duodenojejunal junction, the presence of jejunal loops in the right side of the peritoneal cavity, and a malpositioned cecum.

Surgical intervention is indicated in all infants with symptomatic malrotation. If accompanied by volvulus, this presents one of the most urgent emergencies in neonatal surgery. Any infant with symptoms of intestinal obstruction and findings suggestive of malrotation with volvulus should undergo prompt laparotomy. Immediate resuscitation should be undertaken but not hamper progress toward the operating room, because delayed surgical intervention may allow irreversible infarction of the intestine to occur. With volvulus about the superior mesenteric vascular pedicle, the ischemic intestine can extend from the mid-duodenum to the transverse colon. Laparotomy with detorsion of the volvulized intestine can restore normal blood flow into the compromised intestine (Fig. 33-8). Under ideal circumstances normal perfusion returns after reduction of the volvulus. After prolonged ischemic episodes prompt reperfusion may not occur, and ischemic necrosis of the intestine must be excluded. Infants with short segments of ischemic intestine can undergo resection at the time of primary laparotomy if sufficient viable intestine remains. When long segments of intestine appear questionably viable, the abdomen should be closed and a "second-look" laparotomy planned in 12 to 18 hours. Persistently ischemic intestine should be resected at this later date. At the time of definitive surgical correction, Ladd's procedure, incising the anterior surface of the mesenteric pedicle

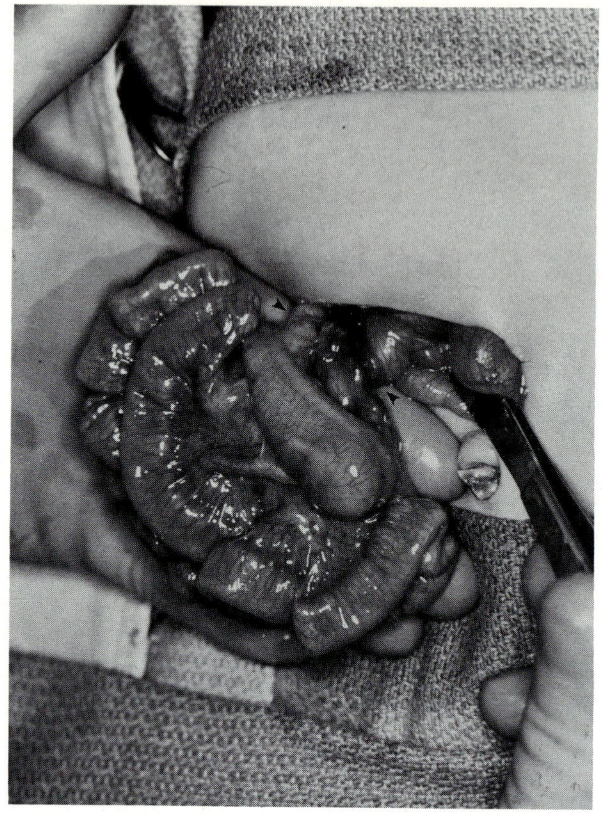

Fig. 33-8. Malrotation with midgut volvulus demonstrating the narrowed mesenteric pedicle *(arrows)* with 360 degrees of torsion. (Photograph courtesy R.J. Stevenson, M.D.)

and laterally displacing the superior mesenteric artery and vein should be undertaken. This widens the vascular pedicle to relieve lymphatic and vascular obstruction. Any retroperitoneal bands attached to the displaced cecum compressing the duodenum (Ladd's bands) should be divided. The duodenum then is positioned along the right pararenal gutter, and the cecum is positioned in the left lateral upper abdomen. An appendectomy is done in all infants without cecal compromise.

Controversy exists concerning the necessity of surgical fixation of the malrotated intestine. The merits of either method of management are not universally accepted. Bill found a higher incidence of chronic abdominal pain and constipation in the group in which surgical fixation was not undertaken. However, similar studies by other authors have not confirmed this finding. Recurrent volvulus has been seen following both methods.

The correct management of the infant with an asymptomatic malrotation discovered after contrast radiographs is less clear. Some authors view malrotation with volvulus as a developmental anomaly that occurs in utero with the age of presentation determined by the tightness of the twist in the mesentery. Postpartum spontaneous volvulus would then be extremely rare, and the mere presence of a malrotation would not indicate surgical intervention. However, cases where volvulus occurred after the repair of congenital diaphragmatic hernia and omphalocele seem to question this concept. At present all infants with symptomatic malrotation and those with volvulus should undergo Ladd's procedure. Those asymptomatic patients discovered in later life with no volvulus have been successfully followed without complication in selected instances.

Certain congenital anomalies have been associated with a high incidence of malrotation. Congenital diaphragmatic hernias, abdominal wall defects, and Beckwith's syndrome should alert the physician to this possibility, and any episode of vomiting or obstructive symptoms should be vigorously pursued. Malrotation has also been associated with chylous ascites resulting from lymphatic hypertension and lymphatic rupture or transudation.

Jejunoileal atresia

Jejunoileal atresias are equally distributed between the jejunum and ileum and are usually single, although multiple atresias have been noted in 6% to 20% of cases. In a review by the Surgical Section of the American Academy of Pediatrics the atresia was found in the proximal jejunum in 31%, the distal jejunum in 20%, the proximal ileum in 13%, and the distal ileum in 36%. Jejunoileal atresia occurs more frequently than duodenal or colonic atresia with a ratio of 4:2:1. Males and females are equally affected. Infants with jejunoileal atresia are often small for gestational age; one third of infants have jejunal atresia, one fourth have ileal atresia, and more than one half of those with multiple atresias are of low birth weight.

The clinical presentation of jejunoileal obstruction includes bilious vomiting, abdominal distension, and failure to pass meconium in three fourths of infants. Polyhydramnios is seen is one third of patients with jejunal atresia but rarely with ileal atresia. Jaundice occurs in one third of those with proximal lesions but only one fifth of those with distal ileal atresias. Generalized abdominal distension increases as the level of obstruction progresses into the more distal intestine. The degree of abdominal distension also increases for the first 12 to 24 hours as gas accumulates within the proximal intestinal tract.

The diagnosis of jejunoileal atresia is easily confirmed by supine and lateral decubitus abdominal radiographs. Multiple air-fluid levels in dilated loops of bowel are characteristic (Fig. 33-9). The level of obstruction can be anticipated by the amount of distended intestine. Peritoneal calcifications are suggestive of meconium peritonitis secondary to in utero intestinal perforation, whereas a single large air-fluid level can represent a localized meconium pseudocyst. There is usually little indication to perform an upper gastrointestinal contrast study when standard radiographs show the characteristic pattern. A contrast enema will demonstrate a microcolon and can help exclude an associated colonic atresia before surgical correction.

The cause of jejunoileal atresia appears to be in utero mesenteric vascular occlusion. The frequent association of jejunoileal atresia with antenatal intussusception, midgut volvulus, internal hernias, or abdominal wall defects supports this etiology.

Simplification of the classification of jejunoileal atresia was proposed by Martin and Zerella and recently modified to include:

Type I. Intraluminal diaphragm occlusion (~20%)

Type II. Cordlike atresia with an intact mesentery (~35%)

Type III. a. Atresia with intestinal discontinuity associated with a mesenteric defect (~35%)

b. Atresia with an extensive mesenteric defect with the distal blood supply being the ileocolic artery ("apple peel" or "Christmas tree" deformity) (~11%)

Type IV. Multiple atresias (~6%)

Occasional familial cases of multiple atresias from the stomach to the rectum suggesting autosomal recessive modes of transmission have been reported. Combinations of jejunoileal and colonic atresias are uncommon but do occur.

The surgical correction of jejunal and ileal atresia depends upon the location of the lesion and the overall length of involved intestine. Experience has taught that retention of the bulbous dilated proximal intestine at the point of the atresia often leads to prolonged intestinal peristaltic dysfunction, whereas side-to-side reconstructions can develop blind loop syndrome. Resection of the distended intestine and selective use of a tapering enteroplasty can avoid many of these problems. Proximal jejunal atresia should be reconstructed by resecting the dilated intestine to the point where normal dimensions are reached, often at or above the ligament of Treitz. An end-to-oblique side anastomosis is then used. When the entire proximal gut is dilated, a progressive tapering enteroplasty constructed over a no. 22 french catheter should be performed. Distal atresias should also be resected to the point of normalization of the intestinal diameter. In type IV atresias where multiple atretic segments are encountered, sequential end-to-end anastomoses are necessary to salvage an adequate total intestinal length. Minimal resection should be undertaken with type III b apple peel atresias because of the extremely short gut often present at the initial operation. At the time of primary recontruction documentation of distal bowel patency by intraluminal saline irrigation is necessary to exclude additional distal atresias. A direct

A B C

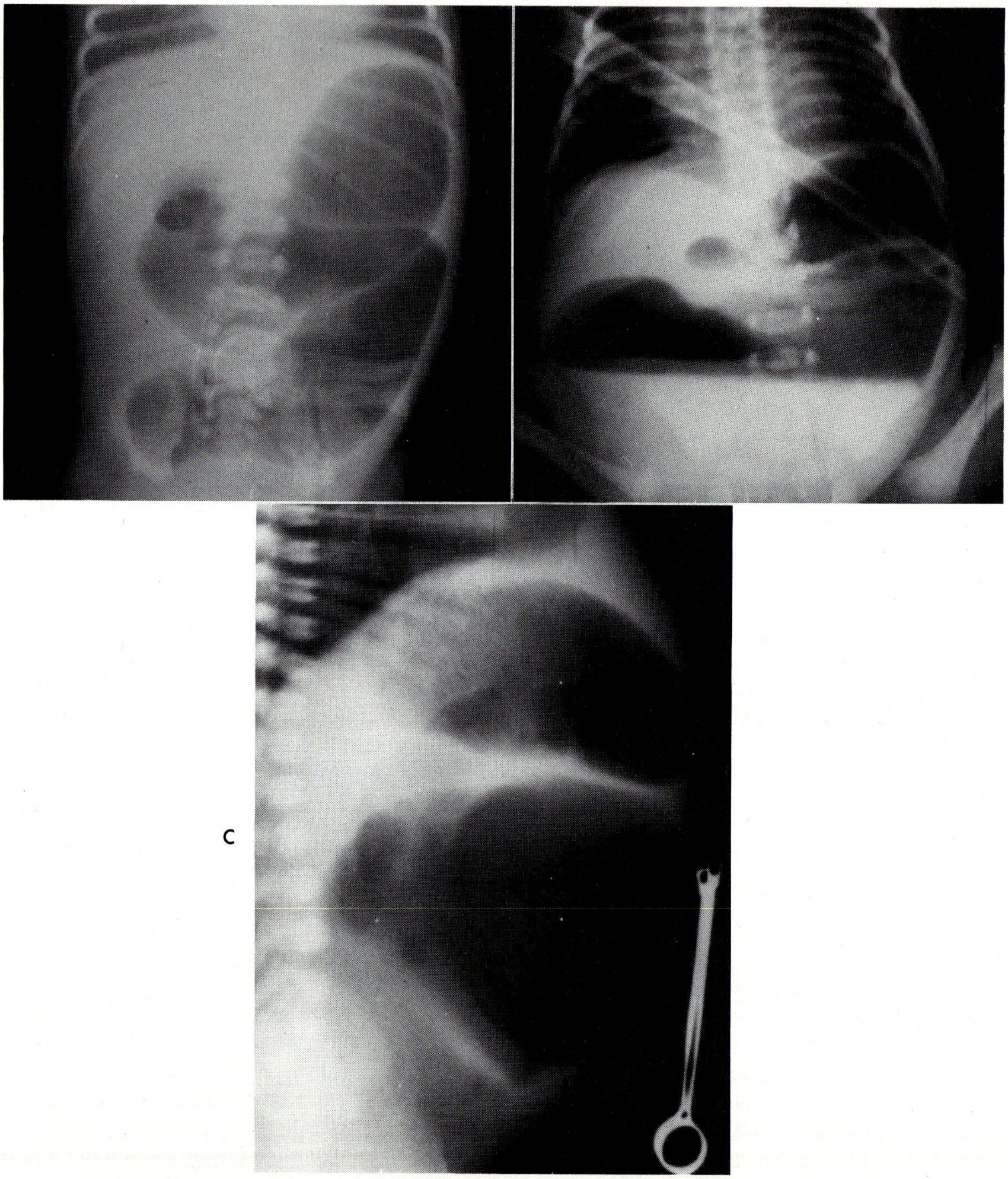

Fig. 33-9. A, 1-day-old infant with high jejunal atresia. Proximal massively dilated air filled jejunum is present with no distal intestinal gas visible. **B** and **C,** Massively distended jejunum with air fluid levels present in a 2-day-old infant with midjejunal atresia. No distal intestine is visualized.

measurement of intestinal length after reconstruction is also helpful for further therapeutic planning.

Primary reconstruction is not indicated in infants with intestinal atresia complicated by volvulus if the intestine is ischemic, or following perforation with associated bacterial peritoneal contamination. Use of a Mikulicz enterostomy for temporary diversion allows reconstruction to be undertaken at a later time under ideal conditions.

Prolonged intestinal dysfunction is often a problem after reconstruction of type III b and IV atresias. Early institution of hyperalimentation in these patients has been lifesaving. Use of a feeding jejunostomy placed through the gastrostomy and directed distal to the anastomosis at the time of operation has been beneficial to those infants with high jejunal or duodenal atresia.

Survival in intestinal atresia is decreased in infants with proximal lesions, complex type III b and IV atresias, short gut syndrome, and in those patients with cystic fibrosis. Additional factors include associated abdominal wall defects, gut perforation, and peritonitis.

Meconium syndromes

Meconium ileus

Meconium ileus in the newborn period occurs almost invariably in infants suffering from cystic fibrosis. These infants have intraluminal obstruction from inspissated meconium, which forms a tenacious putty-like obstruction within the terminal ileum. Meconium ileus is a symptom in 10% to 15% of infants with cystic fibrosis, which is transmitted as an autosomal recessive trait with a heterozygote carrier incidence of 1 in 25, making it the most common potentially lethal genetic disorder in the Caucasian race. Cystic fibrosis is uncommon in blacks and virtually absent in Mongolians.

Intestinal obstruction in infants with meconium ileus occurs as a result of hyperviscous secretions from the mucous glands of the small intestine producing meconium with low water content. This meconium is abnormally sticky and adheres to the intestinal mucosal lining. In addition to hyposecretion of water and electrolytes by the intestine and pancreas, the meconium formed contains abnormally elevated concentrations of albumin and macroproteins. Intrinsic pancreatic disease also affects infants in fetal life with ductal obstruction, leading to atrophy of the acinar cells and advanced pancreatic dysfunction by infancy. Although there is a deficiency or absence of pancreatic enzymes within the duodenal secretions of infants, it appears to be the abnormal intestinal mucous secretions rather than pancreatic insufficiency that leads to the meconium ileus syndrome. Intestinal obstruction from meconium ileus is uncommon in premature infants and seems to reach clinical significance with fetal maturation.

Intestinal obstruction from meconium ileus can exist in two subtypes:

1. *Simple meconium ileus* occurs in two thirds of affected infants. The usual clinical presentation includes midileal obstruction with proximal dilated intestine containing thick, dark green, tarry, tenacious meconium, and a markedly narrowed distal ileum with multiple grapelike pellets of rubbery, inspissated meconium. These inspissated meconium pellets often extend into the proximal portion of the unused narrow microcolon. The clinical picture is that of small bowel obstruction with symptoms occurring within 24 to 48 hours, consisting of failure to pass meconium, abdominal distension, bilious vomiting, and palpable, rubbery loops of bowel. Radiographic examination will disclose multiple dilated loops of intestine of variable size and a characteristic absence of air-fluid levels. A coarse, granular appearance of air within the inspissated meconium is characteristic. The contrast enema discloses a small unused colon, and reflux into the terminal ileum will silhouette the inspissated meconium pellets (Fig. 33-10).

2. *Complicated meconium ileus* exists when volvulus,

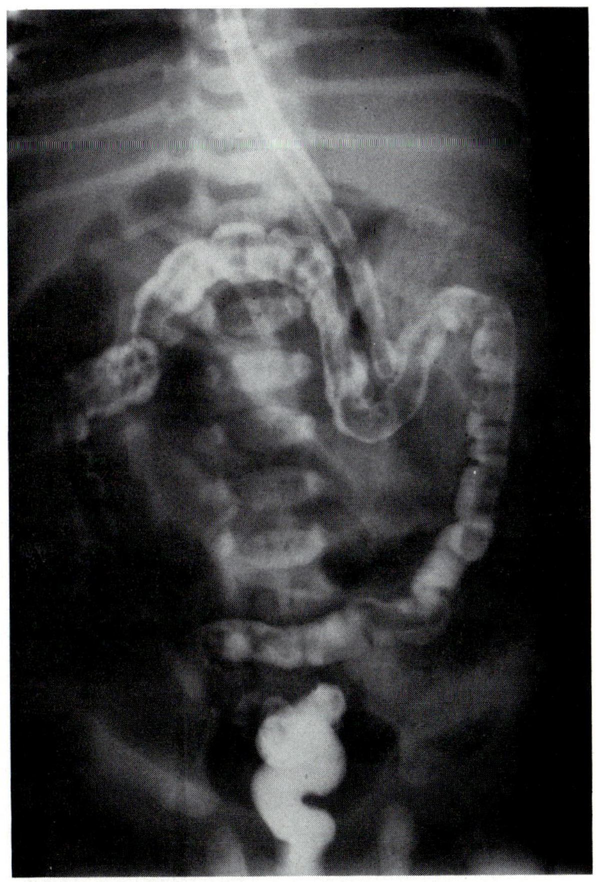

Fig. 33-10. Newborn infant with simple meconium ileus. Contrast enema demonstrates a small caliber unused colon. Multiple dilated small intestinal loops are visualized but not filled with contrast. Inspissated meconium pellets are outlined by contrast within the colon.

intestinal necrosis and perforation, meconium peritonitis, or meconium pseudocyst formation complicates a previous meconium ileus obstruction. These mechanical complications of terminal ileal obstruction occur after progressive distension or volvulus of the dilated proximal intestinal loops. Volvulus may be followed by concentric ischemic strictures when the intervening volvulized segment remains viable, or can lead to complete dissolution of the volvulized intestine with formation of intestinal atresia with or without a giant meconium cyst. Signs of bacterial or chemical peritonitis are interposed on the clinical picture of intestinal obstruction seen with simple meconium ileus. Calcification within the abdomen is indicative of in utero perforation with meconium peritonitis and can be identified on plain radiographs (Fig. 33-11). Scrotal or inguinal canal calcifications are also occasionally seen. A meconium pseudocyst may be seen as an area of increased density surrounded by a rim of calcification displacing the surrounding dilated intestinal loops. Postnatal perforation leads to the characteristic finding of pneumoperitoneum. However, in up to one third of cases, no diagnostic features of complicated meconium ileus can be recognized on plain abdominal radiographs.

Nonsurgical management of meconium ileus was initially described by Noblett in 1969. It remains the primary mode of therapy for infants with simple meconium ileus. Use of hypertonic contrast enema (gastrograffin or hypaque) has been successful as the hyperosmolarity draws fluid into the intestine disimpacting the meconium. This method is successful in disimpacting the meconium obstruction and allowing the establishment of intestinal activity in approximately 60% of patients. Before undertaking nonsurgical management, the following criteria outlined by Noblett must be met:

1. The diagnostic contrast enema should exclude other causes of distal intestinal obstruction.
2. Complications such as volvulus, atresia, perforation, or peritonitis must be excluded.
3. The enema must be undertaken under strict fluoroscopic control.
4. Intravenous antibiotics should be administered.
5. The patient should be seen by a pediatric surgeon who is in attendance during the evaluation.
6. The patient should be fully fluid resuscitated and prepared for imminent operation should complications occur during nonoperative therapy.

Hypertonic contrast is then administered carefully through the microcolon and refluxed into the terminal ileum until it reaches the gas-filled, dilated ileal segment. Evacuation is allowed, and radiographs are repeated after the contrast examination and in 12 to 24 hours to assess progress and exclude late perforation. The enema may be repeated if necessary, recognizing that the risk of

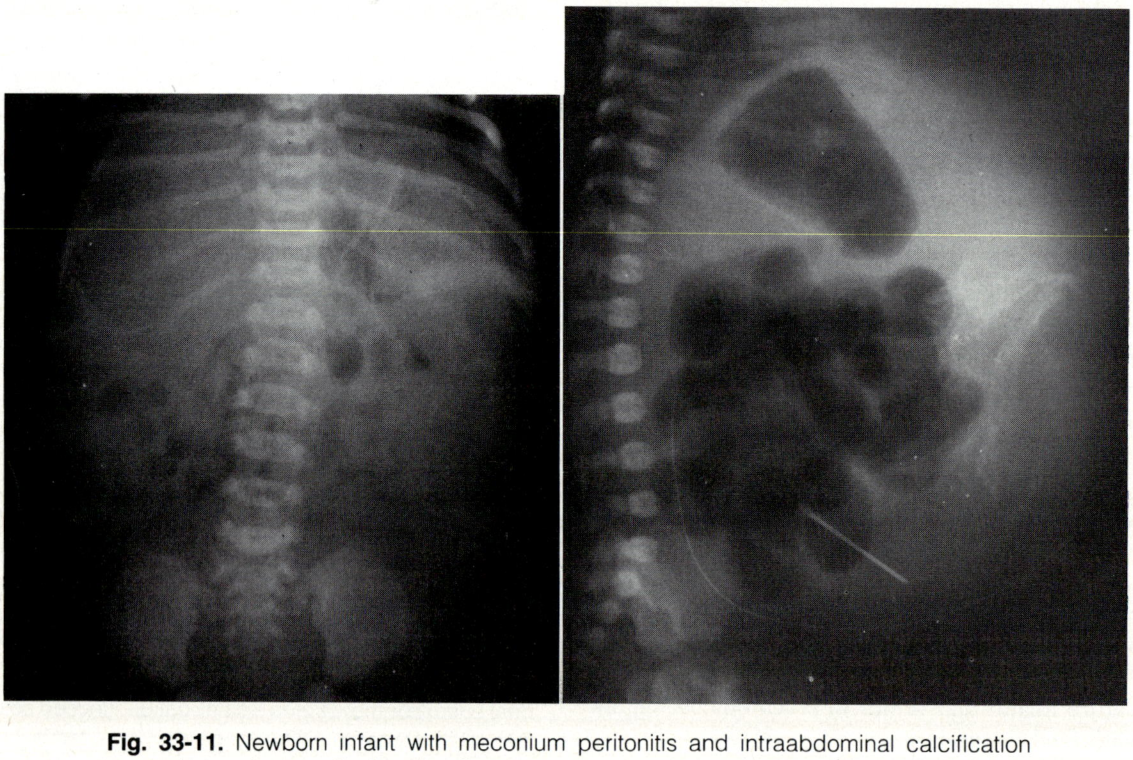

Fig. 33-11. Newborn infant with meconium peritonitis and intraabdominal calcification secondary to in utero ileal perforation.

perforation increases with successive attempts at nonsurgical therapy. Failure to pass meconium, increasing radiographic signs of obstruction, or progressive intestinal distension necessitate immediate operation, not repeat contrast examination. Complications after nonsurgical therapy include hypovolemic shock resulting from inadequate fluid resuscitation and intestinal perforation. Perforation of the microcolon can occur acutely at the time of contrast administration or 12 to 48 hours after enema administration. Factors increasing the risk of perforation include distension of the colon from fluid influx and injury to the mucosa from the wetting agent (polysorbate 80) and gastrograffin.

Surgical therapy of simple meconium ileus is undertaken when nonsurgical enema management fails or when suitable personnel to safely undertake nonsurgical reduction are not available. Irrigation of the involved ileum through an enterotomy placed in the dilated ileum allows removal of the obstruction meconium. Irrigation with 2% to 4% N-acetyl-L-cysteine will facilitate the removal of the tenacious meconium. Any compromised intestine should be resected. Reconstruction with primary end-to-end anastomosis is preferred when the bowel viability is normal. In infants where primary reconstruction of intestinal continuity is unwise, a diverting ostomy is used, allowing later reanastomosis. In our hands the Mikulicz double-barreled enterostomy is preferred although the distal chimney (Bishop-Koop) or proximal chimney (Santulli) ostomies are also acceptable. Division of the Mikulicz enterostomy common wall 5 to 7 days after the primary surgical procedure allows early reestablishment of intestinal continuity.

Complicated meconium ileus always requires surgical therapy. Careful dissection to preserve all viable intestine and identify sites of obstruction and perforation is necessary while all nonviable bowel is excised. Temporary intestinal diversion using the Mikulicz double stoma with early clamp division of the common wall is the safest method of treatment. Gastrostomy tube placement will facilitate postoperative intestinal decompression and allow gradual institution of enteral feedings in infants with diminished gut length. Before undertaking intestinal reanastomosis, a distal contrast study is performed to document removal of all inspissated meconium from the distal intestine.

Postoperative management of patients with meconium ileus should include irrigation of the proximal and distal intestine with 2% to 4% N-acetyl-L-cysteine on a daily basis. When feedings are reinstituted, Pregestimil supplemented with pancreatic enzyme preparations will allow adequate absorption during the period of gut adaptation after intestinal resection.

Surgical mortality rates have now dropped from well over 50% to 10%. Recent progress using early aggressive medical therapy for the pulmonary complications of cystic fibrosis makes vigorous care of infants with meconium ileus a hopeful proposition.

Meconium peritonitis

Meconium peritonitis occurs after in utero perforation of the intestine. Although the perforation usually occurs as a complication of meconium ileus, other causes, such as intestinal atresia, volvulus, internal hernias, congenital peritoneal bands, in utero intussusception, or gastroschisis have also been implicated. Almost all cases are associated with intestinal obstruction or mesenteric vascular occlusion, which must be identified and treated at the time of primary therapy.

Meconium peritonitis has been subdivided into four distinct clinical varieties by Martin and associates.

1. *Meconium pseudocyst* results when a fibrinous wall develops and surrounds an accumulation of meconium. The pseudocyst is surrounded by relatively uninvolved loops of intestine, and the cyst wall may be calcified. This represents the accumulation of meconium over a prolonged period with local containment.

2. *Adhesive meconium peritonitis* results from widespread contamination of the peritoneal cavity by meconium several days to weeks before birth. Scattered calcifications can be detected on abdominal films, and dense vascular adhesions are encountered during operative therapy. Intestinal obstruction often occurs from the primary disease or secondary to adhesions from chemical peritonitis (Fig. 33-10).

3. *Meconium ascites* results when perforation occurs only a few days prior to delivery. Massive amounts of meconium stained ascitic fluid are characteristically present with an absence of intraperitoneal calcification (Fig. 33-12).

4. *Infected meconium peritonitis* results when the intestinal perforation is not sealed and organisms from the colonized intestine invade the peritoneal cavity. This may occur following any of the preceding types of meconium peritonitis when persistent perforation occurs.

In an occasional infant when the perforation has sealed, progressive peritonitis does not ensue and there is no associated intestinal obstruction, making operation unnecessary. However, most cases require surgical intervention. Indications for surgery include intestinal obstruction, persistent peritonitis, an enlarging abdominal mass, abdominal wall cellulitis, and signs of sepsis. At the time of surgery specific operative management appropriate for the primary disease (e.g., volvulus, atresia, and meconium ileus) should be undertaken. Special attention to preserving adequate bowel length is necessary in these infants whose primary intestinal problem may have compromised their intestinal length before surgical intervention. In the absence of bacterial contamination

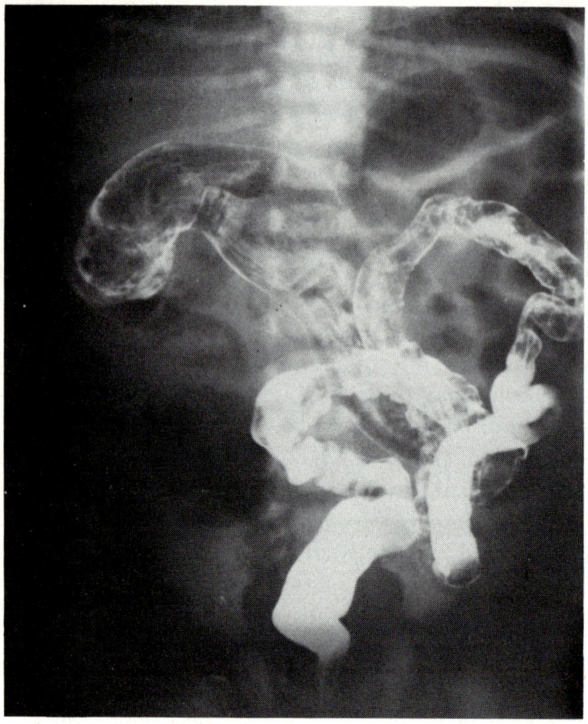

Fig. 33-12. A 2-day-old infant with meconium plug syndrome. Note the normal rectal size associated with intraluminal filling defects at the site of the meconium plug. A small left colon and relative dilation of the proximal right and transverse colon complete the characteristic picture.

primary intestinal reanastomosis can be undertaken. Bacterial peritonitis mandates primary exteriorization and later intestinal reconstruction.

A sweat chloride examination to exclude cystic fibrosis is mandatory in all patients with meconium peritonitis.

Meconium plug syndrome

Meconium plug syndrome represents a spectrum of neonatal colonic dysmotility syndromes, including both true meconium plug obstruction and neonatal small left colon syndrome. Although previous theories stressed the importance of abnormal meconium in forming an obstructing plug, the syndrome now appears to be a functional obstruction resulting from diminished colonic motility and meconium clearance rather than mechanical intraluminal obstruction.

The pathogenesis of the meconium plug syndrome is poorly understood but commonly associated with several circumstances. Infants of diabetic mothers make up roughly one half of the patients with meconium plug obstruction (chapter 37, part one). The hypoglycemia characteristic of these infants is believed to produce increased glucagon production, leading to bowel hypomotility. Infants with hypermagnesemia after treatment for eclampsia have reduced acetylcholine release and subsequent myoneural depression (chapter 37, part two). In addition, systemic sepsis with associated hypoglycemia and sympathomimetic release can cause similar hypomotility. Functional immaturity of the myenteric plexus has also been suggested as an additional etiology.

These syndromes occur with the common finding of low intestinal obstruction appearing during the first 3 days of life. Abdominal radiographs reveal multiple dilated loops of intestine, and a diagnostic contrast enema often outlines the intraluminal plug associated with partial colonic obstruction (Fig. 33-13). Tertiary contractions are absent within the narrow left colon, and the rectum is characteristically of near normal size.

Relief of the obstruction can be obtained after rectal examination in some infants. A contrast enema will be diagnostic in most cases and frequently precipitates evacuation of the typical long and thick meconium plug. In rare cases surgical intervention is necessary to relieve obstruction when hypertonic enemas have been unsuccessful.

After resolution of the intestinal obstruction a rectal biopsy is necessary to exclude Hirschsprung's disease. Sweat chloride examination is also necessary, because 14% to 25% of patients with meconium plugs have been identified as having cystic fibrosis.

Colonic obstructions

Imperforate anus

Imperforate anus anomalies include a wide spectrum of abnormalities of anorectal development, spanning from anal stenosis with otherwise normal pelvic anatomy to agenesis of the entire distal anorectum with associated anomalies of genitourinary development and abnormalities in the continence mechanism. The incidence of imperforate anus varies widely, averaging 1 in 5,000 live births. Although imperforate anus has occasionally followed both recessive and dominant inheritance patterns, in most cases there is no preceding family history. Other associated congenital anomalies occur in over one half of the patients, with genitourinary tract malformations seen in 28%, gastrointestinal in 13%, cardiac in 7%, and skeletal or central nervous system anomalies seen in 6% of affected patients. When these occur in close association, the VATER constellation of anomalies should be excluded. Of significance in the long-term outcome of patients with high imperforate anus is the presence of skeletal deformities or agenesis of the sacrum with their frequently associated deficit in neural innervation to the perineum, hence the musculature responsible for continence. Careful investigation for and recognition of these anomalies is necessary in the early perinatal period to appropriately plan the long-term surgical approach in the patients with complex symptoms.

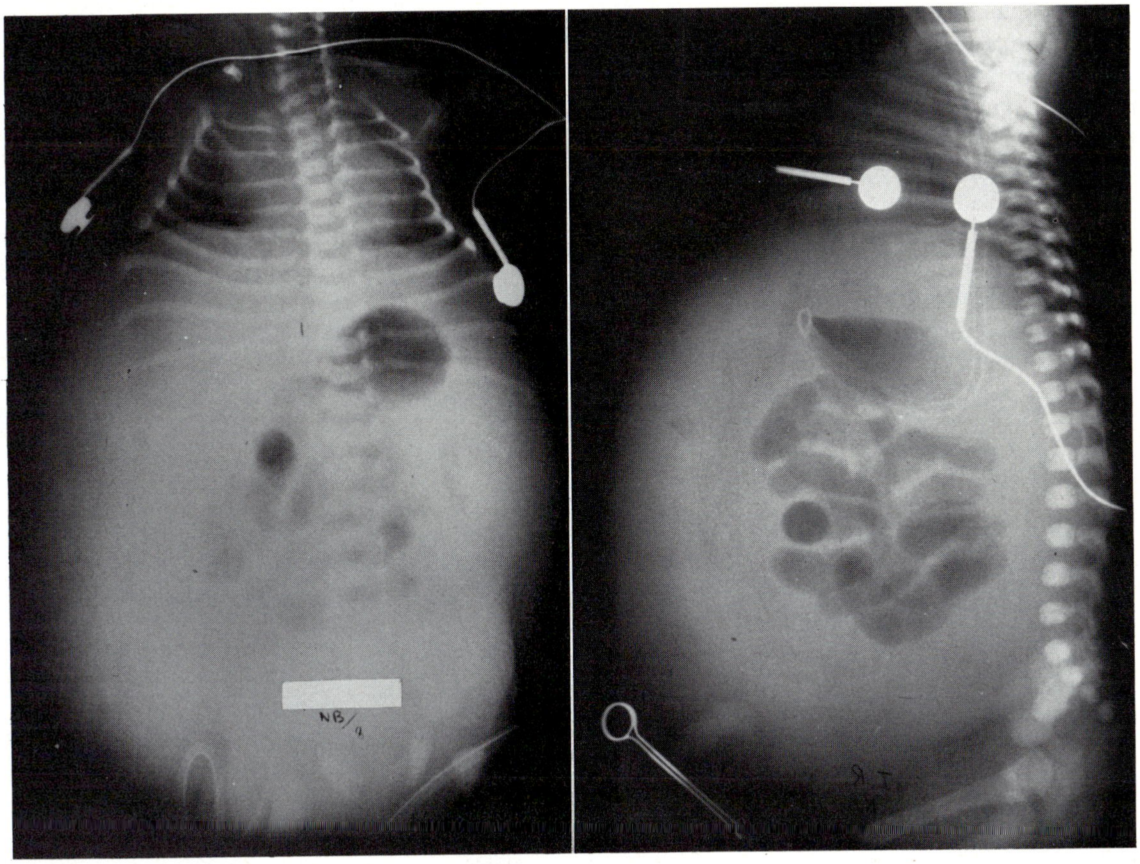

Fig. 33-13. Newborn female with meconium ileus complicated by ileal perforation. Massive meconium ascites is suggested by centralization of bowel loops and was confirmed on paracentesis.

The embryologic development of the anorectum from the primitive cloaca involves division into an anterior urogenital sinus and a posterior intestinal canal by the urorectal septum and the lateral folds during the fourth to sixth weeks of gestation. Perforation of the anal plate allows communication of the developing intestinal tract with the amnionic environment. Failure of this complex separation process at any point in embryologic development will result in one of the many constellations of anatomic findings associated with imperforate anus abnormalities.

Imperforate anus abnormalities are best understood and classified on an anatomic basis. Division of defects into primarily supralevator or high lesions and infralevator or low lesions, with an intermediate group between these two extremes, facilitates preoperative care and surgical intervention. The revised International Classification of Imperforate Anus is included in Table 33-2.

The diagnosis and appropriate management of imperforate anus depends on its early recognition and appropriate staging. Physical examination characteristically shows an absent external anal opening, although infants

Table 33-2. Classification of anorectal malformations

Level	Male	Female
High	Anorectal agenesis with recto-prostatic-urethral fistula	Anorectal agenesis with rectovaginal fistula
	without fistula	without fistula
	Rectal atresia	Rectal atresia
Intermediate	Recto-bulbar-urethral fistula	Rectovestibular fistula
		Rectovaginal fistula
	Agenesis without fistula	Agenesis without fistula
Low	Anocutaneous fistula	Anovestibular fistula
	Anal stenosis	Anocutaneous fistula
		Anal stenosis
		Cloaca
	Rare malformations	Rare malformations

From Stephens, F.D., and Smith, E.D.: Pediatr. Surg. Int. **1**:200, 1986.

with anal stenosis or imperforate anal membrane may have a nearly normal-appearing perineum and are often first recognized when a rectal temperature is attempted. Infralevator anal agenesis occurs with a perineal fistula in slightly over one half of males or posterior fourchette/perineal body fistula in nearly all females. High supralevator and intermediate lesions occur with no anal opening and no perineal fistula. Fistulas in intermediate cases often involve the urethra from the introitus to the bladder or may not be present. In cases of rectal atresia the perineum will appear normal.

The clinical staging of imperforate anus is confirmed radiographically employing the brow-down Wangensteen-Rice invertogram. Air within the distal rectal pouch, present by 6 to 12 hours of age, allows an estimation of the level of the atresia. The pubococcygeal (PC) line, drawn from the inferior margin of the pubis to the inferior margin of the lower sacral segment, has been used to divide high from low lesions. The muscle (M) point can also be identified at the junction of the upper two thirds and the lower one third of the pear-shaped ischium. This point is slightly inferior to the PC line and represents the inferior portion of the puborectalis muscle sling (Fig. 33-14). The puborectalis muscle sling is the most important anatomic structure for anorectal continence, and descent of the distal anal pouch through this muscular sling distinguishes low lesions from high imperforate anal lesions. In intermediate level lesions the distal intestine is within but does not penetrate beyond the puborectalis sling. The highest radiographic level in relations to the PC line and M point should be used for staging, because Valsalva maneuvers and crying may transiently depress the pelvic floor and make an otherwise high lesion appear to descend below the PC line. In questionable cases metrizamide may be administered by mouth, or water-soluble contrast can be instilled into the distal anorectal pouch though a needle inserted into the perineum. Ultrasonography can be used to measure the distance from the perineal dimple to the distal anorectal pouch, but it cannot accurately identify the puborectalis sling. Air within the bladder is indicative of a genitourinary fistula. In selected cases retrograde urethrography or vaginography can be of great value in delineating the presence of a fistula to a genitourinary tract and visualizing the level of the imperforate anorectal pouch by indirect contrast administration.

Surgical correction is determined by the level of the anorectal pouch. Infralevator lesions can generally be corrected in neonates. Anal stenosis is uncommon but responds to immediate dilation with gradual enlargement of the anus to normal size. Imperforate anal membranes can be simply excised and followed by anal dilations. Infralevator anal agenesis in the male is treated by perineal anoplasty with excision of the rectoperineal fistula

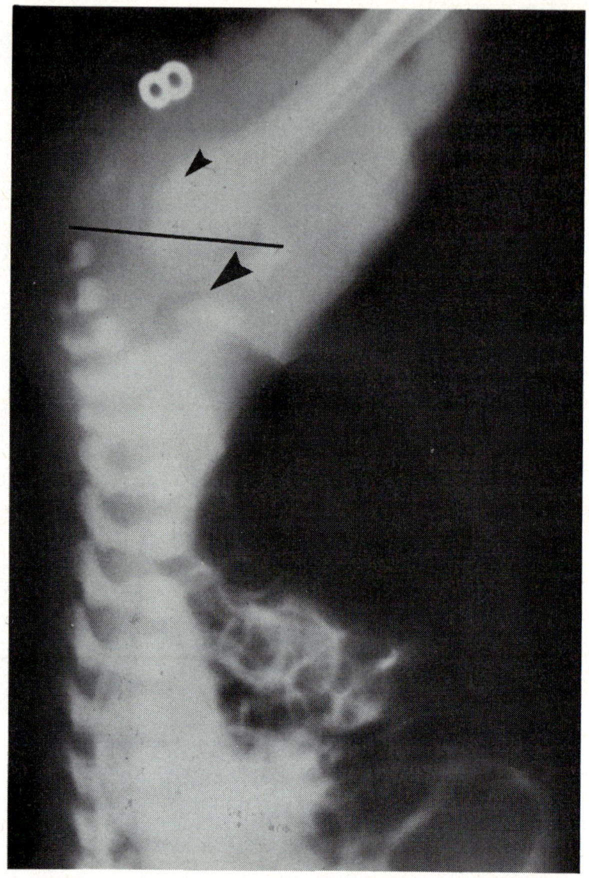

Fig. 33-14. Wangensteen-Rice invertagram in a patient with high supralevator imperforate anus. The PC line and M point *(small arrow)* define the level and staging of the anomaly. The distal rectal pouch ends at the large arrow.

when it is present. In the female a perineal fistula is almost invariably present. Three therapeutic choices are available in female patients: (1) Dilation of the fistula tract can be employed to allow establishment of an adequate lumen from the rectum. With progressive perineal body growth the proximity of the anal fistula and the vagina diminishes. This alternative should only be used when minimal anterior displacement of the anus has occurred. (2) A "cut-back" procedure is accomplished by incising the fistula tract along its posterior midline course and reapproximating the exposed skin and mucosal edges, enlarging the anal opening. Any moist rectal mucosa along the fistula tract is fulgurated. (3) Perineal anoplasty involves transposing the anteriorly directed imperforate anus and fistula to the normal location on the perineum with circumferential reconstruction of the anorectum and reconstruction of the perineal body. This affords the best cosmetic result but risks possible retraction of the mobilized anorectum into the perineum and stricture formation. After perineal anoplasty in males or females, postoperative dilation should be initiated 14 days after anoplasty and continued until an anorectal size is established.

Infants with intermediate and high supralevator lesions should be initially treated with colostomy. A divided colostomy prevents fecal contamination of the distal imperforate segment, decreasing the risk of urinary tract infection in patients with urorectal fistulas. Elective repair of supralevator imperforate anus should be undertaken at 6 to 12 months of age. At the time of repair the bowel must be carefully passed through the puborectalis muscle sling to achieve fecal continence. Direct visualization of this muscle and the pelvic sling has been achieved by two approaches. The sacro-abdominal-perineal pull-through modified by Kiesewetter to include endorectal dissection of the distal blind segment and direct transsacral visualization of the puborectalis sling have been the traditional surgical approach. Recently, a direct transsacral muscle–dividing approach has been advocated by Pena. Both procedures emphasize careful anatomic dissection of the perineum and meticulous placement of the imperforate intestine within the puborectalis-pelvic muscle sling. Perineal anoplasty completes both procedures.

Supralevator rectal atresia can occasionally be treated by dilations if a small perforation is present in the obstructing diaphragm. If complete atresia is present, preliminary sigmoid colostomy should be used in infancy. At approximately 1 year of age the atretic segment can be reconstructed either with a primary anastomosis or after an endorectal dissection with abdominoperineal pull-through.

In spite of meticulous efforts at anatomic reconstruction of the anorectum significant discrepancies still exist in functional results after surgical repair. Low defects achieve good-to-excellent results in almost all cases; however, high imperforate anus continues to have good-to-fair results in only 50% of cases with continence achieved only after extensive periods of anorectal training. Persistent incontinence occurs in approximately 10% of individuals after surgical intervention. Reoperation for poor functional results should be delayed until adolescence, when motivational factors often allow maintenance of continence. Carefully selected refractory cases may be benefited by reoperation with improved continence in two thirds of cases.

Hirschsprung's disease

Hirschsprung's disease, or congenital aganglionic megacolon, is a congenital absence of the parasympathetic innervation to the distal intestine associated with an absence of ganglion cells in the affected areas within both Meissner's and Auerbach's plexus. This absence of normal parasympathetic innervation prevents gut peristalsis, leading to functional constipation. The proximal normally ganglionated intestinal wall becomes thickened secondary to work hypertrophy while attempting to overcome the functional obstruction. A transition zone exists between the normal and abnormal aganglionic intestine, which can often be recognized by its conical tapering appearance. The aganglionic intestine is thin, collapsed, often spastic, and small. Although the aganglionosis may extend proximally to involve the entire intestinal tract, in most cases it is confined to the rectum and rectosigmoid colon. This characteristic distal intestinal involvement occurs secondary to failure of complete distal migration of neural crest cells from a cranial to caudal direction during the eighth to tenth week of fetal life. Complete aganglionosis then exists distal to the transition zone, with the exception of extremely rare instances where skip lesions are identified. In each of these cases classical distal aganglionosis was found in association with a more proximal skip lesion.

The incidence of Hirschsprung's disease is approximately 1 in every 5,000 live births, 80% of patients are male. In 75% to 80% only rectosigmoid involvement is present, and 10% of patients have total colonic involvement.

Failure to pass meconium in the first 24 hours of life is often the earliest symptom of congenital Hirschsprung's disease. Delayed meconium passage beyond 48 hours in an otherwise full-term, healthy infant strongly suggests aganglionic megacolon. Although complete intestinal obstruction is seen in some infants, others are relatively asymptomatic until several weeks of age when progressive constipation or diarrhea associated with abdominal distension occurs. Obstructive abdominal distension may be preceded by or accompanied by vomiting, which is usually of a bilious nature. Diarrhea, when it occurs in infants with aganglionic megacolon, characteristically shows foul-smelling, liquid stools and abdominal distension, differentiating it from the usual infantile diarrhea. In addition, protein-losing enteropathy and failure to thrive can occur secondary to persistent partial intestinal obstruction. Urinary obstruction with hydronephrosis and recurrent urinary tract infection may occur secondary to mechanical compression of the ureters, bladder, and urethra by a massively distended distal rectosigmoid colon.

The most feared and serious complication of Hirschsprung's disease is acute bacterial enterocolitis. These infants have rapidly progressive distention, profuse vomiting, and passage of large amounts of foul-smelling, often bloody stools. Ulceration of the intestinal mucosa with ischemic necrosis of the bowel wall can lead to systemic septicemia, intestinal pneumatosis, intestinal perforation, pericolic abscess formation, and peritonitis. In addition, hemolysis, thrombocytopenia, and protein-losing enteropathy from mucosal loss complicate the septic picture. Mortality still reaches 25% to 30% from entercolitis with unrecognized Hirschsprung's disease in the neonatal period, emphasizing its serious and lethal nature.

Infants with less severe symptoms may develop only periodic bouts of obstruction relieved by digital rectal examination or by enema administration. These infants often remain chronically ill with failure to thrive and persistent constipation. The routine use of laxatives or enema administration to relieve constipation may delay their recognition.

The diagnosis of Hirschsprung's disease is suggested by the physical findings and radiographs but can only be confirmed by rectal biopsy, which will demonstrate absence of ganglion within the distal intestine and/or abnormal pattern of acetylcholinesterase histochemical stain. Radiographic demonstration of diffuse intestinal and colonic distension accompanied by an absence of air within the rectum in a neonate is suggestive of Hirschsprung's disease; however, contrast studies are necessary to definitively demonstrate a "transition zone" (Fig. 33-15). Repeated rectal examinations or enema administration may effectively evacuate the proximal distended bowel and distend the distal aganglionic segment, making recognition of the transition zone difficult if not impossible. The characteristic roentgenographic finding of a normal caliber rectum with funnel-shaped dilation at the level of the transition zone and marked dilation of the proximal colon may not be present until several weeks of age. Retention of barium within the colon 24 hours after contrast examination is, however, very suggestive of Hirschsprung's disease in the neonate.

Anorectal manometric examination in Hirschsprung's disease shows contraction of the internal anal sphincter in response to transient rectal distension. In normal individuals transient rectal distension causes relaxation of the internal anal sphincter. The presence of normal anorectal manometrics is helpful in excluding Hirschsprung's disease during outpatient screening, but at the present time manometrics alone should not be considered diagnostic.

The definitive diagnosis of Hirschsprung's disease can be made only after a histologic confirmation of the absence of ganglia and the presence of excess nonmyelin-

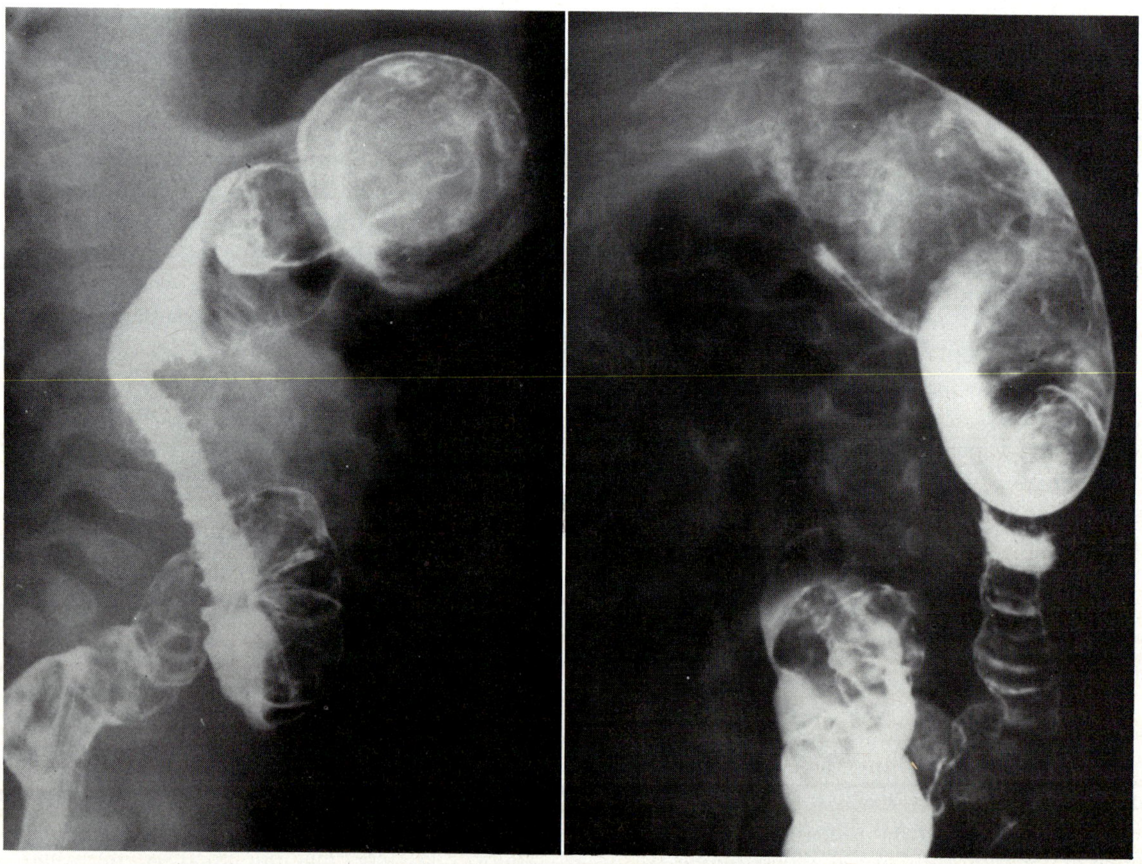

Fig. 33-15. Hirschsprung's disease demonstrating a descending colon transition zone with proximal obstruction, sawtooth pattern within the involved intestine, and a collapsed rectum.

ated nerves within the distal rectum on a rectal biopsy specimen. Since the aganglionic segment begins at the anorectal junction and extends proximally, it is important that the lowest biopsy be obtained within 1 cm of the apex of the anal column. A suction rectal biopsy, including the mucosa and a small portion of submucosa, is an adequate sample to definitively diagnose Hirschsprung's disease when routine pathologic and acetylcholinesterase staining methods are employed. This biopsy may be easily obtained on infants cared for within an incubator or as an outpatient procedure for newborns and young children. Open rectal biopsy should be reserved for infants with equivocal suction rectal biopsies and those children with a previous surgical procedure who have persistent symptoms.

The differential diagnosis of Hirschsprung's disease in the newborn period is limited. On examination and plain radiographs Hirschsprung's disease can be confused with distal ileal and colonic atresia or meconium ileus. However, contrast enema examination will show a microcolon in these cases where Hirschsprung's disease shows a normal or dilated colon. Meconium plug syndrome can result in delayed passage of meconium, however, contrast examination should allow visualization of the meconium plug. Delayed passage of meconium can also occur with neonatal sepsis, adrenal insufficiency, CNS injuries, hypothyroidism, and hypomotility induced by hypermagnesemia and maternal narcotic administration. In each of these cases, when Hirschsprung's disease cannot be excluded, suction rectal biopsy will be definitive.

After the diagnosis of Hirschsprung's disease, mechanical obstruction of the distal colon must be relieved. Although an exceptionally rare patient may be treated with daily enemas and laxatives to prevent colonic obstruction, as a rule all individuals with diagnosed Hirschsprung's disease should undergo diverting colostomy in normally ganglionated bowel proximal to their transition zone. This would ideally be located in the intestine just proximal to the aganglionic gut. However, this requires frozen section examination during the surgical procedure by a skilled pathologist to assure normal ganglionated intestine at the time the colostomy is performed. Placement of a colostomy just proximal to the level of the transition zone is also important in infants who appear on radiographic examination to have a high transition zone at or proximal to the splenic flexure. Placement of the colostomy just above the transition zone allows a definitive pull-through to be undertaken and the colostomy closed as a single surgical procedure when this is preferred. When the ganglionated intestine is extremely dilated just above the level of the transition zone, a colostomy at that level becomes impractical and dangerous to construct. In addition, infants with enterocolitis should not be subjected to the prolonged anesthetic risk and often sequential biopsies necessary to identify the precise transition zone. In these cases a right upper quadrant simple loop colostomy is preferred. The definitive pull-through is then undertaken while the fecal stream remains diverted, the colostomy being closed as a third surgical procedure.

Definitive surgical intervention for Hirschsprung's disease should be postponed until the infant has reached adequate size to allow careful anatomic reconstruction. This should be undertaken at 1 to 1½ years of age or when the infant has reached 10 kg in weight. Attempts at early surgical intervention with or without preliminary decompression have been abandoned in recent years in favor of the better long-term results of definitive surgery in the older child.

Three surgical procedures undertaken for Hirschsprung's disease have continued to enjoy popularity. The Swenson operation involves abdominoperineal sphincter-saving proctectomy and end-to-end anastomosis at the level of the rectum. The Duhamel procedure establishes an oblique end-to-side anastomosis between the proximal ganglionic colon and the anterior aganglionic anorectal wall, which constitutes the front half of the new rectum. The posterior half of the colonic wall contains ganglion cells from the pulled-through intestine. The surgical procedure preserves important pelvic nerves supplying the bladder and ejaculatory mechanism by avoiding any dissection within the anterior pelvis. The third surgical procedure—the Soave operation—uses an endorectal mucosal dissection, removing the rectal mucosa but preserving the aganglionic rectal muscular cuff. The proximal ganglion-containing colon is then drawn through the retained muscular sleeve and anastomosed to the anorectum. Good results should be achievable in approximately 90% of cases.

After surgical correction of Hirschsprung's disease careful attention must be paid to the development of recurrent enterocolitis. Infants who had enterocolitis during the neonatal period are more likely to experience recurrent disease, perhaps related to recurrent mild obstruction associated with anastomotic edema. The avoidance of definitive pull-through in infants who underwent diversion during a bout of enterocolitis for at least 6 months should allow complete healing of the inflammatory process and further diminish the risk of recurrence.

Genetic counseling should be offered to all families with an infant with Hirschsprung's disease. Although the exact hereditary pattern is unclear, over one third of our patients have been found to have a relative born with a similar condition. Familial inheritance increases as the length of aganglionic intestine increases. Down's syndrome has been associated with approximately 10% of children with Hirschsprung's disease. In addition, other hamartomatous, dysgenetic, and neoplastic conditions associated with neural crest maldevelopment should be recognized as being associated in occasional cases with Hirschsprung's disease. These include pheochromocytoma, neuroblastoma, neurofibromatosis, medullary carcinoma of the thyroid gland, carcinoid tumors, and perigangliomas. Sensorineural deafness has also been associated with Hirschsprung's disease, and careful screening tests should be undertaken during the neonatal period to document the presence of normal hearing.

Total colonic aganglionosis is seen in approximately 5% of infants with Hirschsprung's disease. In a smaller percentage the distal small intestine is also devoid of ganglion cells. In these infants radiographic examination discloses a normal-appearing colon but refluxed contrast material will often demonstrate a dilated small intestine. The diagnosis can be established by rectal biopsy, but serial seromuscular biopsies at the time of laparotomy for intestinal diversion are necessary to establish the level of aganglionosis. These infants require surgical diversion at the lowest level of normal ganglionated intestine at the time of diagnosis and definitive surgical intervention at 1 to 1½ years of age. Martin has devised a long side-to-side anastomaosis between the distal aganglionic colon to the level of the splenic flexure and the functional ganglionated small intestine. This surgical reconstruction combines the reabsorptive capacity of the colon with the peristaltic potentiation of the small intestine. Although these infants require a rather prolonged period of bowel accommodation after their definitive surgical procedure, the surgical risks have been minimal with normal growth and development established for most children. This procedure is recommended for infants with total colonic aganglionosis, as well as those in whom the aganglionic segment involves as much as half of the small intestine.

DIAPHRAGMATIC HERNIA

Herniation of the intestinal tract through a defect in the diaphragm results in intestinal obstruction and severe respiratory compromise in most infants, although the symptoms may not be recognized for some time in less severely affected children. The diaphragmatic defect occurs through failure of closure of the pleuroperitoneal canal during the eighth week of fetal life. This most frequently occurs at the left posterolateral lumbocostal triangle, also referred to as the foramen of Bochdalek. With return of the herniated midgut into the abdomen, a persistent defect at this area allows displacement of the intestine into the involved hemithorax. The defect can vary from several centimeters to complete absence of the involved hemidiaphragm, and occurs on the left in 85% of cases. Bilateral hernias are uncommon (1%) and usually fatal. The defect may have an associated hernia sac in 21% to 47% of cases, but this does not seem to limit the amount of herniated intestine.

The severe life-threatening symptoms of diaphragmatic hernias are attributed to the associated pulmonary compromise, not the hernia per se. Large defects with extensive intestinal herniation are associated with congenital hypoplasia of the ipsilateral lung with decreased size and number of bronchi, lung saccules, and alveoli (Chapter 28, part five). Milder forms of hypoplasia are also frequently seen in the contralateral lung. A corresponding decrease in the pulmonary vascular bed is also seen. In utero compression of the ductus arteriosus may increase the pulmonary flow and pressure, resulting in muscular hypertrophy of the pulmonary arteries and leading to persistent pulmonary hypertension in the newborn infant. The clinical spectrum can vary from severe bilateral hypoplasia and fatal outcome to uniform survival in infants with minimal herniation or late onset of lung compression. During the neonatal period most infants (95%) have varying degrees of cyanosis, respiratory distress, a scaphoid abdomen, and mediastinal displacement. Approximately 5% of infants do not demonstrate symptoms as neonates and develop later signs of intestinal obstruction with vomiting, abdominal pain, and repetitive respiratory symptoms. Long-term survival in these infants is determined by their age at time of symptoms and severity of symptoms. Those who require respiratory support at the time of delivery or within the first hours of life and those who are less than 33 weeks' gestational age or 1,000 gm rarely survive. Those with symptoms after 8 hours of life with adequate blood gases have sufficient pulmonary development to allow a good survival rate.

Associated anomalies are uncommon in infants with diaphragmatic hernias with the exception of malrotation and nonfixation of the gut.

Meticulous management of the infant before surgical correction is essential for survival in severely affected infants. Early intubation and placement of a nasogastric tube will diminish air accumulation in the herniated intestine with thoracic encroachment. Mask ventilation should be avoided. Positive pressure ventilation should be instituted only when spontaneous efforts are inadequate, because pneumothorax is a constant risk both in the affected lung and in the contralateral lung.

Correction of acidosis and establishment of adequate perfusion may require both intravenous fluids and pressor agents, dopamine being preferred. Inability to correct the pH above 7.0, Po_2 above 80 mm Hg, and Pco_2 below 50 mm Hg have predicted almost uniform mortality, whereas correction to pH greater than 7.2, Po_2 greater than 100 mm Hg, and Pco_2 less than 50 mm Hg have had improved survival.

Surgical correction should be undertaken expeditiously when the infant has been resuscitated, although stability can often never be achieved. Transabdominal reduction of the herniated intestine and primary closure of the defect is possible in most cases. When prosthetic patch closure is necessary, Dacron or gortex material that is incorporated into the healing tissues should be used. A Ladd's procedure should be undertaken in infants who are stable after diaphragmatic closure to release any obstructing bands from the associated malrotation. Abdominal wound closure is undertaken with care not to compromise venous return, employing the principles used with abdominal wall defects. Adequate nasogastric or gastrostomy tube intestinal decompression is necessary. A chest tube is placed in the involved hemithorax before closure and connected to water seal without suction.

Postoperative care in these infants requires careful pulmonary and ventilatory management and maintenance of adequate perfusion. Rapid frequency low pressure ventilation has often been successful in maintaining mild alkalosis and adequate oxygenation in an effort to avoid pulmonary vasoconstriction and "persistent fetal circulation." Use of paralysis and fentanyl narcosis has also been advocated. In infants who develop progressive right-to-left shunting at the ductus arteriosus and foramen ovale, the use of pulmonary vasodilators can be of benefit occasionally when systemic perfusion pressures are maintained in the normal range with dopamine or dobutamine. Tolazoline, chlorpromazine, nitroprusside, nitroglycerine, and morphine have all been used with variable success. In the infant who fails to respond to these conventional methods, use of temporary extracorporeal cardiopulmonary bypass (ECMO), employing a membrane oxygenator can achieve survival in up to 75% of infants with otherwise certain mortality. (See Chapter 28, part three.)

Survival depends on the infant's preoperative status. Infants with respiratory insufficiency in the first 8 hours of life have a survival of 40% to 60%. Most infants with later onset of symptoms survive. Long-term results demonstrate radiographic hyperinflation of the involved lung over the first year of life. Static lung volumes return to normal, although the dynamic indexes tend to be approximately 20% below normal. Pectus excavatum can occur after survival of severely affected infants. However, in spite of these abnormalities the patients show normal exercise tolerance and are clinically normal when compared to their childhood peers.

Frederick C. Ryckman
William F. Balistreri

BIBLIOGRAPHY

Abdominal wall defects

Allen, R.G., and Wrenn, E.L., Jr.: Silon as a sac in the treatment of omphalocele and gastroschisis, J. Pediatr. Surg. **4**:3, 1969.

Binnington, H.B., Keating, J.P., and Ternberg, J.: Gastroschisis, Arch. Surg. **108**:455, 1974.

Cantrell, J.R., Haller, J.A., Jr., and Ravitch, M.M.: A syndrome of congenital defects involving the abdominal wall, sternum, diaphragm, pericardium, and heart, Surg. Gynecol. Obstet. **107**:602, 1958.

Filippi, G., and McKusick, V.A.: The Beckwith-Wiedemann syndrome, Medicine **49**:279, 1970.

Filler, R.M., and others: Total intravenous nutrition: an adjunct to the management of infants with a ruptured omphalocele, Am. J. Surg. **121**:454, 1971.

Free, E., and Takamoto, R.: Measurement of inferior vena cava pressure at the time of closure of omphaloceles, Z. Kinderchir. **5**:279, 1967.

Gilbert, M.G., and others: Staged surgical repair of large omphaloceles and gastroschisis, J. Pediatr. Surg. **3**:702, 1968.

Gray, S.W., and Skandalakis, J.E.: Embryology for surgeons, Philadelphia, 1972, W.B. Saunders Co.

Greenwood, R.D., Rosenthal, A., and Nadas, A.S.: Cardiovascular malformations associated with omphalocele, J. Pediatr. **85**:818, 1974.

Grosfeld, J.L., and Clatworthy, H.W.: Intrauterine midgut strangulation in a gastroschisis defect, Surgery **67**:519, 1970.

Hollabaugh, R.S., and Boles, E.T., Jr.: The management of gastroschisis, J. Pediatr. Surg. **8**:263, 1973.

Izant, R.J., Jr., Brown, F., and Rothman, B.F.: Current embryology and treatment of gastroschisis and omphalocele, Arch. Surg. **93**:49, 1966.

Martin, L.W., and Torres, A.M.: Omphalocele and gastroschisis, Surg. Clin. North Am. **65**:1035, 1985.

Raffensperger, J.G., and Jona, J.Z.: Gastroschisis, Surg. Gynecol. Obstet. **138**:230, 1974.

Rickham, P.P., Lister, J., and Irving, I.M.: Neonatal surgery, London, 1978, Butterworth & Co.

Rubin, S.Z., and Ein, S.H.: Experience with 55 Silon pouches, J. Pediatr. Surg. **11**:5, 1976.

Schuster, S.R.: A new method for the staged repair of large omphaloceles, Surg. Gynecol. Obstet. **125**:837, 1967.

Schuster, S.R.: Omphalocele-gastroschisis. In Kiesewetter, W.M., editor: Symposium on long-term follow-up in congenital anomalies, Children's Hospital of Pittsburgh, Sept. 14-15, 1979.

Schuster, S.R.: Omphalocele and gastroschisis. In Welch, K., and others, editors: Pediatric surgery, ed. 4, Chicago, 1986, Year Book Medical Publishers.

Swartz, K.R., and others: Ventral hernia in the treatment of omphalocele and gastroschisis, Ann. Surg. **201**:347, 1985.

Touloukian, R.J., and Spackman, T.J.: Gastrointestinal function and radiographic appearance following gastroschisis repair, J. Pediatr. Surg. **6**:427, 1971.

Intestinal duplications

Cooksey, G., and Wagget, J: Tubular duplication of the rectum treated by mucosal resection, J. Pediatr. Surg. **19**:318, 1984.

Dickinson, W.E., Weinberg, S.M., and Vellios, F.: Perforating ulcer in a duodenal duplication, Am. J. Surg. **122**:418, 1971.

Fallon, M., Gordon, A.R.G., and Lendrum, A.C.: Mediastinal cysts of foregut origin associated with vertebral abnormalities, Br. J. Surg. **41**:520, 1954.

Favara, B.E., Franciosi, R.A., and Akers, D.R.: Enteric duplications, thirty-seven cases: a vascular theory of pathogenesis, Am. J. Dis. Child. **122**:501, 1971.

Gardner, C.E., Jr., and Hart, D.: Enterogenous cysts of the duodenum, JAMA **104**:1809, 1935.

Grosfeld, J.L., O'Neill, J.A., Jr., and Clatworthy, H.W., Jr.: Enteric duplications in infancy and childhood, Ann. Surg. **172**:83, 1970.

Gross, R.E.: The surgery of infancy and childhood, Philadelphia, 1953, W.B. Saunders Co.

MacLeod, J.H., and Purves, J.K.B.: Duplications of the rectum, Dis. Colon Rectum **13**:133, 1970.

Mellish, R.W.P., and Koop, C.E.: Clinical manifestations of duplication of the bowel, Pediatrics **27**:397, 1961.

Niesche, J.W.: Duplications of the small bowel with peptic visceration, Ann. New Zealand J. Surg. **42**:356, 1973.

Parker, B.C., and others: Gastric duplications in infancy, J. Pediatr. Surg. **7**:294, 1972.

Ravitch, M.M.: Hindgut duplications, doubling of colon and genital urinary tracts, Ann. Surg. **137**:588, 1953.

Ravitch, M.M.: Duplications of the alimentary canal. In Ravitch, M.M., and others, editors: Pediatric surgery, Chicago, 1979, Year Book Medical Publishers.

Ravitch. M.M.: Duplications of the intestinal tract. In Welch, K., and others, editors: Pediatric surgery, ed. 4, Chicago, 1986, Year Book Medical Publishers.

Rios Dalenz, J.L., Kress, J.W., and Montgomery, L.G.: Duplication of small intestine with perforated peptic ulcer in ectopic gastric mucosa, Arch. Surg. **91**:863, 1965.

Ryckman, F.L., Glenn, J.D., and Moazam, F.: Spontaneous perforation of a colonic duplication, Dis. Colon Rectum, **26**:287, 1983.

Sieber, W.K.: Alimentary tract duplication, Arch. Surg. **73**:383, 1956.

Smith, E.D.: Duplication of the anus and genitourinary tract, Surgery **66**:909, 1969.

Soper, R.T.: Tubular duplication of colon and distal ileum, Surgery **63**:998, 1968.

Soper, R.T., and Selke, A.C.: Duplication cyst of the duodenum, Surgery **68**:562, 1970.

Wrenn, E.L., Jr.: Tubular duplication of the small intestine, Surgery **58**:494, 1962.

Intestinal obstruction

Preampullary obstruction of the intestine: gastric antral mucosal webs and pyloroantral atresia

Berdon, W.E., Baker, D.H., and Santulli, T.V.: Microcolon in newborn infants with intestinal obstruction, Radiology **90**:878, 1968.

Bishop, H.: Small bowel obstruction in the newborn, Surg. Clin. North Am. **56**:329, 1976.

Bjorgvinsson, E., Rudzki, C., and Lewicki, A.M.: Antral web, Am. J. Gastroenterol. **79**:663, 1984.

Carty, H., and Brereton, R.J.: The distended neonate, Clin. Radiol. **34**:367, 1983.

Feliciano, D.V., and Van Heerden, J.A.: Pyloric antral mucosal webs, Mayo Clin. Proc. **52**:650, 1977.

Ghory, M.J., and Sheldon, C.A.: Newborn surgical emergencies of the gastrointestinal tract, Surg. Clin. North Am. **65**:1083, 1985.

Lloyd, J.R., and Clatworthy, H.W., Jr.: Hydramnios as an aid to the early diagnosis of congenital obstruction of the alimentary tract: a study of the maternal and fetal factors, Pediatrics **21**:903, 1958.

Mitchell, K.G., McGowan, A., and Gillespie, G.: Pyloric diaphragm, antral web, congenital antral membrane—a surgical rarity, Br. J. Surg. **66**:572, 1979.

Mucvihill, S.J., and Fonkalsrud, E.W.: Pylorospasm in infancy and childhood, J. Pediatr. Surg. **18**:930, 1983.

Olsen, L., and Gratte, G.: Congenital pyloric atresia: report of a familial occurrence, J. Pediatr. Surg. **11**:181, 1976.

Hypertrophic pyloric stenosis

Ball, T.I., Atkinson, G.O., Jr. and Gay, B.B., Jr.: Ultrasound diagnosis of hypertrophic pyloric stenosis: real-time application and the demonstration of a new sonographic sign, Radiology **147**:499, 1983.

Belding, H.H., and Kernohan, J.W.: A morphologic study of the myenteric plexus and musculature of the pylorus, Surg. Gynecol. Obstet. **97**:322, 1953.

Benson, C.D.: Infantile pyloric stenosis, Progr. Pediatr. Surg. **1**:63, 1970.

Benson, C.D.: Infantile hypertrophic pyloric stenosis. In Welch, K., and others, editors: Pediatric surgery, Chicago, 1986, Year Book Medical Publishers.

Carter, C.O., and Evans, K.A.: Inheritance of congenital pyloric stenosis, J. Med. Genet. **6**:233, 1969.

Dodge, J.A.: Abnormal distribution of ABO blood groups in infantile pyloric stenosis, J. Med. Genet. **8**:468, 1971.

Friesen, S.R., Boley, J.O., and Miller, D.R.: The myenteric plexes of the pylorus: its early normal development and its changes in hypertrophic pyloric stenosis, Surgery **39**:21, 1956.

Ravitch, M.M.: The story of pyloric stenosis, Surgery **48**:1117, 1960.

Touloukian, R.J., and Higgins, E.: The spectrum of serum electrolytes in hypertrophic pyloric stenosis, J. Ped. Surg. **18**:394, 1983.

Yip, W.C., Tay, J.S., and Wong, H.B.: Sonographic diagnosis of infantile hypertrophic pyloric stenosis: critical appraisal of reliability and diagnostic criteria, JCU **13**:329, 1985.

Gastric volvulus

Campbell, J.R.: Other conditions of the stomach. In Welch, K., and others, editors: Pediatric surgery, ed. 4, Chicago, 1986, Year Book Medical Publishers.

Cole, B.C., and Dickinson, S.J.: Acute volvulus of the stomach in infants and children, Surgery **70**:707, 1971.

Sieber, W.K.: The stomach. In Holder, T., and Ashcroft, K., editors: Pediatric surgery, Philadelphia, 1980, W.B. Saunders Co.

Gastric perforation

Bell, M.J.: Perforation of the gastrointestinal tract and peritonitis in the neonate, Surg. Gynecol. Obstet. **160**:20, 1985.

Emanuel, B., Zlotnik, P., and Raffensperger, J.: Perforation of the gastrointestinal tract in infancy and childhood, Surg. Gynecol. Obstet. **46**:926, 1978.

Graivier, L., and others: Neonatal gastric perforation and necrosis: ninety-five percent gastrectomy with colon interposition and survival, Ann. Surg. **177**:428, 1973.

Kadowski, H., and others: Neonatal gastric perforations: a diagnostic clue in preperforative phase, Jpn. J. Surg. **13**:446, 1983.

Parrish, R.A., Sherman, R.T., and Wilson, H.: Spontaneous rupture of the gastroenteric tract in the newborn: a report of 13 cases and description of characteristic x-ray finding, Ann. Surg. **159**:244, 1964.

Quak, S.H., and others: Neonatal total gastrectomy, Clin. Pediatr. **23**:507, 1984.

Shashmikumar, V.L., and others: Spontaneous gastric rupture in the newborn: a clinical review of nineteen cases, Ann. Surg. **182**:22, 1975.

Shaw, A., and others: Spontaneous rupture of the stomach in the newborn: a clinical and experimental study, Surgery **58**:561, 1965.

Postampullary obstruction: intrinsic duodenal obstruction

Aitken, J.: Congenital intrinsic duodenal obstruction in infancy, J. Pediatr. Surg. **1**:546, 1966.

Campbell, D.P., Van Houtte, J.J., and Smith, E.I.: Partially obstructing antral web—a distinct clinical entity, J. Pediatr. Surg. **8**:723, 1973.

Dineen, J.P., and Redo, S.F.: Pyloric obstruction due to mucosal diaphragm, Surgery **53**:674, 1963.

Fonkalsrud, E.W., DeLorimier, A.A., and Hays, D.M.: Congenital atresia and stenosis of the duodenum: a review compiled from the members of the surgical section of the American Academy of Pediatrics, Pediatrics **43**:79, 1969.

Gerber, B.C.: Prepyloric diaphragm: an unusual abnormality, Arch. Surg. **90**:472, 1965.

Jona, J.Z., and Belin, R.P.: Duodenal anomalies and the ampulla of Vater, Surg. Gynecol. Obstet. **143**:565, 1976.

Lynn, H.B.: Duodenal obstruction: atresia, stenosis and annular pancreas. In Ravitch, M.M., and others, editors: Pediatric surgery, Chicago, 1979, Year Book Medical Publishers.

Richardson, W.R., and Martin, L.W.: Pitfalls in the surgical management of the incomplete duodenal diaphragm, J. Pediatr. Surg. **4**:303, 1969.

Rowe, M.I., Buckner, D., and Clatworthy, H.W., Jr.: Windsock web of the duodenum, Am. J. Surg. **116**:444, 1968.

Schnaufer, L.: Duodenal atresia, stenosis and annular pancreas. In Welch, K., and others, editors: Pediatric surgery, ed. 4, Chicago, 1986, Year Book Medical Publishers.

Stauffer, U.G., and Irving, I.: Duodenal artesia and stenosis—long-term results, Prog. Pediatr. Surg. **10**:49, 1977.

Extrinsic duodenal obstruction: malrotation

Bill, A.: Malrotation and failure of fixation of the intestinal tract. In Holder, T., and Ashcroft, K., editors: Pediatric surgery, Philadelphia, 1980, W.B. Saunders Co.

Bill, A.H.: Malrotation of the intestine. In Ravitch, M.M., and others, editors: Pediatric surgery, Chicago, 1979, Year Book Medical Publishers.

Bill, A.H., and Grauman, D.: Rationale and technique for stabilization of the mesentery in cases of nonrotation of the midgut, J. Pediatr. Surg. **1**:127, 1966.

Bill, A.S.: Malrotation. In Kiesewetter, W.M., editor: Symposium on long-term follow-up in congenital anomalies, Children's Hospital of Pittsburgh, Sept. 14-15, 1979.

Brennom, W.S., and Bill, A.H.: Prophylactic fixation of the intestine for midgut nonrotation, Surg. Gynecol. Obstet. **138**:181, 1974.

Filstron, H.C., and Kirks, D.R.: Malrotation—the ubiquitous anomaly, J. Pediatr. Surg. **16**:614, 1981.

Kiesewetter, W., and Smith, J.W.: Malrotation of the midgut in infancy and childhood, AMA Arch. Surg. **77**:483, 1958.

Schwartz, D.L., and others: Recurrent chylous ascites associated with intestinal malrotation and lymphatic rupture, J. Pediatr. Surg. **18**:177, 1983.

Smith, E.I.: Malrotation of the intestine. In Welch, K., and others, editors: Pediatric surgery, ed. 4, Chicago, 1986, Year Book Medical Publishers.

Stauffer, U.G., and Herrmann, P.: Comparison of late results in patients with corrected intestinal malrotation with and without fixation of the mesentery, J. Pediatr. Surg. **15**:9, 1980.

Jejunoileal atresia

DeLorimier, A.A., Fokalsrud, E.W., and Hays, D.M.: Congenital atresia and stenosis of the jejunum and ileum, Surgery **65**:819, 1969.

Dickson, J.A.S.: Apple peel small bowel: an uncommon variant of duodenal and jejunal atresia, J. Pediatr. Surg. **5**:595, 1970.

Grosfeld, J.L.: Jejunoileal atesia and stenosis. In Welch, K., and others, editors: Pediatric surgery, ed. 4, Chicago, 1986, Year Book Medical Publishers.

Grosfeld, J.L., Ballantine, T.V.N., and Shoemaker, R.: Operative management of intestinal atresia and stenosis based on pathologic findings, J. Pediatr. Surg. **14**:368, 1979.

Haller, J.A., et al.: Intestinal atresia, Am. J. Surg. **49**:385, 1983.

Hays, D.M.: Intestinal atresia and stenosis, Curr. Probl. Surg. Oct. 1969.

Martin, L.W., and Zerella, J.T.: Jejunoileal atresia: a proposed classification, J. Pediatr. Surg. **11**:399, 1976.

Nixon, H.H., and Tawes, R.: Etiology and treatment of small intestinal atresia: analysis of a series of 127 jejunoileal atresias and comparison with 62 duodenal atresias, Surgery **69**:41, 1971.

Santulli, T.V., Chin, C.C., and Schullinger, J.N.: Management of congenital atresia of the intestine, Am. J. Surg. **119**:542, 1970.

Touloukian, R.J.: Intestinal atresia and stenosis. In Holder, T., and Ashcroft, K., editors: Pediatric surgery, Philadelphia, 1980, W.B. Saunders Co.

Zerella, J.T., and Martin, L.W.: Jejunal atresia with absent mesentery and a helical ileum, Surgery **80**:550, 1976.

Meconium syndromes: meconium ileus and meconium peritonitis

Benson, C.D., and Adelman, S.: Neonatal colonic problems: meconium plug and left colon syndrome. In Ravitch, M.M., and others, editors: Pediatric surgery, ed. 3, Chicago, 1979, Year Book Medical Publishers.

Berdon, W.E., and others: Microcolon in newborn infants with intestinal obstruction: its correlation with the level and time of onset of obstruction, Radiology **90**:878, 1968.

Bishop, H.C., and Koop, C.E.: Management of meconium ileus: resection, Roux-en-Y anastomosis and ileostomy irrigation with pancreatic enzymes, Ann. Surg. **145**:410, 1957.

Danis, R.K., Brodeur, E.A., and Shield, S.J.: The danger of hydrogen peroxide as a colonic irrigating solution, J. Pediatr. Surg. **2**:131, 1967.

Di Sant'Agnese, P.A., Dische, A., and Danilczenko, A.: Physiochemical differences of mucoproteins in duodenal fluid of patients with cystic fibrosis of pancreas and controls: clinical aspects, Pediatrics **19**:252, 1957.

Frech, R.S., and others: Meconium ileus relieved by 40 percent water-soluble contrast enemas, Radiology **94**:341, 1970.

Gross, R.E.: Intestinal obstruction in the newborn resulting from meconium ileus. In The surgery of infancy and childhood, Philadelphia, 1953, W.B. Saunders Co.

Hartman, A.W., and Hills, W.J.: Rupture of the colon in infants during barium enema: report of two cases, Ann. Surg. **145**:712, 1957.

Heetderks, D.R., Jr., and Berbrugge, G.P.: Healed meconium peritonitis presenting as a scrotal mass in an infant, J. Pediatr. Surg. **4**:363, 1969.

Holsclaw, D.S., Eckstein, H.B., and Nixon, N.H.: Meconium ileus: a 20-year review of 109 cases, Am. J. Dis. Child. **190**:101, 1965.

Kalayoglu, M., and others: Meconium ileus: a critical review of treatment and eventual prognosis, J. Pediatr. Surg. **6**:290, 1971.

Lloyd, D.A.: Meconium ileus. In Welch, K., and others, editors: Pediatric surgery, ed. 4, Chicago, 1986, Year Book Medical Publishers.

Martin, L.: The small intestine: meconium peritonitis. In Ravitch, M.M., and others, editors: Pediatric surgery, ed. 3, Chicago, 1979, Year Book Medical Publishers.

Meeker, I.A., Jr., Hill, J.H., and Kincannon, W.N.: Meconium ileus: inspissated meconium with intestinal obstruction in the newborn, Surg. Clin. North Am. **44**:1483, 1964.

Meeker, I.A., Jr., and Kincannon, W.N.: Acetylcysteine used to liquefy inspissated meconium causing intestinal obstruction in the newborn, Surgery **56**:419, 1964.

Moore, T.C.: Giant cyst in meconium peritonitis, Ann. Surg. **157**:566, 1963.

Moore, T.C.: Internal hernia with high jejunal obstruction in infancy due to adhesions from antenatal meconium peritonitis, J. Pediatr. Surg. **8**:971, 1973.

Noblett, H.: Meconium ileus. In Ravitch, M.M., and others, editors: Pediatric surgery, ed. 3, Chicago, 1979, Year Book Medical Publishers.

O'Neill, J.A., Jr., and others: Surgical treatment of meconium ileus, Am. J. Surg. **119**:99, 1970.

Randolph, J.G., Zollinger, R.M., Jr., and Gross, R.E.: Mikulicz resection in infants and children: a 20-year survey of 196 patients, Ann. Surg. **158**:481, 1963.

Rickham, P.P., and Boeckmann, C.R.: Neonatal meconium obstruction in the absence of mucoviscidosis, Am. J. Surg. **106**:173, 1965.

Santulli, T.V.: Perforation of the rectum or colon in infancy due to enema, Pediatrics **23**:972, 1959.

Schutt, W.H., and Isles, T.E.: Protein in meconium from meconium ileus, Arch. Dis. Child. **43**:178, 1968.

Shaw, A.: Safety of N-acetylcysteine in treatment of meconium obstruction of the newborn, J. Pediatr. Surg. **4**:119, 1969.

Swenson, O.: Meconium ileus and peritonitis. In Pediatric surgery, ed. 3, New York, 1969, Appleton-Century-Crofts.
Wagget, J. Bishop, H.C., and Koop, C.E.: Experience with Gastrografin enema in the treatment of meconium ileus, J. Pediatr. Surg. **5**:649, 1970.
Wiener, E.S.: Meconium peritonitis. In Welch, K., and others, editors: Pediatric surgery, ed. 4, Chicago, 1986, Year Book Medical Publishers.

Meconium plug syndrome

Beardmore, H.E.: The large intestine: the meconium plug syndrome. In Mustard, W.T., and others, editors: Pediatric surgery, ed. 2, Chicago, 1969, Year Book Medical Publishers.
Clatworthy, H.W., Jr., Howard, W.H.R., and Lloyd, J.: The meconium plug syndrome, Surgery **39**:131, 1956.
Cooney, D.R., Rosevear, W., and Grosfeld, J.L.: Maternal and postnatal hypermagnesemia and the meconium plug syndrome, J. Pediatr. Surg. **11**:167, 1976.
Davis, W.S., and Campbell, J.B.: Neonatal small left colon syndrome occurrence in asymptomatic infants of diabetic mothers, Arch. Dis. Child. **129**:1024, 1975.
Ellis, D.G., and Clatworthy, H.W., Jr.: The meconium plug syndrome revisited, J. Pediatr. Surg. **1**:54, 1966.
Philippart, A.I., Reed, J.O., and Georgenson, K.E.: Neonatal small left colon syndrome: intramural not intraluminal obstruction, J. Pediatr. Surg. **10**:733, 1975.
Rosenstein, B.J.: Cystic fibrosis presenting with the meconium plug syndrome, Am. J. Dis. Child. **132**:167, 1978.
Sokal, M.M., and others: Neonatal hypermagnesemia and the meconium plug syndrome, N. Engl. J. Med. **286**:823, 1972.
Stewart, D.R., and others: Neonatal small left colon syndrome, Ann. Surg. **186**:741, 1977.
VanLeeuwen, G., and others: Meconium plug syndrome with aganglionosis, Pediatrics **40**:665, 1967.

Colonic obstruction: imperforate anus

Bil, A.H., Jr.: Pathology and surgical treatment of "imperforate anus," JAMA **166**:1429, 1958.
Bill, A.H., Jr., and Johnson, R.J.: Failure of migration of the rectal opening as the cause for most cases of imperforate anus, Surg. Gynecol. Obstet. **106**:643, 1958.
deVries, P.A.: The surgery of anorectal anomalies: its evolution, with evaluations of procedures, Curr. Probl. Surg. **21**:1, 1984.
deVries, P., and Cox, K.: Surgery for anorectal anomalies, Surg. Clin. North Am. **65**:1139, 1985.
deVries, P.A., and Pena, A.: Posterior sagittal anorectoplasty, J. Pediatr. Surg. **17**:638, 1982.
Hiller, R.I.: The anal sphincter and the pathogenesis of anal fissure and fistula, Surg. Gynecol. Obstet. **52**:921, 1931.
Kiesewetter, W.B.: Imperforate anus. In Holder T., and Ashcroft, K., editors: Pediatric surgery, Philadelphia, 1980, W.B. Saunders Co.
Kiesewetter, W.B.: Imperforate anus: the role and results of the sacro-abdomino-perineal operation, Ann. Surg. **164**:655, 1966.
Kiesewetter, W.B.: Imperforate anus, II. The rationale and technique of the sacro-abdominoperineal operation, J. Pediatr. Surg. **2**:106, 1967.
Kiesewetter, W.B.: Rectum and anus. In Ravitch, M.M., and others, editors: Pediatric surgery, Chicago, 1979, Year Book Medical Publishers.
Kiesewetter, W.B., and Chang, J.H.T.: Imperforate anus: a five to thirty year follow-up perspective, Prog. Pediatr. Surg. **10**:111, 1977.
Kiesewetter, W.B., and Hoon, A.: Imperforate anus: an analysis of mortalities during a 25-year period, Prog. Pediatr. Surg. **13**:211, 1979.
Kiesewetter, W.B., and Nixon, H.H.: Imperforate anus. I. Its surgical anatomy, J. Pediatr. Surg. **2**:60, 1967.
Santulli, T.V., Kiesewetter, W.B., and Bill, A.H.: Anorectal anomalies: a suggested international classification, J. Pediatr. Surg. **5**:281, 1970.
Scott, J.E.S.: The anatomy of the pelvic autonomic nervous system in cases of high imperforate anus, Surgery **45**:1013, 1959.
Smith, E.D.: Urinary anomalies and complications in imperforate anus and rectum, J. Pediatr. Surg. **3**:337, 1968.
Stephens, F.D., and Smith, E.D.: Ano-rectal malformations in children, Chicago, 1971, Year Book Medical Publishers.
Templeton, J.M., and O'Neill, J.A.: Anorectal malformations. In Welch, K., and others, editors: Pediatric surgery, ed. 4, Chicago, 1986, Year Book Medical Publishers.
Wiener, E.S., and Kiesewetter, W.B.: Urologic abnormalities associated with imperforate anus, J. Pediatr. Surg. **8**:151, 1973.

Hirschsprung's disease

Duhamel, B.: Retrorectal and transanal pull-through procedure for the treatment of Hirschsprung's disease, Dis. Colon. Rectum. **7**:455, 1964.
Jordan, F.T., Coran, A.G., and Wesley, J.R.: Modified endorectal procedure for management of long segment aganglionosis, Ann. Surg. **194**:70, 1981.
Martin, L.: Hirschsprung's disease, Surg. Clin. North Am. **65**:1171, 1985.
Martin, L.: Hirschsprung's disease. In Holder, T., and Ashcroft, K., editors: Pediatric surgery, Philadelphia, 1980, W.B. Saunders Co.
Martin, L.W.: Surgical management of total colonic aganglionosis, Ann. Surg. **176**:343, 1972.
Martin, L.W.: Surgical management of Hirschsprung's disease involving the small intestine, Arch. Surg. **97**:183, 1986.
Martin, L.W., and Altemeier, W.A.: Clinical experience with a new operation (modified Duhamel procedure) for Hirschsprung's disease, Ann. Surg. **156**:678, 1962.
Martin, L.W., and Caudill, D.R.: A method for elimination of the blind rectal pouch in the Duhamel operation for Hirschsprung's disease, Surgery **62**:951, 1967.
Martin, L.W., and others: Hirschsprung's disease with skip area (segmental aganglionosis), J. Pediatr. Surg. **14**:681, 1979.
Morikawa, Y., Donahoe, P.K., and Hendren, W.H.: Manometry and histochemistry in the diagnosis of Hirschsprung's disease, Pediatrics **53**:865, 1979.
Okamoto, E., Satini, M., and Kuwata, K.: Histologic and embryologic studies on the innvervation of the pelvic viscera in patients with Hirschsprung's disease, Surg. Gynecol. Obstet. **155**:823, 1982.
Saul, R.A., Sturner, R.A., and Burger, P.C.: Hyperplasia of the myenteric plexus: its association with early infantile megacolon and neurofibromatosis, Am. J. Dis. Child. **136**:852, 1982.
Sieber, W.K.: Hirschsprung's disease. In Ravitch, M.M., and others, editors: Pediatric surgery, Chicago, 1979, Year Book Medical Publishers.
Sieber, W.K.: Hirschsprung's disease. In Welch, K., and others, editors: Pediatric surgery, ed. 4, Chicago, 1986, Year Book Medical Publishers.
Soave, F.: Hirschsprung's disease: a new surgical technique, Arch. Dis. Child. **39**:116, 1964.
Swenson, O., and Bill, A.H.: Resection of rectum and rectosigmoid with preservation of the sphincter for benign spastic lesions producing megacolon: an experimental study, Surgery **24**:212, 1948.
Swenson, O., and others: The treatment and postoperative complications of congenital megacolon with a 25 year follow-up, Ann. Surg. **182**:266, 1975.
Valcek, F.T., and others: Operative failure and secondary repair in Hirschsprung's disease, J. Pediatr. Surg. **17**:779, 1982.

Diaphragmatic hernia

Adzick, N.S., Harrison, M.R., and Glick, P.L.: Diaphragmatic hernia in the fetus: prenatal diagnosis and outcome in 94 cases, J. Pediatr. Surg. (In press).

Ashcraft, K.W., and others: Diagnosis and treatment of right Bochdalek hernia associated with group B streptococcal pneumonia and sepsis in the neonate, J. Pediatr. Surg. **18**:480, 1983.

Bartlett, R.H., and others: Extracorporeal membrane oxygenation (ECMO): cardiopulmonary support in infancy, Trans. Am. Soc. Artif. Intern. Organs **22**:80, 1976.

Boix-Ochoa, J., and others: The important influence of arterial blood gases on the prognosis of congenital diaphragmatic hernia, World J. Surg. **1**:783, 1977.

Boles, E.T., and Anderson, G.: Diaphragmatic hernia. In Kiesewetter, W.M., editor: Symposium on long-term follow-up congenital anomalies, Children's Hospital of Pittsburgh, Sept. 14-15, 1979.

Boles, E.T., Jr., and Anderson, G.: Diaphragmatic hernia in the newborn: mortality, complications and long-term follow-up observations. In Kieswetter, W.B., editor: Symposium on long-term follow-up in congenital anomalies, Children's Hospital of Pittsburgh, Sept. 14-15, 1979.

Booker, P.D.: Congenital diaphragmatic hernia in children, Arch. Dis. Child. **56**:253, 1981.

Chu, J., and others: The pulmonary hypoperfusion syndrome, Pediatric **35**:733, 1965.

Collins, D.: Diaphragmatic hernia. In Holder, T., and Ashcroft, K., editors: Pediatric surgery, Philadelphia, 1980, W.B. Saunders Co.

Collins, D.L., and others: A new approach to congenital posterolateral diaphragmatic hernia, J. Pediatr. Surg. **12**:149, 1977.

Cullen, M., Klein, M., and Philippart, A.: Congenital diaphragmatic hernia, Surg. Clin. North Am. **65**:1115, 1985.

Dibbins, A.W., and Wiener, E.S.: Mortality from neonatal diaphragmatic hernia, J. Pediatr. Surg. **9**:653, 1974.

Gibson, C., and Fonkalsrud, E.W.: Iatrogenic pneumothorax and mortality in congenital diaphragmatic hernia, J. Pediatr. Surg. **18**:555, 1983.

Gillespie, D.J.: High frequency ventilation: a new concept in mechanical ventilation, Mayo Clin. Proc. **58**:187, 1983.

Gray, S.W., and Skandalakis, J.E.: Embryology for surgeons, Philadelphia, 1972, W.B. Saunders Co.

Gross, R.E.: The surgery of infancy and childhood, Philadelphia, 1953, W.B. Saunders Co.

Grotte, G., and others: Posterolateral diaphragmatic hernia—long-term results, Prog. Pediatr. Surg. **10**:35, 1977.

Hansen, J., and others: The decreasing incidence of pneumothorax and improving survival in infants with congenital diaphragmatic hernia, J. Pediatr. Surg. **19**:385, 1984.

Harris, M.C., and others: Group B streptococcal septicemia and delayed onset diaphragmatic hernia, Am. J. Dis. Child. **135**:723, 1981.

Harrison, M.R., and de Lorimier, A.A.: Congenital diaphragmatic hernia, Surg. Clin. North Am. **61**:1023, 1981.

Harrison, M.R., and others: Congenital diaphragmatic hernia: the hidden mortality, J. Pediatr. Surg. **13**:227, 1978.

Hislop, A., and Reid, L.: Persistent hypoplasia of the lung after repair of congenital diaphragmatic hernia, Thorax **31**:450, 1976.

Holder, T.M., and Ashcraft, K.W.: Diaphragmatic hernia. In Ravitch, M.D., and others, editors: Pediatric surgery, ed. 3, Chicago, 1979, Year Book Medical Publishers.

Johnson, D.G., Deaner, R.M., and Koop, C.D.: Diaphragmatic hernia in infancy: factors affecting the mortality rate, Surgery **62**:1082, 1967.

Kittagawa, M., and others: Lung hypoplasia in congenital diaphragmatic hernia: a quantitative study of airway, artery and alveolar developments, Br. J. Surg. **58**:342, 1971.

Klein, M.D., and others: Venovenous perfusion in ECMO for newborn respiratory insufficiency: a clinical comparison with venoarterial perfusion, Ann. Surg. **201**:520, 1985.

Krummel, T.M., and others: Alveolar-arterial oxygen gradients versus the neonatal pulmonary insufficiency index prediction of mortality in ECMO candidates, J. Pediatr. Surg. **19**:380, 1984.

Levin, D.L.: Morphologic analysis of the pulmonary vasculature in congenital left-sided diaphragmatic hernia, J. Pediatr. **92**:805, 1978.

Levin, D.L., and others: Persistent pulmonary hypertension of the newborn, J. Pediatr. **89**:626, 1976.

Levy, J.L., Jr., and others: Bilateral congenital diaphragmatic hernias through the foramina of Bochdalek, J. Pediatr. Surg. **4**:557, 1969.

Levy, J.L., and others: Bilateral congenital diaphragmatic hernia through the foramen of Bochdalek, J. Pediatr. Surg. **4**:557, 1969.

Levy, R.J., and others: Persistent pulmonary hypertension in a newborn with congenital diaphragmatic hernia. Successful management with tolazoline, Pediatrics **60**:740, 1977.

Maisels, M.J., and others: Pulmonary vascular resistance in diaphragmatic hernia: response to tolazoline, Pediatr. Res. **10**:427, 1976.

Manthei, U., Vaucher, Y., and Crowe, C.P.: Congenital diaphragmatic hernia: immediate preoperative and postoperative oxygen gradients identify patients requiring prolonged respiratory support, Surgery **93**:83, 1983.

Mentzer, R.M., Alegre, C.A., and Nolan, S.P.: The effects of dopamine and isoproterenol on the pulmonary circulation, J. Thorac. Cardiovasc. Surg. **71**:807, 1976.

Mishalany, H.G., Nakada, K., and Woolley, MM.: Congenital diaphragmatic hernias: eleven years' experience, Arch. Surg. **114**:1118, 1979.

Moore, T.C., et al.: Congenital posterolateral diaphragmatic hernia in the newborn, Surg. Gynecol. Obstet. **104**:675, 1957.

Priebe, C.J., Jr., and Wicher, W.A.: Ventral hernia with a skin covered Silastic sheet for newborn infants with a diaphragmatic hernia, Surgery **82**:569, 1977.

Raphaely, R.C., and Downes, J.J.: Congenital diaphragmatic hernia: prediction of survival, J. Pediatr. Surg. **8**:815, 1973.

Reynolds, M., Luck, S.R., and Lapper, R.: The "critical" neonate with diaphragmatic hernia: a 21 year perspective, J. Pediatr. Surg. **19**:364, 1984.

Rowe, M.I.: and Uribe, F.L.: Diaphragmatic hernia in the newborn infant: blood gas and pH considerations, Surgery **70**:758, 1971.

Ruff, S.J., and others: Pediatric diaphragmatic hernia: an 11 year experience, Am. J. Surg. **139**:641, 1980.

Simpson, J.S.: Ventral silon pouch: method of repairing congenital diaphragmatic hernia in neonates without increasing intra-abdominal pressure, Surgery **66**:798, 1969.

Stauffer, U.G., and Rickman, P.P.: Congenital diaphragmatic hernia and eventration of the diaphragm. In Rickham, P.P., Lister, J., and Irvings, J.M., editors: Neonatal surgery, London, 1978, Butterworths.

Wells, L.J.: Development of the human diaphragm and pleural sacs, Contrib. Embryol. **35**:109, 1954.

Wohl, M.E., and others: Lung growth and function following repair of congenital diaphragmatic hernia, Pediatr. Res. **7**:424, 1973.

Necrotizing enterocolitis and gastrointestinal hemorrhage

NECROTIZING ENTEROCOLITIS

Necrotizing enterocolitis (NEC) is an acquired gastrointestinal disease affecting primarily premature infants, which in its extreme form is characterized by diffuse or patchy areas of necrotic small and large intestine with or without perforation, leading to significant morbidity and mortality.

The overall incidence of NEC is between 1% to 5% of all admissions to neonatal intensive care units, with an increasing percentage during periodic epidemics of the disease. The incidence increases markedly at lower gestational ages.

Various factors have been associated with the development of NEC, including infectious agents, hypertonic feedings, asphyxia, hypovolemia, hypothermia, and exaggerated shunting reflexes, resulting in irreversible ischemic gastrointestinal injury.

Evidence of an infectious contribution to the pathophysiology of NEC has accumulated. In many nurseries a low background incidence of NEC occurs on which epidemics are superimposed. Meticulous adherence to hand washing and isolation of affected infants—measures designed to interrupt transmission of infectious agents—seems to abort some epidemics. Other findings also implicate a bacterial contribution to the disease. Pneumatosis intestinalis—intramural cysts containing 30% hydrogen gas—is a hallmark of NEC, yet the origin of the gas remains controversial. The only known source of hydrogen in humans is bacterial fermentation of a carbohydrate substrate. It would seem that in NEC enteric bacteria ferment a carbohydrate, usually formula, to produce the hydrogen. Bacteria may interact with numerous other agents to synergistically damage the immature GI tract. What we recognize as NEC is the final expression of that damage.

A

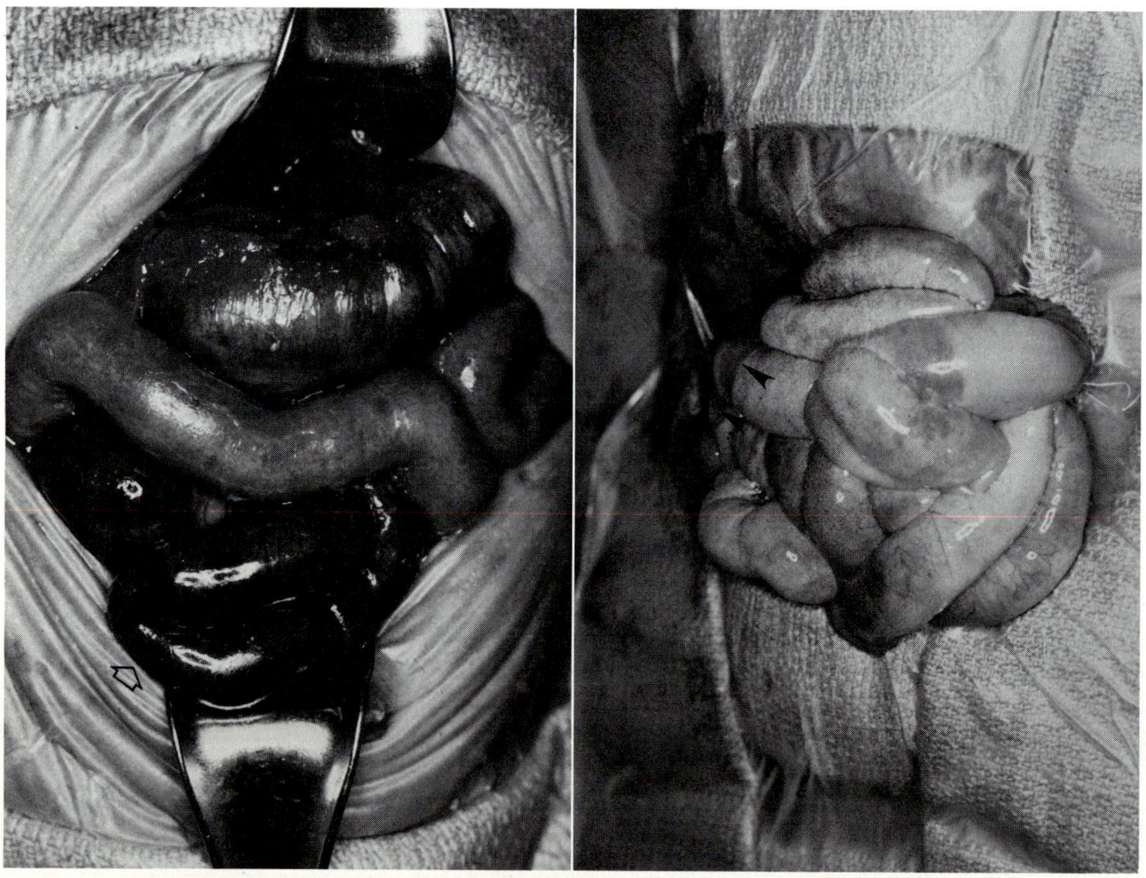

B

Fig. 33-16. Necrotizing enterocolitis. **A,** Focal hemorrhagic lesions are superimposed on the generalized ischemic small intestine *(open arrow)* and colon *(closed arrow)*. A central small intestinal loop shows early focal hemorrhagic lesions. **B,** Diffuse ischemic necrosis of the entire intestine with subserosal pneumatosis *(arrow)*. (Photograph courtesy R.J. Stevenson, M.D.)

NEC affects all segments of the gastrointestinal tract with primary involvement of the jejunum, ileum, and colon. Grossly distended loops of intestine with spotty intramural hemorrhage and areas of necrosis associated with subserosal gas collections are seen (Fig. 33-16). Cloudy-to-turbid peritoneal fluid is common. Microscopically, the earliest recognizable lesion is coagulation necrosis of the mucosa. The more severe lesions reveal a progression from coagulation necrosis to superficial mucosal ulceration, submucosal hemorrhage, and pseudomembrane formation. Later lesions can progress to transmural ischemic perforation of the intestinal wall.

The signs and symptoms of NEC are quite variable, ranging from feeding intolerance to evidence of a fulminant intraabdominal catastrophe with sepsis, shock, peritonitis, perforation, and death. The usual presentation includes abdominal distension, gastric aspirates, bilious vomiting, and bloody stools. Lethargy, apnea, and hypoperfusion also may be prominent features. The onset of symptoms is usually between the third and tenth day of life, and 90% to 95% of infants have received enteral feedings. Physical findings on serial examination allow recognition of abdominal masses associated with localized perforation or signs of progressive peritoneal irritation. However, these physical findings may be minimal and misleading even in infants with progressive disease leading to perforation.

Laboratory evaluation reflects signs of sepsis, including leukocytosis, thrombocytopenia, electrolyte imbalance, acidosis, hypoxia, and hypercarbia. Pneumatosis intestinalis, indicating air within the subserosal bowel wall, is the radiographic hallmark of NEC (Fig. 33-17). Air within the portal venous system has been considered to portend rapid progression; however, this need not be a poor prognosis (Fig. 33-18). Pneumoperitoneum is indicative of intestinal perforation.

Early and aggressive treatment of NEC should be undertaken; this should include vigorous intravenous fluid resuscitation, correction of the hematocrit, bowel rest with nasogastric decompression, and correction of thrombocytopenia.

Empiric intravenous antibiotics directed against enteric flora are started and usually include a semisynthetic penicillin such as ticarcillin and an aminoglycoside. Antibiotic therapy is modified as needed when results of stool, blood, and CSF cultures become available. Re-

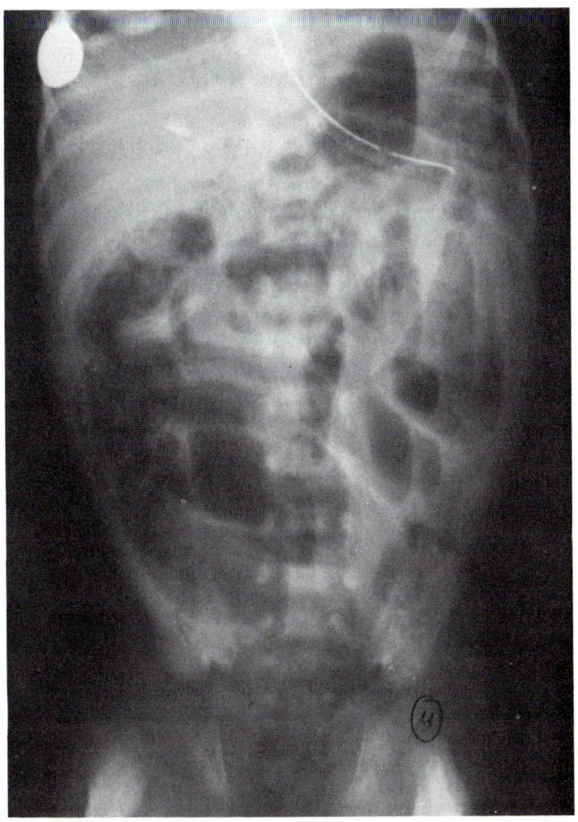

Fig. 33-17. A 1-week-old infant with necrotizing enterocolitis. Pneumatosis intestinalis occurs throughout the colon and multiple dilated proximal intestinal loops are seen.

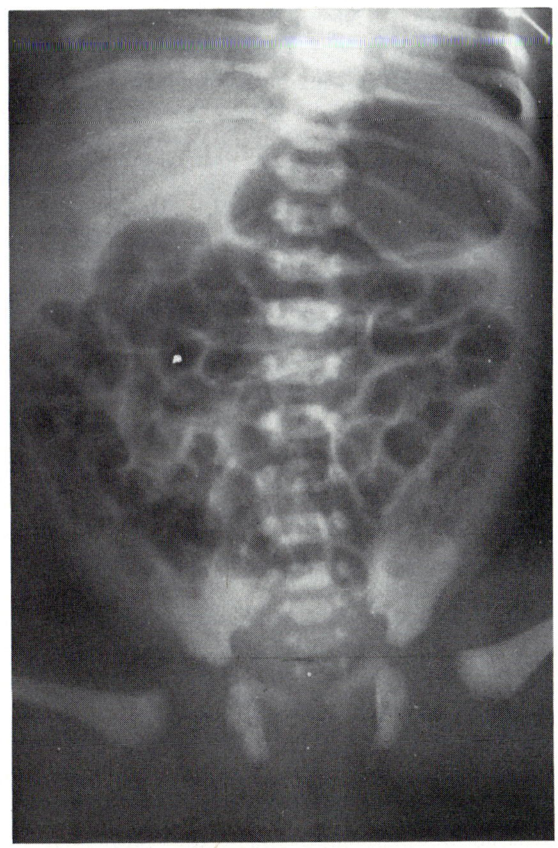

Fig. 33-18. Infant with necrotizing enterocolitis associated with diffuse colonic pneumatosis intestinalis and diffuse portal venous air.

spiratory support including intubation and ventilation is often required. Serial abdominal radiographs every 6 to 8 hours are performed to detect progressive intestinal obstruction and possible perforation. When the disease progresses in spite of maximal medical support, surgical intervention may be necessary.

Indications for surgical intervention differ between centers. The hallmark of successful surgical therapy is the anticipation of impending intestinal necrosis, allowing timely intervention before perforation to prevent gross peritoneal contamination. Unfortunately, there is no absolute indication of imminent perforation. Evidence of progressive deterioration in the form of worsening metabolic acidosis, thrombocytopenia, progressive shock from third-space losses, and increasing abdominal distension indicate ongoing necrosis. Although diagnostic paracentesis has been advocated by Kosloske and Lilly, it does not seem to be helpful in our experience. Radiographic evidence of fixed dilated intestinal loops accompanied by intestinal distension may be indicative of necrotic intestine and may be a harbinger of perforation. Indications for immediate surgical intervention are pneumoperitoneum and abdominal wall erythema or edema. Portal venous air may be indicative of severe and progressive disease but does not mandate immediate surgical intervention. Careful clinical follow-up allows surgical intervention before perforation in most cases.

The basic surgical principles of intestinal decompression, resection of necrotic bowel, and diversion of the proximal fecal stream have formed the cornerstone of surgical therapy for NEC. Nasogastric or gastrostomy tube drainage will allow optimal intestinal decompression and allow later controlled institution of feedings. A central venous line is established for hyperalimentation when clinical stability is achieved, usually several days after the primary surgical procedure.

Use of peritoneal drainage under local anesthesia in selected infants with severe NEC has been advocated by Janik and Ein to allow stabilization and later surgical intervention when required. This seems to be beneficial only in infants less than 1,000 gm in weight under carefully selected instances and cannot be universally used. Progressive sepsis after local drainage mandates laparotomy. Intestinal resection with primary anastomosis has also been advocated for selected infants with localized disease by Harberg; however, the margins of inflammation and ischemia are often poorly demarcated, and primary repair of this abnormal intestine makes stricture formation or intestinal anastomotic leak more likely. Both of these techniques should be used only in carefully selected instances.

After an adequate period of healing intestinal reanastomosis is undertaken. Ischemic stricture formation can best be distinguished from inflammatory narrowing after 4 to 6 months of intestinal diversion. A contrast radiograph of the distal and defunctionalized intestine is essential before reanastomosis to recognize the 25% to 36% of patients who develop strictures within the diverted intestine after NEC.

NEC is the most common cause of death in neonates undergoing surgery. The average mortality is 30% to 40% with a range of up to 60%. Stricture formation occurs in 25% to 35% of survivors after both medical and surgical therapy. Short gut syndrome, abscess formation, cholestasis, sepsis, and occasional recurrence of the disease are all seen as a consequence of the ischemic process or its ongoing therapy.

Attempts to prevent NEC revolve around minimizing the multiple contributing factors in a susceptible host. Correction of hypovolemia and hyperviscosity, and allowing adequate time for homeostatic mechanisms to become intact are important before enteral feeding challenge is begun. Most advocate cautious initiation of enteral feedings in a very small premature infant and in infants who have suffered perinatal asphyxia. Enteral feedings, when initiated, are started slowly using formulas of low volume (possibly dilute) while the child is carefully monitored for signs of feeding intolerance, increase in gastric aspirates, abdominal distension, and guaiac-positive stools. Evidence of feeding dysfunction mandates close observation and may require reinstitution of intravenous support and intestinal decompression.

GASTROINTESTINAL HEMORRHAGE

Over one half of the infants who have gastrointestinal bleeding, even of massive proportions, will have no identifiable cause. The overall prognosis is however very good. The diagnostic possibilities differ greatly from those causes of gastrointestinal bleeding occurring in an older child. The bleeding has frequently been attributed to stress-induced alteration of the stomach or duodenum; however, there is very little definitive data. Typically an apparently normal newborn will have bleeding between the first and fourth days of life. Of the nonidiopathic variety, swallowed maternal blood, anorectal fissures, intestinal ischemia, colitis, and hemorrhagic disorders account for approximately 10% to 15% each. The amount of bleeding is severe enough to require transfusion in many of these patients; however, radiographic and hematologic evaluation will be unrewarding, since no cause will be found in the majority of cases. Spontaneous remission without recurrence is the rule. The mortality in this group is low, and treatment consists of adequate blood replacement and monitoring during the acute hemorrhagic phase.

Hematemesis

Emesis of blood 12 to 24 hours after birth is often due to swallowed maternal blood. Because of rapid intestinal transit, hematochezia may also be present. The child is clinically well. Diagnosis is made with the Apt-Downey test, in which the specimen is mixed with tap water (1 part to 5 parts), centrifuged, and 1 ml of 0.25M sodium hydroxide added to 5 ml of the supernatant. Brown-yellow color indicates adult hemoglobin, and pink indicates fetal hemoglobin.

Hemorrhagic disease of the newborn may occur with gastrointestinal bleeding. Excessive bleeding from puncture sites or from the umbilicus is often present. Congenital clotting disorders, disseminated intravascular coagulation (often associated with sepsis or meningitis), or liver disease may also occur in this fashion. Coagulation studies are diagnostic.

Stress ulceration (with or without perforation of the duodenum or stomach) can lead to hematemesis. The vast majority of these infants have significant underlying illnesses (sepsis, prematurity, diarrheal dehydration, birth asphyxiation, central nervous system abnormalities, malnutrition). The problem can develop as early as the first 3 days of life. The diagnosis can be made endoscopically—via upper gastrointestinal radiograph—or, if perforation occurs, it is made at the time of surgery.

Hemorrhagic gastritis is most often seen in critically ill infants. It has been reported in association with use of drugs (tolazoline) but may be related to the fact that these children are all extremely ill. Diagnosis is confirmed with endoscopy.

Gastric volvulus, duplications, and hiatal hernia can occur with small amounts of hematemesis and are diagnosed via upper gastrointestinal series.

Rectal bleeding

As with hematemesis, swallowed maternal blood, hemorrhagic disease of the newborn, stress ulceration, and hemorrhagic gastritis can occur with rectal bleeding. Anorectal fissures can lead to bright red blood per rectum or blood-streaked stools and can be demonstrated by inspection and infant proctoscopy. The amount of blood loss is small. Bloody stools associated with vomiting and abdominal distention are seen with disorders associated with ischemia such as malrotation with midgut volvulus, intussusception, and intestinal duplications. An abdominal mass on examination or evidence of intestinal obstruction on abdominal x-ray film are the usual presenting features. Much more frequently seen—especially in the premature infant—is NEC, which presents with bloody stools, vomiting, abdominal distension, and sepsis. Pneumatosis intestinalis or perforation is seen on abdominal x-ray film.

Infectious diarrhea with colitis may also cause bloody stools and can be evaluated with stool cultures. Antibiotic-associated colitis is a quite rare possibility. *Clostridium difficile* and toxin are found in the stool, but one must remember that nearly 30% of healthy neonates harbor *C. difficile;* some have the toxin without clinically apparent consequences.

Milk-protein (cow's milk and/or soy protein) induced colitis can be a source of bleeding from the rectum, usually presenting 2 to 3 weeks after exposure to milk protein. Proctoscopy should be performed for diagnostic purposes, as well as for exclusion of other possible sources of bleeding such as a rectal fissure before committing the child to a more expensive casein hydrolysate-based formula. On rare occasions a breast-fed infant may bleed secondary to cow's milk in the mother's diet.

Bright red blood per rectum may occur in a child with hemangiomatosis or from bowel telangiectasia associated with the Rendu-Osler-Weber, Klippel-Trenaunay-Weber, or Turner syndrome, but it more often occurs outside of the neonatal period. The diagnosis can often be suspected on the basis of the clinical examination or family history.

Treatment

Improvements in fiberoptic endoscopy with the development of smaller caliber instruments now make it possible to study neonates. Endoscopy may be performed safely, although it is not frequently necessary. However, as expertise increases the number of infants with "idiopathic" upper gastrointestinal hemorrhage, as well as the number of infants undergoing laparotomy for superficial ulceration or gastritis, will decrease. Careful physical examination and abdominal roentgenograms are usually sufficient to rule out the majority of surgically correctable disorders. Even when massive, most instances of gastrointestinal hemorrhage in a neonate without other gastrointestinal symptoms will stop spontaneously after adequate supportive care.

Supportive therapy to prevent shock and maintain normal electrolyte balance and hematologic status is given. Vitamin K and fresh frozen plasma are necessary in patients with defective coagulation. Insertion of a nasogastric tube can evaluate the presence of upper gastrointestinal bleeding and decompress the gastrointestinal tract while also allowing administration of antacids. Use of H_2-blocking agents (e.g., cimetidine) in the neonate is controversial, primarily because of concern about toxicity of a drug that is excreted principally in the urine. Reduced dosages of 10 mg/kg/day have been used in most reports with careful monitoring of renal function. Serial evaluations of preprandial gastric acidity may be useful in estimating the lowest drug dose necessary to maintain the pH between 5 and 6.

In disorders associated with intestinal ischemia, surgical therapy is often necessary, but it is otherwise rarely indicated in treatment of neonatal gastrointestinal hemorrhage.

Anorectal fissures are treated by assuring passage of frequent soft stools. Milk-protein colitis can be treated with a casein hydrolysate-based formula such as Nutramigen or Pregestimil after other possible causes for the bleeding have been investigated.

Karen D. Crissinger
Frederick C. Ryckman
William F. Balistreri

BIBLIOGRAPHY

Necrotizing enterocolitis

Amoury, R.A.: Necrotizing enterocolitis. In Holder, T., and Ashcroft, K., editors: Pediatric surgery, Philadelphia, 1980, W.B. Saunders Co.

Bell, M., Shackelford, P., and Molleston, J.: Hypothesis: neonatal necrotizing enterocolitis is caused by the acquisition of a pathogenic organism by a susceptible host infant, Surgery **97**:350, 1985.

Bell, M.J., Ternberg, J.L., and Bower, R.J.: The microbial flora and antimicrobial therapy of neonatal peritonitis, J. Pediatr. Surg. **15**:569, 1980.

Bell, M.J., and others: Intestinal stricture in necrotizing enterocolitis, J. Pediatr. Surg. **11**:319, 1976.

Bell, M.J., and others: Neonatal necrotizing enterocolitis therapeutic decisions based on clinical staging, Ann. Surg. **187**:1, 1978.

Brown, E.G., and Sweet, A.Y.: Neonatal necrotizing entercolitis, Pediatr. Clin. North Am. **29**:1149, 1982.

Cikrit, D., and others: Necrotizing enterocolitis: factors affecting mortality in 101 surgical cases, Surgery **96**:648, 1984.

Harberg, F.J., and others: Resection with primary anastomosis for necrotizing enterocolitis, J. Pediatr. Surg. **6**:743, 1983.

Janik, J.S., Ein, S.H., and Mancer, K.: Intestinal stricture after necrotizing enterocolitis, J. Pediatr. Surg. **16**:438, 1981.

Kliegman, R.M., and Fanaroff, A.A.: Necrotizing enterocolitis, N. Engl. J. Med. **310**:1093, 1984.

Kosloske, A.M.: Necrotizing enterocolitis in the neonate, Surg. Gynecol. Obstet. **148**:259, 1979.

Kosloske, A.M., Burstein, J., and Barton, S.A.: Intestinal obstruction due to colonic stricture following neonatal necrotizing enterocolitis, Ann. Surg. **192**:202, 1980.

Kosloske, A.M., and Goldthorn, J.F.: Paracentesis as an aid to the diagnosis of intestinal gangrene: experience in 50 infants and children, Arch. Surg. **117**:571, 1982.

Kosloske, A.M., and Ulrich, J.A.: A bacteriologic basis for the clinical presentations of necrotizing enterocolitis, J. Pediatr. Surg. **15**:558, 1980.

Martin, L.W., and Neblett, W.W.: Early operation with intestinal diversion for necrotizing enterocolitis, J. Pediatr. Surg. **16**:252, 1981.

O'Neill, J. and Holcomb, G.W.: Surgical experience with neonatal necrotizing enterocolitis, Ann. Surg. **189**:612, 1979.

O'Neill, J.A.: Neonatal necrotizing enterocolitis, Surg. Clin. North Am. **61**:1013, 1981.

O'Neill, J.A., Jr.: Necrotizing entercolitis. In Falkner, F., Kretchmer, N., and Rossi, E., editors: Modern problems in paediatrics, vol 23, Basel, Switzerland, 1985, Karger.

Rowe, M.I.: Necrotizing enterocolitis. In Welch, K., and others, editors: Pediatric surgery, ed. 4, Chicago, 1986, Year Book Medical Publishers.

Schwartz, M.Z., and others: Intestinal stenosis following successful management of necrotizing entercolitis, J. Pediatr. Surg. **15**:809, 1980.

Schwartz, M.A., and others: A prospective evaluation of intestinal stenosis following necrotizing enterocolitis, J. Pediatr. Surg. **17**:764, 1982.

Walsh, M.C., and Kliegman, R.M.: Necrotizing enterocolitis: treatment based on staging criteria, Pediatr. Clin. North Am. **33**:179, 1986.

Gastrointestinal hemorrhage

Apt, L., and Downey, W.S., Jr.: "Melena" neonatorum, the swallowed blood syndrome: a simple test for the differentiation of adult and fetal hemoglobin in bloody stools, J. Pediatr. **47**:6, 1955.

Bell, M.J., and others: Perforated stress ulcers in infants, J. Pediatr. Surg. **16**:993, 1981.

Chhattriwalla, Y., and others: The use of cimetidine in the newborn, Pediatrics **65**:301, 1980.

Eastham, E.J., and Walker, W.A.: Adverse effects of milk formula ingestion on the gastrointestinal tract: an update, Gastroenterology **76**:365, 1979.

Hyams, J.S., and others: Recent advances in diagnosis and treatment of gastrointestinal hemorrhage in infants and children, J. Pediatr. **106**:1, 1985.

Powell, G.K.: Milk- and soy-induced enterocolitis of infancy: clinical features and standardization of challenge, J. Pediatr. **93**:553, 1978.

Stillman, A.E., and others: Diffuse neonatal hemangiomatosis with severe gastrointestinal involvement, Clin. Pediatr. **22**:589, 1983.

Viscidi, R.P., and Bartlett, J.G.: Antibiotic-associated pseudomembranous colitis in children, Pediatrics **67**:381, 1981.

Ziemniak, J.A., and others: The pharmacokinetics and metabolism of cimetidine in neonates, Dev. Pharmacol. Ther. **7**:30, 1984.

PART FOUR

Upper gastrointestinal disorders

DISORDERS OF SUCKING AND SWALLOWING

The ability of the fetus to coordinate and integrate sucking, swallowing, and breathing is not well developed until late in gestation (33 to 34 weeks); however, the sucking response can be elicited by the sixteenth week of intrauterine life, and the fetus has been documented to swallow at this time. In the postnatal period there is significant individual variation in the ability to coordinate these mechanisms. This may persist until approximately the sixth month of age. When first fed, the mature infant will have short bursts of three to five sucks followed by single swallows. The sucking pattern rapidly evolves to consist of approximately 30 sucks followed by swallowing. This is the more mature response in which the lips and jaws exert pressure on the nipple and combine with negative intraoral pressure to bring fluid into the mouth. At this time the dorsum of the tongue is elevated against the soft palate to form a seal, preventing milk from entering the pharynx and also forcing milk from the posterior pharynx into the esophagus. Therefore the mouth is separated from the pharynx, and the infant is able to breathe during this phase of swallowing. The tongue forces the milk to the back of the pharynx, and the muscles of the soft palate contract and bring the palate upward and backward to close the connection with the nose. The epiglottis closes the entry to the larynx; together these mechanisms inhibit breathing. The tongue then is thrust forward, the epiglottis rises, and the infant can once again breathe. When the bolus of fluid passes the

Table 33-3. Conditions associated with or causing disorders of sucking and swallowing

Absent or diminished suck	Mechanical factors interfering with sucking	Disorders of the swallowing mechanism (not including esophageal abnormalities)
Maternal anesthesia or analgesia	Macroglossia	Choanal atresia
Anoxia or hypoxia	Cleft lip	Cleft palate
Prematurity	Fusion of gums	Micrognathia
Trisomy 21	Tumors of mouth or gums	Postintubation dysphagia
Trisomy 13	Temporomandibular ankylosis or hypoplasia	Palatal paralysis
Hypothyroidism		Pharyngeal tumors
Neuromuscular abnormalities		Pharyngeal diverticula
Kernicterus		Familial dysautonomia
Werdnig-Hoffmann disease		
Neonatal myasthenia gravis		
Congenital muscular dystrophy		
Infections of the CNS		
Toxoplasmosis		
Cytomegalovirus infection		
Bacterial meningitis		

Modified from Gryboski, J.: Gastrointestinal problems in the infant, Philadelphia, 1983, W.B. Saunders Co.

posterior pharynx and enters the esophagus, the pharyngoesophageal sphincter relaxes and then closes to initiate peristalsis in the esophagus. The normal esophageal peristaltic wave is large and monophasic, but in premature infants the wave may be biphasic and there may be nonperistaltic segmental contractions of the esophagus.

Despite the presence of a well-developed and intricate mechanism for sucking and swallowing, when semisolid foods are first given, the infant will often force the foods back out of the mouth and not swallow them. Abnormalities of the sucking and swallowing reflex occur in premature infants. These may be secondary to maternal anesthesia and may be found in infants who are anoxic or hypoxic at birth or may be the first manifestation of CNS disorders. Infants who have had prolonged orotracheal or nasotracheal intubation may have transient incoordination of sucking and swallowing (Table 33-3).

ESOPHAGEAL DUPLICATIONS AND CYSTS

Duplication of the esophagus occurs most frequently as an expanding posterior mediastinal mass, which may cause cyanosis and respiratory difficulties. Progressive expansion of the duplication may compress the posterior tracheobronchial wall and pulmonary parenchyma and cause the infant to have intermittent vomiting and discomfort with feedings or develop recurrent episodes of pneumonia.

Esophageal cysts usually have a muscular wall and are lined with ciliated or squamous epithelium. They may, however, be lined with *gastric* epithelium, which may be associated with acid secretion and peptic hemorrhage, bleeding, or erosion into a bronchus or lung. Abnormalities associated with duplications include variations of the cervical or upper thoracic vertebrae and intrathoracic anomalies such as agenesis of the lung or tracheoesophageal fistulas and intraabdominal cysts. The diagnosis can be made by barium swallow with attention to lateral and oblique positions. The differential diagnosis includes bronchogenic cysts, tumors of neurogenic origin, teratomas, and abscesses. Treatment is surgical removal of the duplication; this should include a careful search for communication with intraabdominal cysts.

GASTROESOPHAGEAL REFLUX

An area of much contemporary concern is gastroesophageal reflux; this is an extremely common problem in newborns, especially in those born prematurely. At maturity the distal esophagus manifests a physiologic sphincter pressure at the esophageal vestibule, the proximal end of which lies in the thorax, the midportion in the esophageal hiatus of the diaphragm, and the distal end in the abdomen. It is approximately 0.5 cm long in the infant and is much shorter than that of the older child or adult. The esophageal mucosa is lined by columnar epithelium, which is resistant to acid-pepsin digestion, has no acid or pepsin secreting cells, and is firmly attached to the underlining musculature. A cuff of muscle encloses the mucosa and is joined to the diaphragm by the phrenoesophageal membrane. This cuff of muscle and the mucosal anatomy permit opening and closing of the vestibule and would normally serve to prevent retrograde flow of gastric contents into the esophagus. This portion of the terminal esophagus has a higher pressure than that of the stomach below and of the esophagus above. The lower esophageal sphincter (LES) pressure falls after deglutition; opening of the vestibule is related to deglutition and not necessarily to the stripping peristaltic wave of the esophagus. The vestibule opens from above downward and closes in the same manner; both occur very rapidly in the infant. The interval between swallowing and the opening of the vestibule is very short and increases in duration with age. The pressure in full-term infants is usually less than 2.5 mm Hg and remains low until adult pressures (5 to 6 mm Hg) are then attained at 1 to 2 months. Because of the low LES pressure, the prolonged relaxation of the LES itself, and the poor coordination of esophageal motility in the neonate, the majority of normal infants will have regurgitation of some proportion of their feedings. This can be documented by several methods, including barium swallow, measurement of intraesophageal pH, and scintigraphic methodology. In most instances gastroesophageal reflux is a temporary phenomenon that is not associated with adverse clinical consequences and will resolve with age. In the presence of persistent regurgitation, which is associated with poor weight gain or aspiration, specific therapy may be indicated.

The initial treatment of all infants with gastroesophageal reflux is medical. Use of upright positioning, thickened formula feedings, and occasionally metaclopramide to achieve normal gastric emptying will improve almost all infants. As the lower esophageal sphincter tone increases over the first 6 months of life, reflux symptoms often resolve. The onset of symptoms later than 6 months and symptomatic reflux in a child with neurologic impairment both decrease the chances of successful medical therapy.

Indications for surgical intervention include (1) failure to thrive, (2) recurrent pneumonia, (3) anemia caused by esophageal bleeding, (4) persistent vomiting, and (5) a large hiatus hernia or paraesophageal hernia.

Two surgical techniques are used in infants with reflux in the majority of cases, the Nissen fundoplication or the Thal repair. The Nissen operation involves placing the esophagogastric junction within the abdomen and wrapping the fundus 360 degrees around the esophagus for a distance of 3 to 4 cm. The fundus is sutured to itself and the underlying esophageal wall. The vagus nerves are included within the wrap, and the wrap is sutured to the diaphragm to prevent displacement into the chest. The esophageal hiatus is closed to fit snugly around, but not restrict, the esophagus. This repair is used by most surgeons and reliably relieves reflux in 85% of cases. The Thal repair also mobilizes the esophagogastric junction into the abdomen and closes the esophageal hiatus. It forms an anterior wrap of the fundus, encircling 180 degrees of the esophagus.

Both surgical repairs afford excellent control of reflux, reliably prevent recurrent aspiration, and improve weight gain. However, complications of surgery can be significant. Small bowel obstruction requiring reoperation is noted in 5% to 7%, wrap displacement into the chest occurs in 2% to 8%, and disruption of the wrap occurs in from 3% to 10% of patients. Postoperative death is uncommon and occurs almost exclusively in neurologically damaged children. However, these complications mandate the careful selection of individuals for surgical intervention.

Gastroesophageal reflux in a neurologically damaged infant and child represents a significant problem. These infants are often not diagnosed until their symptoms are severe; failure to thrive is common. Their severe esophagitis and malnutrition can be greatly improved by short-term preoperative hospitalization, resuscitative alimentation with vigorous antacid administration, and therapy for any underlying pulmonary disease. Careful attention to the gastric emptying scan will allow recognition of those with underlying delayed gastric emptying who would benefit from a pyloroplasty at the time of fundoplication. Gastrostomy tube placement is especially important to allow good gastric decompression in these aerophagic infants and gradual introduction of incremental or continuous drip feedings. The overall complication rate when repair is undertaken in these children has been reported to be as high as 40%; however, their benefits after surgery still offset this risk.

Reflux strictures of the esophagus are present in up to 10% of all patients undergoing surgical repair. Intraoperative dilation with Hagar or Tucker dilators before Nissen fundoplication is coupled with postoperative dilations through the gastrostomy site using Tucker dilators. Retrograde dilations are preferred because of the high incidence of infants with previous tracheoesophageal fistula repairs in this group.

Special reference should be made to the infant undergoing evaluation for a feeding gastrostomy. All of these infants must have reflux excluded before undergoing gastrostomy placement. However, Jolley has shown that 64% of those infants with no reflux on preoperative evaluation will develop reflux and persistent vomiting after gastrostomy placement, presumably because of changes in esophagogastric orientation. Most of these patients in infancy have neurologic impairment. Although they advocate antireflux repairs for all infants with neurologic impairment undergoing gastrostomy, this policy should be selectively implemented but carefully considered before routine gastrostomy placement is undertaken in these infants.

TRACHEOESOPHAGEAL FISTULA

Tracheoesophageal fistula (TEF) continues to be a relatively common and challenging problem in pediatric surgery. When recognized and treated early, primary repair allows complete reconstitution of normal esophageal continuity. When complicated by aspiration pneumonia or major associated anomalies, it remains a life-threatening malformation. A high index of suspicion allowing early diagnosis and selective management will optimize reconstructive efforts.

TEF occurs with an incidence of approximately 1 in

4,500 live births. The anomaly usually occurs in an isolated form with only rare familial or sibling cases reported. It is, however, often associated with multiple coexisting anomalies composing the Vater syndrome, which includes TEF, as well as vertebral abnormalities, anal anomalies, renal malformations, and limb dysplasias of the radius. These multiple associated anomalies would suggest a common teratogen, although none has been identified.

An anatomically descriptive classification of TEF abnormalities is greatly preferred to the numerous numeric or alphabetic staging systems. Esophageal atresia with a distal TEF makes up the most common subtype, representing 85% of cases. Isolated esophageal atresia without TEF and TEF (H-fistula) without esophageal atresia both make up approximately 5% to 7% of cases in most series. Esophageal atresia with proximal TEF or esophageal atresia with both proximal and distal TEF is rare.

Infants with TEF primarily have symptoms of esophageal obstruction or secondary respiratory complications. In patients with esophageal atresia, polyhydramnios is common (Chapter 6). Involved infants are often described as "mucousy" and frequently cough or choke on their copious oral secretions. Intermittent attacks of cyanosis are characteristic. Abdominal distension occurs when a communication between the trachea and distal esophagus exists. In these infants crying and coughing lead to rapid distension of the gastrointestinal tract with air and gastroesophageal pneumonic reflux of acidic gastric contents. Bile-stained aspirate from the posterior pharynx can be seen after significant aspiration episodes. Recurrent reflux leads to the progressive development of chemical and bacterial aspiration pneumonia. When esophageal atresia exists in the absence of TEF, respiratory symptoms occur only if the diagnosis is delayed and aspiration of upper pouch secretions occurs. Patients without a distal TEF and those with pure esophageal atresia have a gasless abdomen.

The diagnosis of TEF, although suspected from the clinical course, can be rapidly confirmed by placing a no. 10 (Replogle) nasogastric suction catheter. In the presence of esophageal atresia the catheter cannot be passed beyond approximately 10 cm. An AP and lateral radiograph of the chest including the neck will show the catheter within the upper esophageal pouch. Lateral radiographs also often identify the distal TEF and air-filled distal esophagus if exposed during crying. In the presence of these diagnostic findings a proximal pouch contrast study is not necessary to confirm the diagnosis. In cases where the diagnosis is unclear, the possibility of esophageal stenosis rather than atresia is suggested, or a proximal fistula is suspected, 1 to 2 ml of barium can be placed in the upper pouch under fluoroscopic guidance. This should be rapidly aspirated from the upper pouch to prevent subsequent regurgitation and tracheal aspiration following the radiograph. An AP abdominal pelvic radiograph to examine the lumbosacral spine and selected radiographs of the upper extremity when malformed are also mandatory.

In all infants with tracheoesophageal malformations vigorous protective medical management is undertaken while appropriate surgical staging decisions are made. Infants requiring transport to a major pediatric surgical setting should be positioned in a 30-degree upright position, administered supplemental oxygen, and should have an effective upper pouch–suction catheter in position before transport. Meticulous attention to posterior pharyngeal and airway suction is necessary to prevent the development of pneumonitis. Associated life-threatening anomalies that significantly affect treatment decisions and survival should be recognized before surgery. Between 30% to 40% of infants with esophageal atresia have significant coexisting anomalies, with a high proportion of these being cardiovascular. In these infants cardiac investigation, renal ultrasound, and careful review of the skeletal system is necessary. Other non-life threatening but significant anomalies such as cleft palate, duodenal atresia, imperforate anus, and hydrocephalus should also be excluded. Preoperative ultrasound evaluations of the heart and kidneys are indicated on a routine basis.

The surgical management of infants with TEF can be divided into three types: primary repair, delayed primary repair, and staged management.

Primary esophageal anastamosis is the optimal method of treatment of infants who are without associated life-threatening abnormalities, who have minimal to no respiratory compromise or pneumonia, and who weigh greater than 2,000 gm. Delayed primary anastamosis is employed in full-term infants who have established pneumonia at the time of diagnosis or other coexisting problems requiring investigation before correction of the TEF. In these infants a preliminary decompressive gastrostomy should be placed at the time of diagnosis to allow gastric decompression and minimize ongoing pulmonary contamination. Infants with hyperbilirubinemia, sepsis, or other metabolic abnormalities, as well as coexisting cardiac or renal anomalies requiring additional investigation, are best handled in this manner. Staged management is most appropriately directed toward infants with prematurity, established pneumonia, associated life-threatening anomalies, those with a long gap between the two esophageal segments, or those who deteriorate during primary surgical intervention. In these infants ligation of the TEF to prevent ongoing pulmonary contamination is combined with gastrostomy tube placement for subsequent enteral feeding. In patients with "long gap" esophageal atresia and those with no distal TEF the stomach and intestinal tract will often be quite small, and careful positioning of the gastrostomy tube will be necessary. Use of gastrostomy tube decompression with central venous hyperalimentation without ligation of the TEF can allow continuous pulmonary contamination in conjunction with cholestasis from hyperalimentation, often making the care of premature infants with TEF more complicated and dangerous than the risk of thoracotomy for fistula ligation.

Surgical correction is best undertaken through the right hemithorax unless a right aortic arch is present. A retropleural approach is preferred at the time of esophageal reanastomosis to avoid contaminating the hemithorax should an esophageal leak occur. Extensive mobilization of the proximal esophageal pouch is possible because of its longitudinal submucosal blood supply, which is derived from the thyrocervical trunk. In contrast, mobilization of the distal esophagus should be minimized because of its delicate segmental aortic blood supply. A primary end-to-end anastomosis without placing the suture line under tension is the key to successful esophageal reconstruction. In the presence of inadequate esophageal length a circular myotomy of the proximal pouch will often allow a tension-free anastomosis. Closed thoracic drainage will prevent accumulation of any potential secretions should esophageal leak occur. The end-to-end esophageal reconstruction of Salumma has been associated with an inordinately high incidence of recurrent fistula and should not be employed.

Meticulous postoperative care is essential for successful recovery after esophageal reconstruction. Nasotracheal intubation with low pressure ventilation will protect the tracheal suture line while maintaining a good evacuation of tracheal secretions. Extubation should be undertaken at a time when respiratory function is returned to normal. It must be followed by careful and frequent suctioning of the posterior pharynx to prevent secretion accumulation. Poor swallowing associated with postintubation and anastomotic edema makes accumulation of secretions and subsequent aspiration and pulmonary collapse inevitable in the absence of skilled nursing care. Gastrostomy tube feedings may be cautiously begun on the seventh postoperative day if a water-soluble contrast swallow demonstrates the absence of an esophageal leak.

Complications after tracheoesophageal repair include anastomotic complications and respiratory compromise. Anastomotic disruption is suggested by the presence of saliva in the chest tube or the development of an unexpected pneumothorax. These most often occur between the second and sixth postoperative day. In the presence of a small leak with adequate drainage through the thoracostomy tube, healing can be expected with intravenous hyperalimentation, antibiotic support, thoracic drainage, and gastrostomy tube decompression. In patients who deteriorate with mediastinal sepsis, reexploration for adequate thoracic drainage and a diverting cervical esophagostomy, and distal esophageal ligation can be lifesaving. This, however, often mandates esophageal replacement at a later date.

Development of an esophageal stricture after esophageal reconstruction is often associated with anastomotic ischemia from excessive tension on the suture line and is regularly seen following esophageal leaks. Esophageal strictures are most frequently recognized 2 to 3 weeks into the postoperative period by the presence of increasing dysphagia and feeding intolerance. A barium esophagram is diagnostic. Placement of transanastomotic string, followed by retrograde dilation, will allow most anastomoses to be satisfactorily dilated and esophageal continuity preserved. Dilation may be begun safely after 4 postoperative weeks. An occasional stricture remains refractory to dilation and requires resection and reanastomosis.

Controversy exists concerning the use of single- or two-layer anastomotic techniques in esophageal reconstruction. Multiple surveys have demonstrated that esophageal leak is slightly more common in single-layer anastomoses than in their double-layer counterpart; however, esophageal stricture is more common after the two-layer Haight reconstruction. Both complications are greatly increased in premature infants who weigh less than 2,000 gm.

Recurrent TEF is an uncommon complication after TEF repair. Recurrence of shortness of breath, choking, wheezing, and pneumonia herald its development, with the symptoms evolving in porportion to the size of the recurrent fistula. Diagnosis by barium cine esophagram in the prone position is definitive. Reconstruction of the esophagus with esophageal reanastomosis after resection of the recurrent fistula is necessary. In difficult cases a transtracheal approach to recurrent fistulas can be employed.

After tracheoesophageal repair many infants will have stridor, a brassy "TEF" cough, and bronchospastic airway symptoms. Less commonly, apnea, cyanosis, and syncope can result from acute episodic airway obstruction. This syndrome has been associated with innominate artery compression of the anterior, often softened, tracheal wall. A lateral cervical thoracic radiograph demonstrates anterior compression of the trachea, and bronchoscopy shows an anterior pulsatile compression. Anterior aortic arch suspension to the posterior sternum relieves these compression symptoms and has been necessary in approximately 4% of all TEF cases in our experience.

Gastroesophageal reflux associated with recurrent pneumonia or increasing respiratory symptoms has been commonly seen after TEF repair. This important complication must also be excluded in all patients with esophageal strictures that are resistent to dilation or develop late in the course of therapy. Foreign body impaction at the anastomotic site can also occur at the time solid food is instituted.

Esophageal atresia without esophageal fistula occurs with "long gap" esophageal absence and requires selective care. An upper pouch contrast study to exclude a proximal fistula is necessary. Gastrostomy placement should be undertaken early with careful positioning to spare the greater curvature should gastric tube reconstruction be necessary in the future. The small stomach in patients with no distal esophageal communication makes this procedure particularly difficult. Daily bougienage of the proximal and distal pouch, as well as electromagnetic bougienage and multiple circular myotomies, have been used to reconstruct primary esophageal continuity in the occasional patient in whom the gap can be shortened. Most individuals with esophageal atresia ultimately require esophageal replacement at approximately 1 year of age.

Isolated TEF without esophageal atresia (H-type fistula) must be suspected in all infants with coughing during feedings and recurrent pneumonitis. This fistula is best diagnosed by cine-esophagram, using selective esophageal injection to isolate the site of the fistula. In cases where radiographs are inconclusive, esophagoscopy and bronchoscopy are diagnostic. The H-type fistula can almost invariably be reconstructed via a cervical approach. Thoracotomy is rarely necessary.

Success and survival after surgical repair are directly related to the patient's age, preoperative weight, and associated anomalies. In full-term infants with no related associated anomalies survival approaches 100% in most large series. In premature infants with associated congenital abnormalities survival as low as 50% has been regularly reported. Careful preoperative staging, appropriate and judicious use of primary esophageal reconstruction, and vigorous treatment of associated anomalies have greatly improved the survival of these complex infants.

Frederick C. Ryckman
William F. Balistreri

BIBLIOGRAPHY
Disorders of the esophagus

Gastroesophageal reflux

Ashcraft, K.W., and others: The Thal fundoplication for gastroesophageal reflux, J. Pediatr. Surg. **19**:480, 1984.

Balistreri, W.F., and Farrell, M.K.: Gastroesophageal reflux in infants, N. Engl. J. Med. **309**:790, 1983.

Berlatzky, Y., and others: Surgical treatment of gastroesophageal reflux with esophageal stricture in infancy and childhood, Am. J. Surg. **143**:205, 1982.

Byrne, W.J., and others: Gastroesophageal reflux in the severely retarded who vomit: criteria for and results of surgical intervention in twenty-two patients, Surgery **91**:95, 1982.

Byrne, W.J., and others: A diagnostic approach to vomiting in severely retarded patients, Am. J. Dis. Child. **137**:259, 1983.

Fonkalsrud, E.W., Ament, M.E., and Berquist, W.: Surgical management of the gastroesophageal reflux syndrome in childhood, Surgery **97**:42, 1985.

Fonkalsrud, E.W., and others: Gastroesophageal fundoplication for the management of reflux in infants and children, J. Thorac. Cardiovasc. Surg. **76**:655, 1978.

Guggenbichler, J.P., and Menardi, G.: Conservative treatment of gastroesophageal reflux and hiatus hernia, Prog. Pediatr. Surg. **18**:78, 1985.

Johnson, D.G.: Current thinking on the role of surgery in gastroesophageal reflux, Pediatr. Clin. North Am. **32**:1165, 1985.

Johnson, D.G., and Jolley, S.G.: Gastroesophageal reflux in infants and children: recognition and treatment, Surg. Clin. North Am. **61**:1101, 1981.

Jolley, S.G., Smith, E.I., and Tunell, W.P.: Protective antireflux operation with feeding gastrostomy: experience with children, Ann. Surg. **201**:736, 1985.

Johnson, D.G., and others: Surgical selection of infants with gastroesophageal reflux, J. Pediatr. Surg. **16**:587, 1981.

Jolley, S.G., and others: The accuracy of abbreviated esophageal pH monitoring in children, J. Pediatr. Surg. **6**:848, 1984.

Kim, S.H., and Donahoe, P.K.: Gastroesophageal reflux and hiatus hernia in children: experience with 70 cases, J. Pediatr. Surg. **15**:443, 1980.

Leape, L.L.: Gastroesophageal reflux. In Holder, T., and Ashcroft, K., editors: Pediatric surgery, Philadelphia, 1980, W.B. Saunders Co.

Mollitt, D.L., Golladay, E.S., and Seibert, J.J.: Symptomatic gastroesophageal reflux following gastostomy in neurologically impaired patients, Pediatrics **75**:1124, 1985.

O'Neill, J.A., and others: Surgical management of reflux strictures of the esophagus in childhood, Ann. Surg. **196**:453, 1982.

Pennell, R.C., and others: Management of severe gastroesophageal reflux in children, Arch. Surg. **119**:553, 1984.

Randolph, J.: Experience with the Nissen fundoplication for correction of gastroesophageal reflux in infants, Ann. Surg. **198**:579, 1983.

Reyes, H.M., and Ostrovsky, E.: Diagnosis and treatment of gastroesophageal reflux in infants and children, Ann. Surg. **15**:61, 1983.

Scharli, A.F.: Gastroesophageal reflux and severe mental retardation, Prog. Pediatr. Surg. **18**:84, 1985.

Spitz, L., and Kirtane, J.: Results and complications of surgery for gastroesophageal reflux, Arch. Dis. Child. **60**:743, 1985.

Tunell, W.P., Smith, E.I., and Carson, J.A.: Gastroesophageal reflux in childhood: the dilemma of surgical success, Ann. Surg. **197**:560, 1983.

Wesley, J.R., and others: The need for evaluation of gastroesophageal reflux in brain damaged children referred for feeding gastrostomy, J. Pediatr. Surg. **16**:866, 1981.

Tracheoesphageal fistula

Ashcroft, K.W., and Holder, T.M.: Esophageal atresia and tracheoesophageal malformations. In Holder, T.M., and Ashcroft, K.W., editors: Pediatric surgery, Philadelphia, 1980, W.B. Saunders Co.

Benjamin, B., Cohen, D., and Glasson, M.: Tracheomalacia in association with congenital tracheoesophageal fistula, Surgery **79**:504, 1976.

David, T.J., and O'Callaghan, S.E.: Cardiovascular malformations and esophageal atresia, Br. Heart J. **36**:559, 1974.

deLorimier, A.A., and Harrison, M.R.: Long gap esophageal atresia: primary anastomosis after oesophageal elongation by bougienage and esophagomyotomy, J. Thorac. Cardiovasc. Surg. **79**:138, 1980.

Ein, S.H., and others: Recurrent tracheoesophageal fistulas: Seventeen-year review, J. Pediatr. Surg. **18**:436, 1983.

German, J.C., Mahour, G.H., and Woolley, M.M.: Esophageal atresia and associated anomalies, J. Pediatr. Surg. **11**:299, 1976.

Hendren, W.H., and Hale, J.R.: Electromagnetic bougienage to lengthen esophageal segments in congenital esophageal atresia, N. Engl. J. Med. **293**:428, 1975.

Holder, T.M., and Ashcraft, K.W.: Developments in the care of patients with esophageal atresia and tracheoesophageal fistula, Surg. Clin. North Am. **61**:1051, 1981.

Holder, T.M., and others: Esophageal atresia and tracheoesophageal fistula: a survey of its members by the Surgical Section of the American Academy of Pediatrics, Pediatrics **34**:542, 1964.

Howard, R., and Myers, N.A.: Esophageal atresia: a technique for elongating the upper pouch, Surgery **58**:725, 1965.

Ito, T., Sugito, T., and Nagaya, M.: Delayed primary anastomosis in poor-risk patients with esophageal atresia associated with tracheoesophageal fistula, J. Pediatr. Surg. **19**:243, 1984.

Jolley, S.G., and others: Patterns of gastroesophageal reflux in children following repair of esophageal atresia and distal tracheoesophageal fistula, J. Pediatr. Surg. **15**:857, 1980.

Livaditis, A.: Esophageal atresia: a method for overbridging large segmental gaps, Z. Kinderchir. **13**:298, 1973.

Livaditis, A., and Eklof, O.: Esophageal atresia with tracheoesophageal fistula: results of primary anastomosis in infants, Z. Kinderchir. **12**:32, 1943.

Livaditis, A., Radberg, L., and Odensjo, G.: Esophageal end-to-end anastomosis: reduction of anastomotic tension by circular myotomy, Scand. J. Thorac. Cardiovasc. Surg. **6**:206, 1972.

Mahour, G.H., Woolley, M.M., and Gwinn, J.L.: Elongation of the upper pouch and delayed anastomotic reconstruction in esophageal atresia, J. Pediatr. Surg. **9**:373, 1974.

Martin, L.W., and Alexander, F.: Esophageal atresia, Surg. Clin. North Am. **65**:1099, 1965.

Myers, N.A., and Aberdeen, E.: Congenital esophageal atresia and tracheoesophageal fistula. In Ravitch, M.M., et al., editors: Pediatric surgery, Chicago, 1982, Year Book Medical Publishers.

Orringer, M.D., Kirsch, M.M., and Sloan, H.: Long-term esophageal function following repair of esophageal atresia, Ann. Surg. **186**:436, 1977.

Randolph, J.G., Altman, R.P., and Anderson, K.D.: Selective surgical management based upon clinical status in infants with esophageal atresia, J. Thorac. Cardiovasc. Surg. **74**:335, 1977.

Schwartz, M.Z., and Filler, R.M.: Tracheal compression as a cause of apnea following repair of tracheoesophageal fistula: treatment by aortopexy, J. Pediatr. Surg. **15**:842, 1980.

Soave, F.: Discussion in Hoffman, D.G., and Moazam, F.: Transcervical myotomy for wide-gap esophageal atresia, J. Pediatr. Surg. **19**:680, 1984.

Vizas, D., Ein, S.H., and Simpson, J.S.: The value of circular myotomy for esophageal atresia, J. Pediatr. Surg. **13**:357, 1978.

Woolley, M.M.: Discussion in Janik, J.S., and Filler, R.M.: Long-term follow-up of circular myotomy for esophageal atresia, J. Pediatr. Surg. **15**:840, 1980.

PART FIVE

Disorders of digestion

MALDIGESTION

Normal digestive physiology

Even in the neonate, the process of digestion begins in the mouth where salivary enzymes including lipase and amylase are active. The stomach secretes hydrochloric acid, pepsin, and mucus to continue the breakdown of lipids and carbohydrates and begin the degradation of proteins. In addition, the stomach dilutes the ingested food to provide an isotonic mixture to the small intestine. The acidic nature of the gastric discharge into the duodenum stimulates the secretion of cholecystokinin-pancreozymin (CCK-PZ), secretin, and enterokinase. These hormones in turn trigger the secretion of the pancreatic enzymes (or precursors), as well as bile, to complete digestion.

In the neonate lipase and proteases are adequate for the digestion of milk, which contains little polysaccharide. The relative paucity of polysaccharide in the diet is of importance because amylase activity is decreased over the first 3 to 6 months of life.

PANCREATIC INSUFFICIENCY

Pancreatic insufficiency in the newborn manifests itself with watery diarrhea and steatorrhea, beginning shortly after birth.

Direct measurement of pancreatic function is technically difficult in the small infant. Therefore an indirect measurement of pancreatic function is often first performed. Blood tests for immunoreactive trypsinogen show some promise in detecting insufficiency. A measurement of "72-hour fecal fat loss" is simple; if the diet is unvaried, it may be accomplished in 24 or 48 hours. In the small infant steatorrhea is considered to be present when more than 10% of the ingested fat is found in the stool. The stool also can be tested for trypsin activity by using undeveloped x-ray film. A 1:5 dilution of stool and water is made and centrifuged. Serial dilutions (total volume, 1 ml) of this supernatant are incubated with long, narrow strips of undeveloped x-ray film, in test tubes, at 37 degrees C for 1 hour. A simultaneous control stool specimen should digest the gelatin from the film at a titre of 1:100 or greater. In the infant over 1 to 2 months of age a pilocarpine iontophoresis (sweat test) can be performed to rule out cystic fibrosis, which is the leading cause of pancreatic exocrine insufficiency in this age group.

When the results of indirect pancreatic function tests are equivocal, measurement of unstimulated duodenal fluid bicarbonate, amylase, trypsin, and pH may provide sufficient information to exclude absolute pancreatic insufficiency. Where further information is required, the pancreozymin-secretin test may be useful. After an overnight fast, a 3-lumen, double balloon duodenal tube is positioned under fluoroscopy, such that the first balloon is near the ligament of Treitz, and the second balloon is in the first part of the duodenum. The stomach pump is set to suction to prevent dilution of duodenal contents. Duodenal fluid is collected at rest for 20 minutes and then CCK-PZ is given (2 units/kg) by slow intravenous

Table 33-4. Pancreatic function after secretin-pancreozymin tests

	Birth	24 hours after feedings	1 week	1 month	Normal children	Cystic fibrosis	Pancreatic insufficiency
Volume (ml/kg/50 min)							
Premature	4.4 (4-15)	5.9 (1.5-9.8)	8.2 (1.6-16.8)	8.96 (3.4-18.7)	3.9 (1.8-81)	0.3-2.7	1.8-3.9
Term	5.39 (1.6-9.7)	3.29 (9.6-80)	4.3 (9.6-10.4)				
HCO_3^- (mEq/L/50 min)				0.19	0.001-0.04 (0.08-0.37)	0.008-0.19	
Trypsin (μg/kg/50 min)							
Premature	60 (0-482)	43.1 (1.6-148)	233.3 (5-660)	196.1 (0.9-660)	765 (215-2,100)	0-450	0.9-320
Term	66.1 (1.2-350)	26.3 (5-67.8)	96.6 (5-230)				
Lipase (IU/kg/50 min)							
Premature	77.4 (3-343)	65.9 (2.4-209)	328.8 (7.2-1,249)	283.6 (11-730)	1,464 (350-5,000)	0-270	0-68
Term	143.9 (2.2-785)	31.7 (4.9-67.4)	39.9 (6.2-125)				
Chymotrypsin (μg/kg/50 min)					860 (252-1,900)	0-126	0-105
Amylase (IU/kg/50 min)							
Premature	0.88 (0-3.6)	0.62 (0.2-1.4)	2.07 (0.2-8.2)	1.67 (0-4.6)	665 (160-2,150)	0-117	0-31
Term	3.20 (0.1-9.8)	0.38 (0.2-0.5)	1.29 (0.1-3.0)				
Carboxypeptidase A (IU/kg/50 min)					724 (141-2,480)	0-204	0-149

From Gryboski, J.: Gastrointestinal problems in the infant, Philadelphia, 1983, W.B. Saunders Co.

injection, followed in 20 minutes by secretin (2 units/kg). Skin tests should be done before giving the secretagogues systemically, and pulse and blood pressure should be monitored during the test. The samples are collected in 10-minute blocks for 50 minutes, and volume, HCO_3^- concentration, pH, lipase activity, amylase, trypsin, chymotrypsin, and carboxypeptidase A activity are measured (Table 33-4).

SCHWACHMAN'S SYNDROME

Patients with pancreatic insufficiency, normal sweat chloride test, and bone marrow dysfunction have Schwachman's syndrome. These patients have diarrhea, neutropenia, bone marrow hypoplasia, and marked growth retardation. Metaphyseal dysostosis is seen in 10% to 15% of patients with this syndrome. Neutropenia, which may be cyclic, is common. The sweat test is normal, since the defect involves only pancreatic enzyme deficiency with normal water and bicarbonate secretion. Despite the fact that many older patients are able to compensate for their pancreatic insufficiency and they may experience decreasing requirements for replacement enzymes, these patients continue to grow poorly and are much less than the third percentile for height.

CYSTIC FIBROSIS

The gastrointestinal and hepatic manifestations of cystic fibrosis are both varied and common. The incidence of cystic fibrosis is about 1 in 2,500 live births among Caucasians. It is fifty times less common in American blacks.

Pathogenesis

Although the primary defect is unknown, the unifying problem of clinical importance in cystic fibrosis is the presence of thick, viscid mucus, which becomes inspissated in the lumen of ductular structures—especially the pancreas and lungs—but also the intestine (meconium ileus), biliary tract, and appendix.

Clinical manifestations

Meconium ileus is the most common presentation of cystic fibrosis in the newborn. Associated intestinal atresia may be found in 20% to 30% of patients with meconium ileus and may be caused by in utero obstruction. Symptoms usually begin in the first 1 to 2 days of life with delayed passage of meconium, abdominal distension, and vomiting, which may become bilious.

The patient who does not have meconium ileus may,

at 4 to 6 weeks of age, have diarrhea, edema, hypoproteinemia, and a failure to thrive. Vitamin K malabsorption may result in hypoprothrombinemia and the clinical manifestation of a bleeding diathesis. Vitamin E, another fat soluble vitamin, may become deficient, and hypocalcemia may result from the saponification of calcium with unabsorbed fats.

Cholestasis resulting from bile stasis and mucus plugging may occur in the first few weeks of life. This may be the initial manifestation of cystic fibrosis; it is why all children with unexplained neonatal cholestasis should be sweat tested.

Although pancreatic exocrine insufficiency is present in 80% of newborns affected with cystic fibrosis, the islets of Langerhans are not affected early in the patient's life, and pancreatic endocrine insufficiency occurs only as a later complication. As the infant matures pulmonary complications are of prime importance. Additional manifestations in infancy and later childhood include biliary cirrhosis and portal hypertension, rectal prolapse, nasal polyps, peptic ulcer disease, pancreatitis, and the pulmonary complications of infection, fibrosis, and cor pulmonale.

Laboratory manifestations

The *sine qua non* of cystic fibrosis is an elevated sweat chloride. The pilocarpine iontophoresis is the most accurate method of collection. Cystic fibrosis is associated with sweat chloride values equal to or greater than 50 mEq/L. However, in neonates it may not be possible to collect the requisite 40 to 100 mg of sweat.

Children may also have hyponatremic dehydration and hypochloremic metabolic alkalosis secondary to the increased losses of electrolytes in the sweat. Manifestations of meconium ileus and peritonitis are discussed earlier.

NESIDIOBLASTOSIS

Excess and unregulated pancreatic endocrine function in the neonatal period, occurring as refractory hypoglycemia, is often due to nesidioblastosis. This disorder, a result of disorganized pancreatic islet cells, may be inherited as an autosomal dominant trait or be found in association with Beckwith syndrome. Medical therapy (glucose, diazoxide, glucagon, somatostatin) can be used to temporize until a curative surgical, near-total pancreatectomy is performed.

MALABSORPTION AND DIARRHEA

In infants the problem of malabsorption is especially critical because (1) the infant is deprived of nutrients at a critical stage of central nervous system development, and (2) the infant tends to lose large amounts of fluid and can become profoundly dehydrated. Older infants and children with malabsorption may have normal, bulky, or watery stools, but the neonate will have almost exclusively watery diarrhea and on occasion vomiting. The causes of malabsorption include:

- I. Abnormalities of intestinal mucosa
  - A. Infectious diarrhea (e.g., enterotoxigenic *E. coli*, *Salmonella* organisms, *Campylobacter* organisms, rotavirus)
  - B. Physical, chemical, or toxic agents
    1. Antibiotics
    2. Other medications
    3. Narcotic withdrawal
  - C. Specific enzymatic or biochemical abnormalities
    1. Monosaccharide malabsorption
    2. Disaccharide malabsorption
    3. Chloridorrhea
    4. Primary hypomagnesemia
    5. Acrodermatitis enteropathica
    6. Abetalipoproteinemia
    7. Amino acid malabsorption (e.g. phenylketonuria, maple syrup urine disease)
    8. Primary bile acid malabsorption
    9. Specific vitamin malabsorption (B_{12}, folate)
  - D. Acquired defects of the bowel
    1. Massive resection of the small bowel
    2. Necrotizing enterocolitis
- II. Congenital anomalies of the intestine
  - A. Hirschsprung's disease
  - B. Stenosis, duplication, malrotation
- III. Abnormalities of pancreatic secretion
  - A. Cystic fibrosis
  - B. Schwachman's syndrome
- IV. Abnormalities of liver function
  - A. Neonatal hepatitis
  - B. Biliary atresia
  - C. Congenital cholestatic syndromes
- VI. Immunologic disorders
- VII. Hormonal disorders
- VIII. Allergic disorders
  - A. Cow's milk protein sensitivity
  - B. Soy-protein sensitivity

Loose stools in normal infants

Loose stools are common in the breast-fed and the preterm infant and are not necessarily a sign of disease. Loose stools may disappear with time and without either intervention or multiple formula changes.

Infectious diarrhea

Infectious diarrhea is the most common cause of severe diarrhea and malabsorption in the neonatal period. Rotavirus and enterotoxigenic *E. coli* are the most common pathogens. Salmonella, campylobacter, and enteropathogenic, enterohemorrhagic, as well as enteroadherent *E.*

coli, are frequently found. *Giardia* and *Shigella* organisms, which may cause diarrhea in the older infant, are not usually associated with diarrhea in the neonate.

Stool cultures, assay for rotavirus antigen, and tests for occult blood and fecal leukocytes are useful in identifying infectious diarrhea.

Physical and chemical agents

Antimicrobial agents, hyperosmotic liquid medications, and incorrect formula dilutions can all cause diarrheal disease. Many antimicrobial agents are associated with the infrequent complication of pseudomembraneous colitis. *C. difficile*, the causative agent of pseudomembraneous colitis, is also carried by many healthy children under 1 year of age. However, the presence of bloody diarrhea in a patient harboring the organism and toxin is sufficient evidence to warrant treatment (i.e., withdrawal of the antibiotic and if severe, treatment with vancomycin).

Narcotic withdrawal is also marked by jitteriness, hyperreflexia, tachypnea, poor suck, and diarrhea (Chapter 37, part four).

Carbohydrate malabsorption

Primary or secondary carbohydrate intolerance is also a common form of malabsorption seen in the neonate. Acquired forms of carbohydrate malabsorption are much more common than congenital forms and are usually secondary to other disease states that may damage the intestinal mucosa. Sugar that fails to undergo hydrolysis and remains in the intestinal lumen may act as an osmotically active agent. Furthermore, in the colon bacteria act on the sugar to produce both organic acids, such as lactic acid and hydrogen (which can be measured in breath). Organic acids further increase the osmotic diarrhea in the colon and also exert an irritative effect, resulting in the passage of more fluid. Many affected infants have abdominal distension and vomiting.

The presence of a reducing sugar can be detected in the stool with a Clinitest tablet and color chart. Since sucrose is not a reducing sugar, to detect sucrose the test is modified by diluting the stool with an equal volume of 1N HCl instead of water and boiling gently for a few minutes.

Oral carbohydrate tolerance tests, using 2 gm/kg of the sugar and measuring glucose at 0, 20, 40, 60 and 90 minutes may be helpful in detecting intolerance. A normal infant should have a rise of 20 mg/dl above the fasting level, whereas an affected patient has little if any rise in the glucose level and also develops abdominal pain and diarrhea. The offending sugar and increased concentrations of organic acids are found in the stool, as well as a low stool pH.

Breath hydrogen tests are particularly useful in detecting carbohydrate malabsorption in the older infant. This noninvasive technique can be modified for use in the neonate by using a nasal prong technique, but it is somewhat difficult to standardize in this age-group.

Direct measurement of intestinal disaccharidase activity, in mucosa obtained by peroral jejunal biopsy, may be necessary to confirm the diagnosis.

Congenital lactose malabsorption (lactase deficiency) is rare, but secondary lactose intolerance is common. After mucosal damage, lactase is one of the first enzymes to decrease in activity and one of the last enzymes to return to normal activity during the healing process. Treatment consists of removing lactose from the diet until lactase activity returns.

In contrast, sucrose-isomaltose malabsorption is most commonly due to a congenital absence or marked decrease in activity of both sucrase and isomaltase. Secondary sucrose intolerance has been found after severe enteritis. Treatment consists of removing sucrose, as well as dextrins and starch, from the diet.

Congenital glucose-galactose malabsorption is a rare autosomal recessive disorder. Both the intestinal microvilli and the renal tubular cell are unable to bind either glucose or galactose. Treatment is extremely difficult and consists of providing specially prepared formulas with fructose (which is normally absorbed) as the sole carbohydrate.

Transient malabsorption of monosaccharides also has been encountered in infants and usually follows severe gastroenteritis or massive resection of the small intestine. These infants cannot tolerate a 1% to 2% glucose solution and may also not tolerate fructose. Prolonged intravenous alimentation may be necessary.

Congenital chloridorrhea

Congenital alkalotic diarrhea is thought to be secondary to an inability of the infant to absorb chloride, especially in the ileum and colon. The infant usually has severe diarrhea in the first weeks of life with massive losses of water and electrolytes, especially potassium and chloride. The diagnosis is made by finding increased concentrations of chloride in the stool, absent to very low concentration of chloride in urine, and a hypochloremic, hypokalemic alkalosis. This condition represents a prototype of a congenital defect in ion transport.

As the infant matures complications include growth retardation, secondary hyperaldosteronism, urinary tract infection, and degenerative renal changes. Prompt treatment with supplemental potassium chloride (2 to 14 mEq/kg/day) is required.

Abetalipoproteinemia

Abetalipoproteinemia is an autosomal recessive trait marked by abdominal distension, failure to thrive, hypotonia, and steatorrhea. There is a decreased ability to synthesize betalipoprotein, and therefore chylomicra. Complications include neurologic degeneration secondary to vitamin E deficiency, retinitis pigmentosa, and acanthocytosis. A low-fat diet with supplementary medium-chain triglycerides decreases steatorrhea and improves weight gain. Whether this form of therapy has any effect on the neurologic damage to the infant is uncertain. In some infants with severe diarrhea and malabsorption resulting from other causes, hypolipoproteinemia, hypocholesterolemia, and acanthocytosis may be secondarily encountered.

Other inborn errors

See also Chapter 36.

Other specific enzymatic or biochemical abnormalities that may occur very early in life with diarrhea include amino acid malabsorption (phenylketonuria, maple syrup urine disease), primary bile acid malabsorption, specific vitamin malabsorption (B_{12}, folate), disorders of magnesium and zinc absorption (acrodermatitis enteropathica), and lysosomal lipid storage disease (Wolman's disease).

Immunologic disorders

See also Chapter 30.

Immunodeficiency with thrombocytopenia and eczema (Wiskott-Aldrich syndrome) and thymic dysplasia, both X-linked recessive traits, can occur with diarrhea. In addition, patients with specific IgA deficiency may have frequent viral or parasitic enteritides later in infancy.

Hormonal abnormalities

Patients with salt-losing congenital adrenal hyperplasia have projectile vomiting and diarrhea. Virilization and hyperkalemia are also seen.

Neural crest tumors, especially ganglioneuroma or ganglioneuroblastoma, may secrete vasoactive intestinal peptide and cause a secretory diarrhea.

Neonatal thyrotoxicosis can also be associated with a watery diarrhea.

Allergic disorders

The most common allergic gastroenteropathy in the neonatal period is cow's milk protein intolerance. Soy protein has also been shown to be highly sensitizing. Infants may have a wide variety of signs and symptoms, including diarrhea, anemia, hematochezia, edema, vomiting, eczema, leukocytosis, and thrombocytopenia. A characteristic jejunal biopsy with inflammatory changes, eosinophilic infiltration, and lacteal dilation can be seen. Most symptomatic children have an abnormal biopsy. Symptoms usually begin within the first 6 months of life and often improve rapidly when the formula is changed to a non-cow's milk or hydrolyzed protein formula (Nutramigen or Pregestimil). Although one need not necessarily rely on the strict criteria of Goldman, which involves three separate clinical remissions and exacerbations associated with the removal and reintroduction of milk, it is clear that cow's milk protein intolerance is overdiagnosed when the diagnosis rests solely on the symptomatic improvement of any perceived digestive disturbance after removal of milk from the diet. A majority of infants will be able to tolerate milk within 4 to 6 months, which often corresponds to a chronologic age of 9 to 12 months. Prevention is best afforded by not introducing cow's milk until at least 6 months of age and preferably later. Breast-feeding itself has not been shown to be preventative, and sensitization has been reported in breast-fed infants whose mothers are consuming milk.

CONGENITAL ABNORMALITIES OF THE INTESTINE

Intestinal lymphangiectasia is characterized by dilation and abnormalities of the lymphatics of the intestine, protein-losing enteropathy, and unilateral or bilateral lymphedema. In early to late infancy diarrhea, abdominal distension, ascites, and generalized edema may be found. The measurement of alpha-1-antitrypsin in the stool may be useful to demonstrate the protein loss. Small bowel biopsy or lymphangiography may be needed to confirm the diagnosis. Therapy consists of maintaining the patient on a low-fat diet with supplemental medium-chain triglycerides.

Hirschsprung's disease may be an occult cause of diarrhea and malabsorption. In addition, it may occur in infancy as a colitis with bloody diarrhea. This is the reason that all infants with unexplained colitis should have a rectal biopsy to exclude Hirschsprung's disease.

Malrotation, congenital intestinal stenosis, and enteric duplication cysts may also occur with diarrhea in the first few months of life.

SHORT GUT SYNDROME

One of the most frustrating problems is the management of the neonate who has had massive resection of the small intestine. The removal of even a small section of the intestine in the neonatal period may result in severe diarrhea and failure to thrive. The median length of small intestine in the neonate is approximately 250 cm. However, there is considerable individual variability. Infants with as little as 15 cm of small intestine and an intact ileocecal valve have been reported to survive. Two or three times that length of residual small bowel is probably required if the ileocecal valve has been lost. The marked decline in mortality rates that has occurred in the past few years is due in large part to the improved use and understanding of parenteral nutrition.

The ability of the intestine to adapt appropriately and the subsequent survival of the infant after massive intestinal resection are related to:

1. Maturity of the infant at the time of resection
2. Length of the remaining intestine
3. Presence of distal small intestine
4. Presence of the ileocecal valve
5. Presence of an intact colon
6. Intactness of pancreatic and liver function
7. General condition of the infant and absence of other complicating congenital anomalies

Although the jejunum plays an important role in digestion and absorption, infants with resection of the jejunum tend to fare much better than those in whom the ileum is removed. Perhaps this is because loss of the ileum may result in diminished bile acid absorption. This can decrease the bile acid pool sufficiently to impair lipid absorption. In addition, the presence of unabsorbed bile acids in the colon can cause a secretory diarrhea with additional fluid and electrolyte loss.

An intact ileocecal valve delays intestinal transit time, thereby allowing more time for digestion and absorption. Furthermore, the ileocecal valve acts as a barrier to prevent overgrowth of colonic bacteria in the small intestine.

Similarly, the intact colon is also important because the colon functions as a route for water and electrolyte salvage. The neonatal colon may also have an expanded role in the absorption of nutrients.

Other factors that have a positive effect on intestinal adaptation include exposure of the residual bowel to nutrients, biliary and pancreatic secretions, and enteric hormones. Adaptation can occur even in the absence of oral intake and may continue for as long as 1 to 1½ years after the resection. However, the most effective way to promote adaptive change is to feed the infant whenever possible.

Other complications of the short gut syndrome include (1) transient gastric hypersecretion as a result of either increased secretion or decreased catabolism of gastrin, (2) secondary bacterial overgrowth resulting from stasis or blind loop syndrome, (3) vitamin B_{12} deficiency as a result of bacterial overgrowth and/or less than 15 cm of residual ileum, and (4) lactic acidosis as a result of bacterial overgrowth.

Treatment of the short gut syndrome is difficult primarily because it may take weeks or even months for the infant to be able to digest and absorb adequate calories, even when less than 50% of the intestine is resected. Parenteral nutrition must be initiated soon after surgery and continued through the prolonged phase of refeeding. Enteral feedings, usually beginning with an elemental formula (casein hydrolysate, glucose, medium-chain triglyceride) and often using continuous enteral infusion, are begun slowly with very gradual increases in concentration or volume to prevent distension, vomiting, and diarrhea. Nonetheless, the process of refeeding is often complicated by these symptoms as a result of dietary intolerance, bacterial overgrowth, or intercurrent gastroenteritis.

Medications such as loperamide, diphenoxylate, codeine, and phenothiazines have been used with success in individual patients to help control the diarrhea when the loss of fluid and electrolytes has been severe. Cholestyramine (a bile acid binder) may be helpful if bile acid mediated-diarrhea is suspected; this can be initiated as a brief (24 to 48 hour) trial. Treatment of bacterial overgrowth includes the use of either nonabsorbable antibiotics, trimethoprim-sulfamethoxazole, or metronidazole, as well as surgical correction of a blind loop or stagnant section.

INTRACTABLE DIARRHEA

Intractable diarrhea of infancy is still a life-threatening disorder, although recent advances in enteral and parenteral nutrition have significantly decreased the mortality from its initial rate of 70% to 90% to the current rate of approximately 5% to 10%. This syndrome is most often seen as an idiopathic complication of severe infectious diarrhea in infancy. There have been specific associations with enteropathogenic and enteroadherent *E. coli*. However, several other conditions that can occur with intractable diarrhea include:

1. Cow's milk or soy-protein sensitivity
2. Cystic fibrosis
3. Congenital chloridorrhea
4. Glucose-galactose malabsorption
5. Immunodeficiency
6. Increased secretion of gastrin, vasoactive intestinal peptide, or pancreatic polypeptide
7. Abetalipoproteinemia
8. Pseudomembraneous enterocolitis
9. Primary bile acid malabsorption
10. Familial hypoplastic villus atrophy
11. Hirschsprung's disease with enterocolitis
12. Short gut syndrome (acquired or congenital)
13. Congenital anomalies of the intestine (lymphangiectasia, stricture, duplication)
14. Renal tubular acidosis

Clinical manifestations

Diarrheal disease lasting more than 2 to 3 weeks in the neonate or infant may lead to severe malnutrition, dehydration, and acidosis. The inability to provide adequate protein and calories during this period not only delays repair of the damaged gastrointestinal tract but also puts the infant at increased risk for infectious complications including sepsis.

oratory manifestations

Evaluation for viral, parasitic, and bacterial entero- pathogens may provide an etiology for the diarrheal syndrome or identify secondary infections resulting from compromise of the gastrointestinal tract. Measuring the reducing sugar content of the stool will provide information on the presence and degree of carbohydrate malabsorption. White blood count and differential may suggest an allergic etiology (eosinophilia) or secondary infection (leukocytosis). The presence of acanthocytes in the peripheral blood smear suggests abetalipoproteinemia, which can be confirmed on a serum lipoprotein electrophoresis. Urine pH determination, as well as blood pH and serum bicarbonate concentration, will identify the rare patient with renal tubular acidosis who will have intractable diarrhea. A sweat chloride determination may rule out cystic fibrosis but may be inaccurate in the presence of severe malnutrition. Analysis of the chloride content of serum, urine, and stool will exclude the uncommon case of congenital chloridorrhea. Serum immunoglobulin electrophoresis will enable evaluation for immunodeficiency. In the patient with a profuse secretory diarrhea evaluation of catecholamines, serum gastrin, and vasoactive intestinal peptide may be helpful. Patients with primary bile acid malabsorption will have elevated fecal bile acids and low serum levels of bile acids resulting from interruption of the enterohepatic circulation and depletion of the bile acid pool.

Proctosigmoidoscopy and biopsy are simple and useful in detecting enterocolitis (Hirschsprung's or pseudomembraneous). Small bowel biopsy is extremely useful in detecting cow's milk or soy-protein enteropathy, familial villus atrophy, intestinal lymphangiectasia, and abetalipoproteinemia. Small bowel biopsy is less useful as a predictor of the severity or duration of disease. Radiographic contrast studies of the small and large bowel will demonstrate the amount of residual intestine, as well as congenital anomalies of the intestine.

Management

The management of intractable diarrhea is rooted in the dedication to providing adequate protein and caloric intake by combining enteral and parenteral nutrition. In less severe cases use of an elemental infant formula such as Pregestimil may be sufficient to overcome the problem of nutrient delivery. Careful titration of the volume and concentration of the formula to the child's weight, electrolyte balance, stool output, and presence of reducing sugars in the stool is necessary. Therapy often requires the initial use of quarter- or half-strength formula to provide 25 to 50 Cal/kg/day in the form of enteral nutrition. The remainder of the calories is provided by parenteral nutrition and is decreased while slow but gradual advances in the enteral component (e.g., increments of 10 to 20 Cal/kg/every other day) are obtained by increases in the volume or concentration of the formula. This is continued until enteral nutrition adequate for growth is achieved.

Infants who do not tolerate nipple feedings are often successfully managed by continuous nasogastric gavage. This technique has enabled us to avoid central venous hyperalimentation lines in all but the most severe cases of intractable diarrhea. The same process, described above, of gradual increases in the volume or concentration of formula is used with a continuous nasogastric infusion. When full caloric requirements are met and weight gain is beginning to occur, increasing the infusion rate and providing increasing periods of "time off" enable a return to gavage feeding and eventual nipple feeding.

It should be stressed that even if the infant is not receiving enteral nutrition per os, nonnutritive (e.g., pacifier) sucking should be promoted. This avoids the problem of the infant forgetting how to suck. Furthermore, lingual lipase secreted during non-nutritive sucking may aid in digestion of nasogastrically infused nutrients.

In severe cases the use of central venous alimentation is lifesaving. Attempts at refeeding should be retried as the infant grows. If at all possible some enteral nutrition should be provided, even as little as 10% of the caloric requirement, for its possible trophic effects on gastrointestinal adaptation.

Mitchell B. Cohen
William F. Balistreri

BIBLIOGRAPHY

Maldigestion

diSantAgnese, P.A., and Talamo, R.C.: Pathogenesis and physiopathology of cystic fibrosis of the pancreas, N. Engl. J. Med. **277**:1287, 1967.

Durie, P.R., and others: Immunoreactive cationic trypsinogen in cystic fibrosis: a sensitive indicator of exocrine pancreatic dysfunction. Pediatr. Res. **15**:1351, 1981.

Gryboski, J., and Walker, W.A.: Gastrointestinal problems in the infant, Philadelphia, 1983, W.B. Saunders Co.

Henning, S.J.: Postnatal development: coordination of feeding, digestion and development, Am. J. Physiol. **241**:G199, 1981.

Park, R., and Grand, R.: Gastrointestinal manifestations of cystic fibrosis: a review, Gastroenterology **81**:1143, 1981.

Rosenstein, B.J., and Langbaum, T.S.: Incidence of meconium abnormalities in newborn infants with cystic fibrosis, Am. J. Dis. Child. **134**:72, 1980.

Schwachman, H., and others: The syndrome of pancreatic insufficiency and bone marrow dysfunction, J. Pediatr. **65**:645, 1964.

Malabsorption and diarrhea

Bohane, T.D., and others: A clinical study of young infants after small intestinal resection, J. Pediatr. **94**:552, 1979.

Feldman, E.J., Dowling, R.H., and MacNaughton, J.: Effect of oral versus intravenous nutrition on intestinal adaptation after small bowel resection, Gastroenterology **70**:712, 1976.

Gouttebel, M.C., and others: Total parenteral nutrition needs in different types of short bowel syndrome, Dig. Dis. Sci. **31**:718, 1986.

Tilson, D.M.: Pathophysiology and treatment of short bowel syndrome, Surg. Clin. North Am. **60**:1273, 1980.

Vanderhoof, J.A., and others: Effect of high percentage medium chain triglyceride on mucosal adaptation following massive small bowel resection in rats, J. Parenter. Enteral Nutr. **8**:685, 1984.

Zurser, R.B., and others: Use of medium chain triglyceride in the management of patients with massive resection of the small intestine, N. Engl. J. Med. **274**:490, 1966.

Intractable diarrhea

Ament, M.E.: Management of chronic diarrhea with parenteral nutrition and enteral infusion techniques, Pediatr. Ann. **14**:53, 1985.

Avery, G.B., and others: Intractable diarrhea in early infancy, Pediatrics **41**:712, 1968.

Balistreri, W.F., Partin, J.C., and Schubert, W.K.: Bile acid malabsorption—a consequence of terminal ileal dysfunction in protracted diarrhea of infancy, J. Pediatr. **89**:21, 1977.

Dorney, S.F.A., Byrne, W.J., and Ament, M.E.: Case of congenital short small intestine: survival with use of long-term parenteral feeding, Pediatrics **77**:386, 1986.

Fagundes, N.U., Viarro, T., and Lifshitz, F.: Tolerance to glucose polymer in malnourished infants with diarrhea and disaccharide intolerance, Am. J. Clin. Nutr. **42**:228, 1985.

Fitzgerald, J.F.: Management of the infant with persistent diarrhea, Pediatr. Infect. Dis. **4**:6, 1985.

Goldgar, C.M., and Vanderhoof, J.A.: Lack of correlation of small bowel biopsy and clinical course of patients with intractable diarrhea of infancy, Gastroenterology **90**:527, 1986.

Hyams, J.S., and others: Correlation of lactose breath hydrogen test, intestinal morphology, and lactase activity in young children, J. Pediatr. **97**:608, 1980.

Lifshitz, F.: Perspectives of carbohydrate intolerance in infants with diarrhea. In Lifshitz, F., editor: Carbohydrate intolerance in infancy, New York, 1982, Marcel Dekker, Inc.

Lo, C.W., and Walker, W.A.: Chronic protracted diarrhea of infancy: a nutritional disease, Pediatrics **72**:786, 1983.

Soeparto, P., Stobo, E.A., and Walker-Smith, J.A.: Role of chemical examination of the stool in diagnosis of sugar malabsorption in children, Arch. Dis. Child. **47**:50, 1972.

CHAPTER 34

Jaundice and liver disease

PART ONE

Unconjugated hyperbilirubinemia

The yellow discoloration of the skin and other organs caused by accumulation of bilirubin and designated as *jaundice*, or *icterus*, is generally considered a sign of a serious clinical pathologic condition in the older child and adult. The challenge of neonatal jaundice is to distinguish normal physiology from pathosis and the benign situation from the threatening one.

CLASSIFICATION OF NEONATAL JAUNDICE

Bilirubin exists in four different forms in serum: (1) unconjugated bilirubin reversibly bound to serum albumin; this form comprises the major portion of unconjugated bilirubin in serum, (2) a relatively minute fraction of unconjugated bilirubin not bound to serum albumin ("free"), (3) conjugated bilirubin (mainly monoglucuronides and diglucuronides) readily excretable through the renal or biliary system, and (4) conjugated bilirubin covalently bound to serum albumin ("delta" bilirubin); it has a rate of decay similar to that of serum albumin. The latter two forms give a "direct" reaction with standard diazo reagents, while the former two yield an "indirect" reaction. "Delta" bilirubin appears to be virtually absent in the normal newborn but is found in significant amounts in normal older infants and children and in those with conjugated hyperbilirubinemia resulting from various liver disorders. Hyperbilirubinemia characterized by the retention of indirect-reacting unconjugated bilirubin is by far the most common type of hyperbilirubinemia in the neonate; unconjugated bilirubin is the type of pigment found in "physiologic jaundice" and in the pathologic states in which there is increased production, decreased hepatic conjugation, or decreased hepatic uptake of bilirubin. Conjugated hyperbilirubinemia is far less common in the neonate and most often denotes a serious derangement of hepatic function, particularly interference with excretion of bilirubin from the liver into bile or obstruction of the flow of bile in the biliary tree.

Jaundice and hepatic disease in the newborn period, as in the older child and adult, can best be classified according to the type of bilirubin retained. Classification of hyperbilirubinemia as conjugated or unconjugated requires a determination of serum bilirubin concentration that distinguishes between direct- and indirect-reacting pigments. Direct spectrophotometric techniques fail to distinguish direct- from indirect-reacting pigment and are not recommended but may serve as backup in emergency situations or screening. The prototype of colorimetric methods is the van den Bergh test, a modification of the Ehrlich diazo reaction. A method currently utilized because of its precision and sensitivity is that of Jendrassik and Grof, which is used in the automated techniques available in most hospital laboratories. Unconjugated hyperbilirubinemia in the human, regardless of age, is defined as an elevation of the indirect-reacting serum bilirubin concentration to greater than 1 or 1.5 mg/dl, depending on the standard used in calibration of the van den Bergh reaction. Nearly all adults and older children will have indirect-reacting bilirubin concentrations in serum of less than 0.8 mg/dl. Conjugated hyperbilirubinemia is defined as an elevation of the direct-reacting fraction in the van den Bergh reaction to greater than 1.5 or 2 mg/dl, or as existing when this fraction accounts for more than 10% of the total serum bilirubin concentration. The latter portion of the definition is added to guard against overinterpretation of direct reactions in newborns with markedly elevated indirect-reacting bilirubin concentrations, because up to 10% of the unconjugated pigment will behave as direct-reacting pigment in the van den Bergh reaction. Clinical situations in which the direct-reacting serum bilirubin concentration is equal or close to the total bilirubin concentration are extremely rare, especially in the newborn period. In the usual clinical situation with conjugated

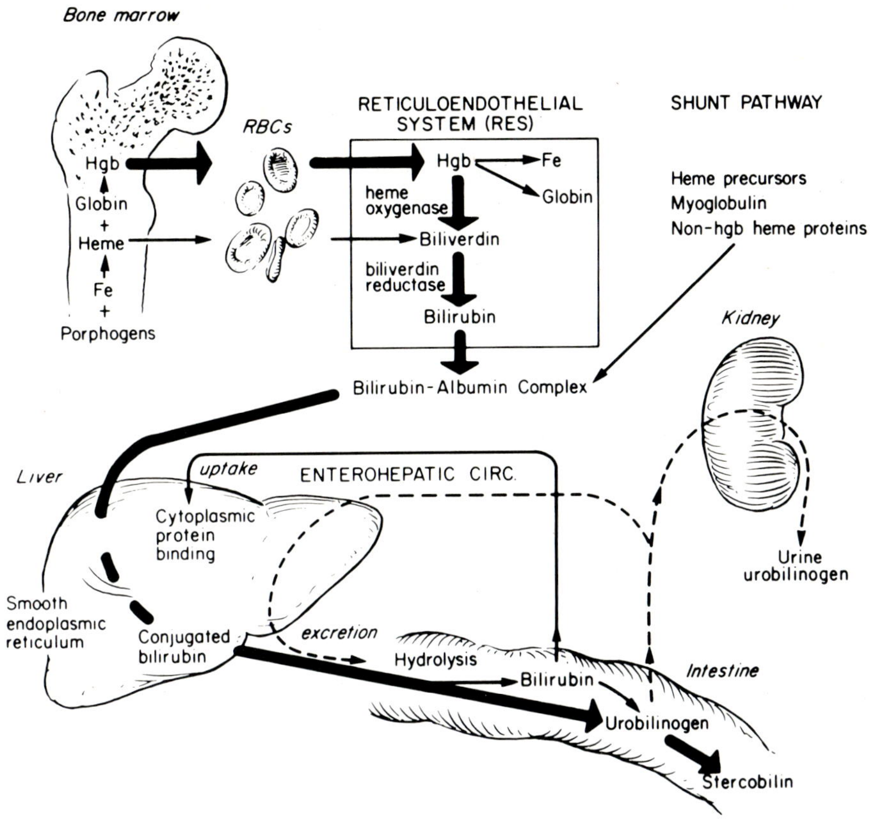

Fig. 34-1. The pathways of bilirubin synthesis, transport, and metabolism. (From Assali, N.S.: Pathophysiology of gestation, New York, 1972, Academic Press, Inc.)

hyperbilirubinemia, the elevated direct-reacting fraction accounts for 20% to 70% of the total pigment. This "mixed" hyperbilirubinemia should be considered primarily under the classification of conjugated hyperbilirubinemia, since the significant pathosis will usually relate to interference with hepatic cell excretion and bile transport rather than to abnormalities of increased bilirubin production or deficient hepatic bilirubin uptake or conjugation.

When compared with the values of direct bilirubin obtained by high-performance liquid chromatography, the values obtained by the Jendrassik and Grof method are falsely high. The older nonspecific diazo reaction methods for measuring direct-reacting bilirubin tend to cause positive bias, whereas the delta bilirubin fraction is underestimated. The ideal method for determination of bilirubin fractions, high-performance liquid chromatographic technique, is impractical for routine clinical laboratory use and the above definition for conjugated hyperbilirubinemia should remain until an improved method is utilized. Kodak Company has recently introduced a novel method (Kodak Ektachem slides), a two-film system for measurements of total and subfractions (indirect, direct, and covalently albumin-bound delta) of bilirubin for general clinical laboratory use. The upper limit of normal for total serum bilirubin by the new method is 1.3 mg/dl and for conjugated fraction, 0.3 mg/dl, of which two thirds is in the form of delta biliubin.

PHYSIOLOGY

Bilirubin synthesis

The pathways of bilirubin systhesis, transport, and metabolism are summarized in Fig. 34-1. In the normal adult, bilirubin is derived primarily from the degradation of heme contained in the circulating erythrocyte when senescence of the red cells results in their lysis in the reticuloendothelial cells of the body. Erythrocyte precursors and nonhemoglobin heme proteins (mainly cytochromes) normally contribute about 20% of the bilirubin excreted into bile. In the newborn, total bilirubin production is increased severalfold as a result of a shortened circulating erythrocyte life span (reduced to 70 to 90 days as compared with 120 days in the adult), increased heme degradation from the very large pool of hematopoietic tissue that ceases to function shortly after birth, and possibly increased turnover of cytochromes. In addition to increased synthesis, increased bilirubin is presented to the liver as a result of enhanced absorption of unconjugated bilirubin by the intestinal mucosa with transport to the liver by way of the enterohepatic circulation. Intestinal absorption in the newborn may be enhanced by starvation, absence of intestinal bacteria necessary for the conversion of bilirubin to colorless urobilinogens and pigmented stercobilins, the large bilirubin pool that exists in meconium, and slow intestinal motility.

The pathway by which hemoglobin, an iron-porphyrin complex bound to a globin, is converted to bilirubin in the reticuloendothelial cell is not fully known. Reticuloendothelial cells contain a microsomal enzyme, heme oxygenase, that is capable of oxidizing the alpha-methene bridge carbon of the heme molecule to form the green pigment biliverdin. The single carbon atom lost from the heme molecule is converted quantitatively to carbon monoxide. The carbon monoxide thus formed is excreted unchanged by the lung. Although there are other potential endogenous and exogenous sources of carbon monoxide, quantitative estimation of its excretion or synthesis offers a reasonably accurate assessment of the rate of heme degradation from all sources and, thus, of bilirubin synthesis. It is believed that nonhemoglobin heme undergoes the same degradative process. Biliverdin, a water-soluble pigment, is rapidly reduced by the cytosolic enzyme biliverdin reductase and by nonenzymatic reducing agents in the reticuloendothelial cell to form bilirubin. The degradation of 1 gm of hemoglobin forms 34 mg of bilirubin.

Bilirubin transport in plasma

The unconjugated bilirubin released into the circulation by the reticuloendothelial cell is rapidly bound to albumin, since the nonpolar pigment is almost totally insoluble in water at pH 7.4. Studies indicate that the solubility of bilirubin is less than 0.01 mg/dl. Each molecule of adult albumin is capable of binding at least two molecules of bilirubin; the first molecule is more tightly bound than the second. Additional binding sites with weaker affinities also may exist but are probably of little clinical importance. Newborns have been found to have a lower plasma binding capacity for bilirubin because of reduced albumin concentrations and reduced molar binding capacities as compared with the adult or older child. Binding of unconjugated bilirubin to albumin is believed to be of some importance in determining and evaluating the risk to the newborn for bilirubin encephalopathy (kernicterus). Unconjugated bilirubin is reversibly bound to albumin, unlike the portion of conjugated bilirubin covalently bound to albumin ("delta" bilirubin).

Hepatic uptake of bilirubin

The hepatocyte is the only cell in the body capable of removing significant quantities of unconjugated bilirubin from the circulation and converting it, by conjugation with other substances, into a form that either the liver cell or the kidney can excrete into bile or urine. Bilirubin enters the liver cell by a process of carrier-mediated diffusion, with ligandin (Y protein) of the liver cell cytoplasm as the major intracellular transport protein; Z protein, another hepatic cytoplasmic carrier, also binds bilirubin but with a lower affinity. Bilirubin dissociates from circulating albumin before it enters the liver cell. Ligandin also binds corticosteroids and exogenous substances, including sulfobromophthalein. The balance between the rates of bilirubin entry into the circulation, hepatic cell uptake, and conjugation of bilirubin determines the serum unconjugated bilirubin concentration under normal circumstances. The rate of bilirubin entry into the plasma pool is the product of both de novo bilirubin synthesis and intestinal bilirubin absorption.

Conjugation of bilirubin

Bilirubin excretion into bile requires conversion of the nonpolar unconjugated bilirubin into a more polar water-soluble substance. In the adult human this is accomplished almost entirely by conjugation of each molecule of bilirubin with two molecules of glucuronic acid by a two-step conjugation process. (Phototherapy achieves a similar result, that is, conversion of bilirubin to a more polar water-soluble substance, but by isomerization of the bilirubin molecule without conjugation.) In the normal adult glucuronide conjugation accounts for the disposal of approximately 95% of all bilirubin. The remaining portion is converted to water-soluble substances by conjugation with substances other than glucuronic acid or by oxidation, hydroxylation, or reduction.

Bilirubin is presumed to be transported from the liver cell plasma membrane by hepatic ligandin (Y protein) to the endoplasmic reticulum, the site of the conjugating enzyme uridine diphosphoglucuronyl (UDP-glucuronyl) transferase. This enzyme catalyzes the transfer of one glucuronic acid molecule from the activated uridine diphosphoglucuronic acid (UDPGA) to one of the two propionic side groups on one of the central pyrrole rings of bilirubin to form bilirubin monoglucuronide. UDPGA is synthesized by the soluble cytoplasmic enzyme uridine diphosphoglucose dehydrogenase, from uridine diphosphoglucose, which, in turn, is synthesized from free glucose. The total capacity of UDP-glucuronyl transferase to form the monoglucuronide of bilirubin has been estimated to be a hundredfold greater than the normal load of bilirubin presented to the liver for disposal. Thus only with reduction in enzyme activity to less than 1% of normal would unconjugated bilirubin retention result.

Although bilirubin monoglucuronide is water soluble and capable of being excreted into bile without further alteration, approximately two thirds of the total bilirubin excreted into bile in adult humans is found to be in the form of a diglucuronide. The addition of the second glucuronide is catalyzed either by the same glucuronyl transferase on the endoplasmic reticulum or by UDP-glucuronate glucuronyl transferase (transglucuronidase), a second enzyme located in the canalicular portion of the hepatocyte plasma cell membrane. The role of the "second enzyme" remains controversial. The substrate for the canalicular transglucuronidation is believed to be bilirubin monoglucuronide itself; the enzyme transfers one molecule of glucuronic acid from one molecule of bilirubin monoglucuronide to another, resulting in the formation of one molecule of bilirubin diglucuronide, which is then excreted from the cell, and one molecule of unconjugated bilirubin, which is then returned to the endoplasmic reticulum for subsequent reconjugation. Under circumstances in which increased loads of bilirubin are delivered to the liver, resulting in retention of conjugated bilirubin, as with severe chronic hemolysis, the retained pigment is bilirubin monoglucuronide.

Conjugates of bilirubin also can be formed with glucose, xylose, and possibly other carbohydrates, sulfates, and taurine. These nonglucuronide conjugates account for no more than 10% of the total bilirubin conjugates excreted in bile in humans.

Bilirubin excretion

The transfer of bilirubin from hepatocyte into bile can occur only after nonpolar bilirubin IXα has been converted to a more polar water-soluble compound, usually by the process of conjugation in the liver just described. The excretory process itself appears to be an energy-dependent concentrative process in which bile bilirubin concentrations are approximately a hundredfold greater than hepatocyte cytoplasmic bilirubin concentrations. The physiology of hepatic bilirubin excretion is discussed further in Part two.

Enteric bilirubin absorption

The monoglucuronides and diglucuronides of bilirubin are relatively unstable conjugates that are readily hydrolyzed to unconjugated bilirubin both nonenzymatically under the influence of mild alkaline conditions, as in the duodenum and jejunum, and enzymatically by the enteric mucosal enzyme β-glucuronidase. Unconjugated bilirubin may then be reabsorbed across the intestinal mucosa to return to the liver via the portal circulation. Although quantitative estimates of the disposal of bilirubin have been performed only for adult humans, these data indicate that approximately 25% of the total bilirubin excreted into the intestine is reabsorbed as unconjugated bilirubin. Approximately 10% of the total is excreted in stool as unaltered bilirubin, whereas the remaining pigment is converted to urobilinoiden, the majority of which is excreted in stool, and a small portion is reabsorbed in the colon and subsequently excreted by both the liver and the kidney.

PHYSIOLOGIC JAUNDICE OF THE NEWBORN

Unconjugated hyperbilirubinemia of the newborn regardless of cause can be understood only in the context of physiologic jaundice of the newborn, since this is a visible demonstration of developmental limitations of bilirubin metabolism and transport in the newborn period. All other abnormal situations are superimposed on these developmental processes.

Physiologic jaundice in the full-term infant

In the full-term neonate physiologic jaundice is characterized by a progressive rise in serum unconjugated bilirubin concentrations from approximately 2 mg/dl in cord blood to a mean peak of 6 mg/dl between 60 and 72 hours of age, followed by a rapid decline to approximately 2 mg/dl by the fifth day of life (Fig. 34-2). This early period of physiologic jaundice has been designated phase I physiologic jaundice. During the period from the fifth to tenth days of life, serum bilirubin concentrations decline very slowly, reaching the normal adult value of approximately 1 mg/dl by the end of that period. This later period of minimal, slowly declining hyperbilirubinemia has been designated phase II physiologic jaundice. Studies in the newborn rhesus monkey, an animal with a pattern of neonatal physiologic jaundice similar to the human, show that phase I results from the combination of a sixfold increase in the load of bilirubin presented to the liver and a marked deficiency in hepatic bilirubin glucuronyl transferase activity. The presence of either of these factors alone would not result in retention of unconjugated bilirubin. Hepatic uptake and excretion of bilirubin are also deficient during this period but are not rate-limiting steps in transport of bilirubin from plasma into bile. The very large increase in bilirubin load appears to result primarily from increased enteric reabsorption of unconjugated bilirubin. Increased de novo synthesis of bilirubin both from circulating and precursor erythrocytes and from nonhemoglobin heme degradation also contributes to this load. In the newborn monkey the markedly increased load persists for 3 to 6 weeks; similar data are not yet available for the human neonate. Deficient conjugation of bilirubin may result from insufficient enzyme synthesis, inhibition of enzymatic activity by naturally occurring substances, deficient synthesis of the glucuronide donor UDPGA, or a combination of these factors. In the human being bilirubin UDP-glucuronyl transferase activity is extremely low in the fetal

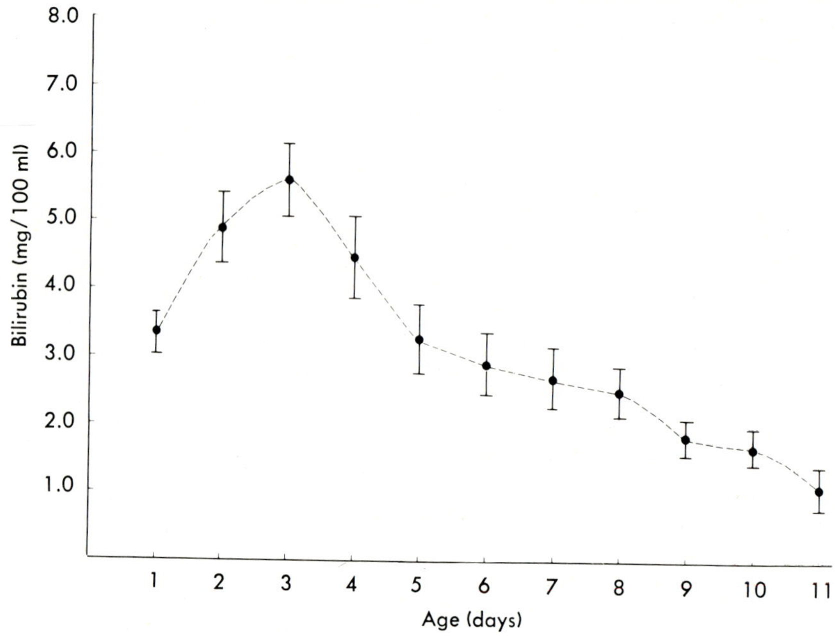

Fig. 34-2. Mean total serum bilirubin concentrations in 22 full-term normal infants during the first 11 days of life.

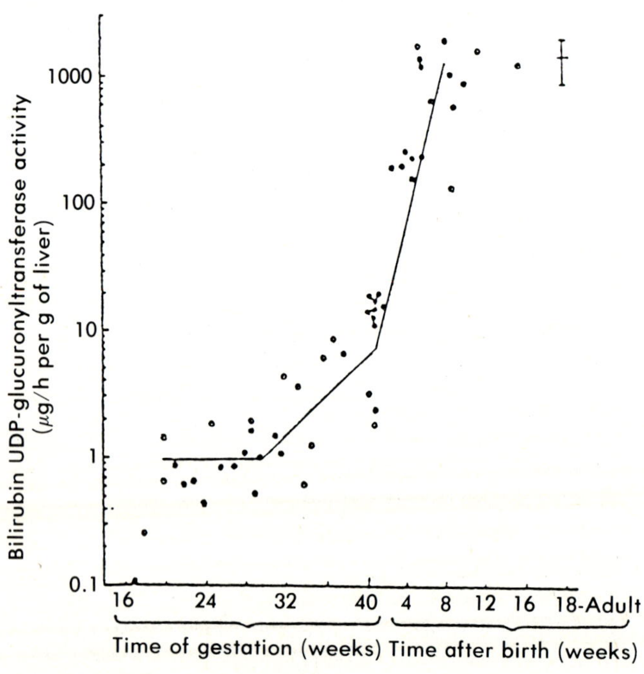

Fig. 34-3. Developmental pattern of hepatic bilirubin UDP glucuronyl transferase activity in humans. (From Kawade, N., and Onishi, S.: Biochem. J. **196:**257, 1981. Reprinted by permission of The Biochemical Society, London, © 1981.)

period, about 0.1% of adult activity before 30 weeks of gestation, gradually increasing to approximately 1.0% at term. After birth, activity increases initially at an exponential rate, reaching the adult level by 6 to 12 weeks of age (Fig. 34-3). Phase II physiologic jaundice appears to result from an imbalance in which hepatic uptake of bilirubin remains reduced and the increased bilirubin load persists. Developmental deficiency of ligandin may contribute to deficient uptake of bilirubin.

Despite the development of physiologic jaundice of some degree in nearly every newborn, only approximately half of all full-term newborns are visibly jaundiced during the first 3 days of life; serum bilirubin concentrations of less than 5 mg/dl usually are not reflected in cutaneous icterus in the newborn, unlike the situation in the older child and adult in whom jaundice will be noticeable in the sclerae and skin at serum bilirubin concentrations as low as 2 mg/dl. Variations in duration of hyperbilirubinemia and in skin color and perfusion may account for these differences. Since routine daily serum bilirubin determinations are not usually performed on full-term or even premature newborns, careful scrutiny of the nursery population several times a day by experienced personnel is essential to detect significant hyperbilirubinemia requiring further investigation. Lack of knowledge and the inherently complex developmental nature of physiologic jaundice prevent one from defining it simply by a serum bilirubin concentration above a specific level. For practical reasons having to do with risks of bilirubin encephalopathy and the likelihood of finding a superimposed explanation for the hyperbilirubinemia, a serum concentration exceeding 5 mg/dl during the first 24 hours of life should alert the physician to a potential need for further investigation.

Physiologic jaundice in the premature infant

Physiologic jaundice in the premature infant is more severe than in the full-term infant, with mean peak concentrations reaching 10 to 12 mg/dl by the fifth day of life. This delay in reaching the maximum concentration as compared with the full-term infant reflects the delay primarily in maturation of hepatic glucuronyl transferase activity in the premature infant. Since mean peak unconjugated bilirubin concentrations of 10 to 12 mg/dl may be associated with bilirubin encephalopathy in certain low birth weight infants, all degrees of visible jaundice in premature infants should be monitored closely and investigated fully. Although bilirubin UDP-glucuronyl transferase activity in premature infants is less than that in term infants, the activity increases rapidly, far exceeding the expected maturational rate noted in utero (Fig. 34-4). This observation indicates that there are two components of the maturation of bilirubin UDP-glucuronyl transferase: (1) chronologic maturation and (2) accelerated maturation related to birth. Nevertheless, normal serum bilirubin concentrations in premature infants may not be reached in many cases until the end of the first month of life.

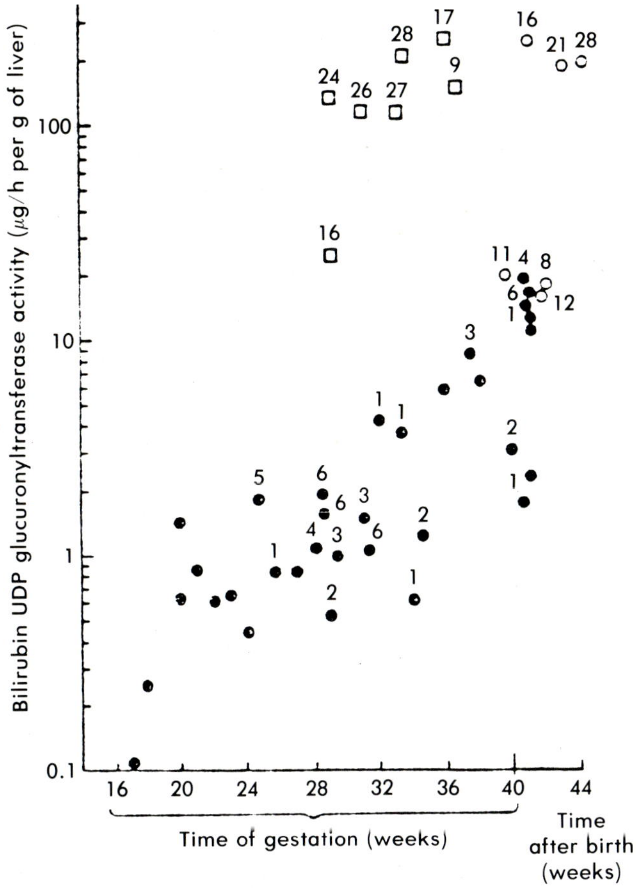

Fig. 34-4. Effect of premature birth on development of hepatic bilirubin UDP glucuronyl transferase activity in humans. Numbers beside symbols represent age (days) at which activities were measured. Symbols represent enzyme activities for premature (□) and full-term (○) infants who lived more than 8 days after birth and for fetuses and premature and full-term infants who died within 7 days of delivery (●). (From Kawade, N., and Onishi, S.: Biochem, J. **196:**267, 1981. Reprinted by permission of The Biochemical Society, London, © 1981.)

Physiologic jaundice in the postmature infant

Nearly all postmature infants and approximately half of all small for dates full-term infants may be expected to have little or no physiologic jaundice, with peak serum bilirubin concentrations less than 2.5 mg/dl. The mechanism for this acceleration of hepatic maturation is unknown. Similarly, infants of mothers treated with phenobarbital, a drug known to stimulate hepatic glucuronyl transferase activity, and those of heroin users have less than the anticipated severity of physiologic jaundice. Other drugs, less well investigated, also may have similar effects.

Conjugated hyperbilirubinemia may occur in combination with physiologic jaundice when excretory mechanisms are unable to cope with the quantity of bilirubin presented to, and conjugated by, the liver. Severe uptake or conjugating deficiency, however, may mask excretory defects for a brief period by preventing sufficient conjugated pigment from reaching the excretory transport step and thus preventing retention and regurgitation of conjugated pigment despite a defect in hepatic excretion.

Bilirubin transport in the fetus

In the fetus synthesized unconjugated bilirubin is transferred rapidly across the placenta into the maternal circulation for excretion by the maternal liver. Small amounts of bilirubin apparently are excreted by the fetal liver into a sluggish bile flow, since meconium accumulates significant amounts of bilirubin during the course of gestation. Unconjugated bilirubin also may be transferred from the maternal circulation into the fetus. In those rare situations in which a pregnant woman has significant unconjugated hyperbilirubinemia, a similar degree of hyperbilirubinemia may be anticipated in cord blood. Conjugated pigment is not transferred in either direction across the placenta. Therefore conjugated hyperbilirubinemia in the mother, as in hepatitis or recurrent jaundice of pregnancy, will not be reflected in the cord blood. It has been recognized that severe hemolytic disease in the fetus results in small but significant increases in amniotic fluid bilirubin concentrations. It is not known how bilirubin enters the amniotic fluid pool, but suggestions have ranged from transfer directly across the placenta from the maternal circulation, to transudation of pigment across the amniotic membranes or cord vessels, to secretion of bilirubin from the fetal lung into the amniotic fluid. The measurement of bilirubin concentrations in amniotic fluid by the optical density technique has markedly improved management of the erythroblastotic infant (Chapter 5).

Genetic and ethnic influences on physiologic jaundice

The severity of physiologic jaundice differs greatly between oriental and other ethnic populations. Mean maximal serum unconjugated bilirubin concentrations in Chinese, Japanese, Korean, and American Indian full-term newborns are between 10 and 14 mg/dl, approximately double those of the non-Oriental populations. The incidence of bilirubin toxicity as defined by autopsy-proven kernicterus also is increased significantly in Oriental neonates. There is no evidence for increased hemolysis in Oriental newborns to account for these dramatic differences. Glucose-6-phosphate dehydrogenase (G6PD) deficiency is far more common in Orientals than in whites; however, it does not relate directly to the increased severity of physiologic jaundice.

Certain geographic isolates also demonstrate a markedly increased incidence of neonatal unconjugated hyperbilirubinemia without associated hemolysis. The most dramatic of these are from certain islands off the coast of Greece, especially the islands of Lesbos and Rhodes. As in the Oriental populations, the incidence of G6PD deficiency in these populations also is markedly increased compared with the incidence in the rest of the world and with the remainder of the Greek population, but this does not directly account for most of those infants with increased serum bilirubin concentrations. The incidence of kernicterus also is much greater in the newborns from these Greek islands than in those of the mainland population.

It has been suggested that the increased incidence of neonatal unconjugated hyperbilirubinemia in Oriental and geographically identifiable populations may result either from environmental influences, such as the maternal ingestion of certain ethnically characteristic herbal medications or foods, or from a genetic predisposition to slower maturation of hepatic bilirubin metabolism. Oriental groups living in the United States appear to have the same severity of neonatal jaundice as those in the Orient, suggesting that the geographic factors alone are not determinant. The question of drugs or foods and that of genetic factors remain to be investigated. Hemolysis, ecchymoses, and other factors that increase bilirubin synthesis in the newborn are particularly likely to produce severe hyperbilirubinemia in these high-risk populations.

PATHOLOGIC STATES OF UNCONJUGATED HYPERBILIRUBINEMIA

Superimposed on the physiologic limitations that result in physiologic jaundice are several specific disorders that may further increase serum unconjugated bilirubin concentrations, prolong unconjugated hyperbilirubinemia beyond the normal period of physiologic jaundice, or both. Most disorders causing exaggerated unconjugated hyperbilirubinemia can be classified in a functional manner according to the step in the pathway most severely affected; that is, (1) bilirubin production, (2) hepatic uptake, or (3) hepatic conjugation. The level of the serum bilirubin concentration does not in itself indicate whether the cause is physiologic or pathologic. Moderate hemolytic disease in one infant with very poor hepatic uptake and conjugation of bilirubin may result in a very rapid rise in the serum bilirubin concentration to 20 mg/dl, whereas the same degree of hemolysis in an infant with much greater hepatic bilirubin uptake and conjugating capacity may result in a slowly rising serum bilirubin concentration that reaches only 6 mg/dl in the same period. Since the balance between bilirubin load and hepatic bilirubin transport processes is so delicate, a small increase in bilirubin production may result in a very marked rise in the serum concentration. Thus it is often very difficult to distinguish between severe physiologic limitations and minor pathologic states.

Increased bilirubin production

Although increased bilirubin production could result from pathologic states in which degradation of nonhemoglobin heme (such as cytochromes) and erythrocyte hemoglobin precursor heme is increased because of specific disease states, such disorders have in fact not been identified in the newborn period. Destruction of circulating erythrocytes is the largest single category of disorders leading to exaggerated unconjugated hyperbilirubinemia in the newborn period. These disorders, which are listed in the box on the facing page, are discussed in more detail in Chapter 32.

Rh erythroblastosis

Rh erythroblastosis was at one time the leading cause of bilirubin encephalopathy and a frequent and serious clinical problem (Chapter 5). With the introduction of high-titer anti-D immunoglobulin G for prophylactic treatment of all unsensitized Rh-negative mothers during pregnancy and after delivery of an Rh-positive infant or performance of an abortion, the incidence of Rh disease has been greatly reduced. Mothers sensitized before the development of immune serum prophylaxis and those without access to preventive treatment still continue to deliver affected infants. Jaundice is only one of many problems affecting the infant with Rh erythroblastosis.

Destruction of erythrocytes and production of large amounts of bilirubin begin in utero, but erythroblastotic infants are not icteric at birth because serum bilirubin concentrations are kept below 5 mg/dl by transfer of unconjugated bilirubin across the placenta. Jaundice may appear, however, within 30 minutes after delivery. Classically the serum bilirubin is all indirect reacting, although small amounts of conjugated bilirubin have been noted. In recent years, with survival of some very severely affected fetuses, particularly those receiving intrauterine transfusions (see Chapter 5), moderate to marked conjugated hyperbilirubinemia has been seen in cord blood or during the first days of life. Total cord bilirubin concentrations may be as high as 40 mg/dl, with at least 80% direct-reacting bilirubin; conjugated bilirubin is not transported across the placenta. The reason for the development of direct-reacting bilirubin in sera is unknown, but it has been suggested that hepatic conjugation may mature more rapidly than usual as a result of chronic exposure to bilirubin in utero, whereas excretory function lags behind. Hepatic excretory function in severe erythroblastosis also may be adversely affected by development of hepatic swelling resulting from heart failure and by congestion caused by severe extramedullary hematopoiesis in liver, anemia, and poor hepatic perfusion and oxygenation.

The risk of kernicterus in states of severe hemolysis, as in Rh erythroblastosis, may be greater than in nonhemolytic hyperbilirubinemia of the same degree. This is suggested both by the increased incidence of brain damage in association with Rh hemolytic disease and by studies suggesting disproportionately decreased albumin binding of bilirubin in association with hemolytic disease.

Conditions associated with increased erythrocyte destruction

A. Isoimmunization
   1. Rh incompatibility
   2. ABO incompatibility
   3. Other blood group incompatibilities
B. Erythrocyte biochemical defects
   1. G6PD deficiency
   2. Pyruvate kinase deficiency
   3. Hexokinase deficiency
   4. Congenital erythropoietic porphyria
   5. Other biochemical defects
C. Structural abnormalities of erythrocytes
   1. Hereditary spherocytosis
   2. Hereditary elliptocytosis
   3. Infantile pyknocytosis
   4. Other
D. Infection
   1. Bacterial
   2. Viral
   3. Protozoal
E. Sequestered blood
   1. Subdural hematoma/cephalohematoma
   2. Ecchymoses
   3. Hemangiomas

ABO hemolytic disease

See also Chapter 32.

Infants with group A or B erythrocytes may have increased hyperbilirubinemia, hemolysis, and positive Coombs' tests because of transfer of maternal anti-A or anti-B antibody into the fetal circulation. Although similar to Rh disease, the disorder may occur in the firstborn without prior sensitization of the mother and symptoms are generally milder and of shorter duration; however, it may also cause severe hemolysis, jaundice, and kernicterus.

Other causes of increased bilirubin production

These include erythrocyte enzyme deficiencies (G6PD deficiency and others), infection, sequestered blood, and structural abnormalities of erythrocytes. The clinical manifestations may be extremely subtle with little or no detectable decrease in hematocrit levels, elevation of reticulocyte count, or clearly definable abnormality of the erythrocyte on microscopic examination of the peripheral smear. A relatively small decrease in erythrocyte life span may enhance bilirubin production sufficiently to raise serum bilirubin concentrations to dangerous levels. No currently available clinical laboratory tool will assist in defining the contribution to hyperbilirubinemia of increased hemolysis of such small degree. Measurement of carbon monoxide production rates may permit quantitative assessments of heme degradation, but it has not been used as a routine clinical procedure.

Glucose-6-phosphate dehydrogenase deficiency

See also Chapter 32.

This deficiency is marked by genetic heterogeneity, such that the majority of infants with the deficiency will not demonstrate exaggerated neonatal jaundice. In the American black population G6PD deficiency is a relatively mild disorder, and exaggerated jaundice in the newborn is unusual and occurs generally only in association with exposure to certain known inciting agents, such as naphthalene or high-dose synthetic vitamin K (K_3). Mediterranean and Oriental types of G6PD deficiency are more often readily apparent, with exaggerated jaundice more common and an associated high incidence of kernicterus. In the more severe form of the disease jaundice may not become apparent until the second or third day of life and may then persist into the second and even third weeks, in association with obvious hemolysis. Those infants developing hemolysis later in the newborn period either may have relatively less hyperbilirubinemia, reflecting their maturing hepatic bilirubin metabolism, or may have significant elevations of direct-reacting bilirubin in sera, indicating that hepatic uptake and conjugation of bilirubin have matured relatively more rapidly than the excretory pathway, resulting in retention of conjugated bilirubin.

Severe neonatal jaundice may be associated with erythrocyte pyruvate kinase deficiency, 2,3-diphosphoglycerate mutase deficiency, 6-phosphogluconic dehydrogenase deficiency, and probably many other enzymatic defects yet to be defined. Although extremely rare, the recessively inherited congenital erythropoietic porphyria may be present with mixed hyperbilirubinemia, splenomegaly, and anemia at birth and may be suspected by the pink reddish–brown urine that fluoresces readily under ultraviolet light.

As in the case of the red blood cell enzyme defects, structural defects of erythrocytes may or may not cause exaggerated neonatal jaundice. *Hereditary spherocytosis* (Chapter 32) is associated with neonatal jaundice in approximately half the cases and must be differentiated from ABO incompatibility, since the latter disorder also is characterized by increased numbers of spherocytes in the peripheral smear. Coombs' testing and examination of parents and other family members for evidence of spherocytes help distinguish the two disorders. Since the disease is inherited as an autosomal dominant trait in most cases, the diagnosis may be suspected more strongly when one parent has either splenomegaly or a history of splenectomy. In some patients, however, differentiation cannot be made, and only continued examination of the peripheral smear beyond the newborn period will determine whether hereditary spherocytosis is the correct diagnosis. *Hereditary elliptocytosis* rarely causes hemolysis in the newborn (Chapter 32). A transient abnormality of erythrocyte morphology associated with hemolysis and neonatal jaundice is the disorder known as *infantile pyknocytosis*. Small, irregular, dense red blood cells with spiny projections are seen in the peripheral smear and account for more than 5% of the total red cell population. Anemia and hemolysis persist throughout the first month of life and often into the second and third months. Jaundice is most severe during the first 2 weeks of life. This disorder was recognized with greater frequency some years ago and now has become quite rare. In vitro studies of erythrocytes and plasma from these infants suggested that the abnormality resided in an extracorpuscular factor. The changing incidence of this disorder suggests that it may be a manifestation of an unknown exogenous toxic factor.

All the aforementioned disorders that may cause exaggerated hemolysis will result in more severe hyperbilirubinemia in the premature infant than in the full-term infant. Although more severe neonatal jaundice is characteristic of the premature infant, efforts should be made to detect abnormalities of erythrocytes in all jaundiced low birth weight infants. Since G6PD deficiency is by far the most common enzymatic defect, all infants with severe hyperbilirubinemia should have determinations of G6PD enzyme levels on pre-exchange transfusion blood specimens. Smears of the peripheral blood always should be examined as part of the evaluation of all infants with serum total bilirubin concentrations greater than 12 mg/dl.

Exaggerated unconjugated hyperbilirubinemia often is cited as a sign of bacterial sepsis; the mechanism is thought to be related to increased red cell destruction. There are, however, no convincing studies supporting this association or the frequency of this association. A work-up for sepsis as part of the investigation of unconjugated hyperbilirubinemia may not be indicated when there are no other signs to suggest sepsis. More clearly related to bacterial sepsis, especially with *Escherichia coli*, *Proteus* organisms, and pneumococci, is the development of conjugated hyperbilirubinemia; this is believed to be a result of inhibition of hepatic excretion of bilirubin by bacterial toxins (Chapter 31).

Hepatic uptake deficiency

Defective hepatic uptake of bilirubin has been suggested as one of the possible contributing causes of chronic unconjugated hyperbilirubinemia in adults (Gilbert's syndrome). Aside from animal studies that suggest that physiologic jaundice of the newborn may result from defective bilirubin uptake, there are no data to suggest that exaggerated hyperbilirubinemia of the newborn results from a specific defect in hepatic bilirubin uptake.

Deficient conjugation of bilirubin

Inherited defects

Two genetically and functionally distinct disorders associated with inherited lifelong deficiency of hepatic glucuronyl transferase activity have been described.

Crigler-Najjar syndrome. This is the rarest and most severe of these chronic nonhemolytic unconjugated hyperbilirubinemias and has been designated type I glucuronyl transferase deficiency. Only approximately 100 infants with type I glucuronyl transferase deficiency have been reported.

Clinical manifestations. Inherited as an autosomal recessive trait, in the homozygous form severe unconjugated hyperbilirubinemia develops during the first 3 days of life and progresses in an unremitting fashion to reach serum concentrations of 25 to 35 mg/dl during the first month of life. Kernicterus occurs commonly during the early neonatal period, although recently there have been some survivors without neurologic sequelae. Stools are pale yellow, and bile bilirubin concentrations will be less than 10 mg/dl (normal, 50 to 100 mg/dl), with total absence of bilirubin glucuronide in bile. Bilirubin glucuronide formation measured in vitro with liver obtained by biopsy is absent. Formation of most nonbilirubin glucuronides is either severely reduced or absent. With either direct hepatic enzymatic assay or indirect measurement of glucuronide formation, both parents are found to have partial defects (approximately 50% normal), but their serum bilirubin concentrations are normal. During the first week of life the recognition of this disorder may be difficult because of confusion with other types of exaggerated unconjugated hyperbilirubinemia. Persistence of unconjugated hyperbilirubinemia at concentrations exceeding 20 mg/dl beyond the first week of life in the absence of obvious hemolysis should alert one to consider this syndrome. In the nursing newborn the much more common disorder of breast milk jaundice also must be considered, but management of breast-feeding, as outlined later, will rapidly differentiate the two.

The diagnosis may be strongly suggested by the persistence of unconjugated hyperbilirubinemia, but it can be definitively established only by direct measurement of hepatic glucuronyl transferase activity. Open surgical biopsy to obtain a specimen of liver should be avoided, since anesthesia and physiologic alterations associated with surgery may precipitate kernicterus. The diagnosis can be strongly supported by identifying partial defects in conjugation in both parents in the absence of jaundice. Duodenal intubation by which bile is obtained that contains little bilirubin is strong circumstantial evidence of the diagnosis, but dilutional effects may be confusing. Direct collection of bile from the gallbladder or common duct with concentrations below 10 mg/dl would be diagnostic, but the surgical intervention necessary is an unwarranted risk. Differentiation from type II glucuronyl transferase deficiency may be achieved by the failure of patients with type I to respond to a week of phenobarbital administration with a marked decline in serum bilirubin concentration. This failure to respond to phenobarbital suggests that the basic defect in the type I disorder is the synthesis of a structurally defective enzyme.

Treatment. The management of these infants requires maintenance of serum bilirubin concentrations below 20 mg/dl during at least the first 2 to 4 weeks of life. Under certain circumstances serum bilirubin concentrations should be kept even lower. The risk of kernicterus persists in adult life, but the serum bilirubin concentrations required to produce brain injury beyond the newborn period are considerably higher, perhaps above 35 mg/dl. Exchange transfusion may be the preferred method for reducing the serum bilirubin concentration in these infants, but repeated frequent exchange transfusions would be required. For this reason most of the infants have been placed under phototherapy either after one or more exchange transfusions or before it was indicated. Phototherapy generally has been continued throughout the early years of life in the hope that this will prevent the development of kernicterus. In recent years patients indeed have survived the neonatal period without apparent brain damage. Whether this is because of the use of phototherapy or related to improved general newborn care is not known. In the older infants and children phototherapy has been used mainly at night, during sleep periods, permitting the children to have normal activity during the daytime. Despite attempts to expose the older children to phototherapy of the highest intensities and longest durations possible, increasingly poorer responses of the serum bilirubin concentration to phototherapy have been observed with aging. This may result from increased skin thickness or a changing distribution of the bilirubin pool. Prompt management of all intercurrent infections, febrile episodes, and other types of illness may help prevent later development of kernicterus. Kernicterus may develop at any age if serum bilirubin concentrations increase to 45 to 55 mg/dl. Despite vigorous efforts to reduce serum bilirubin concentrations, all patients with type I disease have developed severe kernicterus at or before achieving young adulthood, even when they were neurologically normal throughout childhood.

Glucuronyl transferase deficiency type II. This disorder may be manifested in a manner similar to that of the type I syndrome, or it may be a much less severe disorder, even without neonatal manifestations.

Clinical manifestations. In those infants in whom the disorder becomes apparent during the newborn period, unconjugated hyperbilirubinemia generally appears during the first 3 days of life, with serum bilirubin concentrations that may be either in a range compatible with physiologic jaundice (less than 12 mg/dl) or exaggerated. Characteristically, however, bilirubin concentrations will remain more elevated than expected (greater than 3 mg/dl) into the third week of life, and these elevations will persist thereafter, ranging from minimal elevations of greater than 1.5 mg/dl to as high as 22 mg/dl. There may be uncertainty for some period as to whether chronic hyperbilirubinemia has developed. Although kernicterus has been reported in two patients with type II syndrome, its occurrence is unusual. Evidence of hemolytic disease is absent (although it may occur coincidentally), stool color is normal, and the infants are otherwise healthy.

Since this disorder is inherited as an autosomal dominant trait with marked variability of penetrance, one of the parents may be minimally to severely icteric or at least demonstrate a defect in bilirubin conjugation when tested for this function. Other members of the family also may either appear icteric or have detectable low-grade unconjugated hyperbilirubinemia. Screening of the parents and other close relatives for hyperbilirubinemia is a useful method for supporting the diagnosis when it is suspected. A definitive diagnosis can be made only by direct or indirect testing of the infant and the parents for the capacity to form glucuronides of bilirubin or other suitable substances (such as menthol or salicylamide). Bilirubin glucuronide formation can be tested in vitro by performance of a percutaneous liver biopsy. Administration of substances conjugated as glucuronides in liver and excreted in urine, such as menthol or salicylamide, obviates the need for liver biopsy but is unfortunately less specific and accurate. Regardless of the method used, the levels of conjugation are extremely low and not distinguishable from those found in the type I syndrome. Once a deficiency in conjugation is established, it is necessary to distinguish between types I and II. Although examination of gallbladder bile will demonstrate that type I cases have extremely low bilirubin concentrations and type II cases have nearly normal concentrations (50 to 100 mg/dl), this would necessitate surgical exploration, a dangerous procedure for any severely jaundiced infant. Genetic studies may indicate that only one parent and family members from that parent's lineage are affected, suggesting that the infant has type II syndrome, but such studies are not always possible or definitive. Jaundiced infants and adults with the type II syndrome respond readily to oral administration of phenobarbital with a sharp decline in serum bilirubin concentrations to 2 to 3 mg/dl within 7 to 10 days. Individuals with type I syndrome demonstrate no change in serum bilirubin concentration. The response to phenobarbital may be used as a simple clinical tool to differentiate the two syndromes. A dosage of 5 mg/kg/day given once a day is sufficient for infants and young children.

Treatment. The response to phenobarbital administration may be used not only as a diagnostic test but also, when chronically administered, for long-term reduction of bilirubin concentrations for cosmetic and psychosocial reasons. At the serum bilirubin concentrations observed in patients with type II disease, there should be no long-term risk of kernicterus, unless there is coincidental hemolytic disease.

Pregnancy in the patient with either the type I conjugating defect or more severe forms of type II syndrome may present a special hazard to both the mother and fetus. During pregnancy serum bilirubin concentrations may rise, and bilirubin binding by albumin may be altered, thus increasing the risk to the mother of neurologic manifestations of severe unconjugated hyperbilirubinemia. Unconjugated bilirubin crosses the placenta in both directions. With severe unconjugated hyperbilirubinemia in the mother, markedly elevated unconjugated bilirubin concentrations may be anticipated in the fetus, raising the theoretical possibility of congenital kernicterus, a syndrome that has not been observed thus far.

Acquired defects

Late-onset breast milk jaundice. A small cohort of breast-fed infants develop a syndrome characterized by the relatively late onset of exaggerated unconjugated hyperbilirubinemia at a time when jaundice would normally be abating. The estimated incidence is approximately 1 per 100 breast-fed infants. A normal or an exaggerated pattern of physiologic jaundice is observed during the first 3 days of life, following which the serum bilirubin concentrations rise to reach maximum unconjugated bilirubin concentrations of 10 to 27 mg/dl by the tenth to fifteenth days of life in the absence of hemolysis and other evidence of illness. Weight gain and bowel function are characteristically normal. Often the infants are not noted by the parents or other caregivers to be abnormal in any way. Interruption of nursing and substitution with artificial feeding or nursing by another woman for 2 to 4 days result in a prompt decline of the serum bilirubin concentration to approximately half or less of the original level. Resumption of nursing by the mother results in a small but significant increase in serum-indirect bilirubin concentrations of 1 to 3 mg/dl in most infants or arrest of the decline in bilirubin concentrations in others. Failure to respond in this manner indicates that the infant's jaundice is unrelated to breast-feeding, and other causes should be sought. It should be emphasized that interruption of nursing is not recommended as a routine procedure in all jaundiced breast-fed infants but should be reserved for those infants whose serum bilirubin concentrations approach levels considered dangerous for development of kernicterus. Since this syndrome is most commonly seen in full-term, otherwise normal infants, serum bilirubin levels that remain below 20 mg/dl in these infants may be considered to be safe during the first 4 weeks of life, and nursing could but need not necessarily be interrupted. The rare inherited defects in hepatic bilirubin metabolism (type II especially) may occur in breast-fed infants, leading to the erroneous diagnosis of breast milk jaundice. It will become clear, however, that a chronic disorder exists when, after termination of nursing for weeks or even months, unconjugated hyperbilirubinemia persists. Since persistence of low-grade unconjugated hyperbilirubinemia poses no threat to the newborn or older infant, delay in recognition of the defect poses no hazard. The breast milk jaundice syndrome may be anticipated when there is a history of prolonged unconjugated hyperbilirubinemia in other breast-fed infants of the mother, since approximately 70% of the nursed infants of these women may be expected to have the syndrome. Similarly, in the artificially fed infants of these same mothers, prolonged, severe jaundice is rare.

This syndrome was attributed in earlier studies to the presence of an isomerically abnormal progesterone metabolite, pregnane-3α,20β-diol, in milk. This steroid metabolite had been shown to be a competitive inhibitor of glucuronyl transferase in vitro. More recent studies have indicated that the milk associated with this syndrome also contains high concentrations of nonesterified long-chain fatty acids. This led to the suggestion that certain of these fatty acids act as inhibitors of hepatic glucuronyl transferase, resulting in retention of unconjugated bilirubin. This mechanism has not, however, been demonstrated in vivo. Although the presence of both pregnane-3α,20β-diol and increased amounts of nonesterified fatty acids in this human milk has been amply confirmed, the role of these agents in pathophysiology of this syndrome remains uncertain. A recent study on enterohepatic circulation of bilirubin in the rat suggests that milk from mothers of infants with this syndrome enhances enteric reabsorption of bilirubin, increasing the hepatic bilirubin load.

Early onset breast milk jaundice. The relationship between accentuated unconjugated hyperbilirubinemia in the first week of life and breast-feeding has not been fully established. This entity frequently is claimed to be seen by many clinicians but has never been adequately documented. In some hospital nurseries it is said to be the single most frequent cause of neonatal jaundice in full-term newborn infants. It is clear that this is not a universal finding. Two prospective studies failed to show any significant differences between serum bilirubin concentrations of breast- and bottle-fed infants during the first 3 days of life. The possible difference in the incidence of this entity between hospitals may be related to differences in breast-feeding practices. In many hospital settings breast-feeding mothers are not encouraged to nurse their infants with sufficient frequency (at least every 2 hours in the early days of lactation) to permit rapid and effective development of lactation. Frequency of nursing has been shown to correlate inversely with serum bilirubin concentrations on the third day of life. Poor advice and inappropriate supplementation with water and/or formula also may serve to inhibit lactation. Starvation or reduced caloric intake is known to produce elevated unconjugated serum bilirubin levels in many animal species, including humans. The mechanism by which starvation may induce unconjugated hyperbilirubinemia in the neonate has not been explored. Recent studies reveal that a close relationship exists between serum bilirubin concentration and time of meconium passage, bilirubin content in stools, or amount of stools. These observations suggest that the pathologic mechanism for the syndrome of early onset breast milk jaundice may also be related to increased bilirubin reabsorption from the intestine.

Since it is clear that not all jaundice in the breast-fed neonate is a result of breast-feeding, the clinician is faced with the difficult dilemma of whether breast-feeding should be interrupted when the serum bilirubin concentration is rising or markedly elevated. There is unfortunately no firm clinical experience or studies on which to base a recommendation. Breast-feeding should not be interrupted routinely but only when serum bilirubin concentrations are at or near potentially toxic levels.

Transient familial neonatal hyperbilirubinemia. This is a rare syndrome in which every infant of certain mothers may be expected to develop severe unconjugated hyperbilirubinemia during the first 48 hours of life, with bilirubin concentrations usually reaching 20 mg/dl or greater. Many of these infants develop kernicterus unless exchange transfusions are performed. Hemolysis is absent, and the infants are otherwise healthy. The sera of these infants and their mothers are found to contain high concentrations of an unidentified inhibitor of glucuronyl transferase when tested in vitro. The inhibitor is present in maternal sera during the second and third trimesters of pregnancy and in both maternal and newborn sera at the time of delivery. Although sera from normal pregnant women and newborns also inhibit glucuronyl transferase activity to a small degree, sera from these mothers and infants are 4 to 10 times as inhibitory. The serum inhibitory effect gradually declines after delivery to become normal by approximately 14 days post partum. Coincident with the decrease in inhibition, there is a gradual decline in serum bilirubin concentrations in the newborn.

Pyloric stenosis. This disorder is associated with the development of unconjugated hyperbilirubinemia in 10% to 25% of the infants at the time vomiting begins, usually during the second or third week of life (Chapter 33). There is no relationship between the development of jaundice and the degree of dehydration or electrolyte imbalance. Hepatic glucuronyl transferase activity is markedly depressed in the jaundiced infants but not in anicteric infants with pyloric stenosis. The mechanism of diminished glucuronyl transferase activity is unknown but may relate to the presence of an inhibitory substance elaborated in the intestinal tract. Duodenal and jejunal obstruction also is associated with exaggerated unconjugated hyperbilirubinemia. Surgical relief of the obstructive enteropathy results in return of serum bilirubin concentrations to normal within 2 to 3 days. Lower intestinal obstruction, as in Hirschsprung's disease, also may result in unconjugated hyperbilirubinemia, although usually of milder degree than the upper intestinal tract disease. In this situation, as well as in upper intestinal tract obstructions, hyperbilirubinemia may result from increased reabsorption of unconjugated bilirubin from the intestine as a result of enteric stasis, which may also lead to increased hydrolysis of bilirubin glucuronide to unconjugated bilirubin, with enhancement of reabsorption by intestinal mucosa.

Drugs administered to newborns must be considered as potential agents that may exaggerate unconjugated hyperbilirubinemia not only by initiating hemolysis in certain metabolic defects of erythrocytes (G6PD deficiency) but also by inhibition of hepatic glucuronyl transferase activity. Many drugs that have been used in neonatal therapy (such as streptomycin and chloramphenicol) are capable of inhibiting the enzyme in vitro, but only novobiocin (an old and now clinically discontinued antibiotic) has ever been demonstrated to actually produce unconjugated hyperbilirubinemia. Novobiocin is a noncompetitive inhibitor of glucuronyl transferase. The use of any new drug in the neonate should alert the staff to the need to observe for increased jaundice.

Exaggerated neonatal jaundice with undefined mechanisms

Maternal diabetes is associated with an increased incidence of exaggerated and prolonged unconjugated hyperbilirubinemia in the offspring (see Chapter 3). This is unrelated to the severity and duration of the maternal diabetes. Exaggerated jaundice often is attributed to the prematurity of the infant of the diabetic mother. However, even when one compares infants of identical gestational age, there is an increased incidence, duration, and severity of jaundice in the infant of the diabetic mother. Increased red cell mass resulting in increased catabolism of heme has been suggested as a cause of exaggerated jaundice.

Hypothyroidism in the newborn is another disorder in which exaggerated unconjugated hyperbilirubinemia has been observed (Chapter 37, part three). Approximately 10% of hypothyroid infants may be expected to have prolonged and exaggerated jaundice. Treatment with thyroid hormone will promptly alleviate the hyperbilirubinemia. Congenital hypothyroidism often is difficult to diagnose in the newborn, and persistence of unconjugated hyperbilirubinemia should suggest the possibility of thyroid insufficiency.

BILIRUBIN TOXICITY

Kernicterus

The recognition that unconjugated bilirubin has the capability of entering the brain cell under certain circumstances and causing the death of neurons is the reason for the urgency in carefully observing every jaundiced newborn and treating neonatal jaundice.

Pathology

The major pathologic consequence of bilirubin encephalopathy is the result of the yellow staining and necrosis of neurons. The areas of the brain most commonly affected are the basal ganglia, hippocampal cortex, subthalamic nuclei, and cerebellum. The cerebral cortex generally is spared. Only unconjugated bilirubin enters neurons. Although the diagnosis of kernicterus at autopsy has always relied on the grossly yellow staining of the brain tissue and the accompanying neuronal necrosis, recent animal studies have suggested that significant impairment of brain function may result from hyperbilirubinemia even when there is no obvious staining or histologic evidence of cell damage. This suggests that very small quantities of bilirubin may be transiently or permanently cytotoxic.

Approximately half of all infants with kernicterus observed at autopsy have extraneural lesions of bilirubin toxicity. These include necrosis of renal tubular cells, intestinal mucosa, and pancreatic cells in association with intracellular crystals of bilirubin. Gastrointestinal hemorrhage may accompany these lesions.

Clinical manifestations

In the classic presentation of bilirubin encephalopathy, the newborn progressively develops lethargy, rigidity, opisthotonos, high-pitched cry, fever, and convulsions over a period of up to 24 hours. This is followed by death in approximately half the infants so affected. Premature infants with autopsy-proven kernicterus generally have none of these characteristic clinical findings. Survivors of neonatal manifestations of bilirubin encephalopathy often demonstrate choreoathetoid cerebral palsy, high-frequency deafness, and, less often, mental retardation during later infancy and childhood. These sequelae of kernicterus also may develop in infants who never manifest clinical signs of bilirubin encephalopathy during the newborn period. In addition, some infants may have sequelae of subclinical bilirubin encephalopathy characterized only by the later development of mild disorders of motor function or abnormal cognitive function or both, collectively called *minimal brain dysfunction*. Premature infants are particularly susceptible to this type of subtle bilirubin-related brain damage. (See Chapter 27, part six.)

Pathogenesis

The pathogenesis of bilirubin encephalopathy is complex and poorly understood. Although certain sequelae (such as choreoathetoid cerebral palsy and upward gaze palsy) are specific, most sequelae are not and could as well be the result of hypoxic, vascular, or infectious injury. Furthermore, both clinical and laboratory studies have indicated that certain neonatal risk factors that in themselves produce brain damage also increase the likelihood that kernicterus will develop in the presence of mild to moderate unconjugated hyperbilirubinemia. Leading among these factors is hypoxia. The relationship between brain hypoxia and kernicterus is so close that some investigators have suggested that kernicterus will not develop in the absence of some degree of CNS hypoxia. The theory of this relationship may be particularly valid for those clinical situations in which kernicterus develops at relatively low serum bilirubin concentrations (less than 15 mg/dl), as in a very immature infant. Other factors that enhance the development of kernicterus are hypoglycemia, acidosis, bacterial infection (sepsis and meningitis), hypothermia, moderate to severe hemolysis, administration of certain drugs (sulfonamides), hypoalbuminemia, and deficient albumin binding of bilirubin. The mechanism (or mechanisms) by which each of these pathologic states enhances the development of kernicterus is, in part, speculative. Nevertheless, the recognition of the importance of these factors has led to their inclusion in virtually every schema for establishing criteria for treatment of neonatal hyperbilirubinemia (see section on management and Table 34-1).

In the pathogenesis of kernicterus unconjugated bilirubin moves from the plasma pool into the neuron. This movement results either from (1) a reduction in the quantity or quality of binding of bilirubin by the circulating albumin or (2) a major alteration in a membrane function of the epithelial capillary cell or the brain cell that normally excludes bilirubin from entry (the so-called blood-brain barrier). In most clinical situations both factors are operative. The human albumin molecule is capable of binding at least two molecules of bilirubin; the first molecule is more tightly bound than the second. Additional classes of binding sites, if operative in vivo, have much lower affinities than the first two. At a molar ratio of 1, each gram of human albumin binds 8.4 mg of bilirubin. Thus, at an average serum albumin concentration of 3.5 gm/dl, the first binding site should be capable of binding 29.4 mg bilirubin per 100 ml serum. The second binding site should be capable of binding an additional 29.4 mg/dl, for a total binding capacity of 58.8 mg/dl. Various techniques are available to measure albumin binding of bilirubin, but their application and interpretation in clinical management are not generally accepted. The dye-binding methods utilizing 2-(4-hydroxybenzeneazo) benzoic acid and Direct-Yellow-7 are based on the measurement of reserve binding sites on the albumin molecule and should be capable of indicating impending risk; the column chromatographic methods (Sephadex G-25), the salicylate displacement spectrophotometric method (saturation index), the red cell uptake method, and the oxidation technique (peroxidase method) all should be capable of detecting either small amounts of unbound bilirubin ("free" bilirubin) or "loosely bound" bilirubin. In general there is an increased risk of developing kernicterus when there is either an increase in "loose" or "free" bilirubin in the circulation or when binding capacity approaches dangerously close to saturation; however, present data are insufficient to permit a recommendation as to the use of either a single method or combination of methods or numeric standards for the application of any of these methods. The critical point at which the risk of kernicterus is probably significantly increased is when the first binding site on albumin is saturated.

Table 34-1. Maximum total serum bilirubin concentration (mg/dl)* allowed before exchange transfusion

Birth weight category (gm)†	Uncomplicated course	Complicated course‡
Less than 1,000	10	10
1,000-1,249	13	10
1,250-1,499	15	13
1,500-1,999	17	15
2,000-2,499	18	17
2,500 and up	20	18

*Direct-reacting bilirubin concentrations are not subtracted unless they amount to more than 50% of the total serum bilirubin concentration applicable during the first 28 days of life.

†Equivalent gestational age categories may be used in lieu of birth weight for small for gestational age infants.

‡Complications include perinatal asphyxia and acidosis, postnatal hypoxia and acidosis, significant and persistent hypothermia, hypoalbuminemia, hemolysis, hypoglycemia, and proven or suspected bacterial infection.

Some of the factors implicated as increasing the risk of kernicterus in the newborn may operate by direct alteration of albumin binding of bilirubin. Thus acidosis, of even mild degree, the sulfonamide drugs, and possibly sodium benzoate (a preservative in certain drugs) may diminish the binding of bilirubin by albumin; hemolysis may interfere with binding by release of heme pigments into the circulation that may compete with bilirubin for albumin binding sites; hypoglycemia and sepsis may act similarly by increasing free fatty acid concentrations in plasma. Free fatty acids may interfere with binding either by direct competitive displacement of bilirubin, by binding to non-bilirubin binding sites on albumin to produce conformational changes of the albumin molecule with consequent weakening of bilirubin binding, or by complex formation with bilirubin to form a freely circulating pigment not bound to albumin. The increased risk of kernicterus in the newborn and particularly in the premature infant, as compared with the adult, and the demonstration of significantly reduced binding capacity for bilirubin by albumin in the newborn have led to the additional suggestion that a fetal type of albumin, with reduced binding affinity, may exist. Kernicterus has been reported to occur in adults with type I glucuronyl transferase deficiency but only when serum bilirubin concentrations have reached 45 to 55 mg/dl. This contrasts with the situation in the full-term newborn in which an increased incidence of kernicterus may be anticipated at concentrations above 20 mg/dl. There are some suggestions that even at concentrations below 20 mg/dl, full-term infants may develop bilirubin encephalopathy. Abnormal evoked auditory brainstem responses have been reported in full-term infants with serum bilirubin concentrations as low as 15 mg/dl. Immediate improvements in this response have been noted after exchange transfusion. Minimal brain dysfunction has been reported in infants with peak bilirubin levels below 20 mg/dl. In seriously ill premature infants, kernicterus has been repeatedly demonstrated at far lower concentrations, even below 10 mg/dl.

Many mechanisms have been proposed to explain both the entrance of bilirubin into the neuron and the resultant damage to cellular metabolism. Unconjugated bilirubin is a lipid-soluble substance with almost no aqueous solubility. Passage into the lipid moieties of cell membranes and from there into lipids of subcellular organelles (mitochondria) to block critical steps in transport or energy metabolism is possible. Binding to specific proteins in cell membranes or within the cell is also possible. Although it appears to the pathologist that kernicterus is an irreversible form of brain damage, transient or reversible states of bilirubin intoxication have been suggested by clinical observations of increasing lethargy with increasing bilirubin concentrations and awakening after exchange transfusion. Recent evidence of improvement in evoked auditory brainstem responses after exchange transfusion suggests the concept of reversibility of bilirubin encephalopathy. These reversible states remain to be confirmed, but the suggestion of a significant, otherwise unexplained change in the neurobehavioral status of a jaundiced newborn should be considered sufficient basis for institution of immediate exchange transfusion regardless of serum bilirubin concentration or the results of binding studies.

MANAGEMENT OF UNCONJUGATED HYPERBILIRUBINEMIA

Diagnostic clinical and laboratory studies

After appropriate diagnostic tests to establish the cause of the unconjugated hyperbilirubinemia are performed, the clinician is faced with two major decisions: when to institute therapy and which technique (or techniques) to use. Diagnostic studies to determine the presence of hemolytic diseases should be undertaken in full-term infants who become clinically icteric during the first 24 hours of life or whose bilirubin concentrations exceed 12 mg/dl thereafter. All hospitals should routinely determine the maternal blood group and Rh type at the time of the onset of labor and infant blood group, Rh type, and direct Coombs' test immediately after delivery. Additional tests should include hemoglobin or hematocrit determinations, smear of peripheral blood for erythrocyte morphology, and reticulocyte count. In the presence of significant icterus with a potential ABO incompatibility (type O mother and type A, B, or AB infant), the direct Coombs' test should be repeated at least once when originally negative, since initial false-negative results have been seen. If evidence of hemolysis develops or if the infant requires an exchange transfusion, blood should be sent for determination of erythrocyte G6PD activity. A careful history from the parents may reveal familial patterns of neonatal hyperbilirubinemia or anemia or ethnic patterns associated with severe neonatal jaundice. Observation of the parents for jaundice and even determination of serum bilirubin concentrations in them also may be useful in the diagnosis of familial types of hemolytic disease or inherited hepatic dysfunction. Pattern of feeding (time of onset, frequency of breast-feeding) also may be of importance. More extensive studies for rarer forms of hemolytic disease and enzyme assays for glucuronyl transferase activity may be deferred until the chronicity of the disease has been established; this is usually after the first month of life.

Studies for hepatocellular disease (such as hepatitis and obstructive biliary disease), including serum glutamic-oxaloacetic transaminase (SGOT), serum glutamic-pyruvic transaminase (SGPT), alkaline phosphatase, and cholesterol, need to be performed only when there is a significant elevation of conjugated serum bilirubin. A careful physical examination with special attention to liver and spleen size, skin appearance, and neurobehavioral status should be performed frequently in the evaluation of a jaundiced infant. Skin color cannot be relied on for estimation of serum bilirubin concentrations, and it is essential that serum bilirubin determinations be performed on every infant at the time jaundice is first observed and as frequently thereafter as needed to establish the pattern of increase. Recent development of reflectance photometers permits more precise measurement of bilirubin levels than is possible by visual inspection, but cutaneous determinations should be used only for screening purposes. Precise serum bilirubin methods should be used in confirmation. In most patients a repeat determination in 4 to 8 hours will be necessary on the first day of jaundice and at least daily thereafter until a clear pattern of decline is observed. In some patients serum bilirubin concentrations may be monitored on an ambulatory basis, eliminating the need for prolonged hospitalization only for the purpose of obtaining serum bilirubin concentrations. In most cases, a hematocrit should be determined simultaneously with each bilirubin determination. Conjugated bilirubin concentrations should be determined at the time of the first bilirubin estimation and at least daily thereafter.

The method of management chosen for an individual infant will determine in part the serum bilirubin concentration at which therapy is instituted. It is essential therefore that every newborn nursery and neonatal intensive care unit have an established policy regarding the methods to be used and criteria for initiation of therapy.

Exchange transfusion

Exchange transfusion is the standard mode of therapy for treatment of hyperbilirubinemia to prevent kernicterus and for correction of anemia in erythroblastosis fetalis (see Chapter 32). With this technique approximately 85% of the circulating red blood will be replaced when the equivalent of two infant blood volumes (160 ml/kg body weight) is used in aliquots not to exceed 10% of the total blood volume. Serum bilirubin concentrations usually will be reduced by 50%. Although it is a relatively safe procedure in experienced hands, it carries a mortality risk of 0.1% to 1% and a significant morbidity, especially in very low birth weight infants. Apart from complications of the procedure itself and of the blood employed during exchange transfusion, disorders of electrolyte (especially calcium) concentrations and acid-base balance must be avoided. The procedure usually takes 1 to 2 hours to complete. Slower exchanges theoretically should increase the quantity of bilirubin removed by permitting equilibration of pigment from tissue, but the differences are too small to justify the increased risk of prolonging the duration of manipulation. The indications for exchange transfusion should be individualized to some extent and might be based on a variety of criteria that include serum bilirubin concentrations, albumin concentrations, and measurements of albumin binding of bilirubin. Since the latter two techniques still require evaluation for routine clinical use, the conservative indications contained in Table 34-1 are recommended. These criteria are proposed largely on the basis of clinical observations and represent the judgment of a number of neonatologists participating in a controlled clinical trial of phototherapy under the auspices of the National Institute of Child Health and Human Development. Conjugated bilirubin is not subtracted from the total unless the direct-reacting portion exceeds 50% of the total bilirubin. Although direct-reacting bilirubin does not enter the CNS and does not in itself cause kernicterus, it is not known whether direct-reacting bilirubin can partially displace unconjugated bilirubin from albumin binding sites to increase the risk of kernicterus. The same criteria are used on the first day of life as on subsequent days, but in the face of rapidly rising serum bilirubin concentrations, as may be seen in Rh erythroblastosis or other types of hemolytic disease, the decision to perform the exchange should anticipate the rise (from previous serum bilirubin concentrations, hemoglobin concentrations, and reticulocyte count) so that the exchange is under way by the time the critical level is reached. In the severely affected, hydropic or nonhydropic erythroblastotic infant, clinical judgment rather than laboratory data should primarily be used to decide whether the infant requires immediate transfusions after delivery. In this situation a partial exchange transfusion with packed blood cells coupled with measures to ensure adequate ventilation and correction of acidosis and shock often will be life-saving (Chapters 6 and 22). In most exchange transfusions fresh whole or reconstituted, citrate phosphate dextrose–anticoagulated blood should be used (Chapter 32). If blood older than 5 days must be used, the pH should be checked and sodium bicarbonate added to correct the pH to 7.1; correction to pH 7.4 may result in later excessive rebound alkalosis as the citrate is metabolized. Use of heparinized blood avoids additional osmolar loads and may obviate the need to administer calcium or correct for acidosis but may result in hypoglycemia and markedly increased free fatty acid concentrations.

The administration of salt-poor albumin (1 gm/kg) to infants 1 to 2 hours before exchange transfusion to increase the efficiency of bilirubin removal by shifting more tissue-bound bilirubin into the circulation has been advocated and shown to increase the bilirubin removed by 40%. Since the total amount of bilirubin removed during an exchange transfusion is only a small portion of the total body pool of bilirubin, this increase may not significantly alter subsequent bilirubin concentrations or the need for additional exchange transfusions. Although probably benign, the transient increase in serum bilirubin concentration after albumin administration theoretically could increase the risk of kernicterus rather than reduce it if there are local phenomena at the brain level that alter albumin binding of bilirubin.

The potential complications of umbilical catheterization for exchange transfusion are discussed in Chapter 22 and Chapter 24, Part four. Preparations for emergency situations should be made before initiation of the procedure.

Phototherapy

In recent years phototherapy has emerged as the most widely used form of therapy for the treatment and prophylaxis of neonatal unconjugated hyperbilirubinemia. In nearly all infants phototherapy reduces or blunts the rise of serum bilirubin concentrations, regardless of maturity, presence or absence of hemolysis, or degree of skin pigmentation. The initial report from the Collaborative Study on the Effectiveness and Safety of Phototherapy, undertaken under the auspices of the National Institute of Child Health and Human Development, reveals that infants receiving phototherapy require significantly fewer exchange transfusions. They have an incidence of gross kernicterus that is not different from that of infants who did not receive phototherapy but had exchange transfusions alone to control hyperbilirubinemia. Phototherapy has been used in Europe and Latin America for the last 15 to 20 years and in the United States since the early 1970s. No serious long-term side effects have been reported.

In many centers phototherapy is typically begun when bilirubin levels are 5 mg/dl below exchange levels for a given infant, as derived from Table 34-1. At our medical center phototherapy is being used prophylactically for all very low birth weight infants. In contrast, in full-term infants phototherapy is largely reserved for those with a high risk for encephalopathy or rapidly rising bilirubin and those with prolonged hyperbilirubinemia after the first exchange transfusion. In very low birth weight infants prophylactic phototherapy is being so widely used because of the excessive morbidity and mortality observed during exchange transfusions. In the great majority of full-term infants serum bilirubin concentrations already are declining by the time phototherapy is initiated. Furthermore, in full-term, otherwise well infants with hyperbilirubinemia, phototherapy is used very selectively, because exchange transfusion is well tolerated with almost no risk of death and institution of phototherapy in this group may actually prolong hospitalization.

Three independent mechanisms have been proposed to explain the action of phototherapy in reducing serum bilirubin concentrations in newborn infants. The first and the major pathway is geometric photoisomerization of unconjugated bilirubin IXα (Fig. 34-5). Unconjugated bilirubin IXα is usually in the 5Z,15Z configuration. In this form the -COOH group of each carboxymethyl side chain interacts via three hydrogen bonds with the C = O and N—H group of the pyrrole rings in the opposite half molecule. As a result, the ionization of the two COOH groups is inhibited, and therefore the molecule is nonpolar and water insoluble. In vitro, unconjugated bilirubin undergoes Z to E isomerization when illuminated. With tetrapyrrolic bilirubin IXα, either one or both of the bridge double bonds can undergo isomerization, yielding 5E, 15Z, 5Z, 15E, and 5E,15E isomers. The E configuration spatially precludes hydrogen bonding of the molecule, which therefore becomes free to ionize, thereby rendering the E isomer more polar than the Z isomer.

At least two pairs of geometric photoisomers have been identified in vivo. The first pair, photoisomers IA and IB, is presumably the two possible E,Z isomers. The second pair, photobilirubins IIA and IIB, is most likely two rotamers of the 5E,15E isomer. Both pairs presumably are formed rapidly in the skin, subcutaneous tissue, and in their capillaries. Being more polar, all of these isomers partition into the plasma, continuously shifting the equilibrium to promote more isomer formation. These isomers are rapidly taken up by the liver and transported into bile. The photoisomers are destabilized by bile acids, rapidly reverting to native unconjugated bilirubin IXαZZ. The rotameric isomers remain mostly intact and are the major polar photoproducts found in bile. This photoisomerization pathway may be responsible for more than 80% of the augmented bilirubin elimination during phototherapy. Geometric photoisomerization is not the only isomerization pathway open to a photoexcited bilirubin, however. The proximity of the side chain double bond at C-3 to the adjacent pyrrole ring allows an intramolecular cyclization, again rendering the bilirubin molecule more polar (Fig. 34-5, *B*). This structural isomer of bilirubin is called *lumirubin* and is also excreted into bile without hepatic conjugation.

The third pathway of phototherapy involves a variety of oxidation reactions with bilirubin, resulting from an autosensitized reaction involving singlet oxygen. The products formed by these reactions are multiple but include biliverdin, dipyrroles, and monopyrroles. Many of these products are colorless, nonreactive in the van den Bergh test, and presumably excreted by the liver and kidney without need for conjugation. Compared with the photoisomerization pathway, the oxidation mechanism appears to play a minor role in photocatabolism of unconjugated bilirubin in vivo.

In applying phototherapy, banks of 8 to 10 fluorescent lamps are placed approximately 12 to 16 inches above an unclothed infant lying in an open bassinet or an incubator. A shield of the corrective type of Plexiglas should be placed between the lamps and the infant to absorb the small amount of ultraviolet light emitted by most fluorescent lamps and to guard against injury from lamp explosion. Various kinds of fluorescent lamps have been used for phototherapy, including daylight, cool white, blue, and special blue types. Bilirubin absorbs light maximally in the blue range (from 420 to 500 nm), with peak absorption for albumin-bound bilirubin at 460 nm and for unbound bilirubin at 440 nm. Daylight and cool white lamps have a spectral peak between 550 and 600 nm and thus are less effective than special blue lamps, which have a narrow spectral range and peak between 420 and 480 nm.

Effective phototherapy must provide irradiance well above the levels that have been determined to be minimally effective in producing bilirubin degradation, while not exceeding levels beyond which no significant increases in response are evident. A standard phototherapy

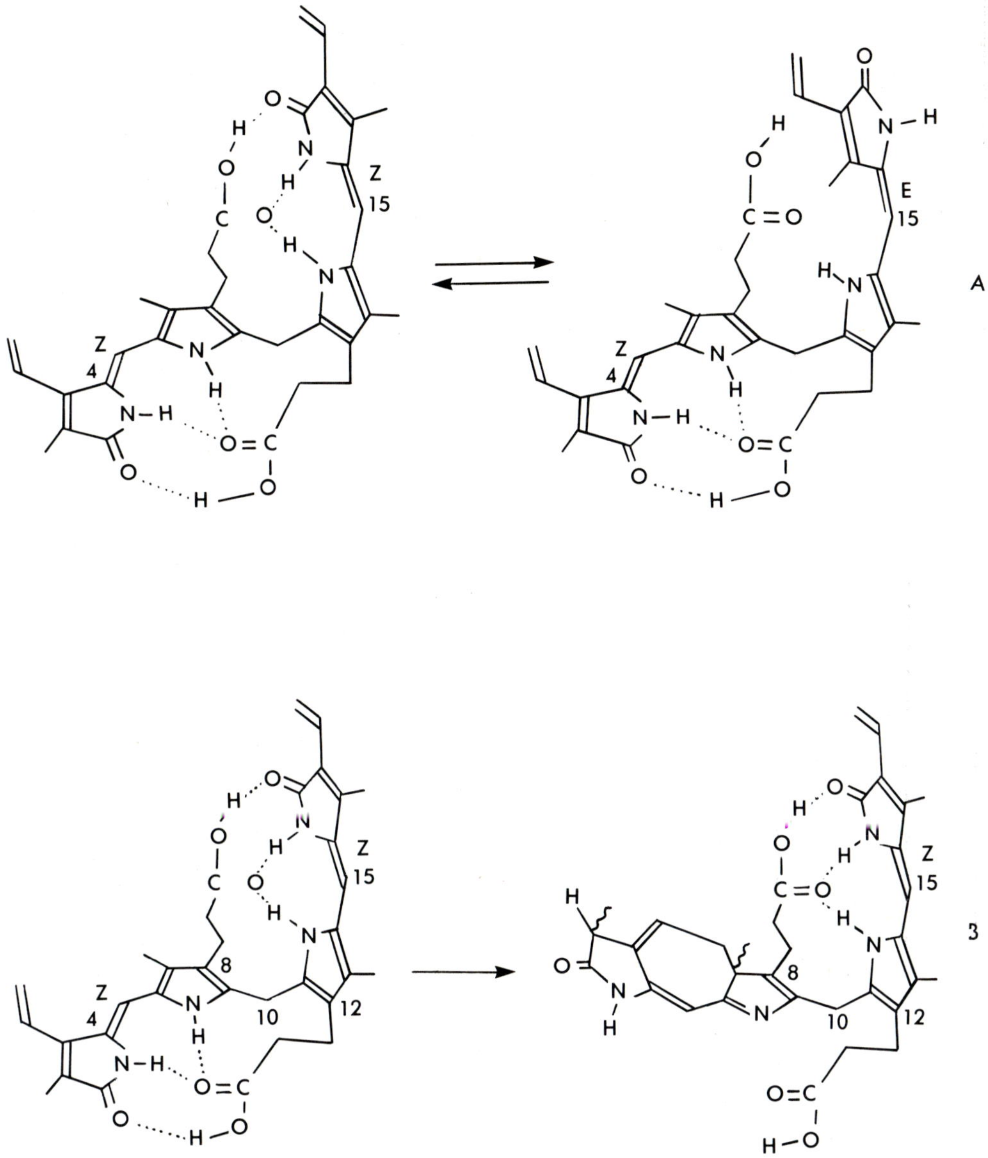

Fig. 34-5. Isomerization pathways for bilirubin during phototherapy. **A,** Z-E carbon-carbon double bond configurational isomerization of bilirubin. **B,** Intramolecular cyclization of bilirubin to form lumirubin. (Modified from McDonagh, A., and Lightner, D.A.: Pediatrics **75:**443, 1985.)

unit with eight new daylight lamps operating under optimal conditions would provide clinically significant, minimally effective levels of phototherapy (approximately 0.9 μW/cm²/nm). According to current knowledge, a saturation point for bilirubin degradation appears to correspond to the energy output provided by a standard phototherapy unit with four daylight and four special blue lamps (approximately 0.9 μW/cm²/nm). Increasing the distance from the lamp to the skin surface of the infant will result in a diminution of light energy by a factor equal to the square of the increase in distance. Thus doubling the distance from 12 to 24 inches will reduce the light energy reaching the infant to one fourth the original energy. The greater the surface area exposed, the greater the effectiveness of phototherapy will be. Skin pigmentation does not reduce the effectiveness of phototherapy. With time in use, fluorescent lamps reduce the energy output to a degree that varies from one type of lamp to another. A meter for monitoring lamp energy output should be used routinely during treatment. Commercially available photometers have been found to measure the same amount of irradiance with some variations. This is because of variations in peak absorptions and absorption band widths of the individual meters. For this reason comparative data have to be established when a new meter is introduced to the service.

The effect of high-intensity light exposure on the eyes of newborn human infants is uncertain, but animal studies indicate that retinal degeneration may occur after several days of continuous exposure. It is essential therefore that the eyes of all newborns exposed to phototherapy be covered with sufficient layers of opaque material to ensure against the possibility of damage. There is an increased insensible and intestinal water loss during phototherapy, which must be compensated for by an increase of about 25% in the fluid volume offered to treated infants (Chapter 25, part two). In addition, stools are slightly looser and more frequent. Phototherapy does not retard growth.

A well-recognized side effect of phototherapy is the bronze baby syndrome. In this disorder the serum, urine, and skin become brown-black (bronze) several hours or more after an infant is placed under the phototherapy lamps. In nearly all patients conjugated hyperbilirubinemia has been noted either before light exposure or after the syndrome has developed. In most patients some evidence of hepatocellular disease has been suggested from chemical or histologic determination. Increased hemolysis was suggested in one patient. In the only patient to die kernicterus was observed at autopsy in association with the bronze baby syndrome. All other patients have recovered without apparent sequelae. The nature of the bronze pigment is unknown, and its development after exposure to high-intensity light may represent an inborn error of metabolism, a preexisting hepatic excretory defect leading to retention of a pigment that would otherwise have been eliminated in bile, or a pigment derived from red blood cell destruction. Since it is not clear at this time whether this is a benign cosmetic response to phototherapy, a sign of impending liver or subclinical liver disease, or a true toxicity to phototherapy, it is essential that conjugated bilirubin concentrations be determined before phototherapy is instituted. If significant elevation of direct-reacting pigment is found, phototherapy should not be used.

Congenital erythropoietic porphyria is another syndrome in which phototherapy is contraindicated, since it may lead to death. This rare disorder is characterized by hemolysis, splenomegaly, and pink to red urine that fluoresces orange under ultraviolet light. Exposure to visible light of moderate to high-intensity and of wavelengths between 400 and 500 nm (blue) will produce severe bullous lesions on the exposed skin and may produce hemolysis. Mixed hyperbilirubinemia with a significant direct-reacting fraction also may be seen in this disease.

It also has been suggested that phototherapy may alter albumin binding of bilirubin by photooxidative damage of albumin; this has not been confirmed in vivo. Other possible dangers of phototherapy include overheating of the infant, electrical shock from poorly grounded or defective equipment, and unproved potential long-term effects on endocrine and sexual maturation, on DNA repairing mechanism of skin epithelial cells, and even on development of skin cancer.

Pharmacologic management

Phenobarbital is one of a large group of drugs that stimulate protein synthesis in general and hepatic glucuronyl transferase and hepatic ligandin synthesis specifically. Chlorophenothane (DDT), ethanol, heroin, and certain antihistamines act similarly. After the demonstration that phenobarbital administration to a child with type II glucuronyl transferase deficiency reduced serum bilirubin concentrations, phenobarbital administration to pregnant mothers and their offspring was shown to reduce by approximately 50% peak serum bilirubin concentrations caused by physiologic jaundice. Studies in newborn rhesus monkeys have demonstrated that the major effect of this therapy is to increase hepatic glucuronyl transferase activity and the conjugation of bilirubin. It also may enhance hepatic uptake of bilirubin in the newborn. The administration of phenobarbital to newborns at the time jaundice is first observed or even immediately after delivery is much less effective than its administration to the mother during pregnancy for at least 2 weeks before delivery. The drug is, however, much less effective in premature infants. As a prophylactic measure, it would be necessary therefore to administer phenobarbital to large numbers of pregnant women for prolonged times during pregnancy, since the time of delivery could not be predicted with certainty. Even then the premature infants most susceptible to the toxic effects of hyperbilirubinemia would receive little or no beneficial effect. The drug is potentially addicting, may lead to excessive sedation of the newborn, and has other potent metabolic effects in addition to those on bilirubin metabolism. For these reasons the use of phenobarbital has not achieved wide application but has been reserved largely for very specific high-risk populations. For example, in the unexplained severe hyperbilirubinemia of the newborns from the Greek coastal islands, the frequency of kernicterus has been significantly reduced by general administration of phenobarbital to pregnant women during the last trimester. A dosage of 60 mg/day is sufficient for maternal administration and 5 mg/kg/day for neonatal treatment. Phenobarbital also is useful in the differentiation between types I and II glucuronyl transferase deficiency. Combining phenobarbital treatment with phototherapy has no advantage, the effect being no greater than that of phototherapy alone.

Enteric reabsorption of unconjugated bilirubin may be a major source of increased bilirubin in the newborn period. Frequent milk feeding (cow or human) prevents the rise of serum bilirubin and enhances the bilirubin-reducing effect of phototherapy. Oral administration of nonabsorbable substances that bind bilirubin in the intestinal lumen and presumably reduce enteric absorption of bilirubin may reduce peak serum bilirubin concentrations in physiologic jaundice by about 50%. Activated charcoal has been used but is effective only when administered during the first 12 hours of life. Agar also has been shown to be effective. Further study of this type of therapy is needed before recommendations can be made regarding clinical applications.

Sn-protoporphyrin has recently come under investigation for clinical use in neonatal unconjugated hyperbilirubinemia. Sn-protoporphyrin is a synthetic heme analog that potently inhibits the activity of heme oxygenase, the rate-limiting enzyme for the degradation of heme to bile pigment. Administration of this compound has been shown to decrease serum bilirubin concentrations in newborn rats, neonatal rhesus monkeys, adult rats with hemolytic anemia, and patients with primary biliary cirrhosis. Precise details on alterations in heme catabolism and its potential side effects are not fully known at this time and must await further animal and human trials. Finally, a novel method for enzymatic removal of bilirubin from blood also has been reported. Hyperbilirubinemic blood is passed through a filter containing immobilized bilirubin oxidase. More than 90% of the bilirubin is degraded in a single pass through a filter. Again, before it is used clinically further refinement of the technique and investigation for potential side effects are required.

Lawrence M. Gartner
Kwang-Sun Lee

BIBLIOGRAPHY

Physiology

Berk, P.D., and others: Comparison of plasma bilirubin turnover and carbon monoxide production in man, J. Lab. Clin. Med. **83**:29, 1974.

Fleischner, G.M., and Arias, I.M.: Structure and function of ligandin and Z protein in the liver; a progressive report. In Popper, H., and Schaffner, F., editors: Progress in liver disease, vol. 5, New York, 1976, Grune & Stratton, Inc.

Gartner, L.M., Lane, D.L., and Cornelius, C.E.: Bilirubin transport by liver in adult *Macaca mulatta*, Am. J. Physiol. **220**:1528, 1971.

Heirwegh, K.P.M., and Brown, S.B., editors: Bilirubin, vol. 2, Metabolism, Boca Raton, Fla., 1982, CRC Press, Inc.

Jansen, P.L.M., and others: Enzymatic conversion of bilirubin monoglucuronide by rat liver plasma membranes, J. Biol. Chem. **252**:2710, 1977.

Jendrassik, K., and Grof, P.: Vereinfachte photometrische methoden zur Bestimmung des Blut-Bilirubins, Biochem. Z. **297**:81, 1939.

Lee, K.S., and Gartner, L.M.: Spectrophotometric characteristics of bilirubin, Pediatr. Res. **10**:782, 1976.

Schmid, R.: Bilirubin metabolism: state of the art, Gastroenterology **74**:1307, 1978.

Schmid, R., and McDonagh, A.F.: Formation and metabolism of bile pigments in vivo. In Dolphin, D., editor: The porphyrins, vol. 6, New York, 1979, Academic Press, p. 258.

Wu, T.W.: Bilirubin analysis—the state of the art and future prospects, Clin. Biochem. **17**:221, 1984.

Physiologic jaundice of the newborn

Bernstein, R.B., and others: Bilirubin metabolism in the fetus, J. Clin. Invest. **48**:1678, 1969.

Cashore, W.J., and Stern, L.: Neonatal hyperbilirubinemia, Pediatr. Clin. North Am. **29**:1191, 1982.

Gartner, L.M., and others: Development of bilirubin transport and metabolism in the newborn rhesus monkey, Pediatrics **90**:513, 1977.

Kawade, N., and Onishi, S.: The prenatal and postnatal development of UDP-glucuronyltransferase activity towards bilirubin and the effect of premature birth on this activity in the human liver, Biochem. J. **196**:257, 1981.

Levi, A.J., Gatmaitan, Z., and Arias, I.M.: Deficiency of hepatic organic anion-binding protein, impaired organic anion uptake by liver and "physiologic" jaundice in newborn monkeys, N. Engl. J. Med. **283**:1136, 1970.

Levine, R.L., and Maisels, M.J., editors: Hyperbilirubinemia in the newborn. Report of the Eighty-Fifth Ross Conference on Pediatric Research, Columbus, Ohio, 1983, Ross Laboratories.

Maisels, M.J.: Bilirubin on understanding and influencing its metabolism in the newborn infant, Pediatr. Clin. North Am. **19**:447, 1972.

Maisels, M.J., and Gifford, K.: Breast-feeding, weight loss, and jaundice, J. Pediatr. **102**:117, 1983.

Vaisman, S.L., Lee, K.S., and Gartner, L.M.: Various bilirubin conjugates in pregnant and nonpregnant rats with and without phenobarbital treatment, Pediatr. Res. **10**:111, 1976.

Pathologic states of unconjugated hyperbilirubinemia

Beck, P.D., Wolkoff, A.W., and Berlin, N.I.: Inborn errors of bilirubin metabolism, Med. Clin. North Am. **59**:803, 1975.

Gartner, L.M., and Arias, I.M.: Studies of prolonged neonatal jaundice in the breast fed infant, J. Pediatr. **68**:54, 1966.

Jaffe, E.R.: Hereditary hemolytic disorders and enzymatic deficiencies of human erythrocytes, Blood **35**:116, 1970.

Liley, A.W.: The use of amniocentesis and fetal transfusion in erythroblastosis fetalis, Pediatrics **35**:836, 1965.

Luzzatto, L.: Genetic heterogeneity and pathophysiology of G6PD deficiency, Br. J. Haematol. **28**:151, 1974.

Meyer, U.A., and Schmid, R.: Congenital erythropoietic prophyria. In Stanbury, J.B., Wyngaarden, J.B., and Fredrickson, S.S., editors: The metabolic basis of inherited disease, ed. 4, New York, 1978, McGraw-Hill Book Co.

Nakamura, H., and others: Auditory nerve and brainstem responses in newborn infants with hyperbilirubinemia, Pediatrics **75**:703, 1985.

Odievre, M.: Breast feeding and hyperbilirubinemia. In Berenberg, S.R., editor: Liver diseases of infancy and childhood, The Hague, 1976, Martinus Nijhoff Medical Division.

Orzalezi, M., and others: ABO system incompatibility: relationship between direct Coombs test positivity and neonatal jaundice, Pediatrics **51**:288, 1973.

Peevy, K.J., and others: Hyperbilirubinemia in infants of diabetic mothers, Pediatrics **66**:417, 1980.

Poland, R.L., and others: High milk lipase activity associated with breast milk jaundice, Pediatr. Res. **14**:1328, 1980.

Scheidt, P.C., and others: Toxicity to bilirubin in neonates: infant development during first year in relation to maximum neonatal serum bilirubin concentration, J. Pediatr. **91**:292, 1977.

Smith, D.W., and others: Congenital hypothyroidism: signs and symptoms in the newborn period, J. Pediatr. **87**:958, 1975.

Windfield, C.R., and MacFaul, R.: Clinical study of prolonged jaundice in breast- and bottle-fed babies, Arch. Dis. Child. **53**:506, 1978.

Woolley, M.M., and others: Jaundice, hypertrophic pyloric stenosis, and hepatic glucuronyl transferase, J. Pediatr. Surg. **9**:359, 1974.

Wysowski, D.K., and others: Epidemic neonatal hyperbilirubinemia and use of a phenolic disinfectant detergent, Pediatrics **61**:165, 1978.

Bilirubin toxicity

Cashore, W.J., and others: Clinical application of bilirubin binding determinations: current status, J. Pediatr. **93**:827, 1978.

Cowger, M.L.: Bilirubin encephalopathy. In Gaull, G., editor: Biology of brain dysfunction, vol. 2, New York, 1973, Plenum Publishing Corp.

Diamond, I.: Bilirubin binding and kernicterus. In Schulman, I., editor: Advances in pediatrics, vol. 16, Chicago, 1969, Year Book Medical Publishers, Inc.

Diamond, I., and Schmid, R.: Experimental bilirubin encephalopathy; the mode of entry of bilirubin-14C into the central nervous system, J. Clin. Invest. **45**:678, 1966.

Gartner, L.M., and Lee, K.S.: Bilirubin binding, free fatty acids and a new concept for the pathogenesis of kernicterus. II. Bilirubin metabolism in the newborn, Birth Defects **12**:264, 1976.

Gartner, L.M., and others: Kernicterus: high incidence in premature infants with low serum bilirubin concentrations, Pediatrics **45**:906, 1970.

Kim, M.H., and others: Lack of predictive indices in kernicterus: a comparison of clinical and pathologic factors in infants with and without kernicterus, Pediatrics **66**:852, 1980.

Lee, K.S., and Gartner, L.M.: Bilirubin binding by plasma proteins: a critical evaluation of methods and clinical implications, Rev. Perinatal Med. **2**:319, 1978.

Lee, K.S., Gartner, L.M., and Vaisman, S.L.: Measurement of bilirubin-albumin binding. I. Comparative analysis of four methods and four human serum albumin preparations, Pediatr. Res. **12**:301, 1978.

Lucey, J.F., and others: Kernicterus in asphyxiated newborn rhesus monkeys, Exp. Neurol. **9**:43, 1964.

Mustafa, M.G., and King, T.E.: Binding of bilirubin with lipids; a possible mechanism of its toxic reactions in mitochondria, J. Biol. Chem. **245**:1084, 1970.

Naeye, R.L.: Amniotic fluid infections, neonatal hyperbilirubinemia and psychomotor impairment, Pediatrics **62**:497, 1978.

Odell, G.B., Storey, G.N.B., and Rosenberg, L.A.: Studies in kernicterus. III. The saturation of serum proteins with bilirubin during neonatal life and its relationship to brain damage at 5 years, J. Pediatr. **76**:12, 1970.

Pearlman, M.A., and others: Absence of kernicterus in low-birthweight infants from 1971 through 1976; comparison with findings in 1966 and 1967, Pediatrics **62**:460, 1978.

Silverman, W.A., and others: A difference in mortality rate and incidence of kernicterus among premature infants allotted two prophylactic antibacterial regimens, Pediatrics **18**:614,1956.

Tukel, S.B., and others: Lack of identifiable risk factors for kernicterus, Pediatrics **66**:502, 1980.

Management of unconjugated hyperbilirubinemia

Bowman, J.M.: Neonatal management. In Queenan, J.T., and others, editors: Modern management of the Rh problem, ed. 2, New York, 1977, Harper & Row Publishers, Inc.

Clark, C.F., and others: The "bronze baby" syndrome: postmortem data, J. Pediatr. **88**:461, 1976.

Committee on Phototherapy in the Newborn: Final report of the Committee on Phototherapy in the Newborn, Washington, D.C., 1974, Division of Medical Sciences, National Research Council, National Academy of Sciences.

De Carvalho, M., and others: Fecal bilirubin excretion and serum bilirubin concentrations in breast-fed and bottle-fed infants, J. Pediatr. **107**:786, 1985.

Ennever, J.F., and others: Phototherapy for neonatal jaundice: in vivo clearance of bilirubin products, Pediatr. Res. **19**:205, 1985.

Lavin, A., and others: Enzymatic removal of bilirubin from blood: a potential treatment for neonatal jaundice, Science **230**:543, 1985.

Lee, K.S., and others: Unconjugated hyperbilirubinemia in very low birth weight infants, Clin. Perinatol. **4**:305, 1977.

McDonagh, A.F., and Lightner, D.A.: "Like a shrivelled blood orange"—bilirubin, jaundice, and phototherapy, Pediatrics **75**:443, 1985.

Moller, J.: Agar ingestion and serum bilirubin values in newborn infants, Acta Obstet. Gynecol. Scand. **53**:61, 1974.

National Institute of Child Health and Human Development: Randomized, controlled trial of phototherapy for neonatal hyperbilirubinemia (multiple articles reporting the various results), Pediatrics **75**(suppl.):385, 1985.

Panagoponlos, G., Valaes, T., and Doxiadis, S.A.: Morbidity and mortality related to exchange transfusions, J. Pediatr. **74**:247, 1969.

Simionatto, C.S., and others: Studies on the mechanism of Sn-protoporphyrin suppression of hyperbilirubinemia: inhibition of heme oxidation and bilirubin production, J. Clin. Invest. **75**:513, 1985.

Strange, M., and Cassady, G.: Neonatal transcutaneous bilirubinometry, Clin. Perinatol. **12**:51, 1985.

Vaisman, S.L., and Gartner, L.M.: Pharmacologic treatment of neonatal hyperbilirubinemia, Clin. Perinatol. **2**:37, 1975.

Valaes, T., and others: Effectiveness and safety of prenatal phenobarbital for the prevention of neonatal jaundice, Pediatr. Res. **14**:947, 1980.

Wallin, A., and Boreus, L.O.: Phenobarbital prophylaxis for hyperbilirubinemia in preterm infants. A controlled study of bilirubin disappearance and infant behavior, Acta Paediatr. Scand. **73**:488, 1984.

PART TWO

Conjugated hyperbilirubinemia

Jaundice in the neonatal period may be associated with a rise in the direct-reacting fraction of serum bilirubin. This is indicative of a defect or insufficiency in bile secretion or biliary flow or both and therefore is commonly accompanied by a rise in serum levels of other constituents of bile, such as bile salts and phospholipids. It frequently is referred to as obstructive jaundice, although the term is inaccurate, since it implies mechanical blockage, which is present in only the minority of cases. The designation *cholestasis,* meaning a reduction in bile flow, more precisely describes this group of disorders. Conjugated hyperbilirubinemia may result from primary defects either in the hepatocellular phase of bile excretion or in canalicular or ductal function or from loss of patency of these structures.

PATHOPHYSIOLOGY

The *hepatocellular phase* involves the transport of conjugated bilirubin across the hepatic cell membrane. This passage occurs at a specific site in the hepatocyte referred to as the biliary pole. Structurally the cytoplasm at this pole is distinguished by a paucity of mitochondria and ribosomes and by the presence of a network of microfilaments, visible with the electron microscope and demonstrated to represent the contractile protein actin. The cell membrane at the biliary pole is differentiated to form microvilli and becomes one facet in the usually multifaceted bile canaliculus formed by several adjacent hepatocytes (Figs. 34-6 and 34-7). An intact pericanalicular actin meshwork is necessary for normal canalicular contraction, an important step in generation of intrahepatic bile flow. The junction between hepatocytes bordering the bile canaliculus is called the "tight junction" and under normal circumstances forms an efficient barrier preventing the contents of the bile canaliculus from reaching the perisinusoidal space of Disse or the vascular compartments. The bile canaliculus, the smallest of the conduits for bile, is therefore an integral part of the hepatocyte. It follows that injury to the hepatocyte may result in impairment of the cellular phase of bile excretion and breakdown of the tight junctions, leading to the clinical and laboratory findings of cholestasis. If cellular damage is extensive, hyperbilirubinemia may be associated with other laboratory abnormalities that reflect impairment of other hepatocellular functions. On the other hand, injury may be limited to the processes responsible for bile transport at the biliary pole, thus resulting in the isolated laboratory finding of conjugated hyperbilirubinemia. A liver biopsy taken in the early stages of one of the diseases caused by hepatocellular defect in bile secretion characteristically would show bile pigment granules in hepatocytes and bile in canaliculi: thus *intracellular* and *intracanalicular* cholestasis. Bile pigment granules are not seen in normal hepatocytes, and the lumens of bile canaliculi are not clearly visualized in routine histologic preparations of normal liver tissue (Fig. 34-6). When examined with the electron microscope, the canalicular lumen is normally small and contains no bile. It is partially obliterated by the projecting microvilli (Fig. 34-7). On rare occasions liver biopsies

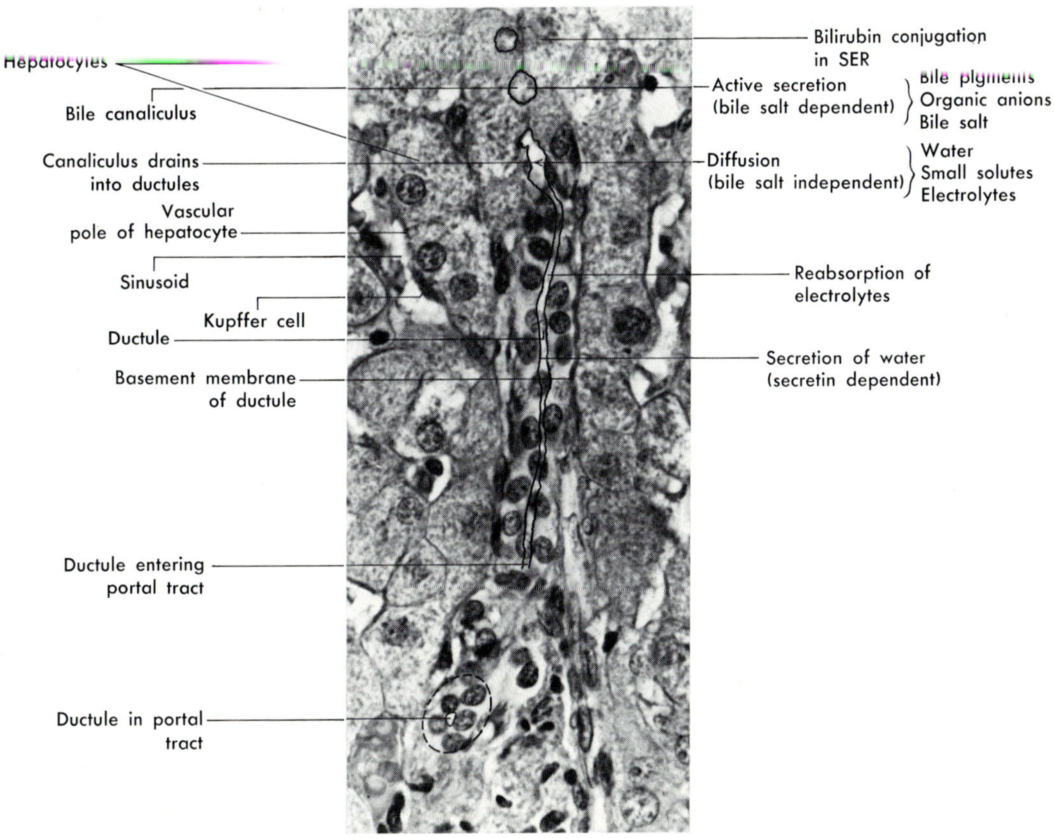

Fig. 34-6. Microscopic section of normal liver depicting transition between bile canaliculus and bile ductule entering portal tract. Anatomic structures are identified to left of illustration, and corresponding physiologic events are listed on right.

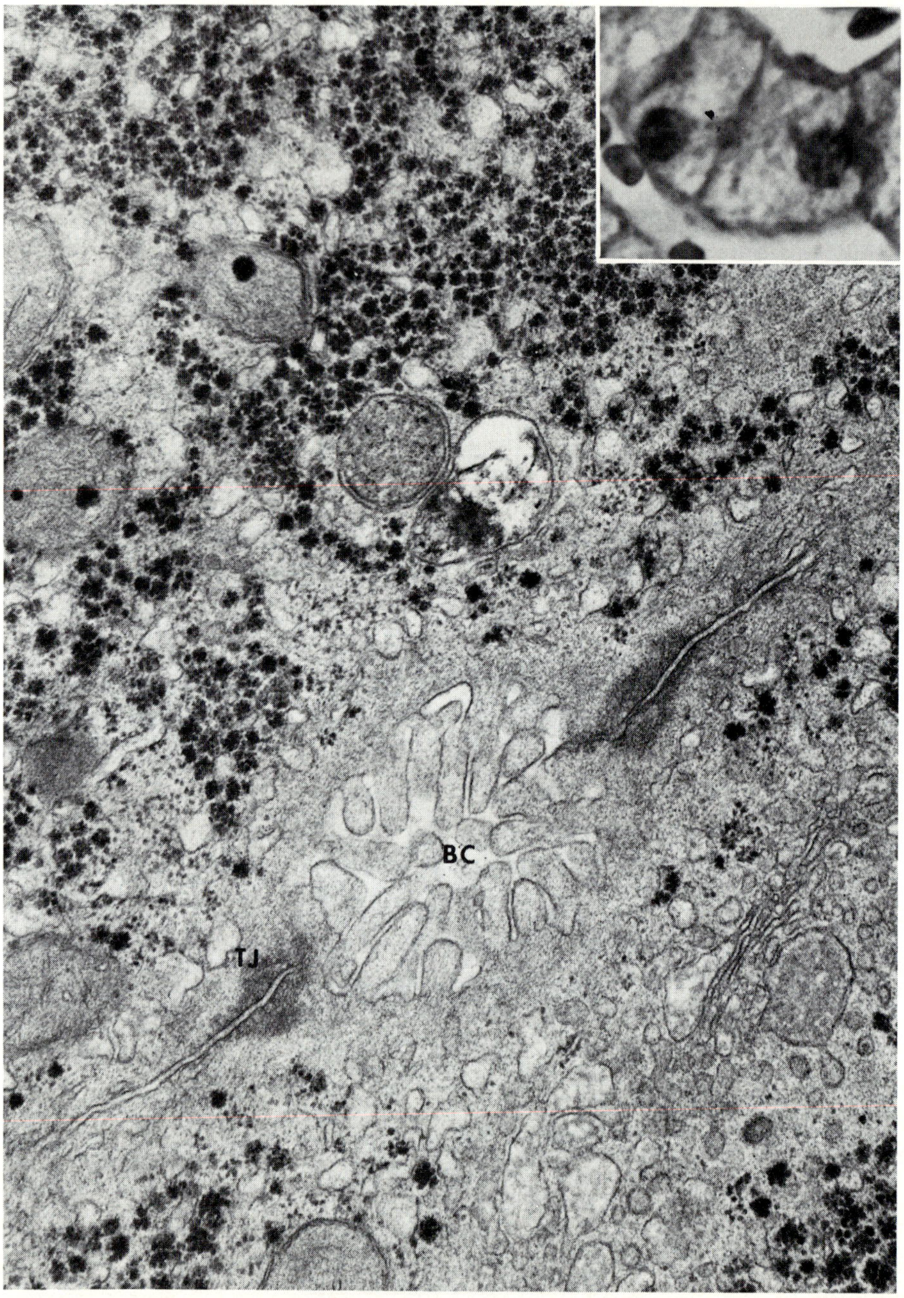

Fig. 34-7. Electron micrograph of two adjacent normal hepatocytes. Note the microvillar surface of the bile canaliculus *(BC)*. Tight junctions *(TJ)* bordering the canaliculus. Insert illustrates a high-power view of two adjacent hepatocytes as seen in the light microscope. In such preparations bile canaliculi appear as poorly defined condensations of the cell membrane. (Courtesy Dr. L. Biempica, Albert Einstein College of Medicine.) (Epon-embedded; ×6,000.)

from patients with conjugated hyperbilirubinemia fail to show any abnormalities when examined with the light microscope.

The *ductal phase* of bile excretion includes those events that take place in the biliary system distal to the bile canaliculus (Fig. 34-6). The intrahepatic component comprises the bile ductules (the initial portion of which is frequently referred to as the canal of Hering); the interlobular (portal) bile ducts, always associated with a vein and an arteriole; and the right and left hepatic ducts, which in some individuals may partially extend beyond the liver capsule. The extrahepatic component includes the common hepatic duct, the cystic duct, the gallbladder, and the common bile duct (choledochus). Most diseases affecting the *extrahepatic* bile ducts are associated with segmental or diffuse luminal obliteration and are expressions primarily of mechanical disturbance in bile flow. Diseases involving the *intrahepatic* ducts are complex and probably result from mechanical obstruction to the flow of bile, abnormalities of the biochemical pathways involved in the process of bile secretion, and in some cases a probable persistence of infectious viruses or viral antigens. A characteristic tissue response to complete mechanical obstruction of a major bile duct is dilatation and proliferation of the proximal portions of the intrahepatic biliary system, including the ductules and canals of Hering, structures that are outside the confines of the portal tracts. The stimulus responsible for this proliferation is unknown. A constant accompaniment to bile duct proliferation is an increase in connective tissue, which leads eventually to biliary cirrhosis. Although bile secretory defects initially may be either cellular or ductal, any long-standing abnormality in the flow of bile leads to hepatic parenchymal cell damage.

The boxed outline lists diseases that may be seen as conjugated hyperbilirubinemia in the neonatal period. They are divided into those primarily caused by a defect in the hepatocellular phase of bile secretion and those caused by ductal disturbances. In most of these disorders direct-reacting bilirubin accounts for 50% to 90% of total serum bilirubin. A small amount of indirect-reacting bilirubin is always present, reflecting mild hemolysis, defective uptake and excretion, or hydrolysis of conjugated bilirubin. Early in the onset of conjugated hyperbilirubinemia in the neonate the direct-reacting portion may account for only 10% to 25% of the total serum bilirubin. As hepatic conjugation and uptake of bilirubin mature, the indirect-reacting portion usually decreases, whereas the direct portion increases.

Diseases that may be seen as conjugated hyperbilirubinemia in the neonatal period

A. Hepatocellular disturbances in bilirubin excretion
    1. Primary hepatitis
        a. Neonatal idiopathic hepatitis (giant cell hepatitis)
        b. Hepatitis caused by identified infectious agents
            (1) Hepatitis B (HB_sAG)
            (2) Rubella
            (3) Cytomegalovirus
            (4) *Toxoplasma* organisms
            (5) Coxsackievirus
            (6) Echovirus 14 and 19
            (7) Herpes simplex and varicella-zoster
            (8) Syphilis
            (9) *Listeria* organisms
            (10) Tubercle bacillus
    2. "Toxic hepatitis"
        a. Systemic infectious diseases
            (1) *E. coli* (sepsis or urinary tract)
            (2) Pneumococci
            (3) *Proteus* organisms
            (4) *Salmonella* organisms
            (5) Idiopathic diarrhea
        b. Intestinal obstruction
        c. Parenteral alimentation
        d. Ischemic necrosis
    3. Hematologic disorders
        a. Erythroblastosis fetalis (severe forms)
        b. Congenital erythropoietic porphyria
    4. Metabolic and heredofamilial disorders
        a. $Alpha_1$-antitrypsin deficiency
        b. Galactosemia
        c. Tyrosinemia
        d. Fructosemia
        e. Glycogen storage disease type IV
        f. Lipid storage diseases
            (1) Niemann-Pick disease
            (2) Gaucher's disease
            (3) Wolman's disease
        g. Cerebrohepatorenal syndrome (Zellweger's syndrome)
        h. Trisomy E
        i. Fibrocystic disease
        j. Familial idiopathic cholestasis: Byler's disease
        k. Hemochromatosis
        l. Idiopathic hypopituitarism
B. Ductal disturbances in bilirubin excretion
    1. Extrahepatic biliary atresia
        a. Without associated malformations
        b. Associated with trisomy E (18)
        c. Associated with polysplenia-heterotaxia syndrome
    2. Intrahepatic biliary atresia (nonsyndromatic paucity of bile ducts)
    3. Alagille syndrome (arteriohepatic dysplasia)
    4. Intrahepatic atresia associated with lymphedema
    5. Extrahepatic stenosis and choledochal cyst
    6. Bile plug syndrome
    7. Fibrocystic disease
    8. Tumors of the liver and biliary tract
    9. Periductal lymphadenopathy

SPECIFIC DISORDERS

Biliary atresia and neonatal hepatitis

Biliary atresia and idiopathic neonatal hepatitis occur with approximately similar frequency and together account for 60% to 80% of all cases of neonatal cholestasis. *Biliary atresia* includes a group of diseases in which there is luminal obliteration or apparent absence of all or segments of the biliary duct system. Involvement may be limited to the major extrahepatic bile ducts or, much more rarely, may involve intrahepatic branches located in portal tracts. The latter situation usually is designated as paucity of intrahepatic bile ducts, or intrahepatic biliary atresia. In rare instances atresia of the major bile ducts coexists with absence or paucity of intrahepatic bile ducts. *Idiopathic neonatal hepatitis,* as used here, includes those infants with prolonged conjugated hyperbilirubinemia without apparent stigmata of generalized viral illness, evidence of an identifiable infectious agent, or etiologically specific metabolic abnormality. On liver biopsy this group is characterized by extensive transformation of hepatocytes into multinucleated giant cells and is therefore sometimes referred to as neonatal giant cell hepatitis. This term is misleading since giant cell transformation of hepatocytes is not specific for any etiologic factor and is observed in various metabolic and infectious disorders. In addition, in some patients with neonatal hepatitis, liver biopsy shows no evidence of giant cells. Necrosis and inflammation are probably always present but are transient, and therefore their absence at any given time does not exclude the diagnosis.

Differentiation between these two groups of diseases may be difficult in the early stages; however, an early accurate diagnosis is essential for the choice of proper clinical management. Extrahepatic biliary atresia, the most frequent form of atresia, requires early surgical intervention. Unrelieved by surgery, the defect inevitably leads to death from biliary cirrhosis in the first 3 years of life. The prognosis in neonatal hepatitis is uncertain. A significant number either die of hepatic insufficiency or progress to chronic liver disease, whereas some recover without sequelae.

Etiology and pathogenesis

The cause of biliary atresia and of neonatal hepatitis remains undetermined. The long-held view that biliary atresia represents a congenital developmental anomaly is now thought untenable. In the majority of cases biliary atresia and neonatal hepatitis occur as isolated abnormalities, and both are considered representative of acquired conditions, probably caused by the same or similar factors. Viral agents are strongly suspected. In support of the acquired nature of biliary atresia is the absence of reported cases in stillborn fetuses and the rare association with other malformations. Similarly, clinical evidence of total obstruction to the flow of bile (such as acholic stools or colorless meconium) is not detected in the early stages of jaundice. The onset of conjugated hyperbilirubinemia and acholic stools is frequently delayed until 2 weeks of life or even later. Microscopic changes observed in the extrahepatic biliary system or its fibrous remnant removed during the Kasai procedure (see under treatment) strongly suggest a sequence of changes reflecting an injury progressing from epithelial necrosis and inflammation to fibrosis and scarring (see Fig. 34-9). Clinical pathologic observations over a long period indicate that some patients fulfill all known criteria for neonatal hepatitis, including surgical demonstration of patent biliary ducts in the early stages of jaundice, and then go on to develop extrahepatic biliary atresia. Landing has proposed the concept of "infantile obstructive cholangiopathy" to include neonatal hepatitis, biliary atresia, and choledochal cyst. According to his theory injury may occur either in utero or in the perinatal period, but the consequences of such injury and therefore clinically manifested disease are delayed until sometime after birth. Injury, regardless of its nature, affects primarily structures involved in bile secretion. It is likely that, in all patients with neonatal hepatitis or any of the forms of biliary atresia, both hepatocytes and the biliary epithelium are involved. Clinical manifestations and outcome may depend on the severity, dominance, and persistence of lesions in a specific location. Thus primary damage to hepatocytes may result in clinical manifestations of neonatal hepatitis, whereas injury to portal radicles of the biliary duct system may result in paucity of intrahepatic ducts, and injury to major bile ducts and gallbladder may result in extrahepatic atresia. Choledochal cyst may represent the mildest form of extrahepatic atresia, in which injury involves only a short segment of the bile duct and results in dilatation or cyst formation of the proximal portion. Reovirus type 3 (Reo 3) recently has been implicated as an etiologic factor in extrahepatic biliary atresia as well as neonatal hepatitis, thus supporting the hypothesis of a common infectious etiology for these two disorders. Serologic studies indicate that more than 60% of infants with extrahepatic biliary atresia and more than 50% with neonatal hepatitis have antibodies to Reo 3 virus in the first year of life, whereas less than 12% of age-matched controls have these antibodies. In addition, a hepatobiliary disease bearing strong resemblance to human biliary atresia can be experimentally induced in very young mice by infection with Reo 3.

No information is available as yet concerning a possible association between intrahepatic bile duct paucity or choledochal cyst and Reo 3 infection. On the other hand cytomegalovirus infection was implicated in intrahepatic bile duct injury and paucity. Patients currently classified as having idiopathic neonatal hepatitis constitute a heterogenous group that undoubtedly includes various as yet undefined metabolic disorders. For example, before neonatal cholestasis was observed in alpha$_1$-antitrypsin deficiency, patients with this disorder were included in the group of idiopathic neonatal hepatitis.

Associated conditions

Most patients with neonatal hepatitis and biliary atresia represent isolated cases without familial incidence or associated anomalies. Neonatal hepatitis has a familial incidence of 10% to 15%, while no familial cases of extrahepatic biliary atresia have been observed. Rare occurrences of concurrent neonatal hepatitis and biliary atresia in two siblings have been reported. Both neonatal hepatitis and biliary atresia occur more frequently in patients with trisomy E (trisomy 18) than in the general population. Biliary atresia has been observed in 50% of reported patients with the polysplenia-heterotaxia syndrome. This syndrome is characterized by situs inversus of abdominal organs, intestinal malrotation, multiple spleens, centrally placed liver, and a variety of cardiac, pulmonary, and vascular malformations. The inferior vena cava is frequently absent and renders these patients unsuitable for liver transplantation when they have inoperable biliary atresia. Familial occurrence of intrahepatic paucity of bile ducts has been described in association with other abnormalities. One familial syndrome includes cholestasis, paucity of intrahepatic bile ducts, and lymphedema of the lower extremities. Most patients in this group are from families of Norwegian extraction. Another syndrome described by Alagille includes cholestasis, paucity of intrahepatic bile ducts in the presence of patent extrahepatic ducts, unusual facies, vertebral anomalies, peripheral pulmonic stenosis with cardiac murmur, posterior embryotoxon, and retarded mental, physical, and sexual development. This syndrome is referred to as Alagille's syndrome or arteriohepatic dysplasia. It is important to recognize this condition since surgical excision of hypoplastic but patent extrahepatic bile ducts and portoenterostomy are contraindicated.

Clinical and laboratory manifestations

Early clinical manifestations of both biliary atresia and neonatal hepatitis may be limited to jaundice. In a small proportion of patients, especially among those who later develop neonatal hepatitis, jaundice may be apparent at birth, documented by increased concentrations of conjugated bilirubin in umbilical cord blood. No case of extrahepatic biliary atresia has ever been described in which elevation of *direct-reacting* bilirubin was found in the cord blood. In most patients with either hepatitis or atresia, jaundice becomes apparent between the second and sixth weeks of life. The dark yellow staining of diapers from the presence of bilirubin in the urine often prompts the parents to seek medical advice. Jaundice is frequently first noted by the physician during a "well baby" visit. Hepatomegaly may be present in both neonatal hepatitis and biliary atresia. Splenomegaly is more frequently present in neonatal hepatitis, but this is not a constant finding. Its presence in biliary atresia usually signifies cirrhosis. Total obstruction to the flow of bile is reflected by acholic stools and may be observed in both neonatal hepatitis and biliary atresia. It is always transient and incomplete in neonatal hepatitis, but its duration is variable and may extend beyond the crucial period during which an accurate diagnosis must be established if surgical correction is needed. Routine clinical and laboratory findings usually will not distinguish between extrahepatic biliary atresia and neonatal hepatitis. A routine series of diagnostic laboratory tests is suggested, however, to establish the severity of hepatic involvement and to screen for possible causes (see box on p. 972). In patients with intrahepatic paucity of bile ducts early clinical manifestations and laboratory findings are identical to those observed in patients with extrahepatic biliary atresia. Later in the first year of life, however, intrahepatic paucity of bile ducts is characterized by rising serum cholesterol concentrations well beyond those observed in other forms of infantile liver disease. Levels over 1,000 mg/dl may be seen as early as the third month of life. Cutaneous xanthomata are prominent in the later stages of this disease, usually after 1 year of age. The failure of routine laboratory tests to distinguish between neonatal hepatitis and biliary atresia has led to continued search for other distinguishing biochemical characteristics. Lipoprotein X is found in the sera of all patients with significant cholestasis, and therefore a qualitative analysis is not helpful in the differential diagnosis. After cholestyramine treatment is administered, however, there may be a decrease in the level of lipoprotein X in patients with neonatal hepatitis and an increase in patients with atresia. Alphafetoproteins are frequently present in the sera of patients with neonatal hepatitis but may be absent in patients with biliary atresia.

A reliable method for the evaluation of patency of extrahepatic bile ducts is isotope scan using ^{99m}Tc-IDA or IDA derivatives such as paraisopropyl iminodiacetic acid or diisopropyliminodiacetic acid. These compounds are efficiently extracted by hepatocytes and are excreted with bile into the intestines. When complete obstruction exists no activity is detected in the intestines. Pretreatment with phenobarbital for 7 days before testing promotes excretion of isotope in infants with severe intrahepatic cholestasis and thus reduces the chance for a mistaken diagnosis of extrahepatic obstruction. Phenobarbital is given orally at a dose of 5 mg/kg/day. Patients are given nothing by mouth for 1 hour before and 2 hours after injection of radiotracer in order to avoid gallbladder contraction and dilution of radiotracer excreted into the intestines.

Ultrasonography has also been applied in the evaluation of neonatal cholestasis. It is particularly valuable in the diagnosis of choledochal cysts. Although the dem-

Recommended laboratory tests for evaluation of neonatal conjugated hyperbilirubinemia

A. Liver function tests
   1. Total and direct-reacting serum bilirubin, total serum protein, and serum protein electrophoresis
   2. SGOT, SGPT, alkaline phosphatase (and 5′-nucleotidase if alkaline phosphatase elevated), and gamma glutamyl transpeptidase
   3. Cholesterol
   4. Serum and urine bile acid concentrations if available
   5. Alpha$_1$-antitrypsin
   6. Technetium 99m iminodiacetic acid (^{99m}Tc-IDA) scan
   7. Alpha-fetoprotein and lipoprotein X(?)

B. Hematologic tests
   1. Complete blood count, smear, and reticulocyte count
   2. Direct Coombs' test and erythrocyte G6PD
   3. Platelet count
   4. Prothrombin time and partial thromboplastin time

C. Tests for infectious diseases
   1. Cord blood IgM
   2. VDRL, FTA-ABS, complement fixation titers for rubella, cytomegalovirus, and herpesvirus, and Sabin's dye titer for toxoplasmosis
   3. HB$_s$AG (Australia antigen) in both infant and mother
   4. Viral cultures from nose, pharynx, blood, stool, urine, and cerebrospinal fluid

D. Urine tests
   1. Routine urinalysis, including protein and reducing substances
   2. Urine culture
   3. Bilirubin and urobilinogen
   4. Amino acid screening

E. Liver biopsy
   1. Light microscopy
   2. Specific enzyme assay (if indicated)

F. Radiologic/ultrasound studies as indicated

G. Additional specific diagnostic studies for metabolic disorders to be performed as indicated or suspected.

onstration of a normal gallbladder is usually indicative of an intrahepatic cause for cholestasis, it may be seen in extrahepatic biliary atresia and is therefore not a reliable sign. Since intrahepatic bile ducts are not dilated in extrahepatic biliary atresia, their presence should suggest another etiology.

Liver biopsy

Histopathologic examination of the liver is an integral part of the evaluation of any patient with persistent conjugated hyperbilirubinemia. It is best performed and analyzed after all other pertinent laboratory data have been gathered. A percutaneous liver biopsy usually yields adequate tissue for microscopic and, if desired, electron microscopic and virologic studies. In experienced hands it is a safe procedure, and in the majority of patients (90% to 95%) it establishes or confirms the correct diagnosis, sparing the infant with neonatal hepatitis an unnecessary surgical procedure. Before the biopsy, however, it must be ascertained that the prothrombin time is within 3 to 5 seconds of normal and that the platelet count is greater than 100,000. A prolonged prothrombin time may be corrected in some patients by administration of vitamin K. In some situations in which a biopsy is urgently required, fresh-frozen plasma may be administered before and 6 hours after percutaneous biopsy. Postoperatively infants must be observed closely for vital signs or clinical changes that indicate significant bleeding, bile peritonitis, or pneumothorax, the rare but significant complications of the procedure. In the final analysis the isotope scan and a percutaneous liver biopsy are the only reliable means available without surgical exploration to distinguish between neonatal hepatitis and extrahepatic biliary obstruction.

Interpretation of liver biopsy

Biliary atresia. The most critical information to be derived from the liver biopsy is the determination of the presence or absence of changes indicative of mechanical blockage in the major bile ducts. It has been shown in patients and in animal experiments that, soon after obstruction of the common bile duct, ducts and ductules in portal tracts and in the periportal zones begin to proliferate. This phenomenon involves most, if not all, portal tracts and is present even at the periphery of the liver, far removed from the site of obstruction. At least three portal tracts should be available for examination. In biliary atresia all tracts will show some degree of proliferation (Fig. 34-8). Minimal and rare proliferation of bile ductules, frequently limited to just one portal tract in a needle biopsy, may be seen in idiopathic neonatal hepatitis and probably reflects a localized or incomplete block caused by bile inspissation. In early stages of biliary atresia ductular proliferation may be present without fibrosis, which will regularly develop later. Ducts frequently appear distorted (Fig. 34-9) because of a discrepancy between the rate of proliferation of biliary epithelium and that of the surrounding fibrous tissue. An associated inflammatory exudate is occasionally seen around proliferated ductules, but a true cholangitis with necrosis of epithelium and intramural inflammation is only rarely encountered. Other changes within portal tracts include dilated lymphatics and, occasionally, tortuous and thick-walled arterioles. In later stages of extrahepatic biliary atresia, ductular epithelium may dis-

A B

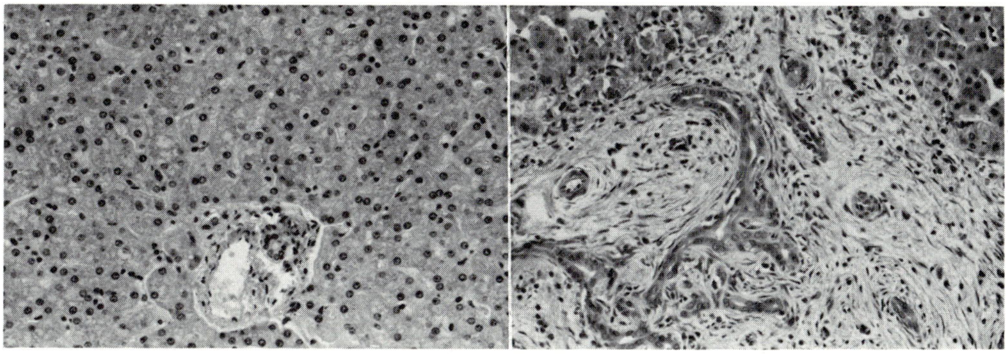

Fig. 34-8. A, Portal tract of normal infant, containing a large, thin-walled vein and single cross section of bile duct. **B,** Portal tract from infant with biliary atresia. Note marked enlargement of tract from fibrosis that surrounds multiple elongated bile ducts. (Both micrographs ×60.)

A B C D

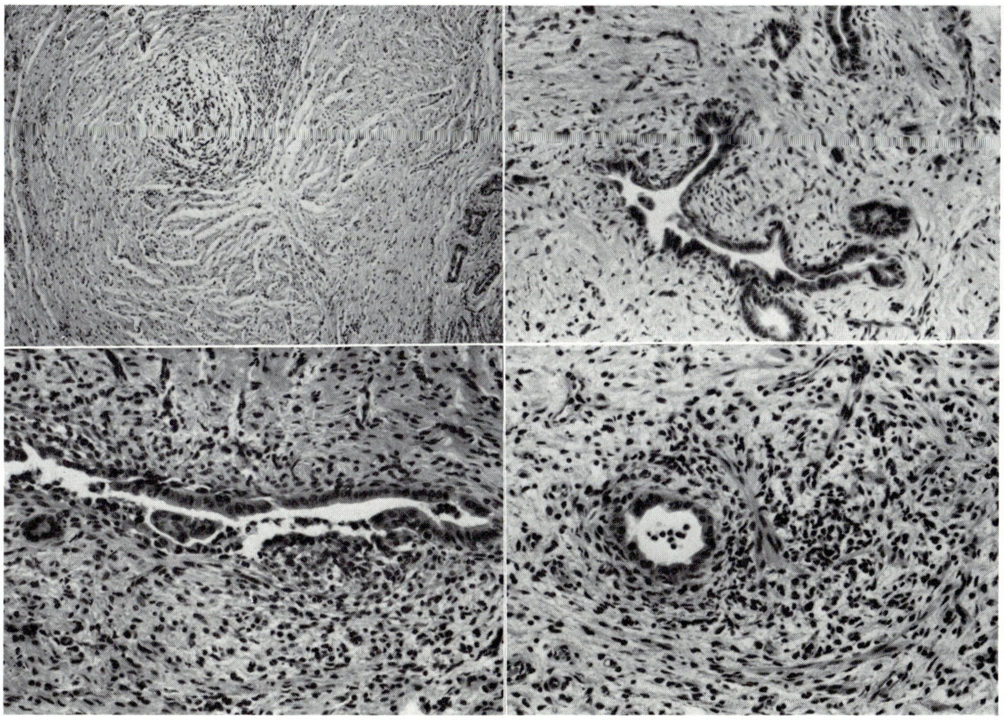

Fig. 34-9. Microscopic preparations of "fibrous remnant" of extrahepatic biliary system resected during Kasai procedure for biliary atresia. **A,** Most distal portion of specimen, showing complete obliteration of lumen by fibrous tissue. **B** to **D,** More proximal segments illustrating a spectrum of changes that includes necrosis of lining epithelium, acute and chronic inflammation, mural fibrosis with distortion of lumen, and great variation in size of ductlike structures. (All micrographs ×60.)

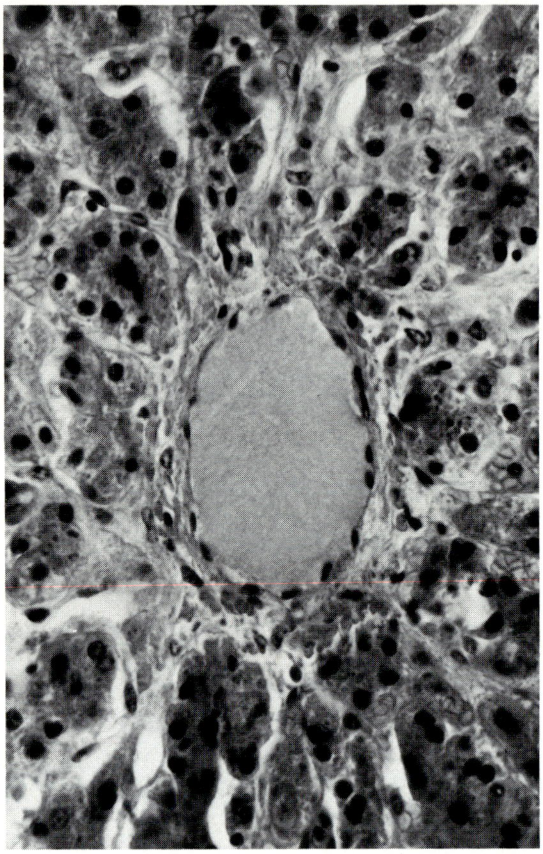

Fig. 34-10. Extrahepatic biliary atresia. Central vein surrounding hepatocytes. Intracanalicular bile plugs are present. In addition, hepatocytes contain intracytoplasmic bile pigment granules. (Paraffin embedding and hematoxylin-eosin staining.)

appear, having been replaced by collagen fibers, and may lead to a secondary paucity of portal bile ducts. A liver biopsy is considered to present paucity of intrahepatic bile ducts when the ratio between the number of ducts and the number of portal tracts is less than 0.9. Five to ten portal tracts must be examined for accurate evaluation. Extensive paucity (atresia) of portal bile ducts, whether primary or secondary, is associated with a clinical syndrome resembling that observed in primary biliary cirrhosis, or sclerosing cholangitis, with hypercholesterolemia, xanthomata, and pruritis. The liver parenchyma in biliary atresia shows intracanalicular and intracellular cholestasis with the intracanalicular component predominating (Fig. 34-10). In one third of all patients with biliary atresia, there is giant cell transformation of hepatocytes. In most cases this transformation is limited to the centrilobular areas and is not accompanied by necrosis and inflammation. Extramedullary hematopoiesis also may be present.

Neonatal hepatitis. This disorder is characterized by marked irregularity in the size of hepatocytes and in some cases by numerous giant cells (Figs. 34-11 and 34-12). Giant cells may contain from 4 to 100 nuclei. The cytoplasm of these giant cells is usually foamy and contains bile pigment. Intracanalicular cholestasis is less prominent than in biliary atresia. Bile canaliculi appear to be reduced in number when giant cells are abundant. Necrosis and inflammation are usually present. Kupffer cells are swollen and contain iron, bile pigment, lipofuscin, and phagocytosed debris of destroyed liver cells. Extramedullary hematopoiesis is almost always present. Although all these findings also may be seen in some cases of biliary atresia, it is the absence of portal bile duct proliferation that distinguishes neonatal hepatitis from biliary atresia (Figs. 34-8 and 34-11). In some cases of neonatal hepatitis there is evidence of inflammatory injury to portal bile ducts, with epithelial reduplication reflecting regenerative activity.

Treatment of neonatal hepatitis

Clinical management of neonatal hepatitis consists of supportive measures, since no specific therapy is known. Many infants have transient but significant reduction in bile flow and often require replacement of fat-soluble vitamins, particularly D and K. Subclinical rickets is common in these infants and may contribute to the increase in serum levels of alkaline phosphatase. Persistence of acholic or very pale stools without significant lowering of direct-reacting serum bilirubin concentrations after 1 month should be viewed as an indication for repeat clinical study, including liver biopsy. This practice will permit detection of patients who sclerose their bile ducts after an initial phase of hepatitis and who are therefore suitable candidates for exploratory laparotomy and corrective surgery. On rare occasions patients with neonatal hepatitis and complete obstruction, as evidenced by acholic stools, may recover rapidly after operative cholangiography that shows normal extrahepatic ducts. This phenomenon is probably a result of "flushing out" of inspissated bile in the extrahepatic biliary system, with consequent relief of obstruction.

Fluctuations in stool color should alert the clinician to the possible existence of a choledochal cyst. This can usually be diagnosed with ultrasound and treated surgically.

There are no early reliable criteria on which the prognosis of a particular patient can be based.

Treatment of extrahepatic biliary atresia

When the clinical evaluation indicates complete biliary obstruction or proves inconclusive, the patient should undergo an exploratory laparotomy. On entry of the abdomen after initial scrutiny of the biliary system, an operative cholangiogram should be performed to confirm

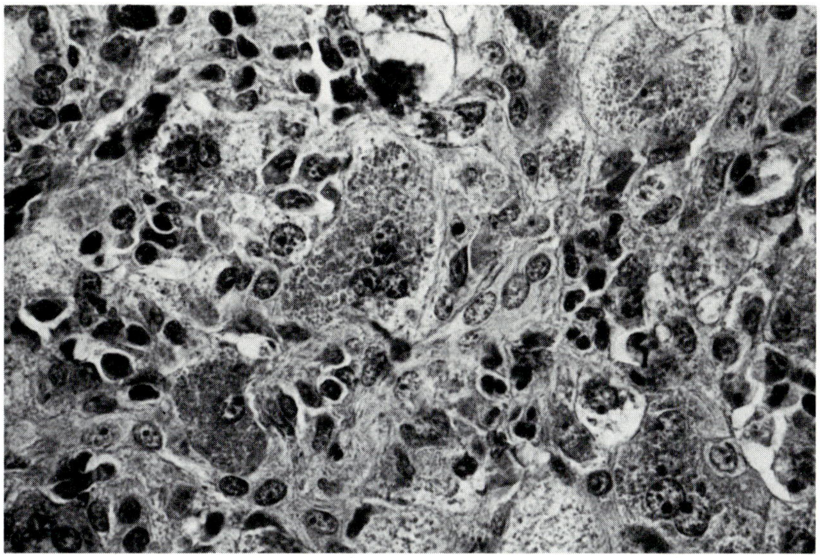

Fig. 34-11. Neonatal hepatitis. Note the marked cellular irregularity obliterating the normal orderly plate arrangement. Intracanalicular bile is present. Small cells in sinusoids represent Kupffer cells and elements of extramedullary hematopoiesis. (Paraffin embedding and hematoxylin-eosin staining; ×60.)

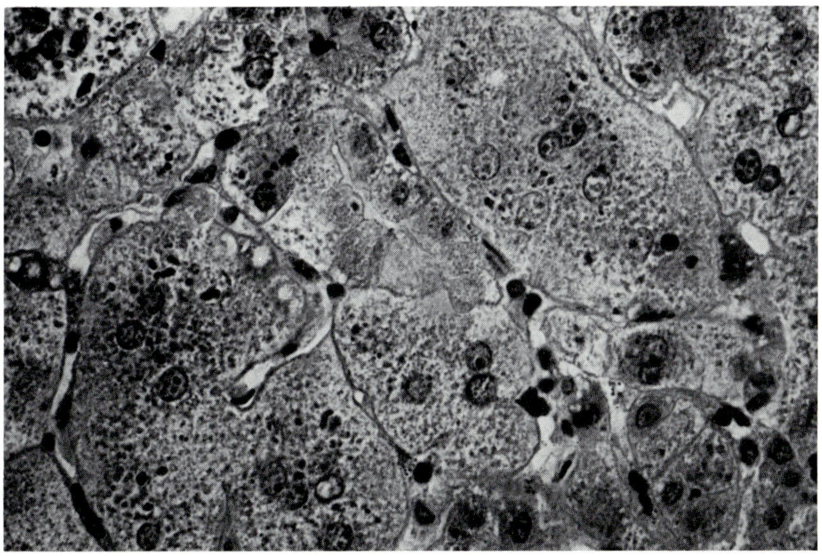

Fig. 34-12. High-power view of transformed giant hepatocytes. Most of the intracytoplasmic granules represent bile pigment. (Paraffin embedding and hematoxylin-eosin staining; ×200.)

and characterize the extrahepatic lesion and define its extent. Operative examination of these infants should be performed only by surgeons prepared to proceed with corrective procedures if necessary. Reoperation after an exploratory laparotomy increases the technical difficulties and delays the institution of corrective measures.

Reconstitution of normal biliary drainage by direct anastomosis of existing bile ducts to the GI tract is possible in only a very small proportion of patients with biliary atresia (estimated at 5% to 10%). These include the rare cases of choledochal cyst and occlusion of a short segment of the common bile duct by a valve, membrane, or fibrosis. In most patients with biliary atresia there are no grossly visible ducts proximal to the atretic segment; in the past all these patients were considered inoperable. Untreated patients, although jaundiced, often appear clinically well in the first few months of life but deteriorate rapidly after cirrhosis develops with clinical manifestations of portal hypertension, ascites, hypersplenism, infection, and hemorrhage.

In 1968 Kasai and associates described an operative procedure in which the transected fibrous tissue of the porta hepatis is anastomosed to a Roux-en-Y loop of small intestine (portoenterostomy). Kasai's portoenterostomy, or variations of this procedure, are currently performed in most medical centers. The immediate goal for surgical correction is the reestablishment of bile drainage. This is now achieved in the majority of infants operated on before 10 weeks of life, with progressively poorer results in older infants and almost no success in infants operated on later than 3 months of age. Cure rate, however, is still poor. In the majority of operated patients liver fibrosis increases with time and eventually progresses to cirrhosis despite adequate bile drainage. It is currently unclear if progressive liver fibrosis represents continuation of injury responsible for the obliterative fibrosis in extrahepatic ducts or if it is the result of ascending cholangitis complicating portoenterostomy. In addition to the age at the time of surgery, other factors that influence the outcome include the size and patency of the microscopic ducts in the porta hepatis. Liver transplantation has been done in patients with biliary atresia or neonatal hepatitis in whom advanced cirrhosis has developed. The results of transplantation since 1981, when cyclosporine and steroid therapy were introduced, are encouraging. Many children survive with normal liver function for 2 years after surgery. Long-term results are as yet unknown.

Bile plug syndrome

Mechanical obstruction of a major bile duct may be caused by precipitated bile and mucus within the lumen. The cause is obscure, although in a few patients it may be associated with cystic fibrosis. Clinical and pathologic findings are identical to those observed in biliary atresia and choledochal cyst. Diagnosis is made at surgery, and the bile plug usually can be removed. The condition is not known to recur.

Hepatitis caused by known infectious agents

See also Chapter 31, part two.

In a small proportion of infants with neonatal hepatitis a specific infectious agent may be identified either by direct isolation and culture or by serologic tests that detect specific antibodies. In some patients viral antigen may be demonstrated with liver biopsy using various immunocytochemical methods. Among infectious agents reported in association with neonatal hepatitis are bacteria such as *Treponema pallidum* and *Listeria* organisms and viruses such as rubella virus, Coxsackievirus, the herpesviruses (herpes simplex and varicella-zoster), cytomegalovirus, and adenovirus. The protozoon *Toxoplasma gondii* also has been reported. Fetal infection may take place in utero either by transplacental spread or by an ascending infection of the amniotic fluid, usually after rupture of membranes. In some cases infection may occur during delivery by aspiration of vaginal contents. Clinically patients in this group may appear sick and fail to thrive and also may have evidence of CNS and other organ involvement. In many patients there are stigmata of generalized infection. Laboratory findings are similar to those seen in idiopathic neonatal hepatitis, but stools are not acholic, and therefore biliary atresia usually is not suspected.

Liver biopsy may be helpful in the diagnosis, especially in infections with the herpesviruses. These DNA viruses replicate in the nucleus, resulting in intranuclear inclusion bodies that can be seen with the light microscope. Cytomegalic inclusion disease is characterized by marked enlargement of hepatocytes and biliary epithelium caused by large intranuclear as well as intracytoplasmic inclusions. In some cases, however, the virus has been isolated from patients in whom liver biopsy results were typical of neonatal giant cell hepatitis with no evidence of inclusions.

Hepatitis B surface antigen may be transmitted from mother to infant, probably by aspiration of vaginal contents or blood during delivery. With few exceptions infants born to HB_sAg positive mothers show no antigenemia in cord blood or in the first month of life. Repeated serologic tests indicate that HB_sAg appears in the serum of these infants between 5 and 7 weeks of life and reaches a peak at 10 weeks. Antigenemia in the newborn may be associated with liver injury, and both may persist for many months or possibly years. It is necessary therefore to closely observe all infants of HB_sAg-positive mothers for many years for clinical and laboratory evidence of chronic liver disease. Severe and even fulminant neonatal hepatitis associated with HB_sAg has been described in infants of chronic carriers and after neonatal transfusions. Prophylaxis with concurrent administration of hepatitis B immune globulin (HBIG) and HG vaccine is recommended. HBIG (0.5 ml intramuscularly) should be given within 12 hours of birth. In addition, 0.5 ml (10 μg) of vaccine should be given intramuscularly within 7 days of birth and repeated at 1 and 6 months of age. Concurrent use of HBIG and vaccine does not seem to interfere with vaccine efficacy.

Neonatal liver injury in metabolic disorders

See also Chapter 36.

Several metabolic disorders result in hepatocellular injury and give rise to a clinical pathologic syndrome that may resemble neonatal hepatitis or biliary atresia. The most commonly observed conditions are $alpha_1$-antitrypsin deficiency, galactosemia, tyrosinemia, and cystic fibrosis.

$Alpha_1$-antitrypsin deficiency in the homozygous state (PiZZ) may be manifested by neonatal liver injury. It is estimated that only 10% to 20% of all individuals with this abnormality will have liver disease. The majority of PiZZ individuals never develop clinical evidence of liver disease but may develop pulmonary emphysema as adults. Patients with $alpha_1$-antitrypsin deficiency may show all the signs and symptoms of neonatal hepatitis or biliary atresia, including acholic stools. Liver biopsy also may show changes consistent with either one of the aforementioned conditions; bile duct proliferation may be so pronounced that exploratory laparotomy is performed. In some patients hepatocytes, particularly in the periportal zone, contain intracytoplasmic inclusions that give a positive reaction with periodic acid–Schiff stain. When frozen liver sections are incubated with fluorescein-tagged antibodies against $alpha_1$-antitrypsin, they bind with these inclusions, thus identifying them as $alpha_1$-antitrypsin. Similar identification of the intracytoplasmic inclusions can be carried out in paraffin-embedded tissue using the immunoperoxidase technique. In many infants neonatal cholestasis may regress before the age of 6 months and reappear in later childhood or adolescence when the patient becomes cirrhotic. The pathogenesis of liver disease associated with this anomaly is not understood.

In *galactosemia* and *tyrosinemia* the infants fail to thrive and appear sick (see Chapter 36). Liver biopsy shows marked fatty accumulation in hepatocytes associated with fibrosis that may be quite extensive even in the first weeks of life. If there is no restriction of intake of foods containing galactose or tyrosine, cirrhosis develops and may lead to death in early infancy.

Cystic fibrosis may be associated with neonatal liver injury that clinically mimics neonatal hepatitis or biliary atresia. Injury is apparently caused by inspissation of mucus and bile in bile ducts. Such inspissation in a major extrahepatic duct may be responsible for the bile plug syndrome described previously. When smaller ducts are partially or completely obstructed by the inspissated material, a localized proliferation of bile ducts and associated fibrosis may develop and leads to a condition known as focal biliary cirrhosis. In some infants the dominant histologic abnormality consists of intracanalicular bile stasis and giant cell transformation of hepatocytes.

Liver injury associated with parenteral alimentation

See Chapter 25, part one.

Total parenteral alimentation (TPN) is being used with increasing frequency, particularly in low birth weight neonates. Following prolonged use (several weeks or longer) many infants show evidence of conjugated hyperbilirubinemia, which may persist for some time after cessation of this mode of feeding. Liver biopsy shows evidence of hepatocellular injury with swelling of hepatocytes, necrosis, cholestasis, and occasional giant cell transformation. Continuation of TPN in the presence of liver injury may cause progression to cirrhosis.

Other causes of conjugated hyperbilirubinemia

Sepsis occasionally is associated with conjugated hyperbilirubinemia in the neonatal period. In some patients generalized bacterial infection may induce hemolysis, whereas in other cases hemolysis cannot be demonstrated, and toxic phenomena may induce functional cholestasis. Postmortem examinations of neonates with severe sepsis have shown centrilobular bile stasis, focal hepatocellular necrosis, and giant cell transformation in some patients. In others no hepatic lesions can be demonstrated. Severe urinary tract infection, particularly with coliform bacilli, is associated with this syndrome; in this case generalized septicemia is not an essential feature, and cholestasis may be caused by massive endotoxin release. Antibiotic treatment is followed by prompt relief of hyperbilirubinemia.

Isolated cases of conjugated hyperbilirubinemia have been described in association with storage diseases, such as *Niemann-Pick disease* and *Gaucher's disease*, and with a familial disorder characterized by extreme *fatty liver*. Bland focal hepatic ischemic necrosis, typically with little or no inflammatory response, has been described in patients with *hypoplastic left-heart syndrome*, severe internal *hemorrhage*, and rarely in association with *umbilical vein catheterization*.

Conjugated hyperbilirubinemia associated with *cerebrohepatorenal syndrome*, *glycogenosis (type IV)*, and *familial recurrent cholestasis*, including *Byler's disease*, usually occurs beyond the neonatal period. *Indian child-*

hood cirrhosis and *congenital hepatic fibrosis* (with or without infantile polycystic disease of kidneys) rarely are seen with significant conjugated hyperbilirubinemia in the neonatal period. Additional rare causes of conjugated hyperbilirubinemia include tumors, such as *metastatic neuroblastoma* and primary *hepatoblastoma*. In these cases development of jaundice is usually delayed until after 2 months of age. Tumors and enlarged periductal lymph nodes also may obstruct the extrahepatic biliary ducts. A familial lethal form of hemochromatosis associated with neonatal cholestasis recently has been described.

Rachel Morecki
Lawrence M. Gartner
Kwang-Sun Lee

BIBLIOGRAPHY

Pathophysiology

Andres, J.M., and others: Developmental hepatology and mechanism of liver dysfunction, part I. J. Pediatr. **90**:686, 1977.

Blitzer, B.L., and Boyer, J.L.: Cellular mechanisms of bile formation, Gastroenterology **82**:346, 1982.

Erlinger, S.: Hepatocyte bile secretion: current views and controversies, Hepatology **1**:352, 1981.

French, S.W.: Role of canalicular contraction in bile flow (editorial), Lab. Invest. **53**:245, 1985.

French, S.W., and Davies, P.L.: Ultrastructural localization of actin-like filaments in rat hepatocytes, Gastroenterology **68**:765, 1975.

Phillips, M.J., and others: Microfilament dysfunction as a possible cause of intrahepatic cholestasis, Gastroenterology **69**:48, 1975.

Popper, H., and Schaffner, F.: Pathophysiology of cholestasis, Hum. Pathol. **1**:1, 1970.

Biliary atresia and neonatal hepatitis

Aagenaes, O.: Hereditary recurrent cholestasis with lymphoedema; two families, Acta Paediatr. Scand. **63**:465, 1974.

Aagenaes, O., van der Hagen, C.B., and Refsum, S.: Hereditary recurrent intrahepatic cholestasis from birth, Arch. Dis. Child. **43**:646, 1968.

Aagenaes, O., and others: Neonatal cholestasis in alpha-1-antitrypsin deficient children, Acta Paediatr. Scand. **61**:632, 1972.

Alagille, D.: Cholestasis in the first three months of life, Prog Liver Dis. **6**:471, 1979.

Alagille, D., and others: Hepatic ductular hypoplasia associated with characteristic facies, vertebral malformations, retarded physical, mental and sexual development and cardiac murmur, J. Pediatr. **86**:63, 1975.

Alpert, L.I., Strauss, L., and Hirschhorn, K.: Neonatal hepatitis and biliary atresia associated with trisomy 17-18 syndrome, N. Engl. J. Med. **280**:16, 1969.

Altman, R.P.: The portoenterostomy procedure for biliary atresia: A five year experience, Ann. Surg. **188**:351, 1978.

Altman, R.P., Chandra, R., and Lilly, G.R.: Ongoing cirrhosis after porticoenterostomy in infants—biliary atresia. J. Pediatr. Surg. **10**:685, 1975.

Balistreri, W.F.: Neonatal cholestasis, J. Pediatr. **106**:171, 1985.

Ballow, M., and others: Progressive familial intrahepatic cholestasis, Pediatrics **51**:998, 1973.

Bangaru, B., and others: Comparative studies of biliary atresia in the human newborn and Reovirus 3 induced cholangitis in weanling mice, Lab. Invest. **43**:456, 1980.

Brent, R.L., and others: Persistent jaundice in infancy, J. Pediatr. **61**:111, 1962.

Brough, A.J., and Bernstein, J.: Conjugated hyperbilirubinemia in early infancy: a reassessment of liver biopsy, Hum. Pathol. **5**:507, 1974.

Campbell, D.P., Poley, J.R., and Alauporic, P.: Determination of serum lipoprotein X for the early differentiation between neonatal hepatitis and biliary atresia, J. Surg. Res. **18**:385, 1975.

Chandra, R.S.: Biliary atresia and other structural anomalies in the congenital polysplenia syndrome, J. Pediatr. **85**:649, 1974.

Chandra, R.S., and Altman, R.P.: Ductal remnants in extrahepatic biliary atresia: a histopathologic study with clinical correlation, J. Pediatr. **93**:196, 1978.

Craig, J.M., and Landing, B.H.: Form of hepatitis in neonatal period simulating biliary atresia, Arch. Surg. **54**:321, 1952.

Dahms, B.B., and others: Arteriohepatic dysplasia in infancy and childhood: a longitudinal study of six patients, Hepatology **2**:350, 1982.

Danks, D.M.: Studies of the etiology of neonatal hepatitis and biliary atresia, Arch. Dis. Child. **52**:360, 1977.

Danks, D.M., and Bodian, M.: A genetic study of neonatal obstructive jaundice, Arch. Dis. Child. **38**:378, 1963.

Danks, D.M., and others: Prognosis of babies with neonatal hepatitis, Arch. Dis. Child. **52**:368, 1977.

Finegold, M.J., and Carpenter, R.J.: Obliterative cholangitis due to cytomegalovirus: A possible precursor of paucity of intrahepatic bile ducts, Hum. Pathol. **13**:662, 1982.

Gautier, M., and Elliot, N.: Extrahepatic biliary atresia: morphological study of 98 biliary remnants, Arch. Pathol. Lab. Med. **105**:397, 1981.

Gerhold, J.P., and others: Diagnosis of biliary atresia with radionuclide hepatobiliary imaging, Radiology **146**:499, 1983.

Glaser, J.H., and others: The role of Reovirus type 3 in neonatal cholestasis, J. Pediatr. **105**:912, 1984.

Greco, M.A., and Finegold, M.J.: Familial giant cell hepatitis, report of two cases and review of the literature, Arch. Pathol. **95**:240, 1973.

Haas, J.: Bile duct and liver pathology in biliary atresia, World J. Surg. **2**:561, 1978.

Haas, L.: Intrahepatic cholestasis in the newborn, Arch. Dis. Child. **43**:438, 1968.

Hitch, D.C., Shikes, R.H., and Lilly, G.R.: Determinants of survival after Kasai's operation for biliary atresia using actuarial analysis, J. Pediatr. Surg. **14**:310, 1979.

Howard, E.R., and others: Results of surgery in 88 consecutive cases of extrahepatic biliary atresia, J. R. Soc. Med. **75**:408, 1982.

Javitt, N.B., and others: Cholestatic syndromes in infancy; diagnostic value of serum bile acid pattern and cholestyramine administration, Pediatr. Res. **7**:119, 1973.

Kasai, M., Watanabe, I., and Ohi, R.: Follow-up studies of long-term survivors after hepatic portoenterostomy for "non-correctable" biliary atresia. J. Pediatr. Surg. **10**:173, 1975.

Kasai, M., and others: Surgical treatment of biliary atresia. J. Pediatr. Surg. **3**:665, 1968.

Kasai, M., and others: Technique and results of operative management of biliary atresia, World J. Surg. **2**:571, 1978.

Kattamis, C.A., Demetrios, D., and Matsaniotis, N.S.: Australia antigen and neonatal hepatitis syndrome, Pediatrics **54**:1257, 1974.

Kobayashi, A., and Ohbe, Y.: Choledochal cyst in infancy and childhood; analysis of 16 cases, Arch. Dis. Child. **52**:121, 1977.

Kobayashi, A., and others: Bone disease in infants and children with hepatobiliary disease, Arch. Dis. Child. **49**:641, 1974.

Landing, B.H.: Considerations of the pathogenesis of neonatal hepatitis, biliary atresia and choledochal cyst; the concept of infantile obstructive cholangiopathy, Prog. Pediatr. Surg. **6**:113, 1974.

Lawson, E.E., and Boggs, J.D.: Long-term follow-up of neonatal hepatitis; safety and value of surgical exploration, Pediatrics **53**:650, 1974.

Madj, M., Reba, R.C., and Altman, R.P.: Effect of phenobarbital on 99mTc-IDA scintigraphy in the evaluation of neonatal jaundice, Semin. Nucl. Med. **11**:194, 1981.

Madj, M., and others: Hepatobiliary scintigraphy with ^{99m}Tc-PIPIDA in the evaluation of neonatal jaundice, Pediatrics **67**:140, 1981.

Morecki, R., and others: Serologic evidence of Reovirus type II infection in biliary atresia, N. Engl. J. Med. **307**:481, 1982.

Morecki, R., and others: Detection of Reovirus type 3 in the porta hepatis of an infant with extrahepatic biliary atresia: ultrastructural and immunocytochemical study, Hepatology **4**:1137, 1984.

Mowat, A.P., Pscharopoulos, H.T., and Williams, R.: Extrahepatic biliary atresia versus neonatal hepatitis, a review of 137 prospectively investigated infants, Arch. Dis. Child. **51**:763, 1976.

Odievre, M.: Long term results of surgical treatment of biliary atresia, World J. Surg. **2**:589, 1978.

Psacharopoulas, P., and others: Extrahepatic biliary atresia: preoperative assessment and surgical results in 47 patients, Arch. Dis. Child. **55**:851, 1980.

Riely, C.A., and others: Arteriohepatic dysplasia: A benign syndrome of intrahepatic cholestasis with multiple organ involvement, Ann. Intern. Med. **91**:520, 1979.

Sharp, H.L., and Krivit, W.: Hereditary lymphedema and obstructive jaundice, J. Pediatr. **78**:491, 1971.

Sharp, H.L., and others: Cholestyramine therapy in patients with a paucity of intrahepatic bile ducts, J. Pediatr. **71**:723, 1967.

Valman, H.B., France, N.E., and Wallis, P.G.: Prolonged neonatal jaundice in cystic fibrosis, Arch. Dis. Child. **46**:805, 1971.

Witzleben, C.A., and others: Studies on the pathogenesis of biliary atresia, Lab. Invest. **38**:525, 1978.

Zeltzer, P.M., and others: Differentiation between neonatal hepatitis and biliary atresia by measuring serum alpha-fetoprotein, Lancet **1**:373, 1974.

Hepatitis caused by known infectious agents

Allen, L., and Murphy, W.R.: Listeriosis, South. Med. J. **51**:1454, 1958.

Beckett, R.S., and Flynn, F.J.J.: Toxoplasmosis; report of two new cases with classification and demonstration of organisms in the human placenta, N. Engl. J. Med. **249**:345, 1953.

Center for Disease Control: Recommendation for protection against viral hepatitis, Ann. Intern. Med. **103**:391, 1984.

Chiba, S., and others: Primary cytomegalovirus infection and liver involvement in early infancy, Tohoku J. Exp. Med. **117**:143, 1975.

Delaplane, D., and others: Fatal hepatitis B in early infancy: the importance of identifying HB-Ag-positive pregnant women and providing immunoprophylaxis to their newborns, Pediatrics **72**:176, 1983.

Desmonts, G., and Couvreur, J.: Congenital toxoplasmosis, a prospective study of 378 pregnancies, N. Engl. J. Med. **290**:1110, 1974.

Dupuy, J.M., Frommel, D., and Alagille, D.: Severe viral hepatitis type B in infancy, Lancet **1**:191, 1975.

Dupuy, J.M., and others: Hepatitis in children, study of 80 cases of B-type acute and chronic hepatitis, J. Pediatr. **92**:17, 1978.

Escobedo, M.B., and others: The frequency of jaundice in neonatal bacterial infections, Clin. Pediatr. **13**:656, 1974.

Hamilton, J.R., and Sass-Kortsak, A.: Jaundice associated with severe bacterial infection in young infants, J. Pediatr. **63**:121, 1963.

Hughes, J.R., and others: Ecovirus 14 infection associated with fatal neonatal hepatic necrosis, Am. J. Dis. Child. **123**:61, 1972.

Kattamis, C.A., and others: Australia antigen and neonatal hepatitis syndrome. Pediatrics **54**:1257, 1974.

Lake, A.M., and others: Enterovirus infections in neonates. J. Pediatr. **89**:787, 1976.

Nahmias, A.J., and others: The TORCH complex—perinatal infections associated with toxoplasma, rubella, cytomegalo- and herpes simplex viruses, Pediatr. Res. **5**:405, 1971.

Newman, C.G.H.: Perinatal varicella, Lancet **2**:1159, 1965.

Oppenheimer, E.H., and others: Congenital syphillis in the newborn infant: clinical and pathologic observations in recent cases, John Hopkins Med. J. **129**:63, 1971.

Philip, A.G.S., and Larson, E.J.: Overwhelming neonatal infection with ECHO 19, J. Pediatr. **82**:391, 1973.

Pugh, R.C.B., Newns, G.H., and Dudgeon, J.A.: Hepatic necrosis in disseminated herpes simplex, Arch. Dis. Child. **29**:60, 1954.

Rotthauwe, H.W.: Viral hepatitis in infancy and childhood, Clin. Gastroenterol. **3**:437, 1974.

Schweitzer, I.L., and others: Hepatitis and hepatitis associated antigen in 56 mother-infant pairs, JAMA **220**:1092, 1972.

Scott, R.B., Wilkins, W., and Kessler, A.: Viral hepatitis in early infancy; report of three fatal cases in siblings simulating biliary atresia. Pediatrics **13**:447, 1954.

Steven, C.E., and others: Perinatal hepatitis B virus transmission in the United States: prevention by passive-active immunization, JAMA **253**:1740, 1985.

Strauss, L., and Bernstein, J.: Neonatal hepatitis in congenital rubella, Arch. Pathol. **86**:317, 1968.

Zuckerman, A.J.: Viral infections of liver in childhood, Postgrad. Med. J. **50**:338, 1974.

Bile plug syndrome

Bernstein, J., Brayland, R., and Brough, J.: Bile plug syndrome; a correctable cause of obstructive jaundice in infants, Pediatrics **43**:273, 1969.

Liver injury associated with parenteral alimentation

Bernstein, J., and others: Conjugated hyperbilirubinemia in infancy associated with parenteral alimentation. J. Pediatr. **90**:361, 1977.

Pallares, R., and others: Cholestasis associated with parenteral nutrition, Lancet **1**:758, 1983.

Sinatra, F.R., and Merritt, R.J.: Cholestatic liver disease associated with total parenteral nutrition, J. Calif. Perinatal Assoc. **2**:98, 1981.

Tovloukian, R., and Seashore, J.H.: Hepatic secretory obstruction with total parenteral nutrition in the infant, J. Pediatr. Surg. **10**:353, 1974.

Metabolic disorders and other causes

Aagenaes, O., and others: Pathology and pathogenesis of liver disease in alpha-1-antitrypsin deficient individuals, Postgrad. Med. J. **50**:365, 1974.

Alagille, D., and others: Hepatic ductular hypoplasia associated with characteristic facies, vertebral malformations, retarded physical, mental, and sexual development, and cardiac murmur, J. Pediatr. **86**:63, 1975.

Cottrall, K., Cook, J.L., and Mowat, A.P.: Neonatal hepatitis syndrome and alpha-1-antitrypsin deficiency; an epidemiologic study in South-east England, Postgrad. Med. J. **50**:376, 1974.

Crocker, A.C., and Farber, S.: Niemann-Pick disease; a review of 18 patients, Medicine **37**:1, 1958.

Dunn, P.M.: Obstructive jaundice and haemolytic disease of the newborn, Arch. Dis. Child. **38**:54, 1963.

Genz, J., Jagenburg, R., and Zetterström, R.: Tyrosinemia, J. Pediatr. **66**:670, 1965.

Goldfischer, S., and others: Idiopathic neonatal iron storage involving the liver, pancreas, and endocrine and exocrine glands, Hepatology **1**:58, 1981.

Hardwick, D., and Dimmick, J.: Metabolic cirrhoses of infancy and early childhood, Perspect. Pediatr. Pathol. **3**:103, 1976.

Herman, S.P., and others: Liver dysfunction and histologic abnormalities in neonatal hypopituitarism, J. Pediatr. **87**:892, 1975.

Howell, R.R.: The glycogen storage diseases. In Stanbury, J.B., and Wyngaarden, J.B., editors: Metabolic basis of inherited disease, ed. 4, New York, 1978, McGraw-Hill Book Co., p. 137.

LaDu, B.N., and Gjessing, L.R.: Tyrosinosis and tyrosinemia. In Stanbury, J.B., and Wyngaarden, J.B., editors: Metabolic basis of inherited diseases, ed. 4, New York, 1978, McGraw-Hill Book Co., p. 256.

Lieberman, E., and others: Polycystic disease of kidneys and liver; clinical radiologic and pathologic correlation, Medicine **50**:277, 1971.

McAdams, A.J., Hug, G., and Boue, K.E., Glycogen storage disease, type I to X; criteria for morphologic diagnosis, Hum. Pathol. **5**:463, 1974.

Nadler, H.L., and others: Congenital galactosemia: a study of 55 cases. In Hsia, DY-Y, editor: Galactosemia, Springfield, 1969, Charles C. Thomas, p. 127.

Nayak, N.C., and Ramalingaswami, V.: Childhood cirrhosis. In Becker, F.F., editor: The liver; normal and abnormal functions. B. The biochemistry of disease, series no. 5, New York, 1975, Marcel Dekker, Inc.

Odievre, M., and others: Alpha-1 antitrypsin deficiency in liver disease in children; phenotypes, manifestations and prognosis, Pediatrics **57**:226, 1976.

Oppenheimer, E.H., and Esterly, J.B.: Hepatic changes in young infants with cystic fibrosis; possible relation to focal biliary cirrhosis, J. Pediatr. **86**:683, 1975.

Perkins, K.W., and others.: Idiopathic hemochromatosis in children. Report of a family, Am. J. Med. **39**:118, 1969.

Laurendau, T., Hill, J.E., and Manning, G.B.: Idiopathic neonatal hemochromatosis in siblings, Arch. Pathol. **72**:48, 1961.

Porter, C.A., and others: α_1-Antitrypsin deficiency and neonatal hepatitis, Br. Med. J. **3**:435, 1972.

Ragazzini, F., Bartolozzi, G., and Ciampolini, M.: Neonatal cholestasis. In Gentilini, P., and others, editors: Intrahepatic cholestasis, New York, 1975, Raven Press.

Sass-Kortsak, A.: Management of young infants presenting with direct-reacting hyperbilirubinemia. Pediatr. Clin. North Am. **21**:777, 1974.

Sharp, H.L.: Current status of alpha-1-antitrypsin, Gastroenterology **70**:611, 1976.

Sveger, T.: Liver disease and alpha-1 antitrypsin deficiency detected by screening of 200,000 infants, N. Engl. J. Med. **294**:1316, 1976.

Valman, H.B., and others: Prolonged neonatal jaundice in cystic fibrosis, Arch. Dis. Child. **46**:805, 1971.

Walker, W., and Mathis, R.K.: Hepatomegaly; an approach to differential diagnosis, Pediatr. Clin. North Am. **22**:929, 1975.

Weber, A.M., and others: Severe familial cholestasis in North American Indian children: a clinical model of microfilament dysfunction? Gastroenterology **81**:653, 1981.

CHAPTER 35

The kidney and urinary tract

RENAL FUNCTION AND ITS MORPHOLOGIC CORRELATES

During intrauterine life the function of the nephric system is minimal; homeostasis of the fetus depends on the placenta, as evidenced at birth by the absence of abnormalities in fluid and electrolyte balance in newborns with bilateral renal agenesis. Formation and excretion of urine are essential, however, for the maintenance of an adequate amount of amniotic fluid. Moreover, urine formation plays a role in the embryogenesis of the urinary system.

At birth the kidneys have a combined weight of about 25 gm compared with 40 gm at 3 months of age and 270 to 300 gm in the adult. The combined volume of the two kidneys in the term newborn ranges from 20 to 25 ml as determined by roentgenography and ultrasonography. The kidneys often retain a fetal lobular structure and are easily palpable.

Nephrogenesis is centrifugal and ceases when the fetus reaches a length of 46 to 49 cm and a weight of 2,100 to 2,500 gm. At term the medullary and juxtamedullary zones of the kidney are still thicker than the outer cortex, and each kidney contains its definitive complement of 800,000 to 1,000,000 nephrons. Both glomerular and tubular size are, however, much smaller than that in the child and the adult as are their functional capacities. In addition, there is a marked anatomic and functional nephronal heterogeneity related principally to the differences between the more mature inner cortex and the less mature outer cortex. Size and function are not directly proportional. For instance, the neonatal kidney has the capacity to reabsorb efficiently sodium, glucose, and phosphate, whereas the reabsorption of certain amino acids and bicarbonate is limited when compared with that of the adult.

In the human the kidney of a fetus above 150 gm body weight receives approximately 3% of the cardiac output as compared with about 5% in the newborn and 20% in the adult. Renal autoregulation is present, albeit limited, during late gestation and the newborn period, even though blood pressure is very low. The sympathetic nervous system does play a part in the regulation of fetal renal circulation, and renal prostaglandins have been shown to blunt the vasoconstrictive effects of hypoxia. The renin-angiotensin system is known to respond adequately to intrauterine hemorrhage.

Glomerular filtration rate (GFR) increases in fetal lambs from 1.2 ml/min at 100 days gestation to 3.2 ml/min close to term. However, the ratios of GFR to body weight and kidney weight change very little during gestation, indicating that the intrauterine increase in absolute GFR is mainly the result of nephrogenesis. The GFR of the premature and term newborn is lower than that of the child and adult, even when correction is made for body weight or surface area (Fig. 35-1). There is a substantial increase in GFR after 34 weeks' gestation, whether development takes place in or outside the uterus. In low birth weight (LBW) infants, GFR is 1.07 ± 0.12 ml/min/kg at birth, a value similar to that observed in fetal lambs. Thereafter GFR increases at a more rapid rate than body weight, mainly as a consequence of the increase in glomerular capillary surface area and in the ultrafiltration pressure. The extrauterine environment accelerates the rise in GFR. Consequently, in infants of the same gestational age GFR is higher among those born prematurely than among those born at term (Fig. 35-2). The GFR of the neonate, and of LBW infants in particular, is much more sensitive than that of children and adults to the depressing effects of severe dehydration and, to a lesser degree, to the enhancing effects of extracellular volume expansion.

Fetal urine is hypotonic to plasma, although its osmolality does increase with gestational age. Arginine vasopressin (AVP) is present in the fetus and its concentration increases with gestational age. Even though the AVP receptors in the collecting duct are present and the

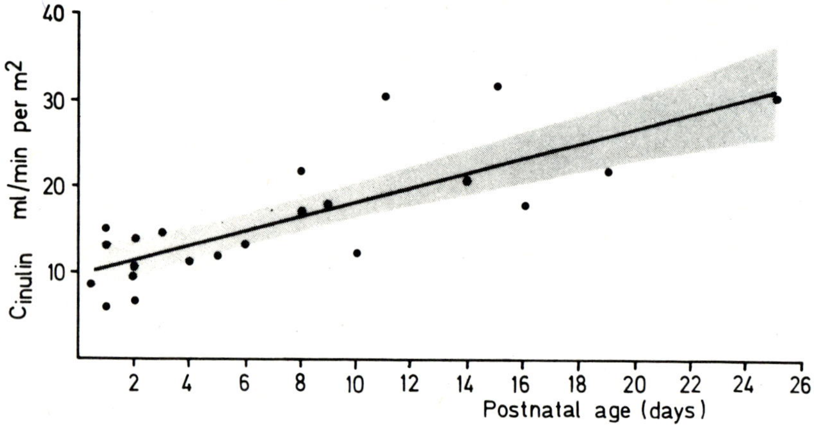

Fig. 35-1. Changes in GFR measured by inulin clearance (C_{inulin}) with postnatal age. The data represent individual values. The line and the shaded area represent the regression line and the 95% confidence limit, respectively ($y = 9.6 + 0.88x$, $r = 0.79$, $p < 0.01$, $n = 22$). (From Guignard, J.P.: J. Pediatr. **87:**268, 1975.)

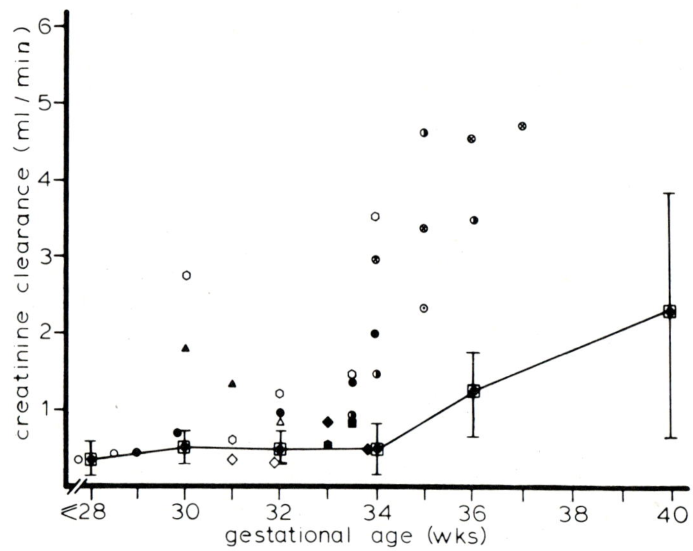

Fig. 35-2. Relationship between creatinine clearance and conceptional age (gestational plus postnatal ages). The line connects values of infants studied at birth, whereas the mass plot represents values obtained in infants studied at later dates. Measurements done in one infant at various ages are marked with the same symbol.

mechanisms for AVP secretion are operative, the response of the fetus and LBW infant to AVP is blunted. The urine/plasma (U/P) ratio of creatinine, an indicator of the concentration capacity of the kidney, rises progressively throughout gestation, reaching a 5:1 value prenatally. This contrasts markedly with the ratio of 20:1 observed after birth; the 5:1 ratio nonetheless indicates a tubular reabsorption of approximately 80% of the filtered water.

During the first week of life of term newborns, blood AVP levels are high, although maximum urinary concentration is only a little above that of plasma, ~350 mOsm/kg water. Within 4 to 6 weeks after birth a urinary osmolality of 600 mOsm/kg water may be reached. This level is similar to that observed in a full-term newborn and less than half that observed in the adult, which is reached by the second year of life. A low urinary osmolality, although quite appropriate to the neonates who have proportionately high fluid intake, renders them vulnerable to abnormal extrarenal losses. A LBW newborn, for instance, will be unable to adapt to an excess fluid loss of 4 to 6 ml/kg/hour or to a supplementary intake of 50 to 70 ml/kg/day. Stresses of this magnitude are easily tolerated by full-term babies. The limited ability to concentrate the urine observed in the premature and term newborn is due to several factors, including the shortness of the loops of Henle, the width of the peripapillary fornices, and the high protein anabolism of the healthy newborn, which accounts for the low urinary urea content and thus, at least in part, for the low osmolality of the medullary interstitium.

The kidney of the newborn is capable of diluting the urine down to 30 mOsm/kg. The clearance of free water prorated to GFR is very high in term newborns. Even LBW infants above the gestational age of 30 weeks are capable of diluting their urine well; however, the very low GFR severely limits their capacity to excrete rapidly a load of water.

Sodium clearance is higher in the fetus than in the term newborn, and urinary Na^+/K^+ ratios decrease with gestational age. The inability of the fetal kidney to conserve sodium may be due to structural and enzymatic immaturity of the renal tubule, to the relatively high extracellular fluid volume, and to a relative insensitivity of the tubule to aldosterone. Nevertheless, the bulk of sodium chloride and bicarbonate is reabsorbed by the fetal animal kidney, and the sodium content of fetal urine decreases from an initial value of about 80 mEq/L at the middle of gestation to 20 to 30 mEq/L at its end.

Term infants conserve sodium avidly, mostly through an enhanced reabsorption in the distal segments of the nephron. Prematurely born and LBW infants, on the other hand, are unable to retain sodium even under conditions of sodium depletion, and thus fractional excretion of sodium is as high as 5% for the first 1 or 2 weeks of life. Plasma renin activity is high in the fetus and has been found to increase adequately in response to sodium loss in both the fetus and newborn; however, the inadequate adrenal production of aldosterone and the relative unresponsiveness of the distal nephron to aldosterone limit the compensatory capacity of the distal nephron and cannot prevent inappropriately high rates of sodium excretion. Haycock and associates have found a negative sodium balance in all very low birth weight (VLBW) infants born before 30 weeks' gestation, in 70% of those 30 to 32 weeks' gestation, in 46% of infants whose gestational age was 33 to 35 weeks, and in none above 36 weeks' gestation. The negative sodium balance causes a contraction of the extracellular volume, a rise in plasma renin activity (PRA) and plasma AVP, hyponatremia, and low serum osmolality in association with moderately concentrated urine. The hyponatremia limits sodium delivery to the distal nephron, causing metabolic acidosis and hyperkalemia and occasionally CNS disturbances. A similar situation may be present in sick term neonates with hypoxia, sepsis, and acute renal failure. The sodium content of breast milk, which is adequate for term infants, therefore needs to be supplemented in LBW and VLBW infants as well as in some sick neonates to the amount of 3 to 10 mEq/kg/day. Because of the very low GFR, the LBW infants are also limited in their ability to excrete a sodium load. Consequently, a newborn is prone to develop hypernatremia and intracerebral hemorrhage, whereas long-term water and salt excess may cause hypervolemia, edema, increased intracranial pressure, congestive heart failure, and the persistence of a patent ductus arteriosus (PDA) (Chapter 25, part 3).

In term newborns, the fraction of filtered sodium reabsorbed in the distal nephron is and remains high even under conditions of sodium loading, thus severely limiting their capacity to excrete an excess of sodium. The significant drain on extracellular sodium resulting from the deposition of sodium in cells (particularly in bone) stimulates the renin-angiotensin-aldosterone axis and may account for the enhanced distal reabsorption and for the absence of the "escape" phenomenon observed in adults. Sodium excretory capacity improves with time, and by the second year of life, the child is fully capable of adjusting to sudden changes in sodium intake.

Urinary excretion of potassium increases with gestational age. This is probably due to the progressive increase in Na^+-K^+-ATPase activity and in the tubular responsiveness to aldosterone. At birth, urinary potassium excretion and urinary K^+/Na^+ ratio is lower in the LBW infant than in the term neonate. The K^+/Na^+ ratio of breast milk, which is 1:1 during the first few days after birth, rises to 3:1 within the first month of postnatal life. This may account in part for the relative hyperkalemia and the high plasma renin and aldosterone levels at this age. The mild metabolic acidosis of the neonate may also contribute to the high K^+/Na^+ values observed. Hyperkalemia is usually of little clinical significance in newborns except under catabolic conditions, when the further rise in serum K^+ concentration and the inability of aldosterone to stimulate K^+ secretion (even in term newborns) may result in life-threatening conditions.

The level of serum bicarbonate is controlled by its renal threshold: up to a certain serum level, all bicarbonate that is filtered is reabsorbed by the renal tubule; above this level, reabsorption is incomplete and some bicarbonate is excreted in the urine. The renal bicarbonate threshold is low in fetal lambs and correlates well with the weight of the fetal kidney. The renal threshold for bicarbonate is also low in term newborns when compared with children and adults, resulting in a low serum bicarbonate concentration and a low buffering capacity of the serum. This low threshold in both fetal and neonatal periods may be due to the relatively high extracellular fluid volume of the fetus and newborn, to the immaturity of the proximal tubule, and the low Na^+-K^+-

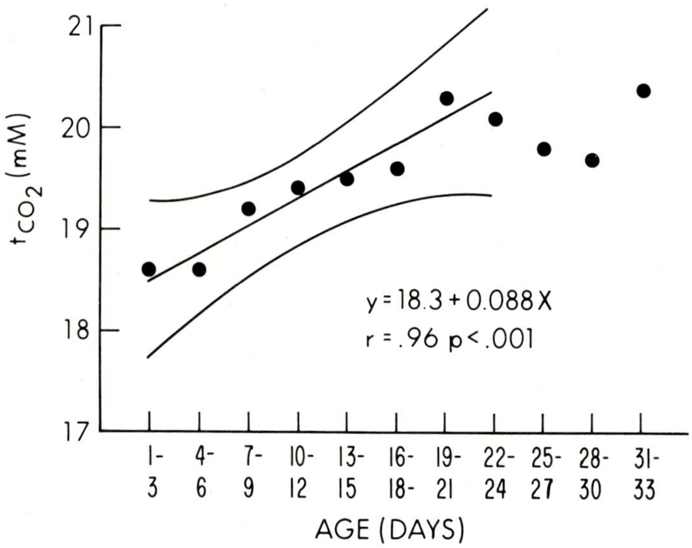

Fig. 35-3. Regression line and confidence limits of plasma total CO_2 (tCO_2) in low birth weight infants as a function of age. The points represent the mean value for each age interval. (From Schwartz, G.J., and others: J. Pediatr. **95:**102, 1979.)

ATPase activity. LBW (Fig. 35-3) and sick infants with hypoxia, sepsis, and renal failure are found to have even lower levels of serum bicarbonate than their normal counterparts and are thus at greater risk of developing the many complications of acidemia. The low bicarbonate threshold is not due to carbonic anhydrase deficiency, which rises appropriately in response to stimuli such as hypokalemia and extracellular volume contraction.

In spite of their low bicarbonate threshold, normal neonates are usually in H^+ balance and thus capable of growth. Excretion of titratable acid and ammonium prorated to body weight and renal weight is low in the fetus and in the neonate. However, both respond adequately to an acid load (such as ammonium chloride) by lowering urine pH. Although their urinary ammonium excretion is limited, possibly caused by an age-related deficiency in glutaminase, the ingestion of milk containing large amounts of phosphate (cow's milk) enhances the capacity to excrete titratable acid. The initial postnatal period, however, is fraught with danger because of limitations in the ability of the collecting duct to establish a lumen-to-blood H^+ gradient and thus to excrete acid in the urine (Chapter 25, part 3).

There seems to be an active transport of calcium from mother to fetus, accounting for the high serum calcium in fetal lambs. Cholecalciferol and 25, hydroxycholecalciferol are also transported from mother to fetus, whereas 1-25,dihydroxycholecalciferol is synthesized both by the placenta and by fetal proximal tubules.

Within the first 3 days of extrauterine life, serum calcium falls from its initial high normal value and then returns progressively over several weeks to a low normal value. The initial fall is more pronounced in LBW infants. The administration of oral glucose solutions to term neonates has been shown to cause a drop in serum calcium, magnesium, and phosphate unrelated to the dilutional effect, or to a parathyroid hormone (PTH) response. This observation emphasizes the need to closely monitor serum calcium in LBW infants, infants of diabetic mothers, and neonates with asphyxia or respiratory distress syndrome (RDS) (Chapter 37, part 2).

Urinary calcium excretion is minimal at birth and rises within several weeks to 3.5 mmol/1.73 m^2/day. In LBW infants 2 to 3 weeks of age one may observe a transient rise in urinary excretion of calcium compatible with a state of relative phosphate depletion, which does not permit normal mineralization of bones. Under physiologic conditions, however, renal excretion plays only a minor role in the calcium homeostasis of the neonate.

Serum phosphorus levels are higher in the fetus than in the mother, and fetal urine contains very little phosphate. At birth, serum phosphorus is above 6 mg/dl and decreases slowly thereafter. The phosphate intake of a normal newborn ranges from 0.5 to 1 mmol/kg/day. Infants are capable of responding to a dietary phosphate load by enhancing the renal phosphate clearance, although a concomitant rise of serum phosphate may occur. Tubular reabsorption of phosphate (TRP) is lower in LBW infants during the first few days of life and rises thereafter to 90% to 95% or above of the filtered load, a level present in the full-term infant right after birth. This compares with a value of 85% to 80% in the older child and the adult. This avidity for phosphorus reabsorption is characteristic of a growing organism. Fetal PTH levels are low, but fetal PTH excretion does rise during hypocalcemia. After birth, PTH rises to normal childhood values within 2 days in term neonates. The administration of PTH to the fetus and the newborn, however, has only a minor phosphaturic effect while causing a marked increase in tubular calcium reabsorption. This blunted tubular response to PTH in the face of normal rises in cyclic adenosine monophosphate (cAMP) may point to a transient dissociation between the production of cAMP and the luminal transport of phosphate in the fetal and neonatal period.

There is an active transfer of magnesium of 3 to 4 mg/kg/day from mother to fetus. The urinary excretion of magnesium in term newborns is very low, about 0.1 to 0.3 mg/kg/day, but fractional excretion of magnesium increases with postnatal age, as proximal tubular reabsorption decreases.

The renal glucose threshold increases in the fetus, reaching 200 mg/dl at the time of birth in the fetal lamb. At birth, maximal glucose reabsorption (T_mG) is higher in the human newborn than in the adult. As a result, urine is usually devoid of glucose.

The filtered load of uric acid increases with gestational age, particularly from the thirty-fourth week onward. Fractional excretion of uric acid is, however, inversely related to gestational age, being over 70% at 30 weeks, just over 50% at term, and declining progressively thereafter as net tubular transport of uric acid matures. The high basal excretion rates of uric acid in infants may predispose them to the risk of uric acid nephropathy when excretion demands are increased.

In summary, the immature kidney is characterized by low rates of glomerular filtration that limit the ability to dispose rapidly of a fluid or solute load. The even greater limitations in tubular reabsorption may result in inappropriate loss in urine of substances present in the glomerular filtrate such as certain amino acids and bicarbonate. On the other hand, the newborn has the tendency to retain glucose, sodium, and phosphate. Although none of these limitations has a detrimental effect in a healthy neonate, they restrict the ability of the newborn to respond to stress.

REACTION OF THE IMMATURE KIDNEY TO INJURY

The tissue reaction of the newborn to suppuration, ischemic necrosis, and hemorrhage incorporates a greater proliferative or regenerative component than that in the adult. After injury, epithelial cells undergo dedifferentiation and apparent multiplication to form distinctive glomerular and tubular forms that mimic a fetal appearance. Such epithelial patterns incorporate both regressive transformation and failure of differentiation. Although commonly seen in dysplastic kidneys, they do not in themselves signify a developmental anomaly, nor do they constitute evidence of an underlying congenital abnormality in an otherwise diseased kidney. These epithelial abnormalities, both glomerular and tubular, often coexist with involutional changes. For example, glomerular hyalinization, sometimes referred to as *congenital glomerulosclerosis*, is a process common enough to be regarded as normal. Ten percent of glomeruli will show histologic evidence of glomerulosclerosis and obsolescence, although we do not understand either the pathogenesis or the significance of the finding. Such changes are found in increased numbers as a consequence of renal necrosis, ischemic damage, and urinary tract obstruction as well as in premature infants and in those with congenital heart disease.

Glomerulosclerosis frequently is accompanied by focal glomerular cyst formation; variable tubular atrophy and tubular cyst formation also may be present. In autosomal trisomy D and E syndromes, sclerotic glomeruli, incorporating both primitive and cystic changes, often are found in the peripheral cortex. Tiny cystic glomeruli are found in the peripheral cortex as subcapsular microcysts in many syndromes of multiple congenital malformations. The cysts are rarely of functional consequence and should not be confused with polycystic disease. It is not known if they are truly abnormalities of renal development and morphogenesis or if they are acquired changes of formed nephrons resulting from undefined metabolic, nephrotoxic influences. Cyst formation seems to be a common response of the fetal or neonatal kidney to severe forms of injury. Congenital urinary tract obstruction may be associated with cystic tubular dilation, an uncommon effect of obstruction in later life.

An important aspect of the reaction of immature kidneys to injury is the effect on subsequent renal growth. Parenchymal disease beginning very early in life may lead to very small, end-stage kidneys, probably because subsequent growth and development are impaired by extensive epithelial damage, fibrosis, and vascular changes. In localized or unilateral diseases, on the other hand, the uninvolved parenchyma is capable of considerable compensatory hypertrophy and functional adaptation. This may relate to the great capacity of the immature fetal kidney for proliferation. All changes, at least in full-term newborns, take place in the existing nephrons, and no new ones are formed.

DIAGNOSIS OF RENAL DISEASE

Clinical evaluation of the kidneys must include assessment of both morphologic status and functional capacity.

Morphologic evaluation

Gross morphologic characteristics can be investigated by a variety of imaging techniques.

A plain film of the abdomen often delineates the edge of the kidney, providing information concerning renal size and shape. In the neonate a small kidney almost always reflects a developmental abnormality rather than the effects of acquired disease. An irregular contour may be indicative of scarring following vascular obstruction or infection. This should be differentiated from fetal lobulation, which often persists into extrauterine life.

Ultrasonography (echography, sonography) allows identification of an abnormal abdominal mass, such as a hydronephrotic kidney, or of the absence of a normal structure, as in unilateral renal agenesis. It also can distinguish cystic from solid formation. The noninvasive nature of this technique and the fact that it allows identification of structural anomalies regardless of the functional status make it very suitable for the investigation of the urinary tract in the newborn (Chapter 12). The renal cortex in the neonate has a higher echogenicity than in the adult. This probably reflects the relatively large contribution of glomeruli to the volume of the outer cortex of the neonate. Prenatal diagnosis of enlarged, ectopic, or cystic kidneys can be made by ultrasonography of the pregnant mother. The findings should be confirmed postnatally and treatment should be deferred to that period.

Radioisotopic methods such as the renal scan and the renogram have the advantage of requiring much lower irradiation than the usual roentgenographic technique. The renal scan is of value in locating anomalous kidneys, determining kidney size, and demonstrating abnormalities in blood flow distribution. Quantitative scanning can also provide information about the relative contribution of each kidney to the overall renal function.

Excretory urography is still a widely used and valuable method of roentgenographic investigation of the kidney (Chapter 13). The usual dose of 50% diatrizoate (Hypaque) sodium given to a child is 1 ml/kg, but in infants a dose of 3 ml/kg (up to a total of 20 ml) is used. For evaluation of a mass in the neonate as much as 5 ml/kg may be given. Since 50% diatrizoate has an osmolarity of 1,000 mOsm/L and a sodium concentration of 50 mEq/L, the material should be used with caution in dehydrated infants and in those with cardiac failure or renal insufficiency. Films taken shortly after the injection of contrast material reveal a "bodygram" effect from opacification of the vascular space. As a consequence, organs or other masses that are highly vascular are opaque, whereas avascular structures such as cysts are translucent and surrounded by a dark shadow. Since the renal parenchyma is visualized during the same phase, the resulting nephrogram can be used for measurement of kidney size and cortical thickness. Subsequent films permit visualization of the entire urinary tract and serve to define the status of the calyceal system, pelves, ureters, and bladder.

Voiding cystourethrography should be considered an essential part of the roentgenologic examination whenever vesicoureteric reflux is suspected or urinary tract infection has been documented. It may also allow visualization of the collecting system when glomerular filtration is compromised and reflux is present. A 12% to 15% solution of a water-soluble contrast medium is instilled into the bladder through a catheter lubricated with an antibiotic ointment (a no. 5 feeding tube is adequate for the newborn). The catheter is removed when complete filling of the bladder is evidenced by leakage around the tube. Films of the urethra during voiding and of the bladder and ureters toward the end of voiding are essential.

Aortography and selective renal angiography are used rarely in the differential diagnosis of abdominal masses in infants. The inferior venacavogram may be of great help in the diagnosis of renal vein thrombosis. However, at least 30% of normal newborns fill the azygos and the hemiazygos septa during this procedure, and this finding therefore should not be considered diagnostic of obstruction. The diagnosis of Wilms' tumor usually can be confirmed by an intravenous urogram; although most of these tumors have a distinctive vascular pattern, some are avascular, and an angiogram may not help in the differentiation from an abscess or hydronephrosis. Angiography is of value in the diagnosis of vascular anomalies, such as segmental hypoplasia and arterial obstruction.

The microscopic morphologic characteristics of the kidney can be investigated by examining tissue obtained by *needle biopsy*. This procedure is used in the diagnosis of parenchymal renal disease; in expert hands the risk of complications is minimal. Although indications for performing a renal biopsy in the newborn are limited, it is an extremely valuable procedure in appropriate patients.

Functional evaluation

Examination of a *freshly voided specimen of urine* provides immediate, invaluable information regarding the condition of the kidney. Although the neonate excretes a higher fraction of filtered protein in urine than does the older child, the concentration usually does not exceed 5 to 10 mg/dl of urine; as a consequence, protein is not detected by conventional methods of testing, such as Albustix or 10% sulfosalicylic acid.

Microscopic examination of the sediment obtained by centrifugation of a 10 ml aliquot of urine for 5 minutes should reveal less than 2 or 3 white blood cells (WBC) per high-power field and usually no red blood cells (RBC) and no casts or bacteria. Large numbers of leukocytes are usually interpreted as indicative of infection. It should be realized, however, that leukocyturia occurs in many noninfectious conditions as well, including obstructive uropathy and a number of types of glomerulonephritis. More than a few cellular casts in the urinary sediment suggest renal parenchymal disease or severely compromised perfusion such as in dehydration or shock. RBC casts are the hallmark of glomerulonephritis.

The *Addis count* provides quantitative information on the rate of excretion in the urine of cells, casts, and protein. In addition, it can serve as a test of concentrating ability if appropriate restriction of fluid intake is imposed before and during the collection period. Since an accurately timed collection is essential for this determination, the test is difficult to perform in the infant. Moreover, data from which the normal range can be established are extremely limited; up to 100,000 WBCs and 75,000 RBCs are considered normal. Detection of casts is unusual in the absence of disease. The amount of protein should not exceed 5 to 10 mg/12 hours. After an overnight thirst, older children normally have a concentrated urine of at least 900 mOsm/L. After the first few weeks of life, an osmolality of 700 or more is expected in infants' urine under the same conditions.

Since the elimination from the blood of certain substances, such as *urea* and *creatinine*, depends on the rate of glomerular filtration, their *plasma concentrations* serve as indicators of the level of renal function. However, the relationship between their concentrations in plasma and GFR is described by a hyperbola, so that until renal function is severely impaired, the increase in plasma urea and creatinine concentrations is relatively small, and their concentrations still may fall within the normal range. Furthermore the concentration of these substances in healthy infants is much lower than it is in older children. A creatinine concentration of 0.6 mg/dl, for instance, which is well within the normal range for older children and adults, might represent a 100% increase over normal value in a newborn and signify therefore a 50% reduction in GFR. Technical difficulties in accurately measuring creatinine in concentrations below 0.5 mg/dl further complicate interpretation of the results. Finally, the concentration of urea in plasma is markedly affected by the intake and rate of anabolism of protein.

A more precise assessment of the functional capacity of the kidney is made by measuring GFR by one of a variety of *clearance methods*. The renal clearance is the amount of plasma that would need to be totally cleared of a particular substance by the kidney per unit of time to account for its rate of excretion in urine. The mathematic expression is $C = (U \times V)/P$, in which C is renal clearance, U is concentration in urine of the substance under study, V is volume of urine per unit of time, and P is the concentration in plasma of the substance under study. Conventionally clearances are expressed as milliliters per minute per 1.73 m^2 of body surface area. If a substance is freely filterable through the glomerular membrane, is physiologically inert, and is neither reabsorbed nor secreted, its clearance is equal to GFR. Inulin, a polymer of fructose, is such a substance. Its clearance remains the best determinant of GFR. However, since a continuous infusion of inulin must be given to maintain an adequate blood concentration during the test, and since the measurement of inulin involves a tedious chemical procedure, the clearance of inulin is not measured routinely. Nevertheless with this method GFR has been shown to be 25 to 30 ml/minute/1.73 m^2 during the first few days of life and 50 ml/minute/1.73 m^2 by the end of the first month. It must be emphasized, however, that individual variation and variability related to the method make interpretation of isolated results difficult unless they are clearly abnormal.

To obviate the need for continuous infusion, the clearance of some substances normally present in blood such as urea and creatinine may be used to estimate GFR. The advantage of the urea clearance is the high concentration of urea in blood and urine and the ease of its chemical determination. The disadvantage is the dependence of its excretion on the rate of urine flow because urea is variably reabsorbed during passage through the nephron. At moderate rates of urine flow (2 to 6 ml/minute/1.73 m^2) approximately 60% of the filtered urea is excreted in the urine, and thus the clearance of urea represents approximately 60% of the actual GFR. The main advantage of the creatinine clearance is its relative independence of rate of urine flow. However, the low concentration of creatinine in the plasma of infants and young children makes the laboratory determination difficult. Since creatinine is excreted by tubular secretion as well as by glomerular filtration, its clearance may overestimate true GFR. Nevertheless the clearance of creatinine remains the best and most widely used method for measurement of GFR under usual clinical circumstances.

Recent progress in the mathematical analysis of multicompartmental models has made the calculation of GFR possible from the plasma disappearance curve of a substance injected intravenously as a single bolus. Substances excreted by glomerular filtration that can be labeled with isotopes, such as ^{125}I-iothalamate sodium and ^{51}Cr-labeled EDTA, as well as compounds that can be measured accurately by chemical methods, such as inulin, can be employed. This method obviates the need for the continuous infusion and timed urine collections that are so difficult to obtain in infants and small children. The amount of radioactivity provided by a single procedure is negligible. It appears, however, that the method overestimates the true GFR by approximately 30% during the first 2 weeks of life.

A reasonably accurate estimate of GFR can be calculated from the plasma concentration of creatinine by using empirically derived formulas. For preterm infants, the formula is: GFR = 0.33 L/Pcr, and for term infants it is: GFR = 0.45 L/Pcr, where GFR is given in milliliters per minute/1.73 m^2 of the body surface area, L is body length in centimeters, and Pcr is plasma creatinine concentration in milligrams per deciliter.

Many clinical situations require assessment of *renal acidifying mechanisms*. This is done by a determination of urinary pH and rates of excretion of titratable acid and ammonium during spontaneous metabolic acidosis or after administration of ammonium chloride and by performance of a bicarbonate titration. After the first few days of life, healthy infants are able to achieve a urinary pH as low as 5. In the presence of acidemia higher pH values cannot be considered normal.

PRESENTING SIGNS AND SYMPTOMS

It is characteristic of the seriously ill newborn to have nonspecific signs of disease, such as fever, irritability, vomiting, poor feeding, and failure to thrive. In such infants disease of the kidneys and urinary tract must be considered in the differential diagnosis. Certain signs that point directly toward urinary tract disease are discussed in this section.

Disorders of micturition

Ninety-two percent of healthy infants pass urine within the first 24 hours after birth and 99% by 48 hours. Often the first micturition takes place in the delivery room and goes unnoticed. If a newborn does not urinate within 72 hours, serious consideration should be given to the possibility of bilateral renal agenesis, urinary tract obstruction, or a renovascular accident. Of these possibilities, the most important to diagnose is obstructive uropathy, since it is amenable to surgical correction. Perinatal asphyxia has also been implicated as a cause of urinary retention in the newborn. Abnormalities in the volume of urine passed by the newborn each 24 hours are practically impossible to assess unless special attention is directed to the urinary system. The frequency of micturition varies from 2 to 6 times during the first and second days of life and from 5 to 25 times during the subsequent 24 hours. The daily urinary volume is 30 to 60 ml during the first and second days, 100 to 300 ml during the following week, and 30 to 50 ml/kg/24 hours subsequently.

Oliguria (urinary output below 15 to 20 ml/kg/24 hours) is most often a consequence of poor renal perfusion caused by shock, dehydration, hypoxia, and rarely renovascular accident. Oliguria or anuria also can result from malformation or urinary tract obstruction. Oliguria of prerenal origin, as in association with diarrheal disease, maternal diabetes, or RSD, usually can be identified by the high solute content of the urine, whereas in oliguria of true renal insufficiency urinary osmolality is low. Urinary retention can mimic anuria of renal origin. This retention can result from asphyxia, neurologic abnormalities such as meningitis or disturbances in the innervation of the bladder (e.g., meningomyelocele), or from obstruction resulting from phimosis, posterior urethral valves, balanoposthitis, or vulvovaginitis. Palpation of the urinary bladder and, if necessary, bladder catheterization may establish the diagnosis. *Polyuria* is most often the result of a defect in concentrating capacity, resulting from medullary abnormalities in renal dysplasia, from renal hypoplasia, or from nephronophthisis or medullary cystic disease. It also is seen in association with lack of antidiuretic hormone or nephrogenic diabetes insipidus.

Proteinuria

Small amounts of protein ordinarily pass through the semipermeable glomerular basement membrane. Although the concentration of these proteins in the proximal tubular fluid probably does not exceed 1 to 2 mg/dl, it can account for a significant loss of protein through the urinary tract. Under normal circumstances more than 95% of this protein is reabsorbed in the proximal tubule. The remainder of the nephron is also able to reabsorb protein, allowing only very small amounts to appear in the final urine. The protein content of the normal urine may be as high as 10 to 25 mg/24 hours in children: de Luna and Hullet reported a mean urinary excretion in newborns of 45 mg/24 hours. However, no more than 10% of full-term and 20% of premature babies have proteinuria in excess of 25 mg/24 hours. The average rates of protein excretion in newborns of various gestational ages are shown in Table 35-1. The usual semiquantitative methods of measurement do not detect concentrations of protein below 5 to 10 mg/dl; as a consequence, significant amounts of protein can pass unnoticed under conditions of diuresis.

Protein excretion in 12- to 24-hour urine collections should be determined whenever renal disease is suspected. Documentation of proteinuria is only the first step in the diagnosis of kidney disease, however, because

Table 35-1. Proteinuria in the newborn

Gestational age (weeks)	Number	Amount of protein ($mg/m^2/hour$)	
		Mean	Range
<28	5	0.86	0.2-1.3
30	12	2.08	0-9.4
32	15	2.32	0-5.2
34	15	2.48	0-13.1
36	17	1.27	0-4.6
40	26	1.29	0-6.1

nearly any form of injury, whether glomerular or tubular, can result in an increase in the excretion of protein. Furthermore nonrenal disorders such as cardiac insufficiency, venous obstruction, pulmonary edema, and fever may also be accompanied by transient proteinuria.

Hematuria

Blood can enter the urine at any point of the urinary system from the kidney to the urethra. In the normal newborn the excretion of RBCs in urine does not exceed 100/minute, or 75,000/12 hours. Red urine usually indicates hematuria, but it may also be caused by the presence of bile pigments, porphyrins, urate, or hemoglobin. The differential diagnosis between hemoglobinuria and hematuria is easy to make if the urine is examined soon after collection. After standing, RBCs may hemolyze, especially in hypotonic urine, and no longer appear as formed elements. When hematuria is diagnosed, its origin must be determined. Extraurinary sources must be excluded. The next step is to determine if the RBCs originate from the upper or the lower urinary tract. The presence of red cell or other types of casts is pathognomonic of parenchymal renal disease. Hematuria in the newborn may result from perinatal asphyxia, a renovascular accident, cortical and medullary necrosis, neoplasia, obstructive uropathy, infection, nephritis, or coagulopathy.

Leukocyturia

Leukocyturia is the presence of an abnormal number of WBCs in the urine. We do not expect to detect more than two to three WBCs per high-power field in a centrifuged specimen of urine. Littlewood found that bag specimens of well-mixed, uncentrifuged urine obtained from 600 newborns on the sixth or seventh day of life contained five or less WBCs per cubic millimeter in 98% of boys but only 56% of the girls. When urine was obtained by a clean-catch technique, only 6% of girls had abnormally high numbers of WBCs in the urine, suggesting perineal contamination of the bag specimens. The most common cause of leukocyturia is urinary tract infection. Increased rates of excretion of WBCs can accompany nephritis and nephrosis and can be indicative of any type of inflammatory process within the urinary tract. The number of WBCs in a urine specimen also varies with urinary flow rate, osmolality, and pH.

Edema

Accumulation of fluid in the interstitial space is a common manifestation of renal disease. It can be the consequence of a decrease in the colloid osmotic pressure of the plasma proteins, as in the nephrotic syndrome, or of a marked decrease in GFR, as in the various nephritides, congenital malformations, or the result of capillary damage. Almost invariably the pathophysiologic mechanism is complex, involving, in addition to physical factors, hypersecretion of aldosterone, and possibly inhibition of a natriuretic hormone. At an early stage the retention of fluid can be detected only by repeated accurate measurements of weight. Later swelling becomes obvious. It is generally stated that the edema of renal disease involves primarily the face and is soft, whitish, and painless. None of the characteristics, however, is specific.

Ascites is the intraabdominal accumulation of fluid. It can occur in the nephrotic syndrome, in which case the fluid has the character of an exudate with a protein content that usually does not exceed 500 mg/dl. A more common, although still unusual, cause of ascites in the newborn is obstruction of the lower urinary tract, particularly in association with posterior urethral valves. The ascitic fluid represents urine that has leaked through a ruptured pelvis or calyx. The differential diagnosis includes chylous ascites, ascites caused by syphilis, hepatobiliary obstruction, ruptured intraabdominal cyst, meconium peritonitis, and bile ascites.

Edema is found occasionally in premature babies during the first few days of life and results from shifts of fluid between body water compartments. *Late edema* develops among some newborns with birth weights below 1,300 gm and a young gestational age. It is frequently associated with cardiorespiratory problems. A difference is observed in the distribution of fluids between various body compartments, with the extracellular compartment being larger than normal in the edematous babies. Some of these cases have been shown to be associated with vitamin E deficiency and anemia (Chapter 32). Unusual causes of edema in the newborn include primary lymphedema (Milroy's disease), congenital lymphedema with gonadal dysgenesis, the syndrome of inappropriate antidiuretic hormone secretion, hyperaldosteronism, congenital analbuminemia, severe protein deficiency, protein-losing gastroenteropathy, scleredema, syphilis, erythroblastosis fetalis, and hereditary angioneurotic edema. The differential diagnosis also includes maternal diabetes (see Chapter 6).

Abdominal masses

Examination of the abdomen by palpation usually can be performed easily during the first 48 hours after birth, before air moves and fills the entire gut and before the tone of the abdominal muscles increases. For the rest of the first week of life, deep abdominal palpation may still be performed relatively easily after the relaxation of the abdominal musculature is induced by evoking the sucking reflex. The kidneys of the newborn are in a lower position than they are later in life, the right usually being lower than the left. The technique of examination de-

Table 35-2. Renal anomalies found in 56 of 10,000 newborn infants

Findings	Infants (number)	Percent of total
Horseshoe kidney	16	29
Renal agenesis, unilateral	15	27
Left	10	
Right	5	
Pelvic kidney	9	17
Left	5	
Right	4	
Hypoplastic kidney, unilateral	3	6
Renal agenesis, bilateral	2	4
Polycystic kidney	2	3
Multicystic kidney	2	3
Crossed renal ectopia	2	3
Double kidney, unilateral	2	3
Double collecting system, unilateral	1	2
Enlarged kidneys, bilateral	1	2
Wilms' tumor	1	2

scribed by Mussels and associates led to the suspicion of renal anomalies in 77 of 10,000 infants; 56 of these anomalies were confirmed by intravenous pyelography (Table 35-2). Conditions accounting for an apparently large kidney are hydronephrosis, tumor, thrombosis of the renal vein, cystic disease and rarely adrenal hemorrhage. A smooth mass is more likely to be the result of hydronephrosis or renal venous thrombosis, whereas an irregular surface suggests malformation or cystic disease. Ultrasonogram, renal scintiscan, cystoureterogram, or intravenous pyelogram is often helpful in the differential diagnosis. A renal venacavogram may be necessary when renal venous thrombosis is suspected.

RENAL INSUFFICIENCY AND RENAL FAILURE

Inadequacy of renal function may be a consequence of developmental anomalies, may arise from prerenal factors such as dehydration and shock, or may be the result of acquired disease of the kidneys. The following are the most common causes of acute renal failure in the newborn.

A. Prerenal
   1. Hypoxemia/asphyxia
   2. Hypotension
   3. Cardiac failure
   4. Hemorrhage
   5. Sepsis
   6. Hypokalemia
B. Renal
   1. Vascular accidents
   2. Nephrotoxins
   3. Pyelonephritis
   4. Nephritis
   5. Hypoplasia/dysplasia
   6. Renal agenesis
C. Postrenal
   1. Neurogenic bladder
   2. "Asphyxiated bladder"
   3. Obstructive uropathy

Clinical manifestations

Renal insufficiency often is suspected on the basis of oliguria or anuria, or it may be detected from biochemical examination of the blood. Urinary output less than 15 to 20 ml/kg/24 hours in the newborn (beyond the first few days of life) is oliguria. It is vital to determine if the cause of oliguria or anuria is *prerenal* (caused by inadequacy of the blood supply to the kidney), *postrenal* (urine is formed but not voided because of obstructive uropathy or a neurogenic bladder), or *true renal failure* (malfunction of the kidneys caused by intrinsic renal disease). This differentiation is readily made in many instances, but at times it can be rather difficult. The variables that are of help in the differential diagnosis between prerenal and true renal failure are listed in Table 35-3.

Transient renal impairment with oliguria and azotemia has been observed in asphyxiated infants, particularly in premature infants, as well as in infants with RDS, receiving assisted ventilation.

In such patients there is a decrease of circulating blood volume, cardiac output, and stroke volume, which causes a diminished blood flow and renal perfusion pressure and a significant drop in GFR, in the clearance of free water and salt, and in the excretion of hydrogen ions. Fluid retention may ensue causing hyponatremia. The severity of renal impairment reflects that of the respiratory system. Similar complications may be observed following cardiac surgery. When the cardiorespiratory function improves and cardiac output returns to above 70% of the normal value, renal function returns to normal.

Transient renal functional impairment is also seen in newborns with a compromised circulatory function caused by the persistence of a PDA who are treated with indomethacin. The renal effect of indomethacin usually lasts for 12 hours. If very severe, it may be offset by the administration of dopamine. The closure of PDA and discontinuation of the indomethacin are followed by normalization of renal function (Chapter 29).

Tolazoline, administered to infants with pulmonary hypertension, induces an intense vasoconstriction that decreases renal perfusion. The drug is excreted by the renal tubules through the organic base system, which matures rapidly during the postnatal period.

Administration of captopril in the latter weeks of pregnancy can cause in the newborn transient systemic hypotension that responds to vascular repletion. The use

Table 35-3. Differential diagnosis between prerenal and renal failure in newborns

	Prerenal	Renal
Urine sodium (mEq/L)	<10	>25
Fractional excretion of sodium (%)	<1.5	>3.5
Urine/plasma osmolarity	>1.5	<1.1
Urine/plasma creatinine	>30	<10
Urine/plasma urea	>30	<10

of large amounts of contrast agents, which are hypertonic, has caused renal venous thrombosis, renal ischemia, and renal insufficiency. Lower quantities of contrast material and adequate hydration can prevent most of these complications.

Gentamicin nephropathy may occur in neonates when serum gentamicin concentrations rise as a result of a primary renal disease process or when the administration of the drug is excessive. Cytoplasmic inclusion bodies have been observed in the proximal convoluted tubules by electron microscopy. The ability of the normal infant to excrete gentamicin is a function of gestational age. The relationship between gentamicin half-life and gestational age is probably exponential.

Increased numbers of cells and casts are found in the urinary sediment in all the conditions just listed. Tubular necrosis in postmortem material is, however, uncommon, and there has been poor correlation between clinical and pathologic findings. The observations suggest that functional impairment results from poor cortical perfusion and that tubular injury is a reflection of cortical ischemia rather than the cause of functional impairment.

Extensive roentgenologic or urologic investigation may be required to demonstrate the cause of postrenal failure. In prerenal failure, if insufficiency of the vascular volume is suspected, the response to administration of fluid may be helpful; isotonic saline in an amount of 15 to 20 ml/kg over 1 to 2 hours or on rare occasions mannitol (0.5 gm/kg in a 20% solution) in 20 to 30 minutes can be given intravenously. A prompt increase in urinary output suggests that additional fluids may be needed. If there is no response, care must be taken to avoid administration of excessive amounts of fluids to "force" a diuresis.

Treatment

Treatment of renal insufficiency in the neonate is similar to treatment in the older child. Consideration must be given to maintenance of the balance of water, electrolytes, and hydrogen ions and to provision of optimal nutrition. Acute renal insufficiency is treated by providing a fluid intake equal to insensible water loss (25 to 40 ml/kg/24 hours) plus urinary output. In the anuric or severely oliguric patient solute requiring urinary excretion is not given. In addition to withholding potassium, it may be necessary to reduce dangerously high plasma levels. When the concentration in plasma exceeds 5.5 mEq/L, polystyrene sodium sulfonate (Kayexalate), a Na^+/K^+ exchange resin, can be given (by enema or by mouth) in a starting dose of 0.5 to 1.5 gm/kg. This is repeated as needed. Moderate or severe degrees of acidemia are treated by administration of sodium bicarbonate. Peritoneal dialysis may be indicated in the infant with total renal failure lasting more than 7 to 10 days or when severe metabolic disturbances cannot be managed with conservative treatment.

In infants with chronic renal insufficiency adequate nutrition requires special attention. Mild to moderate degrees of renal insufficiency usually can be managed with proprietary formulas, such as PM 60-40 or SMA, as the sole source of nutrition. The usual dose of supplemental vitamins should be given. With lesser degrees of function other specific therapy may be required. Normal level of pH and bicarbonate in the blood should be maintained by administration of sodium bicarbonate. This dosage is adjusted according to the patient, starting with 1 to 2 mEq/kg/day and increasing as needed. Concentrations of calcium and inorganic phosphate in the blood should be measured frequently. Young infants fed low-phosphate diets usually do not develop hyperphosphatemia until they reach advanced stages of renal failure. Then calcium carbonate (100 to 200 mg/kg/day) should be given. Phosphate-binding gels (such as aluminum hydroxide [Amphojel]) are usually poorly tolerated and may produce anemia, osteomalacia, and encephalopathy. If the plasma calcium level falls significantly below normal, supplemental oral calcium (such as calcium gluconate [Calglucon]) is given in a dosage of 10 to 20 mg (of elemental calcium)/kg/day. If these measures are not successful in maintaining normal blood levels of calcium, dihydrotachysterol (DHT) in a dose of 0.125 to 0.5 mg/day or 1,25-dihydroxycholecalciferol (calcitriol), 0.125 to 1 μg/day, should be added to the treatment. Care must be taken to avoid too vigorous therapy and induction of hypercalcemia. The serum calcium × phosphate product should not be allowed to exceed 70.

In infants with severe uremia vomiting may be a most troublesome symptom. Treatment with one of the phenothiazine drugs may be helpful. Hypertension in infants is treated as in older children (Chapter 29). Every effort should be made to maintain normal blood pressure. Treatment is usually initiated with a diuretic, such as hydrochlorothiazide (1 to 2 mg/kg/day), to which hydralazine hydrochloride (1 to 2 mg/kg/day) in four divided doses), or propranolol (0.5 to 1 mg/kg/day in 2 to 4 divided doses) is added. Diazoxide, 5 mg/kg intravenously, is indicated whenever prompt decrease in diastolic pressure is required. Another drug used successfully for the treatment of hypertension in the newborn is labetalol, an α- and β-blocker drug with marked β-blocking preponderance. An initial intravenous dose of 1 to 2 mg/kg/hr given as a bolus followed by a 0.5 to 1.5 mg/kg/hr intravenous perfusion is effective in severe hypertension and can be used as an alternative for intravenous diazoxide. Labetalol may then be given orally for longer periods.

Nifedipine, 0.5 to 1 mg/kg/day orally, is a calcium channel blocker that has been used for the treatment of both hypertension and impaired cardiac function. Captopril, an angiotensin I–converting enzyme inhibitor, is started at 2.5 mg/day and then increased progressively until control of blood pressure is achieved. Since 60% of captopril is eliminated through the kidney, it should be used in lower, further spaced doses in infants with renal insufficiency. These additions to the more classical armamentarium of antihypertensive agents permit an efficient control of blood pressure in practically every patient.

Infants who cannot be maintained in a satisfactory metabolic state by dietary and medical therapy alone are candidates for dialysis. Peritoneal dialysis can be used for short periods but may be inadvisable if prolonged treatment is anticipated. Hemodialysis, although technically difficult, has been done in infants, and candidates for such therapy should be referred to appropriate centers.

Recently, continuous arteriovenous hemofiltration for several days, with low-volume cartridges (15 to 22 ml), has been found to be particularly suited to the small infant. Arterial access is by way of the femoral, brachial, or umbilical arteries, whereas venous return is by way of the jugular or umbilical veins. Flows of 10 to 20 ml/min and ultrafiltration of 1 ml/min can be achieved. Acidosis caused by excessive bicarbonate loss must be controlled during the procedure. Hemofiltration is insufficient in a severely catabolic subject in whom hyperalimentation and correction of the metabolic state must precede the procedure. Renal transplantation has not been successful in the neonate; but as experience is gained and technical problems are solved, it is likely to become available for even the smallest infants.

MALFORMATIONS

Renal maldevelopment

Clinical manifestations of renal maldevelopment in the newborn provide few clues to specific anatomic or etiologic diagnoses. Renal enlargement at times is detectable on abdominal palpation and occasionally causes abdominal distension. An inability to palpate the kidney may be an indication of renal agenesis or hypoplasia. Oliguria is less apparent than anuria, and abnormalities of micturition may be undetected. Unusual delay or difficulty in passing urine is reason for evaluating the renal status of the baby. Less specific clinical abnormalities include poor feeding, fussiness, vomiting, dehydration, and persistent respiratory difficulty. A high degree of suspicion is required to establish the diagnosis within the first few days of life. and clinical examination should include urinalysis, blood chemical determinations, ultrasonography, and excretory urography. Urologic examination may be necessary to evaluate abnormalities of the lower urinary tract. Therapy tends to be supportive rather than curative. Certain lesions are lethal because of irremediable parenchymal malformation or because of severe urinary tract obstruction, which often is associated with severe renal dysplasia. The infant mortality for all genitourinary malformations is approximately 10 per 100,000 live births, with 90% in the first month. Less severe degrees of malformation lead to partial functional impairment with few differentiating features. The objectives of prompt clinical recognition are to arrest and to prevent continuing deterioration, especially by identifying those cases amenable to surgical intervention.

Abnormalities of renal development considered in this section include agenesis (the lack of renal embryogenesis), dysplasia (an altered embryogenesis and abnormal differentiation of metanephric structures), and polycystic disease (a diffuse cystic alteration of the kidney without evidence of other maldevelopment). In renal agenesis one or both kidneys are lacking. The diagnosis of dysplasia rests on the finding of abnormally differentiated metanephric structures. Such abnormalities may affect all or part of a kidney, and examples of dysplasia encompass both extremely small, rudimentary kidneys and greatly enlarged kidneys. Some types are markedly cystic, but they must be differentiated from polycystic disease, even though the kidneys may be diffusely or totally affected. In polycystic disease there is a diffuse alteration of both kidneys without evidence of other maldevelopments.

Bilateral renal agenesis, the complete absence of both kidneys, is a common malformation, occurring in approximately 1 of 10,000 deliveries. This condition is characterized by certain external features, including an abnormal facies with a wizened look, known as Potter's facies (Fig. 35-4). The ears are low set, often with folded helices, the chin is small, and the nose seems to be turned down at the tip. A skin crease characteristically curves around the inner canthus of the eye and runs laterally over the cheek. The legs commonly are bowed and the feet clubbed. These abnormalities and vernix nodules (amnion nodosum) on the placental membranes have been attributed to oligohydramnios (Chapter 6), a state common to several malformations in which fetal production of urine is absent or markedly diminished.

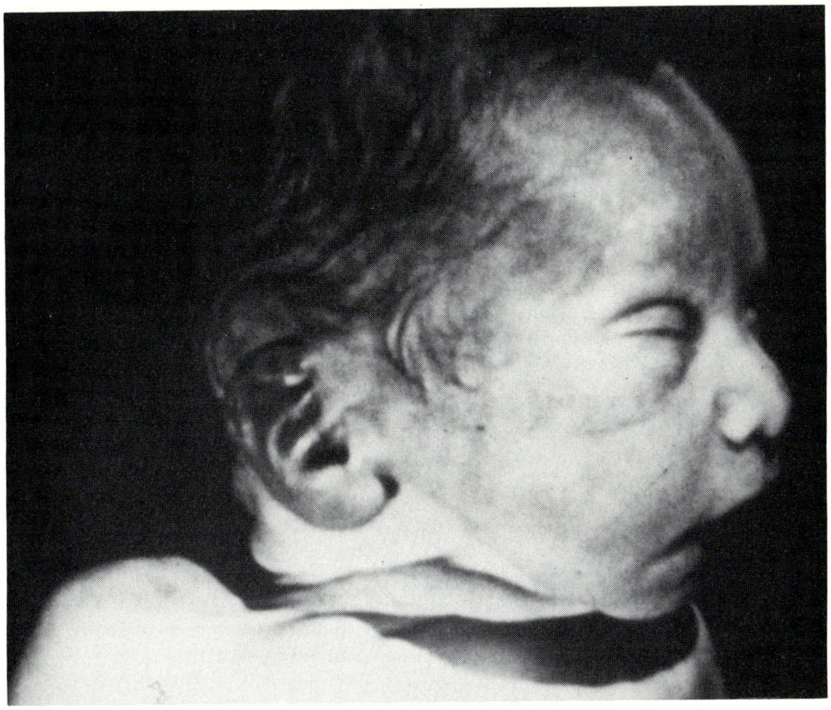

Fig. 35-4. Potter's facies. Characteristic are epicanthal folds, hypertelorism, low-set ears, mongoloid slant of the eyes, crease below the lower lip, and receded chin.

The presence of oligohydramnios, in addition to the failure to detect kidneys and bladder by ultrasonography, can help in the antenatal diagnosis of Potter's syndrome (Chapter 6).

Most cases are sporadic; a few familial instances and the increased incidence of urinary tract malformations among parents and siblings may suggest a genetic origin. The existence of an extra Y chromosome may be one of the predisposing factors, but most studies have shown normal karyotypes. Males are affected considerably more often than females. Infants with bilateral renal agenesis are often born prematurely by breech delivery and show evidence of intrauterine growth retardation. A large number of affected infants, perhaps 40%, are stillborn, and most of the others die shortly after birth. Severe respiratory distress caused by pulmonary hypoplasia with pneumothorax is the usual cause of death (Chapter 28). The lung may weigh as little as half the expected amount and often appears histologically to be underdeveloped. Occasionally infants surviving for several days appear to have died of renal failure.

Other frequently associated internal abnormalities include anal, duodenal, and esophageal atresia, colonic agenesis, and Meckel's diverticulum. The internal genitalia derived from the paramesonephric duct are usually defective or lacking (vas deferens and seminal vesicle in the male and the uterus and upper vagina in the female). The absence of one umbilical artery is often observed. Malformations of the caudal region of the fetus and sirenomelia have been described with some frequency; monsters characteristically have renal agenesis. Unilateral agenesis is a problem in newborns only in the event of injury, malformation, or disease of the remaining kidney.

Renal dysplasia, a condition of abnormal metanephric differentiation, is also a relatively frequent renal problem in the newborn. Severe bilateral dysplasia, like agenesis, is associated with oligohydramnios, Potter's facies, and death from respiratory distress or renal insufficiency within the first few days of life. Morphologic studies reveal two common anatomic forms of dysplasia: (1) aplastic kidneys, which are extremely small, sometimes barely recognizable buttons of tissue, or (2) multicystic kidneys, which are enlarged and grossly cystic. The two conditions are structurally similar, except for the cysts, and form the two ends of a spectrum of parenchymal malformation. The essential anatomic features are structural disorganization and histologic evidence of altered metanephric differentiation (i.e., metaplastic cartilage and abnormal ductal and nephronic elements). Cysts arise as terminal dilations of collecting tubules (Fig. 35-5). Since cyst formation is variable, the two conditions cannot always be sharply separated. Unilateral multicystic dysplasia is the most common form of cystic renal disease in the new-

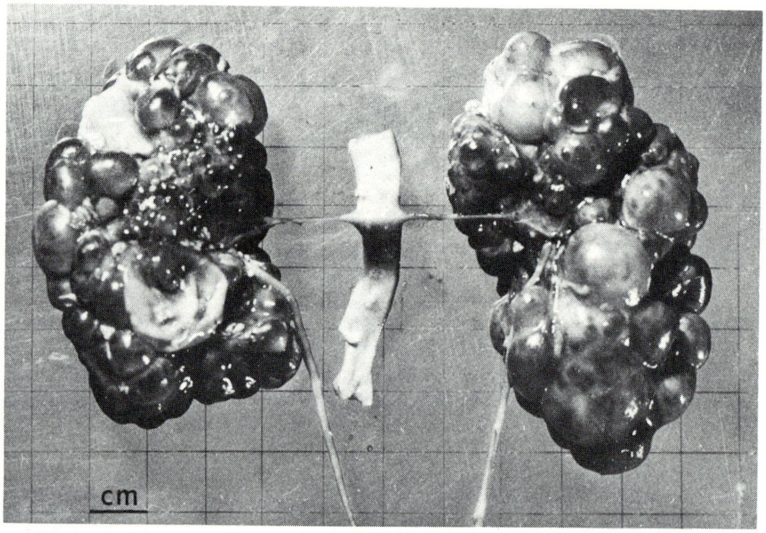

Fig. 35-5. Bilateral multicystic dysplasia in a newborn. The kidneys are enlarged and irregularly cystic, and the usual reniform configuration is barely apparent. Both ureters are atretic, and the renal arteries are extremely small. This condition is a cause of total renal nonfunction.

born, and bilateral multicystic dysplasia in our experience has been more common than polycystic disease. The condition is only rarely familial; it does occasionally occur in association with chromosome abnormalities such as trisomy D and trisomy E.

Renal dysplasia must be differentiated from *hypoplasia*, in which the parenchyma is deficient although normally formed. Simple renal hypoplasia without evidence of parenchymal maldevelopment is seldom severe enough to cause renal insufficiency during the neonatal period. The abnormality was reported to occur in the fetal alcohol syndrome. Oligonephronic hypoplasia, which also becomes clinically apparent in older children, is characterized by a decreased number but markedly increased size of nephrons.

Renal dysplasia is associated commonly with other anomalies of the urinary tract, with a frequency approximating 90%. Our experience has shown multicystic kidneys to be associated invariably with ureteral atresia and pyelocalyceal occlusion. The state of the ureter in renal aplasia has been more variable, partly because of the difficulty in drawing a sharp line between aplasia and less severe degrees of malformation. Consequently, descriptions of ureteral stenosis, ectopy, and dilation are not uncommon in reports of renal aplasia. With bilateral aplastic or multicystic kidneys, abnormalities of the lower urinary tract, such as small bladders and constricted or occluded urethras, may reflect the lack of urine production. Malformations of other systems, particularly cardiovascular and gastrointestinal, are common. The frequency of renal involvement in newborns with multiple malformations is high.

Both aplastic and multicystic kidneys can be unilateral. Unilateral aplasia is asymptomatic, and its disclosure in newborns is usually an incidental finding in the study of another condition. The differential diagnosis of unilateral nonvisualization includes agenesis and severe hypoplasia. Unilateral multicystic kidney, on the other hand, frequently appears as a flank mass, more often on the left side and more often in males. Enlargement is usually moderate, although cystic kidneys can weigh several hundred grams and cause fetal dystocia. Ultrasonography is at present the best tool for diagnosis both before and after birth. Prenatal diagnosis should be confirmed postnatally. Excretory urography usually fails to visualize the kidney, but high-dose urography ("total body opacification") may show selective concentration of contrast medium and partial opacification of the abnormal kidney. Endoscopic examination may reveal absence of an ureteral orifice or nonpatency of the ureter. Although the lesion seems to be relatively innocuous with only rare reports of associated hypertension, most of these kidneys are removed, perhaps unnecessarily. The risk of a malignant nephroblastoma, often cited to justify surgery, is very remote. The prognosis in very young infants is uncertain, mainly because the contralateral kidney is hypoplastic or hydronephrotic in more than one third of patients. A careful assessment is mandatory, therefore, to identify abnormalities correctable by reconstructive surgery. The lesion of multicystic dysplasia is not, however, a progressive disease to which the other kidney will eventually succumb. The contralateral kidney often is hypertrophied and seems to be unduly susceptible to infection and lithiasis later on in life.

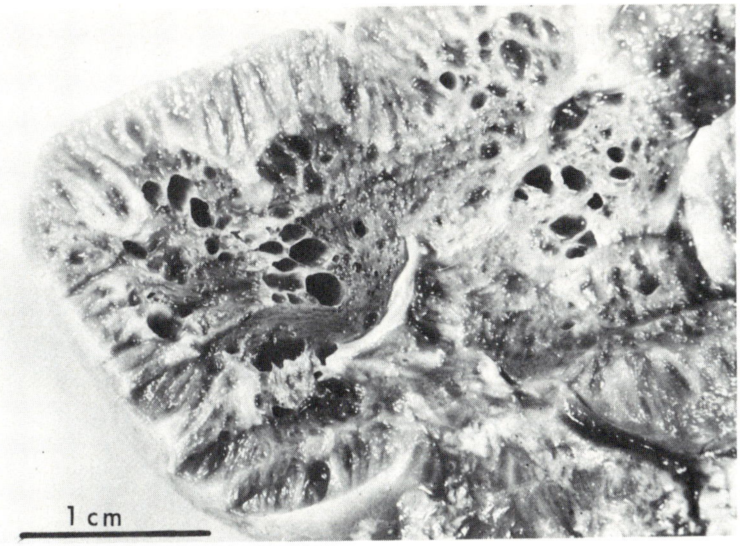

Fig. 35-6. Infantile polycystic disease in a newborn, showing the preservation of lobar structure and cortical-medullary differentiation. The cortex is thickened and spongy, and the medullary pyramids contain grossly apparent cysts; the latter are sometimes visible radiographically. (From Elkin, M., and Bernstein, J.: Clin. Radiol. **20:**68, 1969.)

An uncommon form of severe cystic dysplasia has been observed in newborns also suffering from cerebral malformation with encephalocele, eye anomalies, cleft palate, congenital heart disease, and polydactyly (an assortment of congenital abnormalities known as *Meckel's syndrome*). The clinical manifestations are nonspecific, and the severity of renal involvement is highly variable. The lesion superficially resembles polycystic disease in that the kidneys are enlarged and spongy, they retain a reniform configuration, and the pelves and ureters are patent. Gross examination, however, does reveal a lack of medullary differentiation and demarcation. Histologic examination discloses large numbers of cystic collecting tubules with little metanephric differentiation. Infants with less severe degrees of parenchymal maldevelopment with patent urinary tracts retain limited capacity to function; they have different clinical and pathologic implications because they can excrete urine and concentrate contrast media to some degree. Cortical dysplasia with variable functional impairment has been observed in association with *Jeune's syndrome* and *Zellweger's cerebrohepatorenal syndrome*. Trifling cortical cystic lesions in syndromes of multiple malformations do not affect the function of the kidneys.

Cystic dysplasia must be differentiated from *polycystic disease*, which occurs in autosomal recessive and autosomal dominant forms. Autosomal recessive disease is by far the more common in newborns and has long been known as *infantile* polycystic disease (IPCD). The typical *adult* polycystic disease (APCD) is autosomal dominant with a very high, although variable, degree of penetrance. Even though APCD is usually a disease of middle age, it may occur at any time throughout life and has been recognized recently to account for symptomatic neonatal disease with severe renal enlargement. Either type of polycystic disease can appear sporadically or can affect multiple siblings. The clinical features on occasion may suffice to differentiate the two, and renal biopsies are often decisive, but a carefully taken family history commonly provides the best clue of all.

IPCD appears in newborns as bilaterally, often asymmetrically enlarged, diffusely spongy kidneys. There is dilation of collecting tubules with relatively little fibrosis. IPCD is differentiateed from cystic dysplasia by the preservation of renal shape and landmarks and by the absence of dysplasia (Fig. 35-6). Microdissection has shown that the principal site of dilation is in the collecting tubules. Other portions of nephrons, including glomeruli, are variably dilated, and medullary collecting ducts are characteristically ectatic. In about one third of the patients polycystic changes are also present in the liver and only rarely in other organs.

Many affected infants are stillborn, and the majority of those born alive die within the first few days of life. The condition can be diagnosed clinically in infants with Potter's facies, abdominal enlargement, and a history of oligohydramnios. Abdominal distension at times has been severe enough to cause fetal dystocia. Respiratory distress and congestive heart failure are common. Electrocardiograms show left ventricular hypertrophy and left ventricular strain. Some infants have less severe renal insufficiency and survive the neonatal period. Ultraso-

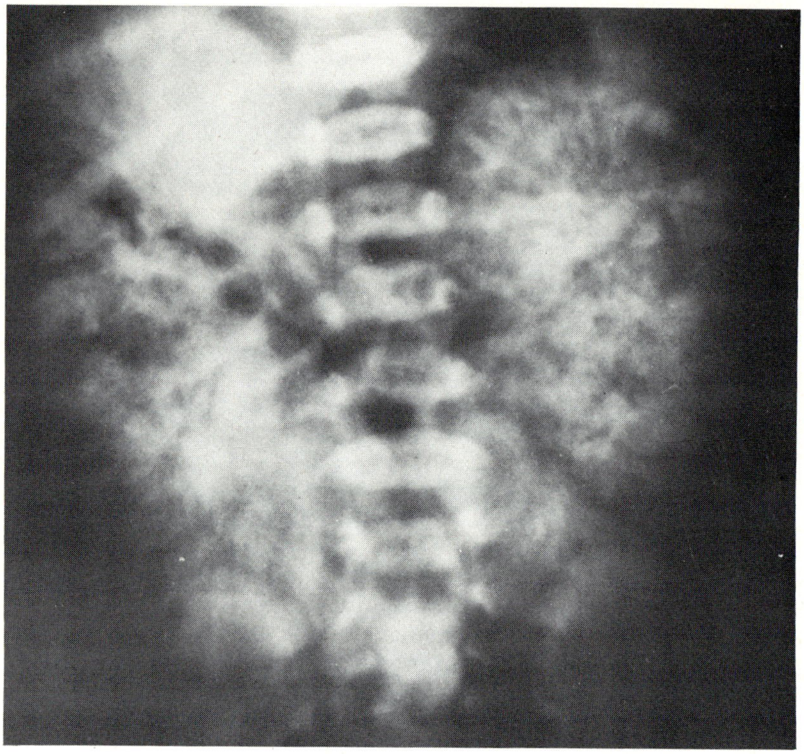

Fig. 35-7. Radiologic presentation of infantile polycystic disease. The irregular renal contour is caused by the presence of cysts.

nography should be diagnostic. Excretory urography discloses delayed concentration of dye, a mottled nephrogram, and retention of contrast medium in small cysts (Fig. 35-7). Urograms in infants with better preservation of renal function show medullary ductal ectasia, the characteristic roentgenographic picture of IPCD.

Variation in clinical expression and in anatomic findings is probably related to the natural history and progression of a single disease. It has also been suggested, however, that IPCD consists of several age-related, genetically different entities with somewhat differing morphologic characteristics and clinical expression. Infants surviving the neonatal period exhibit progressive renal insufficiency. Hypertension usually appears. Children also develop hepatic fibrosis and portal hypertension as part of the clinical spectrum of IPCD.

In adult polycystic disease the roentgenographic pattern is irregular; some babies with APCD *seem* to have had mild medullary ductal ectasia. The cysts reside in nephrons, and cortical involvement may be very patchy. Severe neonatal involvement is associated with severe glomerular dilation. Glomerular cysts cannot be regarded as synonymous with or pathognomonic of APCD, since they do occur in many other conditions, but symptomatic neonatal disease with glomerular cysts carries a presumptive diagnosis of APCD. The disease is always bilateral, although dysynchronous development may account for an initial temporary unilateral, asymmetric involvement. Urographic and ultrasonic studies of the parents of such babies have revealed typical APCD. There is a suggestion that the disease may stabilize in infants surviving the neonatal period, to progress in a more typical fashion during later childhood and early adulthood. Treatment of both forms of polycystic disease is supportive, with measures to avoid the lethal complications of hypertension and maintain a good nutritional status. Patients that survive the first year of life are candidates for kidney transplantation.

Urinary tract obstruction

Obstruction of the urinary tract produces dilation above the site of the lesion, and a retrograde rise in hydrostatic pressure may result in hydronephrosis and impairment of renal structure and function. Severe cases of obstruction are usually first seen in infancy, whereas milder ones are detected later in childhood. The presenting symptoms (such as failure to thrive, respiratory distress, abdominal distension, and vomiting) often are not specific, being a consequence of urinary tract infection or of renal insufficiency.

A distended bladder or a hydronephrotic kidney, when palpated, is the clue to diagnosis. Ultrasonography usually will provide confirmatory evidence.

Urinary obstruction in early fetal life may be a cause

of renal parenchymal maldevelopment. An example is the condition known as ectopic ureterocele, encountered mostly in females. The kidney and ureter are duplicated, and one of the ureters, generally the one that drains the upper pole of the duplex kidney, opens ectopically in the trigone or bladder neck, commonly terminating in an intravesical cyst. The obstructed segment of kidney is usually dysplastic and the normally draining segment usually is normally developed. On excretory urography the diagnosis is suggested by the duplication of the collecting system and a poorly visualized upper pole of the kidney. Visualization of only the lower pole reveals the "drooping lily" sign, with little or no evidence of function in the upper pole. Cystography, when done with a minimum of contrast material, discloses a filling defect in the bladder, corresponding to the ureterocele and the characteristic reflux into the lower ipsilateral urinary system. The diagnosis can be confirmed by cystoscopy. Treatment consists of heminephrectomy, ureterectomy, excision or uncapping of the ureterocele, and often reimplantation of the refluxing ipsilateral ureter.

Stricture of the ureteropelvic junction may cause giant hydronephrosis, which may be evident in the first month of life. Severe hydronephrosis often is associated with dysplastic parenchymal changes. On occasion the kidney associated with ureteral or ureteropelvic stricture is normally formed and merely hydronephrotic. In such instances we have theorized that the obstructive ureteral lesion was acquired relatively late in gestation, perhaps shortly before birth, since many of these specimens are only moderately hydronephrotic despite a complete ureteral obstruction, suggesting a course of short duration. Corrective surgery may preserve adequate renal function in the children with mild hydronephrosis, although the roentgenologic appearance of the collecting system scarcely improves with time.

When hydronephrosis is extreme and there is practically no functioning parenchyma, nephrectomy is indicated. In some of these patients, a hitherto discrete stricture of the ureteropelvic junction in the contralateral kidney may become apparent after nephrectomy.

Lower urinary tract obstruction is more common in the newborn and occurs almost exclusively in males. The most frequent cause is valvular obstruction of the posterior urethra; other obstructive lesions with similar effects of varying severity are urethral atresia, cysts of the verumontanum, and urethral diverticula. Clinical findings of outlet obstruction early in life relate to urinary retention and infection. Fetal ascites also has been described. Mild degrees of obstruction may go undetected for years, and severe obstruction results in vesical dilation, hydroureter, and hydronephrosis. Respiratory distress, abdominal distension, vomiting, and poor feeding are frequent complaints. Urethral obstruction occasionally is associated with aplasia or absence of the abdominal

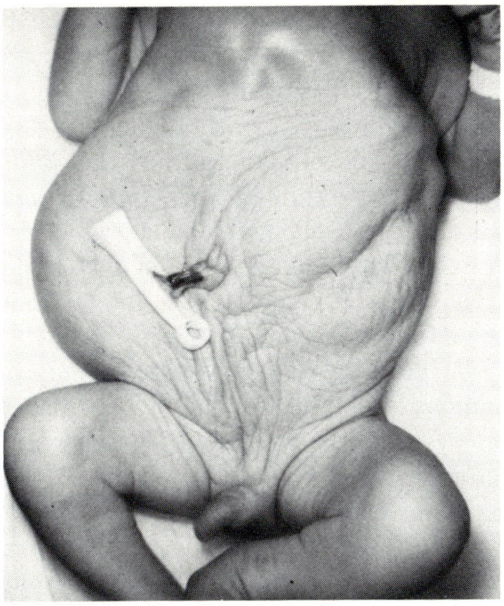

Fig. 35-8. Prune-belly syndrome. Note the distended, flabby abdomen wrinkled like a prune.

musculature, the "prune-belly" syndrome (Fig. 35-8).

Flank and midline suprapubic masses in a male infant are usually evidence of bladder neck or urethral obstruction, rather than of cystic kidneys. Poor urinary stream, dribbling, and other abnormalities in micturition are apparent early in life. There may be complete obstruction, with failure to pass urine at birth. Roentgenographic studies show the obstruction usually as a dilated prostatic urethra ending abruptly at cusplike valves. The bladder is heavily trabeculated, there is evidence of secondary hypertrophy, and vesicoureteral reflux is common. Infection is frequent, particularly after instrumentation. Obstructing valves are most often exaggerations of two mucosal folds that are normally continuous with the lower end of the verumontanum. Supraverumontanal folds and mucosal diaphragms are less common. Obstruction results not just from coaptation of the folds but also from a narrow, stenotic orifice between them. Infants with an obstruction severe enough to be apparent in the newborn period frequently have associated renal parenchymal maldevelopment, presumably resulting from the effect of obstruction on the developing kidney in utero. Renal dysplasia is much less often associated with milder degrees of obstruction apparent later in life. A case where there is evidence of bladder outflow obstruction should be considered an emergency, and immediate steps should be taken to establish the cause and remedy it. Any surgical procedure beyond catheterization of the bladder should await correction of fluid and electrolyte abnormalities. Some of these babies may need peritoneal dialysis before surgery. Removing the urethral obstruction is only part of the treatment. Ureteral dilation and tortuosity are additional causes of obstruction, frequently requiring draining of the upper urinary tract. Infection must be treated vigorously to prevent continuing renal damage, but the impairment imposed by parenchymal malformation cannot be reversed.

The condition known as the *prune-belly syndrome*, or *congenital absence of the abdominal musculature*, is first seen as a distended, flabby abdomen, which is creased like a prune (Fig. 35-8). Female infants comprise less than 5% of cases. The condition is rarely familial, and no cytogenetic abnormality has been detected. Failure of testicular descent is characteristic. Other congenital malformations, such as pulmonary hypoplasia, intestinal malrotation, and imperforate anus, also may be present. The ureters are dilated and tortuous, and the kidneys are hydronephrotic and often dysplastic, suggesting that a generalized developmental defect of abdominal parietes and mesenchyma is responsible for the entire syndrome. The bladder is large, dilated, and hypertrophied, indicating that infravesical obstruction also might be a causative factor. Aplasia or agenesis of the abdominal musculature has been seen in association with urethral atresia, urethral diverticulum, and posterior urethral valves. The bladder, however, is not trabeculated, despite its large capacity, and complete emptying can often be observed roentgenographically. The posterior urethra, also characteristically dilated, tapers at the membranous urethra, but evidence of increased resistance is lacking. Prostatic hypoplasia and sacculation of the prostatic urethra have been described in a series of male infants with the Eagle-Barrett triad—a synonym for the prune-belly syndrome, that is, abdominal muscular atrophy, cryptorchidism, and urinary tract malformation. The sacculation of the prostatic urethra may explain the secondary dilation of the urinary tract with its attendant nonspecific (dysplastic) effects on nephrogenesis. The transient intrapartum appearance of ascites common in obstructive nephropathies, as well as the reverse severe ectasia of the urinary tract, could cause an extreme abdominal distension that could be responsible for the characteristic severe muscular atrophy affecting mainly the muscles of the lower abdomen and the wrinkled appearance of the abdomen after resorption of the ascites. Prognosis is related to the degree of obstruction, the extent of associated renal dysplasia, and the control of infection. Reconstructive surgery has been of limited help, and vigorous antibacterial therapy is critical to prolonging survival. Drainage of the upper tract may be necessary to control infection and prevent continuing damage to kidneys that are frequently dysplastic. When there is associated urethral atresia, the prognosis is poor.

The Ochoa syndrome is also characterized by lower urinary tract obstruction in association with a peculiar facies. The condition is probably transmitted as an autosomal dominant trait.

Other abnormalities of the newborn, such as *exstrophy of the bladder*, *epispadias*, and *neurogenic bladder* caused by meningomyelocele (Chapter 27), are problems of urologic management and require careful control of infection.

Vesicoureteral reflux

The prevalence of vesicoureteral reflux (VUR) among healthy newborns is unknown but appears to be low. None was detected in one series of 26 full-term and 66 premature newborns. A review of the literature revealed a rate of 0.4% among 1,015 normal infants and children. However, the number increases sharply in newborns with urinary tract infection. Among 160 newborns subjected to roentgenologic investigation because of bacteriuria, 61 were found to have VUR, 46 of a moderate or severe degree. In 77% of the 41 children monitored, the reflux disappeared spontaneously, in most of them during the first year of life. The long-term prognosis of infants with VUR depends on the severity of the abnormality and its association with pyelonephritis. Renal scarring, hypoplasia of the kidney, and hypertension are commonly encountered among children with severe grades of reflux. There is a good likelihood that segmental hypoplasia (Ask-Upmark kidney) is a form of reflux nephropathy. Based on current knowledge a voiding cystourethrogram is indicated in any newborn with bacteriuria associated with fever or persisting beyond 1 week of age. Because of a high familial incidence of VUR, there are some who advocate screening in siblings of children with a history of reflux. The treatment of VUR may be medical (prophylaxis of urinary tract infection) in the mild and moderate degrees of reflux and must be surgical in severe forms.

NEPHRITIS

Acute glomerulonephritis can occur in the neonatal period. Its principal cause today is congenital syphilis, a disease of resurgent clinical importance. Congenital luetic nephritis may result in the nephrotic syndrome in newborns and young infants. Other infants may have the clinical findings of hemorrhagic nephritis with hematuria, cylindruria, and moderate azotemia, accompanied by mild to moderate proteinuria. Pathologic studies have shown a proliferative glomerulonephritis with extramembranous deposits of immunoglobulin and complement. Mesangial proliferation may be minimal, despite immune deposits corresponding to a membranous nephropathy. The glomerular lesion is frequently accompanied by prominent cortical infiltrates of plasmacytes and lymphocytes, which may be strong clues to the diagnosis in renal biopsies. The clinical diagnosis is usually based on the demonstration of other stigmata of syphilis and on positive serologic tests (Chapter 31). Antibiotic therapy is ordinarily effective in treating the disease and in reversing the nephrotic syndrome. A proliferative glomerulonephritis with subendothelial deposits of immunoglobulin has been described in congenital toxoplasmosis. It too has been associated with the nephrotic syndrome. Congenital systemic infection with cytomegalovirus, herpesvirus, or rubella virus may cause an interstitial nephritis with tubular lesions of little clinical importance. Glomerular necrosis has been described in cytomegalic inclusion disease.

Chronic glomerulonephritis has been described in several necropsy studies. The patients were severely ill newborns, and in at least one report a rapidly progressing anemia suggested a hemolytic-uremic syndrome. Although studies of renal function have been lacking, it is presumed that the infants suffered from renal insufficiency. In some infants the lesion has been associated with the nephrotic syndrome. The glomeruli were either sclerosed or affected by severe epithelial proliferation and crescent formation. Tubular atrophy and cast formation, interstitial inflammation, fibrosis, and vascular sclerosis complete the picture. The lesion must be differentiated from *congenital glomerulosclerosis*, a process of glomerular involution and hyalinization that takes place in many and perhaps all newborns. Some cases reported as chronic glomerulonephritis may have been examples of severe diffuse mesangial sclerosis, as described in the section on congenital nephrotic syndrome. The number of sclerotic glomeruli found incidentally in newborns dying of diseases other than renal has been as high as 20%, although a figure of 5% to 10% is most commonly accepted. These glomerular changes may be associated with slight focal tubular atrophy; more extensive changes reflect some other disease.

THE NEPHROTIC SYNDROME

The characteristic features of the nephrotic syndrome—proteinuria, hypoproteinemia, hyperlipidemia, and edema—are encountered rarely during the neonatal period. When present, they are usually the expression of the congenital nephrotic syndrome, a familial disease with an autosomal recessive mode of inheritance.

Congenital nephrotic syndrome

Clinical manifestations

Most of the cases of congenital nephrotic syndrome have been reported in Finland, where at least 130 families have been identified. Some 24 families, comprising 40 children, have been reported from the United States, and many other questionable cases have been described. The onset of the disease occurs during intrauterine life, as evidenced by large and abnormal placentas, qualitative similarity between protein content of the amniotic fluid and fetal urine, delivery of small for gestational age and premature babies in about 90% of the cases, faulty intrauterine calcification of the bones, erythroblastosis, and polycythemia (probably reflecting intrauterine anoxia). About 95% of the cases become clinically manifest during the first 8 weeks of life, with most of the children showing proteinuria from the very first day. Pallor, mottling of the skin, cyanosis, and respiratory distress are accompanying symptoms. Protein electrophoresis shows low levels of albumin and IgG and high levels of α-globulin, mostly α_1-macroglobulin.

Prenatal diagnosis is possible because the concentration of alpha-fetoprotein is elevated in amniotic fluid and in maternal serum.

Pathology

The characteristic lesion of the Finnish type of congenital nephrotic syndrome is the so-called microcystic kidney, which has been seen in approximately one third to one fourth of reported cases (Fig. 35-9). The cysts consist of dilated tubules located near the corticomedullary junctions; there is no evidence that they represent a primary abnormality in renal tubular development. Although initially the glomeruli may be only minimally altered, except for ultrastructural evidence of fusion of the foot processes, they undergo progressive sclerosis. Immunofluorescent studies have been generally negative. Another type of lesion found in early infantile nephrotic syndrome is diffuse mesangial sclerosis; the glomeruli are small and compact, containing increased ma-

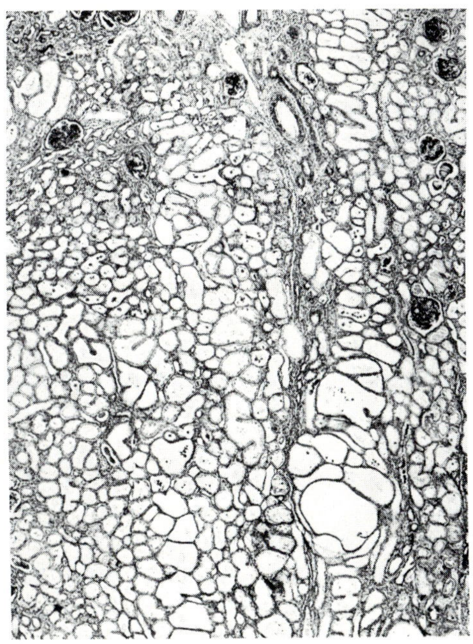

Fig. 35-9. Congenital nephrotic syndrome. Microscopic examination discloses sclerotic and proliferative changes in the glomeruli. The collecting tubules, particularly those near the corticomedullary junction, are dilated to microcystic proportions. (PAS stain; ×40.)

trix with few patent capillary loops, and eventually undergo complete sclerosis. In some patients the glomerular lesions are similar to those seen in later childhood and include minimal change, segmental glomerulosclerosis, and membranous nephropathy. Such patients respond to therapy much like older children do.

Etiology

The cause of the congenital nephrotic syndrome is unknown. Toxic factors such as mercury and phenol, infectious agents such as *Escherichia coli* and *Toxoplasma*, and drugs such as corticosteroids have been considered but never confirmed. An immunologic process has been incriminated in the pathogenesis. Skin transplanted from infants born with this disease to their mothers undergoes accelerated rejection, suggesting intrauterine sensitization to the fetus. However, this response could be the consequence of fetal-maternal transfusion resulting from placental damage. In nine patients with the congenital nephrotic syndrome, γ-globulin and complement were demonstrated by immunofluorescent techniques in renal tissue obtained by biopsy or autopsy. These results have been challenged by Hoyer and associates and by Rapola and Savilahti.

Treatment

The condition is resistant to all forms of therapy. Approximately 75% of the patients succumb, most to infection, during the first 6 months of life. Isolated children have been reported with longer survival times. Recent attempts have been made to perform dialysis and transplants in these children.

Other forms of the nephrotic syndrome

Congenital syphilis, congenital toxoplasmosis, and cytomegalic inclusion disease are associated with a nephrotic syndrome in early life. A heterogeneous group of patients has been included under the name atypical familial nephrosis.

Congenital syphilis accounts for an increasing number of newborns with the nephrotic syndrome. The clinical presentation and the morphologic changes in the kidney are described in Chapter 31. Important differences from congenital nephrosis, which must be considered in the differential diagnosis, are the high levels of IgG in the serum (in contrast to the low levels encountered in congenital nephrosis) and the good response to antibiotic therapy. Congenital syphilis also must be differentiated from *congenital toxoplasmosis*, in which serum immunoglobulin values may be normal.

Cytomegalovirus infection has been associated occasionally with a nephrotic syndrome. None of the patients manifested symptoms of cytomegalic inclusion disease, such as jaundice, petechiae, or central nervous system disturbances.

Atypical familial nephrotic syndrome includes children with the nephrotic syndrome who are within the age range of congenital nephrosis but show a benign course, and children who have the onset of the disease later in life but show changes characteristic of the congenital type of nephrosis. No such case has been described in Finland. Many children with this syndrome are offspring of related parents; some of them are identical twins; and in all families more than one sibling has shown signs of the disease.

ANOMALIES OF RENAL TUBULAR FUNCTION

Dysfunction of the renal tubule can result from a primary defect in the transport ability of the renal tubular membrane or can be a result of a systemic disorder or disease. Primary defects include conditions such as renal glucosuria, renal tubular acidosis (RTA), renal phosphaturia, and the renal aminoacidurias. The latter group includes, among others, cystinosis, glycogen storage disease, Wilson's disease, galactosemia, heavy metal poisoning, hyperglobulinemia, and idiopathic and secondary hypercalcemia. The causes of most of these anomalies of renal tubular transport are unknown; some are inherited, a few are self-limited, many are inconsequential, some have a serious impact on growth and development, and some are amenable to therapy. This is a heterogeneous group of conditions that have as their common denominator one or more disturbances in the function of the renal tubule.

Cystinuria, Hartnup disease, familial iminoglycinuria, hereditary glycinuria, glucoglycinuria, and congenital lysinuria, although present from birth, usually become symptomatic beyond the newborn period. The same is true for tubular disorders, such as hereditary hypophosphatemia (familial vitamin D–resistant rickets), pseudohypoparathyroidism, and most forms of the Fanconi syndrome, including cystinosis. The availability of screening tests for these anomalies makes possible their early recognition and treatment. Only some of the major syndromes particularly pertinent to the newborn period are discussed here.

Renal glucosuria

Glucose does not appear in the urine unless its concentration in blood reaches a level that is about twice normal. In patients with renal glucosuria the renal threshold for this substance is diminished, and glucose is excreted in the urine at normal or slightly elevated blood concentrations. Depending on the level of the threshold, glucose is found in the urine either at all times or only after a load of carbohydrates. Two forms of renal glucosuria are described. In type A the defect involves a depression in both the threshold and the maximum capacity to reabsorb glucose (T_mG). Type B is characterized by a low threshold and a normal T_mG. Since the blood level at which T_mG is observed is far removed from the threshold, the magnitude of the glucosuria relates little to the level of the T_mG. No evidence exists regarding a defect in the intestinal transport of glucose in patients with renal glucosuria, although such an association has been documented in the familial glucose-galactose malabsorption syndrome.

The defect in renal glucosuria is present from birth and may account for otherwise unexplained episodes of hypoglycemia. The inheritance in most patients is autosomal dominant, although an autosomal recessive mode of transmission also has been described. Results of examination of the renal tubular structures by light microscopy are normal; alterations in the mitochondria have been found on electron micrographs. No therapy is necessary other than recognition of the condition, avoidance of confusion with diabetes mellitus, and provision of a normal intake of carbohydrates.

Several patients with renal glucosuria have developed diabetes mellitus later on in life.

The aminoacidurias

The amino acids normally present in the glomerular filtrate are actively reabsorbed, almost completely, in the proximal tubule. The fraction that escapes reabsorption can be detected in the urine by paper or column chromatography. The excretory pattern varies with age, both quantitatively and qualitatively. In normal full-term infants ranging in age from 16 days to 4 months there is a relatively high fractional excretion of threonine, serine, proline, glycine, and alanine, suggesting immaturity of only certain transport mechanisms.

An abnormal excretion of amino acids in urine can result from (1) an increase in the filtered load that exceeds the reabsorptive capacity of the tubule, (2) competition of two or more amino acids for the same transport site, or (3) a selective or generalized defect of the transport system. In renal aminoacidurias plasma amino-acid concentrations are normal. Five specific systems for the tubular transport of amino acids have been described. The first system carries dibasic amino acids (lysine, arginine, and ornithine) and is defective in a condition known as *hyperdibasic aminoaciduria*. In *cystinuria*, in addition to these amino acids, excessive amounts of cystine are excreted. The second transport mechanism is responsible for reabsorption of the acidic amino acids (glutamic and aspartic acids). No human defect in the renal transport of glutamic acid has been identified, but a few patients with aspartyl-glycosaminuria have been described. The third pathway transports imino acids (proline and hydroxyproline) and glycine and is defective in *familial iminoglycinuria*. The remainder of the neutral amino acids share a common transport site, as evidenced by the fact that they are all excreted in excess in *Hartnup disease*. Studies of patients with β-alaninemia have served to define the fifth transport system, that for the β-amino compounds, such as β-alanine, β-isobutyric acid, and taurine.

A number of conditions are characterized by the excretion in the urine of abnormal amounts of most, if not all, amino acids. In patients with Fanconi's syndrome the impairment in proximal tubular reabsorption extends to other substances, such as glucose, phosphate, bicarbonate and uric acid. In most cases the diagnosis of aminoaciduria cannot be made safely before 4 months of age, because the excretion of amino acids is high in early postnatal life. Nevertheless, their existence can be suspected, particularly when the disease is present in family members. In some instances a prenatal diagnosis can be made by amniocentesis. Many of these abnormalities are inherited as autosomal recessive traits, and a few are X linked.

Cystinosis

Cystinosis, inherited as an autosomal recessive trait, is characterized by accumulation of cystine in the lysosomal fraction of metabolically active cells. Plasma cystine levels are normal. The symptoms result from involvement of several organ systems. The infantile form, which is the most severe, has been detected as early as the first month of life by the presence of aminoaciduria in apparently normal siblings of affected children. Thirst, vomiting, diarrhea, dehydration, unexplained fever, and failure to thrive usually become evident much later in infancy. If the child does not die of infection, acidosis, or hypokalemia, renal insufficiency ultimately occurs.

A reliable method of making a positive diagnosis is the determination of the cystine content of peripheral leukocytes, which in the infantile form of the disease is markedly elevated (up to 100 times normal). Treatment is symptomatic. Observation of patients who have undergone kidney transplantation indicates deposition of cystine in the renal interstitium and not in the tubular cells, as is characteristic of cystinosis.

Oculocerebrorenal dystrophy (Lowe's syndrome)

Lowe's syndrome is characterized by multiple tubular dysfunctions, mental retardation, and severe congenital ocular anomalies. The condition is transmitted by a sex-linked recessive gene; all but four of the affected subjects reported were males. The female cases probably represent a different entity. The time of onset varies from the first few months to late childhood. Cataracts, frequently coexisting with glaucoma, are prominent features. The involvement of the nervous system is manifested by severe mental retardation, muscular hypotonia, and tendinous areflexia. Cryptorchidism is common. The renal disorder is characterized by proteinuria, aminoaciduria, and sometimes glucosuria. Therapy is symptomatic. Prognosis depends on the severity of the mental retardation.

Pseudohypoaldosteronism

Pseudohypoaldosteronism results from unresponsiveness of the renal tubule to aldosterone. The consequence is abnormal loss of sodium, hyponatremia, hyperkalemia, and metabolic acidosis. Plasma renin activity and aldosterone concentration are high. The mode of inheritance is sex linked. The symptoms (anorexia, vomiting, failure to thrive) appear 2 to 3 weeks after birth. Differentiation from the salt-losing form of adrenal hyperplasia is made by appropriate investigation of steroid metabolism (Chapter 37, part five). In pseudohypoaldosteronism the excretion of 17-ketosteroids and 17-hydroxysteroids is normal, whereas the excretion of aldosterone is very high. Treatment is urgent and consists of administration of large quantities of sodium chloride. The need for salt supplementation is very significant in premature infants with this condition, but it seems to diminish with age.

Nephrogenic diabetes insipidus

Nephrogenic diabetes insipidus is characterized by insensitivity of the renal tubule to vasopressin. Most of the homozygotes are male, suggesting a sex-linked mode of inheritance. However, asymptomatic females have been reported. Symptoms appear shortly after birth; dehydration, unexplained fever, and failure to thrive are prominent. Polyuria and polydipsia are usually detected later. A significant delay in psychomotor development often occurs, apparently caused by chronic dehydration. The pathogenesis is unknown. Differential diagnosis should include absent or defective antidiuretic hormone, bilateral renal hypoplasia, hydronephrosis, medullary cystic disease, oligomeganephronia, hypercalciuria and hypercalcemia, hypokalemia, and hyperkaliuria. Laboratory tests reveal hyperelectrolytemia with dilute urine. Vasopressin is ineffective. A water-deprivation test should be avoided.

The prognosis is good if the diagnosis is made early in life. Therapy consists of administration of sufficient fluids to maintain normal hydration. In infants the need for water can be minimized by giving a solute-poor milk. Thiazide diuretics have been shown to be effective in decreasing urinary volume and improving concentrating ability, although their mechanism of action remains unclear. Indomethacin, an inhibitor of prostaglandin synthesis, was reported to improve the concentrating ability and act synergistically with chlorothiazide.

A variant of Bartter's syndrome with prenatal onset, polyhydramnios, and premature labor has been described recently. Failure to thrive, hyperthermia, vomiting, and diarrhea are associated with urinary potassium wastage, hypokalemia, hypercalciuria, and nephrocalcinosis. These infants have a markedly elevated urinary secretion of both prostaglandin E_2 and prostaglandin F_2; however, they differ from the infants with the classical Bartter's syndrome in having a normal tubular reabsorption of chloride. Treatment with indomethacin and with fluid and eletrolyte replacement markedly improve the status of the patients. An autosomal recessive mode of heredity has been postulated.

Renal tubular acidosis

Renal tubular acidosis (RTA) is a defect in the reabsorption of bicarbonate or in the secretion of hydrogen ion that is not related to a decrease in GFR. RTA has three forms: the *proximal* type, resulting from the inability of the kidney to maintain a normal threshold for bicarbonate; the *distal* type, resulting from the inability of the kidney to establish an adequate gradient of secretion of hydrogen; and a *mixed* form.

Proximal renal tubular acidosis

Proximal RTA can appear as an isolated defect or coexist with other proximal tubular anomalies, as in some variant of Fanconi's syndrome or oculocerebrorenal syndrome. The primary form is characterized clinically by failure to thrive and chemically by hyperchloremic acidosis. The great majority of patients are male. A transient form of proximal RTA has also been observed in newborns during or following acute infections. This is self-limited but can account for transitory, "unexplained" metabolic acidosis.

The nature of the defect is unknown. The diagnosis is made by demonstration of a low renal threshold for bicarbonate and a normal renal acidifying capacity. The former is determined by a study of bicarbonate reabsorption during continuous infusion of increasing amounts of bicarbonate. There is normal variation in threshold with age; the infant has a bicarbonate threshold of 20 to 22 mmol/L, whereas in the adult the threshold is 24 to 26 mmol/L. The threshold in the premature infant appears to be lower, perhaps 18 to 20 mmol/L. The ability of the kidney to acidify the urine is tested by administration of an acid load (ammonium chloride) and a test of the pH of the urine. Although during the first few days of life the newborn may not be able to lower urinary pH below 6.5 or 6.0, beyond this period urinary pH should reach a value of at least 5.0 after an acid load.

Children with primary proximal RTA do not have a defect in urinary concentration and do not show evidence of rickets, urolithiasis, or nephrocalcinosis.

Therapy consists of administration of sodium citrate or bicarbonate, usually in amounts exceeding 5 mEq/kg/day. The solution should be administered at frequent intervals, since bicarbonate will leak into the urine shortly after being administered, as soon as the plasma bicarbonate exceeds the renal threshold. The condition is self-limited; most patients with primary RTA recover by 2 to 3 years of age.

Distal renal tubular acidosis

Distal RTA is a persistent defect in urinary acidification that usually occurs in isolated cases but may be inherited as an autosomal dominant trait.

The condition affects females predominantly and tends to become overt after the age of 2 years. However, the onset often can be traced to the first months of life by a history of vomiting, anorexia, constipation, polyuria, dehydration, and failure to thrive. Beyond infancy, polyuria, growth retardation, nephrocalcinosis, nephrolithiasis, and interstitial nephritis are the prevailing features. Rickets or osteomalacia, commonly encountered in adults with distal RTA, occurs rarely in children.

The nature of the defect that prevents the kidney from establishing an adequate gradient of hydrogen ion between peritubular blood and tubular fluid is unknown. Evidence that the defect is intrinsic to the renal tubular epithelium is provided by the normal behavior of the transplanted kidney in 15 patients with distal RTA.

The diagnosis is made by observation of a urinary pH consistently above 6.5 or 7.0, despite spontaneous or induced metabolic acidosis.

Therapy consists of administration of sodium bicarbonate, usually in amounts of 1 to 3 mEq/kg/day. The dose may need to be higher in the newborn. Some patients may require supplemental potassium as well. The dose is adjusted to maintain blood pH and bicarbonate within normal limits to ensure a maximum opportunity for normal growth. In addition, therapy is directed toward prevention of nephrocalcinosis; the dose should be sufficient to keep the excretion of calcium in urine below 2 mg/kg/24 hours.

Although primary distal RTA is a permanent defect, when it is correctly treated, the prognosis for growth and prevention of renal insufficiency is good.

RTA type IV and pseudohypoaldosteronism

Severe metabolic acidosis in the neonatal period may also be the result of an enzymatic defect in mineralocorticoid synthesis, pseudohypoaldosteronism (renal tubular unresponsiveness to aldosterone) and a variety of other forms of renal tubular acidosis grouped under the term of RTA type IV. In the more severe forms of RTA type IV, sodium wasting, dehydration, hyperchloremic metabolic acidosis, and hyperkalemia may be fatal unless treatment is initiated with sodium bicarbonate, sodium chloride, and, where indicated, mineralocorticoids. Idiopathic pseudohypoaldosteronism, a disease that affects predominantly males, usually improves with age. An autosomal recessive form of combined proximal and distal RTA in infants with carbonic anhydrase II deficiency has been described. It is associated with osteopetrosis, facial and dental anomalies, cerebral calcification, mental retardation, and restrictive lung disease. Intrauterine growth and prenatal ultrasound are normal. Severe acidosis appears within a few weeks followed by osteopetrosis. The obligatory heterozygotic parents have a 50% deficiency of the carbonic anhydrase measured in RBC hemolysates.

INFECTION OF THE URINARY TRACT

See also Chapter 31.

Asymptomatic bacteriuria has been found in less than 1% of apparently healthy full-term infants; there may be a slight male preponderance. By contrast, studies in premature infants have demonstrated bacteriuria, confirmed by suprapubic puncture, in 2% to 5%. A lower incidence of urinary tract infection has been observed in circumcised than in uncircumcised males younger than 1 month of age (0.11% versus 1.12%).

Diagnostic methods

A variety of methods are available for collection of urine from the newborn for urinalysis and bacteriologic examination. Measures must be taken to avoid cellular and bacterial contamination. The simplest method involves careful cleansing of the external genitalia with soap and water, thorough rinsing to ensure removal of all soap residue, and application of a *sterile plastic bag;* Lincoln and Winberg also have suggested irrigation of the preputial folds of male infants. After application of the bag the baby is checked every 10 to 15 minutes so that the bag can be removed shortly after urination has occurred. If a stool is passed, or if the bag has been in place for more than 1 hour, the bag is removed, the baby is cleansed again, and a fresh bag is affixed.

Catheterization of the bladder is difficult to perform in the neonate because of the normally occurring phimosis of the male and the obscure position of the urethral orifice in the female. If a "bag" specimen is inadequate, a urine specimen should be obtained by suprapubic puncture of the bladder rather than by bladder catheterization.

Suprapubic aspiration of urine from the bladder is easily performed with 24- or 25-gauge, 1-inch needle. The needle is directed perpendicular to the skin, in the midline, 1 inch above the symphysis. In 10% to 15% of attempts no specimen will be obtained because insufficient urine is present in the bladder. Minimum degrees of hematuria are observed transiently in some infants and should be of no concern. This method may be contraindicated for infants with bleeding or clotting disorders.

There are insufficient data on what level of bacterial concentration in a clean-voided, or "bag," urine represents the statistical dividing line between contamination and true bacteriuria in infants. Most workers have viewed counts in excess of 10^4 organisms/ml with suspicion, requiring that repeated examinations consistently demonstrate equal or greater numbers of the same organism to confirm the diagnosis. We have had the experience, however, of meeting these criteria only to find sterile urine from a suprapubic aspirate. Initial screening therefore should be performed on bag urine; those with bacterial counts in excess of 10^4/ml should be repeated, and those found again to be in excess of 10^4/ml should be examined by suprapubic aspiration. Examination of urine collected by the bag technique will reveal no bacterial growth or less than 10^4 organisms/ml in 70% to 90% of cases, thus excluding these infants from further consideration. Infants with bacterial counts above 10^4/ml are candidates for repeat examination, although with this method even counts above 10^5/ml most often prove to be caused by contamination. It is assumed that any bacterial growth in urine obtained by suprapubic aspiration represents true bacteriuria, thus obviating the need for quantitation. Nevertheless, since most infected urines contain bacteria in excess of 10^5 or even 10^6/ml, quantitation of bacteria in suprapubic aspirates can be helpful in that concentrations below 10^4/ml or 10^3/ml must be viewed as possibly representing contamination, despite the technique of collection. The great majority of cultures from infected infants reveal one organism; mixed cultures therefore are also suggestive of contamination.

In the infant about to be treated with antibiotics, urine should be collected by suprapubic aspiration rather than by bag technique, since the former technique yields the most reliable results; once antibiotic therapy is initiated, there is no further opportunity to distinguish between true and false positive results. If the clinical circumstances permit repeated examination of the urine before institution of antibiotic therapy, the simpler bag technique is acceptable, since positive results then can be confirmed or refuted by examination of a suprapubic aspirate.

Unfortunately, it is difficult to determine what amount of leukocyturia is normal in the newborn. Houston found 76% of uninfected infants and children to have 0 to 10 leukocytes/mm^3 of urine, with another 20% falling within the range of 11 to 50. Lincoln and Winberg concluded on the basis of a survey of 500 newborns that normal males should have less than 25 and normal females less than 50 WBCs/mm^3 in clean-catch urine specimens. In contrast, Littlewood found less than 5 leukocytes/mm^3 in clean-catch urine specimens in 97% of male and 94% of female infants. However, Gower and associates reported that the presence of even more than 10 WBCs/mm^3 in suprapubic aspirates usually was not associated with a positive culture. There is a strong association between leukocyturia and bacteriuria in infants. Nevertheless, most infants with leukocyturia do not have bacteriuria; conversely, significant bacteriuria can occur in the absence of leukocyturia. Therefore the final diagnosis of urinary tract infection in the neonate lies in the demonstration of bacteriuria.

Etiology

The spectrum of organisms that has been cultured from the urine of infants is similar to that from the urine of older children with urinary tract infection. *E. coli* predominates, but *Aerobacter*, *Klebsiella*, *Pseudomonas*, and *Proteus* organisms, coliform bacteria, and enterococci are encountered more frequently in infants than in older children (Chapter 31, part one).

Candida infection of the urinary tract may occur in infants, particularly in premature infants being given intravenous hyperalimentation and antibiotic therapy. The fungus may appear as masses obstructing the collecting system with resulting hydronephrosis and/or as fungal vascular thrombi in the cortex, with increased cortical echogenicity. Oliguria, anuria, and renal insufficiency may ensue. Treatment consists of systemic administration of antifungal drugs such as amphotericin B and fluorocytosine, as well as the instillation of amphotericin B into the obstructed kidney by means of a nephrostomy tube (Chapter 31, part three).

Pathogenesis

The majority of urinary tract infections in older infants and children represent ascending infections, that is, entry of organisms through the urethra, migration into the bladder, and then in certain instances, extension to the kidney. Information concerning the route of entry in neonates is not available. Infants found on routine screening to have significant bacteriuria may well have a simple cystitis, which represents a pathogenesis similar to that observed in older subjects. Although proof is lacking, at least some if not all instances of pyelonephritis that occur in the newborn in the absence of urologic malformation represent cases of blood-borne infection, with organisms lodging in the kidney during the course of bacteremia. Many infants with pyelonephritis, diagnosed during life or after death, do have associated septicemia. It is difficult to determine, however, whether the septicemia preceded or occurred as a consequence of the pyelonephritis. Pyelonephritis has been reported to occur three to four times more commonly in male than in female infants.

In the majority of neonates with urinary tract infection urologic-roentgenologic examination reveals structurally normal kidneys and collecting systems. This finding is in striking contrast to infants diagnosed as having urinary tract infection during the remainder of the first year of life in whom the prevalence of urologic malformation has been reported to be as high as 50% to 80%.

Pathology

Postmortem studies of acute pyelonephritis have shown pus-containing tubules and ductules, interstitial edema progressing to fibrosis, and interstitial cellular infiltrates. Proliferative glomerular changes, seen occasionally, have been regarded as reactive. The lesion seems to be capable of complete resolution, unless suppuration and fibrosis supervene. Chronic and recurrent pyelonephritis, commonly associated with hydronephrosis, is accompanied by fibrosis, tubular atrophy, and glomerulosclerosis. Changes once regarded as localized nephronic malformations predisposing the infant to infection may be secondary sclerotic vascular changes; they are common and often are associated with hypertension.

Clinical manifestations

The majority of infants with urinary tract infection are asymptomatic; even in the sick infant there may be little clinical evidence to suggest infection of the urinary tract. The low incidence of asymptomatic bacteriuria in healthy full-term infants suggests that routine screening in this age group is not a profitable undertaking. In contrast, the infant with any evidence of illness is an excellent candidate for covert recurrent urinary tract infection. Screening of apparently healthy premature infants has detected significant bacteriuria in 2% to 5%, with some reports showing the incidence to be considerably higher than this. Repeated screening of premature infants during their stay in the nursery is worthwhile.

Neonates with pyelonephritis may exhibit relatively little evidence of serious infection, or they may appear as toxic, septic, desperately ill infants. A syndrome of pyelonephritis, hepatomegaly, hemolytic anemia, and jaundice (direct- and indirect-reacting bilirubin) has been described in several reports. Other features include poor feeding, lethargy, irritability, occasional vomiting and diarrhea, and azotemia. Hemolysis may be severe enough to require transfusion. The pathogenesis of this syndrome is unknown. The organisms most commonly cultured are the low-numbered serotypes of *E. coli*, especially 04:H5. As in presumptive septicemia (Chapter 31), treatment is urgent and cannot await the results of cultures. The response to antibiotic therapy usually is prompt, with a return of the blood urea to normal, resolution of hepatomegaly, clearing of jaundice, and cessation of hemolysis.

Treatment

See Chapter 31 for discussion of specific antibiotic therapy.

Treatment should be followed by appropriate investigation: ultrasound, a voiding cystourethrogram, and when these show abnormalities, an intravenous urogram. Of utmost importance is the long-term follow-up monitoring, with repeated examination of the urine for possible recurrence of infection.

VASCULAR DISORDERS OF THE KIDNEY

Circulatory disturbances of the kidney include arterial obstruction, venous thrombosis, cortical necrosis, medullary necrosis, and tubular necrosis. These lesions constitute the most common group of acquired renal diseases in the newborn. All of them are believed to be related to obstruction or diversion of renal blood flow, and the ensuing renal necrosis relates in part to the extent, type, and location of the circulatory abnormality. The degree of renal injury is, however, quite variable; renal venous thrombosis, for example, is associated with complete cortical infarction in one case and inconsequential alteration in another. The clinical triad of renal enlargement, hematuria, and azotemia applies to almost the entire group of disorders of the kidney. The clinical identification of a specific condition or anatomic lesion is seldom possible. In general, therapy tends to be conservative and consists principally of maintaining adequate hydration. Anticoagulation appears not to have been helpful. Peritoneal dialysis has been used with some success in newborns.

Arterial obstruction

Arterial obstruction is usually acute and most often the result of thromboembolism. The embolus may originate from a thrombus arising in the ductus arteriosus. Thrombosis developing as a complication of umbilical artery catheterization has become more common in recent years. The renal arteries can be obstructed by an embolus or by a large thrombus occluding the aortic lumen. The ensuing renal infarction may be unilateral or bilateral and total or segmental, depending on the number and distribution of emboli. Embolic lesions also appear in the extremities, gastrointestinal tract, and head. Renal infarction results in an enlarged kidney and either oliguria and hematuria or anuria. There may be vomiting and abdominal tenderness. Infants also develop severe, acute hypertension and may be seen in congestive heart failure without obvious cause. Serum creatinine and blood urea nitrogen levels are elevated. Plasma renin activity is usually in excess of 100 mg/ml/hour, and renal scans indicate a diminution of the renal blood flow. Arteriography may be needed to confirm the location of the vascular obstruction. An important consequence of unilateral or segmental arterial occlusion is subsequent renal atrophy with chronic hypertension. Segmental hypoplasia should be considered in the differential diagnosis. Hypertension may be transient and thus manageable by medical means, but it also can be severe and persistent, necessitating a nephrectomy. Hydralazine, 0.1 and 0.15 mg/kg, or diazoxide, 3 to 5 mg/kg, given intravenously, has been used successfully to control hypertension. The reason for surgery should be the persistence of the hypertension rather than the extent of the infarction, since the capacity of the kidney to recover functionally is impossible to predict in the early stages of the disease (Chapter 29).

Thrombosis of the renal veins

Thrombosis of the renal veins has been more common than arterial occlusion, although its frequency may have declined in recent years as the result of better fluid management and rehydration of distressed infants.

Clinical manifestations

Approximately half of over 300 reported cases have been in infants under 2 months of age. The most important factor in its pathogenesis appears to be dehydration, a mechanism that can account for cases of both antenatal and postnatal thrombosis. Other factors in newborns include relative polycythemia, relatively low renal blood flow and blood pressure, hypoxia, and birth injury. Babies born to diabetic mothers seem to be particularly susceptible, perhaps as the result of glucosuria, polyuria, and dehydration or as the result of extravascular fluid shifts, hypovolemia, and effective dehydration. The intrauterine origin of the lesion has been amply demonstrated. We have observed organizing venous thrombi in a newborn with anencephaly, another condition that may be associated with polyuria and intrauterine dehydration. Renal venous thrombosis may occur as a complication of diarrheal disease of the newborn.

The vascular lesion occurs with or without renal infarction. Venous infarction can result in considerable renal enlargement and anuria or oligohematuria. Thrombocytopenia and depletion of clotting factors are frequent findings, suggesting intravascular consumption, but disseminated coagulation has not been clearly demonstrated. Vomiting, lethargy, anorexia, fever, shock, and associated findings may be related to the initiating causes as much as to the renal lesion. Excretory urography usually discloses nonopacification or slight, diffuse opacification. An ultrasound or a venogram may demonstrate vena caval thrombosis. As a later phenomenon, the intrarenal thrombi undergo calcification and occasionally are visible roentgenographically as radially oriented markings.

Treatment

The lesion can be unilateral or bilateral, the former occurring more frequently. Prompt nephrectomy has been advocated in the past in the treatment of unilateral disease to prevent rapid progression and death. However, medical therapy developed in relation to bilateral venous thrombosis now has been applied successfully to unilateral involvement. This consists mainly of supportive therapy, rehydration, and possible anticoagulation. The results of this approach are as good as those obtained with surgery.

Prognosis

Survival probably depends on the severity of the morbid state that precipitates the renal lesion and on the presence or absence of renal infarction, which cannot be corrected by either form of therapy. Heparin therapy for anticoagulation is potentially dangerous because of bleeding, and its effectiveness has not been established.

The thrombosed kidney will often undergo symmetric involution within several months. Early tubular dysfunction, vesicoureteric reflux, and late-onset hypertension are additional possible consequences of renal venous thrombosis.

Cortical and medullary necrosis

Cortical and medullary necrosis overlap clinically and often coexist pathologically. The frequency of the lesions seems to be increasing relative to renal vein thrombosis, perhaps because of longer survival of severely ill newborns in intensive care nurseries.

Clinical manifestations

The clinical findings are nonspecific and include renal enlargement, anuria or oliguria, and hematuria. Both cortical and medullary necrosis in newborns have been associated with severe anemia and asphyxia. Blood loss in anemic shock has been attributed to twin-twin transfusion, fetal-maternal transfusion, uteroplacental hemorrhage, and severe hemolytic disease. Asphyxial shock commonly is associated with maternal toxemia, and advanced cortical necrosis has been seen in stillborn infants. It has been argued that in hemorrhagic and asphyxial shock renal cortical perfusion is diminished to the point of ischemic tissue necrosis, a mechanism similar to that producing tubular necrosis. Some infants also have thrombocytopenia, and small arteriolar, glomerular, and venular thrombi in the kidney have been interpreted as evidence of disseminated intravascular coagulation. Few patients with documented disseminated intravascular coagulation have had renal cortical necrosis, however, and the local vascular changes may be a result of severely altered renal circulation. Cortical necrosis also occurs in association with sepsis, diarrhea, and dehydration and is common among infants with congenital hypoplastic left heart syndrome. Medullary necrosis in infants with congenital heart disease has been related to the toxicity of large doses of angiographic contrast medium, and medullary necrosis in infants with severe hyperbilirubinemia and kernicterus seems to be a result of the direct toxic effects of unconjugated bilirubin concentrated in the renal medulla.

Pathology

Both cortical necrosis and medullary necrosis are usually bilateral, but involvement may be patchy or focal. The lesion is a bland, coagulative, ischemic necrosis. Medullary necrosis is commonly hemorrhagic and accompanied by variable cortical involvement. Both conditions are accompanied by focal necrosis in other organs: the liver, adrenal gland, intestines, and brain. Necrotic cortical tissue undergoes calcification, producing within weeks a characteristic pattern of bilateral, symmetric cortical calcification. There may be poor renal visualization by excretory urography because of cortical damage and impaired function. Medullary necrosis may be recognized roentgenographically by a deformed pyelocalyceal system with evidence of papillary necrosis and cavitation (Fig. 35-10). Both cortical and medullary necrosis are associated with distinct ultrasonographic images.

Treatment

The clinical differentiation of these two conditions from renal vein thrombosis may be very difficult, but in all three the clinical management is similar, consisting of careful control of fluids and seldom treatment of renal failure.

Prognosis

The prognosis is related to the underlying causes as well as to the severity of the renal lesion. As the result of improved supportive care and improved handling of renal failure, relatively long survival has been described. Prolonged survival may be complicated by severe hypertension. Sparing of juxtamedullary nephrons through collateral circulation in the inner cortex may account for relatively good tubular function despite severe glomerular insufficiency in surviving infants. Percutaneous renal

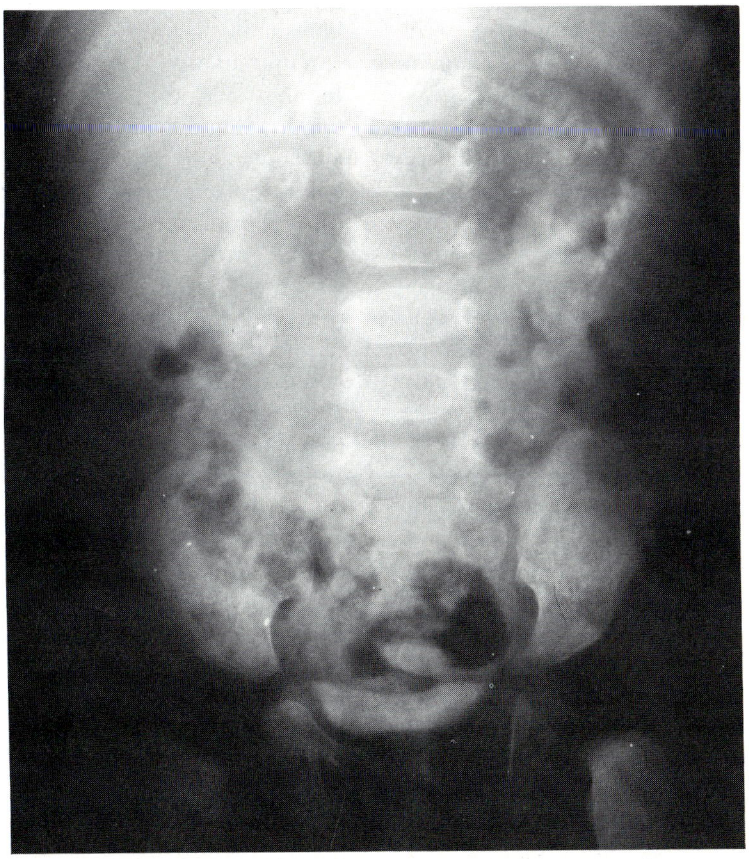

Fig. 35-10. Healing renal cortical necrosis at 9 weeks of age. An intravenous pyelogram at 10 minutes showing a faint nephrogram and faint opacification of the left renal pelvis and bladder. Bilateral renal cortical and adrenal calcification are evident. (From Leonidas, J.C., Berdon, W.E., and Gribetz, D.: J. Pediatr. **79:**623, 1971.)

biopsy may be of value in judging the severity of cortical damage.

TUMORS OF THE KIDNEY

Renal tumors in the newborn are uncommon, although they constitute the largest group of malignant neoplasms in childhood. The majority of neonatal renal tumors are leiomyomatous masses, sometimes referred to as *hamartomas* or *congenital mesoblastic nephromas*. Wilms' tumors, when they do occur, may be well differentiated and consist of cystic and tubular structures. Other renal neoplasms, including renal cell carcinoma, lymphoma, and teratoma, are medical rarities in the newborn. In general, renal tumors occurring early in infancy offer a considerably better outlook than do those in later childhood. The difference is in large measure a result of the relative frequency of mesoblastic nephroma and of well-differentiated Wilms' variants, which carry a good prognosis. Sarcomatous tumors have a poorer prognosis, even in young children. Only a few mesoblastic nephromas, perhaps 1% to 2%, have shown aggressive behavior, and the occurrence of true malignancy with distant metastases has been denied. Cystic Wilms' tumors and nephroblastomas with tubular differentiation are also rarely malignant. However, the rare typical Wilms' tumor in the newborn may pursue the usual malignant course.

Clinical manifestations

In newborns, as in older infants, the initial finding is usually that of abdominal swelling or a palpable mass, often detected by the parents. There may be a history of vomiting and fever, and laboratory examination may disclose hematuria and an elevated erythrocyte sedimentation rate. Older infants frequently have hypertension; it does occur in newborns, but its incidence is unknown.

Wilms' tumors have been associated with several nonrenal malformations, among them congenital aniridia and hemihypertrophy, which has also been associated with adrenal and hepatic tumors, visceral hemangiomas, and pigmented nevi. Aniridia occurs as part of a syndrome that includes cataracts, microcephaly, mental retardation, growth retardation, misshapen ears, and cryptorchidism. A syndrome that encompasses male pseudohermaphroditism with occasional agonadism, glomerulonephritis with nephrotic syndrome, renal failure, and hypertension has also included Wilms' tumor. The Beckwith-Wiedemann syndrome of omphalocele and visceromegaly is also associated with subsequent development of Wilms' tumor (Chapter 37, part one). The external malformations are seen at birth; the tumors develop later. These syndromes, despite their infrequency, should alert physicians to the risk of subsequent malignancy in affected patients.

Pathology

Congenital mesoblastic nephromas are morphologically distinctive, differing grossly and microscopically from typical nephroblastomas. The tumors are usually solitary, unencapsulated, and firm or rubbery. The cut surface has a whorled appearance, resembling uterine leiomyoma, and cysts are variably present. Histopathologic examination shows the tumor to be composed of sheets and intertwined bands of spindle, fibrous, and muscular cells, among which are nests and clusters of atypical and distorted glomeruli and tubules. The contained nephronic elements may be either (1) initially normal parenchyma entrapped within the expanding tumor, or (2) renal elements differentiating out of the metanephric mesenchyme that constitutes the tumor. Foci of rhabdomyomatous differentiation, angiomatous differentiation, cartilaginous differentiation, and hematopoietic infiltration may be seen. Cysts frequently are lined by epithelial cells that appear to have differentiated out of the adjacent stroma. Mitotic activity usually is meager. Increased mitotic activity and cellular atypia may be clues to the rare case that recurs or metastasizes; criteria of aggressive behavior have not been clearly established.

Differentiated Wilms' tumors contain masses of cysts, tubules, and even glomeruli, with little intervening undifferentiated stroma. The degree of epithelial differentiation along the tubules may be variable, but an embryonal appearance usually predominates. More typical nephroblastomas consist of undifferentiated mesenchyme, with only focal muscular and epithelial differentiation. Nephroblastomas usually are discrete, compressing the adjacent kidney tissue into a relatively fibrous capsule. True encapsulation is lacking, however, and the tumor invades the adjacent kidney, renal veins, and contiguous organs. Metastases are principally hematogeneous: lungs, liver, bones, and the opposite kidney.

The *multilocular cystic nephroma* is a benign renal tumor that consists of large cysts separated by fibrous septa. The solid portions of the tumor are usually poorly cellular, but cellular forms that are intermediates between obviously benign types and cystic Wilms' tumors do exist. These tumors thus are regarded as part of the spectrum of neoplasms arising from metanephric blastema, a spectrum that includes the multilocular cystic nephroma, the well-differentiated tubular nephroblastoma, and the typical Wilms' tumor.

An interesting condition is the occurrence within the outer renal cortex of both kidneys of small nodules of undifferentiated tissue that resemble nephroblastoma. Such nodules are commonly seen in trisomy E, and they have been reported in syndromes of fetal gigantism and hemihypertrophy. When small and grossly inapparent, they have been referred to as *nodular blastema*. When the cortex is distorted by large masses of blastematous tissue, the condition is referred to as *nephroblastomatosis*. These two abnormalities are frequently found in kidneys resected because of Wilms' tumor, and Wilms' tumors on a few occasions have been reported to coexist with bilateral nephroblastomatosis. They may provide a link between the malformations and the subsequent development of Wilms' tumor in the syndromes previously noted.

Diagnosis

The differential diagnosis of abdominal masses in the newborn includes neuroblastomas, adrenal hemorrhages, retroperitoneal tumors and cysts, splenomegaly, hepatic tumors, ovarian cysts and tumors, intestinal duplications, and a variety of renal abnormalities. A multicystic dysplastic kidney is the most common cause of abdominal and flank masses in the neonate, followed closely by unilateral (or bilateral) hydronephrosis caused by ureteropelvic junction stricture, hydronephrosis caused by vesicoureteric reflux, and polycystic kidneys. Roentgenography and sonography are important in localizing the lesion to the kidney; in excluding hydronephrosis and polycystic disease; and in identifying ectopic, fused, and solitary kidneys. Scintigraphy has been shown to distinguish between mesoblastic nephroma and nephroblastoma (Wilm's tumor). Excretory urography commonly shows flattening and distortion of the pyelocalyceal system, a finding common to all intrarenal masses. Excretion of contrast medium, however, may be so impaired by infiltrating tumor or by secondary vascular obstruction that the roentgenograms show only a nonfunctioning renal mass. Arteriography may be of additional help in identifying and localizing the tumor, but the characteristically abnormal vasculature is common to mesoblastic nephroma, Wilms' tumor, and multilocular cyst. The leiomyomatous and cystic tumors tend to be less vascular. During the nephrographic phase of the arteriogram the denser renal tissue is seen to be displaced by the tumor. Occasional Wilms' tumors are avascular, perhaps because of hemorrhagic or cystic degeneration, and differentiation from cystic lesions may then be difficult. Renal angiography is also of value in defining the extent of neoplastic involvement and in evaluating the contralateral kidney before surgery.

Bilaterality in nephroblastomas (all ages) occurs in approximately 4% of patients; its frequency in newborns is obscured by other developmental abnormalities, particularly nephroblastomatosis. Wilms' tumors also may coexist with other renal abnormalities, including cystic disease, duplication, fusion, and ectopia, thus complicating roentgenologic interpretation. Wilms' tumors also have occurred with greater than expected frequency in horseshoe-shaped and solitary kidneys.

Treatment

Definitive therapy should be instituted promptly after the diagnosis has been confirmed. The presence of a localized intrarenal mass necessitates surgical exploration. Primary treatment is nephrectomy. Benign mesenchymal tumors require no postoperative therapy. The malignant tumors are treated for 2 to 3 years, with initial postoperative or preoperative radiotherapy in conjunction with repeated courses of chemotherapy in accordance with well-established protocols. Secondary damage from irradiation may supervene, affecting particularly the dorsolumbar spine and the bowel.

Prognosis

The prognosis in neonatal renal tumors is good; this estimate takes into account the benign variants of early infancy. The survival of all infants younger than 1 year may be 70% to 80%. Infants of this age with typical Wilms' tumor, however, may have no better prognosis than do older children. Clinical staging is of help in determining outcome; tumors confined to the kidney have an excellent prognosis, but progressively poorer results can be anticipated with tumors that extend into the renal fossa and vessels.

Adrian Spitzer
Jay Bernstein
Chester M. Edelmann, Jr.
Hayim Boichis

BIBLIOGRAPHY

Renal function and its morphologic correlates

Aldahhan, J., and others: Sodium homeostasis in term and preterm neonates. I. Renal aspects, Arch. Dis. Child. **58**:335, 1983.

Aperia, A., and Elinder, G.: Distal tubular sodium reabsorption in the developing rat kidney, Am. J. Physiol. **240**:F487, 1981.

Aperia, A., and others: Developmental study of the renal response to an oral salt load in preterm infants, Acta Pediatr. Scand. **63**:517, 1974.

Aperia, A., and others: Glomerular tubular balance in preterm and full term infants, Acta Paediatr. Scand. Suppl. **305**:70, 1983.

Aperia, A., and others: Renal hemodynamics in the perinatal period, Acta Physiol. Scand. **99**:261, 1977.

Arant, B.S.: Developmental patterns of renal functional maturation compared in the human neonate, J. Pediatr. **92**:705, 1978.

Aschinberg, L.D., and others: Neonatal changes in renal blood flow distribution in puppies, Am. J. Physiol. **228**:1453, 1975.

Care, A.D., and Ross, R.: Fetal calcium homeostasis, J. Dev. Physiol. **6**:59, 1984.

Coulthard, M.G., and Hey, E.M.: Effect of varying water intake on renal function in healthy preterm babies, Arch. Dis. Child. **60**:614, 1985.

Daniel, S.S., and others: Role of vasopressin in fetal homeostasis, Am. J. Physiol. **242**:F740, 1982.

Daniel, S.S., and others: Excretion of vasopressin in the hypoxic lamb: comparison between fetus and newborn, Pediatr. Res. **18**:227, 1984.

Drukker, A., and others: The renin angiotensin system in newborn dogs: developmental patterns and response to acute saline loading, Pediatr. Res. **14**:304, 1980.

Fetterman, G.H., and others: The growth and maturation of human glomeruli and proximal convolutions from term to adulthood, Pediatrics 35:601, 1965.

Gomez, R.A., and others: Developmental aspects of the renal response to hemorrhage during fetal life, Pediatr. Res. 18:40, 1984.

Guignard, J.P.: Renal function in the newborn infant, Pediatr. Clin. North Am. 29:777, 1982.

Iwamoto, H.S., Oh, W., and Rudolph, A.M.: Renal metabolism in fetal and newborn sheep, Pediatr. Res. 19:641, 1985.

Iwamoto, H.S., and Rudolph, A.M.: Effects of angiotensin II on the blood flow and its distribution in fetal lambs, Circ. Res. 48:183, 1981.

Jose, P.A., and others: Autoregulation of renal blood flow in the puppy, Am. J. Physiol. 229:983, 1975.

Kleinman, L.I., and Banks, R.D.: Segmental nephron sodium and potassium reabsorption in newborn and adult dogs during saline expansion, Proc. Soc. Exp. Biol. Med. 173:231, 1983.

Leake, R.D., Trygstad, C.W., and Oh, W.: Insulin clearance in the newborn infant: relationship to gestational and postnatal age, Pediatr. Res. 10:759, 1976.

Lelievre-Pegorier, M., and Geloso, J.P.: Ontogeny of sugar transport in fetal rat kidney, Biol. Neonate 38:16, 1980.

Lelievre-Pegorier, M., and others: Developmental pattern of water and electrolyte transport in rat superficial nephrons, Am. J. Physiol. 245:F15, 1983.

Matson, J.R., Stokes, J.B., and Robillard, J.E.: Effects of inhibition of prostaglandin synthesis on fetal renal function, Kidney Int. 20:621, 1981.

McCance, R.A., andWiddowson, E.M.: Renal function before birth, Proc. Roy. Soc. Bull. 141:488, 1953.

McCance, R.A., and Widdowson, E.M.: The response of the newborn puppy to water, salt, and food, J. Physiol. 141:81, 1958.

Merlet-Benichou, C., and others: Functional and morphologic patterns of renal maturation in the developing guinea pig, Am. J. Physiol. 241:F618, 1981.

Moore, E.S., and others: Effect of Na_2SO_4 on urinary acidification in the fetal lamb, Am. J. Physiol. 223:167, 1972.

Moore, E.S., and others: Renal phosphate clearance in fetal lambs, Pediatr. Res. 12:1066, 1978.

Moore, E.S., and others: Ontogeny of intrarenal solute gradients in fetal life. In Spitzer, A., editor: The kidney during development: morphology and function, New York, 1982, Masson Publishers.

Rees, L., and others: Hyponatremia in the first week of life in preterm infants. Part I. Arginine vasopressin secretion, Arch. Dis. Child. 59:414, 1984.

Rees, L., and others: Sodium and water balance. Part II. Arch. Dis. Child. 59:423, 1984.

Reitz, R.E., and others: Calcium, magnesium, phosphorus and parathyroid hormone interrelationships in pregnancy and newborn infants, Obstet. Gynecol. 50:701, 1977.

Robillard, J.E., and others: Maturational changes in the fetal glomerular filtration rate, Am. J. Obstet. Gynecol. 122:601, 1975.

Robillard, J.E., and others: Influence of fetal extracellular volume contraction on renal reabsorption of bicarbonate in fetal lambs, Pediatr. Res. 11:649, 1977.

Robillard, J.E., and others: Maturation of the glucose transport process by the fetal kidney, Pediatr. Res. 12:680, 1978.

Robillard, J.E., and others: Developmental aspects of renal tubular reabsorption of water and fetal renal response to arginine vasopressin. In Spitzer, A., editor: The kidney during development: morphology and function. New York, 1982, Masson Publishers.

Rudolph, A.M., and Heymann, M.A.: Circulatory changes during growth in the fetal lamb, Circ. Res. 26:289, 1970.

Spitzer, A.: Factors underlying the increase in glomerular filtration rate during postnatal development. In Spitzer, A., editor: The kidney during development: morphology and function. New York, 1982, Masson Publishers.

Spitzer, A.: The role of the kidney in sodium homeostasis during maturation, Kidney Int. 21:539, 1982.

Spitzer, A., and Brandis, M.: Functional and morphological maturation of the superficial nephrons: relationship to total kidney function, J. Clin. Invest. 53:279, 1974.

Stapleton, F.B.: Renal uric acid clearance in human neonates, J. Pediatr. 103:290, 1983.

Suda, T., and Kurokawa, K.: Characteristic localization of 25-hydroxyvitamin D_3 1-hydroxylase along the fetal nephron. In Holick, M.F., Anast, C.S., and Gray, T.K., editors: Perinatal calcium and phosphorus metabolism, New York, 1983, Elsevier.

Sulyok, E., and others: Postnatal development of renal sodium handling in premature infants, J. Pediatr. 95:787, 1981.

Sulyok, E., and others: Relationship between the postnatal development of the renin-angiotensin-aldosterone system and electrolyte and acid-base status of the NaC1-supplemented premature infant. In Spitzer, A., editor: The kidney during development: morphology and function, New York, 1982, Masson Publishers.

Sulyok, E., and others: Late hyponatremia in premature infants: role of aldosterone and AVP, J. Pediatr. 106:990, 1985.

Weismann, Y., and others: 1,25-dihydroxyvitamin D_3 and 24,25 dihydroxyvitamin D_3 in vitro synthesis by human decidua and placenta, Nature 281:317, 1979.

Wintur, E.M., and others: Regulation of urine osmolality in fetal sheep, J. Exp. Physiol. 67:427, 1982.

Diagnosis of renal disease

Angella, J.J., Prieto, E.N., and Fogel, B.J.: Hemoglobinuria associated with hemolytic disease of the newborn infant, J. Pediatr. 71:530, 1967.

Brion, L., and others: Importance of deep abdominal palpation in the perinatal diagnosis of urologic malformations, Biol. Neonate 46:215, 1984.

Cywes, S., Wynne, J.M., and Louw, J.H.: Urinary ascites in newborn: with a report of two cases, J. Pediatr. Surg. 3:350, 1968.

deLuna, M.B., and Hullet, W.H.: Urinary protein excretion in healthy infants, children and adults, Proc. Am. Soc. Nephrol. 16:16, 1967.

Emanuel, B., and Aronson, N.: Neonatal hematuria, Am. J. Dis. Child. 128:204, 1974.

Gruikshand, G., and Edmond, E.: "Clean catch" urines in the newborn: bacteriology and cell excretion patterns in the first week of life, Br. Med. J. 4:705, 1967.

Haugstvedt, S., and Lundberg, J.: Kidney size in normal children measured by sonography, Scand. J. Urol. Nephrol. 14:251, 1980.

Houston, I.B.: Urinary white cell excretion in childhood, Arch. Dis. Child. 40:313, 1965.

Hricak, H., and others: Neonatal kidneys: sonographic anatomic correlations, Radiology 147:699, 1983.

Klare, B., and others: Radiologic kidney size in children without kidney disease, Pediatr. Radiology 9:153, 1980.

Lawson, T.L., and others: Ultrasonic evaluation of fetal kidneys, Radiology 138:153, 1988.

Lincoln, K., and Winberg, J.: Studies of urinary tract infection in infancy and childhood. III. Quantitative estimation of cellular excretion in unselected neonates, Acta Pediatr. Scand. 53:447, 1964.

Littlewood, J.M.: White cells and bacteria in voided urine of healthy newborns, Arch. Dis. Child. 46:167, 1971.

Longio, L.A., and Martin, L.W.: Abdominal masses in the newborn infant, Pediatrics 21:596, 1958.

MacLaurin, J.C.: Changes in body water distribution during the first two weeks of life, Arch. Dis. Child. 41:286, 1966.

Moskowitz, P.S., Carroll, B.A., and McCoy, J.M.: Ultrasonic renal volumetry in children: accuracy and simplicity of method, Radiology **134**:61, 1980.

Mussels, M., Gaudry, C.L., and Bason, W.M.: Renal anomalies in the newborn found by deep palpation, Pediatrics **47**:97, 1971.

Peterson, P.A., Evrin, P., and Berggard, L.: Differentiation of glomerular, tubular, and normal proteinuria: determinations of urinary excretion of beta-2-macroglobulin, albumin, and total protein, J. Clin. Invest. **48**:1189, 1969.

Sorulf, H., Nordmark, J., and Jonsson, A.: Kidney size in infants and children assessed by area measurements, Acta Radiol. Diag. **19**:154, 1978.

Renal insufficiency and renal failure

Adelman, R.D., and Zakauddin, S.: Urinary enzyme activity in children and neonates receiving gentamicin therapy, Dev. Pharmacol. Ther. **1**:325, 1980.

Barratt, T.M.: Renal failure in the first year of life, Br. Med. Bull. **27**:115, 1971.

Bennett, W.M.: Aminoglycoside nephrotoxicity: experimental and clinical considerations, Mineral Electr. Metab. **6**:277, 1981.

Braumlich, H.: Excretion of drugs during postnatal development, Pharmacol. Ther. **12**:299, 1981.

Chan, K.W., and Na, W.I.: Gentamicin nephropathy in a neonate, Pathology **17**:514, 1985.

Chesney, R.W., and others: Acute renal failure: an important complication of cardiac surgery in infants, J. Pediatr. **87**:381, 1975.

Cifuentes, R.F., Olley, P.M., and Balfe, J.W.: Indomethacin and renal function failure in premature infants with persistent patent ductus arteriosus, J. Pediatr. **51**:313, 1962.

Dahl Palu, C., and others: Intravenous labetalol in severe hypertension, Br. J. Clin. Pharmacol. **13**(suppl. 1):975, 1982.

Griswold, W.R., and others: Propranolol as an antihypertensive agent in children, Arch. Dis. Child. **53**:594, 1978.

Gruskin, A.B., and others: Effect of angiography on renal function and histology in infants and piglets, J. Pediatr. **76**:41, 1970.

Guignard, J.P., and others: Renal function in respiratory distress syndrome, J. Pediatr. **88**:845, 1976.

Holliday, M.A., Potter, D.E., and Dobrin, R.S.: Treatment of renal failure in children, Pediatr. Clin. North Am. **18**:613, 1971.

Mathew, O.P., and others: Neonatal renal failure: usefulness of diagnostic indices, Pediatrics **65**:57, 1980.

Moore, E.S., and others: Effects of positive pressure ventilation on intrarenal blood flow in infant primates, Pediatr. Res. **8**:792, 1974.

Norman, M.E., and Asadi, F.K.: A prospective study of acute renal failure in newborn infants, Pediatrics **63**:475, 1974.

Priebe, H.J., Heiman, J.E., and Hedley-Whyte, J.: Mechanisms of renal dysfunction during positive and expiratory pressure ventilation, J. Appl. Physiol. Respir. Envir. Exercise Physiol. **50**:643, 1981.

Ronco, C., and others: Treatment of acute renal failure in newborns by continuous arteriovenous hemofiltration, Kidney Int. **29**:908, 1986.

Seyberth, H.W., and others: Evaluation of adverse renal reactions to prolonged indomethacin therapy in preterm infants with persistent ductus arteriosus, Pediatr. Pharmacol. **3**:259, 1983.

Trompeter, R.S., Chantler, C., and Haycock, G.B.: Tolazoline and acute renal failure in the newborn, Lancet **1**:1219, 1981.

Tulassay, T., and others: Effect of continuous positive airway pressure on renal function in prematures, Biol. Neonate **43**:152, 1983.

Vidt, D.G., Bravo, E.L., and Fouad, F.M.: Drug therapy: captopril, N. Engl. J. Med. **306**:214, 1982.

Waal Manning, H.J., and Simpson, F.O.: Review of long term treatment with labetalol, Br. J. Clin. Pharmacol. **13**(suppl. 1):15, 1982.

Zinner, S.H., and others: Factors affecting blood pressures in newborn infants, Hypertension **2**(suppl):99, 1980.

Malformations

Acton, C.M., and Drew, J.H.: Vesicoureteral reflux in the neonatal period. In Hodson, J., and Kincaid-Smith, P., editors: Reflux nephropathy, New York, 1979, Masson Publishers.

Aperia, A., and others: Effect of vesico-ureteral reflux on renal function in children with recurrent urinary tract infection, Kidney Int. **9**:418, 1976.

Atwell, J.D., and Vijay, M.R.: Renal growth following reimplantation of the ureter for reflux, Br. J. Urol. **50**:367, 1978.

Aubry, M.C.: Diagnostic antenatal des annomalies du tractus urinaire. Prog. Neonatol. **3**:17, 1983.

Bailey, R.R.: Alternative methods of defining vesicoureteric reflux. In Hodson, J., and Kincaid-Smith, P., editors: Reflux nephropathy, New York, 1979, Masson Publishers.

Bailey, R.R.: Sterile reflux: is it harmless? In Hodson, J., and Kincaid-Smith, P., editors: Reflux nephropathy, New York, 1979, Masson Publishers.

Bailey, R.R.: Vesicoureteric reflux in healthy infants and children. In Hodson, J., and Kincaid-Smith, P., editors: Reflux nephropathy, New York, 1979, Masson Publishers.

Bain, A.D., and Scott, J.S.: Renal agenesis and severe urinary dysplasia: a review of 50 cases with particular reference to associated anomalies, Br. Med. J. **1**:841, 1960.

Bengtsson, U., Hedman, L., and Svalander, C.: Adult type of polycystic kidney disease in a newborn child, Acta Med. Scand. **197**:447, 1975.

Bernstein, J.: Developmental abnormalities of the renal parenchyma: renal hypoplasia and dysplasia. In Sommers, S.C., editor: Pathology annual 1968, New York, 1968, Appleton-Century-Crofts.

Bernstein, J.: Heritable cystic disorders of the kidney; the mythology of polycystic disease, Pediatr. Clin. North Am. **18**:435, 1971.

Bernstein, J.: The morphogenesis of renal parenchymal maldevelopment (renal dysplasia), Pediatr. Clin. North. Am. **18**:395, 1971.

Bernstein, J., Brough, A.J., and McAdams, A.J.: The renal lesion in syndromes of multiple congenital malformations; cerebrohepatorenal syndrome, Jeune asphyxiating thoracic dystrophy; tuberous sclerosis: Meckel syndrome. In Bergsma, D., editor: Birth defects, vol. 10, Baltimore, 1974, The Williams & Wilkins Co.

Blaufox, M.D., and others: Radionuclide scintigraphy for detection of vesico-ureteral reflux in children, J. Pediatr. **79**:239, 1971.

Boal, D.K., and Littlewood Teele, R.: Sonography of infantile polycystic kidney disease, Am. J. Roentgenol. **135**:575, 1980.

Boichis, H., and others: Congenital hepatofibrosis and nephronophthisis, Q. J. Med. **42**:221, 1973.

Buchta, R.M., and others: Familial bilateral renal agenesis and hereditary renal dysplasia, Z. Kinderheikd. **115**:111, 1973.

Burke, E.C., Shin, M.H., and Kelalis, P.P.: Prune-belly syndrome; clinical findings and survival, Am. J. Dis. Child. **117**:668, 1969.

Cain, D.R., and others: Familial renal agenesis and total dysplasia, Am. J. Dis. Child. **128**:377, 1974.

Chevalier, R.L., Garland, T.A., and Buschi, A.J.: The neonate with adult-type autosomal polycystic kidney disease, Int. J. Pediatr. Nephrol. **2**:73, 1981.

Donaldson, M.D.C., and others: Familial juvenile nephronophthisis, Jeune's syndrome, and associated diseases, Arch. Dis. Child. **60**:426, 1985.

Elejalde, B.R.: Genetic and diagnostic considerations in those families with abnormalities of facial expression and congenital urinary obstrucation; the Ochoa syndrome, Am. J. Med. Genet. **3**:97, 1979.

Elkin, M., and Bernstein, J.: Cystic diseases of the kidney, radiological and pathological considerations, Clin. Radiol. **20**:65, 1969.

Fanconi, G., and others: Die familiare juvenile nephronopthise, Helv. Paediatr. Acta **6**:1, 1951.

Haddock, F.P., and others: Sonography of fetal urinary tract anomalies, Am. J. Radiol. **137**:261, 1981.

Johannessen, J.V., Haneberg, B., and Moe, P.J.: Bilateral multicystic dysplasia of the kidneys, Betr. Pathol. **148**:290, 1973.

Josephson, S.: Experimental obstructive hydronephrosis in newborn rats. III. Long term effects on renal function, J. Urol. **129**:396, 1983.

Josephson, S., Ericson, A.C., and Sjoquist, M.: Experimental obstructive hydronephrosis in newborn rats. VI. Long term effects on glomerular filtration and distribution, J. Urol. **134**:391, 1985.

Kelley, R.I.: Review: the cerebrohepatorenal syndrome of Zellweger, morphologic and metabolic aspects, Am. J. Med. Genet. **16**:503-517, 1983.

Kyaw, M.M.: Roentgenologic triad of congenital multicystic kidney, Am. J. Roentgenol. Radium Ther. Nucl. Med. **119**:710, 1973.

Leibowitz, R.L., and Teele, R.L.: Fetal and neonatal hydronephrosis, Urol. Radiol. **5**:185, 1983.

Leonidas, J.C., Strakuss, L., and Krasna, I.H.: Roentgen diagnosis of multicystic renal dysplasia in infancy by high dose urography, J. Urol. **108**:963, 1972.

Lieberman, E., and others: Infantile polycystic disease of the kidneys and liver; clinical, pathological and radiological correlations and comparison with congenital hepatic fibrosis, Medicine **50**:277, 1971.

Lundin, P.M., and Olow, I.: Polycystic kidneys in newborns, infants, and children: a clinical pathological study, Acta Paediatr. **50**:185, 1961.

Machin, G.A.: Urinary tract malformations in the XYY male, Clin. Genet. **14**:370, 1972.

Milutinovic, J., and others: Autosomal dominant polycystic kidney disease: early diagnosis and data for genetic counseling, Lancet **1**:1203, 1980.

Moerman, S., and others: Pathogenesis of the prune belly syndrome: afunctional urethral obstruction caused by prostate hypoplasia, Pediatrics **73**:470, 1984.

Newman, L., and others: unilateral total renal dysplasia in children, Am. J. Roentgenol. Radium Ther. Nucl. Med. **116**:778, 1972.

North, A.F., Jr., Eldredge, D.M., and Tapley, W.B.: Abdominal distention at birth due to ascites associated with obstructive uropathy, Am. J. Dis. Child. **111**:613, 1966.

Passarage, E., and Sutherland, J.M.: Potter's syndrome: chromosome analysis of three cases with Potter's syndrome or related syndrome, Am. J. Dis. Child. **109**:80, 1965.

Peters, P.C., Johnson, D.E., and Jackson, J.H.: The incidence of vesicoureteral reflux in the premature child, J. Urol. **97**:159, 1967.

Potter, E.L.: Bilateral absence of ureters and kidneys: a report of 50 cases, Obstet. Gynecol. **25**:3, 1965.

Proesmans, W., Van Damme, B., and Macken, J.: Nephronophthisis and tapeto retinal degeneration associated with liver fibrosis, Clin. Nephrol. **3**:160, 1975.

Proesmans, W., and others: Autosomal dominant polycystic kidney disease in the neonatal period, Pediatrics **70**:971, 1982.

Qazi, W., and others: Renal anomalies in fetal alcohol syndrome, Pediatrics **63**:886, 1979.

Ransely, P.G., and Risdon, R.A.: Renal papillary morphology in infants and young children, Urol. Res. **3**:111, 1975.

Ransely, P.G., and Risdon, R.A.: Reflux nephropathy: effect of antimicrobial therapy on the evolution of the early pyelonephritic scar, Kidney Int. **20**:733, 1981.

Risdon, R.A.: Renal dysplasia. I. A clinico-pathological study of 76 cases, J. Clin. Pathol. **24**:57, 1971.

Risdon, R.A.: Renal dysplasia. II. A necropsy study of 41 cases, J. Clin. Pathol. **24**:65, 1971.

Risdon, R.A., Young, L.W., and Chrispin, A.R.: Renal hypoplasia and dysplasia: a radiological and pathological correlation, Pediatr. Radiol. **3**:213, 1975.

Rolleston, G.L., Shannon, F.T., and Utley, W.L.F.: Follow-up of vesico-ureteric reflux in the newborn, Kidney Int. **8**(suppl.):S59, 1975.

Ross, D.G., and Tavers, H.: Infantile presentation of adult-type polycystic disease in a large kindred, J. Pediatr. **87**:760, 1975.

Rubenstein, M., Meyer, R., and Bernstein, J.: Congenital abnormalities of the urinary system. I. A postmortem survey of developmental anomalies and acquired congenital lesions in a children's hospital, J. Pediatr. **58**:356, 1961.

Warsaw, B.L., Hymes, L.C., and Woodard, J.R.: Long term outcome of patients with obstuctive uropathy, Pediatr. Clin. North Am. **29**:815, 1982.

Nephritis

Claireaux, A.E., and Pearson, M.G.: Chronic nephritis in a newborn infant, Arch. Dis. Child. **30**:366, 1955.

Collins, R.D.: Chronic glomerulonephritis in a newborn child, Am. J. Dis. Child. **87**:478, 1954.

Kaplan, B.S., and others: The glomerulopathy of congenital syphilis: an immune deposit disease, J. Pediatr. **81**:1154, 1972.

Shahin, M.D., Papadopoulou, Z.L., and Henis, E.H.: Congenital nephrotic syndrome associated with congenital toxoplasmosis, J. Pediatr. **85**:366, 1974.

Taitz, L.S., Isaacson, C., and Stein, H.: Acute nephritis associated with congenital syphilis, Br. Med. J. **2**:152, 1961.

Wiggelinkhuizen, J., and others: Congenital syphilis and glomerulonephritis with evidence for immune pathogenesis, Arch. Dis. Child. **48**:375, 1973.

Yuceoglu, A.M., and others: The glomerulopathy of congenital syphillis: a curable immune-deposit disease, JAMA **229**:1085, 1974.

Nephrotic syndrome

Aula, P., and others: Prenatal diagnosis in congenital nephrosis in 23 high-risk families, Am. J. Dis. Child. **132**:984, 1978.

Chandra, M., and others: Familial nephrotic syndrome and focal segmental glomerulo-sclerosis, J. Pediatr. **98**:556, 1981.

Habib, R., and Bois, E.: Heterogenite des syndromes nephrotiques a debut precoce du nourrisson (syndrome nephrotique "infantile"): etude anatomo-clinique et genetique de 37 observations, Helv. Paediatr. Acta **28**:91, 1973.

Hallman, N., Norio, R., and Rapola, J.: Congenital nephrotic syndrome, Nephron **11**:101, 1973.

Hoyer, J.R., and others: The nephrotic syndrome of infancy: clinical, morphologic, and immunologic studies of four infants, Pediatrics **40**:233, 1967.

Hoyer, J.R., and others: Successful renal transplantation in 3 children with congenital nephrotic syndrome, Lancet **1**:1410, 1973.

Huttunen, N.P.: Congenital nephrotic syndrome of Finnish type: study of 75 patients, Arch. Dis. Child. **51**:344, 1976.

Huttunen, N.P., Hallmann, N., and Rapola, J.: Glomerular basement membrane antigens in congenital and acquired nephrotic syndrome in childhood, Nephron **16**:401, 1976.

Huttunen, N.P., and others: Proteinuria in congenital nephrotic syndrome of the Finnish type, Clin. Nephrol. **13**:12, 1980.

Kaplan, B.S., Bureau, M.A., and Drummond, K.N.: The nephrotic syndrome in the first year of life: is a classification possible? J. Pediatr. **85**:615, 1974.

Kleinknecht, C., and others: Coexistence of antenatal, infantile and juvenile nephrotic syndrome in a single family, J. Pediatr. **98**:938, 1981.

Kouvalainen, K.: Immunological studies on the congenital nephrotic syndrome, Am. J. Dis. Child. **104**:554, 1962.

McDonald, R., Wiggelinkhuizen, J., and Kaschila, R.O.C.: The nephrotic syndrome in very young infants, Am. J. Dis. Child. **122**:507, 1971.

Medearis, D.N.: Cytomegalic inclusion disease: an analysis of the clinical features based on the literature and six additional cases, Pediatrics **19**:467, 1957.

Paatela, M.: Renal microdissection in infants with special reference to the congenital nephrotic syndrome, Ann. Paediatr. Fenn. **9**(suppl. 21):1, 1963.

Papaioannou, A.C., Ascrow, G.G., and Schuckmell, N.H.: Nephrotic syndrome in early infancy as a manifestation of congenital syphilis, Pediatrics **27**:636, 1961.

Seppala, M., and others: Congenital nephrotic syndrome: prenatal diagnosis and genetic counseling by estimation of amniotic-fluid and maternal serum alpha-foetoprotein, Lancet **2**:123, 1976.

Walker, C.H.M., and others: Hemodialysis in infantile nephrotic syndrome, Am. J. Dis. Child. **106**:479, 1963.

White, R.H.R.: The familial nephrotic syndrome: I.A. European survey, Clin. Nephrol. **1**:215, 1973.

Wiggelinkhuizen, J., and others: Alpha fetoprotein in the antenatal diagnosis of the congenital nephrotic syndrome, J. Pediatr. **89**:452, 1976.

Anomalies of renal tubular function

Arant, B.S., and others: Effect of chronic salt and water loading on the tubular defects of a child with Fanconi syndrome (cystinosis), Pediatrics **58**:370, 1976.

Bartter, F.C.: On the pathogenesis of Bartter's syndrome, Mineral Electrol. Metab. **3**:61, 1980.

Bell, N.H., and others: Demonstration of a defect in the formation of adenosine 3′,5′-monophosphate in vasopressin-resistant diabetes insipidus, Pediatr. Res. **8**:223, 1974.

Blachard, Y., and others: The effect of inhibition of prostaglandin synthesis on free water and osmolar clearances in patients with hereditary nephrogenic diabetes insipidus, Mayo Clin. Proc. **49**:188, 1974.

Brodehl, J., and Gellissen, K.: Endogenous renal transport of free amino acids in infancy and childhood, Pediatrics **42**:395, 1968.

Broyer, M., and others: La cystinose infantile, reevaluation des symptomes precoces et tardifs. In Actual. Nephrol. Hop. Necker, Paris, 1980, Flammarion.

Cheek, D.B., and Perry, J.N.: A salt wasting syndrome in infancy, Arch. Dis. Child. **33**:252, 1958.

Dillon, M.T., and others: Pseudohypoaldosteronism, Arch. Dis. Child. **97**:813, 1959.

Donnell, G.N., Litman, N., and Roldan, M.: Pseudohypoadrenalcorticism: renal sodium loss, hyponatremia, and hyperkalemia due to renal tubular insensitivity to mineralocorticoid, Am. J. Dis. Child. **97**:813, 1959.

Chisolm, J.J., Jr., and Harrison, H.E.: Aminoaciduria, Pediatr. Clin. North Am. **7**:333, 1960.

Chisolm, J.J., Jr., and Harrison, H.E.: Aminoaciduria in vitamin D deficiency states, in premature infants and older infants with rickets, J. Pediatr. **60**:206, 1962.

Gill, J.R., Jr.: Bartter's syndrome, Annu. Rev. Med. **31**:405, 1980.

Girardin, E.P., DeWolfe, M.S., and Crocker, J.F.S.: Treatment of cystinosis with cysteamine, J. Pediatr. **94**:838, 1979.

Houston, I.B., Boichis, H., Edelmann, C.M., Jr.: Fanconi syndrome with renal sodium wasting and metabolic alkalosis, Am. J. Med. **44**:638, 1968.

Lowe, C.U., Terrey, M., and MacLachlan, E.A.: Organoaciduria, decreased renal ammonia production, hydrophthalmos, and mental retardation, a clinical entity, Am. J. Dis. Child. **83**:164, 1952.

McSherry, E.: Renal tubular acidosis in childhood, Kidney Int. **20**:799, 1981.

McSherry, E., Portale, A., and Gates, J.: Non-azotemic, non-hyporeninemic type 4 tubular acidosis observed in early childhood, Kidney Int. **14**:796, 1978 (Abstract).

McSherry, E., Sebastian, A., Morris, R.C., Jr.: Renal tubular acidosis in infants: the several kinds including bicarbonate-wasting, classic renal tubular acidosis, J. Clin. Invest. **51**:499, 1972.

Monasterio, G., and others: Renal diabetes as a congenital tubular dysplasia, Am. J. Med. **37**:44, 1964.

Monn, E.: Prostaglandin synthetase inhibitions in the treatment of nephrogenic diabetes insipidus, Acta Paediatr. Scand. **70**:39, 1981.

Morris, R.C.: Renal tubular acidosis: mechanisms, classification and implications, N. Engl. J. Med. **281**:1405, 1969.

Morris, R.C., Jr., and Sebastian, A.: Disorders of the renal tubule that cause disorders of fluid, acid-base, and electrolyte metabolism. In Maxwell, M.H., and Kleeman, C.R., editors: Clinical disorders of fluid and electrolyte metabolism, ed. 3, New York, 1980, McGraw-Hill Book Co.

Nash, M.A., and others: Renal tubular acidosis in infants and children: clinical course, response to treatment and prognosis, J. Pediatr. **80**:738, 1972.

Oetliker, O.H., and Zurbrugg, P.R.P.: Renal tubular acidosis in salt loading syndrome of congenital adrenal hyperplasia (CAH), J. Clin. Endocrinol. Metab. **31**:447, 1970.

Ohlsson, A., and others: A variant of Bartter's syndrome associated with hydramnios, prematurity, hypercalciuria and nephrocalcinosis, Acta Pediatr. Scand. **73**:868, 1984.

Pallisgaard, G., and Goldschmidt, F.: The oculo-cerebro-renal syndrome of Lowe in four generations of one family, Acta. Paediatr. Scand. **60**:146, 1971.

Petersen, S., and others: Pseudohypoaldosteronism: clinical, biochemical and morphological studies in long term follow-up, Acta Paediatr. Scand. **67**:255, 1978.

Pruzansky, W.: Cystinuria and cystine urolithiasis in childhood, Acta Pediatr. Scand. **55**:97, 1966.

Rodriguez-Soriano, J., and Edelmann, C.M., Jr.: Renal tubular acidosis, Ann. Rev. Med. **20**:363, 1969.

Rodriguez-Soriano, J., Vallo, A., and Garcia-Fuentes, M.: Distal renal tubular acidosis in infancy: a bicarbonate wasting state, J. Pediatr. **86**:524, 1975.

Rodriguez-Soriano, J., and others: Proximal renal tubular acidosis: a defect in bicarbonate reabsorption with normal urinary acidification, Pediatr. Res. **1**:81, 1967.

Rosenberg, L.E., Durant, J.L, and Elsas, L.J.: Familial iminoglycinuria: an inborn error of renal tubular transport, N. Engl. J. Med. **278**:1407, 1968.

Rosler, A., and others: Metabolic responses to administration of angiotensin II, K and ACTH in two salt wasting syndromes, J. Clin. Endocrinol. Metab. **44**:292, 1977.

Rosler, A., and others: The nature of the defect of a salt wasting disorder of Jews of Iran, J. Clin. Endocrinol. Metab. **44**:279, 1977.

Schneider, J.A., and Schulman, J.D.: Cystinosis: a review, Metabolism **26**:817, 1977.

Schneider, J.A., and others: Prenatal diagnosis of cystinosis, N. Engl. J. Med. **290**:878, 1974.

Schotland, M.G., Grumbach, M.M., and Strauss, J.: The effect of chlorothiazides in nephrogenic diabetes insipidus, Pediatrics **31**:741, 1963.

Ulick, S., and others: Syndrome of apparent mineralocorticoid excess associated with defects in the peripheral metabolism of cortisol, J. Clin. Endocrinol. Metab. **49**:757, 1979.

Seyberth, H.W., and others: Congenital hypokalemia with hypercalcemia in infants: a hyperprostaglandinuric tubular syndrome different from Bartter's syndrome, J. Pediatr. **107**:69, 1985.

Soriano, J.R., and others: Bartter's syndrome presenting with features resembling renal tubular acidosis, Helv. Paediatr. Acta. **33**:141, 1978.

Spitzer, A., and others: Short stature, hyperkalemia and acidosis: a defect in renal transport of potassium, Kidney Int. **3**:251, 1973.

States, B., and others: Prenatal diagnosis of cystinosis, J. Pediatr. **87**:558, 1975.

Turi, S., Merth, I., and Sztrha, L.: Indomethacin treatment of children suffering from nephrogenic diabetes insipidus or secondary tubulopathy associated with severe polyuria, Int. J. Pediatr. Nephrol. **2**:263, 1981.

Whelan, D.T., and Scriver, G.R.: Hyperdibasic aminoaciduria: an inherited disorder of amino acid transport, Pediatr. Res. **2**:525, 1968.

Infection of the urinary tract

Abbot, G.D.: Neonatal bacteriuria: a prospective study in 1460 infants, Br. Med. J. **1**:267, 1972.

Claesson, I., and others: Radiologic demonstration of compensatory growth of renal parenchyma in children with urinary tract infection and unilateral scarring: an epidemiological study, Kidney Int. **20**:759, 1981.

Dechelette, E., and others: L'infection urinarie du nouveau-ne: a propos de 140 cas, J. Agreg. **13**:485, 1980.

Drew, J.H., and Acton, C.M.: Radiological findings in newborn infants with urinary infection, Arch. Dis. Child. **51**:620, 1976.

Edelmann, C.M., Jr., Ogwo, J., and Fine, B.P.: The prevalence of bacteriuria in full-term and premature newborn infants, J. Pediatr. **82**:125, 1973.

Gower, P.E., and others: Urinary infection in two selected neonatal populations, Arch. Dis. Child. **45**:259, 1970.

Houston, J.B.: Pus cell and bacterial counts in the diagnosis of urinary tract infections in childhood, Arch. Dis. Child. **38**:600, 1983.

Johnston, J.H., and Mix, L.W.: The Ask-Upmark kidney: a form of ascending pyelonephritis? Br.J. Urol. **48**:393, 1976.

Kirpekau, M., and others: Ultrasound in the diagnosis of systemic candidiasis (renal and cranial) in very low birth weight premature infants, Pediatr. Radiology **66**:17, 1986.

Lincoln, K., and Winberg, J.: Studies of urinary tract infections in infancy and childhood. II. Quantitative estimation of bacteriuria in unselected neonates with special reference to the occurrence of asymptomatic infections, Acta. Paediatr. Scand. **53**:307, 1964.

Lincoln, K., and Winberg, J.: Studies of urinary tract infections in infancy and childhood. III. Quantitative estimation of cellular excretion in unselected neonates, Acta Paediatr. Scand. **53**:447, 1964.

Littlewood, J.M.: White cells and bacteria in voided urine of healthy newborns, Arch. Dis. Child. **46**:218, 1972.

Pappu, L.D., and others: Primary renal candidiasis in two premature neonates: report of cases and review of literature on renal candidiasis in infancy, Am. J. Dis. Child. **138**:923, 1984.

Seeler, R.A., and Hahn, K.: Jaundice in urinary tract infection in infancy, Am. J. Dis. Child. **118**:553, 1969.

Smellie, J.M., Normand, I.C.S., and Katz, G.: Children with urinary infection: a comparison of those with and those without vesicoureteric reflux, Kidney Int. **20**:717, 1981.

Smellie, J.M., and others: Effect of vesico-ureteral reflux on renal growth in children with urinary tract infection, Arch. Dis. Child. **56**:593, 1981.

Winberg, J., and others: Clinical pyelonephritis and focal renal scarring: a selected review of pathogenesis, prevention and prognosis, Pediatr. Clin. North Am. **29**:801, 1982.

Wiswill, T.E., Smith, F.R., and Bass, J.W.: Decreased incidence of urinary tract infection in circumcised male infants, Pediatrics **75**:901, 1985.

Vascular disorders of the kidney

Adelman, R.D., and others: Nonsurgical management of renovascular hypertension in the neonate, Pediatrics **62**:71, 1978.

Arneil, G.C., and others: Renal venous thrombosis, Clin. Nephrol. **1**:119, 1973.

Bauer, S.B., and others: Neonatal hypertension: a complication of umbilical-artery catheterization, N. Engl. J. Med. **293**:1032, 1975.

Belman, A.B., and King, L.R.: The pathology and treatment of renal vein thrombosis in the newborn, J. Urol. **107**:852, 1972.

Belman, A.B., and others: Nonoperative treatment of unilateral renal vein thrombosis in the newborn, JAMA **211**:1165, 1970.

Bernstein, J., and Meyer, R.: Congenital abnormalities of the urinary system. II. Renal cortical and medullary necrosis, J. Pediatr. **59**:657, 1961.

Brough, A.J., and Zuelzer, W.W.: Renal vascular disease, Pediatr. Clin. North Am. **11**:533, 1964.

Chesney, R.W., and others: Acute renal failure: an important complication of cardiac surgery in infants, J. Pediatr. **87**:381, 1975.

Demarquez, J.L., and others: Thrombose de la veine renale chez le noveau-ne; traitement par l'urokinase, Arch. Fr. Pediatr. **32**:281, 1972.

Dimmick, J.E., Hardwick, D.F., and Ho-Yuen, B.: A case of renal necrosis and fibrosis in the immediate newborn period: association with the twin-to-twin transfusion syndrome, Am. J. Dis. Child. **122**:345, 1971.

Ford, K.T., Teplick, S.K., and Clark, R.E.: Renal artery embolism causing neonatal hypertension: a complication of umbilical artery catheterization, Radiology **113**:169, 1974.

Groshong, T.D., and others: Renal function following cortical necrosis in childhood, J. Pediatr. **79**:267, 1971.

Gruskin, A.B., and others: Effects of angiography on renal function and histology in infants and piglets, J. Pediatr. **76**:42, 1970.

Halvorsen, J.F., and Moe, P.J.: Renal vein thrombosis in neonates: report of three cases treated with nephrectomy, Acta Pediatr. Scand. **64**:373, 1975.

Leonidas, J.C., Berdon, W.E., and Gribetz, D.: Bilateral renal cortical necrosis in the newborn infant: roentgenographic diagnosis, J. Pediatr. **79**:623, 1971.

Mauer, S.M., and others: Bilateral renal vein thrombosis in infancy: report of a survivor following surgical intervention, J. Pediatr. **83**:933, 1973.

McDonald, P., and others: Some radiologic observations in renal vein thrombosis, Am. J. Roentgenol. Radium. Ther. Med. **120**:368, 1974.

Siegel, S.R., Fisher, D.A., and Oh, W.: Renal function and serum aldosterone levels in infants with respiratory distress syndrome, J. Pediatr. **83**:854, 1973.

Stark, H., and Geiger, R.: Renal tubular dysfunction following vascular accidents of the kidneys in the newborn period, J. Pediatr. **83**:933, 1973.

Takeuchi, A., and Benirschke, K.: Renal venous thrombosis of the newborn and its relation to maternal diabetes, Biol. Neonate **3**:237, 1961.

Tumors of the kidney

Bar-Ziv, J., Hirsch, M., and Perlman, M.: Bilateral nephroblastomatosis, Pediatr. Radiol. **3**:85, 1975.

Beckwith, J.B., and Plamer, N.F.: Histopathology and prognosis of Wilms' tumor: results from the first National Wilms' tumor study, Cancer **41**:1937, 1978.

Berdon, W.E., Wigger, H.J., and Baker, D.H.: Fetal renal hamartoma, a benign tumor to be distinguished from Wilm's tumor: report of 3 cases, Am. J. Roentgenol. Radium Ther. Nucl. Med. **118**:19, 1973.

Birch, J.M., Mardsen, H.B., and Swindell, R.: Incidence of malignant disease in childhood: a 24 year review of the Manchester Childrens tumor registry, Br. J. Cancer **42**:215, 1980.

Bolande, R.P.: Congenital and infantile neoplasia of the kidney, Lancet **2**:1497, 1974.

Breslow, N.E., and others: Wilms' tumor: prognostic factors for patients without metastases at diagnosis: results of the National Wilms' Tumor Study, Cancer **41**:1577, 1978.

Brown, J.M.: Cystic partially differentiated nephroblastoma, J. Pathol. **115**:175, 1975.

D'Angio, G.J., and others: The treatment of Wilms' tumor: results of the second National Wilms' Tumor Study, Cancer **47**:2302, 1981.

Drash, A., and others: A syndrome of male pseudohermaphroditis, Wilms' tumor, hypertension, and degenerative renal disease, J. Pediatr. **76**:585, 1970.

Eklof, O., and Ringertz, H.: Kidney size and growth in unilateral renal agenesis and in the remaining kidney following nephrectomy for Wilms' tumor, Acta. Radiol. (Diagn.) **17**:601, 1976.

Fowler, M.: Differentiated nephroblastoma: solid, crystal, cystic, or mixed, J. Pathol. **105**:215, 1971.

Hung, R., and Kinser, J.: Ultrasonic diagnosis of Wilm's tumor, Am. J. Radiol. **117**:119, 1973.

Joshi, V.V., and others: Congenital mesoblastic nephroma of infancy: report of a case with unusual clinical behavior, Am. J. Clin. Pathol. **60**:811, 1973.

Kumar, A.P.M., and others: Treatment strategy for nodular renal blastema and nephroblastomatosis associated with Wilms' tumor, J. Pediatr. Surg. **13**:281, 1978.

Liban, E., and Kozenitzky, I.L.: Metanephric hamartomas and nephroblastomatosis in siblings, Cancer **25**:885, 1970.

Mankad, V.N., Gray, G.F., Jr., and Miller, D.R.: Bilateral nephroblastomatosis and Klippel Trenaunay syndrome, Cancer **33**:1462, 1974.

Maria, J.E., and others: Renal transplantation in patients with bilateral Wilms' tumor, J. Pediatr. Surg. **14**:577, 1979.

Maurer, H.S., and others: The role of genetic factors in the etiology of Wilms' tumor: two pairs of monozygous twins with congenital abnormalities (aniridia, hemihypertrophy) and discordance for Wilms' tumor, Cancer **43**:205, 1979.

Perlman, M., Levin, M., and Wittels, B.L.: Syndrome of fetal gigantism, renal hamartomas, and nephroblastomatosis with Wilms' tumor, Cancer **35**:1212, 1975.

Sacko, G., and others: Scintigraphic and sonographic diagnosis of neonatal mesoblastic nephroma-case report, Clin. Nucl. Med. **8**:252, 1983.

Telander, R.L., and others: Bilateral massive nephroblastomatosis in infancy, J. Pediatr. Surg. **13**:163, 1978.

CHAPTER 36

Inborn errors of metabolism

It is not possible to review in a chapter each of the hundred or so inborn errors of metabolism that have been reported to cause clinical disease in the affected newborn infant. Therefore this chapter limits itself to the less uncommon diseases that have clinical manifestations in the neonatal period, to those for which therapy has been advised even though clinical manifestations are lacking, and to those diseases, however rare, that contribute to our understanding of metabolic disease in the newborn infant.

In the recognition of inborn errors of metabolism in the newborn period the most important clue is the history of a sibling affected by a metabolic disorder. There are few specific signs of these diseases. Most affected infants are products of normal pregnancies and are clinically normal at birth. At varying intervals after birth they may develop lethargy, poor feeding, and persistent vomiting, generally with some evidence of depression of central nervous system function. Seizures may occur. Frequently myoclonic, the seizures also may be major and either generalized or focal. Although some affected infants have normal or increased muscle tone, the majority show rather profound hypotonia. The tachypnea and hyperventilation of metabolic acidosis may be noted. In a number of diverse disorders prolonged and unusually severe neonatal jaundice has been observed.

The initial laboratory evaluation of an infant suspected of having metabolic disease should include (1) complete blood count, including leukocyte differential and platelet counts, (2) urinalysis with tests for glucose, reducing substance, ketones, and acids reactive with 2,4-dinitrophenylhydrazine, (3) measurement of arterial (or arterialized capillary) pH, P_{CO_2}, and P_{O_2} (or oxygen saturation), and (4) measurement of plasma glucose, sodium, potassium, chloride, bicarbonate, calcium, magnesium, and ammonia.

If the results obtained in this evaluation are normal, and the infant shows clear-cut neurologic deterioration, quantitative analysis of amino acids in cerebrospinal fluid (CSF) should also be done.

All of these initial steps, with the possible exception of quantitative amino acid analysis in CSF, can be carried out rapidly, leading to a rational approach to further investigation and to management. Other necessary components in the overall assessment of the suspect infant include:

1. Quantitative analysis of plasma amino acids
2. Quantitative analysis of amino acids and organic acids in urine
3. Skin biopsy for establishment of fibroblast cultures for subsequent biochemical analysis; such cultures can be established from material obtained at autopsy

If a diagnosis is established in a surviving infant, there are four general approaches to management:

1. If efficacy of any therapeutic measure has not been demonstrated, one may elect to employ no specific management.
2. One may restrict the intake of the metabolite that accumulates in the disorder. This approach is effective in classic phenylketonuria but may not be generally applicable. For example, in some disorders it is possible that adequate levels of the normal product of the blocked reaction are dependent in part on stimulation of residual enzyme activity by high levels of the precursor metabolite.
3. One may increase the intake of the normal metabolite that is not produced because of the metabolic error. This approach has produced chemical remission in orotic aciduria. It requires that the administered metabolite be absorbed and transported effectively to the site of need.
4. One may administer large amounts of the cofactor(s) that participates in the blocked reaction (megavitamin therapy). This form of management has been dramatically effective in some cases—generally, although not always, in disorders involving vitamin metabolism.

It is frequently necessary in practice to institute management of a seriously ill infant before the results of specific tests are known. In such circumstances general

Table 36-1. Some vitamins employed in megavitamin therapy

Vitamin	Recommended allowance (mg/day)	100 × (mg/day)	1,000 × (mg/day)	Toxicity
Pyridoxine	0.3	30	300	None
Thiamine	0.3	30	300	None
Riboflavin	0.4	40	400	None
Niacinamide	6	600	6,000	None (short term)
Cobalamin*	0.0005	0.05	0.5	None
Folic acid	0.03	3	30	Loss of seizure control
Ascorbic acid	35	3,500	35,000	None
Biotin†	0.035	3.5	35	None
Pantothenic acid	2	200	2,000	None

*Recommended megavitamin dose: hydroxocobalamin 2 mg/day IM.
†Recommended megavitamin dose: biotin 10 to 40 mg/day PO.

principles of management are as follows: specimens for the studies previously outlined must be collected as a first priority, both for patient management and for future genetic counseling. Catabolic stress should be minimized by providing the infant with 30 gm of glucose/kg/day (120 kcal/kg/day) for the first few days of management. Megavitamin therapy may be therapeutically effective (Table 36-1). Exchange transfusion or peritoneal dialysis may ameliorate the condition sufficiently to allow definitive diagnosis and management.

NEONATAL SCREENING TESTS

Screening tests for inherited diseases are widely employed in neonatal nurseries. The specific disorders are discussed in detail later in the chapter.

The general usefulness of any given test is a function of its sensitivity and specificity on the one hand, and the possibility of effective intervention on the other. Given current obstetric practice, the former consideration means that the disease must be expressed sufficiently on the third day of life to allow its detection, and that the test employed must be positive in virtually 100% of affected infants and negative in virtually 100% of nonaffected infants. Effectiveness of intervention is to some extent a matter of judgment. All would agree that congenital hypothyroidism detected by screening can be effectively treated. Many would not agree that cystic fibrosis can be more effectively treated because it is detected by neonatal screening, but the issue becomes more complex when genetic counseling is included as a major component of the total process of intervention.

Since neonatal screening is generally government funded, an element of practicality is added: a screening program should be cost effective (i.e., should result in a lowering of the cost to government of medical care for its citizens). Hence a disease for which screening is employed should be common enough and disabling enough to impose a reasonably large associated cost on society, and this cost should be significantly lowered by detection and treatment in the neonatal period.

Another practical consideration involves both the type of sample to be used for screening and the laboratory techniques to be employed. What has evolved as most effective is collection of whole blood obtained by heelstick on filter paper strips and transport of the dried strips to central laboratories, where automated methods of testing can be used at relatively little cost.

The following diseases are generally included in neonatal screening programs in the United States:

1. Congenital hypothyroidism affects roughly 1 in 5,000 infants, can be efficiently detected in dried blood spots, and can be effectively treated at low cost with great reduction in morbidity. (See Chapter 37, part three.)
2. Phenylketonuria affects 1 in 16,000 infants, can be efficiently detected, and can be treated effectively at a cost that is high but much lower in both human and monetary terms than the cost of not screening for and treating the disease.
3. Galactosemia affects 1 in 50,000 to 100,000 infants. The screening assay for galactose in blood (Paigen) is relatively efficient, but the disease is so severe in many neonates that the result of the screening test may be reported too late. Treatment of the disease is very effective and not costly.
4. Maple syrup urine disease affects approximately 1 in 200,000 infants. The screening test is quite reliable but may not be reported in time to prevent life-threatening illness in some affected infants. Treatment is very costly, its success dependent in significant part on the severity of the chemical defect.
5. Homocystinuria affects approximately 1 in 100,000 infants. The screening test currently used measures the level of methionine in whole blood: it is not very sensitive, although relatively specific under current feeding practices. Pyridoxine-responsive homocystin-

uria is effectively treated at low cost. If treatment requires a diet with altered amino acid composition, the cost of treatment rises significantly, and effectiveness is somewhat less predictable.

It is obvious from this discussion that large-scale neonatal screening for phenylketonuria and congenital hypothyroidism is easily justified, that a reliable cribside test for galactosemia would be preferable to large-scale screening, and that large-scale neonatal screening for maple syrup urine disease and homocystinuria has limited usefulness. Screening programs are in a state of evolution, and tests will be added or deleted as their merits dictate.

DISORDERS OF AMINO ACID METABOLISM

Disorders of the metabolism of phenylalanine and tyrosine

Phenylketonuria

Clinically there are two forms of phenylketonuria. The first, classic phenylketonuria, is the result of a deficiency of phenylalanine hydroxylase and responds both chemically and clinically to a diet restricted in phenylalanine. The second form, sometimes called (inappropriately) malignant hyperphenylalaninemia, is the result of defective metabolism of the coenzyme for phenylalanine hydroxylase, tetrahydrobiopterin. In this form of the disorder, dietary restriction of phenylalanine results in lowering of plasma phenylalanine without affecting the neurologic consequences of the disease.

Etiology and pathogenesis. It has been repeatedly demonstrated that phenylalanine hydroxylase activity is absent or nearly so in classic phenylketonuria. The pathogenesis of the clinical disease is unclear but is without doubt related to accumulation in tissues and body fluids of unmetabolized phenylalanine, since restriction of dietary phenylalanine is therapeutically effective.

In the normal growing infant dietary phenylalanine is in part used for protein synthesis and in part hydroxylated to form tyrosine (Fig. 36-1). In the latter reaction tetrahydrobiopterin, the cofactor, is oxidized to dihydrobiopterin. Tetrahydrobiopterin then is regenerated in a NADPH-dependent reaction catalyzed by dihydrobiopterin reductase. Not a vitamin, tetrahydrobiopterin is synthesized de novo from guanosine triphosphate in a series of reactions that are at present being elucidated.

Although neither phenylalanine nor tyrosine can be synthesized de novo, phenylalanine can spare the dietary requirement for tyrosine. Tyrosine cannot be converted back to phenylalanine. This irreversibility is also significant for the interpretation of laboratory data. Defects in metabolism of tyrosine have no direct effect on the level of phenylalanine in plasma; individuals with hereditary tyrosinosis characteristically exhibit normal plasma levels of phenylalanine. Therefore an elevation of plasma phenylalanine occurring under normal dietary conditions in-

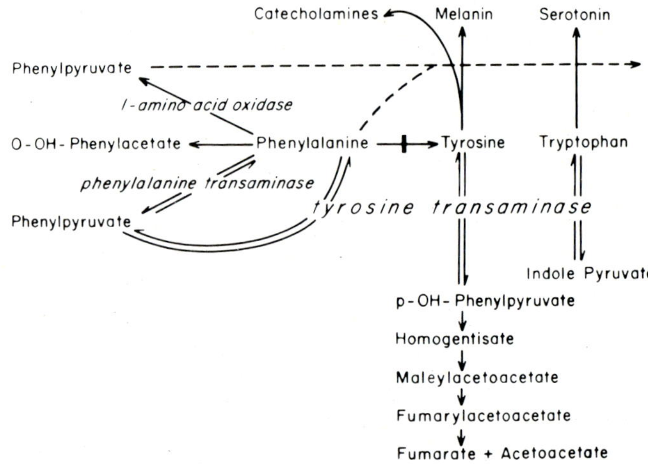

Fig. 36-1. Schematic representation of the metabolism of phenylalanine, tyrosine, and tryptophan. Solid crossbar indicates the metabolic block demonstrated in phenylketonuria, whereas broken crossbars indicate postulated secondary metabolic blocks.

dicates an impairment in phenylalanine hydroxylation. The degradation of tyrosine is initiated in the liver by tyrosine transaminase, an enzyme that also catalyzes the transamination of phenylalanine and tryptophan. In the experimental animal any of these three aromatic amino acids is capable of inducing increased activity of tyrosine transaminase.

In a quantitative sense the metabolic pathway of phenylalanine and tyrosine evolves during the latter part of gestation. As a result, premature infants are likely to show elevations in both phenylalanine and tyrosine in plasma. Full-term infants do so less frequently. This condition commonly is called *transient tyrosinemia*. The elevations in both phenylalanine and tyrosine can be extreme, more than 20 times normal, and indeed may not be without risk of neurologic sequelae. In this regard it should be noted that identification of transient tyrosinemia occurred during an era when infants commonly received formulas that contained four times as much protein per ounce as human milk does. One recent study of a small group of premature infants showed no elevations above normal in plasma phenylalanine and tyrosine when dietary intake simulated that provided by human milk. The quantitative aspects of phenylalanine metabolism are thus relatively simple, but the physiologic ramifications of impairments in the pathway also involve considerations of both the neurochemical metabolism of phenylalanine and the interrelationships of the metabolism of the three aromatic amino acids: phenylalanine, tyrosine, and tryptophan. Phenylalanine and tyrosine are precursors of epinephrine, norepinephrine, dopamine, and octopamine, and tryptophan is a precursor of serotonin (Fig. 36-2). Because the aromatic amino acids have

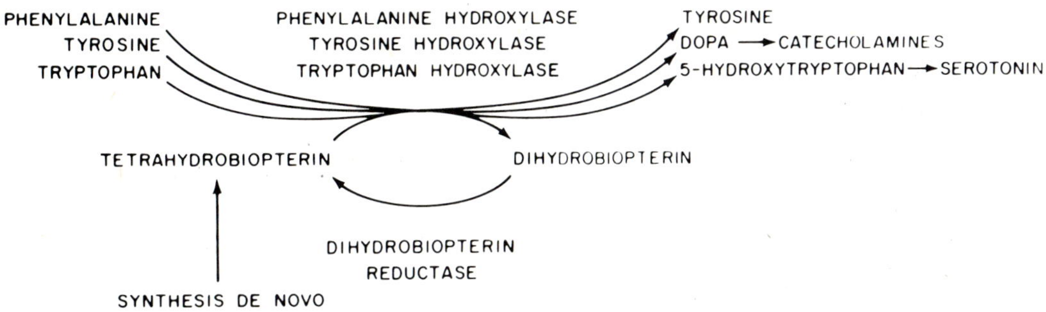

Fig. 36-2. Biopterin metabolism and its relationship to the synthesis of neurotransmitters.

analogous structures and share enzymatic pathways, it can be expected that great excesses in tissue levels of one, for example, phenylalanine, can impair the conversion of the others, for example, tyrosine and tryptophan, into neurally active compounds. Furthermore the hydroxylations of phenylalanine to form tyrosine, of tyrosine to form dopa, and of tryptophan to form 5-hydroxytryptophan all require tetrahydrobiopterin. In the two inborn errors of biopterin metabolism now defined—the first a deficiency of dihydrobiopterin reductase, the second a failure in de novo synthesis of tetrahydrobiopterin—hyperphenylalaninemia occurs together with reduced amounts of neurotransmitters whose synthesis is dependent on the availability of tetrahydrobiopterin.

It is a simplifying and attractive hypothesis, as yet unproven, that the neurologic disorder in phenylketonuria of whatever cause occurs as a result of impaired or disordered synthesis of neurotransmitters. In the classic disease phenylalanine accumulations in excess of 20 times normal interfere with the normal metabolism of tyrosine and tryptophan. In the variant disorder deficiency of tetrahydrobiopterin interferes with normal metabolism of all three aromatic amino acids, although not with the degradative pathways for tyrosine and tryptophan.

Clinical manifestations. There are no reliable clinical manifestations of phenylketonuria in the neonatal period. Feeding difficulties, choking spells, and vomiting occur in some patients. Hypertrophic pyloric stenosis has been diagnosed in a number of patients, and the association may well be more than coincidental. Since the definition of phenylketonuria caused by defective cofactor metabolism, it has become apparent that clinical difficulties in the neonatal period are more likely to occur in this form of the disease than in classic phenylketonuria. Poor muscle tone and impaired feeding have been reported from birth in the variant form, but it does not appear that neonatal neurologic development can be clearly distinguished from normal in any of the forms of phenylketonuria.

Diagnosis. Although urinary phenylpyruvic acid is the hallmark of phenylketonuria, its appearance cannot be relied on in the neonatal period. The classic criterion for the diagnosis of phenylketonuria in the neonatal period is plasma phenylalanine of 20 mg/dl or more associated with low or normal plasma tyrosine, both values obtained while the infant is receiving normal feedings. This criterion was established in studies of classic phenylketonuria, which accounts for 98% of affected subjects. The number of patients known to have cofactor-related disease is now large enough to define a disturbingly wide range of values for plasma phenylalanine associated with these diseases. Suffice it to say that minor elevations in plasma phenylalanine are consistent with the diagnosis, and normal plasma phenylalanine in the first weeks of life does not exclude cofactor-related disease.

It has been proposed that the response of plasma phenylalanine to test doses of tetrahydrobiopterin be used to define cofactor-related disease in hyperphenylalaninemic infants. Lack of response indicates absence of phenylalanine hydroxylase, whereas a fall in plasma phenylalanine indicates either defective de novo synthesis or defective regeneration of tetrahydrobiopterin. Theoretically it is possible that, in the presence of deficient but not absent phenylalanine hydroxylase, a great excess of tetrahydrobiopterin could stimulate hydroxylation of phenylalanine, thus lowering plasma phenylalanine. Quantitation of pterins (metabolites of the biopterin pathway) also has been proposed as a means of defining the presence or absence of cofactor-related disease. At this writing these techniques are becoming widely available in the United States.

Treatment of classic phenylketonuria. The evidence regarding diet therapy in phenylketonuria clearly indicates that restriction of phenylalanine intake is beneficial and also that overrestriction of dietary phenylalanine is detrimental to the health of these infants. The objective of therapy as currently practiced is to reduce plasma phenylalanine to a level that allows normal intellectual development while giving amounts of dietary phenylalanine adequate enough to ensure against phenylalanine deficiency. The usual requirement for phenylalanine in the neonatal period is 60 to 80 mg/kg/day. Infants diagnosed as having treatable hyperphenylalaninemia therefore are given a low-phenylalanine formula (3 mg phenylalanine per ounce of prepared formula) together with enough cow's milk (50 mg phenylalanine per ounce of prepared formula) to provide 70 mg phenylalanine/kg/day. Plasma phenylalanine is monitored and dietary phenylalanine adjusted to achieve an appropriate level of phenylalanine in plasma. Adequate growth cannot be achieved unless plasma phenylalanine is allowed to remain several milligrams per deciliter above the normal fasting level. Our clinic strives to maintain the plasma phenylalanine level at 8 to 10 mg/dl with consistently negative reactions to urinary ferric chloride tests. Solid food is added at appropriate intervals, according to a diet plan such as that ordered by a manufacturer of low phenylalanine formula.

The hazards of a treatment program for phenylketonuria cannot be overemphasized. Points of particular concern are given in the following sections.

Accuracy of diagnosis. The criteria previously given are appropriate for a single point in time only. Apparent phenylalanine tolerance, as manifested by plasma phenylalanine levels, may change markedly with time. Borderline patients not selected for treatment should be observed closely. Those subjected to treatment should be assessed periodically for accuracy of diagnosis. For this purpose a trial of unlimited phenylalanine intake is preferred over an abrupt test of phenylalanine tolerance.

Overtreatment: phenylalanine deficiency. Rouse has documented the hazards of prolonged inappropriate restriction of phenylalanine in the diet of infants not having phenylketonuria. Hackney and co-workers suggested that disappointing results in dietary treatment may in part be the result of unrecognized phenylalanine deficiency. In young infants both phenylalanine requirement and phenylalanine intake may fluctuate widely over short periods of time under ideal conditions. Stress, such as infection, accentuates such fluctuations. It is therefore necessary to monitor plasma phenylalanine at very frequent intervals. The following schedule is suggested:

0 to 6 months	Twice weekly
6 months to 1 year	Once weekly
1 year to 18 months	Twice monthly
18 months until cessation of therapy	Once monthly

The analyses must be promptly performed and the results immediately applied to management.

Growth. Many appropriately treated patients do not grow normally. The distinction between impairment of growth caused by phenylalanine deficiency and that caused by the effects of a largely synthetic diet is sometimes difficult to make.

Treatment for cofactor-related phenylketonuria. For variant phenylketonuria in which tetrahydrobiopterin metabolism is defective, it would seem appropriate to treat with tetrahydrobiopterin. Such therapy may indeed lower plasma phenylalanine, obviating the need for a phenylalanine-restricted diet. However, it seems clear that the dose of tetrahydrobiopterin necessary to reduce plasma phenylalanine is much lower than that required to correct the defects in the metabolism of neurotransmitters in the brain, if in fact tetrahydrobiopterin alone can achieve this primary therapeutic goal. As a result, treatment at present involves the administration of L-dopa, 5-hydroxytryptophan, and carbidopa in addition to management of plasma phenylalanine. The use of tetrahydrobiopterin and its analogs is under intense investigation at this time. Monitoring of the response to therapy involves not only measurement of phenylalanine in blood but also assessment of neurotransmitter levels in CSF, and hence cannot be accomplished without sophisticated laboratory support. Amelioration of neuromuscular manifestations and improvement in sensorium have been demonstrated in older infants treated with various combinations of the agents noted above.

Treatment of hyperphenylalaninemia. Infants whose serum phenylalanine is greater than 10 mg/dl but less than 20 mg/dl are best managed initially by restricting dietary protein to 2 gm/kg/day. Serum phenylalanine generally falls to concentrations less than 10 mg/dl with this management. Should it fail to do so, it is best to use a regimen of specific phenylalanine restriction as in classic phenylketonuria.

Genetics. Classic phenylketonuria is inherited as an autosomal recessive disease. Reasonably accurate differentiation between heterozygous and normal individuals has been achieved by measurement of phenylalanine and tyrosine in blood, but the techniques employed are not useful except in studies of populations. Information concerning the inheritance of cofactor-related disease is all consistent with autosomal recessive transmission. It must be noted that as many as nine distinct varieties of hyperphenylalaninemia have been defined. Some are quite rare, and one of these may be transmitted as a sex-linked character.

Tyrosinosis

Tyrosinosis is a rare disorder in which plasma and urinary tyrosine are greatly increased. The only known clinical abnormality that is consistently present is the Richner-Hanhart syndrome (keratoconjunctivitis palmoplantaris). Conjunctival irritation has been noted in the neonatal period. Deficiency of hepatic mitochondrial tyrosine aminotransferase (TAT) in this disease has been demonstrated (see Fig. 36-1), as has the clinical efficacy of dietary restriction of phenylalanine and tyrosine.

Neonatal tyrosinemia, acute tyrosinemia, chronic tyrosinemia, and hypermethioninemia

These terms were in the past applied to a chemically

heterogeneous group of disorders that had in common elevation of plasma tyrosine with or without concomitant elevation of plasma methionine. The clinical manifestations are predominantly those of acute and chronic liver disease, renal tubular dysfunction, and impairment of central nervous system development.

Etiology and pathogenesis. A number of infants seen within the first year of life, primarily with manifestations of severe hepatic dysfunction, have been shown to have striking elevations of plasma tyrosine or methionine or both. Enzymatic defects in the metabolic pathways for the affected amino acids have been clearly documented in these infants; the most prominent defect being markedly reduced activity of parahydroxy phenylpyruvic acid oxidase (see Fig. 36-1). It is now clear that liver disease causes these enzymatic defects and not vice versa. Tyrosinemia and methioninemia can be seen in a number of diseases that result in diffuse hepatocellular damage, for example, neonatal hepatitis, hereditary fructose intolerance, galactosemia, and fructose-1,6-diphosphatase deficiency.

However, it has become clear over the last decade that the majority of infants who have clinically severe liver disease and elevations of plasma tyrosine and/or methionine suffer from an inherited defect in the last step in the catabolism of phenylalanine and tyrosine, that is, the hydrolysis of fumarylacetoacetic acid to fumaric and acetoacetic acids (Fig. 36-3). Although the exact chemical consequences of this defect are not known, it seems likely that fumarylacetoacetic acid and its by-products are extremely toxic to the liver and the kidney.

Clinical manifestations. The manifestations of this syndrome in the neonatal period are largely those of acute hepatic dysfunction with or without evidence of renal tubular dysfunction. Listlessness, vomiting, diarrhea, abdominal enlargement with hepatomegaly, splenomegaly, and ascites are prominent clinical features. Bleeding disorders are common, and coma may evolve in the course of this disorder. Mortality is high in the neonatal period.

It is readily apparent that the manifestations described above are those of neonatal hepatitis, neonatal septicemia, and the inborn errors of metabolism listed above, all of which enter into the differential diagnosis.

Laboratory manifestations. Moderate to striking elevations of plasma tyrosine or methionine or both are present. In neonatal tyrosinemia, tyrosyluria is a constant finding. Hyperphenylalaninemia and elevation of other plasma amino acids may be seen. Hypoglycemia, hypophosphatemia, and galactosuria have been noted. The results of the usual tests of hepatic function are grossly abnormal. Anemia, thrombocytopenia, and leukopenia are common. In infants with fumarylacetoacetic acid hydrolase deficiency, succinyl acetone is always present in the urine, whereas in other conditions it is apparently absent. Measurement of succinyl acetone, a by-product of the altered metabolism of fumarylacetoacetic acid, requires sophisticated chromatographic techniques. Because delta-amino-levulinic acid is likely to be excreted in excess by these infants, its measurement may be useful in differential diagnosis.

Treatment. Some patients with acute tyrosinemia have responded favorably to a diet restricted in tyrosine and phenylalanine (and methionine, if methioninemia is present). Dietary treatment could be expected to be effective if it resulted in a clinically significant reduction in the production of maleylacetoacetic acid (Fig. 36-3). However, there is some evidence that significant liver damage occurs without elevation of plasma tyrosine. This is consistent with the poor long-term outlook for patients with a known deficiency of fumarylacetoacetic acid hydrolase. Given the mortality of the condition in the neonatal period and the difficulty in differential diagnosis, it is probably wise both to employ low-phenylalanine, low-tyrosine (low-methionine) feedings and to alter the carbohydrate source to glucose.

Prognosis. The disorder may be fatal early, enter a chronic phase, or remit completely; the result is probably dependent on both cause and management. For infants with chronic tyrosinemia caused by a deficiency of fu-

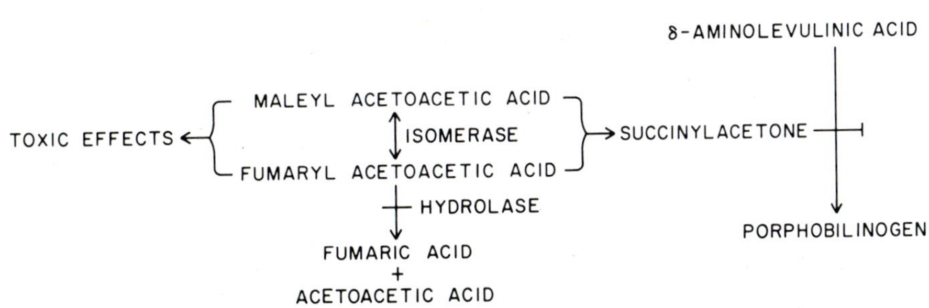

Fig. 36-3. Metabolism of maleylacetoacetic acid. Hydrolysis of fumarylacetoacetic acid by fumarylacetoacetate hydrolase is blocked as indicated in most instances of neonatal tyrosinemia. Secondary block in synthesis of porphobilinogen is also a component of the metabolic error.

marylacetoacetic acid hydrolase, the long-term outlook is not good; many of these infants develop hepatocellular carcinoma during late childhood.

Genetics. When tyrosinemia is the result of an inborn error of metabolism, the usual mode of inheritance is autosomal recessive, whatever the nature of the metabolic error.

Alcaptonuria

Alcaptonuria, a disorder of the oxidation of homogentisic acid (see Fig. 36-1), leads to the excretion of large amounts of homogentisic acid in the urine. The only manifestation of the disorder in the neonatal period is the darkening of diapers on standing. This reaction is the basis for the diagnostic test in which sodium hydroxide is added to freshly voided urine or dropped onto a freshly wet diaper. The production of a blackish brown stain is almost immediate and is virtually diagnostic of alcaptonuria. Plasma tyrosine and phenylalanine are normal in alcaptonuria.

Although a low-phenylalanine, low-tyrosine diet has been recommended in this condition to prevent the deposition of melanin-like by-products in joint cartilage, there is little justification for the imposition of such an abnormal diet in children with this disorder.

Alcaptonuria is inherited as an autosomal recessive disease.

Homocystinuria

Homocystinuria is a disorder of the metabolism of sulfur-containing amino acids that is associated with a progressive clinical syndrome involving the eye, the integument, the bones and connective tissues, the blood vessels, and the central nervous system.

Etiology and pathogenesis. The fundamental defect in homocystinuria is marked reduction in the activity of cystathionine synthetase (Fig. 36-4). This defect leads to the accumulation of homocystine in blood and urine and generally of methionine in the blood. The synthesis of cystine also is impaired. It is generally believed that homocystine and/or the products of its altered metabolism are responsible for the slowly evolving clinical syndrome. Although the results of therapy support this view, the pathogenesis of the disease is by no means clear. Mechanisms have been proposed whereby homocystine, homocysteine, and homocysteic acid could alter the tertiary structure of connective tissue proteins, damage vascular endothelium, alter platelet function, and otherwise inappropriately activate the clotting mechanism. A number of these mechanisms are quite attractive intellectually, but as yet none are proven.

Extensive research into the fate of homocystine has shown that a substantial fraction of homocysteine produced in the metabolism of methionine is reconverted into methionine. A number of disorders of this reconversion have been described. They are much less common than classic homocystinuria; but they are of clinical interest for two reasons. First, several of them involve the metabolism of cobalamin or folic acid and are possibly subject to megavitamin therapy. Second, a number of these defects have resulted in megaloblastic anemia in early infancy. In these disorders, hypermethioninemia is, obviously, not to be expected.

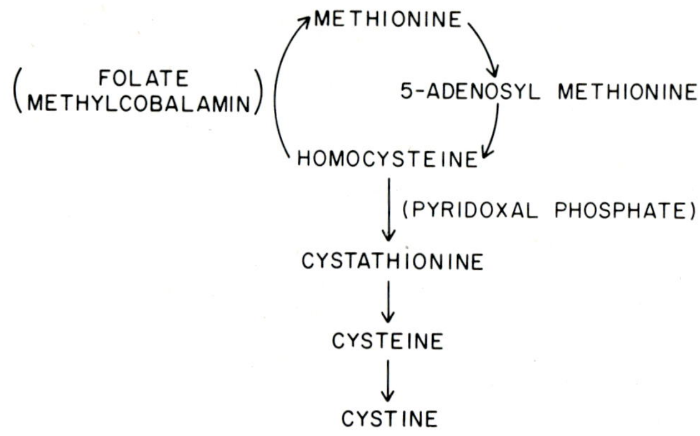

Fig. 36-4. Schematic representation of the pathway of metabolism for the production of cystine from methionine. In classic homocystinuria the synthesis of cystathionine is impaired. Failure of resynthesis of methionine from homocysteine can also result in homocystinuria.

Clinical manifestations. Infants with homocystinuria are normal at birth and remain so throughout the neonatal period. The clinical manifestations are progressive. Most characteristic is ectopia lentis, which commonly appears between 2½ and 3⅓ years of age. Many affected individuals develop constitutional features of Marfan's syndrome, malar flush, and livedo reticularis of the lower extremities. About half the patients have intellectual deficits. Thrombotic episodes involving both small and large arteries and veins are a constant threat to the older homocystinuric individual.

Laboratory manifestations. The characteristic laboratory manifestation of homocystinuria is the presence of homocystine in the urine. This substance can be readily detected by the cyanide-nitroprusside test for compounds containing —S—S— or —S—H groups. Confirmation of the diagnosis is best obtained by column chromatography of amino acids from plasma or urine. The amount of free homocystine in homocystinuric plasma is relatively small. Because homocystine reacts readily with plasma protein, the diagnosis can be missed if plasma samples are allowed to stand for long periods prior to analysis. Rarely homocystine appears in the blood and urine of subjects who have other metabolic disorders. It is therefore worthwhile to exclude both cystathioninuria with secondary homocystinuria and defective cobalamin metabolism giving rise to both homocystinuria and methylmalonic aciduria.

Treatment. The goal of management in homocystinuria is the normalization of plasma homocystine, methionine, and cystine. In about half the affected subjects this goal can be approached effectively by the administration of large doses of pyridoxine, a cofactor for cystathionine synthetase. Effective dosages have ranged from 25 to 1,000 mg/day in older subjects, the wide range reflecting both genetic heterogeneity and in all likelihood the presence of unrecognized folate depletion in some of the treated subjects. For those whose response to megavitamin therapy is less than ideal, a diet low in methionine and enriched in cystine should be employed. With this scheme of management reasonable control of plasma homocystine can be achieved with lowering of plasma methionine. Plasma cystine has proved more refractory to therapy. In any case the available, albeit limited, evidence suggests clinical efficacy.

Genetics. Homocystinuria is inherited as an autosomal recessive disease.

Nonketotic hyperglycinemia

Nonketotic hyperglycinemia is a familial disorder of glycine metabolism in which profound dysfunction of the nervous system is noted shortly after birth. A large percentage of affected infants die within the first 2 weeks of life, and most of the remainder exhibit severe motor and mental retardation.

Etiology and pathogenesis. Of the many pathways of glycine metabolism noted in Fig. 36-5, only glycine cleavage is known to be affected in nonketotic hyperglycinemia, and this appears to be the primary phenomenon in the pathogenesis of this disorder. The mechanism through which the profound clinical effects of the disease are produced is unclear. Extreme elevation in plasma glycine, seen in infants undergoing total parenteral nutrition, has no apparent clinical effect. No forceful argument can be made at this time that abnormalities in gluconeogenesis and methyl group metabolism, occurring as secondary effects of the defect in glycine cleavage, are clinically significant. On the other hand, Perry has pointed out that the clinical manifestations of hyperglycinemia correlate with the concentration of glycine in cerebrospinal fluid, not with concentration in plasma, and that such elevations of glycine in cerebrospinal fluid are seen only in nonketotic hyperglycinemia. The hypothesis that glycine excess in the central nervous system produces the clinical disease by altering neurotransmission gained some support from the observation that two affected infants showed clinical improvement when treated with strychnine, an antagonist to glycine in neurotransmission. Other patients so treated have shown no clinical response.

Clinical manifestations. Almost all patients with this disorder show serious abnormalities within the first few days of life. Poor feeding, lethargy, and hypotonia progressing to coma and apnea have been noted regularly. Seizures, both myoclonic and generalized, are common. Physical examination reveals lack of responsiveness, hypotonia, and diminished Moro and deep tendon reflexes.

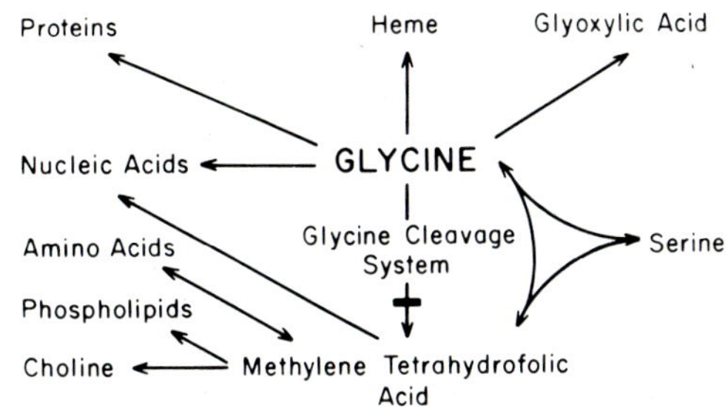

Fig. 36-5. Schematic representation of the metabolism of glycine. Crossbar indicates the metabolic block in nonketotic hyperglycinemia.

In severely affected infants who survive the first 2 weeks of life, a waxing and waning course evolves in which prolonged periods of muscle spasm alternate with brief periods of relaxation. Seizures, typically myoclonic, occur both singly and in bursts. Poor feeding occurs for protracted periods, and motor and mental development is profoundly retarded.

Laboratory manifestations. The essential laboratory finding in nonketotic hyperglycinemia is striking elevation of glycine in cerebrospinal fluid. Plasma and urinary glycine levels are almost always elevated, but the abnormality in blood and urine is much less specific than that in cerebrospinal fluid. Arterial P_{CO_2} may be increased and P_{O_2} decreased as a result of respiratory depression.

Treatment. Aside from the previously noted reports of the efficacy of strychnine therapy in two patients, no effective management of nonketotic hyperglycinemia has been achieved. Dietary therapy and the use of sodium benzoate, methionine, and alanine have been attempted without clinical success. Diazepam has been reported to ameliorate the neuromuscular manifestations.

Genetics. Nonketotic hyperglycinemia is inherited as an autosomal recessive disease.

Histidinemia

Histidinemia is a disorder of the catabolism of histidine caused by lack of histidase activity. It is characterized by the excretion of imidazolepyruvic acid, which gives positive reactions to ferric chloride and 2,4-dinitrophenylhydrazine tests on urine samples, similar to the reactions obtained in phenylketonuria. Plasma histidine is generally four to ten times normal.

Although there may be considerable genetic heterogeneity in histidinemia, there is no clear evidence at present that it is a harmful condition. There are no neonatal manifestations other than the laboratory findings noted above. Although dietary therapy has been proposed for affected neonates because a substantial number of histidinemic patients are mentally retarded, prospective data, obtained on the basis of neonatal screening, do not support this recommendation.

Sulfite oxidase deficiency

Sulfite oxidase deficiency, with or without concomitant deficiency of xanthine dehydrogenase, has been reported in a number of infants. When both deficiencies are present, the defect is lack of the molybdenum cofactor for both reactions. The disease is manifest by seizures—both tonic-clonic and myoclonic—beginning shortly after birth, together with poor feeding and hypertonia. Dislocated lenses are a feature of the disease, and enophthalmos and nystagmus may be present. When xanthinuria is present, urinary xanthine stones may form.

The diagnosis can be made by finding sulfite in the urine, but a more practical test is that for urinary thiosulfate, which is present in the urine in large amounts in sulfite oxidase deficiency, but only in trace amounts normally.

Allopurinol has been employed to reduce xanthine excretion. The major clinical problems are related to deficiency of sulfite oxidase, for which dietary treatment has been given with chemical, but not significant clinical, effect.

DISORDERS OF THE UREA CYCLE

Disorders of the urea cycle severe enough to cause clinical disease in the neonate have as their hallmarks profound encephalopathy and striking elevation of blood ammonia. In the past it was thought that all infants exhibiting these signs were lethally affected. Developments over the past decade now indicate that some potentially lethal inborn errors of the urea cycle can be treated simply and effectively and that lethal hyperammonemic encephalopathy can occur both as a secondary phenomenon early in the course of treatable disorders of the propionate pathway and also as a self-limited phenomenon in infants who have no definable inborn disorder of metabolism. These discoveries clearly mandate an aggressive approach to the management of hyperammonemic encephalopathy in the neonate.

Etiology and pathogenesis

Urea accounts for two thirds of the total urinary nitrogen excreted by the neonate and thus is clearly the major excretory product in nitrogen metabolism. From a quantitative standpoint urea is produced by the liver alone. Its synthesis occurs in five reactions (Fig. 36-6), the first two of which are mitochondrial and energy requiring. The last three reactions occur in the cytosol. Functionally the smooth flow of nitrogen into urea also requires integrity of the hepatic circulation, of transmembrane transport systems, and of general mitochondrial function. Although urea is an end product in that it is not metabolized by mammals, it is a dynamic metabolite functionally. A substantial fraction of the total urea pool is broken down by intestinal microorganisms. The nitrogen, liberated as ammonia, returns to the liver via the portal circulation, where it is either incorporated into amino acids or reincorporated into urea. That human metabolism is oriented toward ammonia fixation is reflected in the normal values for the concentration of ammonia in peripheral blood—25 μmol/L, compared with 500 μmol/L for blood urea nitrogen. Nitrogen destined for excretion in peripheral tissues is transported to the liver predominantly as glutamine and alanine. Chemical hyperammonemia of mild degree can occur in a variety of stressful conditions, but severe hyperammonemia of clinical significance is indicative of a profound disruption in hepatic function, be it circulatory or caused by hepatocellular destruction or deficient activity of one or more of the urea cycle enzymes. Chemically these disorders can be defined as hepatic inability to clear the blood of preformed ammonia and of glutamine.

Clinical manifestations

In the neonate severe hyperammonemia is manifested by a progressive illness beginning with poor feeding, with the evolution of hyperpnea, seizures that may be generalized or focal, waxing and waning consciousness, and ultimately coma and death. Muscle tone may be

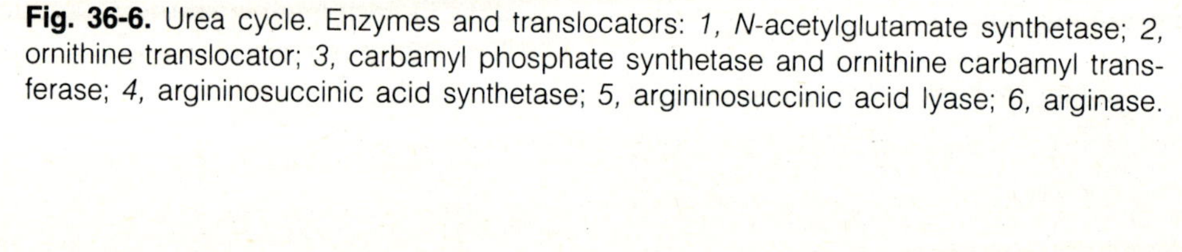

Fig. 36-6. Urea cycle. Enzymes and translocators: *1,* *N*-acetylglutamate synthetase; *2,* ornithine translocator; *3,* carbamyl phosphate synthetase and ornithine carbamyl transferase; *4,* argininosuccinic acid synthetase; *5,* argininosuccinic acid lyase; *6,* arginase.

increased early, or there may be alternating hypertonia and hypotonia. Ultimately there is profound hypotonia. Primitive reflexes are progressively lost. A number of affected infants (including some with inherited defects in the urea cycle) have had pulmonary hemorrhage without apparent primary respiratory disease. Clinical hyperammonemia also has developed within the context of neonatal respiratory distress syndrome (RDS).

Specific entities

Idiopathic, self-limited, neonatal hyperammonemia

This entity has been described only within the last decade. Affected infants generally but not always have been prematurely born. Some have shown signs of fetal distress, and some have had RDS. Signs of encephalopathy—poor feeding, disturbed respiratory pattern, and seizures—generally have appeared within the first 24 to 48 hours of life. Plasma ammonia values have ranged from 170 to 3,000 μmol/dl. When measured, plasma glutamine has been increased as well. Analyses of urea cycle enzymes and of urinary organic acids have been unrevealing. Exchange transfusion has been recommended as preferable to peritoneal dialysis in the management of hyperammonemia. I concur with this recommendation with regard to this specific entity. Depression of central nervous system function often has been severe enough to necessitate ventilatory assistance. Nonetheless not all survivors have shown long-term neurologic deficits.

Reye's syndrome (encephalopathy and fatty degeneration of the viscera)

Reye's syndrome has been reported to occur in the neonate. However, fatty metamorphosis of viscera and encephalopathy are common findings in diverse inborn errors of metabolism causing lethal disease in neonates. An acute, acquired disease of this type, superimposed on a normal metabolic substrate, has not been demonstrated in the neonate.

Deficiency of N-acetylglutamate synthetase

N-Acetylglutamate is required for synthesis of carbamyl phosphate in vitro, and its synthesis has been shown to correlate with carbamyl phosphate synthesis in vivo. Although only one patient with this disorder has been described, the condition is noted because the patient has responded very well to carbamyl glutamate, supplemental arginine and a low-protein diet.

Carbamylphosphate synthetase deficiency (Fig. 36-6)

A number of patients with deficiency of carbamylphosphate synthetase and apparently adequate activity of other urea cycle enzymes have been reported. Some of these patients had complex clinical and chemical disorders, suggesting that the enzyme deficiency was not the primary lesion. In infants with apparent primary carbamylphosphate synthetase deficiency, severe hyperammonemia is the associated clinical disorder. Chemical findings are nonspecific. A variant of this disorder has been described in a number of older infants, who exhibit hyperammonemia, hyperornithinemia, and homocitrullinuria. The defect appears to be failure of transport of ornithine into mitochondria. Because ornithine is a major stimulator of carbamylphosphate synthesis, a reduction in intramitochondrial ornithine can be expected to reduce the synthesis of carbamylphosphate.

Sex-linked hyperammonemia: ornithine carbamyltransferase deficiency (Fig. 36-6)

Ornithine carbamyltransferase deficiency is unique among these disorders in that it shows sex-linked inheritance. The majority of patients recognized thus far have been females, with reduced but not absent enzyme activity. Mother-to-daughter transmission has been demonstrated. Affected males have shown either a variant enzyme or absence of enzyme activity. Absence of enzyme activity is lethal within the first week of life in affected males, if untreated.

Surviving patients with ornithine carbamyltransferase deficiency generally show elevations in plasma and urinary glutamine and alanine. Most have excreted large amounts of orotic acid, apparently synthesized in response to diminished use of carbamylphosphate for citrulline synthesis. Diagnosis is made by enzyme assay of liver tissue.

Argininosuccinicaciduria (Fig. 36-6)

Unique among these disorders is the peculiarly friable hair seen even within the neonatal period in infants with argininosuccinicaciduria. Inheritance in argininosuccinicaciduria is of the autosomal recessive type. Definitive diagnosis may be established by finding large amounts of argininosuccinic acid in the urine or by enzyme assay.

Arginase defiency (Fig. 36-6)

Arginase deficiency has only infrequently been recognized, and it generally has no neonatal manifestations. On the basis of family history, it has been recognized chemically, and treated by diet with success, in a neonate. Diagnosis is made by enzyme assay.

Lysine intolerance with hyperammonemia (Fig. 36-6)

A single instance of lysine intolerance with hyperammonemia has been recorded, without neonatal manifestations. It is postulated that in this disease an impairment in lysine catabolism results in elevated tissue levels of lysine and that the elevated tissue lysine competitively inhibits the hydrolysis of arginine by arginase.

Management. The management of hyperammonemia involves reduction in the load of metabolic nitrogen destined for excretion as both a short-term and long-term goal and removal of free ammonia and its precursors from the body as a short-term goal. Therefore initial management of the sick neonate includes sterilization of the intestine with colistin or neomycin (short-term), cessation of protein feedings (short-term), provision of high carbohydrate intake (100 to 120 kcal/kg/day) by continuous intravenous infusion, and exchange transfusion or peritoneal dialysis (short-term). During the initial phase of management, citrullinemia and argininosuccinicacidemia must be ruled out. The presence of either disease is an indication for the immediate initiation of therapy with arginine in dosages of 2 to 4 mmol/kg/day. When a stable clinical state is achieved, protein feedings can be resumed. It is advisable to administer 0.25 to 0.5 gm/kg/day of a high-quality protein with a total caloric intake of 120 kcal/kg/day. The protein can be increased slowly (no more often than every fourth day) to achieve the best attainable balance between neurologic state and growth. In all primary disorders of the urea cycle except arginase deficiency arginine can be considered an essential amino acid, and sufficient arginine should be administered to maintain normal plasma arginine concentrations. In citrullinemia and argininosuccinicaciduria additional arginine is likely to be beneficial in that it provides a source of ornithine to be used in the synthesis of citrulline and argininosuccinic acid, which are obligatory end products of nitrogen metabolism in these conditions.

The results of long-term management are determined in large part by the degree to which nitrogen elimination is impaired. If the impairment is extremely severe, the aforementioned long-term management will not suffice. For such cases formulas containing either crystalline amino acids or mixtures of amino acids and keto acid analogs of amino acids have been employed successfully. Because the catabolic stress associated with minor infections has led to lethal hyperammonemia in many patients so treated, long-term usefulness of this form of management is questionable at this time.

Brusilow and his associates have devised a system of management with benzoic acid and phenylacetic acid that employs alternative pathways of nitrogen excretion to relieve the metabolic burden on the urea cycle. Although the results of treatment appear to be better than those achieved with conventional management, devastating and lethal hyperammonemic crises have occurred in some patients so managed.

DISORDERS OF ORGANIC ACID METABOLISM

This large group of diseases, each of which is rare, accounts for a small but significant fraction of neonatal clinical illness. In each of these disorders the metabolism of one or more organic acids is disturbed, leading to accumulation of affected acids in the body. Because they are strong acids, their urinary excretion places a heavy burden on the renal acidification mechanism. The accumulated acids have, in addition, a variety of effects on chemical physiology, some of which are clinically devastating. Manifestations vary from patient to patient and are dependent on the nature and severity of the defect, dietary intake, the presence or absence of intercurrent infection, and so forth. Hyperpnea caused by metabolic acidosis is the most common manifestation, but feeding difficulties, vomiting, and depression of central nervous system function, with or without seizures, are also prominent. Chemically, in addition to metabolic acidosis, there may be hypoglycemia, hyperammonemia, and disturbances in serum electrolytes (hypocalcemia, hypokalemia), all of which are poorly understood. In the clinical application of readily available laboratory tests the most valuable sign of organic acidosis is an increase in the undetermined anion fraction in plasma. When defined as serum Na^+ − (serum Cl^- + serum bicarbonate), this value is normally 10 to 15 mEq/L. Slight increases occur in dehydration because of decreased glomerular filtration, but values greater than 17 mEq/L in well-hydrated infants and greater than 20 mEq/L under any circumstances are highly suspicious. It must be recognized, however, that hypoxemia and poor perfusion of tissues can give rise to organic acidosis without an underlying enzymatic defect. In such cases the predominant acid accumulated is lactic acid, although a number of others may be present in both blood and urine.

Carnitine deficiency

Recently it has become apparent that in many of the disorders of organic acid metabolism, carnitine deficiency occurs as a result of the excretion of the carnitine esters of organic acids whose catabolism is impaired. Carnitine, like tetrahydrobiopterin, is not a vitamin but is synthesized in sufficient quantities to carry out its role in the oxidation of fatty acids. In this role, carnitine is esterified to fatty acids, allowing their transport across the mitochondrial membrane, from which point the fatty acids are released and oxidized. Preliminary evidence indicates that loss of unmetabolized carnitine esters in the urine can so deplete carnitine reserves as to impair the oxidation of fatty acids, resulting in lethargy, muscle weakness, impairment of cardiac function, and hypoglycemia. Some, but not all, patients having evidence of carnitine deficiency in the context of organic acidosis have responded favorably to replacement of carnitine. Primary carnitine deficiency, either limited to muscle or systemic, has also been described, though not in the neonatal period.

Acyl-CoA dehydrogenase deficiency

Much of the preliminary evidence concerning carnitine depletion has arisen in the course of investigations of the oxidative metabolism of fatty acids. There are at least four dehydrogenases involved in the oxidation of fatty acids of various lengths and configurations. With the exception of glutaric aciduria type II, diseases involving these pathways are not known to produce clearly defined manifestations in the neonatal period. An evolving hallmark of these disorders is hypoglycemia without ketosis, a situation to be expected in circumstances in which fatty acid catabolism cannot spare glucose through either oxidation or the production of ketone bodies.

Maple syrup urine disease

Maple syrup urine disease, or branched-chain aminoaciduria, is the result of an impairment in the decarboxylation of the keto acid derivatives of the three branched-chain amino acids: leucine, isoleucine, and valine (Fig. 36-7). Profound depression of the central nervous system and death early in life occur in the vast majority of untreated patients. A variant of the disease has been described that is intermittent, and another that shows spontaneous amelioration during infancy.

Etiology and pathogenesis

The transamination of the branched-chain amino acids occurs normally in maple syrup urine disease, but the keto acids produced by transamination are not oxidized normally. Because the transamination reaction is freely reversible, accumulation of these keto acids leads to a corresponding increase in the levels of the branched-chain amino acids. The clinical manifestations of the disease are correlated with elevations in plasma leucine and α-ketoisocaproic acid, but not with accumulations of isoleucine, valine, and their keto acid analogs. The metabolic acidosis sometimes observed in this disease is only in part explained by the excretory load of these specific organic acids. The mechanism by which the profound disturbance of the central nervous system is produced remains unknown. On postmortem examination the brains of affected infants exhibit defective myelinization and spongy degeneration of the white matter. Although hypoglycemia and excessive glycogen deposition in the liver have been noted in these patients, the central nervous system manifestations cannot be explained solely on the basis of hypoglycemia.

Clinical manifestations

Affected infants appear normal at birth. Onset of clinical manifestations generally occurs very early; most patients exhibit profound illness within a week. Initially there may be rapid, shallow respirations, soon followed

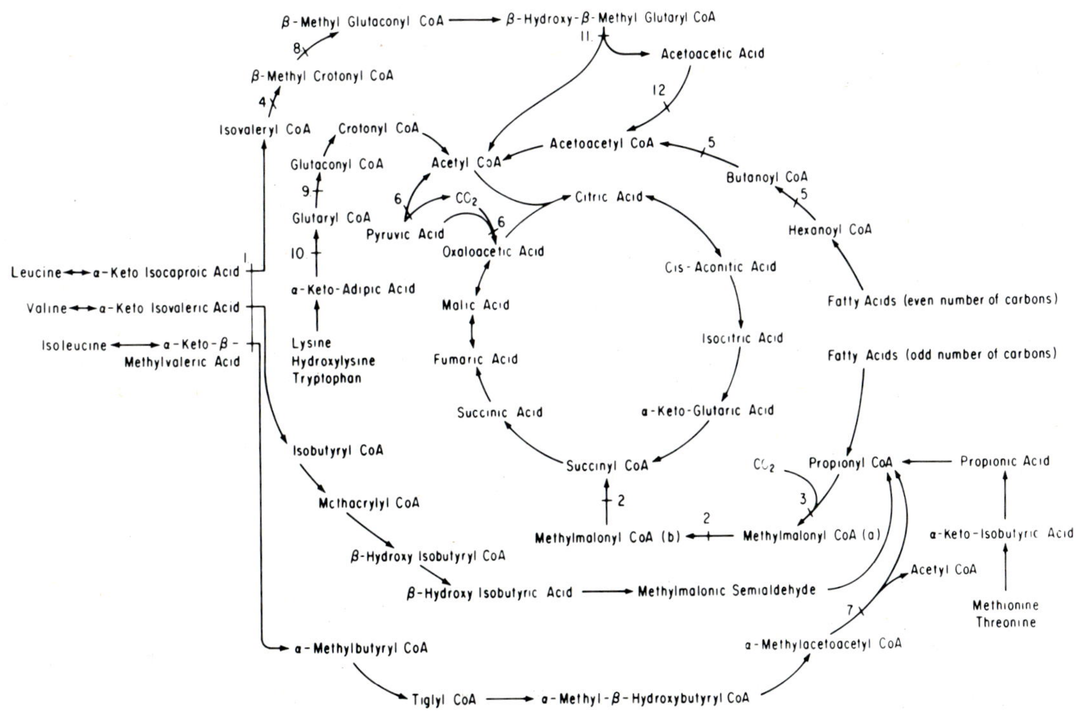

Fig. 36-7. Some pathways of organic acid metabolism. Inborn errors are numbered as follows: *1,* maple syrup urine disease; *2,* methylmalonic acidemia; *3,* propionic acidemia; *4,* isovaleric acidemia; *5,* acyl CoA dehydrogenase; *6,* lactic acidosis; *7,* β-ketothiolase deficiency; *8,* β-methyl crotonylglycinuria; *9,* glutaric aciduria type I; *10,* α-keto adipic aciduria; *11,* 3-hydroxy-3-methylglutaric aciduria; *12,* succinyl-CoA; 3-ketoacid CoA-transferase deficiency.

by profound alteration in consciousness. The infant appears apathetic and characteristically develops alternating hypertonia and hypotonia, accompanied by brief tonic seizures. The odor of maple syrup usually is detected at the time of clinical illness but occasionally has not been noted in fatally affected infants. The untreated disease is rapidly progressive, and death occurs within the neonatal period generally from respiratory failure, with or without complicating bronchopneumonia.

Laboratory manifestations

The presence of α-keto organic acids in the urine, as detected by the 2,4-dinitrophenylhydrazine test, is characteristic of the untreated disease and strongly suggests the diagnosis in infants whose clinical presentation is compatible with the disorder. The diagnosis is confirmed by finding striking elevations of leucine, isoleucine, and valine in plasma. These amino acids also are excreted in the urine in abnormal amounts. Alloisoleucine, an enantiomer of isoleucine, is also present in plasma. This amino acid was identified erroneously as methionine in early descriptions of the disorder. Hypoglycemia usually occurs, as a result of impairment of gluconeogenesis.

Treatment

Restriction of dietary leucine, isoleucine, and valine has been employed with some degree of success. Dietary treatment requires frequent monitoring of plasma leucine, isoleucine, and valine to provide sufficient amounts of these essential amino acids for growth and development while avoiding the severely deleterious effects of excessive administration. Crises with central nervous system dysfunction and metabolic acidosis are associated not only with dietary indiscretion but also with infections and other forms of stress. Dietary therapy must be continued for life.

Crises have been treated successfully by peritoneal dialysis. This therapy also has been suggested for neonates who have become severely affected prior to the institution of dietary therapy.

A thiamine-responsive form of the disease has been described.

Prognosis

Even with early institution of therapy the prognosis for both life and normal intellectual development is guarded. An intermittent form of the disease has been reported in which typical crises occur in children who are otherwise clinically normal. The metabolic defect appears to be similar to but less severe than that found in the classic form of the disease. The relation of the intermittent variety of clinical disease in the neonate has not been elucidated.

Genetics

The disease shows autosomal recessive inheritance.

Disorders of propionate pathway

Disorders of the propionate pathway—β-ketothiolase deficiency, propionic acidemia, and methylmalonic acidemia—all give rise to the ketotic hyperglycinemia syndrome: protein intolerance with ketonuria, ketoacidosis, hypoglycemia, hyperammonemia, hyperglycinemia, neutropenia, thrombocytopenia, and anemia. Manifestations generally are noted during the neonatal period.

Genetically determined enzymatic defects have been described for each of the processes involved in the pathway from α-methyl acetoacetyl CoA to succinyl CoA (Figs. 36-7 and 36-8). The most distal defect, β-ketothiolase deficiency, involves primarily the degradation of isoleucine. The other enzyme defects also impair the

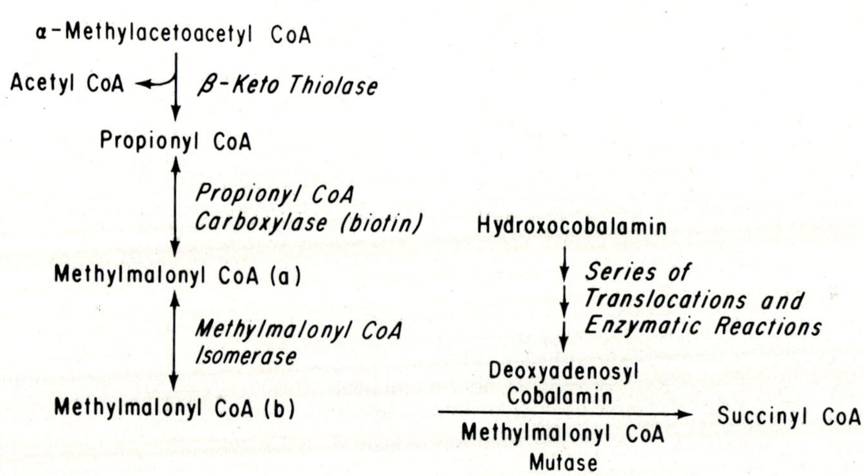

Fig. 36-8. Propionate pathway. Inborn errors of every process indicated have been described.

catabolism of methionine, valine, possibly threonine, cholesterol, and fatty acids with odd numbers of carbon atoms.

Intestinal microorganisms contribute significantly to the load of compounds that are metabolized in the propionate pathway. The pathway is thus a major one whose disruption can be expected to be profoundly deleterious. However, the mechanism by which each of the components of the ketotic hyperglycinemia syndrome is produced remains unknown.

Of great practical importance is that deficiencies in propionyl CoA carboxylase activity in some cases are caused by defective metabolism of the cofactor biotin and are responsive to biotin therapy (Fig. 36-8). Similarly methylmalonic acidemia may be caused by a number of defects in cobalamin metabolism (Fig. 36-8). Such defects may respond to cobalamin therapy.

Clinical manifestations

Although slowly developing clinical disease occurs in association with these enzymatic defects, clinical presentation in the neonatal period is more common. Lethargy, poor feeding, vomiting, and hyperpnea are likely to progress to frank coma, the clinical disease being exacerbated by protein feedings. Seizures are uncommon.

Laboratory manifestations

Laboratory findings in the neonatal period are disturbingly protean. A striking but frequently overlooked clue to the diagnosis is ketonuria. Even in the presence of ketonuria there may be no acidosis but rather hyperammonemia of such degree as to suggest a primary defect in urea cycle function. In a number of affected infants ketoacidosis has been profound, occurring at times together with grossly elevated blood ammonia (greater than 300 μmol/L). The combination of neonatal ketoacidosis and extreme hyperammonemia is virtually diagnostic of a defect in the propionate pathway. Neutropenia, thrombocytopenia, and anemia are only intermittently present, as is hyperglycinemia. Hypoglycemia is very common, particularly during exacerbations of ketoacidosis. The diagnosis is forwarded by determination of the specific pattern of organic acids in blood and/or urine and definitively made by demonstration of the specific enzymatic defect.

Treatment

Initial management is directed toward (1) correction of hypoglycemia if present, (2) management of hyperammonemia (see section on defects of the urea cycle), and (3) management of metabolic acidosis. Sterilization of the intestine is beneficial in that it reduces the absorption of intermediates in the pathway produced by intestinal microorganisms. Glucose infusions sufficient to supply total caloric need are also helpful in that they retard the breakdown of protein. Large doses of sodium bicarbonate may be required initially (20 mEq/kg/day). Once appropriate samples of blood and urine have been collected, it is advisable to employ megavitamin therapy; biotin, 10 mg/day orally, and hydroxycobalamin, 2 mg/day intramuscularly. Once stabilization has been achieved, oral feedings can be instituted employing a diet high in carbohydrates and low in protein (0.5 gm/kg/day). Protein intake then can be liberalized gradually to achieve the best possible clinical state. Throughout the course of the illness, but particularly during crises, careful attention must be paid to the hematologic abnormalities. Severe infection is a serious risk during episodes of neutropenia, and transfusion of whole blood and of platelet concentrates may be required for management of anemia and thrombocytopenia.

Prognosis

Defects in the propionate pathway may be lethal in spite of optimal management, but a number of infants, critically ill at diagnosis, have responded well to treatment. Intellectual and motor development is likely to be delayed but not necessarily profoundly so.

Genetics

Autosomal recessive inheritance is indicated in each of the disorders of the propionate pathway.

Congenital lactic acidosis

Lactic acidosis is most commonly encountered as the result of hypoxemia and/or poor perfusion of tissues. It also can be seen as a complication of a number of metabolic disorders in which the known primary defect does not involve lactate metabolism (hereditary fructose intolerance, fructose-1,6-diphosphatase deficiency, and glycogenosis type I). In a third group of patients lactic acidosis is so dominant a characteristic of the illness as to assume primary importance in nomenclature: hence the term *congenital lactic acidosis*.

Etiology and pathogenesis

The metabolism of lactate is essentially that of pyruvate, with which both lactate and alanine are in equilibrium. Quantitatively pyruvate is catabolized through pyruvate dehydrogenase (with thiamine pyrophosphate and lipoic acid as cofactors) and the citric acid cycle. This pathway seems normally to predominate under conditions of glucose excess. Alternatively pyruvate can be carboxylated to form oxaloacetate in a reaction catalyzed by pyruvate carboxylase, a biotin-requiring enzyme. Oxaloacetate can be used catalytically in the tricarboxylic acid cycle and quantitatively for the synthesis of glucose via phosphoenolpyruvate and reverse glycolysis. The latter sequence of reactions seems to be most active when

Table 36-2. Pyruvate dehydrogenase complex

Enzyme	Substrates	Products
Pyruvate dehydrogenase (E_1)	Pyruvate Thiamine pyrophosphate (TPP)	CO_2 Hydroxyethyl TPP
Dihydrolipoyl transacetylase (E_2)	Hydroxyethyl TPP Lipoic acid CoA SH	TPP Dihydrolipoic acid Acetyl CoA
Dihydrolipoyl dehydrogenase E_3	Dihydrolipoic acid FAD NAD	Lipoic acid FAD NADH + H^+
TOTAL COMPLEX	Pyruvate + CoA SH + NAD	CO_2 + Acetyl CoA + NADH + H^+

glucose is in limited supply. The flow of pyruvate through one or the other pathway, however, is dependent on the integrity of other systems. If the function of the electron transport chain is impaired, as, for example, by anoxia, the action of pyruvate dehydrogenase is slowed. Furthermore, because both pyruvate dehydrogenase and pyruvate carboxylase are mitochondrial enzymes, structural and functional integrity of mitochondria is necessary for their proper functions. In fact, then, lactic acidosis could be accounted for in any number of ways, and indeed infants with lactic acidosis as the predominant manifestation of congenital metabolic disease are a heterogeneous group. Only in the past decade has a systematic effort been made to examine the activities of the pyruvate dehydrogenase complex and of pyruvate carboxylase in these infants. The pyruvate dehydrogenase system is extremely intricate in a technical sense, and its clinical investigation has been most difficult (Table 36-2). The electron transport chain, which is also technically difficult, has been studied in a number of patients with lactic acidosis. The beginning of a systematic classification of defects is visible, but only a beginning. In general it can be said: (1) most infants with congenital lactic acidosis tolerate excess glucose well (not to be expected with pyruvate dehydrogenase deficiency); (2) most are normoglycemic or nearly so (not to be expected with pyruvate carboxylase deficiency); (3) brain damage in most tends to be severe; (4) some have neuropathologic findings of subacute necrotizing encephalomyelitis and, because of the resemblance of these anatomic findings to those of experimental thiamine deficiency, are thought to have defects of pyruvate dehydrogenase.

Robinson reviewed the biochemical investigations of 40 infants and children, all of whom had lactic acidosis, and none of whom had primary glycogenosis or primarily disordered fructose metabolism. In 12 patients, a primary defect in pyruvate metabolism could be identified, and in another 2, the area of difficulty was indicated. In the remaining 28, no defect was identified. It is likely that a number of these had defects in electron transport, which was not analyzed in this study. From his studies, Robinson has concluded the following. First, neonatal lactic acidosis associated with pyruvate dehydrogenase (E_1) deficiency is essentially always lethal. Affected infants frequently show structural brain damage indicating active disease in utero. Second, defects of the E_3 component (lipoamide dehydrogenase) of the pyruvate dehydrogenase complex are associated not only with lactic acidosis but also with the excretion of α-ketoglutaric acid and the keto acid analogs of the branched-chain amino acids. The latter metabolites rise in tissues because their decarboxylation also requires the participation of E_3. Third, pyruvate carboxylase deficiency manifests itself generally in the neonatal period. Absence of the enzyme protein produces not only lactic acidosis and hypoglycemia, as expected, but also hyperammonemia and citrullinemia. The impairment in detoxification of ammonia can be explained by failure to synthesize oxaloacetate, which, through transamination to aspartic acid, is necessary for the operation of the urea cycle. Production of an abnormal pyruvate dehydrogenase results in neonatal lactic acidosis in most cases, but hypoglycemia is not a constant finding and impairment of ammonia metabolism is not noted. Both forms of lactic acidosis are highly lethal.

Lactic acidosis in association with disorders of the electron transport chain has been reported in infants, the most notable syndrome being one of myopathy and renal tubular dysfunction accompanying cytochrome *c* oxidase deficiency. A form of neonatal myopathy has also been described in which cytochrome *c* oxidase deficiency resolves spontaneously over a period of months.

Clinical manifestations

The majority of infants with congenital lactic acidosis are undoubtedly acidotic from birth. In many instances the acidosis is manifest only by mild hyperpnea and poor feeding and is not recognized until some weeks later when intercurrent infection precipitates a severe acidotic crisis. As a group, these infants are profoundly hypotonic and inattentive. They do not follow, and many show optic atrophy early. Although physically normal at birth, they tend to become obese early. Seizures are relatively common and tend to be myoclonic in type. When generalized seizures occur, there is a strong likelihood of hypoglycemia. Tetany has been reported and is thought to be secondary to the formation of calcium lactate complexes in plasma. Development tends to be extremely retarded. Befitting the heterogeneous nature of the disorder, some infants have been hypertonic, and some have shown spontaneous improvement.

Laboratory manifestations

The undetermined anion fraction of plasma electrolytes is increased, with the increase largely accounted for by lactate. Oxygen saturation and Po_2 are normal, and Pco_2 is decreased. Pyruvate and alanine are increased in plasma, and urine contains excessive lactate, pyruvate, and alanine. Blood glucose is generally normal, but hypoglycemia has been noted in some cases. When profound depression of the central nervous system occurs, Po_2 may fall and Pco_2 may rise as a result of hypoventilation. Thus the infant, who is cyanotic and comatose when first examined, may have either decreased oxygenation with secondary lactic acidosis or intrinsic lactic acidosis with secondary hypoventilation. For the former, providing adequate oxygenation results in relatively prompt ameliorization of the lactic acidosis.

Treatment

Initial management is directed toward correction of the metabolic acidosis. Adequate oxygenation of tissues must be ensured. Intravenous sodium bicarbonate generally is required, sometimes in dosages as high as 20 mEq/kg/day. Because of the need for such large amounts of sodium in therapy, edema and hypernatremia are constant threats, requiring careful attention to sodium and water balance with judicious use of diuretics. After appropriate specimens have been obtained for diagnostic purposes, megavitamin therapy is indicated.

Biotin, 10 mg/day, and thiamine, 50 to 200 mg/day, generally are employed (dosages used have been variable). Lipoic acid (which was successful in one case), pantothenic acid, and niacin also have been used. For most patients it can be expected that diet therapy will have little influence on the clinical course of the disease. In a few patients glucose administration has been associated with increased lactate in plasma, suggesting that pyruvate dehydrogenase is specifically affected and that a high fat, low carbohydrate diet may be beneficial. However, transfusion with citrated blood also has precipitated acidotic crises in some patients, suggesting that these individuals have deficiencies in activity of both pyruvate dehydrogenase and α-ketoglutarate dehydrogenase, which is closely related to pyruvate dehydrogenase and a key enzyme in the citric acid cycle. For such individuals glycolysis may be an important source of energy. Thus carbohydrate restriction probably is not indicated and may be deleterious. Patients with presumed pyruvate carboxylase deficiency may have impaired production of oxaloacetic acid. It is possible that supplementation of the diet of such patients with aspartic acid, which can be transaminated to oxaloacetic acid, would increase their ability to use both carbohydrates and fats as sources of energy.

If stabilization of the infant on feedings can be achieved, oral sodium bicarbonate therapy is likely to be required. The dose needed to maintain acid-base homeostasis varies both from individual and from day to day. To avoid alkalosis, I have employed a regimen in which the pH of freshly voided urine is monitored and bicarbonate supplements administered only when urine pH falls below 7.

Prognosis

The outlook for infants with congenital lactic acidosis undoubtedly depends primarily on the nature of the enzyme defect and its responsiveness to cofactor therapy. Severe developmental retardation, with or without death in early infancy, is most likely, but a few patients have done relatively well.

Genetics

The relatively small number of patients studied adequately, the technical difficulty of the biochemical studies, and the clinical and chemical heterogeneity of the condition all conspire against definitive statements regarding genetics. Suffice it to say that the author is unaware of any evidence of sex-linked inheritance for primary lactic acidosis.

Isovaleric acidemia (sweaty feet syndrome)

Isovaleric acidemia is similar clinically to disorders of the propionate pathway.

Etiology and pathogenesis

An enzymatic defect in the catabolic pathway for leucine is responsible for this disease and generally gives rise to metabolic acidosis, depression of the central nervous system, and pancytopenia early in life. Although all these manifestations are common in the presence of accumulations of short-chain fatty acids, the pathogenetic mechanisms are unclear.

Clinical manifestations

Clinically normal at birth, the affected infant characteristically develops tachypnea within the neonatal period. In reported cases the odor of sweaty feet generally has been noted early. Seizures and central nervous system depression with respiratory impairment are not unusual, and serious infection, presumably caused by anemia and neutropenia, frequently has complicated the neonatal course of the illness.

Laboratory manifestations

Metabolic acidosis with an increase in the undetermined anion fraction is a constant finding. Ketosis is found during acidotic crises. Depression of erythrocytes, neutrophils, and platelets is common.

Treatment

As in other organic acidoses, large doses of sodium bicarbonate and even peritoneal dialysis may be required to achieve initial stabilization. Vigorous supportive therapy, including antibiotics and transfusion, also may be required. By analogy with methylmalonic acidemia, sterilization of the intestine is likely to be beneficial. Long-term management entails a high-calorie diet low in protein (perhaps specifically restricted as to leucine) and supplemental sodium bicarbonate as indicated. There is evidence that glycine supplementation, by increasing the formation of isovaleryl glycine, also may be of benefit.

Prognosis

Mortality in the neonatal period has been high in the past, as a result of both depression of central nervous system function and complications associated with pancytopenia. In survivors some degree of developmental retardation can be anticipated.

Genetics

The disease shows autosomal recessive inheritance.

Other disorders of organic acid metabolism

β-Methyl crotonylglycinuria

A number of instances of this entity have been described. Manifestations have included metabolic acidosis, amyotonia syndrome, and mucocutaneous candidiasis. At this point it would appear that most affected individuals suffer from a defect in biotin metabolism, leading to deficient activity of a number of biotin-requiring enzymes. In most reported patients the therapeutic response to biotin, 10 mg/day, has been dramatic. In most instances the disorder has shown autosomal recessive inheritance.

α-Ketoadipic aciduria

This disorder is apparently rare but has been reported to produce intermittent metabolic acidosis in the neonatal period. Levels of plasma and urinary α-aminoadipic acid are increased, as might be expected, and increase further when a lysine load is administered. Specific therapy has not been reported. The mode of inheritance is unknown.

3-OH,3-Methylglutaric aciduria

This recently described defect in leucine catabolism can give rise to both metabolic acidosis and profound hypoglycemia in the neonatal period. In later infancy, the clinical presentation is that of recurrent Reye's syndrome. Of interest, this disorder results in hypoketonemic hypoglycemia, and as a result enters into the differential diagnosis of hyperinsulinism and of carnitine deficiency. Plasma amino acids (including leucine) are normal.

D-Glyceric aciduria

A single infant, with clinical manifestations similar to those of nonketotic hyperglycinemia, was found to have elevated D-glyceric acid in urine and blood. The elevations were not sufficient to cause metabolic acidosis. Serum glycine was increased, but the concentration of glycine in cerebrospinal fluid was not reported.

Glutaric aciduria type I

This rare disorder probably causes no clinically recognizable disease in the neonate but gives rise in later months to a progressive movement disorder characterized by delayed motor development, dystonia, and choreoathetosis. Laboratory findings include increased urinary excretion of glutaric, glutaconic, and hydroxyglutaric acids, and deficiency of glutaryl-CoA dehydrogenase.

Glutaric aciduria type II

Several infants, all of whom died within the neonatal period, were found to excrete in urine large amounts of glutaric acid along with other organic acids, particularly lactic, butyric, isobutyric, and isovaleric acids. The molecular defect in this disorder appears to reside in the electron transport system that links several dehydrogenases to coenzyme Q. There is clear evidence for sex-linked transmission of neonatal glutaric aciduria type II in at least one family, though this may not be the only mode of inheritance. A chemically similar disorder, with onset later in life and a milder course, shows autosomal recessive inheritance.

Succincyl CoA: 3-keto acid CoA-transferase deficiency

At least two infants are known to have been affected by this disorder. Ketoacidosis was evident early in both infants, one of whom died at 6 months and the other at 21 months. Genetic transmission seems assured on the basis of family histories.

DISORDERS OF MONOSACCHARIDE METABOLISM

Neonatal diabetes mellitus

Carbohydrate intolerance to an extent requiring insulin therapy has been noted with some frequency in the neonatal period. The disorder may be temporary or permanent.

Etiology and pathogenesis

The cause of diabetes mellitus, when it occurs in the neonate, is unknown. No consistent abnormalities of pancreatic tissue have been noted in autopsy material from infants with this disorder. Plasma insulin levels have not shown a consistent pattern in the few subjects in whom measurements have been made.

There is some association between the development of diabetes mellitus in the neonatal period and postmaturity and low birth weight, neonatal hypoglycemia, and steroid therapy early in the neonatal period.

Clinical manifestations

The age of patients at detection of this disorder has varied from 4 to 44 days. The most prominent manifestations have been weight loss and dehydration in association with polyuria. Characteristically the affected infant maintains a good oral intake and does not become comatose. The vast majority probably have some degree of metabolic acidosis, but severe ketonuria is not the rule.

Laboratory manifestations

In the excellent review of this disorder by Gentz and Cornblath blood sugar was noted to range from 245 to 2,300 mg/dl in affected infants. Hypernatremia was common, and ketonuria was variable, but metabolic acidosis was detected in most subjects whose acid-base status was evaluated.

Treatment

All patients with this disorder require careful attention to fluid and electrolyte balance. The dose of insulin required to achieve carbohydrate homeostasis varies markedly from patient to patient and from day to day in individual patients. Except for the severely ill infant, insulin therapy should be gradually instituted. Initially one-fourth unit of regular insulin per kilogram of body weight should be administered and the blood sugar should be monitored for 12 hours to assess the insulin sensitivity of the patient. It is not always possible to establish a stable insulin regimen. For many patients coverage with regular insulin on the basis of degree of glycosuria or hyperglycemia is optimal management for the first several months of life. Dietary allowances of protein and carbohydrate should be liberal. Because the risk of insulin-induced hypoglycemia with secondary brain damage is high in the early months of life, it is best not to attempt to achieve aglycosuria. Monitoring of blood glucose, using micro–skin puncture and glucose oxidase strips, is very desirable in the management of this disorder; blood glucose should not be allowed to fall below 130 mg/dl.

Prognosis

Gentz and Cornblath found that 30 of 50 patients with neonatal diabetes had temporary disorders requiring treatment for a mean period of 65 days. For those neonates with permanent diabetes there is no indication that prognosis is worse than it is for individuals who develop diabetes later in life.

Genetics

There is a relatively high incidence of diabetes mellitus in the families of affected infants but no clearly defined inheritance pattern for the disorder.

DISORDERS OF GALACTOSE METABOLISM

Galactokinase deficiency

Deficient activity of galactokinase results in disordered metabolism of galactose and the development of cataracts.

Etiology and pathogenesis

The initial step in the metabolism of dietary galactose is the phosphorylation of galactose, a reaction catalyzed by galactokinase. When this reaction is impaired, ingested galactose is either excreted in the urine or metabolized by unusual pathways. Marked reduction in activity of galactokinase thus results in postprandial galactosuria and in the production of galactitol by enzymatic reduction of galactose. There is substantial evidence to suggest that galactitol, acting as a nondiffusible osmotic agent within the lens, causes swelling of the lens fibers and ultimately distortion of the architecture of the lens. In addition, the reduction of galactose to galactitol drains the lens of compounds that are able to act as hydrogen donors in the stabilization of sulfhydryl-containing proteins. The instability of affected proteins, coupled with the osmotic effects of galactose, finally leads to cataract formation.

Clinical manifestations

In individuals homozygous for galactokinase deficiency cataract formation occurs early in life and has been noted within the neonatal period. Cataract formation in the third and fourth decades of life has been reported in individuals apparently heterozygous for this disorder. Dysfunction of liver and kidney are not seen in galactokinase deficiency, nor is hypoglucosemia produced by galactose ingestion. Pseudotumor cerebri, however, has been reported to occur early in the course.

Laboratory manifestations

The diagnosis is established by demonstration of reduction of activity of galactokinase in red blood cells. Measurement of galactose in blood and urine in the postprandial state can be employed as a screening procedure. Increased urinary galactitol is a more constant finding in this disorder than is either galactosuria or galactosemia.

Treatment

Elimination of galactose from the diet is the treatment of choice. Resorption of cataracts has been reported in some individuals so treated. It appears that galactose restriction should be lifelong in this disorder.

Prognosis

The prognosis for general health is excellent, the only morbidity associated with this condition being visual impairment caused by cataracts.

Galactosemia

Galactosemia is a hereditary disorder of the metabolism of galactose-1-phosphate that is analogous to hereditary fructose intolerance, in which manifestations of renal disease and liver dysfunction follow the ingestion of galactose. Cataracts and some degree of mental retardation are also features of galactosemia.

Etiology and pathogenesis

The biochemical lesion in galactosemia is lack of activity of galactose-1-phosphate uridylyltransferase. This impairment of function leads to the accumulation within cells of galactose-1-phosphate; galactose accumulates both intracellularly and extracellularly. Cataract formation presumably occurs by the mechanism proposed for the development of cataracts in patients with galactokinase deficiency. The disorders of hepatic and renal function appear to be well correlated with the intracellular levels of galactose-1-phosphate. Like hereditary fructose intolerance, hypoglucosemia occurs promptly on administration of galactose, and renal function shows impairment during the course of a galactose tolerance test. Although galactose-1-phosphate is known to inhibit phosphoglucomutase in vitro, the precise mechanism by which hypoglucosemia occurs is not completely understood. The cerebral, renal, and hepatic lesions of galactosemia have not been satisfactorily explained.

Clinical manifestations

Infants with galactosemia are physically normal at birth, although their birth weights may be somewhat lower than those of unaffected siblings. Clinical manifestations may be fulminant, with death occurring within the first few days of life or delayed until some weeks after birth. Vomiting and diarrhea, hepatosplenomegaly, and jaundice, frequently associated with anemia, are the cardinal manifestations. Renal tubular acidosis may occur. Cataracts are usually but not invariably present in the neonatal period. The clinical manifestations that occur early within the neonatal period are strikingly similar to those of neonatal septicemia, and in a number of instances the coexistence of these two entities has been demonstrated. In those infants whose disease has a more insidious onset, clinical manifestations may be predominantly those of failure to thrive associated with hepatomegaly. The major clinical risk to life is progressive liver dysfunction complicated by cirrhosis.

Laboratory manifestations

The diagnosis of galactosemia is made by finding absence or near absence of activity of galactose-1-phosphate uridylyltransferase in red blood cell hemolysates. Some genetic variants of the disorder have been described in which the activity of the enzyme is reduced or unusually unstable. Therefore in some instances it may be necessary to obtain clarification of the diagnosis by measurement of red blood cell galactose-1-phosphate. The normal value of red blood cell galactose-1-phosphate is less than 1 mg/gm of hemoglobin. Untreated galactosemia is always accompanied by marked elevation in red blood cell galactose-1-phosphate. This gauge is also useful in monitoring dietary therapy; most clinics restrict galactose to the extent necessary to maintain red blood cell galactose-1-phosphate at 4 mg/gm of hemoglobin or less.

Measurement of blood and urinary galactose has some value in screening but cannot be depended on to exclude the diagnosis of galactosemia in an infant who is so ill as to have little intake of galactose.

The galactose tolerance test has no place in the diagnosis of neonatal galactosemia. It is potentially dangerous and offers no advantage over the assay of red blood cell galactose-1-phosphate uridylyltransferase and galactose-1-phosphate.

Treatment

Prompt and progressive improvement follows the elimination of galactose from the affected infant's diet. Non-lactose-containing formulas, such as Nutramigen, Prosobee, and several other formulas, may be used for this purpose. The very ill neonate may require vigorous supportive therapy, including transfusion and antibiotics for infection, in addition to elimination of dietary galactose. The appropriate duration of dietary treatment is not exactly known. It appears that the risk of severe liver and renal damage and of cataracts is limited to infancy and that tolerance for dietary galactose increases with age.

If the diagnosis of galactosemia is suspected in a very

ill neonate, the proper course of action is to institute a galactose-free diet, obtaining blood for enzymatic evaluation whenever this is feasible. The elimination of galactose from the diet does not invalidate the enzyme assay, irrespective of the duration of elimination of dietary galactose.

Prognosis

The mortality of individuals with galactosemia symptomatic in the neonatal period is approximately 20%. This is thought to be related to delay in the institution of therapy but may be related in part to concomitant severe bacterial infection. For patients successfully treated in the neonatal period the prognosis for general health is good. Appropriate treatment generally is associated with complete resolution of the hepatic and renal lesions and occasionally even of cataracts. Cataract formation does not progress after the institution of therapy.

Statistically there is an inverse relationship between the age at onset of therapy and intellectual achievement. However, some galactosemic infants recognized at birth and treated promptly have shown inadequate intellectual development when compared with their siblings. Furthermore there is a high incidence of behavioral and learning disorders in the population of galactosemic infants, whether treated or untreated.

Genetics

Galactosemia is inherited as an autosomal recessive disease. Since there is considerable heterogeneity within the population of galactosemic individuals, enzymatic evaluation of the parents of the galactosemic infant is advisable.

Uridine-diphospho-galactose 4-epimerase deficiency

Both the catabolism of galactose and its synthesis from glucose are dependent in large part on the interconversion of uridine-diphospho-glucose and uridine-diphospho-galactose, which is catalyzed by an epimerase.

Deficiency of the epimerase in erythrocytes, but not in liver, has been noted several times. Affected subjects show no clinical disease. One infant with deficiency of the enzyme in liver as well as erythrocytes had typical clinical galactosemia. Presumed to be unable either to synthesize or catabolize galactose, the infant was treated with galactose restriction, not galactose elimination, and responded well to this management.

DISORDERS OF FRUCTOSE METABOLISM

Deficiency of fructose kinase: essential fructosuria

Essential fructosuria, an asymptomatic disorder that results in fructosuria after the ingestion of fructose by affected subjects, is caused by an inborn deficiency in the enzymatic phosphorylation of fructose. It has no apparent clinical significance.

Hereditary fructose intolerance

Hereditary fructose intolerance is a serious disorder of carbohydrate metabolism; the ingestion of fructose produces hypoglycemia, abdominal pain, vomiting, and severe liver and kidney dysfunction.

Etiology and pathogenesis

In hereditary fructose intolerance there is a marked decrease in the activity of fructose-1-phosphate aldolase and usually a reduction in the activity of fructose-1,6-diphosphate aldolase. Since the two enzymatic activities are closely related chemically, it appears possible that the disorder is related to an abnormality in a single protein. In affected subjects the ratio of fructose-1-phosphate aldolase to fructose-1,6-diphosphate aldolase is almost always found to be greater than 2, whereas the normal ratio of these activities is less than 2.

In response to fructose ingestion or infusion, patients exhibit a variable rise in blood fructose and a prompt and striking fall in blood glucose. Plasma inorganic phosphate falls, whereas plasma magnesium rises somewhat. Serum glutamic oxaloacetic transaminase (SGOT) and serum glutamic pyruvic transaminase (SGPT) also rise on the ingestion of fructose, and there is a marked increase in the excretion of amino acids. The exact mechanism responsible for these findings is not entirely understood, although generally it is considered to be related to the impairment in the metabolism of phosphorylated hexose. In vitro fructose-1-phosphate inhibits glycogenolysis. Clinically the hypoglycemia of hereditary fructose intolerance does not respond to glucagon.

Clinical manifestations

Affected infants are normal at birth. Clinical manifestations occur only when the infants receive formulas containing fructose or sucrose. When such formulas are fed, vomiting, sometimes accompanied by diarrhea, promptly develops. There may be postprandial seizures. With continued ingestion of fructose evidence of liver dysfunction appears, with hepatomegaly, jaundice of the obstructive type, and bleeding. At the same time renal function is impaired, with a substantial number of patients developing renal tubular acidosis. If fructose is not eliminated from the diet, progressive deterioration and death may occur within the neonatal period.

Affected infants who survive the early months of life frequently develop a striking aversion to sweets.

Laboratory manifestations

Definitive evidence of this disorder is reduction in the level of activity of fructose-1-phosphate aldolase, together with elevation of the ratio of fructose-1-phosphate aldolase to fructose-1,6-diphosphate aldolase in liver tissue obtained by biopsy. An alternative method of diagnosis requiring less elaborate laboratory facilities is provided by the fructose tolerance test. Fructose, 0.2 gm/kg body weight, is injected intravenously over a few minutes. In the presence of hereditary fructose intolerance there is a striking reduction in blood glucose and plasma phosphate levels. If the question of hereditary fructose intolerance arises in the neonate, fructose should be eliminated from the diet as a therapeutic trial. Definitive tests may be delayed for a year or two if the fructose-free diet proves effective.

Elevations of plasma tyrosine and methionine have been noted in an infant with hereditary fructose intolerance.

In addition to evidence of impaired renal acidification, urinary abnormalities in hereditary fructose intolerance include generalized aminoaciduria, tyrosyluria, intermittent fructosuria, and occasionally galactosuria.

Treatment

The acute manifestations of fructose intolerance are ameliorated by the infusion of glucose. Definitive management is the elimination of fructose from the diet. Supportive measures may be necessary for acutely ill infants. In the management of these patients it is good to remember that orally administered medications sweetened with sucrose or fructose are contraindicated.

Prognosis

For those patients who survive early infancy, the prognosis is excellent. The vast majority of affected adults show no clinical disease but retain a rigid aversion to dietary fructose. Interestingly, dental caries are virtually absent in persons with hereditary fructose intolerance.

Genetics

In general, family histories of hereditary fructose intolerance are compatible with autosomal recessive transmission. However, the disorder appears to have shown dominant inheritance in several families.

Fructose-1,6-diphosphatase deficiency

Fructose-1,6-diphosphatase catalyzes a critical step in the reversal of the glycolytic pathway. Deficiency of the enzyme is associated not only with hypoglycemia but also with overproduction of pyruvic and lactic acids and alanine.

Clinical manifestations

Limited information on the neonatal presentation suggests that hyperpnea, poor feeding, vomiting, and depression of the central nervous system predominate as manifestations. The liver is characteristically enlarged.

Laboratory manifestations

In addition to lactic acidosis and hypoglycemia, there is characteristically ketosis. The liver shows fatty infiltration and, in addition, may have increased glycogen. Fructose-1,6-diphosphatase activity in the liver is markedly reduced or absent.

Treatment

Correction of lactic acidosis should be carried out vigorously with sodium bicarbonate and with sufficient glucose to both correct the hypoglycemia and suppress gluconeogenesis. Long-term management with a low-protein, fructose-free diet has been advised. In older children with deficiency of fructose-1,6-diphosphatase, folic acid therapy has been reported to increase the activity of the enzyme and ameliorate symptoms.

Prognosis

For infants with neonatal disease, the prognosis must be guarded, but most surviving infants have done reasonably well on follow-up.

Genetics

Autosomal recessive inheritance is probable.

GLYCOGENOSES

Glycogenoses (Table 36-3 and Fig. 36-9) can be made somewhat less bewildering if the disorders are divided into three groups that reflect the associated clinical diseases: (1) disorders that directly affect glucose homeostasis (types I, III, VI, and VIII), (2) disorders that affect primarily general hepatic function without directly involving glucose homeostasis (type IV), and (3) disorders that primarily affect neuromuscular function (types II and V). For the physician caring for newborn infants a further simplification can be made by considering those disorders which can be expected to have clinical manifestations during the neonatal period. All the disorders that affect glucose homeostasis fall into this category at least in theory. Of the disorders that primarily affect neuromuscular function, only type II has neonatal manifestations. Since this disease is a disorder of lysosomal function, it is discussed in the section on lysosomal disorders. In the second group, which contains only type IV, there is no neonatal manifestation; the disease is manifested by hepatomegaly at several months of age, followed by progressive cirrhosis, hepatic dysfunction, and death within the first few years of life.

Disorders affecting glucose homeostasis

Etiology and pathogenesis

During fetal life glycogen storage is greatly predominant over glycogenolysis. As a result, fetuses having glycogenoses affecting glucose homeostasis can be expected to be normal, or nearly so, at the end of gestation.

Table 36-3. Glycogenoses

Cori type	Eponym	Deficient enzyme	Affected tissue
I	von Gierke	Glucose-6-phosphatase	Liver, platelets Kidney Gastrointestinal tract
II	Pompe	Acid maltase	All tissues
III	Forbes	Debrancher	Liver, RBC, WBC Muscle variably
IV	Andersen	Brancher	All tissues
V	McArdle	Muscle phosphorylase	Muscle
VI	Hers	Liver phosphorylase	Liver, WBC
VII	Tarui	Muscle phosphofructokinase	Muscle, RBC
VIII	Hug and Schubert	Phosphorylase kinase	Liver, WBC, all other tissues

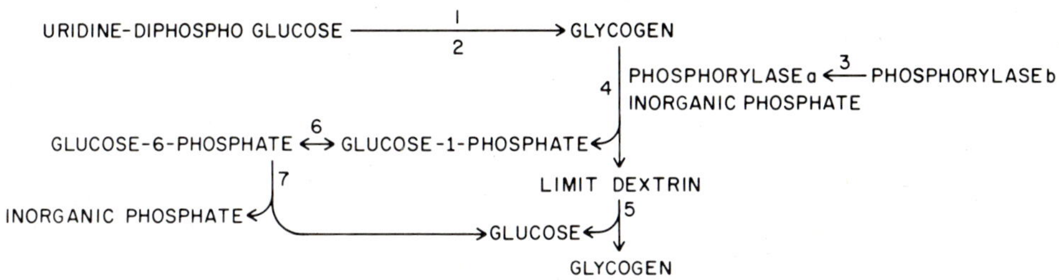

Fig. 36-9. Glycogen synthesis and breakdown: *1,* glycogen synthetase; *2,* brancher enzyme; *3,* phosphorylase b kinase; *4,* glycogen phosphorylase; *5,* debrancher enzyme; *6,* glucose 6 phosphatase.

Abnormality can be anticipated only when glycogenolysis is required for fuel homeostasis. Although such a requirement may occur during gestation, it certainly occurs during the stress of labor, delivery, and the adaptation to extrauterine life. In the normal infant the energy needs associated with this stress are met in part by glucose released from stored glycogen and in part by the release of free fatty acids from adipose tissue. Surprisingly most infants with inborn errors in the release of glucose from glycogen do not manifest illness during the neonatal period. Too few affected infants have been studied in the neonatal period to allow a proven explanation, but some tentative conclusions can be drawn from the physiology of these disorders in later life. First, the disorders of the breakdown of glycogen itself, debrancher deficiency and defects in the phosphorylase cascade, tend to be clinically mild. Hypoglycemia is generally of modest degree and, if severe, accompanied by ketosis. Gluconeogenesis proceeds normally. Thus a metabolic fuel is generally available. Second, patients with severe clinical disease, a minority of the total, almost always have type I glycogenosis, deficiency of glucose-6-phosphatase. This disease is more frequently manifested in the neonatal period, has high rates of mortality and morbidity, and is potentially treatable.

In type I glyogenosis the degradation of glycogen proceeds normally, but the resultant glucose-1-phosphate cannot be converted to free glucose. The accumulation of phosphorylated glucose results in increased glycolysis with the production of excessive amounts of lactate. For reasons that are as yet unclear, the release of free fatty acids and the production of ketone bodies are suppressed. Because gluconeogenesis proceeds through phosphorylated intermediates, it too is lacking. Blood glucose tends to fall to very low levels without a concomitant rise in free fatty acids. Plasma lactate can rise rapidly, producing severe metabolic acidosis. Lactate becomes the major circulating fuel, apparently used effectively by some affected infants but not by others.

The excess of glucose-6-phosphate in type I disease also leads to excessive synthesis of lipids, occasionally associated with xanthomatosis. Hyperuricemia also occurs, in part because of the effect of lactate on uric acid excretion but also because of an increase in uric acid synthesis.

Clinical manifestations

As indicated previously, the affected infant is likely to be physically normal at birth. In disorders other than type I glycogenosis progressive enlargement of the liver with or without hypoglycemia and ketosis is the likely course of the illness. In type I disease early neonatal hypoglycemia is common, with associated hyperpnea caused by lactic acidosis. These can occur prior to enlargement of the liver. Hypoglycemic seizures may be prominent, or the infant may be depressed, waking only for feedings.

Laboratory manifestations

Blood glucose concentration is variable but in type I disease tends to fall precipitously in the after-absorptive state, with lactate in plasma rising concomitantly. Ketonuria sometimes is noted and generally is indicative of a disorder other than type I. The most important single laboratory test in the evaluation of this group of patients is measurement of the response of blood glucose and lactate to the intravenous administration of glucagon (100 μg/kg). This test should be performed 2 hours after feeding, with measurement of blood glucose and lactate made 30 minutes, 15 minutes, and immediately before the administration of the hormone and at 15-minute intervals for an hour thereafter. Failure to respond to glucagon with a rise in blood glucose of 4 mmol/L (72 mg/dl) can be considered diagnostic of glycogenosis. Coupled with this diagnostic result, a sharp rise in plasma lactate in response to glucagon is diagnostic of type I glycogenosis.

Inferences can be made by analyses of erythrocytes, leukocytes, and platelets for both amount and structure of glycogen and for the various enzymatic activities, but refinement of diagnosis is best accomplished by enzymatic analysis of liver tissue obtained by percutaneous biopsy. Although geneal liver function is not seriously affected in these infants, defects of coagulation should be looked for and corrected, if present, before biopsy. Platelet dysfunction has been noted in type I glycogenosis.

A variant of type I, called type Ib, has been shown to be caused not by deficiency of glucose-6-phosphatase but by failure of function of the translocater that permits entry of glucose-6-phosphate into microsomes where the enzyme is localized. Subjects affected by type Ib have neutropenia in addition to the other manifestations of type I disease.

Treatment

Treatment is directed toward prevention of hypoglycemia by frequent feedings and toward minimization of glycogen accumulation by employing only glucose and its polymers as the carbohydrate in the diet. It may be necessary to give feedings every 2 hours during the day and night. Alternatively continuous intragastric feedings can be employed at night, with frequent normally administered feedings during the day. This regimen has achieved notable success in the management of type I glycogenosis. Acidotic crises in type I glycogenosis may be quite severe, requiring both sufficient glucose to suppress glycogenolysis and massive doses of sodium bicarbonate. During more quiescent periods small oral doses of bicarbonate suffice to control the lactic acidosis. Hyperuricemia may require allopurinol therapy. Hyperlipidemia with xanthomatosis has been reported to respond to substitution of medium-chain triglycerides for the ordinary fat in the diet. In older infants, it has been possible to employ suspensions of uncooked cornstarch, administered orally, to maintain control of blood glucose.

Prognosis

For patients with disorders other than type I the prognosis is quite good; most show mild disease in infancy with progressive improvement in later childhood. Although the prognosis of patients with type I disease has greatly improved with the introduction of continuous nocturnal intragastric feedings, and the use of cornstarch as noted above, the outlook must remain guarded. Sudden death from an overwhelming crisis is not unusual. Irreversible cerebral damage may occur before the disorder is recognized. Retardation of growth, persistent hypotonia, and delay in sexual maturation remain problems, as does the development of hepatic adenomata.

DISORDERS OF LIPID METABOLISM

Hyperlipoproteinemia

In recent years evidence has accumulated that links premature atherosclerotic cardiovascular disease with inborn errors of lipid metabolism (Table 36-4). Although xanthomatosis may appear in the neonatal period in these diseases, the life-threatening cardiovascular manifestations do not appear for years to decades after birth. In some instances even the abnormalities of plasma lipids, which appear to be genetically determined, are not manifested during childhood. The demonstration that dietary manipulation, with or without the addition of drugs such

Table 36-4. Hyperlipidemia

Frederickson type	Plasma triglycerides	Cholesterol	Xanthomata	Synonym
I	Increased (milky plasma)	Increased	Present	Familial hyperchylomicronemia
II	Slightly increased (clear plasma)	Increased	Present	Familial hypercholesterolemia
III	Normal	Normal	Absent	"Floating beta" disorder
IV	Normal	Normal	Absent	Familial endogenous hyperlipemia
V	Normal	Normal	Absent	Familial endogenous and exogenous hyperlipemia

as cholestyramine and clofibrate, can cause the plasma lipids of some diseased subjects to return to normal or near normal levels has led to an interest in the prevention of the clinical manifestations of these disorders by similar therapy instituted early in infancy.

Type I hyperlipoproteinemia

Type I hyperlipoproteinemia, a rare disorder, is the result of the failure of release of lipoprotein lipase activity in response to the ingestion of fat. This failure leads to the accumulation in plasma of a large number of chylomicrons, giving the plasma a "cream of tomato soup" appearance. The hyperlipoproteinemia is accompanied by hypercholesterolemia and in many cases by the development of xanthomata. Although this disease is not a lysosomal storage disorder, hepatosplenomegaly with infiltration by foam cells is common in early childhood. Affected individuals develop episodes of abdominal pain that sometimes are associated with evidence of pancreatitis. Premature cardiovascular disease of the atherosclerotic type apparently is not a feature of this disorder.

The lactescence of plasma develops quite soon after the dietary intake of fat is established, and xanthomata have been reported within the neonatal period. Elimination of fat from the diet causes prompt remission in the hyperlipidemia.

A diet containing adequate amounts of essential fatty acids and medium-chain triglycerides rather than the usual dietary fat may be of benefit to patients with this disorder. No systematic trial of this management has been made, nor is any likely considering the rarity of the condition. Type I hyperlipoproteinemia is inherited as an autosomal recessive disease, and heterozygous individuals have no abnormality detectable by present methods.

Type II hyperlipoproteinemia

Type II hyperlipoproteinemia, or familial hypercholesterolemia, is a genetic disorder that has clinical manifestations in both heterozygous and homozygous individuals. The pathogenesis of type II hyperlipoproteinemia has been established as deficiency of the cellular receptor for low-density lipoprotein cholesterol. This leads to failure to clear plasma cholesterol normally, leading in turn to the formation of atheromata and xanthomata early in life. Failure of cellular uptake of cholesterol also impairs the feedback regulation of cholesterol synthesis, resulting in overproduction of cholesterol.

Clinical manifestations in the neonatal period are not common, but xanthomata have been noted at birth. Hypercholesterolemia is present in cord blood in a large number of affected subjects. Individuals homozygous for this disease characteristically exhibit plasma cholesterol levels in excess of 500 mg/dl, whereas heterozygous individuals have elevated levels but to a lesser degree. Hypertriglyceridemia, although present, is not striking, and fasting plasma is clear.

Homozygous subjects have an extremely high mortality from atherosclerotic cardiovascular disease in the first 3 decades of life. The prognosis for the heterozygous state is somewhat better, although these individuals are subject to premature atherosclerotic cardiovascular disease. The management of homozygous subjects has been attempted by both surgical and medical techniques. Portacaval anastomosis, ileal bypass, and repeated plasmapheresis, with and without the use of cholestyramine, clofibrate, and nicotinic acid, have been employed with varying success. There is no clear treatment of choice. For heterozygous individuals control of cholesterol intake and the use of a sequestering agent such as cholestyramine have been advised. Recent studies using inhibitors of cholesterol synthesis show promise for improved management of the heterozygous state. Neither efficacy nor safety of treatment in early life has been established.

The other types of hyperlipoproteinemia have neither clinical manifestations nor detectable laboratory abnormalities in the neonatal period.

Congenital lipodystrophy

Congenital lipodystrophy is a rare disorder, characterized by the absence of fat deposits in skin and viscera.

Etiology and pathogenesis

Concepts concerning the pathogenesis of congenital lipodystrophy have undergone considerable change in recent years. It now seems likely that the effect of insulin on the adipocyte is inhibited, leading both to failure of activation of lipoprotein lipase and to impairment of fat storage. In some older subjects with lipodystrophy, antibodies to insulin receptors have been demonstrated. In other patients the inhibition may be mediated through some as yet unidentified hormonal molecule, perhaps secreted by the hypothalamus. In any case serum insulin levels are consistently elevated, and insulin resistance can be demonstrated.

Clinical manifestations

Affected infants are long and thin at birth, already exhibiting an absence of subcutaneous fat. The face is typically wrinkled. Hepatomegaly, which is always present in later life, is not a prominent finding in neonates. No disability has been attributed to the disorder in early life. The fully developed clinical picture of lipodystrophy—insulin-resistant diabetes mellitus, acanthosis nigricans, hepatomegaly, and hyperchylomicronemia—evolves over the first decade of life.

Laboratory manifestations

There may be no laboratory abnormality in the affected neonate, with hyperlipidemia and glucose intolerance developing only with time. Hypoglycemia has been noted early in the course of the disorder in one patient.

Treatment

There is no specific treatment for this disorder, although the hyperlipidemia generally responds to a low-fat diet.

Prognosis

The prognosis for life and general health is good during the early years. The disorder is disfiguring and in about half the patients is associated with mental deficiency. Acanthosis nigricans is characteristic of later stages, as is diabetes mellitus with its accompanying microangiopathy. Fatty infiltration of the liver, accompanied by fibrosis, is invariably present in the fully developed disorder, and liver dysfunction may result.

Genetics

Current evidence strongly suggests autosomal recessive inheritance.

DISORDERS OF PEROXISOMAL FUNCTION

Zellweger's syndrome, neonatal adrenoleukodystrophy, and infantile Refsum's syndrome

The three entities named above serve as reference points in a rapidly evolving area of pathophysiologic research involving dysfunction of the peroxisome, a tiny intracellular organelle, first identified in 1960, and considered vestigial until 1973, when absence of peroxisomes was noted in tissues from patients suffering from Zellweger's syndrome.

Etiology and pathogenesis

Peroxisomes contain a number of enzymes, both membrane-associated and soluble, that are involved in the synthesis of plasmalogens, the catabolism of lysine, the synthesis of bile acids, and the β-oxidation of very long chain fatty acids. The exact consequences of the failure to carry out any one or all of these functions are unknown. Furthermore, it is likely that peroxisomes carry out other, as yet undefined, functions that are of vital importance in cellular physiology. Because of the technical difficulty of separating peroxisomes from other cellular organelles, it is also possible that functions assigned in earlier studies to these other organelles are actually performed by peroxisomes.

Clinical syndromes associated with peroxisomal dysfunction

Zellweger's syndrome, described in 1964, comprises a broad spectrum of diverse congenital morphologic defects, among which high forehead, widely open fontanels, and flat orbital ridges are constant findings. Camptodactyly, micrognathia, and genital defects are common. Enlargement of the liver is constantly present at autopsy, whether or not it is recognized during life. All affected infants are hypotonic. Failure to thrive from birth is common but not always present. Seizures and nystagmus (with oculogyric crises) together with developmental delay are nearly constant features of the evolving clinical picture. Death occurs within the first year. At autopsy, the liver shows extensive fibrosis and extreme degrees of iron storage. The kidneys are small with multiple small cysts. The brain shows polymicrogyria, pachygyria, and increased water content. In almost all patients with the clinical disorder, no peroxisomes are found on microscopic examination of tissues.

In neonatal adrenoleukodystrophy central nervous system function is similarly affected, with hypotonia, nystagmus, and poor development, but there is no dysmorphism, and the liver and kidneys are not involved.

Infantile Refsum's syndrome, in which phytanic acid accumulates abnormally, comprises retinitis pigmentosa, sensorineural deafness, developmental delay, and hepatomegaly, all appearing within the first year of life.

Laboratory manifestations

Routine laboratory tests are not useful in the diagnosis of these diseases. General tests of liver function are nonspecifically abnormal in Zellweger's syndrome. In both Zellweger's syndrome and neonatal adrenoleukodystrophy marked elevation in the concentration of very long chain fatty acids is found. In all three diseases, phytanic acid oxidase activity in cultured fibroblasts is reduced, although only in infantile Refsum's syndrome is phytanic acid consistently elevated in blood. Plasma pipecolic acid is always increased in Zellweger's syndrome, and it is usually increased in neonatal adrenoleukodystrophy.

Treatment

No specific therapy is available for either Zellweger's syndrome or neonatal adrenoleukodystrophy. Restriction of phytanic acid in the diet is indicated in infantile Refsum's syndrome, but efficacy has not been established given the rarity of the infantile form of the disease.

Genetics

Autosomal recessive inheritance of these disorders is reasonably well established.

DISORDERS OF LYSOSOMAL FUNCTION

Over the past two decades investigations employing electron microscopy and the cytochemistry of subcellular particles have resulted in both the discovery and simultaneous explanation of a large number of "new" storage diseases and also the reexamination of the older, largely clinical descriptions of storage diseases. The process is by no means complete but at this writing has produced a much more orderly and systematic classification of storage diseases, which are now so numerous as to bewilder all but the specialist. This review attempts to put these disorders into perspective and to single out for brief discussion those which can be recognized clinically in the neonatal period.

Etiology and pathogenesis

An increasing number of storage diseases are being classified as disorders of lysosomal function. The lysosome is an intracellular organelle whose role is the isolation of molecules from the cytosol and the degradation of these molecules. Under the electron microscope the lysosome is seen as a cytoplasmic membrane enclosing various cellular constituents. It is characterized by its high acid phosphatase activity.

Hers suggested the following criteria for disorders of lysosomal function: (1) the disease is characterized by storage of material within lysosomes; (2) the stored material can be degraded by a mixture of normal lysosomal enzymes; and (3) an enzymatic activity necessary for this degradation is absent from affected tissues.

Subsequent studies have expanded the original concept: if several hydrolytic enzymes share a common protein subunit, a genetic defect in the synthesis of that subunit can impair the activities of all the enzymes sharing the subunit. The inborn defect may involve a hydrolytic enzyme whose function is necessary not only for the degradation of molecules but also for the modification of other hydrolytic enzymes so that they can be accumulated within the lysosome. The function of lysosomes includes not only assimilation of hydrolytic enzymes but also the modification of these enzymes to the forms found ultimately in chemical analysis of lysosomes. Transport across the lysosomal membrane includes not only the hydrolytic enzymes but also the substrates and products formed during lysosomal catabolism of the substrates. Lysosomal storage may also occur as a secondary phenomenon when there is excessive production of a substance normally accumulated by lysosomes. Storage disorders also may be induced by drugs.

It is beyond the scope of this chapter to review all the lysosomal disorders that can be diagnosed at or before birth by appropriate chemical analysis. This discussion concerns only those diseases that can be expected to produce clinical manifestations during the early weeks of life. It must be borne in mind that all the storage diseases are progressive; clinical manifestations appear when accumulated material has grossly distorted morphologic characteristics or function or both. Factors such as the normal rate of turnover of the stored material, the degree of deficiency of the enzymes involved, and the degree of awareness of the observer determine the time of initial manifestation or recognition. Not only the pathogenesis of storage diseases but also their treatment have been the subject of intense investigation. A number of schemes for enzyme replacement have been developed. Some of these are promising, although none to my knowledge is unequivocally effective. The question of therapy should be investigated thoroughly at the time any of these diseases is diagnosed.

Amino acid storage disease

Cystine storage disease, more commonly referred to as the De Toni-Faconi syndrome, is associated with storage of cystine within lysosomes in a number of tissues. Current evidence suggests that the basis of the disease may be failure of normal transport for cystine across the lysosomal membrane. The disease does not produce clinical manifestations within the first month of life, though it can be diagnosed in the neonatal period by appropriate laboratory studies. An infant having evidence of gross renal tubular dysfunction in this period should be investigated for primary renal tubular disease, galactosemia, hereditary fructose intolerance, and glucose-6-phosphatase deficiency.

Polysaccharide storage disease

Glycogen storage disease type II

Pompe's disease, or type II glycogen storage disease, has been observed to produce clinical abnormalities from birth, although this observation is not necessary for the diagnosis.

Etiology and pathogenesis. Pompe's disease is the prototype for diseases of lysosomal function. The causative biochemical lesion is absence of activity of a lysosomal hydrolytic enzyme, acid maltase (acid α-glucosidase). The cytoplasmic enzymes of glycogen synthesis and degradation—those responsible for glucose homeostasis—are present in normal amounts and function normally. However, two factors prevent hydrolysis of glycogen engulfed by lysosomes. The first is the absence of the hydrolytic enzyme that normally accomplished the function. The second is that the glycogenolytic enzymes of cytoplasm cannot catalyze this hydrolysis in the hostile lysosomal environment. For reasons as yet obscure the devastating effects of the disease occur in the neuromuscular system, even though lysosomal accumulation of glycogen can be demonstrated in many other tissues, including liver and kidney. Mechanical distortion of cellular architecture has been incriminated in the malfunction of nerve and muscle.

Clinical features. Clinical manifestations can appear at any time during the first few months of life. The single most constant finding is profound muscular hypotonia, with diminution of reflexes but without loss of muscle mass. The muscles are firm to the touch. Cardiac failure as a result of myocardial involvement in the disease is very common as the initial complaint. Cardiomegaly is massive, and no murmur suggesting a congenital malformation is present. Hepatomegaly, when present, probably is related to congestive heart failure. Alertness is unaffected. The initial response to cardiotonic measures is generally good, but the overall course of the disease is one of relentless progression. Death is usually the result of respiratory failure, with or without complicating bronchopneumonia.

Laboratory studies. Results of all tests of hepatic glycogen release are normal, as is the structure of the glycogen stored by these patients. The electrocardiogram characteristically shows very large QRS deflections, a shortened PR interval, and a leftward axis. The electromyogram shows typical and virtually diagnostic myotonic discharges. Nerve conduction is slowed.

Confirmation of the diagnosis may be made by demonstration of typical lysosomal inclusions of glycogen in white blood cells, liver, or muscle. Enzymatic confirmation also may be obtained using these tissues, although some patients with Pompe's disease with normal levels of acid maltase in white blood cells have been reported.

Treatment. Attempts have been made to treat such patients by infusing an appropriate enzyme mixture obtained from cultures of *Aspergillus niger*. Beneficial effects have been noted in serial electron micrographs of material obtained by liver biopsy, but no substantive clinical benefit has been shown. Therapy at this time is only supportive.

Prognosis. In general, patients with cardiac involvement as a primary manifestation die within the first year of life, whereas those whose clinical disease does not involve the myocardium may survive for several years.

Genetics. Evidence suggests an autosomal recessive inheritance, although there is a preponderance of males among the reported patients.

Neutral lipidoses

Wolman's disease

Wolman's disease is a disorder of the storage of cholesterol and triglycerides, involving viscera much more than the central nervous system and leading to death within the first few months of life.

Etiology and pathogenesis. The absence of an acid lipase activity leads to the accumulation of cholesterol and triglycerides within intracellular membranous cytoplasmic bodies throughout the body. The liver, spleen, adrenal glands, and gastrointestinal tract are most prominently involved. The nervous system shows definable but less striking abnormalities.

Clinical manifestations. Infants with Wolman's disease show failure to thrive from birth. Vomiting and diarrhea are prominent manifestations, as is progressive abdominal distention with hepatosplenomegaly of massive proportions. The infants show progressive inanition, with maintenance of apparently normal alertness until very late in the course of the disease.

Laboratory manifestations. The most important diagnostic sign is the presence of enlarged calcified adrenal glands on the abdominal roentgenogram. Vacuolated leukocytes are prominent in peripheral blood smears and foam cells in the bone marrow are characteristic. The diagnosis is established by the demonstration of abnormal accumulation of triglycerides and cholesterol in biopsy tissue; the liver is the preferred organ for biopsy. Confirmation by assay of acid lipase activity is useful and may become an essential diagnostic technique.

Treatment. Although several agents known to influence cholesterol metabolism have been used to treat this disorder, no success has been reported. Because of the involvement of the adrenal cortex, replacement therapy with adrenal steroids may be indicated. Such therapy has not altered the course of the disease.

Prognosis. The prognosis is uniformly poor, and death usually occurs within the first 6 months.

Genetics. Wolman's disease is inherited as an autosomal recessive character.

Mucopolysaccharidoses

It is likely that the classic mucopolysaccharidoses (Hurler's, Hunter's, Sanfilippo's, Morquio's, Scheie's, and Maroteaux-Lamy syndromes) cannot be detected clinically in the neonatal period. "Congenital" cases reported in previous years now are generally thought to be examples of more profound lysosomal dysfunction, currently classified as mucolipidoses. To the original six mucopolysaccharidoses, there has been added a seventh with which neonatal clinical disease has been associated.

β-Glucuronidase deficiency (mucopolysaccharidosis VII)

Only a few patients with this disease have been described. There is considerable genetic heterogeneity among them. Some have had clinical disease in the neonatal period.

Etiology and pathogenesis. As its name implies, the disease is caused by deficiency of lysosomal β-glucuronidase. It must be presumed that the defect is more profound in those affected subjects who are clinically abnormal at birth.

Clinical manifestations. The affected infant may exhibit the Hurler syndrome at birth: hepatosplenomegaly, dysostosis multiplex, and hernias. Corneal clouding has not been noted early and may not always occur. Motor and mental development is variably affected.

Laboratory manifestations. Roentgenologic changes of dyostosis are present early. Inclusions are present in granulocytes. Excretion of mucopolysaccharides in urine is increased, although not dramatically so. The diagnosis is made by demonstration of the specific enzyme defect in leukocytes or fibroblasts. Treatment is supportive, but enzyme replacement should be considered.

Genetics. Autosomal recessive inheritance has been demonstrated.

Complex lipidoses

Farber's disease

Farber's disease is an infantile disorder of ceramide storage that is characterized by the accumulation of this material in granulomatous lesions, which involve the skin, subcutaneous tissues, joints, larynx, liver, and central nervous system. It is generally lethal within the first 2 years of life.

Etiology and pathogenesis. The biochemical basis of Farber's disease is, in all likelihood, deficiency of acid ceramidase. Ceramide accumulates in foam cells in many tissues in this disorder, and these foam cells accumulate within granulomas, which appear to evolve into the hyaline fibrotic masses characteristic of the disease. The inflammatory character of Farber's disease is unique among the storage diseases.

Clinical manifestations. Painful swelling of multiple joints, hoarseness, and stridor may appear at any time during the first few weeks of life. Palpable nodules develop in skin and subcutaneous tissue, particularly over the joints. Hepatomegaly and deterioration of central nervous system function, with the evolution of retinal cherry-red spots, form the remainder of the fully developed disease.

Laboratory manifestations. Roentgenographic examination reveals generalized demineralization of bone, destruction of normal joint relationships, erosion of bones at the articular surfaces, and soft tissue calcification. Routine laboratory studies are not helpful in diagnosis, although occasional lipid-laden cells may be found in the bone marrow. Microscopic examination of a nodule obtained by biopsy is the best means currently available to confirm the clinical diagnosis, although it may well be supplanted in the near future by assay of acid ceramidase.

Treatment. Although antiinflammatory agents may provide some symptomatic relief, there is no truly effective therapy for this condition.

Prognosis. The prognosis is uniformly poor; death characteristically occurs within the first 2 years.

Genetics. The disease shows autosomal recessive inheritance.

Gaucher's disease: malignant infantile form

The malignant form of Gaucher's disease is caused by the widespread storage of glucosyl cerebroside in brain, liver, spleen, and other tissues. It is a progressive disorder, with severe central nervous system dysfunction and death generally occurring within the first year of life.

Etiology and pathogenesis. The fundamental biochemical lesion in malignant infantile Gaucher's disease is marked reduction in the activity of glucosyl cerebrosidase. The consequent accumulation of glucosyl cerebroside is considered to be responsible for the clinical findings, although the pathogenetic mechanisms have not been elucidated. There is some degree of neuronal loss on pathologic examination of the brain.

Clinical manifestations. The clinical features of the disease can develop at any time within the first few years of life. In one case, hepatosplenomegaly and ascites were present at birth, but the presentation is not usually this dramatic. Feeding difficulties, vomiting, hepatosplenomegaly, and muscular hypertonia are found in various combinations. Cough and respiratory difficulty are also common. Deterioration of central nervous system function is characteristic, with the evolution of a vegetative state. Retinal cherry-red spots do not develop.

Laboratory manifestations. The serum acid phosphatase is elevated to a striking degree. Absolute confirmation of the diagnosis requires demonstration of the enzymatic deficiency in leukocytes or tissue obtained by biopsy. Microscopic examination of bone marrow and of other tissue generally reveals cellular characteristics specific enough to establish the diagnosis.

Treatment. Treatment is supportive.

Genetics. Gaucher's disease is inherited as an autosomal recessive disorder.

Gaucher's disease: chronic nonneuronopathic form

Although the chronic nonneuronopathic form of Gaucher's disease seldom is recognized in the early months and years of life, it seems likely that the visceral manifestations noted in malignant Gaucher's disease in early life are in fact present at similar ages in the nonneuronopathic disease. The striking differences are the normal neural function and much better prognosis of the nonneuronopathic disease.

Ganglioside storage disease

Tay-Sachs disease

Tay-Sachs disease is a progressive infantile disease of neurologic function, characterized by regression of development, blindness, spasticity, and ultimate fatality. It exhibits no characteristic clinical manifestations outside the nervous system.

Etiology and pathogenesis. Tay-Sachs disease is a result of a deficiency of activity of hexosaminidase A, which is necessary for the degradation of ganglioside GM_2. Although the accumulation of ganglioside GM_2 probably is generalized in a chemical sense, clinically significant accumulation is limited to the nervous system and predominantly to the gray matter of the central nervous system. The precise mechanism by which clinical disease occurs is unknown. Infants dying very early have shrunken brains showing enlarged lateral ventricles and gliosis; those dying late in the disease have enlarged brains with small ventricles, the result of progressive storage of ganglioside.

Clinical manifestations. The onset of clinical manifestations is generally within the first 8 months of life, but onset prior to 3 months of age is unusual. There is gradual deterioration of cortical function. The most characteristic clinical manifestation is hyperacusis, a striking extensor response to sharp sounds. Lack of normal awareness, poor muscle tone, and spasticity also are noted frequently. The retinal cherry-red spots that eventually develop in nearly all patients with Tay-Sachs disease are not present in the neonatal period. Seizures, which may be myoclonic, focal, or generalized, have occurred in the neonatal period but are unusual early in the course of the disease.

Laboratory manifestations. The absence of hexosaminidase A activity in any of several tissues, including white blood cells, liver, and skin fibroblasts, is diagnostic of Tay-Sachs disease. Reduction in the activity of fructose-1-phosphate aldolase in the red blood cells has been documented, but the measurement of this activity cannot be considered a substitute for the assay of hexosaminidase A.

Therapy. No specific therapy is available.

Prognosis. The course is relentlessly progressive, and death generally occurs 13 to 30 months after the onset of clinical manifestations.

Genetics. Tay-Sachs disease shows autosomal recessive inheritance. The disease occurs predominantly in Ashkenazi Jews.

Neimann-Pick disease type A

Infantile Neimann-Pick disease is a progressive disease associated with the storage of sphingomyelin in the nervous system and viscera.

Etiology and pathogenesis. Severe deficiency of sphingomyelinase in all tissues leads to the intracellular accumulation of sphingomyelin within membranous cytoplasmic bodies. The predominant clinical effects are in the nervous system.

Clinical manifestations. Neimann-Pick disease usually is recognized after the neonatal period. Persistent neonatal jaundice and hepatosplenomegaly have been noted retrospectively in a number of patients. The retinal cherry-red spots develop quite early in many cases but are not reliably present within the neonatal period. Neurologic deterioration usually occurs after the neonatal period.

Laboratory manifestations. Vacuolated leukocytes may be observed in blood smears, and Niemann-Pick cells (lipid-laden macrophages) can be seen in the bone marrow. The level of plasma acid phosphatase occasionally is elevated. Specific diagnosis depends on the demonstration of sphingomyelin accumulation and of markedly reduced activity of sphingomyelinase in tissue obtained by biopsy or in tissue cultures of skin fibroblasts or bone marrow. The enzymatic defect also has been demonstrated in peripheral leukocytes.

Therapy. No specific therapy is available.

Genetics. The disorder exhibits autosomal recessive inheritance. A preponderance of reported cases have occurred in Jews, but no racial or ethnic group appears to be spared.

Niemann-Pick disease type B

Type B Niemann-Pick disease is different from type A disease only in that the nervous system is spared in type B disease. Visceral manifestations are similar in the two disorders, but the prognosis is better in type B; the course resembles that of chronic Gaucher's disease.

Mucolipidoses (Table 36-5)

The term *mucolipidoses* was coined to describe diseases combining elements of mucopolysaccharidosis (e.g., dysostosis multiplex) and elements of lipidosis (e.g., macular cherry-red spots). The diseases so classified include a number of entities that are clinically evident in the neonatal period. Most, but not all, are lethal early in life. The excretion of mucopolysaccharide in the urine generally is not increased. However, in a number of these diseases, smaller urinary polysaccharides containing excess sialic acid (*N*-acetyl neuraminic acid) have been found in abnormal amounts. Thus a subgroup, the sialidoses, has evolved. While primary neuraminidase deficiency seems causative in some sialidoses, in others sialic aciduria occurs as a result of a general phenomenon involving a number of hydrolytic enzymes. The segregation of the sialidoses is only part of a trend toward ending the classification of diseases as mucolipidoses. There is considerable scientific reason for doing this, but the use of the classification has distinct clinical merit.

Table 36-5. Mucolipidoses*

Disorder	Defective enzyme	Alternate names
Mucolipidosis I		
Infantile	Neuraminidase	Sialidosis, nephrosialidosis
"Adult"	Neuraminidase	Cherry-red spot-myoclonus syndrome
Mucolipidosis II	Phosphotransferase	I-cell disease
Mucolipidosis III	?	Pseudo-Hurler polydystrophy
Mucolipidosis IV	Ganglioside neuraminidase	Sialolipidosis

*Spranger's classification. Other disorders are classified as mucolipidoses by Spranger without being given systematic names different from those used by other investigators.

Generalized gangliosidosis

Generalized gangliosidosis is a disorder combining the morphologic features of Hurler's syndrome with a clinical course similar to that of the infantile cerebral lipidoses.

Etiology and pathogenesis. Ganglioside GM_1 is the major storage material, but there is also storage of mucopolysaccharides. Assays of lysosomal enzymes have revealed marked deficiency of activity of β-galactosidases A_1, A_2, and A_3. The enzymes share a common polypeptide.

Clinical manifestations. It seems likely that cases reported as neonatal or congenital Hurler's syndrome represent instances of generalized gangliosidosis or other mucolipidoses. Hurler's facies, hepatosplenomegaly, and skeletal abnormalities may be seen at birth or very shortly thereafter. Tense ascites at birth has been described. Developmental retardation is manifested very early, and there is profound failure to thrive. Macular cherry-red spots appear in approximately 50% of cases.

Laboratory manifestations. The excretion of mucopolysaccharides in the urine is normal. However, 10% to 80% of leukocytes contain Reilly bodies, and bone marrow examination reveals finely vacuolated histiocytic cells. Similar evidence of storage is seen in biopsy material from various tissues, particularly the liver. Definitive diagnosis requires demonstration of marked deficiency in β-galactosidases A_1, A_2, and A_3.

Treatment. There is no specific treatment.

Prognosis. The prognosis is uniformly poor. Death usually occurs prior to 2 years of age as a result of pulmonary complications.

Genetics. Autosomal recessive inheritance occurs.

Neuraminidase deficiency (mucolipidosis I)

Currently, there are two clearly defined clinical syndromes associated with generalized neuraminidase deficiency. The first is the cherry-red spot myoclonus syndrome, which has no infantile manifestations. The second is severe infantile neuraminidase deficiency, which characteristically declares itself at birth or shortly thereafter. The two disorders are obviously different chemically, as well as clinically, but the chemical differences are not as yet defined.

Etiology and pathogenesis. That there is a profound disturbance in lysosomal function in mucolipidosis I is not in doubt, nor is there any question that the excretion of oligosaccharides rich in neuraminic acid is the result of deficient neuraminidase activity. What the physiologic substrate for the deficient activity is, is not known, nor is it known whether the inborn defect affects the structure and function of other lysosomal enzymes.

Clinical features. There is heterogeneity in the presentation of even the severe infantile form of neuraminidase deficiency. Some infants have been fatally ill at birth with massive hepatosplenomegaly, anasarca, and poorly developed lungs. Others have been considered normal at birth, but shown the development of dystosis multiplex, cataracts, corneal clouding, macular cherry-red spots, and hepatosplenomegaly over the ensuing months. This latter group, with more slowly progressive infantile disease, probably includes infants previously described as having nephrosialidosis, a clinically similar disorder in which massive proteinuria supervened with time.

Laboratory manifestations. Lymphocytes are vacuolated, and oligosaccharides containing sialic acid are abundant in the urine. As indicated above, some affected infants have shown proteinuria. Definitive diagnosis requires the demonstration of neuraminidase deficiency, since at least one patient with sialic aciduria associated with this clinical syndrome has been reported to have normal lysosomal neuraminidase activity.

Treatment. Treatment is supportive.

Prognosis. The disease is rapidly lethal in infants who are severely affected at birth, but in those with onset later in the first months of life, longevity approaching that of Hurler's disease is not unexpected. The disparity in clinical presentation and outlook indicates that two disorders are involved, but their chemical separation has not yet been accomplished.

Genetics. Autosomal recessive inheritance is indicated by all available data.

I-cell diseases (mucolipidosis II)

I-cell disease is a disorder of lysosomal function characterized by rapid accumulation of heterogeneous material within lysosomes, onset of clinical disease during fetal life, and rapid progression of disease postnatally.

Etiology and pathogenesis. I-cell disease was once considered to be a sialidosis because of the accumulation of sialic acid–rich macromolecules among the stored material. This accumulation is now known to result from a deficiency of lysosomal neuraminidase that occurs as part of a widespread deficiency of lysosomal hydrolases. The enzymes affected are in fact synthesized normally but are not concentrated within lysosomes. The defect has now been shown to be failure of a posttranslational modification of the enzymes necessary for the recognition of the enzymes by receptors on membranes. In electrophoretic and binding studies, the enzymes show structural abnormalities which indicate that failure to interact normally with receptors interferes with other steps (presumably intralysosomal) in the production of the enzymes as they are found in the normal lysosome.

Clinical manifestations. Affected infants have low birth weights and subsequent growth failure. These infants are quiet from birth and show severe developmental retardation early in life. The skin may be somewhat thickened and tight. There is no hepatosplenomegaly, and corneas are clear. Although Hurler-like bony abnormalities are not recognizable clinically, careful examination of roentgenograms will reveal their presence.

Laboratory manifestations. The usual tests of mucopolysacchariduria give normal results, but thin-layer chromatography reveals excessive excretion of smaller saccharides containing sialic acid. No inclusions are seen in leukocytes. The diagnosis is established by finding typical inclusions within cultured fibroblasts.

Treatment. No specific treatment is known for I-cell disease. The prognosis is poor.

Mannosidosis

Mannosidosis is a recently described storage disease in which hepatosplenomegaly, skeletal changes, central nervous system dysfunction, and marmoration of skin may appear within weeks after birth.

The absence of acid α-mannosidase has been demonstrated. Vacuolated lymphocytes and polymorphonuclear inclusions are seen in the bone marrow. Although considered by Spranger in his early classification to be one of the mucolipidoses because of the combination of dysostosis multiplex, absence of mucopolysacchariduria, and presence of inclusion bodies in lymphocytes, there is actually little, if any, lipid storage, and the clinical course is that of rapidly progressive Hurler's syndrome with rather mild dysostosis. There is no specific treatment, and the prognosis is poor.

Mucolipidosis IV

Mucolipidosis IV is relatively slowly progressive but is of interest in that corneal clouding without dysostosis or organomegaly is apparent within the first few weeks of life. Deficiency of a neuraminidase specific for gangliosides has been demonstrated, and hence the name "sialolipidosis" has been suggested for this entity.

Uncategorized storage disorders: stiff skin syndrome

Four patients have been described who have stiff skin and limitation of joint mobility; clinical manifestations have been noted in the newborn period. Histologic changes in the skin suggest mucopolysaccharide storage.

Neonatal iron storage disease

Several infants have exhibited massive lysosomal storage of iron in parenchymal organs shortly after birth. The liver is strikingly affected. The disease has been rapidly fatal in all infants, and it has been commonly preceded by massive hemorrhage.

John F. Nicholson

BIBLIOGRAPHY

General

Cornblath, M., and Schwartz, R.: Disorders of carbohydrate metabolism in infancy, ed. 2, Philadelphia, 1978, W.B. Saunders Co.

Danks, D.M.: Management of newborn babies in whom serious metabolic illness is anticipated, Arch. Dis. Child. **49**:576, 1974.

Nayman, R., and others: Observations on the composition of milk-substitute products for treatment of inborn errors of amino acid metabolism. Comparisons with human milk. A proposal to rationalize nutrient content of treatment products, Am. J. Clin. Nutr. **32**:1279, 1979.

Scriver, C.R., and Rosenberg, L.E.: Amino acid metabolism and its disorders, Philadelphia, 1973, W.B. Saunders Co.

Stanbury, J.B., and others, editors: The metabolic basis of inherited disease, ed. 5, New York, 1983, McGraw-Hill Book Co.

Phenylketonuria

Dhondt, J.L.: Tetrahydrobioterin deficiency: preliminary analysis from an international survey, J. Pediatr. **104**:501, 1984.

Hackney, I.M., Davidson, W., and Linsao, L.: Phenylketonuria: mental development, behavior, and termination of low phenylalanine diet, J. Pediatr. **72**:646, 1968.

Kang, E.S., Sollee, N.D., and Gerald, P.S.: Results of treatment and termination of the diet in phenylketonuria (PKU), Pediatrics **46**:881, 1970.

Kennedy, J.L., and others: The early treatment of phenylketonuria, Am. J. Dis. Child. **113**:16, 1967.

Mamunes, P., and others: Intellectual deficits after transient tyrosinemia in the term neonate, Pediatrics **57**:675, 1976.

O'Flynn, M.E., and others: The diagnosis of phenylketonuria: a report from the collaborative study of children treated for phenylketonuria, Am. J. Dis. Child. **134**:769, 1980.

Rouse, B.M.: Phenylalanine deficiency syndrome, J. Pediatr. **69**:246, 1966.

Snyderman, S.E., and others: The phenylalanine requirement of the normal infant, J. Nutr. **56**:253, 1955.

Tyrosinosis, acute tyrosinosis, and chronic tyrosinemia

Bakker, H.D., and others: Fructose-1, 6-diphosphatase deficiency: another enzyme defect which can present itself with the clinical features of "tyrosinosis," Clin. Chim. Acta **55**:41, 1974.

Fallstrom, S.P., Lindblad, B., and Steen, G.: On the renal tubular damage in hereditary tyrosinosis and on the formation of succinylacetoacetate and succinylacetone, Acta Paediatr. Scand. **70**:315, 1981.

Gaull, G.E., and others: Biochemical observations on so-called hereditary tyrosinosis, Pediatr. Res. **4**:337, 1970.

Grant, D.B., Alexander, F.W., and Seakins, J.W.T.: Abnormal tyrosine metabolism in hereditary fructose intolerance, Acta Paediatr. Scand. **59**:432, 1970.

Hostetter, M.K., and others: Evidence for liver disease preceding amino acid abnormalities in hereditary tyrosinemia, N. Engl. J. Med. **308**:1265, 1983.

Kvittingen, E.A., Halvorsen, S., and Jellum, E.: Deficient fumarylacetoacetate fumarylhydrolase activity in lymphocytes and fibroblasts from patients with hereditary tyrosinemia, Pediatr. Res. **17**:541, 1983.

Sandberg, H.O.: Bilateral keratopathy and tyrosinosis, Acta Ophthalmol. **53**:760, 1975.

Scriver, C.R., Larochelle, J., and Silverberg, M.: Hereditary tyrosinemia and tyrosyluria in a French Canadian geographic isolate, Am. J. Dis. Child. **113**:41, 1967.

Yu, J.S., Walker-Smith, J.A., and Burnard, E.D.: Neonatal hepatitis in premature infants simulating hereditary tyrosinosis, Arch. Dis. Child. **46**:306, 1971.

Nonketotic hyperglycinemia

Arneson, D., and others: Strychnine therapy in nonketotic hyperglycinemia, Pediatrics **63**:369, 1979.

Matalon, R., and others: Nonketotic hyperglycinemia: treatment with diazepam—a competitor for glycine receptors, Pediatrics **71**:581, 1983.

Perry, T.L., and others: Studies of the glycine cleavage enzyme system in brain from infants with glycine encephalopathy, Pediatr. Res. **11**:1192, 1977.

Homocystinuria

Hagberg, B., and Iambraeces, L.: Some aspects of the diagnosis and treatment of homocystinuria, Dev. Med. Child. Neurol. **10**:470, 1968.

Harvey, J.P., and others: Homocystinuria caused by 5, 10-methylene tetrahydrofolate reductase deficiency: a case in an infant responding to methionine, folinic acid, pyridoxine and vitamin B_{12} therapy, J. Pediatr. **98**:275, 1981.

Mudd, S.H., and others: The natural history of homocystinuria due to cystathionine beta-synthase deficiency, Am. J. Hum. Genet. **73**:1, 1985.

Sahuh, S., and others: Homocystinuria and megaloblastic anemia responsive to vitamin B_{12} therapy: an inborn error of metabolism due to a defect in cobalamin metabolism, N. Engl. J. Med. **310**:686, 1984.

Histidinemia

Scriver, C.R., and Levy, H.L.: Histidinemia. Part I. Reconciling retrospective and prospective findings, J. Inherited Metab. Dis. **6**:51, 1983.

Thalhammer, O., Schreibenreiter, S., and Pantlitschko, M.: Histidinemia: detection by routine newborn screening and biochemical observations on three unrelated cases, Z. Kinderheilkd. **109**:279, 1971.

Sulfite oxidase deficiency

Desjacques, P., and others: Combined deficiency of xanthine oxidase and sulfite oxidase: diagnosis of a new case followed by an antenatal diagnosis, J. Inherited Metab. Dis. **8**(suppl. 2):117, 1985.

Shih, V.E., and others: Sulfite oxidase deficiency: biochemical and clinical investigations of a hereditary metabolic disorder in sulfur metabolism, N. Engl. J. Med. **297**:1022, 1977.

Disorders of the urea cycle

Bachman, C., and others: *N*-Acetylglutamate synthetase deficiency: a disorder of ammonia detoxification, N. Engl. J. Med. **304**:543, 1981.

Brusilow, S.W., Valle, D.L., and Batshaw, M.: New pathways of nitrogen excretion in inborn errors of urea synthesis, Lancet **2**:452, 1979.

Hudak, M.L., Jones, M.D., Jr., and Brusilow, S.W.: Differentiation of transient hyperammonemia of the newborn and urea cycle enzyme defects by clinical presentation, J. Pediatr. **107**:712, 1985.

Msall, M., and others: Neurologic outcome in children with inborn errors of urea synthesis, N. Engl. J. Med. **310**:1500, 1984.

Packman, S., and others: Severe hyperammonemia in a newborn infant with methylmalonyl-CoA mutase deficiency, J. Pediatr. **92**:759, 1978.

Saudubray, J.M., and others: Hyperammonemia secondary to hereditary organic acidurias: a study of 29 cases, Adv. Exp. Med. Biol. **153**:135, 1982.

Terheggen, H.G., and others: Familial hyperargininemia, Arch. Dis. Child. **50**:57, 1975.

van der Zee, S.P.M., and others: Citrullinemia with rapidly fatal neonatal course, Arch. Dis. Child. **46**:847, 1971.

Disorders of organic acid metabolism

Bakkaren, J.A.J.M., and others: Organic aciduria in hypoxic premature newborns simulating an inborn error of metabolism, Eur. J. Pediatr. **127**:41, 1977.

Duran, M., and others: Octanoic acidemia and octanoylcaritine excretion with dicarboxylic aciduria due to defective oxidation of medium-chain fatty acids, J. Pediatr. **107**:397, 1985.

Engel, A.G., and Rebouche, C.J.: Carnitine metabolism and inborn errors, J. Inherited Metab. Dis. **7**(suppl. 1):38, 1984.

Saudubray, J.M., and others: Neonatal management of organic acidurias, J. Inherited Metab. Dis. **7**(suppl. 1):2, 1984.

Maple syrup urine disease

Goodman, S.I., and others: The treatment of maple syrup urine disease, J. Pediatr. **75**:485, 1969.

Mantovani, J.F., and others: MSUD: presentation with pseudotumor cerebri and CT abnormalities, J. Pediatr. **96**:279, 1980.

Sallan, S.E., and Cottom, D.: Peritoneal dialysis in maple syrup urine disease, Lancet **2**:1423, 1969.

Scriver, C.R., and others: Thiamine-responsive maple-syrup-urine disease, Lancet **2**:310, 1971.

Snyderman, S.E.: The therapy of maple syrup urine disease, Am. J. Dis. Child. **113**:68, 1967.

Defects in the propionate pathway

Brandt, I.K., and others: Propionic acidemia (ketotic hyperglycinemia): dietary treatment resulting in normal growth and development, Pediatrics **53**:391, 1974.

Hsia, Y.E., Lilljeqvist, A.C., and Rosenberg, L.E.: Vitamin B12-dependent methylmalonicaciduria: amino acid toxicity, long chain ketonuria, and protective effect of vitamin B12, Pediatrics **46**:497, 1970.

Keating, J.P., and others: Hyperglycinemia with ketosis due to a defect in isoleucine metabolism: a preliminary report, Pediatrics **50**:890, 1972.

Nyhan, W.L., and others: Response to dietary therapy in B12 unresponsive to methylmalonic acidemia, Pediatrics **57**:539, 1973.

Congenital lactic acidosis

Brunette, M.G., and others: Thiamine responsive lactic acidosis in a patient with deficient low-Km pyruvate carboxylase activity in liver, Pediatrics **50**:702, 1972.

DiMauro, S., and others: Benign infantile mitochondrial myopathy due to reversible cytochrome c oxidase deficiency, Ann. Neurol. **14**:226, 1983.

Greene, H.L., Schubert, W.K., and Hug, G.: Chronic lactic acidosis of infancy, J. Pediatr. **76**:753, 1970.

Hartmann, A.F., Sr., and others: Lactate metabolism; studies of a child with a serious congenital deviation, J. Pediatr. **61**:165, 1962.

Lie, S.O., and others: Fatal congenital lactic acidosis in two siblings. I. Clinical and pathological findings, Acta Paediatr. Scand. **60**:129, 1971.

Matalon, R., and others: Lipoamide dehydrogenase deficiency with primary lactic acidosis: favorable response to treatment with oral lipoic acid, J. Pediatr. **104**:65, 1984.

Robinson, B.H., and Sherwood, W.G.: Pyruvate dehydrogenase phosphatase deficiency: a cause of congenital chronic lactic acidosis in infancy, Pediatr. Res. **9**:935, 1975.

Robinson, B.H., and Sherwood, W.G.: Lactic acidemia, J. Inherited Metab. Dis. **7**(suppl. 1):69, 1984.

Robinson, B.H., Taylor, J., and Sherwood, W.G.: The genetic heterogeneity of lactic acidosis: occurrence of recognizable inborn errors of metabolism in a pediatric population with lactic acidosis, Pediatr. Res. **14**:956, 1980.

van Biervliet, J.P., and others: Hereditary mitochondrial myopathy with lactic acidemia, a de Toni-Fanconi-Debre syndrome, and a defective respiratory chain in voluntary striated muscles, Pediatr. Res. **11**:1088, 1977.

Isovaleric acidemia

Kelleher, J.F., Jr., and others: The pancytopenia of isolvaleric acidemia, Pediatrics **65**:1023, 1980.

Krieger, I., and Tanaka, K.: Therapeutic effects of glycine in isovaleric acidemia, Pediatr. Res. **10**:25, 1976.

Levy, H.L., and others: Isovaleric acidemia; results of family study and dietary treatment, Pediatrics **52**:83, 1973.

Newman, C.G.H., and others: Neonatal death associated with isolvaleric acidemia, Lancet **2**:439, 1967.

Other disorders of organic acid metabolism

Bartlett, K., and others: Enzyme studies in biotin-responsive disorders, J. Inherited Metab. Dis. 8(suppl. 1):46, 1985.

Coude, F.X., and others: Neonatal glutaric aciduria type II: an X-linked recessive inherited disorder, Hum. Genet. **59**:263, 1981.

Cowan, M.J., and others: Multiple biotin-dependent carboxylase deficiencies associated with defects in T-cell and B-cell immunity, Lancet **2**:115, 1979.

Pryzyrembel, H., and others: Alpha-ketoadipic aciduria, a new inborn error of lysine metabolism; biochemical studies, Clin. Chim. Acta **58**:257, 1975.

Schutgens, R.B.H., and others: Lethal hypoglycemia in a child with a deficiency of 3-hydroxy-3-methyl glutaryl coenzyme-A-lyase, J. Pediatr. **94**:89, 1979.

Stokke, O., and others: Beta-methylcrotonyl-Co-A carboxylase deficiency: a new metabolic error in leucine degradation, Pediatrics **49**:726, 1972.

Tildon, J.T., and Cornblath, M.: Succinyl-Co-A: 3-CoA: 3-ketoacid CoA-transferase deficiency, J. Clin. Invest. **51**:493, 1972.

Wolf, B., and others: Biotinidase deficiency: a novel vitamin recycling defect, J. Inherited Metab. Dis. 8(suppl. 1):53, 1985.

Neonatal diabetes mellitus

Gentz, J.C.H., and Cornblath, M.: Transient diabetes in the newborn, Adv. Pediatr. **16**:345, 1969.

Disorders of galactose metabolism

Holton, J.B., and others: Galactosemia: a new severe variant due to uridine diphosphate galactose-4-epimerase deficiency, Arch. Dis. Child. **56**:885, 1981.

Huttenlocher, P., Hillman, R., and Hsia, Y.: Pseudotumor cerebri in galactosemia, J. Pediatr. **76**:902, 1970.

Kelly, S.: Septicemia in galactosemia, JAMA **216**:330, 1971.

Komrower, G.M., and Lee, D.H.: Long-term follow-up of galactosemia, Arch. Dis. Child. **45**:367, 1970.

Litman, N., Kanter, A., and Finberg, L.: Galactokinase deficiency presenting as pseudotumor cerebri, J. Pediatr. **86**:410, 1975.

Monteleone, J.A., and others: Cataracts, galactosuria and hypergalactosemia due to galactokinase deficiency in a child, Am. J. Med. **50**:403, 1971.

Disorders of fructose metabolism

Baerlocher, K., and others: Hereditary fructose intolerance in early childhood: a major diagnostic challenge, Helv. Paediatr. Acta **22**:465, 1978.

Greene, H.L., Stifel, F.B., and Herman, R.H.: Ketotic hypoglycemia due to hepatic fructose-1, 6-diphosphatase deficiency, Am. J. Dis. Child. **124**:415, 1972.

Pagliara, A.S., and others: Hepatic fructose-1, 6-diphosphatase deficiency, J. Clin. Invest. **51**:2115, 1972.

Steinmann, B., and Gitzelmann, R.: The diagnosis of hereditary fructose intolerance, Helv. Paediatr. Acta **36**:297, 1981.

Glycogenoses

Burr, I.M., and others: Comparison of the effects of total parenteral nutrition, continuous intragastric feedings, and portacaval shunt on a patient with type I glycogen storage disease, J. Pediatr. **85**:792, 1974.

Dunger, D.B., and Leonard, J.V.: Value of the glucagon test in screening for hepatic glycogenosis, Arch. Dis. Child. **57**:384, 1982.

Fernandez, J.: The effect of disaccharrides on the hyperlactacidemia of glucose-6-phosphatase-deficient children, Acta Paediatr. Scand. **63**:695, 1974.

Fernandez, J., and Pikaar, N.A.: Ketosis in hepatic glycogenosis, Arch. Dis. Child. **47**:41, 1972.

Perlman, M., Aker, M., and Slonim, A.E.: Successful treatment of severe type I glycogen storage disease with neonatal presentation by nocturnal intragastric feeding, J. Pediatr. **94**:772, 1979.

Smit, G.P., and others: The dietary treatment of children with type I glycogen storage disease with slow release carbohydrate, Pediatr. Res. **18**:879, 1984.

Disorders of lipid metabolism

Seip, M.: Generalized lipodystrophy, Ergeb. Inn. Med. Kinderheilkd. **31**:59, 1971.

Disorders of peroxisomal function

Borst, P.: Animal peroxisomes (microbodies), lipid biosynthesis and the Zellweger syndrome, Trends Biochem. Sci. **8**:269, 1983.

Opitz, J.M., and others: The Zellweger syndrome (cerebo-hepato-renal syndrome), British Defects **2**:144, 1969.

Poulos, A., and others: Cerebro-hepato-renal (Zellweger) syndrome, adrenoleukodystrophy and Refsum's syndrome: plasma changes and skin fibroblast phytanic acid oxidase, Hum. Genet. **70**:172, 1985.

Disorders of lysosomal storage

General references

Spranger, J.W., and Wiedeman, H.-R.: The genetic mucolipidoses; diagnosis and differential diagnosis, Humangenetik **9**:113, 1970.

Specific references

Crandall, B.F., and others: Review article: mucolipidosis IV, Am. J. Med. Genet. **12**:301, 1982.

Clement, D.H., and Godman, G.C.: Glycogen disease resembling mongolism, cretinism, and amyotonia congenita, J. Pediatr. **36**:11, 1950.

Dean, M.F., and others: Enzyme replacement therapy by fibroblast transplantation: long-term biochemical study in three cases of Hunter's syndrome, J. Clin. Invest. **63**:138, 1979.

Esterly, N.B., and McKusick, V.A.: Stiff skin syndrome, Pediatrics **47**:360, 1971.

Gillian, J.E., and others: Congenital ascites as a presenting sign of lysosomal storage disease, J. Pediatr. **104**:225, 1984.

Goldfischer, S., and others: Idiopathic neonatal iron storage involving liver, pancreas, heart and endocrine and exocrine glands, Hepatology **1**:58, 1981.

Hers, H.G.: Inborn lysosomal diseases, Gastroenterology **48**:625, 1965.

Humbel, R., and Collart, M.: Oligosaccharides in urine of patients with glycoprotein storage diseases. I. Rapid detection of thin-layer chromatography, Clin. Chim. Acta **60**:143, 1975.

Kelly, T.E., and others: Mucolipidosis I (neuraminidase deficiency): three cases and delineation of the phenotype, Am. J. Dis. Child. **135**:703, 1981.

Kjellman, B., and others: Mannosidosis: a clinical and histopathologic study, J. Pediatr. **75**:366, 1969.

Leroy, J.G., and others: I-cell disease: a clinical picture, J. Pediatr. **79**:360, 1971.

Moser, H.W., and others: Farber's lipogranulomatosis, Am. J. Med. **47**:869, 1969.

Rosenstein, B.: Glycogen storage disease of the heart in a newborn infant, J. Pediatr. **65**:126, 1964.

Schneider, J.A., Wong, J., and Seegmiller, J.E.: The early diagnosis of cystinosis, J. Pediatr. **74**:114, 1969.

Sly, W.S., and others: Beta glucuronidase deficiency; report of clinical, radiologic and biochemical features of a new mucopolysaccharidosis, J. Pediatr. **82**:249, 1973.

von Bassewitz, D.B., and others: Vacuolated lymphocytes in type II glycogenosis, Eur. J. Pediatr. **127**:1, 1977.

Wolman, M., and others: Primary familial xanthomatosis with involvement and calcification of the adrenals, Pediatrics **28**:742, 1961.

CHAPTER 37

Metabolic and endocrine disorders

PART ONE

Carbohydrate disorders

Emerging from an intrauterine environment, where nutritional needs are continuously provided by the maternal circulation and regulated by placental exchange, the newborn must effect major physiologic and metabolic changes over a short period to adjust to intermittent enteral feeding. During intrauterine life, *readjustments* in maternal metabolism are required to provide for the progressively increasing demands of the growing fetus. The fetus prepares for extrauterine survival by increasing energy stores and developing enzymatic processes for rapid mobilization of stored energy. As carbohydrate stores become depleted postnatally, the neonate must develop the capacity for hepatic glucose production from other sources. However, abnormalities in the maternal or placental environment may modify the postnatal development of glucose homeostasis.

METABOLIC ADJUSTMENTS DURING PREGNANCY

When food is withheld from a pregnant woman, the use of endogenous fuel occurs more rapidly than in a nonpregnant state, since the mother must supply not only her own needs but also those of the growing fetus. The following biochemical differences are found between gravid and nongravid women following an overnight fast: (1) plasma glucose values are lower, and hypoglycemia may supervene if fasting is prolonged; (2) plasma amino acids are lower, and aminoaciduria is present; (3) muscle catabolism and activation of gluconeogenesis occur more rapidly; (4) maternal lipolysis is increased with elevated values for free fatty acids and ketones; (5) plasma insulin concentration may be lower during the first trimester, but during late pregnancy, insulin is increased even though blood sugar is lower.

In addition to alterations during fasting, maternal metabolism is significantly changed following food ingestion. The response to exogenous glucose in late pregnancy is accompanied by an excessive outpouring of insulin. However, the hypoglycemic action of exogenous insulin is significantly diminished. Thus pregnancy is characterized by augmentation of insulin release concomitant with increased peripheral resistance. Since more insulin is needed during late pregnancy for maintenance of carbohydrate homeostasis, the inability to provide compensatory hyperinsulinism results in gestational diabetes (Chapter 3). The rapid reversibility of glucose intolerance in gestational diabetes suggests that the fetoplacental unit exerts this critical stress.

The placenta may exert its influence on maternal metabolism in two ways: (1) it may play a role in the extraction and degradation of maternal hormones, such as insulin, and (2) it is a site of production of hormones, such as human placental lactogen, estrogens, and progesterone, that may affect carbohydrate metabolism. Human placental lactogen is similar to growth hormone and exerts a significant antiinsulin action; it also increases lipolysis. Human placental lactogen secretion is increased with progressive fetoplacental growth, and at the end of pregnancy its concentration is 750 times that of growth hormone. Although it is difficult to assign relative importance to individual hormones, in concert they effect an enhanced turnover of fat in adipose tissue, cause pancreatic hyperplasia, and increase the amount of insulin required for glucose disposition.

Serum cortisol, which exerts peripheral insulin antagonism, also is increased during pregnancy. However, most of the increase is attributable to biologically inactive protein-bound hormone, which is elevated under the influence of estrogen. Serum growth hormone concentration is not increased during pregnancy and may even be decreased. Plasma glucagon concentration, after an overnight fast, is the same in pregnant women during late gestation as in normal controls and is therefore not responsible for the increased insulin resistance.

During periods of food ingestion, mechanisms exist that selectively favor maternal repletion and anabolism. For example, a larger proportion of the ingested glucose is converted to triglyceride, and there is greater suppression of glucagon following exogenous glucose ingestion; thus a more conducive intrahepatic setting for glycogen deposition is provided.

PLACENTAL TRANSPORT OF NUTRIENTS AND HORMONES

Maternal glucose crosses the placenta to the fetus by facilitated diffusion (Fig. 37-1). Glucose concentration in amniotic fluid decreases with increasing gestational age; fetal urine is probably the major source of this glucose, and, as maturation of kidney tubules results in greater glucose reabsorption, less appears in amniotic fluid. Evidence suggests that the placenta is capable of producing lactate and that lactate is then provided to the fetus in sufficient quantities to account for 25% of fetal oxidative metabolism. Amino acids are actively transported to the fetus against a transplacental gradient with maintenance of amino acids at levels of 1.1 to 4.3 times those in maternal plasma. There is more rapid transport of L-amino acids than D-isomers. Transplacental passage of esterified and free fatty acids is limited; however, ketone bodies readily cross the placenta. In contrast, there is an effective physiologic barrier to the transport of insulin, glucagon, growth hormone, and placental lactogen in the human placenta; there is dissociation of fetal and maternal levels, and equilibrium across the placenta does not occur with any of these hormones. However, all the lipid-soluble steroid hormones are transported freely across the placenta.

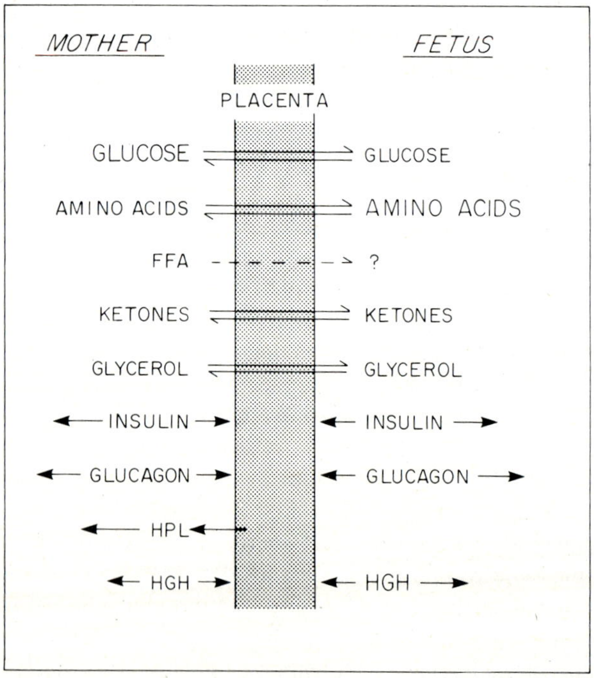

Fig. 37-1. Placental permeability and the relationship between maternal and fetal fuels and hormones. (From Freinkel, N., and Metzger, B.E. In Pregnancy metabolism, diabetes and fetus, CIBA Foundation Symposium no. 63, Amsterdam, 1979, Excerpta Medica.)

FETAL GLUCOSE METABOLISM

See also Chapter 7.

Energy source and stores

The rate of glucose uptake by the fetus via the umbilical circulation is related to the maternal blood glucose level. The concentration of glucose in fetal blood is approximately one third lower than that in maternal blood. Glucose is the major source of energy throughout fetal life; however, in sheep, amino acids and lactate also provide a significant amount of the fuel for fetal oxygen consumption during late gestation. Fetal hepatic glycogen stores have been identified by the ninth week of gestation and at term are three times (150 mg/gm liver) those of a well-fed adult; skeletal muscle glycogen is three to five times that of adults, and cardiac muscle glycogen is 10 times the adult value. Another source of stored energy resides in fetal adipose tissue triglycerides that accumulate in the last trimester. This accumulation of adipose tissue is predominantly a result of synthesis from glucose, since there is limited transfer of free fatty acids from the mother.

During hypoxia the fetus may meet metabolic requirements primarily by glucose production from glycogenolysis and glycolysis. In chronic sheep preparations, total maternal starvation causes a prompt fall in maternal and fetal blood glucose levels for the first 48 hours, but a stable plateau is reached subsequently; the fetus then increases amino acid catabolism, which accounts for most of the fetal oxygen consumption. The human fetus has the potential to replace substrate glucose with β-OH-butyrate for energy during periods of maternal starvation and glucose deprivation.

Fetal hormones

Proinsulin separated from human fetal pancreatic extracts comprises 0.1% to 1.6% of the total insulin values regardless of the age of the fetus, a proportion similar to that in the adult. Immunoreactive insulin has been demonstrated in both plasma and pancreatic tissue as early as 8 weeks' gestation; the source appears to be the fetal pancreas, since the placenta is impermeable to insulin. At 13 to 18 weeks' gestation, fetal insulin response to sustained maternal hyperglycemia is negligible. At term, however, the fetus is capable of a significant response to prolonged hyperglycemia, although to a lesser degree than are adults. When the fetus receives appropriate glucose from the mother, there is minimal requirement for insulin response. With repeated episodes of hyperglycemia, as in maternal diabetes, greater insulin response is seen, indicating that β-cell sensitivity is being induced or enhanced. That insulin may modify the growth rate in utero has been shown by the positive correlation between fetal plasma insulin concentration and fetal weight.

Human growth hormone has been measured as early as 9 weeks' gestation and increases rapidly between the eleventh and sixteenth weeks. Since the transplacental transfer of human growth hormone is negligible, the fetal pituitary appears to be its source in the fetus. At term, fetal plasma human growth hormone levels are higher than those of maternal plasma. Unlike those of adults, fetal human growth hormone levels are not suppressed during hyperglycemia and actually show a paradoxic rise.

The pancreatic α-cells are detectable at approximately 8 to 11 weeks' gestation and constitute 30% of the islet cells at term. Circulating glucagon has been found in fetal plasma as early as the fifteenth week. Fetal pancreatic and circulating glucagon must be of fetal origin, since maternal glucagon does not cross the placenta. Peak concentrations of glucagon in the pancreas are reached at 24 to 26 weeks' gestation and are approximately two or three times higher than those of the adult human pancreas. Similar to those of human growth hormone, glucagon levels fail to diminish during constant glucose infusion. Although the physiologic function of fetal glucagon is unknown, its effect on fetal carbohydrate metabolism is probably minimal. Cortisol is synthesized in a cooperative effort between mother and fetus, involving the fetal zone of the adrenal cortex and progesterone secreted by the placenta as substrate. The fetal adrenal gland can also synthesize cortisol from acetate.

Fetal enzymes

Metabolism in the fetus in large part reflects its dependence on maternally derived substrates. Glucose for energy is continually provided and need not be synthesized. The fetus actively incorporates amino acid into protein and synthesizes triglycerides from glucose. The human fetal liver has the enzymatic capacity for gluconeogenesis and glycogenolysis as early as the third month of gestation. However, if maternal glucose provision is adequate and placental transfer normal, there is no requirement for fetal gluconeogenesis. Nevertheless, during early human fetal life the absolute levels of gluconeogenic enzymes are 10% to 70% of adult values. This does not necessarily mean that these enzymes are rate limiting under these conditions, since early fetal liver may produce glucose from pyruvate. In contrast to its potential role as a provider of glucose, under normal states of maternal nutrition fetal hepatic glycogen content actually increases linearly at this early gestational age. Because of fetal dependence on glucose metabolism, one would also expect high activity of important glycolytic enzymes. Indeed, hexokinase and pyruvate kinase are high in fetal rat tissues and decrease at birth. As the rat fetus approaches term, a marked increase occurs in glycogen synthetase and phosphorylase with a predominance of synthetase, thus facilitating deposition of hepatic glycogen.

NEONATAL GLUCOSE METABOLISM

The newborn must supply its own substrate to meet the energy requirements for maintenance of body temperature, respiration, muscular activity, and regulation of blood glucose.

The concentration of glucose in mixed arteriovenous cord blood is approximately 80% to 90% of that in the mother. Glucose values fall immediately after birth and reach their lowest values by 1 to 1½ hours after birth. In normal, full-term neonates born to healthy mothers, the values stabilize by 3 to 4 hours; mean plasma glucose values from 4 to 72 hours are 60 to 70 mg/dl, and from 73 to 168 hours, mean values are 80 mg/dl. These values are higher than those previously reported, probably because of earlier and more aggressive feeding techniques and studies limited to normal term infants. Glucose values in low birth weight (LBW) infants have not been evaluated recently, but previous studies suggest that the levels are lower than those of infants greater than 2,500 gm and that they stay lower during the first month of life.

Intense lipid mobilization begins within a few minutes after birth and is reflected by a rapid rise in glycerol and free fatty acid. The respiratory quotient declines from levels approaching 1.0 to levels of 0.7 by the third postnatal day, suggesting a changeover from a predominantly carbohydrate to a predominantly fat metabolism at a time when liver glycogen and blood glucose are decreasing. Furthermore, a progressive rise in blood ketones occurs within a few hours after birth and reaches a peak in 2 to 3 days, indicating increased oxidation of free fatty acids. Lipolysis is probably initiated by activation of the autonomic nervous system secondary to cold stimulation of the skin at birth or to clamping of the cord.

Blood glucose concentration is normally maintained at a relatively constant level by a fine balance between hepatic glucose output and peripheral glucose uptake. The latter is influenced by factors such as body temperature, muscular activity, and insulin concentration. Normal neonates have a low capacity for removal of a rapidly injected glucose load, as demonstrated by glucose disappearance rates between 1.0% and 1.3% during the first 24 hours of life. By 5 to 7 days of age, however, glucose disappearance rates are significantly higher than during the first 24 hours of life.

Several groups have begun to study glucose kinetics in infants using the Steele steady state infusion technique with stable isotope tracers. Glucose production is higher in the newborn than in the adult. Kalhan and associates, using glucose-1-^{13}C in normal term infants at 2 to 4 hours of age and prior to feeding found glucose production rates of 4.4 ± 0.4 (mean ± SD) mg/kg/minute. Adult values are approximately half those reported in normal neonates.

Hepatic glucose output depends on (1) adequate glycogen stores, (2) sufficient supplies of endogenous gluconeogenic precursors, (3) a normally functioning hepatic gluconeogenetic and glycogenolytic system, and (4) a normal endocrine system for modulating these processes. At birth the neonate has glycogen stores that are greater than those in the adult. However, because of a twofold greater basal glucose utilization, these stores are rapidly depleted and begin to decline within 2 to 3 hours after birth, remain low for several days, and then gradually rise to adult levels. Muscle and cardiac carbohydrate levels fall more slowly. During asphyxia, energy requirements are met by anaerobic glycolysis, an inefficient mechanism that results in a limited amount of energy and rapid depletion of glycogen stores. In premature infants there is marked reduction of both total carbohydrate and fat content, and depletion of liver carbohydrate occurs within 12 hours after birth. Endogenous gluconeogenic substrate availability probably is not a limiting factor, since the concentration of plasma amino acids is increased at birth as a consequence of active placental transport. Similarly, other gluconeogenic precursors, such as lactate, pyruvate, and glycerol, also are increased.

The fall in blood glucose that normally occurs after birth is accompanied by an elevated level of human growth hormone, a relatively low concentration of immunoreactive insulin, and an increase in plasma glucagon. The neonate shows an attenuated but significant insulin response to a variety of stimuli. Following oral administration of glucose, the insulin response in the normal neonate is similar to that in adults with chemical diabetes, that is, a lag in insulin response and a delayed peak. The premature infant has a minimal and variable insulin response, but the values are markedly increased by intravenous administration of glucose plus amino acids. The physiologic role of human growth hormone has not been defined; human growth hormone values are high during the first 48 to 72 hours and gradually decline but are still elevated at 8 weeks of age. In addition, the newborn shows a paradoxical rise in human growth hormone following glucose infusion. Plasma glucagon values at birth are similar to or slightly higher than maternal levels. A surge in glucagon release is seen within hours after birth, which is probably mediated via adrenergic mechanisms and not as a response to hypoglycemia. Glucagon and human growth hormone are not suppressed during hypoglycemia. In healthy newborns, intravenous and oral alanine feedings raise plasma glucagon and glucose levels. The adrenal medulla secretes little epinephrine at birth and is not a significant regulator of neonatal blood glucose concentration. Nevertheless, hypoglycemia stimulates epinephrine secretion, probably through increased activity of the sympathetic plexus mediated by the splanchnic nerve. The newborn adrenal cortex rapidly establishes independent cortisol production controlled by pituitary adrenocorticotropic hormone (ACTH).

Adaptation to prolonged starvation in adult human beings is facilitated by the ability of the brain to derive much of its energy through oxidation of ketone bodies; this decreases the need for gluconeogenesis and spares muscle protein. Enzymes involved in ketone body utilization pathways are present in brain tissue of human fetuses and in newborns. That ketone bodies are used by the brains of infants and children has been shown by measurements of arteriovenous differences across the brain.

THE CLINICAL PROBLEM OF HYPOGLYCEMIA

Definitions

Ideally hypoglycemia should be defined as a state of glucose insufficiency at the level of the central nervous system. Some studies even suggest that glucose levels may need to be maintained at higher levels than previously considered in the presence of seizures. Sophisticated electroencephalographic and scanning techniques that demonstrate functional abnormalities during hypoglycemia or hyperglycemia may be helpful. At present, however, there are no means of determining tissue glucose insufficiency except for the variable and inconsistent symptoms attributable to low glucose levels. Since the significance of low glucose concentrations without symptoms is not well understood, symptoms cannot be used as sole criteria in determining tissue glucose insufficiency.

The chemical definition of hypoglycemia has classically been based on studies performed in the 1960s, when the concept of gestational age was not well appreciated and early feeding practices not generally accepted. These studies have recently been repeated in normal full-term neonates born to healthy mothers and fed formula from 3 to 4 hours after birth. Using mean and 95% confidence intervals (Fig. 37-2), the authors recommended that plasma glucose values in term neonates be considered

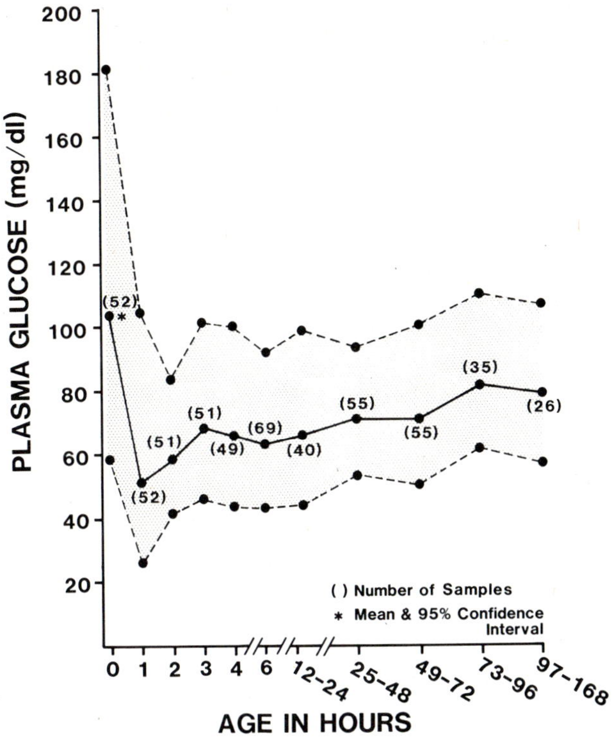

Fig. 37-2. Plasma glucose levels in healthy term neonates delivered vaginally with birth weights between 2.5 and 4.0 kg. (From Srinivasan, G., and others: J. Pediatr. **109:**114, 1986.)

low if two values were less than 35 mg/dl in the first 3 hours, less than 40 mg/dl from 4 to 24 hours, and less than 45 mg/dl from 24 hours to 7 days of age. Ten percent of the infants had one value less than 35 mg/dl in the first 3 hours, but the infants were asymptomatic and glucose values rose spontaneously within the next ½ hour. Others have recommended that serum values less than 35 mg/dl in the first 24 hours and less than 45 mg/dl from 24 to 48 hours be considered hypoglycemic in full-term neonates.

Studies in LBW infants are difficult to perform because of the widespread use of parenteral fluids in these infants. Therefore the definition currently used is similar to that originally recommended, that is, two glucose values less than 25 mg/dl during the first 72 hours after birth (two plasma values, one cerebrospinal fluid and one plasma, or one test strip and one plasma value).

Symptomatic versus asymptomatic hypoglycemia

It is important to determine whether an infant is symptomatic because it has been shown that symptomatic infants are more likely to suffer central nervous system morbidity. Unfortunately clinical manifestations of hypoglycemia are nonspecific (see boxed material).

Clinical signs often associated with neonatal hypoglycemia*

- Tremors or jitteriness
- Irritability
- Exaggerated Moro reflex
- Apneic spells
- Cyanotic spells
- Seizures
- Limpness
- Lethargy
- Hypothermia
- High-pitched or weak cry
- Refusal to feed
- Vomiting
- Cardiac failure
- Cardiac arrest
- Sweating

*The clinical sign should be alleviated with concomitant correction of the glucose level.

Measurement of glucose

Factors that are frequently overlooked in the interpretation of a glucose concentration are the type of sample and the method of analysis. Whole blood includes red cells, which, because of their lower water content, have a glucose concentration lower than that of plasma. Plasma glucose values are higher than those of whole blood by about 14%; the percent difference may be greater at very low (less than 30 mg/dl) values because of a greater probability of laboratory error. Whole blood glucose also varies in accordance with the hematocrit value; in addition, neonatal red blood cells contain high concentrations of glycolytic intermediates such as reduced glutathione. Thus whole blood must be deproteinized with zinc hydroxide before analysis. Capillary blood samples should be collected from a warm heel and taken to the laboratory on ice, since the rate of in vitro glycolysis is increased in neonatal red blood cells; the whole blood glucose level may drop 18 mg/dl/hour if the sample is allowed to stand at room temperature.

Many enzymatic and chemical methods are currently used for glucose determinations. Those that employ reducing methods may give falsely elevated glucose values, since non-glucose reducing substances may range up to 60 mg/dl in newborn blood. In normal infants reducing methods can be used, since galactose and fructose levels are usually minimal. However, enzymatic procedures using glucose oxidase or glucose-6-phosphate dehydrogenase, which specifically measure glucose, are preferable.

The most frequently used method for glucose determination is a system that measures the rate of change in oxygen consumption. When a sample is injected into an enzyme reagent solution, β-D-glucose from the sample combines with dissolved oxygen from the solution, according to the reaction:

$$\beta\text{-D-Glucose} + O_2 \xrightarrow[H_2O]{\text{Glucose oxidase}} \text{Gluconic acid} + H_2O_2$$

At all times during the reaction the rate of oxygen consumption measured by an oxygen electrode is directly proportional to the glucose concentration.

In many nurseries rapid assessment of whole blood glucose concentrations is accomplished by a glucose oxidase-peroxidase chromagen test strip method, either alone or with a reflectance colorimeter (e.g., Dextrostix/Ames Meter or Chemstrip bG/Stat Tek Meter). If whole blood glucose concentration is estimated to be 60 mg/dl by a rapid test strip method, the clinician can be 95% confident that the true value lies between 34 and 86 mg/dl. Another study found that at low glucose levels, Dextrostix overestimated blood glucose concentration and that Chemstrip bG correlated better than Dextrostix to true blood glucose levels. However, in both studies the readings were done by only a limited number of observers. How true would any of these findings have been if multiple observers had been used, as is the clinical reality? In addition, glucose values determined by these techniques are influenced by hematocrit, and appropriate corrections are necessary. The use of plasma may obviate some of these problems. Borderline values should be checked in the laboratory; the likelihood of falsely low values, however, is much greater than for falsely high values.

Interestingly, whereas both hypoxia and hypoglycemia are damaging to the central nervous system, clinical priorities still dictate that blood gases be performed promptly and frequently, and plasma glucose levels in most nurseries are still determined by the inaccurate test strip methods. Since the amount of plasma required in a glucose autoanalyzer is less than 10 μL (0.010 ml) and the procedure takes only a few minutes to perform, the inaccurate test strip should be replaced by an accurate glucose autoanalyzer, particularly for high-risk infants.

Differential diagnosis

Hypoglycemia may be caused by a wide variety of pathologic conditions and is a common finding in many hereditary disorders of carbohydrate and amino acid metabolism, as shown in the following outline. Discussion of individual entities is limited to disorders of carbohydrate metabolism that occur in the neonatal period.

A. Asymptomatic (transient)
B. Symptomatic (transient, idiopathic)
C. Specific etiology
  1. Hyperinsulinism
    a. Maternal diabetes
    b. Erythroblastosis
    c. Beckwith-Wiedemann syndrome
    d. Infant giants
    e. β-Cell nesidioblastosis-adenoma spectrum
    f. Functional β-cell hyperplasia
    g. Leucine sensitivity
    h. Maternal drugs
  2. Endocrine disorders
    a. Panhypopituitarism
    b. Isolated growth hormone deficiency
    c. Cortisol deficiency
      (1) ACTH unresponsiveness
      (2) Isolated glucocorticoid deficiency
      (3) Maternal steroid therapy
      (4) Adrenal hemorrhage
      (5) Adrenogenital syndrome
    d. Hypothyroidism
    e. Glucagon deficiency
  3. Hereditary defects in metabolism
    a. Carbohydrate metabolism
      (1) Galactosemia
      (2) Glycogen storage disease type 1
      (3) Fructose intolerance
    b. Amino acid metabolism
      (1) Maple syrup urine disease
      (2) Propionicacidemia
      (3) Methylmalonic acidemia
      (4) Hereditary tyrosinemia
D. Associated with other neonatal problems
  1. Iatrogenic
    a. Excessive dextrose fluids in intrapartum period
    b. Maternal starvation before delivery
    c. Following abrupt cessation of intravenous fluids
    d. Following exchange transfusion
    e. Hypothermia
    f. Malpositioned umbilical artery catheter
  2. Miscellaneous
    a. Intravenous indomethacin
    b. Neonatal infection
    c. Cardiac malformation
    d. Hypothermia
    e. Hyperviscosity
    f. Chronic diarrhea
    g. Antiinsulin antibodies
    h. Central nervous system abnormalities

Asymptomatic transient neonatal hypoglycemia

Asymptomatic hypoglycemia may be seen frequently before onset of feedings, especially in premature or small for gestational age (SGA) infants. The true incidence of asymptomatic hypoglycemia is impossible to ascertain, since its presence has usually been determined by chance sampling. Some studies have suggested that this be considered as early transitional or adaptive hypoglycemia following the withdrawal of substrate supplied from the mother. Infants in this category are not necessarily SGA, but appropriate for gestational age (AGA) and large for gestational age (LGA) babies have similar problems. There is no sex predilection; perinatal hypoxia, prematurity, maternal toxemia and diabetes, twinning, and delayed feedings may contribute to the hypoglycemia. If symptoms are present, they may be caused by the underlying disease, especially if they are not alleviated by glucose. Hypoglycemia is of short duration and rarely recurs. The infants may respond spontaneously to oral feedings or to relatively low concentrations of constant glucose infusions. Extensive long-term follow-up data are not available, but current data indicate that the prognosis is more favorable than in patients with symptomatic hypoglycemia.

Symptomatic transient idiopathic neonatal hypoglycemia

Incidence and etiology

The incidence of idiopathic transient symptomatic neonatal hypoglycemia varies between 1.3 and 3 per 1,000 live births. Twice as many male as female infants are affected. Among LBW infants, 5.7% may be affected; the incidence rises to 15% in LBW infants who are symptomatic and below the fiftieth percentile for gestational age. The smaller of twins who weighs less than 2.0 kg and is discordant by 25% in weight when compared with the larger twin has a 70% chance of developing symptomatic hypoglycemia (Fig. 37-3).

Clinical and laboratory manifestations

The infants may be born before term, at term, or after term, although preterm infants predominate. Intrauterine growth retardation, manifested by a birth weight below the tenth percentile for gestational age on the Lubchenco intrauterine growth curve, is present in about 75% of the infants (Fig. 37-4). Postterm neonates need not be below the tenth percentile; instead, intrauterine growth retardation is exhibited by a disproportionately low weight-length ratio and clinical signs of dysmaturity. In general, weight is affected to a greater degree than length and head circumference; however, the latter two are below the tenth percentile in a significant number of infants. Decreased head circumference also may indicate microcephaly, which in some patients may be the primary etiologic factor causing hypoglycemia.

Maternal age is not a significant factor, but toxemia is found in a high proportion of mothers. No correlation exists between hypoglycemia and duration of labor, premature rupture of membranes, or the type of analgesia or anesthesia. Birth hypoxia is frequently present.

Symptoms begin within the first 24 hours in about 40% of the infants and after 72 hours in 14%. Associated laboratory features include polycythemia, a frequent observation in intrauterine malnutrition, and hypocalcemia (less than 7.0 mg/dl), which has been found in 20% of the infants and is probably related to prematurity, toxemia, or birth anoxia rather than to intrauterine malnutrition. Cardiomegaly was demonstrated on roentgenogram in 12 and cardiac failure in 4 of 76 infants in one study. The cause of cardiomegaly is unknown, but cardiac

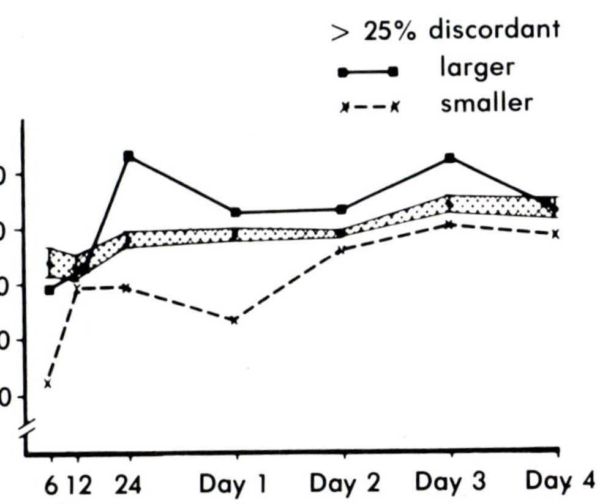

Fig. 37-3. Mean blood glucose values in twins whose birth weights were discordant by more than 25%. Mean ± SD of 100 pairs of twins is shown by stippling. (From Pildes, R.S., and others: Pediatrics **40:**69, 1967.)

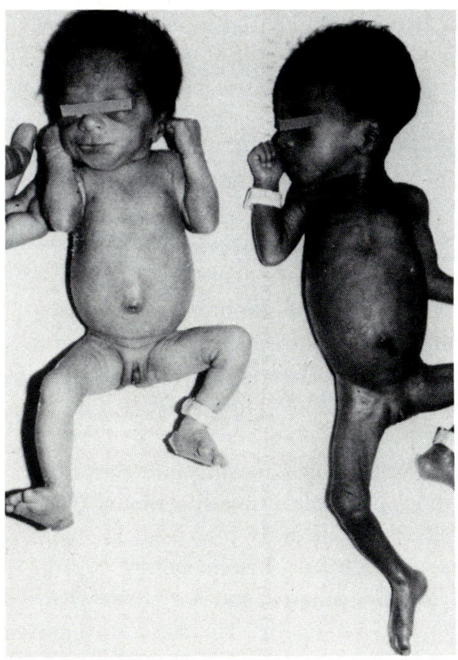

Fig. 37-4. SGA infant, 40 weeks' gestation and 1,100 gm at birth, compared with an AGA infant of 32 weeks' gestation. The SGA infant had asymptomatic hypoglycemia.

congenital anomalies need not be present, and cardiomegaly recedes after carbohydrate homeostasis is established. Polycythemia is a frequent finding in SGA infants and may be a factor in the pathogenesis of cardiomegaly. However, cardiomegaly and congestive failure also have been found in hypoglycemic infants with normal hematocrit values.

Pathogenesis

The association of hypoglycemia with intrauterine growth retardation has led to many studies of carbohydrate homeostasis in SGA infants. Hypoglycemia is not uniformly present in SGA infants, and factors other than intrauterine growth retardation may be necessary to precipitate hypoglycemia in some SGA infants (see following outline). Since SGA infants have experienced nutritional restriction during gestation, it seems reasonable to expect reduced amounts of hepatic glycogen and total body fat. Supportive evidence includes low hepatic carbohydrate levels at postmortem of SGA infants as compared with AGA full-term infants and stillbirths. Normoglycemic SGA infants may show adequate glucagon response to exogenous glucose, but hypoglycemic SGA infants have a reduced glycemic response with rapid improvement following therapy. A relative decrease in liver glycogen available per unit of brain weight may be inferred from the disproportionately increased brain-liver weight ratio in SGA infants. Decreased gluconeogenesis has been suggested because of increased blood levels of alanine and lactate in SGA as compared with AGA infants. In hypoglycemic SGA newborns, levels of gluconeogenic amino acids entering at pyruvate, such as proline, glycine, and valine, are significantly higher than in normoglycemic SGA infants. Decreased gluconeogenesis is also indicated by the poor glycemic response to intravenous and oral alanine of SGA neonates compared with that of normal neonates. Administration of hydrocortisone results in a hyperglycemic response to alanine, which may have been facilitated by lowering plasma insulin levels or by increasing gluconeogenesis from alanine. Animal models suggest that the induction of phospho*enol*pyruvate carboxykinase (PEPCK) is delayed in growth retardation and thus contributes to the hypoglycemia.

Glucose utilization following intravenous glucose administration, particularly in full-term SGA hypoglycemic newborns, is significantly increased as compared with that in normal controls. Insulin values, appropriately depressed in SGA infants, may be elevated in some hypoglycemic SGA neonates. This suggests that β-cell function usually adapts itself to intrauterine starvation but that the adaptation may not be universal in all hypoglycemic SGA infants. The importance of glucagon in the etiology of hypoglycemia is unknown. Human growth hormone secretion appears normal, deficient secretion of catecholamines has been implicated, and a low cortisol production rate has been reported. Finally, the finding of hypoglycemia in microcephalic neonates suggests a defective central nervous system mechanism for glucose homeostasis in some infants.

The following is an outline of the pathogenesis of symptomatic transient neonatal hypoglycemia:

A. Inadequate production of glucose
   1. Decreased glycogen and fat stores
   2. Defective gluconeogenesis
   3. Decreased glucose-sparing substrates, such as:
      a. Ketones
      b. Glycerol
   4. Delayed induction of PEPCK

B. Excessive utilization
   1. Increased peripheral glucose disappearance in some infants
   2. Inadequate counterinsulin hormones
   3. Increased needs
      a. Increased oxygen consumption in SGA infants
      b. Anoxia
      c. Large brain-liver ratio
   4. Hyperinsulinism

Pathology

Evidence that neuronal glucose deprivation specifically damages nerve cells is difficult to substantiate, since hypoxia, acidosis, and other underlying factors typically coexist with severe hypoglycemia. Adult rhesus monkeys subjected to gross insulin hypoglycemia have evidence of damage to the neocortex. In newborn rat pups made hypoglycemic with insulin once per day for 18 days, there was generalized diminution of brain weight, cellularity, and protein content. Widespread neuronal damage has been described in three of six infants who had prolonged hypoglycemia and died in the first week of life.

Prognosis

Untreated hypoglycemia may result in severe neurologic deficit or death. In a long-term prospective follow-up of a group of 39 treated hypoglycemic infants and 41 matched normoglycemic high-risk control neonates, mean height and weight were similar in the two groups at 5 to 7 years of age. However, head circumference, which had been significantly smaller at birth in the hypoglycemic newborns, remained smaller. Abnormal neurologic development could not be ascribed solely to hypoglycemia, except in 2 of 30 infants who had repeated evaluations. Convulsions in the neonatal period were associated with increased neurologic abnormalities and with recurrent nonhypoglycemic seizures. A greater number of hypoglycemic neonates had IQ scores below 86 than did the controls (Fig. 37-5), although the mean

IQ scores were not significantly different. Thus, although treatment resulted in less severe damage than had been expected from previous reports, these studies suggest that treatment of symptomatic infants should be even more aggressive to improve the prognosis.

The hypoglycemia is usually self-limited, but recurrences may be common during the first few days as intravenous fluids infiltrate or are too rapidly discontinued before oral feedings are well tolerated. Recurrent hypoglycemic episodes also occur during the first few months in a few of these infants. In children with ketotic hypoglycemia, retrospective studies show an increased incidence of neonatal hypoglycemia.

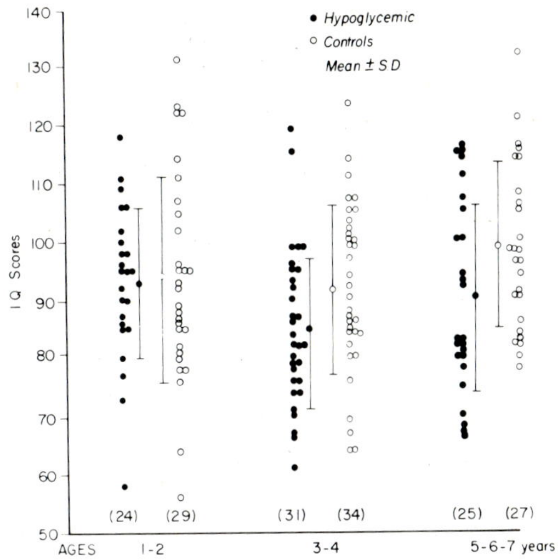

Fig. 37-5. Individual IQ scores in hypoglycemic neonates compared with those of equally high-risk but normoglycemic controls. (From Pildes, R.S., and others: Pediatrics **54:**5, 1974.)

Persistent hypoglycemia: specific etiology

The incidence of all entities in the third category, persistent hypoglycemia with specific etiology, is significantly less than 1 per 1000 live births if hyperinsulinism secondary to maternal diabetes is excluded. These disease states represent hormone excess or deficiency or enzyme deficiency and are not primary substrate problems. Of these, the hyperinsulinism diseases predominate. Most diseases associated with hyperinsulinism, with the exception of β-cell nesidioblastosis-adenoma spectrum and leucine sensitivity, are self-limited, and recurrences tend to be infrequent within a few days. The remaining hormone and enzyme deficiencies need specific hormone replacement or dietary restriction to control the hypoglycemia. Thus their control somewhat depends on how rapid the diagnosis is made.

Infant of the diabetic mother

See also Chapter 3.

Clinical and laboratory manifestation

Infants of diabetic mothers (IDMs) may be LGA but physiologically immature (Fig. 37-6). They need not be large; diabetic mothers with severe vascular disease may give birth to SGA infants. In our nursery most IDMs are AGA; the incidence of LGA infants occurs in about 20% to 40% of class A, B, C diabetic pregnancies. Typically the infant of an uncontrolled diabetic mother has a round, cherubic face and appears plethoric. Hypertrichosis on the pinnae has recently been added to the list of characteristic clinical features. The excessive weight results from increased body fat and enlargement of viscera, primarily liver, adrenals, and heart. The umbilical cord and placenta are also enlarged. Skeletal length is increased in proportion to weight, but the brain appears disproportionately small because it does not increase in size abnormally. The development of ossification centers does not correspond to weight and length but rather to gestational age (or even less than the infant's gestational age). There is considerable reduction in total and extra-

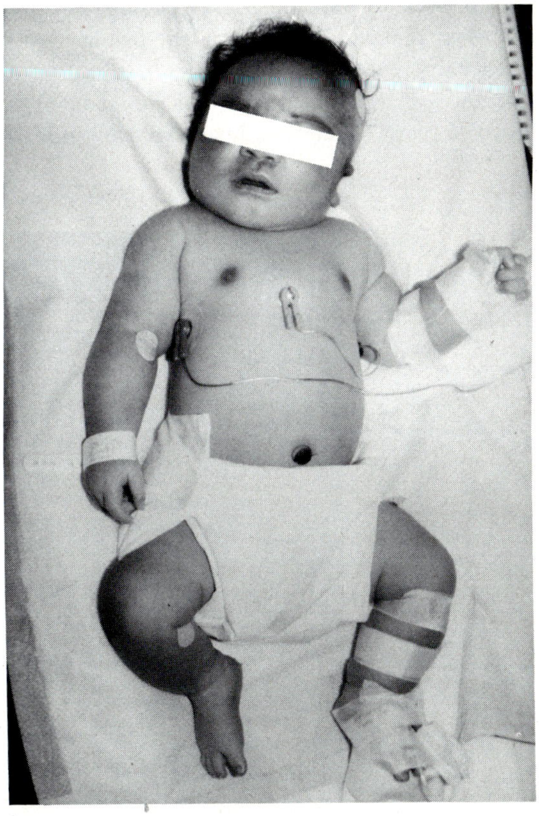

Fig. 37-6. Infant of gestational diabetic mother born at 40 weeks' gestation with birth weight of 4.6 kg. The infant developed persistent hypoglycemia and was treated with intravenous glucose through two separate sites.

cellular water. Skinfold thickness and adipose cell diameter correlate significantly with maternal blood glucose during the third trimester. Maternal glycohemoglobin concentration (Hb A_{1c}) as well as cord blood (Hb F_{1c}) have been shown to correlate with birth weight in infants of class A, B, C diabetic mothers in some but not all studies. Clinical problems in the neonate are extremely variable. In retrospective studies the risk for developing respiratory distress syndrome (RDS) was five to six times greater in IDMs than in infants of comparable gestational age regardless of mode of delivery until 38½ weeks' gestation. Evaluation of lung maturity is therefore essential in preventing hyaline membrane disease in IDMs who are delivered early. The lecithin/sphingomyelin (L/S) ratio of 2.0 or greater, a useful predictor of lung maturity in normal pregnancies, is falsely positive in 20% of IDMs. However, the presence of phosphatidylglycerol (PG) in amniotic fluid increases the probability that the infant will not have respiratory distress from surfactant deficiency. PG is not present in some IDMs unless the L/S ratio is greater than 3.0; thus PG is a better index of lung maturity than L/S ratio alone. In our nursery the incidence of respiratory distress in infants of both gestational and insulin-dependent diabetic mothers is 30% to 40%, but RDS is rare; "wet lung" syndrome or transient tachypnea is the primary cause of respiratory distress (Chapter 28).

Increased cardiothymic shadow is found in approximately 35% and congestive heart failure, judged by tachypnea, tachycardia, and hepatomegaly, in 5% to 17% of the infants (Fig. 37-7). Poor control of maternal diabetes and inclusion of different classes of diabetes may be responsible for the differences in incidence of congestive failure in various centers. Electrocardiograms may be abnormal and show marked right ventricular hypertrophy, combined ventricular hypertrophy, and, rarely, left ventricular hypertrophy. Echocardiographic studies have emphasized the presence of a wide spectrum of hypertrophic cardiomyopathy. Disproportionate septal hypertrophy and abnormal ventricular wall thickening, at times resulting in obstruction of the left ventricle outflow tracts, have been reported. The findings may be indistinguishable from those of hypertrophic subaortic stenosis, but the the natural history appears to be benign. Septal hypertrophy usually resolves within a few months. Cardiac output decreases with advancing septal thickness but is normal by the end of the first week after birth. No consensus exists about the indices of left ventricular performance, although decreased ventricular function has also been very transient. Transient pulmonary hypertension demonstrated by increased right ventricular PEP/ET ratios may explain some of the cardiopulmonary symptoms. Digitalis is contraindicated if heart failure is caused by hypertrophic cardiomyopathy; propranolol may be used to increase ventricular contractility.

Immediately after birth, blood glucose levels fall precipitously to levels lower than those in normal infants. A nadir is reached between 1 and 3 hours of age; by 4

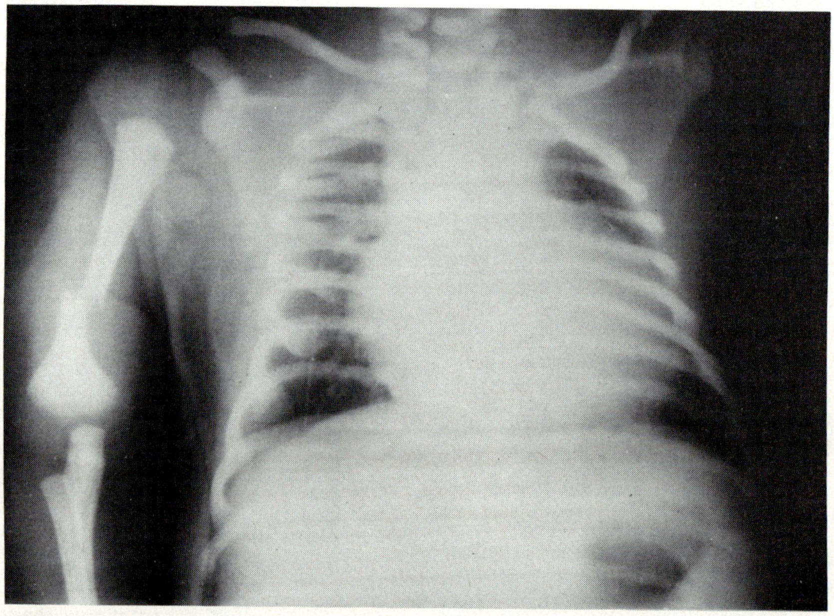

Fig. 37-7. Chest roentgenogram of a vaginally delivered full-term infant (4.7 kg) of a diabetic mother. The infant had cardiomegaly, hepatomegaly, congested lung fields, and fractures of the right humerus and left clavicle.

to 6 hours spontaneous recovery usually has occurred. Plasma glucose levels below 35 mg/dl occur in 30% of IDMs, but the infants are usually asymptomatic; symptomatic hypoglycemia occurs in a small percentage of these infants. The frequency of this complication is greater in infants born to insulin-dependent mothers, in infants whose mothers are poorly controlled during pregnancy, in those whose mothers receive large doses of intravenous glucose during labor or at delivery, and in infants whose mothers had high glucose levels at delivery. Some centers are beginning to report that infants of insulin-dependent diabetic mothers are having less neonatal complications than those of gestational diabetic mothers, presumably because the gestational diabetic mother may not be diagnosed until late in pregnancy, whereas the insulin-dependent diabetic mother is closely followed during her pregnancy.

Hypocalcemia is prevalent in IDMs, even when gestational age and perinatal complications are taken into consideration. Since symptoms of hypocalcemia are similar to those of hypoglycemia, the former must be taken into consideration when therapy for hypoglycemia is ineffective. In general, hypoglycemia is seen during the first hours after birth; hypocalcemia occurs between 24 and 36 hours of age. If initial treatment of hypocalcemia is unsuccessful, then hypomagnesemia should be suspected. In many infants, however, jitteriness remains and cannot be explained by hypoglycemia, hypocalcemia, or hypomagnesemia. Other problems include nonhemolytic hyperbilirubinemia, polycythemia, increased platelet aggregration, neonatal small left colon syndrome (Fig. 37-8), and, rarely, renal vein thrombosis. Infants with renal vein thrombosis usually have unilateral or bilateral flank masses and hematuria. Management consists of adequate hydration as long as renal function is maintained and fluid restriction if renal failure supervenes. The use of heparin is of questionable benefit. Removal of the kidney is not indicated unless hypertension occurs during follow-up. Neonatal small left colon syndrome presents with failure to pass meconium, abdominal distension, and bile-stained vomitus (Fig. 37-8). Contrast enemas show a markedly diminished caliber of the left colon from the splenic flexure. The syndrome is transient, and immature ganglion cells may be present in the intermyenteric plexus.

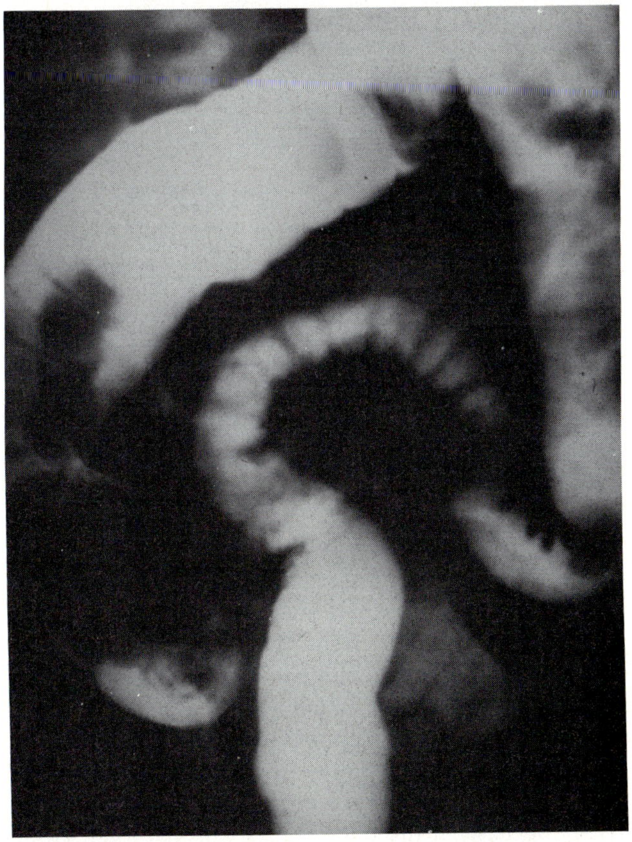

Fig. 37-8. Infant of diabetic mother who developed abdominal distension on day 2, had no passage of meconium, and developed bilious vomiting. A barium enema demonstrated a left microcolon up to the splenic flexure.

Congenital anomalies are two to four times more frequent among IDMs than among normal controls and more often affect multiple organ systems; cardiovascular, central nervous system, and genitourinary malformations predominate (Table 37-1).

The types of anomalies do not appear to be specific, with the possible exception of the caudal regression syndrome (Fig. 37-9). Anomalies are no more frequent in the offspring of diabetic fathers and prediabetic mothers than among those of nondiabetic parents. This is consistent with the hypothesis that anomalies may be the result of metabolic disturbances. Recent studies suggest that

Table 37-1. Collaborative perinatal project: frequency of major malformations in children of diabetic pregnancies

System	%	Diabetic-nondiabetic ratio*
CNS	2.29	3.4
Musculoskeletal	5.29	1.5
Sensory	0.35	1.5
Cardiovascular	2.47	5.6
Respiratory	1.94	2.7
Genitourinary	3.35	3.6
Alimentary	3.53	1.8

From Chung, C.S., and Myrianthopoulos, N.C.: Effect of maternal diabetes on congenital malformations. In Bergsma, D., editor: Factors affecting risks of congenital malformations, Florida: Symposia Specialists for The National Foundation–March of Dimes, BD:OAS **XI**(10):23, 1975.

*Nondiabetic mothers: n = 47,408; diabetic mothers: n = 567.

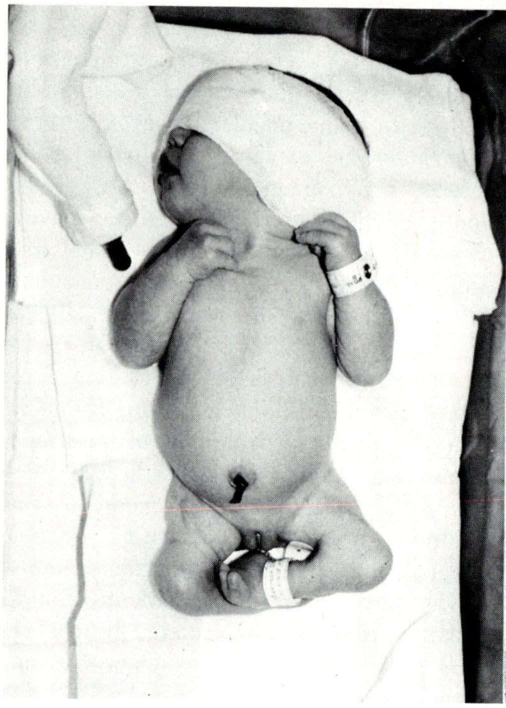

A

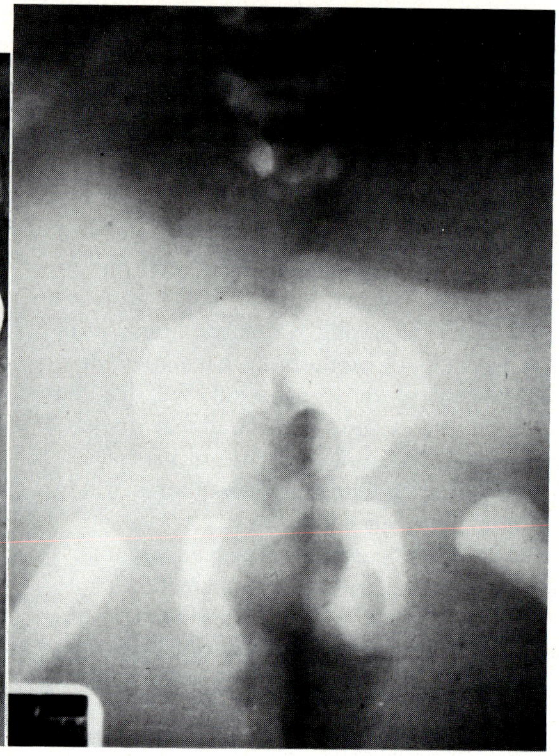

B

Fig. 37-9. A, Infant of diabetic mother with caudal regression syndrome (sacral agenesis). **B,** Roentgenogram of lumbar spine and pelvis of another infant with sacral agenesis shows L2 is hypoplastic. L3 to L5 and sacrum are absent; ilia are hypoplastic; and pubic bones are widely separated.

intensive metabolic control of insulin-dependent diabetic women starting before conception and continuing during the first weeks of pregnancy can prevent congenital malformations in IDMs.

IDMs are often hyptonic and suck poorly even in the absence of hypoxia or metabolic abnormalities. There have been few ultrasound or computed tomography (CT) examinations of the brain, but electroencephalograms and sleep-pattern studies suggest physiologic immaturity of the brain. However, peripheral nerve conduction velocities are generally consistent with gestational age, indicating normal myelinization.

Pathogenesis

The Pedersen hypothesis is now well accepted as the pathogenic sequence responsible for hypoglycemia, macrosomia, and other aberrations that may result from hyperinsulinism. Pedersen suggested the following: maternal hyperglycemia causes fetal hyperglycemia and hypertrophy of the fetal pancreatic islets, leading to fetal hyperinsulinism. An expanded Pedersen hypothesis has been proposed as a result of metabolic changes found in even the mildest of gestational diabetic mothers. These include increased levels of glucose, selected amino acids, lipids, and ketones ("mixed nutrients"). Thus a surfeit of "mixed nutrients" is available to the fetus as long as vascular complications are not present. In addition, the β-cells may be more sensitive to the insulinogenic action of amino acids. The combination of hyperinsulinism and increased mixed nutrients causes increased hepatic glucose uptake and glycogen synthesis, accelerated lipogenesis, and augmented protein synthesis, thus leading to the characteristic macrosomia of these infants. Pathologic correlates include hypertrophy and hyperplasia of the pancreatic islets with a disproportionate increase in the percentage of β-cells. In addition, there is myocardial hypertrophy, an increased amount of cytoplasm in the liver cells, and extramedullary hemopoiesis. The separation of the placenta suddenly interrupts glucose infusion into the neonate without affecting insulin concentration proportionately; this causes hypoglycemia during the first hours after birth.

Hyperinsulinemia has been difficult to document in IDMs because of placental transfer of maternal antiinsulin antibodies, which interfere with the radioimmunoassay of insulin. However, hyperinsulinism has been substantiated from measurements of immunoreactive insulin from infants of gestational diabetic mothers and from infants whose mothers have had few or no insulin antibodies. In addition, oral glucose tolerance tests in infants of gestational diabetic mothers and in normal newborns have demonstrated a significantly higher fasting plasma insulin level in the infants of gestational diabetic mothers despite similar glucose levels; infants of gestational diabetic mothers responded with a prompt elevation of plasma insulin and assimilated the glucose load more rapidly. Measurement of C-peptide, which is released by the β-cells in amounts equimolar with insulin, has confirmed the presence of hyperinsulinism in infants of insulin-dependent mothers. C-peptide levels were increased in cord blood of IDMs as compared with normal controls and were directly related to the severity of maternal diabetes. Higher cord levels of C-peptide were significantly associated with neonatal hypoglycemia and macrosomia, whereas no correlation was found with RDS. Cord levels of C-peptide in IDMs were also elevated at less than 34 weeks' gestation. In addition, IDMs show a prompt C-peptide increase within 2 minutes following an intravenous bolus of glucose, in contrast to the delayed response of normal newborns. Further supports for hyperinsulinemia are the findings of increased glucose disappearance rates of endogenous and exogenous intravenous glucose and the enhanced plasma insulin response following arginine administration as compared with that in normal newborns.

Hepatic glucose production rates in IDMs are significantly lower than in control infants, providing additional evidence for suppression of hepatic glucose output during hyperinsulinemic states. Plasma free fatty acid and D-β-hydroxybutyrate levels during the first 60 minutes of postnatal life are lower in IDMs than in normal controls, another manifestation of the hyperinsulinemia. However, plasma glycerol levels are increased. The lower free fatty acid levels, despite increased glycerol levels, have been explained by an increased rate of reesterification of free fatty acid with α-glycerophosphate derived from glycogen within adipose tissue.

Although hyperinsulinism is probably the principal cause of hypoglycemia, deficient catecholamine and glucagon responses also have been demonstrated and may contribute to hypoglycemia by facilitating insulin action. However, cortisol and human growth hormone levels are similar in IDMs and in normal infants; thus these hormonal responses are appropriate and adequate. Insulin appears to be the important growth factor in fetal development. This may be caused by direct action on cell proliferation or indirectly through stimulation of amino acid and glucose uptake into fetal tissues. On the other hand, there is delay of pulmonary functional maturity, which may reflect insulin-induced alterations in lung growth and substrate flow. In rabbit fetal lung cultures the addition of insulin abolished the stimulatory effect of cortisol on lecithin synthesis. Insulin delayed the appearance of lamellar bodies in type II cells and increased glycogen content of the alveolar lining cells (Chapter 28).

The pathogenic mechanisms responsible for the multiple congenital malformations are most likely secondary to the maternal metabolic milieu during embryogenesis. This has been demonstrated in human beings through studies of Hb A_{1c} that indicate decreased malformations in patients with Hb A_{1c} less than 8.5 during the first trimester as compared to those with Hb A_{1c} greater than 8.5. In diabetic rats administered streptozocin, spinal fusions in the offspring could be prevented through early treatment of the mother with insulin. Glucose as well as D-mannose in rat embryo cultures have been shown to produce teratogenic effects.

It has also been postulated that the mechanisms by which glucose causes teratogenic effects is mediated by a functional deficiency of arachidonic acid or *myo*-inositol at a critical period of organ differentiation.

Treatment

Tight glycemic control during pregnancy based on home blood glucose monitoring and frequent changes in insulin dosage leads to improved survival among IDMs. Periconception metabolic control may decrease the incidence of congenital malformations. Prevention of ketoacidosis and recognition and treatment of toxemia and urinary tract infection are particularly important. Attempts should be made to maintain fasting plasma glucose values below 80 mg/dl and postprandial blood sugar values below 120 mg/dl. Despite these precautions, 10% of intrauterine deaths defy explanation; moreover, some mothers appear predisposed to recurrent stillbirths.

To determine the optimum time to deliver the infant, the possibility of extrauterine survival must be weighed against that of intrauterine death. Hospitalization of diabetic patients is not mandatory unless there are complications such as preeclampsia, acute or chronic polyhydramnios, infections, or poor metabolic control. Ultrasonography done at 18, 28, and 34 weeks' gestation for determination of congenital malformations, polyhydramnios, growth retardation, amniotic fluid volume, and placental grading are useful adjuncts for decision making. At 34 weeks, twice-weekly nonstress heart rate testing and daily fetal movement monitoring are recommended by some investigators. If either is abnormal, then a fetal biophysical profile and oxytocin contraction stress testing may be useful. Amniotic fluid is assayed for phosphatidylglycerol to evaluate pulmonary maturity if delivery becomes an option before the patient goes into spontaneous labor. Many fetuses can be carried to term, thus preventing the complications of prematurity. Vaginal delivery is preferred, but obstetric factors may justify termination of pregnancy by cesarean section.

During labor the rate of glucose infusion should not exceed 200 ml/hour of a 5% dextrose solution to prevent a precipitous fall in neonatal blood glucose.

Delivery should take place in a hospital where the newborn can be carefully monitored. Glucose values are checked during the first 3 to 4 hours after birth and when symptoms are present. Feedings can be started as soon as the infant is stable, usually within 2 to 4 hours after birth, and continued at 3- to 4-hour intervals. The first feeding is human milk or 20 cal/oz formula. If nipple feedings are not tolerated, continuous nasogastric milk infusions can be administered. Treatment is then directed at individual clinical problems.

Prognosis

Perinatal mortality has improved in all series as a result of early identification and good control of diabetes, coupled with delayed delivery to prevent low birth weight. Detection of excessive size and fetal monitoring during labor should lead to prevention of birth trauma and fetal asphyxia. Postneonatal mortality is higher than in normal controls, primarily because of an increased proportion of IDMs with congenital anomalies who survive the newborn period.

Physical growth during childhood and adolescence has been studied by several investigators. Children of diabetic mothers whose birth weight index was greater than or equal to 1.5 had greater weight/height indices at follow-up examination 1 to 19 years later. In another study 40% of LGA newborns of diabetic mothers were obese at age 7 years with a weight/height ratio exceeding 1.2, whereas AGA infants of diabetic mothers did not exhibit the same tendency. Macrosomia at birth may be associated with increased number or size of fat cells and predisposes the infant to subsequent obesity. Thus the tendency to obesity in the IDM is probably secondary to birth weight and not necessarily caused by persistently abnormal metabolism.

The incidence of subsequent overt diabetes varies between 0.5% and 1.0% in most studies, but rates of 7% and 11% have also been reported. These rates are related to genetic factors and not a result of fetal life during maternal diabetes. The risk of subsequent diabetes is higher in infants of diabetic fathers (6.1%) than in those of diabetic mothers (1.3%). In all series the rate is 10 to 30 times higher than in the normal population. Abnormal glucose tolerance tests have been observed in 12% to 14% of children studied.

Neurologic and developmental outcomes of IDMs are indefinite because of the lack of large prospective studies and because most studies do not encompass the period of improved antenatal, intrapartum, and neonatal management of the last decade. Psychomotor development was followed in 749 IDMs for 1 to 26 years by Yssing in Denmark; major cerebral handicaps were seen in 18% of the patients, and cerebral palsy and epilepsy were three to five times more common than in the normal population. Major determinants of poor outcome were poor control, early onset of diabetes and vascular complications, low birth weight and prematurity, and perinatal complications. Maternal acetonuria also has been associated with delayed psychomotor development. SGA infants appear to have a greater incidence of borderline to low IQ values. Mental subnormality unrelated to neonatal hypoglycemia was noted by Haworth in 30% of 37 IDMs at 4½ years of age. However, more recent studies in 73 infants of well-controlled diabetic mothers reveal normal physical and mental development at 5 years of age. Thus it is expected that future prospective studies will continue to demonstrate improved perinatal outcome as well as improved quality of survival.

Erythroblastosis fetalis

See also Chapter 5.

Hypoglycemia is a significant complication of severe erythroblastosis fetalis (Chapter 32, part one). The incidence varies from 17.8% of infants with cord hemoglobin concentrations below 10 gm/dl to 1.9% of those with higher cord hemoglobin values and 31% of infants after exchange transfusions. Although the condition is often asymptomatic, the diagnosis of symptomatic hypoglycemia may be overlooked because the symptoms are ascribed to the primary disease. Hyperinsulinemia has been demonstrated before and during exchange transfusion. Histologically the total number of α- and β-cells are proportionally increased because of hyperplasia of the pancreatic islets; this in turn leads to increased total extractable pancreatic insulin and elevated insulin concentration in cord blood. Plasma and urine insulin values are elevated, and plasma free fatty acid levels are decreased. The α-cell proliferation results in a significant decrease in plasma glucagon following an intravenous bolus of glucose. It is not known how the hemolytic disease influences the development of the endocrine pancreas. Inhibition of insulin activity in vitro by hemolysates, such as glutathione reductase, suggests that products of hemolysis may inactivate circulating insulin, thus stimulating compensatory islet cell hyperplasia. Hypoglycemia, as a late sequela, has been reported in two siblings, ages 7 and 25 months, who had severe erythroblastosis as neonates; this suggests that the disturbance in carbohydrate metabolism may persist for some years.

Beckwith-Wiedemann syndrome (hyperplastic fetal visceromegaly)

The most frequent features of Beckwith-Wiedemann syndrome are macroglossia, omphalocele, and visceromegaly (Fig. 37-10). Of the numerous additional anom-

A

B

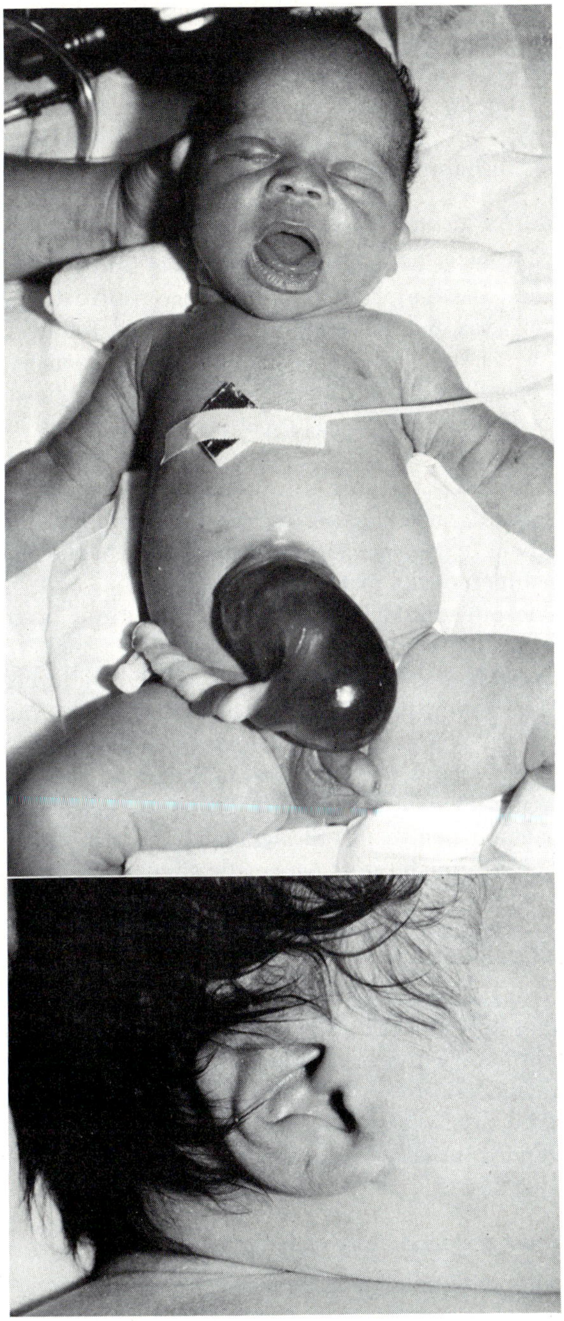

Fig. 37-10. Newborn infant weighing 3.8 kg with Beckwith-Wiedemann syndrome showing **(A)** macroglossia and omphalocele and **(B)** vertical earlobe grooves.

alies recorded, those occurring most consistently include facial nevus flameus, abnormal ear lobe grooves, microcephaly, visceromegaly, renal medullary dysplasia, cytomegaly of the adrenal cortex, and hyperplasia of many organs. Somatic overgrowth may be asymmetric, resulting in hemihypertrophy; advanced physical development may be striking. These patients, along with those having incomplete forms of Beckwith-Wiedemann syndrome, are also at higher risk of developing intraabdominal neoplasia, particularly nephroblastoma.

Symptomatic hypoglycemia occurs in one third to one half of all patients; symptoms usually start within the first 24 hours after birth but may be delayed up to the third day. The hypoglycemia may be severe, difficult to control, and may persist for several months. It is likely that many of the fatalities in patients who have been diagnosed retrospectively were caused by the unrecognized hypoglycemia. Intelligence is normal in many patients, although mild to moderate retardation was a regular feature with Beckwith's orginal series. Mental retardation may partly result from undetected hypoglycemia in the neonatal period or during infancy. However, ultrasound or CT scans should be performed to rule out central nervous system anomalies. Neonatal polycythemia and hypocalcemia also have been observed. Pathologically, islet cell hyperplasia has been demonstrated. Basal hyperinsulinemia and hyperresponsiveness of insulin secretion to glucose and tolbutamide have been demonstrated.

The syndrome is found in siblings, although in some affected individuals only minor anomalies are present. An autosomal dominant mode of inheritance with incomplete penetrance and variable expressivity has been postulated, although the syndrome also has been considered autosomal recessive. Patients are usually cytogenetically normal, but partial duplication of chromosome 11p has been found in a few patients.

Severe hypoglycemia also has been observed in infants of extremely high birth weights who do not have the congenital anomalies noted in the Beckwith-Wiedemann sydnrome. These infants have been referred to as *infant giants;* their birth weights range from 3.8 to 5.3 kg. Pancreatic hyperplasia has been described in some of these infants.

β-Cell nesidioblastosis-adenoma spectrum

Although rare, β-cell nesidioblastosis-adenoma spectrum must be considered in any neonate with persistent symptomatic hypoglycemia in whom no immediately apparent cause can be found. The neonates are usually AGA or LGA, lack any positive physical findings, have a noncontributory maternal history, and have severe hypoglycemia resistant to conventional medical management.

Typically these infants have high blood insulin levels, and, even if in the normal range, insulin levels are likely to be inappropriately elevated in the presence of greatly decreased blood glucose. C-peptide measurements may be useful because C-peptide has double the half-life of insulin. Tolerance tests may be difficult to perform because of the inability to have the patient fast even for short periods. Metabolic studies performed during continuous glucose infusions followed by abrupt cessation of infusate may prove useful but are dangerous. Definitive therapy for infants with hypoglycemia in the nesidioblastosis-adenoma spectrum is early subtotal (85%) or total (95%) pancreatectomy. Recently total pancreatectomy has been advocated as the procedure of choice, although some infants who had recurrent hypoglycemia after subtotal pancreatectomy have been treated successfully with Alloxan (mesoxalyl urea). Zinc protamine glucagon as intramuscular injections or orally administered starch (tapioca starch) have also been used postoperatively. Infants with nesidioblastosis-adenoma spectrum have a high incidence of neurologic damage, which is probably a reflection of the severity of hypoglycemia and the delay in diagnosis. In most instances preoperative medical therapy consisting of various combinations of glucose infusion, corticosteroid, epinephrine, diazoxide, glucagon, and phenytoin fails to control the hypoglycemia. Continuous somatostatin infusion with the addition of glucagon to correct the somatostatin-induced hypoglucagonemia has been used for temporary preoperative medical control, but prolonged trials during which the patient has repeated hypoglycemic attacks are not justified.

β-Cell nesidioblastosis can be differentiated from islet cell adenoma or from functional islet cell hyperplasia only at surgery. However, diffuse lesions (β-cell nesidioblastosis) are common in the newborn, and localized lesions (islet cell adenoma) are more common in older children. If an islet cell tumor is not found, subtotal or total pancreatectomy is performed. The pancreatic tissue should be stained with an insulin-specific stain.

Nesidioblastosis is not simple β-cell hyperplasia, but rather involves all islet cell types and is characterized by disorganization and proliferation of islet cells. It is differentiated from localized adenoma, in which the pathologic finding of "nesidioblastosis" is confined to the tumor. Familial nesidioblastosis suggestive of autosomal recessive inheritance has been reported. Reports have also linked nesidioblastosis with some cases of sudden infant death.

Leucine-induced hypoglycemia

Patients with leucine sensitivity have hyperresponsiveness to the amino acid L-leucine. Leucine sensitivity may be seen with various disorders associated with increased insulin release. Symptoms may be present from birth or appear later in the first year of life. Classically, symptoms occur within 30 minutes of a high-protein meal but may occur after a prolonged fast. Symptoms may be mild at first but increase in severity and result in permanent neurologic impairment if unrecognized and untreated. To make the diagnosis, a significant fall in blood glucose (50%) should occur within 20 to 45 minutes following oral administration of L-leucine. Similar results, however, may be obtained in 70% of patients with insulinomas, since nonspecific increased insulin release may be induced by leucine. Therapy consists of a low-leucine diet and postprandial and bedtime carbohydrate supplements. Prompt recognition and treatment may prevent psychomotor retardation. The hypoglycemia tends to improve spontaneously by 4 to 6 years of age.

Maternal drugs

The antidiabetic drugs tolbutamide and chlorpropamide cross the placenta and produce pancreatic β-cell hyperplasia and increased insulin release. Tolbutamide has a markedly prolonged half-life in the neonate and has been found in higher concentrations in the newborn after delivery than in maternal blood. Protracted hypoglycemia may occur when maternal glucose supply is interrupted. Exchange transfusion has been required in one infant whose mother received chlorpropamide and in whom hypoglycemia was unresponsive to all conventional methods of management.

Benzothiadiazide diuretics may also cause postneonatal hypoglycemia either by stimulation of fetal β-cells or secondary to elevation of maternal glucose levels.

Oral β-sympathomimetic tocolytic drugs have caused sustained hypoglycemia and elevated cord blood insulin levels in infants delivered within 2 days of termination of tocolytic therapy (Chapter 9). These agents may cause neonatal hypoglycemia through maternal hyperglycemia but also through direct pancreatic stimulation of insulin release.

Hypoglycemia and pituitary deficiency

Neonatal hypoglycemia associated with anterior pituitary hypofunction may represent a series of separate syndromes, with defects ranging from no structural abnormalities in the brain to anencephaly. Although considered rare, the true incidence is unknown, since the disorder is usually unrecognized because of the absence of characteristic physical findings.

Clinical and laboratory manifestations

Symptoms of hypoglycemia may begin during the first hours of postnatal life and are marked by their severity. They include sudden and profound limpness, convulsions, apnea, cardiovascular collapse, and cardiac arrest. The infants are of normal length and weight, born at term or after term. Males predominate in a ratio of 2:1, and five of the six neonates in our series were male. Physical examination may be unrevealing; however, some male infants have a small phallus, poorly developed scrotum, and/or small undescended testes (Fig. 37-11). In a few patients, facial abnormalities consisting of cleft lip and palate, poorly developed nasal septum, and hypotelorism have been described. Although the infants are of normal size at birth, growth retardation and delayed bone age may be found by 6 to 8 weeks of age.

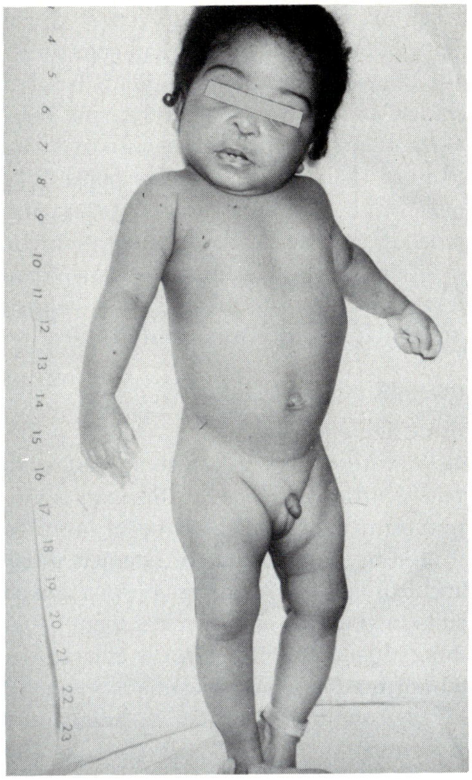

Fig. 37-11. Thirteen-month-old infant with pituitary hypofunction showing repaired cleft lip, delayed growth (59 cm), and small phallus and scrotum.

Tolerance tests and other studies are sometimes difficult to perform because the severity and persistence of symptoms require immediate glucose therapy and frequently steroids. However, determinations of glucose, insulin, and human growth hormone during continuous glucose infusions may be helpful. Normal neonates show an increased, albeit attenuated, insulin response and an elevated basal human growth hormone level that are not suppressed by hyperglycemia. Low human growth hormone and insulin values that do not rise during hyperglycemia suggest pituitary hypofunction. Cord blood human growth hormone levels in normal newborns are markedly elevated but in congenital hypopituitarism are in the normal adult range. Further studies with an intravenous bolus of glucose, glucagon, arginine, or L-dopa provide confirmatory evidence. Because tolbutamide or insulin may provoke severe hypoglycemia, these tests are not indicated. Specific growth hormone deficiency, without other associated endocrine abnormalities, has been described. However, repeated careful evaluation by radioimmunoassay techniques may reveal associated endocrine hypoadrenalism and hypothyroidism. In patients with pituitary "aplasia," thyrotropin (thyroid-stimulating hormone, TSH), thyroxine (T_4), and prolactin were low and did not show a significant increase after stimulation by thyroid-releasing hormone (TRH). Others have shown a rise in TSH following stimulation with TRH, suggesting a primary hypothalamic defect. Other evidence for deficient hypothalamic releasing hormones includes increased prolactin levels and poor luteinizing hormone (LH) response following stimulation with releasing hormones. The adrenals respond to ACTH stimulation, but a deficiency of ACTH may be demonstrated by the use of metyrapone. Although thyroid function studies may be normal at first, abnormalities can be seen later in infancy.

Pathology

At postmortem examination the pituitary gland may be hypoplastic or aplastic, the thyroid and adrenal glands small, and the cellular architecture of the adrenals disorganized, with atrophy or absence of the fetal cortex. In three infants, multiple congenital anomalies of the central nervous system, including holoprosencephaly and arrhinencephaly, were found. A pneumoencephalogram of another infant demonstrated absence of the septum pellucidum and massa intermedia. In one of our infants with cleft lip and palate (Fig. 37-11), the pneumoencephalogram was normal. Hypoplasia or aplasia of the adenohypophysis without cerebral or facial anomalies also may occur. Different expressions of the same syndrome may occur, depending on the extent of pituitary hypoplasia or other central nervous system anomalies or both.

Pathogenesis

The underlying pathogenic mechanisms remain unclear, although aplasia of the anterior pituitary was found in siblings of three patients and in two patients with familial history of consanguinity. This is consistent with a possible autosomal recessive inheritance. A familial history could not be obtained in any of our six patients; the infant with cleft lip and palate, however, has seven normal siblings. Whether the disorder is caused by failure of the pituitary to form or degeneration of the pituitary is unknown. It is also possible that abnormalities of the hypothalamus with a deficiency of hypophysiotropic releasing hormones are responsible for the multiple endocrinopathies observed in these infants. The pathophysiologic relationships among pituitary hypoplasia, the central nervous system anomalies, and the other pituitary hypofunctions are unknown.

Treatment

Therapy consists of replacement with human growth hormone (1 to 2 mg intramuscularly three times weekly), thyroid hormone if hypothyroidism is documented, and physiologic doses of hydrocortisone (5 mg twice daily) for proven hypoadrenalism. Although human growth hormone administration does not always improve physical growth, hypoglycemia is corrected. Bone age may remain retarded, and continuous evaluation of thyroid function should be undertaken even if this was normal at the outset. Testosterone cream (5%) applied topically twice a day or testosterone enanthate (25 or 50 mg) given in three monthly injections has been used to increase the size of the corpora of the penis.

Prognosis

Many patients die in early infancy, and others may have severe physical and mental retardation. It is therefore imperative that early recognition and prompt therapy be instituted.

Cortisol deficiency

ACTH unresponsiveness is a hereditary disorder in which the adrenal glands fail to produce adequate cortisol, but aldosterone secretion is normal and ACTH levels are elevated. Feeding problems, failure to thrive, and regurgitation occur in the neonatal period; hypoglycemia, convulsions, and shock or death may occur in infancy or early childhood. The syndrome is characterized by hyperpigmentation, normal serum electrolyte concentrations, and an unusually severe untoward response to illness or stress. There is often a history of affected siblings, and an autosomal recessive mode of inheritance has been suggested. The pathogenesis of this syndrome is poorly understood. Differentiation of the zones of adrenal cortex in utero require ACTH, except for the zona glomerulosa, which is primarily under renin-angiotensin control. Histologic examination of the adrenal glands of patients with ACTH unresponsiveness has revealed an intact zona glomerulosa and atrophy of the fasciculata and reticularis zones. Migeon and associates have postulated an abnormality at the site (or sites) of ACTH action or cortisol biosynthesis.

Familial isolated glucocorticoid deficiency also has been described in a family of five siblings; in two of the infants glucocorticoid production was normal initially and deficient at a later age. This suggests that in some families there may be a degenerative process in the adrenal gland.

Maternal steroid therapy resulting in neonatal subclinical adrenal insufficiency was reported in an infant having cushingoid facies, transient hypoglycemia, and poor response at 20 hours to intravenous corticotropin.

Adrenal hemorrhage is discussed in Chapter 20.

Adrenogenital syndrome is discussed in Chapter 37, part five.

Hypothyroidism

See Chapter 37, part three.

Congenital glucagon deficiency

Two male infants have been reported with glucagon deficiency; the disorder became evident on the second to third day of postnatal life with repeated convulsive movements, hypotonia, weak cry, and poor suck. In both infants the diagnosis was based on a low basal glucagon concentration and a strong hyperglycemic response to glucagon. In one of the infants response to glucagon was lacking. In one there was a lack of response to hypoglycemia and alanine infusion. Parents of this infant were closely related and had partly deficient glucagon secretion; two siblings of this infant died before 5 months of age with probable hypoglycemia. Thus an autosomal recessive inherited disorder is suggested.

Galactosemia

See also Chapter 36.

Infants with hereditary galactose intolerance are usually normal at birth. Evidence that the fetus is susceptible to the untoward effects of galactose in utero has been demonstrated by the presence of cataracts as early as 7 days after birth in some neonates. Postnatal exposure to milk results in vomiting and diarrhea, poor weight gain, and prolonged jaundice. The liver is enlarged, smooth, firm, and not tender. Hypoglycemia is not a consistent finding. If the condition is untreated, lamellar or zonular cataracts develop and there is a progressive mental retardation and cirrhosis. A milder course has been described in some infants, with failure to thrive as the most constant feature. The cause of the hypoglycemia is unknown, but it may be inhibition of phosphoglucomutase by galactose, which results in decreased hepatic output of glucose. Galactosemia screening programs should identify neonates who have no clinical symptoms.

Glycogen storage disease type I (Von Gierke's disease)

Of the many liver glycogen storage diseases, type I glucose-6-phosphatase deficiency is the most likely to present in the neonatal period (Chapter 36). The genetic defect is autosomal recessive; the heterozygote cannot be detected biochemically, and amniotic fluid analysis is not helpful in predicting the disease. In the most severe form the syndrome may manifest itself in the first days or weeks after birth with profound hypoglycemia (blood glucose level less than 10 mg/dl) and acidosis. The infant appears ill and agitated and has deep, rapid respirations. Recurrent acidosis is the most common cause of readmission to the hospital. Hypoglycemia, although profound, may be asymptomatic. The only physical stigma of glycogen storage disease type I in the neonate is moderate hepatomegaly. The relatively normal appearance shortly after birth suggests that the disease is well controlled in utero. This could be expected, since the fetus is receiving therapeutic total parenteral nutrition from the mother. However, with time the characteristic physical findings appear: short stature, fat doll-like facies, and a protuberant abdomen occupied by an enlarged, firm smooth liver that may reach the iliac crest. Splenomegaly and cardiomegaly are absent. Easy bruising and bleeding tendancies, especially nasal and gastrointestinal, frequently occur.

Laboratory findings following an overnight fast show hypoglycemia, elevated lactate and pyruvate levels, metabolic acidosis, hyperlipidemia, ketonuria and ketonemia, and elevated uric acid concentrations. Serum electrolyte levels may be falsely low because of lipid displacement. Bleeding time is prolonged, and there is reduced platelet adhesion and defective collagen and epinephrine-induced aggregation, suggesting an intrinsic defect in platelet release. The diagnosis may be inferred from the absence of glucose rise and elevated lactate and pyruvate levels during glucagon and galactose tolerance tests. Absence of glucose-6-phosphatase enzymatic activity in liver biopsies provides confirmatory evidence.

Therapy is primarily aimed at maintaining normal glucose concentration, since most of the metabolic abnormalities and growth retardation can be corrected when blood glucose levels are normalized. The various therapies that have been used include total parenteral nutrition, portacaval shunts, continuous nocturnal infusions of glucose-containing fluids, and frequent daytime feedings high in carbohydrates. Uncooked cornstarch suspensions given orally every 6 hours have been recently reported as an alternate effective therapeutic regimen.

Prognosis in early infancy is guarded, but survival beyond adolescence is often associated with improvement of symptoms. Growth retardation continues, but mental retardation is not a constant feature despite profound hypoglycemia; the brain of patients with glycogen storage disease may be capable of using alternate substrates, such as ketone bodies.

Fructose intolerance

Hereditary fructose intolerance may occur in the neonatal period if the susceptible infant is fed a sucrose-containing formula or is given table sugar, fruits, or fruit juices. Symptoms include vomiting, failure to thrive, excessive sweating, and unconsciousness or convulsions. Hypoglycemia is frequent, as are fructosemia and fructosuria, following ingestion of fructose.

Hereditary defects in amino acid metabolism

See Chapter 36.

Hypoglycemia associated with other neonatal problems

Iatrogenic causes

Hypoglycemia during the first hours after birth is usually caused by maternal hyperglycemia even in the absence of diabetes. Excessive fluid administration, especially during induction of anesthesia for cesarean delivery, is the most common cause of maternal hyperglycemia at delivery. Srinivasan and associates reported that glucose levels in cord blood are significantly lower in infants delivered vaginally than in those delivered by cesarean section. Moreover, two normal term neonates who developed symptoms and glucose values less than 25 mg/dl at 1 hour after birth had greatly elevated cord blood glucose values. At the opposite extreme, maternal starvation for a prolonged period before delivery may also be associated with neonatal hypoglycemia.

Reactive hypoglycemia may follow abrupt cessation of hypertonic glucose infusions or exchange transfusions. Acid-citrate-dextrose and citrate-phosphate-dextrose blood contains a significant quantity of glucose, which may stimulate insulin release and cause subsequent hypoglycemia 2 to 3 hours after exchange transfusion is discontinued. Heparinized blood does not contain glucose and may cause hypoglycemia during the exchange. On the other hand, heparin may elevate free fatty acid levels, which secondarily causes hypoglycemia after the exchange. Marked variability of blood glucose values also may occur as a result of changing rates of glucose infusions. Refractory hypoglycemia has been associated with an umbilical artery catheter positioned near the origin of the vessels supplying the pancreas (T11 to L1). Direct glucose infusion into the vessels of the pancreas resulted in a reactive hyperinsulinemic response and hypoglycemia.

Intravenous indomethacin infusion in premature infants with patent ductus arteriosus causes a drop in glucose to potentially hypoglycemic levels (Fig. 37-12). The indomethacin-induced drop in glucose starts as early as 1 hour and lasts at least during the first 24 hours following intravenous indomethacin administration.

Infection

Hypoglycemia, both symptomatic and asymptomatic, has been described in neonatal sepsis caused primarily by gram-negative bacilli. Glucose disappearance rates were significantly increased in the infected, as compared with healthy, neonates; hyperinsulinism could not be demonstrated.

Congenital cardiac malformations

The mean blood glucose concentration in neonates and older children with congenital cyanotic heart disease may be lower than in healthy controls. Glucose disappearance rates and fasting insulin and growth hormone values are normal, but glucose values following glucagon administration are lower than in healthy children. Although the mechanism is unknown, chronic hypoxia leading to decreased glycogen stores may be a contributing factor. Hypoglycemia may also lead to cardiomegaly and congestive heart failure in the absence of congenital malformations.

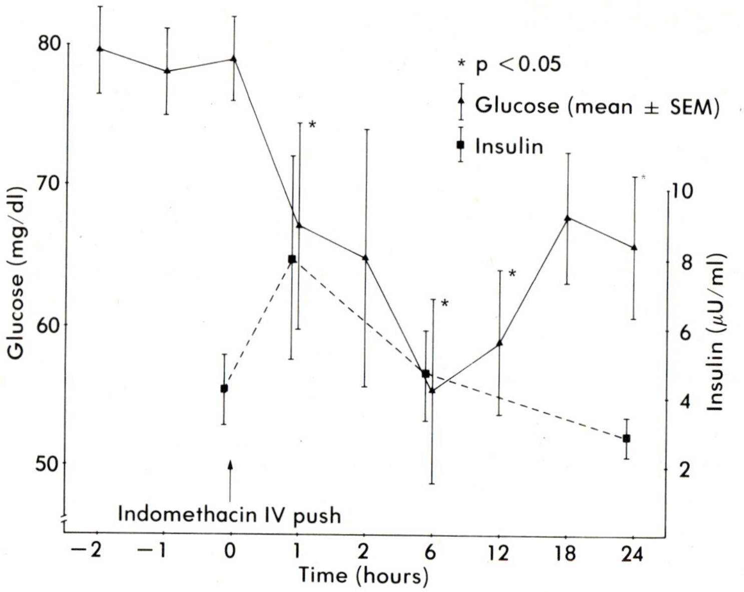

Fig. 37-12. Plasma glucose and insulin changes before and after intravenous indomethacin administration. (From Lilien, L.D., and others: Pediatr. Pharmcol. [New York] **5:**73, 1985.)

Hypothermia

The occurrence of hypothermia secondary to hypoglycemia has been well documented and is a useful clinical sign. Studies in adults using 2-deoxy-D-glucose suggest that hypoglycemia, directly or secondarily, may affect a central thermoregulatory center in the hypothalamus that is sensitive to glucose. Hypoglycemia also may be secondary to hypothermia. The normal core temperature in the neonate is from 36.5° to 37.5° C (97.7° to 99.5° F). If body temperature falls, heat production is increased several times the basal level, resulting in a more rapid depletion of energy stores. Hypoglycemia has been reported in neonates with severe cold injury after prolonged exposure to cold with rectal temperatures below 32° C (89.6° F).

Hyperviscosity

An increased rate of glucose disposal without hyperinsulinemia is part of the syndrome of hyperviscosity and responds to partial exchange transfusion (Chapter 32).

Acute and chronic diarrhea

Hypoglycemia occurs in children with acute diarrheal disease resulting from typhoid, cholera, shigellosis, chronic malnutrition, and kwashiorkor. We have seen four infants, 4 to 8 weeks of age, with hypoglycemia associated with severe diarrhea and secondary malnutrition; glucagon tolerance tests performed in two infants did not show a rise in blood glucose, suggesting that hepatic glycogen stores had been depleted.

DIAGNOSTIC EVALUATION OF NEONATAL HYPOGLYCEMIA

A detailed history and a meticulous physical examination are of utmost importance to avoid numerous provocative stimulatory studies. In most instances of neonatal hypoglycemia the underlying disease process is obvious, and further studies are not necessary. Important maternal historic factors include family history of diabetes, blood group incompatibility, toxemia, hypertension, drug intake, familial history of hypoglycemia, unexplained stillbirth and infant deaths, and the amount of dextrose solution administered before delivery. Physical examination will determine if the infant is SGA or LGA, is postmature, has erythroblastosis, or is an infant of a prediabetic or diabetic mother. Further diagnostic studies are not required unless hypoglycemia is persistent. Macrosomia, abnormal umbilicus, and protuberant tongue are diagnostic features of the Beckwith-Wiedemann syndrome. The presence of chubby, doll-like facies and hepatomegaly without a maternal diabetic history may indicate glycogen storage disease. Cataracts, jaundice, failure to thrive, hepatomegaly, and reducing substances in the urine suggest galactosemia. Abnormalities of the genitalia are associated with pituitary deficiency. Similarly, cleft lip or palate or other facial anomalies may be associated with central nervous system abnormalities and pituitary hypoplasia; roentgenograms in infants with pituitary hypofunction may reveal delayed bone age. The absence of any positive family history association with a normal-appearing AGA neonate is highly suggestive of an insulinoma. In neonates, hypoglycemia is usually associated with the fasting state; therefore a history of symptoms shortly after milk intake suggests leucine sensitivity or galactosemia.

In older infants and children, a 24- to 36-hour fast is recommended for assessment of the various parameters involved in carbohydrate homeostasis. The time required for the development of hypoglycemia in a normal neonate, however, is significantly less, and a prolonged fast may have serious consequences. We have seen one infant with human growth hormone deficiency become limp, bradycardiac, and apneic and have a blood glucose level of 9 mg/dl after a 6-hour fast. Initial baseline laboratory determinations when the diagnosis is not readily apparent should include glucose, insulin, human growth hormone, cortisol, and, if glycogen disease is a consideration, lactate, pyruvate, ketones, pH, and buffer base. Samples should be drawn at least 3 to 4 hours after a feeding or at the time of hypoglycemia. Provocative tolerance tests depend on the results of these studies coupled with the physical findings. Not all tolerance tests are indicated; moreover, it is frequently difficult to obtain sufficient blood for a variety of studies. Selectivity is therefore essential. Glucagon tolerance tests after a cautious 6- to 8-hour fast, for example, are indicated if glycogen storage disease is considered. Glucagon tolerance tests, however, are not of value for pituitary hypofunction or hyperinsulinism. Studies of thyroid and adrenal function are necessary when human growth hormone deficiency has been established or a clinical picture consistent with hypothyroidism or congenital adrenal hyperplasia is present. If hypoglycemia is intractable, biochemical determinations can be done during continuous glucose infusion followed by abrupt cessation of the infusate over a 90- to 120-minute period. It is mandatory that an intravenous line be kept open and a constant vigil maintained by the physician of any infant undergoing prolonged starvation or tolerance tests that are likely to produce hypoglycemia.

TREATMENT OF NEONATAL HYPOGLYCEMIA

The management of neonatal hypoglycemia requires identification of the infants at risk for developing hypoglycemia, initiation of oral feedings within 3 to 4 hours after birth, and minimization of caloric expenditures by decreasing environmental stress. Management also entails monitoring for clinical symptoms of hypoglycemia and performing glucose level determinations in infants at risk for developing hypoglycemia. Infants at risk include (1) those weighing less than 2,500 gm or greater than 4,000 gm at birth, (2) infants less than 37 weeks or greater than 42 weeks of gestational age, (3) infants of diabetic mothers, (4) SGA or dysmature infants, and (5) those who have neonatal problems such as birth asphyxia, respiratory distress, and hypothermia. In high-risk infants, prefeeding glucose levels should be determined within the first 3 hours of birth in asymptomatic infants or whenever symptoms are observed. If glucose screening is done by such methods as Dextrostix or Chemstrip bG, abnormal or borderline levels (≤45 mg/dl) should be checked in the laboratory.

Approximately 10% of even normal, healthy term infants will have an abnormally low glucose level during the first 3 hours after birth and recover spontaneously. If the infant is asymptomatic, a second glucose value is drawn and oral dextrose solution or formula feedings are started. Very low birth weight infants are routinely started on parenteral dextrose solutions at concentrations of 4 to 5 mg/kg body weight/minute.

Hypoglycemia that is confirmed by two separate glucose determinations or by the presence of symptoms and one low value should be treated promptly. A second specimen is drawn before starting therapy to confirm the diagnosis. We use 2 ml/kg of 10% dextrose in water (200 mg/kg) given over 1 minute followed by continuous dextrose infusion of 8 mg/kg/minute via volumetric pump (Fig. 37-13). Glucose levels are monitored hourly until stable above 70 mg/dl. The aim of therapy is to maintain plasma glucose values greater than 40 to 45 mg/dl and preferably closer to the appropriate mean expected for age. Thus dextrose concentration is increased by 2 mg/kg/minute every 4 to 6 hours (or sooner) until glucose levels are stabilized. Two peripheral intravenous sites are used to ensure uninterrupted dextrose infusion in case of infiltration (see Fig. 37-6).

Feedings are given by continuous nasogastric drip feeding and not by bolus feeding unless the hypoglycemia is mild and corrects rapidly. With continuous nasogastric drip feeding and uninterrupted intravenous glucose infusion, glucose levels are more likely to reach a steady state without the peak and trough levels that are expected with bolus carbohydrate intake. Glucose levels therefore, can then be checked at any time and without concern whether the sample was drawn at peak or trough times.

Repeat hypoglycemic episodes should again be treated with a minibolus followed by continuous dextrose infusion at a higher concentration than previously used. Infants who require more than 12 mg/kg/minute usually have hyperinsulinism or other specific etiologic factors. The proper workup should be initiated and corticosteroids started as described in the following discussion.

Once the infant has stabilized at 70 to 100 mg/dl, dextrose concentration in the infusate is decreased gradually by 2 mg/kg/minute every 6 to 12 hours. Glucose determinations are performed before and after each change is made. This is particularly important when hyperinsulinemia is present.

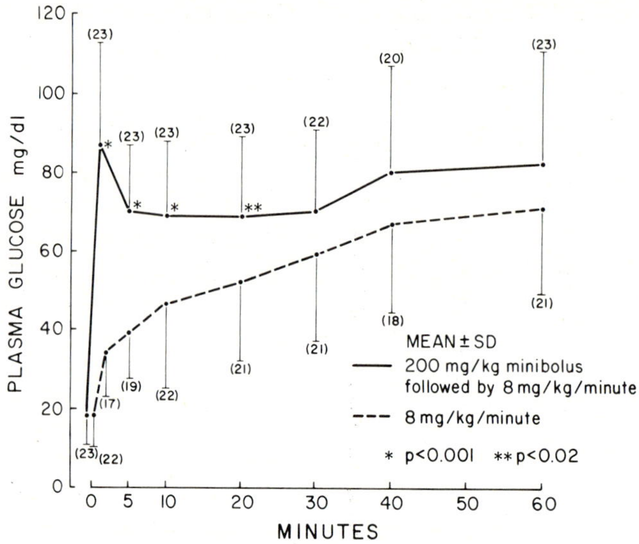

Fig. 37-13. Treatment of 23 hypoglycemic neonates with 200 mg/kg glucose minibolus followed by 8 mg/kg/minute constant glucose infusion, compared with treatment of 22 hypoglycemic neonates with only 8 mg/kg/minute constant glucose infusion. (From Lilien, L.D., and others: J. Pediatr. **97:**295, 1980.)

Hydrocortisone

Hydrocortisone, 10 mg/kg/day given in two doses intravenously, intramuscularly, or orally is administered (1) if plasma glucose values are not above 40 mg/dl despite adequate intravenous dextrose therapy, (2) if hypoglycemia recurs, or (3) if dextrose concentrations greater than 12 mg/kg/minute are required. Hydrocortisone has been shown to (1) reduce peripheral glucose utilization, (2) increase the effects of exogenous glucagon, and (3) enhance gluconeogenesis. When normoglycemia has been maintained for several days, intravenous fluids are tapered first and hydrocortisone is continued until the infant is stable for 48 hours after intravenous fluids have been discontinued. Hydrocortisone is usually necessary for 5 to 7 days. Infants who do not respond to hydrocortisone may need additional or alternate therapy, depending on the etiology of hypoglycemia.

Epinephrine

A trial dose of epinephrine 1:1,000 (0.01 ml/kg) is administered subcutaneously if a hypoglycemic infant does not respond to intravenous glucose plus hydrocortisone. If this trial dose is successful, then a maintenance dose of epinephrine 1:200 in 25% glycerine solution (Sus-Phrine), 0.005 to 0.01 ml/kg/6 hours, is administered subcutaneously or ephedrine sulfate, 0.05 mg/kg/3 hours, is given orally. Epinephrine mobilizies stored fuels from the liver by glycogenolysis, stimulates gluconeogenesis, stimulates lipolysis in adipose tissue, augments glucagon secretion, and suppresses insulin excretion. Because of insulin suppression, epinephrine has been recommended for infants of diabetic mothers. However, epinephrine may have adverse effects by raising lactate levels in the blood.

Diazoxide

This drug (10 to 15 mg/kg/day in three divided doses), a nondiuretic thiazide given intravenously or orally, suppresses pancreatic insulin release and may be effective in protracted hypoglycemia resulting from hyperinsulinism. Failure to respond to diazoxide should not be used as an argument that an infant is not suffering from hyperinsulinemic hypoglycemia. Side effects include hyperglycemia, hirsutism, ketosis, thrombocytopenia, leukopenia, depressed immunoglobulin levels, sodium retention, and hypotension. To prevent the hypotensive side effects, intravenous diazoxide should be given slowly to allow for adequate serum protein binding. The drug has not been investigated widely and should not be used except when all other medical management is ineffective.

Glucagon

Glucagon is a single chain of 29 amino acids and has a mass of approximately 3,500 daltons. Glucagon, 0.3 mg/kg/intravenously or intramuscularly, is not useful in the treatment of neonatal hypoglycemia except as specific therapy for glucagon deficiency (for maintenance therapy in glucagon deficiency, zinc protamine glucagon, 0.1 to 0.5 mg/kg/12 hours intramuscularly) or in combination with somatostatin in β-cell nesidioblastosis-adenoma spectrum. Glucagon raises blood sugar through glycogenolysis and gluconeogenesis and is therefore not effective in SGA neonates who may have depletion of glycogen stores or defective gluconeogenesis. Since glucagon may also stimulate insulin release and concomitant rebound hypoglycemia, it should be accompanied by continued glucose infusion.

Human growth hormone

Human growth hormone is a single chain of 191 amino acids, has a molecular weight of approximately 22,000, and has two disulfide bonds. Human growth hormone, 1 to 2 mg/day intramuscularly three times per week, is effective in infants with hypoglycemia secondary to growth hormone deficiency.

Somatostatin

Somatostatin is a single chain of 14 amino acids, has a molecular weight of approximately 1,000, and has one disulfide bond. Somatostatin, 3.5 to 48 μg/kg/hour by continuous intravenous infusion, suppresses insulin as well as glucagon secretion. It has been of benefit for preoperative control in infants with suspected nesidioblastosis-adenoma spectrum. Some reports have advocated the addition of constant infusion of glucagon to correct the somatostatin induced hypoglucagonemia. Somatostatin may cause a bleeding diathesis.

Pancreatectomy

Removal of 85% to 95% of the pancreas is recommended in persistent cases of hypoglycemia secondary to β-cell nesidioblastosis-adenoma spectrum when workup suggests the diagnosis and aggressive medical treatment has failed. In these cases surgery should be performed within 1 to 3 weeks after the onset of hypoglycemia because severe brain damage is a common finding at follow-up. In many infants who undergo subtotal (85%) pancreatectomy, there is postsurgical recurrence of hypoglycemia. In some of these infants the hypoglycemia improves spontaneously; some have responded to treatment with Alloxan (mesoxalyl urea); and some have required a second procedure entailing near-total (95%) pancreatectomy. Because of the recurrence of hypoglycemia following subtotal pancreatectomy, more recent recommendations favor total pancreatectomy as the initial surgery.

HYPERGLYCEMIA

Definition

The definition of hyperglycemia, as with hypoglycemia, is based on statistical studies of whole blood glucose values in a large population of neonates. An early study recommended that blood glucose values greater than 125 mg/dl be considered hyperglycemic, since these values represented less than 2% of the infants studied. Since plasma glucose values are approximately 15% higher than those in whole blood, most authors have accepted plasma glucose values greater than 145 mg/dl or 150 mg/dl as hyperglycemic. Recent studies in normal, full-term healthy neonates suggest that the ninety-fifth percentile for plasma glucose after a 3-hour fast ranges from 90 to 110 mg/dl, but postprandial values are not available.

Definitions based on statistical studies do not take into account biologic variability and are not based on studies of very low birth weight (VLBW) infants, who are surviving in increasing numbers. The possibility of hyperglycemia should be considered, for example, when weight loss and diuresis are present despite plasma glucose levels that seem only moderately elevated.

Clinical significance

Hyperglycemia in premature infants is a more frequent problem than hypoglycemia (Fig. 37-14). Hyperglycemia has been associated with increased mortality, increased incidence of intraventricular hemorrhage, and increased incidence of major handicaps in VLBW infants. Unfortunately it is difficult to evaluate hyperglycemia as a single independent factor. One study found no significant difference in mortality when stressed hyperglycemic neonates were compared to stressed euglycemic neonates. No study to date has sufficient data to make definitive conclusions regarding the role of hyperglycemia in central nervous system (CNS) hemorrhage, much less the level of glucose at which untoward CNS effects may be detected.

The mechanisms by which hyperglycemia could be a causative factor in CNS hemorrhage have been inferred from studies on hyperosmolarity. Hyperosmolarity of greater than 300 mOsm/L usually leads to osmotic diuresis and possible dehydration. Hyperosmolarity also causes water to shift from the intracellular to the extracellular compartment; contraction of the intracellular volume, particularly in the brain of VLBW infants, may thus predispose the brain to cerebral hemorrhage. Each 18 mg/dl rise in glucose concentration results in an increase in serum osmolarity of 1 mOsm/L. Serum glucose values would therefore have to be approximately 400 mg/dl before significant hyperosmolarity would occur, assuming a normal osmolarity of 280 mOsm/L. On the other hand, in the rat model hyperglycemia decreases regional cerebral blood flow that cannot be explained by increased serum osmolarity.

The extent to which hyperglycemia may contribute to handicaps in the neonate have not been well delineated. In adults, as well as in adult animal models, hyperglycemia before cerebrovascular accidents augments the size of cerebral infarcts and accentuates hypoxic-ischemic brain damage. The immature animal appears to be pro-

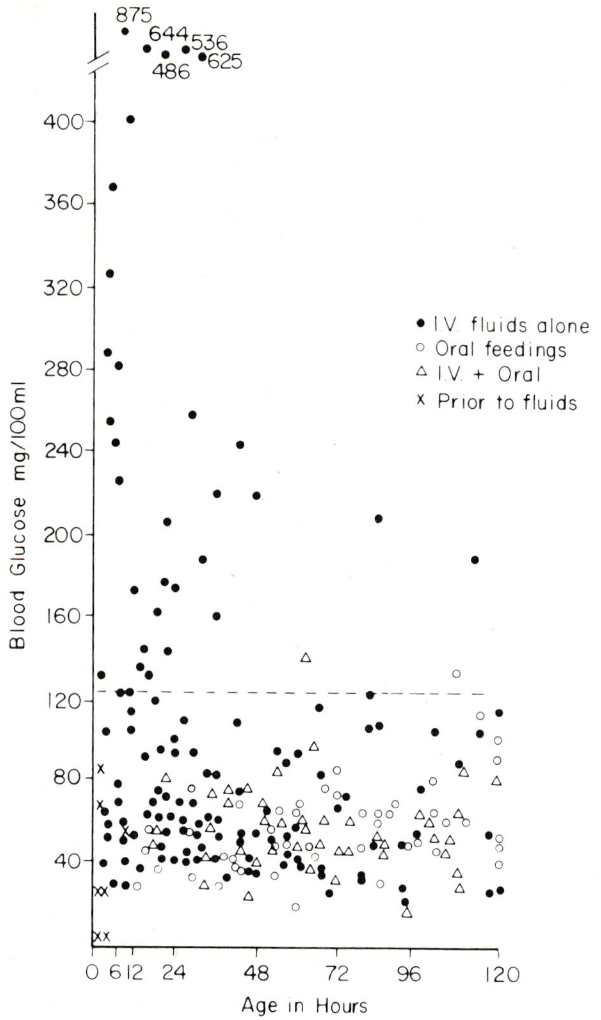

Fig. 37-14. Blood glucose values in infants less than 2,000 gm during the first 5 days of postnatal life. Hyperglycemia was common in infants who were given glucose infusions, 3 to 7 mg/kg/minute. (From Zarif, M., Pildes, R.S., and Vidyasagar, D.: Diabetes **25:**428, 1976.)

tected from increased injury, perhaps because of low activity of hexokinase. Regional cerebral blood flow studies have not been done in the immature animal.

Etiologic factors

Parenteral fluids containing glucose, particularly during the first few days of postnatal life (Fig. 37-14), provide the most common exogenous factor in the etiology of hyperglycemia. In one study hyperglycemia was found in 56% of infants who weighed less than 1,100 gm and were given dextrose infusions at rates greater than 6.6 mg/kg/minute. However, hyperglycemia occurs even when dextrose is infused at rates less than 4 mg/kg/minute. Moreover, premature infants are more likely to develop hyperglycemia when given dextrose-containing fluids if they are VLBW, have low Apgar scores, have respiratory distress, or are septic.

Lipid infusions give rise to sustained increases in serum glucose concentrations; the mean increment in glucose rise is 24% above baseline when 10% intralipid at 0.25 gm/kg/hour is given over 2 hours and 65% when the rate is 0.5 gm/kg/hour. For this reason, as well as to prevent acute increases in triglyceride levels, we usually give lipid infusions continuously over 12 to 24 hours.

The use of methylxanthines, specifically theophylline and caffeine, in premature infants with apnea and the maternal use of diazoxide have been associated with neonatal hyperglycemia. Intravenous theophylline, given as a loading dose of 5 mg/kg over 10 or 20 minutes, is associated with significant increases in plasma glucose during the first hour of study. Oral administration of theophylline for 10 days has been shown to cause increased glucose values, which return to baseline when theophylline is discontinued.

Sepsis caused by group B *Streptococcus* and *Escherichia coli* has also been associated with hyperglycemia in several premature infants.

Finally, hyperglycemia up to 600 mg/dl has been noted in neonates undergoing elective surgery under general anesthesia despite maintaining constant dextrose infusion of 4 mg/kg/minute and replacement of fluid losses with solutions not containing dextrose. Glucose levels began to rise with the induction of anesthesia, increased further by the end of the surgical procedure, and remained elevated for 6 to 12 hours postoperatively. Postsurgical glucose values had a negative correlation with weight of infants at the time of study. Thus smaller infants are at even higher risk for postsurgical hyperglycemia.

Hyperglycemia is also seen in neonates with diabetes mellitus. Although permanent diabetes mellitus has been reported in several neonates, the more commonly observed syndrome is *transient diabetes mellitus*. Onset is from 1 day to 6 weeks of age, and the infants are usually SGA. A variety of syndromes have been described: pancreatic aplasia; pancreatic hypoplasia with both endocrine and exocrine insufficiency; macroglossia and transient diabetes. Intrauterine growth retardation has been the cardinal feature. Presenting symptoms are hyperglycemia or failure to thrive, dehydration, and fever. Infection or underlying CNS lesions occur in one third of the infants. Blood glucose levels range from 250 to 2,300 mg/dl, and minimal ketones are present in the urine. Insulin values are low and do not increase following an intravenous bolus of glucose. With recovery of the patient, insulin values increase and return to normal. Treatment usually consists of adequate hydration. Exogenous insulin may be given if hyperglycemia persists, but the requirements are usually low because these infants are quite sensitive to insulin. Complete recovery is the rule, and permanent diabetes mellitus has not been seen in long-term follow-ups. However, 10% of these infants may be mentally retarded, possibly from an underlying CNS hemorrhage or secondary to overzealous treatment with insulin and resultant hypoglycemia.

Pathogenic mechanisms

Hyperglycemia in very VLBW babies without obvious known factors is generally considered to be caused by persistent endogenous hepatic glucose production despite significant elevations in plasma insulin. Why the liver is insensitive to insulin is unknown. Other hormonal studies have not been helpful; marked variability in catecholamine responses and contradictory results on glucagon occur, and growth hormone and cortisol do not appear to play significant roles.

Lipid infusions elevate blood glucose levels through enhanced gluconeogenesis secondary to increased fatty acid oxidation.

Hypoxia may cause hyperglycemia through stimulation of α-adrenergic receptors, which in turn diminish insulin responses. Sepsis has also been associated with deficient insulin responses.

Hyperglycemia during surgery may be mediated through catecholamine secretion; cortisol plays a significant role at the end of surgery but does not explain the rise in glucose following induction of anesthesia. Insulin responses are not decreased but may be inadequate in view of the massive increases of plasma glucose. Anand (1987) hypothesized that the hyperglycemia is due to glycogenolysis in term and to gluconeogenesis in preterm neonates and that hyperglycemia can be suppressed by giving fentanyl anesthesia.

A genetic basis for diabetes mellitus has been proposed from observations of permanent diabetes in a neonate whose mother also developed permanent diabetes as an infant and from observations of pancreatic hypoplasia and other variants in siblings.

Finally, an abnormal maternal metabolic milieu demonstrated by flat glucose tolerance tests and hypoinsulinemia during pregnancy is associated with intrauterine growth retardation and transient diabetes mellitus. It would appear that delay in maturation of fetal pancreatic cells may be secondary to inadequate in utero stimulation.

Therapy

Primary therapeutic goals in hyperglycemia are prevention and early detection to avoid the need for aggressive intervention. Prevention while providing adequate nutrition is not an easy task, and some degree of hyperglycemia may need to be tolerated. Most infants accommodate to a gradual increase in the amount of dextrose infused. Fluids should be delivered to these high-risk neonates via volumetric infusion pumps capable of delivering very small amounts at a constant, steady rate. Minimizing fluid losses through use of a closed incubator, heat shield, plastic wrapping, or other modes is essential to decrease the need to provide large quantities of dextrose-containing fluids. Fluid losses in infants undergoing surgical procedures should be replaced with lactated Ringer's solution or half-strength saline.

Infants at risk of hyperglycemia need frequent monitoring of plasma glucose levels while receiving parenteral fluids and particularly during the first week after birth. Glucose levels should also be measured following exchange transfusions, after surgical procedures, and in the presence of stress (patent ductus arteriosus, intraventricular hemorrhage, hyaline membrane disease) or infection. Urine glucose testing is helpful in screening for hyperglycemia, but total urinary output and glucose concentration monitoring should be done if osmotic diuresis is suspected.

Treatment is determined by whether the hyperglycemia is transient or persistent and whether an underlying specific etiology exists. In general, transient plasma glucose values less than 200 mg/dl do not require aggressive intervention unless weight loss or significant osmotic diuresis is present. Decreasing parenteral glucose by decreasing rate or concentration usually suffices to correct hyperglycemia. This should be done in a gradual orderly fashion by decreasing the concentration by 2 mg/kg/minute every 4 to 6 hours until glucose values in the ideal range are reached. Solutions not containing dextrose may be used for short periods if plasma glucose values exceed 300 mg/dl, but frequent glucose monitoring is necessary to prevent a precipitous decline.

The potential dangers of using hypotonic solutions have to be considered as well as the methods used to dilute the fluid; solutions containing less than 2.5% dextrose should be avoided. The pharmacy should be consulted to prevent drastic changes in pH or stability whenever such mixtures are contemplated.

Parenteral galactose therapy as an alternate source of nutrition has been found effective in normalizing glucose values, but excessively high plasma galactose concentration develops. The potential dangers therefore preclude its use at this time.

Insulin may be administered if plasma glucose exceeds 300 mg/dl despite lowering the amount of glucose. In one study 10 infants with a mean weight of 875 gm who had hyperglycemia and osmotic diuresis were successfully treated with continuous insulin infusions of 0.01 units/kg/hour; the insulin dosage had to be increased to a maximum of 0.16 units/kg/hour. Other infants have not shown any improvement despite massive doses of insulin in the infusate. We prefer to use crystalline insulin when hyperglycemia persists after other methods have failed;

we use 0.1 to 0.2 units/kg subcutaneously and repeat the dose every 6 hours as needed. Usually one dose is sufficient to lower glucose values, which then can be maintained through proper intravenous fluid therapy.

Rosita S. Pildes
Lawrence D. Lilien

BIBLIOGRAPHY

Adam, P.A.J., and others: Oxidation of glucose and D-β-OH-butyrate by the early human fetal brain, Acta Paediatr. Scand. **64**:17, 1975.

Anand, K.J.S., Sippell, W.G., and Ainsley-Green, A.: Randomized trial of fentanyl anesthesia in preterm babies undergoing surgery: effects on the stress response, Lancet **8524**:62, 1987.

Anand, K.J.S., and others: Can the human neonate mount an endocrine and metabolic response to surgery? J. Pediatr. Surg. **20**:41, 1985.

Anderson, J.M., Milner, R.D.G., and Stritch, S.J.: Effects of neonatal hypoglycemia on the nervous system: a pathological study, J. Neurol. Neurosurg. Psychiatry **30**:295, 1967.

Anderson, O., and others: Influence of the maternal plasma glucose concentration at delivery on the risk of hypoglycemia in infants of insulin-dependent diabetic mothers, Acta Paediatr. Scand. **74**:268, 1985.

Baker, L., and others: Diabetic embryopathy: mechanism involves myo-inositol and arachidonic acid (abstr.) Pediatr. Res. **20**:326A, 1986.

Barrett, C.T., and Oliver, T.K., Jr.: Hypoglycemia and hyperinsulinism in infants with erythroblastosis, N. Engl. J. Med. **278**:1260, 1968.

Beckwith, J.B.: Extreme cytomegaly of the adrenal fetal cortex, omphalocele, hyperplasia of the kidneys and pancreas and Leydig-cell hyperplasia: another syndrome? Paper presented to the Western Society for Pediatric Research, Los Angeles, 1963.

Benedetti-Massi, F., and others: Blood glucose and plasma insulin and glucagon response during intravenous glucose tolerance test in newborn infants affected by erythroblastosis fetalis, Acta Paediatr. Scand. **64**:113, 1975.

Bennett, P.H., Webner, C., and Miller, M.: Congenital anomalies and the diabetic and prediabetic pregnancy. In Pregnancy metabolism, diabetes and the fetus, CIBA Foundation Symposium no. 63, Amsterdam, 1979, Excerpta Medica, p. 207.

Benzing, G., and others: Simultaneous hypoglycemia and acute congestive heart failure, Circulation **40**:209, 1969.

Bier, D.M., and others: Glucose production rate in infancy and childhood, Pediatr. Res. **10**:405, 1976.

Block, M.B., and others: C-peptide immunoreactivity (CPR); a new method for studying infants of insulin-treated mothers, Pediatrics **53**:923, 1974.

Bloom, S.R., and Johnston, D.I.: Failure of glucagon release in infants of diabetic mothers, Br. Med. J. **4**:453, 1972.

Bloomgarden, Z.T., and others: Treatment of intractable neonatal hypoglycemia with somatostatin plus glucagon, J. Pediatr. **96**:148, 1980.

Bommen, M., and others: Plasma C-peptide in hyperinsulinaemic hypoglycaemia, Arch. Dis. Child. **59**:1096, 1984.

Brazy, J.E., and Pupkin, M.J.: Effects of maternal isoxsuprine administration on preterm infants, J. Pediatr. **94**:444, 1979.

Burd, L.I., and others: Placental production and foetal utilization of lactate and pyruvate, Nature **254**:710, 1975.

Burstein, R.L., Papile, L., and Greenberg, R.E.: Mechanisms of hyperglycemia in small premature infants (abstr.), Pediatr. Res. **14**:568, 1980.

Bussey, M.E., Finley, S., and Ogata, E.S.: Hypoglycemia in the newborn rat: delayed phosphoenolpyruvate carboxykinase despite increased glucagon availability, Pediatr. Res. **19**:363, 1985.

Chen, Y.T., Cornblath, M., and Sidbury, J.B.: Cornstarch therapy in type I glycogen storage disease, N. Engl. J. Med. **310**:171, 1985.

Christiansen, R.O., and Johnson, J.D.: Studies of insulin secretion in infantile hypoglycemia, Pediatr. Res. **8**:157, 1975.

Chung, G.S., and Myrianthopoulos, N.C.: Factors affecting risks of congenital malformations, Birth Defects **11**(10):23, 1975.

Churchill, J.A., Berendes, H.W., and Nemore, J.: Neuropsychological deficits in children of diabetic mothers: a report from the collaborative study of cerebral palsy, Am. J. Obstet. Gynecol. **105**:257, 1969.

Cochrane, W.A., and others: Familial hypoglycemia induced by amino acids, J. Clin. Invest. **35**:411, 1956.

Collins, J.E., and Leonard, J.V.: Hyperinsulinism in asphyxiated and small-for-dates infants with hypoglycaemia, Lancet **2**:311, 1984.

Cornblath, M., Parker, M.L., and Reisner, S.H.: Secretion and metabolism of growth hormone in premature and full-term infants, J. Clin. Endocrinol. Metab. **25**:209, 1965.

Cornblath, M., and Schwartz, R.: Carbohydrate metabolism in the neonate, ed. 2, Philadelphia, 1976, W.B. Saunders Co.

Cowett, R.M.: Pathophysiology, diagnosis, and management of glucose homeostasis in the neonate, Curr. Probl. Pediatr. **15**:6, 1985.

Cowett, R.M.: Mechanism(s) of glucose disequilibrium in perinatal hypoxia, Pediatr. Res. **20**:408A, 1986.

Cowett, R.M., and others: Glucose disposal of low birth weight infants: steady state hyperglycemia produced by constant intravenous glucose infusion, Pediatrics **63**:389, 1979.

Cowett, R.M., and others: Glucose kinetics in infants of diabetic mothers, Am. J. Obstet. Gynecol. **146**:781, 1983.

Cummins, M., and Norrish, M.: Follow up of children of diabetic mothers, Arch. Dis. Child. **55**:259, 1980.

Daniel, R.R., and others: Carbohydrate metabolism in pregnancy. XI. Response of plasma glucagon during normal pregnancy and in gestational diabetes, Diabetes **23**:771, 1974.

Davidson, D.C., Blackwood, M.J., and Fox, E.G.: Neonatal hypoglycemia with congenital malformation of pancreatic islets, Arch. Dis. Child. **49**:151, 1974.

Davidson, P.M., and others: Alloxan therapy for nesidioblastosis, J. Pediatr. Surg. **19**:87, 1984.

Davis, W.S., and Campbell, J.B.: Neonatal small left colon syndrome, Am. J. Dis. Child. **129**:1024, 1975.

Driscoll, S.G., and Steinke, J.: Pancreatic insulin content in severe erythroblastosis fetalis, Pediatrics **39**:448, 1967.

Elseweidy, M.M., Fadel, H.E., and Abraham, E.C.: Glycosilated hemoglobin and plasma protein in newborns of normal and diabetic women, Pediatr. Res. **18**:767, 1984.

Epstein, M., Nicholls, E., and Stubblefield, P.G.: Neonatal hypoglycemia after beta-sympathomimetic tocolytic therapy, J. Pediatr. **94**:449, 1979.

Farquhar, J.W.: Prognosis for babies born to diabetic mothers in Edinburgh, Arch. Dis. Child. **44**:36, 1969.

Feldman, F., and others: Glycosilated fetal hemoglobin: correlation with hyperglycemia and birth weight in infants of diabetic mothers, Diabetes **33**:81, 1984.

Fiser, R.H., and others: Insulin-glucagon substrate interrelationships in the neonatal sheep, Am. J. Obstet. Gynecol. **120**:944, 1974.

Freinkel, N., and Metzger, B.E.: Pregnancy as a tissue culture experience: the critical implications of maternal metabolism for fetal development. In Pregnancy metabolism, diabetes and the fetus, CIBA Foundation Symposium No. 63, Amsterdam, 1979, Excerpta Medica.

Fuhrann, K., and others: Prevention of congenital malformations in infants of insulin-dependent diabetic mothers, Diabetes Care **6**:219, 1983.

Gács, G., Kun, E., and Berend, K.: Hypoglycemia in infants and children with cyanotic congenital heart disease, Acta Paediatr. Acad. Sci. Hung. **4**:105, 1973.

Grajwer, L.A., Lilien, L.D., and Pildes, R.S.: Neonatal subclinical adrenal insufficiency—result of maternal steroid therapy, JAMA **238**:1279, 1977.

Grasso, S., and others: Insulin secretion in the premature infant: response to glucose and amino acids, Diabetes **22**:349, 1973.

Gross, I., and Smith, G.J.: Insulin delays the morphological maturation of fetal rat lung in vitro, Pediatr. Res. **11**:515, 1977.

Grylack, L.J., Chu, S.S., and Scanlon, J.W.: Use of intravenous fluids before cesarean section: effects on perinatal glucose, insulin, and sodium homeostasis, Obstet. Gynecol. **63**:654, 1984.

Hakanson, D.O., and Sunderji, S.G.: HbA_{1c} and newborn skinfold thickness: reflection of maternal diabetic control (abstr.), Pediatr. Res. **14**:573, 1980.

Haworth, J.C., Dilling, L.A., and Van Woert, M.: Blood glucose determination in infants and children: the reflectance meter-enzyme test strip system, Am. J. Dis. Child. **123**:469, 1972.

Haworth, J.C., Dilling, L.A., and Vidyasagar, D.: Hypoglycemia in infants of diabetic mothers: effect of epinephrine therapy, J. Pediatr. **82**:94, 1973.

Haworth, J.C., McRae, K.N., and Dilling, L.A.: Prognosis of infants of diabetic mothers in relation to neonatal hypoglycemia, Dev. Med. Child. Neurol. **18**:471, 1975.

Hay, W.W.: Fetal and neonatal glucose homeostasis and their relation to the small for gestational age infant, Semin. Perinatol. **8**:101, 1984.

Hay, W.W., and Sparks, J.W.: Placental, fetal and neonatal carbohydrate metabolism, Clin. Obstet. Gynecol. **28**:473, 1985.

Haymond, M.W., Karl, I.E., and Pagliara, A.S.: Increased gluconeogenic substrates in the small-for-gestational age infant, N. Engl. J. Med. **291**:322, 1974.

Heck, L.J., and Erenberg, A.: Serum glucose levels during the first 48 hours of life in the healthy full-term neonate, Pediatr. Res. **17**:317A, 1983.

Herrera, A.J., and Hsiang, Y.: Comparison of various methods of blood sugar screening in newborn infants, J. Pediatr. **102**:769, 1983.

Hintz, R.L., Menking, M., and Sotos, J.F.: Holoprosencephaly with endocrine dysgenesis, J. Pediatr. **72**:81, 1968.

Humbart, J.R., and Gotlin, R.W.: Growth hormone levels in normoglycemia and hypoglycemia infants born small for gestational age, Pediatrics **48**:190, 1971.

James, T., Blessa, M., and Boggs, T.R.: Recurrent hyperglycemia associated with sepsis in a neonate, Am. J. Dis. Child. **133**:645, 1979.

Johnson, J.D., and others: Hypoplasia of the anterior pituitary and neonatal hypoglycemia, J. Pediatr. **82**:634, 1973.

Kalhan, S.C., Savin, S.M., and Adam, P.A.J.: Measurement of glucose turnover in the human newborn with glucose-1-^{13}C, J. Clin. Endocrinol. Metab. **43**:704, 1976.

Kalhan, S.C., Savin, S.M., and Adam, P.A.J.: Attenuated glucose production rate in newborn infants of insulin-dependent diabetic mothers, N. Engl. J. Med. **296**:375, 1977.

Kaye, R., and others: Catecholamine excretion in spontaneously occurring asymptomatic neonatal hypoglycemia, Pediatr. Res. **4**:295, 1970.

King, K.C., and others: Insulin response to arginine in normal newborns and infants of diabetic mothers, Diabetes **23**:816, 1974.

Kitson, H.F., and others: Somatostatin treatment of insulin excess due to β-cell adenoma in a neonate, J. Pediatr. **96**:145, 1980.

Koivisto, M., Blanco-Sequiros, M., and Krause, N.: Neonatal symptomatic and asymptomatic hypoglycemia: a follow-up study of 151 children, Dev. Med. Child. Neurol. **14**:603, 1972.

Kollee, L.A., and others: Persistent neonatal hypoglycaemia due to glucagon deficiency, Arch. Dis. Child. **53**:422, 1978.

Knip, M., and others: Relation of enteroinsular hormones at birth to macrosomia and neonatal hypoglycemia in infants of diabetic mothers, J. Pediatr. **103**:603, 1983.

Kornhauser, D., Adam, P.A.J., and Schwartz, R.: Glucose production and utilization in the newborn puppy, Pediatr. Res. **4**:120, 1970.

Landau, H., and others: Persistent neonatal hypoglycemia due to hyperinsulinism: medical aspects, Pediatrics **82**:440, 1982.

Langer, J.C., and others: Surgical management of persistent neonatal hypoglycemia due to islet cell dysplasia, J. Pediatr. Surg. **19**:786, 1984.

LeDune, M.A.: Intravenous glucose tolerance and plasma insulin studies in small-for-dates infants, Arch. Dis. Child. **47**:111, 1971.

LeDune, M.A.: Response to glucagon in small-for-dates hypoglycemic and non-hypoglycemic newborn infants, Arch. Dis. Child. **47**:754, 1972.

Lendrum, B., and others: Echocardiographic studies in infants of diabetic mothers, Pediatr. Res. **12**:385, 1978.

Lilien, L.D., Grajwer, L.A., and Pildes, R.S.: Treatment of neonatal hypoglycemia with continuous intravenous glucose infusions, J. Pediatr. **91**:779, 1977.

Lilien, L.D., and others: Hyperglycemia in stressed small premature neonates, J. Pediatr. **94**:454, 1979.

Lilien, L.D., and others: Treatment of neonatal hypoglycemia with minibolus and intravenous glucose infusion, J. Pediatr. **97**:295, 1980.

Lilien, L.D., and others: Decreased plasma glucose following indomethacin therapy in premature infants with patent ductus arteriosus, Pediatr. Pharmacol. (New York) **5**:73, 1985.

Lovinger, R.D., Kaplan, S.L., and Grumbach, M.M.: Congenital hypopituitarism associated with neonatal hypoglycemia and microphallus: four cases secondary to hypothalamic hormone deficiencies, J. Pediatr. **87**:1171, 1975.

Lubchenco, L.O., and Bard, H.: Incidence of hypoglycemia in newborn infants classified by birth weight and gestational age, Pediatrics **47**:831, 1971.

Mann, T.P., and Elliot, R.I.K.: Neonatal cold injury due to accidental exposure to cold, Lancet **1**:229, 1957.

Martin, L., Ryckman, F.C., and Sheldon, C.A.: Experience with 95% pancreatectomy and splenic salvage for neonatal nesidioblastosis, Ann. Surg. **200**:355, 1984.

Mestyan, J., and others: Hyperaminoacidemia due to accumulation of gluconeogenic amino acid precursors in hypoglycemic small-for-gestational age infants, J. Pediatr. **87**:409, 1975.

Metzger, B.E., and others: Effects of gestational diabetes on diurnal profiles of plasma glucose, lipids and individual amino acids, Diabetes Care **3**:402, 1980.

Migeon, C.J., and others: The syndrome of congenital adrenocortical unresponsiveness to ACTH: report of six cases, Pediatr. Res. **2**:501, 1968.

Milsap, R.L., and Auld, P.A.M.: Neonatal hyperglycemia following maternal diazoxide administration, JAMA **243**:144, 1980.

Moncrieff, M.W., Hill, D.S., and Arthur, L.J.H.: Congenital absence of pituitary gland and adrenal hypoplasia, Arch. Dis. Child. **47**:251, 1972.

Nakagawa, S., and others: A new type of hypoglycemia in a newborn infant, Diabetologia **9**:367, 1973.

Nejad, S.A., and Senior, B.: A familial syndrome of isolated aplasia of the anterior pituitary, J. Pediatr. **84**:79, 1974.

Nitzan, M., and Groffman, H.: Hepatic gluconeogenesis and lipogenesis in experimental intrauterine growth retardation in the rat, Am. J. Obstet. Gynecol. **109**:623, 1971.

Obenshain, S.S., and others: Human fetal insulin response to sustained maternal hyperglycemia, N. Engl. J. Med. **283**:566, 1970.

Pedersen, J.: The pregnant diabetic and her newborn: problems and management, ed. 2, Baltimore, 1977, The Williams & Wilkins Co.

Perelman, R.H., and others: Comparative analysis of four methods for rapid glucose determination in neonates, Am. J. Dis. Child. **136**:1051, 1982.

Perlman, M., Aker, M., and Slonim, A.E.: Successful treatment of severe type 1 glucogen storage disease with neonatal presentation by nocturnal intragastric feeding, J. Pediatr. **94**:772, 1979.

Perrine, S.P., Greene, M.F., and Faller, D.V.: Delay in the fetal globin switch in infants of diabetic mothers, N. Engl. J. Med. **312**:334, 1985.

Persson, B.: Carbohydrate and lipid metabolism in the newborn infant, Acta Anaesthesiol. Scand. **55**:50, 1974.

Persson, B., and Gentz, J.: Follow-up of children of insulin-dependent and gestational diabetic mothers, Acta Paediatr. Scand. **73**:349, 1984.

Persson, B., and Tunell, R.: Influence of environmental temperature and acidosis on lipid mobilization in the human infant during the first two hours after birth, Acta Paediatr. Scand. **60**:385, 1971.

Persson, B., Gentz, J., and Moller, E.: Follow-up of children of insulin-dependent (type I) and gestational diabetic mothers, Acta Paediatr. Scand. **73**:778, 1984.

Persson, B., Settergren, G., and Dahlquist, G.: Cerebral arteriovenous differences of acetoacetate and D-β-hydroxybutrate in children, Acta Paediatr. Scand. **61**:273, 1972.

Pildes, R.S.: Insulin in normal and pathological pregnancies and its effects on the fetus and newborn, Pediatr. Adolesc. Endocrinol. **5**:213, 1979.

Pildes, R.S., and Pyati, S.: Hypoglycemia and hyperglycemia in <1000 gm infants. In Clinics in perinatology, Philadelphia, 1986, W.B. Saunders Co.

Pildes, R.S., Patel, D.A., and Nitzan, M.: Glucose disappearance rate in symptomatic neonatal hypoglycemia, Pediatrics **75**:91, 1973.

Pildes, R.S., and others: The incidence of neonatal hypoglycemia: a completed survey, J. Pediatr. **70**:76, 1967.

Pildes, R.S., and others: Plasma insulin response during oral glucose tolerance tests in newborns of normal and gestational diabetic mothers, Pediatrics **44**:76, 1969.

Pildes, R.S., and others: A prospective controlled study of neonatal hypoglycemia, Pediatrics **54**:5, 1974.

Pollak, A., and others: Glucose disposal in low-birth-weight infants during steady-state hyperglycemia: effects of exogenous insulin administration, Pediatrics **61**:546, 1978.

Procianoy, R.S., and Pinheiro, C.E.: Neonatal hyperinsulinism after short-term maternal beta sympathomimetic therapy, J. Pediatr. **101**:612, 1982.

Rahier, J., and others: The basic structural lesion of persistent neonatal hypoglycaemia with hyperinsulinism: deficiency of pancreatic D cells or hyperactivity of B cells? Diabetologia **26**:282, 1984.

Räihä, N.C.R., and Lindros, K.O.: Development of some enzymes involved in gluconeogenesis in human liver, Ann. Med. Exp. Biol. Fenn. **47**:146, 1969.

Raivio, K.O., and Osterlund, K.: Hypoglycemia and hyperinsulinemia associated with erythroblastosis fetalis, Pediatrics **43**:217, 1969.

Rastogi, G.K., Letarte, J., and Fraser, T.R.: Proinsulin content of pancreas in human fetus of healthy mothers, Lancet **1**:7, 1970.

Reid, M.M., and others: Cardiomegaly in association with neonatal hypoglycemia, Acta Paediatr. Scand. **60**:295, 1970.

Robert, M.F., and others: Association between maternal diabetes and the respiratory distress syndrome in the newborn, N. Engl. J. Med. **294**:357, 1976.

Rose, S.R., and others: Management of postoperative nesidioblastosis with zinc protamine glucagon and oral starch, J. Pediatr. **108**:97, 1986.

Sann, L., and others: Effect of intravenous hydrocortisone administration on glucose homeostasis in small for gestational age infants, Acta Paediatr. Scand. **68**:113, 1979.

Schiff, D., and Lowy, C.: Hypoglycemia and excretion of insulin in urine in hemolytic disease of the newborn, Pediatr. Res. **4**:280, 1970.

Schiff, D., Stern, L., and Leduc, J.: Chemical thermogenesis in newborn infants: catecholamine excretion and the plasma non-esterified fatty acid response to cold exposure, Pediatrics **37**:577, 1966.

Schiff, D., and others: Metabolic effects of exchange transfusions, J. Pediatr. **78**:603, 1971.

Schiff, D., and others: Metabolic aspects of the Beckwith-Wiedemann syndrome, J. Pediatr. **82**:258, 1973.

Schwartz, S.S., and others: Familial nesidioblastosis: severe neonatal hypoglycemia in two families, J. Pediatr. **95**:44, 1979.

Senior, B., and others: Benzothiadiazides and neonatal hypoglycemia, Lancet **2**:377, 1976.

Senterre, J., and Karlberg, P.: Respiratory quotient and metabolic rate in normal full term and small for date newborn infants, Acta Paediatr. Scand. **59**:653, 1970.

Shah, M.P.K., and Farquhar, J.W.: Children of diabetic mothers—subsequent weight. In Camerini-Davalos, R.A., and Cole, H.A., editors: Early diabetes in early life, New York, 1975, Academic Press, Inc.

Simmons, M.A., and others: Fetal metabolic response to maternal starvation, Pediatr. Res. **8**:830, 1974.

Smith, B.T., and others: Insulin antagonism of cortisol action on lecithin synthesis by cultured fetal lung cells, J. Pediatr. **87**:953, 1975.

Snyder, R.D., and Robinson, A.: Leucine-induced hypoglycemia, Am. J. Dis. Child. **113**:566, 1967.

Sokoloff, L.: Metabolism of ketone bodies by the brain, Annu. Rev. Med. **24**:271, 1973.

Soltész, G., Mestyán, J., and Schultz, K.: Glucose disappearance rate and changes in plasma nutrients after intravenously injected glucose in normoglycemic and hypoglycemic underweight newborns, Biol. Neonate **21**:184, 1972.

Sosenko, I.R., and others: The infant of the diabetic mother—correlation of increased cord C-peptide levels with macrosomia and hypoglycemia, N. Engl. J. Med. **301**:859, 1979.

Sotelo-Avila, C., Gonzalez-Crussi, F., and Fowler, J.W.: Complete and incomplete forms of Beckwith-Wiedemann syndrome: their oncogenic potential, J. Pediatr. **96**:47, 1980.

Sperling, M.A., DeLamater, P.V., and Phelps, D.: Spontaneous and amino-acid stimulated glucagon secretion in the immediate postnatal period, J. Clin. Invest. **53**:1159, 1974.

Srinivasan, G., and others: Plasma glucose changes in preterm infants during oral theophylline therapy, J. Pediatr. **103**:473, 1983.

Srinivasan, G., and others: Plasma glucose values in normal neonates: a new look, J. Pediatr. **109**:114, 1986.

Srinivasan, G., and others: Carbohydrate homeostasis during anesthesia and surgery in infants, Pediatr. Surg., 1986. (In press.)

Stern, L., Ramos, A.D., and Leduc, J.: Urinary catecholamine excretion in infants of diabetic mothers, Pediatrics **42**:598, 1968.

Tsang, R.C., and others: Parathyroid function in infants of diabetic mothers, Pediatrics **86**:399, 1975.

Urbach, J., and others: Neonatal hypoglycemia related to umbilical artery catheter malposition, J. Pediatr. **106**:825, 1985.

van Assche, F.A., and others: The endocrine pancreas in erythroblastosis fetalis, Biol. Neonate **15**:176, 1970.

Vaucher, Y.E., Walson, P.D., and Morrow, G.: Continuous insulin infusion in hyperglycemic very low birth weight infants, J. Pediatr. Gastroenterol. Nutr. **1**:211, 1982.

Vidnes, J., and Oyasaeter, S.: Glucagon deficiency causing severe neonatal hypoglycemia in a patient with normal insulin secretion, Pediatr. Res. **11**:943, 1977.

Vileisis, R., Cowett, R.M., and Oh, W.: Glycemic response to lipid infusion in the premature neonate, J. Pediatr. **100**:108, 1982.

Vohr, B., Lipsitt, L.P., and Oh, W.: Obesity in children of diabetic mothers with reference to birth size, J. Pediatr. **97**:196, 1980.

Walter, F.J., and others: Cardiac output in infants of insulin-dependent mothers, J. Pediatr. **107**:109, 1985.

Warram, J.H., and others: Differences in risk of insulin-dependent diabetes in offspring of diabetic fathers, N. Engl. J. Med. **311**:149, 1984.

Waziri, M., and others: Abnormality of chromosome 11 in patients with features of Beckwith-Wiedemann syndrome, J. Pediatr. **102**:873, 1983.

Widness, J.A., and others: Glycohemoglobin (HbA_{1c}): a predictor of birth weight in infants of diabetic mothers, J. Pediatr. **92**:8, 1978.

Williams, P.R., and others: Effects of oral alanine feeding on blood glucose, plasma glucagon and insulin concentrations in small-for-gestational age infants, N. Engl. J. Med. **292**:612, 1975.
Yen, S.S.C.: Endocrine regulation of metabolic homeostasis during pregnancy, Clin. Obstet. Gynecol. **16**:130, 1973.
Yeung, C.Y., Lee, V.W.Y., and Yeung, C.M.: Glucose disappearance rates in neonatal infection, J. Pediatr. **82**:486, 1973.
Yssing, M.: Long-term prognosis of children born to mothers diabetic when pregnant. In Camerini-Davalos, R.A., and Cole, H.A., editors: Early diabetes in early life, New York, 1975, Academic Press, Inc.
Zarif, M., Pildes, R.S., and Vidyasagar, D.: Insulin and growth hormone responses in neonatal hyperglycemia, Diabetes **25**:428, 1976.
Zucker, P., and Simon, G.: Prolonged symptomatic neonatal hypoglycemia associated with chlorpropamide therapy, Pediatrics **42**:824, 1968.

PART TWO

Disorders of calcium and magnesium metabolism

CALCIUM PHYSIOLOGY

Recent developments in the understanding of normal calcium physiology have provided a basis for reexamining the pathophysiologic considerations in disordered neonatal calcium homeostasis. Current research has confirmed the complex interrelationships of calcium (Ca) with phosphate (P), magnesium (Mg), and acid-base status, and with the three major Ca regulatory hormones: parathyroid hormone, vitamin D, and calcitonin (Table 37-2).

Ca in blood circulates as three important fractions: (1) protein bound, (2) complexed, and (3) ionized. Complexed Ca (complexed with bicarbonate, phosphate, or citrate) and ionized Ca are also termed *ultrafilterable* Ca (or *non-protein-bound* Ca). Ionized Ca is the only physiologically active fraction of blood Ca. Total Ca concentrations in blood might be reduced as the result of low plasma protein; however, if the ionized Ca remains normal, there may be no physiologic changes. On the other hand, total Ca concentrations may be unchanged when chelating agents are used, such as the citrate in acid-citrated blood; in this instance ionized Ca is lowered, with potentially significant physiologic effects. There are problems in the use of the McClean-Hastings nomogram for prediction of ionized Ca from the total Ca and protein values. Whenever possible, direct measurement of the ionized Ca with an ion-selective electrode would be preferable. In general, however, total and ionized Ca do correlate over a wide range of Ca values in the newborn, although the predictability of ionized Ca from total Ca alone is poor. The same considerations apply to the use of electrocardiographic determinations of the QT or Q_0T interval; although there is a correlation with ionized Ca, the predictability is as low as that for total Ca.

Table 37-2. Biochemical and hormonal effects on calcium and phosphate concentrations

Factors	Usual effect on serum Ca	Usual effect on serum P
BIOCHEMICAL		
Ca	Increase	—
P	Decrease	Increase
Mg	Increase	—
Alkalosis	Decrease	—
HORMONAL		
Parathyroid hormone	Increase	Decrease
Vitamin D	Increase	Increase
Calcitonin	Decrease	Decrease

Calcium balance

During pregnancy Ca is rapidly transferred from mother to fetus via an active placental pump. In the last trimester of pregnancy there is a net transfer of Ca of 100 to 150 mg/kg of fetal body weight. Radiocalcium balance studies in the pregnant rat have shown that about 30% of the total fetal bone is derived from the maternal skeleton; the remainder is from maternal dietary sources. In human beings, serum parathyroid hormone and serum 1α,25-dihydroxycholecalciferol concentrations are elevated in the last trimester of pregnancy, which would facilitate maternal intestinal Ca absorption and increased retention of Ca. In late pregnancy ionized Ca levels in the blood of mammalian fetuses are high and nearly always greater than that of the mother. At birth an abrupt termination of the maternal to fetal Ca supply occurs. To maintain serum Ca homeostasis at this time, it is estimated that an increase of 16% to 20% of Ca flux from fetal bone to extracellular space would be required, unless sufficient exogenous intake of Ca could be achieved. Since dietary Ca in the first few days of life is significantly less than the amount normally received through maternal to fetal transfer, a fall in serum Ca would be expected to occur. However, if normal physiologic processes are operative, compensatory mechanisms would be activated to restore Ca equilibrium immediately. In sick neonates even greater deprivation of Ca is common because of the conventional withholding of milk feeding and the substitution of Ca-free intravenous feeding. In premature infants, infants with birth asphyxia, and infants of diabetic mothers (IDMs), serum Ca concentrations are generally correlated with the amount of oral Ca intake.

Phosphate

Active placental P transport occurs in utero from mother to fetus, with fetal serum P concentrations being significantly greater than maternal values. At birth endogenous breakdown of tissue glycogen occurs with release of P into the extracellular space, further increasing the P load of the infant. Neonatal renal excretion of P is low because of decreased glomerular filtration rate or possibly low parathyroid hormone production initially (decreased parathyroid hormone results in increased renal tubular reabsorption of P). Decreased responsiveness of the renal tubules to parathyroid hormone has been proposed as a reason for low P excretion in the human neonate, although the kidneys of fetal sheep are responsive to the action of parathyroid hormone. Excess P with hyperphosphatemia is a well-known cause of hypocalcemia. Hypocalcemia occurs because of deposition of Ca in bone and soft tissue, blunting of parathyroid hormone activity at the bone site, and augmentation of calcitonin action at the bone site. High endogenous P loading has been proposed as a factor in the cause of early neonatal hypocalcemia (see later discussion on hypocalcemia). This type of hypocalcemia is generally associatied with hyperphosphatemia, which is not derived from exogenous sources, since milk intake is minimal at this age. In late neonatal hypocalcemia, excessive exogenous dietary P is an important factor causing hypocalcemia. The use of cow's milk types of formula (evaporated milks) and the early introduction of cereals to infants (which generally have a high P content) may lead to hypocalcemia. Most proprietary formulas have P contents higher than that of breast milk (although less than that of evaporated milk), tend to cause some degree of hyperphosphatemia, and also have been reported as an infrequent but potential cause of hypocalcemia.

Acid-base status

Acute changes in acid-base status directly affect Ca homeostasis. Decreases in pH increase ionized Ca, and increases in pH decrease ionized Ca. In adults the decrease in ionized Ca in acute alkalosis stimulates the activity of the parathyroid glands. Chronic changes in acid-base status also may affect Ca balance. In chronic acidosis there is mobilization of Ca from bone to the extracellular space, and in chronic alkalosis the reverse occurs. Several reports have documented the clinical association of early neonatal hypocalcemia in sick infants with the amount of bicarbonate administered for the correction of acidosis. It is not clear, however, whether the bicarbonate correction of acidosis adversely affects serum Ca or whether the severity of the illness adversely affects serum Ca. In later infancy, when metabolic acidosis of diarrheal dehydration has been corrected by alkali administration, postacidotic hypocalcemic tetany can result. Ca metabolism in the neonatal period can also affect acid-base status. In the rapidly growing premature infant, deposition of Ca into bone releases hydrogen ions into the extracellular space and is a possible contributing cause of the late metabolic acidosis of prematurity (Chapter 25, part three).

Parathyroid hormone

The parathyroid glands are the most important organs in the control of Ca homeostasis. Parathyroid hormone increases serum Ca primarily by increasing bone resorption of Ca (an action that requires vitamin D), by decreasing renal excretion of Ca, and by increasing intestinal absorption of Ca (through its effect on the production of the final metabolite of vitamin D, 1α,25-dihydroxycholecalciferol). Concurrently, its phosphaturic action removes the P released into the circulation by its bone action, minimizing the possible adverse effect of hyperphosphatemia on Ca homeostasis.

Parathyroid hormone production is regulated by the ionized Ca that reaches the parathyroid glands. Decreases in ionized Ca stimulate, and increases suppress, the production of parathyroid hormone, providing a sensitive feedback mechanism for the control of Ca homeostasis. Acute decreases in Mg also stimulate, and increases suppress, parathyroid hormone production. Paradoxically, however, Mg deficiency reduces parathyroid hormone secretion, most likely by altering the Ca-sensitive, Mg-dependent adenylate-cyclase system involved in parathyroid hormone secretion. More recently, many other factors have been identified that stimulate parathyroid hormone production, such as epinephrine and β-adrenergic agents and decreases in strontium. The parathyroid hormone that is secreted from the parathyroid glands has a molecular weight of 9,500 and contains the biologically active *N*-terminal group. Fragments circulating in the blood include a 7,500 molecular weight moiety (biologically inactive, containing the inactive *C*-terminal) and 4,500 molecular weight and smaller fragments, some of which have biological activity. Radioimmunoassays currently available for the assay of parathyroid hormone concentrations vary in their ability to recognize the *N*- or *C*-terminal, or middle or whole molecule, of the hormone.

Human fetal parathyroid glands are functionally active as early as 12 weeks' gestation, as demonstrated by their ability to resorb bone. In sheep the fetal parathyroid glands can respond to appropriate acute hypocalcemic challenges despite probable suppression of function by the high ionized Ca levels in utero. Parathyroid hormone probably does not cross the placental barrier in either direction. However, *maternal hyperparathyroidism* has been shown to affect the parathyroid function of the fetus adversely. The sequence is probably as follows: maternal hyperparathyroidism results in the maternal hypercalcemia, which leads to fetal hypercalcemia and suppression of the fetal parathyroids. Conversely, *maternal hypoparathyroidism* has resulted in fetal and neonatal hyperparathyroidism. The suggested sequence is as follows: maternal hypoparathyroidism, if untreated, leads to maternal hypocalcemia, fetal hypocalcemia, and secondary fetal and neonatal hyperparathyroidism. A similar pattern has been observed in untreated maternal pseudohypoparathyroidism, resulting in maternal hypocalcemia but normal or elevated concentration of maternal parathyroid hormone.

After birth, decreases in serum Ca are precipitated by the abrupt termination of Ca supply and the imposition of an endogenous P load from tissue breakdown that cannot be excreted by the kidneys. Normally the parathyroid glands should respond by appropriate increases in production of parathyroid hormone, which would act appropriately on target organs to increase and normalize serum Ca concentrations. It was previously proposed that the target organs in the neonate might not be responsive to parathyroid hormone. Later studies, however, indicate that the neonate shows an appropriate calcemic response when challenged with parathyroid hormone. On the other hand, the ability of the neonatal parathyroids to produce parathyroid hormone may be diminished in some infants. In normal full-term infants, when serum Ca concentrations fall slightly after birth, parathyroid hormone concentrations increase appropriately. However, in preterm infants and IDMs there is a variable change in parathyroid hormone concentration in response to marked decreases in serum Ca. The reason for the state of functional hypoparathyroidism in some infants is unclear but may be related in part to the high levels of ionized Ca in utero, which could have suppressed the fetal parathyroids. With time, all infants apparently increase their serum parathyroid hormone concentrations, even to hyperparathyroid levels, presumably in response to the hypocalcemic stress.

Vitamin D

The sequence for vitamin D metabolism in the body is as follows: vitamin D is synthesized in the skin under ultraviolet irradiation (cholecalciferol, or vitamin D_3) or absorbed from dietary sources in the jejunum and duodenum (vitamin D_2, also called ergocalciferol; or vitamin D_3). The metabolism of vitamin D_2 is similar to that of vitamin D_3, and both are described here under the term *vitamin D*. Transport of vitamin D_3 to the liver results in a 25-hydroxylation step to 25-hydroxycholecalciferol (25-hydroxy-D); the latter metabolite is the major circulating vitamin D metabolite in the body (in adults, 25-hydroxy-D concentrations range from 10 to 65 ng/ml). 25-Hydroxy-D is transported to the kidney for 1α-hydroxylation to 1α,25-dihydroxycholecalciferol; this last metabolite is the most active of the vitamin D metabolites. The main factors increasing the rate of conversion of 25-hydroxycholecalciferol to 1α,25-dihydroxycholecalciferol are hypocalcemia, parathyroid hormone (possibly through its hypophosphatemic effect), and hypophosphatemia.

Vitamin D metabolites act (1) on the intestine to absorb Ca and P; (2) on the bone, together with parathyroid hormone, to mobilize Ca and P from bone; and (3) on the kidney to conserve Ca and P. Thus vitamin D sufficiency is necessary for maintenance of normal Ca and P homeostasis. In rats vitamin D and 25-hydroxycholecalciferol cross the placenta from mother to fetus. Limited quantities of 1α,25-dihydroxycholecalciferol appear to cross the monkey placenta. During human pregnancy maternal serum 1α,25-dihydroxycholecalciferol concentrations are elevated, but low cord blood concentrations have been reported. The importance of vitamin D metabolites in utero is uncertain. However, some Indian subcontinent immigrants to the United Kingdom who are vitamin D deficient have offspring who are more prone to late neonatal hypocalcemia. The etiology of the hypocalcemia is uncertain, although it appears to be prevented by vitamin D supplementation in pregnant women. In some preterm infants there may be low serum 25-hydroxycholecalciferol concentrations. No specific evidence, however, shows that decreased vitamin D stores play a role in the hypocalcemia of prematurity. In term infants serum 1α,25-dihydroxycholecalciferol concentrations are low at birth but increase to normal ranges by 24 hours of life, possibly reflecting the need for optimum intestinal calcium and phosphorus absorption (Fig. 37-15). In extremely preterm infants end-organ resistance to 1α,25-dihydroxycholecalciferol may exist and theoretically could contribute to hypocalcemia.

Calcitonin

Calcitonin is produced mainly by the C cells of the thyroid gland, which are embryologically derived from neural crest tissue. Calcitonin is a 32–amino acid molecule that acts at the bone site to antagonize the effect of parathyroid hormone by decreasing the amount of Ca and P released from bone; at the kidney site calcitonin has both calciuric and phosphaturic effects. Thus the overall effect of calcitonin is to decrease serum Ca and P. Factors that increase the production of calcitonin include increases in circulating calcium and magnesium and increases in the gastrointestinal (GI) hormones: gastrin, glucagon, and pancreozymin. These hormones are released secondary to food in the GI tract; for example, glycine and gastric distention stimulate gastrin release, intraduodenal glucose stimulates enteroglucagon, and intraduodenal fat stimulates pancreozymin. Thus it is suggested that this GI-thyroid–C cell system serves to prevent marked increases in serum Ca during food ingestion. In utero, calcitonin-secreting C cells are functionally active. In ovine, porcine, and bovine fetuses given Ca infusions, appropriate increases in calcitonin secretion are produced. Calcitonin activity at the bone site is also present in fetal life. High concentrations of serum calcitonin occur in fetal animals and newborn human beings. After birth serum calcitonin concentrations further increase in newborns. The physiologic impor-

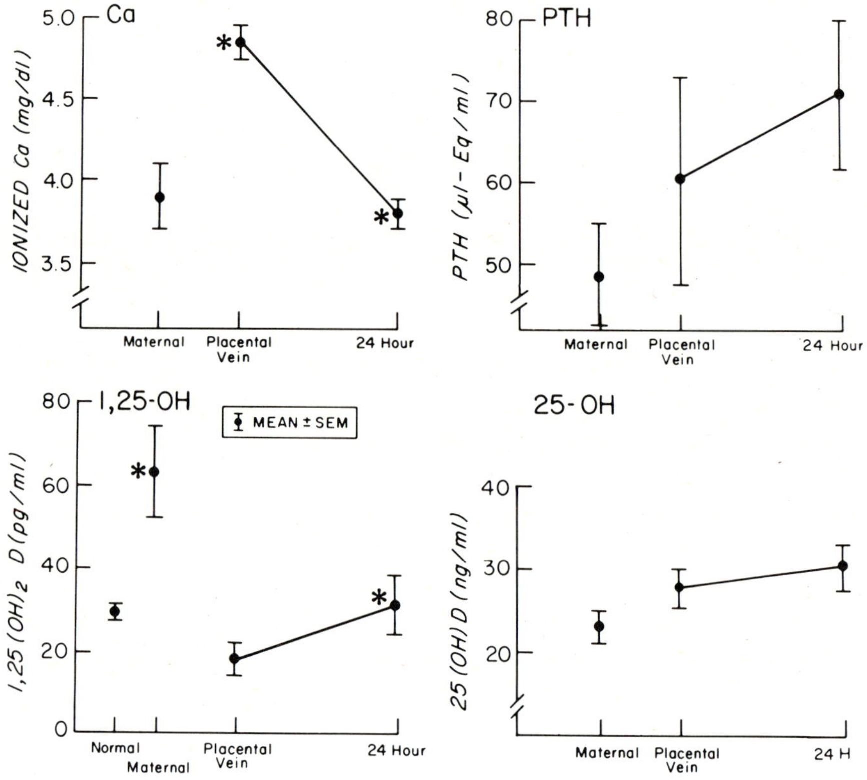

Fig. 37-15. Calcium and 1α,25-dihydroxycholecalciferol in normal full-term infants. Placental vein ionized calcium levels are higher than maternal values and fall after birth. Serum 1α,25-dihydroxycholecalciferol values in mothers are significantly higher than values in normal adults and in the placental vein. Placental vein 1α,25-dihydroxcholecalciferol concentrations are lower than those in adults at birth but revert to normal values at 24 hours. Serum parathyroid hormone and 25-hydroxy vitamin D concentrations in this study were not significantly changed after birth. (Reprinted by permission of the New England Journal of Medicine; from Steichen, J.J., and others: N. Engl. J. Med. **302:**315, 1980.)

tance of this increase in serum calcitonin is unclear. On theoretic grounds calcitonin would be advantageous for infants in protecting the skeleton from excessive bone resorption; however, this could lead to decreases in serum Ca and serum P. It is uncertain whether calcitonin plays any specific role in neonatal hypocalcemia; excess calcitonin would not explain the hyperphosphatemia associated with hypocalcemia. Increased serum calcitonin concentration recently has been documented after birth asphyxia; theoretically calcitonin elevation may contribute to neonatal hypocalcemia following asphyxia.

CLINICAL CONDITIONS OF CALCIUM DISTURBANCE

Hypocalcemia

"Early" neonatal hypocalcemia

Neonatal hypocalcemia that occurs in the first few days of life is the most common type of neonatal hypocalcemia. Neonatal hypocalcemia has been variously and arbitrarily defined as a total serum concentration less than 7 to 8 mg/dl. Hypocalcemia would be best defined by a direct measurement of ionized Ca, the biologically important fraction of Ca. However, limited information exists regarding ionized Ca concentrations in newborn infants. Using traditional ion-selective electrodes, an ionized Ca concentration below 3 to 3.5 mg/dl has been considered indicative of hypocalcemia. Using modern ion-selective electrodes, these numbers will most likely need to be revised upward, but insufficient data are available to be specific. In the absence of this information, for practical purposes we suggest a cutoff point of total Ca concentration of 8 mg/dl in full-term infants and 7 mg/dl in preterm infants.

Prematurity. About 30% of preterm infants develop neonatal hypocalcemia. Serum Ca values after birth, in the first few days of life, correlate directly with gestational age (Fig. 37-16). Thus less mature infants have a greater probability of developing hypocalcemia. Hypocalcemia in premature infants is related in part to decreased Ca intake from decreased milk intake, increased endogenous P loading, and transient functional hypoparathyroidism. Birth asphyxia in some infants com-

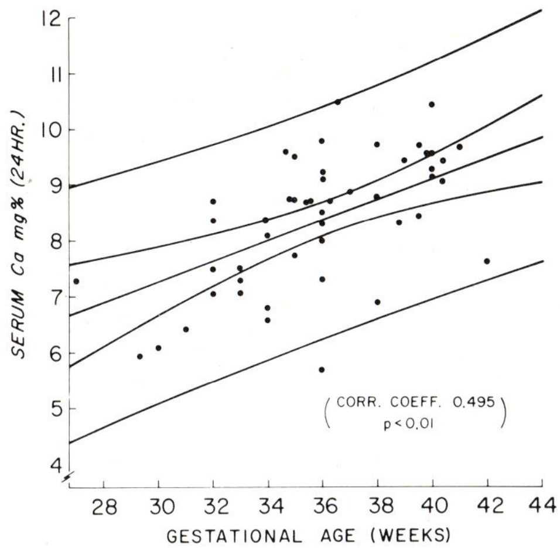

Fig. 37-16. Serum Ca in relation to gestational age at 24 hours of age. (From Tsang, R.C., and others: J. Pediatr. **82:**423, 1973.)

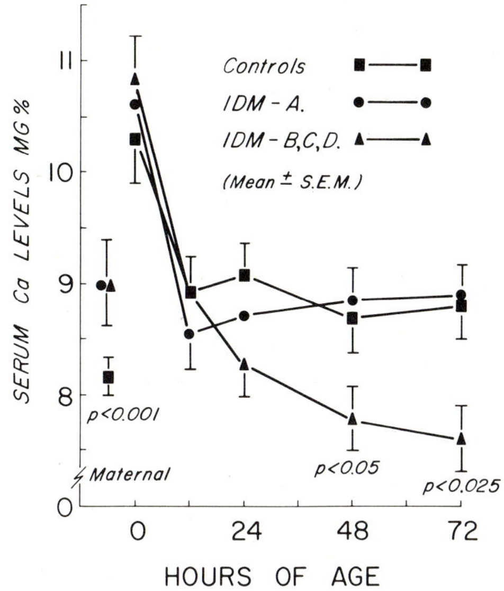

Fig. 37-17. Serum Ca levels in infants of class B, C, D diabetic mothers and infants of class A diabetic mothers compared with levels in control infants matched for sex, gestational age, and presence or absence of birth asphyxia. (From Tsang, R.C., and others: J. Pediatr. **80:**384, 1972.

pounds the problems. Other etiologic factors that have been suggested as causes of hypocalcemia include the correction of acidosis with alkali, decreased circulating vitamin D metabolites, and end-organ resistance to 1α,25-dihydroxycholecalciferol. Gestational age rather than birth weight appears to be an important determinant of neonatal Ca homeostasis. Small for gestational age (SGA) infants are not at high risk for hypocalcemia unless they are also gestationally premature or have birth asphyxia (see following section on asphyxia.)

Neonatal hypocalcemia in preterm infants is associated with hyperphosphatemia and generally occurs at an age (24 to 48 hours) when blood pH, (which is generally low in the first few hours after birth in these infants), has reverted to normal. In nearly all instances hypocalcemia is temporary and shows a gradual reversion toward normal after 1 to 3 days. Factors that contribute to the restoration include improvement in Ca intake when milk feeding increases, increased excretion of P, and restoration of parathyroid function. Ca supplementation may hasten the restorative process.

Infants of diabetic mothers. Neonatal hypocalcemia occurs in about 50% of IDMs. These infants are often delivered prematurely and often have birth asphyxia. Since prematurity and birth asphyxia are significantly associated with hypocalcemia, decreased serum Ca in IDMs relates in part to these two complications. In a prospective matched controlled study, however, neonatal hypocalcemia in IDMs was significant even after controlling for the complicating variables of prematurity and birth asphyxia (Fig. 37-17). The degree of hypocalcemia also varies directly with the severity of maternal diabetes, classified by White's criteria (Chapter 3). Other factors that adversely affect serum Ca in IDMs are the limitation of food and Ca intake because of illness (e.g., respiratory distress and poor feeding) and endogenous P loading from increased tissue glycogen breakdown. Hypocalcemia in IDMs appears to be related to hypomagnesemia and decreased parathyroid hormone secretion. It has been speculated that maternal hypomagnesemia, caused by urinary Mg losses in diabetes, leads to fetal Mg deficiency and secondary fetal functional hypoparathyroidism. Calcitonin also may play a role, since serum calcitonin rises after birth in IDMs to a degree similar to infants of nondiabetic mothers. Hypocalcemia lasts for only a few days, with spontaneous resolution hastened by factors outlined in the discussion of hypocalcemia of prematurity.

Birth asphyxia. Many infants with birth asphyxia are gestationally immature and thus may have decreased serum Ca. However, matched controlled observations have demonstrated that birth asphyxia and gestational immaturity are two separate factors influencing the incidence of hypocalcemia in the immediate neonatal period (Fig. 37-18). In birth asphyxia the factors of decreased Ca intake and increased endogenous P loading appear important, as well as increased serum calcitonin concentrations observed recently in infants with asphyxia. Correction of acidosis with alkali may further aggravate hypocalcemia, theoretically by inducing a decrease of Ca

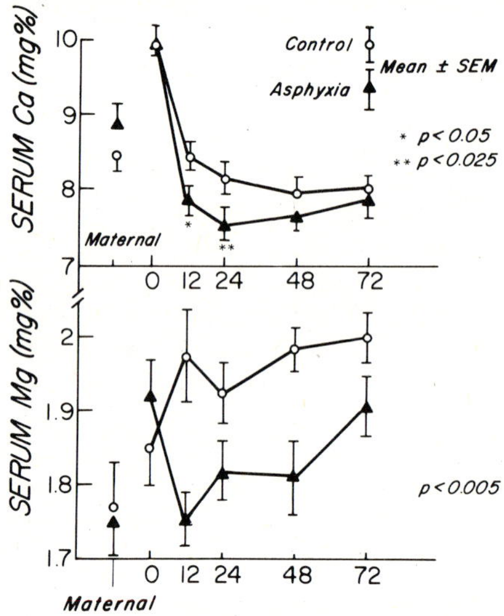

Fig. 37-18. Serum Ca and Mg levels in infants with birth asphyxia compared with levels in control infants matched for sex and gestational age. Serum Mg levels in infants with birth asphyxia were significantly lower from 12 to 72 hours of age. (From Tsang, R.C., and others: J. Pediatr. **84:**428, 1974.)

flux from bone to extracellular space. The hypocalcemia of birth asphyxia often occurs in association with hypomagnesemia and hyperphosphatemia and is generally of a transitory nature.

Infants of epileptic mothers. Anticonvulsant drugs such as phenobarbital and phenylhydantoin increase the hepatic catabolism of vitamin D and its metabolites, and epileptic patients treated with these drugs may develop osteomalacia in the absence of appropriate vitamin D supplementation. Infants of epileptic mothers theoretically may be at risk for developing early hypocalcemia; a prospective study supplementing pregnant mothers receiving antiepileptic drugs with vitamin D (1,000 IU/day) appeared to prevent neonatal hypocalcemia.

"Late" neonatal hypocalcemia

Hypocalcemia occurring in neonates beyond the first 2 to 4 days of life is termed *late* neonatal hypocalcemia. The term is often reserved for infants with cow's milk–induced hypocalcemia, who constitute in some geographic areas the largest group of infants with late hypocalcemia. In some cases, however, the clinical distinction between early and late hypocalcemia may not be clear.

Calcium deficiency. Any intestinal malabsorption syndrome, such as celiac disease or shortened bowel syndromes, can lead to malabsorption of Ca, since Ca absorption is carried out primarily in the small intestine. Concomitant malabsorption of vitamin D or Mg will further disrupt Ca balance.

Phosphate loading. In areas of the world where modified cow's milk with high P content (e.g., evaporated milk) is given to neonates, hypocalcemia is often observed. The greatly reduced number of infants in the United States currently seen with this disorder may be related to the introduction of proprietary formulas with P contents lower than that in cow's milk and the continuation of breast milk feeding (low P content). P-induced hypocalcemia commonly occurs at the end of a week of relatively high P feeding. It is thought that hyperphosphatemia leads to hypocalcemia by increasing tricalcium phosphate deposition in bone and soft tissues, enhancing the hypocalcemic effect of calcitonin or inhibiting the calcemic response to parathyroid hormone. In Asian immigrants to the United Kingdom, maternal vitamin D deficiency appears to be an additional etiologic factor in this condition. The parathyroid glands become hyperplastic in response to P-induced hypocalcemia in an attempt to correct the hypocalcemia. Early introduction of cereals to infants carries with it the potential risk of hypocalcemia because of the generally high P content of commercial cereals.

Hypomagnesemia. Hypomagnesemia, particularly from intestinal Mg malabsorption, generally has accompanied hypocalcemia. Hypocalcemia will not be corrected unless the Mg disturbance is first rectified (see later discussion on Mg disturbances).

Acid-base disturbances. Infants with acidosis secondary to diarrhea who receive alkali therapy to correct their acidosis may develop *postacidotic tetany* with decreases in total and ultrafiltrable Ca. Infants with chronic respiratory disease who become alkalotic because of hyperventilation with mechanical respirators or overcorrection with alkali infusions also may develop decreases in ionized Ca and signs of hypocalcemia.

Parathyroid disorders. The term *transient congenital idiopathic hypoparathyroidism* is applied to a group of infants who resemble infants with early neonatal hypocalcemia. Biochemically, there is hypocalcemia, hyperphosphatemia, and target organ responsiveness to parathyroid hormone. The diagnosis, however, may be delayed beyond the first few days of life, and the disease lasts for a few days to a few weeks, resolving either spontaneously or with short courses of vitamin D. This condition may simply represent an extension of early neonatal hypocalcemia that was not recognized in the immediate neonatal period. True *congenital hypoparathyroidism* can be inherited as an X-linked or autosomal dominant trait, in association with ring chromosomes (16 or 18), or as part of DiGeorge syndrome (congenital absence of the thymus and parathyroids). In the last condition, hypocalcemia is associated with thymic-dependent immunologic deficiencies (Chapter 30) and cardiovascular malformations. *Secondary hypoparathyroidism* may occur in offspring of mothers with hyperparathyroidism. The condition is generally transient, lasting for a few days to a few weeks, and supportive therapy with Ca and vitamin D generally suffices. In some instances protracted neonatal hypocalcemia has suggested that a maternal Ca disorder was present. *Pseudohypoparathyroidism,* or target organ unresponsiveness to parathyroid hormone, is a disease of later childhood and generally is not detected in the neonatal period.

Disordered vitamin D metabolism. *Dietary deficiency of vitamin D* is less common in the Western world. Rapidly growing small premature infants who do not receive supplemental vitamin D, other than that contained in their limited intake of milk, have developed radiologic signs of rickets. Infants with vitamin D deficiency have defective intestinal absorption of Ca and P and development of hypocalcemia and hypophosphatemia. In *neonatal liver disease,* including neonatal hepatitis and biliary atresia, disordered hepatic 25-hydroxylation of vitamin D may lead to hypocalcemia, hypophosphatemia, and rickets (Chapter 34, part two). In normal subjects there appears to be active enterohepatic circulation of 25-hydroxycholecalciferol. In liver disease, decreased bile salt secretion may result in decreased absorption of 25-hydroxycholecalciferol, further compounding the disturbance in vitamin D metabolism. In the kidneys of infants with *vitamin D–dependency rickets,* there may be a congenital metabolic block in the conversion of 25-hydroxycholecalciferol to the final 1α,25-dihydroxycholecalciferol. Reduction in the available amount of the final active vitamin D metabolite results in hypocalcemia and rickets. Finally, in *1α,25-dihydroxycholecalciferol target organ unresponsiveness,* a receptor or postreceptor defect for the final active vitamin D metabolite is present. In this syndrome greatly elevated 1α,25-dihydroxycholecalciferol concentrations are associated with alopecia and rickets. In all these conditions parathyroid hyperplasia may develop in an attempt to correct the hypocalcemia associated with disordered vitamin D metabolism. Hyperparathyroidism may worsen the bone picture by increasing bone resorption, although this serves to partially rectify the hypocalcemia. In addition, the hyperparathyroidism results in hyperphosphaturia and aminoaciduria.

Phototherapy. Phototherapy appears to be an additional possible cause of neonatal hypocalcemia, although the mechanism is uncertain. Phototherapy is known to decrease melatonin secretion. In the rat, melatonin decreases bone Ca uptake by enhancing the action of corticosterone on bone. It has therefore been suggested that a decrease in melatonin secretion secondary to phototherapy would increase bone Ca uptake and lead to hypocalcemia (Chapter 34).

Clinical and laboratory manifestations

The classic description of neonatal hypocalcemic tetany—high-pitched cry, Chvostek's sign (facial muscle twitching when stimulated), and Trousseau's sign (e.g., carpal spasm after constriction of the upper arm)—is useful in the older infant but is of little diagnostic value in the first few days of life. In the early neonatal period the main clinical signs are jitteriness (increased neuromuscular irritability and activity), twitching (jerky movements of one or more extremities), and generalized convulsions. However, these signs are not specific of hypocalcemia and may be confused with signs provoked by hypomagnesemia, hypoglycemia, sepsis, central nervous system injury, or narcotic withdrawal. Furthermore, hypocalcemia may be asymptomatic. Thus it is important to document hypocalcemia by blood measurement and to screen infants at risk for hypocalcemia, such as preterm infants, asphyxiated neonates, and IDMs.

In practice the diagnosis of hypocalcemia therefore is made from the determination of serum total Ca. The measurement of serum Mg should be done at the same time, since both conditions may coexist and the signs of hypomagnesemia are similar to those of hypocalcemia. We do not routinely recommend the measurement of serum parathyroid hormone, calcitonin, and vitamin D metabolites, which are mainly indicated when hypocalcemia is prolonged, refractory, or recurrent. Chest roentgenograms for thymic silhouette identification and immunologic studies are indicated when DiGeorge syndrome is suspected. Electrocardiographic determination of the QT_c or Q_0T_c interval may be useful. A corrected QT interval (QT_c, corrected for heart rate) greater than 0.40 second and a corrected Q_0T (or Q_0T_c, origin of Q to origin of T) greater than 0.20 second suggest hypocalcemia, although neither measurement predicts the ionized Ca value. Electrocardiographic monitoring may be used to gauge the response to Ca salt therapy.

Treatment

Treatment of symptomatic hypocalcemia is the administration of Ca salts. Ten percent Ca gluconate, containing 9.4 mg of elemental Ca per milliliter, is preferred to Ca chloride, which may cause metabolic acidosis. In case of seizures, intravenous administration of 10% Ca gluconate, 2 ml/kg body weight (18 mg elemental Ca/kg), should be given into a peripheral vein over 10 minutes with either electrocardiographic or heart rate monitoring. The infusion should be discontinued if bradycardia occurs. When this dose of Ca salts is given to an adult or older child, there is parathyroid suppression, so that usually this amount should not be exceeded. Continued follow-up intravenous supplementation of Ca at the rate of 75 mg elemental Ca/kg/day generally is sufficient to achieve normocalcemia. When normocalcemia is achieved, stepwise reduction of intravenous Ca (37 mg/kg each day, 18 mg/kg for the last day) may help to prevent rebound hypocalcemia. Complications of intravenous Ca therapy include extravasation of Ca into soft tissue with Ca deposition or sloughing of skin, as well as inadvertent rapid infusion with resultant bradycardia or cardiac standstill. Particular care should be exercised when the Ca infusion is given into an umbilical venous catheter tip close to the heart. Intraarterial infusions are inadvisable because of potential vascular complications. Alternatively if infants can tolerate oral fluids, oral administration of Ca gluconate in the same dosage is useful after initial acute correction. The only complication is an increased frequency of bowel movements, especially when the recommended dosage is exceeded. Preparations such as Neo-Calglucon are hypertonic because of their high sugar content and have a potential for necrotizing enterocolitis. We therefore recommend only the use of 10% Ca gluconate for oral administration.

Other experimental approaches have used 1α, 25-dihydroxycholecalciferol, 1α-hydroxyvitamin D (an analog of 1α, 25-dihydroxycholecalciferol), and intravenous parathyroid hormone successfully to treat neonatal hypocalcemia of term and large preterm infants. The side effects of these drugs are uncertain, however, and we do not recommend their routine use.

In asymptomatic hypocalcemia opinions vary as to the need for and intensity of therapy required. Some authors do not favor treatment because (1) in most instances hypocalcemia resolves spontaneously with time; (2) long-term follow-up studies have not shown clear benefit; (3) total serum Ca is a poor predictor of ionized serum Ca; and (4) intravenous Ca infusion may be dangerous (a recent study suggested that Ca infusion is responsible for brain calcifications). However, (1) many studies do not include adequate data; (2) long-term studies are difficult to perform because of many complicating factors; and (3) hypocalcemia has major potential effects on both the cardiovascular and the central nervous systems. In our institution we therefore treat asymptomatic preterm infants with a serum total Ca concentration of 6 mg/dl or less, since ionized Ca concentration is very low in most of these infants. For therapy we use a cutoff point of 7 mg/dl in term asymptomatic infants.

Prevention of hypocalcemia in asphyxiated or preterm infants also has been successful following use of oral or intravenous Ca salts or vitamin D metabolites, but the need for such an approach is controversial, and we do not recommend it routinely.

In hypocalcemic conditions secondary to other disorders, therapy for the primary disease is important. In P-induced hypocalcemia, use of a low-P formula (e.g., Similac PM 60/40) and avoidance of cereals are indicated. The use of aluminum hydroxide gel (Amphojel) to decrease P absorption is effective, but the long-range effects are unknown. Hypomagnesemia generally requires therapy before hypocalcemia can be successfully treated. When hypocalcemia is persistent, the use of vitamin D or one of its metabolites may be helpful, since vitamin D raises serum Ca levels primarily by increasing intestinal absorption of Ca. Dosages of vitamin D are approximately 400 IU for vitamin D deficiency (2,000 to 10,000 IU initially), 2,000 to 10,000 IU for hepatic disease, 10,000 to 100,000 IU for true hypoparathyroidism, and 5,000 to 50,000 IU for vitamin D–dependency rickets. Repeated therapeutic doses of parathyroid extract are inadvisable because of the possibility of antibody production and refractoriness to therapy.

Hypercalcemia

Hypercalcemia is present when total Ca in serum is greater than 10.5 to 11 mg/dl. Hypercalcemia may be asymptomatic but may lead to severe clinical consequences. Polyuria may occur after interference by hypercalcemia with the antidiuretic hormone action on the kidney. Polyuria may cause dehydration, poor feeding, and polydipsia. Because of a direct vasoconstrictive effect of Ca or an increased renin-angiotensin activity, hypertension may develop. Hypertensive encephalopathy, associated with a direct effect of Ca on nerve cells, may lead to vomiting, hypotonia, lethargy, and seizures. Long-term hypercalcemia may lead to metastatic tissue calcifications, primarily nephrocalcinosis.

Parathyroid disorders

Primary hyperparathyroidism. Congenital primary hyperparathyroidism is a rare disorder of diffuse clear cell parathyroid hyperplasia. Adenomas of the parathyroid are not seen in the neonatal period, although they may develop in later childhood. Familial patterns are occasionally reported and are compatible with recessive inheritance. The condition may not be clinically apparent and may be discovered only at autopsy. Alternatively, clinical signs may be present at birth or delayed for 30 months. Laboratory findings include hypercalcemia up to 25 mg/dl, hypophosphatemia, hyperphosphatasia, hypercalciuria, and phosphaturia; aminoaciduria and albuminuria are seen occasionally. Radiography of the long bones may show diffuse demineralization, subperiosteal resorption in the phalanges, and occasionally osteitis fibrosa and spontaneous fractures. Nephrocalcinosis is rarely seen by radiography but may be detected by ultrasonography. The prognosis for patients with untreated primary hyperparathyroidism is poor, with progressive deterioration and death. Definitive treatment is surgical with subtotal parathyroidectomy; success depends on early diagnosis before severe clinical problems occur.

Secondary hyperparathyroidism. *Congenital hyperparathyroidism* secondary to maternal hypoparathyroidism is a rare cause of hypercalcemia in the newborn. The condition is related to poor control of maternal Ca metabolism during pregnancy. Maternal hypocalcemia is thought to lead to fetal hypocalcemia and consequent chronic stimulation of the fetal parathyroid glands. Infants display the clinical, biochemical, or skeletal features of hyperparathyroidism. Hypercalcemia is not a constant manifestation of the condition, which is dominated by the skeletal features. Secondary hyperparathyroidism is transient with a relatively good prognosis, provided supportive measures are instituted.

Other disturbances

Idiopathic infantile hypercalcemia. This usually occurs in the first year of life. Although the condition may be fatal in a few patients, most often it is self-limiting and resolves within a few months to a few years. Idiopathic infantile hypercalcemia (IIH) may be isolated or associated with the features of the Williams syndrome: elfin facies, mental retardation, and supravalvular aortic stenosis. The relation between IIH and Williams syndrome is complex, since some patients with Williams syndrome do not have IIH. It has been suggested that these patients may have had hypercalcemia during the fetal or early neonatal life before the diagnosis of Williams syndrome. IIH may also occur together with the "blue diaper" syndrome, an inborn error of tryptophan metabolism leading to indicanuria.

The etiology of IIH is unknown. Calcium balance studies indicate increased Ca retention, resolving within the first 2 to 4 years of life. Studies have suggested that vitamin D may play a role in the pathogenesis of the syndrome, since IIH and vitamin D intoxication have some similarities. Pregnant rabbits given high doses of vitamin D give birth to offspring with generalized vascular lesions, some of which resemble supravalvular aortic stenosis. An increased incidence of IIH occurred in Great Britain during a period when vitamin D supplementation through fortified commercial milk, infant cereals, and vitamin D supplements could approximate 4,000 IU/day. Williams syndrome also has been found in infants of mothers who had received 500,000 IU of vitamin D during pregnancy in Germany. However, reports of mothers treated with megadoses of vitamin D or other D metabolites for hypoparathyroidism or for vitamin D–dependent rickets showed that infants born to these mothers only developed a hypercalcemia limited in time and intensity. When precise retrospective dietary histories were obtained, intrauterine or early extrauterine vitamin D intoxication could be excluded in most cases of Williams syndrome. Measurements of serum vitamin D activity or of vitamin D metabolites have lead to contradictory reports of normal, decreased, or increased concentrations. Recently an abnormality of calcitonin secretion has been suggested as an etiologic factor. A need exists to study patients with IIH, primarily in the active, hypercalcemic phase of the syndrome.

Subcutaneous fat necrosis. Small areas of subcutaneous fat necrosis are frequently seen in newborns over areas of increased pressure and are usually of little clinical significance (Chapter 20). Occasionally, however, extensive areas of fat are necrotic, particularly over the back and limbs, in infants born of difficult deliveries, in hypothermic infants, or in large IDMs. Fat necrosis usually appears during the first few days of life, and hypercalcemia follows in the next week or weeks. The clinical signs are similar to those of the benign form of idiopathic hypercalcemia and usually begin around 2 months of age with vomiting and failure to thrive, although in severe instances renal calculi, renal insufficiency, and convulsions can be seen. Proposed pathogenic mechanisms include abnormalities in fat metabolism, abnormal regulation of Ca physiology secondary to sudden release of large amounts of Ca from the subcutaneous fat, or abnormal sensitivity to vitamin D.

Miscellaneous causes

Iatrogenic hypercalcemia. Increased serum Ca levels may be seen as a result of overtreatment of hypocalcemia. After exchange transfusions with citrated blood and intermittent intravenous supplementation of Ca, measurements of total Ca in the infant's blood may be deceptively high, although ionized fractions may be low because of citrate complexing effects.

Paraneoplastic syndrome. In older children and adults hypercalcemia may be associated with malignancies. Hypercalcemia may be secondary to nephroblastoma in young infants.

Congenital hypokalemia with hypercalciuria. A curious syndrome has been reported recently involving premature infants with polyhydramnios, failure to thrive, episodes of fever, vomiting and diarrhea, and renal electrolyte and water wastage. The condition is renal tubular in origin and leads to hypokalemia, polyuria, isosthenuria, hypercalciuria, hypercalcemia, and metabolic alkalosis. Nephrocalcinosis and osteopenia may complicate the syndrome. Hyperprostaglandinuria has been documented, and suppression of prostaglandin E_2 hyperactivity by indomethacin has led to significant improvement in the clinical and biochemical features of the syndrome.

Severe infantile hypophosphatasia. This rare disorder is caused by deficient alkaline phosphatase activity in bone, liver, and intestine. Intrauterine death may occur.

The infantile type is inherited in an autosomal recessive manner. Patients have severe rickets at birth. Hypercalcemia, hypercalciuria, and nephrocalcinosis develop, presumably as a result of the failure of Ca to deposit in bone.

Hypercalcemia associated with hypophosphatemia. Preterm infants of low birth weight fed human milk may develop hypophosphatemic hypercalcemia. This condition is believed to be caused by the low P concentration in human milk, which may be insufficient for some very preterm infants. The P deficiency theoretically leads to increased 1α, 25-dihydroxycholecalciferol production and subsequent increased bone resorption, resulting in hypercalcemia, hypercalciuria, and rickets. The condition may be reversed by P supplementation, 30 to 50 mg/kg/day and preferably oral, to maintain serum P concentration between 3 and 5 mg/dl. Oral calcium salts probably should also be administered to prevent phosphate-induced hypocalcemia.

Familial hypocalciuric hypercalcemia. This disorder, transmitted in an autosomal dominant manner, is also called *benign familial hypercalcemia,* since signs of hypercalcemia are usually absent and there is a low frequency of complications. However, chondrocalcinosis and pancreatitis may occur infrequently. The pathogenesis of the condition is unknown but may be related to altered parathyroid hormone response to Ca. A high rate of severe neonatal hyperparathyroidism has been reported in families with familial hypocalciuric hypercalcemia.

Clinical and laboratory manifestations

The history affords the greatest information for the diagnosis and treatment of hypercalcemia. A close questioning of the mother is important to establish any history of excessive vitamin D intakes during pregnancy or in the neonatal period, especially in regard to vitamin D–fortified foods (milks, cereals) and supplements. A history of familial or maternal Ca-P disease should be investigated. The history of a difficult labor may alert the physician to the presence of fat necrosis. The onset of clinical signs in the immediate neonatal period or later gives some idea as to the severity and possible pathogenic mechanisms involved. The clinical signs of hypercalcemia include those related to its etiology, for example, "blue diapers," fat necrosis, and elfin facies. Plasma protein should be measured to rule out increases in total Ca from dysproteinemic states. Ionized Ca determinations are important in some cases. Plasma P determinations are useful in parathyroid disturbances but are of less value in other disorders. Determination of the percent of renal tubular reabsorption of P may help in distinguishing parathyroid disorders (decreased, less than 85%) from nonparathyroid conditions. The mother's Ca-P status should be determined. Measurement of parathyroid hormone concentrations, especially in conjunction with tests stimulating parathyroid hormone release, such as disodium ethylenediamine tetraacetate (EDTA) stimulation tests, will be helpful in differentiating hypercalcemia from parathyroid or nonparathyroid causes. Plasma 25-hydroxy-D determinations may be useful in instances where vitamin D excess is suspected. The electrocardiogram may show shortening of the QT interval. Bone roentgenograms will identify demineralization or osteolytic lesions (parathyroid overactivity) or osteosclerotic lesions (vitamin D excess) consistent with the etiology of the hypercalcemia.

Treatment

Therapy of hypercalcemia includes restriction of dietary Ca, discontinuation of vitamin D intake through the use of breast milk or vitamin D–free formulas or cow's milk, and empiric avoidance of sunlight. In acute hypercalcemia corticosteroids may be useful (prednisone, 2 mg/kg body weight daily) in decreasing intestinal Ca absorption. Furosemide diuretics are effective as calciuretic agents, provided water and electrolyte balance are maintained. Alternative modes of therapy include the intravenous use of EDTA, which chelates calcium and is excreted in urine, or calcitonin, which blocks parathyroid hormone–related Ca mobilization from bone and has a calciuretic action. The potential side effects of these drugs, especially for long-term therapy in the infant, are unknown.

MAGNESIUM PHYSIOLOGY

Sixty-five percent of body Mg is in the mineral phase of the skeleton, 34% is in the intracellular space, and 1% is in the extracellular fluid. Mg is therefore primarily an intracellular rather than an extracellular cation. Tissue Mg depletion may not be associated with decreased blood Mg concentration, and consequently it is difficult to assess Mg stores accurately. Normal serum Mg concentrations in neonates range between 1.6 to 2.8 mg/dl; 35% of serum Mg is bound to proteins. Mg activates many enzymatic systems and is important in energy production and cell membrane function. It also has important roles in regulation of mitochondrial function and in protein and deoxyribonucleic acid (DNA) synthesis. Serum Mg concentration is mainly regulated by the kidney. In normal conditions 95% to 97% of filtered Mg is reabsorbed. An increase in serum Mg leads to decreased reabsorption, whereas in Mg deficiency states or in a low Mg diet, urinary Mg excretion almost disappears. Other factors that increase urinary Mg include hypercalcemia and P depletion.

Parathyroid hormone increases serum Mg concentration by increased Mg mobilization from bone, increased intestinal Mg absorption, and decreased renal Mg excretion. Acute changes in serum Mg mimic the effects of changes of serum Ca on parathyroid hormone secretion. An increase in serum Mg will decrease parathyroid hormone secretion, whereas a decrease in serum Mg will increase parathyroid hormone secretion. However, paradoxically, chronic Mg deficiency reduces parathyroid hormone secretion, most likely through altering the Ca-sensitive, Mg-dependent adenylate cyclase involved in parathyroid hormone secretion. Excessive vitamin D may lead to hypomagnesemia, possibly secondary to increased intestinal Ca absorption, which results in competition for Mg absorption. Calcitonin may decrease serum Mg concentrations. Mg absorption occurs normally in the small intestine. The percentage absorbed is reduced with higher intakes and is normally 55% to 75% of ingested Mg in infants, compared with 45% in adults on a normal diet.

By the end of pregnancy increasing amounts of Mg undergo placental transfer from mother to fetus, averaging 4.5 mg/day. This transfer occurs against a concentration gradient, most likely involving an active transport mechanism. However, in cases of experimental maternal Mg deficiency in rats, normal maternal muscle Mg concentrations are maintained despite maternal hypomagnesemia and fetal Mg deficiency. It is therefore likely that, during deficiency states in pregnancy, Mg may be retained by the mother at the expense of the fetus. In maternal iatrogenic hypermagnesemia the fetus is unprotected and may become hypermagnesemic as well. At birth serum Mg concentration is inversely related to gestational age. After birth the serum Mg concentration rises slightly but gradually over a few days, except in infants fed cow's milk formula with high P load, in whom serum Mg concentrations may fall slightly.

CLINICAL CONDITIONS OF MAGNESIUM DISTURBANCE

Hypomagnesemia

Hypomagnesemia occurs when serum Mg levels fall below 1.6 mg/dl, although clinical signs usually do not develop until serum Mg levels fall below 1.2 mg/dl. Neonatal hypomagnesemia can result from decreased Mg supply, increased Mg loss, or disordered Mg homeostasis.

Decreased magnesium supply

Sporadic primary intestinal Mg malabsorption has been reported in rare instances in infancy, requiring apparent lifelong supplementation with Mg salts. Similarly, surgical procedures that reduce small-intestinal length can lead to Mg deprivation. Hypomagnesemic infants with intrauterine growth retardation and infants born of mothers with hypomagnesemia may represent conditions in which the maternal supply or placental transfer of Mg is possibly deficient. It is suspected that hypomagnesemia observed in IDMs is caused in part by urinary Mg losses in diabetic mothers (see previous discussion on magnesium physiology).

Increased magnesium loss

The increased loss of Mg caused by repeated exchange blood transfusions with acid citrated blood of low Mg content may lead to hypomagnesemia.

Disordered homeostasis

Neonatal hypoparathyroidism may be associated with hypomagnesemia. Hypoparathyroidism may be sporadic, familial, or related to maternal hyperparathyroidism. In these instances hypomagnesemia may be detected in the neonatal period or might not be diagnosed until later childhood. Treatment of hypomagnesemia generally facilitates the management of hypocalcemia.

Conflicting studies have been published regarding the effect of birth asphyxia on neonatal Mg homeostasis. One study suggested that serum Mg concentrations might be high in infants with birth asphyxia. Recent studies of the hypocalcemia of birth asphyxia have demonstrated the association of decreased serum Mg and increased serum P with the hypocalcemia. The differences in results may reflect differences in gestational ages of the infants studied, since an inverse relationship exists between gestational age and neonatal serum Mg levels.

Hyperphosphatemia, in addition to causing hypocalcemia, can also lead to hypomagnesemia. Thus cow's milk feeding has the potential for causing hypomagnesemia in infants.

Hypermagnesemia

The upper limit of normal for serum Mg levels in infancy is 2.8 mg/dl. The most important cause of neonatal hypermagnesia is maternal hypermagnesemia from magnesium sulfate therapy for toxemia of pregnancy or for tocolysis. Neonatal neuromuscular depression (curare-like effect) may occur with hypermagnesemia, and respiratory failure (CNS depression) can occur in extreme cases. It may be difficult to separate the effects of the hypermagnesemia from the effects of birth asphyxia, since birth asphyxia may occur in infants of toxemic mothers who do not receive Mg therapy. Apgar scores after birth do not correlate with the serum Mg concentrations, but neuromuscular depression may correlate with the duration of Mg therapy given to the mother. Neonatal parathyroid function is suppressed by hypermagnesemia. However, serum Ca concentrations appear to be increased in hypermagnesemic infants, possibly related to direct effects of Mg facilitating the release of Ca from bone (Fig. 37-19).

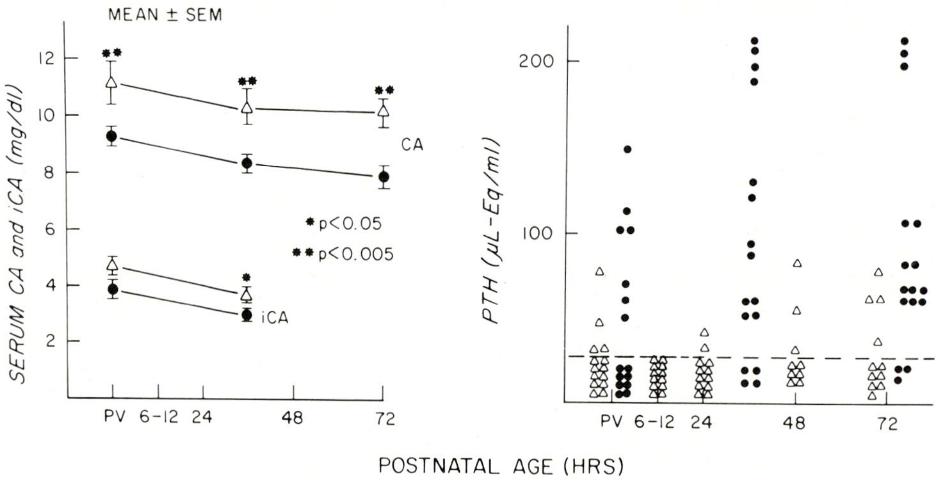

Fig. 37-19. Maternal hypermagnesemia is reflected in neonatal hypermagnesemia. Neonatal hypermagnesemia results in supression of parathyroid hormone, but elevation of serum total and ionized Ca. △, Hypermagnesemic infants; ●, controls. (From Donovan, E.F., and others: J. Pediatr. **96:**305, 1980.)

Clinical and laboratory manifestations

Hypomagnesemia should be considered in any high-risk infant just described and in any infant with hypocalcemia who does not respond clinically or biochemically to Ca or vitamin D therapy. It may occur with the signs of neuromuscular hyperexcitability; muscle twitching; and tonic, clonic, generalized, or focal seizures. Electrocardiographic changes of T wave inversion and ST depression may occur. When hypomagnesemia coexists with hypocalcemia, the determination of the primary defect may be difficult, since hypoparathyroidism may lead to both hypocalcemia and hypomagnesemia, but Mg deficiency may lead to secondary hypoparathyroidism and subsequent hypocalcemia. In this situation we have proposed a test to determine the parathyroid hormone response to an intravenous Mg load of 6 mg elemental mg/kg over 1 hour. An increase in serum parathyroid hormone following the Mg load suggests Mg deficiency with secondary hypoparathyroidism, whereas an absence of parathyroid hormone increase, or even a decrease, suggests hypoparathyroidism unrelated to Mg deficiency.

Hypermagnesemia should be suspected in depressed infants born of mothers who have received magnesium sulfate therapy. Depending on the severity of the hypermagnesemia, the signs may include neuromuscular depression, hypotension (usually at Mg levels above 4 to 6 mg/dl in adults), difficulty in urination (above 5 mg/dl), CNS depression (above 6 to 8 mg/dl), respiratory depression, and coma (above 12 to 17 mg/dl). Electrocardiographic signs include tachycardia or bradycardia and increased atrioventricular and ventricular contraction time.

Treatment

Hypomagnesemia should not be treated with Ca or vitamin D, which may cause a further decrease in serum Mg. Therapy with Mg salt is the treatment of choice. The average amount of magnesium sulfate required in the neonate is 0.25 ml/kg of body weight of a 50% solution (50 mg of elemental Mg/ml) given intramuscularly. Electroencephalographic monitoring during intravenous Mg salt therapy is unlikely to show dramatic changes in electroencephalographic patterns. The dose of Mg can be repeated in conjunction with twice-daily monitoring of serum Mg concentrations during the first few days. Maintenance 50% magnesium sulfate (0.25 ml/kg) may be given orally daily. Four to five times higher doses may be required in malabsorptive states, although diarrhea may ensue with these doses.

In hypermagnesemic conditions supportive therapy is usually sufficient, since the Mg excess is gradually removed through urinary excretion. Adequate hydration is important to ensure adequate urinary flow. In hypermagnesemia associated with neuromuscular depression, diuretic therapy might be attempted, since in adults organic mercurials and ethacrynic acid diuretics increase Mg excretion; this mode of therapy, however, is unproved in the neonate. Exchange blood transfusions with acid-citrated blood may be useful in severe depression by removing the excess Mg from the infant's blood.

RICKETS OF PREMATURITY
Pathophysiology

With the improvement of neonatal survival in very low birth weight infants, rickets of prematurity has become

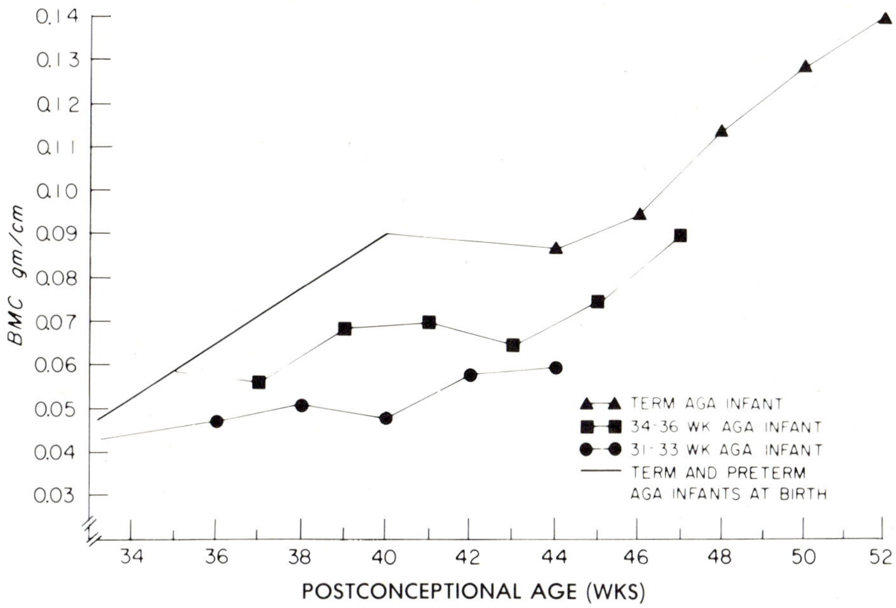

Fig. 37-20. Postnatal bone mineralization in preterm infants on standard proprietary formulas is significantly decreased compared with intrauterine bone mineralization rates. *BMC,* Bone mineral content. (Adapted from data in Minton, S., Steichen, J.J., and Tsang, R.C.: J. Pediatr. **95:**1037, 1979.)

a significant problem. More than 30% of preterm infants may develop radiologic signs of rickets. Very immature and sick infants are at particular risk for development of rickets. Vitamin D deficiency does not appear to be the cause in most cases, and 25-hydroxy-D serum concentrations, the best indicator of vitamin D status, usually are within the normal range. Mineral deficiency is likely to be an important etiologic factor. These infants may have been on total parenteral nutrition (TPN) for extended periods, and their calculated intakes of Ca and P are much lower than the fetal intrauterine requirements, which are normally up to 150 mg Ca/kg/day and 75 mg P/kg/day in the last trimester of pregnancy. Studies using the measurement of bone mineral content (BMC) in these infants by photon absorptiometry have shown that while receiving standard proprietary formula, they have undermineralized bones (Fig. 37-20); when they receive adequate mineral supply, reduced BMC can be prevented in most cases (Fig. 37-21).

It is possible that TPN-induced cholestasis and hypersulfatemia also may play a role in the pathogenesis of rickets of prematurity. More recently aluminum intoxication, a well-known cause of osteopenia, has been suggested as an etiologic factor, since most TPN solutions are contaminated with aluminum. More research, however, is needed to clarify this point. Infants with bronchopulmonary dysplasia or with patent ductus arteriosus may be particularly at risk for rickets if they are submitted to fluid restriction (leading to concomitant inadequate mineral intake) and chronic furosemide therapy. Furosemide has been shown clinically and experimentally to lead to urinary calcium losses and secondary hyperparathyroidism, which may have adverse effects on bone mineralization.

Diagnosis

The diagnosis of rickets may be obvious when fractures exist (up to 30% of very low birth weight infants in a recent study), occurring mainly in the long bones and ribs. In most cases, however, rickets is subclinical, and standard radiographic methods are unable to detect early bone demineralization. Photon absorptiometry allows early detection of osteopenia, but this method is not widely available and is still a research technique not yet validated for clinical usefulness.

Treatment

Prevention of rickets probably is more effective than treatment. Studies using photon absorptiometry have led to the production of *premature infant formulas* fortified with Ca, P, and vitamin D, which allow BMC to stay in the expected intrauterine range.

For infants fed human milk, an additional risk of P deficiency exists. Commercial Ca- and P-fortified powders are available, which may be mixed with human milk. These preparations contain lactose and a cow's milk–derived whey base and are heavily supplemented with Ca, P, and other minerals and trace elements. The efficacy of these powders to prevent rickets, however, is yet to be validated.

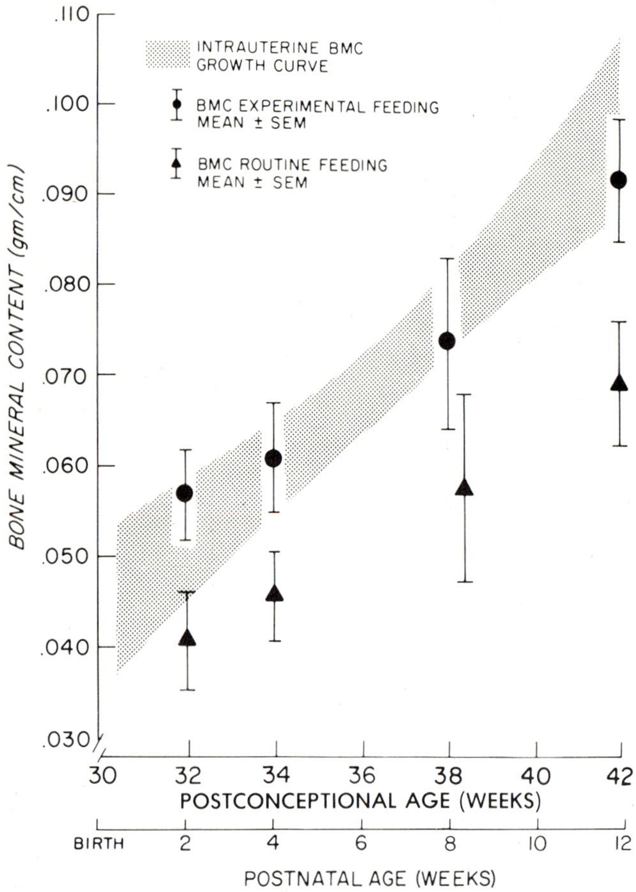

Fig. 37-21. In premature (28 to 32 weeks' gestation) infants fed an experimental formula fortified with calcium (1,260 mg/L) and phosphate (630 mg/L), postnatal bone mineralization is greater than that of premature infants fed standard proprietary formula and approximates the bone mineralization achieved in utero. Similar results are seen in infants of 32 to 35 weeks' gestation. (From Steichen, J.J., Gratton, T.L., and Tsang, R.C.: J. Pediatr. **96:**528, 1980.)

For infants with confirmed rickets of prematurity, the exact requirements of Ca, P, and vitamin D are unknown. We would recommend empirically a daily intake of up to 200 mg Ca/kg, up to 113 mg P/kg, and 400 IU of vitamin D.

Francis Mimouni
Reginald C. Tsang

BIBLIOGRAPHY

Calcium and phosphorus physiology

Anast, C., and others: Evidence for parathyroid failure in magnesium deficiency, Science **177:**606, 1972.

Avioli, L.V., and Haddad, J.G.: Vitamin D: current concepts, Metabolism **22:**507, 1973.

Comar, C.L.: Radiocalcium studies in pregnancy, Ann. N.Y. Acad. Sci. **64:**281, 1956.

Foster, G.V., Byfield, P.G.H., and Gudmundsson, T.V.: Calcitonin, J. Clin. Endocrinol. Metab. **1:**93, 1972.

Garel, J.M., and Dumont, C.: Distribution and inactivation of labelled parathyroid hormone in rat fetus, Horm. Metab. Res. **4:**217, 1972.

Garel, J.M., and Tarlet, M.P.: The effects of calcitonin and parathormone on plasma magnesium levels before and after birth in the rat, J. Endocrinol. **61:**1, 1974.

Garel, J.M., Care, A.D., and Barlet, J.P.: A radioimmunoassay for ovine calcitonin: an evaluation of calcitonin secretion during gestation, lactation, and foetal life, J. Endocrinol. **62:**497, 1974.

Haddad, J.G., Jr., Bousseau, V., and Avioli, L.V.: Placental transfer of vitamin D, and 25-hydroxycholecalciferol in the rat, J. Lab. Clin. Med **77:**908, 1971.

Koo, W., and others: Osteocalcin and calcium response to intravenous 1, 25-dihydroxyvitamin D_2, Pediatr. Res. **18:**301A, 1984.

Levine, B.S., and Coburn, J.W.: Magnesium, the mimic/antagonist of calcium, N. Engl. J. Med. **310:**1253, 1984.

Littledike, E.T., Arnaud, C.D., and Whipp, S.C.: Calcitonin secretion in ovine, porcine, and bovine fetuses, Proc. Soc. Exp. Biol. Med. **139:**428, 1972.

Miller, E.R., and others: Mineral balance studies with the baby pig: effects of dietary vitamin D_2 level upon calcium, phosphorus and magnesium balance, J. Nutr. **85:**255, 1965.

Minton, S.D., Steichen, J.J., and Tsang, R.C.: Bone mineralization in term and preterm appropriate for gestational age infants, J. Pediatr. **95:**1037, 1979.

Omdahl, J.L., and DeLuca, H.F.: Regulation of vitamin D metabolism and function, Physiol. Rev. **53:**327, 1973.

Parsons, J.A., and Potts, J.T.: Physiology and chemistry of parathyroid hormone, J. Clin. Endocrinol. Metab. **1:**33, 1973.

Ramberg, C.F., Jr., and others: Kinetic analysis of calcium transport across the placenta, J. Appl. Physiol. **35:**682, 1973.

Richardson, J.A., and Welt, L.G.: The hypomagnesemia of vitamin D administration, Proc. Soc. Exp. Biol. Med. **118:**512, 1965.

Schedewie, H., and others: Placental crossover and fetal tissue distribution of 1,25 (OH_2) vitamin D in rhesus monkey (abstr.), Pediatr. Res. **14:**580, 1980.

Scothorne, R.J.: Functional capacity of fetal parathyroid glands with reference to their clinical use as homografts, Am. N.Y. Acad. Sci. **120:**669, 1964.

Shami, Y., and Radde, I.C.: The effect of the Ca/Mg concentration on placental (Ca/Mg)-ATPase activity, Biochem. Biophys. Acta **255:**665, 1972.

Smith, F.G., Jr., and others: Fetal response to parathyroid hormone in sheep, J. Appl. Physiol. **27:**276, 1969.

Smith, F.G., Jr., and others: Parathyroid hormone in foetal and adult sheep: the effect of hypocalcemia, J. Endocrinol. **53:**339, 1972.

Steichen, J.J., Gratton, T.L., and Tsang, R.C.: Osteopenia prematurity: the cause and possible treatment, J. Pediatr. **96:**528, 1980.

Steichen, J.J., and others: Vitamin D homeostasis in the perinatal period: 1,25-dihydroxy vitamin D in maternal, cord and neonatal blood, N. Engl. J. Med. **302:**315, 1980.

Steichen, J.J., and others: Elevated serum 1,25 $(OH)_2$ vitamin D concentrations in rickets of prematurity, J. Pediatr. **99:**293, 1981.

Swaminathan, R., and others: The relationship between food gastrointestinal hormones and calcitonin secretion, J. Endocrinol. **59:**2217, 1973.

Venkataraman, P.S., and others: Elevated calcitonin in birth asphyxia and prematurity: role in the pathogenesis of early neonatal hypocalcemia, Pediatr. Res. **18:**352A, 1984.

Venkataraman, P.S., and others: Acute infantile tetany and secondary hyperparathyroidism in infants fed humanized cow milk formula, Am. J. Dis. Child. **139:**664, 1985.

Hypocalcemia

Barak, Y., and others: Response of neonatal hypocalcemia to 1,25-dihydroxyvitamin D_3, Arch. Dis. Child. **64:**642, 1979.

Barr, D.G.D., and others: Chronic hypoparathyroidism in two generations, Helv. Paediatr. Acta **26**:507, 1971.
Brooks, M.N., and others: Vitamin D dependent rickets type II: Resistance of target organs to 1,25-dihydroxyvitamin D, N. Engl. J. Med. **298**:996, 1978.
Chan, G.M., and others: The effect of 1,25$(OH)_2$D vitamin D_3 supplementation in premature infants, J. Pediatr. **93**:91, 1978.
Colletti, R.B., and others: Detection of hypocalcemia in susceptible neonates: the Q_oT_c interval, N. Engl. J. Med. **290**:931, 1974.
Cruikshank, D.P., and others: Altered maternal calcium homeostasis in diabetic pregnancy, J. Clin. Endocrinol. Metab. **50**:264, 1980.
Fleischman, A.R., Rosen, J.F., and Nathenson, G.: 25-Hydroxycholecalciferol for early neonatal hypocalcemia: occurrence in premature newborns, Am. J. Dis. Child. **132**:973, 1978.
Hahn, T.J., and others: Serum 25-hydroxycholecalciferol levels and bone mass in children on chronic anticonvulsant therapy, N. Engl. J. Med. **292**:550, 1975.
Hakanson, D.O., and Bergstrom, W.H.: Prevention of light-induced hypocalcemia by melatonin. In Norman, A.W., editor: Vitamin D, chemical, biochemical and clinical endocrinology of calcium metabolism, New York, 1982, Walter deGruyter & Co.
Harvey, J.C., and others: Third and fourth pharyngeal pouch syndrome, associated with vascular anomalies and hypocalcemic seizure, Clin. Pediatr. **9**:496, 1970.
Hirst, M.A., Hochman, H.I., and Feldman, D.: Vitamin D resistance and alopecia: a kindred with normal 1,25-dihydroxyvitamin D binding, but decreased receptor affinity for deoxyribonucleic acid, J. Clin. Endocrinol. Metab. **60**:490, 1985.
Kooh, S.W., and others: Response of protracted neonatal hypocalcemia to 1,25-dihydroxyvitamin D_3, Lancet **2**:1105, 1976.
Markestad, T., Ulstein, M., and Stranjord, R.E.: Anticonvulsant drug in human pregnancy: effects on serum concentrations of vitamin D metabolites in maternal and cord blood, Am. J. Obstet. Gynecol. **150**:254, 1984.
Moya, F., and others: Total calcium and Q_o-T_c determinations are not useful in the intensive care unit, Pediatrics **74**:317, 1984.
Nervez, C.T., and others: Prophylaxis against hypocalcemia in low birth weight infants requiring bicarbonate infusion, Pediatrics **87**:439, 1975.
Noguchi, A., Eren, M., and Tsang, R.C.: Parathyroid hormone in hypocalcemic and normocalcemic infants of diabetic mothers, J. Pediatr. **97**:112, 1980.
Peden, V.H.: True idiopathic hypoparathyroidism as a sex linked recessive trait, Am. J. Hum. Genet. **12**:323, 1960.
Peterson, S., Christensen, N.C., and Fogh-Andersen, N.: Effect on serum calcium of 1-hydroxy-vitamin D_3 supplementation in infants of low birth weight, infants with perinatal asphyxia and infants of diabetic mothers, Acta Paediatr. Scand. **70**:897, 1981.
Raisz, L.G.: Physiologic and pharmacologic regulation of bone resorption, N. Engl. J. Med. **282**:909, 1970.
Romagnoli, C., and others: Phototherapy induced hypocalcemia, J. Pediatr. **94**:815, 1979.
Rosenbloom, A.L.: Transient congenital idiopathic hypoparathyroidism, South Afr. Med. J. **66**:666, 1978.
Rossier, A., Caldera, R., and Bideau, C.: Neonatal hypocalcemia, Ann. Pediatr. (Paris) **19**:1473, 1972.
Salle, B.L., and others: Early oral administration of vitamin D and its metabolites in premature neonates: effect on mineral homeostasis, Pediatr. Res. **16**:75, 1982.
Schedewie, H.K., and others: Parathormone and perinatal calcium homeostasis, Pediatr. Res. **13**:1, 1979.
Scott, S.M., and others: Effect of calcium therapy in the sick premature infants with early neonatal hypocalcemia, J. Pediatr. **104**:747, 1984.
Stamp, T.C.B.: Effects of long term anticonvulsant therapy on calcium and vitamin D metabolism, Proc. R. Soc. Med. **67**:64, 1979.
Tsang, R.C., Steichen, J.J., and Chan, G.M.: Neonatal hypocalcemia: mechanism of occurrence and management, Crit. Care Med. **5**:56, 1971.
Venkataraman, P.S., and others: Effect of hypocalcemia on cardiac function in very low birthweight preterm neonates: studies of ionized calcium, echocardiography, and cardiac effect of intravenous calcium therapy, Pediatrics **76**:543, 1985.
Venkataraman, P.S., and others: Early neonatal hypocalcemia in very low birth weight infants: high incidence, early onset and refractoriness to supraphysiologic doses of 1,25-dihydroxyvitamin D_3, Am. J. Dis. Child., **140**:1004, 1986.

Hypercalcemia

Black, J.A., Bonham, C., and Carter, R.E.: Association between aortic stenosis and facies of severe infantile hypercalcaemia, Lancet **2**:745, 1963.
Beuren, A.J., and others: Syndrome of supravalvular aortic stenosis, peripheral pulmonary stenosis, mental retardation and similar facial appearance, Am. J. Cardiol. **13**:471, 1964.
Chesney, R.W., DeLuca, H.F., and Gertner, J.M.: Increased plasma 1,25-dihydroxyvitamin D in infants with hypercalcemia and elfin facies, N. Engl. J. Med. **3113**:889, 1985.
Culler, F.L., Jones, K.L., and Deftos, L.J.: Impaired calcitonin secretion in patients with Williams syndrome, J. Pediatr. **107**:720, 1985.
Daiger, S.P., and others: Vitamin D–binding proteins in the Williams syndrome and idiopathic hypercalcemia, N. Engl. J. Med. **298**:687, 1978.
Davies, M., and others: Familial hypocalciuric hypercalcemia and acute pancreatitis, Br. J. Med. **282**:1023, 1981.
Drummond, K.N., and others: The blue diaper syndrome: familial hypercalcemia with nephrocalcinosis and indicanuria, Am. J. Med. **37**:928, 1964.
Fanconi, G., and others: Chronische Hypercalcamie, kombiniert mit Osteosklerose, Hyperazotamie, Minderwuchs and kongenitalen Misbildungen, Helv. Paediatr. Acta **7**:314, 1952.
Fellers, F.X., and Schwartz, R.: Etiology of the severe form of idiopathic hypercalcemia of infancy: a defect in vitamin D metabolism, N. Engl. J. Med. **259**:1050, 1958.
Foley, T.P., and others: Familial benign hypercalcemia, J. Pediatr. **81**:1060, 1971.
Forfar, J.O., and others: Idiopathic hypercalcaemia of infancy: clinical and metabolic studies with special reference to the aetiological role of vitamin D, Lancet **1**:981, 1956.
Fraser, D.: Hypophosphatasia, Am. J. Med. **22**:730, 1957.
Fraser, D., and others: A new look at infantile hypercalcemia, Pediatr. Clin. North Am. **13**:503, 1966.
Friedman, W.F., and Roberts, W.C.: Vitamin D and the supravalvular aortic stenosis syndrome: the transplacental effects of vitamin D on the aorta of the rabbit, Circulation **34**:77, 1966.
Garabedian, M., and others: Elevated plasma 1,25-dihydroxyvitamin D concentrations in infants with hypercalcemia and in elfin facies, N. Engl. J. Med. **312**:948, 1985.
Garcia, R.E.: Idiopathic hypercalcemia and supravalvular aortic stenosis: documentation of a new syndrome, N. Engl. J. Med. **271**:117, 1964.
Goldbloom, R.B., Gillis, D.A., and Prasad, M.: Hereditary parathyroid hyperplasia: a surgical emergency of early infancy, Pediatrics **49**:514, 1972.
Goodenday, L.S., Gordan, G.S.: No risk from vitamin D in pregnancy, Ann. Intern. Med. **75**:807, 1971.
Harrison, H.E., and Harrison, H.C.: Disorders of calcium and phosphate metabolism in childhood and adolescence, Philadelphia, 1979, W.B. Saunders Co.

Kenny, F.M., and others: Metabolic studies in a patient with idiopathic hypercalcemia of infancy, J. Pediatr. **62**:531, 1963.

Lightwood, R.: Idiopathic hypercalcemia with failure to thrive and nephrocalcinosis, Proc. R. Soc. Med. **45**:401, 1952.

Martin, N.D.T., and others: Increased plasma 1,25-dihydroxyvitamin D in infants with hypercalcemia and elfin facies, N. Engl. J. Med. **313**:888, 1985.

Marx, S.J., and others: Normal intrauterine development of the fetus of a woman receiving extraordinarily high doses of 1,25-dihydroxyvitamin D, J. Clin. Endocrinol. Metab. **51**:1138, 1980.

Marx, S.J., and others: An association between neonatal severe primary hyperparathyroidism and familial hypocalciuric hypercalcemia in three kindreds, N. Engl. J. Med. **306**:257, 1982.

Marx, S.J., and others: Familial hypocalciuric hypercalcemia: the relation to primary parathyroid hyperplasia, N. Engl. J. Med. **307**:416, 1982.

Michael, A.F., Hong, R., and West, C.D.: Hypercalcemia in infancy, Am. J. Dis. Child. **104**:235, 1962.

Morgan, H.G., and others: Metabolic studies on two infants with idiopathic hypercalcaemia, Lancet **1**:925, 1956.

Mulivor, R.A., and others: Prenatal diagnosis of hypophosphatasia: genetic, biochemical and clinical studies, Am. J. Hum. Genet. **30**:271, 1978.

Rasmussen, H., and Bartter, F.C.: Hypophosphatasia. In Stanbury, J.B., Wyngaarden, J.B., and Fredrickson, D.S., editors: The metabolic basis of inherited disease, ed. 4, New York, 1978, McGraw-Hill Book Co.

Rowe, J.L., and others: Nutritional hypophosphatemic rickets in a premature infant fed breast milk, N. Engl. J. Med. **300**:293, 1979.

Sagy, M., and others: Phosphate depletion in a premature infant fed human milk, J. Pediatr. **96**:683, 1980.

Schlesinger, B.E., Butler, N.R., and Black, J.A.: Severe type of infantile hypercalcemia, Br. Med. J. **1**:127, 1956.

Seelig, M.S.: Vitamin D and cardiovascular, renal, and brain damage in infancy and childhood, Ann. N.Y. Acad. Sci. **147**:537, 1969.

Seyberth, H.W., and others: Congenital hypokalemia with hypercalciuria in perterm infants: a hyperprostaglandinuric tubular syndrome different from Bartter syndrome, J. Pediatr. **107**:694, 1985.

Stapleton, T., MacDonald, W.B., and Lightwood, R.: Management of "idiopathic" hypercalcaemia of infancy, Lancet **1**:932, 1956.

Taylor, A.B., Stern, P.H., and Bell, N.H.: Abnormal regulation of circulating 25-hydroxyvitamin D in the Williams Syndrome, N. Engl. J. Med. **306**:972, 1982.

Thorgeirsson, U., Costa, J., and Marx, S.J.: The parathyroid glands in familial hypocalciuric hypercalcemia, Hum. Pathol. **12**:229, 1981.

Veldhuis, J.D., and others: Infantile hypercalcemia with subcutaneous fat necrosis: endocrine studies, J. Pediatr. **95**:460, 1979.

Williams, J.C.P., Barratt-Boyes, B.G., and Lowe, J.B.: Supravalvular aortic stenosis, Circulation **24**:1311, 1961.

Magnesium metabolism and disturbances

Alcock, N., MacIntyre, I., and Radde, I.: Determination of magnesium in biological fluids and tissues by flame spectrophotometry, J. Clin. Pathol. **13**:506, 1960.

Anast, C.S.: Serum magnesium levels in the newborn, Pediatrics **33**:969, 1964.

Anast, C.S., and Gardner, D.W.: Magnesium metabolism. In Bronner, F., and Coburn, J.W., editors: Disorders of mineral metabolism: pathophysiology of calcium, phosphorus, and magnesium, New York, 1981, Academic Press, Inc.

Bajpai, E., Sugden, D., and Stern, L.: Serum ionic magnesium in exchange transfusion, J. Pediatr. **70**:193, 1967.

Bajpai, P.C., and others: Serum magnesium levels in the newborn and older children, Arch. Dis. Child. **41**:424, 1966.

Bottini, E., and others: Serum magnesium in icteric newborns undergoing exchange-transfusion with donor's blood collected in ACD solution, Biol. Neonate **12**:102, 1968.

Brady, J.P., and Williams, H.C.: Magnesium intoxication in a premature infant, Pediatrics **40**:100, 1967.

Buckle, R.M., Care, A.D., and Cooper, C.W.: The influence of plasma magnesium concentration on parathyroid hormone secretion, J. Endocrinol. **42**:529, 1968.

Byrne, P.A., and Caddell, J.L.: The magnesium load test. II. Correlation of clinical and laboratory data in neonates, Clin. Pediatr. **14**:460, 1975.

Caddell, J.L., and others: Parenteral magnesium load evaluation of malnourished Thai children, J. Pediatr. **83**:129, 1973.

Carr, C.W., and Woods, K.R.: Studies on the binding of small ions in protein solutions with the use of membrane electrodes. V. The binding of magnesium ions in solutions of various proteins, Arch. Biochem. Biophys. **55**:1, 1955.

Cholst, I.N., and others: The influence of hypermagnesemia on serum calcium and parathyroid hormone levels in human subjects, N. Engl. J. Med. **310**:1221, 1984.

Dancis, J., Springer, D., and Cohlan, S.A.: Fetal homeostasis in maternal malnutrition. II. Magnesium deprivation, Pediatr. Res. **55**:131, 1971.

Davis, J.A., Harvey, D.R., and Yu, J.S.: Neonatal fits associated with hypomagnesemia, Arch. Dis. Child. **40**:286, 1965.

Donovan, E.F., and others: Neonatal hypermagnesemia: effect of parathyroid hormone and calcium homeostasis, J. Pediatr. **96**:305, 1980.

Friedman, M., Hutcher, G., and Watson, L.: Primary hypomagnesemia with secondary hypocalcemia in an infant, Lancet **1**:703, 1967.

Givens, M.H., and Machy, I.G.: The chemical composition of the human fetus, J. Biol. Chem. **102**:7, 1933.

Graham, L.A., Caesar, J.J., and Burgen, A.S.V.: Gastrointestinal absorption and excretion of Mg in man, Metabolism, **9**:646, 1960.

Harris, I., and Wilkinson, A.L.: Magnesium depletion in children, Lancet **2**:735, 1971.

Hutchinson, H.R., and others: Effects of magnesium sulfate on uterine contractility, intrauterine fetus and infant, Am. J. Obstet. Gynecol. **88**:747, 1964.

Jones, K.H., and Fourman, P.: Effects of infusions of magnesium and of calcium in parathyroid insufficiency, Clin. Sci. **30**:139, 196.

Kobayashi, A., and Shiraki, K.: Serum magnesium level in infants and children with hepatic diseases, Arch. Dis. Child. **42**:615, 1967.

Levine, B.S., and Coburn, J.W.: Magnesium, the mimic/antagonist of calcium, N. Engl. J. Med. **310**:1253, 1984.

Lipsitz, P.J.: The clinical and biochemical effects of excess magnesium in the newborn, Pediatrics **47**:501, 1971.

Lipsitz, P.J., and English, I.C.: Hypermagnesemia in the newborn infant, Pediatrics **40**:856, 1967.

MacIntyre, I., Boss, S., and Troughton, V.A.: Parathyroid hormone and magnesium homeostasis, Nature **198**:1058, 1963.

Massry, S.G., Coburn, J.W., and Kleleman, C.R.: Evidence for suppression of parathyroid gland activity by hypermagnesemia, J. Clin. Invest. **49**:1619, 1970.

Mays, J.E., and Keele, D.K.: Serum magnesium levels in healthy children and various disease states, Am. J. Dis. Child. **102**:623, 1961.

Minton, S.D., Steichen, J.J., and Tsang, R.C.: Decreased bone mineral content in small for gestational age infants compared with appropriate for gestational age infants: normal serum 25-hydroxyvitamin D and decreasing parathyroid hormone, Pediatrics **71**:383, 1983.

Paunier, L., and others: Primary hypomagnesemia with secondary hypocalcemia in an infant, Pediatrics **41**:385, 1968.

Rash, D.K., and others: Neuro-behavioral effects of neonatal hypermagnesemia, J. Pediatr. **100**:272, 1982.

Shaul, P., and others: Magnesium infusion as a diagnostic study for Mg deficiency in newborns: response of parathyroid hormone (PTH) and calcitonin (CT), J. Am. Coll. Nutr. **3**:238, 1984.
Skyberg, D., and others: Neonatal hypomagnesemia with selective malabsorption of magnesium—a clinical entity, Scand. J. Clin. Lab. Invest. **21**:355, 1968.
Stone, S.R., and Pritchard, J.A.: Effect of maternally administered magnesium sulfate on the neonate, Obstet. Gynecol. **35**:574, 1970.
Stromme, J.H., and others: Familial hypomagnesemia, Acta Paediatr. Scand. **58**:433, 1969.
Stromme, J.H., and others: Familial hypomagnesemia—a follow-up examination of three patients after 9 to 12 years of treatment, Pediatr. Res. **15**:1134, 1981.
Thoren, L.: Magnesium deficiency in gastrointestinal fluid loss, Acta Chir. Scand. (Suppl.) **306**:5, 1963.
Tsang, R.C.: Neonatal magnesium disturbances, Am. J. Dis. Child. **124**:282, 1972.
Tsang, R.C., and others: Hypomagnesemia in infants of diabetic mothers: perinatal studies, J. Pediatr. **89**:115, 1976.
Wacker, W.E.C., and Parisi, A.F.: Magnesium metabolism, N. Engl. J. Med. **278**:658, 1968.
Willis, M.J., and Sunderman, W.F.: Studies in serum electrolytes. XIX. Nomograms for calculating magnesium ion in serum and ultrafiltrates, J. Biol. Chem. **197**:343, 1952.

Rickets of prematurity

Bosley, A.R.J., Verrier-Jones, E.R., and Campbell, M.J.: Aetiological factors in rickets of prematurity, Arch. Dis. Child. **55**:683, 1980.
Callahan, J., and others: Cholelithiasis in infants: association with total parenteral nutrition and furosemide, Radiology **143**:437, 1982.
Callenbach, J.C., and others: Etiologic factors in rickets of very low birth weight infants, J. Pediatr. **98**:800, 1981.
Cole, D.E.C., and Zlotkin, S.H.: Increased sulfate as an etiological factor in the hypercalciuria associated with total parenteral nutrition, Am. J. Clin. Nutr. **37**:108, 1983.
Davies, D.P., Hughes, C.A., and Moore, J.R.: Rickets in preterm infants, Arch. Dis. Child. **53**:88, 1978.
Greer, F.R., Steichen, J.J., and Tsang, R.C.: Calcium and phosphate supplements in breast milk-related rickets, Am. J. Dis. Child. **136**:581, 1982.
Greer, F.R., Steichen, J.J., and Tsang, R.C.: Effects of increased calcium, phosphorus and vitamin D intake on bone mineralization in very low brith weight infants fed formulas with Polycose and medium-chain triglycerides, J. Pediatr. **100**:951, 1982.
Koo, W.W.K., and others: Skeletal changes in premature infants, Arch. Dis. Child. **137**:1157, 1983.
Koo, W.W.K.: Natural history of rickets and fractures in very low birth weight (VLBW) infants during infancy, Pediatr. Res. **19**:224A, 1985.
Kovar, I.Z., Mayne, P.D., and Robbe, I.: Hypophosphataemic rickets in the preterm infant; hypocalcemia after calcium and phosphorus supplementation, Arch. Dis. Child. **58**:629, 1983.
Kovar, I.Z., Mayne, P., and Wallis, J.: Neonatal rickets in one of identical twins, Arch. Dis. Child. **57**:792, 1982.
Markestad, T., and others: Plasma concentrations of vitamin D metabolites in a case of rickets of prematurity, Acta Paediatr. Scand. **72**:759, 1983.
McIntosh, N., Livesey, A., and Brooke, O.G.: Plasma 25-hydroxyvitamin D and rickets in infants of extremely low birth weight, Arch. Dis. Child. **57**:848, 1982.
Mimouni, F., and Tsang, R.C.: Bone mineralization in infants. In Stern, L., editor: The child at risk of nutrition failure, New York, 1987, Nestle Foundation Publication. (In press.)
Minton, S.D., Steichen, J.J., and Tsang, R.C.: Bone mineral content in term and preterm appropriate for gestational age infants, J. Pediatr. **95**:1037, 1979.
Modanlou, H., Lim, M.O., and Hansen, J.W.: Growth and mineral metabolism in preterm infants receiving a novel human fortifier, Pediatr. Res. **18**:205A, 1984.
Pereira, G.R., and others: Hyperalimentation-induced cholestasis, Am. J. Dis. Child. **135**:842, 1981.
Rowe, J., and others: Hypophosphatemia and hypercalciuria in small premature infants fed human milk: evidence for inadequate dietary phosphorus, J. Pediatr. **104**:112, 1984.
Sato, Y.: Studies on metabolism of calcium in the fetus, Trans. Jpn. Soc. Pathol. **23**:257, 1933.
Sedman, A.B., and others: Evidence of aluminum loading in infants receiving intravenous therapy, N. Engl. J. Med. **312**:1337, 1985.
Seino, Y., and others: Plasma active vitamin D concentration in low birth weight infants with rickets and its response to vitamin D treatment, Arch. Dis. Child. **56**:628, 1981.
Steichen, J.J., Gratton, T.L., and Tsang, R.C.: Osteopenia of prematurity: the cause and possible treatment, J. Pediatr. **96**:528, 1980.
Steichen, J.J., Schell, D., Tsang, R.C.: Effect of soy based or cow milk based formula feeding on bone mineral content, mineral, vitamin D and iron metabolism in term infants, Pediatr. Res. **17**:202A, 1983.
Steichen, J.J., and others: Elevated serum 1,25-dihydroxyvitamin D concentrations in rickets of very low birth weight infants, J. Pediatr. **99**:293, 1981.
Venkataraman, P.S., and others: Secondary hyperparathyroidism and bone disease in infants receiving long term furosemide therapy, Am. J. Dis. Child. **137**:1157, 1983.
Walters, E.G., and others: Vitamin D metabolism in rachitic pre-term infants (letter), Lancet **ii**:629, 1983.

PART THREE

Thyroid disorders

Thyroid disorders of neonates must be considered with regard to many physiologic factors that influence the fetal and neonatal thyroid function. These include embryogenesis of thyroid, action of thyroid hormones, synthesis and transport of these hormones, regulatory mechanisms of thyroid function, fetal-maternal relationships, and the dynamic alteration of thyroid function with birth.

EMBRYOGENESIS

The major portion of human thyroid originates from the median anlage, which arises from the pharyngeal floor and is identifiable in the 17-day-old embryo. Initially the median anlage is in close contact with the endothelial tubes of the embryonic heart. Following the descent of the heart, the rapidly growing median thyroid is progressively pulled caudally until it reaches its definitive level in front of the second to sixth tracheal ring by 45 to 50 days' gestation. The pharyngeal region contracts to become a narrow stalk, the thyroglossal duct, which subsequently atrophies. The descent of the heart may influence the downward movement of thyroid because of its topographic contact. Usually the median anlage grows caudally so that no lumen is left in the tract of its descent. Ectopic thyroid and persistent thyroglossal duct or cyst are the results of abnormalities of the thyroid descent. The lateral parts of the descending median anlage expand to form the thyroid lobes and the isthmus.

The second anlage of the thyroid is composed of a pair of ultimobranchial bodies arising from caudal extension of the fourth pharyngeal pouch. This anlage is initially connected to the pharynx by the ductus pharyngobranchialis IV (late seventh week). Subsequently the pharyngeal connection is lost and the ductal lumen becomes obliterated. The ultimobranchial bodies are incorporated into the expanding lateral lobes of the median anlage. The contribution of ultimobranchial bodies to the ultimate thyroid tissue is small, and its differentiation appears to require the influence of the median anlage. The cells arising from ultimobranchial bodies are identifiable as parafollicular cells or C cells in mammals, and these cells are the source of thyrocalcitonin.

By the latter part of the tenth week the histiogenesis of the thyroid is virtually complete, although the follicles do not contain colloid. A single layer of epithelial cells surrounds the follicular lumen. Thyroxine (T_4) has been detected in the serum of a 78-day-old fetus. Thus the fetal thyroid contributes to the fetal requirement of thyroidal hormones by the beginning of the second trimester.

The anterior pituitary gland is derived from Rathke's pouch. Histologic differentiation of various pituitary cells can be observed by 7 to 10 weeks' gestation, and thyroid-stimulating hormone (TSH) can be detected in the fetal blood by 10 to 12 weeks.

The hypothalamus develops from the ventral portion of the diencephalon. Thyrotropin-releasing hormone (TRH) has been detected in fetal hypothalamus by 8 weeks' gestation, and its concentration thereafter progressively increases.

PHYSIOLOGIC ACTION OF THYROID HORMONES

The principal functions of the thyroid are to synthesize, store, and release the thyroid hormones, T_4 and triiodothyronine (T_3), into the circulation. The major secretory product of the thyroid is T_4. The thyroidal secretion of T_3 accounts for only about 20% of its production. Although T_3 has much greater metabolic activity than T_4 and is the principal active hormone at the cellular level, the physiologic actions of T_4 and T_3 may be considered together because T_4 acts as a prohormone for T_3. Most physiologic effects of thyroid hormones, however, have been described in terms of T_3.

One of the principal actions of thyroid hormone (TH) is to stimulate the rate of cellular oxidation in a large variety of tissues, leading to increased oxygen consumption, liberation of carbon dioxide, and production of heat. Changes in the basal metabolic rate (BMR) in hypothyroidism and hyperthyroidism are well known. The action of TH may be mediated through increased protein synthesis. T_3 binds to nuclear binding sites, leading to enhancement of polymerase activity, which in turn leads to increased cellular messenger ribonucleic acid (mRNA) and the corresponding proteins. Synthesis of membrane sodium-potassium adenosine triphosphatase (ATPase) is enhanced by this mechanism. It should be noted that a large portion of oxygen consumption depends on the sodium pump activity. T_3 can also bind to mitochondrial binding sites, which results in increased mitochondrial respiration. Clinically the calorigenic action of TH affects the circulation by increasing the heart rate, stroke volume, and cardiac output. The pulse pressure is widened mainly by a decrease in the diastolic pressure and by some elevation in the systolic pressure. Circulation time is shortened. In hypothyroidism the ECG may show decreased voltage of all complexes, prolongation of the PR interval, and depression or inversion of the T wave. The effect on the ECG, however, may be secondary to myxedema of the myocardium.

TH affects protein metabolism. Negative nitrogen balance occurs in hyperthyroidism, unless the patient is protected by adequate caloric intake to cover the increased energy requirement. In severe hypothyroidism, deposition of a mucoprotein containing hyaluronic acid occurs in extracellular myxedematous fluid.

TH influences the incorporation of creatine into the phosphocreatine cycle. In hypothyroidism there is an excessive storage of creatine, and in hyperthyroidism the urinary excretion of creatine is increased. However, the total excretion of creatine and creatinine is not affected by TH. Thus TH changes the urinary creatine/creatinine ratio; creatine accounts for 10% to 30% in the normal child, 0% to 10% in hypothyroidism, and 25% to 65% in hyperthyroidism.

The effect of TH on lipid metabolism is seen in the elevated serum cholesterol level in hypothyroidism, except in infants. The total neutral fats, fatty acids, and phospholipids of the serum also are increased in hypothyroidism.

TH also affects the metabolism of carbohydrates, calcium, vitamins, and water and the liver function. The rate of glucose absorption and use is increased by TH. In hypothyroidism, hypercalcemia may occur, the serum carotene level may be high, and the glucuronic acid conjugation mechanism of the liver may be impaired. Retention of water in the extracellular compartment occurs in hypothyroidism, producing the myxedematous fluid. In hyperthyroidism, on the other hand, increased calcium excretion in the urine and feces may lead to demineralization of the bones.

Another principal action of TH is the effect on growth and development. These effects may be tissue specific and may be synergistic with other hormones. Postnatal linear growth is TH- and growth hormone–dependent, which may be mediated through somatomedins. Similar synergistic effects between TH and growth hormone can be observed in skeletal maturation. TH may even exert its effects together with multiple hormones and growth factors. When hypothyroidism occurs in childhood, dental eruption, linear growth, and skeletal maturation are retarded. The retardation of skeletal maturation results in immature skeletal proportions and immature facial contours and contributes to the characteristic body configuration of hypothyroidism, which is different from that seen in stunted growth caused by isolated growth hormone deficiency. Ossification of cartilage is also disturbed in hypothyroidism. This produces the characteristic picture of epiphyseal dysgenesis in roentgenograms of the ossifying epiphyseal centers.

Postnatal growth of the brain is also TH dependent and may be mediated by an interaction between nerve growth factor and TH. Thyroidectomy in neonatal monkeys results in defective growth and development of the brain, and in untreated cretinism, mental retardation often ensues. The degree of mental retardation in cretinism is related to the severity and duration of the hypothyroid state of the infant whose brain is growing. The brain is more susceptible to lack of TH during its rapid growth and development, whereas defective growth and permanent damage do not occur if hypothyroidism begins after morphologic maturation of the brain is completed.

TH also affects the peripheral nerves. In hypothyroidism the relaxation phase of the ankle and knee jerk reflexes is prolonged. In hyperthyroidism sympathetic and autonomic response may be exaggerated.

Production of erythrocytes is regulated by erythropoietin, which in turn is influenced by TH, androgens, estrogens, and growth hormone. The anemia often observed in hypothyroidism can be corrected by administration of TH.

In addition to the classic thyroid hormones, T_4 and T_3, a calcium-lowering principle is found in the thyroid gland: thyrocalcitonin, or calcitonin. Although thyrocalcitonin has hypocalcemic and hypophosphatemic actions when administered to human beings, its physiologic role is not yet clearly understood. Thyroidectomy does not lead to hypercalcemia. Recent evidence suggests, however, that calcitonin deficiency may play a role in the pathogenic process of idiopathic hypercalcemia of infancy (Williams syndrome).

SYNTHESIS, RELEASE, TRANSPORT, AND UTILIZATION OF THYROID HORMONES

The biologically active thyroid hormones, L-thyroxine (T_4) and 3,5,3′-triiodothyronine (T_3), are iodinated amino acids. Their synthesis starts within the follicular cells. Iodine is supplied to the body mainly through dietary intake. However, it can be absorbed readily from the skin and lungs. Thus application of iodine-containing ointment or lotion to the skin can result in misleadingly high protein-bound iodine (PBI) levels. Although some organic iodine compounds, including T_4 and T_3, can be absorbed unchanged from the gastrointestinal tract, most are reduced and absorbed as ionic iodide. Generally, one fourth to one third of ingested iodide is taken up by the thyroid, which constitutes the basis for radioiodine uptake studies. This iodide-trapping mechanism involves an active transport process, an iodide pump that is dependent on oxidative phosphorylation. The iodide pump is present both at the basal and the apical surfaces of follicular cells, the former serving to concentrate iodide into the cells from the extracellular space and the latter serving to pump iodide into the follicular lumen as a secondary reservoir. The mechanism is capable of maintaining the intrathyroidal iodide concentration some 20-fold to 100-fold higher than that of serum. In one type of goitrous cretinism there is a defect in this iodide transport mechanism.

Immediately on entering the follicular cells, iodide is oxidized to an active form for iodination of thyroglobulin, probably by a peroxidase enzyme system. Thyroglobulin, a glycoprotein, is synthesized by the ribosomes of the follicular cells. Iodination of thyroglobulin seems to occur at the cell-colloid lumen interface. Almost all the iodine taken up by the thyroid is rapidly incorporated into the 3-position and the 5-position of the many tyrosyl residues of thyroglobulin to form monoiodotyrosine (MIT) and diiodotyrosine (DIT). Once iodide is organically bound to the tyrosyl residues, it can no longer be released readily from the thyroid. Defects in the iodide organification can be seen in two types of goitrous cretinism.

Synthesis of T_3 requires coupling between MIT and DIT molecules, accompanied by elimination of an alanine residue. T_4 is formed by coupling between two molecules of DIT. These reactions occur within the structure of thyroglobulin and involve oxidative processes, probably catalyzed by thyroid peroxidase as well. Patients with goitrous hypothyroidism caused by a coupling defect have been described.

Secretion of T_4 and T_3 into the circulation requires liberation of these moieties from the peptide bonds. Thyroglobulin molecules pass from the lumen of the follicles into the follicular cells, where proteolysis takes place. Congenital hypothyroidism may occur as a result of abnormal proteolysis of thyroglobulin. Of the approximately 125 tyrosyl residues in the thyroglobulin, only 10 or so form iodothyronines, whereas another 20 consist of MIT and DIT. Following proteolysis of thyroglobulin, the freed MIT and DIT are deiodinated by the iodotyrosine deionidase, and the liberated iodide is reused by the thyroid for iodination. A defective deiodination mechanism of free iodotyrosines results in (1) depletion of iodine as these iodine-containing molecules are released into the circulation and (2) wastage of these compounds as they are subsequently excreted into the urine. This results in goitrous cretinism.

T_4 and T_3 secreted into the circulation are transported by attaching loosely, through noncovalent bonds, to the plasma proteins. Three proteins play a role in the transport system. More than 75% of T_4 is normally bound to thyroxine-binding globulin (TBG). The second carrier protein is the T_4-binding prealbumin (TBPA); only about 15% of T_4 is bound to TBPA. The third protein is the serum albumin, which usually carries less than 10% of the circulating T_4. Whereas T_4 binds with all three proteins, T_3 binds only with TBG and albumin, and its intensity of binding is considerably less than that of T_4. The protein-bound thyroid hormones are biologically inactive and are in equilibrium with active non-protein-bound hormones. Although quantitatively insignificant, the non-protein-bound thyroxine, or free thyroxine (FT_4), concentration more accurately indicates the metabolic status of the individual, since only FT_4 can enter the cells and exert its effect. If the capacity of TBG is increased, a rise in the concentration of total hormone will follow, and the concentration of free hormone will be maintained at the normal level.

FT_4 is taken up by high-affinity binding sites at the cellular membrane. This membrane transport system may play an important role in the delivery of T_4 into the cells, contrary to the previously held view that FT_4 is transported by diffusion. Monodeiodination of T_4 has been shown to occur in many tissues, including the liver, the kidney, the cerebral cortex, and the pituitary gland. This deiodination at peripheral tissues generates 3,5,3′-triiodothyronine (T_3), the metabolically active thyroid hormone, by deiodination of 5′ position of T_4. Thus monodeiodination of T_4 is the principal regulatory mechanism in peripheral thyroid hormone metabolism; 80% of T_3 is produced by monodeiodination of T_4. However, the relative serum levels of T_4 and T_3 do not always reflect the intracellular proportions of the hormones, and the tissue distribution of T_3 may greatly differ from that of T_4 from tissue to tissue. The physiologic action of T_3 is faster than that of T_4, and the plasma half-life of T_3 is shorter: 1.0 day, compared to 6.9 days for T_4. Most T_3 is localized in cells, whereas T_4 is found mainly in the extracellular space. The metabolic effects of T_3 are mediated via attachment to various binding sites, including nuclear, membranous, mitochondrial, and cytosolic sites. However, direct binding of T_4 to nuclear binding sites has also been observed. Peripheral deiodination of T_4 at the 5 position, instead of the 5′, generates reverse T_3 (rT_3). The serum rT_3 concentration parallels that of T_3 in usual circumstances, but not in fetal life or in patients with severe nonthyroidal illness. The rT_3 is metabolically inactive in general, although its nuclear binding activity has been reported.

REGULATORY MECHANISM OF THYROID FUNCTION

The major control mechanism of thyroid function is the hypothalamic-pituitary-thyroid axis. The basophilic cells of the anterior pituitary gland produce and store TSH, which is a glycoprotein capable of rapidly increasing the intrathyroidal cyclic adenosine monophosphate (cAMP). It causes increased uptake of iodine by the thyroid, accelerates virtually all steps of iodothyronine synthesis and release, and increases the size and vascularity of the thyroid gland. These changes are mediated by the increase in cAMP. Human chorionic gonadotropin competes with TSH for receptors on thyroid follicular cells. Similarly, certain autoimmune antibodies—TSH-binding inhibiting antibodies (TBIA) and thyroid-stimulating immunoglobulins (TSI)—found in some patients with autoimmune thyroid diseases competitively bind to TSH receptors. Hyperthyroidism seen in patients with choriocarcinoma and Graves' disease may be explained by this mechanism. The secretion and the plasma level of TSH are inversely related to the levels of free (non-protein-bound) thyroid hormones. The inhibitory feedback action of free iodothyronines involves a direct action of these hormones on the pituitary gland without involving the hypothalamus. Thus the secretion of TSH is directly regulated through an intrinsic mechanism of the pituitary gland that is sensitive to the levels of free iodothyronines. However, the hypothalamus does influence TSH secretion. The hypothalamus secretes TRH, which stimulates the release of TSH by the pituitary gland. TRH is a tripeptide, L-pyroglutamyl-L-histidyl-L-proline-amide. Although the precise anatomic locations of TRH biosynthesis are not known, TRH synthetase is found in the median eminence and ventral and dorsal hypothalamus. When TRH is infused, it rapidly stimulates the release of TSH into the circulation, and the plasma TSH reaches a peak value in 20 to 30 minutes. The plasma half-life of TRH is extremely short and probably does not exceed 4 minutes. Exposure to cold environment increases TRH synthetase activity. TRH synthetase activity is reduced in hypothyroid animals and is increased in hyperthyroid animals. The hypothalamus may regulate the set point of feedback control as a thermostat through TRH, with iodothyronines playing a positive feedback role in TRH synthesis. This control probably operates in neonates whose circulating TSH becomes rapidly elevated after parturition. Administration of TRH stimulates the secretion of prolactin and HGH in addition to the release of TSH. In most children with idiopathic hypopituitarism, TSH release after TRH administration is normal, indicating an impaired TRH secretion rather than a primary TSH deficiency. TRH-mediated TSH release can be augmented by administration of theophylline or estradiol and may be blunted by administration of L-dopa or glucocorticoids. However, clinically significant hypothyroidism rarely, if ever, occurs following prolonged administration of large amounts of glucocorticoids or ACTH.

In addition to the hypothalamic-pituitary regulation, the thyroid is responsive to an intrinsic autoregulatory mechanism, the intrathyroidal iodide, which compensates for the fluctuation in dietary iodine intake. However, iodide trapping by the follicular cells is modulated by variations in dietary iodine intake within the physiologic range.

LABORATORY TESTS USED IN THE DIAGNOSIS OF THYROID DISEASE IN INFANCY AND CHILDHOOD

Concentration of circulating thyroid hormones

With the development of sensitive methods, more tests to determine thyroid function and disease have become available in hospitals and reference laboratories (see boxed material). Concomitantly many previous thyroid function tests have become obsolete. Among those, the PBI determination is still occasionally useful. In the PBI test serum or plasma proteins are precipitated, organic iodine is converted to iodide, and the total iodide is quantitated. Usually T_4 accounts for 80% to 90% of the PBI. Since this test measures the total iodide, it is influenced not only by T_4 levels but also by the levels of inorganic and organic iodine, including MIT and DIT. Therefore a large difference between PBI and T_4 values is often seen in goitrous cretinism caused by an inborn error of T_4 synthesis, in hyperthyroidism, and in thyroiditis because of the release of hormonally inactive iodoproteins into the circulation.

Total plasma or serum T_4, T_3, and rT_3 can be determined by specific radioimmunoassays (RIAs). These procedures require a very small quantity of blood (<50 μL), an advantage exploited for screening neonates for hypothyroidism. Determination of T_4 level is the most routinely used thyroid function test. The plasma pool of T_4 constitutes a large reservoir, and this pool turns over slowly. Thus T_4 measurement usually reflects the adequacy of the hormonal supply. However, it should be kept in mind that more than 99% of circulating T_4 is bound to serum thyroid hormone–binding proteins. Any change or abnormality in the concentration of these proteins, particularly TBG, can affect the T_4 level. Several clinical situations as well as pharmacologic agents can alter the levels of TBG or TBPA, and TBPA can compete with TBG for binding of T_4. Furthermore, certain anticonvulsants are known to not only bind competitively to TBG but also to have a direct suppressive effect on T_4, T_3, FT_4, FT_3, and rT_3 without greatly affecting the TSH level. These include phenytoin, valproate, primidone, carbamazepine, and diphenylhydantoin. Administration of T_3 results in a fall of T_4 as it suppresses the endogenous T_4 secretion. The normal level of T_4 is age dependent in infancy and childhood, particularly during the neonatal period. Serum T_4 concentration reaches its peak shortly after birth and declines slowly, gradually approaching the adult normal range in puberty. The range of normal levels for each age group is also wide. Normal adult values of serum T_4 by RIA are about 8.33 ± 2.42 μg/dl.

The RIA for T_3 requires highly specific antibodies or the separation of T_4 from T_3 before the assay. Only about 20% of T_3 is secreted by the thyroid gland, and the remainder is derived from T_4. This monodeiodination represents 36% to 41% of T_4 disposal. However, the serum concentration of T_3 can vary from day to day. Because of the small quantity of the serum T_3, its level may not fall below the normal range until the concentration of T_4 is critically low. Thus it is not advisable to use the T_3 concentration alone in evaluation of the thyroid status. Serum T_3 levels are physiologically low in the fetus and in the cord blood. It is also low in so-called low T_3 syndrome. The published normal adult levels of serum T_3 range from about 100 to 240 mμg/dl.

Most hormonally inactive rT_3 is derived from deiodination of T_4 and represents a similar order of magnitude of T_4 disposal as that converted to T_3 in normal adults. Its serum half-life is less than one half of that for T_3. The concentration of rT_3 usually parallels that of T_3. However, the levels of rT_3 are disproportionately high in the fetus,

Laboratory tests used for diagnosis of thyroid disorders and assessment of thyroid function in infancy and childhood*

- Concentration of circulating thyroid hormones: PBI, T_4, T_3, rT_3, FT_4, FT_3
- Assessment of thyroid hormone–binding proteins: T_3-resin uptake (T_3U) with free thyroxine index (FT_4I), TBG
- Concentration of circulating TSH
- Assessment of thyroid autoantibodies: antithyroglobulin (ATA), antimicrosomal (AMA), TBIA, TSI
- Measurement of circulating thyroglobulin (TG)
- In vivo tests: radioactive iodine uptake, perchlorate discharge test, TSH stimulation test, TRH stimulation test, T_3 suppression test
- Thyroid imaging: thyroid scan, ultrasonography
- Biopsy: needle, open, tissue culture
- Other tests: assessment of skeletal maturation, ECG, EEG, neck roentgenogram, urinary iodine excretion

*See previous text in this section for identification of abbreviated terms.

in the early neonatal period, and in severe nonthyroidal illness, probably reflecting altered tissue metabolism of T_4. The normal adult serum levels of rT_3 are 30 to 80 mμg/dl.

The minute amounts of FT_4 in the serum can be estimated by equilibrium dialysis. This method depends on the fact that the level of FT_4 is governed by an equilibrium between the levels of binding proteins, protein-bound T_4, and FT_4, following the law of mass action. However, clinically FT_4 does not depend on the T_4-binding capacity as such, since a change in such capacity will soon be compensated by a concordant change in the amount of T_4 released from the thyroid. To estimate the FT_4, serum is equilibrated with a tracer dose of radioactive T_4, which apportions itself between free and bound forms in the same ratio as that of the endogenous hormone. The dialyzable fraction of the labeled T_4 is proportional to the endogenous FT_4. The concentration of FT_4 in the serum is expressed as the product of the total T_4 and the dialyzable fraction. FT_3 levels in the serum can be estimated by a similar method. More recently an RIA for determining the concentration of FT_4 was introduced. The principle of this method is that the rate of binding of labeled hormone to antibodies depends on the FT_4 concentration during a timed incubation. Although the usefulness of FT_4 and FT_3 assays in the diagnosis of thyroid diseases is well established, they cannot be considered as definitive from a theoretic point of view and should not be used for routine screening of thyroid function. The levels of FT_4 and FT_3 do not reflect the thyroid status adequately under all circumstances. The approximate serum values for normal adults are 1.4 to 3.0 mμg/dl for FT_4 and 240 to 620 pg/dl for FT_3. The range of normal values for infants and young children are probably higher than for adults, but the exact ranges have not been established.

Assessment of thyroid hormone–binding proteins

Since the levels of T_4 and T_3 are affected by the levels of thyroid hormone–binding proteins and by the degree of their saturation at the binding site, the T_4 levels must be interpreted with a simultaneous evaluation of these proteins. The most frequently used approach is to determine the T_3-resin uptake (T_3U), which is a rapid, indirect assessment of the binding proteins. In this method a tracer dose of radioactive T_3, which competes for the binding sites with the endogenous hormones, is added to the serum. When the specimen is passed through resin or talc, the unbound radioactive T_3 is absorbed on the resin and can be measured by a radioassay. The amount of radioactive T_3 taken up by the resin is inversely proportional to the unsaturated T_4-binding capacity of the plasma proteins. The value obtained is not necessarily meaningful alone without the knowledge of total hormone concentration. T_3U is often expressed as a ratio (T_3UR) between the T_3U of the patient serum and T_3U of a pool of normal serum. The normal value is about 1.0. This value then is combined with total T_4 value to give an index, the free thyroxine index (FT_4I):

$$FT_4I = \frac{\text{Patient's } T_3U}{\text{Normal } T_3U} \times T_4$$

FT_4I essentially is a corrected T_4 value for the degree of saturation of the thyroid hormone–binding proteins. When the concentrations of TBPA and albumin are close to normal, changes in the degree of saturation of TBG are indicated by the changes of FT_4I from the T_4 value. However, the correlation between FT_4I and FT_4 is not linear. Changes in FT_4I are minimized when the T_4 level is high and are exaggerated when the T_4 level is low.

In general, when TBG is increased in a euthyroid individual, the T_4 will be elevated and T_3U will be low, but the FT_4I will be about normal. A reverse situation will be observed in an individual with low TBG, but again FT_4I will be normal. Administration of a drug that competes with T_4 for the TBG-binding sites will result in a low T_4 and a high T_3U, but FT_4I will be normal, as discussed next.

The serum TBG concentration can be determined by electrophoretic methods or by RIA. These tests are useful in confirming the presence of abnormal levels of TBG. Since the major portion of plasma T_4 is bound to TBG, these measurements give a good approximation of T_4-binding protein capacity. Methods to determine the levels of TBPA have been developed but are not used widely for clinical purposes. The binding capacity of TBG is increased in many clinical situations, including during pregnancy and in neonates. It also may be increased in hypothyroidism, liver disease, and porphyria. Pharmacologic agents that are capable of increasing TBG levels include estrogens, methadone, and heroin. The concentration of TBG may be decreased in preterm infants and in hyperthyroidism, hypercorticoidism, acromegaly, diabetic ketoacidosis, chronic hepatic diseases, alcoholism, nephrotic syndrome and other chronic renal diseases, and protein-calorie malnutrition. Drugs that are capable of decreasing TBG levels include androgens, anabolic steroids, glucocorticoids, and L-asparaginase. Pharmacologic agents that compete with T_4 for TBG binding sites include salicylates, diphenylhydantoin and possibly other anticonvulsants, hypolipidemic agents, sulfonylureas, diazepam, heparin, and fenclofenac. These agents give a falsely low serum T_4 level and a falsely high T_3U. In all these situations the T_3U is inversely related to the available TBG binding capacity for T_4, but FT_4I will give a basically accurate value for the effective T_4 available. Many of the clinical entities that can affect the level of TBG can also affect the level of TBPA. In addition, some drugs, such as salicylates and certain anticoagulants, may compete with T_4 at the TBPA binding sites. However, the effects on TBPA are usually not reflected by a large change in the levels of T_4. The normal values of TBG in adults are about 1.2 to 2.8 mg/dl.

Concentration of circulating thyroid-stimulating hormone

Measurements of serum TSH, together with T_4, have become one of the most important tools for screening thyroid function. Serum concentrations of TSH can be measured by specific RIA methods. The serum TSH values are expressed in microunits per milliliter of the reference standard. The TSH determination is used in neonatal thyroid screening tests, is useful in the diagnosis of hypothyroidism, is an indicator of the adequacy of thyroid hormone replacement therapy, and is used in the TRH stimulation test. The approximate normal adult values are 0.2 to 7.6 μU/ml. TSH is elevated in primary hypothyroidism. A surge of TSH release also occurs at parturition and reaches a peak within 2 hours after birth. TSH in the cord serum and in the serum after the first day of postnatal life is usually less than 20 μU/ml. Thus the TSH assay is useful for screening primary congenital hypothyroidism. Because of the limitation in the sensitivity of the assay, it is not possible to distinguish euthyroid individuals from those with secondary or tertiary hypothyroidism or thyrotoxicosis by the standard TSH assay alone. A highly sensitive RIA for TSH has been developed but is not widely used.

Assessment of thyroid autoantibodies

Numerous methods have been employed for detection of a large variety of thyroid antibodies. Only a few are available for routine use, however, and these assessments are rarely required during the neonatal period and infancy. Assays for antithyroglobulin antibodies (ATA) and antimicrosomal antibodies (AMA) are widely available; these antibodies are found in Hashimoto's thyroiditis. Long-acting thyroid stimulator (LATS), a serum component capable of prolonged stimulation of the thyroid gland, was initially detected in Graves' disease. Since that time several autoantibodies of the immunoglobulin G class have been described in patients with Graves' disease. These antibodies are now often called *thyroid-stimulating immunoglobulins (TSI)*, and appear to act against the TSH receptor in a biologically active fashion.

Rare cases of mothers with atrophic thyroids, in whom either AMA or TBIA was present, have given birth to children with a familial type of congenital hypothyroidism, presumably by transplacental transfer of some form of thyroid autoantibodies.

Measurement of circulating thyroglobulin

Previously it was believed that TG is present only in the thyroid gland. With the development of RIA for TG, it is now known that some TG appears in the circulation. The mean value of TG for normal adults is 4 mμg/ml, with a range of less than 1 to 30 mμg/ml. The mean value for preterm infants at birth is extremely high and rapidly decreases during the first 30 days of life for reasons not yet understood. The mean serum levels of TG for children 7 to 12 years of age is 50 mμg/ml, which progressively decrease to the adult mean value by 20 years of age. In athyroid cretinism the TG level is not detectable. Assessment of TG levels has been shown to be useful in differentiating medullary carcinoma from papillary-follicular carcinoma and in doing follow-up studies of patients treated for the latter type of thyroid carcinoma.

In vivo tests

The classic ^{131}I uptake test has been replaced largely by the use of ^{123}I to reduce radiation to the patient. ^{99m}Tc-pertechnetate also can be used for iodine-trapping studies, since this anion is trapped by the thyroid in similar fashion to iodine. However, pertechnetate is not organified and therefore is discharged early from the thyroid gland. Development of RIA techniques for determination of various thyroid hormones and TSH has largely obviated the need for radioiodine uptake studies in childhood. However, these tests are invaluable for diagnosing iodine-trapping defect and iodine organification defect. In addition to the thyroid gland, the salivary glands, gastric mucosa, uterus, small intestine, and mammary glands are capable of concentrating iodine. In patients with goitrous cretinism caused by iodine-trapping defects, the property of salivary glands to trap iodine can be exploited for diagnostic purposes. The trapping defect is shared by both the thyroid gland and the salivary glands in these patients.

Perchlorate discharge tests are used with the radioiodine uptake test to examine the organification of iodine (see following section on congenital hypothyroidism).

The TSH stimulation and T_3 suppression tests are now rarely used because of the availability of various hormone assays and the development of the TRH stimulation test.

A bolus infusion of TRH in amounts of 7 μg/kg body weight results in an increase of circulating TSH that peaks at 20 to 30 minutes. A peak increment of 10 to 30 μU/ml is seen in healthy children, with a progressive decline to basal levels by 2 to 3 hours. The serum T_3 levels peak at 3 to 4 hours and T_4 levels at 6 to 9 hours after the infusion. Therefore the TRH stimulation test can be used to examine the responsiveness of both TSH to TRH and TH to TSH, when necessary. Common practice, however, involves sampling of blood specimens before and after TRH infusion at 15- to 20-minute intervals up to 60 minutes. Patients with primary hypothyroidism have an exaggerated TSH response. Patients with hyperthyroidism and patients on adequate replacement therapy do not respond to TRH stimulation because of chronic suppression of their TSH by endogenous TH. Patients with secondary hypothyroidism do not respond to the TRH stimulation. Patients with tertiary hypothyroidism usually show a delayed response of TSH to TRH stimulation so that their 60-minute sample has a higher level of TSH than that found after 20 or 30 minutes. The TRH stimulation test is a useful tool in the diagnosis of borderline primary hypothyroidism and hyperthyroidism. Inappropriate response of TSH to TRH stimulation, however, has been observed in patients with malnutrition.

Thyroid imaging

The thyroid scan is usually performed by the use of ^{123}I, ^{125}I, or ^{99m}Tc-pertechnetate. The classic uses of thyroid scan were to localize and delineate functioning or nonfunctioning thyroid nodules and to visualize the irregular uptake pattern within the thyroid in Hashimoto's thyroiditis. This imaging technique is useful in the diagnosis of ectopic thyroid in neonates and infants. However, the risk of using radioisotopes in young children always should be kept in mind. During the first years of life, the thyroid gland is known to be highly sensitive to the radiation effects, resulting in development of thyroid carcinomas many years later.

Ultrasonography of the thyroid gland has been proved useful in distinguishing solid and cystic nodules of the thyroid and is occasionally used to localize the thyroid gland.

Biopsy and other tests

Biopsies and other tests are explained in the following section on congenital hypothyroidism.

THYROID FUNCTION: FETAL-MATERNAL RELATIONSHIP

See also Appendix C.

T_4 is detectable in the fetal serum by the twelfth week of gestation. Thereafter, both the total T_4 and FT_4 increase linearly in relation to the gestational age. The mean cord concentration of T_4 between 20 and 30 weeks' gestation is 5.5 ± 1.6 (SD) μg/dl. At term the T_4 reaches a level of 12.6 ± 4.0 (SD) μg/dl in the umbilical cord serum, which is 10% to 20% lower than the corresponding value in maternal serum. The FT_4 in the cord blood is equal to or higher than that in the maternal blood. Fetal T_4 metabolism differs markedly from that of postnatal life. In the fetus, T_4 is metabolized predominantly to reverse T_3 (rT_3), 3,3′,5′-triiodothyronine, rather than to T_3.

The rT_3 concentration exceeds 250 mμg/dl early in the third trimester and progressively decreases to a level of 150 to 200 mμg/dl at term. After the first 3 to 5 days of life a rapid decrease occurs in the concentration of rT_3, reaching the approximate adult level by 1 to 2 months of life. Reverse T_3 has minimum metabolic activity compared to T_3. Thus serum concentrations and production rates of rT_3 are much higher in the fetus, whereas concentrations of both T_3 and FT_3 in the fetal circulation are lower than in adults. The T_3 and FT_3 levels in the cord blood have been shown to be 30% to 50% of the maternal concentrations at term. TSH is also present in the 12-week-old fetus and rapidly rises thereafter, paralleling the increasing levels of FT_4. It does not correlate with levels of fetal T_4 or the maternal FT_4. The TSH level is higher in the fetus than in the mother, and at term the fetal value is more than twice that found in the mother. This suggests that fetal TSH regulates fetal thyroid function.

T_4-binding proteins also can be detected in the 12-week-old fetus. During early fetal life, T_4 seems to be bound mainly to the TBPA and albumin. The fetal concentration of TBG increases rapidly and by midgestation reaches a level close to that in a full-term infant. During early gestation, the rise of fetal TBG parallels the increase in T_4, and the proportion of T_4 bound to TBG similarly increases during this period. The binding capacity of TBG in premature and full-term infants is close to 1½ times that of the normal adult but is lower than that of the mother. The high level of TBG in the neonate is caused by a transplacental transfer of estrogens from the mother and, to a large extent, accounts for the high T_4 values in these infants. The serum TBG levels remain essentially unchanged during the first 5 days of life. TBPA is low in both newborn and maternal sera. The TBPA probably plays a minor role after midgestation.

Shortly after birth a transient but marked hyperactivity occurs in the thyroid function of neonates (Tables 37-3 and 37-4). Within the first minutes of life a dramatic release of TSH occurs, reaching a peak level of approximately 100 μU/ml at 30 minutes of age. This hypersecretion of TSH persists with decreasing intensity over the following 24 to 72 hours. Evidence shows that this acute rise of TSH may be stimulated, at least in part, by the drop in body temperature of the fetus with birth. In response to the postnatal TSH surge, the levels of T_4, FT_4, T_3, FT_3, and T_3U increase progressively during the first hours of extrauterine life, reaching a peak by about 48 hours of age. The increase in serum T_3 and FT_3 is more marked than that of T_4 and FT_4 during this period. Thus neonates experience a physiologic hyperthyroid state during the first several days of life. Absence of such chemical hyperthyroid state constitutes strong evidence for congenital hypothyroidism. The levels of these thyroid hormones remain elevated during the first 2 weeks of life and gradually fall thereafter, reaching high normal adult values by 4 to 6 weeks of age. True adult levels are not reached until puberty (Table 37-4). The postnatal

Table 37-3. Representative serum values of total and free thyroid hormones, TBG, and TSH in cord blood and early neonatal period compared with adult and maternal values*

References	Source of serum or age of infant	Number of subjects	T_4 (μg/dl)	FT_4 (mμg/dl)	T_3 (mμg/dl)	FT_3 (pg/dl)	TBG (mg/dl)	TSH (μU/ml)
Abuid, Stinson, and Larsen	Cord blood	7-8	12.0 ± 1.6	1.85 ± 0.22	49 ± 6	150 ± 20		
	15 minutes	5-6	13.3 ± 2.5		79 ± 13			
	90 minutes	7	14.1 ± 1.9		191 ± 16			
	24 hours	3-4	22.3 ± 1.6		262 ± 41			
	48 hours	3-4	21.9 ± 1.3		191 ± 37			
	Mothers at term	7-8	12.8 ± 1.4	1.40 ± 0.16	145 ± 12	310 ± 40		
Erenberg and others	Cord blood	26	11.9 ± 0.41	2.9 ± 0.12	50.5 ± 3.6	146 ± 12	5.4 ± 0.47	
	60 minutes	8-12			293	863		
	24 hours	10-21	16.2		419	1260		
	36-48 hours	9		7.0				
	60-72 hours	7-19		6.0	220	620		
	5 days	6	12.6					
	Pregnant women	17	14.3 ± 0.66	2.7 ± 0.15	173.0 ± 8.4	398 ± 30	8.7 ± 0.58	
	Adults	40	8.3 ± 0.38	2.4 ± 0.12	122.0 ± 5.3	378 ± 27	3.5 ± 0.67	
Abuid and others	Cord blood	27-30	10.9 ± 0.3	2.23 ± 0.12	48 ± 3	130 ± 10		8.5 ± 0.7
	3 days	23-26	17.2 ± 0.5	4.87 ± 0.33	125 ± 8	410 ± 20		7.3 ± 1.0
	6 weeks	15	10.3 ± 0.4	2.07 ± 0.08	163 ± 6	400 ± 20		<2.5
	Mothers at term	8	12.8 ± 1.4	1.40 ± 0.16	145 ± 12	310 ± 40		
	Adults	11	8.8 ± 0.5	1.92 ± 0.10	112 ± 5	290 ± 20		

*T_4, T_3, TBG, and TSH were measured by RIA methods, and FT_4 and FT_3 by assessment of the dialyzable fractions. All values are the mean or mean ± standard error of the mean.

Table 37-4. Normal range for T_4, T_3, T_3-resin uptake, TBG, and TSH in infancy and childhood*

	Total T_4 (μg/dl)		Total T_3 (ng/dl)		T_3-resin uptake (%)		TBG (mg/dl)		TSH (μU/ml)	
Age	**Mean**	**Range†**	**Mean**	**Range†**	**Mean**	**Range†**	**Mean**	**Range†**	**Mean**	**Range†**
Cord blood	10.2	7.4-13.0	45	15-75	0.90	0.75-1.05	5.6	—	9.0	<2.5-17.4
1 to 3 days	17.2	11.8-22.6	124	32-216	1.15	0.90-1.40	5.0	—	8.0	<2.5-13.3
1 to 2 weeks	13.2	9.8-16.6	250	—	1.00	0.85-1.15	—	—	—	—
2 to 4 weeks	11.0	7.0-15.0	160	160-240	0.95	0.80-1.15	—	—	4.0	0.6-10.0
1 to 4 months	10.3	7.2-14.4	163	117-209	0.90	0.75-1.05	—	—	<2.5	<2.5
4 to 12 months	11.0	7.8-16.5	176	110-280	0.98	0.88-1.12	4.4	3.1-5.6	2.1	0.6-6.3
1 to 5 years	10.5	7.3-15.0	168	105-269	0.99	0.88-1.12	4.2	2.9-5.4	2.0	0.6-6.3
5 to 10 years	9.3	6.4-13.3	150	94-241	1.00	0.88-1.12	3.8	2.5-5.0	2.0	0.6-6.3
10 to 15 years	8.1	5.6-11.7	113	83-213	1.01	0.88-1.12	3.3	2.1-4.6	1.9	0.6-6.3
Adult	8.4	4.3-12.5	125	70-204	1.01	0.85-1.14	3.5	2.1-5.5	1.8	0.2-7.6

From LaFranchi, S.H.: Pediatr. Clin. North Am. **26:**33, 1979.
*T_4, T_3, TSH, and TBG are measured by RIA.
†Range equals ±2 SD from mean value.

TSH surge occurs even in preterm and small for gestational age neonates, although the changes in serum TSH and in iodothyronines are smaller than those in healthy term infants. In preterm infants the T_4 levels may remain below those of full-term infants during the first weeks of life. However, FT_4 levels are generally in the normal ranges for adults, although low compared with healthy term infants. The T_4 levels in these infants reflect both the low TBG levels and the T_4 levels in relation to their TBG values. The TSH levels return to adult normal values after 3 to 5 days of postnatal life, regardless of gestational age.

Iodine kinetics in infants and children are also different from those in the adult. The thyroid weighs about 2 gm at birth, which is about one tenth of the adult weight. The 24-hour ^{131}I uptake by the thyroid is similar to that of the adult after the first month of age. Thus the concentration of ^{131}I per gram of thyroid tissue in the infant is greater than that in the adult. The thyroid of the infant is more susceptible to damage by radiation. The T_4 turnover rate is also higher in infants and children than in the adult. This accounts for the greater thyroid hormone requirement in children per unit of body weight.

In considering the fetal-maternal relationship, the placenta is of major importance. TSH does not cross the placental barrier, whereas TRH does. The placenta is almost completely impermeable to T_4 during the early stage of pregnancy, and at term the T_4 transport across the placenta is slow and limited. Thus the fetus during the first trimester either does not require T_4 for growth and development or is totally dependent on small amounts of maternal T_4. During the later stages of gestation, the fetus largely depends on its own T_4 production. Iodides cross the placenta readily. Iodides or iodine, when given in a large quantity, produces a transient inhibition of T_4 synthesis by diminishing the iodination process, probably through its effect on thyroidal autoregulation. Thus, in rare instances, iodine given to the mother in large amounts has produced goiter in the offspring.

Other clinically important compounds that can affect the fetal thyroid function by crossing the placenta from mother to fetus are the antithyroid compounds (goitrogens) and the thyroid autoantibodies. The former include perchlorates and thionamide compounds such as thiourea, thiouracil, propylthiouracil, methimazole, and carbimazole. Transplacental transfer of these drugs can result in fetal goiter with or without hypothyroidism. Transfer of TSI across the placenta into the fetus can result in neonatal thyrotoxicosis.

Thyroid hormones can be detected in the amniotic fluid. However, T_4, FT_4, T_3, and TSH levels in the amniotic fluids correlate poorly with maternal or fetal serum levels. In human milk, T_4 is present in insignificant amounts. The concentrations of T_3 and rT_3 in human milk vary considerably from specimen to specimen. However, it is suggested that the T_3 concentration in breast milk is insufficient to prevent the detrimental effects of hypothyroidism, although it may alleviate the symptoms in certain cases.

CONGENITAL HYPOTHYROIDISM (CRETINISM)

Congenital hypothyroidism, or cretinism, is a deficiency of the thyroid believed to have been present at or before birth. Cretinism must be diagnosed promptly because delay in treatment can lead to irreversible brain damage. Yet the overt signs of hypothyroidism are rarely present at birth, and abnormalities of thyroid function may be overlooked during the neonatal period. The dynamic changes in thyroid function following birth, the elevated levels of TBG in neonates, and the sudden deprivation of maternal T_4, however inefficient its transplacental transfer may be, all contribute to the difficulty in establishing a diagnosis.

Etiology and pathogenesis

The etiologic classification of congenital hypothyroidism is shown in the following outline. The term *sporadic cretinism* applies to all forms of primary congenital hypothyroidism, except those caused by dietary iodine deficiency and those caused by inborn errors of hormone synthesis or metabolism.

A. Primary hypothyroidism
   1. Defective embryogenesis of thyroid
      a. Agenesis (athyreosis)
      b. Dysgenesis
         (1) Thyroid remnant in normal location
         (2) Maldescent or ectopic thyroid gland
   2. Inborn error of hormone synthesis or metabolism (familial cretinism)
      a. Iodide-trapping defect
      b. Iodide organification defect
         (1) Without deafness
         (2) With deafness (Pendred's syndrome)
      c. Coupling defect of iodotyrosines
      d. Deiodination defect
         (1) Generalized
         (2) Limited to thyroid gland
         (3) Limited to peripheral tissues
      e. Defect of thyroglobulin
      f. Goiter with calcification
      g. Peripheral tissue unresponsiveness to thyroid hormone
      h. Unresponsiveness of thyroid to TSH
   3. Goitrous cretinism caused by maternal ingestion of goitrogens
   4. Iodine deficiency (endemic goiter)

B. Secondary and tertiary hypothyroidism
   1. TSH deficiency
   2. TRH deficiency

In contrast to the clear-cut preponderance of thyroid disorders in females over males during childhood and adult life, the sex difference in the incidence of congenital hypothyroidism is much less obvious. In North America the female/male ratio is about 2:1, as detected by neonatal screening programs. The relative incidence of each type of cretinism varies widely in different geographic locations.

In the nongoitrous regions, *defective embryogenesis* of the thyroid accounts for 70% to 85% of all cretinism. Failure in the anatomic development of the thyroid gland may be complete or partial. Residual thyroid tissue in the normal position or in ectopic areas is detected in 60% to 80% of infants and children with hypothyroidism. Ectopic thyroid is usually composed of a remnant of undescended thyroid tissue (cryptothyroid) and is situated in the midline. The undescended thyroid is located in the base of the tongue in about half the cases, between the tongue and the hyoid bone in about one fourth, and between the hyoid bone and normal location in the remaining cases. The ectopic tissue is often capable of undergoing compensatory hypertrophy when the hormone production becomes inadequate and may be found as a midline mass. The cause of defective embryogenesis of the thyroid is unknown. Dysgenesis of the thyroid can occasionally be a familial condition. Destruction of the fetal thyroid by maternal thyroid antibodies acquired transplacentally has been suggested as a possible etiologic factor in some instances of sporadic athyreotic cretinism.

Genetically determined *errors of T_4 synthesis or metabolism* involve deficiency of one or more enzymes necessary at various stages of the biosynthetic and metabolic pathways. Impaired hormonal secretion results in hypersecretion of TSH, usually leading to compensatory hyperplasia of the thyroid. Thus familial cretinism is often referred to as *goitrous cretinism*. Hypothyroidism or goiter or both may or may not be present in the newborn and infant, depending on the degree and time of onset of hormonal deficiency. Family members of a goitrous cretin often are found to have less severe defects manifested by goiter without associated hypothyroidism. The exact enzyme defect in some goitrous cretins, including those assumed to result from defects in the coupling mechanism and thyroglobulin synthesis, is still unknown.

Cretins caused by a *defect in the trapping of iodide* can be confused with infants with athyreosis because of the lack of administered radioiodine to concentrate in the neck. However, a goiter is present in these patients, and the saliva fails to concentrate radioiodine. The iodine-trapping defect is an autosomal recessive trait.

There are two types of *defects in the organification of iodide*: one in which iodide peroxidase is deficient or defective, and another in which an iodide transferase is lacking. The former is generally associated with more severe hypothyroidism. The latter is called *Pendred's syndrome* and is associated with congenital deafness and usually a small euthyroid goiter. Both types of iodide organification defects are transmitted as an autosomal recessive trait.

The mode of transmission of other inborn errors of thyroid hormone synthesis or metabolism has not been clearly established, although autosomal recessive inheritance has been suggested for most entities.

In the *coupling defect* of iodotyrosines, T_4 and T_3 are decreased, and MIT and DIT are increased in both the serum and the thyroid gland. In patients with deiodination defects there is a rapid turnover of thyroid iodine and wastage of iodotyrosines into the urine. The defect may be generalized, or it may be limited to intrathyroid or peripheral deiodination.

A *defect in thyroglobulin synthesis* was postulated in patients who had abnormal iodoproteins in their sera. Other unusual types of familial cretinism include a large kindred with goiter characterized by extensive intrathyroid calcification. The transmission pattern in this family suggests an autosomal dominant trait. A family with possible inability of the peripheral tissue to respond to T_4 also has been reported. The affected members of this family had deaf-mutism, goiter, delayed bone maturation, and elevated levels of PBI.

Unresponsiveness of the thyroid to TSH have been reported in two boys who had congenital hypothyroidism without a goiter. The serum TSH was elevated in these individuals, and TSH stimulation test gave no response. A coupling abnormality between the TSH receptor and the TSH receptor–adenylate cyclase system was suggested as the pathogenic process. Resistance to thyroid hormones by peripheral tissues without such resistance by the pituitary has also been reported. The patient was clinically hypothyroid and required huge amounts of thyroid hormone as replacement therapy. However, the test for TSH response to TRH stimulation was normal.

Maternal *ingestion of antithyroid drugs*, especially the thiocarbamides and potassium perchlorate, can cause neonatal goitrous hypothyroidism. Although the correlation between the dosage of drug and the incidence of neonatal goiter is poor, prolonged administration of large doses of these drugs increases the risk of goitrous cretinism. Administration of inorganic iodides to the mother in large amounts, usually for treatment of various respiratory disorders, can also produce a large congenital goiter filled with colloid (Fig. 37-22). Radioiodine treatment given to pregnant women during the second trimester has resulted in hypothyroidism in the offspring. The hypothyroidism was not obvious at birth in most instances.

Endemic goiter occurs in large geographic areas where dietary iodine is deficient. However, the incidence of goiter in neonates is relatively low in these areas, and many individuals living in the same environment do not develop goiter. These observations suggest that other factors may be superimposed on iodine deficiency. Further evidence suggests that iodine deficiency can result in neurologic impairment without manifesting in overt goitrous hypothyroidism *(neurologic endemic cretinism)*. Iodine deficiency results in altered iodine metabolism, and production of T_3 is increased relative to T_4

Secondary and tertiary hypothyroidism have been considered to be extremely rare in neonates. However, an increasing number of such infants have been discovered in recent years through neonatal thyroid screening programs. Most of these patients have TRH deficiency re-

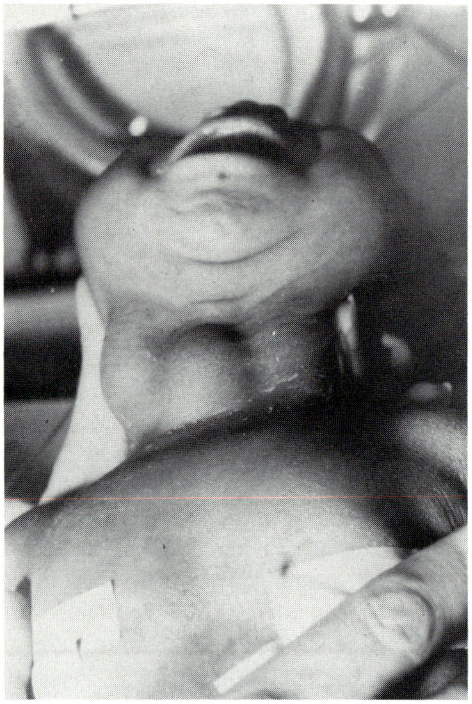

Fig. 37-22. Iodine-induced goiter in a neonate. The lateral bulging of the neck is caused by enlarged lateral lobes of the thyroid.

sulting in low serum levels of T_4 and TSH, but they do respond to TRH infusion by a sharp rise in circulating TSH. TSH deficiency is rare in neonates. Pituitary aplasia, when present, is usually associated with anencephaly or other severe malformations of the brain. These patients rarely survive beyond the neonatal period.

Neonatal screening for hypothyroidism and incidence of congenital hypothyroidism

The availability of highly sensitive and specific RIA systems for T_4 and TSH led to the development of screening programs for neonatal hypothyroidism. During the past decade, several states in the United States and provinces in Canada have mandated such screening through legislation, and screening programs have been established in Europe and Japan.

Most, if not all, programs in the United States use the filter paper spot technique. Capillary blood specimens from a heel stick are obtained at 2 to 5 days of life. The filter paper designed for this purpose bears printed circles. Blood samples are placed in these circular areas so as to fill and saturate the areas. Initially T_4 is measured from these specimens. Specimens that fall in the lowest, approximately third, percentile are subsequently subjected to TSH determinations. This method has the following advantages: (1) it can be easily incorporated into the existing metabolic-genetic screening programs (e.g., phenylketonuria screening); (2) it provides for a comprehensive screening capable of identifying infants with primary hypothyroidism and those at risk for secondary or tertiary hypothyroidism and TBG deficiency; (3) the selectivity is high, since the acute physiologic increase of T_4 at 2 to 5 days of life is lacking in hypothyroid infants; (4) it will detect most cases of compensated hypothyroidism; (5) it has the lowest recall rate of 1% to 2%; and (6) it appears to be capable of detecting nearly all infants with congenital hypothyroidism. Whereas a TSH level greater than 60 μU/ml is highly suggestive of congenital hypothyroidism in these screening tests, a significant number of infants have TSH values that fall between 25 and 50 μU/ml. These infants require close follow-up because many with these levels of TSH will eventually prove to have congenital hypothyroidism.

From various mass screening programs in North America, the overall incidence of congenital hypothyroidism appears to be about 1 in 3,500 to 4,000 births. Significantly, only 2.9% of 277 hypothyroid infants were suspected to be hypothyroid, on the basis of clinical evidence, before the reporting of the screening results in one survey. There is a female preponderance of 2:1 over males in the incidence of congenital hypothyroidism in North America. In the black population the incidence was about 1 in 32,000 births in one area of the United States, suggesting a racial difference in prevalence. The incidence of various types of neonatal hypothyroidism and TBG deficiency, as tabulated from several screening programs, is shown in Table 37-5. An estimate of the incidence of goitrous hypothyroidism is about 1 in 30,000 births in the United States. Infants with secondary (TSH deficiency) or tertiary (TRH deficiency) hypothyroidism comprise about 3% to 5% of the detected cases. Geographic differences exist in the prevalence of transient hypothyroidism, which is related to iodine intake. In areas with adequate iodine supply, most infants with transient hypothyroidism were born of mothers who received goitrogens during pregnancy. However, several infants were found to have idiopathic transient hypothyroidism with an elevated TSH.

Widespread use of screening programs has lead to an increased frequency of diagnosing TBG deficiency. This X-linked trait occurs as frequently as 1 in 10,000 births. The T_4 and TSH concentration will be low, with the T_3U elevated. The diagnosis can be confirmed by a very low TBG concentration measured by a specific RIA. It is important to identify these infants, since they have normal FT_4 levels and should not be treated with thyroid hormone.

Premature infants frequently have low levels of T_4 and FT_4 when compared with the normal range for full-term infants. Serious illness is also associated with low T_4 values. With gestations less than 30 weeks, low TBG may

Table 37-5. Incidence of various neonatal hypothyroidism and TBG deficiency

	Primary hypothyroidism		Secondary and tertiary hypothyroidism	Transient hypothyroidism	TBG deficiency
	1 in 4,254		1 in 68,200	1 in 37,370	1 in 8,913
Aplastic or hypoplastic gland (63%)	Normal or enlarged gland (14%)	Ectopic thyroid tissue (23%)			

be present, but after 30 weeks TBG has reached the level present at term and therefore does not account for the low levels of T_4. In one study 25% of preterm infants had low T_4 and TSH levels. TBG was normal and TSH not elevated. TRH administration produced a rise in TSH and T_4, suggesting that the defect was in the hypothalamus (tertiary hypothyroidism). By 6 months of age all infants had T_4 levels in the normal range, thus documenting the transient nature of the defect. Developmental attainment at 1 year of age was equal to a matched control group that did not have low T_4 levels.

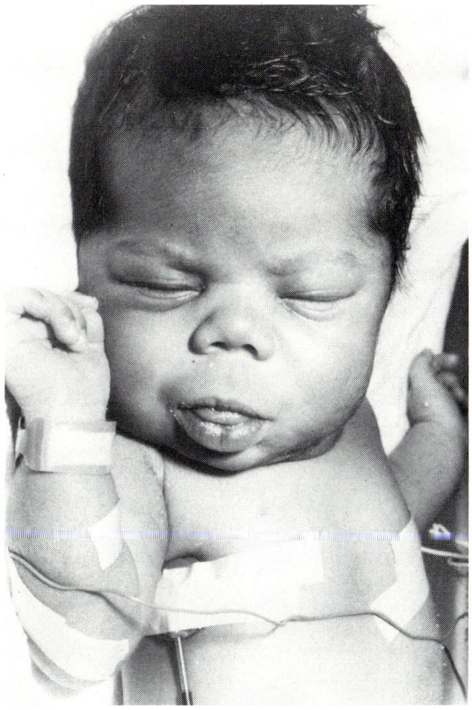

Fig. 37-23. Typical facial features of cretinism.

Clinical manifestations

Even in the athyreotic cretins, the classic clinical features of cretinism are usually absent at birth and appear only gradually over about 6 weeks. In patients with a functional remnant of thyroid tissue and in patients with some types of familial cretinism, the clinical manifestations may be delayed several months or years, depending on the functional state of the thyroid. Nevertheless, signs of hypothyroidism can be detected by careful observation within the first few weeks of life in more severe forms of cretinism. The early manifestations include lethargy, inactivity, hypotonia, large anterior and posterior fontanels, feeding difficulty, respiratory distress, pallor, perioral cyanosis, mottled skin, poor or hoarse cry, constipation, and hypothermia. The feeding difficulty is often first noted by the mother or a nurse as the infant readily falls asleep after sucking for a short period, necessitating repeated stimulation and thus requiring a prolonged period to complete the feeding. The respiratory distress is caused by myxedema of the airway and is characterized by noisy breathing, nasal stuffiness, and intermittent cyanosis, especially in the perioral area. These respiratory symptoms may lead one to suspect congenital anomalies of the airway or congenital heart disease. After the first 2 weeks of life, prolonged physiologic jaundice may be an indication of hypothyroidism. The jaundice may appear to be further prolonged when carotenemia is superimposed after feeding a diet high in carotene.

The classic features of cretinism usually occur after about 6 weeks of life (Fig. 37-23). These include the typical facies, characterized by depressed nasal bridge, relatively narrow forehead, and puffy eyelids, thick, dry, and cold skin; coarse hair, which may appear long and abundant; large tongue; abdominal distension; umbilical hernia, hyporeflexia, bradycardia, hypotension with narrow pulse pressure; anemia; and widely patent cranial sutures.

Lingual thyroid occasionally can be seen in infants and children as a discrete round mass at the base of the tongue, especially when it is hypertrophied from endogenous TSH stimulation (Fig. 37-24). The base of the tongue must be firmly depressed to visualize this mass.

In some instances, sublingual thyroid is palpable as a round midline mass deep under the mandible.

Neonatal goiters may be extremely large, asymmetric, and grotesque and may be confused with a hygroma or other type of mass (Fig. 37-22). Alternatively, the goiter may be quite small and escape notice on a cursory examination.

The onset of symptoms in infants with secondary or tertiary hypothyroidism tends to be gradual because

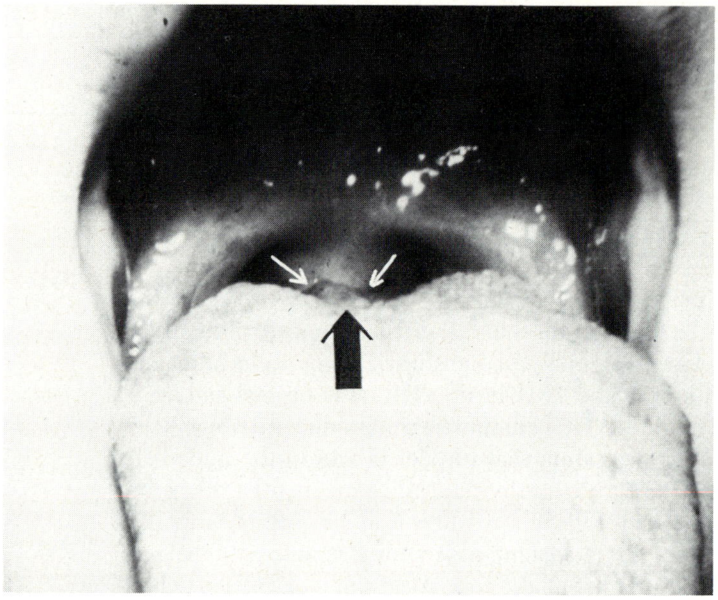

Fig. 37-24. Visualization of a lingual thyroid.

some T_4 production occurs. However, signs of other pituitary hormone deficiencies and/or signs of congenital midbrain defects are typically present. These include neonatal hypoglycemia, small penis, hypospadias, undescended testes, wandering nystagmus, and cleft lip or palate. Growth failure will ensue in these patients.

Laboratory manifestations

No single test exists by which a diagnosis of cretinism can be established. When the diagnosis is suspected, several appropriate thyroid function tests should be employed. It is advisable to assess both the T_4 level and the saturation of T_4-binding proteins. Elevated levels of serum TSH may be a reliable indication of cretinism. However, the TSH level in the cord blood is normally higher than the adult value, and a physiologic TSH surge occurs during the first 48 hours of life, as noted earlier. The results of these tests must be interpreted in combination and in light of the infant's age and the clinical evidence for hypothyroidism. The typical laboratory findings for primary hypothyroidism are low T_4, low T_3U and FT_4I, and elevated TSH. In secondary and tertiary hypothyroidism TSH is low as well as T_4, T_3U, and FT_3I. When these findings are present, further investigation, including assessment of FT_4, T_3, FT_3, and TBG, may or may not be necessary to establish the diagnosis. Many acute and chronic nonthyroidal illnesses, including the respiratory distress syndrome, affect some thyroid function tests but do not produce hypothyroidism. The typical laboratory findings are low serum T_4, FT_4, and T_3, elevated rT_3, and normal TSH. In certain types of hypothyroidism, such as iodine-deficient cretinism, preferential synthesis of T_3 may occur. Therefore normal or high T_3 alone does not exclude hypothyroidism any more than normal T_4 does.

When a confusing situation arises, such as borderline values in the screening tests, the TRH stimulation test is usually helpful (see previous section on in vivo tests).

Severe hyponatremia in association with inappropriate antidiuretic hormone secretion is known to occur in elderly individuals with hypothyroidism. This syndrome has been reported in at least one infant with congenital hypothyroidism.

Retardation of bone maturation is present in about half of the cretins at birth. Thus the assessment of bone age is particularly useful in the newborn. However, roentgenographic examination of the hand and wrist, which is most often used in estimating bone age, is almost totally useless during the neonatal period, since the first ossification center, the hamate, does not appear in the normal infant until 3 to 4 months of age. Retardation of bone maturation in neonates is best assessed by roentgenographic examination of the knee and the foot. The ossification centers of the calcaneus and talus appear at about 26 to 28 weeks' gestation and the distal femur at about 34 to 36 weeks. The proximal tibial epiphyses appear at about 35 weeks' gestation. The absence of the distal femoral epiphyses in a newborn weighing 3,000 gm or more or the absence of the distal femoral and proximal tibial epiphyses in an infant weighing 2,500 to 3,000 gm at birth suggests intrauterine thyroid hormone deficiency.

Ossification of the cartilages of the epiphyses is also disturbed in hypothyroidism. Normally, ossification begins from the center of the cartilage and extends peripherally in an orderly manner. In hypothyroidism cal-

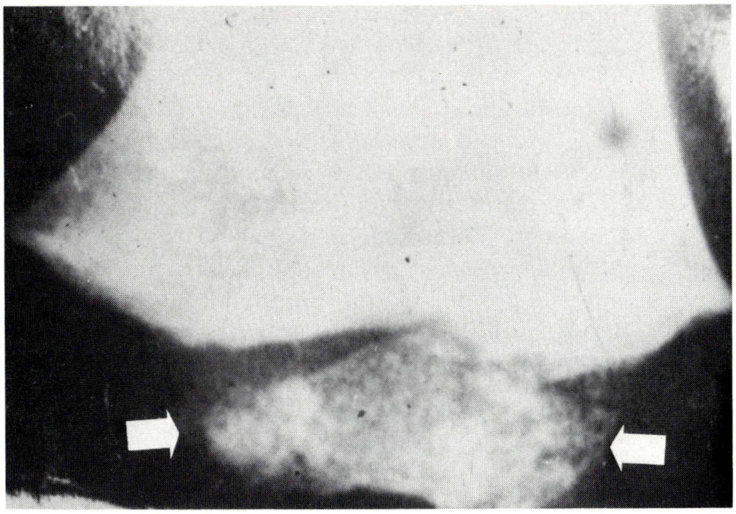

Fig. 37-25. Epiphyseal dysgenesis of the distal femoral center.

cification of epiphyseal centers starts from multiple irregular foci scattered in the developing cartilage. The irregular calcification pattern appears in the roentgenogram as stippled or fragmented ossification centers and is referred to as *epiphyseal dysgenesis* (Fig. 37-25). This finding is highly characteristic of hypothyroidism and provides a strong clue for the diagnosis. A roentgenographic examination of the knee and the foot is useful in detecting epiphyseal dysgenesis during the neonatal period. Abnormal changes occur in the epiphyseal cartilage secondary to thyroid hormone deficiency before calcification, so that even after the hypothyroidism is treated, the characteristic pattern of calcification, epiphyseal dysgenesis, may appear in all centers that normally would have calcified during the period of deficiency.

A goiter and tracheal compression by an enlarged thyroid also may be visualized by roentgenographic examination of the neck.

An estimate of visceral myxedema may be made by detecting a low voltage of all complexes in the ECG and EEG. A roentgenogram of the chest also may reveal the presence of cardiomegaly, reflecting myxedema of the heart.

Measurements of the serum cholesterol levels and the BMR are not reliable diagnostic aids in the assessment of thyroid function during the neonatal period. Tests that use in vivo administration of radioiodine or technetium 99 are unnecessary for the diagnosis of many cretins. However, a radioiodine uptake test can be used to confirm the presence of an agenetic or dysgenetic thyroid. The thyroid 24-hour uptake of radioiodine is variable during the first several weeks and may exceed 90% during the first week of life. A 24-hour uptake of less than 2% is highly suggestive of thyroid agenesis, and if the uptake is less than 10%, presence of a dysgenetic thyroid can be suspected. An ectopic thyroid is usually not detected by the radioiodine uptake test because of the relatively small aperture of the counter used for such a study. In neonates radioiodine should be administered through a nasogastric tube, and the tube should then be flushed with water to prevent any loss of the tracer. To detect an undescended thyroid, a scintillation scan of the pharyngeal area and the neck may be obtained after administration of radioiodine.

The presence of defective iodine-trapping mechanism can be suspected in goitrous cretins when the thyroid fails to concentrate radioiodine within 2 to 4 hours after oral administration of the tracer. The defect can be demonstrated by comparing the radioiodine concentrations in simultaneously obtained samples of the saliva and plasma 1 to 2 hours after the administration of the tracer. In the normal individual the salivary concentration is about tenfold greater than that in the plasma, whereas the salivary glands of patients with defective iodine trapping fail to concentrate radioiodine.

In patients with an iodide organification defect, the iodide taken up by the thyroid is readily released from the gland. When the thyroid uptake of radioiodine is measured at 2, 4, 6, and 24 hours after oral administration of radioiodine in these patients, the uptake may be normal or elevated during the earlier hours. However, the uptake rapidly declines within 24 hours. In normal individuals, on the other hand, the thyroid uptake of radioiodine gradually increases during the first 4 to 6 hours and remains at a plateau level of 15% to 30% of the administered dose at the end of 24 hours. When rapid organification of inorganic iodide fails to take place in the thyroid, an anion such as perchlorate can competitively inhibit the iodine accumulation, and a net loss of iodide from the gland occurs. This property of perchlorate is used in the perchlorate discharge test. This test involves measuring the 2-hour thyroid uptake of radioiodine and then administering sodium or potassium perchlorate orally in amounts of 10 mg/kg body weight. One to 2 hours thereafter, the thyroid uptake is remeasured. If the uptake decreases by more than 10% to 15% of the initial value, the presence of a defect in normal organification of iodide is suggested.

Differentiation among other types of familial cretinism is more difficult and often technically impossible to achieve during infancy. The studies required for the differential diagnosis usually involve administration of radioactive substances in doses greater than considered safe for infants. Studies on iodine kinetics in blood specimens obtained after administration of radioiodine and/or in tissue culture specimens obtained by biopsy may be necessary for the differential diagnosis. Thus, in most instances, patients should be treated for a few years and a definitive study undertaken at a later date. However, secretion of abnormal iodoproteins into the circulation, as would occur in the coupling defect of iodotyrosines, can be suspected when there is a greater than normal discrepancy between the PBI level and the T_4 value.

The diagnosis of cretinism caused by maternal ingestion of goitrogens is usually established from the history and is confirmed by its self-limiting course. The reactions to the perchlorate discharge test are positive in both iodine-induced goiter and following administration of antithyroid drugs. The urinary iodine concentration is elevated in infants with transient hypothyroidism caused by iodine excess.

In iodine deficiency the T_4, T_3, and TSH levels in the cord blood may be normal. Elevation of the TSH levels and a decrease in the T_4 levels may occur only occasionally after birth. The test results from the neonatal thyroid screening program may overlap with the normal range. The urinary concentration of iodine is low (<12 μg/dl) in these infants, and the radioiodine uptake is elevated.

Secondary hypothyroidism may be suspected in infants with both low T_4 and TSH. The TRH infusion test may be employed to distinguish hypothalamic TRH deficiency from pituitary TSH deficiency.

Transient disorders of thyroid function

Several clinical entities of neonates and infants must be distinguished from permanent disorders of thyroid function. The results of neonatal screening tests from these patients may mimic those found in permanent hypothyroidism and lead to an erroneous diagnosis.

Transient primary neonatal hypothyroidism

Transient hypothyroidism may occur in apparently healthy term infants. In geographic areas where dietary supply of iodine is insufficient, transient neonatal hypothyroidism lasting more than several weeks may be seen. The T_4 levels are low and the TSH levels are generally elevated in these infants, but these tests results may overlap with the normal range. In many cases the T_4, T_3, and TSH levels in the cord blood of the affected infants were found to be normal, suggesting that the hypothyroidism developed only after birth. The hypothyroidism and goiter in these infants may be corrected readily by administration of iodine.

Transplacental passage of antithyroid drugs from the mother may cause transient hypothyroidism with a goiter in the neonate. Excessive supply of iodine may also cause transient hypothyroidism. Iodine-containing radiopaque dye injected into amniotic cavity has led to the development of transient neonatal hypothyroidism without a goiter. Excessive application of iodine-containing antiseptics to intact skin has also resulted in transient hypothyroidism in the infant. Transient neonatal hypothyroidism caused by transplacental transfer of maternal TBIA has been reported. In these infants goiter was not present.

The thyroid function reverts to normal either spontaneously or after a short period of therapy in patients with transient primary hypothyroidism. Nevertheless, these patients probably should be treated until their TSH levels revert to and remain within the normal range in order to protect their brain development.

Transient hypothyroxinemia

Transient hypothyroxinemia is seen to some extent in all preterm infants. It is related to an immaturity of the hypothalamic-pituitary axis. The serum T_4 levels are low, but the TSH levels are normal. Low FT_4 and normal TSH responses to TRH stimulation are found in these babies. The serum TBG levels are only slightly low in preterm infants and do not account for the degree of hypothyroxinemia. When the dietary supply of iodine is slightly deficient, low T_4 and FT_4 levels in preterm infants may be accompanied by high TSH levels and exaggerated TSH responses to TRH stimulation. Thus preterm infants living in iodine-deficient areas are exposed to the combined risk of transient tertiary and primary hypothyroidism. The prevalence of transient hypothyroxinemia in one U.S. screening program was 1 in 6,000 births. The T_4 levels on repeated evaluation at 3 to 4 months of age were normal in all the infants in this series. Treatment with thyroid hormones is not indicated in patients with transient hypothyroxinemia.

Transient hyperthyrotropinemia

Transient hyperthyrotropinemia is characterized by elevated serum TSH levels during the neonatal period, despite normal T_4 and FT_4 levels. The elevated TSH levels may persist from a few days to several months. The infants are asymptomatic, and the etiology is unknown. However, these infants must be followed closely to exclude the possibility of impending overt hypothyroidism.

Euthyroid sick syndrome (low T_3 syndrome)

Since the first description of greatly decreased T_3 levels in moribund patients, several investigations have led to the concept that alteration in thyroid hormone occurs as an adaptive response to slow body metabolism in severely ill patients. The syndrome has been variously called euthyroid sick syndrome or low T_3 syndrome and has been recognized in infants and children. These patients may have severe, nonthyroidal illnesses that are either acute or chronic.

The consistent finding is depression of the serum T_3 level, often into the hypothyroid range. This decrease is accompanied by an increase in the rT_3 level in most instances. The Serum T_4 level may be low or normal, and the FT_4 level may be increased or normal, depending on the metabolic clearance rate of the T_4. Serum TBG level may be low or normal, and serum TSH levels are normal. In preterm infants the serum levels of T_4, FT_4, and T_3 are naturally low, and the level of rT_3 is high. Thus preterm infants may present a confusing situation when they are ill from nonthyroid diseases.

In the neonatal period preterm infants with respiratory distress syndrome have been the most frequently encountered patients with euthyroid sick syndrome. In children a variety of nonthyroidal illnesses have been associated with this syndrome. These include severe gastroenteritis, acute leukemia, anorexia nervosa, renal disease, burns, and surgical stress. Alteration in T_4 metabolism to favor production of rT_3 over T_3 appears to occur rapidly under certain stress. Euthyroid sick syndrome has been seen in patients 24 hours after cardiac surgery. The abnormal thyroid function gradually reverts back to normal as their primary illness improves. Treatment with thyroid hormones is not indicated in these patients. However, preterm infants at risk should be followed by serial determinations of T_4, T_3, rT_3, FT_4, TSH, and TBG levels.

Differential diagnosis

Errors in diagnosis of cretinism usually result from a failure to suspect the condition or from diagnosing other disorders as hypothyroidism. These errors typically arise from basing the diagnosis on a few suggestive clinical features and misinterpreting the laboratory data.

During the early neonatal period, respiratory difficulty, pallor, and cyanosis in cretinism must be differentiated from other common causes of respiratory distress and from congenital heart disease. Lethargy, inactivity, hypotonia, and feeding difficulty may be mistaken for manifestations of sepsis or brain damage from a variety of causes. The prolonged jaundice in cretinism must not be confused with icterus caused by hemolytic anemia, septicemia, or hepatic disease. The coarse facial features, macroglossia, and dry skin of cretinism can mislead one to suspect Hurler's syndrome, chondrodystrophy, or mongolism. In rare instances hypothyroidism has been found in patients with mongolism. A large goiter must not be confused with a hygroma, cyst, or tumor of the neck. A lingual thyroid, when visible or obstructing the airway, has been mistaken for a tumor of the pharyngeal area. Although epiphyseal dysgenesis may resemble osteochondritis deformans in its roentgenographic appearance, the latter does not occur during the neonatal period.

Treatment

All hypothyroid infants, with or without goiter, should be rendered euthyroid as promptly as possible by substitution therapy. Neonates with a euthyroid goiter should be regarded as being in a state of impending hypothyroidism and in most instances should be treated. Desiccated thyroid, sodium-L-thyroxine, or triiodothyronine can be used for treatment. Desiccated thyroid has the advantages of being inexpensive and maintaining the T_4 value within the normal range when the patient is rendered euthyroid. Desiccated thyroid has an estimated plasma half-life of 6.9 days in the adult; its latent period, the interval between administration of the drug and the onset of its effect, is longer than that of T_3. One drawback in using desiccated thyroid for replacement has been reported. Daily doses of desiccated thyroid sufficient to maintain a clinical euthyroid state and normal serum T_4 and TSH levels produced serum T_3 levels higher than the normal range in most children and adolescents. Such elevation of T_3 was not induced by appropriate doses of sodium-L-thyroxine. The authors suggest that sodium-L-thyroxine is the drug of choice for treatment of hypothyroidism. Sodium-L-thyroxine is better standardized for its potency than desiccated thyroid but will result in slightly elevated T_4 value.

In the treatment of infants with severe myxedema, possible complications should be kept in mind. Cardiac insufficiency from overtaxing the myxedematous heart by too rapid a mobilization of the myxedema fluid into the circulation is well known in the adult. This complication is prevented by administering a small dose of thyroid hormone at first and gradually increasing the dosage. The infant, however, generally tolerates a rapid restoration to the euthyroid state better than the adult, and some authors have advocated a prompt restoration of T_4 to a normal value. I believe that thyroid hormone should be increased judiciously when evidence of severe myxedema, particularly of the heart, is present. Aspiration of food is another complication of cretins; it may occur after therapy has been started, when the infants begin to feed more vigorously. It results from an impairment in swallowing, caused by myxedema of the pharyngeal area, compounded by increased appetite as the euthyroid state is restored. Therefore, when myxedema is severe, the infant should be fed carefully and slowly by an expert nurse during the early phase of treatment.

There are different views on the exact mode of treatment of severe cretinism. Because of the more rapid action and shorter biologic half-life of T_3, the use of L-thyronine has been favored by some authors. An initial single dose of 0.025 to 0.05 mg/day has been advocated for full-term newborns with congenital hypothyroidism. In preterm infants the starting dose of 0.025 mg/day has been used. However, in severely myxedematous infants it may be wise to start with about one third of these doses, which may be increased every 2 to 3 days until reaching the full replacement dose. It is more convenient to discontinue the L-thyronine and switch to sodium-L-thyroxine once the euthyroid state is achieved so that serum T_4 levels may be used as an accurate indicator of the adequacy of replacement therapy. The average dose of sodium-L-thyroxine required for treatment is about 0.008 mg/kg/day during the first year, 0.005 mg/kg/day from 1 to 6 years of age, and 0.004 mg/kg/day thereafter. Treatment of each patient must be individualized. The dosage should be adjusted so that a clinical euthyroid state and high normal serum T_4 levels can be maintained. The initially elevated serum TSH levels in primary hypothyroidism may not suppress to the normal range for many months despite an adequate replacement therapy. Therefore TSH levels should not be used as the sole criterion for evaluating the adequacy of treatment.

Patients with a euthyroid goiter may be placed on a maintenance dosage of thyroid hormone immediately.

Until hypothyroidism is corrected, the infant should be kept under careful observation, and cardiovascular function should be monitored. Clinical observation should be supplemented by following the growth curve, the maturation of the bones, and the T_4 levels. All congenital hypothyroid patients, except those whose condition was caused by maternal ingestion of goitrogens and by iodine deficiency, require lifetime substitution therapy.

Goitrous cretinism caused by maternal ingestion of goitrogens is a self-limiting condition. The blocking effect of antithyroid drugs usually disappears several days after birth. Therefore, if the goiter is small and the patient is euthyroid, no treatment is required. If the patient is hypothyroid, however, or if the goiter is large, it is safer to treat the infant for several weeks or months. Shrinkage of the goiter may be hastened by substitution therapy, and the treatment can be withdrawn after the thyroid returns to normal size. Occasionally the goiter may be huge, and asphyxia may occur in the neonate from a goiter that encircles the trachea. This complication is most often seen in iodide-induced goiter and constitutes a medical emergency. Antithyroid agents are secreted in breast milk. Therefore, mothers who are taking antithyroid medications should not nurse their infants.

Endemic cretins should be given substitution therapy for an indefinite period, unless iodine prophylaxis can be ensured in the specific geographic location.

Prognosis

Shortly after adequate substitution therapy is instituted, all clinical manifestations of hypothyroidism will disappear, and accelerated linear growth will occur if growth was retarded before the treatment. After a period of "catch-up" growth, an optimum rate of growth will be maintained. Goiter or hypertrophied ectopic thyroid will gradually shrink in size when the patient is properly treated. The coarse hair is gradually lost and is replaced by finer, normal hair over several months. The marked acceleration in bone maturation (catch-up) occurs after a latent period of a few months, and thereafter the osseous development should parallel the chronologic age. When hypothyroidism is treated with a slightly excessive dosage of thyroid hormones for a prolonged period, the bone maturation may gradually exceed the chronologic age, even though the patient may fail to show overt signs of hyperthyroidism or have clearly elevated levels of T_4. With substitution therapy, epiphyseal dysgenesis will appear in centers that failed to calcify while the patient was hypothyroid, and then the calcification will coalesce to form a normal epiphysis.

Although the prognosis for physical recovery is good, the prognosis for normal mental and neurologic performance is uncertain and less favorable. The eventual IQ of severely affected infants with congenital hypothyroidism is inversely related to the duration of thyroid hormone deficiency. Irreversible brain damage can occur from fetal hypothyroidism as well as from postnatal hormone deficiency. Therefore the prognosis for mental development should be guarded, even if the treatment is initiated soon after birth. The mental ability of neonates with marked delay in the bone maturation is likely to be worse than in those with mild or no retardation in bone age. Mental and neurologic competence of cretins is also related to the severity of hypothyroidism. However, even mildly affected patients, treated promptly after birth, may have impairment of arithmetic ability, speech, or fine motor coordination in later life. In infants with congenital hypothyroidism who were started on replacement therapy before 3 months of age, more than 80% had an IQ greater than 85. However, 77% of these infants showed some signs of minimum brain damage.

GOITERS

Most neonatal goiters result from maternal ingestion of goitrogens. Prominent goiter only occasionally is the manifestation of familial goitrous cretinism. Most euthyroid goiters of newborns are caused by compensatory hypertrophy of the thyroid and thus are potentially indicative of impending hypothyroidism. Therefore these goiters should be treated appropriately.

Congenital neoplasms of the thyroid rarely occur. They include Hürthle cell tumor and adenocarcinoma. I have also encountered a teratoma of the thyroid in a newborn that was suggested by calcification within the thyroid. Neoplasm can be suspected when a nodular goiter is present. Radioiodine scintiscan reveals a cold nodular area corresponding to the location of the neoplasm when uptake of radioiodine is lacking. A diagnosis of neoplasm should be confirmed by a biopsy.

THYROTOXICOSIS

Etiology and pathogenesis

Neonatal thyrotoxicosis may occur by transplacental transfer of TSI from the mother. Approximately 50% of patients are born to mothers known to have Graves' disease either before or during the pregnancy. However, neonatal thyrotoxicosis may occur in infants without detectable TSI, and mothers with detectable TSI may give birth to normal infants. Family studies, observation of twins, and age-specific incidence rates suggest that this disease occurs at random in a genetically preselected population. Thus the pathogenesis of congenital Graves' disease has proved elusive, although TSI must play a major role.

Clinical manifestations

When neonatal thyrotoxicosis occurs in the infant born to a mother with untreated active Graves' disease, the clinical manifestations of hyperthyroidism may become apparent within the first 24 hours of life. Infants may be born prematurely from such a mother. Irritability, excessive movement, tremor, flushing of the cheeks, sweating, increased appetite, weight loss or lack of weight gain, supraventricular tachycardia, goiter, and exophthalmos may be observed. Although a goiter is inevitably present in neonatal thyrotoxicosis, its size varies considerably; it may be small and escape notice on a cursory examination, or it may be large enough to cause tracheal compression. Furthermore, the goiter may increase in size during the early neonatal period. Exophthalmos is usually mild when present. Hepatosplenomegaly, thrombocytopenia, and hypoprothrombinemia have been reported in isolated instances. In severe neonatal thyrotoxicosis, hyperthermia, arrhythmias, and cardiac failure may occur; if the condition is untreated, death may ensue.

The course of the syndrome in classic form is self-limited because of the gradual depletion of transplacentally acquired TSI. The signs and symptoms subside spontaneously after 3 to 12 weeks, depending on the severity of the disease, which in turn is probably related to the titer of TSI in the plasma of the neonate. Goiter, however, may persist for some time after all signs of hyperthyroidism disappear. The thyroid gradually returns to normal size. It has been emphasized recently that, in other forms, neonatal thyrotoxicosis may not be a transient disorder and may persist for months or years.

In the infant born to a mother who received antithyroid medications for treatment of Graves' disease during the latter part of pregnancy, the onset of clinical manifestations may be modified by transplacental acquisition of the antithyroid agent as well as TSI. At birth the infant may be euthyroid or even hypothyroid, and the presence of a goiter may be the only abnormal feature. Since the plasma half-life of antithyroid agents is short, the typical manifestations of neonatal thyrotoxicosis may appear several days after birth. If the infant is born in a hypothyroid state, a period of euthyroidism may follow within a few days, and thyrotoxicosis may not occur until 5 to 7 days after birth.

Diagnosis and differential diagnosis

A maternal history of Graves' disease before or during pregnancy is important in the diagnosis of neonatal thyrotoxicosis. Information concerning the treatment of maternal hyperthyroidism also must be obtained. The infant should be examined repeatedly for signs of thyrotoxicosis, and the neck should be palpated carefully to detect a goiter. Determination of FT_4 should be obtained, together with an assessment of T_4-binding protein saturation. The data should be interpreted in relation to the clinical features and age of the neonate. The determination of radioiodine uptake by the thyroid has little value during the neonatal period. A high titer of TSI will strongly support the diagnosis of neonatal thyrotoxicosis. Serial determinations of TSI in the neonate are also helpful.

In the euthyroid or hypothyroid neonate born to a mother who received antithyroid medication during the latter part of pregnancy, it is almost impossible to predict whether thyrotoxicosis will ensue. Therefore serial examinations of the infant must be undertaken during the first 10 days of life.

Although neonatal thyrotoxicosis can be confused with various neurologic disorders, congenital heart disease, or sepsis, a positive maternal history of Graves' disease and the presence of a goiter should readily alert one to the correct diagnosis. In normal neonates and infants the thyroid gland is rarely palpable. Therefore, in general, a palpable thyroid in these individuals should be regarded as a goiter.

Extremely rare cases of thyrotoxicosis are characterized by a total or partial loss of peripheral tissue response to endogenous or exogenous thyroid hormone. The syndrome is called *thyroid hormone resistance*. In these patients the serum level of FT_4 can be elevated without clinical manifestation of hyperthyroidism. When the resistance to circulating thyroid hormone is limited to the pituitary gland, the TSH level is elevated. These patients may have the clinical manifestation of mild hyperthyroidism and are distinguishable by the high levels of TSH.

Treatment

The treatment of thyrotoxicosis in a neonate is similar to that in an older child and involves the use of antithyroid drugs. Care should be exercised not to induce hypothyroidism with excessive medication. Iodine (Lugol's Solution), propylthiouracil, or methimazole is typically used. Lugol's Solution can be given in doses of 1 drop three times daily. Although iodine rapidly inhibits the release of T_4 from the thyroid, its effect tends to disappear after several weeks. Propylthiouracil is given orally in amounts of 10 mg/kg/day in three divided doses at 8-hour intervals. Methimazole is given in amounts of 1 mg/kg/day in three divided doses. Circulating T_4 has a half-life of 6.9 days, and therefore little or no clinical response to antithyroid drugs can be expected during the first few days of therapy. After 1 to 3 months of therapy the dosage of antithyroid drug should be reduced or its administration discontinued to determine whether the disease has a self-limited course.

Most signs and symptoms of hyperthyroidism, including the cardiovascular manifestations, are closely related to increased adrenergic response. Antiadrenergic agents therefore can alleviate many of the untoward manifestations of thyrotoxicosis. In contrast to antithyroid drugs, these agents can rapidly diminish the severity of thyrotoxicity, and their effects are evident within a few hours. Thus reserpine or propranolol hydrochloride, together with iodine or propylthiouracil, may be used in the treatment of severe neonatal thyrotoxicosis. Propranolol hydrochloride is given orally in a dosage of 2 mg/kg/day in two or more divided doses. Digitalization may be necessary in neonates with cardiac failure. Under these circumstances reserpine may be contraindicated or must be used with extreme caution. A large goiter compressing the trachea and resulting in asphyxia must be treated surgically by splitting the isthmus.

The euthyroid or hypothyroid infant born to a mother who received antithyroid medications during pregnancy should be managed as described in the section on congenital hypothyroidism, since these neonates may or may not be kept under close observation. If the infant has already received thyroid hormone, it should be discontinued as soon as thyrotoxic manifestations occur, and appropriate management of hyperthyroidism must be initiated. A mother who is receiving an antithyroid medication should not be allowed to breast-feed the infant, since these agents are secreted into the milk.

Prognosis

Neonatal thyrotoxicosis carries a mortality of about 15% if it is not recognized and treated properly. However, in many instances the syndrome has a self-limited duration and no sequelae have been recognized. A goiter may resolve slowly over several months. Premature closure of all cranial sutures occasionally occurs. It is advisable to obtain a roentgenogram of the skull at 6 to 12 months of age.

FAMILIAL ABNORMALITIES OF THYROXINE-BINDING GLOBULIN

Genetic disorders resulting in either increased or decreased levels of TBG have been reported. Affected individuals are healthy and asymptomatic, since a change in the level of TBG does not lead to an alteration of the FT_4 level. The disorders are usually discovered fortuitously by studying the T_4, which reveals unexpectedly high or low values. The only clinical significance of these conditions, therefore, lies in abnormal T_4 levels possibly leading to erroneous diagnosis.

Decreased TBG

In several families, affected males had no detectable TBG. Moreover, there was no male-to-male transmission of the trait. A female member in one of these families had no detectable TBG and a sex chromosome constitution of XO. Thus, in these families, the trait appeared to be transmitted as an X-linked gene. In another family, however, a deficiency of TBG was found in three males and three females of two generations. The mode of transmission in this family suggested an autosomal dominant trait.

Increased TBG

Studies in two families with increased TBG suggest that the trait was inherited as an autosomal dominant gene. In another family, affected males transmitted the trait to female but not to male offspring, suggesting that the trait was X linked.

The conflicting reports on the mode of inheritance of both the decreased and the increased TBG traits are difficult to reconcile at present. Since the TBG levels were estimated from their binding capacity of T_4, the reported increased TBG may merely reflect an elevated binding capacity of the protein without a quantitative increase in the amount of circulating TBG. Thus the level of TBG may be controlled by more than one gene, one of which could be a regulator gene.

Akira Morishima

BIBLIOGRAPHY

Abuid, J., and others: Total and free triiodothyronine and thyroxine in early infancy, J. Clin. Endocrinol. Metab. **39**:263, 1974.

Abuid, J., Stinson, D.A., and Larsen, P.R.: Serum triiodothyronine and thyroxine in the neonate and the acute increases in these hormones following delivery, J. Clin. Invest. **52**:1195, 1973.

Anderson, H.J.: Hypothyroidism: nongoitrous hypothyroidism. In Gardner, L.I., editor: Endocrine and genetic diseases of childhood, Philadelphia, 1969, W.B. Saunders Co.

Banjerjee, R.K., and others: Effect of thyroxine on the in vitro formation of erythropoietin in kidney medulla slices, Indian J. Biochem. Biophys. **13**:145, 1976.

Bongiovanni, A.M., and others: Sporadic goiter of the newborn, J. Clin. Endocrinol. Metab. **16**:146, 1956.

Braverman, L.E., Ingbar, S.H., and Sterling, K.: Conversion of thyroxine (T_4) to triiodothyronine (T_3) in athyreotic human subjects, J. Clin. Invest. **49**:855, 1970.

Brown, A.L., and others: Racial differences in the incidence of congenital hypothyroidism, J. Pediatr. **99**:934, 1981.

Carter, J.N., and others: Serum T_3 and T_4 levels in sick children, Pediatrics **58**:776, 1976.

Chopra, I.J.: A radioimmunoassay for measurement of thyroxine in unextracted serum, J. Clin. Endocrinol. Metab. **34**:938, 1972.

Chopra, I.J., and Crandall, B.F.: Thyroid hormones and thyrotropin in amniotic fluid, N. Engl. J. Med. **293**:740, 1975.

Chopra, I.J., Sack, J., and Fisher, D.A.: Circulating 3,3′,5′-triiodothyronine (reverse T_3) in the human newborn, J. Clin. Invest. **55**:1137, 1975.

Codaccioni, J.L., and others: Congenital hypothyroidism associated with thyrotropin unresponsiveness and thyroid cell membrane alterations, J. Clin. Endocrinol. Metab. **50**:932, 1980.

Connoll, J.M.C., and others: Changes in circulating thyroid hormones during short-term hepatic enzyme induction with carbamazepine, Eur. J. Clin. Pharmacol. **26**:453, 1984.

Cuestas, P.A., and Engel, R.R.: Thyroid function in preterm infants with respiratory distress syndrome, J. Pediatr. **94**:643, 1979.

Culler, F.L., Jones, K.L., and Deftos, L.J.: Impaired calcitonin secretion in patients with Williams syndrome, J. Pediatr. **107**:720, 1985.

Czernichow, P., and others: Thyroid function studies in paired maternal-cord sera and sequential observations of thyrotropic hormone release during the first 72 hours of life, Pediatr. Res. **5**:53, 1971.

De Groot, L.J., and others: Triiodothyronine stimulates nuclear RNA synthesis, Endocrinology **101**:1690, 1977.

Delange, F., Fisher, D.A., and Malvaux, P., editors: Pediatric thyroidology: pediatric and adolescent endocrinology, vol. 14, New York, 1985, Karger.

Delange, F., and others: Transient hypothyroidism in the newborn infant, J. Pediatr. **92**:974, 1978.

Delange, F., and others: Progress report 1980 on neonatal thyroid screening in Europe, Acta Paediatr. Scand. **70**:1, 1981.

Delange, F., and others: Increased risk of primary hypothyroidism in preterm infants, J. Pediatr. **105**:462, 1984.

De Visscher, M., editor: The thyroid gland, New York, 1980, Raven Press.

Erenberg, A., and others: Total and free thyroid hormone concentrations in the neonatal period, Pediatrics **53**:211, 1974.

Fichsel, H., and Knöpfle, G.: Effects of anticonvulsant drugs on thyroid hormones in epileptic children, Epilepsia **19**:323, 1978.

Fisher, D.A.: Thyroid development and disorders of thyroid function in the newborn, N. Engl. J. Med. **304**:702, 1981.

Fisher, D.A., and Burrow, G.N., editors: Perinatal thyroid physiology and disease, Kroc Foundation Symposia Series, no. 3, New York, 1975, Raven Press.

Fisher, D.A., and Klein, A.H.: Thyroid development and disorders of thyroid function in the newborn, N. Engl. J. Med. **304**:702, 1981.

Fisher, D.A., and Odell, W.D.: Acute release of thyrotropin in the newborn, J. Clin. Invest. **48**:1670, 1969.

Fisher, D.A., Hoath, S., and Lakshmann, J.: The thyroid hormone effects on growth and development may be mediated by growth factors, Endocrinol. Exp. (Bratisl.) **16**:259, 1982.

Fisher, D.A., Oddie, T.H., and Burroughs, J.C.: Thyroidal radioiodine uptake rate measurement in infants, Am. J. Dis. Child. **103**:738, 1962.

Fisher, D.A., and others: Screening for congenital hypothyroidism: results of screening one million North American infants, J. Pediatr. **94**:700, 1979.

Florsheim, W.H., and others: Familial elevation of serum thyroxine-binding capacity, J. Clin. Endocrinol. Metab. **22**:735, 1962.

French, F.S., and Van Wyk, J.J.: Fetal hypothyroidism, J. Pediatr. **64**:589, 1964.

Gershengorn, M.D., and Weintraub, B.D.: Thyrotropin-induced hyperthyroidism caused by selective resistance to thyroid hormone: a new syndrome of "inappropriate secretion of TSH," J. Clin. Invest. **56**:633, 1975.

Goldsmith, R.E., and others: Familial autoimmune thyroiditis: maternal fetal relationship and the role of generalized autoimmunity, J. Clin. Endocrinol. Metab. **37**:265, 1973.

Gorodzinsky, P., and others: Cord serum thyroxine and thyrotropin values between 20 and 30 weeks' gestation, J. Pediatr. **94**:971, 1979.

Greenberg, A.H., and others: Observations on the maturation of thyroid function in early fetal life, J. Clin. Invest. **49**:1790, 1970.

Greene, H.G., and others: Cretinism associated with maternal sodium iodide I^{131} therapy during pregnancy, Am. J. Dis. Child. **122**:247, 1971.

Grumbach, M.M., and Werner, S.C.: Transfer of thyroid hormone across the human placenta at term, J. Clin. Endocrinol. Metab. **16**:1392, 1956.

Hadeed, A.J., and others: Significance of transient postnatal hypothyroxinemia in premature infants with and without respiratory distress syndrome, J. Pediatr. **68**:494, 1981.

Heidemann, P., and Stubbe, P.: Serum 3,5,3′-triiodothyronine, thyroxine, and thyrotropin in hypothyroid infant with congenital goiter and the response to iodine, J. Clin. Endocrinol. Metab. **47**:189, 1978.

Hesch, R.D.: The low T_3 syndrome, New York, 1981, Academic Press, Inc.

Hirsch, P.F., Voekel, E.F., and Munson, P.L.: Thyrocalcitonin: hypocalcemic hypophosphatemic principle of the thyroid gland, Science **146**:412, 1964.

Ingbar, S.H.: Autoregulation in the thyroid: response to iodine excess and depletion, Mayo Clin. Proc. **47**:814, 1972.

Iseki, M., and others: Sequential serum measurements of thyrotropin binding inhibitor immunoglobulin G in transient familiar neonatal hypothyroidism, J. Clin. Endocrinol. Metab. **57**:384, 1983.

Jacobsen, B.B., and others: Serum levels of thyrotropin, thyroxine and triiodothyronine in full-term, small-for-gestational age and preterm newborn babies, Acta Paediatr. Scand. **66**:681, 1977.

Jiang, N-S., and Tue, K.A.: Determination of free thyroxine in serum by radioimmunoassay, Clin. Chem. **23**:1679, 1977.

Kaplan, M.D., Swartz, S.L., and Larsen, P.R.: Partial peripheral resistance to thyroid hormone, Am. J. Med. **70**:1115, 1981.

Kaplan, S.A., editor: Clinical pediatric and adolescent endocrinology, Philadelphia, 1982, W.B. Saunders Co.

Klein, A.H., Agustin, A.V., and Foley, T.P., Jr.: Successful laboratory screening for congenital hypothyroidism, Lancet **2**:77, 1974.

Klein, A.H., and others: Thyroid hormone and thyrotropin responses to parturition in premature infants with and without the respiratory distress syndrome, Pediatrics **63**:380, 1979.

Krenning, E.P., and others: Plasma membrane transport of thyroid hormones: its possible pathophysiological significance, J. Endocrinol. Invest. **6**:54, 1983.

LaFranchi, S.H.: Hypothyroidism, Pediatr. Clin. North Am. **26**:33, 1979.

Landau, H., and others: Amniotic fluid 3,3′,5′-triiodothyronine in the detection of congenital hypothyroidism, J. Clin. Endocrinol. Metab. **50**:799, 1980.

Larsen, P.R., and Broskin, K: Throxine (T_4) immunoassay using filter paper blood samples for screening of neonates for hypothyroidism, Pediatr. Res. **9**:604, 1975.

Larsen, P.R., and others: Immunoassay of thyroxine in unextracted human serum, J. Clin. Endocrinol. Metab. **37**:177, 1973.

Liewendahl, K., Majuri, H., and Helenius, T.: Thyroid function tests in patients on long-term treatment with various anticonvulsant drugs, Clin. Endocrinol. **8**:185, 1978.

Marrow, W.J.: Hurthle cell tumor of the thyroid gland in an infant, Arch. Pathol. **40**:387, 1945.

Marshall, J.S., Levy, R.P., and Steinberg, A.G.: Human thyroxine-binding globulin deficiency: a genetic study, N. Engl. J. Med. **274**:1469, 1966.

Matsuura, N., and others: Familial neonatal transient hypothyroidism due to maternal TSH-binding inhibitor immunoglobulins, N. Engl. J. Med. **303**:738, 1980.

McFaul, R., and others: Neurological abnormalities in patients treated for hypothyroidism from early life, Arch. Dis. Child. **53**:611, 1978.

McKenzie, J.M.: Neonatal Graves' disease, J. Clin. Endocrinol. Metab. **24**:660, 1964.

Mitchell, M.L., and Larsen, P.R.: Screening for congenital hypothyroidism in New England using the T_4-TSH strategy. In Burrow, G.N., and Dussault, J.H., editors: Neonatal thyroid screening, New York, 1980, Raven Press.

Miyai, K., and others: Transient infantile hyperthyrotropinemia: report of a case, Arch. Dis. Child. **54**:965, 1979.

Odell, W.D., Wilber, J.F., and Paul, W.E.: Radioimmunoassay of thyrotropin in human serum, J. Clin. Endocrinol. Metab. **25**:1179, 1965.

Oppenheimer, J.H., and Surks, M.I.: The peripheral action of the thyroid hormones, Med. Clin. North Am. **59**:1055, 1975.

Parker, R.H., and Beierwaltes, W.H.: Thyroid antibodies during pregnancy and in the newborn, J. Clin. Endocrinol. Metab. **21**:792, 1961.

Patel, Y.C., Burger, H.G., and Hudson, B.: Radioimmunoassay of serum thyrotropin: sensitivity and specificity, J. Clin. Endocrinol. Metab. **33**:768, 1971.

Penny, R., and Frasier, S.D.: Elevated serum concentrations of triiodothyronine in hypothyroid patients, Am. J. Dis. Child. **134**:16, 1980.

Perry, R.D., Hodgman, J.E., and Starr, P.: Maternal cord, and serial venous blood: protein-bound iodine, thyroid-binding globulin, thyroid-binding albumin, and prealbumin values in premature infants, Pediatrics **35**:759, 1965.

Petricciani, J.D., and others: Treatment of young cretins with triiodothyronine, Metabolism **20**:678, 1971.

Pyati, S.P., and others: Absorption of iodine in the neonate following topical use of povidone iodine, J. Pediatr. **91**:825, 1977.

Robles-Valdes, C., Mayans, J.A.R., and Lomeli, J.I.A.: Severe hyponatremia in congenital hypothyroidism, J. Pediatr. **94**:631, 1979.

Rodesch, F., and others: Adverse effect of amniofetography on fetal thyroid function, Am. J. Obstet. Gynecol. **126**:723, 1976.

Rootwelt, K., Graves, T., and Johannessen, S.I.: Effect of carbamazepine, phenytoin and phenobarbiton on serum levels of thyroid hormones and thyrotropin in humans, Scand. J. Clin. Lab. Invest. **38**:731, 1978.

Rossi, T., Hirvonen, T., and Toivanen, P.: The concentration of prealbumin in human fetal and infant sera, Scand. J. Clin. Lab. Invest. **26**:35, 1970.

Schultz, R.M., Glassman, M.S., and MacGillivary, M.H.: Elevated threshold of thyrotropin suppression in congenital hypothyroidism, Am. J. Dis. Child. **123**:19, 1980.

Smith, C.S., and Howard, N.J.: Propranolol in treatment of neonatal thyrotoxicosis, J. Pediatr. **83**:1046, 1973.

Smith, T.J., and Edelman, I.S.: The role of sodium transport in thyroid thermogenesis, Fed. Proc. **38**:2150, 1979.

Sokoloff, L., and others: Mechanisms of stimulation of protein synthesis by thyroid hormones in vitro, Proc. Natl. Acad. Sci. U.S.A. **60**:652, 1968.

Spencer, C.A., and Nicoloff, J.T.: Improved radioimmunoassay for human TSH, Clin. Chim. Acta **108**:415, 1980.

Stanbury, J.B., and others: Congenital hypothyroidism with impaired thyroid response to thyrotropin, N. Engl. J. Med. **279**:1132, 1968.

Sterling, K.: Thyroid hormone action at the cell level, N. Engl. J. Med. **300**:173, 1979.

Sullivan, P.R.C., Bollinger, J.A., and Reichlin, S.: Selective deficiency of tissue triiodothyronine: a proposed mechanism of elevated free thyroxine in euthyroid sick, J. Clin. Invest. **52**:83A, 1973.

Sunshine, P., Kusumoto, H., and Kriss, J.P.: Survival time of circulating long-acting thyroid stimulator in neonatal thyrotoxicosis: implications for diagnosis and therapy of the disorder, Pediatrics **36**:869, 1965.

Van Herle, A.J., Vassart, G., and Dumont, J.E.: Control of thyroglobulin synthesis and secretion, N. Engl. J. Med. **301**:239, 1979.

Varma, S.K., and others: Thyroxine, triiodothyronine, and reverse triiodothyronine concentrations in human milk, J. Pediatr. **93**:803, 1978.

Wayne, E.J., Koutras, D.A., and Alexander, W.D.: Clinical aspects of iodine metabolism, Oxford, 1964, Blackwell Scientific Publications Ltd.

Weichsel, M.E.: Thyroid hormone replacement therapy in the perinatal period: neurologic considerations, Pediatrics **92**:1035, 1978.

Weinstein, I.B., and Kitchin, F.D.: Genetic factors in thyroid disease. In Werner, S.C., and Ingbar, S.H., editors: The thyroid, ed. 3, section 26, New York, 1971, Harper & Row, Publishers, Inc.

Wiersinga, M.M., Chopra, I.J., and Solomon, D.H.: Specific nuclear binding sites of triiodothyronine and reverse triiodothyronine in rat and pork liver: similarities and discrepancies, Endocrinology **110**:2052, 1982.

Wilber, J.F.: Thyrotropin releasing hormone: secretion and action, Ann. Rev. Int. Med. **34**:353, 1973.

Wilson, D.M., and others: Serum free thyroxine values in term, premature, and sick infants, J. Pediatr. **101**:113, 1982.

Yeo, P.P.B., and others: Anticonvulsants and thyroid function, Br. Med. J. **i**:1581, 1978.

PART FOUR

Infants of addicted mothers

In the past 2 decades the abuse of both narcotic and nonnarcotic drugs has continued to increase among all social classes. The most often abused drug is marijuana, followed by alcohol and cocaine. Multiple drug use has also increased in the past decade. In 1975 (according to National Institute for Drug Abuse figures) approximately 570,000 to 724,000 narcotic addicts were in the United States, of whom about 24% were in treatment in a methadone maintenance or detoxification program. This number is probably closer to 1 million today. In New York City alone there were about 250,000 addicts, with about

48% in treatment. An estimated 20% to 40% of these addicts are polydrug abusers, consuming additional quantities of alcohol, psychoactive drugs, barbiturates, and other drugs, thereby compounding the drug addiction problem even further. Women comprise 30% of addicts, and 75% are of childbearing age. As a result, an increasing number of babies are born exhibiting the withdrawal syndromes secondary to maternal drug abuse.

HEROIN

Pathology and pathogenesis

Heroin (diacetylmorphine) readily crosses the placenta. It is deacetylated in the liver to monoacetylmorphine and then to morphine. Once in the fetus, heroin is distributed widely and variably throughout the fetal tissues and body compartments. There appear to be significant differences in its distribution between immature infants and adults. Studies of pregnant animals given morphine have shown the concentration in fetal brain was two to three times that in the maternal brain, and similar differences in distribution are likely for heroin.

Fifty percent of infants born to heroin-addicted women are of low birth weight, and 50% of these are small for gestational age (SGA). Postmortem studies of placentas of heroin-addicted mothers have demonstrated that the increased incidence of prematurity may be caused by a high rate of chorioamnionitis or other maternal infection. In addition, autopsies of SGA infants born to narcotic-addicted mothers reveal their organs to be small and consisting of diminished numbers of cells that are of normal size. These autopsy results differ from those obtained from malnourished infants born to nonaddicted mothers, whose organs show a decrease in both number and size of their cells. Therefore it has been postulated that maternal undernutrition is not the only factor responsible for the antenatal growth retardation observed in infants of narcotic addicts; heroin may have a direct growth-inhibiting effect on the fetus.

The incidence of congenital anomalies in infants born to addicted mothers is not higher than in the general population. An increased rate of stillbirths has, however, been reported in those mothers in whom heroin was withdrawn during pregnancy.

Clinical manifestations

Heroin withdrawal symptoms and signs occur in 50% to 75% of infants born to addicted mothers and usually begin within the first 24 to 48 hours of life. The incidence of withdrawal depends on several factors: (1) the dosage of heroin (less than 6 mg/day is associated with no or mild withdrawal symptoms), (2) the duration of maternal addiction (less than 1 year, 55%; greater than 1 year, 73% incidence of withdrawal), and (3) the time of last maternal dose (a higher incidence of withdrawal occurs if heroin is taken within 24 hours of birth). The withdrawal syndrome may consist of a combination of any of the following: irritability, jitteriness, coarse tremors, high-pitched cry, fist-sucking, sneezing, yawning, tachypnea, poor feeding, regurgitation, vomiting, diarrhea, sweating, hypothermia or hyperthermia, hypertonia, hyperreflexia, myoclonus, and, less often, seizures. In addition, an abnormal sleep cycle with absence of quiet sleep and disturbance of active sleep has been described in these infants. Sucking studies have shown a decrease in both the rate and intensity of sucking.

Infants born to heroin addicts have a low incidence of hyperbilirubinemia and respiratory distress syndrome (RDS). The decreased incidence of hyperbilirubinemia probably results from induction of the glucuronyl transferase enzyme system by heroin. The low incidence of RDS may be caused by a direct effect of heroin on lung maturation, with an accelerated production of surfactant, as suggested by animal studies. Respiratory alkalosis may also occur in these infants.

Treatment

Therapy for the heroin withdrawal syndrome is recommended in the following situations: (1) severe irritability and tremors that interfere with feeding and sleep, (2) vomiting and diarrhea, (3) seizures, (4) hyperthermia or hypothermia, and (5) severe tachypnea interfering with feedings. Other causes of these symptoms should be excluded before initiating treatment.

Many neonatal units use a withdrawal evaluation scoring system to decide on the necessity of treatment and its efficacy. Treatment should include one of the following drugs: phenobarbital, paregoric, or diazepam singly or in combination (Table 37-6). The choice of medication varies in individual nurseries. The initial dose of phenobarbital or diazepam should be a high milligram per kilogram of body weight (mg/kg) loading dose followed by a lower maintenance dosage to allow an adequate plasma level and rapid clinical response. While main-

Table 37-6. Dosage schedule for treatment of infants in heroin withdrawal

Drug	Dosage
Phenobarbital*	15-20 mg/kg loading dose IM, then 4-6 mg/kg/day maintenance, q12h PO
Paregoric	4-6 drops every 4-6 hours PO; if no improvement, increase dosage by 2 drops until clinical improvement is apparent
Diazepam (Valium)	0.3-0.5 mg/kg/day (0.9-1.5 mg/kg/day); initial dose IM and then PO q8h
Methadone	0.1-0.5 mg/kg/day every 4-12 hours PO

*Phenobarbital plasma levels should be evaluated frequently to prevent toxicity.

tenance therapy is being given, plasma drug level monitoring is desirable to prevent toxicity. Once a clinical response has been achieved, the medication should be tapered gradually (every other day) and discontinued. The duration of treatment in neonatal heroin withdrawal may vary from 4 days to 6 weeks.

Prognosis

With appropriate management in the neonatal period, the mortality of heroin-addicted infants does not exceed 3% to 4%; in the late 1950s the reported mortality was 34%, with most infants dying of severe dehydration and shock secondary to diarrhea and vomiting. The follow-up of surviving infants often is incomplete because many addicted mothers will not bring their infants for appointments or because the infants have been placed in foster care. Wilson and associates reported on 22 children at 3 to 6 years of age born to heroin addicts. These children demonstrated deficiencies in both height and weight. In addition, 14% had head circumferences less than 3% on the growth chart. Their overall intellectual functioning was not significantly different from that of normal controls, but they exhibited significant difficulties in the general processes of perception and cognition. They also scored significantly lower than controls in tasks requiring attention, concentration, and short-term memory. These children appeared more aggressive, compulsive, and active than their matched controls, often having an uncontrollable temper.

METHADONE

Methadone, a synthetic opiate, has been the therapy of choice for heroin addiction since its introduction for this purpose by Dole and Nyswander in 1965. It blocks the euphoric effects of heroin, thus reducing the craving for the drug. Methadone is metabolized by the liver into two major metabolites and at least five additional metabolites via *N*-demethylation, aromatic ring hydroxylation, and degradation of both side chains. The metabolites are excreted in the urine, feces, and bile. Methadone itself crosses the placenta. The maternal-to-cord plasma ratio of methadone is 2.7:1, and the maternal-to-neonatal plasma methadone ratio at about 1 hour of life is 2.2:1, indicating placental limitation of transport of methadone, rapid tissue binding, or both.

Incidence

An increasing number of infants have been born to methadone-maintained mothers. These mothers seem to have better prenatal care and a somewhat better lifestyle than those taking heroin. However, there is a high incidence of multiple drug abuse, including alcohol, barbiturates, tranquilizers, and other psychoactive drugs; these mothers also are often heavy smokers. The incidence of methadone withdrawal in the infants varies from 70% to 90%, according to most published reports.

Clinical manifestations

Infants born to methadone-maintained mothers are of higher birth weights than infants of heroin addicts and subsequently have a lower incidence of intrauterine growth retardation. According to Kandall and associates, the birth weights of these infants correlate with the first trimester dose of methadone; the higher the methadone dose (at dosage greater than 40 mg/day), the heavier the infant at birth. The mechanism for this is not known. A significantly higher incidence of head circumferences less than the 3% was found in the neonates of mothers on methadone maintenance compared to the control group. This was not associated with SGA infants. No increase in the incidence of congenital anomalies has been reported in children born to methadone-maintained mothers.

Thrombocytosis and increased platelet-aggregating activity have been reported in infants born to mothers receiving methadone maintenance or involved in other polydrug abuse. This phenomenon of unknown etiology occurred after the first week of life and persisted for more than 16 weeks. In addition, abnormal thyroid function (increased triiodothyronine and thyroxine levels) has been described in newborn infants of methadone-treated mothers.

The signs and symptoms of withdrawal in the infant are more severe and prolonged than the withdrawal symptoms seen in infants of heroin-addicted mothers. The clinical manifestations are similar to those described for heroin withdrawal. The incidence of seizures is higher in the infants of methadone-maintained mothers (10% to 20%). When seizures are present, they usually occur between 7 and 10 days of life. The infants have the same disturbances in their sleep cycles as infants of heroin-addicted mothers, that is, no quiet sleep and abnormal REM sleep. The Brazelton Neonatal Behavioral Assessment Scale demonstrated depressed interactive behavior and poor state control, increased tone and tremulousness, and less physical and emotional intimacy. Many of these findings are related to the infant's narcotic abstinence syndrome. However, they may interfere with maternal bonding and care of the infant.

The incidence and severity of withdrawal syndromes in infants of methadone-maintained mothers depend on the maternal and fetal metabolism and excretion of the drug. The higher the level of methadone in maternal plasma and the more rapid the neonatal metabolism and excretion, the higher the incidence of moderate to severe symptoms and signs of withdrawal. The lower the maternal level of methadone and the slower the metabolism and excretion of methadone in the neonate, the less chance the infant has of developing manifestations of drug withdrawal. The time of onset of methadone withdrawal symptoms depends on the time of the last maternal dose. For example, in one study, when the last maternal dose was within 20 hours of delivery, the onset of withdrawal usually occurred between 24 and 52 hours of life; when the maternal dose of methadone was taken more than 20 hours before delivery, the onset of symptoms occurred before 24 hours of life. In addition, the symptomatic infants did not develop the withdrawal syndrome until plasma levels fell below 0.06 μg/ml.

A syndrome of late-onset withdrawal has been described in some infants born to methadone-maintained mothers. This occurs at 2 to 4 weeks of age either with or without previously occurring withdrawal manifestations. The symptoms are similar to those of early withdrawal and often are accompanied by a voracious appetite but poor weight gain. The symptoms may continue for several weeks and require continuing treatment. This late withdrawal syndrome may be the result of the strong tissue binding of methadone and resultant slow excretion, or of the discontinuation of other drugs taken by the mother that are no longer transferred to the infant after delivery.

Systolic hypertension has also been described in infants of mothers on methadone maintenance. This hypertension is found at about 2 weeks of age and may persist for 12 weeks. It was not related to the severity of abstinence syndrome. A higher incidence of sudden infant death syndrome (SIDS) has also been reported in these infants.

Treatment

Therapy for methadone withdrawal includes the same drugs used for heroin withdrawal: phenobarbital, paregoric, and methadone (Table 37-6). The duration of treatment is usually longer than for infants of heroin-addicted mothers (5 days to 4 months).

Prognosis

The few follow-up studies of these infants that are available reveal a higher incidence of hyperactivity, learning and behavior disorders, and poor social adjustment.

In follow-up a higher incidence of infections, especially otitis media and candidal infections, have been found. A continued higher incidence of head circumferences below the third percentile and a higher incidence of neurologic abnormalities, such as developmental delays, poor fine and gross motor coordination, balance problems, delayed language development, and lower scores on developmental testing, have been described. In follow-up at school age, differences in IQ tests were no longer present, but a subgroup of children demonstrated persistent neurologic findings of poor fine motor coordination, balance difficulties, hyperactivity, decreased concentration span, poor task performance, and aggressive behavior. Many of these children demonstrated school problems requiring special attention and referrals.

The outcome of these children appeared to depend on the interrelationships among many factors, including not only intrauterine drug exposure but emotional, familial, and environmental instability that is so frequently associated with the drug culture.

ALCOHOL

An estimated 10 million alcoholics live in the United States today, and about 20% of these are women.

Alcohol crosses the placenta readily and rapidly reaches the fetus. In studies of mothers receiving alcohol for suppression of labor, blood levels of alcohol in the mother and her fetus were similar. After birth, blood alcohol levels are higher in the neonate and are eliminated more slowly than in the mother. Acute alcohol withdrawal has been well documented in the adult, but only a few case reports are available in the pediatric literature, although acute withdrawal has been reported in neonates born to mothers receiving alcohol suppression for premature labor. The syndrome consists of the following: an odor of alcohol on the breath for several hours after birth, a 72-hour phase of hyperactivity, tremors and seizures followed by a 48-hour phase of lethargy, and finally a return to normal activity and responsiveness.

Much attention has focused on the effects of chronic in utero alcohol exposure of infants born to mothers who are moderate to heavy alcohol consumers. Chronic alcohol exposure during pregnancy may result in a multitude of symptoms, varying from mild to severe and consisting of an increased rate of spontaneous abortions and stillbirths, congenital abnormalities, and mental retardation.

Alcohol may interfere with fetal metabolism and endocrine function. Amino acid transport across the placenta is decreased by alcohol. Animal and human studies of the brain have shown decreased brain weight, with suppression of cell division and abnormal morphology of the brain.

The severity and frequency of these effects are related to dosage, pattern of alcohol consumption, time of gestation, and individual susceptibility. The risk of congenital anomalies from chronic in utero alcohol exposure, compared with a population that has only occasional or no alcohol intake, is 10% if the mothers consume more than 1 or 2 oz of absolute alcohol per day, 19% if they consume more than 2 oz, and 40% if they consume more than 5 oz of absolute alcohol per day during pregnancy. The drinking pattern often changes during pregnancy.

Daily alcohol intake decreases, whereas the number of binge drinking days increases.

The *fetal alcohol syndrome* and *alcohol-related birth defects* consist of the following:

1. Central nervous system: microcephaly; withdrawal symptoms, including irritability and tremors; apnea and seizures; abdominal distension; and opisthotonos. The irritability seen in these infants may persist for several months to years with mild to moderate mental retardation
2. Growth deficiency of perinatal onset, continuing postnatally
3. Facial characteristics: short palpebral fissures, hypoplastic philtrum, thinned upper vermilion, and retrognathia
4. A variety of anomalies, including cardiac abnormalities (ventricular septal defect, tetralogy of Fallot), joint defects, limitation of motion of elbow and phalangeal joints, hip dysplasia, anomalies of external genitalia, hypoplasia of labia or hypospadias, and skin hemangiomas

See also Chapter 17.

The frequency of expression of major and minor components of the fetal alcohol syndrome has been reported as 1 or 2 in 1,000 live births. The frequency of a partial expression is 3 to 5 in 1,000 live births.

However, alcohol effects depend not only on the amount of alcohol consumed but on the interaction of quantity, frequency, type of alcohol, and other drug abuse. Other drugs such as cigarettes, caffeine, and marijuana may potentiate the fetal effects of alcohol consumption during gestation.

Birth weight appears to be reduced if absolute alcohol intake exceeds 1 oz/day before pregnancy and during the third trimester of pregnancy. This growth retardation continues through childhood. Studies evaluating human growth hormone, luteinizing hormone, follicle-stimulating hormone, parathyroid hormone, testosterone, and thyroxine, as well as bone age, have shown these all to be within the normal limits. If alcohol consumption is decreased during the third trimester of pregnancy, the effects on birth weight are minimal.

Follow-up studies at 8 and 12 months of age of children of alcohol abusers showed persistent growth retardation. The Bayley Scales of Infant Development scores were significantly lower than those of the control children. The follow-up at age 6 years again found no catch-up growth in these children. They appeared more immature and exhibited poor fine and gross motor coordination, tremors, hyperactivity, poor concentration, and emotional instability. The mean IQ scores were significantly lower than those of the controls. No differences were found in the performance of children raised by foster parents compared to those raised by their biologic parents. No correlation existed between dysmorphogenesis and the intelligence score. The low IQ is thought to reflect central nervous system damage secondary to alcohol and/or its metabolites.

Treatment

The treatment of acute alcohol withdrawal includes the same drugs that are used in the narcotic abstinence syndrome. Prevention of fetal alcohol syndrome or alcohol-related birth defects should center around appropriate management and follow-up of the mother's alcohol intake before and after pregnancy. The recommendation of the National Institute for Alcohol Abuse is not to consume more than an absolute maximum of two drinks per day during pregnancy, that is, 1⅓ oz of absolute alcohol, to prevent any alcohol-associated birth defects or long-term consequences.

MARIJUANA

Marijuana is the most frequently abused drug in the United States. In the past 20 years there has been a 30-fold increase in the use of marijuana, with an estimated 20 million users.

Marijuana, a crude extract from the *Cannabis sativa* plant, contains more than 420 different compounds, many of which are biologically active. Marijuana is quickly absorbed, resulting in a "high" lasting 2 to 3 hours. Although the high is short lasting, elimination of a single dose of marijuana may take several days because of its slow rate of metabolism and slow release from fatty tissues. Marijuana (tetrahydrocannabinol, or THC) is hydroxylated to 11-OH-THC, which is biologically active. This metabolite is then further hydroxylated to inactive metabolites that are excreted in the urine and feces. The half-life after an acute dose is 56 hours and after chronic use is 19 to 28 hours. Depression of the hypothalamic neurotransmitters and defects in the immune system have been reported in heavy marijuana users.

Marijuana crosses the placenta into the fetus. In animal studies the rate of THC metabolism in the fetus is slow. In the human a shortened gestation has been reported with a prolonged, protracted, and arrested labor. A higher incidence of meconium staining has also been reported by some investigators, whereas others have reported no obstetric complications. No higher incidence of congenital complications or effects on physical and growth parameters have been noted. However, in association with moderate to heavy alcohol use, decreased birth weight has been found, as well as a fivefold increased risk of the fetal alcohol syndrome. The Brazelton scale revealed a higher incidence of tremors, altered visual responses, and changes in the regulation of state.

In follow-up at 6 and 12 months of age, no differences were detected on physical and developmental evaluations in general. A subgroup of infants of heavy marijuana smokers scored lower on the Mental Developmental Index of the Bayley evaluation. Visual-evoked potentials performed at 3 to 6 years of age in children of marijuana smokers showed delays in maturation of the visual system compared to control children. Only further follow-up will determine the significance of these findings.

COCAINE

Cocaine is another commonly abused drug in all social classes. It is the most powerfully addictive drug available today. Its use has increased greatly in the past decade, with more than 7 million users in the United States. Cocaine is administered either by snorting, smoking (free-basing), or intravenously. It is frequently used in combination with other drugs of abuse, such as marijuana and alcohol. Cocaine is well absorbed from all sites of administration. In the adult it causes euphoria followed by depression, tachycardia, vasoconstriction, and transient hypertension. It is hydrolyzed by plasma esterases and *n*-dealkylated into various metabolites. It is excreted as free cocaine and metabolites. The half-life of cocaine is dose dependent and varies from 1 to 1½ hours.

In pregnant cocaine users, a higher incidence of spontaneous abortions and abruptio placenta has been reported. These findings may be secondary to the frequent episodes of hypertension. Cocaine crosses into the fetus. In animal studies the concentration of cocaine is less in the fetus than in the mother. Since cocaine causes vasoconstriction, it may decrease its own placental diffusion into the fetus. Cocaine is slowly metabolized by the fetus and neonate, most likely because of immaturity or deficiency of cholinesterase. No congenital anomalies or effects on physical and growth parameters have been described. A case of cerebral infarction in a neonate born to a mother using high doses of cocaine has been reported. The author postulated that this resulted from either intrauterine or postnatal hypertension or from hypotension and bradycardia with cerebral hypoperfusion, both resulting in cerebral hemorrhage. Abnormalities on the Brazelton scale have been described, including depression of the interactive behavior and poor organizational response to environmental stimuli, whereas others have found no early effects of cocaine. No follow-up reports are available.

PHENCYCLIDINE

Phencyclidine hydrochloride (PCP, angel dust), a veterinary immobilizing agent, is one of the most dangerous available drugs of abuse. It may have very unpredictable, bizarre, and violent effects. It can be either smoked, snorted, or orally ingested. PCP acts both as a central nervous system stimulant and depressant. It may affect muscular coordination and speech and give a feeling of drunkenness. Bizarre behavior, including disorientation, hallucinations, and prolonged schizophrenic-like psychosis, have been reported as a result of PCP use. Its use today is not as widespread, but it is frequently misrepresented as another drug of abuse or mixed with other drugs.

PCP (1-[1-*p*henylcyclohexyl]-*p*iperidine) is highly lipid soluble, tissue bound, and well absorbed. It is hydroxylated and conjugated as glucuronides into several metabolites. The excretion and half-life (1 to 3 days) of PCP depend on urinary pH, with acidic urine enhancing its excretion.

PCP crosses the placenta into the fetus. This has been shown both in animal and human studies. In animals the fetal PCP levels were found to be tenfold of the maternal levels, with high levels in the brain and in tissues in both fetus and mother. PCP was also found in breast milk in much higher levels than in the maternal plasma of rabbits. Literature in human neonates is limited. Urine of neonates born to mothers taking PCP has been reported positive for PCP. Growth parameters and physical evaluations in general have been within normal limits, except for one study with two patients. One of the neonates was microcephalic and both exhibited signs and symptoms of narcotic withdrawal syndrome requiring treatment. Another study reported sudden outbursts of agitation, flapping coarse tremors, and facial grimacing with sudden and rapid changes in the level of consciousness. The Brazelton scale demonstrated significant changes in the lability of states and in consolability. At 3 months' follow-up these same infants were within normal limits both in growth and in developmental parameters. The Bayley scales were in the normal range. No further follow-up is available.

AMPHETAMINE

Amphetamine, one of the most potent stimulants available, is frequently used by teenagers and young adults. Tolerance develops quickly, requiring higher and more frequent doses. Its effect may last for several hours.

Amphetamine is a phenylisopropylamine that is well absorbed and quickly localizes in tissues, especially the central nervous system. Its excretion is pH dependent and is enhanced by acidic urine.

The fetal and neonatal effects of maternal use of amphetamines in pregnancy are not very well known. The effects appear to be dose related. In low doses, methamphetamine use has been reported to increase weight gain during pregnancy. If the methamphetamine use was discontinued before 28 weeks' gestation, no fetal effect was found. If the drug use was continued throughout pregnancy, however, a significant decrease in birth weight was described. A study from Sweden on amphetamine abuse during pregnancy showed a higher incidence of perinatal mortality and prematurity. Many neonates exhibited drowsiness, respiratory distress, and jitteriness. On follow-up these infants remained lethargic for several months, with frequent infections and poor weight gain. In early childhood a higher incidence of emotional disturbances and delays in gross and fine motor coordination were reported.

PHENOBARBITAL

Phenobarbital is frequently used in the treatment of seizure disorders and for sedation. It also is a commonly abused drug among patients of all socioeconomic classes. Phenobarbital crosses the placenta readily and is distributed rapidly throughout the fetus, with the greatest concentrations in the liver and brain. Infants of phenobarbital-addicted mothers are usually full term and of appropriate weight for gestational age. Their Apgar scores usually are good. The incidence of phenobarbital withdrawal symptoms is not known. When they do occur, symptoms begin at a median age of 7 days (range, 2 to 14 days) and may last for 2 to 4 months. Desmond and associates described two stages of phenobarbital withdrawal: an acute stage consisting of irritability, constant crying, sleeplessness, hiccups, and mouthing movements, followed by a subacute stage marked by a voracious appetite, frequent regurgitation and gagging, episodic irritability, hyperacusis, sweating, and a disturbed sleep pattern. The second stage may last from 2 to 4 months. The late onset of phenobarbital withdrawal probably results from its slow metabolism and excretion by the newborn. Treatment consists of swaddling, frequent feedings, and protection from noxious external stimuli. If there is no improvement with these methods, the infant should be given phenobarbital and then slowly withdrawn from this drug after control of symptoms.

MISCELLANEOUS DRUGS

Several cases have been reported of neonatal withdrawal syndrome from pentazocine (alone or combined with tripelennamine), a nonnarcotic analgesic that previously was thought to be nonaddictive. Infants born to chronic users of pentazocine have commenced withdrawal symptoms at about 24 hours of age. The symptoms of withdrawal include hypertonia, hyperactivity, tremors, and vomiting. Treatment with phenobarbital for 14 to 17 days has been effective. Infants born to abusing mothers were significantly smaller and also exhibited symptoms and signs of withdrawal.

Other drugs that may cause withdrawal symptoms include codeine, propoxyphene, and diazepam. No reports are available concerning withdrawal from chlordiazepoxide (Librium) and meprobamate, but a fourfold increase in the incidence of malformation has been reported in infants born to mothers taking these drugs during early pregnancy.

URINARY DRUG-SCREENING METHODS

Several methods are available for urinary identification of morphine, methadone, amphetamines, phenothiazines, barbiturates, and sedatives. The methods include fluorometry, ultraviolet spectrophotometry, thin-layer chromatography, gas-liquid chromatography, mass spectrophotometry and immunoassay system. Gas-liquid chromatography and mass spectrophotometry are the most accurate of these and also the most complicated and time consuming. The other methods, which are less accurate but technically easier and less time consuming, are more appropriate for a screening program. The sensitivity of the screening methods is such that a minimum of 1 to 5 μg/ml of these drugs is detectable. The most often used method is thin-layer chromatography with various extraction procedures and chromogenic sprays. The immunoassay system, employing a bacterial antigen-antibody lysosome system, is the simplest and most rapid system available at present but will detect only morphine, methadone, cocaine derivatives, amphetamines, and barbiturates. For a more complete qualitative drug analysis, thin-layer chromatography and mass spectrophotometry can be used. Alcohol is best detected using an autoanalyzer and the enzyme alcohol dehydrogenase. It is sensitive to 0.1 mg alcohol/dl in the blood.

Tove S. Rosen

BIBLIOGRAPHY

Heroin

Cohen, S.: Narcotism: dimensions of the problems in recent developments in chemotherapy of narcotic addiction, Ann. N.Y. Acad. Sci. **311**:4, 1978.

Ingall, D., and Zuckenstatter, M.: Diagnosis and treatment of the passively addicted newborn, Hosp. Pract., 1970.

Kahn, E.J., Newmann, L.L., and Polk, G.A.: The course of heroin withdrawal syndrome in newborn infants treated with phenobarbital and chlorpromazine, J. Pediatr. **75**:495, 1969.

Naeye, R.L., and others: Fetal complications of maternal heroin addiction: abnormal growth, infections and episodes of stress, J. Pediatr. **83**:1055, 1973.

Nathenson, G., and others: The effect of maternal heroin addiction on neonatal jaundice, J. Pediatr. **81**:899, 1972.

Ramenteria, J.L., and Nurrag, N.N.: Narcotic withdrawal in pregnancy: stillbirth incidence with a case report, Am. J. Obstet. Gynecol. **116**:1152, 1973.

Stone, M.L., and others: Narcotic addiction in pregnancy, Am. J. Obstet. Gynecol. **109**:716, 1971.

Taeusch, H.W., Jr., and others: Heroin induction of lung maturation and growth retardation in fetal rabbits, J. Pediatr. **82**:869, 1972.

Wilson, G.S., Desmond, M.M., and Verniaud, W.M.: Early development of infants of heroin-addicted mothers, Am. J. Dis. Child. **126**:457, 1973.

Wilson, G.S., and others: The development of preschool children of heroin addicted mothers: a controlled study, Pediatrics **63**:135, 1979.

Zinberg, N.E., and others: Patterns of heroin use, Ann. N.Y. Acad. Sci. **311**:10, 1978.

Methadone

Anngard, E., and others: Disposition of methadone in methadone maintenance, Clin. Pharmacol. Ther. **14**:194, 1975.

Blinick, G., and others: Methadone assays in pregnant women and progeny, Am. J. Obstet. Gynecol. **121**:617, 1974.

Burstein, Y., and others: Thrombocytosis and increased circulating platelet aggregates in newborn infants of polydrug users, J. Pediatr. **94**:895, 1979.

Herlinger, R.A., Kandall, S.R., and Vaughn, N.G.: Neonatal seizures associated with narcotics withdrawal, J. Pediatr. **91**:638, 1977.

Kandall, S.R., and others: Birth weights and maternal narcotic use. In Senay, E., Shorty, V., and Alkane, H., editors: Development in the field of drug abuse, Proceedings of the 1974 National Association for the Prevention of Addiction to Narcotics, Cambridge, Mass., 1974, Shenkman Publishing Co.

Pierson, P.S., Howard, P., and Kleber, H.D.: Sudden deaths in infants born to methadone-maintained addicts, JAMA **220**:1733, 1972.

Rajegowda, B.K., and others: Methadone withdrawal in newborn infants, J. Pediatr. **81**:532, 1972.

Rosen, T.S., and Pippenger, C.E.: Pharmacologic observations on the neonatal withdrawal syndrome, J. Pediatr. **88**:1044, 1976.

Heroin and methadone

Chasnoff, I.J., Hatcher, R., and Burns, W.J.: Polydrug- and methadone-addicted newborns: a continuum of impairment? Pediatrics **70**:210, 1982.

Hutchings, D.E.: Methadone and heroin during pregnancy: a review of behavioral effects in human offspring, Neurobehav. Toxicol. Teratol. **4**:429, 1982.

Johnson, H.L., Diano, A., and Rosen, T.S.: 24-Month neurobehavioral follow up of children of methadone maintained mothers, Infant Behav. Dev. **7**:115, 1984.

Kaltenbach, K., and Finnegan, L.P.: Developmental outcome of children born to methadone-maintained women: a review of longitudinal studies, Neurobehav. Toxicol. Teratol. **6**:271, 1984.

Kreek, M.J.: Methadone disposition during the perinatal period in humans, Pharmacol. Biochem. Behav. **11**:7, 1979.

Nathenson, G., Golden, G., and Litt, I.F.: Diazepam in the management of the neonatal narcotic withdrawal syndrome, Pediatrics **48**:523, 1971.

Olofsson, M., and others: Investigation of 89 children born by drug-dependent mothers: follow up 1-10 years after birth, Acta Paediatr. Scand. **72**:407, 1983.

Reddy, A.M., Harper, R.G., and Stern, G.: Observation on heroin and methadone withdrawal in the newborn, Pediatrics **48**:353, 1971.

Rosen, T.S., and Johnson, L.H.: Children of methadone-maintained mothers: follow-up to 18 months, J. Pediatr. **101**:192, 1982.

Rosen, T.S., and Johnson, L.H.: Long-term effects of prenatal methadone maintenance. In Pinkert, T.M., editor: Current research on the consequence of maternal drug abuse, NIDA Research Monograph No. 59, 1985, p. 73.

Schulman, C.A.: Alterations of the sleep cycle in heroin addicted and "suspect" newborns, Neuropaediatrie **1**:89, 1969.

Wilson, G.S., Desmond, M.M., and Wait, R.B.: Follow up of methadone treated and untreated narcotic dependent women and their infants: health, developmental and social implications, J. Pediatr. **98**:716, 1981.

Zelson, C., Sook, J.L., and Casalino, M.: Neonatal narcotic addiction, N. Engl. J. Med. **289**:1216, 1973.

Alcohol

Aronson, M., and others: Children of alcoholic mothers: developmental, perceptual and behavioral characteristics as compared to matched controls, Acta Paediatr. Scand. **74**:27, 1985.

Barr, H.M., and others: Infant size at 8 months of age: relationship to maternal use of alcohol, nicotine, caffeine during pregnancy, Pediatrics **74**:336, 1984.

Clarren, S.K., and Smith, D.W.: The fetal alcohol syndrome, N. Engl. J. Med. **298**:1063, 1978.

Clarren, S.K., and others: Brain malformations related to prenatal exposure to ethanol, J. Pediatr. **92**:64, 1978.

Golden, N.L.: Maternal alcohol use and infant development, Pediatrics **70**:931, 1982.

Hanson, J.W., Streissguth, A.P., and Smith, D.W.: The effects of moderate alcohol consumption during pregnancy of fetal growth and morphogenesis, J. Pediatr. **11**:219, 1977.

Jones, K.L., and others: Pattern of malformation in offspring of chronic alcoholic mothers, Lancet **1**:7815, 1973.

Kuzma, J.W., and Sokol, R.J.: Maternal drinking behavior and decreased intrauterine growth, Alcohol Clin. Exp. Res. **6**:396, 1982.

Kyllerman, M., and others: Children of alcoholic mothers: growth, and motor performance compared to matched controls, Acta Paediatr. Scand. **74**:20, 1985.

Mills, J.L., and others: Maternal alcohol consumption and birth weight: how much drinking during pregnancy is safe? JAMA **252**:1875, 1984.

Nichols, M.M.: Acute alcohol withdrawal syndrome in a newborn, Am. J. Dis. Child. **113**:714, 1967.

Ouelette, E.M., and others: Adverse effects on offspring of maternal alcohol abuse during pregnancy, N. Engl. J. Med. **297**:528, 1977.

Peden, V.H., Sammon, J.T., and Downey, D.A.: Intravenously induced infantile intoxication with ethanol, J. Pediatr. **83**:490, 1973.

Pierog, S., Chandavasur, O., and Wexler, O.: Withdrawal symptoms in infants with fetal alcohol syndrome, J. Pediatr. **90**:630, 1977.

Pytkowicz-Streissguth, A., Barr, H.M., and Martin, D.C.: Offspring effects and complications related to self-reported maternal alcohol use, Dev. Pharmacol. Ther. **5**:21, 1982.

Qazi, Q., and others: Factors influencing outcome of pregnancy in heavy drinking women, Dev. Pharmacol. Ther. **4**:6, 1982.

A Report to the Governor of the State of New York on Fetal Alcohol Syndrome by Task Force on FAS/ARBD, Shelia B. Blume, Chairman, New York State Division of Alcoholism and Alcohol Abuse, November 1979.

Reyes, E., and others: Effects of maternal administration of alcohol on fetal brain development, Neurobehav. Toxicol. Teratol. **5**:263, 1983.

Rosett, H.L., and others: Patterns of alcohol consumption and fetal development, Obstet. Gynecol. **61**:539, 1983.

Weiner, L., and others: Alcohol consumption by pregnant women, Obstet. Gynecol. **61**:6, 1983.

Marijuana

Caldwell, J., and Sever, S.: The biochemical pharmacology of abused drugs. III. Cannabis, opiates, and synthetic narcotics, Clin. Pharmacol. Ther. **16**:989, 1974.

Fried, P.: Marijuana use by pregnant women: neurobehavioral effects in neonates, Drug. Alcohol Depend. **6**:415, 1980.

Fried, P.: Postnatal consequences of maternal marijuana use. In Pinkert, T.M., editor: Current research on the consequences of maternal drug abuse, NIDA Research Monograph No. 59, 1985, p. 61.

Greenland, S., and others: The effects of marijuana use during pregnancy. I. A preliminary epidemiologic study, Am. J. Obstet. Gynecol. **143**:408, 1982.

Hingson, R., and others: Effects of maternal drinking and marijuana use on fetal growth and development, Pediatrics **70**:539, 1982.

Petersen, R.C., and Stillman, R.C., editors: Marijuana research findings, 1980, NIDA Research Monograph No. 31, 1980.

Qazi, Q.H., and others: Abnormalities in offspring associated with prenatal marihuana exposure, Dev. Pharmacol. Ther. **8**:141, 1985.

Cocaine

Acker, D., Sachs, B.P., and Tracey, K.J.: Abruptio placentae associated with cocaine use, Am. J. Obstet. Gynecol. **146**:220, 1983.

Chasnoff, I.J., and others: Cocaine use in pregnancy, N. Engl. J. Med. **313**:66, 1985.

Chasnoff, I.J., and others: Perinatal cerebral infarction and maternal cocaine use, J. Pediatr. **108**:456, 1986.

Javaid, J.I., and others: Kinetics of cocaine in humans after intravenous and intranasal administration, Biopharm. Drug. Dispos. **4**:9, 1983.

Madden, J.D., Payne, T.F., and Miller, S.: Maternal cocaine abuse and effect on the newborn, Pediatrics **77**:209, 1986.

Shah, N.S., May, D.A., and Yates, J.D.: Disposition of levo-(3H) cocaine in pregnant and nonpregnant mice, Toxicol. Appl. Pharmacol. **53**:279, 1980.

Phencyclidine

Chasnoff, I.J., and others: Phencyclidine: effects on the fetus and neonate, Dev. Pharmacol. Ther. **6**:404, 1983.

Cook, C.E., and others: Phencyclidine disposition after intravenous and oral doses, Clin. Pharmacol. Ther. **31**:625, 1982.

Goodwin, P.J., and others: Phencyclidine: effect of chronic administration in the female mouse in gestation, maternal behavior, and the neonates, Psychopharmacology **69**:63, 1980.

James, S.H., and Schnoll, S.H.: Phencyclidine tissue distribution in the rat, Clin. Toxicol. **9**:573, 1976.

Nicholas, M.J., Lipshitz, J., and Schreiber, E.C.: Phencyclidine: its transfer across the placenta as well as into breast milk, Am. J. Obstet. Gynecol. **143**:143, 1982.

Petersen, R.C., and Stillman, R.C.: Phencyclidine (PCP) abuse: an appraisal, NIDA Research Monograph No. 21, DHEW Pub. No. 78-228, 1978.

Strauss, A.A., Mondanlow, H.D., and Bosusagba, K.: Neonatal manifestation of maternal phencyclidine (PCP) abuse, Pediatrics **68**:550, 1981.

Amphetamine

Larson, G.: The amphetamine addicted mother and her child, Acta Paediatr. Scand. **278**:7, 1980.

Naeye, R.: Dextroamphetamine and growth of the fetus, Pharmacology **26**:117, 1983.

Ramer, C.M.: The case history of an infant born to an amphetamine addicted mother, Clin. Pediatr. **13**:596, 1971.

Phenobarbital

Bleyer, A.W., and Marshall, R.E.: Barbiturate withdrawal syndrome in a passively addicted infant, JAMA **221**:185, 1972.

Desmond, M., and others: Maternal barbiturate utilization and neonatal withdrawal symptomatology, J. Pediatr. **80**:190, 1972.

Pippenger, C.E., and Rosen, T.S.: Phenobarbital plasma levels in neonates, Clin. Perinatol. **2**:111, 1975.

Miscellaneous drugs

Chasnoff, I.J., and others: Pentazocine and tripelennamine ("T's and Blue's"): effects on the fetus and neonate, Dev. Pharmacol. Ther. **6**:162, 1983.

Chasnoff, I.J., and others: Maternal non-narcotic substance abuse during pregnancy: effects on infant development, Neurobehav. Toxicol. Teratol. **6**:277, 1984.

Gilman, G.A., and others, editors: The pharmacological basis of therapeutics, ed. 7, New York, 1985, MacMillan Publishing Co., Inc.

Goetz, R.L., and Bain, R.V.: Neonatal withdrawal symptoms associated with maternal use of pentazocine, J. Pediatr. **84**:887, 1974.

Klein, R.B., Blatman, S., and Little, G.A.: Probable neonatal propoxyphene withdrawal: a case report, Pediatrics **55**:882, 1975.

Milkovich, B.A., and Van den Berg, B.J.: Effects of prenatal meprobamate and chlordiazepoxide hydrochloride on human embryonic and fetal development, N. Engl. J. Med. **291**:1268, 1974.

Van Leeuwen, G., Guthrie, R., and Stange, F.: Narcotic withdrawal reaction in a newborn infant due to codeine, Pediatrics **36**:635, 1965.

Urinary drug-screening methods

Dole, V.P., and others: Detection of narcotic, sedative and amphetamine drugs in urine, N.Y. State J. Med. **72**:471, 1972.

Inturrisi, C.E., and Verebely, K.: A gas-liquid chromatographic method for the quantitative determination of methadone in human plasma and urine, J. Chromatogr. **65**:361, 1972.

Mule, S.J.: Routine identification of drugs of abuse in human urine. I. Application of fluorometry, thin-layer chromatography and gas-liquid chromatography, J. Chromatogr. **55**:255, 1971.

Rubinstein, K.E., Schneider, R.S., and Ullman, E.F.: Homogenous enzyme immunoassay: a new immunoassay technique, Biochem. Biophys. Res. Commun. **47**:846, 1972.

PART FIVE

Abnormalities of sexual differentiation

Genetic sex is determined at fertilization, but actual sexual differentiation begins at 6 weeks' gestation and is largely completed by 12 to 14 weeks. This section reviews (1) normal fetal sexual differentiation, (2) those disorders that comprise the abnormalities of sexual differentiation, with the major focus being placed on their perinatal manifestations, and (3) an approach to the recognition and diagnosis of neonates who may have an intersex problem, with general principles for their management. An *intersex problem* is defined as a discrepancy in the genetic, gonadal, or genital makeup of an individual.

NORMAL FETAL SEX DIFFERENTIATION

EMBRYOLOGY AND ENDOCRINOLOGY

The embryo and early fetus, regardless of genetic sex (i.e., whether 46,XX or 46,XY), is bipotential with respect to its possible sexual differentiation, having the anatomic and biochemical apparatuses necessary for both male and female development. In the absence of specific genetic directives, the innate tendency of the embryo and early fetus is to differentiate along female lines; that is, female differentiation will occur unless a succession of signals and steps take place to induce male differentiation. Essentially all the control mechanisms affecting fetal sex differentiation involve steps in male differentiation. For normal male differentiation to occur, it is required that all these steps be intact and occur normally. The absence or failure of any one of these control steps will result in the embryo or early fetus differentiating along female lines from that point of differentiation onward.

Fetal sex differentiation begins at 6 weeks with differentiation of the bipotential gonad into either a testis or ovary and ends at 12 to 14 weeks with completion of differentiation of the internal genital ducts and external genitalia along either male or female lines. A description of these events and their control mechanisms follows.

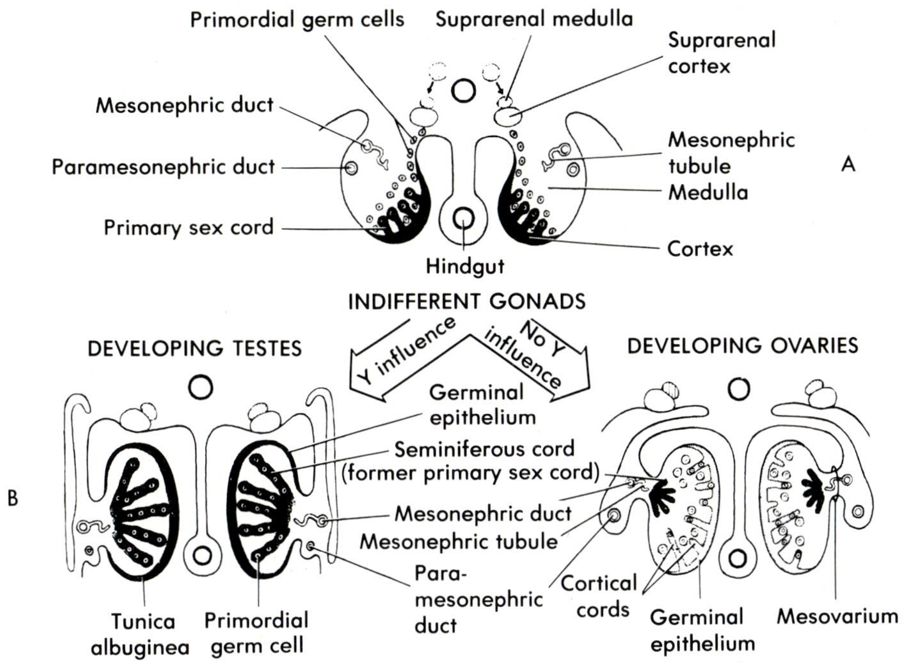

Fig. 37-26. Schematic drawing showing differentiation of the indifferent (bipotential) gonads into testes or ovaries. **A,** The indifferent gonad at 6 weeks' gestation. **B,** Developing testes. Testicular differentiation occurs under the influence of the Y chromosome. The primary sex cords extend into the medulla and differentiate into seminiferous cords at 6 to 7 weeks. The tunica albuginea develops at 7 weeks. **C,** Developing ovaries. Ovarian differentiation occurs in the absence of a Y chromosome. The primary sex cords will form irregular groups in the cortex comprising rapidly dividing oogonia and leading to the formation of primordial follicles between 6½ and 15 weeks. Little development occurs in the medulla, and the tunica albuginea shows only indistinct development. (From Moore, K.L.: The developing human: clinically oriented embryology, ed. 3, Philadelphia, 1982, W.B. Saunders Co., p. 273.)

Gonadal development

The gonads of both sexes differentiate from the indifferent (or bipotential) gonads (Fig. 37-26, *A*). The gonad begins its development at 4 to 5 weeks' gestation as the genital ridge, located on the medial aspect of the mesonephros. Before this, the primordial germ cells are first seen as early as 4½ days' gestation. They migrate from the entoderm of the allantois and yolk sac and reach the genital ridge beginning at 26 or 27 days and later.

Testicular differentiation.

Differentiation of the testis begins in the presence of a Y chromosome at 6 weeks' gestation when the cells of the primitive gonad interact to form the epithelial or primary sex cords and surrounding mesenchymal or interstitial tissue (Fig. 37-26, *B*). The cord cells, thought to be of epithelial origin, become the primitive Sertoli cells, and the primordial germ cells are incorporated into the cords and develop into spermatogonia. In weeks 7 and 8 the cords in the cortex loop to form the seminiferous cords, and in the hilum they anastomose to form the rete cords or rete testis. From 8 weeks on the seminiferous cords become coiled and thickened and contain eight to ten layers of Sertoli cells, whereas the spermatogonia remain located near the basement membrane of the cords. The seminiferous cords and rete testis become lumenized in the second half of gestation.

The fetal testis is characterized by the appearance of Leydig cells in the interstitium between the seminiferous cords beginning at approximately 8 to 8½ weeks, and these may be mesenchymal in origin. Leydig cells increase strikingly in number during the third month, occupy half the volume of the testis by the middle of the fourth month, and then show a significant fall in numbers; some Leydig cells are present postnatally but histologically disappear after 6 months because of a physiologic lowering of gonadotropin stimulation.

As the fetus elongates, the testis descends and occupies a more caudal position. In the sixth and seventh months the cremasteric muscle differentiates in the caudal testicular ligament to form the testicular gubernaculum, which penetrates the inguinal canal and is anchored to the connective tissue of the scrotum. The testis descends behind the peritoneum and reaches the scrotum by the eighth or ninth month; the inguinal canal closes after testicular descent is complete.

Ovarian differentiation

Differentiation of the ovary begins gradually in the absence of a Y chromosome at 6½ to 8 weeks' gestation (Fig. 37-26, *C*). The cord cells become the primitive granulosa cells, which are analogous to the Sertoli cells. The primary sex cords show little development in the medulla or hilum, and epithelioid interstitial cells (analogous to Leydig cells) are not seen. In the cortex, however, the primordial germ cells, now called oogonia, undergo intensive mitotic division during the third month to form a thick zone of mostly oogonia interspersed with a few primitive granulosa cells. Primitive granulosa cells begin to organize around the oocytes to form primordial follicles.

The late fetal ovary (15 to 18 weeks onward) is characterized by the development of primary follicles, which surround follicular cells to form a basement membrane, and each follicle becomes surrounded by connective tissue. At 18 to 22 weeks about 7 million oogonia and oocytes are present, but by birth only 2 million are present, with half of these undergoing degeneration and atresia; only about 400,000 oocytes will persist into reproductive life, of which only approximately 400 are ovulated during the woman's reproductive period.

Development of the genital ducts

The internal genital ducts, unlike the gonads, develop from separate anlagen, from the mensonephric or wolffian ducts in the male and from the parmesonephric or müllerian ducts in the female (Fig. 37-27). The wolffian ducts are formed in 26- to 32-day-old embryos; the müllerian ducts arise at 44 to 48 days and develop in close association with the wolffian ducts, which serve as a guide to the caudal progression of the müllerian ducts. In the absence of wolffian ducts, the müllerian ducts will not develop.

In the male fetus the müllerian ducts begin to undergo regression at 7 to 7½ weeks, shortly after the ipsilateral testicular seminiferous cords have differentiated and preceding the appearance of Leydig cells; regression is completed by 9 to 10 weeks.

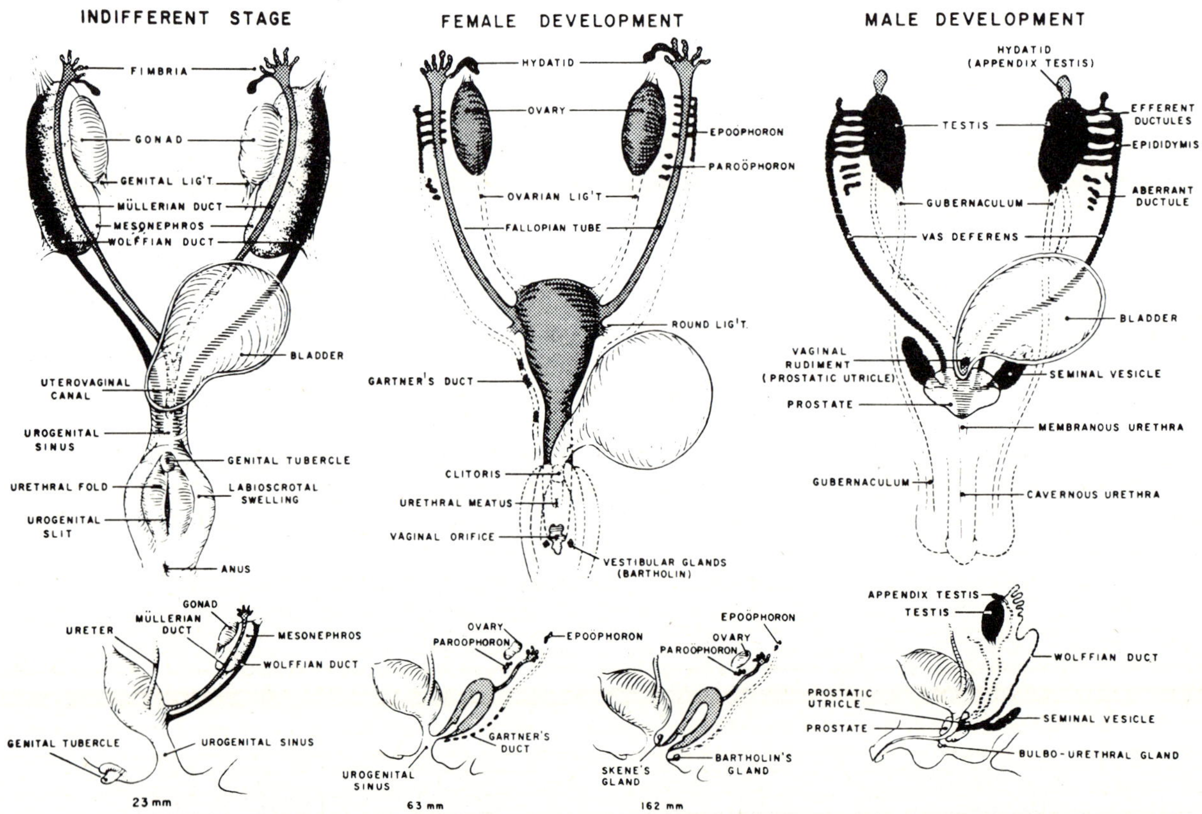

Fig. 37-27. Internal genital duct development. **Left,** Diagram shows the presence of both wolffian and müllerian ducts in a 7½-week-old fetus at the indifferent stage. **Center,** Female fetus beyond 13 weeks. **Right,** Male fetus beyond 14 weeks. (From Grumbach, M.M., and Conte, F.A.: Disorders of sexual differentiation. In Wilson, J.D., and Foster, D.W., editors: Williams textbook of endocrinology, ed. 7, Philadelphia, © 1985, W.B. Saunders Co.)

Differentiation of the wolffian ducts is testosterone dependent and begins at about 8½ weeks. The wolffian ducts differentiate into the epididymis and vas deferens, and beginning at 10½ weeks the seminal vesicles and their ejaculatory ducts develop at the caudal end from lateral outpouchings. The wolffian ducts project into the urogenital sinus just lateral to the termination of the fused müllerian ducts.

The female genital ducts differentiate later than the male genital ducts. In the absence of ipsilateral testes, the müllerian ducts form the fallopian tubes, uterus, and upper portion of the vagina beginning in the third month of gestation. The wolffian ducts, in the absence of local testosterone produced by an ipsilateral testis, rapidly disappear, and by 13 weeks degeneration of these ducts is complete (Fig. 37-27). The fallopian tubes later descend with the ovaries and are included in a fold of peritoneum called the broad ligament. At birth the position of the uterus is vertical, and uterine development is disproportionate in that the uterine cervix is twice as large as the fundus and remains so until puberty. Maternal estrogens probably stimulate uterine growth in utero, so its size at birth is larger than at several months of age; endometrial hyperplasia occasionally may result in transient neonatal uterine bleeding.

The development of the vagina depends on the caudal müllerian ducts having made contact with the entodermal epithelium of the urogenital sinus. At this junction a multilayered, solid epithelial cord known as the vaginal plate is formed; it disintegrates beyond 4 months to form the vaginal lumen. It is not clear whether the lower portion of the vagina is derived from the urogenital sinus and the upper portion is of müllerian origin, or whether the vagina originates entirely from the urogenital sinus. The origin of the hymen is also unclear, but it is thought to be derived from the mesenchyme that separated the vagina from the urogenital sinus.

Development of the external genitalia

The external genitalia in both sexes, as with the gonads, are derived from common anlagen (Fig. 37-28). Their inherent development is along female lines unless systemic androgens, specifically dihydrotestosterone (DHT), induce male differentiation.

In the male fetus the indifferent stage of the external genitalia lasts until the ninth week when, in the presence of systemic androgens, masculinization begins with lengthening of the anogenital distance. The urogenital and labioscrotal folds fuse in the midline, beginning caudally and progressing anteriorly. The urethra develops with fusion of the urogenital folds, which forms both the membranous urethra in the perineum and the penile urethra along the ventral surface of the phallus. Midline fusion of the labioscrotal folds forms the scrotal raphe, whereas the penile raphe represents the fused portions of the urogenital folds. These processes are complete in the 14-week fetus.

In the female fetus at 9 weeks the anogenital distance does not increase, and the urogenital folds and labioscrotal swellings do not fuse. The labioscrotal swellings develop predominantly in their caudal portions, but less so than in male fetuses, and remain unfused as they transform into the labia majora. The urogenital folds develop into the labia minora. The epithelium of the vaginal vestibule between the labia minora and the hymen is en-

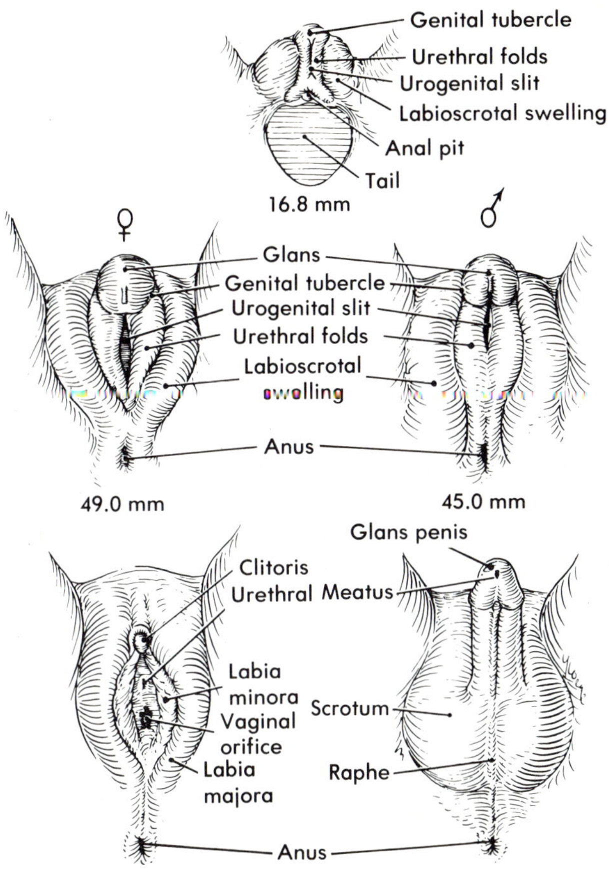

Fig. 37-28. Differentiation of the external genitalia in the male and female fetus from the common primordia. **Top,** The indifferent genitalia are shown at about 48 days. The tail of the embryo has been cut away to uncover the genitalia. **Middle,** The genitalia at about 9½ weeks. In the male, anogenital lengthening and midline fusion have begun. **Bottom,** Newborn genitalia. Genitalia differentiation is complete by about 14 weeks' gestation. However, growth during the second and third trimesters accounts for the difference in phallic size. (From Grumbach, M.M., and Conte, F.A.: Disorders of sexual differentiation. In Wilson, J.D., and Foster, D.W., editors: Williams textbook of endocrinology, ed. 7, Philadelphia, © 1985, W.B. Saunders Co., p. 331.)

todermal, being derived from the urogenital sinus, whereas the epithelium between the labia minora and majora is ectodermal in origin.

Fetal gonadal endocrine function

The fetal testes play a major role in male sex differentiation in producing two hormones, müllerian-inhibiting factor (MIF) and testosterone, which are major determinants of internal and external genital differentiation. The fetal ovaries, on the other hand, play little or no role in female sex differentiation, although they may have some steroidogenic capacity.

MIF, also called müllerian-inhibiting substance and antimüllerian hormone, is a large glycoprotein (molecular weight, 140,000 to 235,000 daltons) produced by the Sertoli cells beginning at 7 to 7½ weeks that induces irreversible involution of the müllerian ducts. It is thought to reverse the differentiation of müllerian mesenchyme and epithelium by altering the state of phosphorylation of critical proteins and possibly by blocking the effect of epidermal growth factor or other differentiating agents. MIF appears to be secreted locally, since it induces only ipsilateral müllerian duct regression. Levels of MIF activity in the human fetal testis decline by late pregnancy and are low at birth, although continued MIF activity may be found in infantile testes up to 9 months to 2 years of age. MIF also may play a role in stimulating testicular descent, since its levels are lower in undescended testes, although this lower level may only reflect impaired production resulting from the nondescent.

The other major hormone produced by the fetal testis is testosterone, a C_{19} steroid (Fig. 37-29). It is synthesized by the Leydig cells beginning at 8½ weeks, and

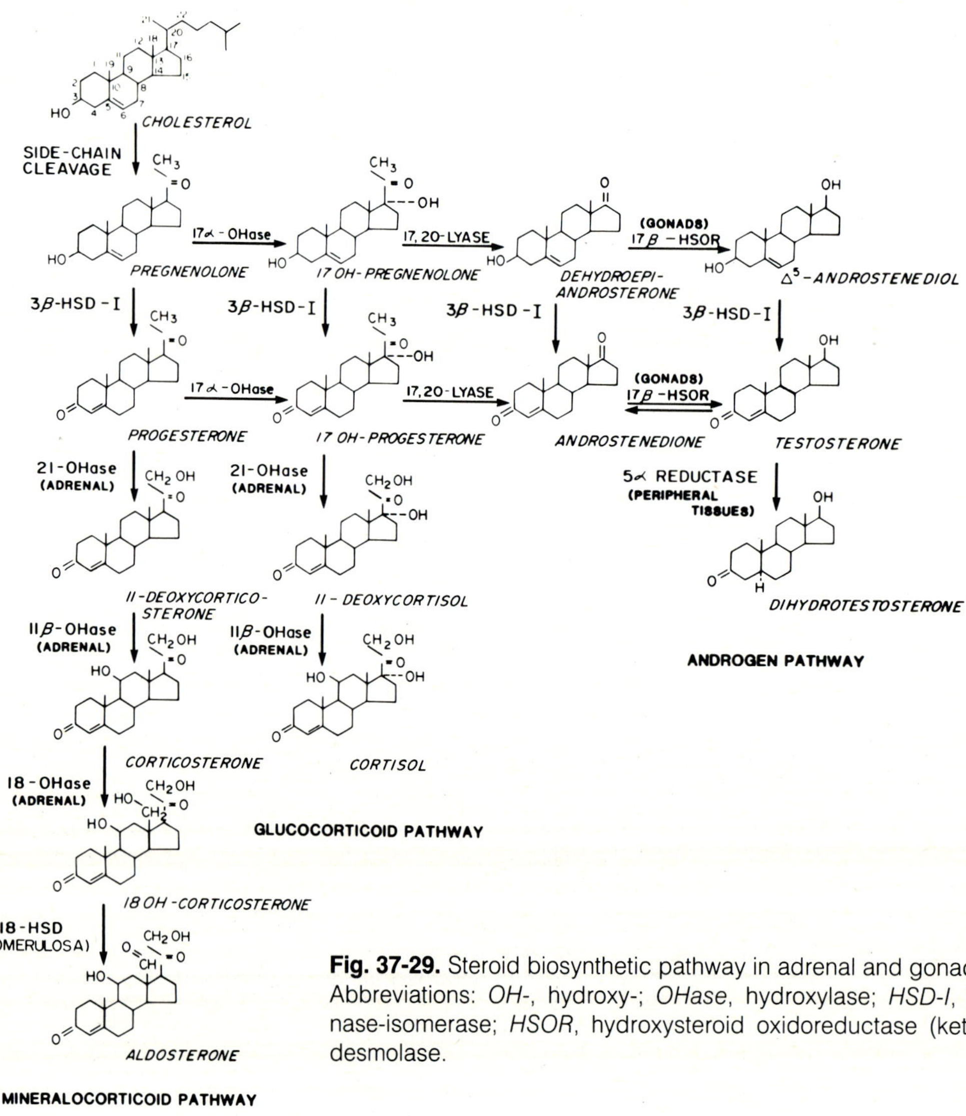

Fig. 37-29. Steroid biosynthetic pathway in adrenal and gonadal (and peripheral) tissues. Abbreviations: *OH-*, hydroxy-; *OHase*, hydroxylase; *HSD-I*, hydroxysteroid dehydrogenase-isomerase; *HSOR*, hydroxysteroid oxidoreductase (ketosteroid reductase); *lyase*, desmolase.

testicular production achieves peak serum testosterone levels at 12 to 18 weeks. In the second half of gestation males show a gradual decline and females a rise in serum testosterone levels, so that by the third trimester males have similar or only slightly higher levels than females (Fig. 37-30).

The major stimulus for testicular secretion of testosterone during the period of genital differentiation is believed to be placental human chorionic gonadotropin (hCG), whereas fetal pituitary luteinizing hormone (LH) is believed to be the principal stimulus during the second half of gestation (Fig. 37-30), when growth of the penis and other genitalia occurs. Fetal serum hCG levels are estimated to be 15 to 150 times lower than maternal levels, suggesting that only a small fraction of placental hCG reaches the fetus. The human fetal kidneys and liver have the capacity to synthesize hCG at midgestation; if production occurs at 8 to 14 weeks, this may represent an alternate source of fetal hCG during sexual differentiation. The fetal testes are able to bind and respond to hCG with production of testosterone. In the second and third trimesters, fetal serum LH levels correlate with the subsequent maintenance and decline in serum testosterone.

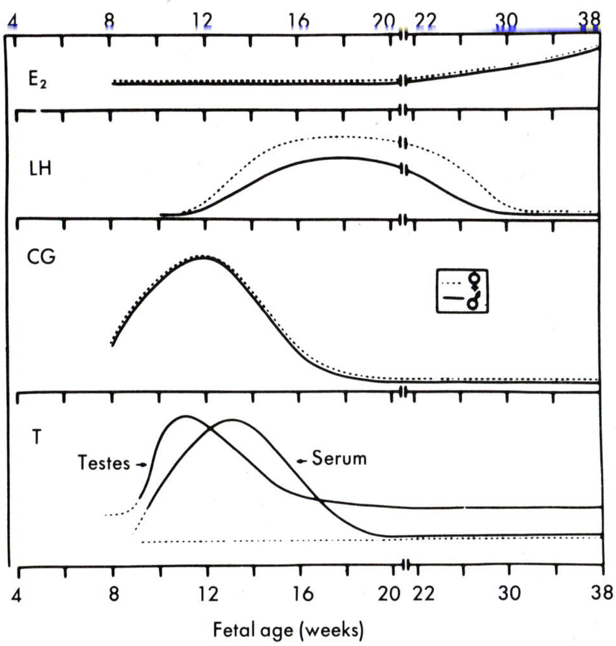

Fig. 37-30. Serum levels of estradiol *(E_2)*, leuteinizing hormone *(LH)*, human chorionic gonadotropin*(hCG)*, and serum and testicular concentrations of testosterone *(T)* throughout fetal life. (From Reyes, F.I., Winter, J.D.S., and Faiman, C.: Gonadotropin-gonadal interrelationships in the fetus. In New, M.I., and Fiser, R.J., Jr., editors: Diabetes and other endocrine disorders during pregnancy and in the newborn, Progress in clinical and biological research, vol. 10, New York, 1976, Alan R. Liss, Inc.)

Starting at 8 weeks' gestation, the fetal ovary becomes capable of converting testosterone or androstenedione to estrone and estradiol. Whether the human fetal ovaries actually produce estradiol or other hormones has not been demonstrated; most estrogen present in the fetus is produced by the placenta. Amniotic fluid levels of estradiol at 12 to 16 weeks, however, are slightly higher in females, which suggests the possibility of ovarian synthesis of estrogen. Estradiol synthesis, possibly stimulated by follicle-stimulating hormone (FSH), if it does occur, could play a local role in ovarian differentiation.

CONTROL OF FETAL SEX DIFFERENTIATION

Gonadal differentiation: role of the H-Y antigen

The Y chromosome is pivotal in determining the differentiation of the bipotential gonad. In the presence of the Y chromosome, the bipotential gonad will differentiate into a testis; if the Y chromosome is absent, ovarian differentiation will then occur. The presence of one, two, or more X chromosomes does not alter this course. The induction of testicular differentiation is exerted during 6 and 7 weeks' gestation, when the Y-bearing somatic (epithelial and mesenchymal) cells of the gonadal blastema and the primordial germ cells interact to form seminiferous cords. Conversely, these same cells lacking a Y chromosome will interact at 6½ to 8 weeks to form primordial follicles.

The differentiation of the Y-chromosomal gonadal cells into seminiferous cords is attributed to the presence of a specific protein on the cell surface membranes, the H-Y (histocompatibility-Y) antigen, which is regulated by the H-Y gene located on the short arm of the Y chromosome. The H-Y antigen is found on all cells having a Y chromosome, but only the gonadal cells of both sexes have specific receptors for the H-Y antigen, which thus permits their interaction or stimulation. The Sertoli cells also can secrete H-Y antigen, and in vitro studies have shown that H-Y antigen can act as a hormone to induce male differentiation of gonadal cells. H-Y antigen is a protein with a molecular weight of 18,000 daltons in monomeric form; it polymerizes readily to form larger aggregates. Probably more than one gene and chromosome regulate H-Y antigen production. The H-Y locus on the short arm of the Y chromosome is probably a regulatory gene; the structural gene is postulated to be on an autosome, and the X chromosome may also contain a gene that represses H-Y antigen production.

The concept of the H-Y antigen explains many disorders of gonadal differentiation. The finding of testicular tissue in the absence of a Y chromosome can be explained by translocation of the H-Y gene to an X chromosome or by mutation of the structural or repressor gene. The absence of testicular tissue in an XY individual can be explained by a selective loss or mutation of the H-Y gene or of the structural gene, or by lack of a normal receptor for the H-Y antigen. As helpful as these concepts are, however, it still remains to be definitely proved that it is the H-Y antigen, and not another closely related genetic product, that is the testis determinant.

In the absence of the H-Y antigen, the indifferent gonad will undergo early ovarian differentiation, regardless of the karyotype. Early ovarian differentiation does not require two X chromosomes and thus is seen in 45,XO fetuses. Whether a specific ovary-inducing factor exists is not known. In later ovarian development the presence of two X chromosomes is required to provide a double dose of certain genes for oocyte differentiation; unlike somatic cells, germ cells do not undergo random inactivation of the second X chromosome. In the absence of part of or all the second X chromosome, ovarian development fails to progress beyond 13 to 15 weeks of fetal age, and the primordial follicles and germ cells degenerate rapidly. The resultant gonad appears as an elongated, whitish streak that microscopically shows whorls of fibrous tissue (appearing as ovarian stroma) lacking in germ cells or epithelial (endocrine) elements. This streak gonad is characteristic for the gonadal dysgenesis syndromes. Y-chromosomal fetuses who fail to undergo testicular differentiation are believed to undergo the same early ovarian differentiation and late degeneration as occurs in the 45,XO fetus. They also have streak gonads postnatally and are categorized as having gonadal dysgenesis, but they carry a high risk for development of gonadal tumors, unlike gonadal dysgenesis patients with X chromosome abnormalities. This may result from the persistence of residual XY germ cells that did not degenerate.

Spermatogonia that lose the Y chromosome are nonviable, suggesting that genes on the Y chromosome are necessary for spermatogenesis. The X chromosome is normally inactivated in the spermatocyte, but the presence of a second X chromosome (e.g., 47,XXY syndrome) will result in meiotic failure, loss of germ cells, and infertility.

Genital differentiation: role of müllerian inhibiting factor and testosterone

In the absence of testes, female sex differentiation occurs regardless of whether an ovary, streak gonad, or no gonad is present; a male fetus castrated early also undergoes female sex differentiation (Fig. 37-31). This is in keeping with the inherent tendency of the fetus to develop along female lines.

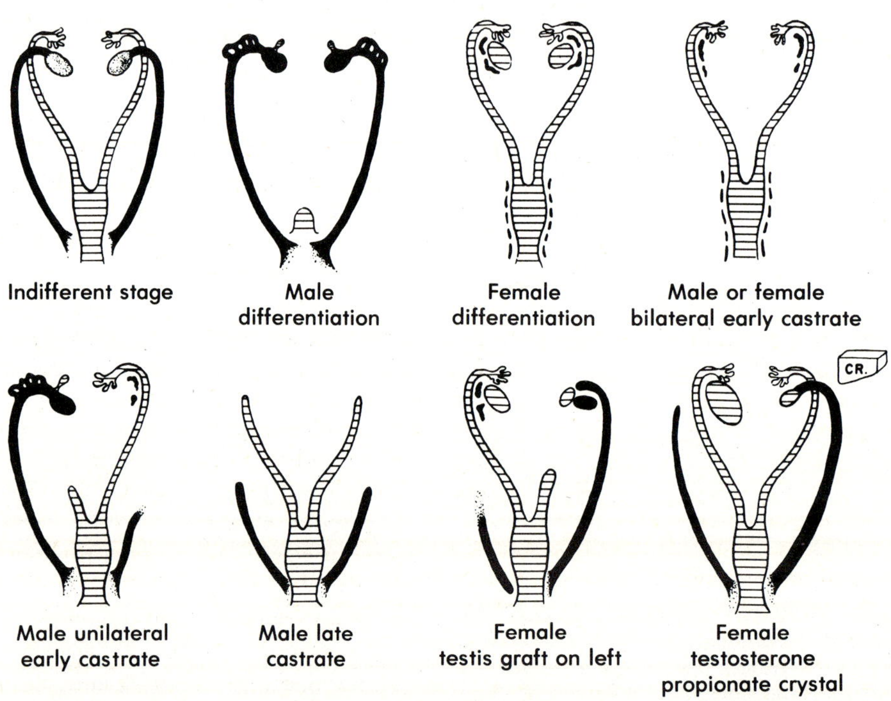

Fig. 37-31. Schematic representation of Jost's studies of the factors controlling genital duct differentiation in the rabbit embryo. These findings also apply to the human embryo. (From Grumbach, M.M., and Conte, F.A.: Disorders of sexual differentiation. In Wilson, J.D., and Foster, D.W., editors: Williams textbook of endocrinology, ed. 7, Philadelphia, © 1985, W.B. Saunders Co.)

Male sex differentiation requires bilateral testes, which produce MIF and testosterone. MIF acts locally to cause regression of the ipsilateral müllerian duct only. If only one testis is present, müllerian duct development will occur on the contralateral side (Fig. 37-31). The entire length of the müllerian duct is not sensitive to MIF at the same time, so its regression occurs sequentially, starting either at its cranial end or at the section adjacent to the caudal end of the testis. Testosterone does not cause müllerian duct regression.

Testosterone secreted by the fetal testis acts locally to stimulate differentiation of the ipsilateral wolffian duct (Fig. 37-31) and also is secreted into the systemic circulation to serve as a prohormone in the masculinization of the external genitalia. If only one testis is present, the contralateral wolffian duct will fail to differentiate, indicating that systemic testosterone is inadequate for stimulation of wolffian differentiation. Thus testosterone derived from maternal sources or from the fetal adrenals, as in congenital adrenal hyperplasia, will not induce wolffian development.

The external genitalia and urogenital sinus undergo male differentiation as a result of the action of DHT, which is produced peripherally within these tissues by the single-step conversion of testosterone by 5α-reductase. DHT in turn must bind to the androgen receptor to induce male differentiation (Fig. 37-32). Testosterone in the external genitalia serves only as a prohormone and, unlike its effect on the wolffian ducts, does not itself induce external genital male differentiation. The source of the systemic testosterone does not matter, so androgens derived from maternal sources or from the fetal adrenals in congenital adrenal hyperplasia also may induce masculinization of the external genitalia when metabolized to DHT. The absence of one testis is usually associated with incomplete masculinization of the external genitalia, suggesting that two testes are generally required to provide adequate systemic levels of testosterone and consequently adequate DHT. If 5α-reductase activity is deficient, DHT will not be produced, and the external genitalia will follow their inherent tendency and differentiate along female lines, with only slight masculinization occurring because this enzyme deficiency is typically not complete. A distal blind vaginal pouch also develops. The period in which DHT may induce male differentiation is limited to before 12 to 14 weeks' gestational age; any deficiency, such as incomplete labioscrotal fusion, cannot be corrected beyond this time. Hypospadias thus may reflect an error in differentiation, for whatever reason, that occurred between 9 and 14 weeks' gestation.

Cells that are stimulated by androgens to undergo differentiation include not only the cells of the wolffian duct, external genitalia, and urogenital sinus, but also the cells of the bone marrow, liver, kidney, and other tissues. The effect of androgens on such target cells is

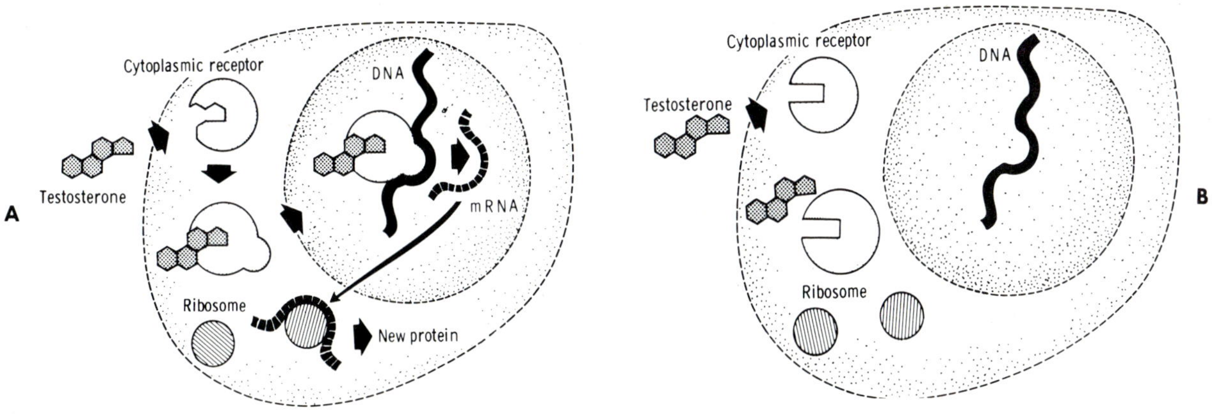

Fig. 37-32. Role of the androgen receptor in mediating testosterone or dihydrotestosterone (DHT) action within peripheral target tissues. **A,** Normal process. Testosterone freely diffuses into the target cell. In the wolffian duct tissues, testosterone itself binds with the androgen receptor, whereas in the external genital tissues, testosterone is first reduced by 5α-reductase to DHT, which then binds in the external genital tissues with the androgen receptor. The steroid-receptor complex then translocates to the nucleus, where it binds to a specific acceptor, leading to the transcription of nuclear messenger ribonucleic acid *(mRNA)* and synthesis of new protein that result in male differentiation. **B,** Consequence of loss of specific binding of testosterone or DHT. A qualitative abnormality of the androgen receptor or of a postreceptor step results in failure of testosterone or DHT to stimulate male differentiation of the target cell. The cell thus behaves as though androgens were absent, that is, in a female manner. (From Imperato-McGinley, J., and Peterson, R.E.: Am. J. Med. **61:**251, 1976.)

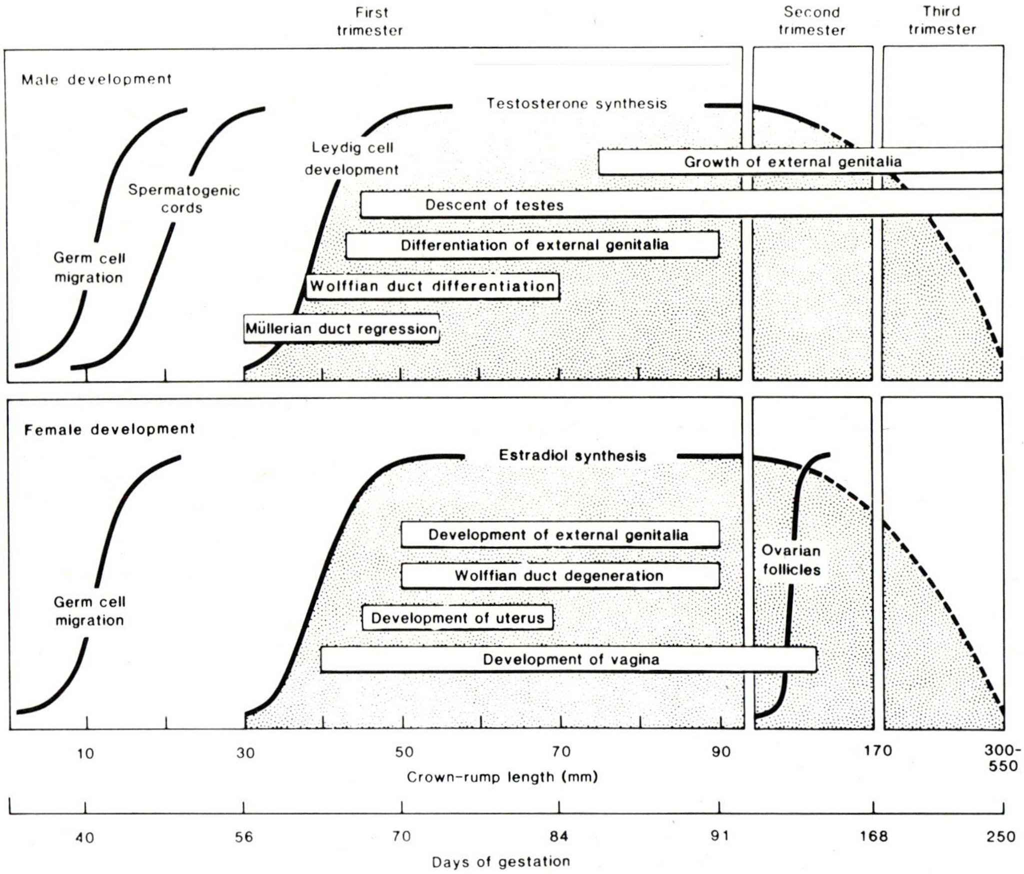

Fig. 37-33. Relationship between gonadal and genital differentiation and development in male *(top)* and female *(bottom)* fetuses from 5 weeks' gestational age to term. (The curve showing estradiol synthesis by the female ovary should be ignored, since there is no evidence for significant estradiol secretion by the human fetal ovary; estradiol also is not considered to be of any importance in fetal sex differentiation.) (From Wilson, J.D., George, F.W., and Griffin, J.E.: Science **211:**1278, 1981. Copyright 1981 by the American Association for the Advancement of Science.)

mediated by a specific protein receptor located in the cytosol or nucleus and a specific acceptor, presumably a nonhistone protein, located in the nucleus. Testosterone enters target cells by passive diffusion and either remains unmetabolized or is reduced via the 5α-reductase enzyme to DHT. Testosterone or DHT then binds to the androgen receptor, and this receptor-steroid complex is translocated to the nucleus, where it interacts with a specific acceptor. This interaction results in transcription of certain genes with consequent production of new messenger ribonucleic acid (mRNA) and synthesis of new proteins, resulting in differentiation of the target cells (Fig. 37-32, *A*). Androgen receptors have been identified in many tissues from various species and in fetuses as early as 8 weeks' gestational age and are present equally in both sexes.

A deficiency of androgen-receptor binding results in androgen insensitivity, which may be partial or complete (Fig. 37-32, *B*). In terms of fetal sex differentiation, the androgen-mediated events of wolffian duct differentiation, masculinization of the external genitalia, and growth of genital stuctures would either be impaired or would completely fail to occur, depending on the extent of receptor deficiency. XY patients with complete androgen insensitivity, also known as testicular feminization syndrome, have bilateral testes and absence of müllerian ducts with failure of formation of wolffian ducts, complete lack of masculinization of the external genitalia, and a distal vaginal pouch, giving them a normal phenotypic female appearance. Patients with partial androgen insensitivity have partial wolffian duct development and partial masculinization of the external genitalia (one example is the pedigree originally described by Reifenstein). In other patients the receptor deficiency may be

Fetal sex differentiation

1. Occurs in the first trimester (6 to 14 weeks) only
2. Is inherently female and does not require ovaries or estrogens
3. As a male requires:
   - H-Y gene, H-Y antigen and its receptor
   - Bilateral testes producing müllerian-inhibiting factor and testosterone
   - 5α-Reductase enzyme (external genitalia)
   - Testosterone and dihydrotestosterone receptor (internal and external genitalia)

so slight as to result only in a micropenis or infertility. The gene responsible for formation of the androgen receptor is located on the X chromosome. Androgen insensitivity also may be caused by an abnormality beyond the androgen receptor step (postreceptor defect), such as a deficiency in the nuclear acceptor or in the events related to transcription of mRNA or new protein formation.

Summary

Fetal sex differentiation occurs between 6 and 12 to 14 weeks of fetal age in a given sequence (Fig. 37-33) and with certain requirements (see boxed material); growth of the genitalia occurs thereafter. The inherent development of the fetus is along female lines. Female sex differentiation between 6 and 14 weeks of fetal age does not appear to require ovaries or estradiol or even two X chromosomes; it does require the absence of male determinants (H-Y antigen, MIF, testosterone). The only abnormalities seen in female sex differentiation are masculinization of the external genitalia following exposure of the female fetus to abnormally elevated levels of androgens between 8 and 14 weeks, as in congenital adrenal hyperplasia, and the abnormalities of ovarian development that occur beyond 13 to 15 weeks gestation, such as in 45,XO Turner's syndrome. Male sex differentiation is more complicated and requires the H-Y gene(s), the H-Y antigen and its receptor, bilateral testes producing MIF and testosterone, peripheral 5α-reductase activity, and intact androgen receptor function in the target cells. Consequently there are many more disorders of male sex differentiation than of female sex differentiation.

ABNORMALITIES OF SEXUAL DIFFERENTIATION

The abnormalities of sexual differentiation are classified in the boxed material on the right and are reviewed in the following discussion.

Classification of abnormalities of sexual differentiation

DISORDERS OF GONADAL DIFFERENTIATION

- True hermaphroditism
- Gonadal dysgenesis
  - X chromosome abnormalities (Turner's syndrome)
  - XX gonadal dysgenesis
  - Y chromosome abnormalities and mixed gonadal dysgenesis
  - XY gonadal dysgenesis
- Testicular dysgenesis
  - Dysgenetic testes (renal disease, Wilms' tumor)
  - Testicular regression
    - Early (XY gonadal agenesis)
    - Late (congenital anorchia)
  - Rudimentary or small testes
  - Seminiferous tubule dysgenesis
    - XXY (Klinefelter's) syndrome and variants
    - XX male

DISORDERS OF TESTICULAR HORMONE SYNTHESIS OR ACTION (MALE PSEUDOHERMAPHRODITISM)

- Deficiencies of müllerian-inhibiting factor
- Testicular unresponsiveness to human chorionic gonadotropin or luteinizing hormone (Leydig cell hypoplasia)
- Inborn errors of testosterone biosynthesis
  - Enzyme defects affecting cortisol and testosterone synthesis (congenital adrenal hyperplasia)
    - Cholesterol side-chain cleavage enzyme deficiency
    - 3β-Hydroxysteroid dehydrogenase deficiency
    - 17α-Hydroxylase deficiency
  - Enzyme defects affecting testosterone synthesis
    - 17,20-Desmolase (17,20-lyase) deficiency
    - 17β-Hydroxysteroid oxidoreductase deficiency
- Disorders of androgen-dependent target tissues
  - 5α-Reductase deficiency
  - Androgen insensitivity syndromes
    - Complete (testicular feminization syndrome)
    - Partial (incomplete testicular feminization)
- Maternally derived progestins

MASCULINZATION OF FEMALE EXTERNAL GENITALIA (FEMALE PSEUDOHERMAPHRODITISM)

- Congenital adrenal hyperplasia
  - 21-Hydroxylase deficiency: simple virilizing and salt-losing forms
  - 11β-Hydroxylase deficiency
  - 3β-Hydroxysteroid dehydrogenase deficiency
- Maternally derived androgenic substances
  - Virilizing ovarian or adrenal tumors
  - Congenital adrenal hyperplasia in mother
  - Androgen, progestin, or estrogen therapy
- Non-androgen-induced genital masculinization
  - Associated with malformations of intestine and urinary tract
  - Isolated genital masculinization

OTHER DISORDERS OF SEXUAL DIFFERENTIATION OR MORPHOGENESIS

- Hypospadias
- Micropenis
- Cryptorchidism
- Müllerian and vaginal dysgenesis

DISORDERS OF GONADAL DIFFERENTIATION

This group of disorders is characterized by the failure of either testes or ovaries to undergo normal anatomic differentiation or development. Most of these disorders result from abnormalities in the genetic control of gonadal differentiation, but in some the cause may result from an embryonic fault or an unrecognized disturbance in gonadogenesis.

True hermaphroditism

True hermaphroditism is defined as the coexistence in an individual of ovarian and testicular tissue in either the same gonad or opposite gonads. The ovarian tissue must contain ovarian follicles or corpora albicantia, since fibrous stroma alone does not define ovarian tissue; for testicular tissue to be definitely diagnosed, it must contain seminiferous tubules or spermatozoa. Several chromosome karyotypes are seen in true hermaphroditism: approximately three fifths of the cases are 46,XX; one fifth are 46,XY or 45,XO/46,XY; and one fifth show mosaicism or chimerism, being 46,XX/46,XY or 46,XX/47,XXY. The most frequently occurring gonadal combinations are an ovary and testis or an ovary and ovotestis; the XX karyotype favors the development of an ovary, the XY karyotype a testis. The ovotestis accounts for 44% of all gonads in this condition, the ovary 34% and testis, 22%; 0.7% of patients may have a unilateral streak gonad or a tumor. Ovarian tissue occurs more often on the left side and testicular tissue more often on the right side.

The internal genital ducts reflect the gonadal constitution. On the side of an ovary a fallopian tube is almost always seen, and on the side of the testis the vas deferens and epididymis are almost always present. On the side of an ovotestis a vas is seen 35% of the time, and a fallopian tube, often closed at the fimbrial end, is seen 65% of the time. A uterus is described in about 86% of patients, but it is usually hypoplastic, unicornuate, or otherwise maldeveloped, being normal in only 10%.

The external genitalia are usually ambiguous, although several cases have been reported with normal male or female appearance. The urethra most often opens on the perineum as a urogenital sinus, giving an appearance of perineal hypospadias. The phallus is usually larger than a normal clitoris (Fig. 37-34) and often has chordee; it often is of sufficient size to give the genitalia a more masculine appearance. Gonads are descended or palpable in 61% of patients, more frequently on the right side; about 60% are ovotestes and most of the remainder are testes, but rarely an ovary may descend. The ovotestis is more likely to descend if it contains a greater proportion of testicular tissue. The ovarian portion of the ovotestis tends to be firm and convoluted and is histologically normal except for a reduction in the number of primordial follicles in infants. The testicular portion tends to be soft, smooth, and histologically normal in infants, but it becomes abnormal in more than 90% of adults, marked by tubular atrophy with undifferentiated germ cells and absence of spermatogenesis. In intact testes, the histiology is similar, with spermatogenesis seen in only 12% of patients. Fertility has been reported in a small number of females and in only one male. The testosterone response to hCG stimulation more often is low but can be normal, depending on the amount of testicular tissue present. Gonadal tumors occur in 2.6% and are more frequent in Y chromosome–positive patients. Renal abnormalities have been noted in 4.6% of 150 cases reviewed.

The incidence of true hermaphroditism is unknown. Most cases occur sporadically, but several affected families have been reported. There are three possible causes of true hermaphroditism: (1) chimerism or mosaicism involving the second X and the Y chromosome, (2) translocation of the H-Y gene locus to an X chromosome or an autosome, or conversely, possible translocation of an ovarian gene locus from the X to the Y chromosome or an autosome, and (3) the possibility of an autosomal gene mutation that causes sex reversal. *Chimerism* refers to the presence of two cell lines that originate from different zygotes, whereas in *mosaicism* the different cell lines originate from a common zygote by nondisjunction.

Most cases of true hermaphroditism are potentially recognizable in the neonatal period because of ambiguous genitalia. If a gonad is an ovotestis, one pole may feel firmer. Most patients will have a palpable uterus. Approximately 70% of cases will be X-chromatin positive on buccal smear; in these individuals it is necessary to rule out female pseudohermaphroditism, particularly congenital adrenal hyperplasia, and an XX male. The definitive diagnosis requires a gonadal biopsy, but this is preferably delayed to beyond the neonatal period because making the diagnosis is not urgent.

The assignment of sex of rearing should be based on the size of the phallus and the likelihood of satisfactorily correcting the external genital abnormalities to give a normal male or female appearance by early childhood. The chances for fertility are extremely poor as a male and only a little better as a female, so this should not be a major factor in deciding the sex of rearing, although the presence of a normal uterus or vagina would be an argument for female assignment. A decision as to sex of rearing should not await a gonadal biopsy. At the time of genital reconstructive surgery, a deep wedge biopsy of both gonads down to the hilum is done. Effort should be made to preserve appropriate gonadal tissue, with removal of unwanted gonadal and genital tissue. The preservation of ovarian tissue is more likely to be successful with regard to later endocrine and fertility function than will preservation of testicular tissue. With an

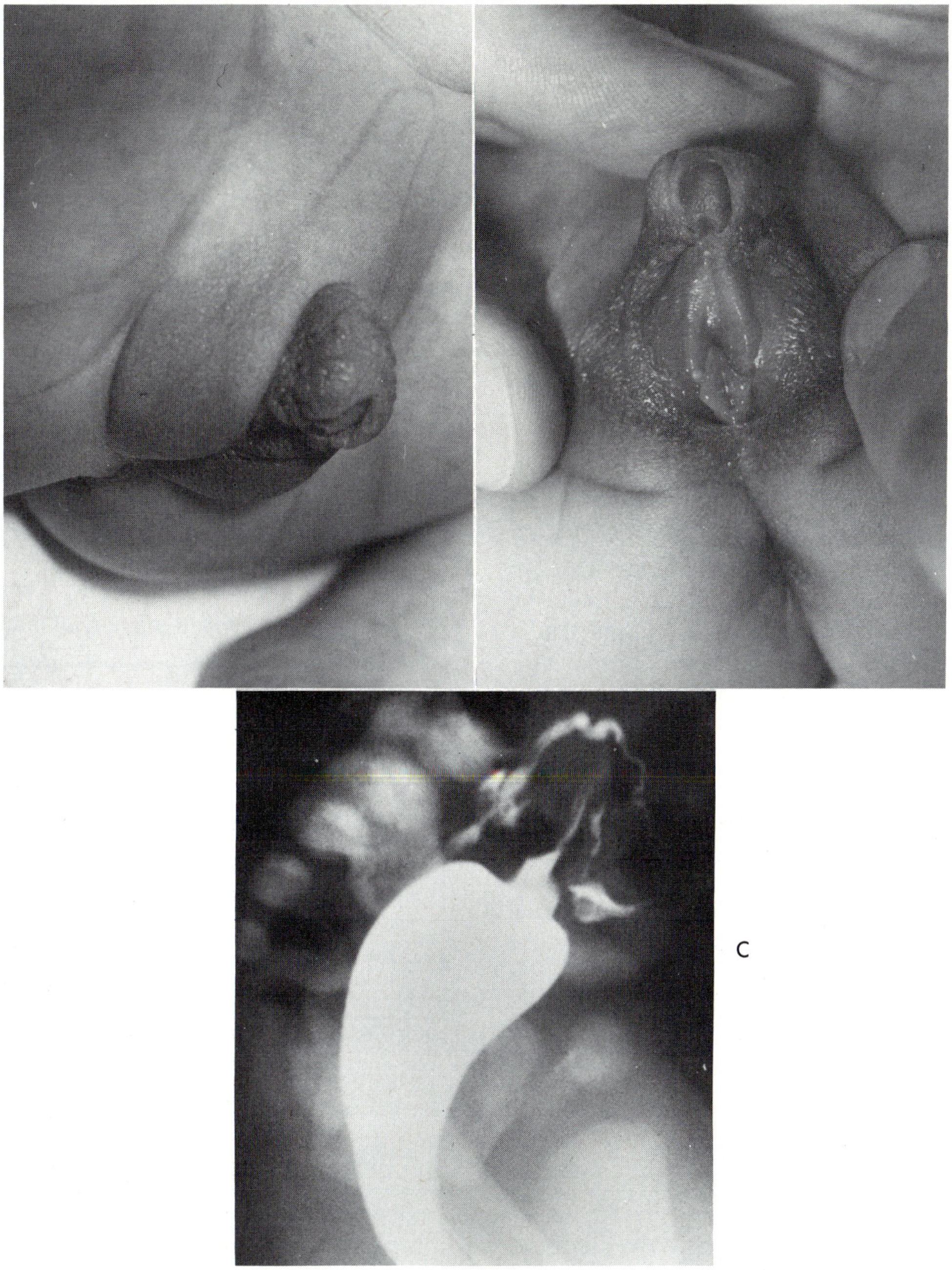

Fig. 37-34. A, A 46,XX neonate with true hermaphroditism was noted at birth to have clitoromegaly (1.8 × 0.8 cm) and slightly rugated and full labia majora. **B,** The genitalia were otherwise those of a normal female; gonads were impalpable, and a uterine cervix was present on rectal examination and endoscopy. **C,** A genitogram showed presence of a 5 cm vagina, above which contrast media entered a uterus and bilateral fallopian tubes. Serum testosterone was high-normal for a female at 60 ng/dl on day 1 of life, was abnormally elevated to 75 ng/dl and 134 ng/dl at ages 2 and 5 weeks, and increased to 389 ng/dl after hCG stimulation. Bilateral gonads spontaneously descended into the inguinal region at age 5 weeks (before hCG stimulation) and were found to be ovotestes on biopsy; ovarian tissue was left behind on one side. Clitoral reduction was performed later in infancy because of a further increase in clitoral size to 2.4 × 1.3 cm.

ovotestis, preservation of the desired portion is sometimes possible, but complete removal is necessary when the ovarian and testicular tissues are not arranged pole to pole, since the testicular tissue is then frequently located in the hilar region. The risk of gonadal tumor development, which is greater for testicular than ovarian tissue, needs to be monitored subsequently.

Gonadal dysgenesis

Gonadal dysgenesis describes a group of disorders marked by the presence of a streak gonad unilaterally or bilaterally in an individual. The streak gonad represents the result of failed gonadal (ovarian or testicular) differentiation. As discussed next, multiple causes exist, the most common resulting from structural abnormalities of the X chromosome (Turner's syndrome).

X chromosome abnormalities (Turner's syndrome)

Turner, in 1938, described a series of phenotypic females who had a triad of somatic features consisting of infantilism (short stature, delayed bone age, absence of secondary sexual development), webbing of the skin of the neck, and deformity of the elbow (cubitus valgus). Other investigators subsequently noted similar patients to have gonadal dysgenesis (manifested as bilateral streak gonads) with elevated gonadotropins; other somatic abnormalities were also frequently associated. In 1959 the cause of this form of gonadal dysgenesis was found to be a loss of the second X chromosome, that is, a 45,XO chromosome karyotype. Variant forms of this syndrome were also recognized in which patients had only partial deletions of the second X chromosome or X chromosome mosaicism such as XO/XX. The somatic abnormalities appear to be controlled by genes located on the X chromosome.

In fetuses with 45,XO gonadal dysgenesis, normal ovarian differentiation occurs up to 13 to 15 weeks' gestation, followed by rapid degeneration and atresia of the primordial ovarian follicles. In affected neonates and infants the late stages of this process are usually evident, with scattered primordial ovarian follicles in varying states of degeneration seen histologically. The streak gonad is the final result and usually appears by childhood; it is an elongated, whitish streak consisting of whorls of connective tissue, suggestive of ovarian stroma, that contains no germinal elements or endocrine or other epithelial elements.

Affected patients have normal müllerian duct development, absence of wolffian ducts, and phenotypically female external genitalia. Since the genitalia are normal, identification of neonates is limited to those who have the accompanying Turner's somatic abnormalities, as listed in the boxed material. The presence of lymphatic

Features of Turner's phenotype in the neonate

Intrauterine growth retardation
Head and facies: low-set ears, low nuchal hairline, asynchronous growth of scalp hair, epicanthus, folds below lower lids, micrognathia, high palate
Lymphatic: lymphedema of dorsa of hands and feet, hypoplasia of nails, loose neck folds (cutis laxa) or cystic hygroma, gross edema, hydrops
Skeletal: short fourth metacarpals, shield chest
Urinary tract: rotated or horseshoe kidneys, renal hypoplasia, duplications
Cardiovascular: coarctation of aorta, aortic stenosis

Modified from Gordon, R.R., and O'Neill, E.M.: Br. Med. J. **1:**483, 1969.

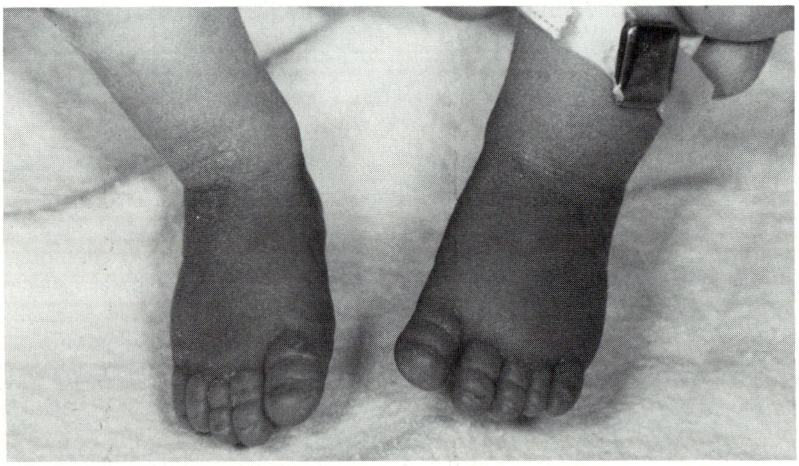

Fig. 37-35. Lymphedema of the dorsa of the feet with hypoplasia of the nails in a newborn with 45,XO gonadal dysgenesis (Turner's syndrome).

(Fig. 37-35) or cardiovascular abnormalities is most useful. Other patients come to medical attention later, usually because of short stature or failure of secondary sexual development.

Patients with X chromosome mosaicism or partial deletion of the second X chromosome tend to have fewer somatic and gonadal manifestations than those with the 45,XO karyotype. In cases of mosaicism, the relative proportion of XX to XO cells may determine the extent to which normal development of gonadal and somatic tissues can occur. Patients having only a partial deletion of the X chromosome may also manifest a modified phenotype, depending on the part of the X chromosome deleted. The combined incidence of 45,XO, partial deletion, and mosaic Turner's syndromes is approximately 1 in 2,000 female newborns.

The cause of monosomy X is unknown. The mean maternal and paternal ages are not raised, so nondisjunction is not thought to be important; a postfertilization abnormality is thought to be most likely. The incidence of the 45,XO karyotype in spontaneous abortuses is very high, generally estimated to be 10%. The mean incidence of living 45,XO newborns, however, is only approximately 1 in 5,000 female births, suggesting that about 99% of XO fetuses abort. The reasons for this high mortality are unclear, but hypoalbuminemia, generalized edema, serous effusions, and renal and cardiovascular abnormalities may play a role.

An infant suspected of having Turner's syndrome may be screened with a buccal smear; the clinician must recognize that false-negative and false-positive results may occur. (In the first few days of life, 46,XX female neonates normally may have a reduced percentage of sex-chromatin–positive nuclei as low as 4%.) Patients with partial deletion or mosaicism of the X chromosome may have a normal buccal smear. A definitive diagnosis requires a karyotype. A high rate of failure occurs in the culture of 45,XO cells, so repeated attempts may be necessary. Banding techniques should be used, and 20 or more cells should be assessed for the possibility of mosaicism. At times, multiple tissues need to be karyotyped before mosaicism may be identified. Serum follicle-stimulating hormone (FSH) is abnormally elevated in infancy and again after age 10 to 12 years, but it is normal in childhood.

The sex of rearing is female. The prognosis is usually for absence of any ovarian functions, but 3% to 5% of patients do show variable secondary sexual development, and a very small number of pregnancies have been reported. Successful pregnancies have also been achieved in gonadal dysgenesis by embryo transfer and hormone support. There is no increased risk of gonadal tumor development. Monitoring of growth, for recurrent otitis media and hearing loss, and for other associated abnormalities is recommended in childhood. The incidence of mental retardation is not increased, although directional sense and space-form recognition are impaired. The antenatal diagnosis of Turner's syndrome has occurred following ultrasound identification of a cystic hygroma early in the second trimester and appropriate karyotyping.

XX gonadal dysgenesis

Patients with XX gonadal dysgenesis have bilateral streak gonads (some have hypoplastic ovaries) with intact müllerian duct structures and female external genitalia. They differ from patients with Turner's syndrome in that they usually have normal stature, absence of Turner's stigmata, no abnormality of the X chromosome, and frequently a familial condition. An abnormality of an autosomal gene that regulates either germ cell migration, formation of the bipotential gonad, or ovarian differentiation is thought to be the cause. Associated defects are seen in some families, including deafness, neurologic abnormalities, and renal disease. Isolated instances of clitoromegaly have been described, resulting from testosterone production by either hilar cells or luteinized gonadal stromal cells in a streak gonad; such patients are likely to be recognized in infancy. The differential diagnosis includes defects in estradiol synthesis.

Y chromosome abnormalities

Patients with Y chromosome abnormalities involving a partial deletion of the Y chromosome may have abnormal gonadal and statural development. These cases have provided some insight as to the possible location of the gene loci for testicular differentiation and growth.

An abnormal or partially deleted Y chromosome will frequently result in chromosome mosaicism, usually XO/XY or XO/XYY. The relative prevalence of the XO and XY cell lines and whether the Y chromosome has retained or lost the H-Y locus results in a wide range of gonadal and somatic phenotypes. At one end of the spectrum, affected individuals largely manifest the 45,XO features and appear identical with 45,XO Turner's syndrome patients. They have bilateral streak gonads and müllerian structures, female external genitalia, short stature, and Turner's somatic abnormalities. However, they differ in also having a 15% to 20% risk of gonadal tumor development and an increased risk of unwanted virilization. At the other end of the spectrum are XO/XY phenotypic males with predominantly 46,XY features. They have almost normal male external genitalia, bilateral testes and wolffian duct development, absence of müllerian structures, normal stature, and absence of Turner's stigmata. Whether they have an increased risk of gonadal tumor formation is unknown.

Individuals toward the middle of the spectrum manifest a mixture of XO and XY features. They have ambiguous genitalia, varying degrees of testicular development (dysgenetic or normal, and unilateral or bilateral), persistence of müllerian structures, and variable presence of short stature or other Turner's stigmata. They also are at high risk for gonadal tumor development and often have a gonadal tumor obscuring the original gonadal architecture. A major subset of this group is the syndrome of mixed gonadal dysgenesis, described next.

Mixed gonadal dysgenesis

Mixed gonadal dysgenesis is used to describe individuals with a unilateral functioning (normal or dysgenetic) testis and a contralateral streak or absent gonad. All have some degree of virilization of the external genitalia, ranging from clitoromegaly or partial labial fusion to almost normal male external genitalia; slightly more than half have a urogenital sinus. All patients have some müllerian development, consisting of an upper vagina, uterus, and a fallopian tube, usually on the side having a streak or absent gonad. An epididymis or vas deferens is present on the testicular side in half the patients, and the testis is most frequently located in the inguinal canal. Variably normal to diminished or absent testosterone responses have been reported with hCG stimulation, and gonadotropins have been normal or elevated. Gonadal tumors occur in 22%, affecting either the testis or the streak gonad; a gonadal tumor has not been described in a scrotal testis. Diagnostic overlap with true hermaphroditism may occur in infants if the "streak gonad" still contains a number of primordial ovarian follicles that suggest ovarian tissue rather than a streak gonad.

Management involves appropriate sex assignment in the newborn period based on functional considerations first and fertility second. The association of short stature with the 45,XO karyotype may influence a decision toward female sex of rearing. Dysgenetic gonads should be removed in infancy or early childhood because of the increased risk of tumor formation. The cause of mixed gonadal dysgenesis is thought to be an abnormality of the Y chromosome. The syndrome provides confirmation that the unilateral testis affects only ipsilateral wolffian and müllerian duct development.

XY gonadal dysgenesis

The syndrome of XY gonadal dysgenesis is characterized by a normal XY karyotype with the presence of bilateral streak gonads, intact müllerian structures, a female phenotype, and absence of the somatic abnormalities of Turner's syndrome. Most cases occur sporadically, but family aggregates have been reported, some involving two or three generations, compatible with either X-linked recessive or autosomal dominant male-limited inheritance. XY gonadal dysgenesis is genetically heterogeneous in that some individuals are H-Y antigen negative, and others are H-Y antigen positive. In the latter, it is postulated that the receptor for the H-Y antigen is abnormally formed or absent.

Clinical recognition of 46,XY gonadal dysgenesis is possible in the newborn period in infants with clitoromegaly; occasional neonates have presented with edema of the feet, and a significant association appears to exist with camptomelic dwarfism. There is a very high risk for the development of gonadal tumors in XY gonadal dysgenesis, approximately 5% in the first decade of life (occurring as early as 3 years of age) and overall about 30%. Prophylactic removal of the streak or dysgenetic gonads is indicated in infancy. The sex of rearing should be female.

The syndrome of XY gonadal dysgenesis has often been categorized with XX gonadal dysgenesis under the general term of *XY and XX pure gonadal dysgenesis* ("pure" because Turner's somatic stigmata are usually absent). This seems inappropriate. The cause of the XY form appears to be related to abnormalities of the H-Y antigen or its receptors, whereas the XX form appears to result from an autosomal mutation that affects ovarian development. The importance of XY gonadal dysgenesis is that it proves Jost's hypothesis that early castration or failure of testicular development will result in a female genital phenotype, regardless of chromosome constitution.

Testicular dysgenesis

In testicular dysgenesis the underlying defect is disordered testicular differentiation or development that results in anatomically or histologically abnormal testes and secondary impairment of hormonogenesis or spermatogenesis.

Dysgenetic testes

Dysgenetic testes are defined by the following characteristics: (1) their failure to induce regression of the ipsilateral müllerian duct structures, (2) their association with incomplete masculinization of the genitalia, (3) their variably abnormal histology, and (4) their increased predisposition to develop tumors originating from the germinal structures. The testes may be of normal or small size and are usually cryptorchid. The chromosome karyotype typically is 46,XY, but other karyotypes are seen. This disorder overlaps with (or may be part of) the Y chromosomal forms of gonadal dysgenesis and mixed gonadal dysgenesis, with distinction made by the presence or absence of a streak gonad(s). Dysgenetic testicular tissue is also seen in true hermaphroditism. The differential diagnosis includes the persistent müllerian duct syndrome caused by a disorder of MIF, as discussed later.

Associated glomerulopathy and Wilms' tumor. A number of patients with dysgenetic testes or Y chromosomal gonadal dysgenesis have had associated severe glomerulopathy (proteinuria, nephrotic syndrome, or renal failure) appearing in the neonatal period or infancy; more than half developed Wilms' tumor around the same age. Most had ambiguous genitalia but some had a female phenotype; müllerian duct structures were usually present. Karyotypes have been 46,XY with one case being 46,XX/46,XY. Aniridia, hypertension, gonadoblastoma, mental retardation, and a deletion of the short arm of chromosome 11 have been reported. End-stage renal disease develops rapidly. The death rate was 68% in a review of 22 cases. Urine testing of patients with dysgenetic testes, monitoring for development of Wilms' tumor in those with renal disease, and prophylactic gonadectomy for the 30% risk of tumor development are recommended. Most cases have been sporadic; defective embryogenesis of the urogenital ridge is postulated to be the cause.

Testicular regression syndromes

Early regression with genital ambiguity (XY gonadal agenesis). These XY patients are characterized by complete absence of testes, including absence of gonadal streaks, associated with almost complete absence of both müllerian and wolffian duct derivatives and female to partially masculinized genitalia (clitoromegaly and posterior labial fusion). Their gonadal and genital features may be explained as being caused by very early regression of the developing fetal testes, between approximately 8 and 10 weeks. Testicular failure must have occurred after the initial production of MIF by Sertoli cells but before the Leydig cells could produce sufficient testosterone for a reasonable time.

Other XY individuals have testes with quite well-developed wolffian structures but incomplete masculinization of external genitalia. Presumably testicular regression occurred slightly later than in those patients completely lacking internal genital ducts. Affected siblings have been reported, raising a possibility of autosomal recessive inheritance. The H-Y antigen has been present in the several cases studied. The differential diagnosis includes testicular insensitivity to hCG or LH (Leydig cell hypoplasia).

Late regression: congenital anorchia (vanishing testes syndrome). Many cases have been reported of cryptorchid 46,XY males who on exploration were found to have bilateral anorchia but with normal wolffian structures, absence of müllerian structures, and normal male external genitalia. The vas deferens ends blindly, often without an epididymis, either in the inguinal canal or upper scrotum (sometimes palpable as a small knot of tissue), retroperitoneally near the usual location of the internal inguinal ring, or in the iliac fossa. Neonates and infants with anorchia fail to show any rise in testosterone during either endogenous LH or exogenous hCG stimulation; serum LH and FSH levels should be abnormally elevated in infancy after age 2 weeks. In the 46,XY individual with a male phenotype, these findings are usually pathognomonic; if uncertainty exists, laparoscopy, computed tomography (CT), or surgical exploration may be necessary. In patients with monorchia (4% of cryptorchid boys), endocrine testing is not helpful in ruling out an abdominal gonad, and surgical exploration is indicated. The cause of congenital anorchia is not established, but the most likely explanation for at least some cases, including those occurring shortly after birth, is vascular occlusion or trauma resulting from testicular hemorrhage, torsion of the testis, breech delivery, or similar events. Infections, teratogens, immune mechanisms, or hereditary factors may play a role. The possibility that bilateral congenital anorchia is part of a continuum with early testicular regression has been suggested.

Rudimentary or small testes

A few 46,XY patients have been described with abnormally small testes associated with either ambiguous genitalia, a micropenis, or hypogonadism in adulthood. They have male internal genital ducts and lack any müllerian structures. Data are not available as to what constitutes a small testis in the neonate. Testes with a longest diameter of 1 cm or more are probably normal; 0.8 cm, low-normal; and 0.6 cm, abnormally small. It is unclear whether rudimentary or small testes represent a distinct entity, an attenuated form of testicular regression, or a variant form of dysgenetic testes. Testosterone levels are low, and LH and FSH levels are normal to high. Associated somatic abnormalities and affected siblings are seen. The differential diagnosis includes gonadotropin deficiency, dysgenetic testes, XXY syndrome, and Leydig cell hypoplasia. The sex of rearing is dictated principally by penile size and the likelihood of adequately correcting the ambiguous genitalia.

Seminiferous tubule dysgenesis

47,XXY (Klinefelter's) syndrome and variants. The major clinical manifestations of Klinefelter's syndrome develop with onset of puberty, and most patients are recognized at this time or beyond. The constant features then are small testes (100%) with azoospermia (93%) and histologic evidence of impaired spermatogenesis (100%). Infants with 47,XXY Klinefelter's syndrome occasionally have small testes or a micropenis that might permit their recognition. In 63 infants detected through chromosome screening programs at seven centers, congenital abnormalities included cleft palate, cryptorchidism, and inguinal hernia. An increased risk of XXY is present among twins. Mental, motor, speech, behavioral, and emotional development are frequently impaired. Testicular histology in the first year of life has varied from normal to extensively abnormal, with decreased to absent spermatogonia. Gonadotropin and testosterone studies of XXY infants in the first year of life have not been published. In one series, LH and FSH levels were normal from age 1 year up to midpuberty and then became elevated. Patients with Klinefelter's syndrome may be predisposed to the development of germ cell tumors, particularly those of extragonadal origin, which have occurred as early as a few months of age.

The incidence of the 47,XXY karyotype in live newborn males is about 1 in 1,000; if Klinefelter's variants are added, the overall incidence is about 1 in 800. Increased maternal age is associated with an additional X chromosome in both male and female offspring, although this effect is not so marked as that seen for autosomal trisomies.

Among the variant forms of Klinefelter's syndrome, patients with 48,XXXY, and 49,XXXXY karyotypes are more likely to be recognized early in life. All have somatic abnormalities and mental retardation, and many have a hypoplastic penis; of those with the 49,XXXXY karyotypes, all also have cryptorchidism and 14% have cardiac defects. Patients with 48,XXYY and 46,XY/47,XXY karyotypes are unlikely to be recognized in infancy.

XX male. These patients have bilateral testes in the absence of a Y chromosome, usually with normal male internal and external genitalia and a male psychosexual orientation. As with Klinefelter's syndome, the detrimental influence of the second X chromosome results in absence of spermatogonia and hyalinization of the tubules in adults; the testicular histology is near normal in the first year of life, but after age 1 to 2 years spermatogonia are lacking. Some 10% to 20% of patients have ambiguous genitalia at birth because of decreased fetal testosterone production; the testes are normal-sized prepubertally but may be cryptorchid. Most, if not all, XX males inherit one maternal and one paternal X chromosome, and all patients tested have been H-Y antigen positive. The cause in most cases may be X-Y interchange; other possible explanations include an autosomal gene mutation causing sex reversal (this may explain some of the familial cases), loss of an X chromosome gene that represses H-Y gene function, or unrecognized mosaicism. The differential diagnosis includes 46,XX true hermaphroditism (which appears to overlap with this syndrome), Klinefelter's syndrome, and female pseudohermaphroditism.

DISORDERS OF TESTICULAR HORMONE SYNTHESIS OR ACTION (MALE PSEUDOHERMAPHRODITISM

Male pseudohermaphroditism is defined as the presence of abnormal differentiation of either the internal genital ducts or the external genitalia in an individual having bilateral testes that contain tubular elements (seminiferous tubules with Sertoli cells and germinal cells). Disordered synthesis or action of MIF or testosterone is the underlying cause of the abnormalities seen. Some cases of dysgenetic testes and rudimentary testes overlap phenotypically with this category, but their underlying cause is testicular dysgenesis and not a primary disorder of the testicular hormones. Clinically, all patients with male pseudohermaphroditism are 46,XY; are familial, except maternally derived progestins; should have normal-sized and histologically normal testes in infancy, except Leydig cell hypoplasia; and lack any müllerian duct development, except persistent müllerian duct syndrome. In those who are severely undermasculinized, a blind distal vaginal pouch is present. It results when a lack of androgen stimulation permits the urovaginal septum to persist.

Deficiencies of müllerian-inhibiting factor (persistent müllerian duct syndrome)

Patients with MIF deficiencies are characterized by the presence of bilateral fallopian tubes and a uterus (occasionally hypoplastic or rudimentary) with an otherwise normal male phenotype, bilateral normal testes, and a 46,XY karyotype. Most have cryptorchidism, usually bilateral. The vas deferens is typically enmeshed with the tubes and uterus, so that the testes are frequently intraabdominal and difficult to bring down into the scrotum. Inguinal hernias occur in 37% and frequently contain a tube or rudimentary uterus; transverse testicular ectopia has been reported in many patients. These findings should enable most cases to be identified in infancy. The cause is believed to be either a deficiency of MIF, synthesis of an abnormal MIF, an MIF receptor defect, or a defect in timing of its secretion. Several familial cases involving brothers are reported, but the mode of inheritance is not known. The differential diagnosis includes dysgenetic testes, mixed gonadal dysgenesis, and true hermaphroditism. Both gonads should be verified as being normal testes. The sex of rearing should be male, and orchiopexy should be performed in infancy; about 5% to 10% of reported patients have developed testicular tumors in adulthood, possibly from either long-standing cryptorchidism or the underlying defect. The müllerian structures do not need to be removed, since they do not develop malignancy and a strong risk of damaging the wolffian duct structures is present. Spermatogenesis and presumably fertility are intact, but the risk of testicular tumor needs to be monitored.

Testicular unresponsiveness to human chorionic gonadotropin or luteinizing hormone (Leydig cell hypoplasia)

Patients with testicular unresponsiveness to hCG or LH have bilateral testes but fail to undergo male genital differentiation because of a failure to respond to hCG. The cause is thought to be a defect in the hCG-LH receptor that prevents binding of hCG and its stimulation of testosterone biosynthesis; primary agenesis or hypoplasia of the Leydig cells is an alternate possible explanation. In the complete absence of hCG binding, a female phenotype with a blind vaginal pouch but no wolffian or müllerian ducts is seen, whereas other patients have shown clitoromegaly, posterior labial fusion or perineal hypospadias (making them identifiable in the newborn period), and good development of the epididymis and vas deferens, suggesting a less than complete defect. The testes are usually cryptorchid and are small postpubertally, although possibly of normal size in infancy. The characteristic findings are a low basal level of testosterone, failure of testosterone response to hCG stimulation, and marked paucity or absence of Leydig cells on biopsy of the testes. The seminiferous tubules and Sertoli cells are normal, but spermatogenic arrest or absence is seen. The differential diagnosis includes XY gonadal agenesis, rudimentary testes, and those forms of male pseudohermaphroditism involving deficient androgen synthesis or action. The sex of rearing should be based on functional considerations. Familial occurrence has been reported.

Inborn errors of testosterone biosynthesis

Five enzymes, present in both the gonads and the adrenals, are involved in the biosynthesis of testosterone from cholesterol. A defect in any one will result in decreased to absent androgen (and estrogen) synthesis and male pseudohermaphroditism. The first three enzymes are also necessary for the adrenal biosynthesis of cortisol: *cholesterol side-chain cleavage enzyme* (20,22-desmolase), *3β-hydroxysteroid dehydrogenase,* and *17α-hydroxylase*. A defect in any of these three enzymes results in accompanying cortisol (with or without aldosterone) deficiency, that is, congenital adrenal hyperplasia. The disorders involving these three enzymes are discussed in the section on congenital adrenal hyperplasia (p. 1144). The remaining two testosterone biosynthetic enzymes, 17,20-desmolase and 17β-hydroxysteroid oxidoreductase, are not needed for cortisol synthesis. Their deficiency primarily causes impaired testosterone synthesis and abnormal male differentiation.

17,20-Desmolase (17,20-lyase) deficiency

17,20-Desmolase is necessary for the C_{21} side-chain cleavage of 17-hydroxypregnenolone and 17-hydroxyprogesterone to form, respectively, the C_{19} steroids, dehydroepiandrosterone (DHA), and androstenedione, which are precursors of both testosterone and estrogens. The 46,XY patients with a deficiency of this enzyme have incomplete masculinization, ranging from mild hypoplasia of male genitalia to significant ambiguity to female-appearing genitalia, depending on the severity of the defect. Some with a female phenotype may be recognized early because of an inguinal or labial gonad(s); otherwise they are diagnosed later because of delayed puberty.

Affected 46,XX patients appear normal in infancy but have delayed puberty because of inadequate estradiol synthesis. The XY patients characteristically show an increased ratio of C_{21}/C_{19} steroids, with abnormally increased levels of 17-hydroxypregnenolone and 17-hydroxyprogesterone (also progesterone and pregnenolone) and low or normal levels of DHA and androstenedione (also DHA and testosterone). Adrenocorticotropic hormone (ACTH) or hCG stimulation may further increase the C_{21}/C_{19} steroid ratios and is diagnostically useful. The elevated levels of progesterone and pregnenolone that are also seen may be caused by accompanying deficiency of 17α-hydroxylase. The activities of both 17α-hydroxylase and 17,20-desmolase are mediated by the single enzyme, P450c17, suggesting that the defect may reside here and thereby affect both enzyme steps. Serum cortisol and ACTH levels are normal, but the adrenal appears to be an important source of the elevated progestogens, since they are suppressible with dexamethasone. The inheritance is autosomal recessive. Prenatal screening in one mildly affected patient showed a modest increase in amniotic fluid levels of 17-hydroxyprogesterone and 17-hydroxypregnenolone and low levels of C_{19} steroids. The differential diagnosis includes other causes of male pseudohermaphroditism.

The decision as to sex of rearing of the affected 46,XY neonate is based on functional considerations and can be made in the first days of life without knowledge of the biochemical findings. The testes should be removed before puberty if the sex of rearing is female.

17β-Hydroxysteroid oxidoreductase (17-ketosteroid reductase) deficiency

This enzyme is necessary for the conversion of androstenedione to testosterone and of estrone (E_1) to estradiol (E_2). It is present in both gonadal and peripheral tissues but to only a very small extent in adrenocortical tissue. Its deficiency is associated primarily with diminished testosterone synthesis, resulting in failure of male differentiation in utero. Most reported 46,XY patients with this enzyme deficiency have had female-appearing or slightly masculinized (clitoromegaly, posterior labial fusion) genitalia, but a few had more masculinization, including one infant with a micropenis. The epididymis and vas deferens are well developed, and in many the testes may be descended in the inguinal canal or labioscrotal folds, which may bring the patient to medical attention. The characteristic biochemical finding is a greatly elevated level of androstenedione with a low to normal level of testosterone (high androstenedione/testosterone ratio; also elevated E_1/E_2 ratio) during periods of endogenous LH or exogenous hCG stimulation. Modest elevations of 17-hydroxyprogesterone, a precursor of androstenedione, may occur. Serum LH levels may be elevated beyond the first or second weeks up to age 4 to 6 months. Unlike the 17,20-desmolase deficiency, the adrenal component in this disorder is negligible, since this enzyme deficiency is essentially limited to the testes. Thus hCG stimulation is necessary to diagnose this defect. The peripheral conversion of androstenedione to testosterone is intact, indicating that the peripheral isoenzyme is under different genetic control, which explains the frequently normal levels of testosterone found. Patients with the female phenotype have sometimes been incorrectly diagnosed as having the androgen insensitivity syndrome. The sex of rearing is based on the size of the phallus in the infant. A striking observation is a change in gender identity from female to male that occurs at puberty in many undiagnosed and untreated patients, reflecting the significant levels of testosterone produced by peripheral conversion of androstenedione. A comparable change in gender identity may be seen with the untreated 5α-reductase deficiency. The testes should be removed early in life in those raised as female. The inheritance is either autosomal recessive (more likely) or X-linked recessive.

Disorders of androgen-dependent target tissues

This group of disorders in androgen-dependent tissues is characterized by an abnormality not of testicular hormone synthesis but of androgen metabolism or action in the peripheral tissues; that is, these disorders represent (1) a failure of the peripheral tissues to metabolize testosterone to dihydrotestosterone (DHT) because of a deficiency in 5α-reductase or (2) a failure in testosterone and DHT action resulting from an androgen receptor or postreceptor defect.

5α-Reductase deficiency

Patients with 5α-reductase enzyme deficiency are unable to convert testosterone to DHT in their peripheral tissues and thus have reduced to negligible production of DHT. The consequence is that male differentiation in utero of the external genitalia fails to occur. Affected males have normally developed testes with male internal ducts (these can be stimulated by testosterone) and absent müllerian duct structures but female-appearing external genitalia. In the cases reported to date, the external genitalia have been partially virilized, presumably because the enzyme deficiency has never been total. At birth most patients are potentially recognizable with clitoromegaly, a single perineal orifice (a urogenital sinus that gives an appearance of perineal hypospadias), and posterior labial fusion in some; a small, distal vaginal pouch is typically present (Fig. 37-36). Most have been reared as females. At puberty, noncastrated individuals show striking virilization brought on by the increase in testosterone, and in many a change in gender identity from female to male occurs. Secondary sexual characteristics induced by DHT, such as acne, body and facial hair, and prostatic enlargement, are reduced or do not appear.

To date no published experience is available concerning the biochemical findings in affected neonates or infants in the first year of life. The characteristic biochemical abnormality seen under gonadotropin (endogenous LH or exogenous hCG) stimulation is an elevated level of serum testosterone (T), and a low level of DHT, causing the T/DHT ratio to be abnormally elevated. Since

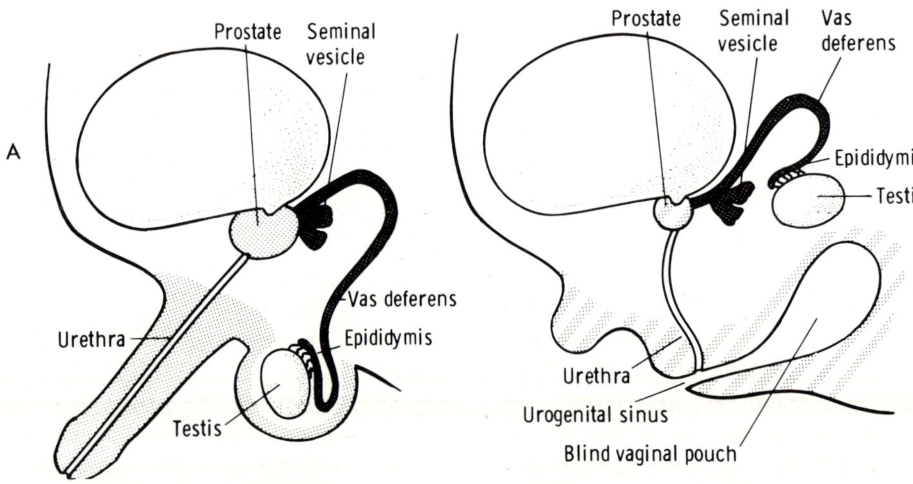

Fig. 37-36. A, Male differentiation of the external genitalia and urogenital sinus structures is DHT-stimulated *(light stippled area)*, whereas wolffian duct differentiation is testosterone-stimulated *(dark stippled area)*. **B,** 5α-Reductase deficiency results in impaired male differentiation of DHT-responsive tissues. The external genitalia appear female, and the vesicovaginal septum develops to create a distal blind vaginal pouch (in this diagram) opening into a urogenital sinus. Wolffian duct differentiation is normal. (From Imperato-McGinley, J., and Peterson, R.E., Am. J. Med. **61**:251, 1976.)

the deficiency of 5α-reductase also involves the liver, both adrenal and gonadal urinary C_{21} and C_{19} steroid metabolites show an abnormally increased 5β/5α ratio; classically the urinary etiocholanolone/androsterone ratio is elevated postpubertally and during hCG stimulation of the testes prepubertally. Serum LH may be abnormally elevated at age 1 to 2 months. In patients with androgen insensitivity, serum DHT may also be low and the T/DHT ratio elevated (5α-reductase activity is stimulated by androgen); urinary 5β/5α steroid ratios will distinguish these disorders. Acquired 5α-reductase deficiency also occurs in hypothyroidism and low triiodothyronine (T_3) states. The inheritance of primary 5α-reductase deficiency is autosomal recessive. Affected 46,XX females have no genital abnormalities and are fertile but do show abnormal urinary 5β/5α steroid ratios. Heterozygotes can be detected by intermediate elevations of urinary 5β/5α metabolites.

Determination of the sex of rearing is difficult in this disorder. Theoretically some prospect for fertility exists, although impaired spermatogenesis with spermatogenic arrest is usually seen. Also, the penile length achieved has been very small, not more than half of normal adult size. There is no experience to show whether early intervention with DHT or high-dose testosterone therapy can provide an adequate penile length either during childhood or by adulthood, but this is doubtful. Phallic length should be used to decide on the sex of rearing in the neonate or young infant.

Androgen insensitivity syndromes

The androgen insensitivity syndromes refer to those disorders in which peripheral tissues are partially to completely incapable of responding to stimulation by any androgen because of an androgen receptor or postreceptor defect (Fig. 37-37). Androgen-mediated events, such as masculine differentiation in utero or virilization during puberty, fail to occur or are impaired to a variable extent, depending on the completeness of the defect.

Complete androgen insensitivity (testicular feminization) syndrome. Affected individuals have a 46,XY karyotype with bilateral testes but failure of wolffian duct development and complete absence of any masculinization of the external genitalia. They have normal female-appearing external genitalia with a distal vaginal pouch, but müllerian structures are absent (microscopic rem-

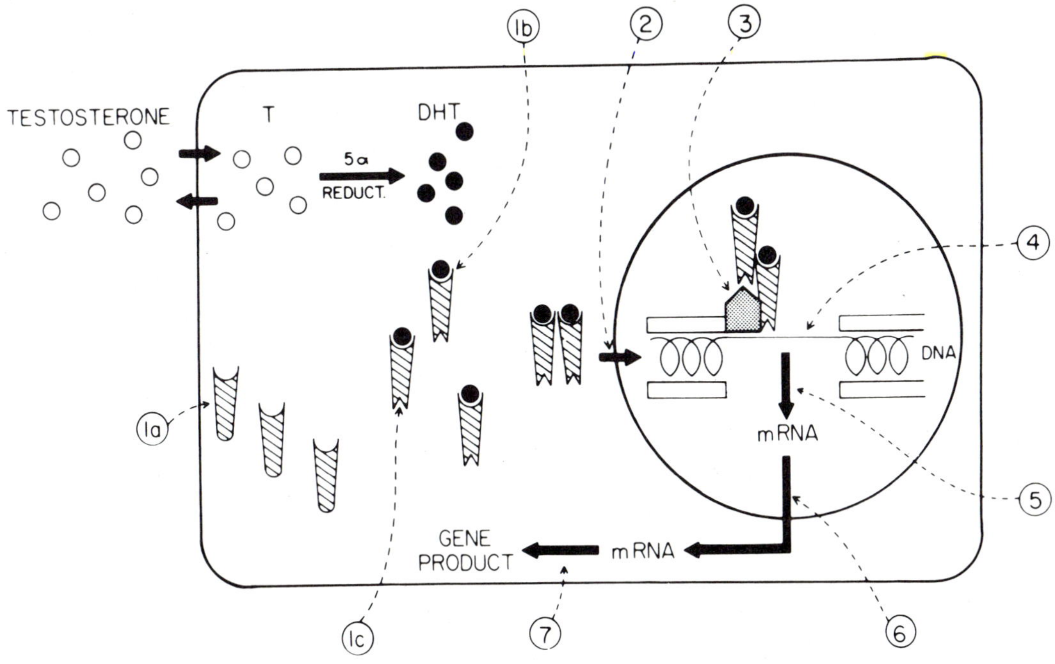

Fig. 37-37. Androgen-dependent target cell showing steroid hormone action. Numbers refer to sites where mutations might result in androgen insensitivity. *1,* Mutations affecting cytosol androgen-receptor protein, including *a,* absent protein, *b,* abnormality of androgen (DHT in this diagram) binding site, *c,* abnormality of acceptor binding site; *2,* defective translocation of androgen-receptor complex to nucleus; *3,* abnormalities of nuclear acceptor site; *4,* abnormal regulatory molecules; *5,* abnormal transcription of nuclear mRNA; *6,* abnormal mRNA processing; *7;* abnormal translation in synthesis of new protein. (From Fichman, K.R., Migeon, B.R., and Migeon, C.J.: Genetic disorders of male sexual development. In Harris, H., and Hirschhorn, K., editors: Advances in human genetics, vol. 10, New York, 1980, Plenum Press.)

nants have been reported, possibly from high, unopposed estrogen interfering with the action of MIF). The testes are of normal size and may be descended into the inguinal canal or labia majora, and more than half have an inguinal hernia, which may lead to clinical recognition in infancy. At puberty these patients undergo normal female breast development and labial growth and acquire a female habitus, but they have primary amenorrhea. Gender identity remains female in adulthood.

The androgen receptor dysfunction in this disorder has several causes: (1) absence of the androgen receptor, (2) a qualitative defect of the androgen receptor, or (3) a postreceptor defect affecting nuclear binding of the androgen receptor–steroid complex or a defect in transcription. Occurrence of the syndrome is familial in 30% of cases, and a family history of many "female" siblings is sometimes found. In the cases caused by an absent or defective androgen receptor, the inheritance is X-linked recessive (the gene for the androgen receptor is located on the X chromosome near the centromere), and mothers or other heterozygous carriers show abnormal androgen receptor function in half their cells studied. Spontaneous mutation is thought to account for the sporadic cases. The genetics of the postreceptor defects is not known.

This syndrome can be screened for in utero by ultrasound examination of the fetal genitalia and determination of the karyotype, and in the neonate by establishing the absence of a uterine cervix via rectal examination or the presence of a Y chromosome. Basal testosterone levels should be in the normal to above-normal male range in the first 36 hours of life and again at 1 to 2 or 3 months of age, when the LH levels are also inappropriately elevated. The differential diagnosis includes other forms of male pseudohermaphroditism; hCG stimulation testing may be needed to rule out these other defects.

The sex of rearing of these individuals should be unequivocally female. There is an increased risk of gonadal malignancy occurring after the first 2 decades, with one case reported at age 14 years. Their testes ideally should be left in the abdomen until the latter part of the second decade before their removal so that they may feminize normally at puberty.

Partial androgen insensitivity (incomplete testicular feminization) syndrome. This disorder is probably the most common cause of male pseudohermaphroditism. Affected 46,XY patients have bilateral testes and absent müllerian ducts but incomplete masculinization of their external genitalia that ranges from female-appearing genitalia with clitoromegaly or posterior labial fusion to phenotypically normal male-appearing genitalia. Many patients have perineal, penoscrotal (Fig. 37-38), or penile hypospadias, and others may have a micropenis. Wolffian duct development also occurs but is often incomplete, although this may not correlate with the extent of external genital masculinization. The underlying cause is similar to that for complete androgen insensitivity except for being a partial or incomplete defect; that is, there is either partial absence of the androgen receptor, a qualitatively abnormal receptor that functions to some extent, or an incomplete postreceptor defect. Although pathophysiologically similar to complete androgen insensitivity, the two disorders are distinct and are not seen together in the same pedigree. Partial androgen insensitivity is either X-linked or sex-limited autosomal dominant. Affected relatives in a pedigree tend to have similar severity of the defect.

Serum levels of testosterone are in the normal to above-normal male range in the first 36 hours of life and again at 0.5 to 2 or 3 months of age, with accompanying abnormally elevated levels of LH in the latter period in the few neonates reported. An abnormally elevated testosterone/DHT ratio resulting from secondary 5α-reductase deficiency (this enzyme is induced by androgen stimulation) may cause diagnostic confusion with primary 5α-reductase deficiency in some patients. Androgen insensitivity may be inferred by poor growth of the phallus in response to a course of testosterone enanthate, 25 mg intramuscularly given every 3 to 4 weeks for up to four doses. Definitive diagnosis remains with the research center and requires demonstration of (1) deficient androgen receptor or postreceptor function in genital skin fibroblasts or (2) impaired nitrogen and phosphorus retention or failed suppression of LH in response to administration of exogenous testosterone or DHT; however, high doses of these androgens will induce nitrogen or phosphorus retention or LH suppression, which is compatible with the partial nature of this disorder. In addition to 5α-reductase deficiency, the differential diagnosis includes other causes of male pseudohermaphroditism; patients with true hermaphroditism, mixed gonadal dysgenesis, or maternal exposure to progestins also may have similar features.

The sex of rearing is determined by the penile size and, if necessary, by the capacity of the phallus to grow in response to testosterone. All patients will be infertile. The risk for development of gonadal tumors is not known, but carcinoma in situ (a precancerous lesion) has been found in three of eight patients with partial androgen insensitivity in one series, at ages 2 months and 13 and 15 years, which raises the need for monitoring these patients if the testes are not removed. High-dose testosterone therapy may be needed in those raised as male to maintain adequate penile growth; it must be given cautiously because other organ systems may be more responsive. The testes are removed in those raised as female.

A

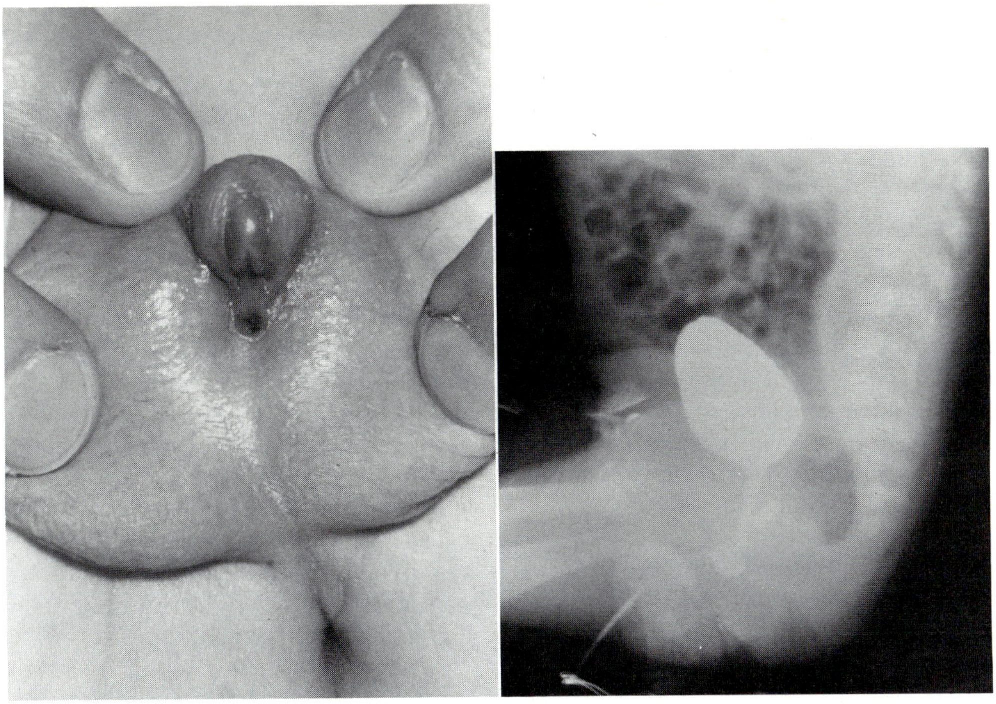

B

Fig. 37-38. A, This 46,XY infant with partial androgen insensitivity had ambiguous genitalia at birth (phallus, 1.8 × 0.8 cm; penoscrotal hypospadias; 1 cm testes in scrotum and absence of a uterine cervix on rectal examination). **B,** Genitogram performed following endoscopy shows presence of 2 cm utriculus or blind pouch opening into the urethra, just below the verumontanum (seminal colliculus); no evidence of a uterus was found. Serum testosterone was elevated up to 475 ng/dl at age 40 hours and 1,517 ng/dl at age 7½ weeks, with elevated serum LH of 23 mIU/ml at age 7½ weeks. Androgen receptor binding in genital skin fibroblasts showed no demonstrable abnormality, as is often found in partial defects. The parents insisted on male sex of rearing. Testosterone therapy did not increase penile size until the dose was increased fourfold above physiologic replacement. Repair of hypospadias was done in infancy. A younger brother was born with a similar defect.

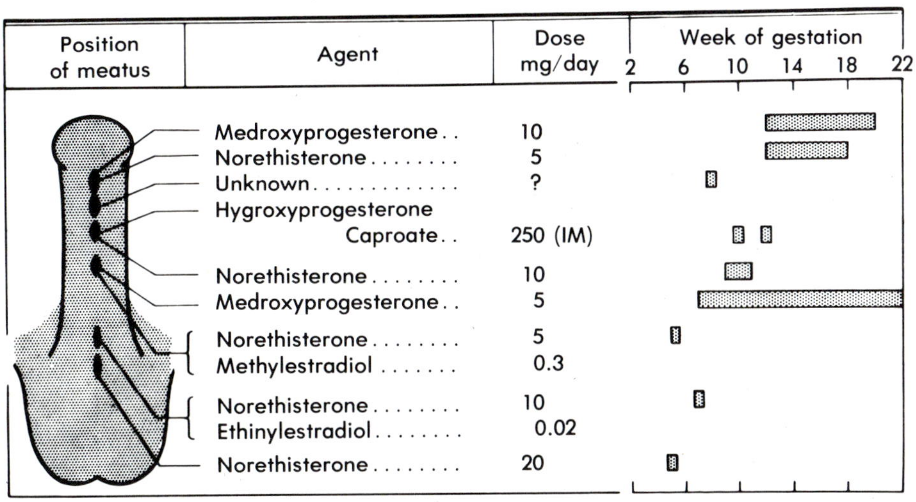

Fig. 37-39. Hypospadias associated with maternal treatment with progestins. Effect of maternal intake of progestins between 5 and 14 weeks' gestation on differentiation of external genitalia in male (46,XY) fetuses. Hypospadias of varying degrees of severity results, depending on the timing and intensity of the exposure. (From Aarskog, D.: N. Engl. J. Med. **300:**75, 1979. Reprinted by permission of The New England Journal of Medicine.)

Maternally derived progestins

Maternal intake of oral progestins between 8 and 14 weeks' gestation has been associated with the development of penile hypospadias of varying degrees of severity, related to the timing and duration of intake (Fig. 37-39). The mechanism by which this may occur has been thought to be either progestogen inhibition of 5α-reductase activity or competitive inhibition at the androgen receptor site, blocking the binding of DHT.

One case of male pseudohermaphroditism occurred in a boy whose mother received high doses of diethylstilbestrol. Other males so exposed have not shown genital ambiguity but have displayed an increased incidence of hypoplastic testes, abnormal semen, epididymal cysts, and meatal stenosis. Whether high-dose estrogens cause male pseudohermaphroditism is not known.

MASCULINIZATION OF FEMALE EXTERNAL GENITALIA (FEMALE PSEUDOHERMAPHRODITISM)

Female pseudohermaphroditism is characterized by normal ovarian and müllerian duct development with ambiguity or variable masculinization of the external genitalia. The external genital ambiguity is almost always androgen induced; most cases are caused by fetal congenital adrenal hyperplasia, and a few cases result from a maternal androgen source. In rare cases, however, a source of androgens is not found, and an error in differentiation is presumed to be the cause (see boxed material on classification of sex differentiation abnormalities, p. 1131).

Androgen exposure between 8 and 12 to 14 weeks' fetal age will result in variable male *differentiation* of the external genitalia, that is, labioscrotal fusion, regression of the urovaginal septum to form a urogenital sinus, ventral displacement of the urethral (urogenital) meatus toward or on the phallus, and male phallus differentiation (Fig. 37-40). Androgen exposure occurring beyond 12 or 14 weeks will produce *growth*, but not differentiation, of the external genitalia, namely, clitoral hypertrophy, defined in the neonate by a clitoral diameter greater than 6 mm. Most female pseudohermaphrodites are identified at birth because of genital ambiguity, but more severely affected neonates may be initially missed, being incorrectly designated as "males" with hypospadias or undescended testes. The major concerns in wanting to identify female pseudohermaphrodites at birth are that (1) congenital adrenal hyperplasia, if present, should be diagnosed promptly, since it is potentially life threatening, and (2) sex assignment should be made correctly, along female lines.

The following discussion reviews congenital adrenal hyperplasia and its manifestations in *both* female and male neonates, not just concerning its role in causing female pseudohermaphroditism.

Congenital adrenal hyperplasia

Congenital adrenal hyperplasia (CAH) is one of the most common inborn errors of metabolism, occurring in 1 in 5,000 to 15,000 births. It consists of a group of autosomal recessive disorders affecting one or more of those enzymes necessary for the biosynthesis of cortisol. The cortisol deficiency that results leads to hypersecretion of ACTH and thus adrenocortical hyperplasia. Depending on which enzyme is deficient, adrenal mineralocorticoid or gonadal androgen-estrogen synthesis may also be affected. The increased production of precursor steroids before the enzyme block also may result in abnormal sex steroid formation or other effects.

The affected enzymes are those involved in the path-

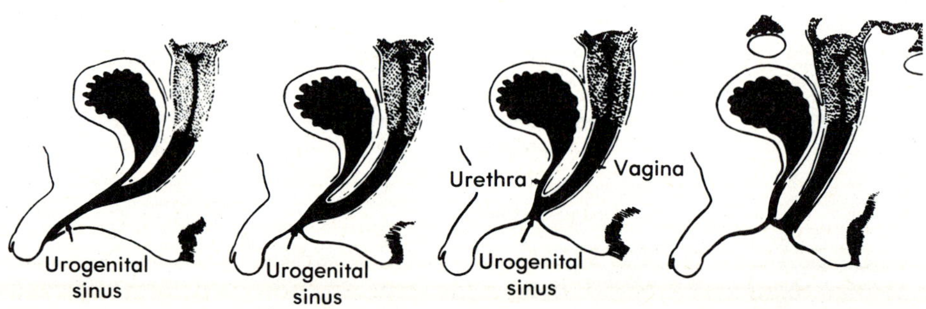

Fig. 37-40. Effects of androgen exposure in utero on external genital development in the 46,XX female. Exposure beginning after 12 to 14 weeks results in clitoromegaly *(left)*, whereas androgen exposure between 8 and 12 to 14 weeks results in variable male differentiation (i.e., urogenital sinus, posterior labial fusion, hypospadiac appearance or even a normal male appearance except for impalpable gonads), depending on the timing intensity and duration of androgen stimulation *(three diagrams on right)*. (From Grumbach, M.M., and Ducharme, J.R.: The effects of androgens on fetal sexual development: androgen-induced female pseudohermaphrodism, Fertil. Steril. **11**:157, 1960. Reproduced with permission of the publisher, The American Fertility Society.)

way leading from cholesterol to cortisol: the cholesterol side-chain cleavage enzyme complex (or 20,22-desmolase), 3β-hydroxysteroid dehydrogenase, 17α-hydroxylase, 21-hydroxylase, and 11β-hydroxylase. Except for 17α-hydroxylase, these enzymes are also necessary for mineralocorticoid (aldosterone) biosynthesis (see Fig. 37-29). The first three enzymes are also present in gonadal tissue, where they are necessary for biosynthesis of the sex steroids. Their deficiency in males results in deficient testosterone synthesis and incomplete male sex differentiation; in females it results in deficient estrogen synthesis, but this is not of clinical significance until puberty.

The 21- and 11β-hydroxylases are found predominantly in the adrenal cortex and only minimally in gonadal tissue, and they are not necessary for the synthesis of sex steroids. Their deficiencies (and to a lesser extent, deficiency of 3β-hydroxysteroid dehydrogenase), however, result in excess formation of precursor steroids, which yield increased production of androgens that induce masculinization of affected female fetuses in utero. By this mechanism, female pseudohermaphroditism occurs and affected females should thus be identifiable at birth by their abnormal genitalia. Affected males having 21- or 11β-hydroxylase deficiency, however, do not manifest recognizable penile enlargement or other virilization at birth, but they will develop these postnatally if untreated. Affected males with 3β-hydroxysteroid dehydrogenase deficiency, on the other hand, do have recognizable genital ambiguity at birth because of testosterone deficiency. Finally, all five enzyme deficiencies are clinically important because of the adrenal (glucocorticoid with or without mineralocorticoid) insufficiency associated with them. This is life threatening and needs to be recognized and managed early.

21-Hydroxylase deficiency

21-Hydroxylase enzyme deficiency is by far the most common cause of CAH, accounting for perhaps 90% to 95% of all cases. Two forms are seen in neonates: a simple virilizing form in which the enzyme deficiency is partial and a salt-losing form in which the enzyme deficiency is more complete. (A third form, late-onset 21-hydroxylase deficiency, does not have clinical manifestations in the fetus, neonate, or infant.) Both forms are characterized by abnormal virilization of the female fetus. In the simple virilizing form the partial enzyme block can be compensated for, so that adrenal insufficiency tends not to occur except in stressful circumstances. In the salt-losing form adrenal insufficiency occurs under basal conditions and tends to manifest in the neonatal period or soon thereafter as an adrenal crisis.

Simple virilizing form. The 21-hydroxylase enzyme is necessary for the conversion of 17-hydroxyprogesterone to 11-deoxycortisol (compound S) and of progesterone to 11-deoxycorticosterone (DOC). Partial deficiency of this enzyme results in an impairment of cortisol and aldosterone biosynthesis, which is compensated for by increased secretion of ACTH and angiotensin. This causes overproduction of the steroids before the enzyme block and a secondary increased secretion of adrenal androgens, which are converted in peripheral tissues to testosterone and DHT, where they cause abnormal virilization (Fig. 37-41).

Affected fetuses produce increased amounts of androgens beginning in the first trimester. In the female fetus this leads to varying degrees of male differentiation of the external genitalia and urogenital sinus, but the internal genital ducts develop normally along female lines without any wolffian duct development. At birth the spectrum of masculinization in females ranges from mild clitoromegaly, usually with some posterior labial fusion, to perineal or penile hypospadias, to occasionally complete male differentiation with the urethra opening at the tip of a male-sized phallus; the latter phenotype may have a normal male appearance except that the gonads are impalpable. In the male the increased secretion of fetal androgens is of little significance in relation to the fetal production of testicular androgens. The external genitalia are usually normal at birth; slight enlargement of the penis may occur, but this is rarely recognizable as such. Female and male neonates may have increased pigmentation of the genitalia or areolae. The extent of male differentiation in female fetuses tends to reflect the severity of the enzyme defect; thus females with the simple virilizing form often show less extensive male differentiation than those with the salt-losing type.

Patients with untreated simple virilizing 21-hydroxylase deficiency continue to produce excessive androgens postnatally, resulting in accelerated growth and skeletal maturation and the appearance of androgen-induced sexual changes. Patients with mild CAH generally do not develop symptoms of adrenal insufficiency unless exposed to major stress or significant salt depletion (reduced salt intake, vomiting, excessive sweating). A few patients with either form have come to medical attention because of recurrent hypoglycemic episodes or seizures, usually occurring during common infections. Associated congenital anomalies, such as renal abnormalities, are occasionally seen in CAH, although their incidence is not greater than occurs in the general population.

Salt-losing form. Severe deficiency of the 21-hydroxylase enzyme results in significant impairment of cortisol and aldosterone synthesis that cannot be compensated for by the increased levels of ACTH and angiotensin. The development of cortisol and aldosterone deficiency, usually in the first weeks of life, results in an acute adrenal crisis and sodium wasting. This characterizes the salt-losing form of CAH and distinguishes it from the simple virilizing form (Fig. 37-41).

The precursor steroids, 17-hydroxyprogesterone and

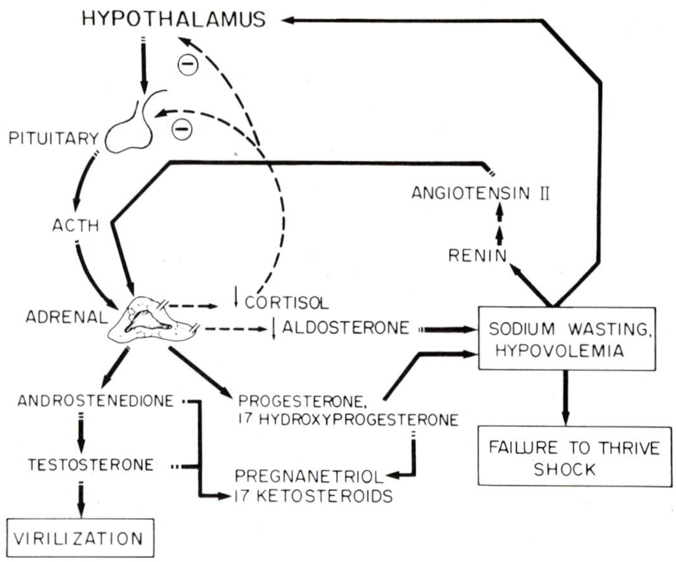

Fig. 37-41. Pathophysiology of 21-hydroxylase deficiency. Impaired cortisol biosynthesis results in increased ACTH stimulation, adrenal hyperplasia, and increased formation of (1) progesterone and 17-hydroxyprogesterone (the precursor steroids before the enzyme block), which induce sodium wasting, and of (2) androgens, which induce masculinization. Impaired aldosterone biosynthesis results in renal sodium wasting. In the simple virilizing form these defects can be compensated for by the increased ACTH and renin-angiotensin stimulation, but in the salt-losing form full compensation does not occur, leading to adrenal insufficiency with sodium wasting, hypovolemia, failure to thrive, and shock if untreated.

progesterone, and 16α-hydroxyprogesterone, a metabolite of progesterone, are produced in increased amounts and have their own adverse effects since they function as salt-losing hormones. They may act directly on the renal tubules to cause sodium wasting, but more likely they act competitively to inhibit aldosterone action at the distal tubule, since they do not cause sodium wasting in the absence of mineralocorticoids. Their presence in a setting of diminished levels of mineralocorticoids has the effect of increasing the severity of the hypoaldosteronism by causing an additional amount of sodium wasting by the kidney. The production of C_{19} androgens also tends to be greater in the salt-losing form because of the more intense ACTH and angiotensin stimulation. Females with the salt-losing form may show more complete masculinization of the external genitalia, and some are incorrectly designated as male at birth (Fig. 37-42). Males generally come to medical attention when they develop adrenal insufficiency.

Symptoms or signs of adrenal insufficiency are not present at birth and rarely occur before 3 to 4 days of age. Approximately half of untreated patients with salt-losing CAH will have onset of adrenal crisis between 6 and 14 days of age, and only a small number will have an earlier onset; by 1 month of age more than three fourths will have developed an adrenal crisis. Less se-

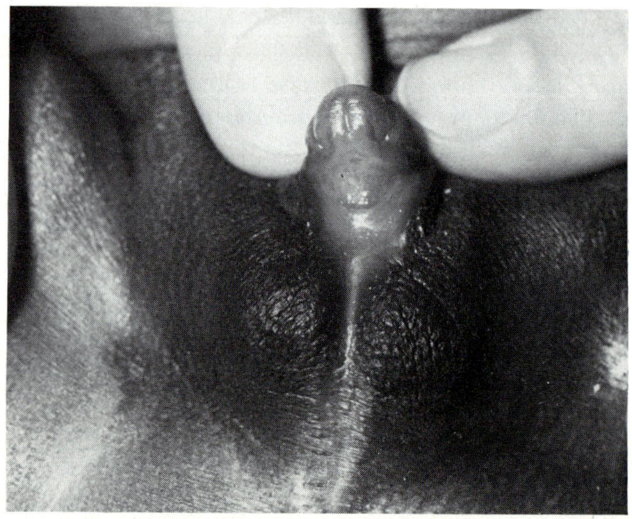

Fig. 37-42. Four-week-old 46,XX neonate with salt-losing 21-hydroxylase deficiency was erroneously thought to be a male with penile hypospadias at birth. However, the associated findings of a small phallus (2.3 × 0.8 cm) and impalpable gonads should have led to suspicion of an intersex problem and immediate evaluation. Serum 17-hydroxyprogesterone at age 3½ weeks was 199 ng/ml (normal value, less than 1.2). Sex reassignment to female was made, replacement therapy instituted, and genital reconstructive surgery performed subsequently.

verely affected individuals may appear in the following months, usually in association with a stressful condition causing decreased salt intake or increased salt losses, and a few escape having any crisis. The early symptoms and signs of adrenal crisis are nonspecific and include lethargy, poor appetitite, regurgitation of feedings, failure to thrive, or weight loss. Hyperkalemia, hyponatremia, and metabolic acidosis may be seen early. The regurgitation of feedings may progress to projectile vomiting. Severe symptoms and signs may occur within 1 to 2 days, including dehydration, hypotension, muscle weakness, obtundation, a gray or cyanotic appearance, cold and clammy skin, hyperkalemic cardiac conduction abnormalities, and hyponatremic or hypoglycemic seizures. The differential diagnosis in the male infant includes sepsis, congenital heart disease, and pyloric stenosis. Pyloric stenosis differs from a salt-losing crisis by the development of metabolic alkalosis rather than metabolic acidosis.

The development of an acute adrenal crisis is partly caused by hypoaldosteronism, which results in renal sodium wasting with depletion of total body sodium, and impaired ability to secrete potassium and hydrogen ions in the distal tubule. The decreased total body sodium results in hyponatremia, hypovolemia, and decreased tissue perfusion, which accounts for many of the early symptoms just described and eventually results in hypotension and shock.

Hypocortisolemia represents the other major component of adrenal insufficiency and results in impairment of cardiovascular, metabolic, and other systemic functions. Among the cardiovascular effects associated with glucocorticoid deficiency are decreased stroke volume and cardiac output, decreased blood pressure, and decreased vascular tone or reactivity. Depletion of renin substrate occurs in the presence of cortisol deficiency and impairs the renin-angiotensin axis, leading to circulatory failure. Norepinephrine raises the peripheral blood pressure only in the presence of cortisol, suggesting that cortisol exerts a permissive action. Impaired ability to concentrate the urine also occurs because of reduced responsiveness of the renal collecting tubules to vasopressin.

Cortisol deficiency is associated with an inability to maintain normal hepatic glycogen stores, which during a period of starvation may lead to hypoglycemia. Fat becomes the primary source of energy, which may lead to lipid depletion. Cortisol is normally important for mobilizing increased glucose production by the liver, both by inducing gluconeogenic enzymes and by its permissive effect on epinephrine- and glucagon-induced glycogenolysis. Cortisol deficiency is associated with impaired muscle activity, a normochromic, normocytic anemia, and eosinophilia.

The mechanism for the delay in adrenal crisis is that newborns normally have a very low aldosterone secretion rate of 9 to 41 μg/24 hours, or mean of 23 μg/24 hours, at age 3 hours to 7 days, which then rises dramatically to 25 to 138 μg/24 hours, or mean of 72 μg/24 hours, at 8 days to 12 months. Plasma aldosterone concentrations are high in the first week, attributed to a low metabolic clearance rate because of neonatal hepatic immaturity. With maturation of the liver, an increased amount of aldosterone must be secreted to maintain adequate plasma levels. The salt-losing patient is thus spared in the first few days of life but is unable to meet the subsequently increased aldosterone secretory requirements. A second reason for the delay is that it typically takes several days of complete glucocorticoid withdrawal for a crisis to develop, and longer if some cortisol is present.

Biochemical findings

Blood. The serum level of cortisol and the cortisol production rate are normal in the untreated simple virilizing form of CAH and can be increased further in response to ACTH administration, although often not to the extent seen in normal individuals. In the salt-losing form of CAH, serum cortisol levels tend to be low-normal or low, and the cortisol production rate is low (Fig. 37-43). An inadequate rise of each of these parameters is seen in response to ACTH administration. ACTH levels in the untreated patients of both forms of CAH are elevated, but more so in the salt-losing patients.

The aldosterone production rate in the patient with simple virilizing CAH is also corrected and actually is elevated, although hyperaldosterone-induced effects (hypokalemia, metabolic alkalosis, hypertension) are not seen. This elevation is thought to be secondary to the presence of increased levels of the salt-losing steroids, 17-hydroxyprogesterone and progesterone, which antagonize mineralocorticoid action at the distal tubules. Plasma renin activity is also elevated, which supports this explanation. In the salt-losing patient, the aldosterone production rate under conditions of normal sodium replacement ranges from low to normal. Unlike the simple virilizing form, however, no increase in aldosterone production is seen in response to sodium restriction or ACTH administration.

Of the steroids preceding the enzyme block, 17-hydroxyprogesterone is the most strikingly elevated. Its serum levels are increased 40 to 400 times above the upper limit of normal, to levels of 40 to 800 ng/ml and occasionally higher, whereas serum progesterone levels are increased six to 75 times. Two principal routes of metabolism of 17-hydroxyprogesterone are by 11β-hydroxylation to form 21-deoxycortisol, and by side-chain cleavage to form the C_{19} androgens. Serum 21-deoxycortisol levels are greatly elevated, ranging from 18 to 169 ng/ml (normal, less than 1 ng/ml). The biochemical

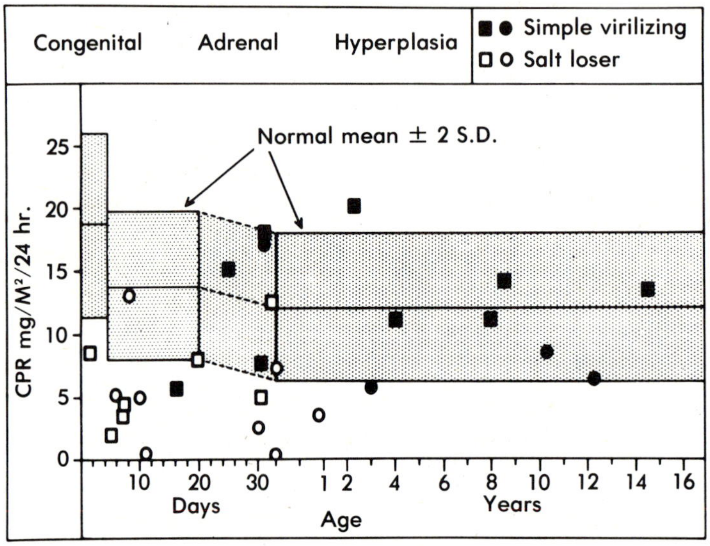

Fig. 37-43. Cortisol production rate (CPR) in patients with untreated simple virilizing and salt-losing forms of 21-hydroxylase deficiency. The former show an ability to compensate with normal CPR during high ACTH stimulation, unlike most of the salt-losing patients, who have abnormally low CPRs. Most with the simple virilizing form, however, cannot further increase their CPR during stress, thereby also placing them at risk for adrenal insufficiency. (From Migeon, C.J.: Diagnosis and treatment of adrenogenital disorders. In DeGroot, L.I., and others, editors: Endocrinology, New York, 1979, Grune & Stratton, Inc. Modified from Migeon, C.J., and Kenny, F.M., J. Pediatr. **69:**779, 1966.)

effects of 21-deoxycortisol, if any, are unknown, but in the routine laboratory assays for cortisol, 21-deoxycortisol may cross-react significantly and cause the cortisol measurements to appear higher than they actually are.

The major C_{19} androgen produced is androstenedione, which is principally derived from the side-chain cleavage of 17-hydroxyprogesterone. Serum levels of androstenedione range from 2.2 to 55 ng/ml (upper normal in the first 2 months, 1.3 ng/ml). Of the other C_{19} adrenal steroids secreted, serum levels of DHA are usually elevated, whereas serum levels of the sulfated and glucuronide esters of androstenedione or DHA are elevated in some but normal in other patients. The adrenal C_{19} steroids have little biologic effect of their own but can serve as prohormones for testosterone synthesis. Approximately 15% of the androstenedione produced is metabolized in peripheral tissues (particularly liver, muscle, skin) to testosterone, with the adrenal synthesizing very little testosterone directly. Serum testosterone levels in affected children range between 1.1 and 6 ng/ml (normal, less than 0.3 ng/ml in females), and the serum androstenedione/testosterone ratios range between 2:1 and 7:1. In female and in male patients, about two thirds and one third of the testosterone produced, respectively, is derived from adrenal-synthesized androstenedione; the remaining portions reflect that amount produced under normal circumstances.

Urine. The steroids produced by the adrenal are ultimately metabolized to physiologically inactive forms by the liver, kidneys, adrenals, and connective tissue. Several steroid metabolites are excreted in the meconium and feces of newborns, but more than 90% of steroid excretion is found in the urine at all ages, chiefly as glucuronide or sulfate conjugates or in hydroxylated forms.

The 24-hour urine steroid pattern in 21-hydroxylase deficiency classically shows significant elevations of pregnanetriol and the 17-ketosteroids. Urine levels of pregnanetriol in these infants are 0.2 to 10 mg/24 hours in the neonatal period (normal, barely detectable to less than 0.1 mg/24 hours), although some infants may have initially normal levels. Urinary free 17-hydroxyprogesterone is also elevated and may be superior to pregnanetriol, particularly in neonates, for the diagnosis of 21-hydyroxylase deficiency. Urinary 17-ketosteroids range between 2 and 40 mg/24 hours in infants, as compared with normal levels of up to 2.5 mg/24 hours in the first 3 to 4 weeks of life. The urinary 17-hydroxycorticosteroids, which reflect cortisol production, are normal or low; urinary free cortisol presumably behaves similarly.

Pathology. The bilateral adrenal glands are characteristically hyperplastic and enlarged, and the surface is convoluted or cerebriform. Microscopically the effects of excessive ACTH stimulation are seen. Most of the ad-

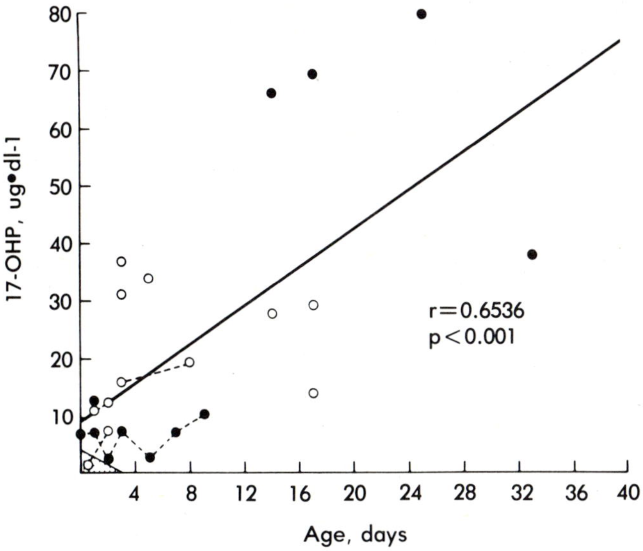

Fig. 37-44. Serum 17-hydroxyprogesterone levels in untreated salt-losing male (•) and female (○) neonates with 21-hydroxylase deficiency show a significant rise with age. Interrupted lines indicate levels obtained on more than one occasion. Overlap with normal levels *(hatched area)* may occur on the first day(s) of life. (From Holcombe, J.S., and others: J. Pediatr. **98:**573, 1981.)

renal cortex is composed of eosinophilic compact cells with finely granular cytoplasm containing fine lipid droplets, which extend from the medulla toward the outer cortex. The zona glomerulosa, from which mineralocorticoids are produced, is less well described; it is two to four times wider in the simple virilizing form of CAH but is either normal or absent in the salt-losing form. In a severely virilized 20-week-old aborted female fetus, however, the adrenals were neither grossly enlarged nor microscopically hyperplastic.

Diagnosis. The diagnosis of 21-hydroxylase deficiency in the neonatal period should be considered in females with any masculinization of the external genitalia (and also in presumed "males" with impalpable gonads or hypospadias), or in either sex if there is a family history of unexplained death in infancy or of CAH, presence of hyperpigmentation, development of symptoms or signs of adrenal insufficiency or crisis, or development of postnatal virilization, which generally appears after the first year of life. The most useful diagnostic test at present is an elevated level of serum 17-hydroxyprogesterone, but caution is needed in interpreting values, particularly in the first week of life. An elevated level of serum 21-deoxycortisol may be the most specific test for 21-hydroxylase deficiency, but its measurement is not readily available and experience is limited. Many affected neonates show normal levels of 17-hydroxyprogesterone on the first day of life and only mild elevation in the first several days before levels become very high (Fig. 37-44). Levels in normal neonates range up to 30 ng/ml in cord serum and are high in peripheral serum in the first 12 hours of life before declining to below 2 ng/ml after 24 hours of age. Levels in premature and sick neonates (e.g., with asphyxia, intraventricular hemorrhage, or sepsis or after major surgery) may reach 40 ng/ml, which overlaps with levels found in many affected infants in the first several days of life. The differential diagnosis also includes 11β-hydroxylase deficiency, 3β-hydroxysteroid dehydrogenase deficiency, pseudohypoaldosteronism, and 17,20-desmolase deficiency, where moderate to marked elevations of 17-hydroxyprogesterone occur. There are several reports of individuals showing evidence for a combined 21- and 11β-hydroxylase deficiency, which may cause diagnostic confusion.

Before the development of serum radioimmunoassays, diagnosis was based on finding elevated levels of 24-hour urinary pregnanetriol and 17-ketosteroids. Overlap with normal neonates may occur, with pregnanetriol being low in some affected neonates in the first week(s) of life, and 17-ketosteroids ranging up to 4 mg/24 hours in normal neonates in the first days of life before declining to less than 0.5 mg/24 hours by 1 month of age. Because serum assays have proved reliable and 24-hour urine collections are very difficult to perform in neonates and infants, urinary studies are not necessary to make a diagnosis.

The diagnosis of the salt-losing form of CAH is based on the clinical course, that is, the development of hyponatremia with hyperkalemia or symptoms or signs of mineralocorticoid deficiency. Measurements of cortisol, aldosterone, or plasma renin activity show considerable overlap with the simple virilizing form and are not diagnostically useful, although a persistently elevated level of plasma renin activity occurring in the presence of full glucocorticoid replacement is diagnostic of the salt-losing form and warrants the addition of mineralocorticoid replacement therapy.

The differential diagnosis of adrenal insufficiency includes the inherited enzyme deficiencies in cortisol or aldosterone synthesis, ACTH deficiency or hypopituitarism, congenital adrenal hypoplasia or aplasia, hereditary ACTH unresponsiveness, pseudohypoaldosteronism, adrenal hemorrhage, Wolman's disease, adrenoleukodystrophy (neonatal or childhood forms), and adrenal suppression following pharmacologic glucocorticoid therapy given to the mother during pregnancy or to the infant. Hyponatremia may occur with inadequate sodium intake or excessive losses, in water overload, inappropriate antidiuretic hormone (ADH), congestive heart failure, cirrhosis, nephrotic syndrome, potassium depletion, or with diuretic therapy.

Treatment. Cortisol replacement, equivalent to the amount secreted daily in normal individuals (12 mg/m^2/

24 hours), is the mainstay of treatment. It suppresses the increased output of ACTH and thereby causes the ACTH-stimulated adrenocortical activity to be decreased. Existing aldosterone secretion is maintained by endogenous angiotensin stimulation, and the reduction in 17-hydroxyprogesterone and progesterone results in a diminished salt-losing tendency. Adrenal androgen secretion is decreased, so that abnormal virilization no longer occurs. Patients with salt-losing CAH additionally require replacement mineralocorticoid therapy, with sodium supplementation often being required in neonates and infants.

Maintenance cortisol replacement therapy may be given either orally or intramuscularly, but allowance must be made for differences in the potency, absorption, and duration of action of the different preparations available. Hydrocortisone is the oral preparation of choice. Because of its short half-life and its partial inactivation by gastric acidity, the maintenance oral hydrocortisone dosage may approach twice physiologic production; replacement doses usually range from 10 to 28 mg/m^2/day given in three divided doses. Prednisone, prednisolone, and dexamethasone are used much less in infants and growing children because they are so much more potent and difficult to adjust and are more likely to cause growth suppression. Cortisone acetate is the intramuscular preparation used; it has a duration of action of 3 days. Its physiologic replacement dosage averages 15 mg/m^2/day or 40 to 50 mg/m^2 every 3 days. The phosphate and succinate esters of hydrocortisone are generally limited to intravenous usage because they have a short duration of action of about 8 hours.

At the initiation of therapy or during periods of stress or illness, two to three times the maintenance dose of glucocorticoid should be given. The levels of 17-hydroxyprogesterone and other abnormally elevated steroids should fall toward normal within several days. The patient's pattern of growth and serum levels of 17-hydroxyprogesterone and androstenedione (or DHAS or testosterone) are used to manage the long-term glucocorticoid therapy.

For infants who require maintenance mineralocorticoid replacement therapy, it is provided orally. 9a-fluorohydrocortisone acetate (Florinef), 0.05 to 0.15 mg or, occasionally, higher doses, are administered on a daily basis. Sodium supplementation (1 to 5 mEq/kg/day) is often needed in the first 1 to 3 years, in part because the renal tubules are less able to conserve sodium. Measurements of the blood pressure and the level of plasma renin activity are used to adjust the mineralocorticoid dosage and need for sodium supplementation.

In acute salt-losing adrenal crisis, fluid replacement (beginning with 20 ml/kg body weight of 0.9% saline and 5% glucose for hypovolemia), sodium replacement, continuous glucose infusion, glucocorticoid therapy at 3 to 4 times maintenance (initially given intravenously as the phosphate or succinate ester of hydrocortisone), and mineralocorticoid replacement (Florinef, 0.1 to 0.2 mg orally every 12 to 24 hours) are needed. Acidosis, hypoglycemia, and hyperkalemia may be present and should be managed, and the patient should be monitored for potassium toxicity. In those patients awaiting diagnosis, glucocorticoid therapy can be withheld until diagnostic tests are completed. However, therapy should be administered if blood pressure or other functions are not correctible with fluid, saline, glucose, and mineralocorticoid replacement.

The cardiac toxicity of hyperkalemia is exacerbated by hypocalcemia, hyponatremia, metabolic acidosis, or rapid elevations of potassium. The latter may occur with the administration of potassium-containing antibiotics, with use of stored blood for transfusion, or by tissue destruction or hemolysis; hypovolemia may cause impaired renal tubular secretion of potassium. Although the treatment of choice of hyperkalemia caused by adrenal insufficiency is mineralocorticoid replacement, mineralocorticoids cannot work in the face of inadequate sodium for exchange with potassium at the renal tubule; thus adequate sodium replacement is important. If hyperkalemic-induced cardiac toxicity is severe, the most rapidly effective therapeutic measure is intravenous calcium infusion (given as 10% calcium gluconate, 0.4 ml/kg); administered slowly (with cardiac monitoring), it will result in a shift of potassium into cells. Overtreatment with sodium or mineralocorticoids can result in hypernatremia, hypertension, metabolic alkalosis, or fluid retention with congestive heart failure or pulmonary edema.

Sex of rearing. The sex of rearing should be female in all 46,XX CAH patients, regardless of the extent of masculinization of their genitalia. This is based on the observation that they have normal ovaries and müllerian structures and have the potential to lead normal, fertile lives as females. Surgical correction of the masculinized external genitalia in female patients is done when a reasonable body size has been achieved, usually toward the end of the first year and preferably no later than 18 months of age. The sex of rearing in male (46,XY) patients is not a problem. Patients maintained under good control with steroid replacement therapy should show normal growth and development and have normal sexual function in adulthood.

Genetics. The 21-hydroxylase deficiency is one of the most common autosomal recessive disorders. Given an estimated incidence of 1 in 5,000 to 15,000 births, the carrier (heterozygote) frequency in the general population is thus 1 in 35 to 60. Heterozygotes have normal basal levels of 17-hydroxyprogesterone but show a significantly greater than normal rise of serum 17-hydroxyprogesterone, 17-hydroxyprogesterone plus progesterone, or 21-deoxycortisol within 30 to 360 minutes of intravenous ACTH stimulation. These studies demonstrate the existence in the heterozygote of a partial biochemical defect that manifests under conditions of maximum ACTH stimulation and provides a means for their identification.

The structural gene that codes for the adrenal 21-hydroxylase protein, or cytochrome P450c21, has been mapped on the short arm of chromosome 6 within the major histocompatibility complex, between the human lymphocytic antigen (HLA)B and DR loci in tandem with a second (liver ?) P450c21 gene and two genes coding for the C4A and C4B proteins (the fourth component of complement). Pedigree analyses have shown 21-hydroxylase deficiency to be HLA linked and C4 linked, which provides another means, in addition to biochemical testing, for identification of homozygotes or heterozygotes in families with an affected offspring. A strong link exists between the HLA-Bw47 haplotype with salt-losing 21-hydroxylase deficiency and between the B14 haplotype with the late-onset form. Initial studies of the P450c21 gene in the salt-losing form have shown it to be either deleted (in patients with the Bw47 haplotype) or converted to an inactive gene; perhaps other alterations of this gene result in the simple virilizing and late-onset forms of 21-hydroxylase deficiency.

Prenatal diagnosis and newborn screening. The prenatal diagnosis of 21-hydroxylase deficiency is made possible by the finding of elevated levels of amniotic fluid 17-hydroxyprogesterone (and androstenedione) from 14 weeks' gestation and beyond. HLA typing of cultured amniotic cells and the blood lymphocytes of the affected sibling and parents provides a second means of diagnosis. The diagnosis of fetuses with the salt-losing form has been reliable in the several cases reported, but one case of the simple virilizing form was missed by both hormone and HLA testing; infrequent errors in identifying normal fetuses also may occur. The in utero treatment of a female fetus having salt-losing 21-hydroxylase deficiency has been reported. To suppress the fetal adrenals, dexamethasone was given to the mother starting in the fifth week of pregnancy, before the onset of fetal external genital differentiation and before the expected rise of adrenal androgens, and was successful in preventing any virilization of the external genitalia. Because of the very limited experience, this treatment should be viewed as experimental.

Newborn screening of newborns for CAH by measurement of 17-hydroxyprogesterone in blood collected on filter paper at a few days of age has been reported by several groups. Justifications for this include the increased mortality that occurs in infants who are missed and die of salt-losing crisis or sudden infant death and the increased morbidity that results from adrenal insufficiency, incorrect sex assignment, and premature virilization.

11β-Hydroxylase deficiency (hypertensive CAH)

Deficiency of 11β-hydroxylase (cytochrome P450c11), which mediates 11β- and also 18-hydroxylation, results in impaired biosynthesis of cortisol and aldosterone, abnormal virilization from increased androgens formed from the cortisol precursors, and low renin hypertension that results from increased formation of 11-DOC, a moderately potent mineralocorticoid. It is the second most common form of CAH, accounting for about 5% to 8.5% (or more) of all cases. It was first recognized in 1951 and 1952 by Wilkins and associates, who reported a group of patients who had virilizing CAH with hypertension that remitted when adrenal activity was suppressed by replacement doses of cortisone.

The clinical presentation of 11β-hydroxylase deficiency is varied, and not all patients develop hypertension. Classically, females are born with virilization ranging from clitoral enlargement to extensive masculinization of the external genitalia that may lead to incorrect sex assignment, whereas males may have a somewhat larger penis, although not routinely clinically recognizable. Both sexes may have hyperpigmentation of the genitalia and areolae. Postnatal virilization affects both sexes, and some males have developed gynecomastia in infancy or childhood. Sodium retention occurs and volume-induced hypertension is present in 50% to 80% of classic cases; it has been observed in affected infants. However, the relative severities of the hypertension, virilization, and biochemical findings do not always correlate. Serum sodium levels tend to be upper-normal to minimally elevated, but hypokalemia is inconsistently present.

In exception to the classic presentations, some affected and untreated neonates have presented with salt-losing disorders, which has led to diagnostic confusion with 21-hydroxylase deficiency. The cause of their salt-losing condition is unclear but may be related to a combination of physiologic renal immaturity in sodium reabsorption, more severe aldosterone deficiency and less adequate DOC, and presence of precursor steroids with mineralocorticoid antagonist properties. A mild form of 11β-hydroxylase deficiency occurs in which affected females show little or no masculinization at birth but have late onset of mild virilization with absent or mild hypertension.

The characteristic biochemical abnormality seen is an elevated level of serum 11-deoxycortisol (compound S), with reported levels ranging between 40 and 400 ng/ml (normal, 7.8 ± 5.3 ng/ml). Serum DOC levels also have been elevated in the few patients measured, ranging between 10 and 180 ng/ml (normal, 0.06 ng/ml). Urinary tetrahydro-11-deoxycortisol (THS) is characteristically elevated, and urinary tetrahydro-11-deoxycorticosterone (THDOC) levels are similarly elevated in patients with the classic form. The aldosterone secretion rate is decreased, but plasma renin activity (PRA) levels are suppressed secondary to the elevated levels of DOC; in the few neonates and young infants studied, however, PRA levels have ranged from suppressed to high-normal or minimally elevated, reflecting variable ability to retain sodium. Serum 17-hydroxyprogesterone is mildly elevated, and androstenedione and urinary 17-ketosteroids are also increased and may cause diagnostic confusion with 21-hydroxylase deficiency. In the mild or late-onset form, basal urinary THDOC levels are normal, and it is suggested that these patients have a limited defect of 11β-hydroxylase affecting only the conversion of 11-deoxycortisol to cortisol, and not that of DOC to corticosterone.

11β-Hydroxylase deficiency should be considered in XX neonates with masculinization of the external genitalia, in any patients beyond the neonatal period with abnormal virilization, in salt-losing neonates, and in all hypertensive patients. The diagnosis is based on finding elevated serum levels of 11-deoxycortisol and DOC and increased urinary levels of THS and in demonstrating their suppressibility with cortisol replacement therapy. The differential diagnosis includes 21-hydroxylase deficiency, other causes of hypertension and, after the neonatal period, a virilizing adrenal or ovarian tumor.

Treatment is with cortisol replacement therapy, as outlined for 21-hydroxylase deficiency. Glucocorticoid replacement reduces ACTH and thus the levels of precursor steroids, toward normal, with cessation of virilization. Decreased DOC formation also occurs, which leads to correction of hypertension in most (although not all) affected patients. A complication of the reduced DOC formation, however, is a diminished sodium-retention ability. This may lead to salt-losing during episodes of gastroenteritis or other illnesses affecting sodium balance, and growth may be impaired. Consequently the addition of 9α-fluorohydrocortisone acetate (Florinef) is advocated if PRA is elevated during adequate glucocorticoid replacement. The sex of rearing should be in agreement with the gonadal sex, since normal sexual function and fertility can be attained. 11β-Hydroxylase deficiency is autosomal recessive, based on examination of pedigrees. Heterozygotes have not been shown to manifest a biochemical abnormality under maximum ACTH stimulation. The disorder is not HLA linked, and the chromosome location of the gene for 11β-hydroxylase has not been determined. Prenatal diagnosis has been successfully accomplished with measurement of THS levels in amniotic fluid and maternal urine.

3β-Hydroxysteroid dehydrogenase deficiency

Bongiovanni first described six patients in 1961 and 1962 with 3β-hydroxysteroid dehydrogenase (3β-HSD) deficiency. Three males had severe penile or perineal hypospadias and three females were minimally virilized at birth with posterior labial fusion and clitoral hypertrophy but normal placement of the urethral meatus. Five had a salt-losing condition, and four of these died in the first months of life despite adequate steroid treatment. In this disorder the salt-losing adrenal crises result from impaired cortisol and aldosterone biosynthesis in the adrenal, and the incomplete male genital differentiation results from decreased testosterone biosynthesis in the testes. The mild prenatal virilization in the females is thought to result from increased precursor steroid formation; that is, the increased amounts of dehydroepiandrosterone (DHA) are probably converted by peripheral 3β-HSD in the liver and other tissues (the peripheral 3β-HSD enzyme is under different genetic control and is thus intact) to biochemically active androgens that induce mild masculinization of the genitalia in the female.

The characteristic biochemical finding in the untreated patient is a marked elevation of serum 17-hydroxypregnenolone. Elevated serum pregnenolone is also found, and the C_{19}, Δ^5-steroids DHA and DHA sulfate are higher in most, but not all, patients. Urinary 17-ketosteroids are elevated. Mildly to markedly elevated levels of 17-hydroxyprogesterone, which result from the peripheral conversion of 17-hydroxypregnenolone, have caused diagnostic confusion with 21-hydroxylase deficiency in a number of cases, although the level of 17-hydroxypregnenolone is inevitably higher than that of 17-hydroxyprogesterone in individuals with 3β-HSD deficiency. Levels of Δ^4-steroids progesterone or testosterone also may be higher than expected and cause diagnostic confusion. Aldosterone levels are low and PRA is elevated.

Clinical heterogeneity occurs in 3β-HSD deficiency as in the 21- and 11β-hydroxylase deficiency disorders. Several patients with abnormal genitalia but without salt-losing disorders have been reported, including one in the original group reported by Bongiovanni. Some of the patients have shown partial defects in aldosterone biosynthesis that could be compensated for, but at least two demonstrated normal aldosterone biosynthesis and evidence that their 3β-HSD defect did not involve the zona glomerulosa. Another form of 3β-HSD deficiency in a brother and sister involved only the C_{21} steroid pathway, resulting in cortisol and aldosterone deficiency with acute adrenal crises in childhood, but with intact 3β-HSD activity in the adrenal and gonadal C_{19} steroid pathway, leading to intact testosterone biosynthesis and normal genitalia in both. A mild form of 3β-HSD deficiency with late onset also occurs, but it is not of clinical significance in infancy.

Treatment is the same as described for 21-hydroxylase deficiency; serum levels of 17-hydroxypregnenolone and DHA serve as guides concerning the adequacy of glucocorticoid replacement. Sex assignment is according to the gonadal sex or is female for XY individuals having too small a penis. The inheritance is autosomal recessive; ACTH stimulation of heterozygotes has yielded an abnormal response in some but not others. Prenatal diagnosis has not been reported.

Cholesterol side-chain cleavage enzyme (20,22-desmolase) deficiency (congenital lipoid adrenal hyperplasia)

Deficiency of the cholesterol side-chain cleavage enzyme complex, which includes P450scc (SCC deficiency), results in impaired synthesis of all adrenal and gonadal steroids. It is a rare but serious disorder; many patients have died within the first several months of life. The clinical course for most cases has been the development of severe adrenal insufficiency, sometimes occurring in the first days of life but in milder cases beginning beyond several weeks of age. Sodium wasting has often been extreme, and hypoglycemia may occur. The XX female patients have had normal female external genitalia; XY male patients have external genitalia that have appeared female or ambiguous, with a blind vaginal pouch frequently being present. Hyperpigmentation and respiratory problems may occur.

The adrenal glands are enlarged with a characteristically enormous accumulation of lipid, giving the name *congenital lipoid adrenal hyperplasia*. Biochemically there is a decreased to absent production of all adrenal steroids, depending on the severity of the defect, and an accumulation of cholesterol and its esters in the adrenal. Serum cholesterol levels have not been elevated, but in one case the urinary cholesterol level was elevated to 0.8 and 0.9 mg/24 hours (normal, 0.11 to 0.35 mg/24 hours).

SCC deficiency should be considered in cases of adrenal insufficiency and in XY males with ambiguous genitalia. The diagnosis is based on demonstrating a deficiency of the glucocorticoids, mineralocorticoids, and androgens. An increase in urinary cholesterol and the presence of bilateral adrenal hyperplasia via ultrasound or CT scan are supportive. In XX females with adrenal insufficiency and no genital abnormalities, the differentiation of SCC deficiency from congenital adrenal hypoplasia is very difficult and depends on demonstrating the presence or absence of the adrenal glands.

Treatment includes cortisol, mineralocorticoid, salt, and replacement therapy, as outlined for 21-hydroxylase deficiency. This needs to be given aggressively in infancy to reduce the high mortality risk. The sex of rearing in XY patients has been along female lines; the decision should be based on phallic size and the chances for achieving normal-appearing genitalia by early childhood. The inheritance of SCC deficiency is probably autosomal recessive. In one patient the P450scc enzyme was absent from adrenal mitochondria, suggesting a gene deletion or mutation. In three other patients, however, the structural gene for P450scc, (which has been located on chromosome 15), was found to be intact, suggesting that another cause was responsible in these patients.

17α-Hydroxylase deficiency

Deficiency of 17α-hydroxylase (P450c17) results in impairment of adrenal synthesis of cortisol and gonadal synthesis of androgens and estrogens. The resultant increased ACTH secretion causes (1) increased formation of the precursor steroid, progesterone; (2) stimulation of the 17-deoxysteroid (mineralocorticoid) pathway in the zone fasciculata to produce increased DOC, corticosterone (B), and 18-hydroxycorticosterone (18-OHB) (aldosterone is not synthesized in the zona fasciculata pathway); and (3) adrenocortical hyperplasia. Clinically this results in hypokalemic alkalosis, borderline hypernatremia, and volume-induced hypertension that is often severe. Such findings have been reported in an infant (electrolytes were normal) and in a 3-year-old child. Adrenal insufficiency may, but usually does not, develop because of the mineralocorticoid and glucocorticoid properties of DOC and B. The XX female patients have normal genitalia at birth, but XY male patients have phenotypically female to sightly masculinized external genitalia, often with a distal vagina or prostatic utricle and variable testicular descent. The internal genital ducts are appropriate for the gonadal sex, although wolffian duct development may be incomplete. The differential diagnosis for XY patients includes androgen insensitivity (testicular feminization) syndrome.

The serum levels and production rates of cortisol are low to low-normal, whereas those for DOC and B are markedly elevated; serum levels of progesterone are also elevated but occasionally have been normal. The serum level and production rate of aldosterone and the level of PRA are low because of the increased DOC. Cortisol replacement therapy corrects these abnormalities, and in most patients aldosterone secretion returns to normal, although in several cases it has remained abnormally low. Serum levels of testosterone are low and show a poor rise following hCG stimulation. Urinary 17-hydroxycorticosteroids and 17-ketosteroids are low to low-normal, whereas the tetrahydro-derivatives of DOC and corticosterone are characteristically elevated; pregnanediol ranges from normal to elevated.

Cortisol replacement is given as described for 21-hydroxylase deficiency, but mineralocorticoid therapy is not necessary unless aldosterone secretion fails to return to normal. The sex of rearing of XY patients should be female unless the genitalia are sufficiently male-sized at birth and surgically correctable. The inheritance is most probably autosomal recessive. The few heterozygotes tested show a partial biochemical defect under maximum ACTH stimulation with abnormal elevation of the 18-OHB/aldosterone ratio; this ratio is greatly elevated in affected homozygotes. Two or more structural genes that code for P450c17 have been identified in the human genome; the adrenal P450c17 gene lies on chromosome 10. It is not known if this gene also encodes for the testicular P450c17 or if a second gene encodes for a specific testicular isoenzyme of P450c17.

Maternally derived androgenic substances

Masculinization of the female fetus occasionally occurs from exposure to androgens or certain other agents derived from the maternal circulation. The extent of masculinization is related to the compound, dosage, and duration and timing of exposure. Exposure at 8 to 14 weeks' gestation may result in midline fusion of the labioscrotal folds, opening of the vagina and urethra into a common urogenital sinus, and in more severe cases development of a prostate and possibly seminal vesicles. Exposure beyond 12 to 14 weeks can only result in clitoromegaly and hypertrophy of the labia majora but no midline fusion and no development of a urogenital sinus. Maternally derived androgens usually do not stimulate wolffian duct development, and the müllerian duct structures and bilateral ovaries develop normally.

Androgen-secreting tumors of the ovary occur rarely in pregnant women, and only one case of virilizing adrenal tumor has been reported. Among the reasons why a considerable portion of female fetuses do not undergo masculinization is that the placenta aromatizes most maternal androgens before they cross over to the fetus, and the high maternal (versus fetal) levels of sex-steroid binding globulin favor concentration of these androgens on the maternal side.

Maternal ingestion of synthetic progestins, androgens, or danazol (a derivative of 17α-ethinyl testosterone) may cause abnormal masculinization of the female fetus. In the male fetus, progestin exposure from 8 to 14 weeks' gestation may result in hypospadias. These substances have been given to pregnant women because of habitual or threatened abortions, as pregnancy-test drugs, as a postcoital "morning-after" pill, as an oral contraceptive, or to "nonpregnant" women for endometriosis, menorrhagia, breast cancer, alopecia, or other problems. Since these medications often have been given for only part of the pregnancy, the extent of clitoral enlargement, urethral displacement, and labioscrotal fusion is often discordant, unlike the other causes of female pseudohermaphroditism. The mother may rarely show mild androgenization. Advanced skeletal maturation occurs in the offspring exposed to the more androgenic substances. Stimulation of the androgen receptor or inhibition of certain steroidogenic enzymes, such as 3β-hydroxysteroid dehydrogenase, are two possible mechanisms.

Paradoxic masculinization of female fetuses has also occurred in a very small number of pregnancies in which diethylstilbestrol (DES) was administered. In contrast, males exposed to DES in utero have had an increased incidence of cryptorchidism and hypoplastic testes. The affected female offspring had clitoromegaly, with midline labioscrotal fusion and formation of a urogenital sinus occurring in those exposed between 8 and 14 weeks' gestation. Inhibition of 3β-hydroxysteroid dehydrogenase with secondarily increased adrenal androgen production is one postulated mechanism. Although DES has been contraindicated in the treatment of pregnancy complications since 1971, it is still used as a postcoital contraceptive and for other medical problems. Females exposed prenatally to DES have an increased incidence of structural abnormalities of the vagina, cervix, and uterine cavity; increased pregnancy wastage, possibly related to the structural abnormalities; and an increased incidence of clear cell adenocarcinoma of the genital tract. The exposed female offspring need to have periodic screening for the development of clear cell adenocarcinoma beginning at age 14 years, or sooner if vaginal bleeding or discharge occurs.

The masculinization of females that occurs with androgen or other drug exposure in utero does not progress postnatally. Biochemical studies show normal levels of androgens or their metabolites and of 17-hydroxyprogesterone. Surgical correction of midline labioscrotal fusion or major clitoromegaly should be done by age 12 to 18 months; mild clitoromegaly may not need to be corrected, since the clitoris will become less prominent with an increase in general body size.

Non-androgen-induced genital masculinization

Female pseudohermaphroditism not caused by androgen exposure is often associated with other congenital malformations. Examples include the VATER (*v*ertebral abnormalities, *a*nal atresia, *t*racheoesophageal fistula with *e*sophageal atresia, *r*adial and renal dysplasia) association, imperforate anus, renal agenesis, duplication or hydronephrosis of the kidneys, or other abnormalities of the lower intestinal or genitourinary tract. The ovaries are usually normal, but there often is accompanying absence or malformation of the müllerian structures. The cause of this form of female pseudohermaphroditism may be a disturbance in morphogenesis. Idiopathic clitoral hypertrophy, with or without labioscrotal fusion, by definition occurs without any evidence for androgen or other drug exposure and without other associated congenital abnormalities. Unrecognized stimulation of the androgen receptor may represent an underlying mechanism.

OTHER DISORDERS OF SEX DIFFERENTIATION OR MORPHOGENESIS

Hypospadias

Hypospadias is a condition of failed male urethral differentiation in which the urethral meatus lies somewhere proximal to the tip of the glans penis, either on the ventral surface of the glans or penile shaft, or in severe cases on the perineum. It is the second most common genital abnormality (after cryptorchidism) in male newborns, with an incidence in different series ranging between 0.25% to 0.82%. It occurs less frequently in blacks (0.39%) than in whites (0.61%). The types of hypospadias seen comprise approximately 87% glanular or coronal, 10% penile, and 3% penoscrotal and perineal, although higher proportions of the latter type have been reported.

Other anomalies frequently accompany the hypospadias. Chordee (ventral curvature of the penis) is usually caused by fibrous tissue growth in the area of failed urethral development. Its location (glanular or midshaft) and severity are easier to assess in the erect penis. The prepuce in the hypospadic penis is usually deficient ventrally and thus appears hooded. Other genital anomalies include meatal stenosis, hydrocele, cryptorchidism in 8% to 10%, and inguinal hernia in 8% of patients. More severe forms of hypospadias are often associated with incompletely translocated labioscrotal folds or a shawl scrotum and with a prostatic utricle. Urinary tract abnormalities are seen in 9% to 28% of cases of hypospadias, with renal ectopia, horseshoe kidneys, and reflux having a higher than normal prevalence. Patients with urinary tract symptoms, family history of reflux, multiple congenital anomalies, or ambiguous genitalia are more likely to have significant abnormalities and should have uroradiographic evaluation. Asymptomatic patients have a 3% to 4% incidence of significant abnormalities and should have a urinalysis and urine culture done to determine the need for other evaluations.

About 7% to 8% of hypospadic patients have a brother or father with hypospadias, reaching 16.7% in individuals with penoscrotal or perineal hypospadias. This familial tendency is thought to result from a polygenic mode of inheritance.

Mild hypospadias (glanular to penile) without other genital abnormalities or dysmorphic features is very unlikely to have an identifiable endocrinopathy, intersex problem, or chromosomal abnormality. Severe hypospadias (penoscrotal or perineal; see Fig. 37-38) is associated with approximately a 15% risk of such problems occurring. The addition of other genital abnormalities (cryptorchidism or abnormally small penis; see Fig. 37-42) increases the risk of occurrence of an intersex problem or endocrinopathy to 35% in mild, and 79% in severe, hypospadias. Hypospadias also occurs in certain rare syndromes, many of which carry a very poor prognosis.

The cause of hypospadias in at least some cases results from a partial deficiency in either testosterone production, in conversion of testosterone to DHT (5α-reductase deficiency), or in the function of the cytoplasmic androgen receptor protein (partial androgen insensitivity). In 4% to 23% of cases, maternal exposure to progestins at 8 to 14 weeks' gestation has been the cause of hypospadias (see Fig. 37-39).

The evaluation of hypospadias in the newborn includes a history for possible maternal progestin or estrogen exposure and a family history of hypospadias, endocrine, or intersex problems; an examination to evaluate the hypospadias, identify somatic or other genital abnormalities, and assess for the presence of a uterus or gross abnormality of the kidneys; and measurement of penile length to be certain that rearing the infant as a male is appropriate. Additional studies are not necessary in infants with mild hypospadias without other abnormalities. Diagnostic studies should be done in hypospadic infants at greater risk for an endocrine or intersex problem.

The immediate concerns in the evaluation of neonatal hypospadias relate to withholding circumcision, identification of possible male or female pseudohermaphrodites, selection of sex of rearing, and recognition of syndromes that may have a poor prognosis. If penile length is found to be abnormally small, assuming that correction has been made for some loss of length caused by chordee, female sex of rearing should be considered. If both gonads are impalpable, the possibility must be seriously considered that the infant has female pseudohermaphroditism, such as CAH (See Fig. 37-42).

Surgical repair of hypospadias is ideally done later in the first year by an experienced surgeon in a pediatric setting. It is important for the boy that his genital appearance be close to normal so that he may develop a normal body image and that he be able to stand to urinate. Multistage procedures may be required for more severe forms of hypospadias, and complication rates may be 10% to 25%. Education of the family and preparation of the patient for these procedures are very important, since psychologic problems are seen in adults who underwent hypospadias repair as children.

Micropenis

A micropenis is arbitrarily defined as a penis with a normally formed urethra that opens at the tip of the glans in which either (1) the stretched length is more than 2.5 standard deviations below the mean for age, or (2) the penile corpora cavernosa are absent or severely deficient in size, resulting in an abnormally thin penis, regardless of penile length. Penile length should be measured fully stretched, with the ruler pressed down against the pubic ramus, depressing the suprapubic fat pad completely, and measuring to the tip of the glans only, ignoring any

A

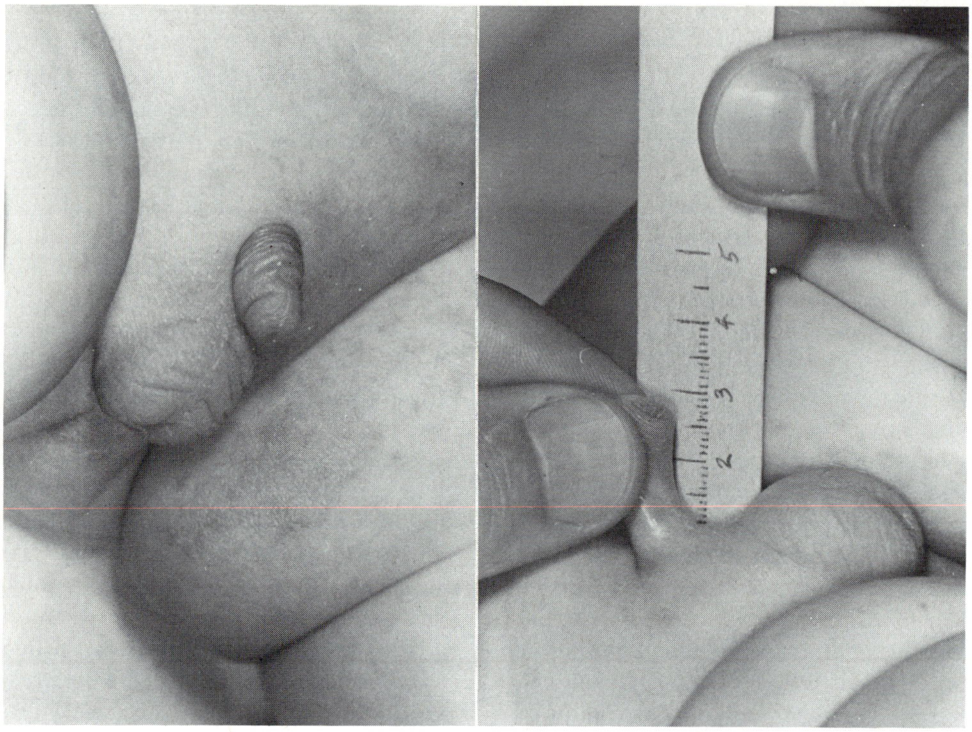

B

Fig. 37-45. A, Two-month-old male with micropenis and cryptorchidism caused by LH and FSH deficiency; the scrotum is compact or "unlived-in," and the testes are inguinal. **B,** Centimeter markings are inked on a wooden tongue blade, which is placed near the penis and depressed down on the pubic ramus. The penis is maximally stretched with measurement made to the tip of the glans (measurement here is 1.7 cm; normal, 3.5 ± 0.4 cm, [mean ± SD]), ignoring the excess foreskin. The width of the stretched penis at midshaft was 0.6 cm (normal, 0.9 to 1.3 cm). hCG stimulation and testosterone therapy increased the penile size to 4.2 × 1.1 cm by age 6 months, and the hCG caused the testes to descend into the scrotum.

excess foreskin (Fig. 37-45). The width is measured at midshaft of the stretched penis.

The cause of most cases of micropenis is endocrinologic and reflects a deficiency of those factors (testosterone or DHT and possibly growth hormone) needed for normal penile growth to occur beyond 14 weeks' gestation. The major causes include hypopituitarism (LH with or without growth hormone deficiency) (30%), primary hypogonadism (25%), partial androgen insensitivity (2%), and idiopathic or undiagnosed (43%). It is unknown whether growth hormone deficiency alone (without LH deficiency) can cause micropenis. The association of micropenis with early neonatal hypoglycemia (growth hormone and ACTH-cortisol deficiency), cryptorchidism (LH deficiency; Fig. 37-45), persistent neonatal jaundice (ACTH-cortisol deficiency), or cleft lip or palate should immediately raise the strong possibility of congenital hypopituitarism. Other congenital malformations, such as septo-optic dysplasia, and chromosome abnormalities are occasionally associated. The diagnostic evaluation of micropenis includes assessment of growth hormone, testosterone, LH, and FSH status. An hCG stimulation test should be done if testosterone elevation is not seen. A karyotype may need to be determined.

The selection of sex of rearing is based principally on penile size, since a correlation exists between the penile size in infancy and its final size in adulthood. The sex of rearing should be female if the stretched penile length is less than 1.5 cm in the term neonate or if the penile corpora cavernosa are severely deficient or absent; the sex should be male if the stretched length is 2.0 cm or more and if penile diameter is adequate. The length criteria should be adjusted for the premature neonate (Fig. 37-46). The administration of a course of testosterone therapy to assess penile responsiveness may be done to exclude significant androgen insensitivity.

Cryptorchidism

Cryptorchidism, or testicular maldescent, is present when one or both testes have failed to descend completely into the scrotum (to a position 4 cm or more below the pubic crest in term males more than 2.5 kg). Since

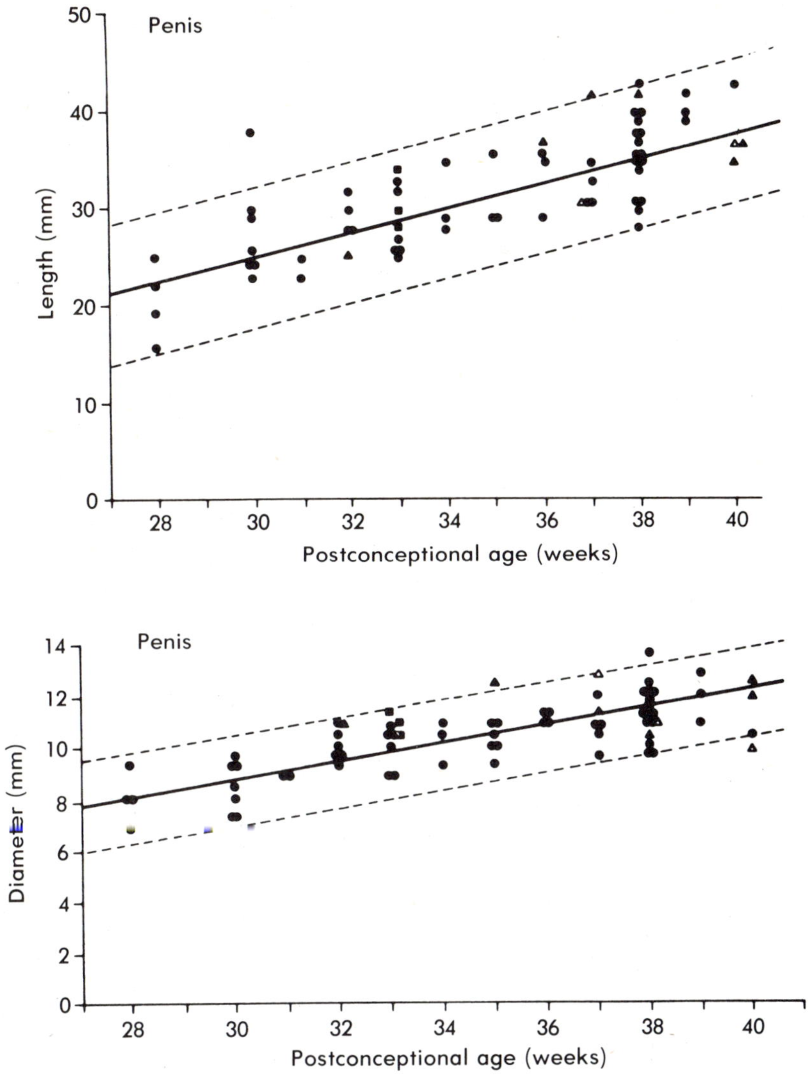

Fig. 37-46. A, Stretched penile lengths (mean ±2SD) and **B,** penile diameters (mean ±2SD) in 63 normal premature and full-term male infants (●), two small for gestational age infants (△), seven large for gestational age infants (▲), and four twins (■). (From Feldman, K.W., and Smith, D.W.: J. Pediatr. **86:**395, 1975.)

the testes normally descend between 7 months of fetal age through the first several months of postnatal age, most affected newborns actually will be found to be normal when reevaluated. The incidence of cryptorchidism at birth is 2.7% in full-term males and about 21% in premature males, approaching 100% in the very premature. In these cryptorchid neonates, however, postnatal completion of testicular descent is seen in 50% of the full-term cryptorchid males by 6 weeks of age and in 67% of the full-term and 73% of the premature cryptorchid males by 3 months of age. A few additional individuals will attain full descent by age 9 months, with the net result being that about 75% of full-term, and about 90% of premature, cryptorchid newborns will have full testicular descent by age 9 months without therapeutic intervention. Spontaneous testicular descent is very rare after age 9 months. The incidence of true cryptorchidism is 0.78% at age 1 year, similar to the incidence observed in older age groups.

The causes of true cryptorchidism are not known, but it frequently occurs with disorders of the hypothalamic-pituitary-testicular hormone axis, in association with intrinsically abnormal testes, and with anatomic defects of the epididymis and the abdominal wall. Cryptorchidism is seen in higher incidence in patients having umbilical hernia (6%), gastroschisis (15%), omphalocele (33%), and prune belly syndrome (100%), in which intraabdominal pressure may be important. It is also seen in meningomyelocele (25%), particularly when the defect is above L2 and affects the genitofemoral nerve, and in cerebral palsy (41%). True cryptorchidism is associated with lower LH and testosterone levels during the pituitary-testicular hormonal surge at age 1 to 3 months and occurs frequently in hypopituitarism or hypogonadotropism, Prader-Willi syndrome, primary hypogonadism, and many intersex disorders. A role for MIF is suggested by the high association with persistence of müllerian ducts. Frequent association is also seen with trisomies 13 and 18 and with Noonan's, Aarskog-Scott, and other syndromes. An increased incidence of cryptorchidism occurs with administration of estrogens to the mother. Familial cases are reported, and cryptorchidism is found in 6.2% of brothers and 1.5% to 4% of fathers.

Associated anomalies include an inguinal hernia in about 90% of patients, abnormal epididymal formation in 36% or 66%, and hypospadias in about 3% (such patients are at a 53% risk for having an intersex problem). Major upper urinary tract anomalies occur in about 3%, but routine invasive diagnostic studies are not essential for all patients; cryptorchidism is noted in 5% of patients with Wilms' tumor.

Complications of cryptorchidism include (1) progressive histologic deterioration with changes beginning after age 6 months, (2) impaired spermatogenesis with a decrease in the number of spermatogonia after the second year of life, (3) increased (20- to 40-fold) risk for cancer in the undescended testis and also in the descended testis in unilateral cryptorchidism, (4) trauma to the testis that is relatively fixed in position, (5) torsion, (6) symptomatic inguinal hernia, and (7) psychologic factors relating to altered body image. The inguinal hernia may require repair in early infancy if large enough to permit abdominal contents to enter or if it is symptomatic.

Torsion of the testis occurs more frequently in cryptorchidism, particularly in the neonatal period and infancy and occasionally in utero. It may be difficult to diagnose, so destruction of the testis often results. If a scrotal testis is involved, the clinical presentation includes a scrotal mass, which is either nontender or only mildly so, with reddish to bluish discoloration of the scrotal skin. The patient is usually otherwise well, and the mildness of symptoms often delays diagnosis. Torsion of the impalpable cryptorchid testis is much more difficult to identify early because pain and irritability may be intermittent; some neonates have had an abdominal mass.

If both testes are impalpable, the differential diagnosis includes anorchia, persistent müllerian duct syndrome, Leydig cell hypoplasia, intraabdominal testes and, most importantly, an XX female with CAH or other severe virilizing disorder. Thorough examination, sex chromosome determination, biochemical studies and, if appropriate, hCG stimulation testing to demonstrate the presence of functioning Leydig cells are done. CT and laparoscopy have been useful in locating intraabdominal testes, but laparotomy with methodic exploration to the ends of the spermatic blood vessels is definitive in cases that are not otherwise resolved.

Because of the early appearance of histologic changes in the cryptorchid testis and the findings that early treatment improves the prospect for fertility and decreases the risk of malignancy, correction of cryptorchidism is recommended in the first 2 years of life, with certain precautions. Spontaneous descent may occur up to 6 to 9 months of age, so that treatment before this time does not seem to be indicated unless the testis is ectopic or has other associated abnormalities. Orchiopexy is the treatment of choice. It optimally should be done by a surgeon with much experience in this age group because the risk for subsequent loss of the testis is high. A more aggressive approach in bilateral cryptorchidism is to first give a course of low-dose hCG, such as 500 to 1,000 units intramuscularly twice weekly for 3 to 6 weeks, or gonadotropin-releasing hormone (or possibly both hormones together) at some time after 7 to 9 months of age to avoid disrupting the normal increase in hypothalamic-pituitary-testicular axis activity seen in the first 6 to 7 months of life. These hormonal therapies have a low rate of success of perhaps 8% to 30% but may offer benefit by inducing appropriate maturation of the testis. The chances for success with hormone treatment are much less in unilateral cryptorchidism, in which inherent abnormalities involving both the undescended and the descended testes are often seen.

Müllerian and vaginal dysgenesis

The association of abnormal to absent müllerian duct structures with vaginal agenesis in 46,XX females with normal ovaries occurs frequently (the eponym *Mayer-Rokitansky-Kuster-Hauser syndrome* is variably used in the literature) and is the second most common cause of primary amenorrhea after Turner's syndrome. Renal abnormalities, including ectopy and agenesis, are seen in about 70% of patients and are major in 15%, including unilateral, horseshoe, and pelvic kidneys. The syndrome has been expanded to include other frequently associated abnormalities (the MURCS association), that is, defects resulting from cervicothoracic somite dysplasia (Klippel-Feil syndrome, hand anomalies) and the occurrence of short stature. Deafness, inguinal hernias, congenital heart and lung lesions, and other defects are also seen. A disturbance in mesodermal organization, in part involving the formation of the caudal segments of the müllerian ducts in the fourth and fifth weeks of embryogenesis, is suggested; the possibilities of both a teratogenic and a pleiotropic genetic cause are raised. The differential diagnosis includes complete androgen insensitivity. Some patients have had an abnormal karyotype. Examination for the vaginal orifice (absent in this disorder) or occasional occurrence of hydrometria or presence of somatic abnormalities would help to identify affected neonates. Vaginal construction is necessary; the extent of the uterine malformation needs to be assessed. Approximately 70% of female patients with unilateral renal agenesis have ipsilateral müllerian duct abnormalities.

IDENTIFICATION, DIAGNOSIS, AND MANAGEMENT OF INTERSEX DISORDERS

IDENTIFICATION OF NEONATES WITH AN INTERSEX PROBLEM

The reasons for wanting to identify and diagnose an intersex problem promptly in the neonatal period or soon after are (1) to designate the correct sex of rearing, (2) to diagnose CAH before the occurrence of adrenal crisis, (3) to identify those at increased risk for developing a gonadal tumor, (4) to provide genetic counseling and the option for prenatal diagnosis in the future, and (5) to correct problems early so that the patient may go through childhood with a normal body image and gender identity.

Most intersex patients have some abnormality of their external genitalia and are thus potentially identifiable at birth. The genitalia do not need to be overtly "ambiguous" to qualify for a diagnostic evaluation. An intersex problem is likely to be present if an individual has (1) two or more abnormalities of the external genital structures, such as penile hypospadias and an undescended gonad, or (2) the presence of certain single genital abnormalities (Table 37-7). Some neonates lack any external

Table 37-7. Characteristics of ambiguous genitalia

Abnormal characteristics	Examples of associated disorder
ABNORMALITY OF ANY TWO OF THE FOLLOWING	
Phallus—size*,†	
Urethral meatus—location	
Labioscrotal folds—fusion	
Gonad(s)—location or size‡	
PRESENCE OF ANY OF THE FOLLOWING ABNORMALITIES	
With male-appearing genitalia:	
Micropenis*	Growth hormone or LH deficiency Testosterone deficiency (in second, third trimester) Partial androgen insensitivity Syndrome; idiopathic
Impalpable gonads	Anorchia Persistent müllerian duct syndrome XX with 21- or 11β-hydroxylase deficiency Cryptorchidism
Small gonads‡	XXY, XX male Dysgenetic or rudimentary testes
Inguinal mass (uterus or tube)	Persistent müllerian duct syndrome, dysgenetic testes
With female-appearing genitalia:	
Clitoromegaly†	XX with 21- or 11β-hydroxylase or 3β-HSD deficiency Other female pseudohermaphroditism True hermaphroditism Gonadal dysgenesis, dysgenetic testes Male pseudohermaphroditism Tumor infiltration of clitoris Premature female; idiopathic
Posterior labial fusion	As for clitoromegaly
Palpable gonad(s)	True hermaphroditism Mixed gonadal dysgenesis, dysgenetic testes Male pseudohermaphroditism
Inguinal hernia or mass	As for palpable gonad(s)

*Length of penis is determined using maximally stretched penis, with ruler depressing suprapubic fat above pubic symphysis and measurement made from base of penis to tip of glans, ignoring excess foreskin. Width of stretched penis is measured at midshaft. Micropenis is defined by a stretched length or width below −2.5 SD of mean for age (Fig. 37-46).
†Clitoris is abnormally enlarged if its width is more than 6 mm in neonate.
‡Gonad is abnormally small if longest diameter is less than 0.8 cm.

Table 37-8. Characteristics of Y chromatin–positive or H-Y antigen–positive intersex disorders

Disorder	External genitalia	Internal ducts	Gonadal tissue	Biochemical*		Fertility	Gonadal tumors	Inheritance‡	Comment
				Testosterone	Other				
DISORDERS OF GONADAL DIFFERENTIATION									
True hermaphroditism (with Y chromosome)	F, A, M	F, M	Ovary, testis or ovotestis	– to Nl		1 case	4.5%	Few familial	
Gonadal dysgenesis									
Y chromosome abnormalities	F, A, M	F, M	Streaks or dysgenetic testes	– to ±		–	15%-20%		
Mixed gonadal dysgenesis	F, A, M	F, M	Streak and testis	– to ±		–; ? possible	22%		
XY Gonadal dysgenesis	F	F	Streaks	–		–	30%	X-linked or ADML; aut rec × 1 family	Camptomelic dwarfism
Testicular dysgenesis									
Dysgenetic testes	A	F, M	Testes, dysgenetic	– to Nl		–; ? possible	+	Few familial	Renal disease, Wilms' tumor
Testicular regression						–	–	Few familial	
Early (gonadal agenesis)	F, A	F; occasionally absent or M	Absent	–; rarely ±					
Late (anorchia)	M	M	Absent	–		–	–	Few familial	
Rudimentary testes	M, A	M	Testes, small	– to ±		Not reported	None reported	Some familial	
XXY (Klinefelter's) syndrome	M	M	Testes, ±small	– to Nl		Absent	–		
XX Male	M, A	M	Testes, ±small	– to Nl		Absent	–	Few familial	
DISORDERS OF TESTICULAR HORMONES (MALE PSEUDOHERMAPHRODITISM)									
Persistent müllerian duct syndrome	M	F and M	Testes, occasionally hypoplastic	Nl		+	5%-10%	Some familial	Cryptorchidism
Unresponsiveness to hCG and LH	F, A	Absent	Testes, small	–		–	None reported	Some familial	
Testicular enzyme deficiencies									
Cholesterol SCC deficiency	F, A	M	Testes	–	+ + Urinary cholesterol	–	–	Aut rec	Addisonian
3β-HSD deficiency	F, A	M	Testes	– to ±	+ + 17OHPe:17OHP + + Pe:P	–	–	Aut rec	Addisonian
17α-Hydroxylase deficiency	F, A	M	Testes	–	+ + DOC,B; + P + + 18OHB:Aldo	–	–	Aut rec	Hypertension
17,20-Desmolase deficiency	F, A	Absent or M	Testes	–	+ + 17OHPe:DHA + + 17OHP:Δ	–	–	X-linked or aut rec	

17β-HSOR deficiency	F, A	M	Testes	–	+ +Δ:T + +E_1:E_2	–	1 case	Aut rec	
Disorders of androgen-dependent target tissues									
5α-Reductase deficiency	F, A	M	Testes	Nl	+ +T:DHT	Possible	–	Aut rec	
Androgen insensitivity									
Complete	F	Absent or M	Testes	Nl or + +	Nl to +T DHT	–	22%-33% >20 yr	X-linked	
Partial	A	M	Testes	Nl or + +	Nl to +T DHT	–	Carcinoma in situ	X-linked	
Maternally derived progestins	A	M	Testes	Nl		Nl	None reported		Hypospadias

Modified from Danish, R.K.: Indian J. Pediatr. **49:**555, 1982.
SCC, Side-chain cleavage; HSD, hydroxysteroid dehydrogenase; HSOR, hydroxysteroid oxidoreductase.
A, Ambiguous; F, female; M, male; Nl, normal; –, decreased to absent; ±, low normal; +, increased.
Aldo, Aldosterone; Δ, androstenedione; B, corticosterone; 180HB, 18-hydroxycorticosterone; DHA, dehydroepiandrosterone; DHT, dihydrotestosterone; DOC, 11-deoxycorticosterone; E_1, estrone, E_2, estradiol; Pe, pregnenolone; 17OHPe, 17-hydroxypregnenolone; P, progesterone; 17OHP, 17-hydroxyprogesterone; T, testosterone.
*"Few familial" or "some familial" indicates that a small or moderate portion of cases have been reported to occur in families; there is insufficient information to indicate whether their inheritance is X linked, autosomal recessive (aut rec), or autosomal dominant, male-limited (ADML).

genital abnormality but have other features that may lead to their diagnosis. Examples include Turner's phenotype—gonadal dysgenesis caused by X and occasionally Y chromosome abnormalities (see boxed material on features of this phenotype, p. 1134); camptomelic dwarfism—bowing and angulation of the lower limbs, flat facies, shortened vertebrae (XY gonadal dysgenesis); hyperpigmentation; sodium wasting or failure to thrive (CAH); and hypertension (11β-hydroxylase and 17α-hydroxylase deficiencies). Finally, some intersex patients do appear phenotypically normal at birth, as in many cases of gonadal dysgenesis or of complete androgen insensitivity syndrome, and will not come to medical attention until an older age. A summary of the clinical findings of the various intersex disorders is provided in Tables 37-8 and 37-9.

Neonates suspected of having an intersex problem should have the pronouncement of their sex deferred. The parents of the neonate should be told something along the following lines: "The genitalia are unfinished in their development, and we will need a few days to perform some studies to determine which sex your baby was intended to be reared as." Most of the diagnostic evaluation can be performed within 2 or 3 days, at which time the appropriate sex of rearing can almost always be determined, often without a definitive diagnosis being known.

Diagnostic evaluation

The evaluation of the neonate suspected of having an intersex problem is outlined in the boxed material on p. 1163. The history, physical examination, and buccal smear for chromatin bodies are done at the outset, and a 10 to 15 ml blood sample is obtained for determination of the karyotype and measurement of steroid hormones. Ideally a blood sample is obtained within the first 36 hours of age, when testosterone levels are physiologically increased if testicular tissue is present (Fig. 37-47). Basal blood samples are also diagnostically useful at 1 to 2 months of age in assessing the peak of pituitary-testicular axis function in infancy (this begins to rise at 1 to 2 weeks and ends by 6 to 7 months of age) and at any age when evaluating adrenocortical function for suspected CAH. ACTH or hCG stimulation testing is frequently needed. A 24-hour urine collection is not necessary if the radioimmunoassays for serum steroids are available. Endoscopy of the urovaginal orifice(s) is done together with retrograde genitography to assess for presence of müllerian duct structures; endoscopy is important to direct where the radiopaque contrast material is to be injected. The gonadal biopsy is necessary only in certain disorders and is preferably deferred until genital corrective surgery is done.

The presence of abnormal genitalia raises the following

Table 37-9. Characteristics of X chromatin–positive intersex disorders

Disorder*	External genitalia	Internal ducts	Gonadal tissue	Biochemical† Testosterone	Biochemical† 17-OH Prog	Biochemical† Other	Postnatal virilization†	Fertility	Gonadal tumors	Inheritance†	Comment
DISORDERS OF GONADAL DIFFERENTIATION											
XX True hermaphroditism	F, A, M	F, M	Ovary, testis, or ovotestis	F to M	Nl		+	Very rarely	1.5%	Few familial	
Gonadal dysgenesis											
X Chromosome abnormalities	F	F	Streaks	–	–		–	–	–		Turner's phenotype
XX Gonadal dysgenesis	F	F	Streaks	–	–		–	–	–	Aut rec	
XX Male	M, occasionally A	M	Testes	M	Nl		+	–	–	Few familial	
MASCULINIZATION OF FEMALE EXTERNAL GENITALIA (FEMALE PSEUDOHERMAPHRODITISM)											
Congenital adrenal hyperplasia											
21-Hydroxylase deficiency	F, A, M	F	Ovaries	++	++	++Δ,17KS, PT	+	Nl	–	Aut rec	Addisonian
11β-Hydroxylase deficiency	F, A, M	F	Ovaries	++	+	++CpdS, DOC, THS, 17KS	+	Nl	–	Aut rec	Hypertension in 70%
3β-HSD Deficiency	F, A	F	Ovaries	– to ±	+	++17OHPe:17OHP ++Pe:P	+	?–	–	Aut rec	Addisonian
(Cholesterol SCC deficiency)	F	F	Ovaries	–	–	++Urinary cholesterol	–	?–	–	Aut rec	Addisonian
(17α-Hydroxylase deficiency)	F	F	Ovaries	–	–	++DOC, B; +P ++18OHB:Aldo	–	?–	–	Aut rec	Hypertension
Maternal androgens	F, A	F	Ovaries	–	–		–	Nl	–	None	
Idiopathic	F, A	F	Ovaries	–	–		–	Nl	–	Some familial	Somatic malformations

Modified from Danish, R.K.: Indian J. Pediatr. **49:**555, 1982.

A, ambiguous, F, female; M, male; Nl, normal; –, decreased to absent ±, low normal; +, increased; Aldo, aldosterone; Δ, androstenedione, B, corticosterone, 18OHB, 18-hydroxycorticosterone, CpdS, compound S or 11-deoxycortisol; DOC, 11-deoxycorticosterone; 17KS, urinary 17-ketosteroids; Pe, pregnenolone, 17OHPe, 17-chydroxypregnenolone; P, progesterone, 17OHP, 17-hydroxyprogesterone; PT, urinary pregnanetriol; THS, urinary tetrahydro-11-deoxycortisol.

*Disorders in parentheses do not have genital ambiguity in female (46,XX) neonates; HSD, hydroxysteroid dehydrogenase, SCC, side-chain cleavage.

†"Few familial" or "some familial" indicates that a small or moderate portion of cases have been reported to occur in families; there is insufficient information to indicate whether their inheritance is X-linked, autosomal recessive (aut rec), or autosomal dominant.

Diagnostic evaluation of intersex problems in the neonate

1. History: maternal androgens, drugs, teratogens; affected relatives; siblings who died in infancy; consanguinity
2. Physical: genitalia, gonads, rectal, hyperpigmentation, Turner's stigmata, dysmorphic features
3. Chromosomes: buccal smear for X and Y chromatin, karyotype
4. Anatomic: endoscopy, retrograde genitogram; ultrasound
5. Biochemical: obtain 10 to 15 ml of blood for following tests (see below for optimum ages)

If patient is:	*Obtain serum levels at appropriate ages for*:*
XX with müllerian ducts	17OHP, CpdS, 17OHPe, T
XX without müllerian ducts	T, E_2, LH, FSH
XY with müllerian ducts	T, E_2, LH, FSH
XY without müllerian ducts	T, DHT, LH, FSH, and: if T/DHT is increased, determine urine etiocholanolone/androsterone ratio, or if T is normal to low, obtain A, DHA, 17OHP, P, and 17OHPe

Basal hormone studies, if done at:

0 to 36 hours—testes are active because of prior in utero hCG stimulation; T and DHT levels are increased

0.5 to 4 months—pituitary-testicular axis is physiologically active; LH, FSH, T, and DHT are increased (peak levels occur at 1 to 2 months in term infant, later in premature infant)

Any age—adrenal steroids are abnormal in untreated congenital adrenal hyperplasia

Hormone stimulation tests:

hCG (500 to 1,500 units intramuscularly every 2 to 4 days over 1 to 2 weeks)—useful to assess for presence or adequacy of testicular (Leydig cell) tissue or to diagnose a testosterone biosynthetic defect after basal testing is done

ACTH—may be useful in 17,20-desmolase deficiency

6. Gonadal biopsy: generally deferred until genital surgery is done at older age and limited to certain diagnoses, e.g., true hermaphroditism, gonadal dysgenesis with a Y chromosome, dysgenetic testes, rudimentary testes, XX male, persistent müllerian duct syndrome, and Leydig cell hypoplasia

*A, Androstenedione; CpdS, compound S or 11-deoxycortisol; DHA, dehydroepiandrosterone; DHT, dihydrotestosterone; E_2, estradiol; FSH, follicle-stimulating hormone; hCG, human chorionic gonadotropin; LH, luteinizing hormone; 17OHP, 17-hydroxyprogesterone; 17OHPe, 17-hydroxypregnenolone; P, progesterone; T, testosterone.

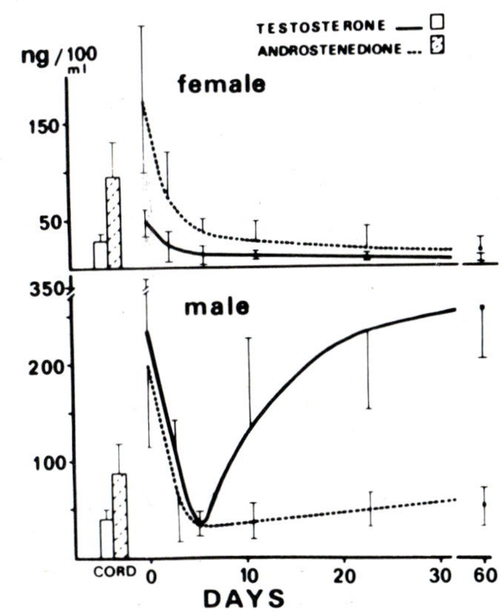

Fig. 37-47. Pattern of testosterone and androstenedione plasma levels during the first month of life in normal neonates. The curves join the mean values (±1 SD) between the different age groups. (From Forest, M.G., and Cathiard, A.M.: J. Clin. Endocrinol. Metab. **41:**977, 1975. © 1975, The Endocrine Society.)

questions: (1) if the infant is 46,XX, why are the genitalia excessively masculinized? and (2) if the infant is 46,XY, why is masculinization of the genitalia incomplete or severely deficient? Assessment of the chromosomal, gonadal, and biochemical status should provide a satisfactory answer.

The chromosomal status can be known within 1 day with reasonable certainty by assessing for both the X and Y chromatin on the buccal smear. The 46,XX neonates may normally show a lowered percentage of X chromatin, as low as 4%, in the first several days of life. The karyotype is the definitive analysis, and some laboratories can provide results within 3 or 4 working days.

The gonadal status can be inferred in the neonatal period from knowledge of the following:

1. *Gonadal descent and size.* For practical purposes, only a gonad containing testicular tissue, that is, a testis or ovotestis, can descend to a position where it is palpable (an ovary virtually never descends); a small gonad may be rudimentary or dysgenetic.
2. *Müllerian duct structures.* Presence of a uterine cervix indicates either one or both gonads did not produce MIF; the presence of bilateral fallopian tubes indicates both gonads failed to produce MIF.

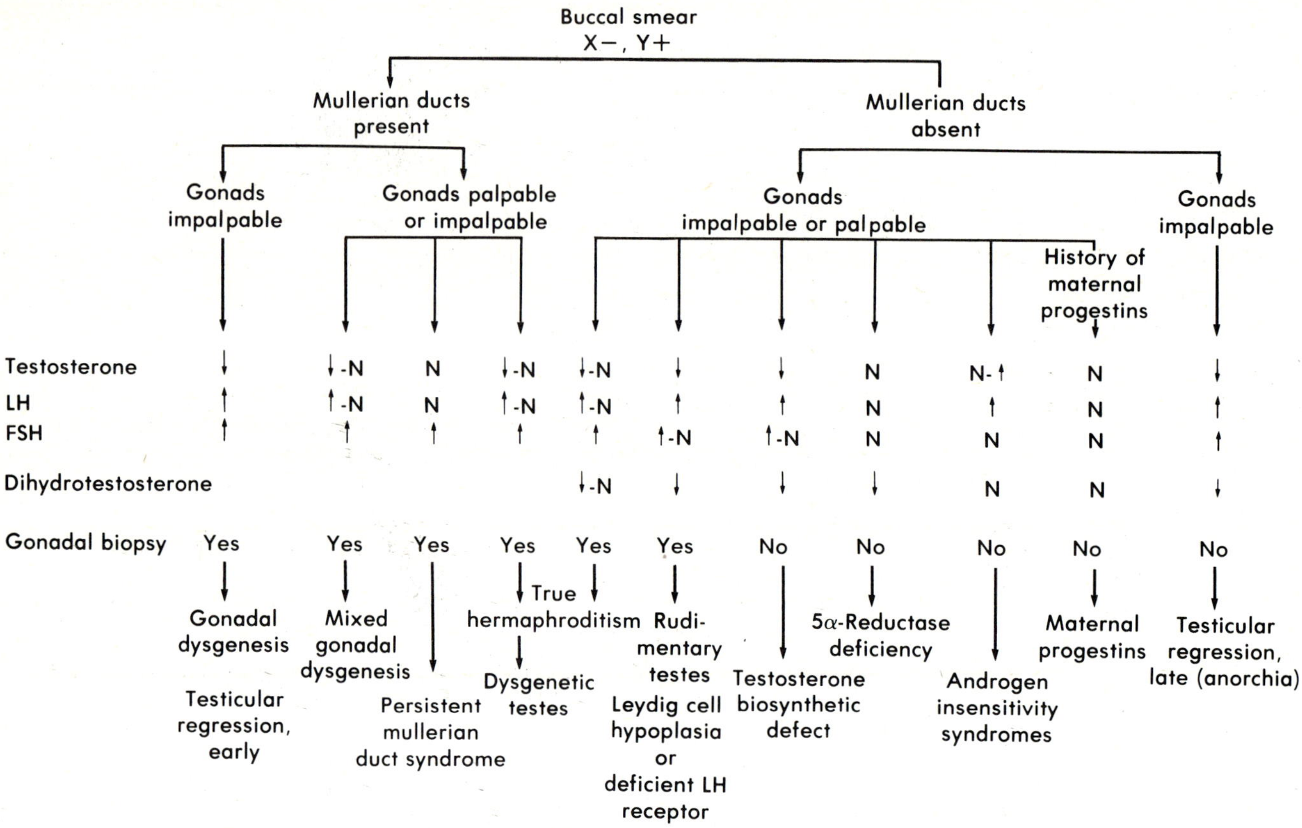

Fig. 37-48. Differential diagnosis of intersex problems: presence of Y chromatin. Flow diagram for the diagnosis of XY or Y chromatin-positive intersex disorders. True hermaphrodites may present with presence or absence of müllerian ducts. *Nl*, Normal range; ↓, decreased; ↑, increased.

3. *Chromosomes*. Bilateral ovaries can be present only if no Y and two X chromosomes are present. Testes, dysgenetic testes, ovotestes, streak gonads, or no gonads may occur with any karyotype.

The biochemical studies will further clarify the gonadal status or may provide a definitive diagnosis in many patients.

1. Elevated levels of testosterone occur physiologically in the neonatal period at 0 to 36 hours and at 0.5 to 4 to 6 months of age in the presence of functioning testes (Fig. 37-47) or may occur abnormally at any time from adrenal secretion of androgens in congenital adrenal hyperplasia; decreased levels of testosterone occur if Leydig cells are deficient or absent, if LH activity is impaired, or if there is a testosterone biosynthetic defect; levels of DHT should follow a pattern similar to those of testosterone, except in 5α-reductase deficiency.
2. An elevated cord or peripheral blood level of 17-hydroxyprogesterone, 11-deoxycortisol (compound S), or 17-hydroxypregnenolone, suggests 21- or 11β-hydroxylase or 3β-hydroxysteroid dehydrogenase deficiencies, respectively, and would imply that any increased levels of testosterone were adrenal and not testicular in origin in a 46,XX patient.
3. Abnormal levels of either C_{21} or C_{19} steroids or abnormally increased steroid precursor/product ratios may suggest a defect in testosterone biosynthesis or its peripheral conversion to DHT.
4. Levels of estradiol in female infants with bilateral ovaries overlap but may be higher (up to 75 pg/ml) than in male infants with testes (up to 35 pg/ml) in the first several months.
5. An elevated level of FSH connotes dysgenetic or absent testicular or ovarian tissue (FSH elevation may not occur until several months of age in some).
6. An abnormally elevated level of LH in males at 2 weeks to 4 to 6 months of age suggests impaired testosterone synthesis or action.

The actual process used to arrive at a final diagnosis is charted in flow diagrams for XY and XX patients, respectively (Figs. 37-48 and 37-49). The appearance of

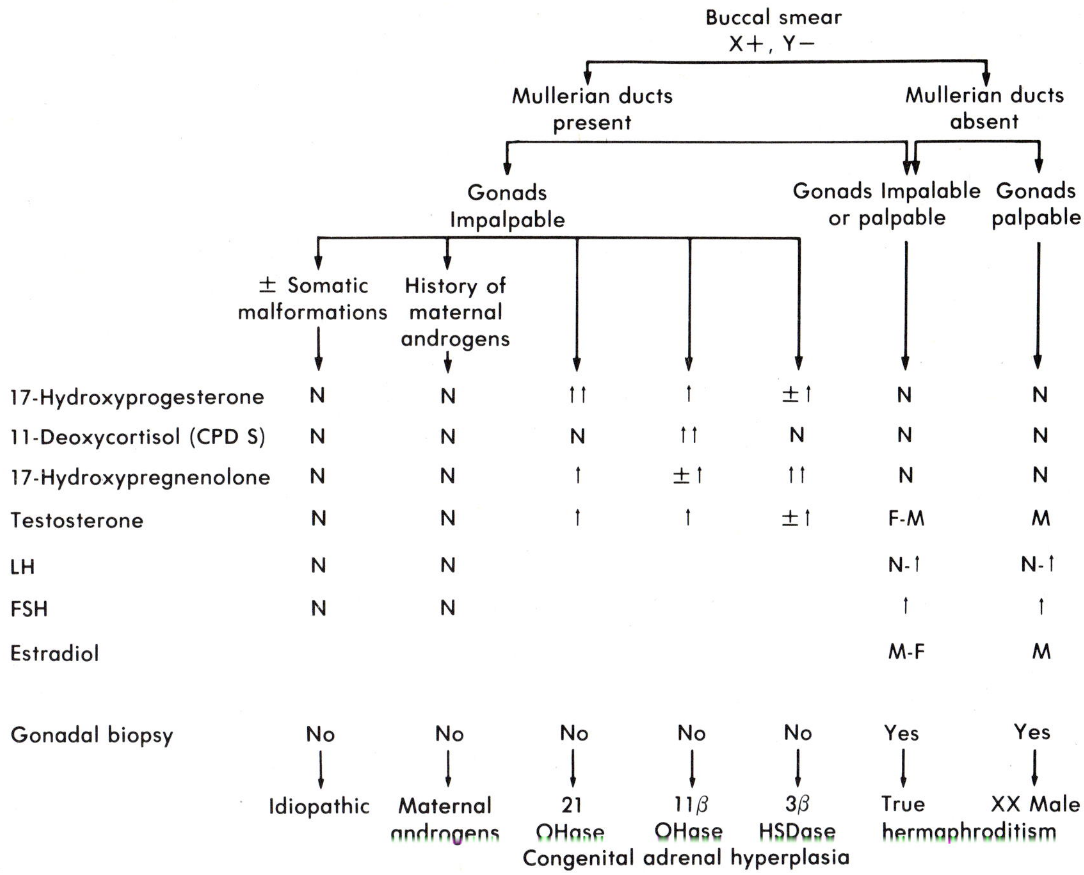

Fig. 37-49. Differential diagnosis of intersex problems: absence of Y chromatin. Flow diagram for the diagnosis of XX or Y chromatin-negative disorders. *F*, Female range; *M*, male range; *Nl*, normal range; ↓, decreased; ↑, increased.

the external genitalia is almost never characteristic for a specific diagnosis and is not diagnostically useful. Since the assay for the androgen receptor is not yet available in commercial laboratories, the diagnosis of the androgen insensitivity syndromes is inferred from the clinical findings and the biochemical and penile growth responses to testosterone therapy. In some cases it may not be possible to distinguish between two or three diagnoses because of overlapping features and unavailability of certain tests.

Sex assignment

The selection of sex of rearing of the intersex neonate is usually made when the chromatin and müllerian duct status is known, or it occasionally may need to be deferred until the biochemical results are returned. The decision is best made in consultation with appropriate specialists. If bilateral ovaries are deduced to be present, the neonate should be reared as female; if bilateral ovaries are not present, the sex of rearing is determined by the length of the penis (see box on p. 1176). It is best to make this decision as early as possible. Infants who were incorrectly sex-assigned at birth may successfully undergo sex reassignment up to 18 months to 2 years of age, but beyond this time it is believed that gender identity is sufficiently fixed and should not be altered.

The reason for rearing all neonates with bilateral ovaries as female, despite many having well-masculinized external genitalia, is that these patients are capable of normal female hormone secretion and are potentially fertile; their genitalia can be reconstructed to a normal female phenotype with only one or two surgical procedures. As males they would require life-long hormonal therapy and would be infertile; hypospadias repair and hysterectomy would be necessary.

If bilateral ovaries are absent, the principal criterion for male sex of rearing is whether one may expect a patient to achieve a normal penile size in both childhood and adulthood. As yet there is no evidence to show that a neonate having an abnormally small penis, for example, a length of 4 standard deviations below the mean, can be treated so that his penile length will reach a normal

Criteria for selection of sex of rearing for intersex disorders

FEMALE SEX OF REARING IF:

Bilateral ovaries are present (regardless of degree of masculinization of genitalia).

or

Stretched penile length or width are more than 2.5 SD below the mean for age.

MALE SEX OF REARING IF:

Ovaries are absent.

and

Stretched penile length and width are above −2.5 SD of the mean for age.

MODIFYING FACTORS:

If stretched penile length is borderline (1.5 to 2.0 cm in a term neonate), female sex of rearing is recommended if the patient has:

1. Partial androgen insensitivity

   or

2. A prospect for very shortened adult height, e.g., mixed gonadal dysgenesis

   or

3. A prospect of poor outcome of surgical repair of genitalia along male lines.

If penile chordee is present, allow for the increase in penile length that will occur when the chordee is corrected.

In premature neonates note that the normal stretched penile lengths and widths are smaller (Fig. 37-46).

size in adulthood, that is, within 2.5 standard deviations of the mean. A trial of testosterone therapy to determine if the penis will respond may be reassuring but is not predictive of whether a normal penile size can be attained in adulthood. If penile length is severely diminished, it is safer for that patient to be reared as a female.

In summary, the underlying aims in selecting the more appropriate sex of rearing are (1) that the genitalia be correctable to a normal size and function by early childhood, so that the child may grow up with a normal body image and gender identity; (2) that the genitalia be normal in size and function in adulthood to permit normal penile-vaginal intercourse; and (3) if the first two goals are feasible, that fertility should be retained.

Management

The most immediate concern in a neonate with abnormal genitalia is whether CAH is present. One may expect the onset of adrenal insufficiency to occur between 3 and 14 days in 50% of affected patients and later in the rest, but not earlier. The specific treatment is described in the section on congenital adrenal hyperplasia.

Infants reared as male with a small penis should be treated with testosterone, administered intramuscularly, to increase penile size into the normal range for age. The bone age needs to be monitored. Topical testosterone therapy is not recommended. If testes are undescended after age 6 to 9 months, a course of gonadotropin-releasing hormone or hCG treatment may bring on testicular descent, particularly if bilateral. Nonresponders should have an orchiopexy done, optimally in infancy and certainly by age 4 to 5 years. Dysgenetic testes should be removed, and prosthetic testes may be placed in the scrotum.

Surgical correction of the ambiguous genitalia in patients reared as female is best done in the first year by an experienced surgeon. Clitoral reduction is preferably done by resection of the corpora cavernosa and suturing the glans to the pubis; clitoral recession or amputation is not recommended. There is debate as to whether vaginal orifice exteriorization should be done in infancy. Construction of a vagina in a patient lacking a vagina is deferred until adulthood when she plans to be sexually active. Wolffian duct structures do not need to be removed.

Surgical correction of ambiguous genitalia in the male should be done in infancy so that he will have a normal genital appearance and be able to stand to urinate. Circumcision of the penis should not be done before hypospadias repair. Plastic surgical attempts to increase penile size are not recommended, since no method is available that can provide a reasonably normal appearing and functional penis. Only androgen therapy is of benefit. Male patients having a vagina that enters a urogenital sinus may have urinary incontinence if the vagina acts as a reservoir, in which case the vagina should be excised. Müllerian duct structures do not necessarily need to be removed because the wolffian ducts may be embedded in its walls and thus unintentionally removed, although occasional cases of uterine cancer have been reported.

The gonads should be removed either (1) if their hormonal production will lead to inappropriate virilization or feminization in patients reared as female or male, respectively, or (2) if they are at increased risk for tumor development. The increased levels of testosterone produced by the testes in the first half year of life are generally not a major problem, and afterward the testes are relatively inactive hormonally until puberty. Ovarian sex steroid production is not clinically important until puberty. Gonadal tissue destined to secrete sex hormones inappropriate for the sex of rearing is removed at some time before the onset of puberty.

Patients with streak or dysgenetic gonads having a Y

chromosome are at greatly increased risk for tumor development, occurring as early as 3 to 5 years of age. Gonadectomy should be performed in the first few years of life, particularly in individuals with a Y gonadal streak. In complete androgen insensitivity syndrome it is considered safe to leave the testes in situ until 15 to 18 years of age. Intersex patients lacking a Y chromosome and testicular tissue do not appear to be at increased risk for gonadal tumor development.

Patients with hypogonadism will require testosterone or estrogen-progesterone replacement therapy at puberty. The sex steroids are not necessary for normal growth before puberty.

Genetic counseling should be provided to the family when the diagnosis is known. Heterozygote detection is available for 21- and 17α-hydroxylase and 5α-reductase deficiencies and androgen insensitivity syndrome. Prenatal diagnosis has been reported for 21- and 11β-hydroxylase and 17,20-desmolase deficiencies and is possible for complete androgen insensitivity syndrome and for gonadal dysgenesis caused by X or Y chromosomal abnormalities. Many families benefit by the involvement of a social worker or psychologist who may assist the family in understanding confusing medical issues and in dealing with their emotions. As the patient grows up, he or she will need to gradually learn the facts of the disorder.

Female patients exposed to increased androgens in utero may show an increase in their level of activity, tomboyishness, greater preference for pursuing career interest, decreased interest in maternal roles, and more male friends. Boys exposed to decreased levels of androgens or increased levels of progesterone in utero may show less typically masculine behavior. Some patients will have learning disability or behavioral or psychologic problems that may be related to their underlying disorder, such as Klinefelter's syndrome, or to abnormalities of body image or gender identity, for which psychologic counseling may be of benefit. The prognosis for most well-managed patients, however, is that they can expect to grow up with a normal body image and gender identity, attain appropriate scholastic and job-related goals, lead a normal social life, become married if they wish, and have normal sexual relations. Since many patients will be infertile, they should expect to have their children by adoption.

Robert K. Danish

BIBLIOGRAPHY

Normal fetal sex differentiation

Brunner, M., and others: On the secretion of H-Y antigen, Cell **37**:615, 1984.

Donahoe, P.K., and others: Müllerian-inhibiting substance: an update, Recent Prog. Horm. Res. **38**:279, 1982.

Forest, M.G., and others: Concentration of 14 steroid hormones in human amniotic fluid of midpregnancy, J. Clin. Endocrinol. Metab. **51**:816, 1980.

Gondos, B.: Development of the reproductive organs, Ann. Clin. Lab. Sci. **15**:363, 1985.

Gordon, J.W., and Ruddle, F.H.: Mammalian gonadal determination and gametogenesis, Science **211**:1265, 1981.

Haseltine F.P., and Ohno, S.: Mechanisms of gonadal differentiation, Science **211**:1272, 1981.

Hutson, J.M., Donahoe, P.K., and Budzik, G.P.: Müllerian inhibiting substance: a fetal hormone with surgical implications, Aust. N.Z. J. Surg. **55**:599, 1985.

Imperato-McGinley, J., and Peterson, R.E.: Male pseudohermaphroditism: the complexities of male phenotypic development, Am. J. Med. **61**:251, 1976.

Jirasek, J.E.: Morphogenesis of the genital system in the human, Birth Defects **13**(2):13, 1977.

Kaplan, S.L., Grumbach, M.M., and Aubert, M.L.: The ontogenesis of pituitary hormones and hypothalamic factors in the human fetus: maturation of central nervous system regulation of anterior pituitary function, Recent Prog. Horm. Res. **32**:161, 1976.

McGregor, W.G., Kuhn, R.W., and Jaffe, R.B.: Biologically active chorionic gonadotropin: synthesis by the human fetus, Science **220**:306, 1983.

Meck, J.M.: The genetics of the H-Y antigen system and its role in sex determination, Perspect. Biol. Med. **27**:560, 1984.

O'Rahilly, R.: The development of the vagina in the human, Birth Defects **13**(2):123, 1977.

Reyes, F.I., Winter, J.S.D., and Faiman, C.: Gonadotropin-gonadal interrelationships in the fetus. In New, M.I., and Fiser, R.H., Jr., editors: Diabetes and other endocrine disorders during pregnancy and in the newborn, Progress in clinical and biological research, vol. 10, New York, 1976, Alan R. Liss, Inc.

Taguchi, O., and others: Timing and irreversibility of müllerian duct inhibition in the embryonic reproductive tract of the human male, Dev. Biol. **106**:394, 1984.

Tapanainen, J., and others: Age-related changes in endogenous steroids of human fetal testis during early and midpregnancy, J. Clin. Endocrinol. Metab. **52**:98, 1981.

Wachtel, S.S.: Human sexual development, J. Endocrinol. Invest. **7**:663, 1984.

Wilson, J.D.: The endocrine control of sexual differentiation, Harvey Lect. **79**:145, 1984.

Wilson, J.D., George, F.W., and Griffin, J.E.: The hormonal control of sexual development, Science **211**:1278, 1981.

Disorders of gonadal differentiation

Aaronson, I.A.: True hermaphroditism: a review of 41 cases with observations on testicular histology and function, Br. J. Urol. **57**:775, 1985.

Aynsley-Green, A., and others: Congenital bilateral anorchia in childhood: a clinical, endocrine and therapeutic evaluation of twenty-one cases, Clin. Endocrinol. **5**:381, 1976.

Bloomgarden, Z.T., and others: Genetic and endocrine findings in a 48,XXYY male, J. Clin. Endocrinol. Metab. **50**:740, 1980.

Bluth, E.I., Maragos, V.A., and Merritt, C.R.B.: Antenatal diagnosis of Turner's syndrome, South Med. J. **77**:1335, 1984.

Bove, K.E.: Gonadal dysgenesis in a newborn with XO karyotype, Am. J. Dis. Child. **120**:363, 1970.

Brosnan, P.G., and others: A new familial syndrome of 46,XY gonadal dysgenesis with anomalies of ectodermal and mesodermal structures, J. Pediatr. **97**:586, 1980.

Connors, M.H., and Styne, D.M.: Familial functional anorchism: a review of etiology and management, J. Urol. **133**:1049, 1985.

Conte, F.A., Grumbach, M.M., and Kaplan, S.L.: A diphasic pattern of gonadotropin secretion in patients with the syndrome of gonadal dysgenesis, J. Clin. Endocrinol. Metab. **40**:670, 1975.

Eddy, A.A., and Mauer, S.M.: Pseudohermaphroditism, glomerulopathy, and Wilms tumor (Drash syndrome): frequency in end-stage renal failure, J. Pediatr. **106**:584, 1985.

Edlow, J.B., and others: Neonatal Klinefelter's syndrome, Am. J. Dis. Child. **118**:788, 1969.

Edman, C.D., and others: Embryonic testicular regression: a clinical spectrum of XY agonadal individuals, Obstet. Gynecol. **49**:208, 1977.

Flannery, D.B., and others: Antenatally detected Klinefelter's syndrome in twins, Acta Genet. Med. Gemellol. (Roma) **33**:51, 1984.

German, J., and others: Genetically determined sex-reversal in 46,XY humans, Science **202**:53, 1978.

Gordon, R.R., and O'Neill, E.M.: Turner's infantile phenotype, Br. Med. J. **1**:483, 1969.

Haddad, H.M., and Wilkins, L.: Congenital anomalies associated with gonadal aplasia: review of 55 cases, Pediatrics **23**:885, 1959.

Harris, J.S., and Heller, R.H.: The detection of Klinefelter's syndrome at birth, Clin. Pediatr. **13**:581, 1974.

Hoefnagel, D., and others: Camptomelic dwarfism associated with XY gonadal dysgenesis and chromosome anomalies, Clin. Genet. **13**:489, 1978.

Jacobs, P.A.: The incidence and etiology of sex chromosome abnormalities in man, Birth Defects **15**(1):3, 1979.

Jarow, J.P., and others: Elevation of serum gonadotropins establishes the diagnosis of anorchism in prepubertal boys with bilateral cryptorchidism, J. Urol. **136**:277, 1986.

Josso, N., and Briard, M.-L.: Embryonic testicular regression syndrome: variable phenotypic expression in siblings, J. Pediatr. **97**:200, 1980.

Karsh, R.B., and others: Congenital heart disease in 49,XXXXY syndrome, Pediatrics **56**:462, 1975.

Kofman, S., and others: Clinical and endocrine spectrum in patients with the 45,X/46,XY karyotype, Hum. Genet. **58**:373, 1981.

Kogan, S.J., and others: Human monorchism: a clinicopathological study of unilateral absent testes in 65 boys, J. Urol. **135**:758, 1986.

Litvak, A.S., and others: The association of significant renal anomalies with Turner's syndrome, J. Urol. **120**:671, 1978.

Muller, J., and others: Carcinoma in situ of the testis in children with 45,X/46,XY gonadal dysgenesis, J. Pediatr. **106**:431, 1985.

Murken, J.-D., and others: Klinefelter's syndrome in a fetus, Lancet **2**:171, 1974.

Najjar, S.S., Takla, R.J., and Nassar, V.H.: The syndrome of rudimentary testes: occurrence in five siblings, J. Pediatr. **84**:119, 1974.

Nihoul-Fekete, C., and others: Preservation of gonadal function in true hermaphroditism, J. Pediatr. Surg. **19**:50, 1984.

Page, D.C., and De La Chapelle, A.: The parental origin of X chromosomes in XX males determined using restriction fragment length polymorphisms, Am. J. Hum. Genet. **36**:565, 1984.

Rajfer, J., and others: Dysgenetic male pseudohermaphroditism, J. Urol. **119**:525, 1978.

Raspa, R.W., Burbige, K.A., and Hensle, T.W.: The sex reversal syndrome (the XX male patient), J. Urol. **134**:152, 1985.

Robinson, A.: Neonatal deaths and sex-chromosome anomalies, Lancet **1**:1223, 1974.

Robinson, A., and others: Summary of clinical findings: profiles of children with 47,XXY, 47,XXX and 47,XYY karyotypes, Birth Defects **15**(1):261, 1979.

Roe, T.F., and Alfi, O.S.: Ambiguous genitalia in XX male children: report of two infants, Pediatrics **60**:55, 1977.

Rosenberg, C., and others: Testicular regression in a patient with virilized female phenotype, Am. J. Med. Genet. **19**:183, 1984.

Rosenthal, A.: Cardiovascular malformations in Klinefelter's syndrome: report of three cases, J. Pediatr. **80**:471, 1972.

Rushton, D.I., and others: The fetal manifestations of the 45,XO karyotype, J. Obstet. Gynaecol. Br. Commonw. **76**:266, 1969.

Salbenblatt, J.A., and others: Pituitary-gonadal function in Klinefelter syndrome before and during puberty, Pediatr. Res. **19**:82, 1985.

Shapiro, L.R., and others: Deceleration of intellectual development in a XXXXY child, Am. J. Dis. Child. **122**:163, 1971.

Shepard, T.H., and others: Lowered plasma albumin concentration in fetal Turner syndrome, J. Pediatr. **108**:114, 1986.

Simpson, J.L.: Gonadal dysgenesis. In Simpson, J.L.: Disorders of sexual differentiation: etiology and clinical delineation, New York, 1976, Academic Press, Inc.

Szpunar, J., and Rybak, M.: Middle ear disease in Turner's syndrome, Arch. Otolaryngol. **87**:34, 1968.

Troche, V., and Hernandez, E.: Neoplasia arising in dysgenetic gonads, Obstet. Gynecol. **41**:74, 1986.

van Niekerk, W.A., and Retief, A.E.: The gonads of human true hermaphrodites, Hum. Genet. **58**:117, 1981.

Warburton, D., and others: Monosomy X: a chromosomal anomaly associated with young maternal age, Lancet **1**:167, 1980.

Weiss, L.: Additional evidence of gradual loss of germ cells in the pathogenesis of streak ovaries in Turner's syndrome, J. Med. Genet. **8**:540, 1971.

Winters, S.J., and others: H-Y antigen mosaicism in the gonad of a 46,XX true hermaphrodite, N. Engl. J. Med. **300**:745, 1979.

Wolf, U.: XY gonadal dysgenesis and the H-Y antigen: report on 12 cases, Hum. Genet. **47**:269, 1979.

Zah, W., Kalderon, A.E., and Tucci, J.R.: Mixed gonadal dysgenesis: a case report and review of the world literature, Acta Endocrinol. **197**(suppl.):1, 1975.

Disorders of testicular hormone synthesis or action (male pseudohermaphroditism)

Beheshti, M., and others: Familial persistent müllerian duct syndrome, J. Urol. **131**:968, 1984.

Berkovitz, G.D., Brown, T.R., and Migeon, C.J.: Androgen receptors, Clin. Endocrinol. Metab. **12**:155, 1983.

Eil, C.: Familial incomplete male pseudohermaphroditism associated with impaired nuclear androgen retention: studies in cultured skin fibroblasts, J. Clin. Invest. **71**:850, 1983.

Eil, C., and others: Leydig cell hypoplasia causing male pseudohermaphroditism: diagnosis 13 years after prepubertal castration, J. Clin. Endocrinol. Metab. **58**:441, 1984.

Forest, M.G., Lecornu, M., and de Peretti, E.: Familial male pseudohermaphroditism due to 17-20-desmolase deficiency. I. In vivo endocrine studies, J. Clin. Endocrinol. Metab. **50**:826, 1980.

Hodgins, M.B., Duke, E.M.C., and Ring, D.: Carrier detection in the testicular feminization syndrome: deficient 5α-dihydrotestosterone binding in cultured skin fibroblasts from the mothers of patients with complete androgen insensitivity, J. Med. Genet. **21**:178, 1984.

Imperato-McGinley, J., Peterson, R.E., and Gautier, T.: Primary and secondary 5α-reductase deficiency. In Serio, M., and others, editors: Sexual differentiation: basic and clinical aspects, New York, 1984, Raven Press.

Imperato-McGinley, J., and others: Hormonal evaluation of a large kindred with complete androgen insensitivity: evidence for secondary 5α-reductase deficiency, J. Clin. Endocrinol. Metab. **54**:931, 1982.

Imperato-McGinley, J., and others: Decreased urinary C_{19} and C_{21} steroid 5α-metabolites in parents of male pseudohermaphrodites with 5α-reductase deficiency: detection of carriers, J. Clin. Endocrinol. Metab. **60**:553, 1985.

Johnson, L., and others: Characterization of the testicular abnormality in 5α-reductase deficiency, J. Clin. Endocrinol. Metab. **63**:1091, 1986.

Josso, N., and others: Persistence of müllerian ducts in male pseudohermaphroditism, and its relationship to cryptorchidism, Clin. Endocrinol. **19**:247, 1983.

Kaufman, F.R., and others: Male pseudohermaphroditism due to 17,20-desmolase deficiency, J. Clin. Endocrinol. Metab. **57**:32, 1983.

Jukier, L., and others: Partial androgen resistance associated with secondary 5α-reductase deficiency: identification of a novel qualitative androgen receptor defect and clinical implications, J. Clin. Endocrinol. Metab. **59**:679, 1984.

Lanes, R., and others: Sibship with 17-ketosteroid reductase (17-KSR) deficiency and hypothyroidism: lack of linkage of histocompatibility leucocyte antigen and 17-KSR loci, J. Clin. Endocrinol. Metab. **57**:190, 1983.

Lee, P.A., and others: Leydig cell hypofunction resulting in male pseudohermaphroditism, Fertil. Steril. **37**:675, 1982.

Migeon, B.R., and others: Studies of the locus for androgen receptor: localisation on the human X chromosome and evidence for homology with the Tfm locus in the mouse, Proc. Natl. Acad. Sci. U.S.A. **78**:6339, 1981.

Muller, J.: Morphometry and histology of gonads from twelve children and adolescents with the androgen insensitivity (testicular feminization) syndrome, J. Clin. Endocrinol. Metab. **59**:785, 1984.

Nagel, R.A., Lippe, B.M., and Griffin, J.E.: Androgen resistance in the neonate: use of hormones of hypothalamic-pituitary-gonadal axis for diagnosis, J. Pediatr. **109**:486, 1986.

Peterson, R.E., and Imperato-McGinley, J.: Male pseudohermaphroditism due to inherited deficiencies of testosterone biosynthesis in sexual differentiation: basic and clinical aspects. In Serio, M., and others, editors: Sexual differentiation: basic and clinical aspects, New York, 1984, Raven Press.

Price, P., and others: High dose androgen therapy in male pseudohermaphroditism due to 5α-reductase deficiency and disorders of the androgen receptor, J. Clin. Invest. **74**:1496, 1984.

Rosler, A., and Kohn, G.: Male pseudohermaphroditism due to 17β-hydroxysteroid dehydrogenase deficiency: studies on the natural history of the defect and effect of androgens on gender role, J. Steroid Biochem. **19**:663, 1983.

Stephens, J.D.: Prenatal diagnosis of testicular feminization, Lancet **2**:1038, 1984.

Ulloa-Aguirre, A., and others: Endocrine and biochemical studies in a 46,XY phenotypically male infant with 17-ketosteroid reductase deficiency, J. Clin. Endocrinol. Metab. **60**:639, 1985.

Ulloa-Aguirre, A., and others: The presence of müllerian remnants in the complete androgen insensitivity syndrome: a steroid hormone-mediated defect? Fertil. Steril. **45**:320, 1986.

Female pseudohermaphroditism and congenital adrenal hyperplasia

Barnes, A.B., and others: Fertility and outcome of pregnancy in women exposed in utero to diethylstilbestrol, N. Engl. J. Med. **302**:609, 1980.

Bongiovanni, A.M.: Androgens, estrogens, and the fetus. In New, M.I., and Fiser, R.H., Jr., editors: Diabetes and other endocrine disorders during pregnancy and in the newborn, Progress in clinical and biological research, vol. 10, New York, 1976, Alan R. Liss, Inc.

Bongiovanni, A.M.: Urinary steroidal pattern of infants with congenital adrenal hyperplasia due to 3-beta-hydroxysteroid dehydrogenase deficiency, J. Steroid Biochem. **13**:809, 1980.

Cara, J.F., and others: Elevated 17-hydroxyprogesterone and testosterone in a newborn with 3-beta-hydroxysteroid dehydrogenase deficiency, N. Engl. J. Med. **313**:618, 1985.

Cavallo, A., and others: The use of plasma androstenedione in monitoring therapy of patients with congenital adrenal hyperplasia, J. Pediatr. **95**:33, 1979.

D'Armiento, M., and others: 17α-Hydroxylase deficiency: mineralocorticoid hormone profiles in an affected family, J. Clin. Endocrinol. Metab. **56**:697, 1983.

David, M., and Forest, M.G.: Prenatal treatment of congenital adrenal hyperplasia resulting from 21-hydroxylase deficiency, J. Pediatr. **105**:799, 1984.

Dean, H.J., Shackleton, C.H.L., and Winter, J.S.D.: Diagnosis and natural history of 17-hydroxylase deficiency in a newborn male, J. Clin. Endocrinol. Metab. **59**:513, 1984.

Del Carmen-Cravioto, M., and others: A new inherited variant of the 3β-hydroxysteroid dehydrogenase-isomerase deficiency syndrome: evidence for the existence of two isoenzymes, J. Clin. Endocrinol. Metab. **62**:360, 1986.

dePeretti, E., and others: Endocrine studies in two children with male pseudohermaphroditism due to 3β-hydroxysteroid (3β-HSD) dehydrogenase defect. In Genazzani, A.R., Thijssen, J.H.H., and Siiteri, P.K., editors: Adrenal androgens, New York, 1980, Raven Press.

Donohoue, P.A., and others: Gene conversion in salt-losing congenital adrenal hyperplasia with absent complement C4B protein, J. Clin. Endocrinol. Metab. **62**:995, 1986.

Finkelstein, M., and Shaefer, J.M.: Inborn errors of steroid biosynthesis, Physiol. Rev. **59**:353, 1979.

Geggel, R.L., DeLuca, K., and Villee, D.B.: Heart failure secondary to iatrogenic systemic hypertension in an infant with congenital adrenal hyperplasia, Clin. Pediatr. **23**:358, 1984.

Griffiths, K.D., and others: Plasma renin activity in the management of congenital adrenal hyperplasia, Arch. Dis. Child. **59**:360, 1984.

Gutai, J.P., Lee, P.A., Johnsonbaugh, R.E.: Detection of the heterozygous state in siblings of patients with congenital adrenal hyperplasia due to 21-hydroxylase deficiency, J. Pediatr. **94**:770, 1979.

Hauffa, B., and others: Congenital adrenal hyperplasia due to deficient cholesterol side-chain cleavage activity (20,22-desmolase) in a patient treated for 18 years, Clin. Endocrinol. **23**:481, 1985.

Haymond, M.W., and Weldon, V.V.: Female pseudohermaphroditism secondary to a maternal virilizing tumor: case report and review of the literature, J. Pediatr. **82**:682, 1973.

Hensleigh, P.A., Carter, R.P., and Grotjan, H.E., Jr.: Fetal protection against masculinization with hyperreaction luteinalis and virilization, J. Clin. Endocrinol. Metab. **40**:816, 1975.

Hinde, F.R.J., and Johnston, D.I.: Hypoglycemia during illness in children with congenital adrenal hyperplasia, Br. Med. J. **289**:1603, 1984.

Hochberg, Z., and others: Requirement of mineralocorticoid in congenital adrenal hyperplasia due to 11-hydroxylase deficiency, J. Clin. Endocrinol. Metab. **63**:36, 1986.

Holcombe, J.H., Keenan, B.S., and Clayton, G.W.: Plasma 17α-hydroxyprogesterone and aldosterone concentrations in infants and children with congenital adrenal hyperplasia—the role of salt-losing hormones in salt wasting, J. Pediatr. **98**:573, 1981.

Holcombe, J.H., and others: Neonatal salt loss in the hypertensive form of congenital adrenal hyperplasia, Pediatrics **65**:777, 1980.

Hurwitz, A., and others: Combined 21- and 11β-hydroxylase deficiency in familial congenital adrenal hyperplasia, J. Clin. Endocrinol. Metab. **60**:631, 1985.

Jones, H.W., and Verkauf, B.S.: Surgical treatment in congenital adrenal hyperplasia: age at operation and other prognostic factors, Obstet. Gynecol. **36**:1, 1970.

Kai, H., and others: Female pseudohermaphroditism caused by maternal congenital adrenal hyperplasia, J. Pediatr. **95**:418, 1979.

Koshimizu, T.: Plasma renin activity and aldosterone concentration in normal subjects and patients with salt-losing type of congenital adrenal hyperplasia during infancy, Clin. Endocrinol. **10**:515, 1979.

Kowarski, A., and others: Aldosterone secretion rate in congenital adrenal hyperplasia: a discussion of the theories on the pathogenesis of the salt-losing form of the syndrome, J. Clin. Invest. **44**:1505, 1965.

Kuhnle, U., Land, M., and Ulick, S.: Evidence for the secretion of an antimineralocorticoid in congenital adrenal hyperplasia, J. Clin. Endocrinol. Metab. **62**:934, 1986.

Kuhnle, U., and others: Virilization without adrenal hyperplasia in 21-hydroxylase deficiency during fetal life, J. Clin. Endocrinol. Metab. **58**:574, 1984.

Lebovitz, R.M., Pauli, R.M., and Laxova, R.: Delayed diagnosis in congenital adrenal hyperplasia: need for newborn screening, Am. J. Dis. Child. **138**:571, 1984.

Lorenzen, F., and others: Studies of the C-21 and C-19 steroids and HLA genotyping in siblings and parents of patients with congenital adrenal hyperplasia due to 21-hydroxylase deficiency, J. Clin. Endocrinol. Metab. **50**:572, 1980.

Matteson, K.J., and others: Study of cholesterol side-chain cleavage (20,22 desmolase) deficiency causing congenital lipoid adrenal hyperplasia using bovine-sequence P450scc oligodeoxyribonucleotide probes, Endocrinology **118**:1296, 1986.

Matteson, K.J., and others: Assignment of the gene for adrenal P450c17 (steroid 17α-hydroxylase/17,20 lyase) to human chromosome 10, J. Clin. Endocrinol. Metab. **63**:789, 1986.

McKenna, T.J., and others: Pregnenolone, 17-OH-pregnenolone, and testosterone in plasma of patients with congenital adrenal hyperplasia, J. Clin. Endocrinol. Metab. **42**:918, 1976.

Migeon, C.J., and Kenny, F.M.: Cortisol production rate. V. Congenital virilizing adrenal hyperplasia, J. Pediatr. **69**:779, 1966.

Murphy, J.F., and others: Plasma 17-hydroxyprogesterone concentrations in ill newborn infants, Arch. Dis. Child. **58**:532, 1983.

New, M.I., and Levine, L.S.: Congenital adrenal hyperplasia, Monogr. Endocrinol. **26**:1, 1984.

Pang, S., and others: Non-salt-losing congenital adrenal hyperplasia due to 3β-hydroxysteroid dehydrogenase deficiency with normal glomerulosa function, J. Clin. Endocrinol. Metab. **56**:808, 1983.

Pang, S., and others: Pitfalls of prenatal diagnosis of 21-hydroxylase deficiency congenital adrenal hyperplasia, J. Clin. Endocrinol. Metab. **61**:89, 1985.

Park, I.J., Jones, H.W., Jr., and Melhem, R.E.: Nonadrenal familial female hermaphroditism, Am. J. Obstet. Gynecol. **112**:930, 1972.

Park, I.J., and others: Special female hermaphroditism associated with multiple disorders, Obstet. Gynecol. **39**:100, 1972.

Riordan, F.A.I., and others: Bloodspot 17α-hydroxyprogesterone radioimmunoassay for diagnosis of congenital adrenal hyperplasia and home monitoring of corticosteroid replacement therapy, Lancet **1**:708, 1984.

Rosenberg, B., Hendren, W.H., and Crawford, J.D.: Posterior urethrovaginal communication in apparent males with congenital adrenocortical hyperplasia, N. Engl. J. Med. **280**:131, 1969.

Rösler, A., and others: Prenatal diagnosis of 11β-hydroxylase deficiency congenital adrenal hyperplasia, J. Clin. Endocrinol. Metab. **49**:546, 1979.

Rovner, D.R., and others: 17α-Hydroxylase deficiency: a combination of hydroxylation defect and reversible blockade in aldosterone biosynthesis, Acta Endocrinol. **90**:490, 1979.

Shackleton, C.H.L.: Congenital adrenal hyperplasia caused by defect in steroid 21-hydroxylase: establishment of definitive urinary steroid excretion pattern during first weeks of life, Clin. Chim. Acta **67**:287, 1976.

Shaw, R.W., and Farquhar, J.W.: Female pseudohermaphroditism associated with danazol exposure in utero: case report, Br. J. Obstet. Gynecol. **91**:386, 1984.

Verhoeven, A.T.M., and others: Virilization in pregnancy coexisting with an (ovarian) mucinous cystadenoma: a case report and review of virilizing ovarian tumors in pregnancy, Obstet. Gynecol. Surv. **28**:597, 1973.

Waldhäusl, W., and others: Combined 17α- and 18-hydroxylase deficiency associated with complete male pseudohermaphroditism and hypoaldosteronism, J. Clin. Endocrinol. Metab. **46**:236, 1978.

White, P.C., New, M.I., and Dupont, B.: HLA-linked congenital adrenal hyperplasia results from a defective gene encoding a cytochrome P-450 specific for steroid 21-hydroxylation, Proc. Natl. Acad. Sci. U.S.A. **81**:7505, 1984.

Zachmann, M., Tassinari, D., and Prader, A.: Clinical and biochemical variability of congenital adrenal hyperplasia due to 11β-hydroxylase deficiency: a study of 25 patients, J. Clin. Endocrinol. Metab. **56**:222, 1983.

Zadik, Z., and others: Salt loss in hypertensive form of congenital adrenal hyperplasia (11β-hydroxylase deficiency), J. Clin. Endocrinol. Metab. **58**:384, 1984.

Hypospadias, micropenis, cryptorchidism, and müllerian and vaginal dysgenesis

Aarskog, D.: Maternal progestins as a possible cause of hypospadias, N. Engl. J. Med. **300**:75, 1979.

Allen, T.D., and Griffin, J.E.: Endocrine studies in patients with advanced hypospadias, J. Urol. **131**:310, 1984.

Buyse, M., and Feingold, M.: Syndromes associated with abnormal external genitalia. In Vallet, H.L., and Porter, I.H., editors: Genetic mechanisms of sexual development, New York, 1979, Academic Press, Inc.

Coulam, C.B., and others: Androgen receptor in human foreskin. II. Characterization of the receptor from hypospadiac tissue, Am. J. Obstet. Gynecol. **147**:513, 1983.

Danish, R.K., and others: Micropenis. II. Hypogonadotropic hypogonadism, Johns Hopkins Med. J. **146**:177, 1980.

deMuinck-Keizer-Schrama, S.M., and others: Double-blind placebo-controlled study of luteinising-hormone–releasing-hormone nasal spray in treatment of undescended testes, Lancet **1**:876, 1986.

Duncan, P.A., and others: The MURCS association: müllerian duct aplasia, renal aplasia, and cervicothoracic somite dysplasia, J. Pediatr. **95**:399, 1979.

Editorial: The undescended testis: is there a role for LHRH? Lancet **1**:1133, 1986.

Garagorri, J.M., and others: Results of early treatment of cryptorchidism with human chorionic gonadotropin, J. Pediatr. **101**:923, 1982.

Gendrel, D., Roger, M., and Job, J.-C.: Plasma gonadotropin and testosterone values in infants with cryptorchidism, J. Pediatr. **97**:217, 1980.

Greene, R.A., and others: MURCS association with additional congenital anomalies, Hum. Pathol. **17**:88, 1986.

Hadziselimovic, F., Herzog, B., and Seguchi, H.: Surgical correction of cryptorchism at 2 years: electron microscopic and morphometric investigations, J. Pediatr. Surg. **10**:19, 1975.

Hadziselimovic, F., and others: The significance of postnatal gonadotropin surge for testicular development in normal and cryptorchid testes, J. Urol. **136**:274, 1986.

Hutson, J.M.: A biphasic model for the hormonal control of testicular descent, Lancet **2**:419, 1985.

Kaplan, L.M., and others: Association between abdominal wall defects and cryptorchidism, J. Urol. **136**:645, 1986.

Lee, P.A., and others: Micropenis. I. Criteria, etiologies and classification, Johns Hopkins Med. J. **146**:156, 1980.

Lee, P.A., and others: Micropenis. III. Primary hypogonadism, partial androgen insensitivity syndrome, and idiopathic disorders, Johns Hopkins Med. J. **147**:175, 1980.

Levitt, S.B., and others: The impalpable testis: a rational approach to management, J. Urol. **120**:515, 1978.

Lovinger, R., Kaplan, S., and Grumbach, M.: Congenital hypopituitarism associated with neonatal hypoglycemia and microphallus: four cases secondary to hypothalamic hormone deficiencies, J. Pediatr. **87**:1171, 1975.

Lutzker, L.G., Kogan, S.J., and Levitt, S.B.: Is routine intravenous urography indicated in patients with hypospadias? Pediatrics **59**:630, 1977.

Mengel, W., and others: Studies on cryptorchidism: a comparison of histological findings in the germinative epithelium before and after the second year of life, J. Pediatr. Surg. **9**:445, 1974.

Money, J., Lehne, G.K., and Pierre-Jerome, F.: Micropenis: gender, heterotosexual coping strategy, and behavioral health in nine pediatric cases followed to adulthood, Compr. Psychiatry **26**:29, 1985.

Rajfer, J., and Walsh, P.C.: The incidence of intersexuality in patients with hypospadias and cryptorchidism, J. Urol. **116**:769, 1976.

Russell, L.J., Weaver, D.D., and Bull, M.J.: The axial mesodermal dysplasia spectrum, Pediatrics **67**:176, 1981.

Salisbury, D.M., and others: Micropenis: an important early sign of congenital hypopituitarism, Br. Med. J. **288**:621, 1984.

Schultz, J.R., Klykylo, W.M., and Wacksman, J.: Timing of elective hypospadias repair in children, Pediatrics **71**:342, 1983.

Sheldon, C.A.: Undescended testis and testicular torsion, Surg. Clin. North Am. **65**:1303, 1985.

Shelton, T.B., and Noe, H.N.: The role of excretory urography in patients with hypospadias, J. Urol. **134**:97, 1985.

Tarry, W.F., Duckett, J.W., and Stephens, F.D.: The Mayer-Rokitansky syndrome: pathogenesis, classification and management, J. Urol. **136**:648, 1986.

Varner, R.E., Younger, J.B., and Blackwell, R.E.: Müllerian dysgenesis, J. Reprod. Med. **30**:443, 1985.

Waaler, P.E., and Maurseth, K.: Cryptorchidism: is routine intravenous pyelography indicated? Arch. Dis. Child. **51**:324, 1976.

Diagnosis and management of intersex disorders

Bartone, F.F., and others: Pitfalls in using human chorionic gonadotropin stimulation test to diagnose anorchia, J. Urol. **132**:563, 1984.

Berkovitz, G.D., and others: Etiologic evaluation of male pseudohermaphroditism in infancy and childhood, Am. J. Dis. Child. **138**:755, 1984.

Chaussain, J.L., and others: Longitudinal study of plasma testosterone in male pseudohermaphrodites during early infancy, J. Clin. Endocrinol. Metab. **49**:305, 1979.

dePeretti, E., and Forest, M.G.: Pitfalls in the etiological diagnosis of congenital adrenal hyperplasia in the early neonatal period, Hormone Res. **16**:10, 1982.

Donahoe, P.K., and Hendren, W.H., III: Perineal reconstruction in ambiguous genitalia infants raised as females, Ann. Surg. **200**:363, 1984.

Fauré, C., Fortier-Beaulieu, M., and Josso, N.: Genitography in intersex conditions concerning 86 cases, Ann. Radiol. **12**:259, 1969.

Feldman, K.W., and Smith, D.W.: Fetal phallic growth and penile standards for newborn male infants, J. Pediatr. **86**:395, 1975.

Fonkalsrud, E.W., Kaplan, S., and Lippe, B.: Experience with reduction clitoroplasty for clitoral hypertrophy, Ann. Surg. **186**:221, 1977.

Forest, M.G.: Pattern of the response of testosterone and its precursors to human chorionic gonadotropin stimulation in relation to age in infants and children, J. Clin. Endocrinol. Metab. **49**:132, 1979.

Forest, M.G., and Cathiard, A.M.: Pattern of plasma testosterone and Δ^4-androstenedione in normal newborns: evidence for testicular activity at birth, J. Clin. Endocrinol. Metab. **41**:977, 1975.

Forest, M.G., and others: Kinetics of the hCG-induced steroidogenic response of the human testis. III. Studies in children of the plasma levels of testosterone and hCG: rationale for testicular stimulation test, Pediatr. Res. **14**:819, 1980.

Gendrel, D., and others: Simultaneous postnatal rise of plasma LH and testosterone in male infants, J. Pediatr. **97**:600, 1980.

Gordon, L.P.: The use of cytogenetic techniques for the diagnosis of endocrine diseases, Clin. Lab. Med. **4**:835, 1984.

Guthrie, R.D., Smith, D.W., and Graham, C.B.: Testosterone treatment for micropenis during early childhood, J. Pediatr. **83**:247, 1973.

Jones, H.W., Jr.: Problems of sex differentiation—surgical correction, Birth Defects **14**(6C):63, 1978.

Lippe, B.M., and Sample, W.F.: Pelvic ultrasonography in pediatric and adolescent endocrine disorders, J. Pediatr. **92**:897, 1978.

Manley, C.B.: Elective genital surgery at one year of age: psychological and surgical considerations, Surg. Clin. North Am. **62**:941, 1982.

Manuel, M., Katayama, K.P., and Jones, H.W., Jr.: The age of occurrence of gonadal tumors in intersex patients with a Y chromosome, Am. J. Obstet. Gynecol. **124**:293, 1976.

Mollard, P., Juskiewenski, S., and Sarkissian, J.: Clitoroplasty in intersex: a new technique, Br. J. Urol. **53**:371, 1981.

Money, J., Hampson, J.G., and Hampson, J.L.: Hermaphroditism: recommendations concerning assignment of sex, change of sex, and psychologic management, Bull. Johns Hopkins Hosp. **97**:284, 1955.

Muram, D., and Dewhurst, J.: Inheritance of intersex disorders, Can. Med. Assoc. J. **130**:121, 1980.

Pang, S., and others: Dihydrotestosterone and its relationship to testosterone in infancy and childhood, J. Clin. Endocrinol. Metab. **48**:821, 1979.

Pang, S., and others: Serum androgen concentrations in neonates and young infants with congenital adrenal hyperplasia due to 21-hydroxylase deficiency, Clin. Endocrinol. **11**:575, 1979.

Reinisch, J.M., and Sanders, S.A.: Prenatal gonadal steroidal influences on gender-related behavior, Prog. Brain Res. **61**:407, 1984.

Riley, W.J., and Rosenbloom, A.L.: Clitoral size in infancy, J. Pediatr. **96**:918, 1980.

Rosenfield, R.L., Lucky, A.W., and Allen T.D.: The diagnosis and management of intersex, Curr. Probl. Pediatr. **10**:10, 1980.

Scully, R.E.: Neoplasia associated with anomalous sexual development and abnormal sex chromosomes, Pediatr. Adolesc. Endocrinol. **8**:203, 1981.

Siebermann, R.E.: The pathology of gonads and adrenal cortex in intersex, Prog. Pediatr. Surg. **16**:149, 1983.

Simpson, J.L., and Photopulos, G.: The relationship of neoplasia to disorders of abnormal sexual differentiation, Birth Defects **12**(1):15, 1976.

Sober, I., Bar-Ziv, Y., and Lieberman, E.: The radiological evaluation of intersex: technique of demonstrating müllerian duct remnants in difficult cases, J. Urol. **123**:439, 1980.

Tapanainen, J., and others: Enhanced activity of the pituitary-gonadal axis in premature human infants, J. Clin. Endocrinol. Metab. **52**:235, 1981.

Tapanainen, J., and others: Effect of gonadotropin-releasing hormone on pituitary-gonadal function of male infants during the first year of life, J. Clin. Endocrinol. Metab. **55**:689, 1982.

Winter, J.S.D., and others: Pituitary-gonadal relations in infancy. 2. Patterns of serum gonadal steroid concentrations in man from birth to two years of age, J. Clin. Endocrinol. Metab. **42**:679, 1976.

CHAPTER 38

The skin

The skin of the newborn may have a variety of lesions: some innocent, temporary, and the result of a physiologic reaction; others the result of episodic disease; and still others indicative of a serious, potentially fatal underlying disorder. The definitive diagnosis of specific skin lesions requires an understanding of the physiologic characteristics and peculiarities of neonatal skin, a recognition of primary skin lesions, and knowledge of their significance.

BIOLOGY OF FETAL AND NEONATAL SKIN

Structure of the epidermis

There has been little documented study of cutaneous development in the human embryo less than 30 days of age. Between 30 and 40 days, the embryonic skin consists of an external layer of cells, the periderm, which not only serves as a cover but may also serve as a nutritional interface with the amniotic fluid.

Human skin has two distinct interdependent components: the epidermis, derived from the fetal periderm, and the dermis, which together provide a regenerating protective coat. The epidermis has marked regional variations in thickness, color, permeability, and surface chemical components. It consists of a highly ordered compact layering of keratinocytes and melanocytes. Intermixed is a third distinct cell type, the Langerhans cell, which is derived from bone marrow precursors and migrates to the primitive epidermis. The Langerhans cell of human epidermis behaves as a monocyte or macrophage able to both synthesize antigens and to recognize and process antigens presented to it at the cell membrane, thus stimulating blastogenesis in immunocompetent T-helper lymphocytes and lymphokine production.

The young keratinocytes are columnar basal cells that produce and contain a filamentous protein, keratin. They lie adjacent to the dermis, separated from it by a narrow basement membrane. Ultrastructurally, the basement membrane has been shown to consist of a number of zones of varying electron density. Immunologically distinct elements of collagen appear to exist within these zones. The basal keratinocytes divide and migrate toward the surface. Their cellular structure is replaced by keratin, and the cells become dehydrated and flattened, forming a tough, resilient, anuclear, relatively impermeable membrane. In infants these cells of the stratum corneum are more uniform in size than those of children or adults.

Another important component of the epidermis is the melanocyte, a cell of neural crest origin capable of producing melanin, which migrates into the dermis and is first visible in the 10-week-old fetus. The melanocytes in the basal layer contain melanin at about the fourth month of fetal age. Melanin protects against ultraviolet radiation damage to vital nuclear elements. Melanin granules (melanosomes) are formed in the cytoplasm of the melanocyte and move via the dentritic processes toward the basal cell. As the basal keratinocyte matures, its melanin is dispersed as a fine intracellular granular dust that may be visualized in the horny layer. Melanin production is low; the newborn is not as pigmented as the older child and is more sensitive to sunlight. Yet there is no significant difference in the number of melanocytes in light, medium, or deeply pigmented skin or in infant or adult skin. The difference in color is a result of the number, size, and distribution of melanosomes and the activity of individual melanocytes. It has recently been postulated that color variations in human skin may not only have a sun-protective function but also may serve as camouflage.

The epidermis is attached to the dermis, in part, by vertically arranged anchoring fibrils composed of collagen. These anchoring fibrils are first identified in the 24-week fetus. The epidermis is less adherent to the dermis in the early weeks of life, resulting in a greater propensity to blister formation in the newborn.

The permeability of the stratum corneum in the newborn appears to vary with the gestational age of the infant. Nachman and Esterly assessed permeability by comparing the skin-blanching response in infants of varying gestational ages to the topical application of a 10% phenylephrine (Neo-Synephrine) solution. The skin of the youngest infants (28 to 34 weeks) had the most rapid

Disorders associated with abnormal amounts and morphologic characteristics of hair

A. Disorders with hypertrichosis
  1. Generalized
    a. Congenital lipodystrophy
    b. Cornelia de Lange syndrome
    c. Craniofacial dysostosis with dental, eye, and cardiac anomalies
    d. Hypertrichosis lanuginosa universalis
    e. Hypertrichosis with gingival fibromatosis
    f. Leprechaunism
    g. Mucopolysaccharidoses
  2. Localized
    a. Congenital hemihypertrophy with hypertrichosis
    b. Hairy ears
    c. Hairy elbows syndrome
    d. Hairy nevi
    e. Ring chromosome E (low hairline)
    f. Trisomy 18 (back and forehead)
    g. Turner's syndrome (low occipital hairline)

B. Disorders with hypotrichosis*
  1. Atrichia with papular lesions
  2. Combined immunodeficiency syndrome with short-limbed dwarfism
  3. Congenital alopecia
  4. EEC syndrome (ectrodactyly, ectodermal dysplasia, cleft lip-palate)
  5. Goltz's syndrome
  6. Hallermann-Streiff syndrome (oculomandibulodyscephaly)
  7. Hidrotic ectodermal dysplasia
  8. Hypohidrotic ectodermal dysplasia
  9. Hypotrichosis, syndactyly, and retinitis pigmentosa
  10. Incontinentia pigmenti
  11. Keratosis follicularis spinulosa decalvans
  12. Ocular-dental-digital dysplasia
  13. Oral-facial-digital syndrome
  14. Progeria
  15. Rothmund-Thomson syndrome
  16. Seckel syndrome
  17. Trisomy A

C. Disorders with hair of abnormal morphology
  1. Structural defects
    a. Arginosuccinicaciduria—trichorrhexis nodosa
    b. Hereditary trichodysplasia (Marie Unna hypotrichosis)—twisted hair
    c. Menkes syndrome
    d. Monilethrix
    e. Netherton's syndrome—multiple defects
    f. Trichothiodystrophy (BIDS syndrome)—multiple defects
    g. Pili annulati
    h. Pili bifurcati
    i. Pili torti
    j. Pili torti and nerve deafness
    k. Trichorrhexis nodosa
    l. Trichoschisis
  2. Abnormal color, caliber, and fragility
    a. Cartilage-hair hypoplasia—small caliber
    b. Citrullinemia—fragile, atrophic bulbs
    c. Congenital trichomegaly with dwarfism, mental retardation, and retinal pigmentation—long brows and lashes
    d. Dyskeratosis congenita—sparse and fine hair
    e. Hartnup disease—fine, fragile hair
    f. Hereditary enamel hypoplasia and kinky hair—abnormal curliness
    g. Homocystinuria—fine, fragile hair
    h. Marinesco-Sjögren syndrome—fragile, brittle, rough hair
    i. Phenylketonuria—fine, light-colored hair
    j. Pierre Robin anomalad—fine, light-colored hair
    k. Trichorhinophalangeal syndrome—thin, sparse hair
    l. Trisomy 21—fine, light-colored, atrophic bulbs
    m. Tyrosinemia—fine, light-colored hair
    n. Woolly hair—abnormal curliness

*A supplementary listing may be found in the review by Muller.

and prolonged response, whereas the skin of full-term infants in most instances failed to blanch even on the first day of life.

The appendages

The appendages derive from invaginations of epidermal germinative buds into the dermis. They include hair, sebaceous glands, apocrine glands, eccrine glands, and nails. The arrector pili muscle is attached to the hair follicle.

Lanugo (fine, soft, immature hair) frequently covers the scalp and brow in the premature infant. The scalp line may be poorly demarcated, and lanugo also may cover the face. Scalp hair is usually somewhat coarser and more mature earlier in dark-haired infants. The growth phases of the hair follicle are usually synchronous at birth; 80% of the follicles are in the resting state. During the first few months of life the synchrony between hair loss and regrowth is disturbed, and hair may become coarse and thick, acquiring an adult distribution, or there may be a temporary alopecia. There are also sex differences in hair growth; boys' hair grows faster than girls' hair. In both sexes scalp hair growth is slower at the crown. The normal pattern of hair growth is disturbed in many chromosomal disorders, resulting in eccentric crown whorls or double- or triple-crown whorls. The box below shows disorders associated with abnormal amounts and morphologic characteristics of hair.

Nails are fully formed at birth. Syndromes associated with nail defects are listed in the boxed material below.

The eccrine sweat glands are coiled structures that form during the first trimester as a downgrowth from epidermal cellular clones. No new glands are formed after birth. They are distributed over the entire body surface and are innervated by a sympathetic cholinergic mechanism. During the first 24 hours of life full-term infants usually do not sweat; at about the third day sweating begins on the face. Palmar sweating begins later. Sweating varies markedly with ambient and body temperature and activities such as crying and eating.

The sebaceous glands differentiate primarily from the epithelial portion of the hair follicle at about 13 to 15 weeks of life and almost immediately produce sebum in all hairy areas. The glands develop as solid outpouchings from the upper third of the hair follicle. These solid buds become filled with liquid centrally where the cells disintegrate; acini and ducts develop, opening most frequently into the canals between the hair follicle wall and hair shaft. Ectopic glands occur occasionally on the lips, buccal mucosa, esophagus, and vagina. The rapid growth and activity of sebaceous glands up to and immediately after birth is governed in part by maternal androgens and possibly also by endogenous steroid production by the fetus. Androgens are the only hormones that unequivocally have a stimulating effect on the sebaceous glands; estrogens depress their growth. Between 2 months and 2 years, the sebaceous glands of the normal infant begin a period of quiescence that lasts until puberty.

The apocrine glands are relatively large organs that originate from and empty into a hair follicle. Embryologically they develop somewhat later than the eccrine glands. Apocrine development is advanced by 7 or 8 fetal months, when the glands begin to produce a milky white fluid containing water, lipids, protein, reducing sugars, ferric iron, and ammonia; in the newborn the acini are well formed. The biologic function of the gland is unknown.

Syndromes associated with nail defects

A. Total or partial absence of nails; nail hypoplasia or dysplasia
   1. Acrodermatitis enteropathica
   2. Anonychia and ectrodactyly
   3. Apert's syndrome (acrocephalosyndactyly)
   4. Cartilage-hair hypoplasia
   5. Deafness and nail dystrophy (Feinmesser; Robinson)
   6. Dyskeratosis congenita
   7. Ellis-van Creveld syndrome
   8. Enamel hypoplasia and curly hair
   9. Epidermolysis bullosa
   10. Fetal hydantoin syndrome
   11. Focal dermal hypoplasia (Goltz syndrome)
   12. Glossopalatine ankylosis, microglossia, hypodontia, and other anomalies of the extremities (Gorlin-Pindborg)
   13. Hypohidrotic ectodermal dysplasia
   14. Incontinentia pigmenti
   15. Larsen syndrome
   16. Long-arm 21 deletion syndrome
   17. Nail-patella syndrome
   18. Popliteal web syndrome
   19. Progeria
   20. Pyknodysostosis (Maroteaux-Lamy)
   21. Rothmund-Thomson syndrome
   22. Skin hypoplasia—nail dystrophy (Basan)
   23. Trisomy 13
   24. Trisomy 18
   25. Turner's syndrome

B. Hypertrophic or abnormally large nails
   1. Congenital hemihypertrophy
   2. Familial hyperpigmentation with dystrophy of the nails (Touraine-Soulignac)
   3. Pachyonychia congenita
   4. Rubinstein-Taybi syndrome
   5. Otopalatodigital syndrome

Data from Gorlin and Pindborg, 1964; Pardo-Costello and Pardo, 1960; Samman, 1972; and Smith, 1976.

Structure of the dermis

The fetal dermis acquires some of the characteristics of adult dermis at about 20 weeks' gestation. However, it is only in the more mature fetus that both the structural and biochemical qualities of the newborn dermis are detectable. The dermis has a symbiotic relation to and may exert a controlling influence on the epidermis. It is a metabolically active tissue that contains fibrous elements, amorphous ground substance, free cells, nerves, blood vessels, and lymphatic vessels. The fibrous elements are collagen and elastic tissue. Collagen of types I and III, and a small amount of V, make up more than 90% of the connective tissue of the dermis. With increasing age, collagen becomes progressively less soluble, and thicker bundles predominate. The morphologic characteristics and chemical and physical properties of cutaneous elastic fibers are different from those of collagen. Histochemically stainable elastic tissue first appears in the 22-week-old fetus. Clinical changes in cutaneous elasticity in aging skin and in some diseases may be related to the spatial arrangement of elastic tissue or collagen fibers in the skin and to a qualitative change in the elastic fiber rather than to the quantity of elastin present in the dermis. The fibroblasts are the most numerous cells of the dermis. They produce collagen and the mucopolysaccharides of the ground substance. Mast cells (which produce heparin and histamine), histiocytes, macrophages, lymphocytes, neutrophils, and an occasional plasma cell and eosinophil are also present in the dermis. The major mucopolysaccharides in the ground substance of skin are hyaluronic acid and dermatan sulfate (chondroitin sulfate B). With an increase in age, there is a shift from hyaluronic acid toward dermatan sulfate and a decrease in water content of the dermis.

The blood and lymphatic vessels

The vascular supply of the skin is closely related to its size and function. Therefore the physiologic requirements of skin vary considerably; skin blood flows range from 0.1 to 150 ml/mm^3 of tissue per minute. The vascular network supplying the skin develops in early embryonic life from the mesoderm. The dermis and epidermis are served by networks of anastomosing arteries of three types: cutaneous, perforating, and segmental. The cutaneous vessels are arranged in the dermis in superficial and deep plexuses and are accompanied by an even more complex venous arrangement. Those capillary vessels found in the papillae enter them perpendicular to the immediately overlying epidermis. This orderly arrangement of vessels in the superficial dermis becomes apparent only 17 weeks after birth. The cutaneous vasculature derives from muscular perforating arteries that supply both muscle and skin. The perforating arteries themselves derive from the segmental (intercostal) vessels of the embryo. Direct cutaneous arteriovenous anastomoses are present in abundance, with glomerular organs probably responsible for thermoregulatory shunting. The appendages have special vascular networks.

Vasomotor tone is controlled by a delicate and complex series of nervous and pharmacologic mechanisms that involve the sympathetic nervous system, norepinephrine, acetylcholine, and histamine and also may involve serotonin, vasoactive polypeptides, corticosteroids, and prostaglandins. The nervous system control of thermoregulation also involves the hypothalamus, higher centers, sympathetic and sensory nerves, and the axon reflex.

Cutaneous innervation

The nerve networks in the dermis develop at a very early embryologic age and appear to be distributed in random fashion. The most superficial nerves have the smallest diameter and are the least myelinated. The nerves conduct stimuli from specialized epidermal cells called Merkel's tactile cells. In addition to the dermal nerve network, which may show considerable regional variation, nerve fibers may serve particular regions or structures, such as hair follicles, eccrine glands, arrector pili muscles, and the subepidermal zone. The sebaceous glands are not innervated.

Cutaneous nerves serve overlapping cutaneous areas; one nerve impulse does not necessarily stimulate one spot on the cerebral cortex. Sensation is probably the product of several factors, including spatial and temporal patterns of nerve stimulation in skin and spinal cord, local chemical factors in the skin, previous experience, conditioning, the state of cortical arousal, and genetic factors relating to nerve stimulation threshold. Special neurologic structures include a dense perifollicular nerve network with exquisite tactile sensory properties and mucocutaneous end organs highly concentrated in erogenous zones. Meissner's tactile organs are found in newborn skin as undeveloped structures that mature after birth. Merkel's corpuscles are important for two-point tactile discrimination on palms and fingertips; they are disk-shaped terminals that are seen during the twenty-eighth week of fetal life. After birth these receptors undergo little alteration. Vater-Pacini corpuscles are found around the digits, palms, and genitals; they are fully formed and numerous at birth.

The arrector pili muscles are innervated by sympathetic nerves, and norepinephrine acts as the neurotransmitter. The eccrine glands are innervated by sympathetic fibers, but acetylcholine acts as the neurotransmitter. Parasympathetic fibers may accompany the sensory nerves in the vessel walls and cause vasodilation. The axon reflex is poorly developed in the newborn; in the neonate of low birth weight, axon reflex sweating may be difficult to elicit.

NORMAL SKIN IN THE NEWBORN

The gross appearance of the skin at birth is related in part to the maturity of the infant. In the normal full-term infant the skin is soft, wrinkled, velvety, and covered with a greasy yellow-white material with a pH of 6.7 to 7.4; this is the vernix caseosa, a mixture of desquamating cells and sebum. Removal of the vernix is followed by desquamation of the epidermis in most infants. The fetal epidermis is rich in glycogen. Glycogen, present in the basal layer at the sixth fetal month, diminishes as normal keratogenesis progresses but may reaccumulate at the site of an injury. Beneath the vernix the pH of newborn skin surface varies from 5.5 to 6.0, depending on the particular site sampled. Skin surface lipids in the first 2 weeks of life are low in cholesterol and high in wax esters compared with childhood values. Free fatty acids and triglycerides slowly decrease during the postnatal period and childhood.

Within a few hours of birth the skin develops an intense red color, which may remain for several hours. With fading of this erythema, bluish mottling (livedo reticularis) becomes evident, particularly when the infant is exposed to a cool environment. Localized mild edema also may be present over the pubis and the dorsa of the hands and feet, possibly an additional manifestation of an unstable peripheral circulation. Although the body surface tends to be less pigmented during the neonatal period than later in life, certain areas such as the linea alba, the areolas, and the scrotum often are deeply pigmented as a result of high circulating levels of maternal and placental hormones. Palpable nodules of breast tissue, active secretion by mammary glands, and a hyperplastic vaginal epithelium are additional normal end organ responses to these hormones.

The premature infant's skin may be readily distinguished from the full-term infant's skin. At birth it is more transparent and gelantinous and tends to be free of wrinkles. The premature infant may be covered with fine lanugo hair, which in the full-term infant has been lost or in some areas replaced by vellus hair. Sexual hormonal effects are less conspicuous in the premature infant; the scrotum is less rugose and pigmented, the labia majora are less prominent, nipples and areolas are less pigmented, and breast tissue is less palpable.

EPHEMERAL CUTANEOUS LESIONS

A number of benign and ephemeral lesions are commonly observed in a normal nursery population.

Milia

About 40% of infants have multiple yellow-white 1 mm cysts (milia) scattered over the cheeks, forehead, nose, and nasolabial folds. These may be few or numerous, but they frequently occur in clusters. Histologically, milia are keratogenous cysts similar to Epstein's pearls, which are distributed along the midpalatal raphe and Bohn's nodules, which occur on the palate and the buccal and lingual aspects of the dental ridges. The intraoral lesions are found in 75% to 80% of newborns. All these cysts exfoliate spontaneously within the first few weeks of life.

Pigmentary lesions

The most frequently encountered pigmented lesion is the mongolian spot, which occurs in over 70% of black, oriental, and American Indian infants and in approximately 5% of white infants. Although most of these lesions are found in the lumbosacral area, occurrence at other sites is not uncommon. The pigmentation is macular and gray-blue, may cover an area 10 cm or larger in diameter, and results from an infiltrate of melanocytes deep in the dermis. Most of these lesions gradually disappear during the first few years of life, but aberrant lesions in unusual sites are more likely to persist. Because of their distinctive color and morphology, mongolian spots are not easily confused with congenital pigmented melanocytic nevi or café-au-lait spots. Lentigines, freckles, melanocytic nevi, and café-au-lait spots have their onset later in infancy or in early childhood, although occasionally the latter two types of lesions may be present at birth.

Abnormal hyperpigmentation of the areolas and genitals may be evidence for the existence of an in utero glucocorticoid insufficiency associated with defects in the biosynthesis of hydrocortisone.

Salmon patches

Salmon patches (vascular macules) are present in 30% to 50% of normal newborns. They are usually found on the nape, the eyelids, and the glabella. In a prospective study of affected infants most of the facial lesions had faded by 1 year of age, but those on the neck were more persistent. Surveys of adult populations confirm the persistence of the nuchal lesions in about one fourth of the population.

Harlequin color change

Harlequin color change is a phenomenon observed in the immediate neonatal period and is more common in the low birth weight infant. A sharp midline demarcation bisects the body longitudinally into pale and intensely red sides. The peak frequency of attacks in one series occurred on the second, third, and fourth days, but episodes were observed during the first 3 weeks of life. These episodes are of no pathologic significance. They have been attributed to a temporary imbalance in the autonomic regulatory mechanism of the cutaneous vessels; there are no accompanying changes in respiratory rate, muscle tone, or response to external stimuli.

Erythema toxicum

Erythema toxicum is a benign and self-limited eruption that usually develops between 24 and 72 hours of age, but lesions may appear until about 3 weeks of age. The incidence of affected full-term newborns in a normal nursery population varies from 30% to 70%. The disorder is less common with decreasing birth weight and gestational age. These lesions may vary considerably in character and number; they may be firm, shotty, 1 to 3 mm, pale yellow to white papules or pustules on an erythematous base or erythematous macules up to 3 cm in diameter. Individual lesions are evanescent, often lasting only a matter of hours. They may be found on any area of the body but occur only rarely on the palms and soles. There are no related systemic symptoms, and their cause is unknown. A microscopic examination of a Wright- or Giemsa-stained smear of the pustules demonstrates numerous eosinophils; Gram stains are negative for bacteria, and cultures are sterile. No treatment is necessary.

Transient neonatal pustular melanosis

Transient neonatal pustular melanosis is a distinctive eruption that consists of two types of lesions: small superficial vesicopustules with little or no surrounding erythema (Fig. 38-1, *A*) and pigmented macules often

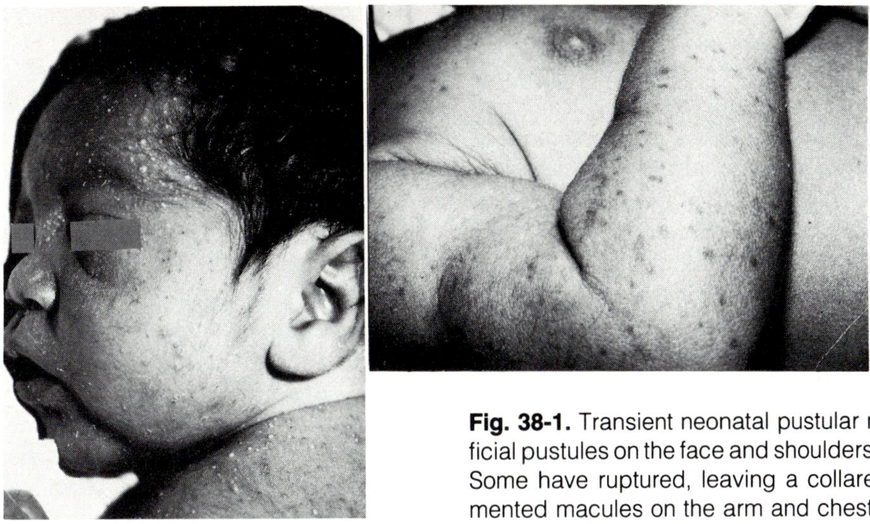

Fig. 38-1. Transient neonatal pustular melanosis. **A,** Superficial pustules on the face and shoulders of a 1-day-old infant. Some have ruptured, leaving a collarette of scale. **B,** Pigmented macules on the arm and chest of a newborn.

encircled by a collarette of fine scale (Fig. 38-1, *B*). Both types of lesions may be present at birth, but the macules are observed more frequently. The lesions may be profuse or sparse and occur on any body surface, including the palms, soles, and scalp. Sites of predilection are the forehead, submental area and anterior neck, and lower back. When intact pustules rupture, a pigmented macule is often discernible central to the collarette of scale, which represents the margin of the unroofed pustule. Presumably the macules result from postinflammatory hyperpigmentation, and those present at birth may be the sequelae of in utero pustular lesions. Pustular melanosis may be confused with erythema toxicum, congenital cutaneous candidiasis, or a staphylococcal pyoderma. Cultures and Gram stains of smears prepared from intact pustules are devoid of organisms; Wright stains of intralesional contents demonstrate cellular debris, polymorphonuclear leukocytes, and a few or no eosinophils, in contrast to erythema toxicum. Although the pustules disappear in 48 hours, the macules may persist for up to 3 months. Neither type of lesion requires therapy, and, although the cause in unknown, parents may be reassured that the disorder is benign and transient.

Miliaria

Miliaria is an eruption resulting from sweat retention. The lesions are of two types: superficial thin-walled vesicles without inflammation (miliaria crystallina) and small, erythematous, grouped papules (miliaria rubra). The eruption most frequently develops in the intertriginous areas and over the face and scalp (Fig. 38-2). It is exacerbated by exposure to a warm and humid environment. Miliaria can sometimes be confused with erythema toxicum; rapid resolution of the lesions when the infant is placed in a cooler environment differentiates them from pyoderma. A Wright-stained smear of vesicular lesions will demonstrate only sparse squames permitting exclusion of infectious vesicular eruptions. No topical therapy is indicated.

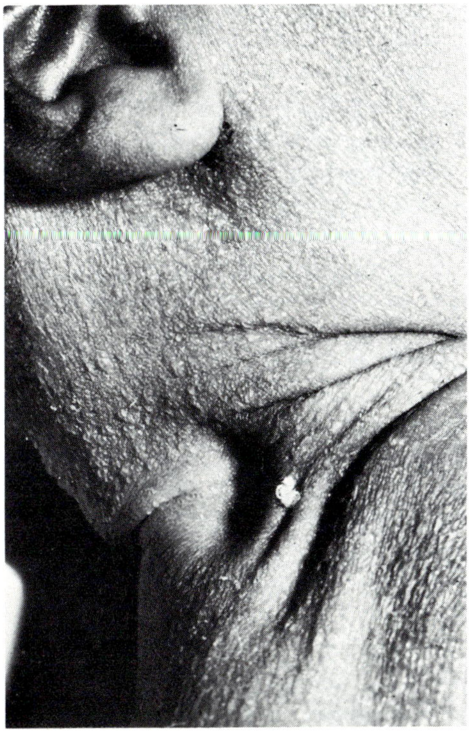

Fig. 38-2. Miliaria crystallina on the neck.

Infantile acne

Infantile acne is an uncommon but distressing facial eruption (usually in male infants) that has its onset during the first few weeks of life. The condition resembles acne in the adolescent patient and is characterized by comedones, papules, pustules, and, rarely, nodules. The duration may vary, but usually the disorder clears spontaneously during the latter portion of the first year of life. This condition probably represents a heightened end organ response to an active androgen metabolism. Conservative treatment with mild topical acne preparations to produce drying and peeling should suffice. Occasionally the infant may be left with pitted scarring. This problem should be distinguished from the much milder and relatively transient follicular plugging, commonly seen on the faces of infants during the first month of life.

THE SCALY BABY

Of the major causes of excessive scaling in the neonate, physiologic desquamation of the normal newborn and the desquamation seen in dysmature infants are not of long-term significance. However, ichthyosis, a less common cause, is a chronic heritable disease.

Physiologic desquamation and dysmaturity

The newborn with accentuated physiologic desquamation usually has a gestational age of between 40 and 42 weeks (Chapter 10); peak shedding occurs about the eighth day of life. These infants are otherwise normal in physical appearance and behavior. In contrast, the dysmature infant (Chapter 7) has distinctive characteristics. The dysmature infant's body is lean with thin extremities and little subcutaneous fat; weight is low in relation to length. The skin is parchmentlike, scaly, and stained with meconium, as are the nails and umbilical cord; the hair is abundant, and the nails are abnormally long. In both the normal infant with accentuated physiologic scaling and the dysmature infant, desquamation is a transient phenomenon, and the integument continues to serve its intended protective function. However, the infant with ichthyosis may have a serious difficulty early in life because of impaired barrier function and the subsequent risks of secondary infection.

Ichthyosis

Of the four major types of ichthyosis, three may be apparent during the first month of life: X-linked ichthyosis, lamellar ichthyosis (nonbullous congenital ichthyosiform erythroderma), and epidermolytic hyperkeratosis (bullous congenital ichthyosiform erythroderma). The diagnosis depends on the morphologic features, the histologic pattern of a skin biopsy, pedigree information, and, in certain instances, electron microscopic studies and enzyme analysis. The fourth type, ichthyosis vulgaris, is the most common and benign form and rarely has its onset before the third month of life. In addition to the aforementioned disorders, two descriptive terms have been used for ichthyotic conditions that occur only in the newborn: *harlequin fetus* and *collodion baby*. Several rare syndromes (e.g., Netherton's syndrome, *k*eratitis, *i*chthyosiform erythroderma, *d*eafness [KID] syndrome, Sjögren-Larsson syndrome) with ichthyosis as a feature may also be manifest in the neonate.

Harlequin fetus

The harlequin fetus represents the most severe form of ichthyosis and is inherited as an autosomal recessive trait. The cause of this disorder is unknown. X-ray diffraction studies have disclosed no consistent abnormalities in the epidermal fibrous proteins. The skin of the harlequin fetus is hard, thick, and gray or yellow, with deep crevices running both transversely and vertically. The fissures are most prominent over the areas of movement. Rigidity of the skin about the eyes results in marked ectropion, although the globe is usually normal. The ears and nose are underdeveloped, flattened, and distorted, and the lips are everted and gaping, thus producing a "fish mouth" deformity. The nails and hair may be hypoplastic or absent. Extreme inelasticity of the skin is associated with flexion deformity of all joints. The hands and feet are ischemic, hard, and waxy in appearance, with poorly developed distal digits. These infants usually do not survive after the first week or two of life. Intrauterine diagnosis by fetoscopy and fetal skin biopsy has been accomplished successfully and can be offered as an option to couples at risk.

Collodion baby

The collodion baby (lamellar exfoliation of the newborn) is less severely affected and occurs more commonly than the harlequin fetus and may represent a phenotypic expression of several genotypes. This disorder usually eventuates in lamellar ichthyosis (recessive type); the literature is controversial regarding the relationship of collodion baby to other types of ichthyosis and some of the syndromal complexes. Rarely, shedding of the collodion-like membrane may reveal a normal underlying integument. A significant number of these babies are premature. The infant is covered with a cellophane-like membrane, which, by its tautness, may distort the facial features and the digits. Less commonly only part of the integument is involved. The membrane is shiny and brownish yellow, resembling an envelope of collodion or oiled parchment, and may be perforated by hair. The presence of ectropion, eclabium, and crumpled ears causes these infants to resemble one another for the first few days of life. Fissuring and peeling begin shortly after birth, and large sheets may desquamate, revealing erythema of variable intensity. Once the membrane has fissured, no respiratory difficulties are encountered. Complete shedding of the collodion membrane may take several months. Pedigree information and histopathologic examination of a skin biopsy are additional aids in the delineation of the specific type of ichthyosis. Despite the apparent thickened skin, these infants have an abnormal epidermal barrier. Major complications include dehydration caused by increased water loss and cutaneous and systemic infection. The infant should be placed in an environment with increased humidity, but prompt attention should be paid to signs of infection. Keratolytic agents should be avoided, since increased permeability may lead to systemic toxicity. A bland emollient will suffice for lubrication during the neonatal period.

X-linked ichthyosis

The patient with X-linked ichthyosis, if affected at birth, may have collodion membranes or only hyperkeratosis. In several studies 17% to 36% of the subjects had manifestations of the disease at birth, and 84% to 94% were affected by 3 months of age. The scales are characteristically large, thick, and dark and are prominent over the neck, anterior trunk, and extensor extremities. Sparing of palms and soles and partial sparing of the flexures are helpful diagnostic features. Usually the axillae or the antecubital fossae or both are involved early in life. Systemic manifestations are generally absent, and complications are rare. Skin biopsy is helpful (although the histologic pattern resembles that of lamellar ichthyosis), showing hyperkeratosis, a well-developed granular layer, hypertrophic epidermis, and a perivascular lymphocytic infiltrate. This form of ichthyosis is present only in males and not in heterozygous females. The cutaneous abnormality has been linked with a steroid sulfatase enzyme deficiency in the somatic tissues of affected males. Deep corneal opacities also have been described as a relatively reliable genetic marker in older boys and men with the disorder, whereas female carriers have this finding inconsistently. Female carriers of the gene for X-linked ichthyosis, when pregnant with an affected male fetus, have a deficiency of placental steroid sulfatase reflected by low maternal urinary estriol excretion and difficult or prolonged labor often requiring intervention.

Lamellar ichthyosis (nonbullous congenital ichthyosiform erythroderma)

A brilliant and generalized erythema often characterizes the scaly infant with lamellar ichthyosis. Affected babies are commonly of low birth weight. Hyperkeratosis is universal, involving the flexural areas and other body surfaces (Fig. 38-3), but scaling in the neonatal period is less prominent than later in childhood. The palms and soles may show only increased skin markings or may be considerably thickened. Ectropion, often severe later in life, is not usually a problem during the neonatal period. Macerated skin in the intertriginous areas may serve as an entry point for bacterial organisms. Lamellar ichthyosis has a recessive mode of inheritance. Since it also can occur as the cutaneous feature of several rare syndromes, affected infants must be thoroughly evaluated, particularly for central nervous system (CNS) abnormalities.

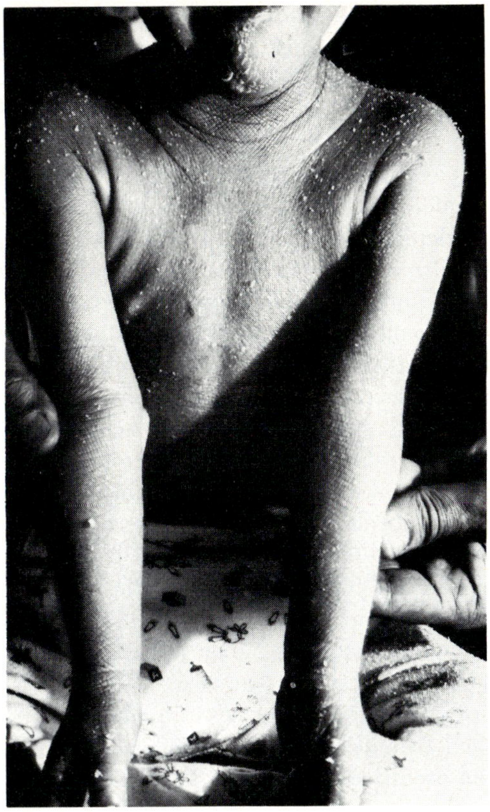

Fig. 38-3. Lamellar ichthyosis. Note generalized scaling including the flexural areas.

Epidermolytic hyperkeratosis (bullous congenital ichthyosiform erythroderma)

The infant with epidermolytic hyperkeratosis has recurrent bullous lesions, erythema, dryness, and peeling. During the neonatal period bullae may occur over widespread areas, resulting in extensive denudation with secondary infection, sepsis, and death. These skin lesions may be confused with those of staphylococcal scalded skin syndrome or epidermolysis bullosa. Antibiotics may be required during the first months of life. The bullous lesions become less prominent as the infant grows older and disappear completely in adulthood. The histopathologic picture in epidermolytic hyperkeratosis is diagnostic and consists of vacuolization of the epidermis; abnormally large, clumped keratin granules; hyperkeratosis; and an increased granular layer. An accurate family history is also critical, since this disorder is inherited as an autosomal dominant trait.

VESICOBULLOUS ERUPTIONS

Blistering eruptions in the neonatal period may be caused by infections, congenital diseases, or infiltrative processes or may be of unknown origin. The proper management of such infants depends on knowledge of the cause of the disease or, when this is not possible, on an understanding of the pathogenesis of the type of blister encountered. The latter often depends on determining at what level within the skin the blister has occurred.

Blister sites may be either epidermal or subepidermal. In the epidermis the blister can be very high (subcorneal), midepidermal, or basal. The midepidermal blister may be formed by primary separation of intercellular contacts (acantholysis), by secondary edematous disruption of intercellular contacts (spongiosis), or by intracellular injury, as seen in viral infections. The diagnosis of a blistering disease usually requires a family history, an immediate past history of the infant and mother, laboratory studies relative to finding an infectious agent, evaluation of the infant's general state of health, consideration of the morphologic characteristics of the eruption, and a biopsy of the involved skin. The biopsy should be obtained from a fresh, typical, small lesion and should include some normal surrounding skin. Treatment of erosive lesions with steroids and antibiotics should be tempered by awareness that knowledge of the metabolism and toxicity of these substances in the neonate is incomplete and that increased permeability of the skin may result in excessive absorption.

BACTERIAL AND YEAST INFECTIONS

The colonization of the newborn's skin begins at birth. The organisms acquired at birth are similar to those found on adult skin. *Staphylococcus epidermidis* (coagulase negative) predominates, but diphtheroids, streptococci, and coliform bacteria are also found. The newborn skin affords an excellent culture medium for *Staphylococcus aureus;* the groin and other skin sites may become colonized before the umbilicus. *Candida albicans* is not usually found on normal skin but may be present in the oral mucosa or in the diaper area as a result of fecal contamination (Chapter 31).

Bullous impetigo

The lesions of impetigo usually appear after the first few days of life. This is in contrast to congenital blistering diseases, which are often present at birth. The blisters vary in size and may appear on any body surface. They soon rupture, leaving a red, moist, denuded area. When the epidermis is shed in large sheets, staphylococcal scalded skin syndrome should be suspected. The organism most frequently involved is *S. aureus,* group 2 phage type. Certain phage types (for example, type 71) usually are associated with these lesions. The diagnosis is made by Gram stain and culture of the blister fluid. Blood cultures should be obtained from affected infants. Contacts and nursery personnel should be investigated for a source of the infecting organism. The infant should be placed in isolation and observed carefully for early signs of sepsis. A high index of suspicion during examination of other infants in the nursery is the most effective means of preventing epidemic spread of this infection (Chapter 31, part one).

Topical therapy consists of compresses of physiologic saline. Systemic antibiotics are indicated to cover the principal etiologic possibilities until the results of culture are available. Fluid and electrolyte replacement therapy may be required if the disease is extensive. Recovery is usually complete in several days, and there is no residual scarring.

Staphylococcal scalded skin syndrome

The scalded skin syndrome is a severe bullous eruption that has been reported at all ages, although it is rare in adults. The eponym *Ritter's disease* has been used for infants up to a few weeks of age but is now obsolete.

The eruption is heralded by a bright erythema that resembles a scald. Flaccid bullae form high in the epidermis (granular layer), and the upper epidermis may be detached by gentle traction with the examining finger (positive Nikolsky's sign). Areas of denudation occur first on the face and in the flexural areas (Fig. 38-4, *A*). The entire epidermis may be shed from the limb like a glove (Fig. 38-4, *B*). Crusting about the mouth and eyes results in a typical facies. Conjunctivitis is common as is hyperemia of the mucous membranes, but oral ulcerations do not occur. Some infants with a milder form of the disease display a scarlatiniform eruption without bullae or denudation.

The infecting organism in scalded skin syndrome is *S. aureus,* usually a group 2 phage type, although other phage types occasionally have been incriminated. These organisms produce an exotoxin, called exfoliatin, that is responsible for the cutaneous manifestations. Purified toxin has been demonstrated to cause scalded skin syndrome in newborn mice and more localized lesions in adult human volunteers. Histologic examination of the skin demonstrates separation at the level of the granular layer with cell death and acantholysis; there is a striking absence of inflammatory infiltrate. Since intact bullae are sterile, cultures should be obtained from the nasopharynx, conjunctival sac, abnormal skin, blood, and any other suspected focus of infection that might have provided a portal of entry for the organism. Treatment consists of prompt systemic administration of penicillinase-resistant semisynthetic penicillin and fluid and electrolyte replacement, if necessary. A flaky desquamation occurs during the healing phase. Scarring never occurs, since the blister cleavage plane is intraepidermal in location.

A

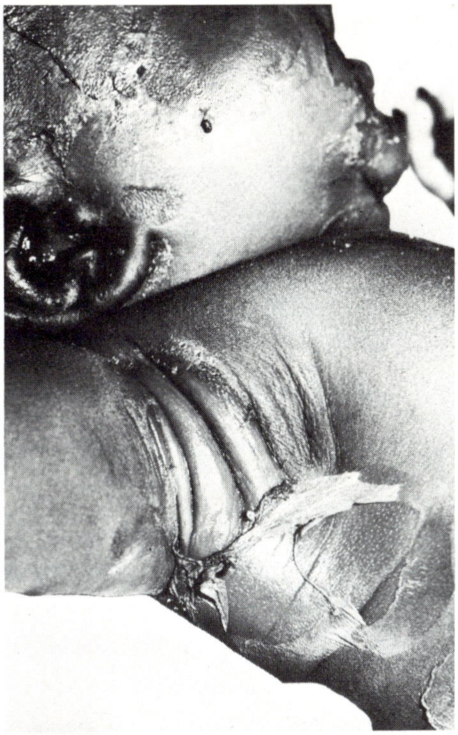

B

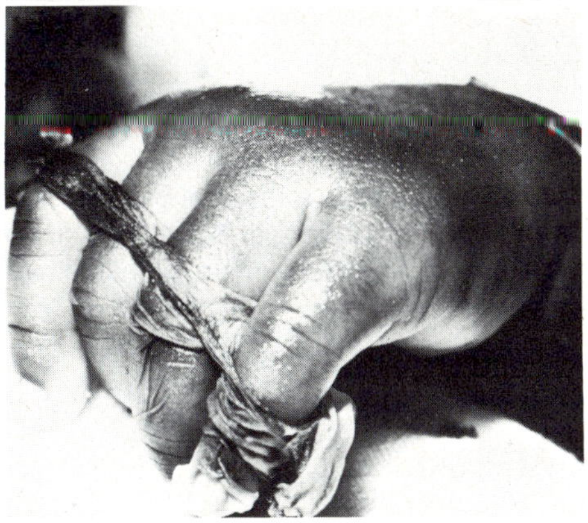

Fig. 38-4. Staphylococcal scalded skin syndrome. **A,** Extensive denudation in the axilla. **B,** Glovelike shedding of the epidermis of the hand.

Viral lesions

The vesicles of variola, vaccinia, varicella, herpes zoster, and herpes simplex have similar histologic patterns (Chapter 31, parts 2 and 3). The vesicle occurs in the midepidermis. Acantholysis and marked destruction of individual cells result in the ballooning type of degeneration characteristic of viral vesicles. Eosinophilic mononuclear and multinucleated giant cells may be seen on a smear carefully prepared by scraping the base of a fresh vesicle and staining with Giemsa or Wright stain (the Tzanck test). These giant cells are always seen in the herpes group (varicella-zoster and simplex) and are uncommon in the pox group (variola and vaccinia). A young viral blister also may be identified according to the type of viral inclusion body found in the degenerated cells.

HEREDITARY BLISTERING DISEASES

Epidermolysis bullosa

Epidermolysis bullosa refers to a group of heterogeneous hereditary defects that are characterized by intraepidermal or subepidermal blisters produced by minor degrees of trauma and heat. Although there may be as many as 16 different variants of this disorder, basically the epidermolysis bullosas can be grouped into two major types: those lesions that result in complete healing without scarring and those that inevitably produce scars. Nonscarring epidermolysis bullosa has two modes of transmission: autosomal recessive (junctional epidermolysis bullosa) and autosomal dominant (epidermolysis bullosa simplex). The term *nonscarring* refers to the manner in which an uncomplicated blister may heal. Unfortunately, in the recessive form, few blisters heal without complications, and scarring may result as a secondary phenomenon.

Junctional epidermolysis bullosa of the Herlitz type is usually present at birth. The epidermis loosens after minimum trauma, and bullae of varying sizes are formed anywhere on the body. The nails are frequently involved. Oral and anal lesions also occur. Many lesions heal spontaneously, but large bullae may fail to heal and result in moist chronic vegetative lesions. Loss of electrolytes and protein via these erosions and a refractory anemia may complicate the clinical course. The life span of most patients is short. The blisters form between the basement membrane of the epidermis and the plasma membrane of the basal cells, lying therefore at the junction between dermis and epidermis. The cause of separation is unknown, although a structural defect in the hemidesmosomal attachments between the basal cells and the basement membrane is a consistent and characteristic finding. Treatment is usually protective and palliative. A benign atrophic variant with relatively mild involvement can also be present at birth.

The autosomal dominant form of nonscarring epidermolysis bullosa (simplex) may be present at birth or may appear shortly thereafter in areas of trauma related to delivery (Fig. 38-5, *A*). The legs, feet, and scalp develop bullae that are often hemorrhagic and that heal rapidly. When the nails are shed, they regrow promptly. In contrast to the severe recessive nonscarring form, the infants are usually in good general health. In all forms of epidermolysis bullosa, blisters may be readily elicited by gentle rubbing. Mild trauma will result in a blister within a few minutes to hours, and the resulting fresh lesions

A

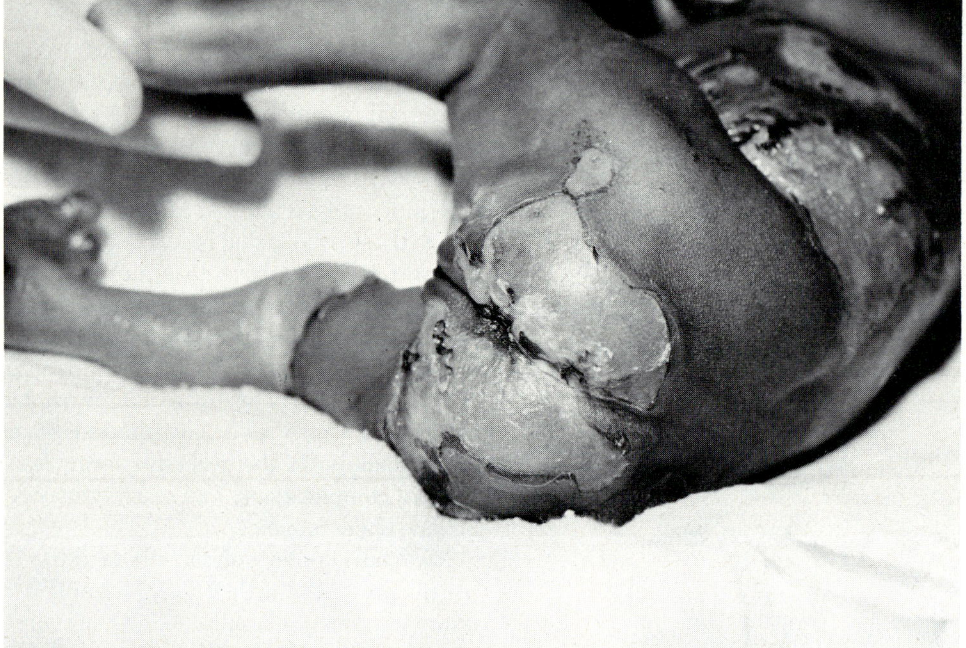

B

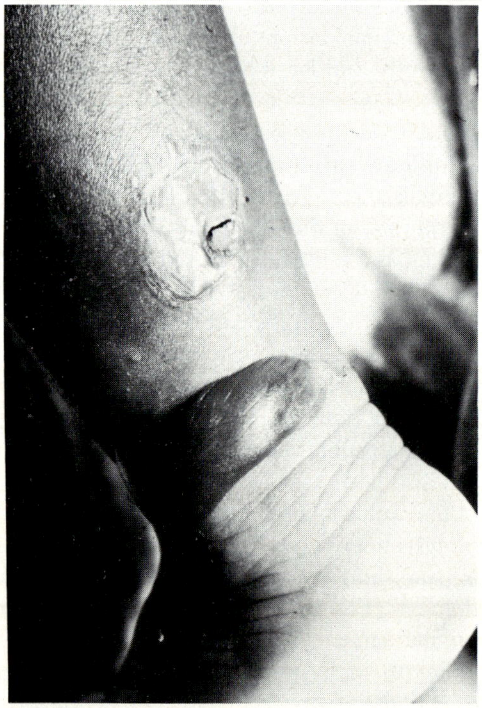

Fig. 38-5. A, Denudation as a result of blistering in an infant with epidermolysis bullosa letalis. **B,** Large intact bulla and ruptured bulla on the leg of an infant with dominant dystrophic epidermolysis bullosa.

may be used for histopathologic examination. The diagnostic blister of the dominant form results from acute disintegration of basal cells. Cytolysis starts in the perinuclear region and spreads centrifugally to involve the entire basal cell. The cause is unknown. Treatment is aimed at protecting the skin from trauma and secondary infection.

Scarring epidermolysis bullosa (dystrophic epidermolysis bullosa) has both a recessive and a dominant form. In recessive scarring epidermolysis bullosa hemorrhagic erosions and blisters may be present at birth, especially about the feet. In contrast to the nonscarring group, milia may mark the site of healed blisters. The toe and finger lesions heal with fusion of digits and loss of nails, which result in a characteristic mittenlike envelope of the hands. As the fingers fuse (this usually takes several years), the hands and arms become fixed in a flexed position, and contractures develop. Repeated episodes of blistering, infection, and scar formation lead to severe deformities, loss of hair, buccal mucosal scarring, dysphagia, and retarded physical and sexual development. Visceral amyloidosis, hyperglobulinemic purpura, and clotting abnormalities are associated with this severe, life-limiting disease.

The dominant form of scarring epidermolysis bullosa is less severe than the recessive type. Lesions may be present at birth, or they appear later and are usually limited to the elbows, knees, hands, feet, and sacrum (Fig. 38-5, *B*). Oral involvement is common but is usually not severe. Nails may be lost, but deforming scars and contractures are infrequent. Red plaques rather than blisters may result from injury. The lesions heal with soft wrinkled scars. Hypopigmentation, hyperpigmentation, and milia often are found at old blister sites. The general health is usually unimpaired.

The electron microscopic changes in all the scarring forms are identical and diagnostic. There is a sharp separation just beneath the basement membrane (subepidermal bulla), and the normal basal layer anchoring fibrils are rudimentary or absent. The defect probably involves the connective tissue of the dermis immediately adjacent to the basement membrane of the epidermis. There are elevated levels of collagenase in the skin of such patients.

Treatment for scarring epidermolysis bullosa is essentially the same as that for the nonscarring forms. In selected patients surgery may be indicated for correction of flexion deformities or fused digits. Iron therapy is necessary to treat the anemia.

Incontinentia pigmenti

Incontinentia pigmenti is a hereditary disorder that affects the skin, skeletal system, eyes, and CNS. Its mode of inheritance is probably as an X-linked dominant trait.

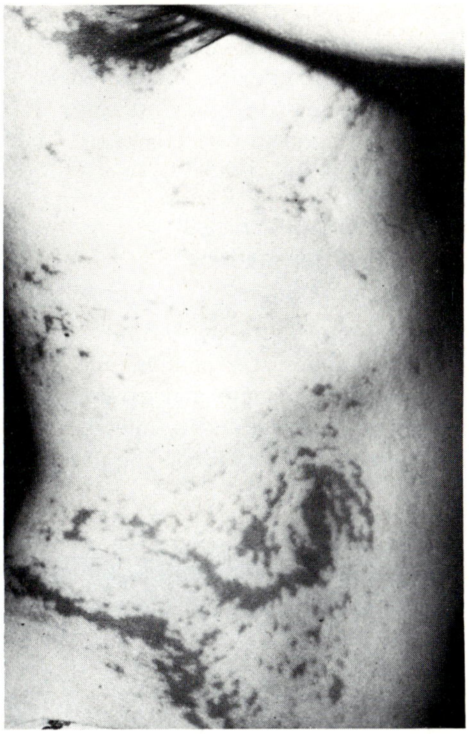

Fig. 38-6. Incontinentia pigmenti. Whorled chocolate-brown macular hyperpigmented lesions on the trunk.

Almost all patients are female, but a few affected males have been reported. The cutaneous lesions are usually present at birth and have three morphologic stages. Initially there are inflammatory vesicles, which are arranged linearly and appear in crops during the first few weeks of life. Pigmented, warty excrescences develop next, usually on the distal limbs. Finally a patterned, macular hyperpigmentation in streaks and whorls appears on the trunk and extremities (Fig. 38-6). These bizarre pigmented lesions represent the third and end stage. Occasionally pigmentation may accompany some of the early lesions.

The vesicular lesions occur on the trunk and limbs and vary in density from few to many. Nail hypoplasia, areas of alopecia, and ocular and skeletal abnormalities may also be detected. There is often peripheral eosinophilia during the vesicular phase of the disease. The diagnosis should be considered when inflammatory vesicles arranged in lines are seen in a newborn female infant. Delayed dentition, partial anodontia, and abnormalities of the CNS can occur but may not be apparent during the neonatal period. Biopsy of a small blister demonstrates a subcorneal vesicle filled with eosinophils. The differential diagnosis includes herpes simplex infection and other blistering diseases. The clinical evolution of the cutaneous process, the demonstration of large numbers of eosinophils in the skin lesion and peripheral blood, and the presence of pigment-laden macrophages in the upper dermis of end-stage lesions establish the diagnosis. No specific therapy is required for the skin lesions; if inflammation becomes excessive during the vesicular phase, treatment with compresses and topical steroids may be helpful.

OTHER BULLOUS DISEASES

Acrodermatitis enteropathica

Acrodermatitis enteropathica, a rare disorder, is inherited as an autosomal recessive trait. It is characterized by acute vesicobullous, eczematous, and psoriasiform eruptions around the mouth and genitals and on the peripheral extremities. Secondary infection with *C. albicans* is a common complication. The onset may be as early as the third week of life, but more frequently it occurs later in infancy. Failure to thrive, hair loss, marked irritability, and paronychial lesions are additional features of the disease. Chronic, severe, and intractable diarrhea is the most serious manifestation and may be life threatening. The disease is caused by a defect in zinc metabolism, and extremely low plasma zinc levels have been documented in untreated patients; the exact nature of the defect is unknown. Oral zinc sulfate is the treatment of choice and has induced dramatic remissions of the disease. A similar eruption has been noted in premature infants maintained on total parenteral nutrition inadequately supplemented with zinc. These infants suffer from relative zinc deficiency caused by high metabolic demands.

A

B

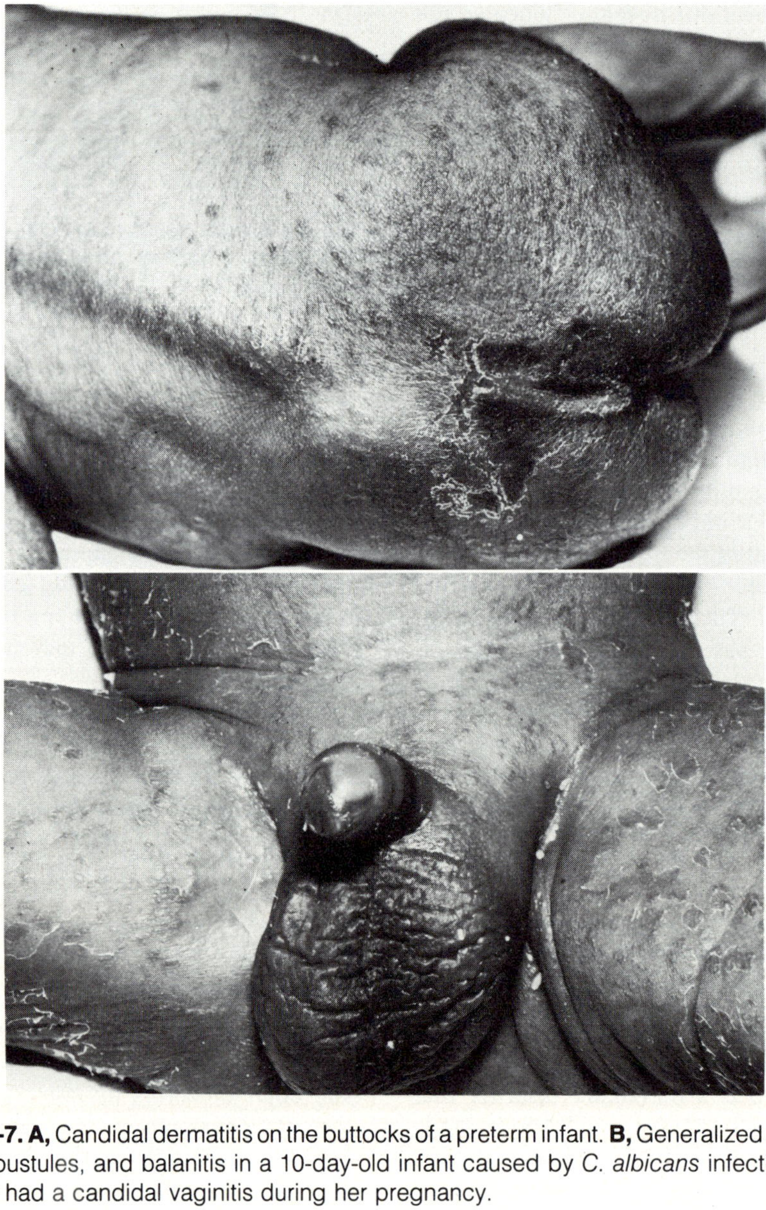

Fig. 38-7. A, Candidal dermatitis on the buttocks of a preterm infant. **B,** Generalized scaling, vesicopustules, and balanitis in a 10-day-old infant caused by *C. albicans* infection. The mother had a candidal vaginitis during her pregnancy.

Candidiasis

See also Chapter 31, part three.

Cutaneous candidiasis in infancy may be a mild episodic disease or a chronic disorder, or it may result in disseminated infection and death. The latter two forms often are associated with multiple endocrinopathies, a defect in the immune response, or both. Candidiasis in the first 4 weeks of life is usually benign and is most often localized to the oral cavity (thrush) or the diaper area (Fig. 38-7). If maternal vaginal organisms are acquired during the birth process, the infant may manifest symptomatic mouth lesions or become an intestinal carrier. Fecal contamination is the usual source of the organism in candidal dermatitis. Paronychial lesions also may occur, particularly in thumb-sucking infants. Rarely, cutaneous or systemic candidiasis may be present at birth as a result of transplacental or ascending infection.

The early cutaneous lesions are vesicular with an areola of erythema; these rapidly become pustular and confluent, forming a moist erosion surrounded by satellite pustules. In the chronic mucocutaneous or granulomatous forms (rare in the neonatal period) the scalp, lips, hands, and nails may be sites of chronically scaling, heaped-up lesions. The diagnosis is aided by identification of budding yeast spores on Gram stain or of spores and pseudohyphae on a potassium hydroxide preparation. Growth of the organism is rapid on Sabouraud's or Mycosel agar.

Treatment depends on the extent of involvement. Specific topical candidicidal agents include nystatin, amphotericin B, and the imidazole group. Systemic administration of amphotericin B or 5-fluorocytosine should be reserved for those patients with evidence of severe disseminated disease involving more than the gastrointestinal tract and skin.

PIGMENTARY ABNORMALITIES

The melanocyte system of the newborn skin is not usually at maximum functional maturity. As a result, all babies, even black, Indian, or oriental, may look pink or tan at birth. Within the first few weeks racial color becomes more evident because melanin production has been stimulated by exposure to light. For purposes of classification it is useful to think of pigmentary changes as diffuse or localized.

Diffuse hyperpigmentation

The intensity of pigmentation must be considered in light of the infant's genetic and racial background. Diffuse hyperpigmentation in the newborn is a very unusual occurrence. It may be caused by a gene whose main effect is on the melanocyte, by a hereditary disease that has secondary pigmentary consequences, by endocrinopathy, by a nutritional disorder, or by hepatic disease. Although in such cases hyperpigmentation may be described as diffuse, in fact it may be accentuated in certain areas, such as the face, over bony prominences, or in the flexural creases.

Localized hyperpigmentation

Flat lesions

Café au lait patches. These pigmented macules, which may be present in the newborn infant (Fig. 38-8, *A*), are light brown in whites and dark brown in blacks. Solitary lesions are found in approximately 19% of normal children and have no significance. Lesions that are greater than 1.5 cm in length, more than six in number, and especially when accompanied by axillary freckling, are strongly suggestive of neurofibromatosis (Fig. 38-8, *B*). The axillary freckles really represent tiny café au lait spots. Café au lait spots are often the first cutaneous lesions to appear in neurofibromatosis, but they may increase so slowly in number that additional genetic and clinical investigations may be required to establish a diagnosis. For example, small pigmented spots (Lisch nodules) may be detected on the iris by slitlamp examination in most patients over the age of 6 years with classic neurofibromatosis. Melanin macroglobules may be identified in the café au lait spots of neurofibromatosis, but they may be found as well in the pigmentary lesions of other disorders. Patients with tuberous sclerosis also may have café au lait spots. They are identical in appearance to those of neurofibromatosis but are usually accompanied by white macules (as discussed later).

McCune-Albright syndrome. In McCune-Albright syndrome the pigmented patch is usually unilateral, elongated, and large (more than 10 cm), with a ragged, irregular ("coast of Maine") border. Melanin macroglobules are less common in the melanocytes of these café au lait spots than in those of neurofibromatosis.

Nevocellular nevi. Approximately 1% to 2% of newborn infants have pigmented nevi of the congenital type. Small lesions (as opposed to giant pigmented nevi) are light to dark brown, often with variegated color or speckling and an accentuated epidermal surface ridge pattern (Fig. 38-9). These lesions vary in site, size, and number but are most often solitary. Histologically many of them are characterized by the presence of nevus cells in the deeper dermis and fat and in perivascular, periappendageal, and perineural sites throughout the dermis. Although there is no clear-cut evidence that the small congenital nevus is a premalignant lesion, it is the prevailing opinion that these lesions pose a significant risk for development of malignant melanoma, mostly during adult life. For this reason, many dermatologists advise removal of these lesions before or about the time of puberty. Should the family elect to observe rather than excise the nevus, periodic evaluation of the lesion for surface changes and associated symptoms should be carried out. Biopsy is

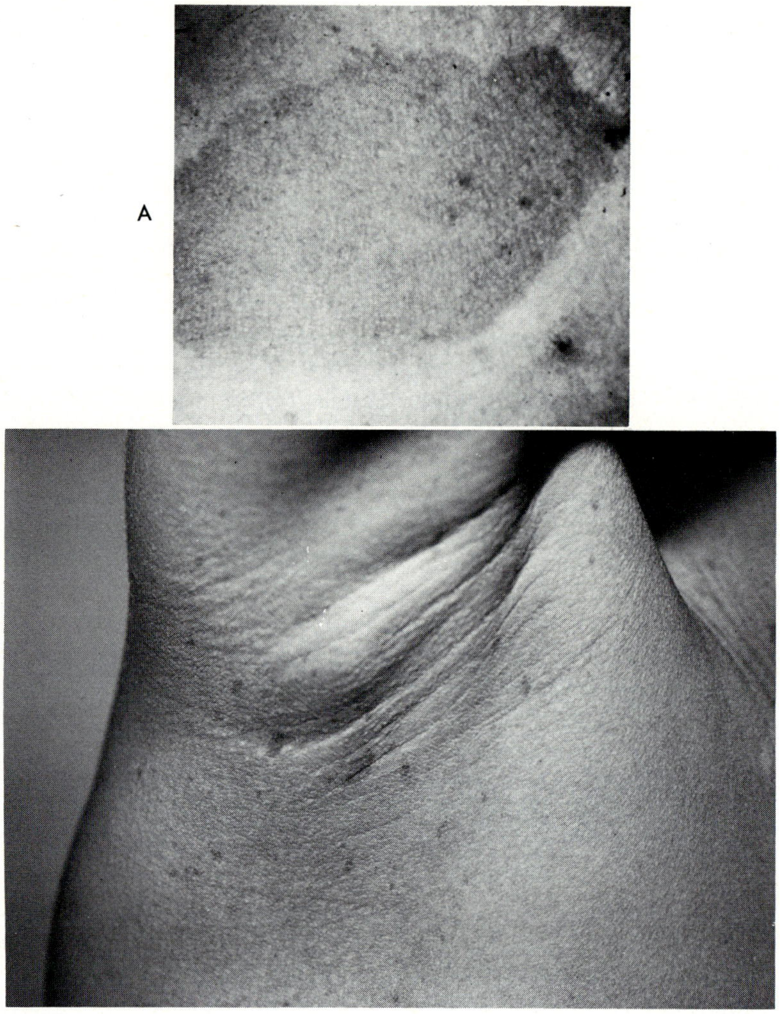

A

B

Fig. 38-8. A, Café au lait patch. **B,** Axillary freckling in neurofibromatosis.

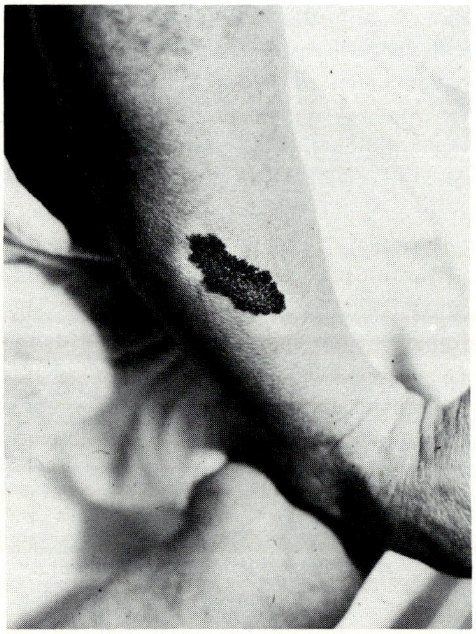

Fig. 38-9. Pigmented nevus on the leg of a newborn.

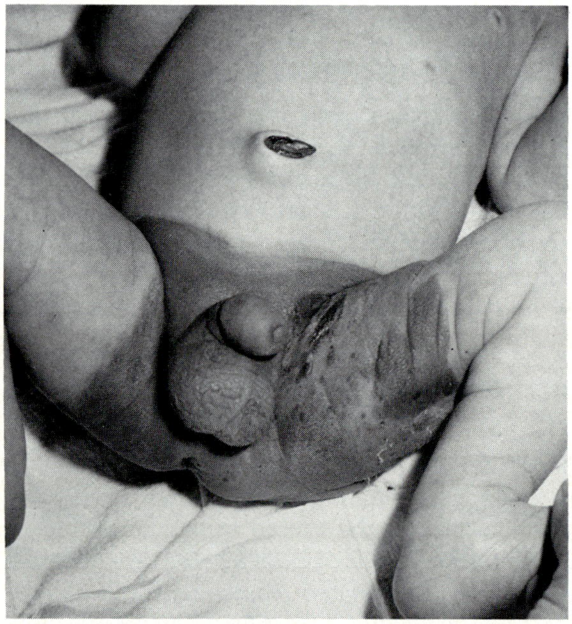

Fig. 38-10. Giant pigmented nevus in the bathing trunk area.

indicated in instances where malignant change is suspected.

Peutz-Jeghers syndrome. The cutaneous lesions of the Peutz-Jeghers syndrome may be present at birth or develop soon thereafter. They consist of pigmented macules, somewhat darker than freckles, that develop around the nose and mouth. The lips and oral mucosa often are involved, as are the hands, fingertips, and nails. Macular hyperpigmentation is the only visible sign of this autosomal dominant disorder until adolescence, when the patient begins to suffer from attacks of intussusception—evidence of coexisting small bowel polyposis.

Xeroderma pigmentosum. Xeroderma pigmentosum is transmitted by an autosomal recessive gene and results in marked hypersensitivity to ultraviolet light. Soon after birth, depending on the rapidity and intensity of light exposure, the infant develops erythema, speckled hyperpigmentation, atrophy, actinic keratoses, and all known types of cutaneous malignancy. The outcome is often fatal by the second decade of life as a result of metastatic disease. The underlying abnormality is a deficiency in an endonuclease that is responsible for the repair of DNA damaged by ultraviolet light. Genetic heterogeneity has been demonstrated in patients with xeroderma pigmentosum who have defective excision repair of DNA. Seven complementation groups have been identified, each with a characteristic range of DNA repair rates. Patients in each of these groups differ with regard to clinical features and epidemiologic patterns. For example, neurologic involvement is usual in certain variants. Protection from ultraviolet light exposure is mandatory, since this will prevent many of the cutaneous abnormalities and tumors. According to Cleaver, prenatal diagnosis of xeroderma pigmentosum is possible by using autoradiography to measure abnormal DNA synthesis of desquamated cells obtained from amniotic fluid.

Postinflammatory hyperpigmentation. Hyperpigmentation may result secondarily from any inflammatory process in the skin and thus may have many causes, including primary irritant dermatitis, infectious processes, panniculitis, and hereditary diseases, such as epidermolysis bullosa. The hyperpigmentation may result from an increase in melanosome production, increased melanin deposits in basal cells, increased numbers of keratinocytes, increase in the thickness of the stratum corneum, or deposits of melanin in dermal melanophages.

Raised lesions

The most important of the congenital pigmented nevi is the *giant hairy (garment) nevus* (Fig. 38-10). About 10% of these patients develop malignant melanoma in the nevus over a lifetime. These nevi may occupy 15% to 35% of the body surface, most often involving the trunk. The pigmentation is often variegated from light brown to black. The affected skin may be leathery in consistency. Almost invariably, numerous pigmented nevi coexist elsewhere on the body. Leptomeningeal melanocytosis has been documented in some of these patients, and this latter complication may be manifested as seizures.

The melanocytic invasion may involve subcutaneous tissue, fascia, or even underlying muscle. Because of the significant incidence of malignant degeneration, the hideous deformity and the intense pruritus that may accompany them, it is desirable when feasible to surgically excise these lesions as soon as possible. The infant should be old enough to withstand major surgery. *Intradermal* or *compound* (involving both epidermal junction and dermis) *nevi,* circumscribed, hairy or nonhairy, and pigmented, may be present at birth. They occur everywhere but on the palms and soles and may be flat or elevated, warty, or dome shaped. Histologically the melanocytic nevus cells are found localized to the upper dermis and around the appendages and contain variable amounts of pigment. Usually the diagnosis presents no problem, nor does their surgical removal.

Occasionally a *blue nevus* (so called because of its Prussian blue color) or dermal melanocytoma may be present at birth. They are usually 1 to 3 cm in diameter, oval, dome-shaped tumors found on the upper half of the body. They grow very slowly and have little tendency to become malignant but may be difficult to differentiate clinically from vascular tumors. Excisional biopsy is diagnostic and curative of the condition.

Incontinentia pigmenti and urticaria pigmentosa (mastocytosis)

Both incontinentia pigmenti and urticaria pigmentosa, which start as blistering diseases, have hyperpigmentation as a prominent feature of the process (see earlier discussion).

Hypopigmentation

Diffuse or localized loss of cutaneous pigment in the neonate may be caused by a heritable or developmental disorder or may be acquired as a result of a nutritional disease or postinflammatory change. Decrease in cutaneous melanin may be caused by an absence or destruction of melanocytes or by a defect in one of four biologic processes: formation of melanosomes, formation of melanin, transfer of melanosomes into keratinocytes, and transport of melanosomes by keratinocytes.

Albinism (complete albinism, oculocutaneous albinism)

Albinism, which occurs in all races, has an incidence of between 1:5,000 to 1:25,000; the phenotypic picture is caused by an autosomal recessive gene. Several forms of this disorder have been delineated. The affected infant usually has markedly reduced skin pigment, yellow or white hair, pink pupils, gray irides, photophobia, and cutaneous photosensitivity. Melanocytic nevi can be present in patients with albinism, and the nevi may or may not be pigmented. In blacks the skin may be tan; the hair may have a yellow or orange color; freckles can appear on exposure to light. The usual eye findings are nystagmus and a central scotoma with reduced visual acuity. Other associated abnormalities reported in albinism are small stature and coagulation disorders.

The biochemical defect responsible for this disorder is a deficiency of tyrosinase, the enzyme responsible for converting tyrosine to dopa, an early step in the formation of melanin (Chapter 36). The range of tyrosinase deficiency correlates well with the spectrum of color seen in affected individuals. Structurally the melanosomes appear to be normal. Treatment is aimed at protection from ultraviolet light, since early actinic keratoses and squamous cell carcinoma are common occurrences in these patients.

Partial albinism (piebaldism)

Partial albinism (better called segmental albinism) is an inherited disease caused by an autosomal dominant gene. It is present at birth but may not be evident in fair-skinned infants because of a lack of contrast in skin color. The differential diagnosis may include vitiligo, achromic nevus, nevus anemicus, and the hypomelanotic macules of tuberous sclerosis. In piebaldism the hair and skin are affected. The amelanotic areas usually involve the widow's peak and anterior scalp, forehead to the base of the nose, the chin, thorax, trunk, back, midarm, and midleg. There are normal islands of pigment within the amelanotic areas, and the distribution pattern is fairly constant. Examination of an affected area by electron microscopy shows an absence of melanocytes or melanocytes with markedly deformed melanosomes. Repigmentation does not take place.

Phenylketonuria

Phenylketonuria, caused by an absence of phenylalanine hydroxylase, results in a variety of neurologic and cutaneous abnormalities, which include mental retardation, seizures, diffuse hypopigmentation, eczema, and photosensitivity (Chapter 36).

Chediak-Higashi syndrome

See also Chapter 32, part one.

The Chediak-Higashi syndrome is a rare, fatal disorder transmitted by an autosomal recessive gene. Its clinical features include diffuse to moderate reduction in cutaneous and ocular pigment, photophobia, hepatosplenomegaly, and recalcitrant, recurrent infections. The leukocytes and other cells contain large granules, and this finding has its parallel in the melanocyte, which produces giant melanosomes. It is not known why there is a clinical pigmentary deficiency, but it appears to have little to do with true albinism. Windhorst and Padgett have speculated that the basic defect is a structural defect in the lipoprotein matrix that gives rise to the melanosome (and granulocytic lysosomes). Thus the melanin granule either is destroyed too easily or cannot be transferred to the keratinocyte (melanocytic impaction). The diagnosis may be made by the characteristic family history, physical findings, laboratory demonstration of abnormal leukocytes and melanosomes, and the usual course, which leads to death in childhood. Death results from a lymphoma-like process or infection. Hodgkin's disease recently has been reported as the fatal outcome in one patient.

Klein-Waardenburg syndrome

Klein-Waardenburg syndrome is inherited as an autosomal dominant condition; the most constant features are lateral displacement of the inner canthi of the eyes, a prominently broad nasal root, confluent eyebrows, variegation of pigment in the iris (heterochromia iridis) and fundus, congenital deafness, a white forelock, and cutaneous hypochromia. The clinical picture is quite striking and the diagnosis usually is not difficult. Although usually limited to small areas, the hypopigmentation may be severe and extensive enough to resemble that of piebaldism.

Nevus anemicus

Nevus anemicus is a permanent pale, mottled lesion that occurs most often on the trunk. The lesions contain normal amounts of pigment. There is no decrease in the number of blood vessels in the affected area, but the vascular tone is increased because of an excess local accumulation of catecholamines. There is no effective treatment.

Nevus achromicus

Present at birth, nevus achromicus is usually a unilateral, somewhat hypopigmented, irregularly shaped, bizarre, streaky lesion. The hypopigmented area is quite uniform in color and, in contrast to nevus anemicus, the vessels within it react normally to rubbing. The melanocytes in the affected epidermis seem to be functioning poorly or not at all. Large areas of nevus achromicus may be associated with an increased incidence of abnormalities, particularly of the musculoskeletal, ocular, and central nervous system (hypomelanosis of Ito).

White spots in tuberous sclerosis

From 50% to 90% of infants with tuberous sclerosis have white macules that become apparent at birth or soon thereafter (Fig. 38-11). In fair-skinned infants the hypopigmented areas may be more easily demonstrated by examining the skin with a Wood's lamp. These lesions

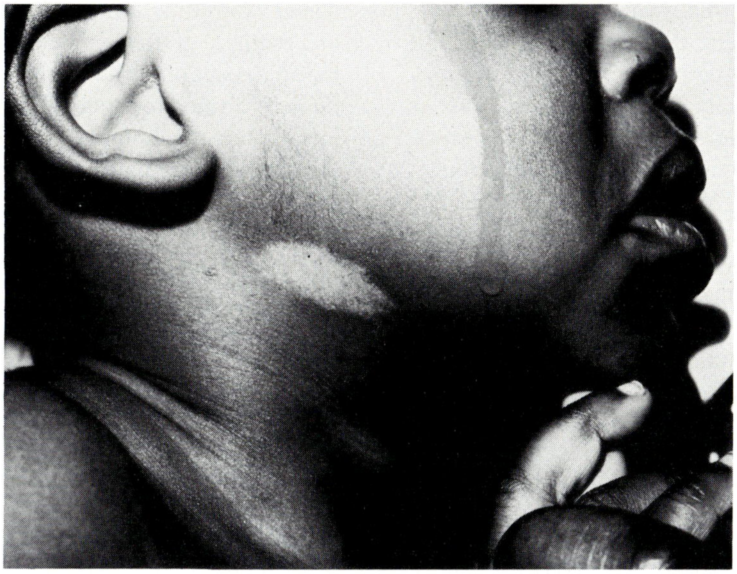

Fig. 38-11. White leaf macule in a child with tuberous sclerosis.

are variable in number and occur more frequently on the trunk and buttocks. The melanocytes within areas of macular hypopigmentation contain poorly pigmented melanosomes.

ANGIOMAS

Cutaneous hemangiomas are common developmental nevoid lesions involving the dermal and subcutaneous vasculature. They are either superficial (approximately 65%), subcutaneous (15%), or mixed (20%). The terms *capillary* and *cavernous* refer to the histopathologic patterns apparent on biopsy. Capillary hemangiomas show only dilated vessels, with or without endothelial proliferation; cavernous hemangiomas have large, dilated, blood-filled cavities with a compressed endothelial lining.

Capillary and cavernous hemangiomas

The strawberry (capillary) hemangioma is a raised, circumscribed, soft, bright red tumor that is lobulated and compressible. When a deeper (cavernous) component is present, it consists of a bluish red mass with less well-defined borders. If the entire nevus is deeply situated, the overlying skin may appear normal or show only a blue discoloration. The histologic pattern will depend on whether the angioma is purely capillary, cavernous, or mixed in type.

Approximately 20% to 30% of raised angiomatous nevi are present at birth (Fig. 38-12, *A*), and roughly 90% are evident by the second month of age. The remainder have their onset between the second and ninth months of life. Girls are affected more often than boys. The most common site is the face, and most infants have a single

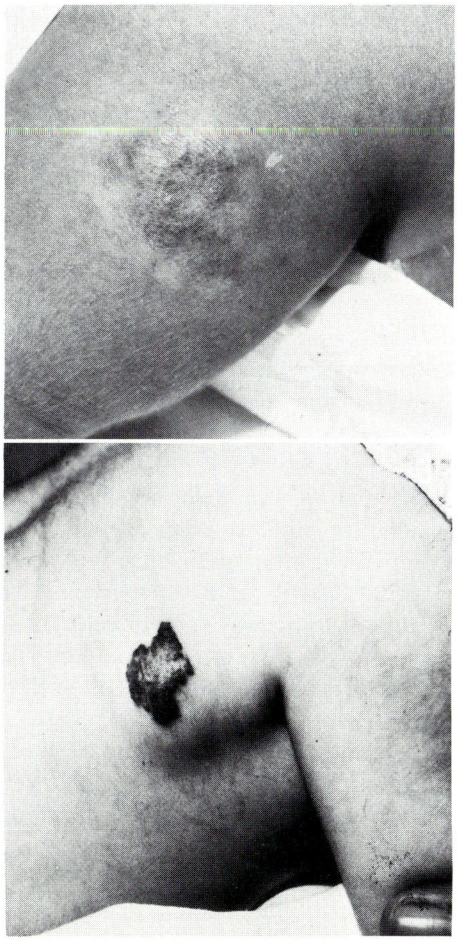

A

B

Fig. 38-12. A, Hemangioma on the thigh of a preterm infant. Areas of pallor, often an initial sign, are still present. **B,** Mixed capillary and cavernous hemangioma on the back.

lesion (Fig. 38-12, *B*). Virtually all these lesions show some increase in size during the first 6 months of life, often with an initial rapid growth spurt. The phase of active expansion, particularly in larger nevi, may result in ulceration, which is usually of no consequence unless complicated by secondary infection or hemorrhage.

If left untreated, most of the hemangiomas in this group will involute spontaneously. Regression may be anticipated when pale gray areas appear on the previously bright red surface of the lesion. Approximately 50% of hemangiomas disappear by 5 years of age and 70% by 7 years of age. Rapidity and completeness of resolution seen unrelated to the size of the lesion or age of appearance. In some patients there are no residual skin changes; others show variable degrees of atrophy and telangiectasia. Lesions that ulcerate tend to scar and therefore may result in a less satisfactory cosmetic appearance. Profuse hemorrhage is rare unless there is an accompanying thrombocytopenia or coagulation defect. Minor degrees of hemorrhage usually can be managed by compression bandages.

The vast majority of patients with strawberry hemangiomas require no treatment other than careful monitoring to detect possible complications and to provide much needed reassurance to parents. However, under certain circumstances, intervention may be indicated. Such situations include rapid growth of a lesion that compromises a vital structure, marked tissue destruction, or associated symptomatic thrombocytopenia. Surgical excision is one means of approach, but an acceptable cosmetic result is not always achieved. A short intensive course of oral corticosteroids may be effective in young infants if severity of involvement warrants such therapy. Alternate-day corticosteroid therapy has been shown to be successful in some infants.

Kasabach-Merritt syndrome

The association of thrombocytopenia, microangiopathic hemolytic anemia, an acute or chronic consumption coagulopathy, and a rapidly enlarging hemangioma is known as the *Kasabach-Merritt syndrome*. This phenomenon is most frequently seen in early infancy, and in one review of 74 cases the median age of hospital admission was 5 weeks. Most but not all of the hemangiomas associated with the coagulopathy are very large. Hematologic evaluation should include clotting studies, fibrinogen level, fibrin split products, and levels of factors II, V, and VIII in addition to the hemoglobin, platelet count, and smear.

In contrast to the infant with a hemangioma and normal hematologic findings, the infant with Kasabach-Merritt syndrome usually needs to be hospitalized and treated promptly. Spontaneous petechiae and ecchymoses, bruising, prolonged bleeding from punctures or orifices, oozing from the umbilicus or circumcision site, or rapid enlargement of the hemangiomatous mass are indications for intervention. The hematologic abnormalities have been attributed to sequestration and destruction of platelets within the hemangioma as well as increased consumption of coagulation factors. Treatment is determined by the clinical and hematologic findings and may include fresh blood, fresh frozen plasma, or platelet-rich transfusions, heparinization, systemic corticosteroid therapy, and inhibitors of platelet function such as aspirin and dipyridamole. Surgical extirpation of the hemangioma, when feasible, will usually result in prompt recovery. A few of these infants have recovered without treatment after spontaneous involution of the hemangioma.

Miliary hemangiomatosis (diffuse neonatal hemangiomatosis)

Miliary hemangiomatosis is a rare disorder in which multiple hemangiomas develop in the skin and viscera, most commonly the gastrointestinal tract, liver, CNS, and lungs. Despite supportive therapy, affected infants can die early in life from intractable high-output failure, gastrointestinal hemorrhage, respiratory tract obstruction, or severe neurologic deficiency caused by extensive compression by CNS angiomas. Corticosteroid therapy has been successful in some instances. Multiple cutaneous hemangiomas can also occur in the absence of visceral lesions. These infants have a benign course and can be observed expectantly.

Blue rubber bleb nevus syndrome

The blue rubber bleb nevus syndrome is a rare disorder consisting of multiple cavernous hemangiomas of the skin and bowel. Cutaneous lesions sometimes are present at birth, and their appearance is characteristic, as the descriptive name of this syndrome suggests. The lesions are blue to purple, rubbery, compressible protuberances that vary from a few millimeters to 3 to 4 cm in diameter. They are diffusely distributed over the body surface and may be sparse or number in the hundreds. Gastrointestinal lesions are common in the small bowel but also may involve the colon. Occasionally lesions in the liver, spleen, and CNS also have been noted. Severe anemia may result from recurrent episodes of gastrointestinal bleeding. Neither the skin nor the bowel lesions regress spontaneously. Surgery is sometimes palliative, but it is frequently impossible to resect all the affected bowel.

Cavernous hemangiomas also have been reported as a congenital feature of Riley-Smith syndrome and Leroy's syndrome (I cell disease). *Maffucci's syndrome* (cavernous hemangiomas and dyschondroplasia) and *Gorham's disease* (cavernous hemangiomas and disappearing bones) are not usually apparent in the neonatal period.

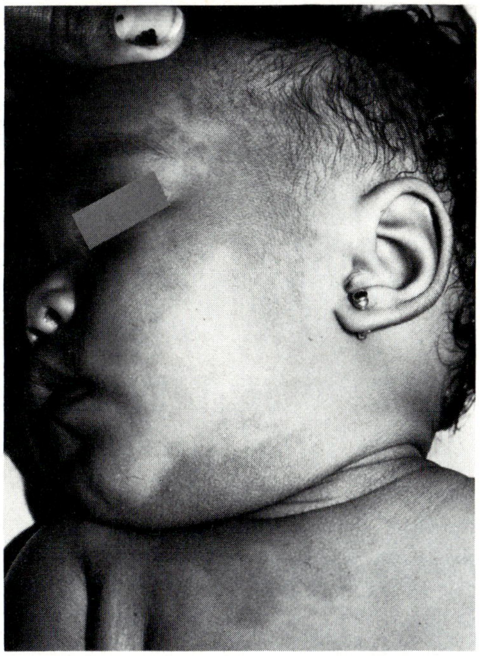

Fig. 38-13. Nevus flammeus on the upper face, chin, neck, and anterior chest. This infant had a similar lesion on the other side of the face.

Port-wine stain (nevus flammeus)

Nevus flammeus is present at birth and should be considered a permanent developmental defect. These lesions may be only a few millimeters in diameter or may cover extensive areas, occasionally involving up to half the body surface. They do not proliferate after birth; the apparent increase in size is caused by growth of the child. A nevus flammeus may be localized to any body surface, but facial lesions are probably the most common (Fig. 38-13). Port-wine nevi usually are sharply demarcated and flat, but they may have a pebbly or slightly thickened surface. Variation in color ranges from pale pink to purple. The most successful modality of treatment in childhood is the use of an opaque cosmetic cream (such as *Covermark* or *Dermablend*) that blends with the surrounding skin. Laser therapy is quite effective in obliterating these nevi after puberty; infants and children are usually not responsive or are prone to hypertrophic scarring.

Most port-wine nevi occur as isolated defects and do not indicate involvement of other organs; however, occasionally the nevus flammeus may be a clue to the presence of certain vascular syndromes.

Sturge-Weber syndrome (encephalofacial angiomatosis)

Sturge-Weber syndrome consists of a facial port-wine nevus, usually in the cutaneous distribution of the trigeminal nerve, leptomeningeal angiomatosis, mental retardation, seizures, hemiparesis contralateral to the facial lesion, and ipsilateral intracortical calcification. Ocular manifestations are frequent and include buphthalmos, glaucoma, angioma of the choroid, hemianoptic defects, and optic atrophy (Chapter 39). Roentgenograms of the skull of the older child show pathognomonic "tramline," double-contoured calcifications in the cerebral cortex on the same side as the nevus flammeus. CT scan may detect the calcifications in the younger child before they are apparent on roentgenograms. Electroencephalography may demonstrate unilateral depression of cortical activity, with or without spike discharges.

The prognosis depends on the extent of cerebral involvement, rapidity of progression, and response to treatment. Anticonvulsant therapy and neurosurgical procedures have been of value in some patients.

Klippel-Trenaunay-Weber syndrome

Klippel-Trenaunay-Weber syndrome is characterized by a cutaneous macular vascular nevus (nevus flammeus), venous varicosities, and overgrowth of the bony structures and soft tissues of the involved part. The vascular lesions are usually apparent at birth. Rarely the hemangioma may be of the capillary or cavernous type and can be associated with arteriovenous shunts or lymphoangiomatous anomalies. Complications include severe edema, phlebitis, thrombosis, and ulceration of the affected area as well as hemangiomatous involvement of the viscera. The prognosis depends on the extent of involvement, which can be assessed by peripheral vascular studies and scans. Surgery may be effective in treating severe limb hypertrophy in some patients. Jobst garments are also helpful in some instances.

Macular vascular nevi also occur with moderate frequency in trisomy 13, Rubenstein-Taybi syndrome (broad thumbs and toes, slanted palpebral fissures, and hypoplastic maxilla), and in the Beckwith-Wiedemann syndrome (macroglossia, omphalocele, macrosomia, and cytomegaly of the fetal adrenal gland) (Chapter 37, part one).

Lymphangiomas

Lymphangiomas are hamartomatous malformations composed of dilated lymph channels that are lined by normal lymphatic endothelium. They may be superficial or cavernous and often are associated with anomalies of the regional lymphatic vessels.

Lymphangioma circumscriptum is probably the most common type of lymphangioma and may be present at birth or appear in early childhood. Areas of predilection are the oral mucosa, the proximal limbs, and the flexures (Fig. 38-14). The tumor consists of clustered, small, thick-walled vesicles resembling frog spawn; it is often

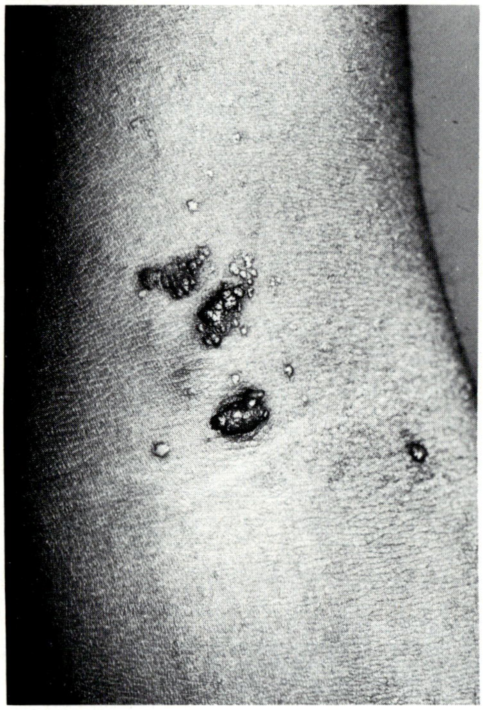

Fig. 38-14. Lymphangioma circumscriptum on the upper arm.

skin colored but may be of a red or purple cast because of a hemangiomatous component. Treatment is by excision with attention to removal of the deep component of the lesion. Large lesions may require full-thickness skin grafting. Recurrence has been noted even in full-thickness grafts.

Simple lymphangioma appears in infancy as a solitary, skin-colored, dermal or subcutaneous nodule. Following trauma it may exude serous fluid. Occasionally it has been associated with more extensive lymphatic involvement. Uncomplicated lesions may be removed by simple excision.

Cavernous lymphangioma is a diffuse, soft tissue mass consisting of large, cystic dilations of lymphatics in the dermis, subcutaneous tissue, and intermuscular septa. Surgery is impractical in most cases.

Cystic hygroma

Cystic hygroma is a benign, multilocular tumor usually found in the neck region. The tumors tend to increase in size and should be treated by surgical excision.

VERRUCOUS (EPIDERMAL OR ORGANOID) NEVI

Verrucous nevi are a group of lesions that are commonly found in the neonatal period. Most of them consist of an overgrowth of keratinocytes and may have an identifiable differentiation toward one of the appendages normally found in skin. They vary considerably in their size, clinical appearance, histologic characteristics, and evolution, depending on the topographic location of the lesion on the body. Lesions occurring in sites normally rich in sebaceous glands (such as the scalp) may look like sebaceous nevi, whereas others, found in areas where the epidermis is thick (e.g., the elbow), look primarily warty in nature (Fig. 38-15).

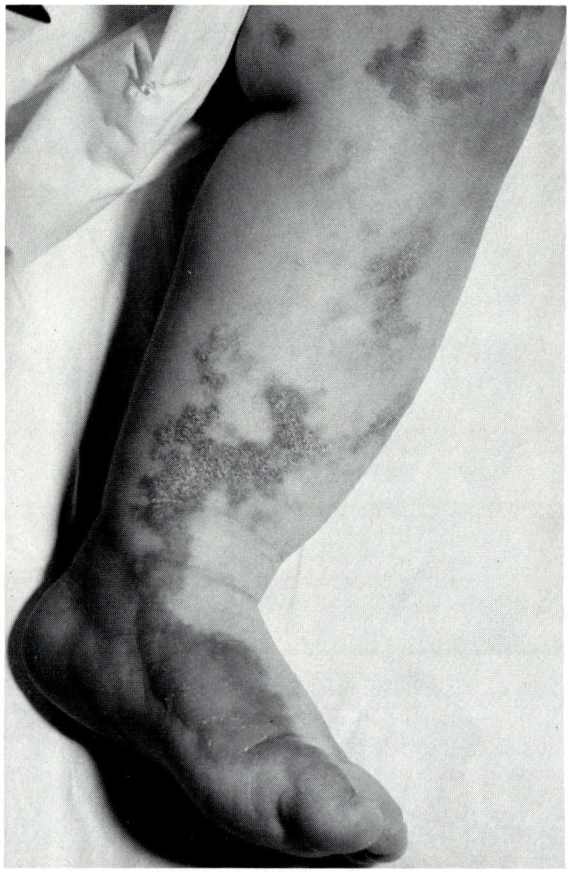

Fig. 38-15. Verrucous epidermal nevus on the leg of an infant.

Most commonly in the newborn period epidermal nevi take the form of a small papillomatous yellow or pink growth on the scalp, forehead, or face (simple sebaceous nevus). Since a significant incidence of basal cell epitheliomas occurs in these lesions after puberty, they should be removed surgically.

The treatment of large verrucous epidermal nevi is generally unsatisfactory. The only effective treatment necessitates removal of the lesion together with its underlying dermis. In localized lesions this may be accomplished by electrodesiccation and plastic repair; but this

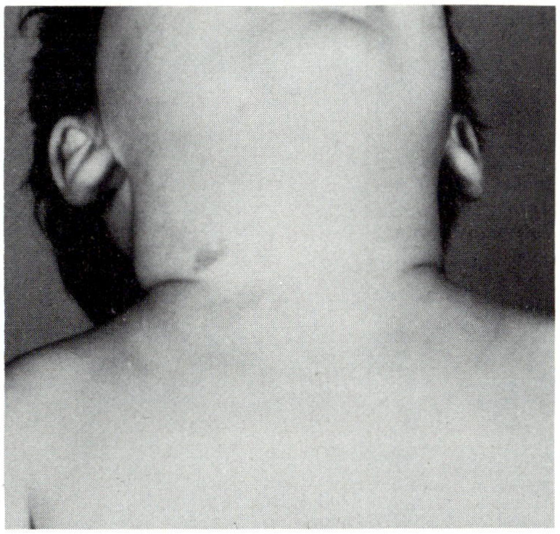

Fig. 38-16. Epidermal nevus on the right side of the neck in a child with hemihypertrophy.

treatment should be delayed beyond the neonatal period, since lesions may develop over a period of years. The scars that result from surgery may be as cosmetically unsatisfactory as the original lesion, and an extension of the nevus may appear beyond the repaired area. In the older child salicylic acid (3% in cold cream) may keep the lesion soft, and water-dispersible bath oils provide some palliative relief. When the nails are involved, no treatment is effective, and aside from trimming or filing the affected nails, none is indicated.

The epidermal nevus syndrome

Solomon and co-workers reviewed the associated findings in 23 patients with large epidermal nevi, including all the types previously described. In more than two thirds of these patients associated skeletal defects, ocular and vascular anomalies, and serious CNS disease were identified. The anomalies found included kyphoscoliosis, vertebral defects, shortened limbs, osseous hypertrophy, angiomas of the skin and CNS, mental retardation, convulsive disorders, ocular complications, Wilms' tumor, and vitamin D–resistant rickets (Fig. 38-16). In one study, the homogenized lesions injected into beagles were found to produce phosphatemia. Recently it has been shown that a parathyroid hormone–like protein may be extracted from cultured human keratinocytes. On discovering the existence of an epidermal nevus, the physician must take a careful family history and perform a thorough physical examination. Particular emphasis should be placed on the musculoskeletal and nervous systems, as well as on the eyes and skin. These infants may require baseline electroencephalographic studies and periodic roentgenographic evaluation of skeletal growth as well as a CT scan of the head. Renal studies to exclude tumor and inappropriate excretion of phosphate may also be indicated.

ECZEMA

The term *eczema* is a source of confusion. For the purposes of this discussion eczema is a "genus" of skin disorder of which there are several species (e.g., eczematous contact dermatitis). There are four phases of eczema, any one of which may persist as the dominant feature, depending on the age of the patient, the local physiologic characteristics of the skin involved, and the persistence of the underlying cause. The initial stage is *erythema*, which proceeds to microvesicle formation, *weeping*, or oozing. The epidermal response to the injurious process then causes a burst of rapid epidermal mitotic activity that leads to *scaling*. Finally, *lichenification* (thickening of the skin) and *pigmentary disturbances* supervene. In the young infant the first three stages predominate; lichenification is not seen.

Although the eczematous eruption itself is not difficult to recognize, it may be quite difficult to distinguish one type of eczema from another, particularly because the histologic features (spongiosis) in most of them are identical. The most common causes of eczema in the adult are least common in the newborn. Eczema is much less common in the neonatal period than in the infant older than 2 months. During the neonatal period eczema may be exogenous or endogenous. The exogenous causes include primary irritant contact dermatitis and infection. The endogenous group may be divided into those causes in which the skin's role is predominant and others in which the eruption reflects a serious systemic disease.

Primary irritancy (as opposed to allergy) is probably the most common exogenous cause of eczema in the newborn. The distribution of the eruption varies somewhat, depending on the precipitating agent. Saliva may be irritating to the face, and fecal excretions may be irritating to the buttocks. Detergent bubble bath, antiseptic proprietary agents, and harsh soaps may cause an acute eczematous diaper dermatitis, which may become generalized. Precise information about what has been applied to the skin is imperative in making an accurate diagnosis.

When exogenous agents have been excluded as a cause of the eruption and the infant is otherwise quite well, several diagnoses may be entertained. One of these is *seborrheic eczema (seborrheic dermatitis)*. This condition is characterized by greasy scaling associated with patchy redness, fissuring, and occasional weeping, usually involving the scalp, ears, axillary and perineal folds (Fig. 38-17). There is controversy as to whether the seborrheic eczema is a distinct entity or whether it presages

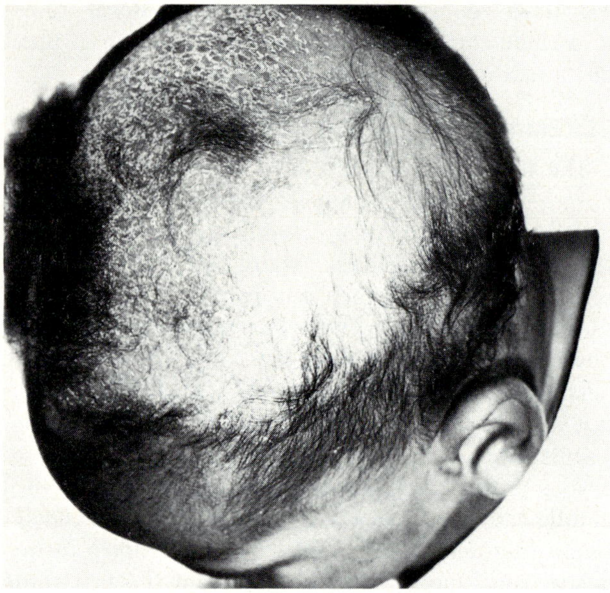

Fig. 38-17. Seborrheic dermatitis on the scalp of an infant resulting in partial alopecia.

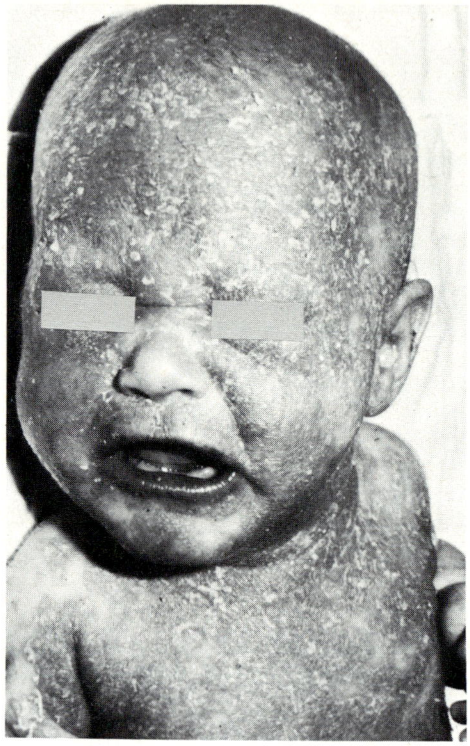

Fig. 38-18. Generalized seborrheic eczema.

the advent of atopic dermatitis. Some infants never progress beyond the seborrheic phase of the dermatitis, which in its classic form rarely is seen in the first month. *Cradle cap* is probably a minor variant of seborrheic eczema. The usual course of seborrheic eczema is one of rapid regression after 1 or 2 weeks of therapy. Occasionally a seborrheic-like process may involve the entire body, resulting in a full-blown exfoliative dermatitis (Fig. 38-18). It has been called *Leiner's disease* when associated with a defect in the function of the fifth component of complement (C5), a condition that is familial and extremely rare. Scaling also may result from staphylococcal scalded skin syndrome or congenital ichthyosiform erythroderma.

From the preceding discussion it should be clear that diaper dermatitis may have a variety of causes. Its proper management should include culture for bacteria and yeast, the discontinuance of all ointments containing irritants, and conservative treatment for 1 or 2 weeks (see later discussion). If no improvement follows, a skin biopsy may be indicated.

Eczema also may be a feature of a number of systemic conditions, including ataxia-telangiectasia, X-linked agammaglobulinemia, phenylketonuria, gluten-sensitive enteropathy, and long-arm 18 deletion syndrome. Most patients with hypohidrotic ectodermal dysplasia have an eczematous eruption identical to atopic dermatitis. Purpura is a frequent additional component of eczema, particularly in histiocytosis X and Wiskott-Aldrich syndrome.

Topical treatment of eczema

When bacterial or fungal infection exists, appropriate antibacterial or antifungal therapy is indicated based on the results of culture and sensitivity studies. Weeping lesions should be treated by compressing or bathing in tepid water; protective ointments, such as simple zinc oxide paste, should be applied after each diaper change; soiled ointments and pastes should be removed with mineral oil. A more extensive eruption may be treated for short periods with 1% hydrocortisone ointment. A scaly eruption in the scalp may be treated by frequent shampooing with a sulfur- or salicylic acid–containing shampoo. Bathing should be done in tepid water containing a water-dispersible oil. Infants with diffuse dermatitis lose heat readily and are intolerant of even mild changes in environmental temperature or humidity. Therefore humidification of the bedroom in winter and air conditioning in summer are desirable. The efficacy of dietary management of atopic eczema remains controversial. Dietary manipulation may add little to the beneficial effects of the treatments just suggested.

SUBCUTANEOUS AND INFILTRATIVE DERMATOSES

Juvenile xanthogranuloma

One fifth of infants with juvenile xanthogranuloma are affected at birth, and two thirds have onset of lesions

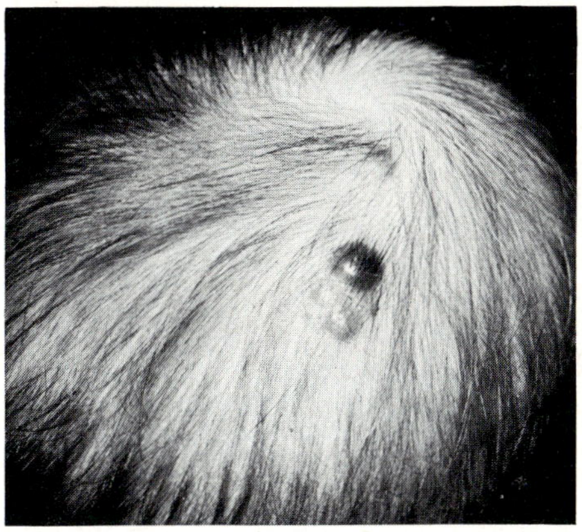

Fig. 38-19. Multiple papulonodular lesions of juvenile xanthogranuloma on the scalp.

before 6 months of age. There is no predilection for race or sex; no familial predisposition has been noted for this self-limited disorder, which usually remains confined to the skin. The skin lesions often are restricted to the head, neck, and upper trunk and typically are reddish yellow, small papules, which may enlarge to become nodules (Fig. 38-19). Involution may leave a flat atrophic pigmented scar. Serum lipids are normal, but histologically the lesions result from an infiltrate of fat-laden histiocytes, giant cells, and mixed inflammatory cells. Ocular lesions are the most frequent complication (although rarely involvement of other organs may occur) and may result in tumors, unilateral glaucoma, hyphema, uveitis, heterochromia iridis, and proptosis. Ophthalmologic consultation is required for management of the ocular lesions, but the best treatment for the skin lesions is expectant observation.

Mastocytosis

Mast cell disease may be present at birth and can result in a solitary mast cell tumor, a disseminated maculopapular or nodular eruption, a bullous eruption, or a diffuse infiltration of the skin. The disseminated form may be complicated by mast cell infiltrates in internal organs. The diagnosis can be made by demonstration of excessive numbers of mast cells on skin biopsy. The most common form noted at birth is the firm, solitary mast cell tumor. These are generally ovoid and pink or tan and rarely exceed 6 cm in diameter. The lesions are conspicuous by their tendency to form wheals when rubbed and, in the newborn, to develop overlying blisters. Solitary lesions involute spontaneously within months to years. The maculopapular and nodular eruptions often develop later in infancy. Systemic manifestations of histamine release in the form of flushing attacks or generalized pruritus are due to mechanical or chemical factors or overheating. Treatment is usually not necessary but in symptomatic patients distressing cutaneous symptoms, such as dermographism and pruritus, may be palliated with oral antihistamines. Hot water bathing and vigorous toweling must be avoided as well as histamine releasers such as codeine, morphine and its derivatives, aspirin, and polymyxin B. The prognosis for most patients with mastocytosis, even in its disseminated cutaneous form, is good. The genetics of this condition are unclear. A few pedigrees have been reported with multiple affected family members.

Subcutaneous fat necrosis and sclerema neonatorum

Both subcutaneous fat necrosis and sclerema neonatorum occur within the first 3 months of life. Recently it has been suggested that they may be variants of the same basic disorder of fat metabolism. Sclerema neonatorum usually affects the preterm or debilitated newborn. It is manifested by diffuse hardening of the subcutaneous tissue, resulting in a tight, smooth skin that feels bound to the underlying structures. The skin is cold and stony hard. The joints become immobile and the face masklike. The affected infant also may have multiple congenital anomalies or develop sepsis, pneumonia, or severe gastroenteritis. CNS abnormalities, autonomic dysfunction, and respiratory distress frequently complicate the course of the disease. The mortality is high, but the cutaneous changes rarely last longer than 2 weeks if the infant survives. For those infants who are severely ill, exchange transfusion and systemic administration of steroids have been used; however, their efficacy has not been confirmed.

The lesions of subcutaneous fat necrosis are localized and sharply circumscribed (Chapters 20 and 37, part two). They may appear as small nodules or large plaques and are found on the cheeks, buttocks, back, arms, and thighs. The affected tissue is hard, may appear reddish or violaceous, and occasionally has the texture of orange peel. Histologically there is a granulomatous reaction in the fat, with foreign body giant cells, fibroblasts, lymphocytes, and histiocytes. Resolution of the lesion results in fibrosis. Possible precipitating causes of fat necrosis include cold exposure, trauma, asphyxia, and peripheral circulatory collapse. Usually the lesions resolve in several weeks or months without complications. Rarely calcium may be deposited in the lesion, leading to ulceration and drainage. Careful drainage of calcified areas may lessen subsequent scarring.

Cold panniculitis

Cold-induced fat necrosis of the cheeks may occur in the small infant. Warm, red, indurated plaques appear a few hours to a few days following the episode of cold exposure. The lesions resolve in 2 to 3 weeks. An ice cube applied to normal skin of these patients for 2 minutes will result in formation of a nodule at the site of application. The induced nodule appears in 3 to 72 hours and parallels the course of the spontaneous lesion. The histologic picture is one of perivascular inflammation and aggregation of lipids from rupture of fat cells. Postinflammatory hyperpigmentation may mark the site of a healed nodule.

MISCELLANEOUS CONGENITAL DISEASES AFFECTING THE SKIN

A multitude of hereditary diseases affect the skin. Some of the congenital diseases with prominent cutaneous findings are reviewed.

Focal dermal hypoplasia (Goltz's syndrome)

Focal dermal hypoplasia is a profound mesodermal and ectodermal deficiency syndrome that occurs almost exclusively in females and appears to be inherited as an X-linked or simple dominant gene. The cutaneous lesions consist of linear streaks of atrophy, yellow-brown or red excrescences—some papillomatous and others with the appearance of partially deflated balloons—perioral and perianal papillomas, pigmentary variability, telangiectasia, sweating abnormalities, hyperkeratosis, alterations in the quality and density of hair, and vascular instability. There is almost complete absence of the dermis and its appendages in affected areas of skin; herniations of fat that lie just beneath the epidermis result in the characteristic yellow saclike nodules and papules. Associated with the cutaneous features are skeletal defects (spinal anomalies, microcrania, asymmetry of facial bones, absence of digits, syndactyly, phocomelia, and rib, scapular, clavicular, and pelvic anomalies), ocular anomalies (ranging from enophthalmia to minor pigmentary defects of the iris), dental anomalies, renal defects, CNS defects (mental retardation and seizures), and a variety of other soft tissue abnormalities affecting heart, gastrointestinal tract, and muscle.

Cutis laxa (generalized elastolysis)

There are two major forms of congenital cutis laxa: one inherited as an autosomal dominant trait and the other inherited in an autosomal recessive manner (Fig. 38-20). In both forms of the disease affected infants have diminished resilience of the skin, which hangs in folds and results in a bloodhound appearance, at once pathetic and aged. The joints are not hypermobile, and there is no tendency to increased bruising as in Ehlers-Danlos syndrome. Elastic tissue may be greatly diminished in the dermis and is of poor quality. The collagen has normal tensile properties. In the autosomal dominant form there are few complications, and the life span is usually normal. In the recessive type of cutis laxa, elastic fibers elsewhere in the body are defective, resulting in inguinal, diaphragmatic, and ventral hernias, rectal prolapse, diverticula of the gastrointestinal and genitourinary tracts, pulmonary emphysema, and aortic aneurysms. Cardiorespiratory complications may cause death during childhood.

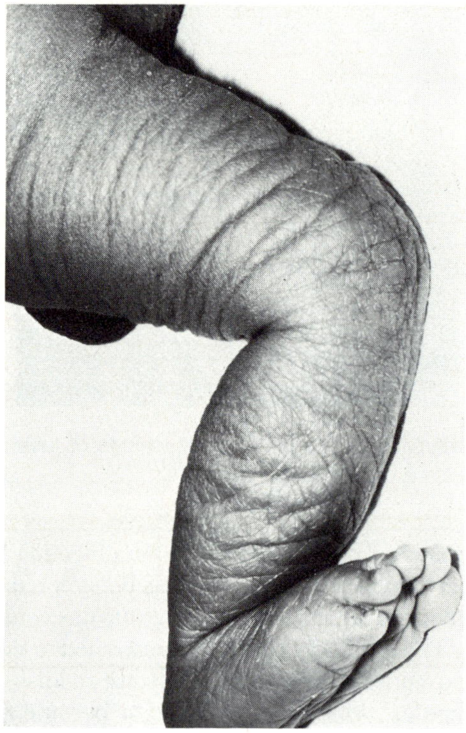

Fig. 38-20. Redundant skin on the leg of a neonate with cutis laxa and dwarfism.

Cutis hyperelastica (Ehlers-Danlos syndrome)

There are ten clinical forms of Ehlers-Danlos syndrome with the common features of hyperextensible skin, joint laxity, and soft tissue fragility. In addition, bleeding episodes and cardiovascular complications are characteristic of some forms of the disorder. The skin of patients with Ehlers-Danlos syndrome is hyperextensible when stretched but snaps back with normal resiliency. In contrast to cutis laxa, the skin does not hang in redundant folds, the joints are hypermobile, and there is a tendency to bruise easily. Associated findings may include short stature, scoliosis, periodontosis, and eye defects. Involvement of the gastrointestinal tract may lead to episodes of acute blood loss. Aortic aneurysms also may develop. All forms of the disease are inherited; some are autosomal dominant traits, others are autosomal recessive, and one form is X-linked. Biochemical studies have confirmed specific enzyme defects for types IV, V, VI, and VII.

THE ECTODERMAL DYSPLASIAS

Anhidrotic (hypohidrotic) ectodermal dysplasia

Absence of sweating, hypotrichosis, and defective dentition are the most striking features of this disorder, which is usually inherited in an X-linked recessive fashion. The existence of females with the full syndrome suggests that an autosomal recessive gene may cause the same phenotype. The facies is distinctive because of frontal bossing and depression of the bridge of the nose. Eyebrows and lashes are absent or sparse. The skin around the eyes is wrinkled and frequently hyperpigmented. The skin elsewhere is thin, dry, and hypopigmented, and the cutaneous vasculature is more visible.The scalp and body hair is sparse and the ears and chin prominent. The lips are thick and everted and may show pseudorhagades. Dental anomalies range from total anodontia to hypodontia with defective teeth.

The most striking physiologic abnormality is the absence of sweating, which can be demonstrated by application to the palm of 1 drop of 5% O-phthalaldehyde in xylene. Absence or hypoplasia of eccrine glands is confirmed by skin biopsy. Other glandular structures also may be absent or hypoplastic. Less constant ancillary findings include conductive hearing loss, gonadal abnormalities, stenotic lacrimal puncta, corneal dysplasia, and cataracts. Mental development is usually normal. Marked heat intolerance is caused by an inability to adequately regulate the body temperature by sweating. Fever occurs with increases in ambient temperature and exercise and should respond quickly to environmental cooling and rest. Some febrile reactions, however, may be caused by recurrent upper respiratory tract infections. Since the respiratory mucosa also may be deficient in mucous-secreting glands, viral respiratory tract infections in these patients tend to linger and become complicated by secondary bacterial infections in the bronchial tree. Every effort should be made to moderate extreme environmental temperatures by air conditioning. Deficient lacrimation can be palliated by the regular use of artificial tears. The nasal mucosa also must be protected by intermittent saline irrigations and application of petrolatum. It is imperative that these children have a thorough dental evaluation during the first years of life, and prostheses should be provided even for toddlers so that adequate nutrition is maintained. Reconstructive procedures can be performed later in life to improve the facial configuration. A wig may be required for patients with scant scalp hair.

The incidence of atopic diseases—asthma, allergic rhinitis, and atopic dermatitis—is increased significantly in patients with anhidrotic ectodermal dysplasia. Atopic manifestations should be managed as they would be in otherwise normal infants and children.

Numerous other types of ectodermal dysplasia have been defined including hidrotic ectodermal dysplasia, the EEC syndrome (ectrodactyly, ectodermal dysplasia, and cleft palate), Rapp-Hodgkin syndrome, and the Ellis-van Creveld syndrome. Isolated lack of sweat glands occurs in congenital familial anhidrosis.

DIAGNOSTIC TECHNIQUES

Punch biopsy technique

Cutaneous punch biopsy may provide valuable information and is a frequently used diagnostic procedure. Biopsy should be avoided around the eyelids and their margins, the tip and bridge of the nose, the cupid's bow of the lips, the columella of the upper lip, and the nipples. Hairy areas should be shaved. The site should be prepared with 70% alcohol and the area infiltrated with 0.5 to 1 ml of 1% lidocaine hydrochloride without epinephrine. A sharp 3 mm punch is pressed firmly against the lesion and gently rotated until a slight give is felt. Considerable gentleness and a sharp punch are required so that the epidermis is not torn away from the dermis in performing the biopsy, particularly in the blistering diseases. It is desirable to obtain some subcutaneous fat with each biopsy. Newborn fat generally will separate quite readily. One may cut the plug away from the underlying tissue with a sharp scissors. The tissue should not be squeezed. Usually no sutures are necessary, and a simple dressing will suffice for the healing period.

The specimen should be placed in a bottle containing 10% aqueous buffered formaldehyde solution (Formalin), and the bottle should be agitated to ensure that the skin plug is immersed in the formaldehyde solution. The bottle then should be labeled as to name, date, and site of biopsy. Clinical information should be included with the specimen sent to the pathologist. It is often desirable in a general pathology laboratory to inform the pathologist that a skin biopsy from an infant is being forwarded so that special care may be taken in the processing. Tiny specimens are easily lost during the gross examination or in automated tissue-processing devices.

PRINCIPLES OF THERAPY

Treatment of the skin of the newborn requires adjustment from the adult dosage of topical medicaments. The following guidelines are useful.

1. Minor fleeting erythematous macular or papular eruptions occur at the end of the first month. Their cause is unknown, and the best treatment is patience.
2. The more severe a dermatitis, the more vulnerable is the skin, and therefore the more conservative should be the topical therapy.
3. To treat appropriately and to induce confidence in the infant's family, one should know the natural course of a skin disease and so advise the parents.
4. Systemic complications of diffuse cutaneous erup-

tions occur more readily in infants; they should be anticipated and treated early.

5. If lesions in different stages are present on different parts of the body surface, the most acute stage should be treated.
6. It is best to know and use a few topical remedies. Plain tap water is one of the safest and most helpful treatments for any acute dermatitis.
7. Pruritus is often more trying for parents than for the infant. Environmental control of temperature and humidity and mild sedation is quite helpful for uncomplicated pruritus.
8. The passage of time is the most effective treatment of small, uncomplicated hemangiomas.
9. Talcum powder is unnecessary for skin care of infants and poses the risk of inhalation.
10. Normal skin does not need extensive lubrication. If lubrication is desirable, it is better to use cream (e.g., hydrophilic ointment) than oil.
11. Removal of a protective paste from the perineal area should be done gently with mineral oil, not by scrubbing with soap and water.
12. Lotions, pastes, and talc should not be used on weeping lesions.
13. Occlusive dressings (such as polyethylene film or plastic wrap) should not be used in this age group.
14. Daily shampoos are not harmful if used to treat seborrheic dermatitis.
15. Exposure to sunlight should be very gradual, especially in fair-skinned infants.
16. Topical anesthetic agents, proteolytic enzymes, and tar ointments are rarely indicated in this age group.

Nancy Burton Esterly
Lawrence M. Solomon

BIBLIOGRAPHY

Alper, J., Holmes, L.B., and Mihm, M.C., Jr.: Birthmarks with serious medical significance: nevocellular nevi, sebaceous nevi, and multiple cafe au lait spots, J Pediatr. **95**:696, 1979.

Arlette, J.P., and Johnston, M.M.: Zinc deficiency dermatosis in premature infants receiving prolonged parenteral alimentation, J. Am. Acad. Dermatol. **5**:37, 1981.

Aschinberg, L.C., and others: Vitamin D–resistant rickets associated with epidermal nevus syndrome: demonstration of a phosphatemic substance in the dermal lesions, J. Pediatr. **91**:56, 1977.

Atherton, D.J., and others: A double blind controlled cross-over trial of antigen avoidance diet in atopic eczema, Lancet **1**:401, 1978.

Baden, H.P., and others: Keratinization in the harlequin fetus, Arch. Dermatol. **118**:14, 1982.

Baran, R., and Dawber, R.P.R.: Diseases of the nails and their management, Oxford, 1984, Blackwell Scientific Publications.

Barman, J.M., and others: The first stage in the natural history of the human scalp hair cycle, J. Invest. Dermatol. **48**:138, 1967.

Beighton, P.: The dominant and recessive forms of cutis laxa, J. Med. Genet. **9**:216, 1972.

Brown, S.H., Jr., Neerhout, R.C., and Fonkalsrud, E.W.: Prednisone therapy in the management of large hemangiomas in infants and children, Surgery **71**:168, 1972.

Carney, R.G., Jr.: Incontinentia pigmenti: a world statistical analysis, Arch. Dermatol. **112**:535, 1976.

Carr, A., and others: Relationship between erythema toxicum and maturity, Am. J. Dis. Child. **112**:129, 1966.

Cataldo, E., and Berkman, M.D.: Cysts of the oral mucosa in newborns, Am. J. Dis. Child. **116**:44, 1968.

Champion, R.H.: Disorders of sweat glands. In Rook, A., Wilkinson, D.S., and Ebling, F.J.G., editors: Textbook of dermatology, ed. 3, Philadelphia, 1979, F.A. Davis Co.

Cleaver, J.E.: Xeroderma pigmentosum; progress and regress, J. Invest. Dermatol. **60**:374, 1973.

Cooper, T.W., and Bauer, E.A.: Epidermolysis bullosa: a review, Pediatr. Dermatol. **1**:181, 1984.

Curran, J.P., Al-Salihi, F.L.: Neonatal staphylococcal scalded skin syndrome: massive outbreak due to an unusual phage type, Pediatrics **66**:285, 1980.

Deutsch, T.A., and Esterly, N.B.: Elastic fibers in fetal dermis, J. Invest. Dermatol. **65**:320, 1975.

Elias, P.M., Fritsch, P., and Epstein, E.H., Jr.: Staphylococcal scalded skin syndrome, Arch. Dermatol. **113**:207, 1977.

Elias, S., and others: Prenatal diagnosis of harlequin ichthyosis, Clin. Genet. **17**:275, 1980.

Fost, N.C., and Esterly, N.B.: Successful treatment of juvenile hemangiomas with prednisone, J. Pediatr. **72**:351, 1968.

Freire-Maia, N., and Pinheiro, M.: Ectodermal dysplasias: a clinical and genetic study, New York, 1985, Alan R. Liss, Inc.

Fromm, A.: Epstein's pearls, Bohn's nodules and inclusion cysts of the oral cavity, J. Dent. Child. **34**:275, 1967.

Gorlin, R.J., and Pindborg, J.J.: Syndromes of the head and neck, New York, 1964, McGraw-Hill Book Co.

Green, M.: Comparison of adult and neonatal skin eccrine sweating. In Masbrich, H.I., and Boisits, E.K., editors: Neonatal skin, New York, 1981, Marcel Dekker.

Griffiths, A.D.: Skin desquamation in the newborn, Biol. Neonate **10**:127, 1966.

Hamada, H.: Age changes in melanocyte distribution of the normal human epidermis, Jpn. J. Dermatol. **82**:223, 1972.

Harris, J.R., and Schick, B.: Erythema neonatorum, Am. J. Dis. Child. **92**:27, 1956.

Holbrook, K.: Basic science. In Hanson, R., and Schachner, L., editors: Pediatric dermatology. (In press.)

Holden, K.R., and Alexander, F.: Diffuse neonatal hemangiomatosis, Pediatrics **46**:411, 1970.

Horsefield, G.J., and Yardley, H.J.: Sclerema neonatorum, J. Invest. Dermatol. **44**:326, 1965.

Hurwitz, S.: The skin and systemic disease in children, Chicago, 1985, Year Book Medical Publishers, Inc.

Illig, L., and others: Congenital nevi less than or equal to 10 cm as precursors to melanoma: 52 cases, a review and a new conception, Arch. Dermatol. **121**:1274, 1985.

Jacobs, A.H., and Walton, R.G.: The incidence of birthmarks in the neonate, Pediatrics **58**:212, 1976.

Katz, D.A., and others: Subcutaneous fat necrosis of the newborn Arch. Dermatol. **120**:1517, 1984.

Kondo, J., Sakurai, S., and Sarai, Y.: New types of exfoliation obtained from staphylococcal strains belonging to phage groups other than group II, isolated from patients with impetigo and Ritter's disease, Infect. Immunol. **10**:851, 1974.

Kraemer, K.H.: Xeroderma pigmentosum; a prototype disease of environmental-genetic interaction, Arch. Dermatol. **116**:541, 1980.

Larregue, M., Bressieux, J.M., and Fournet, J.P.: Collodion baby, Mod. Probl. Pediatr. **20**:40, 1983.

Larregue, M., and others: Le syndrome du naevus epidermique, Ann. Dermatol. Venereol. **101**:45, 1974.

Mackenzie, I.C.: Ordered structure of the epidermis, J. Invest. Dermatol. **65**:45, 1975.

McKusick, V.A.: Heritable disorders of connective tissue, ed. 4, St. Louis, 1972, The C.V. Mosby Co.

Melish, M.E., and Glasgow, L.A.: Staphylococcal scalded skin syndrome: the expanded clinical syndrome, J. Pediatr. **78**:958, 1971.

Menendino, J.J., Jr., and others: A parathyroid-like protein from cultured human keratinocytes, Science **231**:388, 1986.

Merlob, P., Metzker, A., and Reisner, S.H.: Transient neonatal pustular melanosis, Am. J. Dis. Child. **136**:521, 1982.

Mollica, F., Pavone, L., and Nuciforo, G.: Linear nevus sebaceous syndrome in a newborn, Am. J. Dis. Child. **128**:868, 1974.

Mortenson, O., and Strougard-Andresen, P.: Harlequin color change in the newborn, Acta Obstet. Gynecol. Scand. **38**:352, 1959.

Mosher, D.B., Fitzpatrick, T.B., and Ortonne, J.P.: Abnormalities of pigmentation. In Fitzpatrick, T.B., and others, editors: Dermatology in general medicine, New York, 1979, McGraw-Hill Book Co.

Muller, S.A.: Alopecia: syndromes of genetic significance, J. Invest. Dermatol. **60**:475, 1973.

Nachman, R.L., and Esterly, N.B.: Increased skin permeability in preterm infants, J. Pediatr. **79**:623, 1971.

Neild, V.S., and others: Egg and milk exclusion diets in atopic eczema, Br. J. Dermatol. **114**:117, 1986.

Neldner, K.H., and Hambridge, K.M.: Zinc therapy of acrodermatitis enteropathica, N. Engl. J. Med. **292**:879, 1975.

Perera, P., Kurban, A.K., and Ryan, T.J.: The development of the cutaneous microvascular system in the newborn, Br. J. Dermatol. **82**(Suppl. 5):80, 1970.

Ramamurthy, R.S., and others: Transient neonatal pustular melanosis, J. Pediatr. **88**:831, 1976.

Reed, W.B., Lopez, D.A., and Landing, B.: Clinical spectrum of anhidrotic ectodermal dysplasia, Arch. Dermatol. **102**:134, 1970.

Reed, W.B., and others: Giant pigmented nevi, melanoma and leptomeningeal melanocytosis, Arch. Dermatol. **91**:100, 1965.

Robertson, A.F., and Sotos, J.: Treatment of acrodermatitis enteropathica with zinc sulfate, Pediatrics **55**:738, 1975.

Rudolph, N., and others: Congenital cutaneous candidiasis, Arch. Dermatol. **113**:1101, 1977.

Sagebiel, R.W., and Odland, G.F.: Ultrastructural identification of melanocytes in early human embryos. In Riley, V., editor: Pigmentation: its genesis and biologic control, New York, 1972, Appleton-Century-Crofts.

Samman, P.D.: The nails in disease, ed. 2, London, 1972, William Heinemann Medical Books, Ltd.

Schachner, L., and Press, S.: Vesicular, bullous and pustular disorders in infancy and childhood, Pediatr. Clin. North. Am. **30**:609, 1983.

Shapiro, L.G., and others: Enzymatic basis of typical X-linked ichthyosis, Lancet **2**:756, 1978.

Silvers, D.N., Greenwood, R.S., and Helwig, E.B.: Cafe-au-lait spots without giant pigment granules, Arch. Dermatol. **110**:87, 1974.

Simpson, J.R.: Natural history of cavernous haemangiomata, Lancet **2**:1057, 1959.

Smith, D.W.: Recognizable patterns of human malformation, ed. 3, Philadelphia, 1982, W.B. Saunders Co.

Smith, L.T., and Holbrook, K.: Embryogenesis of the dermis in human skin, Pediatr. Dermatol. (In press.)

Solomon, L.M., and Beerman, H.: Cold panniculitis, Arch. Dermatol. **88**:897, 1963.

Somerville, D.A.: The effect of age on the normal bacterial flora of the skin, Br. J. Dermatol. **81**:14, 1969.

Stingl, G., Tamaki, K., and Katz, S.I.: Origin and function of epidermal Langerhans cells, Immunol. Rev. **53**:149, 1980.

Symposium: The management of congenital nevocytic nevi, Pediatr. Dermatol. **2**:143, 1984.

Tromovitch, T.A., Abrams, A.A., and Jacobs, P.H.: Acne in infancy, Am. J. Dis. Child. **106**:230, 1963.

Whitehouse, D.: Diagnostic value of the cafe-au-lait spot in children, Arch. Dis. Child. **41**:316, 1966.

Wilkes, T., and others: The sensitivity of the axon reflex in term and premature infants, J. Invest. Dermatol. **47**:101, 1966.

Williams, M.L.: The ichthyoses—pathogenesis and prenatal diagnosis: a review of recent advances, Pediatr. Dermatol. **1**:1, 1983.

Windhorst, D.B., and Padgett, B.: The Chediak-Higashi syndrome and the homologous trait in animals, J. Invest. Dermatol. **60**:529, 1973.

Witkop, C.J., and others: Ophthalmologic, biochemical, platelet, and ultrastructural defects in various types of oculocutaneous albinism, J. Invest. Dermatol. **60**:443, 1973.

CHAPTER 39

The eye

PART ONE

Diagnosis and evaluation

An infant usually has contact with only one physician during the neonatal period. It is important therefore for the neonatologist or pediatrician to recognize the subtle irregularities of the eye that may help to save the eye or the life of the patient. Emphasis is placed on developing the ability of clinicians to recognize diseases early in their course. Blinding diseases such as congenital glaucoma, exposure of the cornea, or ocular infections will rapidly destroy useful vision unless a diagnosis is made and treatment begun as soon as possible. Early detection and treatment of congenital cataracts are necessary for optimal visual rehabilitation. Malignant orbital tumors and retinoblastomas can threaten the life of the neonate. Ocular findings may lead to a diagnosis of a general pathologic condition such as galactosemia or rubella. A detailed examination is described for the detection of occult ocular disease, and a minimum ocular examination is detailed for all neonates. No attempt is offered to make the examiner an ocular specialist, since ophthalmic consultation is available if important ocular disease is suspected or discovered.

The eyes are not completely developed either anatomically or functionally at birth, and they constantly change during the neonatal period. Thus an ocular reflex or response expected at an early age may be distinctly abnormal at a later, more mature phase. It is important to recognize the normal findings during different stages of the infant's growth to understand what is abnormal.

EXAMINATION OF THE EYE AND ORBIT

Screening eye examination

A brief screening examination should be done on all infants by a pediatrician or attending physician. If eye abnormalities are suspected because of genetic disease, prenatal infection, prematurity, or systemic anomalies, a more detailed evaluation is necessary.

A screening examination should include the following:

A. History (including family history and any perinatal abnormalities)
B. Examination
   1. Reaction to light or visual stimuli
   2. Pupillary size and reaction to light
   3. Extraocular muscles (general alignment and range of movement)
   4. External assessment (symmetry of orbits and lids, size of globe)
   5. Conjunctiva (color, discharge)
   6. Cornea (size, clarity)
   7. Iris
   8. Lens (normal black pupil with direct illumination and clear red reflex through the ophthalmoscope)
   9. Fundus (good red reflex, optic disc and macula)

If a red reflex cannot be obtained, dilation of the pupils with 0.5% tropicamide (Mydriacyl) will facilitate this.

Comprehensive eye examination

The screening examination outlined usually identifies the majority of serious eye problems, such as glaucoma, cataract, infection, and tumor. However, if abnormalities are suspected because of history, the presence of systemic anomalies, or observations on the screening examination, a more detailed ocular evaluation is mandatory.

A comprehensive ocular examination should begin with a careful history, especially of ocular diseases in the family. For example, a family history of retinoblastoma necessitates a thorough, periodic search of the fundus for the onset of this dominantly inherited malignant disease. Important information regarding maternal diseases (for example, rubella), injuries, or unusual medications during the prenatal period should be obtained. It is also important to note the length and abnormalities of pregnancy, labor, and delivery. Premature birth suggests possible retinopathy of prematurity (ROP), and difficult de-

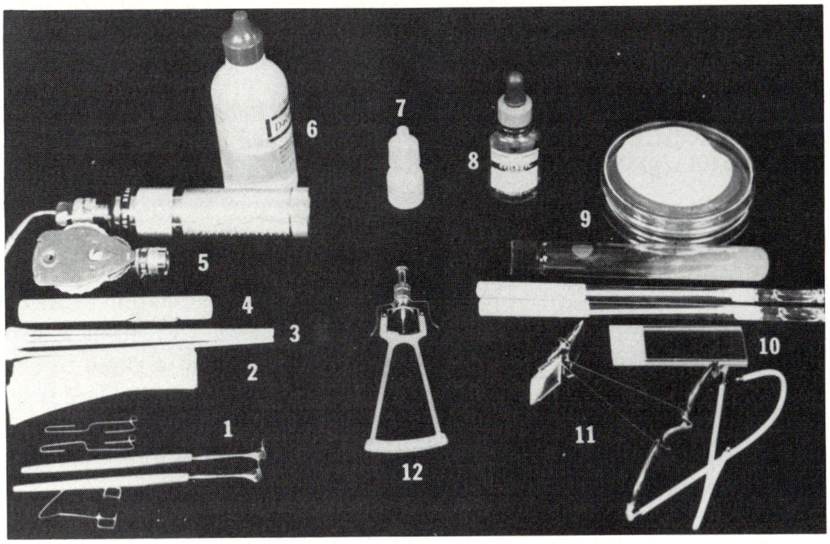

Fig. 39-1. Equipment for ocular examination: *1,* eye speculum, paper clip retractors or Desmarres' retractors; *2,* fluorescein strips; *3,* sterile cotton-tipped applicator; *4,* penlight or otoscope; *5,* ophthalmoscope; *6,* saline or 5% dextrose irrigation; *7,* 2.5% phenylephrine, ophthalmic; *8,* 1% cyclopentolate, ophthalmic; *9,* culture tubes and plates, sterile swabs; *10,* glass microscope slides; *11,* loupe; and *12,* Schiøtz tonometer.

livery with obstetric forceps may result in direct ocular trauma.

The examination should be done under comfortable circumstances with proper equipment (Fig. 39-1). Ideally, the examining surface is as high as the examiner's waist, and the room light is bright but can be darkened easily for intraocular examinations. Have available a blanket to swaddle the infant and a nurse or assistant to hold the infant's head or expose the eye. Irritating and forceful studies should be deferred until all general observations have been made. A great deal can be learned if the examiner takes a few moments initially to observe the infant for spontaneous general and ocular activity. These findings are considerably more reliable while the infant is undisturbed and comfortably held or nursing rather than screaming and crying.

The general facial configuration and the external structure of the orbit are inspected first. The orbital contents should be proportional and symmetric compared with the overall craniofacial configuration. The lids are examined grossly and are compared for symmetry of both horizontal and vertical placement. The spontaneous opening and closing of the eyes are assessed. If ptosis is present particular attention should be directed to the size of the pupils. Miosis (a small pupil) on the side of the ptosis is suggestive of Horner's syndrome. A rapid up-and-down movement of the lid during nursing indicates a jaw-winking phenomenon.

The eyes should be examined for spontaneous range of motion and for conjugate movement. This is best done while the infant is undisturbed and nursing. Fixation and the ability to follow a brightly colored object should be noted for each eye separately and for both eyes together in an older infant but not a neonate. An aversive reaction to a bright light can be observed in infants.

The pupils should be round and equal in diameter. A penlight or ophthalmoscope with a transilluminating head is used to shine direct light at each pupil, one at a time. Normally, each pupil constricts to both direct and contralateral stimulation. First, the reaction of the illuminated pupil is observed. It should constrict briskly (although the response in the neonate may be slower than in an older child) and should remain so as long as the illumination is maintained. If no response is observed the contralateral pupil's reaction to the direct illumination of the first eye is studied. If the contralateral pupil alone constricts the directly illuminated eye must have intact photoreceptors and optic nerve pathways. Failure of constriction in the directly illuminated eye in this instance may result from inflammation or paralysis of the iris, which prevents pupillary movement. If neither the illuminated pupil nor the contralateral pupil constricts on subsequent direct illumination, the first eye is deficient in vision and may be blind. Each eye should be assessed similarly for both direct and consensual reactions.

Direct light stimulation to one eye normally produces direct and consensual pupillary constriction. If the light is rapidly shifted to the opposite eye after pupillary constriction, both pupils should remain constricted for the duration of the stimulation. If, however, the shift of light is followed by dilation of the newly, directly stimulated eye, a relative afferent pupillary defect (the Marcus Gunn pupil) is present. This indicates decreased vision in the mydriatic eye. Rarely, pupillary reflexes may be completely normal, and the child still does not see because of intracranial abnormalities, particularly in the occipital cortex. This phenomenon is termed *cortical blindness*.

The normal neonate frequently has small, 2 mm pupils that may tend to change size symmetrically and rhythmically (hippus). This phenomenon rarely has clinical significance.

The pupillary space should be uniformly black. Any amount of a white reflection is abnormal and indicates an opacity within the lens, vitreous, or retina.

The lid margins should be inspected for regularity of contour and for the presence of lacrimal puncta. The puncta are two minute holes in the lid margins posterior and medial to the lashes and a short distance lateral from the inner corners of the eyes. They should lie next to the globe but should not be turned either in or out.

Palpation is performed to examine the orbital margin, the contents of the upper and lower lids, and the round contour of the globes. The orbital rims should be sharply outlined. In the newborn they are initially round and increase in vertical diameter with normal growth. The area of the lacrimal sac is palpated for abnormal masses or increased size by pressing the sac against the bones of the nose and medial orbital wall. Expression of mucopurulent or purulent material from the lacrimal puncta should be noted.

The examiner should view the lash structures under magnification, either with an ocular loupe (which gives 2× to 3× magnification) or through the ophthalmoscope with the +10-diopter lens in place. Normally, the lashes are directed outward in an orderly row. Abnormalities include distichiasis, an additional row of lashes posterior to the gray line; entropion, an inward turning of the lid; and trichiasis, an inward turning of the lashes. Lashes that contact the cornea are dangerous, for continued irritation eventually will predispose the eye to infection and abrasion of the cornea.

The conjunctival sac is inspected after the lids are separated with the use of a pediatric ocular speculum, lid retractors, or the fingers. All instruments that are introduced into the eye, of course, should be sterilized, and care is taken to avoid a corneal abrasion. The bulbar and palpebral conjunctiva are normally moist and pinkish. Redness or exudate is abnormal and often indicates infection, which can be confirmed by analyzing a smear, scraping, or culture of the tissue. The conjunctiva of the lids overlying the tarsal plates should be examined after the lids are everted. Eversion is usually simple to perform when the lids are separated with fingers, particularly if the infant is attempting to squeeze the lids shut. If the lids cannot be readily everted, further attempts probably should not be pursued unless they are performed by an ophthalmologist, since the delicate lid structures may be stretched or torn.

The normally white sclera is evaluated for changes of color. A bluish coloration, however, is present in premature infants and in other small babies because of their very thin sclera. The cornea is inspected with a penlight. Magnification with a loupe or an ophthalmoscope with the +10-diopter lens in place is again employed. During the first few days of life premature and full-term infants may demonstrate a somewhat less than transparent and slightly hazy cornea. This is thought to be the result of corneal edema, and it soon disappears. The surface of the cornea should have good luster, and the whole cornea should be absolutely transparent. A change in luster usually indicates a break or an unevenness in the anterior surface, as occurs from an abrasion of the cornea or corneal edema. Transparency should extend to the extreme periphery. Any opacity or translucency is abnormal after the first few days of life. Changes in transparency or opacification in the peripheral cornea are associated with a local mesenchymal abnormality, which may be complicated by congenital glaucoma.

The horizontal diameter of the cornea measures approximately 10 mm. However, a number of apparently normal corneas in full-term infants are between 9 and 10 mm. The average adult cornea measures 12 mm in the horizontal diameter; this dimension is achieved during the first year of life. Although the corneas should be equal in size, an accurate measurement usually is unnecessary at this time, unless congenital glaucoma is suspected. Corneal haze or enlargement, photophobia, or tearing requires an accurate measurement of corneal diameter and intraocular pressure in glaucoma suspects.

The anterior chamber should be assessed for clarity and depth. The depth is the distance between the posterior surface of the cornea and the anterior surface of the iris. Normally, the neonate has a moderately shallow chamber. As the eye grows in the first year of life, the iris and lens flatten and the corneal diameter increases, which deepens the anterior chamber.

The irises are usually similar in appearance. Although normally incomplete for the first 6 months of life, pigmentation of both irises develops simultaneously. In a normal infant the iris is often blue or blue-gray for the first few weeks or months of life. However, darkly pigmented white people and the darker races may show pigmentation at birth or within the first week. Heterochromia (dissimilarity in pigmentation between the two eyes) may indicate a normal hereditary pattern, congenital Horner's syndrome, or several syndromes (e.g., Waardenburg), which are discussed later in this chapter. These syndromes may not develop until the end of the neonatal period, or even later in life, when the iris is fully pigmented.

The lens should be clear and appear black in direct light. The red reflex observed through the ophthalmoscope should show no dullness or irregularities.

The fundus examination should be conducted in a dimly lit room with the infant's pupils dilated. Safe dilation in newborn and premature infants can be achieved with one drop of 1% tropicamide (Mydriacyl) and one drop of 2.5% phenylephrine. Phenylephrine 10% solution should not be used, because it may cause an acute rise in blood pressure or cardiac dysrhythmias. It takes dark irises somewhat longer than the average 20 minutes to dilate fully. Drops may be repeated once or twice if the pupils do not dilate well. Infants with cardiac irregularities or those with changing neurologic signs should not have their pupils dilated. In actual practice the vast majority of neonates, especially premature infants, can and should have their pupils dilated. Visualizing the fundus of the newborn eye is difficult under any circumstances and is nearly impossible with undilated pupils.

Each eye should be looked at under the ophthalmoscope with a +10-diopter lens in place, beginning approximately 5 inches in front of the eye. Because this lens gives a sharp plane of focus, only one plane of depth may be studied with the ophthalmoscope at a given distance from the eye. Thus the ophthalmoscope may be used in a tomographic fashion, first to study the cornea, then the anterior chamber and iris, the pupil and lens, and finally the anterior vitreous. Each structure is focused on individually as the examiner moves closer to the patient and decreases the dioptric power of the ophthalmoscope.

After the lenses in the ophthalmoscope have been changed, the posterior vitreous and fundus can be studied in detail. Most neonatal eyes, especially those of premature infants, have short anteroposterior lengths, and their fundi are sharply in focus with plus-diopter lenses.

The optic nerve is the largest and most readily recognized structure in the posterior pole. Its diameter observed through the ophthalmoscope should be approximately half to three fourths of the diameter of the total area illuminated at one time. The optic disc is usually round and sharp in outline. It may be somewhat oval in its vertical diameter. Excessive elongation, especially inferiorly, may indicate a defect or coloboma of the disc. The disc appears to be larger in the myopic infant and smaller in the hyperopic infant. The optic nerve head or disc has been described as being somewhat more pale in the neonate than in the adult.

The retinal vessels should exit from the disc in the superior and inferior quadrants, be smooth in outline as they curve diagonally, and branch dichotomously to cover the full extent of the retina. Branches usually leave the main vessel at an angle of less than 90 degrees. The arterioles and venules of the retinal circulation should be examined for size, regularity, color, and the presence or absence of pulsation. The examiners should follow the course of these vessels from the disc to the periphery, as far as possible in each meridian of the clock. The macular area of the retina, which subserves precise central vision and color vision, is located approximately one and one-half disc diameters temporal to the disc and is identified by a slightly reddish brown color and by a small (0.5 mm) avascular zone. In premature infants the normal macular coloration is usually absent, and all neonates lack the foveal reflex until approximately 4 months of age. The normal reddish brown pigment of the macula should be approximately half of a disc diameter in size and should show uniform regularity. Pigment mottling or stippling in the macula or elsewhere is abnormal.

The examination of the retina should be continued from the macula as far toward the periphery as possible. Attention should be given to the regularity of the normal pink-orange color. The far periphery of the retina, especially in the premature infant, appears pale gray and hazy, often falsely suggesting a retinal detachment. Premature and newborn infants have completely developed pigment epithelium but incompletely developed uveal pigment in the choroid. This immature state gives a pale appearance to the fundus and offers a better view of the choroidal blood vessels, which appear as indistinct, closely packed, red, linear structures. They are broad and randomly interconnected.

Abnormalities of the fundus are located by their anatomic distance from the disc, and size is expressed in fractions or multiples of the disc diameter. Areas of the fundus that appear to be out of focus in comparison with the surrounding fundus may indicate an elevation or tumor of the retina or underlying tumors of the choroid. Rapid rhythmic motions of the fundus during the examination may indicate the presence of nystagmus that was not obvious during external inspection.

NORMAL OCULAR FINDINGS

The eye of the newborn differs from the adult eye primarily in function, although structural differences are also present. The growth of the eye, which parallels that of the brain, continues at a rapid rate for the first 3 years of life, especially during the first year. The anteroposterior dimension of the eye at birth is about 16.5 mm

Table 39-1. Ocular measurements

Measurement	Full-term newborn (mm)	Premature newborn (1,000-1,300 gm) (mm)
Intermedial canthal distance	18-22	12-16
Medial canthus to lateral canthus	17-27	12-16
Anteroposterior diameter of eye at birth	16	10-16
Horizontal diameter of cornea	10 (average) 9 (lower limits)	7.5-8 (lower limits)

and grows to approximately 24 mm in adulthood. Normal values in the neonate fall within a very wide range. Suspected abnormalities in size frequently may be substantiated only by comparing the eye proportionately with nearby structures or by measured values in the fellow eye.

The lid fissures of the full-term infant are usually quite narrow, often being widely separated horizontally by prominent epicanthal folds. The term *telecanthus* indicates a disproportionate increase in distance between the medial canthal angles. It is particularly noticeable in infants with fetal alcohol and Waardenburg syndromes and in a number of other syndromes. Measurements between the two medial canthi may vary from 18 to 22 mm. Hypertelorism is defined as an increase in distance between the orbits, observed clinically as a large interpupillary distance, that is frequently noted in many craniofacial syndromes. Horizontal measurement of the lid fissures has ranged from 17 to 27 mm. These measurements should be symmetric (Table 39-1).

Reflex tearing to irritants is evident shortly after birth. However, emotional tearing starts with the onset of activity of the sebaceous glands of the skin, at about 3 weeks of age, and is developed at 2 to 3 months. The newborn possesses a strong blink reflex to light and to stimulation of the lids, lashes, or cornea. The reflex response to a threatening gesture does not appear until 7 or 8 weeks of age in the full-term infant.

After birth, the eyes should appear straight for the most part. Erratic, purposeless, and independent movements, however, may be observed during the first few weeks of life. Any constant strabismus requires further evaluation.

The macula provides central, precise vision. The center of the macula is termed the *fovea;* movement of the eyes to project the object of regard onto the fovea is called *fixation*. A somewhat unsteady gaze can be maintained shortly after birth, particularly if a strong light stimulus is used. However, the ability to maintain steady gaze or to fixate and follow an object and its movement is only weakly initiated at 5 to 6 weeks of age. At first the eyes pursue a moving visual stimulus extremely weakly and for only a few degrees of eye movement. The infant makes no attempt to locate or direct the eyes toward the target. By 3 months of age the infant can fixate and pursue movements instantaneously in both vertical and horizontal directions. At approximately 4 months of age central fixation is associated with the motor activity of grasping. Binocular fusion with convergence ability, which requires a visual acuity of approximately 20/40 to 20/60, is present at 6 months of age.

Visual acuity cannot be directly measured in the neonatal period. However, the infant's ability to fixate and pursue movements can be an accurate guide to the amount of visual function present. Central, steady fixation requires a visual acuity of at least 20/40 to 20/60. Unsteady fixation indicates an acuity of approximately 20/200 or worse. Inability to fixate on a light, even weakly, suggests a visual acuity of less than 20/400.

A recent technique to measure visual acuity in the infant is called *forced-choice preferential looking*. This method is used as a research tool and in many clinical settings. It is presumed that an infant will look at a striped target in preference to a uniformly gray target. By varying the size of the stripe a quantitative measurement of visual acuity is achieved. The disadvantages to this procedure include the number of people necessary to administer the test, the time involved, and the cooperation of an alert infant.

Another method to assess visual acuity in infancy is visual evoked potential, which measures the cortical response to a visual stimulus, usually a flash or a checkerboard pattern. Electrodes are placed over the occipital cortex to monitor activity in the brain, and a computer-averaged tracing is made from the cortical impulse.

Optokinetic nystagmus describes the reflex ocular response to a moving target. As a target moves across the visual field, a pursuit motion occurs, followed by a rapid return motion in the opposite direction to regain fixation. We experience this response when telephone poles or fence posts are watched from a fast-moving vehicle. Unfortunately, most estimations of acuity rely heavily on adequate motor responses as part of the visual evaluation. Thus immature or underdeveloped motor systems may reduce or interfere with eye or head movements and decrease the accuracy of the visual analysis.

Three distinct ocular rotational reflexes may be elicited in the neonatal period. From birth, a turning of the head

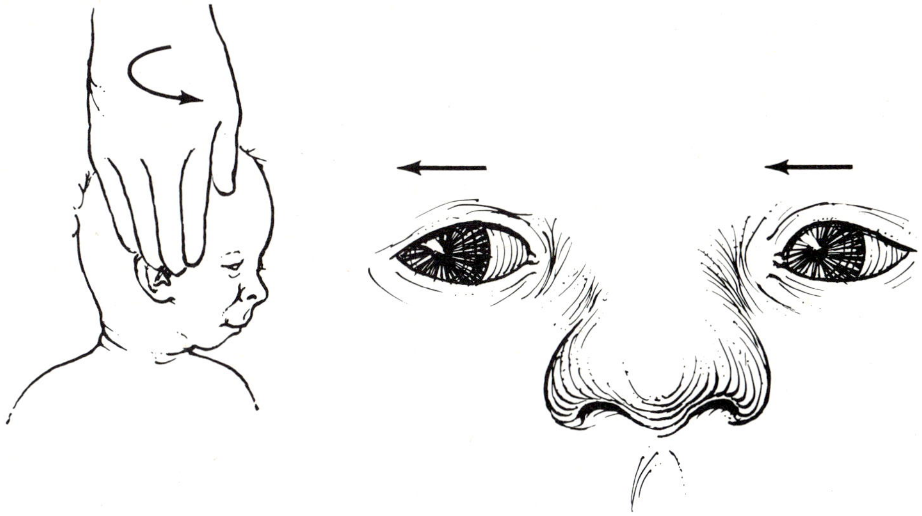

Fig. 39-2. Doll's head rotation. As the head is turned on the shoulders, a tonic neck muscle reflex produces corresponding ocular rotation in the opposite direction, as though the eyes were remaining in their original position as the head moves.

on the shoulders produces an opposite movement of the eyes (Fig. 39-2). This doll's eye movement is a reflex elicited by the stretching of cervical muscles and a response by cranial oculomotor nerves. It may be normal in blind or brain-damaged infants. The vestibuloocular reflex is elicited when the infant is held vertically and rotated on its own long axis (Fig. 39-3). The response is similar to the doll's eye movement, in that the eyes appear to remain stationary while the body moves; longitudinal rotation to the right produces an equal and conjugate ocular rotation to the left. When rotation stops the infant's eyes return slowly to the primary position. This reflex relies on the functioning of higher central nervous system centers and may be reduced in severely brain-damaged infants but normal in blind infants.

A third rotational reflex may be elicited by holding the infant vertically, as in the vestibuloocular reflex. The infant is rotated in an arc on the long axis of the examiner. With the infant's eyes held open the ocular rotation is first in the direction of the movement (the eyes appear to move more rapidly than the infant and in the same direction as the infant's movement). This ocular reflex may be a form of optokinetic nystagmus and appears to be reduced in infants with major defects of the visual system or of the central nervous system. Precise location of this reflex pathway is not known; however, it has been reduced in infants with cortical damage whose doll's eye and vestibuloocular reflexes were retained.

Unfortunately, all such rotary or postrotary responses must rely on functioning saccadic eye movements. Depending in part on the maturation of the motor system, saccadic eye movement may be unpredictable in the neonate, and reduced reflex responses may be the fault of the motor system and not the visual system. Thus predictions of decreased sensory function should be made with some caution.

Whether or not a child can see is occasionally questioned in early infancy because of a lack of visual response or because of other associated abnormalities. While a general assessment of visual function can be made at an early age, it is inadvisable to make pronouncements about total blindness unless one is absolutely confident of the etiologic diagnosis. Many infants may have delayed visual responses caused by prematurity, slower motor development, or other abnormalities. Careful observation and serial appraisal of the infant by an ophthalmologist is the best course to follow when visual impairment or blindness is suspected.

Prematurity

The ocular findings of the premature infant differ from those of the full-term neonate. At 28 weeks' gestation the globe is only 10 to 14 mm in diameter. The anterior and posterior hyaloid vascular systems are frequently present to some degree, although their involution will continue over the next several months (Fig. 39-4). One may see remnants of this system in the form of persistent blood vessels or fibrous strands anterior and posterior to the lens. The main hyaloid artery coursing from the optic disc to the posterior lens surface may be patent or may appear as a white strand in the vitreous. A moderate amount of vitreous haze is often present at this time, interfering with visualization of the fundus.

Transient cataracts have also been reported in the pre-

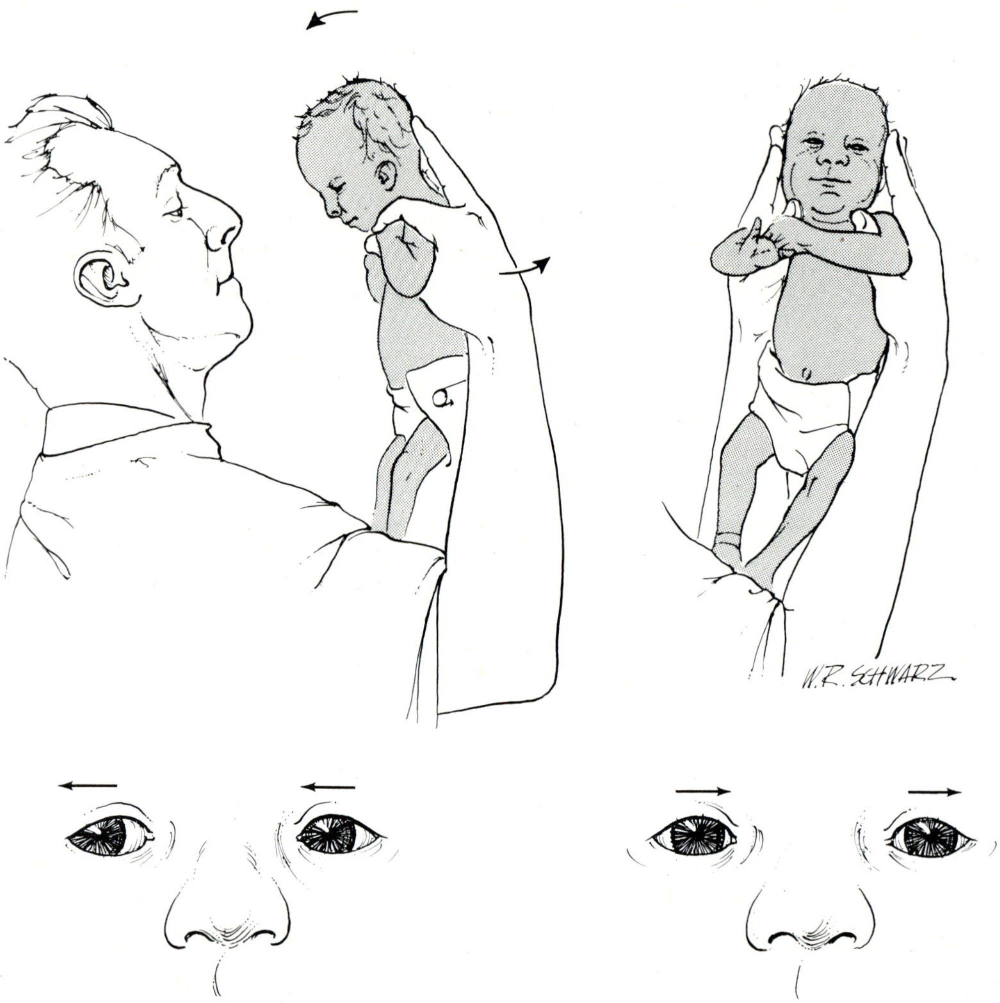

Fig. 39-3. Rotational nystagmus. The infant's head is inclined slightly forward, eyes open. With rotation, the eyes move in the opposite direction, as in doll's head rotation. When rotation stops, the recovery movement occurs in the reverse direction.

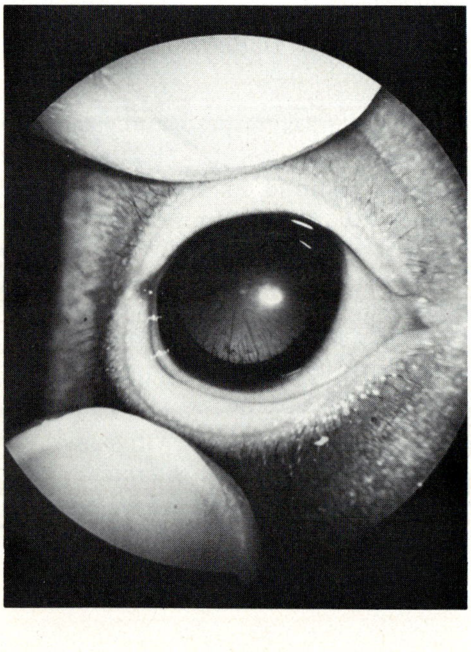

Fig. 39-4. Persistent pupillary membrane in a premature infant. Note the remnants of vascular loops of the anterior hyaloid system anterior to the lens. They will continue to atrophy during the first months of extrauterine life.

mature infant. These lens opacities appear as vacuoles located near the posterior lens capsule. They are usually bilateral and symmetric. Although most regress some can form more advanced cataracts.

Besides these changes noted at birth, premature infants have a high incidence of myopia and strabismus in childhood. Careful follow-up of all children born prematurely is advisable to ensure early detection of these ocular conditions.

REQUESTING OPHTHALMIC CONSULTATION

Routine consultation for all normal infants in the nursery is not recommended. Pathologic ocular findings in normal neonates are sufficiently rare that ophthalmic evaluation should be requested only for those whose ocular examination indicates the presence of an abnormality or who for some reason are at increased risk for ocular problems. Indications for ophthalmic consultation include a family history of congenital cataracts, retinoblastoma, or congenital glaucoma. Intrauterine infectious disease such as rubella, cytomegalovirus, or toxoplasmosis necessitates a thorough eye evaluation. If oxygen therapy has been administered in the neonatal period to a premature infant, ophthalmologic consultation is necessary to rule out retinopathy of prematurity.

Infants who are the products of precipitous or difficult deliveries may require a more thorough indirect ophthalmoscopic examination through dilated pupils if the neonatologist's examination indicates corneal or scleral injury or retinal hemorrhage.

Subdural hematomas and increased cerebrospinal fluid pressure, as in hydrocephalus, do not produce papilledema in neonates unless the cranial sutures have closed prematurely. Infections or other external disease should be promptly evaluated and treated as necessary.

Nancy Anderson Hamming
John E. Read
Marilyn T. Miller

BIBLIOGRAPHY

Apple, D.J., and Rabb, M.F.: Clinicopathologic correlation of ocular disease, St. Louis, 1973, The C.V. Mosby Co.

Duke-Elder, S.: System of ophthalmology, vol. 3, Normal and abnormal development, part 2: Congenital deformities, St. Louis, 1964, The C.V. Mosby Co.

Khodadoust, A.A., Mohsen, A., and Biggs, L.S.: Optic disc in normal newborns, Am. J. Ophthalmol. **66**:502, 1968.

Liebman, S.D., and Gellis, S.S., editors: The pediatrician's ophthalmology, St. Louis, 1966, The C.V. Mosby Co.

Newell, F.W.: Ophthalmology: principles and concepts, ed. 2, St. Louis, 1969, The C.V. Mosby Co.

Parks, M.M.: Growth of the eye and development of vision. In Liebman, S.D., and Gellis, S.S., editors: The pediatrician's ophthalmology, St. Louis, 1966, The C.V. Mosby Co.

Smith, D.W.: Recognizable patterns of human malformations: genetic, embryologic and clinical aspects: major problems in clinical pediatrics, vol. 3, Philadelphia, 1970, W.B. Saunders Co.

PART TWO

Neonatal eye disease

TRAUMA

Birth trauma

See also Chapter 20.

Eye injuries may be associated with the duration of labor and difficulty of delivery. Lid petechiae and hemorrhages, noted more often with face presentations than with vertex presentations, usually resolve quite rapidly without treatment. Subconjunctival hemorrhages also occur frequently and require no treatment. Such findings, however, should increase the suspicion of associated intraocular injuries. Forceps deliveries, particularly when associated with improper application, may produce lacerations of the lid or globe. A forceps mark or lid laceration requires a careful and complete examination of the orbit for associated injuries. Forceps application also may produce ruptures in Descemet's membrane of the cornea. Seen only with magnification, these ruptures appear as diagonal lines in the posterior cornea. They are rapidly followed by excess hydration of the cornea with a subsequent cloudy appearance that must be differentiated from congenital glaucoma, infections of the cornea, or diseases associated with cloudy cornea, such as the mucopolysaccharidoses. Prolonged labor or forceful delivery with forceps also may produce bleeding into the anterior chamber. Retinal hemorrhages are common after delivery. They are usually small, multiple, and scattered throughout the retina like dots. Any hemorrhage near or in the macular area should be noted, since it may be related to subnormal visual acuity and strabismus observed later. Retrobulbar hemorrhage may produce protrusion or proptosis of the globe and must be differentiated from a retrobulbar tumor. Rarely, the eye may be completely prolapsed, especially when the orbit is shallow. This constitutes an emergency owing to corneal exposure and stress on the optic nerve and blood supply.

Ocular injuries

The treatment of ocular injuries requires a full and careful evaluation of the extent of damage, particularly of the globe. Ocular injuries caused by trauma in the neonate must be treated with the same meticulous care that is required in the adult. Because of the diminutive size of the neonate's eye, treatment usually requires microscopic evaluation and repair, with the infant under general anesthesia. Lid lacerations should be repaired carefully to minimize permanent deformity. Involvement of the lacrimal canaliculi, the lid margin, and the lacrimal gland requires special attention. Avulsion or tissue loss of the lids necessitates urgent treatment to prevent exposure injuries to the cornea.

Blunt trauma to the ocular area of the neonate may produce blood in the anterior chamber (hyphema), rupture of the globe, dislocation of the lens, vitreous hemorrhage, contusion cataract, scleral rupture, traumatic retinal detachment, retinal hemorrhages or edema, rupture of the choroid, and arterial or venous occlusion in the retina. Thermal and chemical burns about the eyes must be treated with extreme care. Treatment by an ophthalmologist is required after the usual first-aid measures of cooling and protective covering are performed. Of immediate priority in the first-aid management of a chemical burn of the eye is copious irrigation with a noninjurious fluid such as tap water, milk, or normal saline solution.

Corneal abrasions in the infant, which occur more frequently than is realized, are suggested by a symptom of tearing in one eye. The use of eye bandages during phototherapy has increased the incidence of this complication. Diagnosis is made by staining the cornea with a fluorescein-impregnated paper strip. This is done by moistening a sterile fluorescein strip with a drop of sterile saline solution and touching it to the lower conjunctival fornix. The area of corneal abrasion turns light green in ordinary illumination but is best seen in a light with a cobalt-blue filter. A corneal abrasion also is suggested when a small shadow cast by the irregular epithelium is seen on the iris surface. This shadow follows the movement of the examining light. Treatment required for healing most injured eyes is the instillation of antibiotic drops for a few days.

Lacerations may involve the conjunctiva, the cornea, or the sclera. It should be presumed that all conjunctival lacerations are associated with a laceration of the globe until proved otherwise. Lacerations of the cornea or sclera require immediate evaluation and surgical repair, even tiny ones, as in the case of perforations from a diaper pin.

Orbital or ocular foreign bodies require specialized and precise localization to determine the proper therapeutic approach. Fortunately, they occur rarely in the neonate.

CONGENITAL ANOMALIES OF THE EYE

Chromosomal eye syndromes

See also Chapters 16 and 17.

Any alteration of gene dosage, as may occur in the duplication or deletion syndromes, often results in multiple systemic anomalies. Most ocular abnormalities have been reported in patients with chromosomal aberrations; many are nonspecific and not diagnostic of a specific chromosomal syndrome.

The following are examples of common chromosomal syndromes or chromosomal defects associated with ocular findings of particular importance.

Trisomy 13

Trisomy 13 is manifested by cleft palate and lip, polydactyly, umbilical hernia, renal dysgenesis, and malformations of the heart and of the central nervous system. Ocular findings are microphthalmia or anophthalmia, colobomas of the iris or choroid, corneal opacities, persistent hyperplastic primary vitreous, retinal dysplasia, cataracts, and many low-incidence anomalies.

Trisomy 18

Trisomy 18 is characterized by micrognathia, flexed fingers with the index finger overlapping the third finger, generalized hypertonicity of skeletal muscles, mental retardation, ventricular septal defect, umbilical hernia, "rocker-bottom" feet, and malrotation of the gut. Ocular abnormalities include corneal and lens opacities, ptosis, strabismus, epicanthal folds, abnormal orbital ridges, hypertelorism, microphthalmia, glaucoma, and myopia. Congenital optic atrophy also has been reported.

Trisomy 21

Down's syndrome is a well-recognized entity consisting of typical facies, mental retardation, small obese habitus, large tongue, and cardiac, genitourinary, and gastrointestinal abnormalities. The ocular findings associated with this entity are epicanthus, hypertelorism, upward slant of the palpebral fissures, and congenital or juvenile cataracts. Brushfield's spots may be found on the unusually thin, lightly colored irises. Because strabismus, cataracts, high refractive errors, keratoconus, and blepharitis are also common, these children should be evaluated by an ophthalmologist during infancy. Systemic or topical therapy with atropine may result in unusual and sometimes dangerous systemic responses in infants with Down's syndrome.

Turner's syndrome

Infants with Turner's syndrome may show ptosis, congenital cataracts, and occasionally corneal nebulae and blue scleras in the neonatal period. Strabismus is present in a high percentage of these infants.

Deletion 11p–

Infants with deletion of the short arm of chromosome 11 involving the 11p 13 band may have a syndrome of aniridia, genitourinary abnormalities, and mental retardation (AGR). Wilm's tumor has been noted in a large percentage of children with this deletion.

Deletion of 13q–

Patients with this syndrome have a unique facial configuration often with microcephaly, micrognathia, large malformed ears, a wide nasal bridge with hypertelorism, and protruding upper incisors. Other findings include urogenital, thumb, and congenital cardiac defects. Ocular abnormalities, which may be profound, include epicanthus, microphthalmia, iris and choroidal colobomas, ptosis, cataracts, antimongoloid palpebral apertures, and, most important, retinoblastoma. The gene for expression of esterase D is located near the area on the chromosome responsible for retinoblastoma. Therefore, detecting subnormal levels of esterase D could implicate a small deletion causing the retinoblastoma.

CRANIOFACIAL ANOMALIES AND SYNDROMES

See also Chapter 17.

Eye abnormalities associated with congenital anomalies of the face, skull, or head are briefly reviewed in this section.

Craniosynostosis syndromes

See also Chapter 27, part five.

Premature closure of the cranial sutures may occur in the embryonic period or early childhood. Normally, most cranial sutures do not close until adult life, although there is individual variation. The involved suture determines the shape of the skull, since growth is inhibited perpendicular to the closed suture. Compensatory growth occurs not only at the open sutures but also in weakened areas of the cranial vault. There may be variable patterns of suture closure and a wide spectrum of skull shapes. Mental retardation may occur, but many patients show normal intellectual capacity and function, and the assumption of retardation because of unusual facies may cause significant psychologic problems.

Premature craniosynostosis may exist as a primary isolated anomaly or may be associated with systemic malformations. A metabolic disturbance is a less frequent cause. Two of the most common examples of craniosynostosis syndromes are Crouzon's and Apert's syndromes.

Crouzon's syndrome/disease

Crouzon's disease is an autosomal dominant disorder characterized by maxillary hypoplasia, shallow orbits, parrot-beak nose, moderate hypertelorism, highly arched palate, and a variety of abnormal skull conformations, depending on the pattern of suture involvement. Visual acuity may be reduced owing to optic atrophy either of a primary or secondary type or, in some cases, owing to severe exposure keratitis secondary to exorbitism; strabismus is a less frequent finding. Infrequent anomalies include iris, pupillary, and corneal malformations and cataracts.

Apert's syndrome

Apert's syndrome (acrocephalosyndactyly) is another common craniosynostosis syndrome with abnormally shaped skull, shallow orbits, syndactyly of the hands and feet, midface hypoplasia, strabismus, and moderate hypertelorism. Mental retardation is more prevalent than in Crouzon's disease. Other minor anomalies reported include downward slanting of the palpebral fissure, ptosis, and tortuous retinal vessels. Less frequent findings are keratoconus, cataract, astigmatism, nystagmus, retinal pigmentary changes, and congenital glaucoma. Most cases are sporadic, but a few families have demonstrated autosomal dominant transmission.

Cornelia de Lange syndrome

The typical facial appearance in infants with Cornelia de Lange syndrome is a low hairline, eyebrows that are joined in the middle (synophrys), long eyelashes, and a small upturned nose. Skeletal deformities ranging from syndactyly to phocomelia may be present. Eye disorders, which are less frequently encountered, include hypertelorism and antimongoloid slant, strabismus, nystagmus, ptosis, high myopia, and pupillary abnormalities. Some patients with this diagnosis resemble children with the fetal alcohol syndrome.

Cretinism (congenital hypothyroidism)

Swollen eyelids, hypertelorism, and an enlarged tongue constitute an early suggestive triad.

Ocular hypertelorism

Ocular hypertelorism is a term indicating increased separation between the bony orbits. It is an anatomic description rather than a diagnostic entity. Hypertelorism of mild to moderate severity is found in many syndromes but occurs most frequently and prominently in the median facial cleft syndrome (frontonasal dysplasia) and may be the result of morphokinetic arrest during embryogenesis. Characteristic findings are medial cleft nose, lip, and palate, a widow's peak, and cranium bifidum occultum. The most common ocular abnormality is a nonparetic form of exotropia. Epibulbar dermoids, palpebral fissure changes, and optic atrophy occasionally have been reported.

Hemifacial microsomia

Hemifacial microsomia describes a group of patients with microtia, macrostomia, and mandibular anomalies. Most, but not all, patients show unilateral involvement. Ocular manifestations may range from clinical anophthalmia to minor fissure asymmetry. Goldenhar's syndrome is probably a variant of this group, with characteristic epibulbar dermoids or lipodermoids, usually in the inferotemporal quadrant. Limbal dermoids are reported more frequently than lipodermoids and may occasionally be bilateral. Another common finding is an upper eyelid coloboma almost always on the most affected side.

Mandibulofacial dysostosis (Treacher Collins' or Franceschetti's syndrome)

Mandibulofacial dysostosis, a dominantly inherited syndrome, is characterized by the bilateral occurrence of colobomas or notching of the outer portion of the lower eyelid, malar and mandibular hypoplasia, downward slanting of the palpebral fissures, macrostomia, and ear anomalies. Although anomalies of soft tissues are common, serious ocular anomalies are infrequent and varied.

Hallermann-Streiff syndrome

Oculomandibulofacial dyscephalia is characterized by hypoplasia of the mandibles; a thin, prominent nose, described as a parrot beak; and bilateral cataracts, often associated with microphthalmia or microcornea or both. Glaucoma may complicate the eye findings. Additionally, anomalies that may include atrophy of the facial skin, hypotrichosis, and marked dwarfism with dental and nasal abnormalities give the infant an aged, wrinkled appearance. All cases have been sporadic, and the causative factors are unknown.

TTV-OFM syndrome complex

This is a heterogeneous collection of syndromes with a wide variety of facial and limb anomalies referred to by many authors as *terminal transverse defects with orofacial malformations* (TTV-OFM). They include the aglossia-adactylia syndrome, Handhart's syndrome, ectrodactyly with orofacial malformations, ankyloglossia syndrome, and Möbius' syndrome. The pattern of craniofacial anomalies noted in the TTV-OFM complex include oral and facial clefts, micrognathia, microglossia, pectoral muscle malformations with ipsilateral hand malformations (Poland's syndrome), dental and oral anomalies, and hypoplastic limb anomalies. The pathology in all these syndromes is similar and is caused by a heterogeneous group of genetic and environmental factors.

Pierre Robin anomalad

The Pierre Robin anomalad is characterized by micrognathia, glossoptosis, and cleft palate. The ocular abnormalities occur in a variety of syndromes and include retinal detachment, microphthalmia, congenital glaucoma, cataracts, and high myopia. It is a frequent finding in Stickler syndrome.

Sturge-Weber syndrome

The association of capillary angiomas of the upper part of the face, the eye, and the leptomeninges forms a triad of signs also termed *encephalooculofacial angiomatosis*. The capillary angioma, or port-wine stain of the face (nevus flammeus), is typically unilateral and may or may not be confined to the distribution of the first or second division of the trigeminal nerve. Angiomas that include the forehead and the upper lid are the most frequently implicated in patients with ocular disease. The associated choroidal angioma is frequently located near the disc; it is usually indistinct and difficult to visualize without indirect ophthalmoscopy and fluorescein angiography of the fundus. If present, it may lead to macular edema and decreased visual acuity. There is no apparent hereditary pattern. Congenital glaucoma frequently occurs and, if unrecognized, can lead to irreversible blindness.

Waardenburg syndrome

Waardenburg syndrome is transmitted as an autosomal dominant trait and is associated with lateral displacement of the medial canthi (telecanthus) and puncta; coalescing of eyebrows, frequently in the midline; white forelock; heterochromia iridis; and nerve deafness. The ocular fundus may also show pigmentary changes.

ABNORMAL EYELIDS

Colobomas

Colobomas of the lids are partial-thickness or complete defects that may range from a small notching of the lid borders to involvement of the entire length of the lid. Most lid colobomas occur in the medial aspect of the upper lid (Fig. 39-5). When the lower lid is involved the defect is more often in its lateral aspect. The cause of lid colobomas is unknown. It has been suggested these isolated colobomas may arise from the localized failure of adhesion of the lid folds, resulting in a lag of growth, or from mechanical effects of amniotic bands.

The treatment of lid colobomas is very important when they prevent adequate lid closure and produce corneal exposure. Subsequent thickening, opacification, infection, ulceration, or perforation of the unprotected cornea may occur. Surgical correction of a small coloboma is accomplished by removing a V-shaped wedge that includes the coloboma, with subsequent primary closure of the full-thickness defect. Larger colobomatous defects require more extensive plastic repair.

Congenital blepharophimosis

Blepharophimosis describes eyelids that are too narrow horizontally and vertically (Fig. 39-6). There is usually an associated ptosis, and strabismus is frequently present. Lid fissure measurements commonly are reduced to approximately two thirds of normal, whereas the space between the medial canthi is considerably widened. A relatively rare condition, its cause is usually unknown. Autosomal dominant transmission is frequent. Surgical repair is frequently required, whereby the medial and lateral canthal angles are widened where possible. Ptosis surgery may be used to elevate the upper lid.

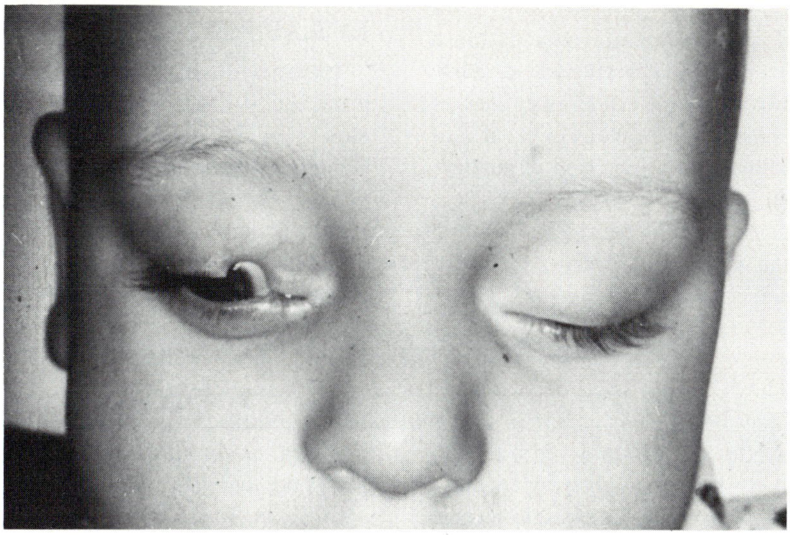

Fig. 39-5. Atypical coloboma of right upper lid.

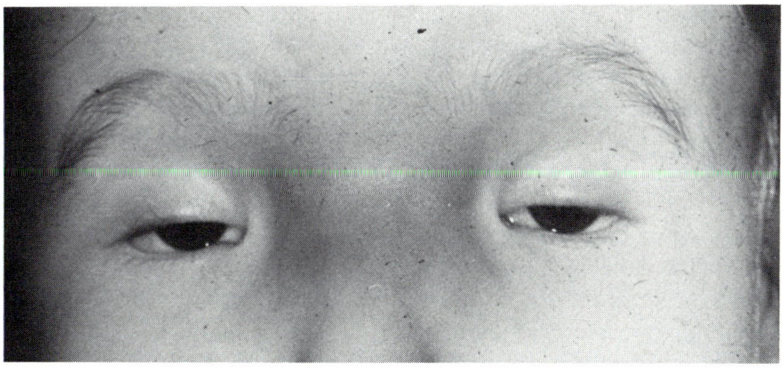

Fig. 39-6. Congenital blepharophimosis, ptosis, and epicanthus inversus (bilateral).

Epicanthus

Epicanthus is the most commonly encountered lid abnormality. A skin fold originating in the upper lid extends over the medial end of the upper lid, the medial canthus, and the caruncle and ends in the skin of the lower lid. It frequently occurs in normal infants in the neonatal period and gradually disappears as the growth of the bridge of the nose obliterates the excess skin in this area, but it may give a false appearance of crossed eyes (pseudostrabismus) for a few years. Epicanthus inversus is similar, except that the predominance of the skin fold arises in the lower lid and runs diagonally upward toward the root of the nose to overlie the medial canthus. A plastic surgical technique may be employed later in life to obliterate this extra skin fold, especially if the fold is sufficiently prominent to simulate the appearance of esotropia.

LID TUMORS

Hemangiomas

Hemangiomas of the lid are relatively frequent in infancy, with an incidence of approximately 1% in full-term newborns. Approximately 20% of hemangiomas are noted at the time of birth, although 95% become apparent by 6 months of age.

Capillary hemangiomas, the most frequently encountered vascular tumor, may progress at a rapid rate during the first 5 to 6 months of life, producing a considerable enlargement and reddish blue discoloration of the upper or lower lid. Such tumors gradually reduce in size and may completely disappear within the first 5 years of life.

Treatment should initially be confined to expectant observation, since resolution is usually the rule. However, some tumors may require therapy because of an occasionally alarming rate of growth that produces a refractive error or obstruction of the pupillary axis. Both complications may result in severe amblyopia within a short period of time. If amblyopia is suspected, early intervention is necessary to prevent visual loss. Glasses and patching may be necessary to prevent or treat amblyopia. Treatment may involve an injection of corticosteroid into the lid lesion.

Another type of hemangioma is the port-wine stain of the face (nevus flammeus) associated with leptomeningeal angiomas in Sturge-Weber syndrome.

Lymphangiomas

Lymphangiomas are slowly progressive, diffuse, soft tumors of the lids that may be present at birth or may gradually develop during the first several years of life. They tend to enlarge slowly and cease growing by early adulthood. Approximately 25% of all lymphangiomas occur in the orbital or periorbital region. Of these, 80% are found in the lids. There may be sufficient vascularization to make differentiation from hemangiomas difficult except by histologic study. Because of edema and hemorrhage lymphangiomas tend to increase in size more dramatically than do hemangiomas. Surgical removal and repair of the tumor are necessary if it is cosmetically unacceptable. Recurrence, however, is frequent.

Dermoid cysts

Of congenital ectodermal origin, dermoid cysts develop in the brow, lid, or orbit at the closure site of an embryonic cleft. They usually occur in the lateral third of the brow or upper lid. The skin overlying the soft cyst is freely movable, although the cyst remains attached to the periosteum at the site of the embryonic cleft. Roentgenograms of the area are important, since the cysts may connect with the cranial cavity, paranasal sinuses, or the orbit. Surgical removal is performed if the lesion is enlarging or cosmetically unacceptable.

Neurofibromatosis

Neurofibromatosis (von Recklinghausen's disease) is a congenital, autosomal dominant disease that produces tumors of proliferating Schwann cells. The presence of café au lait spots in the patient or parents should alert the examiner to the possibility of this disease. Lid involvement rarely occurs in the neonatal period. The characteristic lid tumor is initially small and gradually enlarging, composed of wormlike tissue with overlying elephantiasis of the skin. The periorbital tissue can be massively deformed. Radical excision, done for cosmetic purposes, is usually incomplete, and at times a recurring tumor grows larger than the original lesion. Optic nerve gliomas are found frequently in patients with neurofibromatosis.

ABNORMALITIES OF EYEBROWS AND EYELASHES

Excessive hair on the lids and forehead may occur as a dominant characteristic in male infants and, on occasion, may be extreme. Distichiasis describes an additional row of lashes posterior to the gray line (the tarsal edge or center of the lid margin). This condition usually results in contact of the lashes with the cornea, producing corneal irritation and abrasions. Hypertrichosis involving the eyebrows, forehead, and upper lid appears in the Cornelia de Lange syndrome, a pathologic dwarfism associated with multiple congenital anomalies. Hypertrichosis lanuginosa is transmitted as an autosomal dominant condition. The fetal lanugo persists into adult life, creating an abundant covering of hair on the eyebrows, forehead, eyelids, and other areas of the body.

Congenital ectropion and entropion

Congenital ectropion is an eversion of the lid margin, most commonly of the lower lid. It may be associated with other eyelid or ocular abnormalities. If the ectropion is mild no treatment is necessary. A more severely everted lid may require surgical correction.

Often associated with lid or ocular abnormalities, congenital entropion is an inturning of the lid margin, most often of the lower lid. If the lashes on the lid margin rub on the cornea, surgery is necessary to prevent corneal abrasion and ulceration.

PTOSIS

Ptosis (droopy eyelid) is defined as an upper lid that cannot or does not rise to a normal level (Fig. 39-7). In the position of primary gaze the lids should be elevated to a point at least midway between the pupil and the upper margin of the cornea. Since accurate lid position can be evaluated only in the undisturbed patient, care must be taken to not upset the child when evaluating for ptosis.

Ptosis results from the partial or complete dysfunction of the musculus levator palpebrae superioris. Complete dysfunction is present when no elevation of the lid occurs on upward gaze. Ptosis may be unilateral or bilateral, with any gradation of function in either situation.

Unilateral ptosis (Fig. 39-7) should prompt a comparison of pupillary size to diagnose Horner's syndrome. Congenital Horner's syndrome may result from trauma at birth, although it may be associated with mediastinal or cervical disease. Also, the involved iris is hypopigmented.

Ptosis also may be associated with the jaw-winking phenomenon. The affected patient shows a marked movement of the involved upper lid during nursing activity. The jaw-winking portion of the syndrome is thought to decrease or disappear in early adulthood; how-

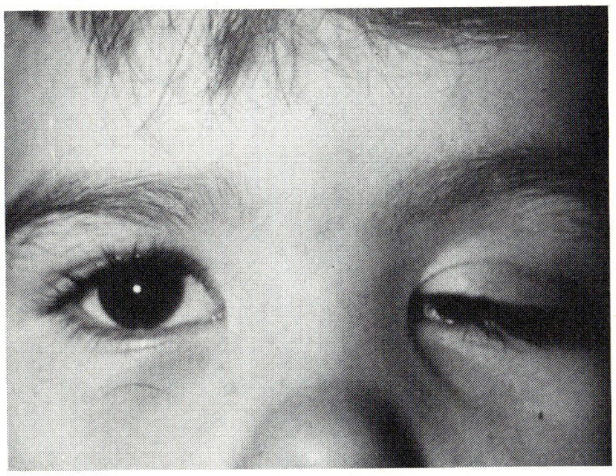

Fig. 39-7. Congenital ptosis of left upper lid.

ever, the ptosis remains. Early surgical correction of the ptosis is frequently unsatisfactory because of the continued presence of the jaw-winking phenomenon, even though shortening the levator palpebrae muscle may improve the ptosis. The syndrome is caused by anomalous innervation of the levator palpebrae muscle (abnormal connections of the motor fibers of the pterygoid, lingual, and levator palpebrae muscles). Thus the levator palpebrae muscle is relatively toneless unless the jaw or tongue is additionally activated.

Two forms of myasthenia gravis (see Chapter 17) may produce ptosis in the neonatal period; one of these may occur in the newborns of mothers with myasthenia gravis. This form presents shortly after birth with weakness in all muscle groups but usually resolves spontaneously within 2 to 4 weeks. Myasthenia congenita, which also presents in the infant shortly after birth, commonly includes ptosis, extraocular muscle palsies, and facial weakness. Generalized weakness is not usual.

A temporary, apparent ptosis (so-called protective ptosis) may occur from corneal or conjunctival irritation or infection and in conditions such as congenital glaucoma. These conditions should always be considered and ruled out before another form of ptosis is diagnosed, since they are the more important and often correctable ocular diseases.

Ptosis rarely occludes the eye to the extent that amblyopia develops. However, patients with ptosis may have strabismus with accompanying amblyopia. Weakness of the superior rectus muscle may also be seen with congenital ptosis.

ABNORMAL GLOBE

Anophthalmia

Anophthalmia is a rare phenomenon in which there is total absence or a minute rudiment of the globe, usually bilaterally. This may occur as a developmental failure of the optic vesicle; is often accompanied by other congenital anomalies, such as central nervous system defects and retardation; and has been observed in chromosomal anomaly syndromes (e.g., trisomy 13). Since lid formation is not dependent on ocular formation, the lids are present with lashes and lacrimal puncta, even though the globe may be absent. However, the lids remain closed or may be partially fused and will be sunken without the support of the eye. The lacrimal gland is present and is capable of producing tears. Anophthalmia occurs sporadically; however, some cases of familial occurrence with varied types of inheritance have been described. Treatment is for cosmetic purposes. Plastic molds of the conjunctival sac of gradually enlarging sizes are used to stretch the lids and sac sufficiently to hold a cosmetic prosthetic shell.

Cryptophthalmos

In cryptophthalmos the eyelids fail to form their normal cleavage, and uninterrupted skin runs from the forehead to the malar area. It may be unilateral. The eyelids and eyelashes usually are absent; however, the eye can be palpated beneath the skin and may even be observed to move with the stimulation of a strong light. The anterior segment of the eye is invariably disorganized into fibrovascular tissue adherent to the subcuticular tissue of the lids. The conjunctival sac is absent. Therefore attempts to separate the lids from the ocular structures are usually unsuccessful, and surgical correction is not advisable in most circumstances. It is frequently associated with systemic anomalies (particularly genitourinary), and the cryptophthalmus syndrome may show an autosomal recessive mode of inheritance.

Microphthalmos

Microphthalmia describes a variety of conditions in which the diameter of the neonatal eye is less than two thirds of the normal 16 mm. Relatively rare is pure congenital microphthalmia, in which the abnormally small eye is the only clinical finding. It is associated with three features of importance: a high degree of hypermetropia, hypoplasia of the macula, and the late occurrence of glaucoma. It has been reported in both recessive and dominant transmissions.

Colobomatous microphthalmia occurs when the embryonic cleft of the optic vesicle fails to close. Typically associated with other ocular anomalies such as colobomas of the iris, ciliary body, choroid, or optic nerve, this form may be transmitted as an autosomal dominant or X-linked trait.

Microphthalmia may also be associated with other ocular and systemic syndromes including intrauterine infections such as rubella and cytomegalovirus, craniofacial anomalies, anterior chamber cleavage syndromes, and chromosomal abnormalities.

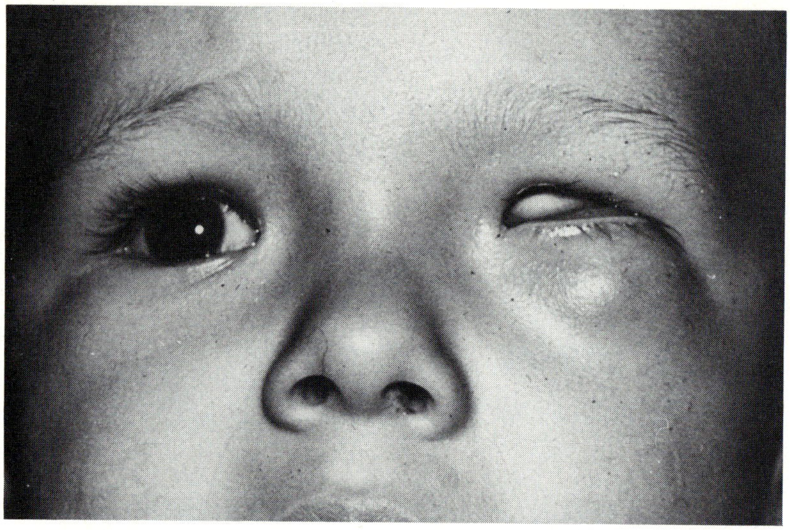

Fig. 39-8. Congenital microphthalmia with large cyst of left eye.

The large eye

The presence of an abnormally enlarged eye in the neonatal period is a rare occurrence but is extremely important to recognize. An apparently enlarged eye may be caused by colobomatous microphthalmia with an associated large cyst (Fig. 39-8), congenital megalophthalmus (congenital macrocornea), or congenital glaucoma. Colobomatous microphthalmia results when the embryonic optic vesicle fails to close. Tissue that originally should have become intraocular is encased in a cystic structure outside the eye in the orbit. If the cyst becomes sufficiently large that proptosis occurs, the microphthalmic eye simulates an enlarged eye.

Macrocornea is an enlarged cornea exceeding 13 mm in diameter. The cornea is usually clear, with distinct margins and thin iris stroma. Macrocornea as an isolated finding is usually inherited in an autosomal dominant manner. Megalophthalmus, which is commonly inherited as an X-linked recessive trait, is characterized by deep anterior chambers, subluxation of the lens, hypoplastic iris, and cataract formation in early adult life. Congenital glaucoma is discussed later in this chapter.

LACRIMAL ABNORMALITIES

The watery eye

Epiphora (excess tearing) frequently does not occur until after the first 3 weeks of life, when the major portion of the lacrimal gland has become functional. With the onset of emotional tearing at 3 to 4 weeks, epiphora is a frequent symptom. Although the usual cause of epiphora is a blockage of the nasolacrimal ducts, the possibility of congenital glaucoma is the most important consideration in the differential diagnosis of this symptom. (Congenital glaucoma is discussed in more detail later in this chapter.) Less commonly, tearing may result from dacryocystitis, an obstruction of the common canaliculus, or from congenital absence of the lid puncta. Congenital absence of the entire lacrimal drainage apparatus is extremely rare.

Epiphora occurs with an obstruction of the lacrimal drainage apparatus, which often results from a persistent membrane or a narrowing of the bony canal at the lower end of the nasolacrimal duct. This condition creates a stagnant pooling of tears in the lacrimal sac, which contributes to chronic or recurrent dacryocystitis. The inflammation is heralded by a purulent exudate in the medial canthal area of the conjunctiva. Severe dacryocystitis may produce a swelling and induration of the lacrimal sac medial and inferior to the medial canthus. Treatment of the nasolacrimal infection consists of the local instillation of antibiotic drops or ointment. If it is especially severe, systemic administration of medication and locally applied heat may be required. Repeated massage of the nasolacrimal sac at the root of the nose, done at home, may serve to encourage the opening of the nasolacrimal duct. If the epiphora continues, a lacrimal probe passed through the nasolacrimal duct to the nose usually creates an adequate opening; recurrent probings are occasionally necessary. If probings are unsuccessful, silicone intubation of the lacrimal system or fracturing the inferior turbinate often provides good results. When the puncta or common canaliculus is absent, or when major obstructions occur in the lacrimal sac, probing is insufficient. A surgical procedure, usually performed later in the child's life, is needed to bypass the tears from the conjunctival sac to the nose. Occasionally, minor surgical unroofing of a congenitally closed punctum will be sufficient.

Reflex tearing may be produced by any stimulation of the fifth cranial nerve. Therefore epiphora may occur as the result of corneal abrasion, corneal foreign body, or nasal and facial lesions that irritate the fifth cranial nerve. Chronic nasal congestion also may produce epiphora by mechanically blocking the nasolacrimal duct.

The dry eye

Recognition of alacrima in the infant is important to prevent corneal abrasions, infections, and perforations, the inevitable results of dry eye. During the first month an infant with alacrima of any cause may not appear to be different from the normal infant, since tear production is minimal during this period. The usual time of discovery is at 6 to 12 months of age or later, after the lack of tears has produced changes such as scarring or ulceration in the corneal epithelium. The tear film is minimal but present with alacrima. At 1 to 2 months of age early symptoms are conjunctival hyperemia and photophobia. Instead of the ample tears expected with conjunctival irritation, a sticky mucoid secretion is noted, and the cornea shows a punctate staining with fluorescein. Treatment includes the frequent use of artificial tears such as 1% methylcellulose (as often as every 15 to 30 minutes), punctal occlusion, or tarsorrhaphy.

Congenital absence of the lacrimal secretion

Isolated congenital lack of tears, usually bilateral, is a rare anomaly. The cause is unknown but has been suggested to be either the result of hypoplasia of the lacrimal gland or the absence of innervation of the lacrimal gland structures. Treatment includes the frequent use of artificial tears and prevention of secondary infection.

Familial dysautonomia

The ocular findings in the Riley-Day syndrome are characteristic and may produce the initial criteria for diagnosis. These include alacrima and corneal anesthesia. These ocular changes, plus constriction of the pupil by instillation of 0.125% pilocarpine, may establish the diagnosis. The onset of major systemic symptoms is at approximately age 2 years. The abnormal swallowing mechanism, inappropriate blood pressure and respiratory control, decreased sensitivity to pain, deficient taste perception, and the ocular findings in this syndrome are the result of sympathetic and parasympathetic imbalance of an undefined type. Additional ocular findings are myopia, anisometropia (different refractive error in the two eyes), exotropia, and occasionally ptosis. Tortuosity of the retinal vessels also has been noted in a majority of the patients examined for this finding. The concomitant alacrima and corneal hypesthesia make the cornea particularly susceptible to corneal abrasion, infection, and ulceration. Thus corneal scarring is a frequent secondary finding in familial dysautonomia.

HYPOTELORISM

Cebocephaly
Ocular-dental-digital dysplasia
Trisomy 13
Scaphocephalism

HYPERTELORISM

Apert's syndrome
Cerebral gigantism
Cerebrohepatorenal syndrome
Chromosome 18p- and 18q- syndromes
Crouzon's disease
Infantile hypercalcemia
Median cleft face syndrome
Smith-Lemli-Opitz syndrome
Chromosome 4p- syndrome
Chromosome 5p- (cri-du-chat) syndrome
Chromosome 13q- syndrome
Chromosome 21q- syndrome

ABNORMAL ORBITS

Abnormal spatial relationships between the two orbits, creating either excessively wide or narrow intraorbital distances, are frequent findings. These abnormalities are caused by a variety of related cranial abnormalities involving the disproportionate growth or lack of development of the body and lesser wing of the sphenoid and ethmoid sinuses and of the maxillary processes (see box). Hypotelorism (a narrowing of the intraorbital distance) may be associated with central nervous system malformation. Hypertelorism (a widening of the intraorbital distance) is normal in the early fetus and may persist as a genetic trait. Hypertelorism may occur as an associated finding in other diseases.

ORBITAL CELLULITIS

Cellulitis of the orbital tissue is rare in the neonate but is a common cause of proptosis in older children and in adults. This infection often originates in the paranasal sinuses and produces massive swelling of the orbital contents. The possibility of its occurrence is enhanced by a highly virulent upper respiratory tract sinus infection or a puncture wound of the orbit. The disease is characterized by the rapid onset of progressive proptosis, often with redness of the lids, chemosis of the conjunctiva, and systemic signs of toxicity and hyperpyrexia. Rapid loss of vision caused by compression of the orbital structures can occur. Diagnosis is made by clinical appearance and by CT of the orbits and sinuses. Treatment includes systemic administration of antibiotics; application of warm, moist compresses; and surgical drainage of the purulent infection, if necessary.

ORBITAL TUMORS

The contents of the orbit are confined to a conical shape by its bony walls. At the posterior apex of the orbit the extraocular muscles originate and the vascular and nerve structures enter the orbit. The bony structures of the lateral wall do not protect the orbital contents as far anteriorly as do the remaining sides of the orbit, which leaves the eye more susceptible to trauma on its lateral side. In the neonate the orbital rims form a circular outline at the anterior base of the cone.

Tumors within the orbital cavity can most easily expand anteriorly, producing proptosis or exophthalmos. Those located within the cone of extraocular muscles produce a symmetric anterior displacement, whereas tumors located outside the cone of extraocular muscles displace the eye out and away from the area of origin of the tumor. Thus a tumor in the inferior portion of the orbit will displace the eye upward and forward, whereas one located medially will displace the eye laterally and forward. Proptosis also may occur from venous engorgement of the orbital cavity, such as that produced by a carotid-cavernous fistula. Unfortunately, a cephalic bruit is often heard in the infant and is thus not pathognomonic of carotid-cavernous sinus fistulas. The diagnosis of proptosis may be confirmed if the examiner sights the infant's eyes and lids from above, over the prominence of the eyebrows. A more anterior protrusion of the orbital contents is observed when compared with the opposite side. The proptotic eye frequently has a widened palpebral fissure.

A false diagnosis of proptosis may occur with a slight ptosis of one eye, which gives the opposite normal eye an appearance of a wide palpebral fissure. Marked enlargement of the eye, as occurs in congenital glaucoma, makes the eye appear proptotic because of the increased size of the globe. Facial abnormalities that produce shallow orbits, as in Crouzon's disease, simulate exophthalmos, because the normal amount of orbital structures appears to protrude in an abnormally shallow orbit. Since the extraocular muscles retract the globe a paralysis of all the extraocular muscles may produce as much as 2 mm of proptosis without a tumor to increase the orbital contents. If a tumor is located anterior to the equator of the globe, it can extend anteriorly into the lids without producing proptosis. A diffuse extensive tumor can produce sufficient general changes to fix the eye, whereas a localized tumor induces proptosis, usually without interfering with rotation of the eye.

Orbital tumors may develop from both ectodermal and mesodermal tissues or may arise by metastasis from distant body tissues. They also may originate from the intracranial cavity or paranasal sinuses and enter the orbit by growing through bony defects in the orbital wall. Roentgenograms are valuable in the diagnosis of orbital disease. Ultrasound, magnetic resonance imaging, and CT are particularly helpful aids.

Orbital hematoma

Bleeding into the orbital contents may result from birth trauma. This bleeding produces a unilateral proptosis that tends to increase gradually in size during the first 3 or 4 hours after birth. Ecchymoses of the lids may be associated findings at birth or may occur 1 to 2 days later. Differential diagnosis includes dermoid cysts, teratoma, and other congenital tumors of the orbit. The hematoma usually absorbs spontaneously over a 1- to 2-week period. It is important during this time to ensure that the cornea is not abraded and that the retinal circulation is not compromised. If examination with the direct ophthalmoscope shows compression of the arterial or venous supply at the disc, a surgical decompression of the orbit is required.

Hemangioma

Capillary hemangioma is the most common primary orbital tumor that produces exophthalmos. In infants the hemangioma usually is not well encapsulated and frequently involves the lower lid as well as the orbit. Although observation of lid involvement assists in making the diagnosis, a biopsy frequently is required to rule out other orbital tumors. Crying or straining by the infant will often cause the mass to increase in size and assume a bluish coloration. Treatment usually is deferred until after the age of 2 years, at which time spontaneous regression frequently occurs. The use of systemic corticosteroid therapy has been advocated when excessive growth has produced dangerous compression of the orbital structures. Local injection of corticosteroids is discussed in the section on lid hemangiomas, which begins on p. 1211.

Lymphangioma

Lymphangiomas are composed of thin-walled vascular channels that may involve the orbit and lids as well as other tissues in the body. The tumors may cause proptosis, ptosis, strabismus, or anisometropia. Amblyopia is common and must be aggressively treated. The lesion itself is difficult to treat, since it does not regress spontaneously or respond to radiation or corticosteroid therapy. Although surgery is the treatment of choice, results are not always satisfactory.

Dermoid cysts

Dermoid cysts are thought to arise from a congenital nest of primitive ectoderm at the site of closure of a fetal cleft. They usually contain connective tissue, sebaceous glands, and hair follicles. Cysts are often located near the orbital rim, where they are attached to bone at suture sites. Cysts located within the orbit produce proptosis and vertical or horizontal displacement of the globe. Roentgenographic examination may document bony erosion where the cyst is attached. Surgical excision is recommended but may prove difficult when the dermoid cyst extends through the bony suture in surrounding structures. Trauma, such as that occurring at birth, may produce a hemorrhage into the dermoid cyst. This occurs rarely, but under such circumstances differentiation from a primary hematoma of the orbit is difficult.

Teratoma

Teratoma is a primary orbital tumor composed of the three embryonic cell layers. It may differentiate into a variety of tissues containing cartilage, connective tissue, skin, hair, and sebaceous glands, or into endodermal epithelium. Bone is a frequent component and may be identified by orbital roentgenograms. Orbital teratomas that are present at birth produce a striking massive proptosis. Treatment is early excision of the orbital contents (exenteration) both for cosmetic value and for the malignant changes that may occur within the tumor.

Rhabdomyosarcoma

Rhabdomyosarcoma is the most common malignant tumor of the orbit in children (Fig. 39-9). Although it may be found in the neonatal period, the average age of occurrence is 6 to 10 years. Rhabdomyosarcoma develops in the orbit more frequently than elsewhere in the body. It produces exophthalmos with vertical or horizontal displacement, frequently with a palpable mass in the lid or the brow and with progressive protrusion of the eye. Diagnosis is made by biopsy. Although surgical exenteration has been used in the past, the present treatment of choice is irradiation and chemotherapy.

Hyperthyroid exophthalmos

This rare neonatal sequela of hyperthyroidism occurs as the result of maternal Graves' disease during the last trimester of pregnancy (Chapter 37, part three). The infant is born with classic hyperthyroidism, including exophthalmos, upper lid retraction, and extraocular muscle development. Symptoms usually subside during the first 2 months of life.

Lymphoma

Proptosis caused by lymphomatous lesions of the orbit is rare in the neonatal period. Diagnosis is made by biopsy, and the prognosis with radiation treatment is usually good.

Neurofibromatosis

Neurofibromatosis (von Recklinghausen's disease) is also rare in the neonate. However, plexiform neuromas of the lids and orbit have been reported in the first 3 months of life. The typical "bag of worms" tissue may produce proptosis and irregular enlargement of one or both lids. The overlying tissue becomes hypertrophic, creating elephantiasis of the skin. Von Recklinghausen's disease also has been associated with glioma of the optic nerve, a slowly growing tumor appearing during the first 10 years of life. Invasion of the optic nerve by the glioma results in loss of vision.

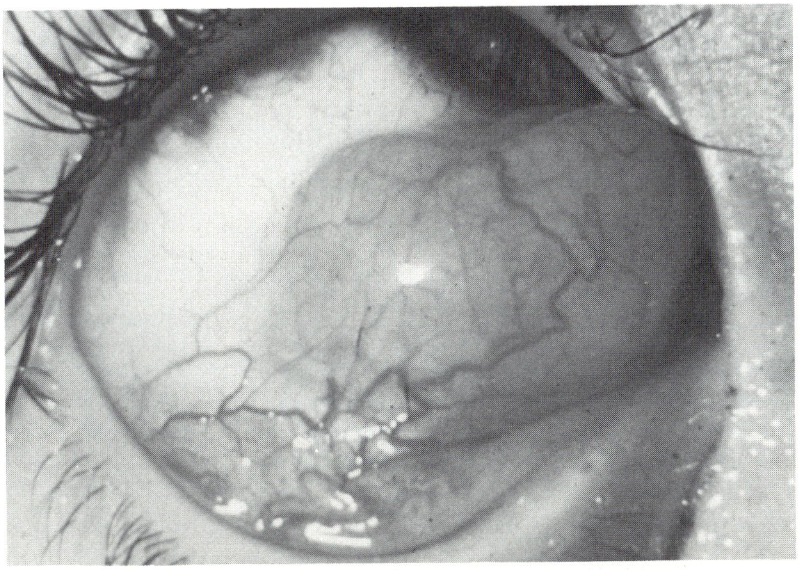

Fig. 39-9. Rhabdomyosarcoma of right orbit.

Letterer-Siwe disease

Letterer-Siwe disease is the most severe of the histiocytosis syndromes. The condition usually affects children under 2 years of age and is nearly always fatal. Reticuloendothelial cells proliferate in the skin, lymph nodes, and spleen, as well as in the tissue of the orbit, producing proptosis. Hepatosplenomegaly and generalized lymphadenopathy with bone lesions and anemia are typical findings. Diagnosis is made from a biopsy of skin lesions or of lymph nodes. Palliative treatment includes corticosteroids, irradiation, and chemotherapy.

Congenital deformities producing proptosis

An orbital encephalocele or meningocele producing proptosis or an orbital cyst may be evident at birth or may be delayed until later years. This abnormality results from a defect in the wall between the cranial cavity and the orbit, usually located at the suture lines. Pressure within the cranium causes herniation of brain tissue or meninges or both into the orbit, most often at the inner angle of the orbit at the root of the nose. Diagnosis is made by identifying the bony defect in association with the area of the orbital cyst. Clinically, an encephalocele is suggested by the presence of a pulsating, fluctuant cyst that can be somewhat reduced with digital pressure or that increases with coughing or crying. Excessive manipulation of the encephalocele may produce slowing of the pulse and respiration or convulsions. Slowly progressive proptosis, demonstrated by pulsation synchronous with the vascular pulse or accentuated with coughing, is diagnostic. Neurosurgical correction is difficult and has high rates of morbidity and mortality.

CONGENITAL GLAUCOMA

The presence of epiphora in the neonate, especially when combined with photophobia, should always suggest the possibility of congenital glaucoma. Congenital glaucoma is fortunately not very common. However, the devastating effects of the uncontrolled pressure that occurs without adequate surgical treatment are sufficiently important to keep this disease uppermost in the mind of the examining physician. The obvious signs of enlarged corneal diameters and a cloudy cornea are not likely to be missed if present at birth. However, the onset of the glaucoma may be sufficiently delayed so that the eyes remain normal for the first weeks or months of life. The usual initial symptoms before corneal changes occur include epiphora, photophobia, and blepharospasm. Persistent symptoms of this nature that do not result from corneal abrasion or a foreign body require specific evaluation for increased intraocular pressure. Early diagnosis is essential and can be made with the precise measurement of corneal diameters, ocular tonometry, and examination of the optic discs.

As the disease progresses, the increased intraocular pressure produces further stretching of the eye, creating increased corneal and ocular diameters. A corneal diameter of more than 12 mm should suggest glaucoma. (The normal corneal diameter at birth is 10 to 11 mm; this increases to about 11.5 or 12 mm at 1 year of age.)

Buphthalmos (an enlarged eye caused by glaucoma) (Fig. 39-10) also may be caused by a variety of diseases that obstruct the aqueous drainage mechanism in the anterior chamber angle. The boxed list includes diseases associated with glaucoma.

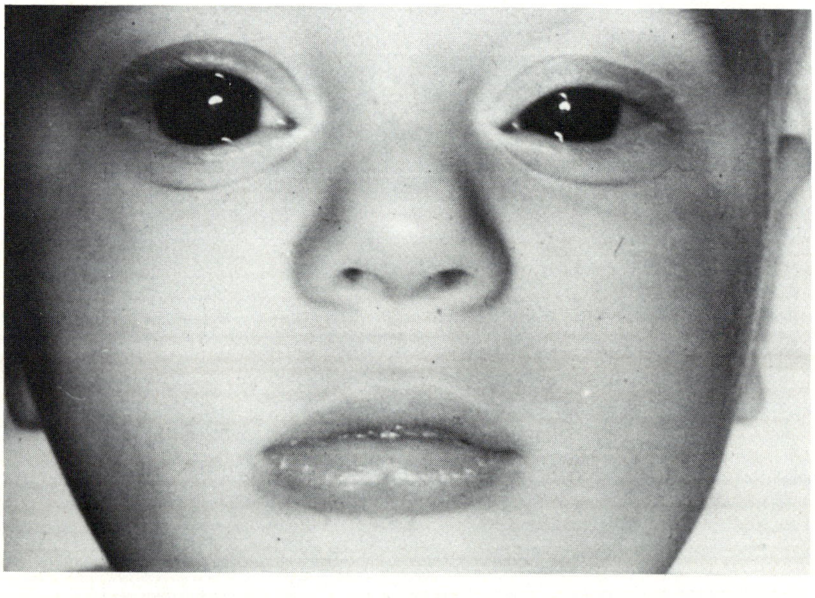

Fig. 39-10. Bilateral congenital glaucoma (buphthalmos), right eye greater than left.

GLAUCOMA

Isolated (congenital)
Rubella syndrome
Hallermann-Streiff syndrome
Rieger's anomaly
Lowe's syndrome
Persistent hyperplastic primary vitreous (rare)
Aniridia
Sturge-Weber syndrome
Homocystinuria (infrequent)
Marfan's syndrome (infrequent)
Weill-Marchesani syndrome (infrequent)
Neurofibromatosis (infrequent)
Ocular-dental-digital syndrome (infrequent)

Once glaucoma is suspected, the infant should be examined under general anesthesia by an ophthalmologist. If the diagnosis is confirmed, a surgical procedure should be performed on the anterior chamber angle (goniotomy) while the infant is still under anesthesia, since medical therapy is ineffective. If congenital glaucoma is diagnosed early in its course, the percentage of successful recoveries is high; however, if the eye is considerably enlarged, the possibility of reducing intraocular pressure and achieving useful vision is greatly decreased.

ABNORMAL CORNEA

Cloudy cornea

The normal premature infant may have a slightly hazy cornea for the first 7 days of life. In the normal full-term infant a similar appearance may be noted for the first 48 hours after delivery. This finding is thought to be caused by a temporary excess hydration of the cornea. A persistently hazy or cloudy cornea should immediately suggest congenital glaucoma. Once this has been ruled out, mesenchymal dysgenesis, corneal dystrophies, or systemic disease should be considered.

Size

Most newborns have a corneal diameter of approximately 10 mm. If this measurement exceeds 12 mm, congenital glaucoma must be considered, especially if corneal haze, tearing, and photophobia are present. If the intraocular pressure is normal, simple macrocornea may be present. This is an autosomal dominantly inherited condition without other ocular abnormalities. Another type of enlarged cornea, which is inherited as an X-linked trait, is associated with other ocular abnormalities, such as subluxed lenses, hypoplastic iris, cataract, and glaucoma.

A corneal diameter of less than 10 mm may be an isolated finding or may be associated with other ocular anomalies. Cases of autosomal dominant and recessive inheritance have been described.

Anterior chamber cleavage syndromes—mesenchymal dysgenesis

A wide spectrum of clinical findings are noted in this group of syndromes, including abnormalities of the cornea, anterior chamber, and iris. Corneal opacities, iris adhesions, and glaucoma have been noted with extensive involvement.

Corneal dystrophies

Most corneal dystrophies become apparent in adolescence or early adult life. However, congenital hereditary corneal dystrophy may be present at birth. This condition is characterized by bilateral cloudy corneas and normal intraocular pressure. An early corneal transplant may be helpful, but the prognosis is guarded.

Corneal manifestations of systemic disease

Corneal opacities and haze can occur owing to inborn errors of metabolism. Most are not associated with corneal opacities in the neonatal period. Systemic diseases that cause corneal opacities include the mucopolysaccharidoses, mucolipidoses, Fabry's disease, hypophosphatasia, cystinosis, and Wilson's disease.

THE ABNORMAL SCLERA

The normal full-term neonate has a glistening white sclera. The overlying conjunctiva and conjunctival vessels superimpose a filmy and vascular pattern. A generalized bluish discoloration of the underdeveloped sclera is normal in premature infants. Rarely, a congenital weakness in a small area of the sclera produces a bulging, or a staphyloma. The light-blue color is caused by thinness of the sclera, which transmits the darker color of the underlying uveal tissue. Osteogenesis imperfecta may be associated with a similar bluish discoloration of the sclera in the full-term neonate because of inadequately developed scleral collagen. Blue sclera may also be seen in other systemic diseases such as Marfan's syndrome, Ehlers-Danlos syndrome, and Crouzon's syndrome.

Pigmentation of the conjunctiva and sclera is common in the darkly pigmented races. Intrascleral nerve loops often appear as darkly pigmented dots approximately 3 to 4 mm from the limbus. Congenital ocular melanosis and oculodermal melanosis (Ota's nevus) present as a unilateral slate-blue pigmentation in infancy. A higher incidence of uveal melanoma may occur in both of these conditions.

IRIS ABNORMALITIES

Aniridia

Aniridia (absence of the iris) is a rare congenital anomaly, usually bilateral, that is almost invariably associated with poor vision and nystagmus. A small rudimentary

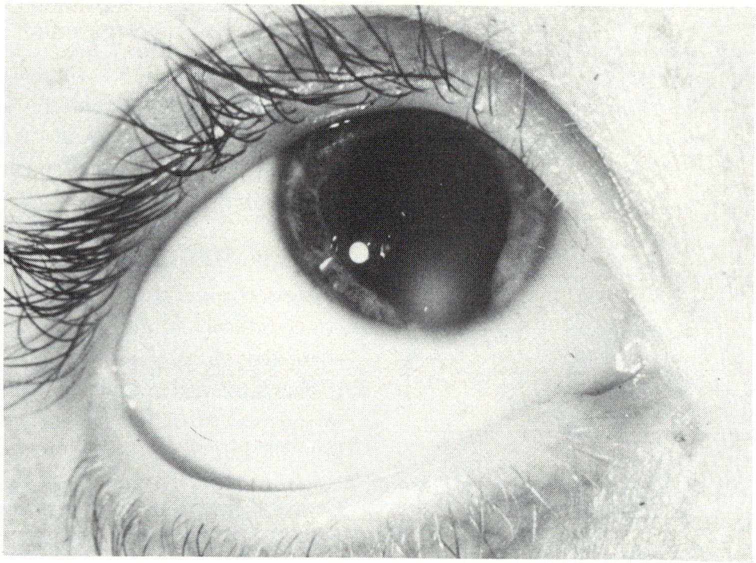

Fig. 39-11. Typical iris coloboma with inferonasal iris defect.

cuff of peripheral iris can be observed grossly or microscopically. Associated ocular findings include congenital glaucoma in more than 50% of cases, corneal pannus, cataract, abnormal optic discs, and foveal hypoplasia. The foveal hypoplasia causes the nystagmus and poor visual acuity. Aniridia may be an autosomal dominant trait or may occur sporadically. The sporadic variety is associated with Wilms' tumor in approximately 20% of cases. Most infants with aniridia and Wilms' tumor have a deletion of the short arm of chromosome 11. Thus all infants with sporadic aniridia should undergo chromosomal analysis to detect small deletions; if a deletion exists the infant has a 90% risk of developing Wilms' tumor.

Coloboma

Iris coloboma is one of the most common congenital abnormalities of the eye. It may occur as a single ocular finding or may be transmitted as an autosomal dominant characteristic. Typical colobomas occur in the inferonasal quadrant where the embryonic fissure closes (Fig. 39-11). Atypical colobomas may arise in any quadrant and rarely may be multiple (see boxed material). Atypical colobomas, which vary from a small notch in the pupil to the absence of an entire segment of the iris, usually are not associated with visual difficulties. Since typical iris colobomas result from an abnormal closure of the embryonic fissure, they also may be associated with a coloboma of the ciliary body, fundus, or optic nerve. When the optic nerve or macula is involved in the coloboma, visual difficulty occurs. Thus it is always wise to evaluate the fundus for a pathologic condition when an iris coloboma is detected.

Syndromes associated with iris colobomas

Congenital colobomatous microphthalmia
CHARGE syndrome
Trisomy 13
Trisomy 18
Rieger's syndrome
Iris coloboma and anal atresia syndrome
Lowe's syndrome (infrequent)
Rubinstein-Taybi syndrome (infrequent)
Chromosome 13q- syndrome

Persistent pupillary membrane

Persistent pupillary membranes are common in the neonate, particularly in the premature infant. The membranes are remnants of the anterior fetal vascular coat of the lens that failed to atrophy in the seventh month of gestation. The filmy lacework of fibers that radiates from the pupillary rim over the center of the lens may persist into adulthood or may continue to atrophy.

The unusually colored iris

Heterochromia indicates a difference in pigmentation between the two irises. Since many infants do not develop iris pigmentation until after the neonatal period, this condition is infrequently seen and is of little diagnostic value in this age group. However, in white infants with darkly colored irises and in the darkly pigmented races, some iris pigmentation is established at birth or

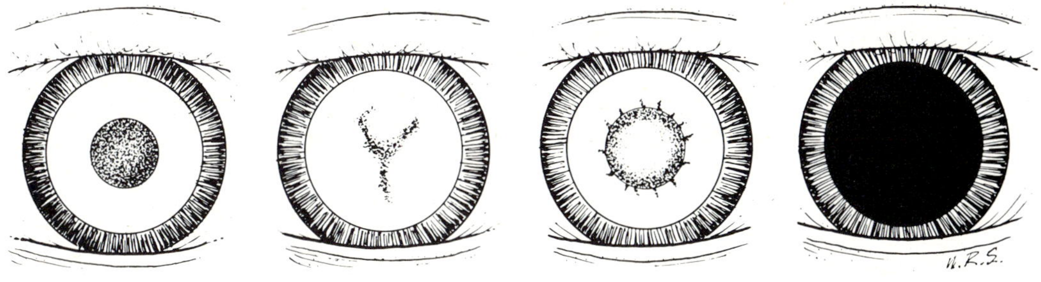

Fig. 39-12. The appearance of the red reflex with various cataracts. With the ophthalmoscope set at +10, the dilated pupil is observed with the examiner standing approximately 1 foot from the infant. The normal eye is seen to have a clear round red reflex. Lens opacities (cataracts) interrupt the red reflex, producing black opacities as shown.

shortly thereafter; these neonates occasionally show abnormalities in pigmentation. Heterochromia may occur as an isolated autosomal dominant trait. It also is associated with several syndromes. The progressive hemifacial atrophy of Romberg occasionally demonstrates a lack of pigmentation on the affected side of the face; Waardenburg syndrome is typically associated with heterochromia; and congenital Horner's syndrome produces heterochromia, usually after the neonatal period, resulting from the failure of normal pigmentation to develop in the iris on the sympathetically denervated side. Aganglionic megacolon (Hirschsprung's disease) may be associated with iris heterochromia.

ABNORMALITIES PRODUCING A WHITE PUPIL—LEUKOKORIA

The white pupil

A white pupil (also called a cat's eye reflex) denotes an ocular abnormality of the lens, vitreous, or fundus. An understanding of the etiology of diseases associated with a white pupil is helpful in searching for genetic factors and in requesting pertinent laboratory data that may be diagnostic, as in galactosemia. Knowledge of available treatment encourages early correction before permanent visual loss occurs or before secondary complications produce irreversible ocular damage.

Examination for the white pupil

Since the infant sleeps much of the time and since the pupils are small, a white pupil often is not noticed until the infant becomes more alert and active. A white or absent fundus reflex provides an early clue that an abnormality exists; therefore an evaluation of the pupil should be basic to all examinations of neonates.

The initial examination may be made with a hand light or the light of an otoscope or ophthalmoscope. With the light source held close to the infant's eye, the pupillary reflex is evaluated for whitish discoloration. If a discoloration is present the percentage of involvement of the pupillary area is estimated. With a +10-diopter lens in the ophthalmoscope a red reflex is obtained by observing the pupillary area from a position approximately 1 foot from the eye. When an extensive pathologic condition of the cornea, lens, or vitreous totally obstructs the reflection of light from the red fundus, the fundus reflex in the pupil is black. With lesser degrees of opacification or less amounts of diseased tissue, the reflex is dull red. Irregular densities, such as those occurring in an incomplete cataract, produce a correspondingly irregular reflex (Fig. 39-12). White lesions in the fundus itself (retina and choroid) provide a white reflex rather than a black or red one. The abnormality often may be localized initially by focusing through the pupil with the ophthalmoscope and the +10-diopter lens. Abnormalities of the lens appear to be in focus immediately adjacent to the plane of the pupil, whereas abnormalities of the vitreous come into focus more posterior to the pupil. By moving slightly to the side while viewing the opacity, the examiner can see that the more deeply it is placed behind the pupil, the greater the apparent relative movement of the opacity in relation to the pupil. Definitive evaluation requires slit-lamp examination and ophthalmoscopy with a dilated pupil. An examination with the infant under anesthesia is occasionally necessary to examine the abnormalities fully.

The lens (cataracts)

A large number of morphologic types of cataracts are known, but only a brief description is presented here. The size and shape of the cataract (lens opacification) depend on the area of the lens that is being formed at the time the damage or developmental defects occur. The lens grows continuously during life, laying down new lens fibers on its external surface, much like an onion. Damage that occurs in the early fetal period produces opacifications in the center of the lens. Such nuclear cataracts have clear layers in the periphery of the lens. Later periods of damage produce ringlike opacifications surrounded by central and peripheral clear areas (zonular cataracts). Recent damage produces peripheral opacifications near the surface of the lens (cortical cataracts). Very dense opacities cause greater visual disturbance, especially if they are located in the central axis, whereas peripheral opacities near the equator or the periphery of the lens produce little or no visual disturbance.

Etiology. Cataracts may be grouped according to cause: idiopathic, genetic, viral, inborn errors of metabolism, trauma, association with other eye malformations, and generalized syndromes. Included herein are the most frequently encountered cataracts for which a cause is known. The remaining causative factors are shown in Table 39-2, with an evaluation as to their frequency of occurrence.

Table 39-2. Neonatal cataracts

Type	Incidence of occurrence in the syndrome
Genetic	
Dominant	
Recessive	
X-linked recessive	
Viral	
Rubella	50% incidence
Cytomegalic inclusion disease	Infrequent
Inborn errors of metabolism	
Galactosemia	50% incidence
Galactokinase deficiency	Frequent
Lowe's syndrome	Frequent
Trauma	
Birth trauma	Infrequent
Blunt trauma	Frequent
Perforating injuries	Frequent
Battered child syndrome	Infrequent
Endocrine	
Congenital hypoparathyroidism	Frequent
Albright's hereditary osteodystrophy	Infrequent
Neurologic	
Marinesco-Sjögren syndrome	Infrequent
Smith-Lemli-Opitz syndrome	Rare
Miscellaneous	
Aniridia (sporadic or associated with Wilms' tumor)	Infrequent
Treacher Collins' syndrome	Infrequent
Pierre Robin anomalad	Infrequent
Rubinstein-Taybi syndrome	Infrequent
Hallermann-Streiff syndrome	Frequent
Chromosomal anomalies	
Trisomy 13	Infrequent
Trisomy 18	Infrequent
Turner's syndrome	Infrequent
Associated with other eye malformations	
Microphthalmia	Frequent
Rieger's anomaly	Infrequent

Genetically determined cataracts often are isolated abnormalities. They are frequently present at birth but occasionally originate during childhood. The primary mode of transmission is autosomal dominant. Recessive and X-linked transmission have been recorded.

The rubella embryopathy syndrome comprises multiple congenital anomalies that result from maternal viremia during the first trimester of pregnancy. Cataracts are present in approximately 50% of these patients (Fig. 39-13). The opacification may be nuclear (confined to the center of the lens) or complete (involving all layers of the lens). The rubella virus may remain dormant in lens material in the offspring for as long as several years. Microphthalmia and anterior uveitis also may be present in the same eye. The pupil is usually small and sometimes difficult to dilate because the iris structures are atrophic. The iris therefore transilluminates abnormally. Congenital glaucoma also occurs in 10% to 25% of patients with congenital rubella; when present at birth it causes an enlarged, hazy cornea. A cloudy, edematous, or white cornea, however, also may be found with normal intraocular pressure as part of the rubella embryopathy. Rubella retinopathy may be detected later in life. It is a pigmentary degeneration of the retina without demonstrable effect on visual function. A TORCH titer should be obtained in all infants with nongenetic congenital cataracts. The acronym TORCH includes assays for toxoplasmosis, rubella, cytomegalic inclusion disease, and herpes simplex.

Galactosemia is a hereditary inborn error of metabolism with deficiency of the enzyme galactose-1-phosphate uridyltransferase and accumulation of galactose-1-phosphate, galactose, and galactitol (Chapter 36). The affected neonate may be normal at birth. Cataracts may appear during the first 2 months of life. The cataracts may be zonular or may appear as the classically described "drop of oil" (vacuoles) in the center of the lens. The latter form results from the inbibition of water that occurs in association with an accumulation of galactose and galactitol in the lens. Diagnosis is made by the finding of galactosuria or the absence of galactose-1-phosphate uridyltransferase in red blood cells. Early diagnosis and a reg-

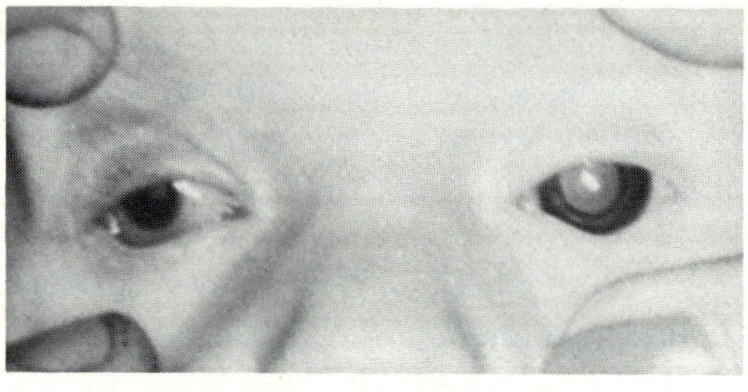

Fig. 39-13. Rubella syndrome with cataract of the left eye and microphthalmia of the right eye.

imen of a galactose-free diet will prevent the development or further progression of cataracts. Resolution of the lens opacity also may occur if the infant receives the appropriate diet. A less severe form of galactosemia may be caused by a deficiency of galactokinase. Such affected children may be otherwise healthy but demonstrate progressive lens opacities, and cataracts may develop at a later age.

Defects in calcium-phosphate metabolism as a result of hypoparathyroidism may cause cataracts but are usually associated with systemic abnormalities.

Treatment. All congenital cataracts require early evaluation by an ophthalmologist. Most dense cataracts are surgically treated to prevent amblyopia or strabismus. Some small central cataracts may be effectively managed by long-term dilation of the pupil to expose the optically clear periphery of the lens. If dilation is inadequate a portion of the iris may be removed surgically (optical iridectomy) for the same purpose. Removal of the lens (as soon as possible if the cataract is complete) followed by contact lens application or spectacle correction may provide the best hope of restoring vision. However, the visual effects of lens extraction without a corrective lens will be no better than leaving the cataract in its original state. If the cataract is monocular the visual prognosis is not as good as when both eyes are affected equally.

Pendular nystagmus may be associated with bilateral cataracts and may continue after surgery. This type of nystagmus is a broad to-and-fro excursion of the eyes that is approximately equal in both directions. It is usually the result, not the cause, of poor visual acuity. Treatment of bilateral, dense congenital cataracts by surgical removal and subsequent correction with glasses or contact lenses may prevent the development of or may reverse pendular nystagmus.

The dislocated lens

The discovery of a dislocated lens (ectopia lentis) in the neonatal period is helpful to identify systemic disease processes that are associated with this abnormality. In the following diseases lens dislocation may be present during the neonatal period or in the first or second decade of life: homocystinuria, sulfite oxidase deficiency, hyperlysinemia, Marfan's syndrome, Ehlers-Danlos syndrome, and Weill-Marchesani syndrome. The dislocation results from a laxity, absence, or defect of the zonular attachments that suspend the lens from the ciliary body. Trauma may also cause a dislocated lens.

Ectopia lentis may be suggested by iridodenesis, or tremulousness, of the iris, which occurs when the posterior surface of the iris lacks the normal support of the lens. The examiner can identify an eccentrically located lens by widely dilating the pupil and visualizing a portion of the equator of the lens in the pupillary space (Fig. 39-14). The dislocated lens usually is not treated during the neonatal period, unless there is the complication of cataract formation or glaucoma. The glaucoma may be caused either by complications of the cataract formation or by blockage of aqueous flow through the pupil.

Diseases of the vitreous and retina producing a white pupil

Diseases of the posterior portion of the neonatal eye that may be sufficiently severe in their involvement of the vitreous or retina to produce a white reflex in the pupil are retinoblastoma, persistent hyperplastic primary vitreous, retinal dysplasia, Norrie's disease, incontinentia pigmenti, vitreous hemorrhage, or retinopathy of prematurity (see part three). Further, any lesion creating a white area in the fundus (e.g., a coloboma or medullated nerve fibers) may produce a white pupillary reflex.

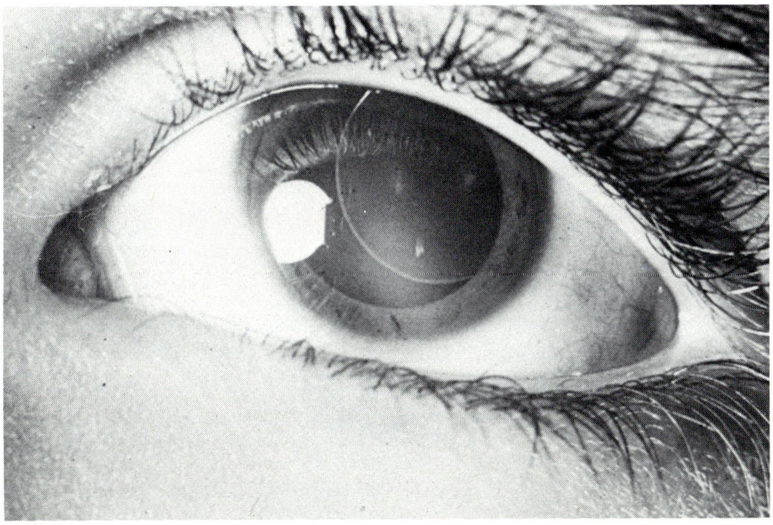

Fig. 39-14. Ectopia lentis (dislocated lens) of the left eye.

Retinoblastoma. Retinoblastoma is the most frequent malignant tumor affecting the neonatal eye. This malignancy usually produces a white pupil only when it involves a large enough area of the posterior segment of the eye.

Retinoblastoma occurs in approximately one of every 25,000 to 30,000 births, with no predilection for race or sex. The tumor arises sporadically or is inherited through an autosomal dominant pattern that exhibits approximately 80% penetrance. Most cases appear to be sporadic. The inherited variety may be gradually increasing in frequency because of a greater survival rate of patients whose retinoblastoma has been treated. Unilateral tumors are usually sporadic and may represent a somatic mutation. Bilateral retinoblastomas are commonly inherited. An affected individual who has survived the hereditary form of retinoblastoma will have about a 40% risk that each offspring will be similarly affected. An individual surviving a sporadic unilateral variety of tumor will have about a 10% chance or less that each offspring will be affected. Those surviving sporadic bilateral involvement appear to have a 40% chance that each offspring will be affected. Empiric risk figures suggest that normal parents with one affected child will have about a 6% chance that a subsequent child will be affected. However, if they have two affected children the risk increases to 40% for each additional child.

The genetic basis for retinoblastoma has been widely studied. Knudson and associates have postulated that two mutational events are necessary for the development of retinoblastoma. Some cases of retinoblastoma have shown abnormalities of chromosome 13.

Clinical manifestations. The tumor originates in the retina and grows anteriorly into the vitreous or posteriorly into the choroid. Early in its course it produces decreased vision and strabismus. With further growth a white pupil (Fig. 39-15) is noted and frequently detected by the parents. Any cross-eyed infant requires a fundus examination with dilated pupils to rule out retinoblastoma. With further enlargement the tumor produces secondary glaucoma, which may be associated with pain and photophobia or symptoms identical to those of congenital glaucoma. With extension into the anterior chamber an opaque layer of white cells (hypopyon) or spontaneous bleeding (hyphema) may occur. The calcification in a retinoblastoma is most easily detected by means of ultrasound or CT.

Diagnosis. The diagnosis of retinoblastoma is supported by the detection of one or more solid white masses in the fundus of the eye. A high percentage of patients have multiple tumors. Small, whitish opacities in the vitreous, representing an anterior seeding of the tumor, may be present. Calcification noted radiologically within the eye (found in 75% of patients) and findings on ultrasound and CT confirm the diagnosis. Aqueous humor levels of lactic acid dehydrogenase may be elevated in comparison with serum values. The differential diagnosis may be exceedingly difficult if the tumor is advanced or atypical and enucleation may be required for histologic study and positive identification. Persistent hyperplastic primary vitreous may be confused with retinoblastoma.

Treatment. The management of retinoblastoma is determined by its size and location. Examination should be performed with the infant under anesthesia, and accurate relationships of all lesions should be plotted on retinal drawings. Reese's classification, which is used to grade the severity and prognosis of the disease, has five groupings. The most favorable, group I, includes small,

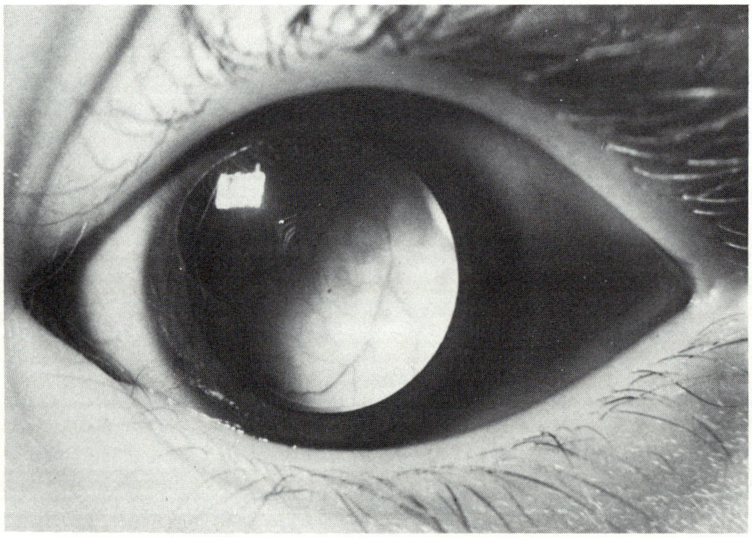

Fig. 39-15. Leukokoria, advanced retinoblastoma.

single or multiple tumors in the posterior half of the fundus. The least favorable, group V, is characterized by tumors involving more than half the retina or seeding of the tumor into the vitreous. Intermediate groups are graded upward in severity according to the tumor's increased size and more anterior location.

The standard treatment of unilateral retinoblastoma has been enucleation. Since direct extension along the optic nerve is one mode by which the disease is spread, it is important to remove as much optic nerve as possible in the process of enucleation. Recently, however, unilateral (and bilateral) tumors in groups I, II, and III have been treated by therapeutic cobalt or linear acceleration x-irradiation. With advanced bilateral disease the more involved eye is usually enucleated for histologic identification, and the remaining eye is treated with supervoltage radiation. Treatment modalities also include radioactive applicators for small, isolated, recurrent tumors in accessible locations. Photocoagulation, cryotherapy, and diathermy also have been used successfully to control localized recurrences. Treatment can effect a total regression in some cases. A reduction in size occurs in large tumors. The color of the tumor changes from pinkish white to grayish or glistening white. A regressed tumor often has the appearance of cottage cheese. Chemotherapeutic agents such as cyclophosphamide, vincristine, and adriamycin have been combined in a palliative way with irradiation for treatment of orbital spread or distant metastases.

Prognosis. The most significant factor in the prognosis is the stage of the disease at the time treatment is instituted. With prompt, adequate treatment group I patients have approximately a 95% chance for 5-year survival. With advanced disease or evidence of extension beyond the globe, the cure rate is markedly reduced (less than a 30% chance for 5-year survival). Although radiation therapy may be effective in curing the retinoblastoma, it unfortunately has its own complications. Children surviving retinoblastoma may develop new malignant disease in the irradiated tissue, cataracts, or radiation retinopathy. Other primary malignancies may also arise. The most common secondary malignancy is osteogenic sarcoma. Abramson and associates have found a 90% incidence of secondary malignancies by age 30 years in patients with retinoblastoma. Thus careful lifelong follow-up of these patients is essential.

Persistent hyperplastic primary vitreous. A congenital anomaly that produces a white pupil at birth or shortly thereafter, persistent hyperplastic primary vitreous (PHPV) results from the failure of the embryonic hyaloid system (the primary vitreous) to reabsorb. The embryonic system develops as a complex network of vessels that grows anteriorly from the disc to surround the developing lens (the tunica vasculosa lentis). This vascular scaffolding supplies the posterior part of the eye and lens during its early formation and is replaced by clear secondary vitreous when the eye further matures. During the fifth to eighth months of gestation the hyaloid vascular system atrophies almost completely, leaving a small, nearly transparent canal running from the disc to the posterior surface of the lens (Cloquet's canal). Failure of this vascular system to atrophy completely may leave a number of possible remnants seen at birth. At the disc a small protrusion of mesodermal tissue, called *Bergmeister's papilla,* extends a short distance into the vitreous. Remnants of the hyaloid artery may be seen extending from the disc to the posterior central area of the lens. A small remnant of the tunica vasculosa lentis on the posterior central area of the lens is called a *Mittendorf dot*. A persistence and hyperplasia of the entire system is called *PHPV*.

Clinical manifestations. At birth, PHPV may appear as a sheet of white tissue immediately behind the lens. It is usually most dense at the center of the lens and thins out toward the periphery. Vessels are frequently seen to radiate from its center. The retrolental mass therefore may be pinkish white. When the pupil is dilated the ciliary processes may be drawn centrally along the posterior surface of the lens toward the central mass.

Almost always unilateral, PHPV occurs in full-term infants without a history of oxygen therapy. The involved eye is commonly microphthalmic. The anterior chamber is frequently shallower than in the fellow eye because fibrous contraction of the primary vitreous pulls the ciliary body centrally, forcing the lens forward. With continued organization and contraction of the primary vitreous, the lens capsule may be involved, and cataracts may form. At this stage in the development of the disease there may be glaucoma, posterior chamber hemorrhages, and hemorrhages into the lens. Retinal detachment occurs in the final stages, with continued vitreous traction. PHPV should be suspected in the neonate with a rapidly progressive unilateral mature cataract.

Diagnosis. Differentiation of PHPV from retinopathy of prematurity (ROP; see part three) is usually possible because of the unilateral involvement and occurrence of PHPV in a full-term infant. ROP usually develops bilaterally in a premature infant who has had oxygen therapy. Differentiation from retinoblastoma is aided by the presence of visible ciliary processes in the periphery of the dilated pupil and the presence of vascular elements in the central portion of the retrolental mass. Also, retinoblastomas do not usually occur in microphthalmic eyes. The absence of roentgenographic evidence of calcification within the eye may be of additional value. A persistent embryonic iris vessel or one that notches the pupil suggests the presence of PHPV, even when an opaque lens obscures its presence. CT and ultrasound may also help in the differentiation.

Treatment. Surgical removal of the lens and vitreous

with optical correction and amblyopia treatment must be attempted very early (within the first few weeks) to achieve any degree of success. Only very mild cases have been reported to have moderate visual success, and the prognosis for visual recovery should be extremely guarded.

Retinal dysplasia. Retinal dysplasia is a congenital anomaly of full-term infants, is usually bilateral, and is associated with microphthalmic eyes. It may occur as part of a group of congenital anomalies, including defects of the central nervous system, cardiovascular system, and skeletal system, of sufficient severity to produce early death of the infant: Trisomy 13 should be considered. When the dysplasia is advanced a white retrolental mass may be produced. Milder forms of dysplasia occur as developmental abnormalities but often are detected only by histologic techniques; results of chromosomal analysis are usually normal.

Norrie's disease. A rare genetic disorder transmitted as an X-linked recessive trait, Norrie's disease is characterized by the presence of bilateral massive retinal detachments, resulting in a white pupil. Organization of the retinal detachment may disrupt the lens, producing cataract, or may affect the anterior chamber angle, producing congenital glaucoma. The usual result is atrophy of the globe (phthisis bulbi).

Other causes of leukokoria

Other lesions that may simulate retinoblastoma are cataract, coloboma of fundus, congenital retinal fold, retinoschisis, organizing vitreous hemorrhage, or scarring from retinopathy of prematurity. There are other causes of leukokoria in children, but some of them present in an older age group, such as nematode endophthalmitis, Coats' disease, and uveitis.

Retinal abnormalities

Observing the neonatal eye should be a routine part of the examination of every infant. With the direct ophthalmoscope the fundus appears as a flat, two-dimensional surface. However, this represents a three-dimensional organization of tissue in which several successive layers are viewed simultaneously as the result of their transparency. The retinal vessels lie near the surface of the retina. Deep to the vessels the retina is nearly transparent, with a sheen to its inner surface. This transparency is disturbed when abnormalities are present. The tissue resembles a pale, ghostlike sheet when it is detached. Retinal edema gives a slightly raised opalescent appearance. Infection obscures the underlying structures with a fuzzy white thickening of the retinal tissue.

During the neonatal period nonvascular structures of the fundus are nearly transparent because uveal pigmentation is lacking. Therefore, in all pathologic processes characterized by either a lack or an excess of pigment, these defects may be only minimally suggested and may become progressively evident as the uveal pigmentation culminates after the first 6 months of life. The choroid is the deepest layer normally visible with the ophthalmoscope. Pathologic processes that prevent its development or that destroy areas of choroid therefore will expose areas of bare sclera, which will appear glistening white with the ophthalmoscope.

Hereditary abnormalities

Retinoschisis is a hereditary abnormality in which the superficial layers of the retina are split from the deeper layers and are elevated into the vitreous. This splitting creates a veil-like appearance in front of the retina. Visual function is absent in the affected tissue. Retinoschisis is a progressive, degenerative disorder that has an X-linked recessive transmission. Macular changes and vitreous hemorrhages can occur as associated findings. Both lead to loss of vision.

Leber's congenital amaurosis often produces symptoms of blindness shortly after birth. Typical findings are a salt-and-pepper appearance of the fundus, with a grayish cast to the retina. Although the fundus may have a normal appearance electroretinography discloses severely deficient retinal function. Children with this disorder may rub their eyes excessively (oculodigital phenomenon). Leber's congenital amaurosis is transmitted as an autosomal recessive disease.

The diagnosis of albinism in the neonatal period is extremely difficult to substantiate because the uveal pigment is normally underdeveloped during this period. The diagnosis may be suggested when pigmentation of the skin, hair, and irises fails to progress during the first several months in comparison with that of parents and siblings. Lack of pigmentation is more apparent earlier in darker races. The fundus remains quite pale, and choroidal vessels are prominent. Photophobia, pendular nystagmus, and abnormal transillumination of the irises are characteristic features of albinism. Moderately to severely reduced vision is characteristic, often secondary to foveal hypoplasia.

Congenital disorders

A retinal fold is a white fold or ridge of retinal tissue running from the disc, typically inferotemporally, to the periphery. The macular area occasionally may be involved.

Congenital grouped pigmentation is an uncommon finding in which small areas of the retina, one disc diameter or less in size, show hyperpigmentation. These areas typically are paired or grouped and are usually kidney shaped. They have no clinical significance but should not be confused with old inflammatory scars.

A coloboma of the fundus is visible as a defect in the

retinal and choroidal layers through which the underlying sclera is visible. A coloboma usually occurs inferonasally, which is the site of the closure of the embryonic fissure. The fissure usually begins to close around the equator and then extends posteriorly toward the optic disc and anteriorly toward the periphery. Any part or all of this region may be involved in the colobomatous defect.

Infectious diseases

Intrauterine ocular infections result from maternal infections that cross the placental barrier (Chapter 31). Chorioretinitis occurs in patients with rubella and, occasionally, in patients with influenza and congenital syphilis. An irregularity of the retinal pigment develops with what appears to be a salt-and-pepper type of distribution. Congenital cytomegalic inclusion disease may include a variety of chorioretinal lesions, from large, whitish, necrotic lesions in the posterior pole to the more typical multiple, small, peripheral, white areas that tend to enlarge or coalesce as the disease progresses. Congenital toxoplasmosis in its severe form may lead to large chorioretinal scars in the macular area. These scars appear as large white areas of exposed sclera, with prominent, darkly pigmented borders. The treatment of ocular manifestations of congenital toxoplasmosis has not been established. When seen in the neonatal fundus, scar formation usually is a sign of the inactive disease. In addition to intrauterine infections, postnatally acquired candidal septicemia may be associated with fluffy retinal and vitreous exudates. TORCH titers should be obtained to help in the diagnosis of chorioretinitis.

Acquired pathologic conditions of the fundus

The retina of the premature infant is incompletely formed at birth and continues to develop during the first few months of neonatal life. The periphery of the fundus, from the equator to the ora serrata (the junction of the retina and the ciliary body), appears pale or grayish. These are normal findings that gradually give way to the reddish pink color of the fundus as the retina progressively differentiates.

Birth trauma may produce a pathologic condition of the retina (Chapter 20); there may be scattered retinal hemorrhages, vitreous hemorrhage, or areas of retinal edema. (ROP is discussed in part three.)

The abnormal macula

Several of the storage diseases alter the appearance of the macula, which may be useful in detecting these disorders (Table 39-3) (Chapter 36). The stored material accumulates in the ganglion cells of the retina, which decreases the transparency of the retina except at the very center of the macula where no ganglion cells exist. Therefore the center of the macula retains its normal cherry-red appearance in sharp contrast to the surrounding grayish fundus. Sphingolipidoses that may produce a cherry-red spot are Tay-Sachs disease, in which a cherry-red spot may be present shortly after birth or may develop during the first year, and Niemann-Pick disease (infantile), in which approximately 50% of patients develop a cherry-red spot in the macula during the neonatal period. Of the so-called mucolipidoses Farber's disease has been noted to show a grayish discoloration of the macula at 6 to 8 weeks of age, and GM_1 generalized gangliosidosis has been found to demonstrate a cherry-red spot in the macula in approximately 30% of patients before 2 months of age. The mucopolysaccharidoses are characterized by the abnormal deposition of mucopolysaccharides in the cornea but the macula appears normal. Neuraminidase deficiency (Goldberg's syndrome) appears to be a mucolipidosis with both a macular cherry-red spot and mild corneal clouding.

Table 39-3. Neonatal macular changes

Condition	Defect
Tay-Sachs disease	Cherry-red spot
Niemann-Pick disease	Cherry-red spot
GM, generalized gangliosidosis	Cherry-red spot
Neuraminidase deficiency	Cherry-red spot and corneal clouding
Farber's disease	Gray macula
Best's vitelliform degeneration	Cystic macula (rare)
Toxoplasmosis	Chorioretinal scar
Coloboma	Absence of retina and choroid

Optic disc abnormalities

All transmission of the visual pathways must exit the eye through the optic disc. Mild degrees of pallor or optic atrophy can be difficult to establish in the neonate. Disc margins should, however, be clear and distinct.

Persistence of hyaloid artery

Persistence of the central hyaloid artery is a common developmental abnormality. Its presence in the premature infant is sufficiently frequent to be considered normal. It occurs in some 3% of full-term infants. It is most frequently a fine thread of nearly transparent tissue; it rarely may be patent and contain blood. The artery commonly continues to atrophy during the neonatal period, with rare persistence into adulthood.

Bergmeister's papilla

The persistence of the mesodermal supporting elements of the hyaloid vascular system at the disc may leave a small protuberance of gray-white tissue extending from the disc forward into the vitreous. A small knuckle of a retinal vessel may course into this area and return to the disc before supplying the normal retina, or the papilla may be associated with one or several small, round, pearl-gray cysts of remaining glial tissue. Vision usually is unimpaired.

Myelinated nerve fibers

Normal myelinization of the optic nerve fibers occurs in fetal development in reverse direction to the growth of the axons themselves. Development of myelin sheaths therefore progresses from the geniculate bodies through the optic tracts, optic chiasm, and optic nerves to end normally just posterior to the optic disc. This process is usually complete at birth or within the first month of extrauterine life. Myelination of the nerve fibers occasionally proceeds through the disc and into the retinal surface as a glistening white, opaque area involving the peripheral portion of the disc and extending into segments of the nearby retina. At times there is no continuity between the disc and the myelinated nerve fibers of the retina. The edges of the myelinated areas are feathered, and the involved areas are sometimes arcuate. This process is stable after the first several months of life, and visual acuity is not often impaired, except for an enlarged area of the blind spot when measured in adults.

Conus or congenital crescent

The sharp margins of the optic disc are created by the abrupt ending of the choroid and pigment epithelium at the disc borders. On occasion these structures fail to extend to the immediate edge of the disc in one quadrant; instead, they stop short in a sloping margin, which is crescent shaped. The underlying sclera is then visible as a whitish crescent adjacent to the disc. This crescent is sometimes bordered by a darkly pigmented line. Two thirds of congenital crescents occur below the disc. Most eyes with congenital crescents have associated defective vision in the form of hypermetropic astigmatism. A congenital conus should be differentiated from a myopic conus, or crescent, in that the former is present at birth, is inferiorly located, and is stationary throughout life; the latter develops as the eye becomes excessively myopic and is usually temporal.

Coloboma of the disc

Coloboma of the disc is formed when the embryonic optic vesicle fails to close adequately. A coloboma of the iris or choroid has a similar pathogenesis. The disc may appear enlarged and elongated, usually inferiorly or temporally. The coloboma may include the macular area. The blood vessels may be distributed normally or may be displaced to the periphery of the disc and appear somewhat disorganized in their initial direction from the disc. Colobomas of the disc frequently are associated with defective vision.

Optic pit

The surface of the optic disc occasionally shows a hole or pit. This pit usually is situated near the lower temporal quadrant of the disc at its border and may vary in size, shape, and depth. It is thought to be a minimal coloboma of the disc. Visual defects frequently are present with this finding. Later in life they are manifested as an enlarged blind spot, sector field defects, or involvement of the papillomacular bundle, with production of a partial paracentral or central scotoma. Moreover, serous fluid may elevate the macula and cause reduction in visual acuity.

Oblique discs

The optic nerve commonly enters the posterior aspect of the eye from a slightly nasal angle. If this angle is accentuated the nerve head or disc may be tilted obliquely, with its temporal margin considerably more posterior than its nasal margin. This gives the disc an ovoid appearance, with its longest diameter in the vertical meridian. This abnormality may be associated with reduced visual acuity.

Hypoplasia of the optic nerve

Hypoplasia of the optic disc is a rare anomaly in which part or all of the optic nerve fibers fail to develop and reach the disc. The optic disc is smaller than normal and may be pale, but the retinal vessels usually are normal. A hypopigmented ring around the hypoplastic nerve creates the so-called double-ring sign. This may occur unilaterally or bilaterally. Visual impairment may range from mild to severe.

Optic nerve hypoplasia may occur as an isolated finding or in association with other ocular or systemic abnormalities. CT of the brain may also reveal midline abnormalities, a disorder referred to as *septooptic dysplasia* (DeMorsier syndrome). Endocrine abnormalities are frequently found in this syndrome.

Congenital optic atrophy

Congenital optic atrophy is a condition of unknown cause in which the nerve fibers have formed and subsequently atrophied. The disc is pale and has a normal size and configuration. The child is usually blind, or vision is exceedingly poor and associated with nystagmus. The condition remains static and often is unassociated with other central nervous system disturbances.

NEUROMUSCULAR ABNORMALITIES

Strabismus

Clinically significant strabismus is recognized less frequently in the neonatal period than in the remainder of the first 5 years of life. Its diagnosis is important, however, since therapy, when indicated, must begin early. Few, if any, patients with, for example, congenitally crossed eyes will spontaneously "grow out" of this problem with the passage of time. Esotropia (crossed eyes) may result from inheritance, paralysis of the lateral rectus muscles, or refractive errors (usually hyperopia) or may be secondary to any type of disease that reduces visual acuity in one eye. Exotropia (wall eyes) is rare in the neonate (except congenital anomalies such as Greig's hypertelorism). The usual forms of exotropia do not appear until 1 to 2 years of age or later.

Strabismus can be diagnosed by the Hirschberg test, which allows the pupillary light reflex to be evaluated on both corneas while the patient fixates binocularly on a small light source that is held before the patient's face and directed toward the pupils. If the patient is properly fixating with both eyes on the light source, the pupillary light reflex should appear in the same part of the pupillary space of each eye. If the light reflex is centered in one eye and deviated to the lateral side of the pupil or cornea of the fellow eye, esotropia is present. A rough estimation of the visual acuity can be made by determining the fixation pattern of each eye while the infant fixates on a light. If only one eye moves to fixate on the light centrally and steadily at all times, the one that does not invariably has poor acuity.

An alternative fixation target is the human face. This may be the most reliable target to assess the very young neonate and may be used for visual evaluation in the same fashion as a light source.

When strabismus is present, a careful ocular examination is required to rule out the possibility of an intraocular pathologic condition. Pathologic conditions that may create esotropia are corneal opacities, cataracts, and diseases of the fundus that have reduced or destroyed macular vision, such as infections (for example, toxoplasmosis) or tumors (for example, retinoblastoma). *Fundus examination with the patient's pupils dilated is mandatory*.

Congenital esotropia may be present while the neonate is still in the nursery or may become evident during the first 2 weeks of life. Results of an ocular examination may be otherwise normal, and visual acuity is usually equal in both eyes. Amblyopia may develop from congenital esotropia, although it is more frequently noted with accommodative esotropia, which appears later in childhood.

Esotropia caused by the paralysis of the lateral rectus muscles may occur as a result of birth trauma; it is diagnosed by failure of an eye to deviate laterally beyond the midline. Lateral rotation is best examined when one eye of the patient is occluded and the opposite eye is observed. Congenital esotropia also shows a weakness of lateral gaze when both eyes are tested simultaneously but normal lateral rotations with one eye occluded.

Pseudostrabismus is used to describe infants who appear cross-eyed because the bridge of the nose is wide and the epicanthal folds on either side cover most of the sclera on the medial side of the cornea. True strabismus is ruled out when the corneal light reflex is found to be symmetrically placed in both pupils.

The treatment of strabismus begins with an adequate ocular examination and a careful cycloplegic refraction. Aims in the treatment of strabismus include the prevention of strabismic amblyopia, the improvement or correction of the cosmetic appearance, and, if possible, the creation of binocular vision. The chances of improving amblyopia and strabismus are better the earlier that therapy is begun. Treatment (drops, patching, glasses, surgery, and so on) should be completed well before the child is of school age to eliminate a visual or cosmetic handicap.

Amblyopia

Amblyopia is a decrease in vision in one or both eyes that is not caused by organic disease. Main classifications are (1) strabismic amblyopia, (2) anisometropic amblyopia, and (3) deprivation amblyopia.

Amblyopia may develop at any time during the "sensitive period" of visual development, which usually occurs during the first 6 years in humans. Any interference in vision, whether secondary to strabismus, refractive error, or occlusion of the visual axis, can lead to amblyopia. Children with a family history of strabismus or amblyopia should be seen by an ophthalmologist early in life and monitored carefully. Any child with a suspected pathologic condition, such as cataracts, ptosis, or lid lesions, should also have a complete ophthalmologic evaluation.

Treatment of amblyopia is accomplished by patching the better-seeing eye. The patching regimen is tapered as visual improvement is noted. If an organic lesion has caused the amblyopia, patching or treatment of the lesion or both may be necessary. If bilateral amblyopia is present because of high refractive error, glasses are prescribed. Visual deprivation secondary to cataracts may necessitate prompt lens extraction.

Nystagmus

Nystagmus refers to an oscillation of one or both eyes; it may occur in a horizontal, vertical or torsional plane. The two main types of nystagmus are pendular and jerk nystagmus. Pendular nystagmus is a to-and-fro movement of the eyes, of equal amplitude in both directions. Jerk nystagmus is characterized by a slow component in one direction and a fast component in the opposite direction. Nystagmus may also be described by its rate (rapid or slow) and by its amplitude (fine or coarse).

Physiologic nystagmus, usually a jerk nystagmus, may be seen in several situations. The optokinetic phenomenon of a target moving past the eyes will cause a slow-moving component as the eyes fixate on an object, followed by a rapid refixation movement in the opposite direction. Vestibular nystagmus occurs with rotation of the body or with irrigation of the ear, causing a movement of the fluid within the semicircular canals. Positional nystagmus is seen in extreme gaze, usually in a horizontal direction.

Pathologic forms of nystagmus may result from ocular, neurologic, or vestibular defects. "Ocular" nystagmus is often pendular. It can be caused by a lesion in the eye or in any of the pathways leading back to the visual cortex. Ocular defects causing congenital nystagmus include optic nerve hypoplasia or atrophy, macular scars, cataracts, aniridia, and albinism. Certain types of hereditary nystagmus also are pendular. A congenital type of jerk nystagmus may be diagnosed early in life. In this form of nystagmus visual acuity may be improved by turning the eyes in one particular direction of gaze; thus a head turn is adopted to maximize vision. An interesting form of nystagmus called *spasmus nutans* usually develops within the first 2 years of life and disappears within months to several years after its onset. The nystagmus of spasmus nutans is often very fine and rapid and may be asymmetric or even monocular. The classical triad of spasmus nutans includes nystagmus, head nodding, and torticollis, although the diagnosis is often made when one or two of the features are absent. A neurologic condition—with much more serious consequences than nystagmus—occasionally may present similar characteristics. Therefore careful follow-up is essential and further diagnostic studies may be advisable.

A posterior fossa lesion or a defect in the motor pathways can present as either a pendular or jerk nystagmus. Seesaw nystagmus, which is often associated with chiasmal lesions, is characterized by an upward movement of one eye and a simultaneous downward movement of the other eye.

Nystagmus can also be caused by a defect in gaze mechanism. This can occur in brainstem or cerebellar disease, in disorders of the medial longitudinal fasciculus, or as a result of medications (such as barbiturates or diphenylhydantoin) or a paresis of an extraocular muscle.

Central or peripheral defects in the vestibular system may cause a jerk nystagmus. Nystagmus that is due to peripheral vestibular disease is usually associated with tinnitus, deafness, and vertigo.

Pupillary abnormalities

Abnormalities of the pupil may be the result of structural disease of the iris or to neurologic abnormalities. Neurologic abnormalities may be described in terms of pupil size (miosis or mydriasis) or abnormal function.

Miosis may result from paralysis of the sympathetic pathways, as in Horner's syndrome, or from irritation of the parasympathetic pathways, as may occur in central nervous system inflammation.

Mydriasis is most often caused by a paralysis of the parasympathetic pathways, which may occur in a third nerve palsy or with increased intracranial pressure. Local trauma, such as may occur during a difficult forceps delivery, may also damage the iris sphincter and result in mydriasis.

Anisocoria describes a difference in the size of the two pupils. When this condition is seen the examiner should evaluate the patient in both bright and dim illumination to determine which is the abnormal pupil. Some normal individuals have a small degree of anisocoria.

An afferent pupillary defect occurs when a defect is present anterior to the lateral geniculate body before synapse in the pretectal region. Both the direct and consensual reflexes should be evaluated. For a more detailed description of pupillary abnormalities, the reader is referred to a textbook on neurology or neuroophthalmology.

NEONATAL INFECTIONS

Conjunctivitis

See also Chapter 31.

Neonatal conjunctivitis may be caused by a variety of agents including chemical, bacterial, chlamydial, and viral. If undiagnosed and untreated, permanent scarring and loss of vision may occur. It is essential to culture the exudate and a conjunctival scraping to look for evidence of bacterial or chlamydial infection.

A common cause of ophthalmia neonatorum is the instillation of 1% silver nitrate into the eyes at birth. In spite of its disadvantages and occasional irritation, the Credé prophylaxis is statistically the most effective, least troublesome method of preventing gonococcal conjunctivitis. However, silver nitrate prophylaxis does not prevent the development of chlamydial conjunctivitis, which is becoming the most common neonatal eye infection. The rate at which chemical conjunctivitis occurs from silver nitrate is approximately 10% in all newborns. The risk of infection is probably enhanced by the prolonged contact of the germicide. This is the only conjunctivitis generally present from the first postnatal day. It is usually unilateral, and the lids are slightly swollen. The conjunctiva is congested and edematous; purulence is not observed. This condition clears spontaneously in 3 to 4 days if no secondary bacterial infection occurs. Eye drops of 10% sodium sulfacetamide, administered four times a day, may be used locally to prevent secondary infection. Secondary bacterial infection is suspected if the disease persists beyond this time or increases in severity. Cultures with sensitivity tests identify the organism and suggest appropriate treatment.

Gonorrheal conjunctivitis

Conjunctivitis caused by *Neisseria gonorrhoeae* is an acute, severe, purulent conjunctivitis with an incubation period of 2 to 5 days (Chapter 31). The rate of occurrence in the United States today is less than 0.03% because silver nitrate or antibiotic instillation are legally required at birth. There have been reports of resistance to the Credé prophylaxis. If *Neisseria gonorrhoeae* is the cause of the conjunctivitis, immediate treatment with intravenous penicillin and topical antibiotics is necessary.

Nongonococcal bacterial conjunctivitis

Ophthalmia neonatorum also may result from other common pathogens, such as staphylococci, pneumococci, streptococci, or gram-negative bacteria. These bacterial infections usually appear several days after birth. Most respond well to topical antibiotics, such as 10% sulfacetamide solution four times a day.

Chlamydial conjunctivitis (inclusion blennorrhea) is currently the most common infection in the neonatal period. The infection is frequently acquired from the mother as the child passes through the birth canal. The usual cultures and Gram staining are unproductive in inclusion blennorrhea. The typical basophilic inclusion bodies in the epithelial cells are demonstrated with Giemsa-stained smears of the conjunctival scraping of the lower lid.

Chlamydial conjunctivitis is treated with the administration of erythromycin or sulfacetamide ointment three times a day for 2 to 3 weeks. Systemic antibiotics may be necessary since chlamydia can cause pneumonia. It is recommended that the child's mother and her sexual contacts be treated with tetracycline or erythromycin, 250 mg, four times a day for up to 1 month.

Any child who has a chronic or recurrent conjunctivitis may have a blocked nasolacrimal duct. The duct will frequently open spontaneously during the first year of life. Treatment with topical antibiotics and massage of the lacrimal sac may help resolve the problem.

Nancy Anderson Hamming
John E. Read
Marilyn T. Miller

BIBLIOGRAPHY

Abbassi, V., Lowe, C.U., and Calecagno, P.L.: Oculocerebro-renal syndromes; a review, Am. J. Dis. Child. **115**:145, 1968.

Abramson, D.H., and others: Treatment of orbital rhabdmyosarcoma, Ophthalmology **86**:1330, 1979.

Baum, J.D., and Bulpitt, C.J.: Retinal and conjunctival hemorrhage in the newborn, Arch. Dis. Child. **45**:344, 1970.

Chimonidou, E., Palmimeris, G., and Velissaropoulos, P.: Retinoblastoma; some aspects concerning diagnosis, heredity, and treatment, J. Pediatr. Ophthalmol. Strabismus **16**:101, 1979.

Cogan, D.G., and Kuwabara, T.: The spingolipidoses and the eye, Arch. Ophthalmol. **79**:437, 1968.

de Venecia, G., and Lobeck, C.C.: Successful treatment of eyelid hemangioma with prednisone, Arch. Ophthalmol. **84**:98, 1970.

Egbert, P.R., and others: Visual results and ocular complications following radiotherapy for retinoblastoma, Arch. Ophthalmol. **96**:1826, 1979.

Ellsworth, R.M.: The practical management of retinoblastoma, Trans. Am. Ophthalmol. Soc. **67**:462, 1969.

Emery, J.M., and others: G_{M1}-gangliosidosis; ocular and pathological manifestations, Arch. Ophthalmol. **85**:177, 1971.

Faris, B.M., and others: The role of cryotherapy in the management of early lesions of retinoblastoma, Ann. Ophthalmol. **85**:177, 1971.

Fontaine, M.: Manifestations ocularies de la prématurité, Arch. Ophthalmol. (Paris) **31**:383, 1971.

Forbes, G.B., and Forbes, G.M.: Silver nitrate and the eyes of the newborn: Credé's contribution to preventive medicine, Am. J. Dis. Child. **121**:1, 1971.

Francois, J.: General anomalies and diseases associated with congenital cataracts. In Congenital cataracts. Springfield, Ill., 1963, Charles C Thomas, Publisher.

Fraumeni, Jr., J.F., and Glass, A.G.: Wilms' tumor and congenital aniridia, JAMA **206**:825, 1968.

Friendly, D.S.: Ocular manifestations of physical child abuse, Trans. Am. Acad. Ophthalmol. Otolaryngol. **75**:381, 1971.

Gitzelmann, R.: Hereditary galactokinase deficiency; a newly recognized cause of juvenile cataracts, Pediatr. Res. **1**:14, 1967.

Goldberg, M.F.: Waardenburg's syndrome with fundus and other anomalies, Arch. Ophthalmol. **76**:797, 1966.

Goldberg, M.F., editor: Genetic and metabolic eye disease, Boston, 1974, Little, Brown & Co.

Goldberg, M.F., Maumenee, A.E., and MuKusick, V.A.: Corneal dystrophies associates with abnormalities of mucopolysaccharide metabolism, Arch. Ophthalmol. **74**:516, 1965.

Goldberg, M.F., Payne, J.W., and Brunt, P.W.: Ophthalmologic studies of familial dysautonomia; the Riley-Day syndrome, Arch. Ophthalmol. **80**:732, 1968.

Goldberg, M.F., and others: Macular cherry-red spot, corneal clouding and β-galactose deficiency; clinical biochemical and electron microscopic study of a new autosomal recessive storage disease, Arch. Intern. Med. **128**:387, 1971.

Haik, B.B., and others: Capillary hemangioma of the lids and orbit. An analysis of the clinical features and therapeutic results in 101 cases, Ophthalmology **86**:760, 1979.

Knudson, Jr., A.G., Hethcote, H.W., and Brown, B.W.: Mutation and childhood cancer: a probabilistic model for the incidence of retinoblastoma, Proc. Natl. Acad. Sci. USA **72**:5116, 1975.

Knudson, Jr., A.G., and others: Chromosomal deletion and retinoblastoma, N. Engl. J. Med. **295**:1120, 1976.

Kushner, B.J.: Local steroid therapy in adnexal hemangioma, Ann. Ophthalmol. **11**:1005, 1979.

McCormick, A.Q.: Transient cataracts in premature infants: a new clinical entity, Can. J. Ophthalmol. **3**:202, 1968.

Reese, A.B.: Tumors of the eye, ed. 2, New York, 1963, Harper & Row, Publishers.

Sagerman, R.H., Cassady, R.J., and Trette, P.: Radiation therapy for rhabdomyosarcoma of the orbit, Trans. Am. Acad. Ophthalmol. Otolaryngol. **72**:849, 1968.

Scheie, H.G., and Albert, D.M.: Adler's textbook of ophthalmology, Philadelphia, 1969, W.B. Saunders Co.

Smith, G.F., Berg, J.M., and McCreary, B.D.: de Lange syndrome. In the First Conference on the Clinical Delineation of Birth Defects. Part II. Birth defects: original article series, vol. 5, White Plains, N.Y., 1969, National Foundation March of Dimes.

PART THREE

Retinopathy of prematurity

This vascular retinopathy develops only in the incompletely vascularized retina of premature infants, leading to a wide range of outcomes from normal vision to total loss of vision. *Retrolental fibroplasia*, as it was called in the early 1940s when it was first described, almost disappeared between 1954 and 1970, when oxygen use was severely restricted, but has returned to plague modern newborn intensive care units (ICUs) as one of the major causes of handicap in surviving infants of extremely low birth weight. An estimated 500 infants annually are virtually blind and another estimated 1,500 have serious retinal scars.

INCIDENCE

Incidence figures for ROP vary strikingly from one neonatal ICU to the next depending on the child's age at first examination, the frequency of examinations, and the definitions of mild ROP that are applied. The risk of ROP rises dramatically from 9% to 34% for premature infants of 1 to 1.5 kg birth weight to 22% to 88% for those weighing less than 1 kg at birth. Gestational age or birth weight or both are the strongest predictors of ROP. Once these parameters are controlled for, the strongest predictors of severe stages of this disease are the requirement for prolonged administration of oxygen and other indicators of a complicated perinatal course (number of blood gas measurements done, number of abnormal blood gas values found, amount of transfusion required, sepsis, and intracranial hemorrhage).

PATHOGENESIS

Only those infants whose retinal vessels have not yet completed their centrifugal growth from the optic disc to the ora serrata develop this disorder of neovascularization. The vessel growth begins at 15 to 18 weeks of gestation as the retina thickens and matures, exceeding the ability of the underlying choroid to supply its needs through diffusion alone. First, primitive future endothelial cells form cords that canalize into a network of evenly spaced capillaries, which further differentiate into primitive and then mature arterioles and venules. Each of these steps can be seen simultaneously at any point in time in the immature retina because they are sequentially proceeding from the disc outward.

If a catastrophe occurs to these vessels the natural progress is arrested. Hyperoxia, shock, asphyxia, hypothermia, vitamin E deficiency, and light exposure have all been advanced as possible reasons for the initial injury. After this initial injury vessel growth can resume normally (no ROP), or for unknown reasons the primitive vessels may pile up within the retina, growing without forward progress and forming a ridge of tissue that can become extremely large. This tissue may then regress, and vessels once again progress toward the periphery, or this condition can worsen through the growth of fibrovascular tissue into the vitreous cavity. When this occurs the tissue may yet regress, but it often begins to contract and form a scar (cicatrix) that pulls and distorts the retina and can lead to a displaced macula, retinal folds, or retinal detachments. In some infants the eye becomes inexplicably inflamed with vitreous haze, exudate along the retinal vessels, and engorgement and tortuosity of the posterior pole vessels and the remnants of the tunica vasculosa lentis in the iris. This process is usually seen preceding partial or total retinal detachment, sometimes as early as 8 to 10 weeks after birth.

Once the initiating event(s) is triggered we have even less understanding of what determines which infants then have cicatrix formation and which experience regression or healing. Preliminary evidence in a very imperfect animal model suggests that chronic hypoxia may contribute to the failure of healing.

The randomized multicenter trial of 1953 inexorably linked oxygen to this disease when it showed that the then common practice of administering greater than 50% inspired oxygen for more than 4 weeks resulted in an incidence of severe retinopathy of 23% in survivors weighing less than 1,500 gm at birth, compared to just 7% in infants given oxygen for cyanosis only. In the era that followed, oxygen use was severely restricted, probably resulting in an increased mortality rate; however, ROP was nearly eliminated for a time. The current resurgence is believed to result from the increased survival of infants with retinas so immature at birth that current cautious use of oxygen is not a significant contributing factor in the disease and that other complications of the perinatal period in addition to the extreme immaturity are responsible.

CLASSIFICATION

In 1984 the International Classification of Acute Retinopathy of Prematurity (ICROP) was published after 2 years of work by ophthalmologists bedeviled by this disorder throughout the world. The novel features of this new classification are three: First, it locates the disease (anterior to posterior) by defining three zones; second, the extent of the disease is described by the number of clock hours involved; and third, the accelerated, inflammatory nature of extremely aggressive disease is identified by the designation *plus disease*. As in previous classifications the degree of vasculopathy at the vascular-avascular transition is divided into stages 1, 2, and 3, with stage 4 being reserved for retinal detachment. Fig. 39-16 demonstrates sketches of two retinas, both with stage 3 disease but differing markedly as described by the ICROP. The ICROP description contains far more information, and as we gain experience with it, it will probably make early prognostication easier.

The ICROP classifies only the proliferative phase of the disease process. In 1985 work began on classification

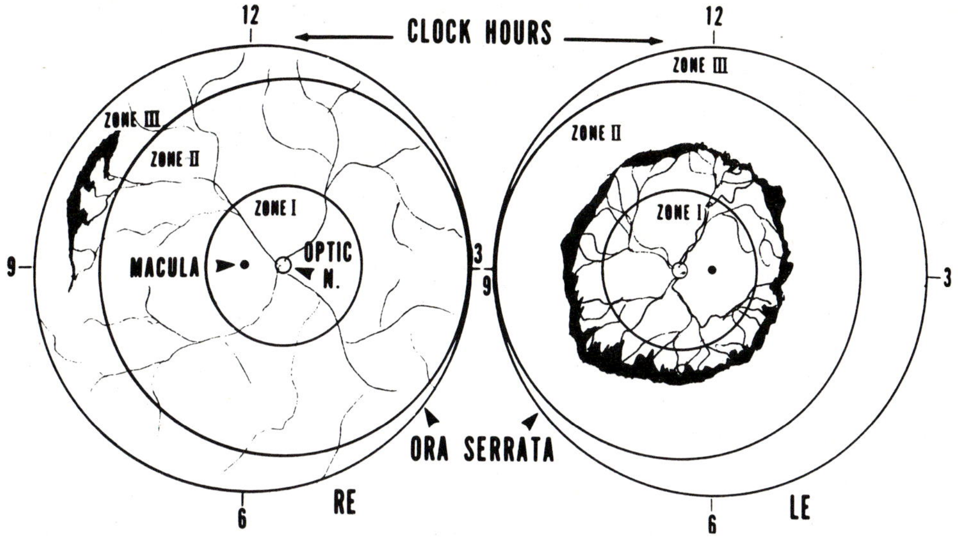

Fig. 39-16. How the ICROP shows the extent and posterior extension of ROP. Stage 3 retinopathy is shown in both retinal sketches made on the diagrams of the three zones on the retina. On the left, however, the disease is in zone 3 and covers only 2 clock hours, whereas on the right the disease is in zone 2 and extends for 12 clock hours.

of the cicatricial stages and retinal detachment, with the goal of developing a clinically useful description.

CLINICAL COURSE

When infants with ROP are examined regularly from 6 weeks of age, they will demonstrate the sequential development of the stages of the disease described above until they reach a turning point when the vessels regress and heal or they go on to advanced disease. Quite variable rates of progression are observed, with the worst forms presenting early (5 to 9 weeks) in zone 1 or 2 (the most immature) and progressing rapidly through the stages to plus disease and exudative retinal detachments by 8 to 20 weeks after birth. In Japan this has been termed *rush disease*. A slower evolution of the disorder to complete resolution or partial cicatrix is more common and may take as long as a year to stabilize, although the outcome of most ROP is apparent by 3 months after birth. The latter type of disease is far less aggressive and usually results in less visual impairment.

Even infants who have only mild ROP (stage 1 or 2 without the plus component) and heal without residual cicatrix have a higher than expected incidence of myopia, strabismus, glaucoma, cataract, amblyopia, and other sequelae. The infants who have residual cicatrix without retinal detachments are also more likely to have any of these problems and, in addition, are at risk for developing very slowly progressive retinal degenerations that can lead to retinal detachments in later decades.

The few infants who do progress to total retinal detachment require close monitoring and support for secondary glaucoma, entropion, infections caused by eye rubbing, and referral to and continued support in the early intervention programs for the visually handicapped.

DIFFERENTIAL DIAGNOSIS

Infants who have been systematically followed through the newborn period present no difficulty in differential diagnosis. However, when an infant first presents with an extensive retinal detachment or a completely white pupil, it can be extremely difficult to differentiate from the other causes of leukokoria (see Part two). One particular entity bears special mention. In recent years several families have been described with familial exudative vitreoretinopathy, an autosomal dominant proliferative retinopathy with variable penetrance that closely simulates ROP. Should a full-term or near-term infant present with what appears to be ROP, it is wise to examine other family members, with this disease in mind.

RECOMMENDATIONS FOR EXAMINATION SCHEDULE

At the present time, there is no proven intervention for ROP; therefore routine screening is indicated only in premature infants to detect those infants with ROP for statistical purposes and to identify those that need regular follow-up examinations for continuing eye care. Because the examinations are informational the first examination, particularly for infants weighing less than 1 kg, should not be delayed until the week of discharge from the hospital, since after long difficult months this is a time of special optimism for the family and a most inappropriate time for the first tidings of possible blindness. We presently use the recommendations shown in the box on p. 1234. (See also Chapter 27, part six.)

Schedule for first indirect fundoscopy in premature infants		
Who:	a.	All infants <32 weeks' gestation at birth
	b.	Infants of 32 to 36 weeks' gestation at birth if oxygen was given for more than 6 hours
When:	a.	Before discharge from the hospital*
	b.	By 6 to 8 weeks after birth

*Note: Examinations done before 6 weeks of age may show only an incompletely vascularized retina that may still develop ROP, thereby necessitating further follow-up. However, many of the larger premature infants will have completely vascularized retinas, even at 2 or 3 weeks of age, and are at no further risk, thus sparing the need for further outpatient follow up.

After the acute process has resolved continued follow-up is dictated by the pathologic condition that has been present. For the reasons described those infants who have had ROP require close observation until it is possible to readily test their vision by conventional means (age of literacy). Those that have significant residual cicatrix require ophthalmologic follow-up for life.

THERAPY

Given present knowledge, the only effective prophylaxis is the prevention of premature deliveries. Continuous transcutaneous oxygen monitoring has not proved efficacious for preventing this disorder, nor has early vitamin E therapy proved to be uniformly effective. We have yet to confirm the possibility that reduced ambient light will lessen the incidence of disease, but even if it should prove to reduce this incidence, it does not eliminate disease.

There are no proven therapies for established ROP; however, investigational procedures are being evaluated. Once ROP is established photocoagulation or cryotherapy of the peripheral avascular retina (which is presumably producing an angiogenic substance that is driving the vessels to grow abnormally) is offering some hope of arresting the progress of severe ROP. In 1986 a multicenter randomized clinical trial of cryotherapy was begun in the United States and should prove or disprove the efficacy and safety of this mode of therapy.

Once total or near total retinal detachment has occurred, the eye is generally considered to have no prognosis for vision. However, total vitrectomy has been applied experimentally to selected infants and young children, with the successful reattachment of the retina in some cases. It is not yet known whether any useful vision has been regained or retained through this process, but it is certainly encouraging to realize that there is great interest concerning ROP and that there is the promise of systematic investigation bringing an answer to these problems.

Dale L. Phelps

BIBLIOGRAPHY

Bancalari, E., and others: Influence of continuous transcutaneous oxygen monitoring on the incidence of retinopathy of prematurity (ROP), Pediatr. Res. **19**:33A, 1985. (Abstr.)

Day, R.L., and others: Interpretation of statistical nonsignificance and retrolental fibroplasia, Pediatrics **63**:342, 1979.

Flower, R.W., and others: Retrolental fibroplasia; evidence for a role of the prostaglandin cascade in the pathogenesis of oxygen-induced retinopathy in the newborn beagle, Pediatr. Res. **15**:1293, 1981.

Gunn, T.R., and others: Risk factors in retrolental fibroplasia, Pediatrics **65**:1096, 1980.

Hindle, N.W., and Leyton, J.: Prevention of cicatricial retrolental fibroplasia by cryotherapy, Can. J. Ophthalmol. **13**:277, 1978.

Hittner, H.M., and others: Retrolental fibroplasia: efficacy of vitamin E in a double-blind clinical study of preterm infants, N. Engl. J. Med. **305**:1365, 1981.

An international classification of retinopathy of prematurity, Pediatrics **74**:127, 1984.

Johnson, L., Schaffer, D., and Boggs, Jr., T.R.: The premature infant, vitamin E deficiency and retrolental fibroplasia, Am. J. Clin. Nutr. **27**:1158, 1974.

Kingham, J.D.: Acute retrolental fibroplasia, Arch. Ophthalmol. **95**:38, 1977.

Kingham, J.D.: Acute retrolental fibroplasia. II. Treatment of cryosurgery, Arch. Ophthalmol. **96**:2049, 1978.

Kingham, J.D.: Retrolental fibroplasia, Am. Fam. Physician **119**:125, 1979.

Kinsey, V.E., Jacobus, J.T., and Hemphill, F.M.: Retrolental fibroplasia: cooperative study of retrolental fibroplasia and the use of oxygen, Arch. Ophthalmol. **56**:481, 1956.

Kinsey, V.E., and others: PaO_2 levels and retrolental fibroplasia; a report of the cooperative study, Pediatrics **60**:655, 1977.

Lucey, J.F., and Dangman, B.: A reexamination of the role of oxygen in retrolental fibroplasia, Pediatrics **73**:82, 1984.

McCormick, A.Q.: Retinopathy of prematurity, Curr. Probl. Pediatr. **7**:11, 1977.

Phelps, D.L.: Retinopathy of prematurity: an estimate of vision loss in the United States—1979, Pediatrics **67**:924, 1981.

Puklin, J.E., and Ehrenkranz, R.A.: Influence on retrolental fibroplasia of intramuscular vitamin E administration during respiratory distress syndrome, Ophthalmology **89**:96, 1982.

Retinopathy of Prematurity Conference syllabus, vols. 1 and 2, Columbus, Ohio, 1981, Ross laboratories.

Schaffer, D.B., Quinn, G.E., and Johnson, L.: Sequelae of arrested mild retinopathy of prematurity, Arch. Ophthalmol. **102**:373, 1984.

Schaffer, D.B., and others: Vitamin E and retinopathy of prematurity: follow-up at one year, Ophthalmology **92**:1005, 1985.

Shahinian, Jr., L., and Malachowski, N.: Retrolental fibroplasia: a new analysis of risk factors based on recent cases, Arch. Ophthalmol. **96**:70, 1978.

Silverman, W.A.: Retrolental fibroplasia: a modern parable, New York, 1980, Grune & Stratton.

Silverman, W.A., and Flynn, J.T., editors: Controversies in fetal and neonatal medicine: retinopathy of prematurity, Boston, 1985, Blackwell Scientific Publications.

Slusher, M.M., and Hutton, W.E.: Familial exudative vitreoretinopathy, Am. J. Ophthalmol. **87**:152, 1979.

Tarkkanen, A., and Mustonen, R.: Retrolental fibroplasia: cases seen at the Helsinki University Eye Hospital 1956-1974, Acta. Ophthalmol. **56**:169, 1978.

Tasman, W.: Late complications of retrolental fibroplasia, Ophthalmology **86**:1724, 1979.

CHAPTER 40

Orthopedic problems

Significant congenital musculoskeletal abnormalities are relatively common, exceeded in frequency only by congenital abnormalities of the central nervous and cardiovascular systems. Specific limb bud abnormalities (such as congenital absence of the radius) may be associated with silent genitourinary tract abnormalities or hematologic disorders (Fanconi's syndrome). An association of other organ system anomalies always should be investigated in the neonate with skeletal abnormalities, as outlined in Chapter 17.

A dramatic new diagnostic tool for use in antenatal diagnosis of dwarfism, fetal age, fetal limb growth, and related skeletal dysplasias has been achieved by ultrasonography (Chapter 12).

The definitive antenatal detection of congenital limb deformities before ultrasound was confined mainly to roentgenography and fetoscopy. Roentgenography is realistic only late in pregnancy and has some risk of radiation to the fetus. Fetoscopy permits direct examination of the fetus but is invasive and has a 3% to 5% fetal mortality.

Ultrasound is noninvasive and can be repeated with safety. The newer, high-resolution, real-time scanning has made it possible to establish a normal parameter for limb length early in gestation (Fig. 40-1). Routine ultrasound examinations are used for the patient at risk for skeletal dysplasias. Many different skeletal dysplasias have been diagnosed in utero. Eight of the most important dysplasias are listed in Table 40-1.

The technique is relatively new and much data are still being accumulated on this topic. This technology is most helpful to the obstetrician and neonatologist in providing a complete prenatal examination of skeletal anomalies in a fetus.

CLASSIFICATION OF CONGENITAL MUSCULOSKELETAL MALFORMATIONS

A classification according to parts that have been affected by certain embryologic failures has been proposed that places all malformations in seven categories. Only four of these categories relate to the neonate: (1) failure of formation of parts, (2) failure of differentiation (separation of parts), (3) duplications, and (4) congenital constriction bands (Chapter 17).

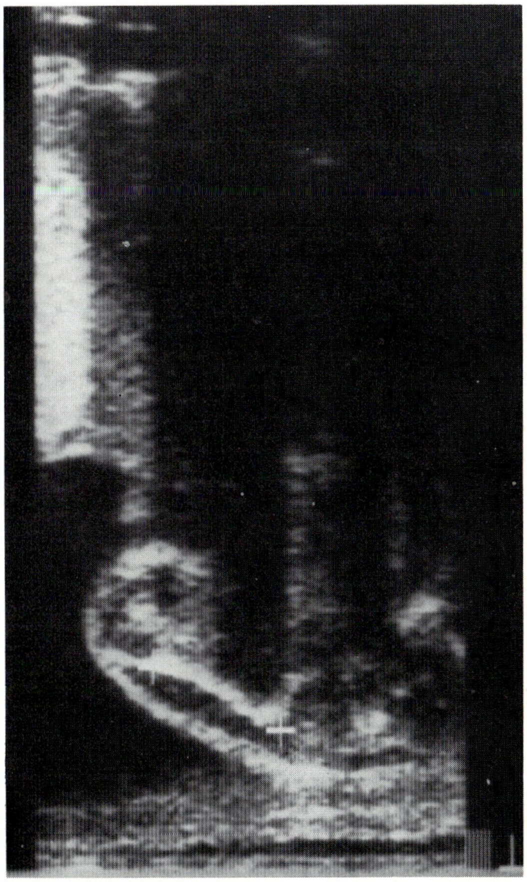

Fig. 40-1. Tibia *(right)* 2 cm, 17 weeks; *(left)* 1.8 cm, 16 weeks. Femur *(right)* 2.4 cm, 16.6 weeks; *(left)* 2.1 cm, 15.6 weeks. Humerus *(right)* 1.7 cm, 15 weeks; *(left)* 2 cm, 16 weeks. Ultrasound indicates that fetal short-limb disease is highly possible. Gestation determined by biparietal diameter is 27.7 weeks. Gestation by femur length is 17.6 weeks.

Table 40-1. Expected ultrasound findings in skeletal dysplasias

Condition	Inheritance	Head	Chest and body	Spine	Limbs
Achondrogenesis I (Parenti-Fraccaro)	AR	Thin, poorly mineralized skull	Short chest and body with thin ribs	Low-level echoes from vertebral bodies	Marked symmetic reduction
Achondrogenesis II	AR	Increased head/body ratio	Short, barrel-shaped thorax	Low-level echoes from vertebral bodies	Symmetric reduction, straight
Achondroplasia	AD	Increased head/chest, biparietal diameter, and head/body ratio, bulging forehead			Short limbs, especially femurs and humeri
Chondroectodermal dysplasia (Ellis-van Creveld syndrome)	AR		Long, narrow chest, congenital heart disease (occasional)		Shortening of both proximal and distal segments; hexadactyly
Diastrophic dysplasia	AR				Short with contractures—"hitchhiker" thumbs
Hypophosphatasia	AR	Very thin, with poor mineralization, sometimes collapsed	Thin, poorly visualized ribs		Short, thin, ribbonlike fractures
Osteogenesis imperfecta					
Blue sclerae, lethal variety	AR	Thin, often collapsed cranium	Rib fractures	(?) Fractures	Short, broad, and angulated with fractures; femurs especially tend to be broad with marked bowing
Normal sclerae	AR	Thin, but not as marked as blue sclerae	Occasional rib fractures	Fractures possible, broad bones, mild bowing, slightly short	
Spondyloepiphyseal dysplasia congenita (Spranger-Wiedemann)	AD		Short, barrel-shaped chest		Proximal shortening

Adapted from Sillence, D.O., Rimoin, D.L., and Lachman, R.: Neonatal dwarfism, Pediatr. Clin. North Am. **25**(3):453, 1978.

Failure of formation of parts

Transverse limb deficiencies (congenital amputations)

Transverse limb deficiencies occur at any level; most commonly they are distal, involving fingertips, toes, metacarpal or metatarsal bones, or the distal aspect of the forearm or tibia. Rarely they occur above the elbow (Figs. 40-2 to 40-4). Treatment consists of early prosthetic fitting between 6 months and 1 year of age.

Longitudinal limb deficiencies

The remaining skeletal limb deficiencies are in this category. They represent absent long bones or parts of long bones (hypoplasia). The most common anomalies are congenital absence of the thumb, radius, fibula, and proximal femur. Treatment of an absent thumb is elective pollicization of the index finger to the absent thumb position (Figs. 40-5 and 40-6). The best timing varies with the surgeon; 18 months is the earliest age, but many surgeons prefer to wait until the child is 4 to 5 years old. The absent radius (congenital clubhand) is rare but produces a dislocation of the hand and wrist if not treated (Fig. 40-7). Plaster casting from the day of birth followed by surgical stabilization at 18 months of age is recommended. An absent fibula produces a shortened extremity without a normal ankle joint and requires significant surgical reconstruction. In the severe cases amputation in preschool years is recommended to achieve satisfactory ambulation (Fig. 40-8). Congenital hypoplasia of the femur (proximal femoral focal deficiency) is a dramatic and significant functional limb loss and shortening (Fig. 40-9). Early custom prosthetic fitting is required at 12 to 18 months; frequently amputation of the foot facilitates a more cosmetic prosthesis.

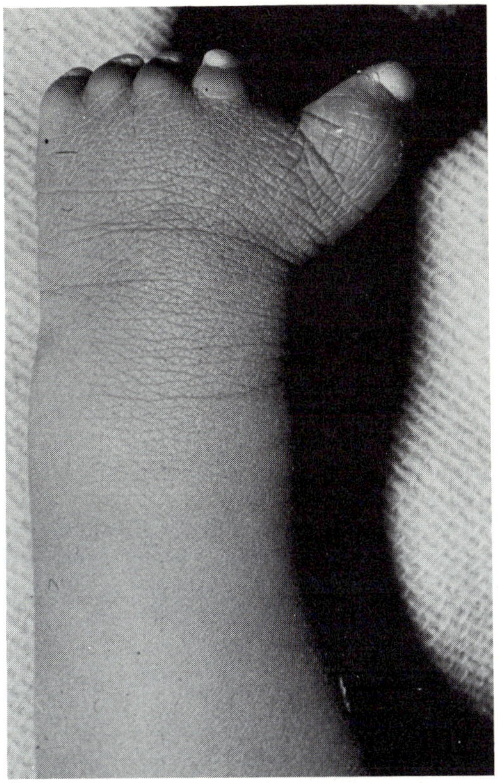

Fig. 40-2. Congenital transverse amputation of fingers at metacarpal level. Note that the thumb, wrist, and forearm are normal.

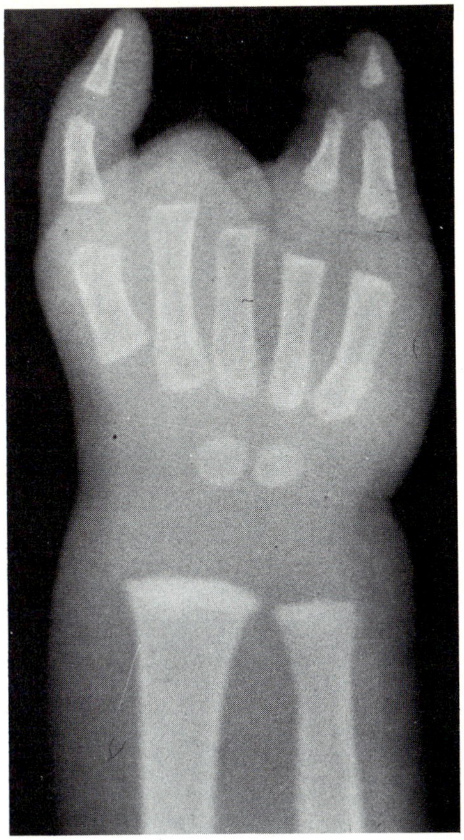

Fig. 40-3. Congenital transverse amputation of fourth and fifth fingers at proximal phalanx level, third and index fingers at metacarpal level. The thumb is normal.

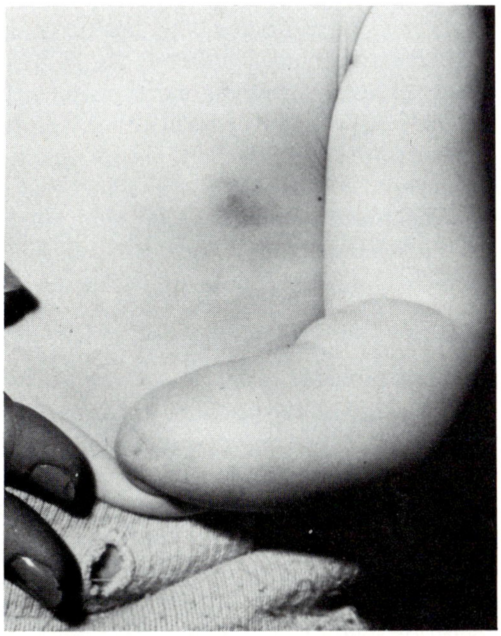

Fig. 40-4. Congenital wrist level (carpus) amputation, normal elbow and shoulder.

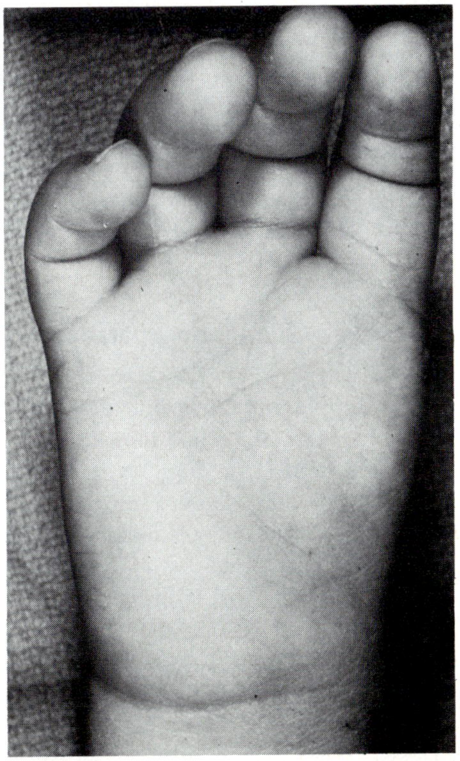

Fig. 40-5. Absence of the thumb with a normal forearm, wrist, and adjacent fingers.

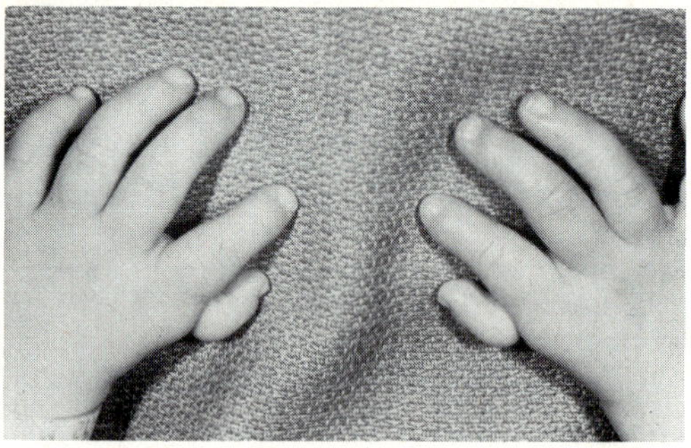

Fig. 40-6. Hypoplasia of the thumb bilaterally. Thumbs are nonfunctional and should be ablated and the bands pollicized at a later age.

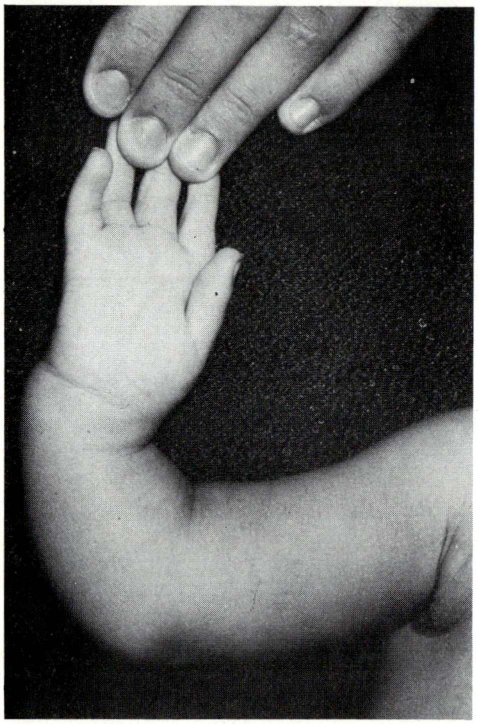

Fig. 40-7. Absent radius in a patient with normal fingers and thumb.

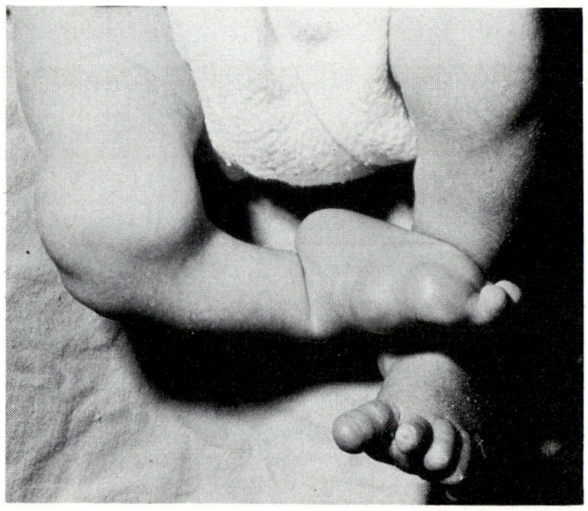

Fig. 40-8. Congenital absence of the tibia. This condition, despite the normal-appearing foot, should be treated by early amputation and fitting of prosthesis.

Failure of differentiation (nonseparation of parts)

There are multiple variations in skeletal differentiation. Only the most common and most functionally significant are presented here. *Synostosis*, or congenital bony fusion across a joint or between two long bones, occurs at the elbow, carpus, and metacarpals but most commonly in the digits (Fig. 40-10). Treatment of synostosis (division and grafting) is primarily indicated for phalangeal synostosis and is performed at 2 to 3 years of age or earlier to prevent angular digital deformity. *Syndactyly* is present when the soft parts are involved without synostosis (Fig. 40-11). The anomalies of syndactyly and synostosis are most commonly seen as isolated findings but also may be associated with genetic syndromes such as Apert's syndrome. Syndactyly also is treated at 2 to 3 years of age by division and supplemental skin grafting. The feet, when involved in either synostosis or syndactyly, are treated on a more elective basis. Congenital soft tissue contracture also is a failure of differentiation. This is represented by *skin webs*, seen in the neck or thumb web space, *arthrogryposis*, *trigger digits*, and *camptodactyly* (joint contracture) (Fig. 40-12).

Duplications

Duplications probably result from a very early insult to the limb bud, so that splitting of the original embryonic part occurs. These defects may range from polydactyly to twinning or mirror bands (Fig. 40-13). The definitive treatment is elective surgical removal of the nonfunctional duplication, although on occasion the nonfunctional duplication is best retained. This procedure should be performed at 18 months; some surgeons prefer to wait until the child is 3 to 4 years old.

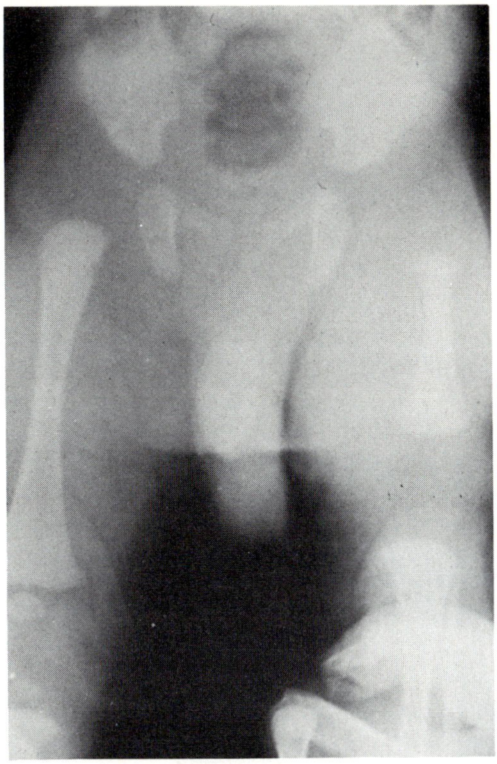

Fig. 40-9. Congenital hypoplasia of the proximal femur, sometimes known as proximal femoral focal deficiency.

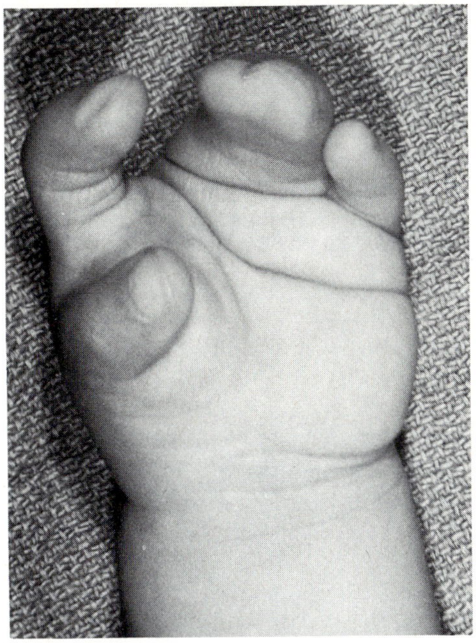

Fig. 40-10. Congenital distal synostosis of phalanges with syndactyly of third and fourth fingers.

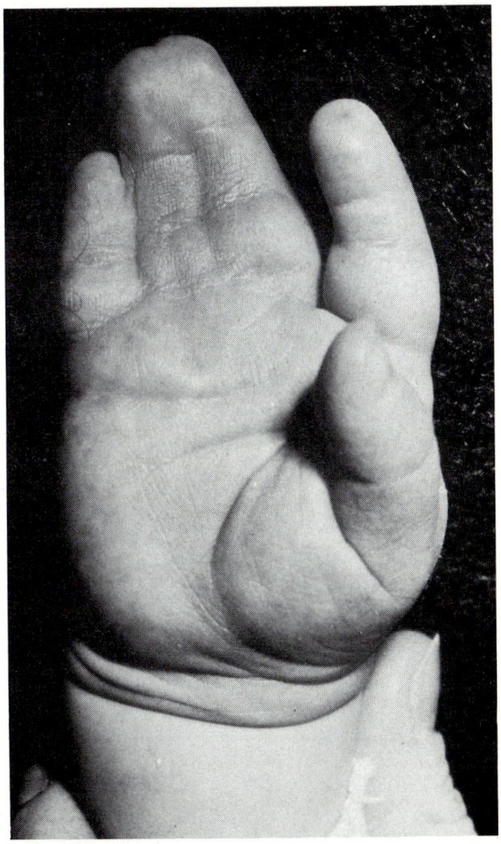

Fig. 40-11. Most commonly involved in simple syndactyly are the third and fourth fingers.

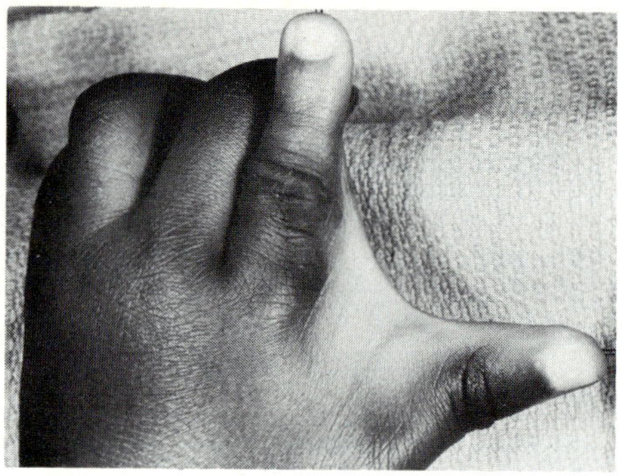

Fig. 40-12. Congenital web of thumb—index finger. Early Z-plasty and skin grafting are recommended.

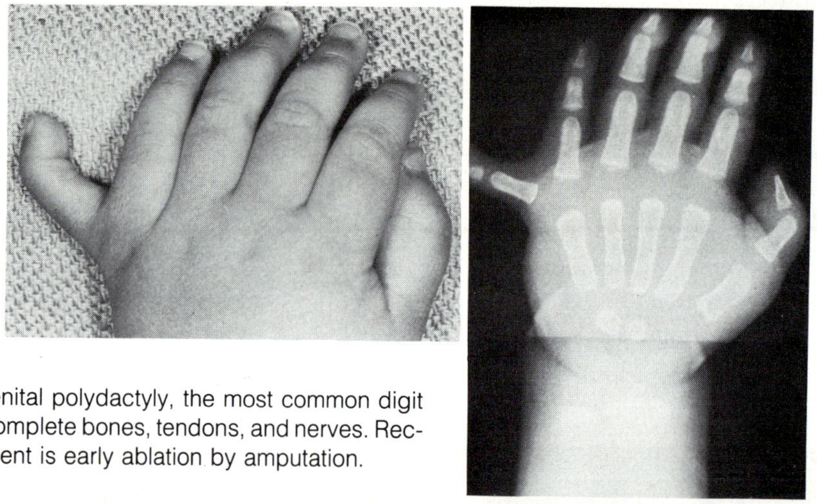

Fig. 40-13. Congenital polydactyly, the most common digit duplication, with complete bones, tendons, and nerves. Recommended treatment is early ablation by amputation.

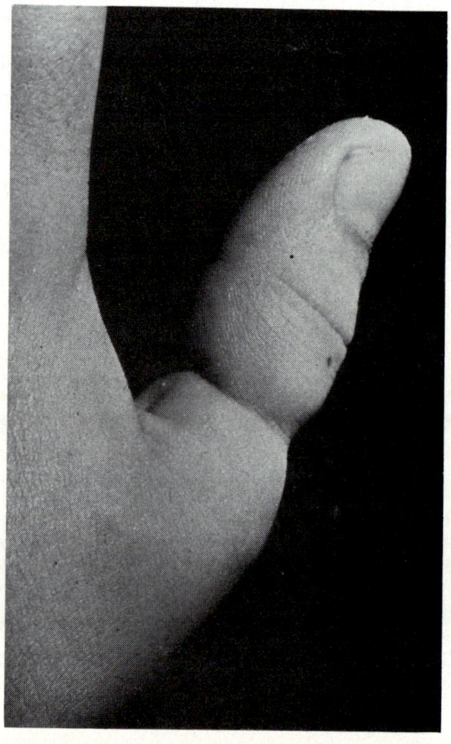

Fig. 40-14. Annular constriction ring present at base of thumb. Early Z-plasty provides successful treatment and normal growth.

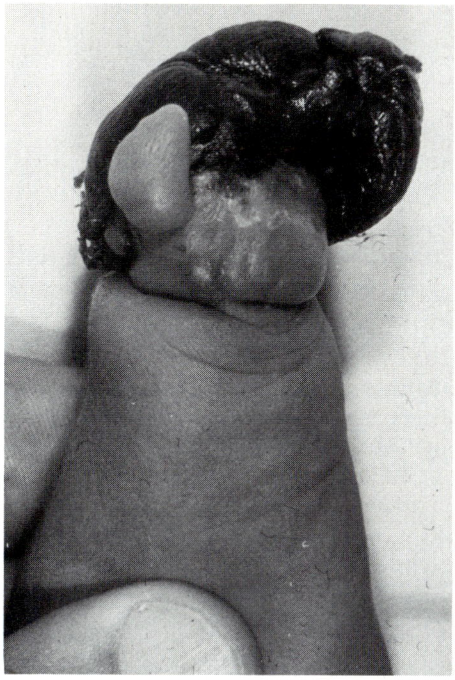

Fig. 40-15. One-week-old infant with evidence of annular band at wrist and intrauterine gangrene with fetal amputation of hand.

Congenital constriction band syndrome

Necrosis of the primordial limb bud mesenchymal tissue may produce focal scarring, which in turn produces annular constriction bands (Chapter 11) or rings (Fig. 40-14). This also may result in intrauterine gangrene and fetal amputations (Fig. 40-15). Healing of infarctions during the stage of separation of the parts may give the appearance of syndactyly. When the constriction band is present on the fully formed digit or extremity, release by multiple Z-plasty is indicated within the first 6 months of life to prevent edema or growth disturbance.

CONGENITAL HIP DISLOCATION

Congenital hip dislocation is one of the most challenging and important congenital abnormalities of the musculoskeletal system. It is almost as common as clubfoot and yet not as obvious at birth. Congenital hip dislocation demands a specific method of examination for its detection; unless treated early and definitively, it will lead to a painful and crippling deformity in adult life. Dislocation (luxation) refers to the femoral head being completely outside the acetabulum but still within the stretched and elongated capsule. Subluxation of the femoral head refers to the head riding on the edge of the acetabulum. The latter defect is easily reduced and is stable when the hip is flexed and abducted but is subluxated when the hip is extended and adducted. When the infant's hip is either dislocated or subluxated, the bony development of the acetabulum becomes progressively abnormal, leading to acetabular dysplasia. This discussion does not focus on the less common teratologic hip dislocation arising as part of a generalized congenital abnormality such as arthrogryposis multiplex and spina bifida.

Incidence

The left hip is affected three times more frequently than the right hip, and the condition is bilateral in only one out of every four children so affected. The disease is rare in the black population. There is considerable variation in the incidence of congenital hip dislocation in different parts of the world. In England and Sweden the frequency is estimated at approximately 1 per 1,000 live births; the incidence in northern Italy, southern France, and Japan is three times as high. The highest incidence is among the Lapps and certain American Indians and may be related to swaddling with hip extended and adducted in the first few months of life.

Etiology

Both environmental and genetic factors play a role in the causation of congenital hip dislocation. The sex ratio is approximately one male to seven females and may be related to estrogenic hormone metabolism. Primary acetabular dysplasia with poor covering of the femoral head may predispose children to congenital hip dislocation. Such dysplasia may be seen on the unaffected side in some 30% of unilateral cases of hip dislocation and is probably present but poorly recognized in many bilateral cases. Acetabular dysplasia may be found in one or both parents of affected children, and its genetic determination is probably multifactorial. Generalized joint laxity with capsular relaxation also has been demonstrated in families of some affected children. The most important environmental factor determining the incidence of congenital hip dislocation relates to the intrauterine breech posture with hips flexed and knees partially extended. There is a significantly higher incidence of congenital hip dislocation in breech presentations.

Pathology

The significant pathologic findings vary with time; initially there is only abnormal laxity of the capsule, elongation of the ligamentum teres, and a femoral head that may be small but of normal configuration. Without therapeutic intervention, growth and weight bearing stimulate further pathologic changes in the infant's hip. The femoral head becomes displaced upward and backward to lie on the ilium. The capsule elongates, extending across the acetabulum, and eventually adheres to the floor of the fossa, while the hip adductor muscles become progressively shortened. The acetabulum becomes shallow and more oblique; with persistent dislocation a secondary or false acetabulum may develop on the ilium posterior to the original fossa. The femoral head also becomes small with persistent dislocation, and its shape changes. All these changes constitute increasing obstacles to subsequent reduction of the congenitally dislocated hip.

Clinical manifestations

Apart from demonstrating definite dislocation or malformation or both, roentgenographic studies have little to offer diagnostically during the neonatal period. Diagnosis depends on clinical evaluation, which will identify more than 95% of infants with congenital hip dislocation. This evaluation, Ortolani's maneuver, is performed by placing the infant on the back with knees bent and hips flexed to 90 degrees and fully abducted. When the hip is reduced by abduction, a click is appreciated as the femoral head slides across the posterior aspect of the acetabulum and enters the socket. With adduction of the hip the femoral head redislocates out of the acetabulum with a palpable click, which can be best appreciated with the thumb on the lesser trochanter and the index finger on the greater trochanter. During this examination the infant should be relaxed and the hip adductors not tight; entry and exit clicks must be differentiated from the clicks associated with a tight iliotibial band or a gluteal tendon sliding over the greater trochanter and the knee click of a subluxating patella or a discoid meniscus.

Although Ortolani's maneuver is diagnostic for congenital hip dislocation, it has several shortcomings that limit its use during the immediate neonatal period: (1) as the hips are abducted and dislocated, the femoral head may slide so smoothly over the low rim of the acetabulum that a click is not appreciated; (2) a truly dislocated hip cannot be reduced and therefore cannot provide the characteristic exit and entrance clicks; and (3) infants with congenitally unstable hips (subluxated or subluxatable) may escape detection only to dislocate in the future. Barlow's test, a modification of Ortolani's maneuver, therefore should be carried out on all newborns and, when combined with the latter maneuver, will detect almost all congenitally abnormal hips. In Barlow's test the infant is placed on the back with hips flexed to 90 degrees and the knees fully flexed. The index finger of each hand is applied over the greater trochanter and the thumbs opposite the lesser trochanter in the femoral triangle. The hips are brought into midabduction, and thumb pressure is applied posteriorly over the lesser trochanter; an unstable hip will dislocate across the posterior lip of the acetabulum. With release of thumb pressure the femoral head will be reduced back into the hip socket (Fig. 40-16).

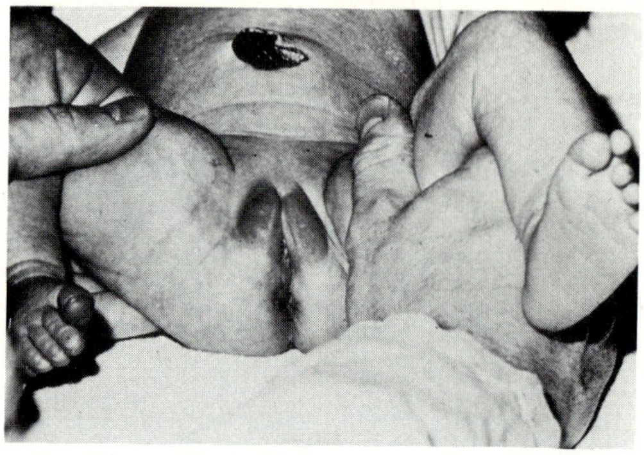

Fig. 40-16. Positioning of the hip in the newborn to perform two diagnostic tests. Ortolani's sign, or click of reduction, is elicited when abducting the hip in this manner. The "reverse" Ortolani, or Barlow, maneuver is performed by bringing the femur into adduction with flexion, causing a click of exit or dislocation.

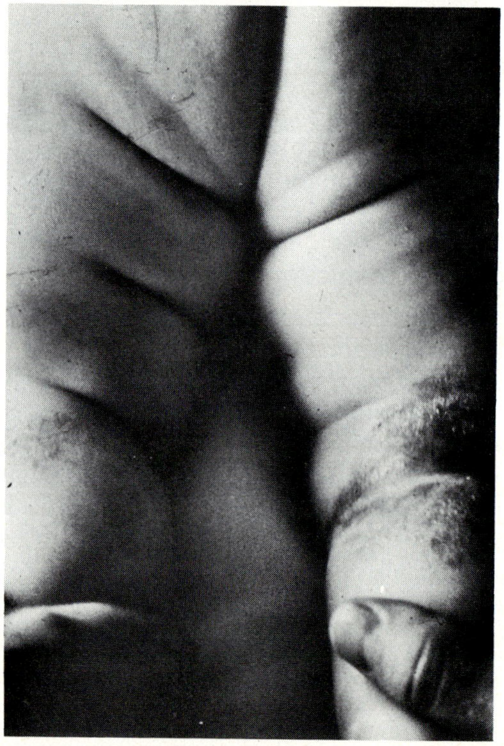

Fig. 40-17. Asymmetric gluteal and thigh folds are not diagnostic but should alert suspicion.

Ultrasound is becoming the imaging modality of choice for both diagnosis and screening. The cartilaginous femoral head can be identified on ultrasound and its relationship to the acetabulum visualized. Radiographs of the hip at this age are difficult to interpret because of the lack of ossification of the proximal femoral head. As well as helping in the diagnosis of congenital hip dislocation, ultrasound also can reduce the number of false-

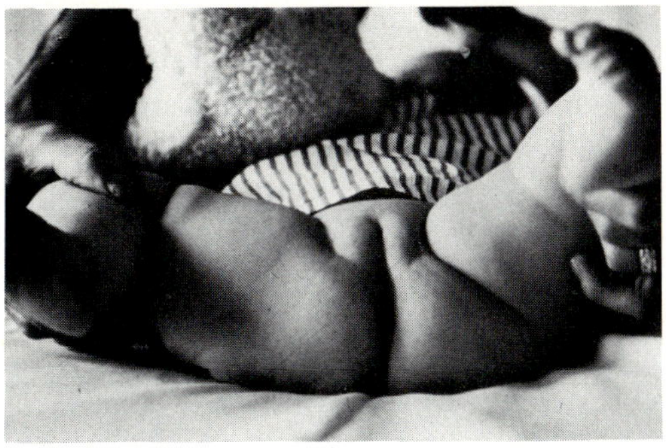

Fig. 40-18. Limitation of abduction of the thighs when hips are flexed at 90 degrees.

positives from the screening programs. Children with a click but a normal ultrasound need not be treated but should be followed carefully with serial ultrasound examinations. Ultrasound examinations also can be performed following reduction of dislocated hips to confirm the surgical reduction.

With the passage of time other physical findings appear. These findings include asymmetry of the skinfolds of the thigh (Fig. 40-17), shortening of the involved extremity, limitation of passive abduction of the hip in the 90-degree flexed position (Fig. 40-18), apparent shortening of the femur as shown by differences in the knee levels with the hips flexed at right angles and the infant in the supine position (Galeazzi's sign), and piston mobility or the telescoping sign.

Treatment

Early diagnosis and appropriate therapeutic intervention are essential to avoid crippling deformity. The orthopedic treatment of congenital dislocation and subluxation of the hip varies with the age of the affected individual; only therapy that is applicable to the neonate is considered here. Initially all unstable hips, either subluxated or dislocated, should be gently reduced, which usually is not difficult at this age, and maintained in a stable position of flexion and abduction by some device, such as the Frejka pillow, orthopedic splints, or multiple diapers. The treatment of the subluxatable (dislocatable) hip is more controversial, since 75% of these hips will revert to normal during the first few weeks of life without therapeutic intervention. However, these hips also should be maintained in a stable position of flexion and abduction. Occasionally a dislocated hip is too unstable to be kept reduced by a simple device, and a plaster hip spica cast is indicated for these infants. A period of 3 to 4 months usually is required before the capsule becomes tighter and the femoral head stimulates development of the acetabulum. The hips should be periodically assessed both clinically and roentgenographically.

Prognosis

The crippling sequelae of congenital dislocation and subluxation of the hip can be virtually eliminated by alert diagnosis and adequate treatment in the neonatal period.

CONGENITAL KNEE DISLOCATION

Congenital knee dislocation is a rare disorder that most often is a manifestation of arthrogryposis. It consists of anterior dislocation of the knee. More commonly congenital hyperextension of the knee (genu recurvatum) occurs without dislocation and is seen in normal infants. Both conditions are more common in the female and after breech presentation, suggesting an etiologic relationship with congenital hip dislocation. The completely dislocated knee usually requires surgical correction, whereas genu recurvatum almost always spontaneously improves. Some orthopedic surgeons have advocated plaster casting for this latter abnormality.

CONGENITAL PATELLA DISLOCATION

Patella dislocation rarely occurs. The patella usually is displaced laterally, and this can occur with or without congenital dislocation of the knee. The abnormality may be bilateral. An attempt should be made to replace the patella and to apply a dressing to maintain it in the correct position. However, early reconstructive surgery frequently is indicated.

CONGENITAL SHOULDER DISLOCATION

Congenital shoulder dislocation is extremely rare. The head of the humerus may lie beneath the spine of scapula, with the arm in a position of abduction and internal rotation. This condition frequently is associated with other congenital malformations. It is often difficult to differentiate between congenital dislocation, dislocation caused by birth trauma, and subluxation resulting from obstetric paralysis. Orthopedic surgical intervention is necessary.

CONGENITAL DISLOCATION OF THE RADIUS

Congenital dislocation of the radius, a rare abnormality, usually is not detected early because there is relatively little deformity and frequently no disability. The radial head dislocates laterally and, as a result of overgrowth, increases in length. Reconstructive surgery has little to offer, since it seldom improves function.

CONGENITAL PSEUDARTHROSIS

Congenital pseudarthrosis is a rare but serious abnormality that most frequently involves the tibia. The tibia, which has failed to grow normally in width, becomes angulated in its lower third, resulting in an anterior bowing of the leg before birth. It is frequently seen in children with neurofibromatosis, but the exact etiologic relationship is unknown. The thin sclerotic bone at the site of the angulation is unstable, and a pathologic fracture occurs at birth or shortly thereafter. Since the abnormal bone is avascular at this site, the fracture fails to unite, and a pseudarthrosis develops, with a resultant increase in the angular deformity. Congenital pseudarthrosis also may affect the clavicle but is often asymptomatic. Extensive orthopedic surgical manipulation is necessary for correction of pseudarthrosis.

CLUBFOOT

Clubfoot may be congenital or acquired and may accompany the oligohydramnios syndrome (Chapter 6). Talipes (Latin, *talus*, ankle bone, and *pes*, foot) is the generic name used to designate these foot and ankle deformities, which are conventionally described according to the position of the foot: (1) varus, or inversion; (2) valgus, or eversion; (3) equinus, or plantar flexion; and (4) calcaneus, or dorsiflexion.

Talipes equinovarus deformities are the most common and represent more than 95% of all congenital clubfeet. This abnormality occurs with a frequency of 1 per 1,000 live births; the condition is more common in males (2:1) and is bilateral in 50% of infants. All degrees of the equinovarus deformity exist, and the condition is often present in the fetus when the foot begins to form. Pathologically the muscles on the posterior and medial aspect of the leg are shortened, and the distal portions of the tibia and fibula usually show slight inward rotation (tibial torsion). In most instances the individual bones of the feet are normal at birth, and only their relationship to each other is affected.

Talipes calcaneovalgus deformities are the second most common variety of clubfoot. This is generally a mild and transient deformity involving a normal foot and is probably a result of intrauterine malposition rather than a true developmental abnormality. Other varieties of clubfeet are extremely rare.

The therapeutic approach to children with clubfeet is similar regardless of the type. It consists of determining whether the abnormality in the foot can be passively brought to the opposite position. If this maneuver proves successful, simple exercises started early in life will correct the deformity. If the foot abnormality is fixed and cannot be passively overcome, orthopedic treatment consisting of plaster cast or splintering or both is indicated. Forceful manipulation and surgery are rarely required.

Talipes varus (metatarsus primus varus) is an adduction deformity of the first metatarsal in relation to the other four metatarsals. The medial border of the forefoot is curved inward, and there is a wide space between the first and second toes. If treated early by the application of a series of corrective plaster casts, the deformity is rapidly corrected.

In *metatarsus varus* (metatarsus adductus) the forefoot, involving all five metatarsals, is adducted and inverted at the tarsometatarsal joint. The normal position of the heel and ankle readily distinguishes this condition from congenital clubfoot. Metatarsus varus usually is associated with internal tibial torsion. This deformity is quite common (2:1,000 live births) and is generally bilateral. In most patients the forefoot deformity is mild and flexible, and the prognosis is good with simple stretching and the avoidance of sleeping in the prone position with the feet curved in. If the deformity is marked and fixed, treatment involves application of a series of plaster casts molding the foot into adduction and pronation.

Harold M. Dick

BIBLIOGRAPHY

Baker, C.J., and Rudolph, A.J.: Congenital ring constrictions and intrauterine amputations, Am. J. Dis. Child. **121**:393, 1971.

Benacerraf, B.R., and Frigoletto, E.D.: Prenatal ultrasound diagnosis of clubfoot, Radiology **155**:211, 1985.

Berman, L., and Klenerman, L.: Ultrasound screening for hip abnormalities: preliminary findings in 1001 neonates, Br. Med. J. **293**:719, 1986.

Carter, C.O., and Wilkinson, J.A.: Genetic and environmental factors in the etiology of congenital dislocation of the hip, Clin. Orthop. **33**:119, 1964.

Ferguson, A.B.: Orthopaedic surgery in infancy and childhood, ed. 5, Baltimore, 1981, The Williams & Wilkins Co.

Filly, R.A., and Golbus, M.S.: Ultrasonography of the normal and pathologic fetal skeleton. In Callen, P.W., editor: Ultrasonography in obstetrics and gynecology, Philadelphia, 1983, W.B. Saunders Co.

Hobbins, J.C., and Mahoney, M.J.: Skeletal dysplasia. In Sanders, R.G., and James, A.E., editors: The principles and practice of ultrasonography in obstetrics and gynecology, ed. 3, Norwalk, Conn., 1985, Appleton-Century-Crofts.

Jeanty, P., and others: Ultrasonic evaluation of fetal limb growth, Radiology **140**:165, 1981.

Kay, W.H., and others: A proposed international terminology for the classification of congenital limb deficiencies: the recommendations of a working group of the International Society for Prosthetics and Orthotics, Orthot. Prosthet. **28**(2):33, 1974.

Mantagos, S., and others: Prenatal diagnosis of diastrophic dwarfism, Am. J. Obstet. Gynecol. **139**:111, 1981.

O'Brien, G.D., Queenan, J.T., and Campbell, S.: Assessment of gestational age in the second trimester by real-time ultrasound measurement of the femur length, Am. J. Obstet. Gynecol. **139**:540, 1981.

O'Brien, G.D., Rodeck, C., and Queenan, J.T.: Early prenatal diagnosis of diastrophic dwarfism by ultrasound, Br. Med. J. **280**:1300, 1980.

Palmen, K.: Preluxation of the hip joint: diagnosis and treatment in the newborn and the diagnosis of congenital dislocation of the hip joint in Sweden during the years 1948-1960, Acta Paediatr. Scand. Suppl. **129**:1, 1961.

Queenan, J.T., O'Brien, G.D., and Campbell, S.: Ultrasound measurement of fetal limb bones, Am. J. Obstet. Gynecol. **138**:297, 1980.

Salter, R.B.: Textbook of disorders and injuries of the musculoskeletal system, ed. 2, Baltimore 1983, The Williams & Wilkins Co.

Sillence, D.O., Rimoin, D.L., and Lachman, R.: Neonatal dwarfism, Pediatr. Clin. North Am. **25**(3):453, 1978.

Torpin, R.: Amniochorionic mesoblastic fibrous strings and amnionic bands: associated constricting fetal malformations or fetal death, Am. J. Obstet. Gynecol. **91**:65, 1965.

von Rosen, S.: Diagnosis and treatment of congenital dislocation of the hip joint in the newborn, J. Bone Joint Surg. **44B**:284, 1962.

APPENDIX A

Blood specimen collection in the newborn

Blood specimens may be obtained from newborns for diagnostic laboratory tests via skin puncture or venous or arterial sampling. The major considerations are specimen volume and potential for injury to the infant. If the samples are obtained frequently for diagnostic tests or in large volumes, iatrogenic anemia may occur. It is recommended that a daily log be kept in each infant's hospital record showing the amount of blood removed and the time of day each specimen is obtained. If an amount exceeding 10% of the infant's blood volume is removed, the infant will generally require a replacement blood transfusion. The currently available state-of-the-art laboratory analyzers require only microquantities of blood to perform multiple laboratory tests, and with these instruments it is no longer necessary to collect large volumes of blood from infants.

SKIN PUNCTURES

When well-defined guidelines are followed, skin puncture is the least hazardous technique for collecting mass screening blood specimens from newborns. Recent increased interest in screening programs for metabolic defects has resulted in the development of new devices for skin puncture blood collection and has stimulated studies to compare the values of constituents in skin puncture, arterial, and venous blood.

In newborns, skin puncture blood may be obtained from the lateral or medial plantar heel surface. Histologic examination shows that uncomplicated skin puncture wounds heal with minimal scarring and without neuroma formation, although foci of calcification in the heel skin have been reported. To prevent calcaneal puncture and the risk of osteochondritis, heel punctures in the newborn should be done (1) on the most medial or lateral portions of the plantar surface of the heel, (2) no deeper than 2.4 mm, (3) not on the posterior curvature of the heel, and (4) not through previous puncture sites that may be infected.

Some commercially available skin puncture lancet blades may be longer than 2.5 mm and may be hazardous if used to puncture the heels of low birth weight premature newborns. However, in term newborns the lancets currently available that have blades equal to or less than 2.4 mm frequently produce punctures that yield very small specimens and require more than one puncture to obtain the needed volume for testing. In full term newborns if the person performing the puncture follows all guidelines except for the 2.4 mm depth, the chances of bone puncture will be remote and lancets equal to or less than 5 mm can be used. There are two reasons for this. (1) In 95% of newborns, the calcaneus does not extend medial to a line drawn posteriorly from the midgreat toe to the heel or lateral to a line drawn posteriorly from between the fourth and fifth toes to the heel. Thus, if the punctures are performed outside these lines, they can be deeper than 2.4 mm and the risk of striking the bone is remote. (2) In term infants the calcaneus is 5 mm or more beneath the skin.

Skin punctures of the finger should not be performed in infants, especially premature ones, since punctures in this site have resulted in local infection and gangrene of the distal phalanx because of the short distance from the skin surface to the underlying bone in newborns.

The skin puncture site must not be swollen, since an accumulation of tissue fluid or blood within the skin will contaminate the blood specimen for diagnostic tests. Before puncture of the skin, the site should be warmed to increase the blood flow to the skin (up to sevenfold). Since the increase is primarily in arterial blood flow, the blood specimen obtained after warming has been called *arterialized skin puncture blood*. This warming step is essential for accurate results when specimens are collected for pH and blood gas determinations, although their use in evaluating arterial Po_2 is extremely limited (Chapter 28, part three). The simplest and least expensive method of warming is to cover the site for 3 minutes with a hot, moist towel at a temperature no higher than 40° C. This warming technique will adequately increase the blood flow but will not burn the skin nor result in a significant change in the values of any chemical constituent routinely measured in a hospital chemistry laboratory.

The chosen skin puncture site should be cleaned with 75% aqueous solution of isopropanol. After cleaning, the skin must be completely dried with a sterile gauze pad before puncture, since any remaining alcohol will cause rapid hemolysis of any blood that contacts it. Povidone-iodine (Betadine) should not be used to clean skin puncture sites because blood contaminated with it may have falsely elevated levels of potassium, phosphorus, uric acid, and bilirubin.

The infant's heel should be grasped with a moderately firm grip, and the skin puncture should be at a slight angle to the skin surface. After the puncture, the first drop of blood should be wiped away with sterile gauze, since it is most likely to contain larger amounts of tissue fluids and not be a representative specimen. The use of heparinized or nonheparinized capillary tubes for collection depends on whether plasma or serum is desired.

After the puncture, the blood will form a drop over the site, and when the tip of the capillary tube is placed against the drop, the blood will flow into the tube by capillary action. Blood flow is enhanced if the puncture site is held downward; a gentle continuous pressure (milking) should not be used, since it may increase hemolysis and tissue fluid in the specimen. If an adequate puncture has been performed, 0.5 to 1 ml of blood can be collected from a single puncture site.

After collection of a specimen for pH and blood gas analysis, a small magnetic mixing bar placed in the bore of the tube allows the blood in the tube to be adequately mixed. Specimens obtained for pH and blood gas analysis should be transported in water containing ice chips to prevent a significant change in blood pH.

VENOUS AND ARTERIAL SAMPLING

The increased availability of microtechniques for laboratory tests has reduced the need for obtaining blood from the neonate via venipuncture. Care should always be exercised in drawing venous blood samples from newborns, especially when deep veins are used. Patient hazards include hemorrhage, venous thrombosis, reflex arteriospasm, damage to surrounding tissues, and infection.

Umbilical arterial catheters offer a convenient and ready source of blood for laboratory tests, especially blood gas determinations. The numerous serious hazards of umbilical catheters are described in Chapters 22 and 24. The ability to sample blood accurately for chemical analysis through a catheter being used for administration of peripheral fluids depends on the size of the catheter and the concentration gradient between the chemical constituents in the blood and the parenteral fluid being administered. It has been shown that, when a 10% glucose solution is infused into the umbilical artery through a no. 5F catheter (0.3 ml capacity), a clinically significant glucose contamination occurs in blood specimens drawn through the catheter even after a volume of blood 10 times the catheter capacity has been shunted. It has been recommended that the amount of blood initially shunted from the catheter (and subsequently returned) to obtain accurate chemical measurements should be the following:

1. If using a 3½F catheter: 3 ml for glucose, 1 ml for sodium and potassium, and 0.4 ml for pH.
2. If using a 5F catheter: 4 ml for glucose, 1 ml for sodium or potassium, and 0.4 ml for pH.
3. If using an 8F catheter: 4 ml for sodium, 2 ml for potassium, 1.2 ml for pH, and an amount greater than 6 ml for glucose.

Solutions that contain *benzyl alcohol* or other preservatives should not be used to flush intravascular catheters, since toxicity may occur in the form of metabolic acidosis, CNS depression, respiratory distress (with gasping), hypotension, renal failure, and even seizures and intracranial hemorrhage.

Blood for coagulation studies, activated partial thromboplastin time, and whole blood partial thromboplastin time can be drawn through 5F heparinized umbilical catheters, and accurate results are obtained if 4 ml of blood is shunted before obtaining the sample.

When it is necessary to obtain an arterial blood sample from a newborn, alternative sites to the umbilical artery are the radial and brachial arteries. Scalp and femoral arteries should be avoided because of the risk of cerebral thrombosis and hip damage, respectively.

DIFFERENCES IN VALUES IN SKIN PUNCTURE BLOOD, VENOUS BLOOD, AND ARTERIAL BLOOD IN NEWBORNS

Blood obtained by skin puncture is not specifically blood from capillaries but is a mixture of blood from arterioles, venules, and capillaries and contains interstitial and intracellular fluids. Chemistry values for 12 constituents simultaneously obtained in skin puncture serum, skin puncture plasma, and venous serum have been compared. The effect of warming the skin before the puncture also was studied. No clinically important differences were found in the concentration of the constituents measured in skin puncture serum and plasma with or without warming the skin before puncture. When the concentration of each of the measured constituents was compared between skin puncture blood and venous serum, there were differences in the concentrations of glucose, potassium, total protein, and calcium, which could be clinically significant. Except for those of glucose, the concentrations in venous serum were higher. The degree of hemolysis reflected by plasma (free) hemoglobin concentration was the same in skin puncture serum and plasma, although the total plasma hemoglobin is higher in skin puncture than in venous specimens.

There is poor correlation of Po_2 values in arterialized skin puncture blood and umbilical artery blood in term and preterm infants with a variety of illnesses. Almost uniformly the Po_2 is lower in skin puncture blood, and if these samples are used to determine Po_2, toxic levels of oxygen may be undetected. Therefore arterial or transcutaneous measurements should be used to monitor arterial Po_2. It is also preferable to measure pH and Pco_2 in newborns with cardiopulmonary abnormalities by using arterial blood (or measuring transcutaneous Pco_2).

Thomas A. Blumenfeld

BIBLIOGRAPHY

Skin puncture

Blumenfeld, T.A., Hertelendy, W.G., and Ford, S.H.: Simultaneously obtained skin puncture serum, skin puncture plasma, and venous serum compared and effects of warming the skin before puncture, Clin. Chem. **23**:1705, 1977.

Blumenfeld, T.A., Turi, G.K., and Blanc, W.A.: Recommended sites and depth of newborn heel skin punctures based on anatomic measurements and histopathology, Lancet **1**:230, 1979.

Blumenfeld, T.A., and others: Standard procedures for the collection of diagnostic blood specimens by skin puncture. TSH 1, Villanova, Pa., 1979, National Committee for Clinical Laboratory Standards.

Gambino, S.R.: Blood pH, pCO_2, oxygen saturation, and pO_2, Chicago, 1967, American Society of Clinical Commission on Continuing Education.

Gandy, G., and others: The validity of pH and pCO_2 measurements in capillary samples in sick and healthy newborn infants. Pediatrics **34**:192, 1964.

Hicks, J.R., Rowland, G.L., and Buffone, G.J.: Evaluation of a new blood collection device (microtainer) that is suited for pediatric use, Clin. Chem. **22**:2034, 1976.

Karna, P., and Poland, R.L.: Monitoring critically ill newborn infants with digital capillary blood samples: an alternative, J. Pediatr. **92**:270, 1978.

Lilien, L.D., and others: Neonatal osteomyelitis of the calcaneus: complication of heel puncture, J. Pediatr. **88**:478, 1976.

Meites, S., and others: Skin puncture and blood-collecting techniques for infants, Clin. Chem. **25**:183, 1979.

Michaelsson, M., and Sjolin, S.: Hemolysis in blood samples from newborn infants, Acta Paediatr. Scand. **54**:325, 1965.

Sell, E.J., Hansen, R.C., and Struck-Pierce, S.: Calcified nodules on the heel: a complication of neonatal intensive care, J. Pediatr. **96**:473, 1980.

Von Steirteghem, A.C., and Young, D.S.: Povidone-iodine (Betadine) disinfectant as a source of error, Clin. Chem. **23**:1512, 1977.

Venipuncture

Blumenfeld, T.A.: Clinical applications of microchemistry. In Werner, M.W., editor: Microtechniques for the clinical laboratory: concept and application, New York, 1976, John Wiley & Sons, Inc.

Differences in values in skin puncture and arterial and venous specimens in newborns

Blumenfeld, T.A., Hertelendy, W.G., and Ford, S.H.: Simultaneously obtained skin puncture serum, skin puncture plasma, and venous serum compared and effects of warming the skin before puncture, Clin. Chem. **23**:1705, 1977.

Christensen, R.D., and Rothstein, G.: Pitfalls in the interpretation of leukocyte counts of newborn infants, Am. J. Clin. Pathol. **72**:608, 1979.

Feusner, J.H., and others: Platelet counts in capillary blood, Am. J. Clin. Pathol. **72**:410, 1979.

Gandy, G., and others: The validity of pH and pCO_2 measurements in capillary samples in sick and healthy newborn infants, Pediatrics **34**:192, 1904.

Langer, P.H., Jr., and Fies, H.L.: Blood sugar values of blood obtained simultaneously from the radial artery, antecubital vein, and the finger, Am. J. Clin. Pathol. **12**:559, 1942.

Michaelsson, M., and Sjolin, S.: Hemolysis in blood samples from newborn infants, Acta Paediatr. Scand. **54**:325, 1965.

Mountain, K.R., and Campbell, D.G.: Reliability of oxygen tension measurements on arterialized capillary blood in the newborn, Arch. Dis. Child. **45**:134, 1970.

Stuart, J., and others: Capillary blood coagulation profile in the newborn, Lancet **2**:1467, 1979.

APPENDIX B

Therapeutic agents

Agent	Dosage		Comments
ADRENERGICS			
Dobutamine	2-50 μg/kg/min		Titrate dose to target effect; in young infants increased heart rate may be the predominant mechanism for increased cardiac output; tolerance may develop with prolonged use (>3 days)
Dopamine	1-4 μg/kg/min		"Renal dose" to promote splanchnic blood flow and cortical redistribution of renal blood flow
	5-8 μg/kg/min		Cardiotonic dose; pharmacodynamic response similar to dobutamine
	>8 μg/kg/min		Pressor dose; vasoconstrictive action both direct and indirect
Epinephrine	1:1,000 aqueous solution; 0.01 ml/kg/dose SC		Repeat every 2-4 hr as needed; may repeat after 15 min
	1:10,000 aqueous solution; 0.1 ml/kg IV, intratracheal, or intracardiac		
	0.05-1.0 μg/kg/min IV		Continuous ECG and blood pressure monitoring necessary
Isoproterenol	0.1-4.0 μg/kg/min IV		Continuous ECG and blood pressure monitoring essential to prevent hypotension and tachycardia
ANTIBACTERIALS			
Amikacin*	0-7 days:	15 mg/kg/day divided every 12 hr IV, IM	Serum concentrations should be monitored and dosage adjusted to achieve peak concentrations ≤40 μg/ml and trough concentrations ≤10 μg/ml
	>7 days:	15-22.5 mg/kg/day divided every 8 hr IV	
Ampicillin	0-7 days:	100 mg/kg/day divided every 12 hr IV, IM	Meningitis doses
		50-100 mg/kg/day divided every 12 hr IV, IM	Other indications
	>7 days:	200 mg/kg/day divided every 6-8 hr IV, IM	Meningitis doses
		100 mg/kg/day divided every 6-8 hr IV, IM	Other indications
Carbenicillin	0-7 days:	200-300 mg/kg/day divided every 8 hr IV, IM	Serum sodium and potassium levels should be carefully monitored
	>7 days:	300-400 mg/kg/day divided every 6-8 hr IV, IM	

*Dosage recommendations for aminoglycoside antibiotics are suggested starting points. A target-concentration strategy should be adopted to ensure their safe and effective use. Serum concentration monitoring and dosage adjustment is part of the physician's commitment to their use.

†Cephalosporins are generally ineffective against *Enterococcus, Listeria monocytogenes,* and anaerobes. Therefore they should seldom be employed as single-agent empiric therapy in newborn infants.

Agent	Dosage	Comments
Cefazolin†	0-7 days: 25-50 mg/kg/day divided every 12 hr >7 days: 25-100 mg/kg/day divided every 8 hr	
Cefotaxime†	100-200 mg/kg/day divided every 6-8 hr	Broad-spectrum cephalosporin; may be useful for gram-negative meningitis
Ceftazidime†	100-200 mg/kg/day divided every 12 hr until 1 mo of age then every 8 hr	Broad-spectrum cephalosporin; only antipseudomonal cephalosporin; may be useful for gram-negative meningitis
Ceftriaxone†	50-100 mg/kg/day divided every 12 hr	Highly potent against group B streptococci, pneumococci, *Staphylococcus aureus, Haemophilus influenzae, Escherichia coli, Klebsiella,* and *Serratia;* high CSF activity and resistance to degradation by β-lactamases
Chloramphenicol	0-7 days: 25 mg/kg/day divided every 12 hr 7-14 days: 25-50 mg/kg/day divided every 8-12 hr >14 days: 25-50 mg/kg/day divided every 8 hr	Serum concentrations should be monitored; the succinate is not predictably cleaved, and doses should be adjusted to yield peak concentrations ≤25 μg/ml, trough concentrations ≤6 μg/ml
Clindamycin	>7 days: 8-20 mg/kg/day divided every 6 hr PO, IV	Not recommended for infants less than 1 month of age
Erythromycin estolate	0-7 days: 20 mg/kg/day divided every 12 hr >7 days: 20 mg/kg/day divided every 6-8 hr PO	
Gentamicin*	0-7 days: 5 mg/kg/day divided every 12 hr IV, IM >7 days: 7.5 mg/kg/day divided every 8-12 hr IV, IM	Serum concentrations should be monitored and doses adjusted to achieve peak concentrations ≤10 μg/ml, trough concentrations ≤2 μg/ml
Kanamycin*	0-7 days: 15-20 mg/kg/day divided every 12 hr IV, IM >7 days: 20-30 mg/kg/day divided every 8 hr IV, IM	
Methicillin	0-7 days: 50-100 mg/kg/day divided every 12 hr IV, IM >7 days: 100-200 mg/kg/day divided every 6-8 hr IV, IM	Not recommended because of increased intestinal nephritis
Metronidazole	10-30 mg/kg/day divided every 8 hr IV or PO	
Mezlocillin	150-300 mg/kg/day divided every 6-8 hr for 3 doses	More potent than carboxypenicillins against gram-negative organisms
Moxalactam	150-200 mg/kg/day divided every 8 hr IV	Reserved for gram-negative infections and not reliably effective for group B streptococci or pneumococcus
Nafcillin	0-7 days: 50-100 mg/kg/day divided every 12 hr IV >7 days: 100-200 mg/kg/day divided every 6-8 hr IV	Greatest CSF penetration of isoxazolyl (antistaphylococcal) penicillins
Oxacillin	0-7 days: 50-100 mg/kg/day divided every 12 hr IV >7 days: 100-200 mg/kg/day divided every 6-8 hr IV	
Penicillin G	0-7 days: 100,000-150,000 units/kg/day divided every 12 hr IV, IM	Meningitis dose
	50,000-100,000 units/kg/day divided every 12 hr IV, IM	Other indications
	>7 days: 150,000-400,000 units/kg/day divided every 6-8 hr IV, IM	Meningitis dose
	75,000-100,000 units/kg/day divided every 8 hr IV, IM	Other indications

Continued.

Agent	Dosage	Comments
Penicillin G benzathine	0-7 days: 50,000 units/kg single dose IM	For treatment of congenital syphilis when CNS is not involved
	>7 days: 50,000 units/kg single dose IM	
	150-300 mg/kg/day divided every 8-12 hr (preliminary recommendation)	More potent than carboxy-penicillins against gram-negative organisms and provides effective single-drug therapy for *Klebsiella, Enterococcus,* and *Bacteroides*
Ticarcillin	0-7 days: <2,000 gm: 150 mg/kg/day divided every 12 hr	Serum sodium and potassium should be carefully monitored
	0-7 days: >2,000 gm: 225 mg/kg/day divided every 8 hr	
	>7 days: 225-300 mg/kg/day divided every 6-8 hr	
Tobramycin*	0-7 days: 5 mg/kg/day divided every 12 hr IV, IM	Serum concentrations should be monitored and doses adjusted to achieve peak concentrations ≤10 μg/ml and trough concentrations ≤2 μg/ml
	>7 days: 7.5 mg/kg/day divided every 8 hr IV, IM	
Trimethoprim with sulfamethoxazole	5-10 mg trimethoprim and 25-50 mg sulfamethoxazole/kg/day divided every 12 hr IV, PO	Sulfamethoxazole can displace bilirubin, but this is less likely than with other sulfonamides, use with caution
	20 mg/kg trimethoprim and 100 mg/kg sulfamethoxazole/kg/day divided every 6 hr IV	Treatment for infections caused by *Pneumocystis carinii*
Vancomycin	0-7 days: 20 mg/kg/day divided every 12 hr IV	Intravenous therapy reserved for *Staphylococcus epidermidis* or methicillin-resistant *Staphylococcus aureus;* dose of 20 μg/kg/day divided every 12 hr may be adequate to achieve peak serum concentrations ≤40 μg/ml and trough concentrations ≤10 μg/ml; IV doses in excess of 30 mg/kg/day may lead to potentially toxic serum concentrations
	10-50 mg/kg/day divided every 12 hr PO	Oral treatment for pseudomembranous enterocolitis
ANTIFUNGALS		
Amphotericin B	0.5-1.0 mg/kg/day IV infusion over 2-4 hr	Patients with *Candida* sepsis generally treated to a total dose of 15-30 mg/kg; serum potassium and creatinine clearance values should be monitored closely; alternate-day therapy may permit better control of electrolyte status
5-Fluorocytosine	50-150 mg/kg/day divided every 6 hr PO 1,500-4,500 mg/m²/day divided every 12 hr IV	Should not be employed as a single agent in the treatment of fungal sepsis
Miconazole	20-40 mg/kg/day IV divided every 8 hr	Titrate dose to yield serum concentrations above the MIC for infecting organism; no data available for newborn infants
Nystatin	400,000 units/day divided every 6-8 hr PO	
ANTITUBERCULOUS AGENTS		
Isoniazid	10 mg/kg/day PO	Prophylaxis
	15-30 mg/kg/day as a single dose PO	Therapeutic
	10 mg/kg/day divided every 8-12 hr IM	Therapeutic
Rifampin	10-20 mg/kg/day as a single dose PO	Use with caution in patients with hepatic dysfunction
Streptomycin	20-40 mg/kg/day divided every 12 hr IM	Use higher dose if tuberculous meningitis is present
ANTIVIRAL		
Acyclovir	500 mg/m²/dose given over 1 hr every 8 hr	May be advantageous in infants because of somewhat greater efficacy and less fluid required for administration
Adenine arabinoside	15-30 mg/kg/day over 12 hr at a concentration not exceeding 0.45 mg/ml of standard intravenous fluid	Efficacy documented only for herpes simplex virus encephalitis

Agent	Dosage	Comments
ANTICOAGULANT		
Heparin	Load with 50-100 units/kg IV and then maintain with 100 units/kg IV every 4 hr or 20,000 units/m^2/day by continuous IV infusion	These dosing recommendations should serve as a starting point; therapy in each patient should be individualized to give a PTT of 1.5 to 2.5 times the control value; remember heparin clearance in infants may be more rapid than in adults
ANTICONVULSANTS		
Carbamazepine	10 mg/kg/day divided twice per day PO for initial therapy	Dose will require a gradual increase because of the "autoinduction" phenomenon; titrate to achieve serum concentrations between 4 and 12 μg/ml (≈20-40 nmol/L); no convenient dosage form available for infants
Paraldehyde	Loading dose: 0.2-0.4 ml/kg IV followed by a continuous IV infusion of 0.1-0.5 ml/kg/hr of a 4% solution 0.3 ml/kg/dose per rectum every 4-6 hr	Infusion rate should be adjusted to control patient's seizures; rapid infusion may cause cardiac depression and pulmonary edema
Phenobarbital	Loading dose: 15-20 mg/kg slow IV push (50 mg/kg maximum) Maintenance dose: 4-6 mg/kg/day IV, IM, or PO as a single dose	Serum concentrations should be monitored and doses adjusted to maintain concentrations between 15 and 30 μg/ml; the long half-life of the drug suggests that single daily doses will be sufficient; little information available on oral absorption in the first month of life
Phenytoin	Loading dose: 15-20 mg/kg IV at a rate not to exceed 50 mg/min (30 mg/kg maximum); may be diluted in 0.9% NaCl only to a concentration of 0.1 mg/ml Maintenance dose: 5-8 mg/kg/day IV, PO	Loading dose should be administered with continuous ECG monitoring; serum concentrations should be monitored and doses adjusted to maintain concentrations between 10 and 20 μg/ml; oral absorption during the first month of life is negligible; the drug displays dose dependent kinetics, so great care must be exercised when making a dosage change
Valproic acid	10-60 mg/kg/day divided every 12 hr PO; initial dose 10-15 mg/kg/day; may be given rectally	Little data available for newborns; optimum seizure control in children reported at serum concentrations between 50 and 100 μg/ml; may be administered rectally
ANTIDOTES		
Atropine	0.01-0.03 mg/kg IV, SC, or endotracheal	
Methylene blue	1.2 mg/kg/dose IV over 5 min	Treatment for methemoglobinemia
Naloxone	0.01-0.1 mg/kg/dose IV	May be repeated every 10-15 min
Protamine	1 mg for every 100 units of heparin in the previous 3-4 hr by IV drip (50 mg/dose maximum)	
BLOOD DERIVATIVES		
Albumin	0.25-1 gm/kg/day IV	May use 5% or 25% if infused over same length of time; maintain serum concentration within physiologic range
Blood, packed cells	5-10 ml/kg/IV	
Blood, whole	10-20 ml/kg IV	
Fibrinogen	50 mg/kg IV	Repeat as needed
Plasma, fresh, frozen	10-20 ml/kg IV	
CARDIOVASCULAR DRUGS		
Captopril	0.2-0.5 mg/kg day divided every 8 hr	Angiotensin-converting enzyme inhibitor; may be effective in high-renin hypertension and severe CHF; must monitor renal function
Diazoxide	3-5 mg/kg IV as a bolus injection; may repeat in 30 min and then every 2-5 hr	Should not be used in treatment of compensatory hypertension such as associated with coarctation of the aorta and arteriovenous shunting; rapid injection not essential

Continued.

Agent	Dosage	Comments
Digoxin	Premature: 0.02-0.04 mg/kg IV	Total digitalizing dose (load with half initially then, one fourth every 6 hr)
	0.01 mg/kg/day divided every 12 hr	Maintenance dose (may be given once daily)
	Full term: 0.04 mg/kg IV	Total digitalizing dose (load with half)
	0.01 mg/kg/day divided every 12 hr PO	Maintenance dose; oral doses (elixir) are 75% as effective as IV doses; based on pharmacokinetics; maintenance dose may be given once daily; serum concentration in infants may be erroneous because of the presence of an endogenous digoxin-like substance (EDLS)
Hydralazine	0.2 mg/kg/dose or 1.7-3.5 mg/kg/day divided every 4-6 hr IV, IM	
	1 mg/kg/day divided every 6 hr to increase as needed up to 7.5 mg/kg/day PO	
Indomethacin	First dose 0.2 mg/kg; then if <2 days, 0.1 mg/kg/dose, 12 hr for 2 doses	Prostaglandin synthetase inhibitor; may be used for PDA closure or to reverse K^+ wasting in Bartter's syndrome
	If 2-7 days, 0.2 mg/kg/dose every 12 hr for 2 doses	
	If 3-8 days, 0.25 mg/kg/dose every 12 hr for 2 doses	Monitor renal function
	IV dosing only; PO not recommended	
Lidocaine	0.5-1.5 mg/kg/dose by slow IV push; may be repeated every 5-10 min as needed	Side effects include hypotension, seizures, respiratory arrest, asystole
	20-50 μg/kg/min by continuous IV infusion	
Neostigmine	2 mg/kg/day divided every 3-4 hr PO	
Nitroglycerin	0.2-60 μg/kg dose IV or SC	May be used as a paste as well
Nitroprusside	0.5-10 μg/kg/min by continuous IV infusion	Must have continuous intraarterial blood pressure monitoring; may produce profound hypotension, metabolic acidosis, thrombocytopenia, and CNS symptoms
Phenoxybenzamine	0.1-5 μg/kg/min	Vasodilator for long-term IV therapy
Phentolamine	0.01 mg/kg/dose IV or SC	May cause profound hypotension owing to blocking action; may be used for local infusion into IV infiltrates owing to catecholamines or calcium
Phenytoin	See anticonvulsant dosage above	Drug of choice for digitalis intoxication
Procainamide	2 mg/kg dose given over 5 min IV	
	40-60 mg/kg/day divided every 6 hr PO	
Propranolol	0.01-0.15 mg/kg/dose by slow IV push; then 0.5-1.0 mg/kg/day divided every 6 hr PO	For dysrhythmias
	Starting dose: 1 mg/kg/day divided every 6 hr PO	For hypertension
	0.15-0.25 mg/kg/dose IV	For tetralogy spells
Pyridostigmine	1-2 mg every 4-12 hr PO	
	0.05-0.15 mg every 4-8 hr IM	
Tolazoline	1-2 mg/kg IV as a test dose; then 1-2 mg/kg/hr by continuous IV infusion	Monitor blood pressure and renal status; may cause gastrointestinal and pulmonary hemorrhages
Verapamil	0.1-0.3 mg/kg by IV infusion over 2 min	Treatment of paroxysmal supraventricular tachydysrhythmias; always have $CaCl_2$ at the bedside when administering
CHOLINERGIC BLOCKING AGENTS		
Atropine	See antidotes	
Belladonna, tincture	0.1 ml/kg/day divided every 6-8 hr PO	Maximum dose 3.5 ml/day
CHOLINESTERASE INHIBITOR		
Edrophonium	Test dose: 1.0 mg IV for neonates; 0.2 mg/kg/dose IV for infants	Give 20% of test dose initially; if no response in 1 min, give remainder in 1 mg increments; keep atropine available, since drug may precipitate cholinergic crisis

Agent	Dosage	Comments
DIURETICS		
Acetazolamide	5 mg/kg/day as a single dose PO, IM	May cause acidosis
Chlorothiazide	20-30 mg/kg/day divided every 12 hr PO	May cause hypokalemia, alkalosis, hyperglycemia
Ethacrynic acid	2-3 mg/kg/day divided every 12 hr PO	Ototoxicity may occur
	0.5-2.0 mg/kg/dose every 6-8 hr PO	Dosage for infants not well established
Furosemide	1-2 mg/kg/dose every 6-8 hr PO	Ototoxicity may occur in renal disease
	0.5-5.0 mg/kg/dose every 12 hr IM or IV	May cause hypokalemia, alkalosis, and dehydration
Spironolactone	1.7-3.3 mg/kg/day divided every 6-8 hr	May require several days of therapy before effect is seen; always monitor urine Na^+/K^+ ratio
ENDOCRINE		
Adrenal		
ACTH	1.6 units/kg/day divided every 6-8 hr IV, IM, SC	
Cortisone	25 mg/m²/day divided every 8 hr	Physiologic replacement
	12 mg/m²/day single dose IM	
Desoxycorticosterone	1-3 mg/day IM	
Hydrocortisone	50 mg/kg IV initial dose, then 50-75 mg/kg/day divided every 6 hr	Treatment for gram-negative shock
Prednisone	1-3 mg/kg/day PO	Every other day therapy advisable to minimize growth retardation
Pancreas		
Glucagon	0.025-0.1 mg/kg/dose SC, IV, IM; may repeat every 20-30 min	Treatment for hypoglycemia (1.0 mg maximum dose); may be an effective inotropic agent in CHF
Insulin	0.01-0.1 unit/kg/hr continuous IV infusion	Titrate rate of infusion to achieve desired serum glucose concentration
Pituitary		
Vasopressin	Aqueous: 1-3 ml/day divided every 8 hr SC	
	Tannate in oil: 0.2 ml/dose every 1-3 days IM	
	Nose drops: 1-2 drops at bedtime and every 4-6 hr as needed	
Thyroid		
Dessicated thyroid	Initial: 8-15 mg/day as a single dose PO	Titrate dosage at weekly intervals to normalize serum T_4; usual maintenance 50-200 mg/day
Lugol's solution	One drop 3 times per day PO	
Methimazole	Initial: 0.4 mg/kg/day divided every 8 hr PO	
	Maintenance: 0.2 mg/kg/day divided every 8 hr	
Propylthiouracil	5-10 mg/kg/day divided every 8 hr	Dosage for infants not well established
Triiodothyronine (T_3)	Calculate dosage as for desiccated thyroid using the equivalent: 65 mg desiccated thyroid = 25 μg T_3	
MINERALS		
Calcium		
Chloride (27% Ca^{++})	250-300 mg/kg/day as a 2% solution divided every 6 hr PO	
	25 mg/kg as a slow IV push	Drug of choice during CPR
Glubionate (90 mg Ca^{++} gm salt)	500 mg/kg/day divided every 4-8 hr PO	High osmotic load
Gluconate (9.4% Ca^{++})	500 mg/kg/day divided every 4-8 hr PO	
	100-200 mg/kg/dose by slow IV infusion	Monitor heart rate when administering IV
Lactate (13% Ca^{++})	500 mg/kg/day divided every 4-8 hr PO	

Continued.

Agent	Dosage	Comments
Iron		
Ferrous sulfate drops (25 mg Fe/ml)	6 mg elemental iron/kg/day divided in 3 doses PO	Treatment of iron-deficiency anemia
	1-2 mg elemental iron/kg/day divided into 2-3 doses	Prophylaxis
Ferrous gluconate (7 mg Fe/ml)	As above	
Magnesium		
Magnesium sulfate	0.05 ml/kg of a 50% solution every 6 hr IV or IM × 3-4 doses initially; then 12-15 mg/100 ml of maintenance IV fluid	For hypomagnesemia, calcium gluconate should be available as an antidote, monitor serum concentrations
NARCOTICS		
Meperidine	6 mg/kg/day divided every 4-6 hr PO, IV, IM, SC as needed	
Morphine	0.05-0.2 mg/kg/dose repeated every 3-4 hr IV, IM as needed	
Paregoric	0.2 ml every 3-4 hr; increase to a maximum dose of 0.5 ml every 3-4 hr	Preparation of choice for neonatal narcotic withdrawal; should be used along with scoring systems
SEDATIVES/TRANQUILIZERS		
Chloral hydrate	10-30 mg/kg/day divided every 6-8 hr IV, IM, PO, PR	Sedative dose
	50 mg/kg as a single dose PO or PR	Hypnotic dose
Chlorpromazine	2.0-2.5 mg/kg/day divided every 6 hr PO, IM	
Diazepam	0.1-3.0 mg/kg/dose IV, PR, PO, never IM; may repeat as needed	May displace bilirubin. Several active metabolites may accumulate with continued use; infants tend to be resistant to the sedative effects and require higher doses than older patients; IV and PR administration may be particularly effective for acute termination of seizures; rapid IV infusion may cause apnea
Promethazine	0.25-1.0 mg/kg/dose divided every 6-8 hr as needed PO, IM	
Secobarbital	2-5 mg/kg/dose every 6-8 hr as needed IV	
VITAMINS (Daily requirements)		
A	250-750 IU PO	
B_1 (thiamine)	Premature: 200 μg PO Full term: 40 μg PO Treatment: 10 mg given every 6-8 hr	
B_2 (riboflavin)	Premature: 400 μg PO Full term: 60 μg PO	
B_6 (pyridoxine)	Premature: 400 μg PO Full term: 35 μg PO	Give 50 mg stat for pyridoxine-dependent seizures
B_{12} (cyanocobalamin)	Premature: 1.5 μg PO Full term: 0.15 μg PO	
C (ascorbic acid)	Premature: 60 mg PO Full term: 600 IU PO	
D	Premature: 600 IU PO Full term: 40-100 IU PO	
E	Premature: 30 IU PO Full term: 4 IU PO	
K	Premature: 15 μg Treatment: 1-10 mg IM	Start with 1 mg and adjust to normalize clotting functions

Agent	Dosage	Comments
MISCELLANEOUS		
Aminophylline	Loading dose: 5-6 mg/kg by slow IV infusion Maintenance dose: 1-2 mg/kg/dose every 8-12 hr IV or PO	Serum theophylline concentrations should be monitored and doses adjusted to achieve peak concentrations between 6 and 13 μg/ml for apnea; caffeine serum concentrations should be monitored
Bethanechol	0.1-0.2 mg/kg PO each meal (up to 60 min before) to 4 doses/day	Caution should be used in patients with esophageal stricture or pulmonary disease
Caffeine	Loading dose: 10 mg/kg IV or PO	Serum caffeine levels in the range 5-20 μg/ml; caffeine may accumulate in the serum of theophylline-treated infants
Chloroquine	10 mg/kg/day PO 5 mg/kg/day IV	
Cimetidine	20-40 mg/kg/day IV, PO divided every 6 hr	
Kayexalate	Calculate dose to desired exchange PO or PR every 6 hr as needed; average is 0.5-1 gm/kg/dose; 1 mEq potassium/1 gm resin	
Mannitol	0.5-2.0 gm/kg IV over 1 hr following a 200 mg/kg IV test dose	
Methadone	0.3-0.4 mg/kg/day PO	
Metoclopramide	0.1-0.5 mg/kg/day divided every 8 hr	May reduce gastric aspirates
Pancuronium bromide (Pavulon)	0.04-0.10 mg/kg/dose repeated as needed IV	Morphine or barbiturate may be considered with Pavulon to ease anxiety

Jeffrey L. Blumer

APPENDIX C

Tables of normal values

PHYSIOLOGIC PARAMETERS

Table 1. Electrocardiographic data in the neonate*

Parameter	Age: 0-24 hours		1-7 days		8-30 days		1-3 months	
Heart rate (beats/min	119	(94-145)	133	(100-175)	163	(115-190)	154	(124-190)
PR interval (sec)	0.1	(0.07-0.12)	0.09	(0.07-0.12)	0.09	(0.07-0.11)	0.1	(0.07-0.13)
P wave amplitude II	1.5	(0.8-2.3)	1.6	(0.8-2.5)	1.6	(0.08-2.4)	1.6	(0.8-2.4)
QRS duration (sec)	0.065	(0.05-0.08)	0.06	(0.04-0.08)	0.06	(0.04-0.07)	0.06	(0.05-0.08)
QRS axis (degrees)	135	(60-180)	125	(80-160)	110	(60-160)	80	(40-120)
R amplitude V_{4R} (mm)	8.6	(4-14.2)	—		6.3	(3.3-8.5)	5.1	(1.1-10.1)
R amplitude V_1 (mm)	11.9	(4.3-21)	—		11.1	(3.3-18.7)	11.2	(4.5-18)
R amplitude V_5 (mm)	10.2	(4-18)	10.7	(3.4-19)	11.9	(3.5-27)	13.6	(7.3-20.7)
R amplitude V_6 (mm)	3.3	(2.3-7)	5.1	(2.2-13.1)	6.7	(1.7-20.5)	8.4	(3.6-12.9)
S amplitude V_{4R} (mm)	3.8	(0.2-13)	—		1.8	(0.8-4.6)	3.4	(0-9.3)
S amplitude V_1 (mm)	9.7	(1.1-19.1)	—		6.1	(0-15)	7.5	(0.5-17.1)
S amplitude V_5 (mm)	11.9	(0-24)	6.8	(3.6-16.2)	4.8	(2.7-12.3)	4.7	(2-12.7)
S amplitude V_6 (mm)	4.5	(1.6-10.3)	3.3	(0.8-9.9)	2.0	(0.6-9)	2.4	(0.8-5.8)

Modified from Liebman, J., and Plonsey, R.: Electrocardiography. In Moss, A.J., Adams, F.H., and Emmanovilides, G.C., editors: Heart disease in infants, children and adolescents, ed. 2, Baltimore, 1977, The Williams & Wilkins Co.

*Mean (5th percentile to 95th percentile)

Table 2. Time of first void in 500 infants

Hours	395 Full-term infants: No. of infants	Cumulative %	80 Preterm infants: No. of infants	Cumulative %	25 Postterm infants: No. of infants	Cumulative %
In delivery room	51	12.9	17	21.2	3	12
1-8	151	51.1	50	83.7	4	38
9-16	158	91.1	12	98.7	14	84
17-24	35	100	1	100	4	100
>24	0	—	0	—	0	—

From Clark, D.A.: Pediatrics **60:**457, 1977. Reproduced by permission of Pediatrics © 1977.

Table 3. Time of first stool in 500 infants

Hours	395 Full-term infants: No. of infants	Cumulative %	80 Preterm infants: No. of infants	Cumulative %	25 Postterm infants: No. of infants	Cumulative %
In delivery room	66	16.7	4	5	8	32
1-8	169	59.5	22	32.5	9	68
9-16	125	91.1	25	63.8	5	88
17-24	29	98.5	10	76.3	3	100
24-48	6*	100	18†	98.8	0	—
>48	0	—	1‡	100	0	—

From Clark, D.A.: Pediatrics **60:**457, 1977. Reproduced by permission of Pediatrics © 1977.

*At 25, 26, 27, 28, 33, and 37 hours.

†Five stooled more than 36 hours after birth at 38, 39, 40, 42, and 47 hours.

‡At 59 hours.

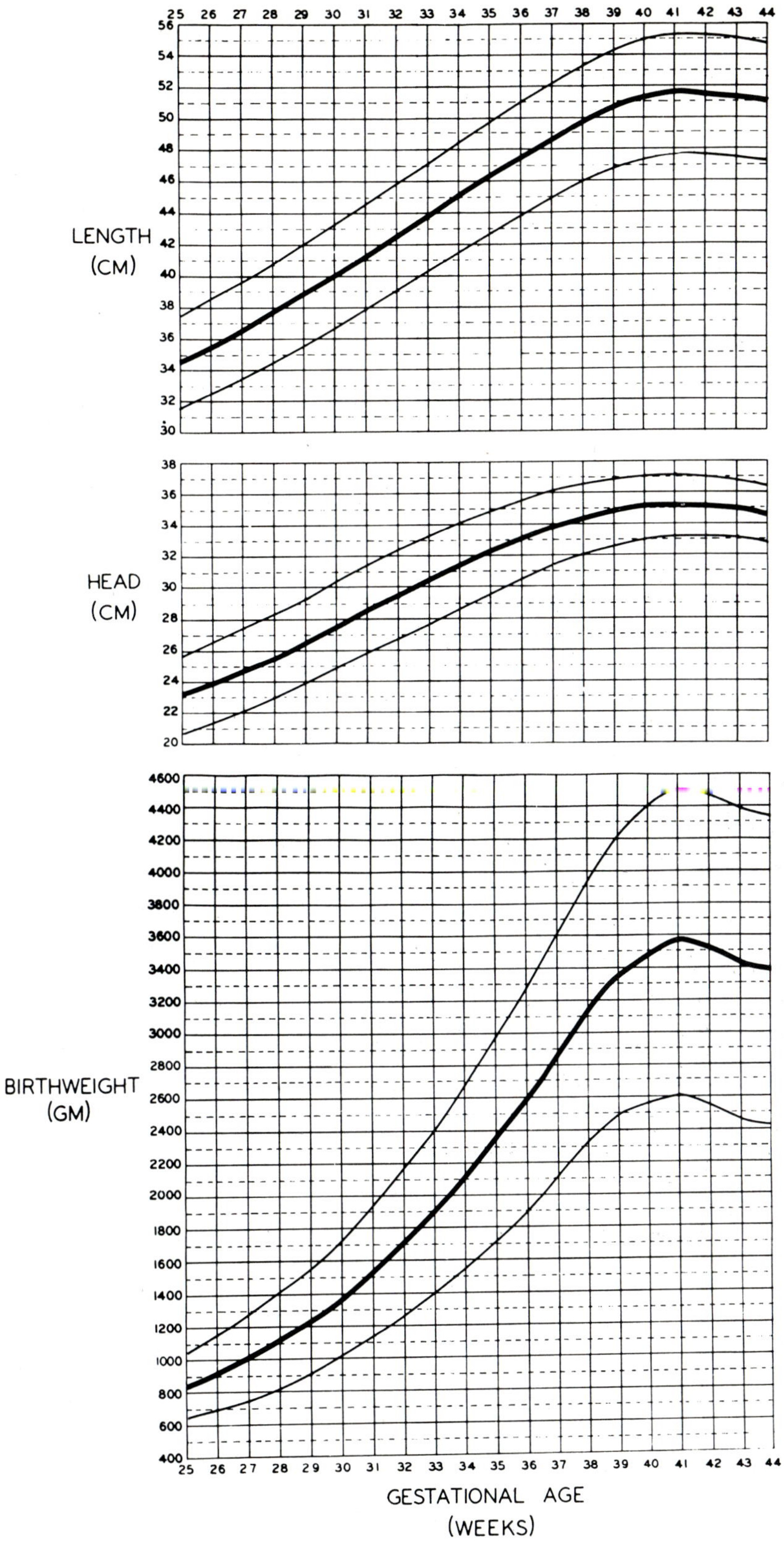

Fig. C-1. Intrauterine growth curves. (From Usher, R., and McLean, F.: J. Pediatr. **74:**901, 1969.)

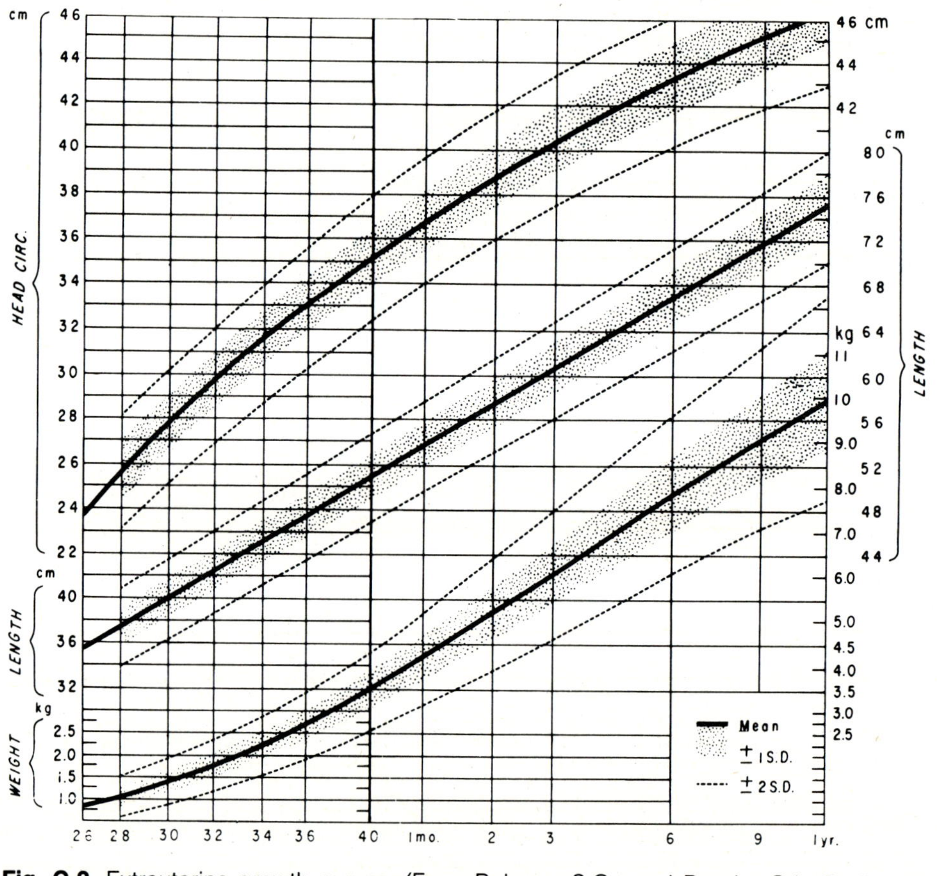

Fig. C-2. Extrauterine growth curves. (From Babson, S.G., and Benda, G.I.: Pediatrics **89:**814, 1976.)

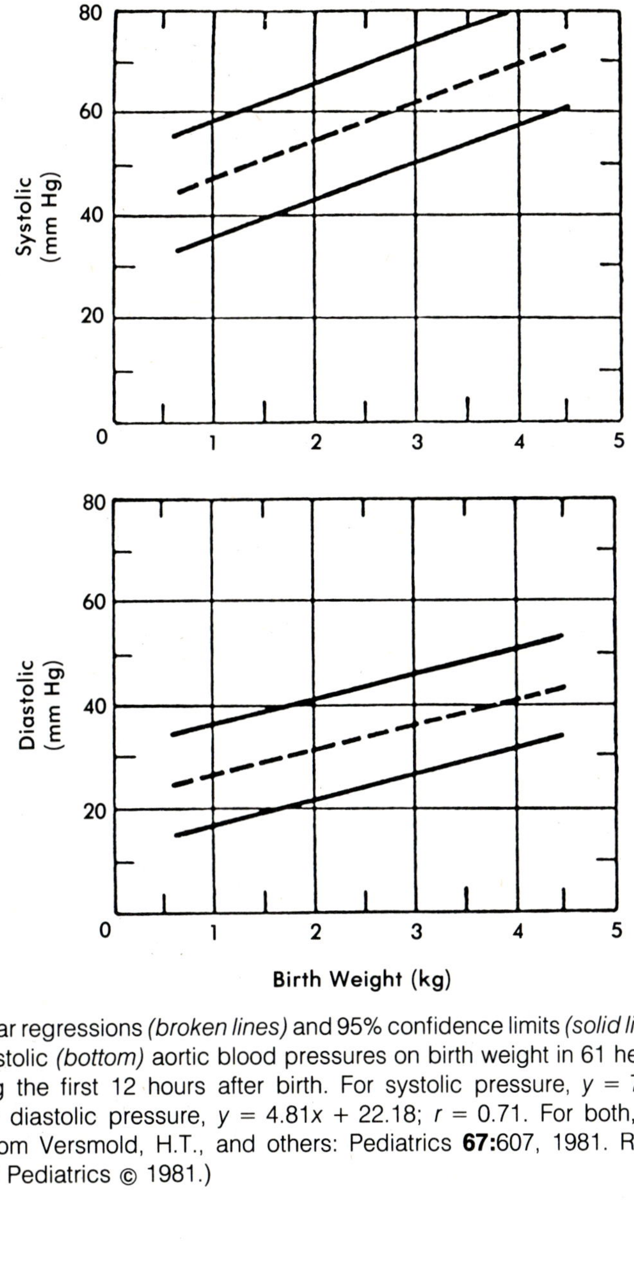

Fig. C-3. Linear regressions *(broken lines)* and 95% confidence limits *(solid lines)* of systolic *(top)* and diastolic *(bottom)* aortic blood pressures on birth weight in 61 healthy newborn infants during the first 12 hours after birth. For systolic pressure, $y = 7.13x + 40.45$; $r = 0.79$. For diastolic pressure, $y = 4.81x + 22.18$; $r = 0.71$. For both, $n = 413$ and $P<0.001$. (From Versmold, H.T., and others: Pediatrics **67:**607, 1981. Reproduced by permission of Pediatrics © 1981.)

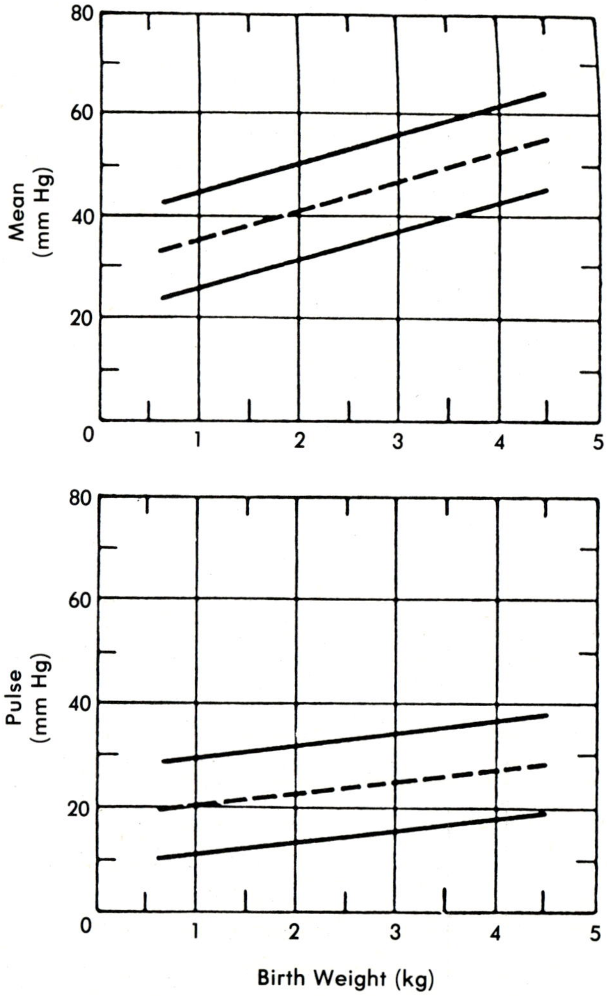

Fig. C-4. Linear regressions *(broken lines)* and 95% confidence limits *(solid lines)* of mean pressure *(top)* and pulse pressure (systolic-diastolic pressure amplitude) *(bottom)* on birth weight in 61 healthy newborn infants during the first 12 hours after birth. For mean pressure, $y = 5.16x + 29.80$; $n = 443$; $r = 0.80$. For pulse pressure, $y = 2.31x + 18.27$; $n = 413$; $r = 0.45$. For both, $P<0.001$. (From Versmold, H.T., and others: Pediatrics **67:**607, 1981. Reproduced with permission of Pediatrics © 1981.)

BLOOD CHEMISTRY VALUES

Table 4. Acid-base status

Determination	Sample source	Birth	1 Hour	3 Hours	24 Hours	2 Days	3 Days
VIGOROUS TERM INFANTS, VAGINAL DELIVERY							
pH	Umbilical artery	7.26					
	Umbilical vein	7.29					
P_{CO_2} (mm Hg)	Arterial	54.5	38.8	38.3	33.6	34	35
	Venous	42.8					
O_2 saturation	Arterial	19.8	93.8	94.7	93.2		
	Venous	47.6					
pH	Left atrial		7.30	7.34	7.41	7.39 (temporal artery)	7.38 (temporal artery)
CO_2 content (mEq/L)	—	—	20.6	21.9	21.4		
PREMATURE INFANTS							
	Capillary (skin puncture)						
pH	<1,250 gm				7.36	7.35	7.35
P_{CO_2} (mm Hg)					38	44	37
pH	>1,250 gm				7.39	7.39	7.38
P_{CO_2} (mm Hg)					38	39	38

From Schaffer, A.J.: Diseases of the newborn, ed. 3, Philadelphia, 1971, W.B. Saunders Co. Data from Weisbort and others: J. Pediatr. **52:**395, 1958; Bucci, G., and others: Biol. Neonate **8:**81, 1965.

Table 5. Serum electrolytes in term infants

Determination	Cord	1-12 Hours	12-24 Hours	24-48 Hours	48-72 Hours
Sodium mEq/L*	147 (126-166)	143 (124-156)	145 (132-159)	148 (134-160)	149 (139-162)
Potassium, mEq/L	7.8 (5.6-12)	6.4 (5.3-7.3)	6.3 (5.3-8.9)	6.0 (5.2-7.3)	5.9 (5.0-7.7)
Chloride, mEq/L	103 (98-110)	100.7 (90-111)	103 (87-114)	102 (92-114)	103 (93-112)
Calcium, mg/dl	9.3 (8.2-11.1)	8.4 (7.3-9.2)	7.8 (6.9-9.4)	8.0 (6.1-9.9)	7.9 (5.9-9.7)
Phosphorus, mg/dl	5.6 (3.7-8.1)	6.1 (3.5-8.6)	5.7 (2.9-8.1)	5.9 (3.0-8.7)	5.8 (2.8-7.6)
Blood urea, mg/dl	29 (21-40)	27 (8-34)	33 (9-63)	32 (13-77)	31 (13-68)
Total protein, gm/dl	6.1 (4.8-7.3)	6.6 (5.6-8.5)	6.6 (5.8-8.2)	6.9 (5.9-8.2)	7.2 (6.0-8.5)
Blood sugar, mg/dl	73 (45-96)	63 (40-97)	63 (42-104)	56 (30-91)	59 (40-90)
Lactic acid, mg/dl	19.5 (11-30)	14.6 (11-24)	14.0 (10-23)	14.3 (9-22)	13.5 (7-21)
Lactate, mmol/L†	2.0-3.0	2.0			

From Schaffer, A.J.: Diseases of the newborn, ed. 3, Philadelphia, 1971, W.B. Saunders Co.
*Acharya, P.T., and Payne, W.W.: Arch. Dis. Child **40:**430, 1965.
†Daniel, S.S., Adamsons, K., Jr., and James, L.S.: Pediatrics **37:**942, 1966.

Table 6. Serum electrolyte values in preterm infants

	Age 1 week			Age 3 weeks			Age 5 weeks			Age 7 weeks		
Constituent	Mean	SD	Range	Mean	SD	Range	Mean	SD	Range	Mean	SD	Range
Na (mEq/L)	139.6	±3.2	133-146	136.3	±2.9	129-142	136.8	±2.5	133-148	137.2	±1.8	133-142
K (mEq/L)	5.6	±0.5	4.6-6.7	5.8	±0.6	4.5-7.1	5.5	±0.6	4.5-6.6	5.7	±0.5	4.6-7.1
Cl (mEq/L)	108.2	±3.7	100-117	108.3	±3.9	102-116	107.0	±3.5	100-115	107.0	±3.3	101-115
CO_2 (mM/L)	20.3	±2.8	13.8-27.1	18.4	±3.5	12.4-26.2	20.4	±3.4	12.5-26.1	20.6	±3.1	13.7-26.9
Ca (mg/dl)	9.2	±1.1	6.1-11.6	9.6	±0.5	8.1-11.0	9.4	±0.5	8.6-10.5	9.5	±0.7	8.6-10.8
P (mg/dl)	7.6	±1.1	5.4-10.9	7.5	±0.7	6.2-8.7	7.0	±0.6	5.6-7.9	6.8	±0.8	4.2-8.2
BUN (mg/dl)	9.3	±5.2	3.1-25.5	13.3	±7.8	2.1-31.4	13.3	±7.1	2.0-26.5	13.4	±6.7	2.5-30.5

From Klaus, M.H., and Fanaroff, A.A.: Care of the high risk neonate, ed. 3, Philadelphia, 1986, W.B. Saunders Co. Adapted from Thomas, J., and Reichelderfer, T.: Clin. Chem. **14:**272, 1968.

Table 7. Selected chemistry values in full-term and preterm infants

Constituent	Preterm	Term	Reference
Ammonia (μg/100 ml)	—	90-150	1
Base, excess (mmol/L)	—	−10 to −2	2
Bicarbonate, standard (mmol/L)	18-26	20-26	2
Bilirubin, total (mg/dl)			
Cord	<2.8	<2.8	2
24 Hours	1-6	2-6	
48 Hours	6-8	6-7	
3-5 Days	10-12	4-6	
≥1 Month	<1.5	<1.5	
Bilirubin, direct	<0.5	<0.5	2
Calcium, total (mg/dl), Week 1	6.0-10.0	7.0-12.0	3
Calcium, ionized (mg/dl), 72 hours	2.5-5.0	2.5-5.0	4
Ceruloplasmin (mg/dl)	—	20-40	
Creatinine phosphokinase			
Day 1	—	44-1150	5
(arb U) Day 4	—	14-97	
Creatinine (mg/dl)			
Birth	Mother's level	Mother's level	1, 6
10 Days	1.3 ± 0.07 (mean ± SD)	0.8-1.4	
1 Month	0.6 ±0.05 (mean ± SD)	—	
Gamma-glutamyl transferase (U/L)	—	14-331	7
Glucose (mg/dl)			
<72 hours	20-125	30-125	8; see also Fig. 33-2
>72 hours	40-125	40-125	
Lactate dehydrogenase (U/L)	—	357-953	7
Magnesium (mg/dl)	—	1.5-2.8	9
Osmolality (mOsm/L)	—	280-295	2
Phosphatase, acid (U/L)	—	7.4-19.4	2
Phosphotase, alkaline (U/L) (mean ± SD)			
26-27 weeks	320 ± 87	164 ± 68	10
28-29	292 ± 87	—	
30-31	281 ± 85	—	
32-33	254 ± 72	—	
34-35	236 ± 62	—	
36	207 ± 60	—	
Phosphorus (mg/dl)			
Birth	5.6-8.0	5.0-7.8	11
Week 1	6.1-11.7	4.9-8.9	
Month 1	6.6-9.4	5.9-9.5	
SGOT (aspartate amino transferase)	—	24-81	7
SGPT (alanine amino transferase)	—	10-33	7
Urea nitrogen (mg/dl)	—	5-25	2
Uric acid (mg/dl)	—	3.0-7.5	2

[1]Meites, S.: Pediatric clinical chemistry: a survey of normals, ed. 1, 1977, American Association of Clinical Chemistry.
[2]Wallach, J.B.: Interpretation of pediatric tests, Boston, 1983, Little, Brown & Co.
[3]Meites, S.: Crit. Rev. Clin. Lab. Sci. **6:**1, 1975.
[4]Brown, D.M., Boen, J., and Bernstein, A.: Pediatrics **49:**841, 1972.
[5]Drummond, L.M.: Arch. Dis. Child. **54:**362, 1979.
[6]Stonestreet, B.S., and Oh, W.: Pediatrics **61:**788, 1978.
[7]Statlan, B.E., and Freer, D.E.: Clin. Chem. **24:**1010(abstract), 1978.
[8]Cornblath, M., and Schwartz, R., editors: Disorders of carbohydrate metabolism, ed. 2, Philadelphia, 1976, W.B. Saunders Co.
[9]Tsang, R.C.: Am. J. Dis. Child. **124:**282, 1972.
[10]Glass, L., and others: Arch. Dis. Child. **57:**373, 1982.
[11]O'Brien, D.: Interpretation of biochemical values. In Kempe, C.H., and Silver, H.K., editors: Current pediatric diagnosis and treatment, ed. 3, Los Altos, Calif., 1974, Lange Medical Publications.

BLOOD PROTEIN VALUES

Table 8. Serum total protein and electrophoresis fractions

Fraction	Age			
	Cord blood	At birth	1 Week	1-3 Months
Total protein	4.78-8.04	4.6-7.0	4.4-7.6	3.64-7.38
Albumin	2.17-4.04	3.2-4.8	2.9-5.5	2.05-4.46
Alpha-1	0.25-0.66	0.1-0.3	0.09-0.25	0.08-0.43
Alpha-2	0.44-0.94	0.2-0.3	0.30-0.46	0.40-1.13
Beta	0.42-1.56	0.3-0.6	0.16-0.60	0.39-1.14
Gamma	0.81-1.61	0.6-1.2	0.35-1.3	0.25-1.05

Data from Meites, S., editor: Pediatric clinical chemistry: a survey of normals, methods and instruments, Washington, D.C., 1977, American Association for Clinical Chemistry; Ellis, E.F., and Robbins, J.B.: Children are different, Columbus, Ohio, 1970, Ross Laboratories.

Table 9. Haptoglobin levels in preterm infants

Gestation (weeks)	Days after birth					
	0	5	10	15	21	28
<32	10 (3)	—	—	—	—	—
32-34	—	18.5 (2)	51.6 (3)	42.6 (3)	12 (1)	12 (1)
34-36	9.8 (9)	14.9 (11)	11.4 (10)	11.6 (9)	7.1 (7)	16.5 (4)
36-38	13.0 (7)	18.3 (3)	16.6 (5)	16.3 (2)	11 (1)	7.5 (1)
38+	9.3 (8)	28.3 (6)	20.9 (4)	10.1 (5)	9.2 (3)	7.0 (1)
TOTALS	10.5 (27)	19.6 (22)	19.5 (22)	16.1 (19)	8.3 (12)	13.2 (7)

From Philip, A.G.S.: Biol. Neonate **19:**322, 1971.
*Haptoglobin levels are measured as mg/dl MetHb binding capacity. Numbers in parentheses indicate number of samples from which mean values were derived

Table 10. Haptoglobin levels in full-term infants

	Birth	Fifth day
Haptoglobin (mg/dl Hgb binding capacity)	23.9 (10.6-50)	52.3 (14.8-100)

Table 11. Plasma IG concentrations in premature infants (25 to 28 weeks' gestation)

Age (months)	*n*	IgG* (mg/dl)	IgM* (mg/dl)	IgA* (mg/dl)
0.25	18	251 (114-552)†	7.6 (1.3-43.3)	1.2 (0.07-20.8)
0.5	14	202 (91-446)	14.1 (3.5-56.1)	3.1 (0.09-10.7)
1.0	10	158 (57-437)	12.7 (3.0-53.3)	4.5 (0.65-30.9)
1.5	14	134 (59-307)	16.2 (4.4-59.2)	4.3 (0.9-20.9)
2.0	12	89 (58-136)	16 (5.3-48.9)	4.1 (1.5-11.1)
3	13	60 (23-156)	13.8 (5.3-36.1)	3 (0.6-15.6)
4	10	82 (32-210)	22.2 (11.2-43.9)	6.8 (1-47.8)
6	11	159 (56-455)	41.3 (8.3-205)	9.7 (3-31.2)
8-10	6	273 (94-794)	41.8 (31.1-56.1)	9.5 (0.9-98.6)

From Ballow, M., and others: Pediatr. Res. **20:**899, 1986.
*Geometric mean.
†The normal ranges in parentheses were determined by taking the antilog of (mean logarithm ± 2 SD of the logarithms).

Table 12. Plasma IG concentrations in premature infants (29 to 32 weeks' gestation)

Age (months)	*n*	IgG* (mg/dl)	IgM* (mg/dl)	IgA* (mg/dl)
0.25	42	368 (186-728)†	9.1 (2.1-39.4)	0.6 (0.04-1)
0.5	35	275 (119-637)	13.9 (4.7-41)	0.9 (0.01-7.5)
1	26	209 (97-452)	14.4 (6.3-33)	1.9 (0.3-12)
1.5	22	156 (69-352)	15.4 (5.5-43.2)	2.2 (0.7-6.5)
2	11	123 (64-237)	15.2 (4.9-46.7)	3 (1.1-8.3)
3	14	104 (41-268)	16.3 (7.1-37.2)	3.6 (0.8-15.4)
4	21	128 (39-425)	26.5 (7.7-91.2)	9.8 (2.5-39.3)
6	21	179 (51-634)	29.3 (10.5-81.5)	12.3 (2.7-57.1)
8-10	16	280 (140-561)	34.7 (17-70.8)	20.9 (8.3-53)

From Ballow, M., and others: Pediatr. Res. **20:**899, 1986.
*Geometric mean.
†The normal ranges in parentheses were determined by taking the antilog of (mean logarithm ± 2 SD of the logarithms).

Table 13. Plasma amino acids in preterm and full-term infants

Amino acid	Premature, first day	Newborn, before first feeding	16 Days-4 months
Taurine	105-255	101-181	
OH-proline	0-80	0	
Aspartic acid	0-20	4-12	17-21
Threonine	155-275	196-238	141-213
Serine	195-345	129-197	104-158
Asp + Glut	655-1155	623-895	
Proline	155-305	155-305	141-245
Glutamic acid	30-100	27-77	
Glycine	185-735	274-412	178-248
Alanine	325-425	274-384	239-345
Valine	80-180	97-175	123-199
Cystine	55-75	49-75	33-51
Methionine	30-40	21-37	15-21
Isoleucine	20-60	31-47	31-47
Leucine	45-95	55-89	56-98
Tyrosine	20-220	53-85	33-75
Phenylalanine	70-110	64-92	45-65
Ornithine	70-110	66-116	37-61
Lysine	130-250	154-246	117-163
Histidine	30-70	61-93	64-92
Arginine	30-70	37-71	53-71
Tryptophan	15-45	15-45	
Citrulline	8.5-23.7	10.8-21.1	
Ethanolamine	13.4-105	32.7-72	
α-Amino-*n*-butyric acid	0-29	8.7-20.4	

Data from Dickinson, J.C., Rosenblum, H., and Hamilton, P.B.: Pediatrics **36:**2, 1965; Dickinson, J.C., Rosenblum, H., and Hamilton, P.B.: Pediatrics **45:**606, 1970.

Table 14. Urine amino acids in normal newborns

Amino acid	μmol/day
Cysteic acid	TR-3.32
Phosphoethanolamine	Tr-8.86
Taurine	7.59-7.72
OH-proline	0-9.81
Aspartic acid	Tr
Threonine	0.176-7.99
Serine	Tr-20.7
Glutamic acid	0-1.78
Proline	0-5.17
Glycine	0.176-65.3
Alanine	Tr-8.03
α-Amino-*n*-butyric acid	0-0.47
Valine	0-7.76
Cystine	0-7.96
Methionine	Tr.0.892
Isoleucine	0-6.11
Tyrosine	0-1.11
Phenylalanine	0-1.66
β-Aminoisobutyric acid	0.264-7.34
Ethanolamine	Tr-79.9
Ornithine	Tr-0.554
Lysine	0.33-9.79
1-Methylhistidine	Tr-8.64
3-Methylhistidine	0.11-3.32
Carnosine	0.044-4.01
Arginine	0.088-0.918
Histidine	Tr-7.04
Leucine	Tr-0.819

Modified from Meites, S., editor: Pediatric clinical chemistry: a survey of normals, methods and instruments, Washington, D.C., 1977, American Association for Clinical Chemistry.

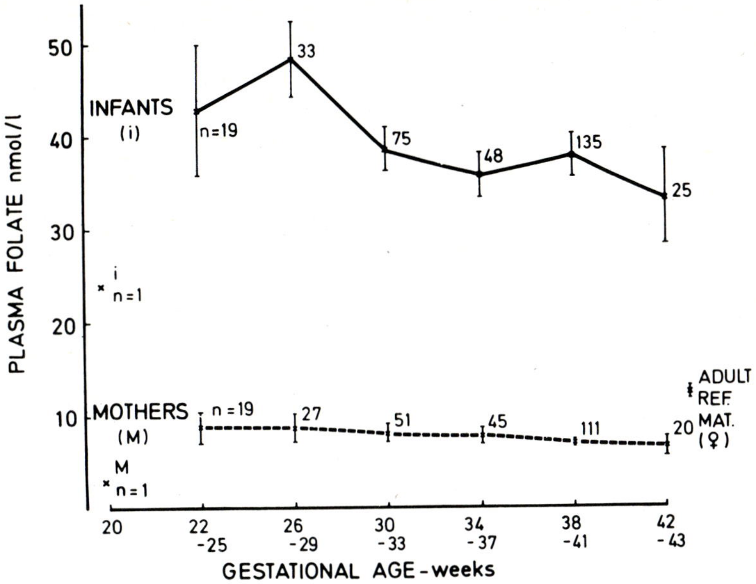

Fig. C-5. Plasma folate (nmol/L). (From Ek, J.: J. Pediatr. **97:**288, 1980.)

CEREBROSPINAL FLUID VALUES

Table 15. Healthy term newborns

	Age			
	0-24 Hours	**1 Day**	**7 Days**	**>7 Days**
Color	Clear or xanthochromic	Clear or xanthochromic	Clear or xanthochromic	
Red blood cells/mm^3	9 (0-1,070)	23 (6-630)	3 (0-48)	
Polymorphonuclear leukocytes/mm^3	3 (0-70)	7 (0-26)	2 (0-5)	
Lymphocytes/mm^3	2 (0-20)	5 (0-16)	1 (0-4)	
Proteins (mg/dl)	63 (32-240)	73 (40-148)	47 (27-65)	
Glucose (mg/dl)	51 (32-78)	48 (38-64)	55 (48-62)	
Lactate dehydrogenase (IU/L)	22-73	22-73 (Birth-7 days)	22-73	0-40

Data from Naidoo, B.T.: S. Afr. Med. J. **42:**932, 1968; Neches, W., and Platt, M.: Pediatrics **41:**1097, 1968.

Table 16. Cerebrospinal fluid cytology in low birth weight and in term infants (findings in 46 neonates)*

Category	Weight, gm	RBCs/ cu mm	WBCs/ cu mm	Polymorphonuclear leukocytes, %	Lymphocytes, %	Macrophages, %
Low birth weight (n = 22)	1,437 (652-2,438)	50 (0-431)	7 (0-28)	16 (0-100)	28 (0-100)	56 (0-100)
Normal birth weight (n = 24)	3,240 (2,665-3,997)	131 (0-478)	11 (1-38)	21 (0-100)	20 (0-100)	59 (0-100)

From Pappu, L.D., and others: Am. J. Dis. Child. **136:**297, 1982. Copyright 1982, American Medical Association.
*Values are given as mean with range in parentheses.

Table 17. Cerebrospinal fluid values in high-risk neonates without meningitis

	Term	Preterm
WBC count (cells/mm³)		
No. of infants	87	30
Mean	8.2	9.0
Median	5	6
SD	7.1	8.2
Range	0-32	0-29
±2 SD	0-22.4	0-25.4
Percentage PMN*	61.3%	57.2%
Protein (mg/dl)		
No. of infants	35	17
Mean	90	115
Range	20-170	65-150
Glucose (mg/dl)		
No. of infants	51	23
Mean	52	50
Range	34-119	24-63
CSF/blood glucose (%)		
No. of infants	51	23
Mean	81	74
Range	44-248	55-105

From Sarff, L.D., and others: J. Pediatr. **88:**473, 1976.
*PMN, Polymorphonuclear cells.

VITAMIN AND MINERAL LEVELS

Table 18. Vitamin A (μg/dl)

Group	Gestation (weeks)	Birth weight (gm)	Vitamin A (μg/dl)	RBP (mg/dl)*	Vitamin A:RBP ratio
Term	39.5 ± 0.2	3260 ± 63	23.9 ± 1.8	3.6 ± 0.2	0.51 ± 0.05
(n = 32)	(37-42)	(2600-4,080)	(13.0-67.6)	(1.7-6.0)	(0.19-1.30)
Preterm	32.1 ± 0.5	1630 ± 111	16.0 ± 1.0	2.8 ± 0.2	0.39 ± 0.02
(n = 39)	(24-36)	(570-2,640)	(1.8-30.0)	(1.1-4.6)	(0.06-0.68)

From Shenai, J.P., and others: J. Pediatr. **99:**302, 1981.
*Retinol binding protein.

Table 19. Vitamin D (ng/ml); plasma concentrations of 25-hydroxyvitamin D(OHD) and 24,25-$(OH)_2D$, and the ratio of 24,25-$(OH)_2D$ to 25-OHD with increasing postnatal age

Age	1 day	3 days	1 week	2 weeks	3-4 weeks	5-10 weeks	Adults
Number of patients	14	14	15	15	14	16	17
25-OHD (ng/ml)							
Median	10.6	11.3	14.6	16.5*	21.4	26.8†	31.8
Range	6.1-29.5	7.6-29.5	6.0-29.9	8.9-39.3	11.7-41.8	15.4-40.6	15.2-42.6
24,25-$(OH)_2D$ (ng/ml)							
Median	0.4‡	0.4	0.4	0.4	0.5	0.5	1.7
Range	<0.3-0.6	<0.3-2.1	<0.3-1.8	<0.3-0.8	<0.3-0.9	0.4-1.1	0.4-2.0
$\frac{24,25\text{-}(OH)_2D}{25\text{-}OHD}$ × 100 (%)§							
Median	3.8	4.0	2.1	2.1‖	1.8	1.7	4.7
Range	1.5-13.0	1.7-7.0	0.7-7.0	0.5-4.8	1.2-3.7	1.1-3.6	2.5-5.9

From Markestad, T., and others: Pediatric Res. **18:**269, 1984.
*$P < 0.02$ compared with the values at 1 day.
†$P < 0.01$ compared with the values at 2 weeks.
‡$P < 0.01$ compared with the adult values.
§Nondetectable concentrations of 24,25-$(OH)_2D$ have arbitrarily been assigned a value of half the detection limit. For each of the age groups 1 day to 3-4 weeks two to four values are thus calculated.
‖$P < 0.01$ compared with the 1 day and adult values.

Table 20. Vitamin E (mg/dl) [mean ± standard deviation]

Weeks	1	2	3	4	5	6	7	8	9	10
<1500 gm	0.40	0.30	0.25	0.25	0.25	0.25	0.25	0.25	0.35	0.45
28-32 weeks	[0.05]	[0.04]	[0.03]	[0.03]	[0.03]	[0.03]	[0.03]	[0.03]	[0.04]	[0.05]
1500-2000 gm	0.45	0.40	0.40	0.45	0.45	0.45	0.50	0.50	0.60	0.70
32-36 weeks	[0.05]	[0.05]	[0.05]	[0.05]	[0.05]	[0.05]	[0.05]	[0.05]	[0.06]	[0.06]
2000-2500 gm	0.50	0.45	0.50	0.60	0.70	0.75	0.75	0.75	0.75	0.80
36-40 weeks	[0.05]	[0.05]	[0.05]	[0.06]	[0.06]	[0.06]	[0.60]	[0.60]	[0.60]	[0.70]
>2500 gm	0.55	0.55	0.55	0.60	0.75	0.80	0.85	0.85	0.85	0.85
Term	[0.60]	[0.60]	[0.60]	[0.60]	[0.70]	[0.70]	[0.80]	[0.80]	[0.80]	[0.80]

From Klaus, M.H., and Fanaroff, A.A.: Care of the high-risk neonate, Philadelphia, 1986, ed. 3, W.B. Saunders Co.

Table 21. Copper (μg/dl) (mean ± standard deviation)*

	Weeks of postconceptual age										
	25-28	29-30	31-32	33-34	35-36	37-38	39-40	41-42	43-44	45-46	47-60
M	28.6	27.1	31.5	36.4	39.2	47.2	52.1	59.6	70.2	65.3	81.8
SD	17.1	14.9	17.5	14.6	13.8	24.1	11.6	21.1	28.1	15.8	18.0
n	16	27	35	43	33	22	20	18	18	9	4

From Hillman, L.S.: J. Pediatr. **98:**305, 1981.
*M, Mean; SD, standard deviation; *n*, number.

Table 22. Iron (μg/dl)

Serum iron (μg/dl)		Total iron-binding capacity (μg/dl)		
Infant	Mother	Infant	Mother	References
173	98	259	470	Hagberg (1953)
147	80	226	446	Laurell (1947)
193 (145-240)	—	240 (147-468)	—	Sturgeon (1954)
159 (106-227)	—	—	—	Vahlquist and others (1941)

From Oski, F.A., and Naiman, J.L.: Hematologic problems in the newborn, ed. 2, Philadelphia, 1972, W.B. Saunders Co.

Table 23. Zinc (μmol); serum zinc concentrations by postconceptional age (PCA)

Weeks (PCA)	29-30 *n* = 10	31-32 *n* = 21	33-34 *n* = 27	35-36 *n* = 22	37-38 *n* = 16	39-40 *n* = 12	41-42 *n* = 6	42-44 *n* = 10	45-46 *n* = 8	47-48 *n* = 6
Zinc (μmol) (mean ± SD)	20.2 ±5.6	15.1 ±3.5	13.0 ±3.5	9.6 ±2.7	9.0 ±2.1	8.9 ±2.1	9.5 ±2.1	9.0 ±1.4	11.0 ±2.6	11.9 ±1.5

From Tyrala, E.E., and others: Acta Paediatr. Scand. **72:**695, 1983.

HORMONES AND STEROID METABOLITES

Table 24. Steroid metabolites

	Age	Male	Female
Plasma and serum			
Follicle-stimulating hormone (FSH)[1]	0-2 years	4-12 IU/L	6-40 IU/L
Luteinizing hormone (LH)[1]	0-2 years	0.6-1.8 IU/L	1.3-3.0 IU/L
Testosterone[1]	0-2 years	4-37 ng/dl	7-18 ng/dl
Human growth hormone (HGH)[2]	Newborn (fasting)	15-40 ng/ml; response to provocation variable	
	After newborn (fasting, resting)	0-5 ng/ml; response to natural and artificial provocation (i.e., arginine, insulin, hypoglycemia) >8 ng/ml	
17-Hydroxyprogesterone[3]	<4 days	<15 μg/L	
	>4 days	<5 μg/L	
Urine			
17-Hydroxycorticosteroids[4,5]	Birth-14 days	0.05-0.3 mg/day	
	15 days-1 year	0.1-0.5 mg/day	
17-Ketosteroids[6]	Birth-14 days	<2.5 mg/day	
	15 days-1 year	<1.0 mg/day	
Pregnanetriol[1]	Birth-14 days	0.0-0.2 mg/day	
	15 days-1 year	0.0-0.1 mg/day	

[1]Meites, S., editor: Pediatric clinical chemistry: a survey of normals, methods and instruments, Washington, D.C., 1977, American Association for Clinical Chemistry.
[2]O'Brien, D., and Rodgerson, D.O.: Interpretation of biochemical values. In Kempe, C.H., Silver, H.K., and O'Brien, D., editors: Current pediatric diagnosis and treatment, ed. 3, Los Altos, Calif., 1974, Lange Medical Publications.
[3]Barnes, N.D., and Atherden, S.M.: Arch. Dis. Child. **47:**62, 1972.
[4]Smith, E.K., Reardon, H.S., and Field, S.H.: J. Pediatr. **64:**652, 1964.
[5]Ulstrom, R.A., and others: J. Clin. Endocrinol. Metab. **20:**1066, 1960.
[6]Mitchell, F.L.: Vitam. Horm. **25:**191, 1967.

Thyroid function in full-term and preterm infants

Table 25. Serum T_4 concentration in premature and term infants

	Estimated gestational age (weeks)				
	30-31	32-33	34-35	36-37	Term
Cord					
Mean	6.5*	7.5	6.7†	7.5	8.2
SD	1.0	2.1	1.2	2.8	1.8
n	3	8	18	17	37
12-72 hr					
Mean	11.5‡	12.3‡	12.4‡	15.5†	19.0
SD	2.1	3.2	3.1	2.6	2.1
n	12	18	17	15	6
3-10 days					
Mean	7.7‡	8.5‡	10.0‡	12.7†	15.9
SD	1.8	1.9	2.4	2.5	3.0
n	7	8	9	9	29
11-20 days					
Mean	7.5†	8.3‡	10.5	11.2	12.2
SD	1.8	1.6	1.8	2.9	2.0
n	5	11	9	9	8
21-45 days					
Mean	7.8‡	8.0‡	9.3†	11.4	12.1
SD	1.5	1.7	1.3	4.2	1.5
n	11	17	13	5	5
46-90 days	(30 to 37 weeks)				
Mean		9.6			10.2
SD		1.7			1.9
n		16			17

From Cuestas, R.A.: J. Pediatr. **92:**963, 1982.
*$P<0.05$.
†$P<0.005$
‡$P<0.001$
for the comparison of premature vs. term infants (t test)

Table 26. Serum-free T_4 index in premature and term infants

	Estimated gestational age (weeks)				
	30-31	32-33	34-35	36-37	Term
Cord					
Mean			5.6	5.6	5.9
SD			1.3	2.0	1.1
n			12	10	14
12-72 hr					
Mean	13.1*	12.9*	15.5†	17.1	19.7
SD	2.4	2.7	3.0	3.5	3.5
n	12	14	14	14	6
3-10 days					
Mean	8.3*	9.0*	12.0‡	15.1	16.2
SD	1.9	1.8	2.3	0.7	3.2
n	6	9	5	4	11
11-20 days					
Mean	8.0§	9.1‡	11.8	11.3	12.1
SD	1.6	1.9	2.7	1.9	2.0
n	5	8	8	4	8
21-45 days					
Mean	8.4§	9.0‡	10.9		11.1
SD	1.4	1.6	2.8		1.4
n	11	17	5		5
46-90 days	(30 to 35 weeks)				
Mean		9.4			9.7
SD		1.4			1.5
n		13			10

From Cuestas, R.A.: J. Pediatr. **92:**963, 1982.
*P 0.001
†P 0.025
‡P 0.01
§P 0.005
for comparison of premature vs term infants (t test)

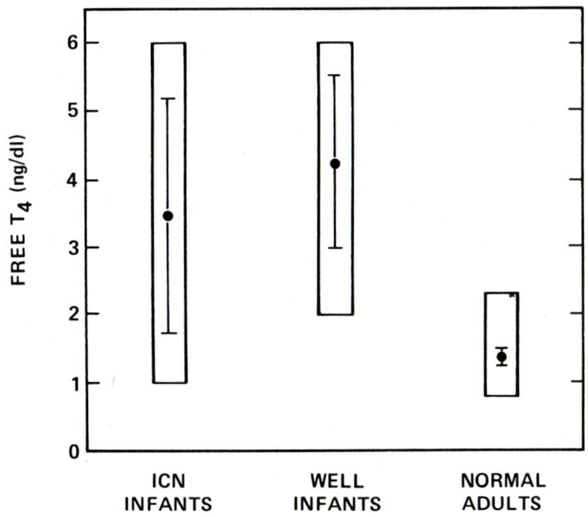

Fig. C-6. Free thyroxine (T_4) levels in sick infants, healthy term infants, and normal adults. The center • represents the mean ± the SD. (From Wilson, D.M., and others: J. Pediatr. **101:**113, 1982.)

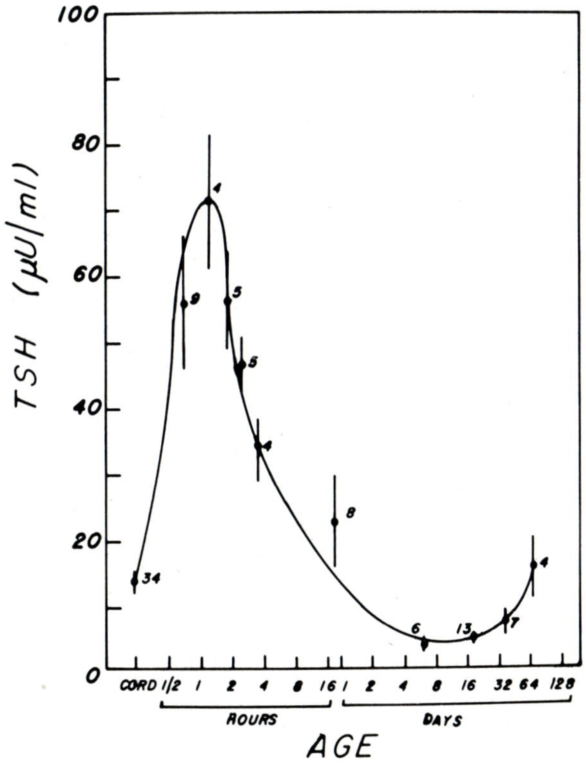

Fig. C-7. Thyroid-stimulating hormone levels in healthy preterm infants. Mean, standard error of the mean, and sample size are shown. (From Cuestas, R.A.: J. Pediatr. **92:**963, 1982.)

Michele C. Walsh

INDEX

Page numbers in *italics* indicate boxed material and illustrations.
Page numbers followed by *t* indicate tables.

C

I

O

S

U

V